OTHER PMIC TITLES OF INTEREST

PRACTICE MANAGEMENT

365 Ways to Manage the Business Called Private Practice
Achieving Profitability with a Medical Office System
Capitation: Tools, Trends, Traps & Techniques
Computerizing Your Medical Office
Critical Concepts in Medical Practice Management
Doctor Business
Encyclopedia of Practice and Financial Management
Getting Paid for What You Do
Health Information Management
The Managed Care Handbook
Managing Costs in the Physician's Office Laboratory
Managing Medical Office Personnel
Marketing Strategies for Physicians
McGraw-Hill Pocket Guide to Managed Care
Medical Marketing Handbook
Medical Office Policy Manual
Medical Practice Forms
Medical Practice Handbook
Medical Practice Pre-employment Tests Book
Medical Staff Privileges
Negotitating Managed Care Contracts
The New Practice Handbook
On-Line Systems: How to Access and Use Databases
Patient Satisfaction
Patients Build Your Practice
A Physician's Guide to Clinical Research Opportunities
Physician's Office Laboratory
Professional and Practice Development
Promoting Your Medical Practice
Starting in Medical Practice
Spanish/English Handbook for the Medical Professional
Surviving a Competitive Health Care Market

MEDICAL REFERENCE AND CLINICAL

Drugs of Abuse
Hematology: A Guide to the Diagnosis and Treatment of Blood Disorders
Medical Care of the Adolescent Athlete
Medical Procedures for Referral
Neurology: Problems in Primary Care
Patient Care Emergency Handbook
Patient Care Flowchart Manual
Patient Care Procedures for Your Practice
Questions and Answers on AIDS
Sexually Transmitted Diseases

AVAILABLE BY CALLING 1-800-MED-SHOP
OR BY VISITING HTTP://PMICONLINE.COM

OTHER PMIC TITLES OF INTEREST

CODING AND REIMBURSEMENT

Codelink® Guides to CPT and ICD-9-CM Code Linkages
Coder's Handbook
Collections Made Easy!
CPT Plus!
CPT & HCPCS Coding Made Easy!
E/M Coding Made Easy!
HCPCS Coders Choice®, Color Coded, Thumb Indexed
Health Insurance Carrier Directory
ICD-9-CM, Coders Choice®, Color Coded, Indexed
ICD-9-CM Coding For Physicians' Offices
ICD-9-CM Coding Made Easy!
Medicare Compliance Manual
Medicare Rules & Regulations
Medical Fees
Reimbursement Manual for the Medical Office
Working with Insurance and Managed Care Plans

FINANCIAL MANAGEMENT

Accounts Receivable Management for the Medical Practice
Business Ventures for Physicians
Financial Planning Workbook for Physicians
Financial Valuation of Your Practice
Pension Plan Strategies
Physician Financial Planning in a Changing Environment
Securing Your Assets
Selling or Buying a Medical Practice

RISK MANAGEMENT

Behavioral Types and the Art of Patient Management
Law, Liability and Ethics for Medical Office Personnel
Malpractice Depositions
Malpractice: Managing Your Defense
Medical Malpractice: A Physician's Guide
Testifying in Court

DICTIONARIES AND OTHER REFERENCE

Health and Medicine on the Interet
Medical Acronyms, Eponyms and Abbreviations
Medical Phrase Index
Medical Word Building
Medico-Legal Glossary
Spanish/English Handbook for Medical Professionals

AVAILABLE BY CALLING 1-800-MED-SHOP
OR BY VISITING HTTP://PMICONLINE.COM

ICD·9·CM

MILLENNIUM EDITION

International Classification of Diseases
9th Revision

Clinical Modification
Sixth Edition

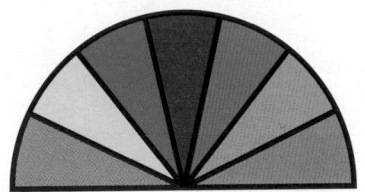

Color Coded

2003

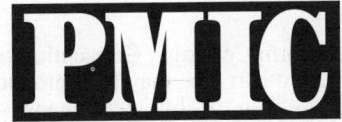

Volumes 1 & 2

ISBN 1-57066-258-4 (Soft cover)
ISBN 1-57066-262-2 (Hard cover)

Volumes 1, 2, & 3

ISBN 1-57066-259-2 (Soft cover)
ISBN 1-57066-261-4 (Timesaver Binder)

Non-indexed versions

ISBN 1-57066-257-6 (Volumes 1 & 2)
ISBN 1-57066-260-6 (Volumes 1, 2, & 3)

Practice Management Information Corporation [PMIC]
4727 Wilshire Boulevard, Suite 300
Los Angeles, California 90010
1-800-MED-SHOP
http://pmiconline.com/

Printed in China

Preface

Health care professionals have long used coding systems to describe procedures, services, and supplies. However, most described the reason for the procedure, service or supply with a diagnostic statement. Of those health care professionals who do code the diagnosis, either due to a requirement for a computer billing system and/or electronic claims filing, many do not code completely or accurately. With the passage of the Medicare Catastrophic Coverage Act of 1988, diagnostic coding using *ICD-9-CM* became mandatory for Medicare claims. In the area of health care reimbursement rules and regulations, the typical progression is that changes required for Medicare are followed shortly by similar changes for Medicaid and private insurance carriers.

To some professionals, the requirement to use diagnostic coding may have seemed like a burden or simply another excuse for Medicare intermediaries to delay or deny payment. However, it is important to understand that the proper use of coding systems for both procedures and diagnoses gives the professional absolute control over his or her billing and reimbursement. Accurate diagnosis coding is not easy. It requires a good working knowledge of medical terminology and a fundamental understanding of *ICD-9-CM*. In addition, the coder must know the rules and regulations required to comply with Medicare requirements for coding.

This edition of the *International Classification of Diseases, 9th Revision, Clinical Modification (ICD-9-CM)* is published by Practice Management Information Corporation in recognition of its responsibility to promulgate this classification throughout the United States for morbidity coding and billing purposes. The *International Classification of Diseases, 9th Revision*, originally published by the World Health Organization (WHO) is the foundation of the *ICD-9-CM* and continues to be the classification employed in cause-of-death coding in the United States.

The *ICD-9-CM* is recommended for use in all clinical settings, but is required for reporting diagnoses and diseases to all U.S. Public Health Service and Health Care Financing Administration programs. This version faithfully follows and contains the same information found in the U.S. Public Health Service and Health Care Financing Administration version of the *ICD-9-CM*.

All official authorized addenda effective October 1, 2002 have been included in this edition. A new revision will be available approximately September 15th of each year. Revised editions may be purchased from:

Practice Management Information Corporation
4727 Wilshire Boulevard, Suite 300
Los Angeles, California 90010
1-800-MED-SHOP

Or by contacting our web site at http://pmiconline.com/

Disclaimer

This publication is identical in content to U.S. Department of Health and Human Services Publication No. (PHS) 91-1260 with the exception that this publication includes special symbols to indicate additions and revisions from the previous edition and special symbols to facilitate identification of diagnostic codes that require 4th or 5th digit specificity, the use of color coding to alert the user to special coding considerations, and thumb indexing to make locating codes easier. This publication is revised annually so that we may present the most current information possible. Though all of the information is carefully researched and checked for accuracy and completeness, the publisher accepts no responsibility with regard to errors, omissions, misuse or misinterpretation.

Table of Contents

Table of Contents

Table of Contents

Table of Contents

Introduction to ICD-9-CM

ICD-9-CM is an acronym for *International Classification of Diseases, 9th Revision, Clinical Modification,* published under different names since 1900. *ICD-9-CM* is a statistical classification system that arranges diseases and injuries into groups according to established criteria. Most *ICD-9-CM* codes are numeric and consist of three, four or five numbers and a description. The codes are revised approximately every 10 years by the World Health Organization and annual updates are published by the Centers for Medicare and Medicaid Services (CMS).

HISTORICAL PERSPECTIVE

The *International Classification of Diseases, 9th Revision, Clinical Modification (ICD-9-CM)* is based on the official version of the *World Health Organization's (WHO) 9th Revision, International Classification of Diseases (ICD-9)*. *ICD-9* is designed for the classification of morbidity and mortality information for statistical purposes, and for the indexing of medical records by disease and operations, and for data storage and retrieval. *ICD-9-CM* replaced the Eighth Revision International Classification of Diseases, Adapted for Use in the United States commonly referred to as *ICDA*.

The concept of extending the International Classification of Diseases for use in hospital indexing was originally developed in response to a need for a more efficient basis for storage and retrieval of diagnostic data. In 1950, the U.S. Public Health Service and the Veterans Administration began independent tests of the International Classification of Diseases for hospital indexing purposes. In the following year, the Columbia Presbyterian Medical Center in New York City adopted the International Classification of Diseases, 6th Revision for use in its medical record department. A few years later, the Commission on Professional and Hospital Activities adopted the International Classification of Diseases for use in hospitals participating in the Professional Activity Study (PAS).

In view of the growing interest in the use of the International Classification of Diseases for hospital indexing, a study was undertaken in 1956 by the American Medical Association and the American Medical Record Association of the relative efficiencies of coding systems for diagnostic indexing. Following this study, the major uses of the International Classification of Diseases for hospital indexing purposes consolidated their experiences and an adaptation was published in December 1959. A revision containing the first "Classification of Operations and Treatments" was published in 1962.

In 1968, following a study by the American Hospital Association, the United States Public Health Service published the Eighth Revision International Classification of Diseases, Adapted for Use in the United States. This publication became commonly known as ICDA, and served as the basis for coding diagnostic data for official morbidity and mortality statistics in the United States.

ICD-9-CM Background

In February 1977, a committee was convened by the National Center for Health Statistics to provide advice and counsel for the development of clinical modification of the ICD-9. The organizations represented on the committee included:

American Association of Health Data Systems
American Hospital Association
American Medical Record Association
Association for Health Records
Council on Clinical Classifications, sponsored by:

American Academy of Pediatrics
American College of Obstetricians and Gynecologists
American College of Physicians
American College of Surgeons
American Psychiatric Association

Commission on Professional and Hospital Activities
Health Care Financing Administration
WHO Center for Classification of Diseases

The resulting *ICD-9-CM* is a clinical modification of the *World Health Organization's International Classification of Diseases, 9th Revision (ICD-9)*. The term "clinical" is used to emphasize the modifications intent; namely, to serve as a useful tool in the area of classification of morbidity data for indexing of medical records, medical care review, ambulatory and other medical care programs, as well as for basic health statistics.

In use since January 1979, *ICD-9-CM* provides a diagnostic coding system that is more precise than those needed only for statistical groupings and trend analysis. Official addenda (updates) to *ICD-9-CM* are issued in October each year by the Health Care Financing Administration.

Use of ICD-9-CM Codes for Professional Billing

Until passage of the Medicare Catastrophic Coverage Act of 1988, health care professionals were not required to report *ICD-9-CM* codes when billing government or private insurance carriers for reimbursement. The exception to this requirement was for those health care professionals who filed insurance claims electronically and those who used "code driven" computer billing services or computer systems.

Most health care professionals simply included the text or description of the injury, illness, sign or symptom that was the reason for the encounter. Insurance carriers who used *ICD-9-CM* coding had to code the diagnostic statements prior to input into their computer systems for reimbursement processing.

A specific requirement of the Medicare Catastrophic Coverage Act of 1988 required health care professionals to include *ICD-9-CM* codes on their Medicare claim forms effective April 1, 1989. A two-month grace period, to June 1, 1989, was allowed at the request of the American Medical Association, to allow health care professionals additional time to develop the knowledge and systems necessary to implement the requirement.

TERMINOLOGY

There are terms used throughout this publication that are important for a proper understanding of *ICD-9-CM*. The following terms are defined specifically as they are used for *ICD-9-CM* with the knowledge that some terms may have other definitions and meanings.

acute	refers to the condition that is the primary reason for the current encounter.
addenda	official updates to *ICD-9-CM* published continuously since 1986, that become effective on October 1st of each year.
adverse	any response to a drug that is noxious and unintended and occurs with proper dosage.
aftercare	an encounter for something planned in advance, for example, cast removal.
AHFS	American Hospital Formulary Service.
alphabetic	the portion of *ICD-9-CM* that lists definitions and codes in alphabetic order. Also called Volume 2.
category	refers to diagnoses codes listed within a specific three-digit category, for example category 250, Diabetes Mellitus.
cause	that which brings about any condition or produces any effect.
chronic	continuing over a long period of time or recurring frequently.
CMS	Centers for Medicare and Medicaid Services (formerly HCFA), the government agency that administers the Medicare and Medicaid programs.
CMS1500	formerly HCFA1500, the uniform health insurance claim form used for billing services to Medicare and other insurance carriers
coding	the process of transferring written or verbal descriptions of diseases, injuries and procedures into numerical designations.
combination	a code that combines a diagnosis with an associated secondary process or complication.
complication	the occurrence of two or more diseases in the same patient at the same time.
concurrent	when a patient is being treated by more than one provider for different care conditions at the same time.
conventions	refers to the use of certain abbreviations, punctuation, symbols, type faces, and other instructions that must be clearly understood in order to use *ICD-9-CM*.
CPT	Current Procedural Terminology. Listing of codes and descriptions for procedures, services and supplies published by the American Medical Association. Used to bill insurance carriers.
diagnosis	a written description of the reason(s) for the procedure, service, supply or encounter.
down coding	the process where insurance carriers reduce the value of a procedure, and the resulting reimbursement, due to either 1) a mismatch of CPT code and description or 2) ICD-9-CM code does not justify the procedure or level of service.

E codes	specific ICD-9-CM codes used to identify the cause of injury, poisoning and other adverse effects.
eponyms	medical procedures or conditions named after a person or a place.
etiology	the cause(s) or origin of a disease.
HCFA	see CMS.
HCFA1500	see CMS1500.
hierarchy	a system that ranks items one above another.
ICD-9-CM	International Classification of Diseases, 9th Revision, Clinical Modification.
ICD-10	International Classification of Diseases, 10th Revision
late effect	a residual effect (condition produced) after the acute phase of an illness or injury has ended.
main term	refers to listings in the Alphabetic Index appearing BOLDFACE type.
manifestation	characteristic signs or symptoms of an illness.
multiple	refers to the need to use more than one ICD-9-CM code to fully identify coding a condition.
primary code	the ICD-9-CM code that defines the main reason for the current encounter.
residual	the long-term condition(s) resulting from a previous acute illness or injury.
rule out	refers to a method used to indicate that a condition is probable, suspected, or questionable but unconfirmed. ICD-9-CM has no provisions for the use of this term.
secondary	code(s) listed after the primary code that further indicate the cause(s) codefor the current encounter or define the need for higher levels of care.
sections	refers to portions of the Tabular List that are organized in groups of three-digit code numbers. For example, Malignant Neoplasm of Lip, Oral Cavity and Pharynx (140-149).
sequencing	the process of listing ICD-9-CM codes in the proper order.
specificity	refers to the requirement to code to the highest number of digits possible, 3, 4 or 5, when choosing an ICD-9-CM code.
sub term	refers to listings appearing in the Alphabetic Index under MAIN TERMS and always indented two spaces to the right.
subcategories	refers to groupings of four-digit codes listed under three-digit categories.
tabular list	the portion of ICD-9-CM that lists codes and definitions in numeric order. Also referred to as Volume 1.
V codes	specific ICD-9-CM codes used to identify encounters for reasons other than illness or injury, for example, immunization.
Volume 1	see TABULAR LIST
Volume 2	see ALPHABETIC INDEX
Volume 3	procedure codes used only for hospital coding. Volume 3 contains both a numeric listing and alphabetic index.

FORMAT OF ICD-9-CM

The *International Classification of Diseases, 9th Revision, Clinical Modification* was originally published as a three volume set (2nd edition). Newer versions of ICD-9-CM are available as either a two-volume set (Volume 1 and Volume 2) or as a three-volume set (Volumes 1, 2 and 3), depending on the publisher. It is also now available on CD-ROM from the U.S. Government.

The Third Edition of ICD-9-CM includes all official addenda from October 1986 through October 1988. The Fourth Edition of ICD-9-CM includes all official addenda from October 1986 through October 1994. This edition of ICD-9-CM includes all official addenda from October 1986 through October 2002.

The Tabular List (Volume 1)

The Tabular List (Volume 1) is a <u>numeric</u> listing of diagnosis codes and descriptions consisting of 17 chapters that classify diseases and injuries, two sections containing supplementary codes (V codes and E codes) and six appendices.

Classification of Diseases and Injuries

The Classification of Diseases and Injuries includes the following 17 chapters:

Chapter 1   Infectious and Parasitic Diseases (001-139)

Chapter 2   Neoplasms (140-239)

Chapter 3   Endocrine, Nutritional and Metabolic Diseases, and Immunity Disorders (240-279)

Chapter 4   Diseases of the Blood and Blood-Forming Organs (280-289)

Chapter 5   Mental Disorders (290-319)

Chapter 6   Diseases of the Nervous System and Sense Organs

Chapter 7   Diseases of the Circulatory System (390-459)

Chapter 8   Diseases of the Respiratory System (460-519)

Chapter 9   Diseases of the Digestive System (520-579)

Chapter 10   Diseases of the Genitourinary System (580-629)

Chapter 11   Complications of Pregnancy, Childbirth, and the Puerperium (630-676)

Chapter 12   Diseases of the Skin and Subcutaneous Tissue (680-709)

Chapter 13   Diseases of the Musculoskeletal System and Connective Tissue (710-739)

Chapter 14   Congenital Anomalies (740-759)

Chapter 15   Certain Conditions Originating in the Perinatal Period (760-779)

Chapter 16   Symptoms, Signs and Ill-defined Conditions (780-799)

Chapter 17   Injury and Poisoning (800-999)

Each chapter of the Tabular List (Volume 1) is structured into four components; namely:

Sections: groups of three-digit code numbers

Categories: three-digit code numbers

Subcategories: four-digit code numbers

Fifth-Digit Subclassifications: five-digit code numbers

Supplementary Classifications

There are two supplementary classifications included in the Tabular List (Volume 1). These are:

V Codes   Supplementary Classification of Factors Influencing Health Status and Contact with Health Services (V01-V83)

E Codes   Supplementary Classification of External Causes of Injury and Poisoning (E800-E999)

Appendices

The Tabular List (Volume 1) includes six appendices. These are:

Appendix 1   Morphology of Neoplasms

Appendix 2   Glossary of Mental Disorders

Appendix 3   Classification of Drugs by American Hospital Formulary Service List Number and their ICD-9-CM Equivalents

Appendix 4   Classification of Industrial Accidents According to Agency

Appendix 5   List of Three-Digit Categories

Appendix 6   Supplementary Classification of External Causes of Injury and Poisoning (E codes)

Specifications for the Tabular List

1. Three-digit rubrics and their contents are unchanged from *ICD-9*.

2. The sequence of three-digit rubrics is unchanged from *ICD-9*.

3. Three-digit rubrics are not added to the main body of the classification.

4. Unsubdivided three-digit rubrics are subdivided where necessary to:

   a) Add clinical detail

   b) Isolate terms for clinical accuracy

5. The modification in *ICD-9-CM* is accomplished by the addition of a fifth digit to existing *ICD-9* rubrics, except as noted under #7 below.

6. Four-digit rubrics are added to subdivided three-digit codes only when there is no other means of achieving desired detail. These codes, unique to *ICD-9-CM* (28 three-digit categories) are marked with the symbol in the Tabular List.

7. The optional dual classification in *ICD-9* is modified.

   a) Duplicate rubrics are deleted:

      1) Four-digit manifestation categories duplicating etiology entries.

      2) Manifestation inclusion terms duplicating etiology entries.

   b) Manifestations of diseases are identified, to the extent possible, by creating five digit codes in the etiology rubrics.

   c) When the manifestation of a disease cannot be included in the etiology rubrics, provision for its identification is made by retaining the *ICD-9* rubrics used for classifying manifestations of disease.

8. The format of *ICD-9-CM* is revised from that used in *ICD-9*.

   a) American spelling of medical terms is used.

   b) Inclusion terms are indented beneath the titles of codes.

   c) Codes not to be used for primary tabulation of disease are printed in italics with the notation, "code also underlying disease."

The Alphabetical Index (Volume 2)

The Alphabetic Index (Volume 2) of ICD-9-CM consists of an alphabetic list of terms and codes, two supplementary Sections following the alphabetic listing, plus two special tables found within the alphabetic listing. The Alphabetic Index (Volume 2) is structured as follows:

MAIN TERMS: appear in **BOLDFACE** type

SUBTERMS: are always indented two spaces to the right under main terms

CARRY-OVER LINES: are always indented more than two spaces from the level of the preceding line

Supplementary Sections

The supplementary sections following the Alphabetic Index are:

TABLE OF DRUGS AND CHEMICALS

This table contains a classification of drugs and other chemical substances to identify poisoning states and external causes of adverse effects.

INDEX TO EXTERNAL CAUSES OF INJURIES & POISONINGS (E-CODES)

This section contains the index to the codes that classify environmental events, circumstances, and other conditions as the cause of injury and other adverse effects.

Special Tables

The two special tables, located within the Alphabetic Index, and found under the main terms as underlined below, are:

HYPERTENSION TABLE

NEOPLASM TABLE

Specifications for the Alphabetic Index

1. Format of the Alphabetic Index follows the format of the *ICD-9*.

2. Main terms in the Alphabetic Index are printed in bold face type.

3. When two codes are required to indicate etiology and manifestation, the optional manifestation code appears in brackets, e.g., diabetic cataract 250.5 *[366.41]*.

Procedures: Tabular List and Alphabetic Index (Volume 3)

Volume 3 consists of two sections, a tabular list of codes and an alphabetic index. These codes define procedures instead of diagnoses. Frequently used incorrectly by health care professionals, codes from Volume 3 are intended only for use by hospitals. The Fourth Edition of ICD-9-CM printed by the U.S. Government Printing Office did not include Volume 3. The Fifth Edition of ICD-9-CM issued by the U.S. Government included Volume 3 on a CD-ROM.

The ICD-9-CM Procedure Classification is a modification of WHO's "Fascicle V, Surgical Procedures," and is published as Volume 3 of ICD-9-CM. It contains both a Tabular List and an Alphabetic Index. Greater detail has been added to the ICD-9-CM Procedure Classification necessitating expansion of the codes from three to four digits. Approximately 90% of the rubrics refer to surgical procedures with the remaining 10% accounting for other investigative and therapeutic procedures.

Tabular List of Procedures

The Tabular List includes 16 chapters containing codes and descriptions for surgical procedures and miscellaneous diagnostic and therapeutic procedures.

Alphabetic Index to Procedures

The Alphabetic Index provides an alphabetic index to the Tabular List of Volume 3

Specifications for the Procedure Classification

1. The *ICD-9-CM* Procedure Classification is published in its own volume containing both a Tabular List and an Alphabetic Index.

2. The classification is a modification of Fascicle V "Surgical Procedures" of the *ICD-9* Classification of Procedures in Medicine, working from the draft dated Geneva, 30 September-6 October 1975, and labeled WHO/ICD-9/Rev. Conf. 75.4.

3. All three-digit rubrics in the range 01-86 are maintained as they appear in Fascicle V, whenever feasible.

4. Nonsurgical procedures are segregated from the surgical procedures and confined to the rubrics 87-99, whenever feasible.

5. Selected detail contained in the remaining fascicles of the *ICD-9 Classification of Procedures in Medicine* is accommodated where possible.

6. The structure of the classification is based on anatomy rather than surgical specialty.

7. The *ICD-9-CM* Procedure Classification is numeric only, i.e., no alphabetic characters are used.

8. The classification is based on a two-digit structure with two decimal digits where necessary.

9. Compatibility with the *ICD-9 Classification of Procedures in Medicine* was not maintained when a different axis was deemed more clinically appropriate.

CONVENTIONS USED IN THE TABULAR LIST

The ICD-9-CM Tabular List (Volume 1) makes use of certain abbreviations, punctuation, symbols, and other conventions that must be clearly understood. The purpose of these conventions is to first, provide special coding instructions, and second, to conserve space.

Abbreviations

NOS
:   Not Otherwise Specified. Equivalent to Unspecified. This abbreviation refers to a lack of sufficient detail in the statement of diagnosis to be able to assign it to a more specific sub division within the classification.

NEC
:   Not Elsewhere Classified. Used with ill-defined terms to alert the coder that a specified form of the condition is classified differently. The category number for the term including NEC is to be used only when the coder lacks the information necessary to code the term to a more specific category.

Punctuation

( ) PARENTHESIS are used to enclose supplementary words that may be present or absent in a statement of disease without effecting the code assignment.

[ ] SQUARE BRACKETS are used to enclose synonyms, alternate wordings or explanatory phrases.

: COLONS are used after an incomplete phrase or term that requires one or more of the modifiers indented under it to make it assignable to a given category. EXCEPTION to this rule pertains to the abbreviation NOS.

{ } BRACES are used to connect a series of terms to a common stem. Each term on the left of the brace is incomplete and must be completed by a term to the right of the brace.

Symbols

• A filled BLACK CIRCLE preceding a code indicates that the code is new to this revision of *ICD-9-CM*. A symbol key appears on all left-hand pages of the Tabular List, Volume 1.

▲ A filled BLACK TRIANGLE preceding a code indicates that there is a revision to the text or notes of an existing code. A symbol key appears on all left-hand pages of the Tabular List, Volume 1.

[4] [5] A circle containing the number 4 or the number 5 preceding a code indicates that a fourth or fifth digit is required for coding to the highest level of specificity. Valid digits are in [brackets] under each code. Definitions of valid fifth digits are found under the major category.

Other conventions

Type Face:

BOLD: Bold type face is used for all codes and titles in the Tabular List.

Italics: Italicized type face is used for all exclusion notes and to identify those rubrics that are not to be used for primary tabulations of disease.

Format: *ICD-9-CM* uses an indented format for ease in reference.

Instructional Notations

Instructional terms define what is, or what is not, included in a given subdivision. This is accomplished by using both inclusion and exclusion terms.

INCLUDES: Indicates separate terms, such as, modifying adjectives, sites and conditions, entered under a subdivision, such as a category, to further define or give examples of, the content of the category.

Excludes: Exclusion terms are enclosed in a box and are printed in italics to draw attention to their presence. The importance of this instructional term is its use as a guideline to direct the coder to the proper code assignment. In other words, all terms following the word EXCLUDES: are to be coded elsewhere as indicated in each instance.

NOTES These are used to define terms and give coding instructions. Often used to list the fifth-digit subclassifications for certain categories.

SEE Acts as a cross reference and, is an explicit direction to look elsewhere. This instructional term must always be followed. (Cross references provide the user with other possible modifiers for a term, or, its synonyms.)

SEE CATEGORY A variation of the instructional term SEE. This refers the coder to a specific category. You must *always* follow this instructional term.

SEE ALSO A direction given to look elsewhere if the main term or subterm(s) are not sufficient to code the information you have.

CODE FIRST This instructional note is used for those codes not intended to be used as a principal diagnosis, or not to be sequenced before the underlying disease. The note requires that the underlying disease (etiology) be coded first with the code the note is applied to being coded second. This note appears only in the tabular list (Vol. 1).

USE ADDITIONAL CODE This instruction is placed in the Tabular List in those categories where the coder may wish to add further information, by using an additional code, to give a more complete picture of the diagnosis or procedure.

Related terms

AND Whenever this term appears in a title, it should be interpreted as "and/or."

WITH When this term is used in a title it indicates a requirement that both parts of the title must be present in the diagnostic statement.

COLOR CODING

All PMIC versions of *ICD-9-CM* include color-coding to alert the user to special coding situations or conditions that require additional attention. The use of color-coding is found in the Tabular List of Volume 1 and the Tabular List of Volume 3. The color is applied as solid rectangular bars over the codes only so that the descriptions remain clear and legible. The color codes and definitions are printed at the bottom of all right-sided pages of Volume 1 and Volume 3.

Volume 1

Three digit codes. Coding to fourth or fifth digit specificity is required.

Unspecified code. Descriptions include the term "unspecified". Use only if a more specific diagnosis is not known or available.

Nonspecific code. Descriptions include the term "nonspecific, unspecified, other specified or other". A report *may* be required by insurance carriers.

Manifestation codes. Used only to code the manifestation of an underlying disease. Code the underlying disease first.

Medicare secondary payer (MSP) alert. Diagnoses that may trigger a post-payment review by Medicare. Medicare is usually the secondary payer for these diagnoses.

Volume 3*

Noncovered operating room procedure. An operating room procedure that is not covered by Medicare.

Non-operating room procedure. A procedure that is not performed in the operating room that affects DRG assignment.

Bilateral procedure.

Valid operating room procedure. Prompts a change in DRG assignment.

Nonspecific operating room procedure. Choose a more precise code if possible.

*These colors appear only in the three-volume edition

MEDICARE REQUIREMENTS FOR ICD-9-CM CODING

The Medicare Catastrophic Coverage Act of 1988 (PL 100-330) requires that health care professionals submit an appropriate diagnosis code, using the *International Classification of Diseases, 9th Revision, Clinical Modification (ICD-9-CM)* for each procedure, service, or supply billed under Medicare Part B.

To comply with the regulations, health care professionals must convert the reason(s) for the procedures, services or supplies, performed or issued, from written diagnostic statements that may include specific diagnoses, signs, symptoms and/or complaints, into ICD-9-CM diagnosis codes. The Health Care Financing Administration (now the Centers for Medicare and Medicaid Services) originally set the implementation date for this requirement as April 1, 1989, however, it was subsequently delayed until June 1, 1989, at the request of the American Medical Association, to give health care providers additional time to prepare for the change.

HCFA Guidelines for Using ICD-9-CM Codes

The Center for Medicare and Medicaid Services (CMS, formerly HCFA) has prepared guidelines for using ICD-9-CM codes and instructions on how to report them on claim forms. In addition, CMS has directed your medicare intermediary to provide you with a written copy of these instructions. The basic guidelines are summarized below, however, it is very important that you obtain a copy of the guidelines from your Medicare intermediary as implementation of CMS requirements varies from one intermediary to another.

1. Indicate on the claim form or itemized statement the appropriate code(s) from the ICD-9-CM code range 001.0 through V83.02 to identify diagnoses, symptoms, conditions, problems, complaints or other reason(s) for the procedure, service or supply provided.

    A. In choosing codes to describe the reason for the encounter, the health care professional will frequently be using codes within the range from 001.0 through 999.9, the section of ICD-9-CM for the classification of diseases and injuries (e.g. infectious and parasitic diseases; neoplasms; signs, symptoms and ill-defined conditions). Codes that describe symptoms as opposed to diagnoses are acceptable if this is the highest level of certainty documented by the physician.

    B. ICD-9-CM also provides codes to deal with visits for circumstances other than a disease or injury, such as an encounter for a laboratory test only. These codes are found in the V-code section and range from V01.0 through V83.02.

2. The ICD-9-CM code for the diagnosis, condition, problem, or other reason for the encounter documented in the medical record as the main reason for the procedure, service or supply provided should be listed first. Additional ICD-9-CM codes that describe any current coexisting conditions are then listed. Do not include codes for conditions that were previously treated and no longer exist.

3.   ICD-9-CM codes should be used at their highest level of specificity.

    A.   Assign three digit codes only if there are no four digit codes within the coding category.

    B.   Assign four digit codes only if there is no fifth digit subclassification for that category.

    C.   Assign the fifth digit subclassification code for those categories where it exists.

Claims submitted with three or four digit codes where four and five digit codes are available may be returned to you by the Medicare intermediary for proper coding. It is recognized that a very specific diagnosis may not be known at the time of the initial encounter. However, that is not an acceptable reason to submit a three digit code when four or five digits are available.

For example, if the patient has chronic bronchitis, ICD-9-CM code 491, and the physician has not yet documented whether the bronchitis is simple, mucopurulent, or obstructive, the code for unspecified chronic bronchitis, ICD-9-CM code 491.9, should be listed.

4.   Diagnoses documented as "probable," "suspected," "questionable," or "rule out" should not be coded as if the diagnosis is confirmed. The condition(s) should be coded to the highest degree of certainty for the encounter, such as describing symptoms, signs, abnormal test results, or other reasons for the encounter.

5.   Chronic disease(s) treated on an ongoing basis may be coded and reported as many times as the patient receives treatment and care for the condition(s).

6.   When patients receive ancillary diagnostic services only during an encounter, the appropriate "V code" for the service should be listed first, and the diagnosis or problem for which the diagnostic procedures are being performed should be listed second.

    A.   V codes will be used frequently by radiologists who perform radiological examinations on referrals. For example, ICD-9-CM code V72.5, Radiological examination, not elsewhere classified, describes the reason for the encounter and should be listed first on the claim form or statement. If the reason for the referral is known, a second ICD-9-CM code that describes the signs or symptoms for which the examination was ordered should be listed.

    B.   Failure to list a second ICD-9-CM code in addition to the V code may result in claim delays or denials. The ICD-9-CM code V72.5, Radiological examination, not elsewhere classified, includes referrals for routine chest x-rays that are not covered by the Medicare program. Medicare intermediaries may establish screening programs to verify that the referrals were not for routine chest x-rays. By supplying a second ICD-9-CM code to describe the reason for the referral, these claims can be clearly identified by the Medicare intermediary as referrals to evaluate symptoms, signs or diagnoses. The mission of a second ICD-9-CM code may lead to requests for additional information from Medicare intermediaries prior to processing the claim.

7. For patients receiving only ancillary therapeutic services during an encounter, list the appropriate V code first, followed by the ICD-9-CM code for the diagnosis or problem for which the services are being performed. For example, a patient with multiple sclerosis presenting for rehabilitation services would be coded using either V57.1 Other physical therapy, or V57.89 Other care involving use of rehabilitation procedures, followed by code 340 Multiple sclerosis.

8. For surgical procedures, use the ICD-9-CM code for the diagnosis for which the surgery was performed. If the postoperative diagnosis is known to be different at the time the claim is filed, use the ICD-9-CM code for the post-operative diagnosis.

9. Code all documented conditions that coexist at the time of the visit that require or affect patient care, treatment or management. Do not code conditions that were previously treated and no longer exist.

Completing the CMS1500 Claim Form

Health care professionals using the Uniform Health Insurance Claim Form, CMS1500, to file claims for services provided to Medicare beneficiaries must list a minimum of one ICD-9-CM code and may list up to four total ICD-9-CM codes on the claim form.

The ICD-9-CM code for the diagnosis, condition, problem or other reason for the encounter is listed first, followed by up to three additional codes that describe any coexisting conditions. At times, there may be several conditions that equally resulted in the encounter. In these cases, the health care professional is free to select the one that will be listed first.

The ICD-9-CM codes are listed in Box 23 of the "old" CMS1500 (10/84) claim form and Box 21 of the "new" CMS1500 (12/90) claim form (see example). In addition, in Box 24 D of both versions of the form, you must indicate by a number from 1 to 4, or combination of numbers, which diagnoses from Box 23 support the procedure, service or supply listed in Box 24 C.

Due to space limitations on the claim form you may use only up to four ICD-9-CM codes for diagnoses, conditions, or signs and symptoms. Frequently the patient may have more than four conditions present at the time of the encounter, however, you must choose only four codes to be listed on the claim form.

If.you strongly believe that additional diagnostic information is needed by the Medicare intermediary for proper claim processing you may attach additional supporting documentation to your manual claim. Keep in mind that in most cases the additional documentation will be ignored by the claims examiners, and, in other cases will result in reimbursement delay while someone reviews your documentation.

Medicare Penalties for Non-compliance

The Medicare Catastrophic Coverage Act of 1988 mandates submission of an appropriate ICD-9-CM diagnosis code or codes for each procedure, service, or supply furnished by the health care professional to Medicare Part B beneficiaries. The Act further specifies that compliance is mandatory and that penalties may be assessed for noncompliance.

The penalties for noncompliance differ depending upon whether or not the health care professional has agreed to accept assignment or not.

1. For health care professionals who accept assignment on a Medicare claim and who fail to include ICD-9-CM codes as required will have their claim(s) returned for proper coding and may be subject to post-payment review by the Medicare intermediary, as well as payment denials.

2. For health care professionals who do not accept assignment, the penalties are more severe.

    A. If the original claim form does not include ICD-9-CM codes as required, and the health care professional refuses to provide the codes promptly on request to the Medicare intermediary, the professional may be subject to a civil monetary penalty in an amount not to exceed $2,000, per claim.

    B. If the health care professional continuously fails to provide ICD-9-CM codes as requested, the professional may be subject to the sanction process described in section 1842 (j) (2) (A), that mandates that the professional may be barred from participation in the Medicare program for a period not to exceed five years.

CODING AND BILLING ISSUES

Diagnosis Codes Must Support Procedure Codes

Each service or procedure performed for a patient should be represented by a diagnosis that would substantiate those particular services or procedures as necessary in the investigation or treatment of their condition based on currently accepted standards of practice by the medical profession.

Place (Location) of Service

The actual setting that the services are rendered in for particular diagnoses plays an important part in reimbursement. Many people became accustomed to using Emergency Rooms for any type of illness or injury. By utilizing highly specialized places of service for conditions that were not true emergencies, third party payer were being billed with CPT codes indicating emergency services were rendered. Since the cost of services rendered on an emergency basis is considerably more expensive than those services in an non-emergency situation, third party payers began watching for those claims with diagnoses that did not indicate that a true emergency existed. Payment then was based on what the cost would have been had the patient been treated in the proper setting.

Level of Service Provided

The patient's condition and the treatment of that condition must be billed according to the criteria, as published by the AMA, for each level of service (i.e., minimal, brief, limited, intermediate, extended, comprehensive). Many practices bill the office visit level that they know will pay better rather than to consider the criteria that must be met to use a particular level of service. Again, the patient's diagnosis enters into this concept as well as it is often the diagnosis that indicates the complexity of the level of service to be used.

Frequency of Services

Many times claims are submitted for a patient with the same diagnosis and the same procedure(s) time after time. When the diagnosis indicates a chronic condition and the claims do not indicate any change in the patient's treatment or, give any indication that the patient's condition has been altered (i.e., exacerbated, other symptomology) the third party payer may deny payment based on the frequency of services for the reported condition.

Down Coding

Down coding is the process of reducing a code from one of a higher value to one of a lower value that results in lowered reimbursement. In the area of procedure coding, this process results in the loss of millions of dollars annually by health care professionals and their patients.

With procedure coding, down coding claims is easily resolved by either providing a procedure description that matches that of Current Procedural Terminology (CPT) exactly, or, even better, by eliminating all procedure descriptions from your claim forms, that forces the insurance carrier to allow full value for your procedure, service, or supply. With diagnosis coding, the issue is not mismatch of description to code, as the description is not required, but that the ICD-9-CM code(s) provide justification for the procedure, service or supply or the level of service provided.

A key point to remember is that if there are any current coexisting conditions that may complicate the treatment for the primary condition, it is very important to include the ICD-9-CM codes for the coexisting conditions that will help to justify the level of service provided.

Concurrent Care

Reimbursement problems often arise when a patient is being treated by different professionals, within the same billing entity (medical group or clinic), for different problems at the same time. This is known as concurrent care. For example, a patient may be hospitalized by a clinic's general surgeon for an operation and may also be seen while hospitalized by the group's cardiologist for an unrelated cardiac condition.

If you submit claims for daily hospital visits by both of the above professionals without explanation, most insurance carriers would reject one daily visit as an apparent "duplication" of service. Prior to publication of the 1992 edition of CPT, the key to obtaining proper reimbursement for concurrent care was first, to use the procedure modifier - 75, Concurrent Care, Services Rendered by More than One Physician, and second, to submit a different *ICD-9-CM* code for the services provided by each physician, that support and justify the need for those services.

Note that modifier -75 was deleted in the 1992 edition of CPT, therefore, when using the new CPT Evaluation and Management codes to bill Medicare, the *ICD-9-CM* code becomes the key factor for proper reimbursement of concurrent care.

ICD-10

Since 1948, the World Health Organization has revised the *International Classification of Diseases* approximately every 10 years, with a modified version appearing in the United States about one to three years following the WHO publication. Based on the regular schedule, *ICD-10* should have been released in 1987. However, due to difficulties in coordinating the international committees, the first volume of *ICD-10*, the Tabular List, was not published until June of 1992.

Implementation of ICD-10 in the United States

Prior to being implemented in the United States, *ICD-10* must be converted to "American" English and pass through a variety of private and government committees, agencies, associations and organizations. As of this printing, the official position of the Centers for Medicare and Medicaid Services (CMS) is that *ICD-10* will not be mandated for Medicare claims for several years.

WHERE TO GET ANSWERS TO QUESTIONS ABOUT ICD-9-CM

Questions regarding the use and interpretation of the *International Classification of Diseases, 9th Revision, Clinical Modification* should be directed in writing to any of the organizations listed below.

Coding Advice/Central Office on ICD-9-CM
American Hospital Association
One North Franklin
Chicago, Illinois 60606

World Health Organization Collaborating Center
for Classification of Diseases in North America
National Center for Health Statistics
Department of Health and Human Services
6525 Belcrest Road
Hyattsville, Maryland 20782

Morbidity Classification Branch
National Center for Health Statistics
Department of Health and Human Services
6525 Belcrest Road, Room 1100
Hyattsville, Maryland 20782

Centers for Medicare and Medicaid Services (CMS)
Division of Prospective Payment System
Mail Stop C4-07-07
7500 Security Blvd.
Baltimore, MD 21244-1850

Comments, questions or suggestions regarding the PMIC version of *ICD-9-CM* should be directed in writing to:

Managing Editor
Practice Management Information Corporation
4727 Wilshire Boulevard, Suite 300
Los Angeles, California 90010
http://pmiconline.com

ICD-9-CM CODING FUNDAMENTALS

Learning and following the basic steps of coding will increase your chances of better and faster reimbursement from third party payers, as well as establish meaningful profiles for future reimbursement rates. To become a proficient coder, two basic principles always must be considered.

First, it is imperative that you use both the Alphabetic Index (Volume 2) and the Tabular List (Volume 1) when locating and assigning codes. Coding only from the Alphabetic Index will cause you to miss any additional information provided only in the Tabular List, such as exclusions, instructions to use additional codes or the need for a fifth-digit.

Second, the level of specificity is important in all coding situations. A three-digit code that has subdivisions indicates you must use the appropriate subdivision code. Also, any time a fifth-digit subclassification is provided, you must use the fifth-digit code.

NINE STEPS FOR ACCURATE ICD-9-CM CODING

1. Locate the main term within the diagnostic statement.

2. Locate that main term in the Alphabetic Index (Volume 2). Keep in mind that the primary arrangement for main terms is by condition in the Alphabetic Index (Volume 2); main terms can be referred to in outmoded, ill-defined and lay terms as well as proper medical terms; main terms can be expressed in broad or specific terms, as nouns, adjectives or eponyms and can be with or without modifiers. Certain conditions may be listed under more than one main term.

3. Remember to refer to all notes under the main term. Be guided by the instructions in any notes appearing in a box immediately after the main term.

4. Examine any modifiers appearing in parentheses next to the main term. See if any of these modifiers apply to any of the qualifying terms used in the diagnostic statement.

5. Take note of the subterms indented beneath the main term. Subterms differ from main terms in that they provide greater specificity, becoming more specific the further they are indented to the right of the main term in 2-space increments; also, they provide the anatomical sites affected by the disease or injury.

6. Be sure to follow any cross reference instructions. These instructional terms ("see" or "see also") must be followed to locate the correct code.

7. Confirm the code selection in the Tabular List (Volume 1). make certain you have selected the appropriate classification in accordance with the diagnosis.

8. Follow instructional terms in the Tabular List (Volume 1). Watch for exclusion terms, notes and fifth-digit instructions that apply to the code number you are verifying. It is necessary to search not only the selected code number for instructions but also the category, section and chapter in which the code number is collapsible. Many times the instructional information is located one or more pages preceding the actual page you find the code number on.

9. Finally, assign the code number you have determined to be correct.

ITALICIZED ENTRIES

During the process of designating a code to identify a principal diagnosis it is important to remember that italicized entries or codes in slanted brackets cannot be used. In these instances, it is required that the etiology code be sequenced first and the manifestation code be listed second even if the physician recorded them in the opposite order.

OTHER AND UNSPECIFIED CODES

Subcategories for diagnoses listed as "Other" and "Unspecified" are referred to as residual subcategories. Remember, the subdivisions are arranged in a hierarchy starting with the more specific and ending with the least specific. In the Tabular List (Volume 1), in most instances, the four-digit subcategory ".8" has been reserved for "Other" specified conditions not classifiable elsewhere and the four-digit subcategory ".9" has been reserved for "Unspecified" conditions. Following is an example demonstrating this principle.

005   Other food poisoning (bacterial)

Excludes:	salmonella infections (003.0-003.9)

               toxic effect of:
                    food contaminants (989.7)
                    noxious foodstuffs (988-0-988.9)

005.0   Staphylococcal food poisoning
           Staphylococcal toxemia specified as due to food

005.1   Botulism
           Food poisoning due to Clostridium botulinum

005.2   Food poisoning due to Clostridium perfringens [C. welchii]
           Enteritis necroticans

005.3   Food poisoning due to other Clostridia

005.4   Food poisoning due to Vibrio parahaemolyticus

005.8   Other bacterial food poisoning

Excludes:	salmonella food poisoning (003.0-003.9)

     005.81   Food poisoning due to Vibrio vulnificus

     005.89   Other bacterial food poisoning
               Food poisoning due to Bacillus cereus

005.9   Food poisoning, unspecified

As you look at Category 005, note that codes 005.0-005.4 indicate that the food poisoning is related to specific types of organisms. Therefore, subcategories 005.0-005.4 are regarded as more specific than subcategory 005.9. Fifth-digit subclassification 005.89 *Other bacterial food poisoning* would include other specific types of <u>bacterial</u> food poisoning not classified elsewhere, as well as <u>bacterial</u> food poisoning NOS. Whereas subcategory 005.9 *Food poisoning unspecified* would be used for a diagnostic statement of "Food poisoning NOS" where the causative organism is not mentioned.

The hierarchy from more specific to less specific is not consistently maintained at the fifth-digit level. The level of specificity at the fifth-digit level is usually (not always) indicated by the use of 0 and 9. The digit 9 identifies the entry for "Other specified" while the digit 0 identifies the "Unspecified" entry. Below is an example.

279   Disorders involving the immune mechanism

> **279.0**   Deficiency of humoral immunity
>
> > **279.00**   Hypogammaglobulinemia, unspecified
> > Agammaglobulinemia NOS
> >
> > **279.01**   Selective IgA immunodeficiency
> >
> > **279.02**   Selective IgM immunodeficiency
> >
> > **279.03**   Other selective immunoglobulin deficiencies
> > Selective deficiency of IgG
> >
> > **279.04**   Congenital hypogammaglobulinemia
> > Agammaglobulinemia:
> > Bruton's type
> > X-linked
> >
> > **279.05**   Immunodeficiency with increased IgM
> > Immunodeficiency with hyper-IgM:
> > autosomal recessive
> > X-linked
> >
> > **279.06**   Common variable immunodeficiency
> > Dysgammaglobulinemia (acquired)
> > (congenital) (primary)
> > Hypogammaglobulinemia:
> > acquired primary
> > congenital non-sex-linked
> > sporadic
> >
> > **279.09**   Other
> > Transient hypogammaglobulinemia of infancy

Notice that the fifth-digit 0 identifies "Unspecified" and the fifth-digit 9 identifies "Other specified."

ACUTE AND CHRONIC CODING

Whenever a particular condition is described as both acute and chronic, code according to the subentries in the Alphabetic Index (Volume 2) for the stated condition. The following directions should be considered.

1.   If there are separate subentries listed for acute, subacute and chronic, then use both codes, sequencing the code for the acute condition first.

2.   If there are no subentries to identify acute, subacute or chronic, ignore these adjectives when selecting the code for the particular condition.

3.   If a certain condition is described as a subacute condition and the index does not provide a subentry designating subacute, then code the condition as if it were acute.

CODING SUSPECTED CONDITIONS

Whenever the diagnosis is stated as "questionable," "probable," "likely," or "rule out," it is advisable to code documented symptoms or complaints by the patient. The reason for this is that you do not want an insurance carrier to include a disease code in the patient's history if in fact the "suspected" condition is never proven.

Keep in mind that there are no "rule out" codes per se in the ICD-9-CM coding system. If your diagnostic statement is "Rule out Breast Carcinoma" and you use code 174.9 *Malignant neoplasm of female breast, unspecified*, the code definition does not state "rule out." Therefore, the insurance carrier processes the code 174.9 as is, which results in the patient having an insurance history of breast cancer.

To avoid what could become a problem for you and your patient (including the potential of litigation), you should use codes for signs and symptoms in these cases. For example, use code 611.72 *Lump or mass in breast*, or 611.71 *Mastodynia (breast pain)* if these symptoms exist and this is the highest degree of certainty you can code to.

If the patient is asymptomatic but there is a family history of breast cancer then you should consider using a V-code, such as V16.3 *Family history of malignant neoplasm, breast* as your diagnosis code. There are also V-codes to indicate screening for a particular illness or disease. In the above example, code V76.1 *Special screening for malignant neoplasm, breast* could also have been used.

It is important to note that when you use a screening code from the V-code section you should also code signs or symptoms. The reason for doing so is because most health insurance carriers do not provide coverage for routine screening procedures or preventive medicine.

COMBINATION CODES

A combination code is used to fully identify an instance where two diagnoses or a diagnosis with an associated secondary process (manifestation) or complication is included in the description of a single code number. These combination codes are identified by referring to the subterms in the Alphabetic Index (Volume 2) and the inclusion and exclusion terms in the Tabular List (Volume 1).

Examples of commonly used combination codes include 034.0 *Streptococcal sore throat* and 404 *Hypertensive heart and renal disease*. Code 034.0 exists because the throat is often infected with Streptococcus and code 404 must be used whenever a patient has both heart and renal disease instead of assigning codes from categories 402 and 403.

Two main terms may be joined together by combination terms listed in the Alphabetic Index (Volume 2) as subterms such as:

associated with   *in*
complicated (by)   *secondary to*
due to   *with*
during   *without*
following

The listing for the above terms advises the coder to use one or two codes depending on the condition.

MULTIPLE CODING

The concept of multiple coding is encouraged when the use of more than one code number will fully identify a given condition. Thus, use of multiple codes allows all the components of a complex diagnosis to be identified. However, the statement of diagnosis must mention the presence of all the elements for each code number used.

When is multiple coding mandatory? Only if the instructional term "Code Also" appears in italics under an italicized subdivision in the Tabular List (Volume 1). In this instance, you should interpret mandatory as....requires the use of both codes, and that these codes must be sequenced with the code for the etiology being listed first and the code identifying the manifestation listed second. You will recognize mandatory multiple coding situations by instructional terms used in the Tabular List (Volume 1). Terms to watch for are: "Code also....," "Use additional code...," and "Note:..."

If you turn to Category 330 in the Tabular List (Volume 1), you will notice the instructional term cited: "Use additional code if desired, to identify associated mental retardation." The phrase "...identify associated mental retardation..." should be interpreted as "...identify associated mental retardation, if stated to be present in the diagnostic statement." With this understood, these diagnostic statements would be coded as below.

Coding Examples

Cerebral degeneration in childhood with mental retardation

    330.9   Unspecified cerebral degeneration in childhood

    319   Unspecified mental retardation

Cerebral degeneration in childhood

    330.9   Unspecified cerebral degeneration in childhood

In the Alphabetic Index (Volume 2), if two codes are listed, the first should be sequenced first with the code in italicized brackets listed second to indicate the additional code. However, the fact that two codes appear after a subterm in the Alphabetic Index does not automatically indicate mandatory multiple coding. It is necessary to verify both code numbers in the Tabular List. If, in the Tabular List, the code number is also in italics as in the Alphabetical Index and, the instructional term "Code also" appears in italics, then both criteria have been met for mandatory multiple coding.

Coding Example

Diabetic neuropathy

    250.60 Diabetes with neurological manifestations

    [357.2] Polyneuropathy in diabetes

    In the Alphabetic Index (Volume 2) under "Diabetes," you will find "Neuropathy" listed followed by the codes 250.6 and [357.2] in brackets.

It should also be noted at this point, that even though mandatory multiple coding is always indicated by the presence of the instructional term "Code first" in italics beneath the italicized code number and title for the manifestation, this does not always hold true under the code number for the etiology. Multiple coding is not to be used in those instances when a combination code accurately identifies all of the elements within the diagnostic statement.

CODING LATE EFFECTS

You use late effects coding when coding diagnostic statements that identify a residual effect (condition produced) after the acute phase of an illness or injury has ended. The proper coding sequence is to list the code number identifying the residual (the current condition) first, with the code number identifying the cause (original illness/injury no longer present in its acute phase but which was the cause of the long term residual condition) listed second.

Coding Example

Hemiplegia due to previous cerebral vascular accident

    342.90 Hemiplegia, unspecified, affecting unspecified side

    438.20 Late effects of cerebrovascular disease, Hemiplegia affecting unspecified side

    The <u>residual</u> for this statement is "Hemiplegia" as it is the long term condition that resulted from a previous acute illness. The <u>cause</u> for this statement is "Cerebral vascular accident" as it is the original illness no longer in its acute phase but which did cause the long term residual condition now present.

How do you recognize when to use late effects coding and when not to? Often, the diagnostic statement will contain key words to help identify a late effects situation. Key words used in defining late effects include:

    late
    due to an old injury
    due to a previous illness/injury
    due to an illness/injury occurring one year or more ago

In cases where these key words (phrases) are not included within the diagnostic statement, an effect is considered to be late if sufficient time has elapsed between the occurrence of the acute illness/injury and the development of the residual effect.

Coding Example

Excessive scar tissue due to third degree burn, right leg

709.2   Scar conditions and fibrosis of skin

906.7   Late effect of burn of other extremities

The previous diagnostic statement does not indicate the time element with any modifying terms as "old" or "previous." The fact that enough time has elapsed for the development of scar tissue indicates that the acute phase of the injury has subsided and the scarring should be coded as a late effect.

If a diagnostic statement only specifies the cause of the late effect and does not indicate the residual, then use the code number for the cause.

Coding Example

Residuals of tuberculosis

137   Late effects of tuberculosis

The above statement does not identify the actual residuals, so you would use the code for the cause.

To find the code for such a statement in the Alphabetic Index (Volume 2), refer to the main term "LATE" and the subterm "EFFECTS OF." The only codes available for causes of late effects are:

137   Late effects of tuberculosis

138   Late effects of acute poliomyelitis

139   Late effects of other infectious and parasitic diseases

268.1   Rickets, late effects

326   Late effects of intracranial abscess or pyogenic infection

438   Late effects of cerebrovascular disease

677   Late effects of complication of pregnancy, childbirth and the puerperium

905   Late effects of musculoskeletal and connective tissue injuries

906   Late effects of injuries to skin and subcutaneous tissues

907   Late effects of injuries to the nervous system

908   Late effects of other and unspecified injuries

909   Late effects of other and unspecified external causes

E999   Late effect of injury due to war operations and terrorism

Be sure to distinguish between a late effect and a historical statement in a diagnosis. Whenever the statement uses the terms "effects of old...," "sequela of...," or "residuals of...," then code as late effects. If the diagnosis is expressed in terms as "history of...," these are coded to personal history of the illness or injury and are coded to the V-Codes (V-10 to V-15).

CODING INJURIES

Injuries comprise a major section of ICD-9-CM. Categories 800-959 include fractures, dislocations, sprains and various other types of injuries. Injuries are classified first according to the general type of injury and within each type there is a further breakdown by anatomical site.

In cases where a patient has multiple injuries, the most severe injury is the principal diagnosis. Where multiple sites of injury are specified in the diagnosis, you should interpret the term "with" as indicating involvement of both sites, and interpret the term "and" as indicating involvement of either or both sites. You will also note that fifth-digits are commonly used when coding injuries to provide information regarding level of consciousness, specific anatomical sites and severity of injuries.

Some general rules to apply when coding fractures follow. Fractures can either be "open" or "closed." An "open" fracture is when the skin has been broken and there is communication with the bone and the outside of the body. Whereas, with a "closed" fracture the bone does not have contact with the outside of the body.

Note the following descriptions as set forth in the ICD-9-CM at the four-digit subdivision level to help distinguish between an "open" and "closed" fracture.

Closed Fractures

comminuted	*simple*
linear	*greenstick*
fissured	*depressed*
spiral	*fractured NOS*
impacted	slipped epiphysis
elevated	

Open Fractures

compound	*with foreign body*
missile	*infected*
puncture	

Anytime that it is not indicated whether a fracture is open or closed, code it as if it were closed. Fracture-dislocations are classified as fractures. Pathological fractures are classified to the condition causing the fracture (i.e. osteoporosis) with the use of an additional code to identify the *Pathological fracture* (733.1).

When coding burns, code only the most severe degree of burns when the burns are of the same site but of different degrees. In cases of burns where it is noted that there is an infection, assign the code for the burn and also the code for the infection (958.3 *Posttraumatic wound infection NEC*).

The percentage of the body surface involved with burns is specified by using Category 948. This code may be used as a solo code when the site of the burn is unspecified. There is also a fifth-digit subclassification included in Category 948 to identify the percentage of the total body surface involved with third degree burns. Use Category 949 only when neither the site nor the percentage of the body surface involved is specified in the diagnosis.

POISONING AND ADVERSE EFFECTS OF DRUGS

There are two different sets of code numbers to use to differentiate between poisoning and adverse reactions to the correct substances properly administered. First, you must make the distinction between poisoning and adverse reaction. Poisoning by drugs includes:

Poisoning

Accidental

1. Given in error during diagnostic or therapeutic procedures.

2. Given in error by one person to another (for example, mother to child).

3. Taken in error by self.

Purposeful

1. Suicide attempt.

2. Homicide attempt.

Adverse Reaction in Spite of Proper Administration of Correct Substance

1. In therapeutic of diagnostic procedure.

2. Taken by self or given to another as prescribed.

3. Accumulative effect (intoxication due to....).

4. Interaction of prescribed drugs.

5. Synergistic reaction (enhancing the effect of another drug).

6. Allergic reaction.

7. Hypersensitivity.

To code poisoning by drugs, use the Alphabetic Index (Volume 2) which contains the Table of Drugs and Chemicals. This table includes one column to identify the poisoning code (960-989) and four columns of External Cause Codes to classify whether the poisoning was an accident, suicide, assault or undetermined.

The column labeled "Therapeutic Use" is not used for poisonings but in coding adverse reactions to correct substances properly administered. The External Cause Codes are optional but may be used if a facility's coding policy requires their use.

Note that in the Alphabetic Index (Volume 2) that the subterm entry "Drug" under the main term of "Poisoning" refers the coder to the Table of Drugs and Chemicals for the code assignment. Because the Table of Drugs and Chemicals is so extensive, it is acceptable to code directly from the Table without verifying the code obtained in Volume 1.

What if the drug which caused the poisoning is not listed in the Table of Drugs and Chemicals?

1. Refer to Appendix C in Volume 1 (American Hospital Formulary Service) and locate the name of the drug.

2. Note the AHFS category number listed.

3. Turn to the Table of Drugs and Chemicals in the Alphabetic Index (Volume 2) of ICD-9-CM.

4. Locate the term "Drug."

5. Refer to the subterm "AHFS List."

6. Look through the list until you find the AHFS Category Number determined in step 2 above. The AHFS Category Numbers are listed in numeric order.

7. Assign the code.

How Do You Identify Poisoning by Drugs?

The statement of diagnosis will usually have descriptive terms that would indicate poisoning. Look for terms such as:

Intoxication	*Toxic effect*
Overdose	*Wrong drug given/taken in error*
Poisoning	*Wrong dosage given/taken in error*

Adverse effects of a medicine taken in combination with alcohol or from taking a prescribed drug in combination with a drug the patient took on his/her own initiative (for example antihistamines) are coded as poisonings. If you wish to code a manifestation of the poisoning as well, this code is always listed second, after listing the code identifying the poison first.

Adverse Effects of Drugs

The World Health Organization (WHO) defines adverse drug reaction as any response to a drug "which is noxious and unintended and which occurs at doses used in man for prophylaxis, diagnosis or therapy." Notice that this definition does not include the terms "overdose" or "poisoning."

Why does ICD-9-CM differentiate between poisoning and adverse drug reaction? Tabulation of statistical data indicates how often a drug reaction occurred because of the drug itself versus how often the drug was either not given or taken properly.

Two codes are required when coding adverse drug reactions to the correct substance properly administered. One code is used to identify the manifestation or the nature of the adverse reaction such as urticaria, vertigo, gastritis, etc. This code is assigned from Categories 001-799 in Volume 1.

Refer to the main term identifying the manifestation in the Alphabetic Index (Volume 2). But remember that the Table of Drugs and Chemicals is not used to locate the code for the manifestation, and the code used to identify the manifestation does not identify the drug responsible for the adverse reaction.

A second code is required to identify the drug causing the adverse reaction. In ICD-9-CM, the only codes provided to identify the drug causing an adverse reaction to a substance properly administered are E930 through E949. Anytime a code is selected from the E930-E949 range, it can never be sequenced first or stand as a solo code.

Locating the Proper E Code

How do you locate the proper E code to identify the drug which was responsible for causing an adverse reaction to a correct substance properly administered? Turn to the Table of Drugs and Chemicals in the Alphabetic Index (Volume 2). Earlier we noted that the column labeled "Therapeutic Use" was not used for coding instances involving poisoning. However, for adverse drug reactions to a correct substance properly administered, the "Therapeutic Use" column is used to find the proper code within the range E930 through E949 to identify the drug.

Drug Interactions Between Two or More Drugs

Drug interactions between two or more prescribed drugs are classified as adverse drug reactions to a correct substance properly administered. This holds true regardless of whether the drugs were prescribed by the same physician or different physicians.

Two types of drug interactions should be noted:

1.   Synergistic interaction. One drug enhances the action of another drug so that the combined effect is greater than the sum of the effects of each used alone.

2.   Antagonistic interaction. One drug represses the action of another drug.

To properly code drug interactions, first code the manifestation. Then code each drug involved in the interaction using the E codes from the column labeled "Therapeutic Use" from the Table of Drugs and Chemicals.

Coding Example

Gastritis due to interaction between Motrin and Procainamide

535.50   Unspecified gastritis and gastroduodenitis
List the manifestation first

E935.8   Other specified analgesics and antipyretics

E942.0   Cardiac rhythm regulators

Coding Example

When a diagnostic statement does not state specifically the manifestation or nature of the adverse reaction, you should use the code provided to identify an adverse drug reaction of unspecified nature, 995.2 *Unspecified adverse effect of drug, medicinal and biological substance.* For example:

Allergic reaction to Motrin, proper dose

995.2   Unspecified adverse effect of drug medicinal and biological substance

E935.8   Other specified analgesics and antipyretics

Note in the above example that the code indicating the manifestation, although unspecified as to the nature, is listed first followed by the E code to identify the drug. When the drug causing an adverse effect is unknown or unspecified, use code E947.9 *Unspecified drug or medicinal substance.*

It is very important to remember that codes in the range 960 through 979 are never used in combination with codes in the range E930 through E949 because codes in the range 960-979 identify poisonings and codes in the range E930-E949 identify the external cause of adverse reactions to the correct substance properly administered.

CODING COMPLICATIONS OF MEDICAL AND SURGICAL CARE

A complication is when you have the occurrence of two or more diseases in the same patient. Recent studies have revealed serious deficiencies in properly coding complications for insurance claims processing. Often the complication is never mentioned. Complications are responsible for many of the procedures that are ordered for patients, therefore the complication should be coded and submitted on your insurance claims.

Postoperative complications that affect a specific anatomical site or body system are classified to the appropriate chapter 1 through 16 of the Tabular Index (Volume 1). Postoperative complications affecting more than one anatomical site or body system are classified in the chapter on injury and poisoning (Chapter 17, Categories 996-999). If the Alphabetic Index (Volume 2) does not provide a specific main term and subterm to identify a postoperative complication, classify the complication to categories 996-999.

Coding Example

Postcholecystectomy syndrome

576.0   Postcholecystectomy syndrome

The Alphabetic Index (Volume 2) specifically classifies the postoperative condition to one of the categories from 001 through 799. See main term "Complication," subterms "surgical procedure" and "postcholecystectomy syndrome."

Coding Examples

Postoperative wound infection

> **998.5**   Postoperative infection
>
> The Alphabetic Index (Volume 2) has a main term "Infection" and subterms "wound, postoperative" for this condition. Note that this code appears in Chapter 17 within categories 996-999.

Postoperative atelectasis

> **997.3**   Respiratory complications
>
> Refer to the main term "Atelectasis" in the Alphabetic Index (Volume 2). Note there is no subterm for postoperative beneath this main term. Therefore, you must presume this complication is classified to one of the categories in the range 969-999. You may also code 518.0 *Pulmonary collapse*, to identify the nature of the respiratory complication for statistical purposes; however, the code for the complication must be listed first.

COMPLICATIONS FROM MECHANICAL DEVICES

Subcategories in the range 996.0 through 996.5 are used to identify mechanical complications of devices. Mechanical complications are the result of a malfunction on the part of the internal prosthetic implant or device. What indicates a mechanical complication? Breakdown or obstruction, displacement, leakage, perforation or protrusion of the devices are all forms of mechanical complications.

Coding Examples

Displacement of cardiac pacemaker electrode

> **996.01**   Mechanical complication of cardiac device, implant, and graft due to cardiac pacemaker (electrode)

Protrusion of nail into acetabulum

> **996.4**   Mechanical complication of internal orthopedic device, implant, and graft

Other complications of devices, such as infection or hemorrhage, are due to an abnormal reaction of the body to an otherwise properly functioning device. All complications involving infection are coded to category 996.7 Other complications of internal prosthetic device, implant and graft.

Coding Examples

Infected arteriovenous shunt

> **996.6**   Infection and inflammatory reaction due to internal prosthetic device, implant, and graft

Anterior chamber hemorrhage due to displaced prosthetic lens

> **996.7** Other complications of internal (biologic) (synthetic) prosthetic device, implant, and graft

CARDIAC COMPLICATIONS

In the case of cardiac complications, ICD-9-CM defines the "immediate postoperative period" as "the period between surgery and the time of discharge from the hospital." This definition is the basis of whether to code cardiac complications under subcategory 997.1 *Cardiac complications affecting specified body systems, not elsewhere classified*, or under subcategory 429.4 *Functional disturbances following cardiac surgery.*

Use 997.1 for a cardiac complication that occurs anytime between surgery and hospital discharge from any type of procedure performed. Use subcategory 429.4 to code long-term cardiac complications resulting from cardiac surgery.

It is important to distinguish between complications and aftercare. Aftercare is usually an encounter for something planned in advance (example, removal of Kirshner wire). Aftercare is classified using codes in the range of V51-V58. An encounter for a complication occurs from unforeseen circumstances, such as wound infection, resulting in complication of the patient's condition.

SPECIAL CODING SITUATIONS

As you become an experienced coder you will encounter situations where the standard rules do not seem to apply, or which require a special understanding in order to code properly. These situations include coding of circulatory diseases, diabetes, mental disorders, infectious diseases, manifestations, neoplasms, and pregnancy and childbirth. The following sections address these specific special coding situations.

CODING CIRCULATORY DISEASES

Because of the variety of terms and phrases used by physicians to identify diseases of the circulatory system, you will often experience difficulty in coding. To accurately code disorders of the circulatory system, it is imperative that the coder carefully read all inclusion, exclusion and "use additional code" notations contained in the Tabular List (Volume 1).

Fifth digit subclassifications are also frequently used to code combination disorders or to provide further specificity in this section. Even those in specialties other than cardiology will frequently find themselves coding circulatory system diagnoses due to the prevalence of circulatory disorders in this country.

Chapter 7 of the Tabular List (Volume 1), titled Diseases of the Circulatory System, contains the following major sections:

Acute Rheumatic Fever (390-392)

Chronic Rheumatic Heart Disease (393-398)

Hypertensive Disease (401-405)

Ischemic Heart Disease (410-414)

Diseases of Pulmonary Circulation (415-417)

Other Forms of Heart Disease (420-429)

Cerebrovascular Disease (430-438)

Diseases of Arteries, Arterioles, and Capillaries (440-448)

Diseases of Veins, Lymphatics, and Ohter Diseases of the Circulatory System (451-459)

Diseases of Mitral and Aortic Valves

Certain diseases of the mitral valve of unspecified etiology are presumed to be of rheumatic origin and others are not. None of the disorders of the aortic valve of unspecified etiology are presumed to be of rheumatic origin. When you have disorders involving both the mitral and aortic valves of unspecified etiology, then they are presumed to be of rheumatic origin.

Coding Examples

Mitral valve insufficiency

424.0   Mitral valve disorders

Refer to the main term "Insufficiency" in the Alphabetic Index (Volume 2). Note the subterm "mitral (valve)."

Mitral valve stenosis

394.0   Mitral stenosis

Refer to the main term "Stenosis" and the sub-term "mitral (valve)" in the Alphabetic Index (Volume 2).

Aortic valve insufficiency

424.1   Aortic valve disorders

Aortic valve stenosis

424.1   Aortic valve disorders

Look up the main term "Stenosis" and the subterm "aortic" in the Alphabetic Index (Volume 2). Remember that aortic valve disorders of unspecified etiology are not considered rheumatic in nature or origin.

Insufficiency of mitral and aortic valves

396.3   Mitral valve insufficiency and aortic valve insufficiency

Under the main term "Insufficiency" in the Alphabetic Index (Volume 2) you will find the subterm "aortic." Further review will locate "with," "mitral valve disease," "insufficiency, incompetence or regurgitation" which directs you to code 396.3

Ischemic Heart Disease

In ischemic heart disease, the manifestations are due to a lack of blood flow to the heart rather than to the anatomical lesion of the coronary arteries. The most common cause of coronary heart disease is coronary atherosclerosis. However, ischemic heart disease can be due to non-coronary disease, such as aortic valvular stenosis, as well. There are many synonyms used to indicate ischemic heart disease such as: coronary artery heart disease, ASHD, and coronary ischemia. Categories in the range 410-414, Ischemic Heart Disease, includes that with mention of hypertension. Use an additional code to identify the presence of hypertension.

Coding Examples

Angina pectoris

413.9   Other and unspecified angina pectoris

As no mention of hypertension is made in the diagnostic statement, a single code is all that is required.

Angina pectoris with essential hypertension

413.9   Other and unspecified angina pectoris

401.9   Essential hypertension, unspecified

In this example, the mention of hypertension in the diagnostic statement requires the use of a second code.

Myocardial Infarction

A myocardial infarction is classified as acute if it is either specified as "acute" in the diagnostic statement or with a stated duration of eight weeks or less. When a myocardial infarction is specified as "chronic" or with symptoms after eight weeks from the date of the onset, it should be coded to subcategory 414.8 *Other specified forms of chronic ischemic heart disease.* If a myocardial infarction is specified as old or healed or has been diagnosed by special investigation (EKG) but is currently not presenting any symptoms, code using category 412 *Old myocardial infarction.*

Coding Examples

Myocardial infarction three weeks ago

410.92   Acute myocardial infarction, unspecified site

Chronic myocardial infarction with angina

    414.8   Other specified forms of chronic ischemic heart disease

    413.9   Other and unspecified angina pectoris

Myocardial infarction diagnoses by EKG, symptomatic

    412   Old myocardial infarction

Arteriosclerotic Cardiovascular Disease (ASCVD)

Arteriosclerotic cardiovascular disease (ASCVD) is classified to subcategory 429.2 *Cardiovascular disease, unspecified*. You should use an additional code to identify the presence of arteriosclerosis when coding ASCVD. For example, the diagnostic statement "generalized arteriosclerotic cardiovascular disease" should be coded using 429.2 followed by 440.9 *Generalized and unspecified atherosclerosis.*

"Other forms of heart disease", categories 420-429, are used for multiple coding purposes to fully identify a stated diagnosis. The exception to this rule is if the Alphabetic Index (Volume 2) or Tabular List (Volume 1) specifically instructs you otherwise.

Coding Examples

Arteriosclerotic heart disease with acute pulmonary edema

    428.1   Left heart failure

    414.0   Coronary atherosclerosis

    Note that the code for ASHD (414.0) is listed second as a possible underlying cause of the acute situation.

Arteriosclerotic heart disease with congestive heart failure

    428.0   Congestive heart failure, unspecified

    414.0   Coronary atherosclerosis

Cerebrovascular Disease

When coding cerebrovascular disease (codes 430-438), you should code the component parts of the diagnostic statement identifying the cerebrovascular disease, unless specifically instructed to do otherwise in the Alphabetic Index (Volume 2) or Tabular List (Volume 1).

Coding Examples

Cerebrovascular arteriosclerosis with subarachnoid hemorrhage

    430   Subarachnoid hemorrhage

    437.0   Cerebral atherosclerosis

Cerebrovascular accident secondary to thrombosis

434.00 Cerebral thrombosis, without mention of cerebral infarction

In this example, you use only one code because of the instructions in the Alphabetic Index (Volume 2). When you look up the main term "Accident" with subterm "cerebrovascular," you are instructed to "(*see also* Disease, cerebrovascular, acute) 436". When you locate the main term "Disease" and subterms "cerebrovascular," "acute" and "thrombotic," you are further instructed to "*see* Thrombosis, brain". This is where you finally locate the single code for this diagnosis, 434.0. When you look up the code in the Tabular List (Volume 1), you are instructed to add a fifth digit "0" if it is without mention of cerebral infarction, and "1" if it is with cerebral infarction.

Whenever there are conditions resulting from the acute cerebrovascular disease, code them if they are stated to be residual(s). If the resulting condition is stated to be transient, do not code them.

Coding Examples

Cerebrovascular accident with residual aphasia

436 Acute, but ill-defined, cerebrovascular disease

784.3 Aphasia

Cerebrovascular accident with transient hemiparesis

436 Acute, but ill-defined, cerebrovascular disease

Hypertensive Disease

As demonstrated earlier with ischemic heart disease, conditions that are classified to cerebrovascular disease (codes 430-438) include that with mention of hypertension, but you must identify the hypertension with another code (401-405) and list it second.

Hypertensive disease is classified to the categories 401-405. The Table of Hypertension is located in the Alphabetic Index (Volume 2) under the main term "Hypertension." This Table contains subterms to identify types of hypertension and complications as well as three columns labeled "malignant," "benign," and "unspecified."

Hypertension is frequently the cause of various forms of heart and vascular disease. However, the mention of hypertension with some heart conditions should not be interpreted as a combination resulting in hypertensive heart disease. The combination is only to be made if there is a cause-and-effect relationship between hypertension and a heart condition classified to subcategories 425.8, 428.0-428.9, 429.0-429.3 and 429.8-429.9.

First you need to be able to make a distinction between conditions specified as "due to" or "with" hypertension. Keep in mind that the phrase "due to hypertension" and the word "hypertensive" are considered synonymous.

Coding Examples

Hypertensive heart disease

    402.90   Hypertensive heart disease, unspecified, without heart failure

Heart disease due to hypertension

    402.90   Hypertensive heart disease, unspecified, without heart failure

Each of the above diagnostic statements indicate clearly a cause-and-effect relationship between hypertension and the condition by specifying that the condition is "due to." Therefore, both statements are coded using 402.90.

If the phrase "with hypertension" is stated or, the diagnostic statement mentions the conditions separately, then you code the conditions separately.

Coding Example

Myocarditis with hypertension

    429.0   Myocarditis, unspecified

    401.9   Essential hypertension, unspecified

As a cause-and-effect relationship is not indicated in the diagnostic statement, the conditions are coded separately.

High Blood Pressure Versus Elevated Blood Pressure

With the ICD-9-CM coding system there is a differentiation made between high blood pressure (hypertension) and elevated blood pressure without a diagnosis of hypertension. If the diagnostic statement indicates elevated blood pressure without the diagnosis of hypertension, it is coded to subcategory 796.2 *Elevated blood pressure reading without diagnosis of hypertension*. If the diagnostic statement indicates high blood pressure or hypertension, it is coded to category 401 *Essential hypertension*.

DIABETES MELLITUS CODING (250)

In 1980, the American Diabetic Association reclassified the types of diabetes mellitus to signify whether or not the patient is dependent on insulin for survival of life. In 1994, additional classifications were added. Note the revisions (bracketed portions) of the statements below for the fifth-digit subclassification.

0   type II [non-insulin dependent type] [NIDDM type] [adult-onset type] or unspecified type, not stated as uncontrolled

       Fifth digit 0 is for use with type II, adult onset diabetic patients, even if the patient requires insulin

1   type I [insulin dependent type] [IDDM] [juvenile type], not stated as uncontrolled

2   type II [non-insulin dependent type] [NIDDM] [adult-onset type] or unspecified type, uncontrolled

Fifth digit 2 is for use with type II, adult onset diabetic patients, even if the patient requires insulin

3   type I [insulin dependent type][IDDM][juvenile type], uncontrolled

Do not assume a patient has insulin-dependent diabetes simply because the patient is receiving insulin, as some non-dependent diabetics may require temporary use when they encounter stressful situations such as surgery or physical or mental illness.

Anytime diabetes is described as "brittle" or "uncontrolled" you should interpret it as diabetes mellitus complicated and assign code 250.9 with the appropriate fifth-digit, 0, 1, 2 or 3. However, if there is also a specific complication present, then assign the code identifying that specific complication, for example, Diabetes mellitus, brittle, with ketoacidosis would be 250.13.

CODING MENTAL DISORDERS

You should be aware of the existence of the glossary of mental disorders in Appendix B of the Tabular List (Volume 1). This glossary is not used for coding purposes but rather as a guide to provide a common frame of reference for statistical comparisons. It is simply an alphabetized listing of mental disorders with definitions.

The coder should choose code assignments based on the terminology used by the physician or psychiatrist and not by the coder's impression of the content of the categories and subcategories. The chapter on mental disorders has many fifth digit subclassifications to watch for when selecting your code.

INFECTIOUS AND PARASITIC DISEASES

There are two categories for identifying the organism causing diseases classified elsewhere. These codes may be used as either additional codes, or as solo codes depending on the diagnostic statement.

     041   Bacterial infection in conditions classified elsewhere and of unspecified site

     079   Viral and chlamydial infection in conditions classified elsewhere and of unspecified site

Coding Examples

Acute UTI due to Escherchia coli

     599.0   Urinary tract infection, site not specified

     041.4   Escherchia coli

Staphylococcus infection

     041.11   Staphylococcus aureus

Bacterial infection

041.9   Bacterial infection, unspecified

The basic coding principles regarding combination codes (one code accurately identifies the components of the condition) applies throughout the chapter on Infectious and Parasitic Diseases.

In the Alphabetic Index (Volume 2), a subterm that identifies an infectious organism takes precedence in code assignment over a subterm at the same indentation level that identifies a site or other descriptive term.

Coding Example

Chronic syphilitic cystitis

095.8   Other specified forms of late symptomatic syphilis

Using the Alphabetic Index (Volume 2) to look up the main term "Cystitis (bacillary)," you will note the subterms "chronic 595.2" and "syphilitic 095.8" at the same indentation level under the main term. Therefore, code 095.8 is assigned to this diagnostic statement, as the organism has precedence over other descriptive terms or anatomical sites.

MANIFESTATIONS

Manifestations are characteristic signs or symptoms of an illness. Signs and symptoms that point rather definitely to a given diagnosis are assigned to the appropriate chapter of ICD-9-CM. For example, hematuria is assigned to the Genitourinary System chapter. However, Chapter 16 *Symptoms, Signs and Ill-Defined Conditions* (780-799), includes ill-defined conditions and symptoms that may suggest two or more diseases or may point to two or more systems of the body, and are used in cases lacking the necessary study to make a final diagnosis.

Conditions allocated to Chapter 16 include:

1.   Cases for which no more specific diagnosis can be made even after all facts bearing on the case have been investigated; for example code 784.0 *Headache*.

2.   Signs or symptoms existing at the time of initial encounter that proved to be transient and whose cause could not be determined; for example code 780.2 *Syncope and collapse*.

3.   Provisional diagnoses in a patient who failed to return for further investigation or care; for example code 782.4 *Jaundice, unspecified, not of newborn*.

4.   Cases referred elsewhere for investigation or treatment before the diagnosis was made; for example code 782.5 *Cyanosis*.

5.   Cases in which a more precise diagnosis was not available for any other reason; for example code 780.4 *Dizziness and giddiness*.

6.   Certain symptoms which represent important problems in medical care and which it might be desired to classify in addition to a known cause; for example, code 780.01 *Coma*.

In the last case, if the cause of a symptom or sign is stated in the diagnosis, assign the code identifying the cause. An additional code may be assigned to further identify this symptom or sign if there is a need to further identify the symptom or sign. In such cases, the code identifying the cause will ordinarily be listed as the principal diagnosis.

CODING OF NEOPLASMS

The coding of neoplasms requires a good understanding of medical terminology. All neoplasms are classified in the Tabular List (Volume 1) in Chapter 2 *Neoplasms* 140-239 which contains the following broad groups:

140-195	Malignant neoplasms, stated or presumed to be primary, of specified sites, except of lymphatic and hematopoietic tissue
196-198	Malignant neoplasms, stated or presumed to be secondary, of specified sites
199	Malignant neoplasms, without specification of site
200-208	Malignant neoplasms, stated or presumed to be primary of lymphatic and hematopoietic tissue
210-229	Benign neoplasms
230-234	Carcinoma in situ
235-238	Neoplasms of uncertain behavior
239	Neoplasms of unspecified nature

Table of Neoplasms

The Table of Neoplasms appears in the Alphabetic Index (Volume 2) under the main term "Neoplasms." This table gives the code numbers for neoplasms of anatomical site. For each anatomical site there are six possible code numbers according to whether the neoplasm in questions is either:

Malignant:
 Primary
 Secondary
 Ca in situ
Benign
Of uncertain behavior
Of unspecified nature

Definitions of Site and Behaviors of Neoplasms

Primary	Identifies the stated or presumed site of origin.
Secondary	Identifies site(s) to which the primary site has spread (direct extension) or metastasized by lymphatic spread, invading local blood vessels, or by implantation as tumor cells shed into body cavities.

In-situ
Tumor cells that are undergoing malignant changes but are still confined to the point of origin without invasion of surrounding normal tissue (non-infiltrating, non-invasive or pre-invasive carcinoma).

Benign
Tumor does not invade adjacent structures or spread to distant sites but may displace or exert pressure on adjacent structures.

Of Uncertain Behavior
The pathologist is not able to determine whether the tumor is benign or malignant because some features of each are present.

Of Unspecified Nature
Neither the behavior nor the histological type of tumors are specified in the diagnostic statement. This type of diagnosis may be encountered when the patient has been treated elsewhere and comes in terminally ill without accompanying information, is referred elsewhere for work-up, or no work-up is performed because of advanced age or poor condition of the patient.

Steps to Coding Neoplasms

1. ICD-9-CM disregards classification of neoplasms by histological type (according to tissue origin) with the exception of lymphatic and hematopoietic neoplasms, malignant melanoma of skin, lipoma, and a few common tumors of bone, uterus, ovary, etc. All other tumors are classified by system, organ or site. The existence of these exceptions makes it necessary to first consult the Alphabetic Index (Volume 2) to determine whether a specific code has been assigned to a specified histological type. For example, *Malignant melanoma of skin of scalp* is coded 172.4 although the code specified in the "Malignant: Primary Column" of the Neoplasm Table for skin of scalp is 173.4.

2. The General Alphabetical Index (Volume 2) also provides guidance to the appropriate column for neoplasms which are not assigned a specific code by histological type. For example, if you look up *Lipomyoma, specified site* in the Alphabetic Index (Volume 2), you will find "*see* Neoplasm, connective tissue, benign."

   The guidance in the Alphabetic Index (Volume 2) can be over-ridden if a descriptor is present. For example, *Malignant adenoma of colon* is coded as 153.9 and not as 211.3 because the adjective "malignant" overrides the entry "adenoma — *see also* Neoplasm, benign."

3. The Neoplasm Table may be consulted directly if a specific neoplasm diagnosis indicates which column of the table is appropriate but does not delineate a specific type of tumor.

4. Sites marked with an asterisk (*), such as buttock NEC* or calf*, should be classified to malignant neoplasm of skin of these sites if the variety of neoplasm is a squamous cell carcinoma or an epidermoid carcinoma and to benign neoplasm of skin of these sites if the variety of neoplasm is a papilloma (of any type).

5.   Primary malignant neoplasms are classified to the site of origin of the neoplasm. In some cases, it may not be possible to identify the site of origin, such as malignant neoplasms originating from contiguous sites.

Neoplasms with overlapping site boundaries are classified to the fourth-digit subcategory .8 "other." For example, code 151.8 *Malignant neoplasm of contiguous or overlapping sites of stomach* whose point of origin cannot be determined.

6.   Neoplasms which demonstrate functional activity require an additional code to identify the functional activity.

Coding Example

Cushing's syndrome due to malignant pheochromocytoma

      194.0   Malignant neoplasm of adrenal gland

      255.0   Disorders of adrenal glands; Cushing's syndrome

Code sequencing depends on the circumstances of the encounter.

7.   Two categories in the malignant neoplasm section represent departures from the usual principles of classification in that the fourth-digit subdivisions in each case are not mutually exclusive. These categories are 150 *Malignant neoplasm of esophagus* and 201 *Hodgkin's disease*. The dual axis is provided to account for differing terminology, for there is no uniform international agreement on the use of these terms.

Coding Example

Malignant neoplasm of the esophagus

      150.0   Cervical esophagus

      150.1   Thoracic esophagus

      150.2   Abdominal esophagus

or using alternate coding

      150.3   Upper third of esophagus

      150.4   Middle third of esophagus

      150.5   Lower third of esophagus

8.   When the treatment is directed at the primary site of the malignancy, designate the primary site as the principal diagnosis, except when the encounter or hospital admission is solely for *Radiotherapy* (V58.0) or, for *Chemotherapy* (V58.1).

9.   When surgical intervention for removal of a primary site or secondary site malignancy is followed by adjunct chemotherapy or radiotherapy, code the malignancy using codes in the 140-198 series, or, where appropriate, in the

200-203 series as long as chemotherapy or radiotherapy is being actively administered. If the admission is for chemotherapy or radiotherapy, the malignancy code is listed second.

10.   When the primary malignancy has been previously excised or eradicated from its site and there is no adjunct treatment directed to that site, and there is no evidence of any remaining malignancy at the primary site, use the appropriate code from the V10 series to indicate the site of the primary malignancy. Any mention of extension, invasion or metastasis to a nearby structure or organ, or to a distant site, is coded as a secondary malignant neoplasm to that site and may be the principal diagnosis in the absence of the primary site.

11.   If the patient has no secondary malignancy and if the reason for admission or for the visit is follow-up of the malignancy, two codes are used and sequenced.

Coding Example

Follow-up of breast cancer treated with chemotherapy. No evidence of recurrence.

   V67.2   Follow-up examination following chemotherapy

   V10.3   Personal history of carcinoma of breast

12.   Malignancies of hematopoietic and lymphatic tissue are always coded to the 200.0-208.9 series unless specified as "in remission." If they are in remission, they are coded as V10.60-V10.79.

13.   If the primary malignant neoplasm previously excised or eradicated has recurred, code it as primary malignancy of the stated site unless the Alphabetic Index (Volume 2) directs you to do otherwise.

Coding Examples

Recurrence of prostate carcinoma

   185   Malignant neoplasm of prostate

Recurrence of breast carcinoma in mastectomy site

   198.2   Secondary malignant neoplasm of other specified sites, skin of breast

   Make sure to code any mention of secondary site(s).

14.   Terminology referring to metastatic cancer is often ambiguous, so when there is doubt as to the meaning intended, the following rules should be used:

   A. Cancer described as metastatic "from" a site should be interpreted as primary of that site.

   B. Cancer described as metastatic "to" a site should be interpreted as secondary of that site.

Coding Examples

Carcinoma in axillary lymph nodes and lungs metastatic from breast

> **174.9**   Malignant neoplasm of female breast, unspecified
>
> **196.3**   Secondary and unspecified malignant neoplasm of lymph nodes of axilla and upper limb
>
> **197.0**   Secondary malignant neoplasm of lung

Adenocarcinoma of colon with extension to peritoneum

> **153.9**   Malignant neoplasm of colon, unspecified
>
> **197.6**   Secondary malignant neoplasm of retroperitoneum and peritoneum

15.   Diagnostic statements when only one site is identified as metastatic:

A. Code to the category for "primary of unspecified site" for the morphological type concerned UNLESS the code thus obtained is either 199.0 or 199.1.

B. If the code obtained in the above step is 199.0 or 199.1, then code the site qualified as "metastatic" as for a primary malignant neoplasm of the stated site EXCEPT for the sites listed below, which should always be coded as secondary neoplasm of the state site:

Bone	Mediastinum
Brain	Meninges
Diaphragm	Peritoneum
Heart	Pleura
Liver	Retroperitoneum
Lymph nodes	Spinal cord

Sites classifiable to 195

C. Also assign the appropriate code for primary or secondary malignant neoplasm of specified or unspecified site, depending on the diagnostic statement you are coding.

Coding Examples

Metastatic renal cell carcinoma of lung

> **189.0**   Malignant neoplasm of kidney, except pelvis
>
> **197.0**   Secondary malignant neoplasm of lung

Metastatic carcinoma of lung

> **162.9**   Malignant neoplasm of bronchus and lung, unspecified
>
> **199.1**   Malignant neoplasm without specification of site, other

This code is assigned to identify "secondary neoplasm of unspecified site" per the instructions in step C above.

Metastatic carcinoma of brain

> **198.3**   Secondary malignant neoplasm of other specified sites, brain and spinal cord
>
> **199.1**   Malignant neoplasm without specification of site, other

In this case, the brain is one of the sites listed in Step B as an exception. So for this diagnostic statement, the code assignment is for secondary neoplasm of the brain and primary malignant neoplasm of unspecified site.

16.   When two or more sites are stated in the diagnostic statement and all are qualified to be "metastatic," you should code as for "primary site unknown" and code the stated sites as secondary neoplasms of those sites.

Coding Example

Metastatic melanoma of lung and liver

> **172.9**   Malignant melanoma of skin, site unspecified
>
> **197.0**   Secondary malignant neoplasm of lung
>
> **197.7**   Secondary malignant neoplasm of liver, specified as secondary

17.   When there is no site specified in the diagnostic statement, but the morphological type is qualified as "metastatic," code as for "primary site unknown." Then assign the code for secondary neoplasms of unspecified site.

Coding Example

Metastatic apocrine adenocarcinoma

> **173.9**   Other malignant neoplasms of skin, site unspecified
>
> **199.1**   Malignant neoplasm without specification of site, other

18.   When two or more sites are stated in the diagnosis and only some are qualified as "metastatic" while others are not, code as for "primary site unknown." However, you should interpret the following sites as secondary neoplasms:

Bone	*Meninges*
Brain	*Peritoneum*
Diaphragm	*Pleura*
Heart	*Retroperitoneum*
Liver	*Spinal Cord*

Sites classifiable to category 195

Coding Example

Carcinoma of lung, metastatic, and brain

198.3 Secondary malignant neoplasm of brain and spinal cord

197.0 Secondary malignant neoplasm of lung

199.1 Malignant neoplasm without specification of site, other

Pregnancy, Childbirth, and the Puerperium

Chapter 11 of the Tabular List (Volume 1) uses fifth-digit subclassifications extensively. In general, the fifth digit is not given in the Alphabetic Index (Volume 2), so each code must be verified in the Tabular List (Volume 1).

The codes for Ectopic and Molar Pregnancy (630-633), do not require the fifth digit. Note also that for the codes 634-638, there is a "common" set of fourth-digit subcategory codes to include complications. Be aware of the use of section marks with categories 634-637 to indicate the need for a fifth digit. All other codes, 640-676 require the use of a fifth digit with the single exception of code 650 *Normal delivery*.

Coding Example

Pregnancy, 3 months gestation complicated by benign essential hypertension

642.03 Benign essential hypertension complicating pregnancy, childbirth, and the puerperium, antepartum condition or complication

Categories 647 and 648 are used for conditions that are usually classified elsewhere, but which have been classified here because they are complications of pregnancy. The interaction of certain conditions with the pregnant state complicates the pregnancy and/or aggravates the non-obstetrical condition (i.e., diabetes mellitus, drug dependence, thyroid dysfunction) and are the main reasons for the obstetrical care provided.

Coding Examples

Rubella in woman, 7 months gestation

647.53 Infectious and parasitic conditions in the mother classifiable elsewhere, but complicating pregnancy, childbirth or the puerperium, rubella, antepartum condition or complication

Pregnancy with diabetes mellitus

648.03 Other current conditions in the mother classifiable elsewhere, but complicating pregnancy, childbirth or the puerperium, diabetes mellitus, antepartum condition or complication

If greater detail is needed for the complication, use an additional code to identify the complication more completely.

Coding Example

Pregnancy with pernicious anemia

> **648.23** Other current conditions in the mother classifiable elsewhere, but complicating pregnancy, childbirth or the puerperium, anemia, antepartum condition or complication
>
> **281.0** Pernicious anemia

Using V Codes

V-codes are used to identify encounters with the health care setting for reasons other than an illness or injury, for example, immunization. V-codes are also used to identify encounters of persons who are injured or ill and whose injury or illness is influenced by some circumstance or problem classified to the V-codes, for example, a person with a functioning pacemaker who requires emergency gastrointestinal surgery. V-codes fall into one of three categories: problems, services or factual.

Problem   These v-codes identify a circumstance or problem that could affect a patient's overall health status but is not itself a current illness or injury. In other words, you may note that a patient has a drug allergy to sulfonamides by using code V14.2 *Personal history of allergy to sulfonamides*. Although this allergy is not considered an illness or a problem in a healthy person, it may affect how the physician will actually care for the patient. You would only use a problem V-code when the problem has a potential effect on the patient's current diagnosis and the physician's treatment plan for management of the illness or injury.

Service   These v-codes describe circumstances other than an illness or injury which prompt the patient's visit. This type of visit often occurs when the patient has a chronic disease but is not acutely ill. An example would be a patient with a known neoplasm that has sought care to receive chemotherapy. In this instance, you would assign V58.1 *Maintenance chemotherapy* as the primary code on your claim and list the code to identify the known neoplasm second.

Factual   These v-codes are used to describe certain facts that do not fall into the "problem" or "service" categories. For example, coding the type of birth using code V30.1 *Single liveborn, born before admission to hospital*.

V-codes can be used as a solo code, a principal code or as a secondary code. It is important to use V-codes properly. If a complication is present, the complication should be coded to categories 001-799 instead of to a V-code.

Coding Example

Colostomy status with colostomy malfunction

569.60 Colostomy and enterostomy complications, unspecified

Code V44.3 *Artificial opening status, colostomy* would not be used in this case because of the complication.

Key words found in diagnostic statements which may result in selection of a V code include:

Admission for	*Health or healthy*
Aftercare	*History (of)*
Attention to	*Maintenance*
Care (of)	*Maladjustment*
Carrier	*Observation*
Checking/checkup	*Problem (with)*
Contact	*Prophylactic*
Contraception	*Replacement (by)(of)*
Counseling	*Screening*
Dialysis	*Status*
Donor	*Supervision (of)*
Examination	*Test*
Fitting of	*Transplant*
Follow up	*Vaccination*

Using E Codes

E-codes permit the classification of environmental events, circumstances and conditions as the cause of injury, poisoning and other adverse effects. The use of E-codes together with the code identifying the injury or condition provides additional information of particular concern to industrial medicine, insurance carriers, national safety programs and public health agencies.

The E-codes may be assigned with any of the codes in the main classification 001-999 to identify the external cause of an injury or condition. E-codes are *never* used as solo codes or as principal diagnostic codes.

When using E-codes, search the Alphabetic Index (Volume 2) for the main term identifying the cause such as "accident," "fire," "shooting," "fall," or "collision." To find the E-code for an adverse reaction to surgical or medical treatment, use the main term "reaction."

Coding Example

Burns to right arm, occurred while burning trash

943.00 Burn of upper limb, except wrist and hand, unspecified degree

E897 Accident caused by controlled fire not in building or structure

E-codes are important for providing the details of an accident to an insurance carrier to enable them to issue faster and more accurate reimbursement. Most insurance carriers want to be sure they reimburse only for services covered under their policy and not for services covered under worker's compensation, automobile or homeowner's insurance. A clear understanding of the circumstances will eliminate questions from the insurance carrier which cause delays in reimbursements.

Coding Example

Fractured ribs due to fall from ladder at home

807.00 Fracture of ribs, closed, unspecified

E881.0 Fall from ladder

E849.0 Place of occurrence, home

Using the above E-codes to provide important information regarding the circumstances of the injury to the insurance carrier eliminates any doubt about the insurer's responsibility for coverage.

When using E-codes always list the E-codes as secondary or supplemental to the code(s) describing the injury.

Anatomical Illustrations

A fundamental knowledge and understanding of basic human anatomy and physiology is a prerequisite for accurate diagnosis coding. While a comprehensive treatment of anatomy and physiology is beyond the scope of this text, the large scale, full color anatomical illustrations on the following pages are designed to facilitate the diagnosis coding process for both beginning and experienced coders.

The illustrations provide an anatomical perspective of diagnosis coding by providing a side-by-side view of the major systems of the human body and a corresponding list of the most common diagnoses categories used to support medical, surgical and diagnostic services performed on the illustrated system.

The diagnostic categories listed on the left facing page of each anatomical illustration are three-digit categories and may not be used for coding. These categories are provided as "pointers" to the appropriate section of the ICD-9-CM Volume 1 where the complete listings, including 4th and 5th digits if appropriate, may be found.

PLATE 1. SKIN AND SUBCUTANEOUS TISSUE - MALE

Viral diseases accompanied by exanthem   050-057

Neoplasms

Malignant melanoma of skin	172
Other malignant neoplasm of skin	173
Malignant neoplasm of male breast	175
Kaposi's sarcoma	176
Benign neoplasm of skin	216
Carcinoma in situ of skin	232

Infections of skin and subcutaneous tissue

Carbuncle and furuncle	680
Cellulitis and abscess of finger and toe	681
Other cellulitis and abscess	682
Acute lymphadenitis	683
Impetigo	684
Pilonidal cyst	685
Other local infections of skin and subcutaneous tissue	686

Other inflammatory conditions of skin and subcutaneous tissue

Erythematosquamous dermatosis	690
Atopic dermatitis and related conditions	691
Contact dermatitis and other eczema	692
Dermatitis due to substances taken internally	693
Bullous dermatoses	694
Erythematous conditions	695
Psoriasis and similar disorders	696
Lichen	697
Pruritus and related conditions	698

Other diseases of skin and subcutaneous tissue

Corns and callosities	700
Other hypertrophic and atrophic conditions of skin	701
Diseases of nail	703
Diseases of hair and hair follicles	704
Disorders of sweat glands	705
Diseases of sebaceous glands	706
Chronic ulcer of skin	707
Urticaria	708
Other disorders of skin and subcutaneous tissue	709
Symptoms involving skin and other integumentary tissue	782

Symptoms, signs and ill-defined conditions   780-799

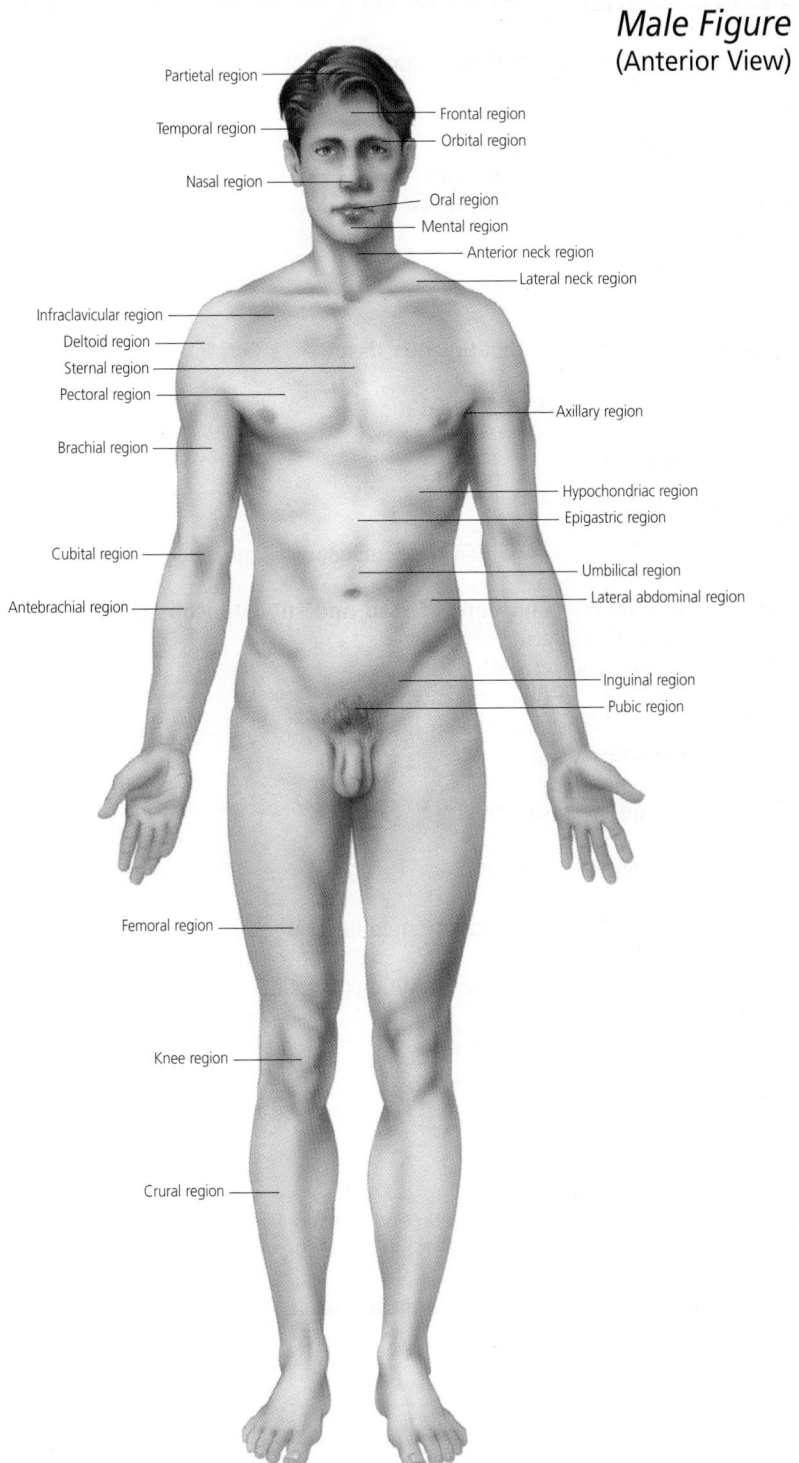

Male Figure
(Anterior View)

Partietal region

Frontal region

Temporal region

Orbital region

Nasal region

Oral region

Mental region

Anterior neck region

Lateral neck region

Infraclavicular region

Deltoid region

Sternal region

Pectoral region

Axillary region

Brachial region

Hypochondriac region

Epigastric region

Cubital region

Umbilical region

Antebrachial region

Lateral abdominal region

Inguinal region

Pubic region

Femoral region

Knee region

Crural region

PLATE 2. SKIN AND SUBCUTANEOUS TISSUE - FEMALE

Viral diseases accompanied by exanthem   050-057

Neoplasms
Malignant melanoma of skin	172
Other malignant neoplasm of skin	173
Malignant neoplasm of female breast	174
Kaposi's sarcoma	176
Benign neoplasm of skin	216
Carcinoma in situ of skin	232

Infections of skin and subcutaneous tissue
Carbuncle and furuncle	680
Cellulitis and abscess of finger and toe	681
Other cellulitis and abscess	682
Acute lymphadenitis	683
Impetigo	684
Pilonidal cyst	685
Other local infections of skin and subcutaneous tissue	686

Other inflammatory conditions of skin and subcutaneous tissue
Erythematosquamous dermatosis	690
Atopic dermatitis and related conditions	691
Contact dermatitis and other eczema	692
Dermatitis due to substances taken internally	693
Bullous dermatoses	694
Erythematous conditions	695
Psoriasis and similar disorders	696
Lichen	697
Pruritus and related conditions	698

Other diseases of skin and subcutaneous tissue
Corns and callosities	700
Other hypertrophic and atrophic conditions of skin	701
Other dermatoses	702
Diseases of nail	703
Diseases of hair and hair follicles	704
Disorders of sweat glands	705
Diseases of sebaceous glands	706
Chronic ulcer of skin	707
Urticaria	708
Other disorders of skin and subcutaneous tissue	709
Symptoms involving skin and other integumentary tissue	782

Symptoms, signs and ill-defined conditions   780-799

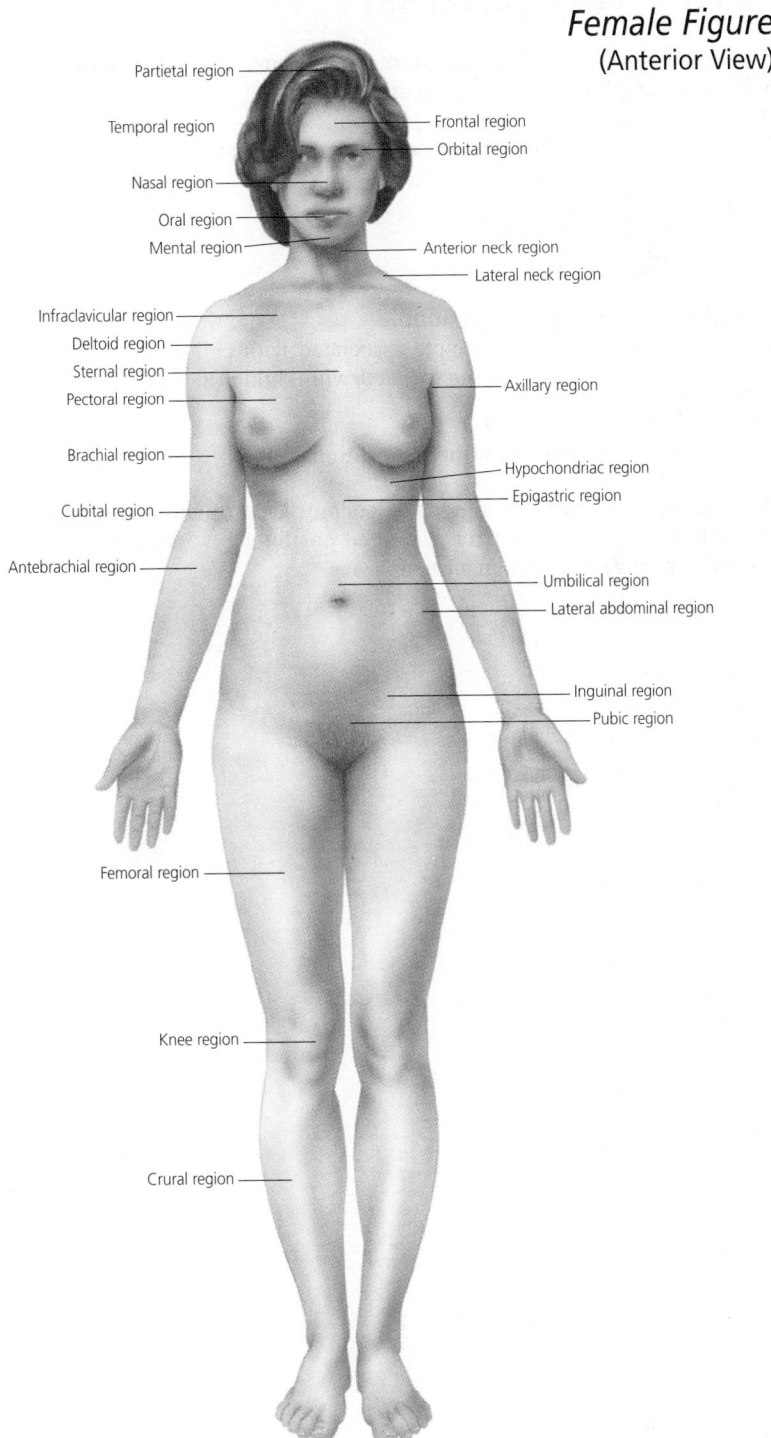

Female Figure
(Anterior View)

Partietal region

Temporal region

Frontal region

Orbital region

Nasal region

Oral region

Mental region

Anterior neck region

Lateral neck region

Infraclavicular region

Deltoid region

Sternal region

Pectoral region

Axillary region

Brachial region

Hypochondriac region

Cubital region

Epigastric region

Antebrachial region

Umbilical region

Lateral abdominal region

Inguinal region

Pubic region

Femoral region

Knee region

Crural region

PLATE 3. FEMALE BREAST

Female Breast

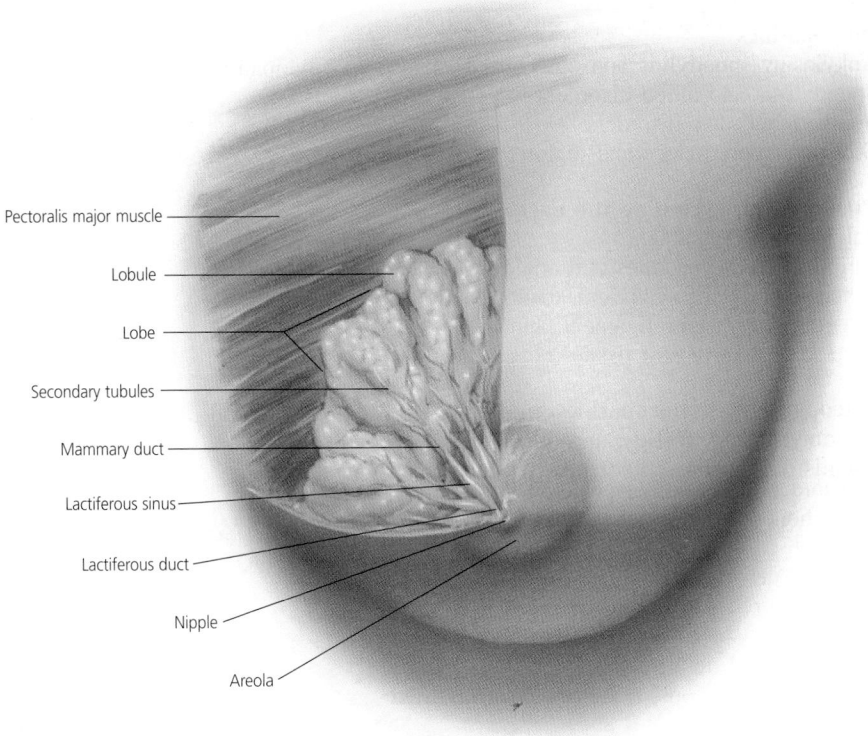

Pectoralis major muscle

Lobule

Lobe

Secondary tubules

Mammary duct

Lactiferous sinus

Lactiferous duct

Nipple

Areola

PLATE 4. MUSCULAR SYSTEM AND CONNECTIVE TISSUE - ANTERIOR VIEW

Muscular System
(Anterior View)

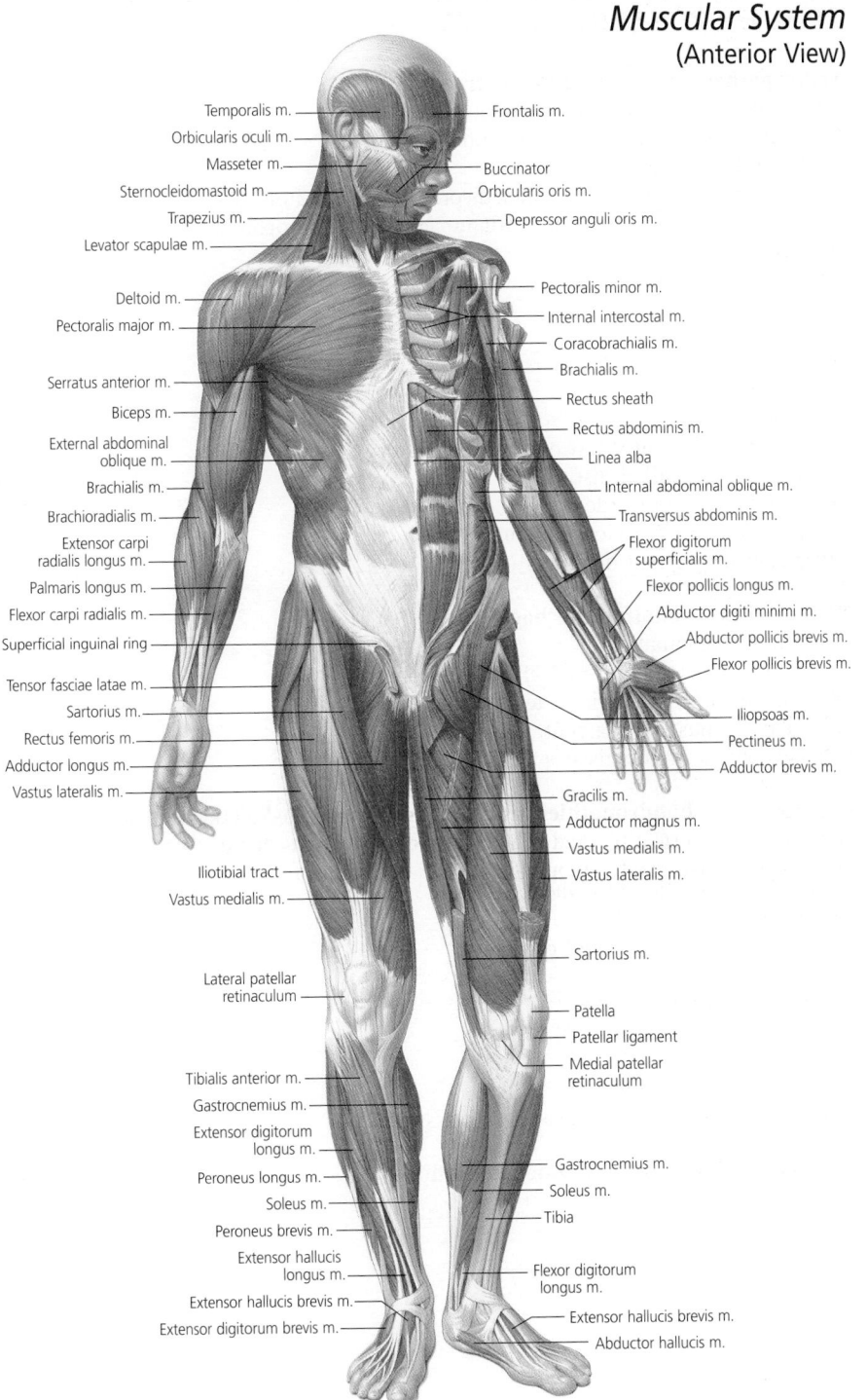

Temporalis m.
Orbicularis oculi m.
Masseter m.
Sternocleidomastoid m.
Trapezius m.
Levator scapulae m.

Frontalis m.
Buccinator
Orbicularis oris m.
Depressor anguli oris m.

Deltoid m.
Pectoralis major m.

Serratus anterior m.
Biceps m.
External abdominal oblique m.
Brachialis m.
Brachioradialis m.
Extensor carpi radialis longus m.
Palmaris longus m.
Flexor carpi radialis m.
Superficial inguinal ring
Tensor fasciae latae m.
Sartorius m.
Rectus femoris m.
Adductor longus m.
Vastus lateralis m.

Pectoralis minor m.
Internal intercostal m.
Coracobrachialis m.
Brachialis m.
Rectus sheath
Rectus abdominis m.
Linea alba
Internal abdominal oblique m.
Transversus abdominis m.
Flexor digitorum superficialis m.
Flexor pollicis longus m.
Abductor digiti minimi m.
Abductor pollicis brevis m.
Flexor pollicis brevis m.
Iliopsoas m.
Pectineus m.
Adductor brevis m.
Gracilis m.
Adductor magnus m.
Vastus medialis m.
Vastus lateralis m.

Iliotibial tract
Vastus medialis m.

Sartorius m.

Lateral patellar retinaculum

Patella
Patellar ligament
Medial patellar retinaculum

Tibialis anterior m.
Gastrocnemius m.
Extensor digitorum longus m.
Peroneus longus m.
Soleus m.
Peroneus brevis m.
Extensor hallucis longus m.
Extensor hallucis brevis m.
Extensor digitorum brevis m.

Gastrocnemius m.
Soleus m.
Tibia
Flexor digitorum longus m.
Extensor hallucis brevis m.
Abductor hallucis m.

PLATE 5. MUSCULAR SYSTEM AND CONNECTIVE TISSUE - POSTERIOR VIEW

Muscular System
(Posterior View)

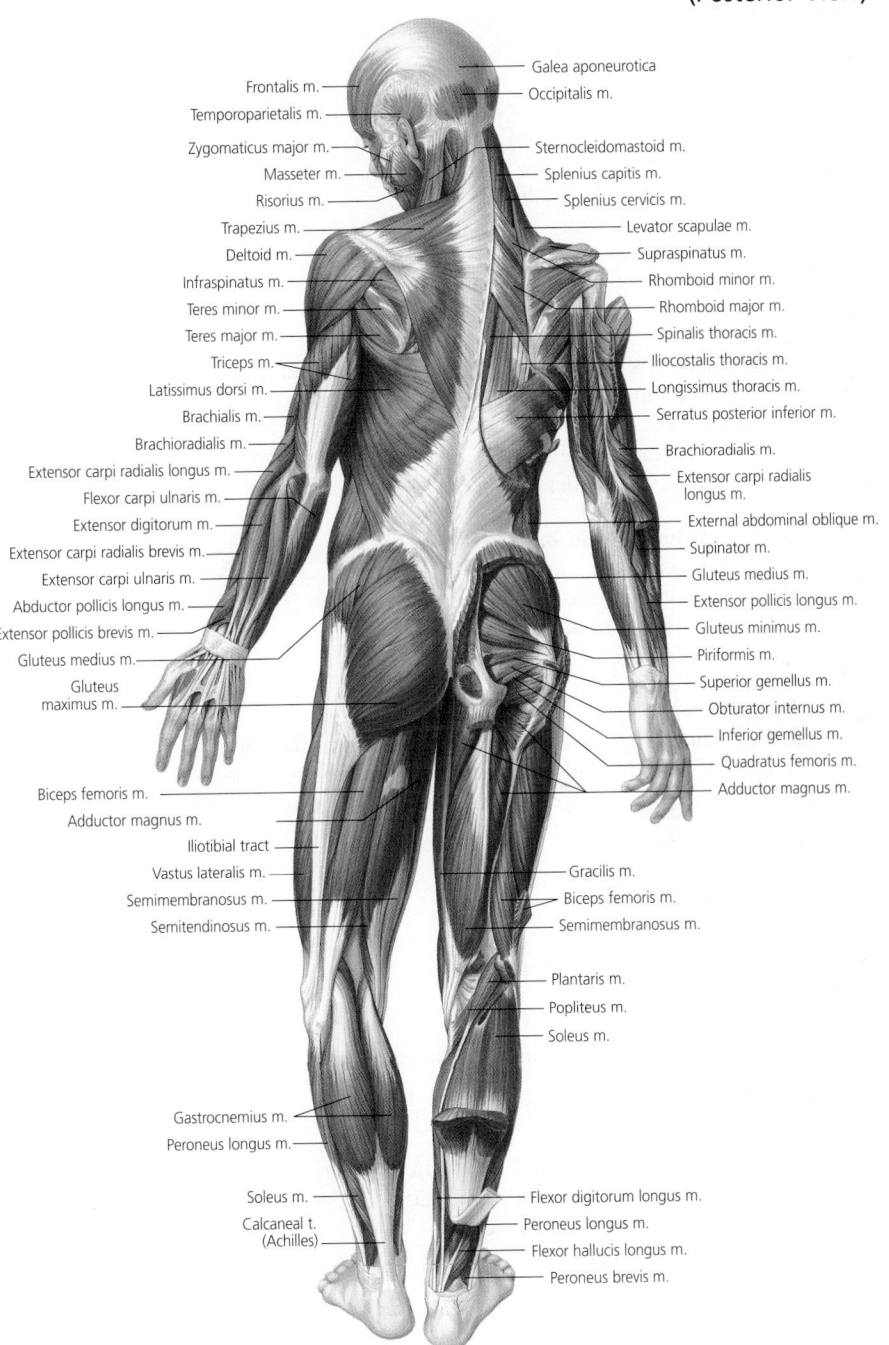

PLATE 6. MUSCULAR SYSTEM - SHOULDER AND ELBOW

Shoulder and Elbow
(Anterior View)

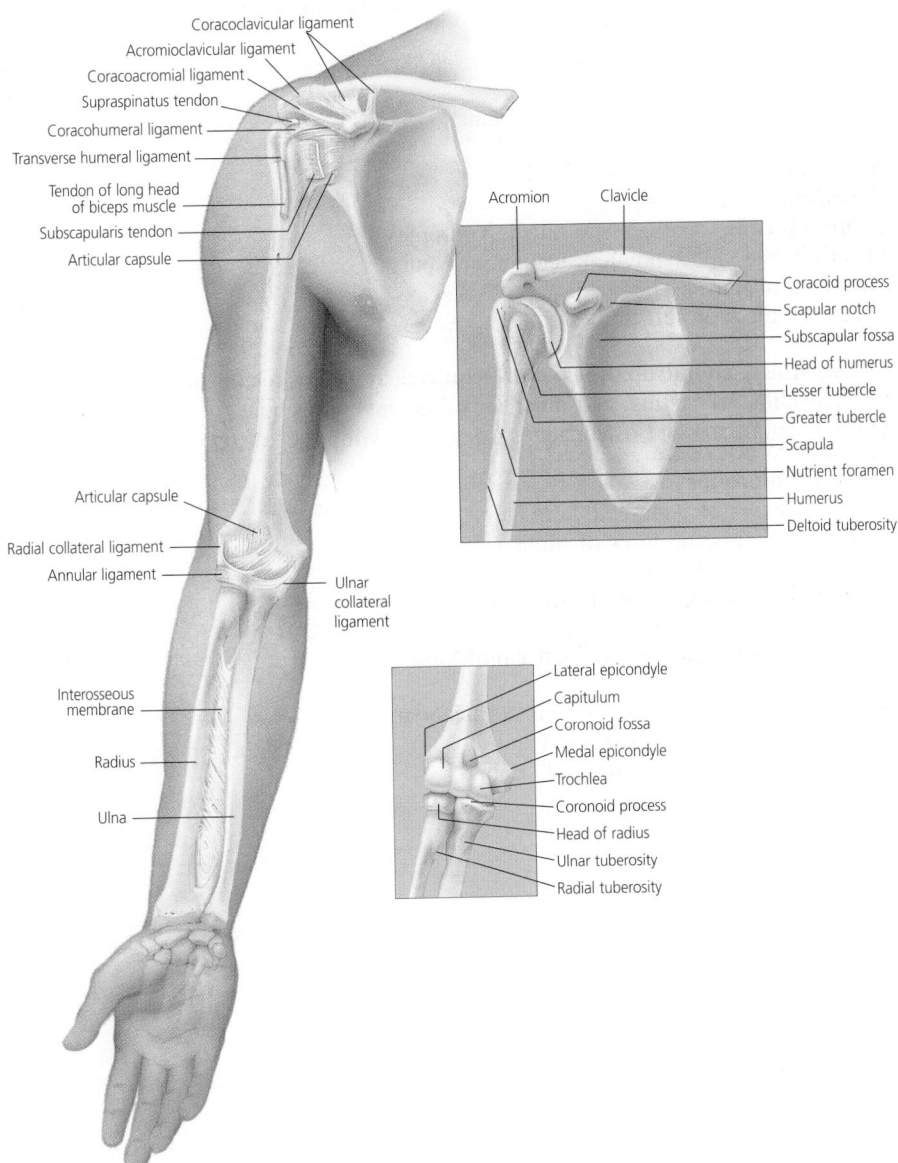

Coracoclavicular ligament
Acromioclavicular ligament
Coracoacromial ligament
Supraspinatus tendon
Coracohumeral ligament
Transverse humeral ligament
Tendon of long head of biceps muscle
Subscapularis tendon
Articular capsule

Acromion
Clavicle
Coracoid process
Scapular notch
Subscapular fossa
Head of humerus
Lesser tubercle
Greater tubercle
Scapula
Nutrient foramen
Humerus
Deltoid tuberosity

Articular capsule
Radial collateral ligament
Annular ligament
Ulnar collateral ligament

Interosseous membrane
Radius
Ulna

Lateral epicondyle
Capitulum
Coronoid fossa
Medal epicondyle
Trochlea
Coronoid process
Head of radius
Ulnar tuberosity
Radial tuberosity

PLATE 7. MUSCULAR SYSTEM - HAND AND WRIST

Arthropathies and related disorders
Diffuse diseases of connective tissue
Arthropathy associated with infections
Crystal arthropathies
Arthropathy associated with other disorders classified elsewhere
Rheumatoid arthritis and other inflammatory polyarthropathies
Osteoarthrosis and allied disorders
Other and unspecified arthropathies
Other derangement of joint
Other and unspecified disorders of joint

710
711
712
713
714
715
716
718
719

Rheumatism, excluding the back
Polymyalgia rheumatica
Peripheral enthesopathies and allied syndromes
Other disorders of synovium, tendon, and bursa
Disorders of muscle, ligament, and fascia
Other disorders of soft tissues

725
726
727
728
729

Osteopathies, chondropathies, and acquired musculoskeletal deformities
Osteomyelitis, periostitis, and other infections involving bone
Osteitis deformans and osteopathies associated with other disorders
   classified elsewhere
Osteochondropathies
Other disorders of bone and cartilage
Other acquired deformities of limbs
Other acquired deformity
Nonallopathic lesions, not elsewhere classified

730

731
732
733
736
738
739

Symptoms, signs and ill-defined conditions

780-799

Sprains and strains of joints and adjacent muscles
Sprains and strains of wrist and hand
Other and ill-defined sprains and strains

842
848

Hand and Wrist

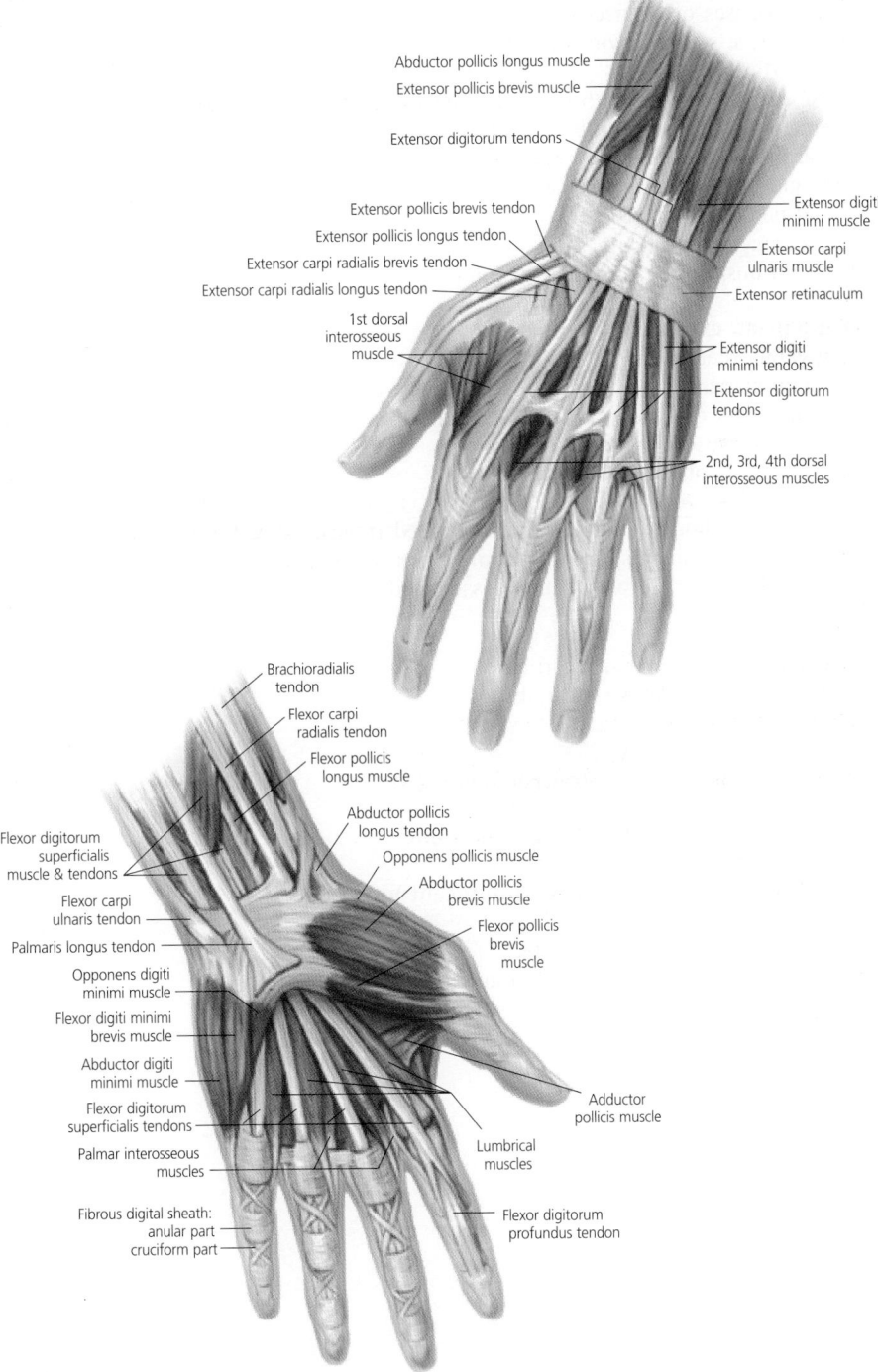

Abductor pollicis longus muscle

Extensor pollicis brevis muscle

Extensor digitorum tendons

Extensor pollicis brevis tendon

Extensor pollicis longus tendon

Extensor carpi radialis brevis tendon

Extensor carpi radialis longus tendon

1st dorsal interosseous muscle

Extensor digiti minimi muscle

Extensor carpi ulnaris muscle

Extensor retinaculum

Extensor digiti minimi tendons

Extensor digitorum tendons

2nd, 3rd, 4th dorsal interosseous muscles

Brachioradialis tendon

Flexor carpi radialis tendon

Flexor pollicis longus muscle

Abductor pollicis longus tendon

Opponens pollicis muscle

Abductor pollicis brevis muscle

Flexor digitorum superficialis muscle & tendons

Flexor carpi ulnaris tendon

Palmaris longus tendon

Opponens digiti minimi muscle

Flexor digiti minimi brevis muscle

Abductor digiti minimi muscle

Flexor digitorum superficialis tendons

Palmar interosseous muscles

Fibrous digital sheath: anular part cruciform part

Flexor pollicis brevis muscle

Adductor pollicis muscle

Lumbrical muscles

Flexor digitorum profundus tendon

PLATE 8. MUSCULOSKELETAL SYSTEM - HIP AND KNEE

Arthropathies and related disorders

Diffuse diseases of connective tissue	710
Arthropathy associated with infections	711
Crystal arthropathies	712
Arthropathy associated with other disorders classified elsewhere	713
Rheumatoid arthritis and other inflammatory polyarthropathies	714
Osteoarthrosis and allied disorders	715
Other and unspecified arthropathies	716
Internal derangement of knee	717
Other derangement of joint	718
Other and unspecified disorders of joint	719

Rheumatism, excluding the back

Polymyalgia rheumatica	725
Peripheral enthesopathies and allied syndromes	726
Other disorders of synovium, tendon, and bursa	727
Disorders of muscle, ligament, and fascia	728
Other disorders of soft tissues	729

Osteopathies, chondropathies, and acquired musculoskeletal deformities

Osteomyelitis, periostitis, and other infections involving bone	730
Osteitis deformans and osteopathies associated with other disorders classified elsewhere	731
Osteochondropathies	732
Other disorders of bone and cartilage	733
Other acquired deformities of limbs	736
Curvature of spine	737
Other acquired deformity	738
Nonallopathic lesions, not elsewhere classified	739

Symptoms, signs and ill-defined conditions   780-799

Sprains and strains of joints and adjacent muscles

Sprains and strains of hip and thigh	843
Sprains and strains of knee and leg	844
Other and ill-defined sprains and strains	848

Hip and Knee
(Anterior View)

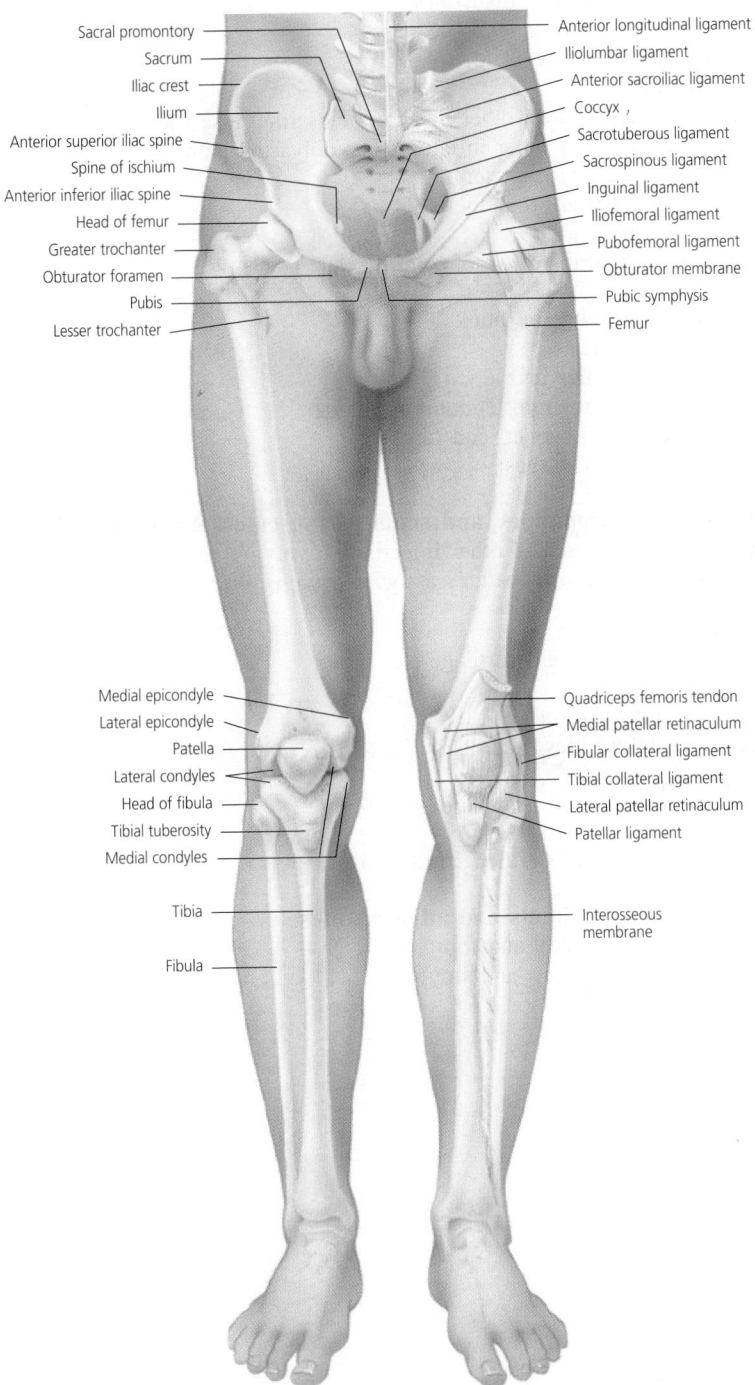

Sacral promontory
Sacrum
Iliac crest
Ilium
Anterior superior iliac spine
Spine of ischium
Anterior inferior iliac spine
Head of femur
Greater trochanter
Obturator foramen
Pubis
Lesser trochanter

Anterior longitudinal ligament
Iliolumbar ligament
Anterior sacroiliac ligament
Coccyx ,
Sacrotuberous ligament
Sacrospinous ligament
Inguinal ligament
Iliofemoral ligament
Pubofemoral ligament
Obturator membrane
Pubic symphysis
Femur

Medial epicondyle
Lateral epicondyle
Patella
Lateral condyles
Head of fibula
Tibial tuberosity
Medial condyles

Tibia

Fibula

Quadriceps femoris tendon
Medial patellar retinaculum
Fibular collateral ligament
Tibial collateral ligament
Lateral patellar retinaculum
Patellar ligament

Interosseous
membrane

PLATE 9. MUSCULOSKELETAL SYSTEM - FOOT AND ANKLE

Arthropathies and related disorders
Diffuse diseases of connective tissue	710
Arthropathy associated with infections	711
Crystal arthropathies	712
Arthropathy associated with other disorders classified elsewhere	713
Rheumatoid arthritis and other inflammatory polyarthropathies	714
Osteoarthrosis and allied disorders	715
Other and unspecified arthropathies	716
Other derangement of joint	718
Other and unspecified disorders of joint	719

Rheumatism, excluding the back
Polymyalgia rheumatica	725
Peripheral enthesopathies and allied syndromes	726
Other disorders of synovium, tendon, and bursa	727
Disorders of muscle, ligament, and fascia	728
Other disorders of soft tissues	729

Osteopathies, chondropathies, and acquired musculoskeletal deformities
Osteomyelitis, periostitis, and other infections involving bone	730
Osteitis deformans and osteopathies associated with other disorders classified elsewhere	731
Osteochondropathies	732
Other disorders of bone and cartilage	733
Flat foot	734
Acquired deformities of toe	735
Other acquired deformities of limbs	736
Other acquired deformity	738
Nonallopathic lesions, not elsewhere classified	739

Symptoms, signs and ill-defined conditions
780-799

Sprains and strains of joints and adjacent muscles
Sprains and strains of ankle and foot	845
Other and ill-defined sprains and strains	848

Foot and Ankle

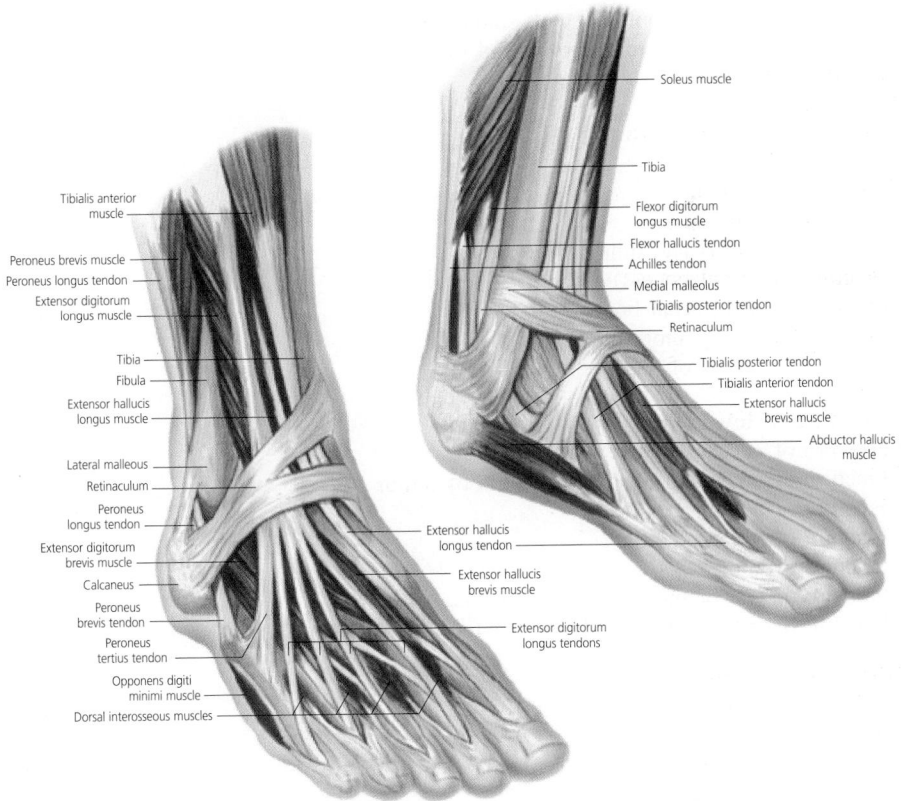

Tibialis anterior muscle

Peroneus brevis muscle
Peroneus longus tendon
Extensor digitorum longus muscle

Tibia
Fibula
Extensor hallucis longus muscle

Lateral malleous
Retinaculum
Peroneus longus tendon
Extensor digitorum brevis muscle
Calcaneus
Peroneus brevis tendon
Peroneus tertius tendon
Opponens digiti minimi muscle
Dorsal interosseous muscles

Extensor hallucis longus tendon

Extensor hallucis brevis muscle

Extensor digitorum longus tendons

Soleus muscle

Tibia

Flexor digitorum longus muscle
Flexor hallucis tendon
Achilles tendon
Medial malleolus
Tibialis posterior tendon
Retinaculum

Tibialis posterior tendon
Tibialis anterior tendon
Extensor hallucis brevis muscle

Abductor hallucis muscle

PLATE 10. SKELETAL SYSTEM - ANTERIOR VIEW

Symptoms, signs and ill-defined conditions   780-799

Fracture of skull
Fracture of vault of skull   800
Fracture of base of skull   801
Fracture of face bones   802
Multiple fractures involving skull or face with other bones   804

Fracture of neck and trunk
Fracture of vertebral column without mention of spinal cord injury   805
Fracture of vertebral column with spinal cord injury   806
Fracture of rib(s), sternum, larynx and trachea   807
Fracture of pelvis   808

Fracture of upper limb
Fracture of clavicle   810
Fracture of scapula   811
Fracture of humerus   812
Fracture of radius and ulna   813
Fracture of carpal bone(s)   814
Fracture of metacarpal bone(s)   815
Fracture of one or more phalanges of hand   816
Multiple fractures of hand bones   817

Fracture of lower limb
Fracture of neck of femur   820
Fracture of other and unspecified parts of femur   821
Fracture of patella   822
Fracture of tibia and fibula   823
Fracture of ankle   824
Fracture of one or more tarsal and metatarsal bones   825
Fracture of one or more phalanges of foot   826

Dislocation
Dislocation of jaw   830
Dislocation of shoulder   831
Dislocation of elbow   832
Dislocation of wrist   833
Dislocation of finger   834
Dislocation of hip   835
Dislocation of knee   836
Dislocation of ankle   837
Dislocation of foot   838

Skeletal System
(Anterior View)

Frontal bone — Parietal bone
Temporal bone — Orbit
Nasal conchae — Zygomatic bone
Maxilla — Nasal septum
Manubrium of sternum — Mandible
— Hyoid bone
Coracoid process
Acromion — Clavicle
Greater tubercle — Coracoclavicular ligament
Head of humerus — Supraspinatus tendon
Scapula — Subscapularis tendon
Humerus — Body of sternum
— Xiphoid process
True ribs (1–7) — Costal cartilages
False ribs (8–12) — Anterior longitudinal ligament
Medial epicondyle — Ulnar collateral ligament
Lateral epicondyle — Radial collateral ligament
Radius — Annular ligament
Ulna — Iliac crest
Sacrum — Anterior sacroiliac ligament
Anterior superior iliac spine — Interosseous membrane
Head of femur — Inguinal ligament
Greater trochanter — Coccyx
— Iliofemoral ligament

L3

A
B — E
C — F
D — G
— H

Metacarpals
Proximal phalanges
Middle phalanges
Distal phalanges

Pubic symphysis

Key to Carpal Bones

A	Scaphoid
B	Trapezium
C	Trapezoid
D	Capitate
E	Lunate
F	Pisiform
G	Triquetral
H	Hamate

Femur

Medial epicondyle — Quadriceps femoris tendon
Lateral epicondyle — Tibial collateral ligament
Patella — Fibular collateral ligament
Head of fibula — Patellar ligament
Tibial tuberosity — Tibia
— Fibula
— Interosseous membrane

Key to Tarsal Bones

J	Intermediate cuneiform
K	Lateral cuneiform
L	Cuboid
M	Talus
N	Navicular
O	Calcaneus
P	Medial cuneiform

J
K — M
L — N
O
P

Medial malleolus
Lateral malleolus

PLATE 11. SKELETAL SYSTEM - POSTERIOR VIEW

Symptoms, signs and ill-defined conditions   780-799

Fracture of skull
Fracture of vault of skull	800
Fracture of base of skull	801
Fracture of face bones	802
Multiple fractures involving skull or face with other bones	804

Fracture of neck and trunk
Fracture of vertebral column without mention of spinal cord injury	805
Fracture of vertebral column with spinal cord injury	806
Fracture of rib(s), sternum, larynx and trachea	807
Fracture of pelvis	808

Fracture of upper limb
Fracture of clavicle	810
Fracture of scapula	811
Fracture of humerus	812
Fracture of radius and ulna	813
Fracture of carpal bone(s)	814
Fracture of metacarpal bone(s)	815
Fracture of one or more phalanges of hand	816
Multiple fractures of hand bones	817

Fracture of lower limb
Fracture of neck of femur	820
Fracture of other and unspecified parts of femur	821
Fracture of patella	822
Fracture of tibia and fibula	823
Fracture of ankle	824
Fracture of one or more tarsal and metatarsal bones	825
Fracture of one or more phalanges of foot	826

Dislocation
Dislocation of jaw	830
Dislocation of shoulder	831
Dislocation of elbow	832
Dislocation of wrist	833
Dislocation of finger	834
Dislocation of hip	835
Dislocation of knee	836
Dislocation of ankle	837
Dislocation of foot	838

Skeletal System
(Posterior View)

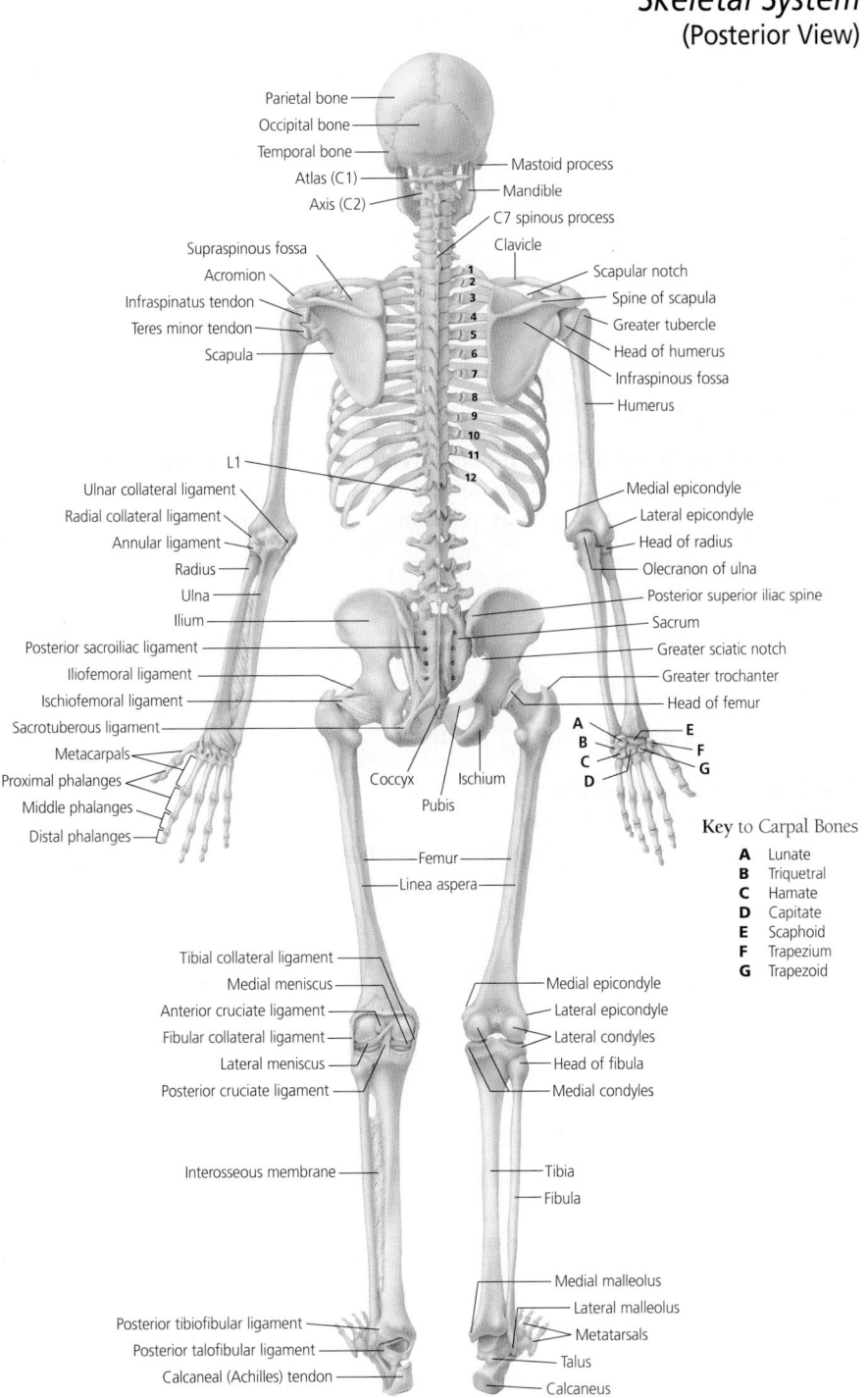

Parietal bone
Occipital bone
Temporal bone
Atlas (C1)
Axis (C2)
Mastoid process
Mandible
C7 spinous process
Clavicle
Supraspinous fossa
Acromion
Infraspinatus tendon
Teres minor tendon
Scapula
Scapular notch
Spine of scapula
Greater tubercle
Head of humerus
Infraspinous fossa
Humerus
L1
Ulnar collateral ligament
Radial collateral ligament
Annular ligament
Radius
Ulna
Ilium
Posterior sacroiliac ligament
Iliofemoral ligament
Ischiofemoral ligament
Sacrotuberous ligament
Metacarpals
Proximal phalanges
Middle phalanges
Distal phalanges
Medial epicondyle
Lateral epicondyle
Head of radius
Olecranon of ulna
Posterior superior iliac spine
Sacrum
Greater sciatic notch
Greater trochanter
Head of femur
Coccyx
Ischium
Pubis
Femur
Linea aspera

A
B
C
D
E
F
G

Key to Carpal Bones

A	Lunate
B	Triquetral
C	Hamate
D	Capitate
E	Scaphoid
F	Trapezium
G	Trapezoid

Tibial collateral ligament
Medial meniscus
Anterior cruciate ligament
Fibular collateral ligament
Lateral meniscus
Posterior cruciate ligament
Medial epicondyle
Lateral epicondyle
Lateral condyles
Head of fibula
Medial condyles
Interosseous membrane
Tibia
Fibula
Medial malleolus
Lateral malleolus
Metatarsals
Posterior tibiofibular ligament
Posterior talofibular ligament
Calcaneal (Achilles) tendon
Talus
Calcaneus

PLATE 12. SKELETAL SYSTEM - VERTEBRAL COLUMN

Arthropathies and related disorders

Diffuse diseases of connective tissue	710
Arthropathy associated with infections	711
Crystal arthropathies	712
Arthropathy associated with other disorders classified elsewhere	713
Rheumatoid arthritis and other inflammatory polyarthropathies	714
Osteoarthrosis and allied disorders	715

Dorsopathies

Ankylosing spondylitis and other inflammatory spondylopathies	720
Spondylosis and allied disorders	721
Intervertebral disc disorders	722
Other disorders of cervical region	723
Other and unspecified disorders of back	724

Osteopathies, chondropathies, and acquired musculoskeletal deformities

Osteomyelitis, periostitis, and other infections involving bone	730
Osteitis deformans and osteopathies associated with other disorders classified elsewhere	731
Osteochondropathies	732
Other disorders of bone and cartilage	733
Curvature of spine	737
Other acquired deformity	738
Nonallopathic lesions, not elsewhere classified	739

Symptoms, signs and ill-defined conditions   780-799

Fracture of neck and trunk

Fracture of vertebral column without mention of spinal cord injury	805
Fracture of vertebral column with spinal cord injury	806

Vertebral Column
(Lateral View)

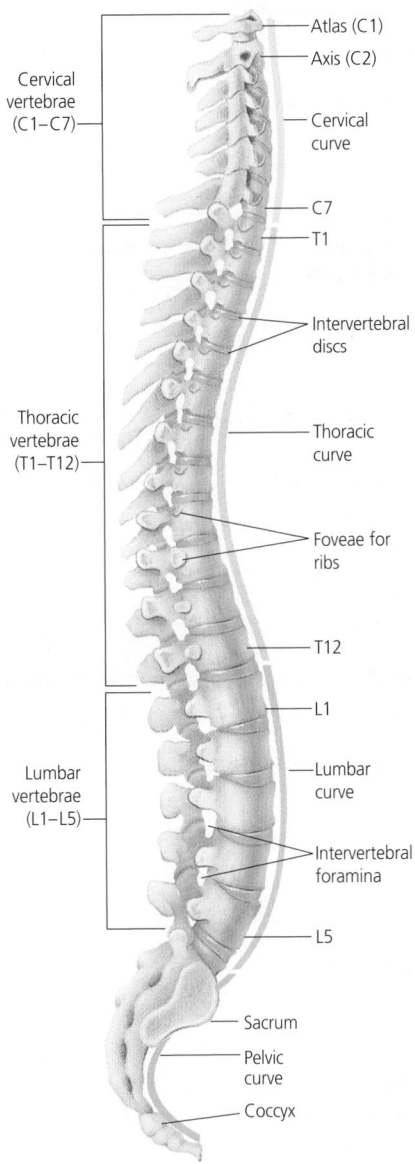

Cervical vertebrae (C1–C7)

Atlas (C1)

Axis (C2)

Cervical curve

C7

T1

Intervertebral discs

Thoracic vertebrae (T1–T12)

Thoracic curve

Foveae for ribs

T12

L1

Lumbar vertebrae (L1–L5)

Lumbar curve

Intervertebral foramina

L5

Sacrum

Pelvic curve

Coccyx

PLATE 13. RESPIRATORY SYSTEM

Respiratory System

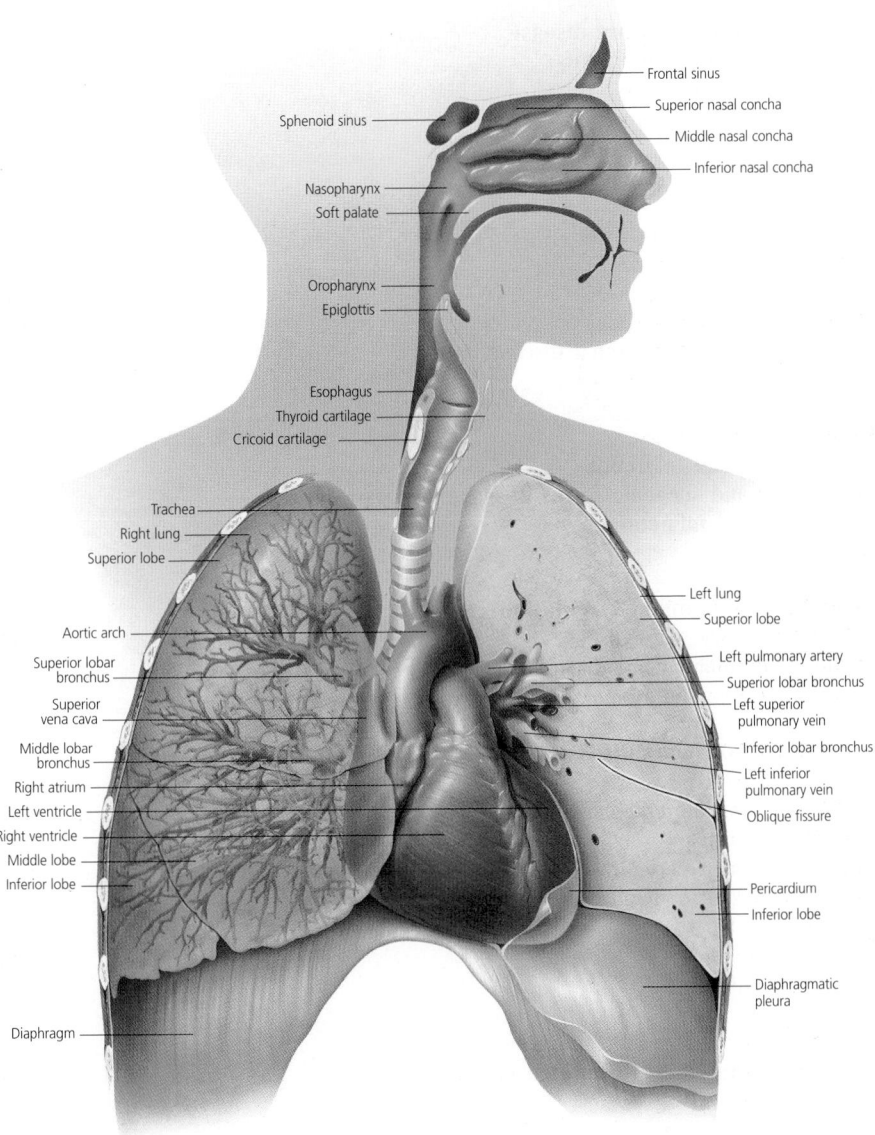

Frontal sinus
Superior nasal concha
Middle nasal concha
Inferior nasal concha
Sphenoid sinus
Nasopharynx
Soft palate
Oropharynx
Epiglottis
Esophagus
Thyroid cartilage
Cricoid cartilage
Trachea
Right lung
Superior lobe
Left lung
Superior lobe
Aortic arch
Left pulmonary artery
Superior lobar bronchus
Superior lobar bronchus
Superior vena cava
Left superior pulmonary vein
Middle lobar bronchus
Inferior lobar bronchus
Right atrium
Left inferior pulmonary vein
Left ventricle
Oblique fissure
Right ventricle
Middle lobe
Inferior lobe
Pericardium
Inferior lobe
Diaphragmatic pleura
Diaphragm

PLATE 14. HEART AND PERICARDIUM

Acute rheumatic fever

Rheumatic fever without mention of heart involvement — 390
Rheumatic fever with heart involvement — 391
Rheumatic chorea — 392

Chronic rheumatic heart disease

Chronic rheumatic pericarditis — 393
Diseases of mitral valve — 394
Diseases of aortic valve — 395
Diseases of mitral and aortic valves — 396
Diseases of other endocardial structures — 397

Hypertensive disease

Essential hypertension — 401
Hypertensive heart disease — 402
Hypertensive renal disease — 403
Hypertensive heart and renal disease — 404
Secondary hypertension — 405

Ischemic heart disease

Acute myocardial infarction — 410
Other acute and subacute forms of ischemic heart disease — 411
Old myocardial infarction — 412
Angina pectoris — 413

Diseases of pulmonary circulation

Acute pulmonary heart disease — 415
Chronic pulmonary heart disease — 416
Other diseases of pulmonary circulation — 417

Other forms of heart disease

Acute pericarditis — 420
Acute and subacute endocarditis — 421
Acute myocarditis — 422
Other diseases of pericardium — 423
Other diseases of endocardium — 424
Cardiomyopathy — 425
Conduction disorders — 426
Cardiac dysrhythmias — 427
Heart failure — 428

Symptoms, signs and ill-defined conditions — 780-799

Heart
(External View)

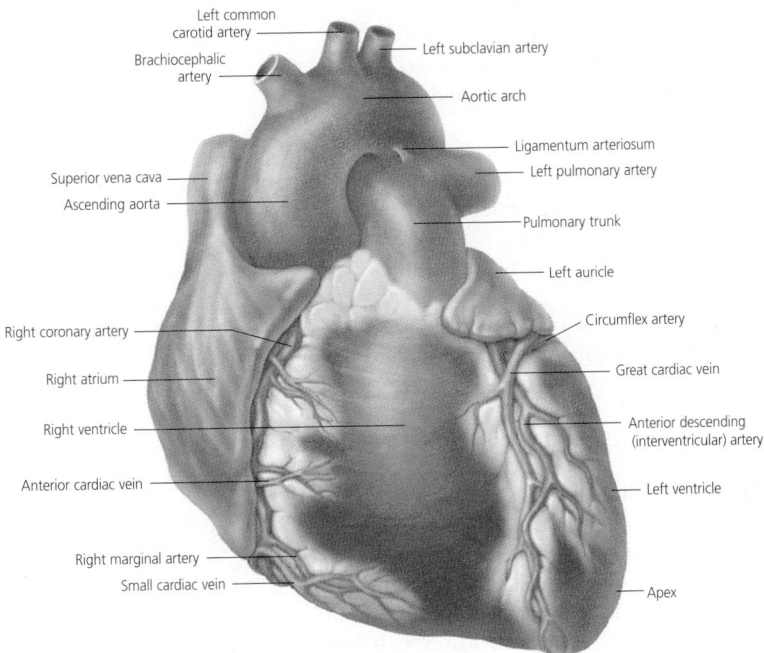

Left common carotid artery

Brachiocephalic artery

Left subclavian artery

Aortic arch

Ligamentum arteriosum

Left pulmonary artery

Superior vena cava

Ascending aorta

Pulmonary trunk

Left auricle

Right coronary artery

Circumflex artery

Great cardiac vein

Right atrium

Right ventricle

Anterior descending (interventricular) artery

Anterior cardiac vein

Left ventricle

Right marginal artery

Small cardiac vein

Apex

Heart
(Internal View)

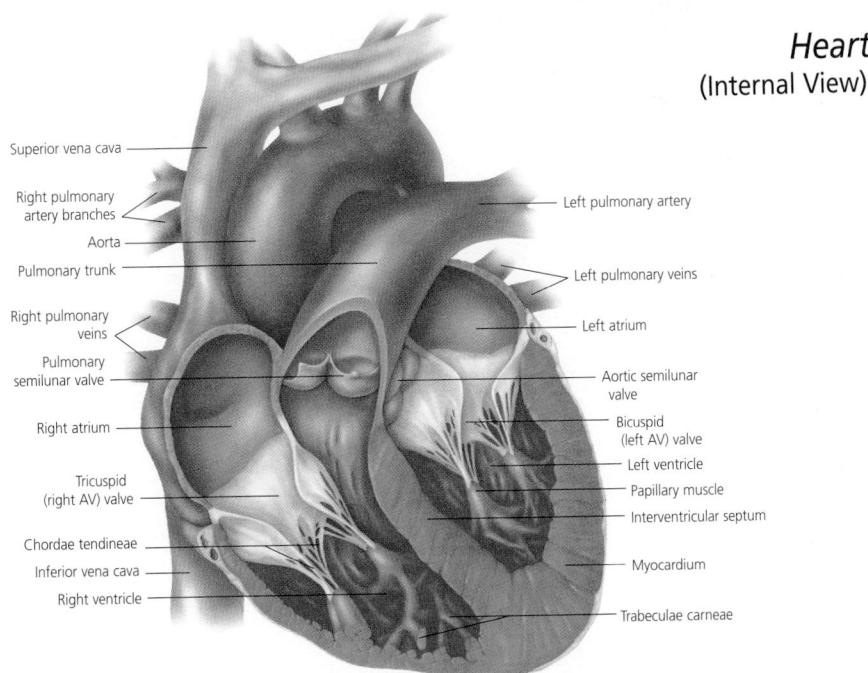

Superior vena cava

Right pulmonary artery branches

Aorta

Pulmonary trunk

Left pulmonary artery

Left pulmonary veins

Left atrium

Right pulmonary veins

Pulmonary semilunar valve

Aortic semilunar valve

Right atrium

Bicuspid (left AV) valve

Left ventricle

Tricuspid (right AV) valve

Papillary muscle

Interventricular septum

Chordae tendineae

Inferior vena cava

Right ventricle

Myocardium

Trabeculae carneae

PLATE 15. CIRCULATORY SYSTEM

Vascular System

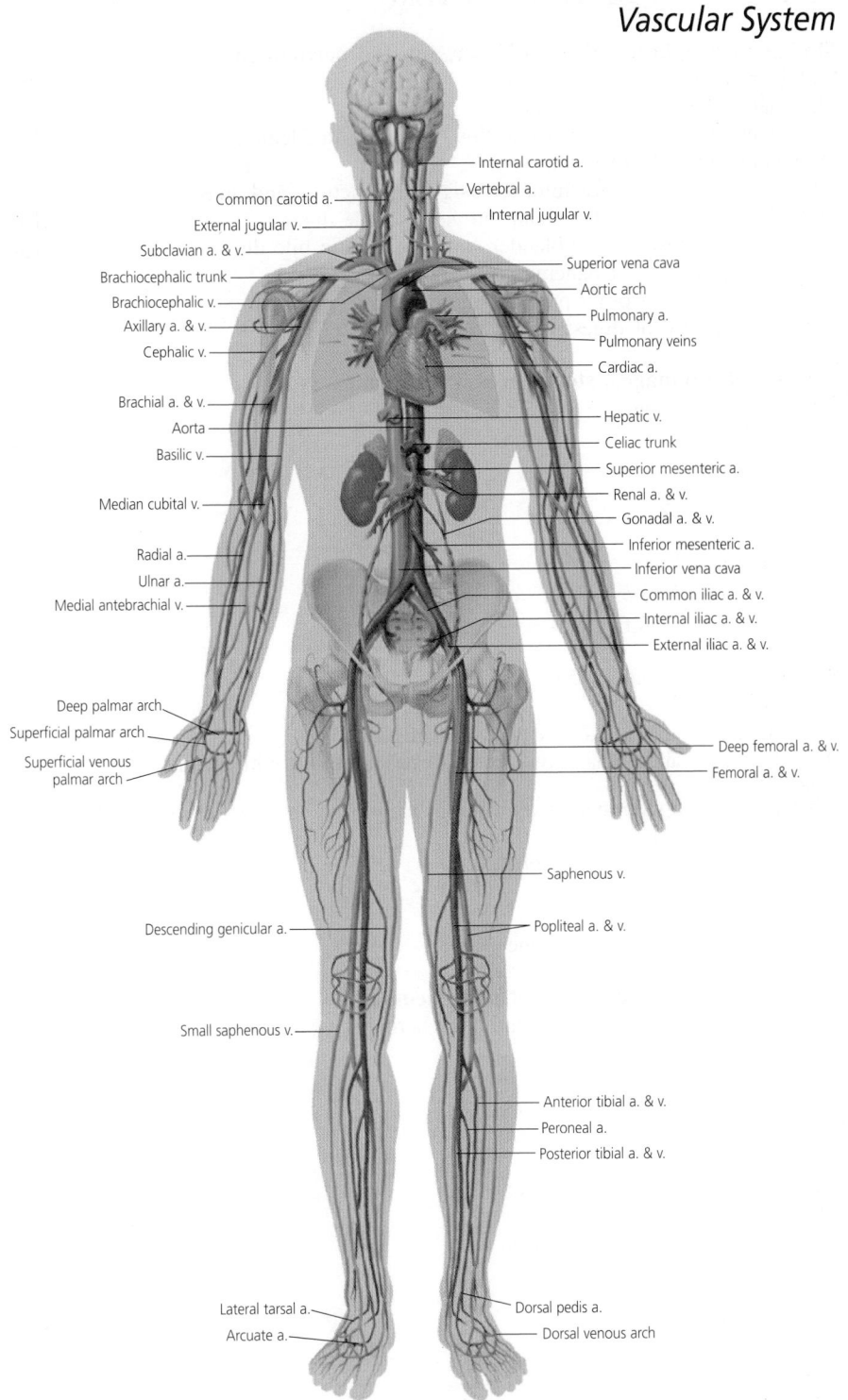

PLATE 16. DIGESTIVE SYSTEM

Malignant neoplasms of digestive organs and peritoneum

Diseases of esophagus, stomach, and duodenum

Appendicitis

Hernia of abdominal cavity

Noninfectious enteritis and colitis

Other diseases of intestines and peritoneum

Other diseases of digestive system

Digestive System

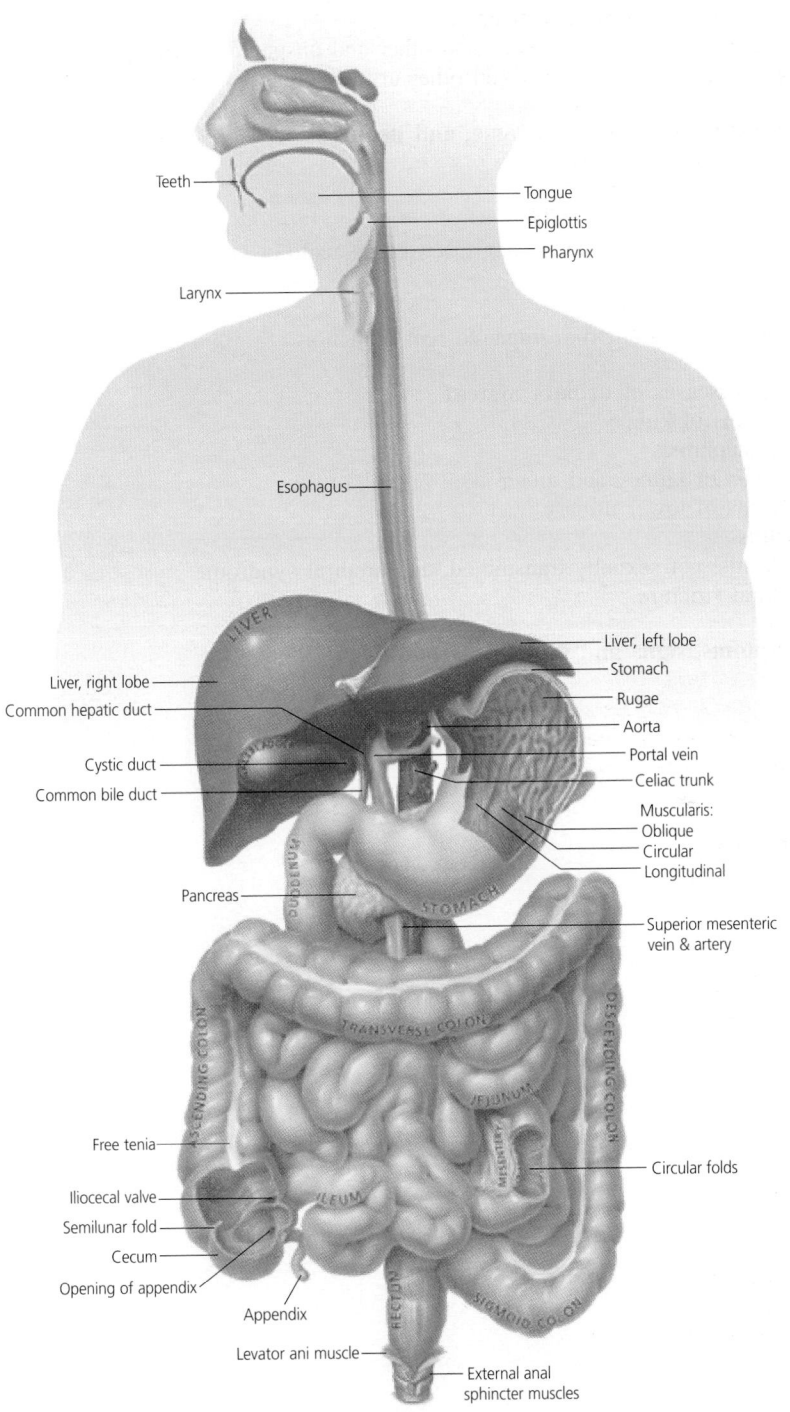

PLATE 17. GENITOURINARY SYSTEM

Urinary System

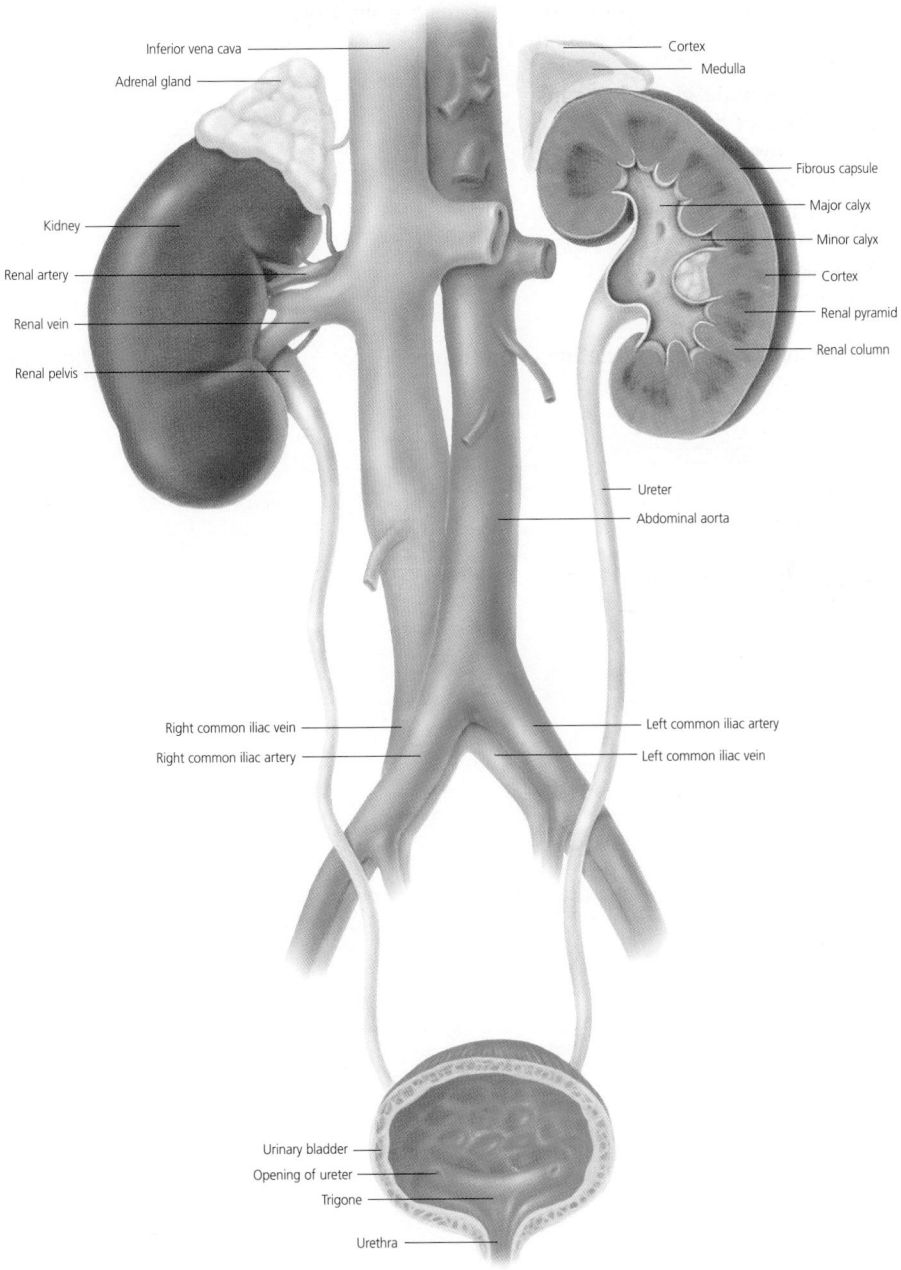

PLATE 18. MALE GENITAL ORGANS

Neoplasms

Malignant neoplasm of prostate	185
Malignant neoplasm of testis	186
Malignant neoplasm of penis and other male genital organs	187
Benign neoplasm of male genital organs	222

Diseases of male genital organs

Hyperplasia of prostate	600
Inflammatory diseases of prostate	601
Hydrocele	603
Orchitis and epididymitis	604
Redundant prepuce and phimosis	605
Infertility, male	606
Disorders of penis	607

Symptoms, signs and ill-defined conditions   780-799

Male Reproductive System

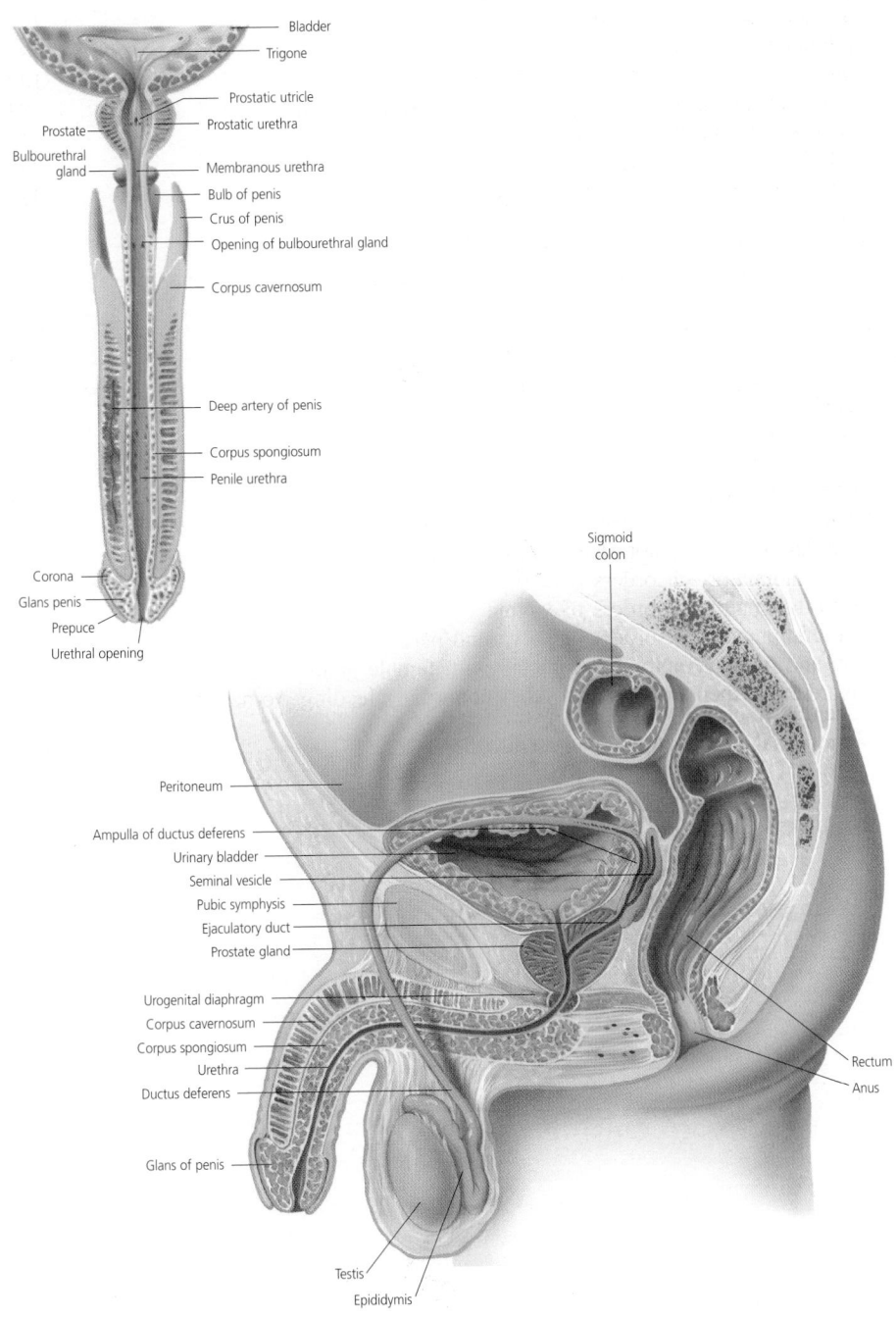

Bladder
Trigone
Prostatic utricle
Prostatic urethra
Prostate
Bulbourethral gland
Membranous urethra
Bulb of penis
Crus of penis
Opening of bulbourethral gland
Corpus cavernosum
Deep artery of penis
Corpus spongiosum
Penile urethra
Corona
Glans penis
Prepuce
Urethral opening

Sigmoid colon
Peritoneum
Ampulla of ductus deferens
Urinary bladder
Seminal vesicle
Pubic symphysis
Ejaculatory duct
Prostate gland
Urogenital diaphragm
Corpus cavernosum
Corpus spongiosum
Urethra
Ductus deferens
Glans of penis
Rectum
Anus
Testis
Epididymis

PLATE 19. FEMALE GENITAL ORGANS

Female Reproductive System

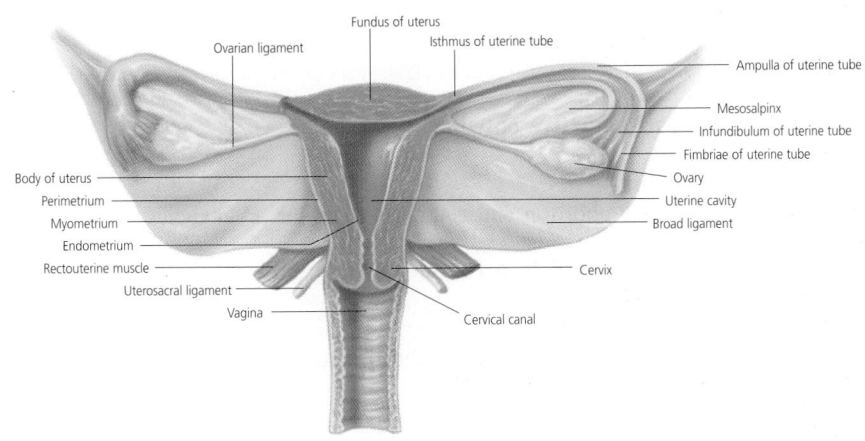

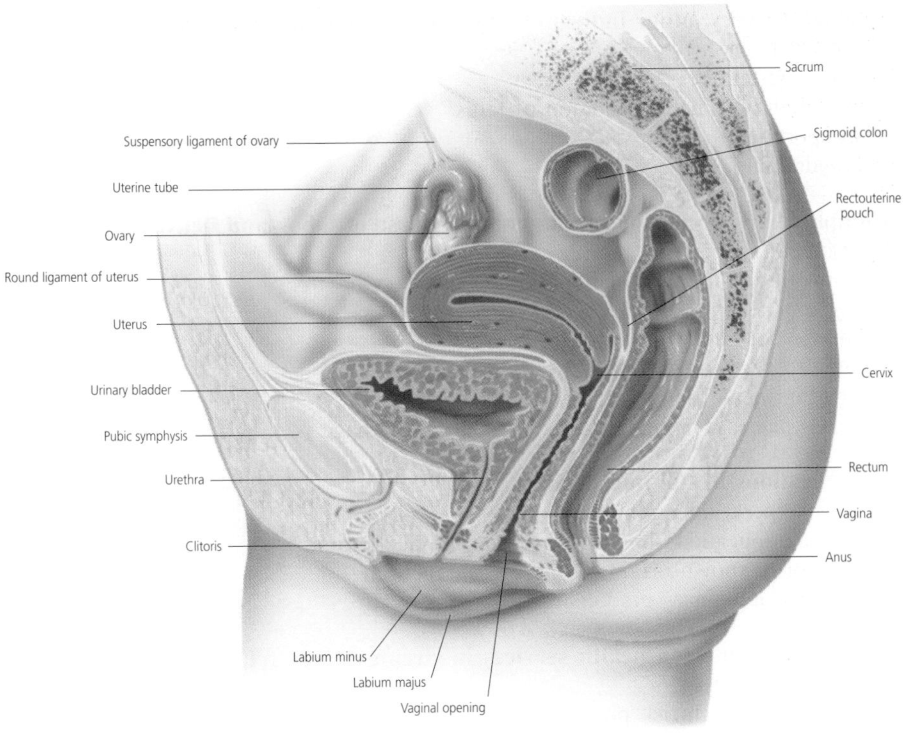

Fundus of uterus
Ovarian ligament
Isthmus of uterine tube
Ampulla of uterine tube
Mesosalpinx
Infundibulum of uterine tube
Fimbriae of uterine tube
Ovary
Body of uterus
Perimetrium
Myometrium
Uterine cavity
Endometrium
Broad ligament
Rectouterine muscle
Uterosacral ligament
Cervix
Vagina
Cervical canal

Sacrum
Suspensory ligament of ovary
Sigmoid colon
Uterine tube
Rectouterine pouch
Ovary
Round ligament of uterus
Uterus
Urinary bladder
Cervix
Pubic symphysis
Urethra
Rectum
Clitoris
Vagina
Anus
Labium minus
Labium majus
Vaginal opening

PLATE 20. PREGNANCY, CHILDBIRTH AND THE PUERPERIUM

Female Reproductive System: Pregnancy
(Lateral View)

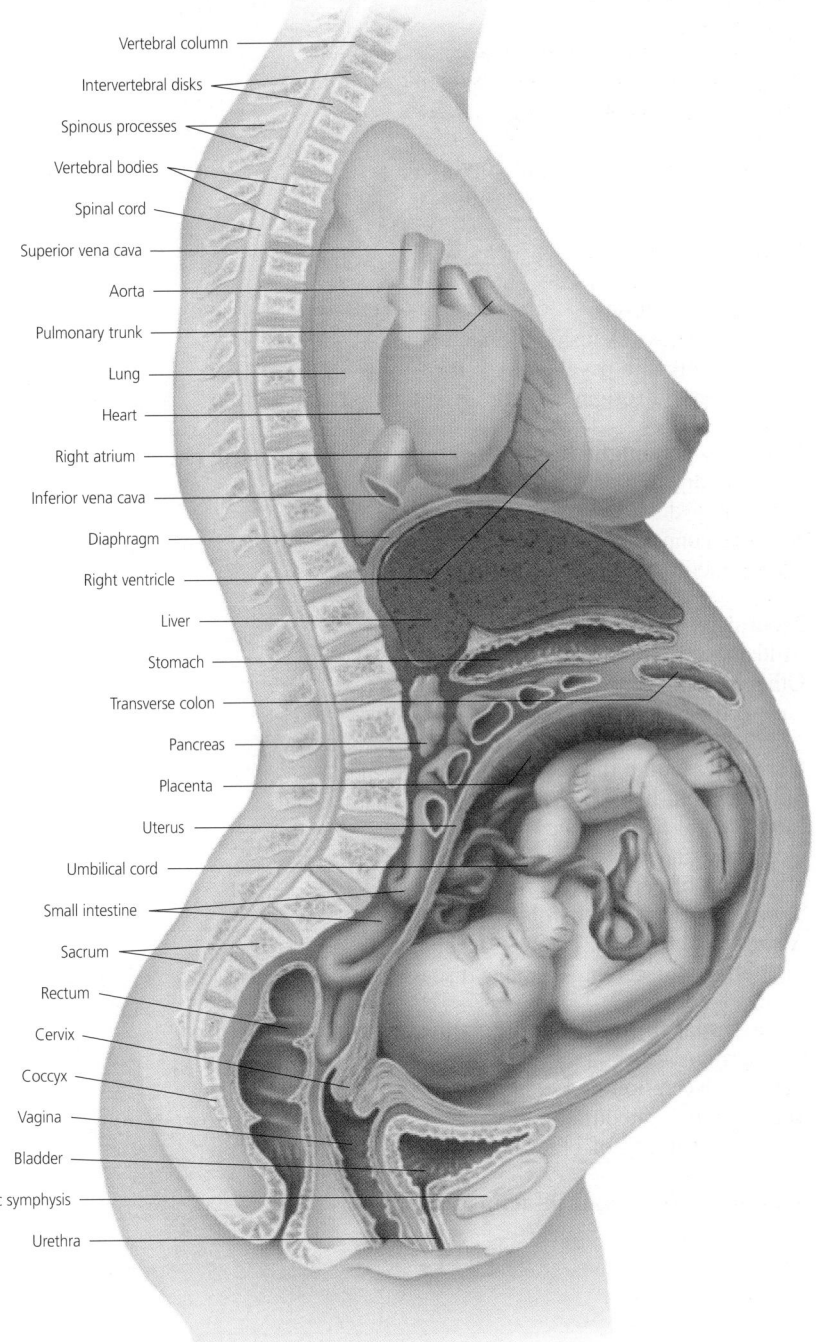

Vertebral column

Intervertebral disks

Spinous processes

Vertebral bodies

Spinal cord

Superior vena cava

Aorta

Pulmonary trunk

Lung

Heart

Right atrium

Inferior vena cava

Diaphragm

Right ventricle

Liver

Stomach

Transverse colon

Pancreas

Placenta

Uterus

Umbilical cord

Small intestine

Sacrum

Rectum

Cervix

Coccyx

Vagina

Bladder

Pubic symphysis

Urethra

PLATE 21. NERVOUS SYSTEM - BRAIN

Neoplasms
Malignant neoplasm of brain ... 191

Organic psychotic conditions
Senile and presenile organic psychotic conditions ... 290
Alcoholic psychoses ... 291
Drug psychoses ... 292
Transient organic psychotic conditions ... 293
Other organic psychotic conditions (chronic) ... 294

Other psychoses
Schizophrenic psychoses ... 295
Affective psychoses ... 296
Paranoid states (Delusional disorders) ... 297
Other nonorganic psychoses ... 298
Psychoses with origin specific to childhood ... 299

Neurotic, personality, and other nonpsychotic disorders
Neurotic disorders ... 300
Personality disorders ... 301
Specific nonpsychotic mental disorders due to organic brain damage ... 310
Hyperkinetic syndrome of childhood ... 314

Mental retardation
Mild mental retardation ... 317
Other specified mental retardation ... 318
Unspecified mental retardation ... 319

Cerebrovascular disease
Subarachnoid hemorrhage ... 430
Intracerebral hemorrhage ... 431
Occlusion and stenosis of precerebral arteries ... 433
Occlusion of cerebral arteries ... 434
Transient cerebral ischemia ... 435
Acute but ill-defined cerebrovascular disease ... 436
Late effects of cerebrovascular disease ... 438

Intracranial injury, excluding those with skull fracture
Concussion ... 850
Cerebral laceration and contusion ... 851
Subarachnoid, subdural, and extradural hemorrhage, following injury ... 852
Intracranial injury of other and unspecified nature ... 854

Symptoms, signs and ill-defined conditions ... 780-799

Brain
(Base View)

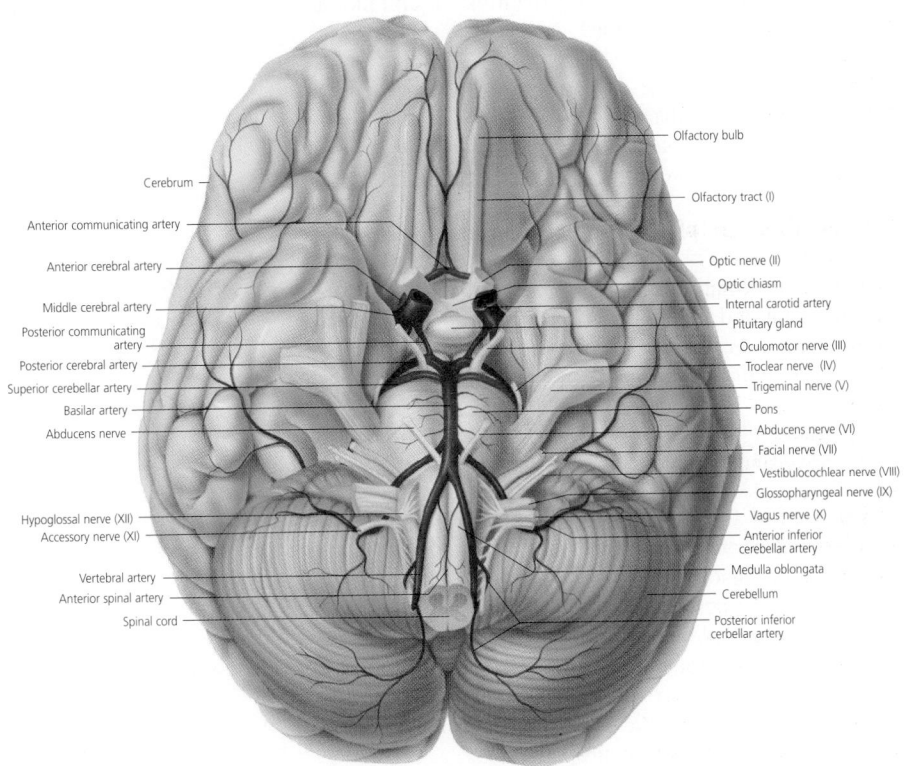

Olfactory bulb

Cerebrum

Anterior communicating artery

Olfactory tract (I)

Anterior cerebral artery

Optic nerve (II)

Optic chiasm

Middle cerebral artery

Internal carotid artery

Posterior communicating artery

Pituitary gland

Oculomotor nerve (III)

Posterior cerebral artery

Troclear nerve (IV)

Superior cerebellar artery

Trigeminal nerve (V)

Basilar artery

Pons

Abducens nerve

Abducens nerve (VI)

Facial nerve (VII)

Vestibulocochlear nerve (VIII)

Glossopharyngeal nerve (IX)

Hypoglossal nerve (XII)

Vagus nerve (X)

Accessory nerve (XI)

Anterior inferior cerebellar artery

Medulla oblongata

Vertebral artery

Anterior spinal artery

Cerebellum

Spinal cord

Posterior inferior cerebellar artery

PLATE 22. NERVOUS SYSTEM

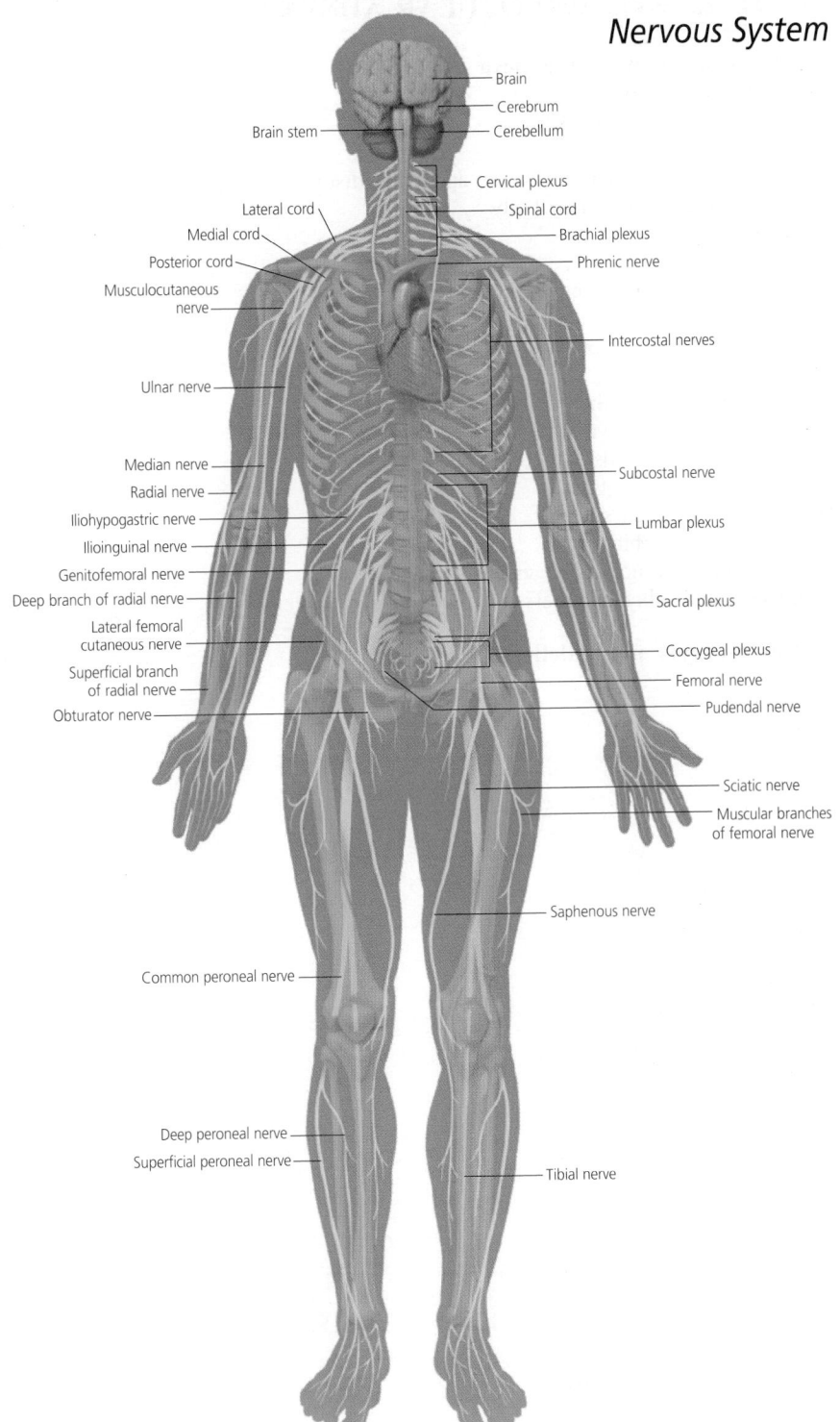

Nervous System

Brain
Cerebrum
Cerebellum
Brain stem
Cervical plexus
Lateral cord
Spinal cord
Medial cord
Brachial plexus
Posterior cord
Phrenic nerve
Musculocutaneous nerve
Intercostal nerves
Ulnar nerve
Median nerve
Subcostal nerve
Radial nerve
Iliohypogastric nerve
Lumbar plexus
Ilioinguinal nerve
Genitofemoral nerve
Deep branch of radial nerve
Sacral plexus
Lateral femoral cutaneous nerve
Coccygeal plexus
Superficial branch of radial nerve
Femoral nerve
Obturator nerve
Pudendal nerve
Sciatic nerve
Muscular branches of femoral nerve
Saphenous nerve
Common peroneal nerve
Deep peroneal nerve
Superficial peroneal nerve
Tibial nerve

PLATE 23. EYE AND OCULAR ADNEXA

Right Eye
(Horizontal Section)

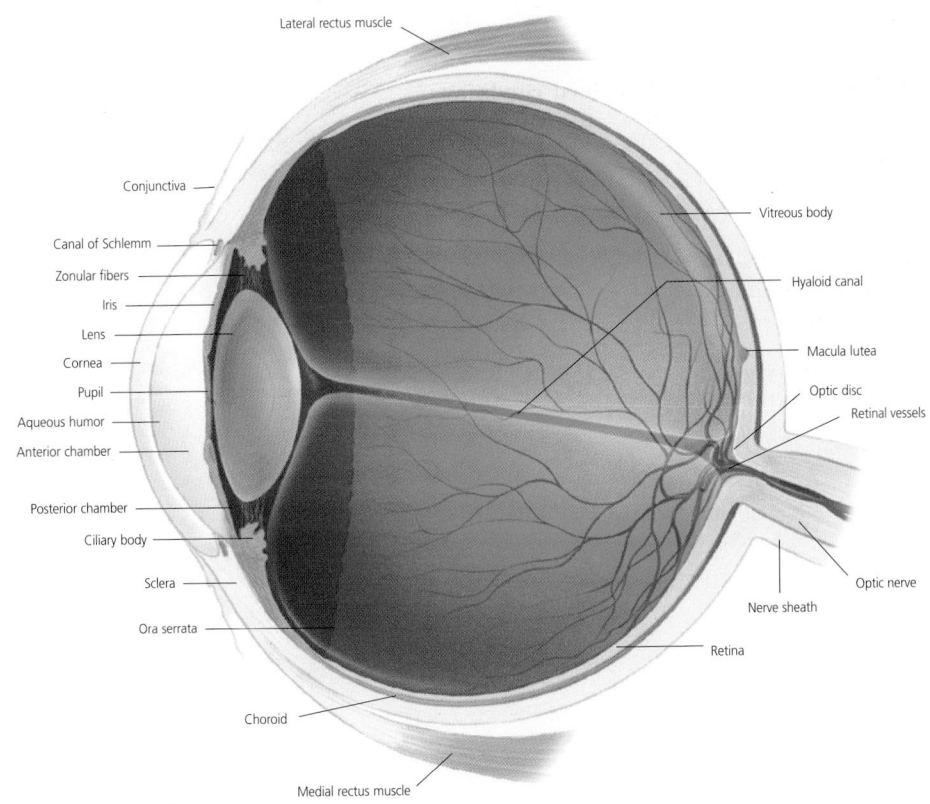

Lateral rectus muscle

Conjunctiva

Canal of Schlemm

Zonular fibers

Iris

Lens

Cornea

Pupil

Aqueous humor

Anterior chamber

Posterior chamber

Ciliary body

Sclera

Ora serrata

Choroid

Medial rectus muscle

Vitreous body

Hyaloid canal

Macula lutea

Optic disc

Retinal vessels

Optic nerve

Nerve sheath

Retina

PLATE 24. AUDITORY SYSTEM

The Ear

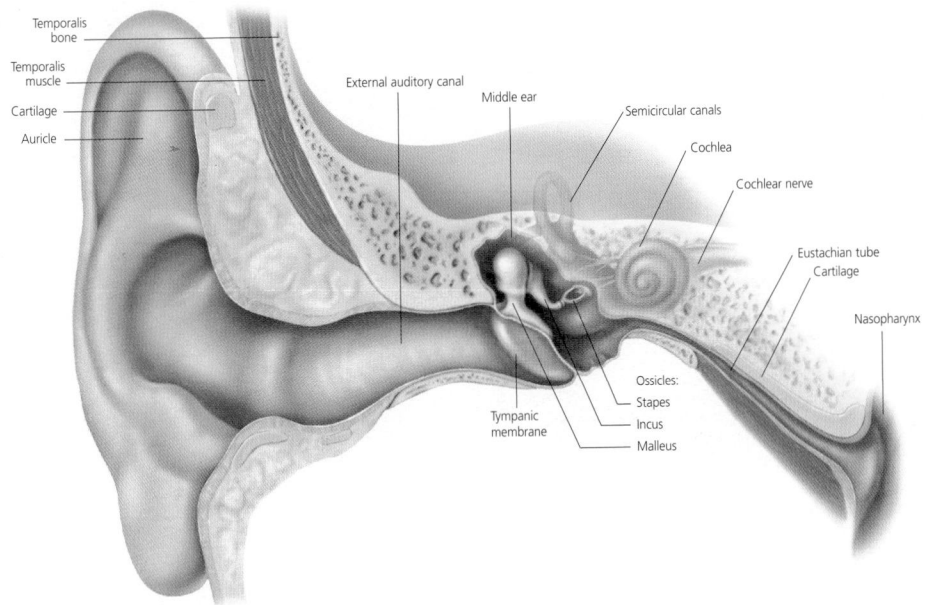

DISEASES: TABULAR LIST

VOLUME 1

1. INFECTIOUS AND PARASITIC DISEASES (001-139)

Note: Categories for "late effects" of infectious and parasitic diseases are to be found at 137-139.

Includes: diseases generally recognized as communicable or transmissible as well as a few diseases of unknown but possibly infectious origin

[Excludes:] *acute respiratory infections (460-466)*
carrier or suspected carrier of infectious organism (V02.0-V02.9)
certain localized infections
influenza (487.0-487.8)

INTESTINAL INFECTIOUS DISEASES (001-009)

[Excludes:] *helminthiases (120.0-129)*

001 Cholera

001.0 Due to Vibrio cholerae

001.1 Due to Vibrio cholerae el tor

001.9 Cholera, unspecified

002 Typhoid and paratyphoid fevers

002.0 Typhoid fever
Typhoid (fever) (infection) [any site]

002.1 Paratyphoid fever A

002.2 Paratyphoid fever B

002.3 Paratyphoid fever C

002.9 Paratyphoid fever, unspecified

003 Other salmonella infections
Includes: infection or food poisoning by Salmonella [any serotype]

003.0 Salmonella gastroenteritis
Salmonellosis

003.1 Salmonella septicemia

[5] **003.2 Localized salmonella infections**

003.20 Localized salmonella infection, unspecified

003.21 Salmonella meningitis

003.22 Salmonella pneumonia

003.23 Salmonella arthritis

003.24 Salmonella osteomyelitis

003.29 Other

003.8 Other specified salmonella infections

003.9 Salmonella infection, unspecified

004 Shigellosis
Includes: bacillary dysentery

004.0 Shigella dysenteriae
Infection by group A Shigella (Schmitz) (Shiga)

004.1 Shigella flexneri
Infection by group B Shigella

004.2 Shigella boydii
Infection by group C Shigella

004.3 Shigella sonnei
Infection by group D Shigella

004.8 Other specified shigella infections

004.9 Shigellosis, unspecified

005 Other food poisoning (bacterial)

[Excludes:] *salmonella infections (003.0-003.9)*
toxic effect of:
food contaminants (989.7)
noxious foodstuffs (988.0-988.9)

005.0 Staphylococcal food poisoning
Staphylococcal toxemia specified as due to food

Add 4th or 5th digit | Nonspecific code | Unspecified code | Manifestation code

005.1 Botulism
Food poisoning due to Clostridium botulinum

005.2 Food poisoning due to Clostridium perfringens [C. welchii]
Enteritis necroticans

005.3 Food poisoning due to other Clostridia

005.4 Food poisoning due to Vibrio parahaemolyticus

⑤ **005.8 Other bacterial food poisoning**

Excludes: *salmonella food poisoning (003.0-003.9)*

005.81 Food poisoning due to Vibrio vulnificus

005.89 Other bacterial food poisoning
Food poisoning due to Bacillus cereus

005.9 Food poisoning, unspecified

006 Amebiasis
Includes: infection due to Entamoeba histolytica

Excludes: *amebiasis due to organisms other than Entamoeba histolytica (007.8)*

006.0 Acute amebic dysentery without mention of abscess
Acute amebiasis

006.1 Chronic intestinal amebiasis without mention of abscess
Chronic:
amebiasis
amebic dysentery

006.2 Amebic nondysenteric colitis

006.3 Amebic liver abscess
Hepatic amebiasis

006.4 Amebic lung abscess
Amebic abscess of lung (and liver)

006.5 Amebic brain abscess
Amebic abscess of brain (and liver) (and lung)

006.6 Amebic skin ulceration
Cutaneous amebiasis

006.8 Amebic infection of other sites
Amebic: Ameboma
appendicitis
balanitis

Excludes: *specific infections by free-living amebae (136.2)*

006.9 Amebiasis, unspecified
Amebiasis NOS

007 Other protozoal intestinal diseases
Includes: protozoal:
colitis
diarrhea
dysentery

007.0 Balantidiasis
Infection by Balantidium coli

007.1 Giardiasis
Infection by Giardia lamblia
Lambliasis

007.2 Coccidiosis
Infection by Isospora belli and Isospora hominis
Isosporiasis

007.3 Intestinal trichomoniasis

007.4 Cryptosporidiosis

007.5 Cyclosporiasis

007.8 Other specified protozoal intestinal diseases
Amebiasis due to organisms other than Entamoeba histolytica

007.9 Unspecified protozoal intestinal disease
Flagellate diarrhea   Protozoal dysentery NOS

● Code new
to this edition

▲ Revision of
existing code

④ ⑤ Fourth or fifth
digit required

008 Intestinal infections due to other organisms
Includes: any condition classifiable to 009.0-009.3 with mention of the responsible organisms

[Excludes:] *food poisoning by these organisms (005.0-005.9)*

[5] **008.0 Escherichia coli [E. coli]**

008.00 E. coli, unspecified
E. coli enteritis NOS

008.01 Enteropathogenic E. coli

008.02 Enterotoxigenic E. coli

008.03 Enteroinvasive E. coli

008.04 Enterohemorrhagic E. coli

008.09 Other intestinal E. coli infections

008.1 Arizona group of paracolon bacilli

008.2 Aerobacter aerogenes
Enterobacter aerogenes

008.3 Proteus (mirabilis) (morganii)

[5] **008.4 Other specified bacteria**

008.41 Staphylococcus
Staphylococcal enterocolitis

008.42 Pseudomonas

008.43 Campylobacter

008.44 Yersinia enterocolitica

008.45 Clostridium difficile
Pseudomembranous colitis

008.46 Other anaerobes
Anaerobic enteritis NOS
Gram-negative anaerobes
Bacteroides (fragilis)

008.47 Other Gram-negative bacteria
Gram-negative enteritis NOS

[Excludes:] *Gram-negative anaerobes (008.46)*

008.49 Other

008.5 Bacterial enteritis, unspecified

[5] **008.6 Enteritis due to specified virus**

008.61 Rotavirus

008.62 Adenovirus

008.63 Norwalk virus
Norwalk-like agent

008.64 Other small round viruses [SRV's]
Small round virus NOS

008.65 Calcivirus

008.66 Astrovirus

008.67 Enterovirus NEC
Coxsackie virus
Echovirus

[Excludes:] *poliovirus (045.0-045.9)*

008.69 Other viral enteritis
Torovirus

008.8 Other organism, not elsewhere classified
Viral:
enteritis NOS
gastroenteritis

[Excludes:] *influenza with involvement of gastrointestinal tract (487.8)*

009 Ill-defined intestinal infections

[Excludes:] *diarrheal disease or intestinal infection due to specified organism (001.0-008.8)*
diarrhea following gastrointestinal surgery (564.4)
intestinal malabsorption (579.0-579.9)
ischemic enteritis (557.0-557.9)
other noninfectious gastroenteritis and colitis (558.1-558.9)
regional enteritis (555.0-555.9)
ulcerative colitis (556)

009.0 Infectious colitis, enteritis, and gastroenteritis

Colitis, septic
Enteritis, septic
Gastroenteritis, septic
Dysentery:
  NOS
  catarrhal
  hemorrhagic

009.1 Colitis, enteritis, and gastroenteritis of presumed infectious origin

[Excludes:] *colitis NOS (558.9)*
enteritis NOS (558.9)
gastroenteritis NOS (558.9)

009.2 Infectious diarrhea

Diarrhea:
  dysenteric
  epidemic
Infectious diarrheal disease NOS

009.3 Diarrhea of presumed infectious origin

[Excludes:] *diarrhea NOS (787.91)*

TUBERCULOSIS (010-018)

Includes: infection by Mycobacterium tuberculosis (human) (bovine)

[Excludes:] *congenital tuberculosis (771.2)*
late effects of tuberculosis (137.0-137.4)

The following fifth-digit subclassification is for use with categories 010-018:

0 unspecified
1 bacteriological or histological examination not done
2 bacteriological or histological examination unknown (at present)
3 tubercle bacilli found (in sputum) by microscopy
4 tubercle bacilli not found (in sputum) by microscopy, but found by bacterial culture
5 tubercle bacilli not found by bacteriological examination, but tuberculosis confirmed histologically
6 tubercle bacilli not found by bacteriological or histological examination but tuberculosis confirmed by other methods [inoculation of animals]

[5] **010 Primary tuberculous infection**

[Excludes:] *nonspecific reaction to tuberculin skin test without active tuberculosis (795.5)*
positive PPD (795.5)
positive tuberculin skin test without active tuberculosis (795.5)

[5] **010.0 Primary tuberculous complex**

[5] **010.1 Tuberculous pleurisy in primary progressive tuberculosis**

[5] **010.8 Other primary progressive tuberculosis**

[Excludes:] *tuberculous erythema nodosum (017.1)*

[5] **010.9 Primary tuberculous infection, unspecified**

[5] **011 Pulmonary tuberculosis**

Use additional code, if desired, to identify any associated silicosis (502)

[5] **011.0 Tuberculosis of lung, infiltrative**

[5] **011.1 Tuberculosis of lung, nodular**

[5] **011.2 Tuberculosis of lung with cavitation**

[5] **011.3 Tuberculosis of bronchus**

[Excludes:] *isolated bronchial tuberculosis (012.2)*

[5] **011.4 Tuberculous fibrosis of lung**

[5] **011.5 Tuberculous bronchiectasis**

● Code new to this edition
▲ Revision of existing code
[4] [5] Fourth or fifth digit required

[5] **011.6 Tuberculous pneumonia [any form]**

[5] **011.7 Tuberculous pneumothorax**

[5] **011.8 Other specified pulmonary tuberculosis**

[5] **011.9 Pulmonary tuberculosis, unspecified**
Respiratory tuberculosis NOS
Tuberculosis of lung NOS

[5] **012 Other respiratory tuberculosis**
[*Excludes:*] *respiratory tuberculosis, unspecified (011.9)*

[5] **012.0 Tuberculous pleurisy**
Tuberculosis of pleura
Tuberculous empyema
Tuberculous hydrothorax
[*Excludes:*] *pleurisy with effusion without mention of cause (511.9)*
tuberculous pleurisy in primary progressive tuberculosis (010.1)

[5] **012.1 Tuberculosis of intrathoracic lymph nodes**
Tuberculosis of lymph nodes:
hilar
mediastinal
tracheobronchial
Tuberculous tracheobronchial adenopathy
[*Excludes:*] *that specified as primary (010.0-010.9)*

[5] **012.2 Isolated tracheal or bronchial tuberculosis**

[5] **012.3 Tuberculous laryngitis**
Tuberculosis of glottis

[5] **012.8 Other specified respiratory tuberculosis**
Tuberculosis of:
mediastinum
nasopharynx
Tuberculosis of:
nose (septum)
sinus [any nasal]

[5] **013 Tuberculosis of meninges and central nervous system**

[5] **013.0 Tuberculous meningitis**
Tuberculosis of meninges (cerebral) (spinal)
Tuberculous:
leptomeningitis
meningoencephalitis
[*Excludes:*] *tuberculoma of meninges (013.1)*

[5] **013.1 Tuberculoma of meninges**

[5] **013.2 Tuberculoma of brain**
Tuberculosis of brain (current disease)

[5] **013.3 Tuberculous abscess of brain**

[5] **013.4 Tuberculoma of spinal cord**

[5] **013.5 Tuberculous abscess of spinal cord**

[5] **013.6 Tuberculous encephalitis or myelitis**

[5] **013.8 Other specified tuberculosis of central nervous system**

[5] **013.9 Unspecified tuberculosis of central nervous system**
Tuberculosis of central nervous system NOS

[5] **014 Tuberculosis of intestines, peritoneum, and mesenteric glands**

[5] **014.0 Tuberculous peritonitis**
Tuberculous ascites

[5] **014.8 Other**
Tuberculosis (of):
anus
intestine (large) (small)
mesenteric glands
rectum
retroperitoneal (lymph nodes)
Tuberculous enteritis

Add 4th or 5th digit — Nonspecific code — Unspecified code — Manifestation code

⑤ **015 Tuberculosis of bones and joints**
>   Use additional code, if desired, to identify manifestation, as:
>   tuberculous:
>   arthropathy (711.4)
>   necrosis of bone (730.8)
>   osteitis (730.8)
>   osteomyelitis (730.8)
>   synovitis (727.01)
>   tenosynovitis (727.01)

⑤ **015.0 Vertebral column**
>   Pott's disease
>   Use additional code, if desired, to identify manifestation, as:
>   curvature of spine [Pott's] (737.4)
>   kyphosis (737.4)
>   spondylitis (720.81)

⑤ **015.1 Hip**

⑤ **015.2 Knee**

⑤ **015.5 Limb bones**
>   Tuberculous dactylitis

⑤ **015.6 Mastoid**
>   Tuberculous mastoiditis

⑤ **015.7 Other specified bone**

⑤ **015.8 Other specified joint**

⑤ **015.9 Tuberculosis of unspecified bones and joints**

⑤ **016 Tuberculosis of genitourinary system**

⑤ **016.0 Kidney**
>   Renal tuberculosis
>   Use additional code, if desired, to identify manifestation, as:
>   tuberculous:
>   nephropathy (583.81)
>   pyelitis (590.81)
>   pyelonephritis (590.81)

⑤ **016.1 Bladder**

⑤ **016.2 Ureter**

⑤ **016.3 Other urinary organs**

⑤ **016.4 Epididymis**

⑤ **016.5 Other male genital organs**
>   Use additional code, if desired, to identify manifestation, as:
>   tuberculosis of:
>   prostate (601.4)
>   seminal vesicle (608.81)
>   testis (608.81)

⑤ **016.6 Tuberculous oophoritis and salpingitis**

⑤ **016.7 Other female genital organs**
>   Tuberculous:
>   cervicitis
>   endometritis

⑤ **016.9 Genitourinary tuberculosis, unspecified**

⑤ **017 Tuberculosis of other organs**

⑤ **017.0 Skin and subcutaneous cellular tissue**

Lupus:	Tuberculosis:
exedens	colliquativa
vulgaris	cutis
Scrofuloderma	lichenoides
	papulonecrotica
	verrucosa cutis

>   Excludes: *lupus erythematosus (695.4)*
>   *disseminated (710.0)*
>   *lupus NOS (710.0)*
>   *nonspecific reaction to tuberculin skin test without active tuberculosis (795.5)*
>   *positive PPD (795.5)*
>   *positive tuberculin skin test without active tuberculosis (795.5)*

● Code new   ▲ Revision of   ④ ⑤ Fourth or fifth
  to this edition   existing code   digit required

[5] **017.1 Erythema nodosum with hypersensitivity reaction in tuberculosis**
Bazin's disease
Erythema:
induratum
nodosum, tuberculous
Tuberculosis indurativa

[Excludes:] *erythema nodosum NOS (695.2)*

[5] **017.2 Peripheral lymph nodes**
Scrofula
Scrofulous abscess
Tuberculous adenitis

[Excludes:] *tuberculosis of lymph nodes:*
bronchial and mediastinal (012.1)
mesenteric and retroperitoneal (014.8)
tuberculous tracheobronchial adenopathy (012.1)

[5] **017.3 Eye**
Use additional code, if desired, to identify manifestation, as:
tuberculous:
chorioretinitis, disseminated (363.13)
episcleritis (379.09)
interstitial keratitis (370.59)
iridocyclitis, chronic (364.11)
keratoconjunctivitis (phlyctenular) (370.31)

[5] **017.4 Ear**
Tuberculosis of ear
Tuberculous otitis media

[Excludes:] *tuberculous mastoiditis (015.6)*

[5] **017.5 Thyroid gland**

[5] **017.6 Adrenal glands**
Addison's disease, tuberculous

[5] **017.7 Spleen**

[5] **017.8 Esophagus**

[5] **017.9 Other specified organs**
Use additional code, if desired, to identify manifestation, as:
tuberculosis of:
endocardium [any valve] (424.91)
myocardium (422.0)
pericardium (420.0)

[5] **018 Miliary tuberculosis**
Includes: tuberculosis:
disseminated
generalized
miliary, whether of a single specified site, multiple sites, or unspecified site
polyserositis

[5] **018.0 Acute miliary tuberculosis**

[5] **018.8 Other specified miliary tuberculosis**

[5] **018.9 Miliary tuberculosis, unspecified**

ZOONOTIC BACTERIAL DISEASES (020-027)

020 Plague
Includes: infection by Yersinia [Pasteurella] pestis

020.0 Bubonic

020.1 Cellulocutaneous

020.2 Septicemic

020.3 Primary pneumonic

020.4 Secondary pneumonic

020.5 Pneumonic, unspecified

020.8 Other specified types of plague
Abortive plague
Ambulatory plague
Pestis minor

020.9 Plague, unspecified

021 Tularemia
Includes: deerfly fever
infection by Francisella [Pasteurella] tularensis
rabbit fever

021.0 Ulceroglandular tularemia

021.1 Enteric tularemia
Tularemia:
cryptogenic
intestinal
typhoidal

021.2 Pulmonary tularemia
Bronchopneumonic tularemia

021.3 Oculoglandular tularemia

021.8 Other specified tularemia
Tularemia:
generalized or disseminated
glandular

021.9 Unspecified tularemia

022 Anthrax

022.0 Cutaneous anthrax
Malignant pustule

022.1 Pulmonary anthrax
Respiratory anthrax
Wool-sorters' disease

022.2 Gastrointestinal anthrax

022.3 Anthrax septicemia

022.8 Other specified manifestations of anthrax

022.9 Anthrax, unspecified

023 Brucellosis
Includes: fever:
Malta
Mediterranean
undulant

023.0 Brucella melitensis

023.1 Brucella abortus

023.2 Brucella suis

023.3 Brucella canis

023.8 Other brucellosis
Infection by more than one organism

023.9 Brucellosis, unspecified

024 Glanders
Infection by:
Actinobacillus mallei
Malleomyces mallei
Pseudomonas mallei
Farcy
Malleus

025 Melioidosis
Infection by:
Malleomyces pseudomallei
Pseudomonas pseudomallei
Whitmore's bacillus
Pseudoglanders

026 Rat-bite fever

026.0 Spirillary fever
Rat-bite fever due to Spirillum minor [S. minus]
Sodoku

026.1 Streptobacillary fever
Epidemic arthritic erythema
Haverhill fever
Rat-bite fever due to Streptobacillus moniliformis

026.9 Unspecified rat-bite fever

027 Other zoonotic bacterial diseases

● Code new to this edition ▲ Revision of existing code ④ ⑤ Fourth or fifth digit required

027.0 Listeriosis
> Infection by Listeria monocytogenes
> Septicemia by Listeria monocytogenes

Use additional code, if desired, to identify manifestation, as meningitis (320.7)

> Excludes: *congenital listeriosis (771.2)*

027.1 Erysipelothrix infection
> Erysipeloid (of Rosenbach)
> Infection by Erysipelothrix insidiosa [E. rhusiopathiae]
> Septicemia by Erysipelothrix insidiosa [E. rhusiopathiae]

027.2 Pasteurellosis
> Pasteurella pseudotuberculosis infection
> Mesenteric adenitis by Pasteurella multocida [P. septica]
> Septic infection (cat bite) (dog bite) by Pasteurella multocida [P. septica]

> Excludes: *infection by:*
> > *Francisella [Pasteurella] tularensis (021.0-021.9)*
> > *Yersinia [Pasteurella] pestis (020.0-020.9)*

027.8 Other specified zoonotic bacterial diseases

027.9 Unspecified zoonotic bacterial disease

OTHER BACTERIAL DISEASES (030-041)

> Excludes: *bacterial venereal diseases (098.0-099.9)*
> > *bartonellosis (088.0)*

030 Leprosy
> Includes: Hansen's disease
> infection by Mycobacterium leprae

030.0 Lepromatous [type L]
> Lepromatous leprosy (macular) (diffuse) (infiltrated) (nodular) (neuritic)

030.1 Tuberculoid [type T]
> Tuberculoid leprosy (macular) (maculoanesthetic) (major) (minor) (neuritic)

030.2 Indeterminate [group I]
> Indeterminate [uncharacteristic] leprosy (macular) (neuritic)

030.3 Borderline [group B]
> Borderline or dimorphous leprosy (infiltrated) (neuritic)

030.8 Other specified leprosy

030.9 Leprosy, unspecified

031 Diseases due to other mycobacteria

031.0 Pulmonary
> Infection by Mycobacterium:
> > avium
> > intracellulare [Battey bacillus]
> > kansasii
> Battey disease

031.1 Cutaneous
> Buruli ulcer
> Infection by Mycobacterium:
> > marinum [M. balnei]
> > ulcerans

031.2 Disseminated
> Disseminated mycobacterium avium-intracellulare complex (DMAC)
> Mycobacterium avium-intracellulare complex (MAC) bacteremia

031.8 Other specified mycobacterial diseases

031.9 Unspecified diseases due to mycobacteria
> Atypical mycobacterium infection NOS

032 Diphtheria
> Includes: infection by Corynebacterium diphtheriae

032.0 Faucial diphtheria
> Membranous angina, diphtheritic

032.1 Nasopharyngeal diphtheria

032.2 Anterior nasal diphtheria

032.3 Laryngeal diphtheria
> Laryngotracheitis, diphtheritic

113

| Add 4th or 5th digit | Nonspecific code | Unspecified code | Manifestation code |

⑤ **032.8 Other specified diphtheria**

    032.81 Conjunctival diphtheria
        Pseudomembranous diphtheritic conjunctivitis

    032.82 Diphtheritic myocarditis

    032.83 Diphtheritic peritonitis

    032.84 Diphtheritic cystitis

    032.85 Cutaneous diphtheria

    032.89 Other

032.9 Diphtheria, unspecified

033 Whooping cough
    Includes: pertussis
Use additional code, if desired, to identify any associated pneumonia (484.3)

033.0 Bordetella pertussis [B. pertussis]

033.1 Bordetella parapertussis [B. parapertussis]

033.8 Whooping cough due to other specified organism
    Bordetella bronchiseptica [B. bronchiseptica]

033.9 Whooping cough, unspecified organism

034 Streptococcal sore throat and scarlet fever

034.0 Streptococcal sore throat

    Septic:
      angina
      sore throat

    Streptococcal:
      angina
      laryngitis
      pharyngitis
      tonsillitis

034.1 Scarlet fever
    Scarlatina

    Excludes: *parascarlatina (057.8)*

035 Erysipelas

    Excludes: *postpartum or puerperal erysipelas (670)*

036 Meningococcal infection

036.0 Meningococcal meningitis
    Cerebrospinal fever
      (meningococcal)

    Meningitis:
      cerebrospinal
      epidemic

036.1 Meningococcal encephalitis

036.2 Meningococcemia
    Meningococcal septicemia

036.3 Waterhouse-Friderichsen syndrome, meningococcal
    Meningococcal hemorrhagic adrenalitis
    Meningococcic adrenal syndrome
    Waterhouse-Friderichsen syndrome NOS

⑤ **036.4 Meningococcal carditis**

    036.40 Meningococcal carditis, unspecified

    036.41 Meningococcal pericarditis

    036.42 Meningococcal endocarditis

    036.43 Meningococcal myocarditis

⑤ **036.8 Other specified meningococcal infections**

    036.81 Meningococcal optic neuritis

    036.82 Meningococcal arthropathy

    036.89 Other

036.9 Meningococcal infection, unspecified
    Meningococcal infection NOS

● Code new
  to this edition
▲ Revision of
  existing code
④ ⑤ Fourth or fifth
    digit required

037 Tetanus

[Excludes:] *tetanus:*
complicating:
abortion (634-638 with .0, 639.0)
ectopic or molar pregnancy (639.0)
neonatorum (771.3)
puerperal (670)

038 Septicemia

[Excludes:] *bacteremia (790.7)*
during labor (659.3)
following ectopic or molar pregnancy (639.0)
following infusion, injection, transfusion, or vaccination (999.3)
postpartum, puerperal (670)
septicemia (sepsis) of newborn (771.81)
that complicating abortion (634-638 with .0, 639.0)

038.0 Streptococcal septicemia

[5] **038.1 Staphylococcal septicemia**

038.10 Staphylococcal septicemia, unspecified

038.11 Staphylococcus aureus septicemia

038.19 Other staphylococcal septicemia

038.2 Pneumococcal septicemia

038.3 Septicemia due to anaerobes
Septicemia due to bacteroides

[Excludes:] *gas gangrene (040.0)*
that due to anaerobic streptococci (038.0)

[5] **038.4 Septicemia due to other gram-negative organisms**

038.40 Gram-negative organism, unspecified
Gram-negative septicemia NOS

038.41 Hemophilus influenzae [H. influenzae]

038.42 Escherichia coli [E. coli]

038.43 Pseudomonas

038.44 Serratia

038.49 Other

038.8 Other specified septicemias

[Excludes:] *septicemia (due to):*
anthrax (022.3)
gonococcal (098.89)
herpetic (054.5)
meningococcal (036.2)
septicemic plague (020.2)

038.9 Unspecified septicemia
Septicemia NOS

[Excludes:] *bacteremia NOS (790.7)*

039 Actinomycotic infections

Includes: actinomycotic mycetoma
infection by Actinomycetales, such as species of Actinomyces, Actinomadura, Nocardia, Streptomyces
maduromycosis (actinomycotic)
schizomycetoma (actinomycotic)

039.0 Cutaneous
Erythrasma
Trichomycosis axillaris

039.1 Pulmonary
Thoracic actinomycosis

039.2 Abdominal

039.3 Cervicofacial

039.4 Madura foot

[Excludes:] *madura foot due to mycotic infection (117.4)*

039.8 Of other specified sites

Add 4th or 5th digit | Nonspecific code | Unspecified code | Manifestation code

039.9 Of unspecified site
Actinomycosis NOS
Maduromycosis NOS
Nocardiosis NOS

040 Other bacterial diseases

Excludes: bacteremia NOS (790.7)
bacterial infection NOS (041.9)

040.0 Gas gangrene
Gas bacillus infection
or gangrene
Infection by Clostridium:
histolyticum
oedematiens
perfringens [welchii]
septicum
sordellii
Malignant edema
Myonecrosis, clostridial
Myositis, clostridial

040.1 Rhinoscleroma

040.2 Whipple's disease
Intestinal lipodystrophy

040.3 Necrobacillosis

⑤ **040.8 Other specified bacterial diseases**

040.81 Tropical pyomyositis

● **040.82 Toxic shock syndrome**
Use additional code to identify the organism

040.89 Other

041 Bacterial infection in conditions classified elsewhere and of unspecified site
Note: This category is provided to be used as an additional code where it is desired to identify
the bacterial agent in diseases classified elsewhere. This category will also be used to
classify bacterial infections of unspecified nature or site.

Excludes: bacteremia NOS (790.7)
septicemia (038.0-038.9)

⑤ **041.0 Streptococcus**

041.00 Streptococcus, unspecified

041.01 Group A

041.02 Group B

041.03 Group C

041.04 Group D [Enterococcus]

041.05 Group G

041.09 Other Streptococcus

⑤ **041.1 Staphylococcus**

041.10 Staphylococcus, unspecified

041.11 Staphylococcus aureus

041.19 Other Staphylococcus

041.2 Pneumococcus

041.3 Friedländer's bacillus
Infection by Klebsiella pneumoniae

041.4 Escherichia coli [E. coli]

041.5 Hemophilus influenzae [H. influenzae]

041.6 Proteus (mirabilis) (morganii)

041.7 Pseudomonas

⑤ **041.8 Other specified bacterial infections**

041.81 Mycoplasma
Eaton's agent
Pleuropneumonia-like organisms [PPLO]

041.82 Bacillus fragilis

041.83 Clostridium perfringens

● Code new
to this edition

▲ Revision of
existing code

④ ⑤ Fourth or fifth
digit required

041.84 Other anaerobes
Gram-negative anaerobes
Bacteroides (fragilis)

[Excludes:] *Helicobacter pylori (041.86)*

041.85 Other Gram-negative organisms
Aerobacter aerogenes
Gram-negative bacteria NOS
Mima polymorpha
Serratia

[Excludes:] *Gram-negative anaerobes (041.84)*

041.86 Helicobacter pylori (H. pylori)

041.89 Other specified bacteria

041.9 Bacterial infection, unspecified

HUMAN IMMUNODEFICIENCY VIRUS (HIV) INFECTION (042)

042 Human immunodeficiency virus [HIV] disease
Acquired immune deficiency syndrome
Acquired immunodeficiency syndrome
AIDS
AIDS-like syndrome
AIDS-related complex
ARC
HIV infection, symptomatic

Use additional code(s) to identify all manifestations of HIV

Use additional code, if desired, to identify HIV-2 infection (079.53)

[Excludes:] *asymptomatic HIV infection status (V08)*
exposre to HIV virus (V01.7)
nonspecific serologic evidence of HIV (795.71)

POLIOMYELITIS AND OTHER NON-ARTHROPOD-BORNE VIRAL DISEASES OF CENTRAL NERVOUS SYSTEM (045-049)

[5] **045 Acute poliomyelitis**

[Excludes:] *late effects of acute poliomyelitis (138)*

The following fifth-digit subclassification is for use with category 045:

0 poliovirus, unspecified type

1 poliovirus type I

2 poliovirus type II

3 poliovirus type III

[5] **045.0 Acute paralytic poliomyelitis specified as bulbar**
Infantile paralysis (acute) specified as bulbar
Poliomyelitis (acute) (anterior) specified as bulbar
Polioencephalitis (acute) (bulbar)
Polioencephalomyelitis (acute) (anterior) (bulbar)

[5] **045.1 Acute poliomyelitis with other paralysis**
Paralysis:
acute atrophic, spinal infantile, paralytic
Poliomyelitis (acute):
anterior, with paralysis except bulbar
epidemic, with paralysis except bulbar

[5] **045.2 Acute nonparalytic poliomyelitis**
Poliomyelitis (acute):
anterior, specified as nonparalytic
epidemic, specified as nonparalytic

[5] **045.9 Acute poliomyelitis, unspecified**
Infantile paralysis, unspecified whether paralytic or nonparalytic
Poliomyelitis (acute):
anterior, unspecified whether paralytic or nonparalytic
epidemic, unspecified whether paralytic or nonparalytic

046 Slow virus infection of central nervous system

046.0 Kuru

046.1 Jakob-Creutzfeldt disease
Subacute spongiform encephalopathy

046.2 Subacute sclerosing panencephalitis
Dawson's inclusion body encephalitis
Van Bogaert's sclerosing leukoencephalitis

046.3 Progressive multifocal leukoencephalopathy
Multifocal leukoencephalopathy NOS

046.8 Other specified slow virus infection of central nervous system

046.9 Unspecified slow virus infection of central nervous system

047 Meningitis due to enterovirus
Includes: meningitis:
abacterial
aseptic
viral

[Excludes:] *meningitis due to:*
adenovirus (049.1)
arthropod-borne virus (060.0-066.9)
leptospira (100.81)
virus of:
herpes simplex (054.72)
herpes zoster (053.0)
lymphocytic choriomeningitis (049.0)
mumps (072.1)
poliomyelitis (045.0-045.9)
any other infection specifically classified elsewhere

047.0 Coxsackie virus

047.1 ECHO virus
Meningo-eruptive syndrome

047.8 Other specified viral meningitis

047.9 Unspecified viral meningitis
Viral meningitis NOS

048 Other enterovirus diseases of central nervous system
Boston exanthem

049 Other non-arthropod-borne viral diseases of central nervous system
[Excludes:] *late effects of viral encephalitis (139.0)*

049.0 Lymphocytic choriomeningitis
Lymphocytic:
meningitis (serous) (benign)
meningoencephalitis (serous) (benign)

049.1 Meningitis due to adenovirus

049.8 Other specified non-arthropod-borne viral diseases of central nervous system
Encephalitis:
acute:
inclusion body
necrotizing
epidemic
Encephalitis:
lethargica
Rio Bravo
von Economo's disease

049.9 Unspecified non-arthropod-borne viral diseases of central nervous system
Viral encephalitis NOS

VIRAL DISEASES ACCOMPANIED BY EXANTHEM (050-057)

[Excludes:] *arthropod-borne viral diseases (060.0-066.9)*
Boston exanthem (048)

050 Smallpox

050.0 Variola major
Hemorrhagic (pustular) smallpox
Malignant smallpox
Purpura variolosa

050.1 Alastrim
Variola minor

050.2 Modified smallpox
Varioloid

050.9 Smallpox, unspecified

● Code new to this edition ▲ Revision of existing code ④ ⑤ Fourth or fifth digit required

051 Cowpox and paravaccinia

051.0 Cowpox
Vaccinia not from vaccination

[Excludes:] *vaccinia (generalized) (from vaccination) (999.0)*

051.1 Pseudocowpox
Milkers' node

051.2 Contagious pustular dermatitis
Ecthyma contagiosum Orf

051.9 Paravaccinia, unspecified

052 Chickenpox

052.0 Postvaricella encephalitis
Postchickenpox encephalitis

052.1 Varicella (hemorrhagic) pneumonitis

052.7 With other specified complications

052.8 With unspecified complication

052.9 Varicella without mention of complication
Chickenpox NOS
Varicella NOS

053 Herpes zoster
Includes: shingles
zona

053.0 With meningitis

[5] **053.1 With other nervous system complications**

053.10 With unspecified nervous system complication

053.11 Geniculate herpes zoster
Herpetic geniculate ganglionitis

053.12 Postherpetic trigeminal neuralgia

053.13 Postherpetic polyneuropathy

053.19 Other

[5] **053.2 With ophthalmic complications**

053.20 Herpes zoster dermatitis of eyelid
Herpes zoster ophthalmicus

053.21 Herpes zoster keratoconjunctivitis

053.22 Herpes zoster iridocyclitis

053.29 Other

[5] **053.7 With other specified complications**

053.71 Otitis externa due to herpes zoster

053.79 Other

053.8 With unspecified complication

053.9 Herpes zoster without mention of complication
Herpes zoster NOS

054 Herpes simplex

[Excludes:] *congenital herpes simplex (771.2)*

054.0 Eczema herpeticum
Kaposi's varicelliform eruption

[5] **054.1 Genital herpes**

054.10 Genital herpes, unspecified
Herpes progenitalis

054.11 Herpetic vulvovaginitis

054.12 Herpetic ulceration of vulva

054.13 Herpetic infection of penis

054.19 Other

054.2 Herpetic gingivostomatitis

054.3 Herpetic meningoencephalitis
Herpes encephalitis Simian B disease

⑤ **054.4 With ophthalmic complications**

> **054.40** With unspecified ophthalmic complication
>
> **054.41** Herpes simplex dermatitis of eyelid
>
> **054.42** Dendritic keratitis
>
> **054.43** Herpes simplex disciform keratitis
>
> **054.44** Herpes simplex iridocyclitis
>
> **054.49** Other

054.5 Herpetic septicemia

054.6 Herpetic whitlow
> Herpetic felon

⑤ **054.7 With other specified complications**

> **054.71** Visceral herpes simplex
>
> **054.72** Herpes simplex meningitis
>
> **054.73** Herpes simplex otitis externa
>
> **054.79** Other

054.8 With unspecified complication

054.9 Herpes simplex without mention of complication

055 Measles
> Includes: morbilli
> rubeola

055.0 Postmeasles encephalitis

055.1 Postmeasles pneumonia

055.2 Postmeasles otitis media

⑤ **055.7 With other specified complications**

> **055.71** Measles keratoconjunctivitis
> Measles keratitis
>
> **055.79** Other

055.8 With unspecified complication

055.9 Measles without mention of complication

056 Rubella
> Includes: German measles
>
> *Excludes:* congenital rubella (771.0)

⑤ **056.0 With neurological complications**

> **056.00** With unspecified neurological complication
>
> **056.01** Encephalomyelitis due to rubella
> Encephalitis due to rubella
> Meningoencephalitis due to rubella
>
> **056.09** Other

⑤ **056.7 With other specified complications**

> **056.71** Arthritis due to rubella
>
> **056.79** Other

056.8 With unspecified complications

056.9 Rubella without mention of complication

057 Other viral exanthemata

057.0 Erythema infectiosum [fifth disease]

057.8 Other specified viral exanthemata
> Dukes (-Filatow) disease
> Exanthema subitum
> [sixth disease]
> Fourth disease
> Parascarlatina
> Pseudoscarlatina
> Roseola infantum

057.9 Viral exanthem, unspecified

● Code new
to this edition

▲ Revision of
existing code

④ ⑤ Fourth or fifth
digit required

ARTHROPOD-BORNE VIRAL DISEASES (060-066)

Use additional code, if desired, to identify any associated meningitis (321.2)

Excludes: *late effects of viral encephalitis (139.0)*

060 Yellow fever

060.0 Sylvatic
Yellow fever:
jungle
sylvan

060.1 Urban

060.9 Yellow fever, unspecified

061 Dengue
Breakbone fever

Excludes: *hemorrhagic fever caused by dengue virus (065.4)*

062 Mosquito-borne viral encephalitis

062.0 Japanese encephalitis
Japanese B encephalitis

062.1 Western equine encephalitis

062.2 Eastern equine encephalitis

Excludes: *Venezuelan equine encephalitis (066.2)*

062.3 St. Louis encephalitis

062.4 Australian encephalitis
Australian arboencephalitis
Australian X disease
Murray Valley encephalitis

062.5 California virus encephalitis
Encephalitis: Tahyna fever
California
La Crosse

062.8 Other specified mosquito-borne viral encephalitis
Encephalitis by Ilheus virus

Excludes: *West Nile virus (066.4)*

062.9 Mosquito-borne viral encephalitis, unspecified

063 Tick-borne viral encephalitis
Includes: diphasic meningoencephalitis

063.0 Russian spring-summer [taiga] encephalitis

063.1 Louping ill

063.2 Central European encephalitis

063.8 Other specified tick-borne viral encephalitis
Langat encephalitis   Powassan encephalitis

063.9 Tick-borne viral encephalitis, unspecified

064 Viral encephalitis transmitted by other and unspecified arthropods
Arthropod-borne viral encephalitis, vector unknown
Negishi virus encephalitis

Excludes: *viral encephalitis NOS (049.9)*

065 Arthropod-borne hemorrhagic fever

065.0 Crimean hemorrhagic fever [CHF Congo virus]
Central Asian hemorrhagic fever

065.1 Omsk hemorrhagic fever

065.2 Kyasanur Forest disease

065.3 Other tick-borne hemorrhagic fever

065.4 Mosquito-borne hemorrhagic fever
Chikungunya hemorrhagic fever
Dengue hemorrhagic fever

Excludes: *Chikungunya fever (066.3)*
dengue (061)
yellow fever (060.0-060.9)

| | Add 4th or 5th digit | | Nonspecific code | | Unspecified code | | Manifestation code |

065.8 **Other specified arthropod-borne hemorrhagic fever**
Mite-borne hemorrhagic fever

065.9 **Arthropod-borne hemorrhagic fever, unspecified**
Arbovirus hemorrhagic fever NOS

066 **Other arthropod-borne viral diseases**

066.0 **Phlebotomus fever**
Changuinola fever   Sandfly fever

066.1 **Tick-borne fever**
Nairobi sheep disease   Tick fever:
Tick fever: Kemerovo
  American mountain   Quaranfil
  Colorado

066.2 **Venezuelan equine fever**
Venezuelan equine encephalitis

066.3 **Other mosquito-borne fever**
Fever (viral):   Fever (viral):
  Bunyamwera   Oropouche
  Bwamba   Pixuna
  Chikungunya   Rift valley
  GuamaR Mayaro   Ross river
  Mucambo   Wesselsbron
  O'nyong-nyong   Zika

Excludes: dengue (061)
          yellow fever (060.0-060.9)

● **066.4** **West Nile fever**
West Nile encephalitis
West Nile encephalomyelitis
West Nile virus

066.8 **Other specified arthropod-borne viral diseases**
Chandipura fever   Piry fever

066.9 **Arthropod-borne viral disease, unspecified**
Arbovirus infection NOS

OTHER DISEASES DUE TO VIRUSES AND CHLAMYDIAE (070-079)

070 **Viral hepatitis**
Includes: viral hepatitis (acute) (chronic)

Excludes: cytomegalic inclusion virus hepatitis (078.5)

The following fifth-digit subclassification is for use with categories 070.2 and 070.3:

0 **acute or unspecified, without mention of hepatitis delta**

1 **acute or unspecified, with hepatitis delta**

2 **chronic, without mention of hepatitis delta**

3 **chronic, with hepatitis delta**

070.0 **Viral hepatitis A with hepatic coma**

070.1 **Viral hepatitis A without mention of hepatic coma**
Infectious hepatitis

⑤ **070.2** **Viral hepatitis B with hepatic coma**

⑤ **070.3** **Viral hepatitis B without mention of hepatic coma**
Serum hepatitis

⑤ **070.4** **Other specified viral hepatitis with hepatic coma**

070.41 **Acute or unspecified hepatitis C with hepatic coma**

070.42 **Hepatitis delta without mention of active hepatitis B disease with hepatic coma**
Hepatitis delta with hepatitis B carrier state

070.43 **Hepatitis E with hepatic coma**

070.44 **Chronic hepatitis C with hepatic coma**

070.49 **Other specified viral hepatitis with hepatic coma**

⑤ **070.5** **Other specified viral hepatitis without mention of hepatic coma**

070.51 **Acute or unspecified hepatitis C without mention of hepatic coma**

070.52 **Hepatitis delta without mention of active hepatits B disease or hepatic coma**

070.53 **Hepatitis E without mention of hepatic coma**

● Code new
to this edition

▲ Revision of
existing code

④ ⑤ Fourth or fifth
digit required

070.54 Chronic hepatitis C without mention of hepatic coma

070.59 Other specified viral hepatitis without mention of hepatic coma

070.6 Unspecified viral hepatitis with hepatic coma

070.9 Unspecified viral hepatitis without mention of hepatic coma
Viral hepatitis NOS

071 Rabies
Hydrophobia
Lyssa

072 Mumps

072.0 Mumps orchitis

072.1 Mumps meningitis

072.2 Mumps encephalitis
Mumps meningoencephalitis

072.3 Mumps pancreatitis

[5] **072.7 Mumps with other specified complications**

072.71 Mumps hepatitis

072.72 Mumps polyneuropathy

072.79 Other

072.8 Mumps with unspecified complication

072.9 Mumps without mention of complication
Epidemic parotitis
Infectious parotitis

073 Ornithosis
Includes: parrot fever
psittacosis

073.0 With pneumonia
Lobular pneumonitis due to ornithosis

073.7 With other specified complications

073.8 With unspecified complication

073.9 Ornithosis, unspecified

074 Specific diseases due to Coxsackie virus
[*Excludes:*] *Coxsackie virus:*
infection NOS (079.2)
meningitis (047.0)

074.0 Herpangina
Vesicular pharyngitis

074.1 Epidemic pleurodynia
Bornholm disease
Devil's grip
Epidemic:
myalgia
myositis

[5] **074.2 Coxsackie carditis**

074.20 Coxsackie carditis, unspecified

074.21 Coxsackie pericarditis

074.22 Coxsackie endocarditis

074.23 Coxsackie myocarditis
Aseptic myocarditis of newborn

074.3 Hand, foot, and mouth disease
Vesicular stomatitis and exanthem

074.8 Other specified diseases due to Coxsackie virus
Acute lymphonodular pharyngitis

075 Infectious mononucleosis
Glandular fever
Monocytic angina
Pfeiffer's disease

076 Trachoma
[*Excludes:*] *late effect of trachoma (139.1)*

076.0 Initial stage
Trachoma dubium

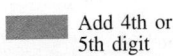

Add 4th or 5th digit | Nonspecific code | Unspecified code | Manifestation code

076.1 Active stage
Granular conjunctivitis (trachomatous)
Trachomatous:
follicular conjunctivitis
pannus

076.9 Trachoma, unspecified
Trachoma NOS

077 Other diseases of conjunctiva due to viruses and Chlamydiae
[*Excludes:*] *ophthalmic complications of viral diseases classified elsewhere*

077.0 Inclusion conjunctivitis
Paratrachoma
Swimming pool conjunctivitis
[*Excludes:*] *inclusion blennorrhea (neonatal) (771.6)*

077.1 Epidemic keratoconjunctivitis
Shipyard eye

077.2 Pharyngoconjunctival fever
Viral pharyngoconjunctivitis

077.3 Other adenoviral conjunctivitis
Acute adenoviral follicular conjunctivitis

077.4 Epidemic hemorrhagic conjunctivitis
Apollo:
conjunctivitis
disease
Conjunctivitis due to enterovirus type 70
Hemorrhagic conjunctivitis (acute) (epidemic)

077.8 Other viral conjunctivitis
Newcastle conjunctivitis

[5] **077.9 Unspecified diseases of conjunctiva due to viruses and Chlamydiae**

077.98 Due to Chlamydiae

077.99 Due to viruses
Viral conjunctivitis NOS

078 Other diseases due to viruses and Chlamydiae
[*Excludes:*] *viral infection NOS (079.0-079.9)*
viremia NOS (790.8)

078.0 Molluscum contagiosum

[5] **078.1 Viral warts**
Viral warts due to Human papillomavirus

078.10 Viral warts, unspecified
Condyloma NOS
Verruca:
NOS
vulgaris
Warts (infectious)

078.11 Condyloma acuminatum

078.19 Other specified viral warts
Genital warts NOS
Verruca:
plana
plantaris

078.2 Sweating fever
Miliary fever
Sweating disease

078.3 Cat-scratch disease
Benign lymphoreticulosis (of inoculation)
Cat-scratch fever

078.4 Foot and mouth disease
Aphthous fever
Epizootic:
aphthae
Stomatitis

078.5 Cytomegaloviral disease
Cytomegalic inclusion disease
Salivary gland virus disease

Use additional code, if desired, to identify manifestation, as:
cytomegalic inclusion virus:
hepatitis (573.1)
pneumonia (484.1)

[Excludes:] *congenital cytomegalovirus infection (771.1)*

078.6 Hemorrhagic nephrosonephritis
Hemorrhagic fever:
epidemic
Korean
Hemorrhagic fever:
Russian
with renal syndrome

078.7 Arenaviral hemorrhagic fever
Hemorrhagic fever:
Argentine
Bolivian
Hemorrhagic fever:
Junin virus
Machupo virus

[5] **078.8 Other specified diseases due to viruses and Chlamydiae**

[Excludes:] *epidemic diarrhea (009.2)*
lymphogranuloma venereum (099.1)

078.81 Epidemic vertigo

078.82 Epidemic vomiting syndrome
Winter vomiting disease

078.88 Other specified diseases due to Chlamydiae

078.89 Other specified diseases due to viruses
Epidemic cervical myalgia
Marburg disease
Tanapox

079 Viral and chlamydial infection in conditions classified elsewhere and of unspecified site

Note: This category is provided to be used as an additional code where it is desired to identify the viral agent in diseases classifiable elsewhere. This category will also be used to classify virus infection of unspecified nature or site.

079.0 Adenovirus

079.1 ECHO virus

079.2 Coxsackievirus

079.3 Rhinovirus

079.4 Human papillomavirus

[5] **079.5 Retrovirus**

[Excludes:] *human immunodeficiency virus, type 1 [HIV-1] (042)*
human T-cell lymphotrophic virus, type III [HTLV-III] (042)
lymphadenopathy-associated virus [LAV] (042)

079.50 Retrovirus, unspecified

079.51 Human T-cell lymphotrophic virus, type I [HTLV-I]

079.52 Human T-cell lymphotrophic virus, type II [HTLV-II]

079.53 Human immunodeficiency virus, type 2 [HIV-2]

079.59 Other specified retrovirus

079.6 Respiratory syncytial virus (RSV)

[5] **079.8 Other specified viral and chlamydial infections**

079.81 Hantavirus

079.88 Other specified chlamydial infection

079.89 Other specified viral infection

[5] **079.9 Unspecified viral and chlamydial infections**

[Excludes:] *viremia NOS (790.8)*

079.98 Unspecified chlamydial infection
Chlamydial infection NOS

079.99 Unspecified viral infection
Viral infection NOS

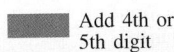

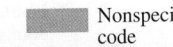

RICKETTSIOSES AND OTHER ARTHROPOD-BORNE DISEASES (080-088)

Excludes: *arthropod-borne viral diseases (060.0-066.9)*

080 Louse-borne [epidemic] typhus

Typhus (fever):
classical
epidemic

Typhus (fever):
exanthematic NOS
louse-borne

081 Other typhus

081.0 Murine [endemic] typhus
Typhus (fever):
endemic
flea-borne

081.1 Brill's disease
Brill-Zinsser disease
Recrudescent typhus (fever)

081.2 Scrub typhus
Japanese river fever
Kedani fever

Mite-borne typhus
Tsutsugamushi

081.9 Typhus, unspecified
Typhus (fever) NOS

082 Tick-borne rickettsioses

082.0 Spotted fevers
Rocky mountain spotted fever
São Paulo fever

082.1 Boutonneuse fever
African tick typhus
India tick typhus
Kenya tick typhus

Marseilles fever
Mediterranean tick fever

082.2 North Asian tick fever
Siberian tick typhus

082.3 Queensland tick typhus

⑤ **082.4 Ehrlichiosis**

082.40 Ehrlichiosis, unspecified

082.41 Ehrlichiosis chafeensis (E. chafeensis)

082.49 Other ehrlichiosis

082.8 Other specified tick-borne rickettsioses
Lone star fever

082.9 Tick-borne rickettsiosis, unspecified
Tick-borne typhus NOS

083 Other rickettsioses

083.0 Q fever

083.1 Trench fever
Quintan fever

Wolhynian fever

083.2 Rickettsialpox
Vesicular rickettsiosis

083.8 Other specified rickettsioses

083.9 Rickettsiosis, unspecified

084 Malaria

Note: Subcategories 084.0-084.6 exclude the listed conditions with mention of pernicious
complications (084.8-084.9).

Excludes: *congenital malaria (771.2)*

084.0 Falciparum malaria [malignant tertian]
Malaria (fever):
by Plasmodium falciparum
subtertian

084.1 Vivax malaria [benign tertian]
Malaria (fever) by Plasmodium vivax

084.2 Quartan malaria
Malaria (fever) by Plasmodium malariae
Malariae malaria

● Code new
to this edition

▲ Revision of
existing code

④ ⑤ Fourth or fifth
digit required

084.3 Ovale malaria
Malaria (fever) by Plasmodium ovale

084.4 Other malaria
Monkey malaria

084.5 Mixed malaria
Malaria (fever) by more than one parasite

084.6 Malaria, unspecified
Malaria (fever) NOS

084.7 Induced malaria
Therapeutically induced malaria

> Excludes: *accidental infection from syringe, blood transfusion, etc. (084.0-084.6, above, according to parasite species)*
> *transmission from mother to child during delivery (771.2)*

084.8 Blackwater fever
Hemoglobinuric: Malarial hemoglobinuria
  fever (bilious)
  malaria

084.9 Other pernicious complications of malaria
Algid malaria
Cerebral malaria

Use additional code, if desired, to identify complication, as:
  malarial:
    hepatitis (573.2)
    nephrosis (581.81)

085 Leishmaniasis

085.0 Visceral [kala-azar]
Dumdum fever   Leishmaniasis:
Infection by Leishmania: dermal, post-kala-azar
  donovani   Mediterranean
  infantum   visceral (Indian)

085.1 Cutaneous, urban
Aleppo boil   Leishmaniasis, cutaneous:
Baghdad boil   dry form
Delhi boil   late
Infection by Leishmania   recurrent
  tropica (minor)   ulcerating
                      Oriental sore

085.2 Cutaneous, Asian desert
Infection by Leishmania tropica major
Leishmaniasis, cutaneous:
  acute necrotizing
  rural
  wet form
  zoonotic form

085.3 Cutaneous, Ethiopian
Infection by Leishmania ethiopica
Leishmaniasis, cutaneous:
  diffuse
  lepromatous

085.4 Cutaneous, American
Chiclero ulcer
Infection by Leishmania mexicana
Leishmaniasis tegumentaria diffusa

085.5 Mucocutaneous (American)
Espundia
Infection by Leishmania braziliensis
Uta

085.9 Leishmaniasis, unspecified

086 Trypanosomiasis
Use additional code, if desired, to identify manifestations, as:
trypanosomiasis:
  encephalitis (323.2)
  meningitis (321.3)

	Add 4th or 5th digit		Nonspecific code		Unspecified code		Manifestation code

086.0 Chagas' disease with heart involvement
American trypanosomiasis with heart involvement
Infection by Trypanosoma cruzi with heart involvement
Any condition classifiable to 086.2 with heart involvement

086.1 Chagas' disease with other organ involvement
American trypanosomiasis with involvement of organ other than heart
Infection by Trypanosoma cruzi with involvement of organ other than heart
Any condition classifiable to 086.2 with involvement of organ other than heart

086.2 Chagas' disease without mention of organ involvement
American trypanosomiasis
Infection by Trypanosoma cruzi

086.3 Gambian trypanosomiasis
Gambian sleeping sickness
Infection by Trypanosoma gambiense

086.4 Rhodesian trypanosomiasis
Infection by Trypanosoma rhodesiense
Rhodesian sleeping sickness

086.5 African trypanosomiasis, unspecified
Sleeping sickness NOS

086.9 Trypanosomiasis, unspecified

087 Relapsing fever
Includes: recurrent fever

087.0 Louse-borne

087.1 Tick-borne

087.9 Relapsing fever, unspecified

088 Other arthropod-borne diseases

088.0 Bartonellosis
Carrión's disease
Oroya fever
Verruga peruana

⑤ **088.8 Other specified arthropod-borne diseases**

088.81 Lyme Disease
Erythema chronicum migrans

088.82 Babesiosis
Babesiasis

088.89 Other

088.9 Arthropod-borne disease, unspecified

SYPHILIS AND OTHER VENEREAL DISEASES (090-099)

[Excludes:] *nonvenereal endemic syphilis (104.0)*
urogenital trichomoniasis (131.0)

090 Congenital syphilis

090.0 Early congenital syphilis, symptomatic
Congenital syphilitic:
- choroiditis
- coryza (chronic)
- hepatomegaly
- mucous patches
- periostitis
- splenomegaly

Syphilitic (congenital):
- epiphysitis
- osteochondritis
- pemphigus

Any congenital syphilitic condition specified as early or manifest less than two years after birth

090.1 Early congenital syphilis, latent
Congenital syphilis without clinical manifestations, with positive serological reaction and negative spinal fluid test, less than two years after birth

090.2 Early congenital syphilis, unspecified
Congenital syphilis NOS, less than two years after birth

090.3 Syphilitic interstitial keratitis
Syphilitic keratitis:
- parenchymatous
- punctata profunda

[Excludes:] *interstitial keratitis NOS (370.50)*

⑤ **090.4 Juvenile neurosyphilis**
Use additional code, if desired, to identify any associated mental disorder

090.40 Juvenile neurosyphilis, unspecified
Congenital neurosyphilis
Dementia paralytica juvenilis
Juvenile:
general paresis
tabes
taboparesis

090.41 Congenital syphilitic encephalitis

090.42 Congenital syphilitic meningitis

090.49 Other

090.5 Other late congenital syphilis, symptomatic
Gumma due to congenital syphilis
Hutchinson's teeth
Syphilitic saddle nose
Any congenital syphilitic condition specified as late or manifest two years or more after birth

090.6 Late congenital syphilis, latent
Congenital syphilis without clinical manifestations, with positive serological reaction and negative spinal fluid test, two years or more after birth

090.7 Late congenital syphilis, unspecified
Congenital syphilis NOS, two years or more after birth

090.9 Congenital syphilis, unspecified

091 Early syphilis, symptomatic
[Excludes:] *early cardiovascular syphilis (093.0-093.9)*
early neurosyphilis (094.0-094.9)

091.0 Genital syphilis (primary)
Genital chancre

091.1 Primary anal syphilis

091.2 Other primary syphilis
Primary syphilis of:
breast
fingers
Primary syphilis of:
lip
tonsils

091.3 Secondary syphilis of skin or mucous membranes
Condyloma latum
Secondary syphilis of:
anus
mouth
pharynx
Secondary syphilis of:
skin
tonsils
vulva

091.4 Adenopathy due to secondary syphilis
Syphilitic adenopathy (secondary)
Syphilitic lymphadenitis (secondary)

[5] **091.5 Uveitis due to secondary syphilis**

091.50 Syphilitic uveitis, unspecified

091.51 Syphilitic chorioretinitis (secondary)

091.52 Syphilitic iridocyclitis (secondary)

[5] **091.6 Secondary syphilis of viscera and bone**

091.61 Secondary syphilitic periostitis

091.62 Secondary syphilitic hepatitis
Secondary syphilis of liver

091.69 Other viscera

091.7 Secondary syphilis, relapse
Secondary syphilis, relapse (treated) (untreated)

[5] **091.8 Other forms of secondary syphilis**

091.81 Acute syphilitic meningitis (secondary)

091.82 Syphilitic alopecia

091.89 Other

091.9 Unspecified secondary syphilis

092 Early syphilis, latent
Includes: syphilis (acquired) without clinical manifestations, with positive serological reaction and negative spinal fluid test, less than two years after infection

Add 4th or 5th digit | Nonspecific code | Unspecified code | Manifestation code

092.0 Early syphilis, latent, serological relapse after treatment

092.9 Early syphilis, latent, unspecified

093 Cardiovascular syphilis

093.0 Aneurysm of aorta, specified as syphilitic
Dilatation of aorta, specified as syphilitic

093.1 Syphilitic aortitis

⑤ **093.2 Syphilitic endocarditis**

093.20 Valve, unspecified
Syphilitic ostial coronary disease

093.21 Mitral valve

093.22 Aortic valve
Syphilitic aortic incompetence or stenosis

093.23 Tricuspid valve

093.24 Pulmonary valve

⑤ **093.8 Other specified cardiovascular syphilis**

093.81 Syphilitic pericarditis

093.82 Syphilitic myocarditis

093.89 Other

093.9 Cardiovascular syphilis, unspecified

094 Neurosyphilis
Use additional code, if desired, to identify any associated mental disorder

094.0 Tabes dorsalis
Locomotor ataxia (progressive)
Posterior spinal sclerosis (syphilitic)
Tabetic neurosyphilis
Use additional code, if desired, to identify manifestation, as:
neurogenic arthropathy [Charcot's joint disease] (713.5)

094.1 General paresis
Dementia paralytica   Paretic neurosyphilis
General paralysis (of the   Taboparesis
insane) (progressive)

094.2 Syphilitic meningitis
Meningovascular syphilis

Excludes: acute syphilitic meningitis (secondary) (091.81)

094.3 Asymptomatic neurosyphilis

⑤ **094.8 Other specified neurosyphilis**

094.81 Syphilitic encephalitis

094.82 Syphilitic Parkinsonism

094.83 Syphilitic disseminated retinochoroiditis

094.84 Syphilitic optic atrophy

094.85 Syphilitic retrobulbar neuritis

094.86 Syphilitic acoustic neuritis

094.87 Syphilitic ruptured cerebral aneurysm

094.89 Other

094.9 Neurosyphilis, unspecified
Gumma (syphilitic) of central nervous system NOS
Syphilis (early) (late) of central nervous system NOS
Syphiloma of central nervous system NOS

095 Other forms of late syphilis, with symptoms
Includes: gumma (syphilitic)
syphilis, late, tertiary, or unspecified stage

095.0 Syphilitic episcleritis

095.1 Syphilis of lung

095.2 Syphilitic peritonitis

095.3 Syphilis of liver

095.4 Syphilis of kidney

● Code new   ▲ Revision of   ④ ⑤ Fourth or fifth
to this edition   existing code   digit required

095.5 Syphilis of bone

095.6 Syphilis of muscle
Syphilitic myositis

095.7 Syphilis of synovium, tendon, and bursa
Syphilitic:
- bursitis
- synovitis

095.8 Other specified forms of late symptomatic syphilis
[Excludes:] *cardiovascular syphilis (093.0-093.9)*
neurosyphilis (094.0-094.9)

095.9 Late symptomatic syphilis, unspecified

096 Late syphilis, latent
Syphilis (acquired) without clinical manifestations, with positive serological reaction and negative spinal fluid test, two years or more after infection

097 Other and unspecified syphilis

097.0 Late syphilis, unspecified

097.1 Latent syphilis, unspecified
Positive serological reaction for syphilis

097.9 Syphilis, unspecified
Syphilis (acquired) NOS

[Excludes:] *syphilis NOS causing death under two years of age (090.9)*

098 Gonococcal infections

098.0 Acute, of lower genitourinary tract
Gonococcal:
- Bartholinitis (acute)
- urethritis (acute)
- vulvovaginitis (acute)

Gonorrhea (acute):
- NOS
- genitourinary (tract) NOS

[5] **098.1 Acute, of upper genitourinary tract**

098.10 Gonococcal infection (acute) of upper genitourinary tract, site unspecified

098.11 Gonococcal cystitis (acute)
Gonorrhea (acute) of bladder

098.12 Gonococcal prostatitis (acute)

098.13 Gonococcal epididymo-orchitis (acute)
Gonococcal orchitis (acute)

098.14 Gonococcal seminal vesiculitis (acute)
Gonorrhea (acute) of seminal vesicle

098.15 Gonococcal cervicitis (acute)
Gonorrhea (acute) of cervix

098.16 Gonococcal endometritis (acute)
Gonorrhea (acute) of uterus

098.17 Gonococcal salpingitis, specified as acute

098.19 Other

098.2 Chronic, of lower genitourinary tract
Gonococcal:
- Bartholinitis specified as chronic or with duration of two months or more
- urethritis specified as chronic or with duration of two months or more
- vulvovaginitis specified as chronic or with duration of two months or more

Gonorrhea:
- NOS specified as chronic or with duration of two months or more
- genitourinary (tract) specified as chronic or with duration of two months or more

Any condition classifiable to 098.0 specified as chronic or with duration of two months or more

[5] **098.3 Chronic, of upper genitourinary tract**
Includes: any condition classifiable to 098.1 stated as chronic or with a duration of two months or more

098.30 Chronic gonococcal infection of upper genitourinary tract, site unspecified

098.31 Gonococcal cystitis, chronic
Any condition classifiable to 098.11, specified as chronic
Gonorrhea of bladder, chronic

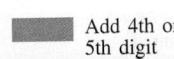

Add 4th or 5th digit | Nonspecific code | Unspecified code | Manifestation code

098.32 Gonococcal prostatitis, chronic
Any condition classifiable to 098.12, specified as chronic

098.33 Gonococcal epididymo-orchitis, chronic
Any condition classifiable to 098.13, specified as chronic
Chronic gonococcal orchitis

098.34 Gonococcal seminal vesiculitis, chronic
Any condition classifiable to 098.14, specified as chronic
Gonorrhea of seminal vesicle, chronic

098.35 Gonococcal cervicitis, chronic
Any condition classifiable to 098.15, specified as chronic
Gonorrhea of cervix, chronic

098.36 Gonococcal endometritis, chronic
Any condition classifiable to 098.16, specified as chronic

098.37 Gonococcal salpingitis (chronic)

098.39 Other

[5] **098.4 Gonococcal infection of eye**

098.40 Gonococcal conjunctivitis (neonatorum)
Gonococcal ophthalmia (neonatorum)

098.41 Gonococcal iridocyclitis

098.42 Gonococcal endophthalmia

098.43 Gonococcal keratitis

098.49 Other

098.5 Gonococcal infection of joint

098.50 Gonococcal arthritis
Gonococcal infection of joint NOS

098.51 Gonococcal synovitis and tenosynovitis

098.52 Gonococcal bursitis

098.53 Gonococcal spondylitis

098.59 Other
Gonococcal rheumatism

098.6 Gonococcal infection of pharynx

098.7 Gonococcal infection of anus and rectum
Gonococcal proctitis

[5] **098.8 Gonococcal infection of other specified sites**

098.81 Gonococcal keratosis (blennorrhagica)

098.82 Gonococcal meningitis

098.83 Gonococcal pericarditis

098.84 Gonococcal endocarditis

098.85 Other gonococcal heart disease

098.86 Gonococcal peritonitis

098.89 Other
Gonococcemia

099 Other venereal diseases

099.0 Chancroid
Bubo (inguinal):
chancroidal
due to Hemophilus ducreyi
Chancre:
Ducrey's
simple
soft
Ulcus molle (cutis) (skin)

099.1 Lymphogranuloma venereum
Climatic or tropical bubo
(Durand-) Nicolas- Favre disease
Esthiomene
Lymphogranuloma inguinale

099.2 Granuloma inguinale
Donovanosis
Granuloma pudendi (ulcerating)
Granuloma venereum
Pudendal ulcer

● Code new to this edition
▲ Revision of existing code
④ ⑤ Fourth or fifth digit required

099.3 Reiter's disease
Reiter's syndrome
Use additional code for associated:
arthropathy (711.1)
conjunctivitis (372.33)

⑤ **099.4 Other nongonococcal urethritis [NGU]**

099.40 Unspecified
Nonspecific urethritis

099.41 Chlamydia trachomatis

099.49 Other specified organism

⑤ **099.5 Other venereal diseases due to Chlamydia trachomatis**

Excludes: *Chlamydia trachomatis infection of conjunctiva (076.0-076.9, 077.0, 077.9)*
Lymphogranuloma venereum (099.1)

099.50 Unspecified site

099.51 Pharynx

099.52 Anus and rectum

099.53 Lower genitourinary sites

Excludes: *urethra (099.41)*

Use additional code, if desired, to specify site of infection, such as:
bladder (595.4)
cervix (616.0)
vagina and vulva (616.11)

099.54 Other genitourinary sites
Use additional code, if desired, to specify site of infection, such as:
pelvic inflammatory disease NOS (614.9)
testis and epididymis (604.91)

099.55 Unspecified genitourinary site

099.56 Peritoneum
Perihepatitis

099.59 Other specified site

099.8 Other specified venereal diseases

099.9 Venereal disease, unspecified

OTHER SPIROCHETAL DISEASES (100-104)

100 Leptospirosis

100.0 Leptospirosis icterohemorrhagica
Leptospiral or spirochetal jaundice (hemorrhagic)
Weil's disease

⑤ **100.8 Other specified leptospiral infections**

100.81 Leptospiral meningitis (aseptic)

100.89 Other

Fever:	Infection by Leptospira:
Fort Bragg	australis
pretibial	bataviae
swamp	pyrogenes

100.9 Leptospirosis, unspecified

101 Vincent's angina

Acute necrotizing ulcerative:	Spirochetal stomatitis
gingivitis	Trench mouth
stomatitis	Vincent's:
Fusospirochetal pharyngitis	gingivitis
	infection [any site]

102 Yaws
Includes: frambesia
pian

102.0 Initial lesions

Chancre of yaws	Initial frambesial ulcer
Frambesia, initial or primary	Mother yaw

Add 4th or
5th digit   Nonspecific
code   Unspecified
code   Manifestation
code

102.1 Multiple papillomata and wet crab yaws
Butter yaws
Frambesioma
Pianoma
Planter or palmer papilloma of yaws

102.2 Other early skin lesions
Early yaws (cutaneous) (macular) (papular) (maculopapular) (micropapular)
Frambeside of early yaws
Cutaneous yaws, less than five years after infection

102.3 Hyperkeratosis
Ghoul hand
Hyperkeratosis, palmer or plantar (early) (late) due to yaws
Worm-eaten soles

102.4 Gummata and ulcers
Nodular late yaws (ulcerated)
Gummatous frambeside

102.5 Gangosa
Rhinopharyngitis mutilans

102.6 Bone and joint lesions
Goundou, of yaws (late)
Gumma, bone, of yaws (late)
Gummatous osteitis or periostitis, of yaws (late)
Hydrarthrosis, of yaws (early) (late)
Osteitis, of yaws (early) (late)
Periostitis (hypertrophic), of yaws (early) (late)

102.7 Other manifestations
Juxta-articular nodules of yaws
Mucosal yaws

102.8 Latent yaws
Yaws without clinical manifestations, with positive serology

102.9 Yaws, unspecified

103 Pinta

103.0 Primary lesions
Chancre (primary) of pinta [carate]
Papule (primary) of pinta [carate]
Pintid of pinta [carate]

103.1 Intermediate lesions
Erythematous plaques of pinta [carate]
Hyperchromic lesions of pinta [carate]
Hyperkeratosis of pinta [carate]

103.2 Late lesions
Cardiovascular lesions, of pinta [carate]
Skin lesions:
- achromic of pinta [carate]
- cicatricial of pinta [carate]
- dyschromic of pinta [carate]

Vitiligo of pinta [carate]

103.3 Mixed lesions
Achromic and hyperchromic skin lesions of pinta [carate]

103.9 Pinta, unspecified

104 Other spirochetal infection

104.0 Nonvenereal endemic syphilis
Bejel
Njovera

104.8 Other specified spirochetal infections
[Excludes:] *relapsing fever (087.0-087.9)*
syphilis (090.0-097.9)

104.9 Spirochetal infection, unspecified

● Code new to this edition
▲ Revision of existing code
④ ⑤ Fourth or fifth digit required

MYCOSES (110-118)

Use additional code, if desired, to identify manifestation, as:
arthropathy (711.6)
meningitis (321.0-321.1)
otitis externa (380.15)

Excludes: *infection by Actinomycetales, such as species of Actinomyces, Actinomadura, Nocardia, Streptomyces (039.0-039.9)*

110 Dermatophytosis
Includes:
infection by species of Epidermophyton, Microsporum, and Trichophyton
tinea, any type except those in 111

110.0 Of scalp and beard
Kerion
Sycosis, mycotic
Trichophytic tinea [black dot tinea], scalp

110.1 Of nail
Dermatophytic onychia   Tinea unguium
Onychomycosis

110.2 Of hand
Tinea manuum

110.3 Of groin and perianal area
Dhobie itch   Tinea cruris
Eczema marginatum

110.4 Of foot
Athlete's foot   Tinea pedis

110.5 Of the body
Herpes circinatus
Tinea imbricata [Tokelau]

110.6 Deep seated dermatophytosis
Granuloma trichophyticum
Majocchi's granuloma

110.8 Of other specified sites

110.9 Of unspecified site
Favus NOS   Ringworm NOS
Microsporic tinea NOS

111 Dermatomycosis, other and unspecified

111.0 Pityriasis versicolor
Infection by Malassezia [Pityrosporum] furfur
Tinea flava
Tinea versicolor

111.1 Tinea nigra
Infection by   Microsporosis nigra
   Cladosporium species   Pityriasis nigra
Keratomycosis nigricans   Tinea palmaris nigra

111.2 Tinea blanca
Infection by Trichosporon (beigelii) cutaneum
White piedra

111.3 Black piedra
Infection by Piedraia hortai

111.8 Other specified dermatomycoses

111.9 Dermatomycosis, unspecified

112 Candidiasis
Includes: infection by Candida species
moniliasis

Excludes: *neonatal monilial infection (771.7)*

112.0 Of mouth
Thrush (oral)

112.1 Of vulva and vagina
Candidal vulvovaginitis
Monilial vulvovaginitis

112.2 Of other urogenital sites
Candidal balanitis

Add 4th or   Nonspecific   Unspecified   Manifestation
5th digit   code   code   code

112.3 Of skin and nails
Candidal intertrigo
Candidal onychia
Candidal perionyxis [paronychia]

112.4 Of lung
Candidal pneumonia

112.5 Disseminated
Systemic candidiasis

⑤ **112.8 Of other specified sites**

    112.81 Candidal endocarditis

    112.82 Candidal otitis externa
       Otomycosis in moniliasis

    112.83 Candidal meningitis

    112.84 Candidal esophagitis

    112.85 Candidal enteritis

    112.89 Other

112.9 Of unspecified site

114 Coccidioidomycosis
Includes: infection by Coccidioides (immitis)
           Posada-Wernicke disease

114.0 Primary coccidioidomycosis (pulmonary)
Acute pulmonary coccidioidomycosis
Coccidioidomycotic pneumonitis
Desert rheumatism
Pulmonary coccidioidomycosis
San Joaquin Valley fever

114.1 Primary extrapulmonary coccidioidomycosis
Chancriform syndrome
Primary cutaneous coccidioidomycosis

114.2 Coccidioidal meningitis

114.3 Other forms of progressive coccidioidomycosis
Coccidioidal granuloma
Disseminated coccidioidomycosis

114.4 Chronic pulmonary coccidioidomycosis

114.5 Pulmonary coccidioidomycosis, unspecified

114.9 Coccidioidomycosis, unspecified

⑤ **115 Histoplasmosis**
The following fifth-digit subclassification is for use with category 115:

    0 without mention of manifestation

    1 meningitis

    2 retinitis

    3 pericarditis

    4 endocarditis

    5 pneumonia

    9 other

⑤ **115.0 Infection by Histoplasma capsulatum**
American histoplasmosis
Darling's disease
Reticuloendothelial cytomycosis
Small form histoplasmosis

⑤ **115.1 Infection by Histoplasma duboisii**
African histoplasmosis
Large form histoplasmosis

⑤ **115.9 Histoplasmosis, unspecified**
Histoplasmosis NOS

116 Blastomycotic infection

● Code new
  to this edition
▲ Revision of
  existing code
④ ⑤ Fourth or fifth
    digit required

116.0 Blastomycosis
Blastomycotic dermatitis
Chicago disease
Cutaneous blastomycosis
Disseminated blastomycosis
Gilchrist's disease
Infection by Blastomyces [Ajellomyces] dermatitidis
North American blastomycosis
Primary pulmonary blastomycosis

116.1 Paracoccidioidomycosis
Brazilian blastomycosis
Infection by Paracoccidioides [Blastomyces] brasiliensis
Lutz-Splendore-Almeida disease
Mucocutaneous-lymphangitic paracoccidioidomycosis
Pulmonary paracoccidioidomycosis
South American blastomycosis
Visceral paracoccidioidomycosis

116.2 Lobomycosis
Infections by Loboa [Blastomyces] loboi
Keloidal blastomycosis
Lobo's disease

117 Other mycoses

117.0 Rhinosporidiosis
Infection by Rhinosporidium seeberi

117.1 Sporotrichosis
Cutaneous sporotrichosis
Disseminated sporotrichosis
Infection by Sporothrix [Sporotrichum] schenckii
Lymphocutaneous sporotrichosis
Pulmonary sporotrichosis
Sporotrichosis of the bones

117.2 Chromoblastomycosis
Chromomycosis
Infection by Cladosporidium carrionii, Fonsecaea compactum, Fonsecaea pedrosoi,
    Phialophora verrucosa

117.3 Aspergillosis
Infection by Aspergillus species, mainly A. fumigatus, A. flavus group, A. terreus
    group

117.4 Mycotic mycetomas
Infection by various genera and species of Ascomycetes and Deuteromycetes, such as
    Acremonium [Cephalosporium] falciforme, Neotestudina rosatii, Madurella grisea,
    Madurella mycetomii, Pyrenochaeta romeroi, Zopfia [Leptosphaeria] senegalensis
Madura foot, mycotic
Maduromycosis, mycotic

Excludes: *actinomycotic mycetomas (039.0-039.9)*

117.5 Cryptococcosis

Busse-Buschke's disease	Pulmonary cryptococcosis
European cryptococcosis	Systemic cryptococcosis
Infection by Cryptococcus neoformans	Torula

117.6 Allescheriosis [Petriellidosis]
Infections by Allescheria [Petriellidium] boydii [Monosporium apiospermum]

Excludes: *mycotic mycetoma (117.4)*

117.7 Zygomycosis [Phycomycosis or Mucormycosis]
Infection by species of Absidia, Basidiobolus, Conidiobolus, Cunninghamella,
    Entomophthora, Mucor, Rhizopus, Saksenaea

117.8 Infection by dematiacious fungi, [Phaehyphomycosis]
Infection by dematiacious fungi, such as Cladosporium trichoides [bantianum],
    Dreschlera hawaiiensis, Phialophora gougerotii, Phialophora jeanselmi

117.9 Other and unspecified mycoses

Add 4th or 5th digit	Nonspecific code	Unspecified code	Manifestation code

118 Opportunistic mycoses

Infection of skin, subcutaneous tissues, and/or organs by a wide variety of fungi generally considered to be pathogenic to compromised hosts only (e.g., infection by species of Alternaria, Dreschlera, Fusarium)

HELMINTHIASES (120-129)

120 Schistosomiasis [bilharziasis]

120.0 Schistosoma haematobium
Vesical schistosomiasis NOS

120.1 Schistosoma mansoni
Intestinal schistosomiasis NOS

120.2 Schistosoma japonicum
Asiatic schistosomiasis NOS
Katayama disease or fever

120.3 Cutaneous
Cercarial dermatitis
Infection by cercariae
  of Schistosoma

Schistosome dermatitis
Swimmers' itch

120.8 Other specified schistosomiasis
Infection by Schistosoma:
  bovis
  intercalatum
  mattheii

Infection by Schistosoma spindale
Schistosomiasis chestermani

120.9 Schistosomiasis, unspecified
Blood flukes NOS

Hemic distomiasis

121 Other trematode infections

121.0 Opisthorchiasis
Infection by:
  cat liver fluke
  Opisthorchis (felineus) (tenuicollis) (viverrini)

121.1 Clonorchiasis
Biliary cirrhosis due to clonorchiasis
Chinese liver fluke disease
Hepatic distomiasis due to Clonorchis sinensis
Oriental liver fluke disease

121.2 Paragonimiasis
Infection by Paragonimus
Lung fluke disease (oriental)

Pulmonary distomiasis

121.3 Fascioliasis
Infection by Fasciola:
  gigantica
  hepatica

Liver flukes NOS
Sheep liver fluke infection

121.4 Fasciolopsiasis
Infection by Fasciolopsis [buski]
Intestinal distomiasis

121.5 Metagonimiasis
Infection by Metagonimus yokogawai

121.6 Heterophyiasis
Infection by:
  Heterophyes heterophyes
  Stellantchasmus falcatus

121.8 Other specified trematode infections
Infection by:
  Dicrocoelium dendriticum
  Echinostoma ilocanum
  Gastrodiscoides hominis

121.9 Trematode infection, unspecified
Distomiasis NOS

Fluke disease NOS

122 Echinococcosis

Includes: echinococciasis
  hydatid disease
  hydatidosis

122.0 Echinococcus granulosus infection of liver

122.1 Echinococcus granulosus infection of lung

● Code new
  to this edition

▲ Revision of
  existing code

④ ⑤ Fourth or fifth
  digit required

122.2 Echinococcus granulosus infection of thyroid

122.3 Echinococcus granulosus infection, other

122.4 Echinococcus granulosus infection, unspecified

122.5 Echinococcus multilocularis infection of liver

122.6 Echinococcus multilocularis infection, other

122.7 Echinococcus multilocularis infection, unspecified

122.8 Echinococcosis, unspecified, of liver

122.9 Echinococcosis, other and unspecified

123 Other cestode infection

123.0 Taenia solium infection, intestinal form
Pork tapeworm (adult) (infection)

123.1 Cysticercosis
Cysticerciasis
Infection by Cysticercus cellulosae [larval form of Taenia solium]

123.2 Taenia saginata infection
Beef tapeworm (infection)
Infection by Taeniarhynchus saginatus

123.3 Taeniasis, unspecified

123.4 Diphyllobothriasis, intestinal
Diphyllobothrium (adult) (latum) (pacificum) infection
Fish tapeworm (infection)

123.5 Sparganosis [larval diphyllobothriasis]
Infection by:
  Diphyllobothrium larvae
  Sparganum (mansoni) (proliferum)
  Spirometra larvae

123.6 Hymenolepiasis
Dwarf tapeworm (infection)
Hymenolepis (diminuta) (nana) infection
Rat tapeworm (infection)

123.8 Other specified cestode infection
Diplogonoporus (grandis) infection
Dipylidium (caninum) infection
Dog tapeworm (infection) infection

123.9 Cestode infection, unspecified
Tapeworm (infection) NOS

124 Trichinosis
Trichinella spiralis infection
Trichinellosis
Trichiniasis

125 Filarial infection and dracontiasis

125.0 Bancroftian filariasis
Chyluria due to Wuchereria bancroftii
Elephantiasis due to Wuchereria bancroftii
Infection due to Wuchereria bancroftii
Lymphadenitis due to Wuchereria bancroftii
Lymphangitis due to Wuchereria bancroftii
Wuchereriasis

125.1 Malayan filariasis
Brugia filariasis due to Brugia [Wuchereria] malayi
Chyluria due to Brugia [Wuchereria] malayi
Elephantiasis due to Brugia [Wuchereria] malayi
Infection due to Brugia [Wuchereria] malayi
Lymphadenitis due to Brugia [Wuchereria] malayi
Lymphangitis due to Brugia [Wuchereria] malayi

125.2 Loiasis
Eyeworm disease of Africa
Loa loa infection

125.3 Onchocerciasis
Onchocerca volvulus infection
Onchocercosis

	Add 4th or 5th digit		Nonspecific code		Unspecified code		Manifestation code

125.4 Dipetalonemiasis
Infection by:
Acanthocheilonema perstans
Dipetalonema perstans

125.5 Mansonella ozzardi infection
Filariasis ozzardi

125.6 Other specified filariasis
Dirofilaria infection
Infection by:
Acanthocheilonema streptocerca
Dipetalonema streptocerca

125.7 Dracontiasis
Guinea-worm infection
Infection by Dracunculus medinensis

125.9 Unspecified filariasis

126 Ancylostomiasis and necatoriasis
Includes: cutaneous larva migrans due to Ancylostoma
hookworm (disease) (infection)
uncinariasis

126.0 Ancylostoma duodenale

126.1 Necator americanus

126.2 Ancylostoma braziliense

126.3 Ancylostoma ceylanicum

126.8 Other specified Ancylostoma

126.9 Ancylostomiasis and necatoriasis, unspecified
Creeping eruption NOS
Cutaneous larva migrans NOS

127 Other intestinal helminthiases

127.0 Ascariasis
Ascaridiasis
Infection by Ascaris lumbricoides
Roundworm infection

127.1 Anisakiasis
Infection by Anisakis larva

127.2 Strongyloidiasis
Infection by Strongyloides stercoralis
Excludes: *trichostrongyliasis (127.6)*

127.3 Trichuriasis
Infection by Trichuris trichiuria
Trichocephaliasis
Whipworm (disease) (infection)

127.4 Enterobiasis
Infection by Enterobius vermicularis
Oxyuriasis
Oxyuris vermicularis infection
Pinworn (disease) (infection)
Threadworm infection

127.5 Capillariasis
Infection by Capillaria philippinensis
Excludes: *infection by Capillaria hepatica (128.8)*

127.6 Trichostrongyliasis
Infection by Trichostrongylus species

127.7 Other specified intestinal helminthiasis
Infection by:
Oesophagostomum apiostomum and related species
Ternidens diminutus
other specified intestinal helminth
Physalopteriasis

127.8 Mixed intestinal helminthiasis
Infection by intestinal helminths classified to more than one of the categories
120.0-127.7
Mixed helminthiasis NOS

● Code new
to this edition   ▲ Revision of
existing code   ④ ⑤ Fourth or fifth
digit required

127.9 Intestinal helminthiasis, unspecified

128 Other and unspecified helminthiases

128.0 Toxocariasis
Larva migrans visceralis
Toxocara (canis) (cati) infection
Visceral larva migrans syndrome

128.1 Gnathostomiasis
Infection by Gnathostoma spinigerum and related species

128.8 Other specified helminthiasis
Infection by:
Angiostrongylus cantonensis
Capillaria hepatica
other specified helminth

128.9 Helminth infection, unspecified
Helminthiasis NOS
Worms NOS

129 Intestinal parasitism, unspecified

OTHER INFECTIOUS AND PARASITIC DISEASES (130-136)

130 Toxoplasmosis
Includes: infection by toxoplasma gondii
toxoplasmosis (acquired)

[Excludes:] *congenital toxoplasmosis (771.2)*

130.0 Meningoencephalitis due to toxoplasmosis
Encephalitis due to acquired toxoplasmosis

130.1 Conjunctivitis due to toxoplasmosis

130.2 Chorioretinitis due to toxoplasmosis
Focal retinochoroiditis due to acquired toxoplasmosis

130.3 Myocarditis due to toxoplasmosis

130.4 Pneumonitis due to toxoplasmosis

130.5 Hepatitis due to toxoplasmosis

130.7 Toxoplasmosis of other specified sites

130.8 Multisystemic disseminated toxoplasmosis
Toxoplasmosis of multiple sites

130.9 Toxoplasmosis, unspecified

131 Trichomoniasis
Includes: infection due to Trichomonas (vaginalis)

[5] **131.0 Urogenital trichomoniasis**

131.00 Urogenital trichomoniasis, unspecified
Fluor (vaginalis), trichomonal or due to Trichomonas (vaginalis)
Leukorrhea (vaginalis), trichomonal or due to Trichomonas (vaginalis)

131.01 Trichomonal vulvovaginitis
Vaginitis, trichomonal or due to Trichomonas (vaginalis)

131.02 Trichomonal urethritis

131.03 Trichomonal prostatitis

131.09 Other

131.8 Other specified sites

[Excludes:] *intestinal (007.3)*

131.9 Trichomoniasis, unspecified

132 Pediculosis and phthirus infestation

132.0 Pediculus capitis [head louse]

132.1 Pediculus corporis [body louse]

132.2 Phthirus pubis [pubic louse]
Pediculus pubis

132.3 Mixed infestation
Infestation classifiable to more than one of the categories 132.0-132.2

132.9 Pediculosis, unspecified

Add 4th or 5th digit | Nonspecific code | Unspecified code | Manifestation code

133 **Acariasis**

133.0 **Scabies**

Infestation by Sarcoptes scabiei

Norwegian scabies
Sarcoptic itch

133.8 **Other acariasis**
Chiggers
Infestation by:
Demodex folliculorum
Trombicula

133.9 **Acariasis, unspecified**
Infestation by mites NOS

134 **Other infestation**

134.0 **Myiasis**
Infestation by:
Dermatobia (hominis)
fly larvae
Gasterophilus (intestinalis)

Infestation by:
maggots
Oestrus ovis

134.1 **Other arthropod infestation**
Infestation by:
chigoe
sand flea
Tunga penetrans

Jigger disease
Scarabiasis
Tungiasis

134.2 **Hirudiniasis**
Hirudiniasis (external) (internal)
Leeches (aquatic) (land)

134.8 **Other specified infestations**

134.9 **Infestation, unspecified**
Infestation (skin) NOS

Skin parasites NOS

135 **Sarcoidosis**
Besnier-Boeck- Schaumann disease
Lupoid (miliary) of Boeck
Lupus pernio (Besnier)
Lymphogranulomatosis, benign
(Schaumann's)

Sarcoid (any site):
NOS
Boeck
Darier-Roussy
Uveoparotid fever

136 **Other and unspecified infectious and parasitic diseases**

136.0 **Ainhum**
Dactylolysis spontanea

136.1 **Behçet's syndrome**

136.2 **Specific infections by free-living amebae**
Meningoencephalitis due to Naegleria

136.3 **Pneumocystosis**
Pneumonia due to Pneumocystis carinii

136.4 **Psorospermiasis**

136.5 **Sarcosporidiosis**
Infection by Sarcocystis lindemanni

136.8 **Other specified infectious and parasitic diseases**
Candiru infestation

136.9 **Unspecified infectious and parasitic diseases**
Infectious disease NOS
Parasitic disease NOS

LATE EFFECTS OF INFECTIOUS AND PARASITIC DISEASES (137-139)

137 **Late effects of tuberculosis**

Note: This category is to be used to indicate conditions classifiable to 010-018 as the cause of late effects, which are themselves classified elsewhere. The "late effects" include those specified as such, as sequelae, or as due to old or inactive tuberculosis, without evidence of active disease.

137.0 **Late effects of respiratory or unspecified tuberculosis**

137.1 **Late effects of central nervous system tuberculosis**

137.2 **Late effects of genitourinary tuberculosis**

137.3 **Late effects of tuberculosis of bones and joints**

137.4 **Late effects of tuberculosis of other specified organs**

● Code new
to this edition

▲ Revision of
existing code

④ ⑤ Fourth or fifth
digit required

138 Late effects of acute poliomyelitis

Note: This category is to be used to indicate conditions classifiable to 045 as the cause of late effects, which are themselves classified elsewhere. The "late effects" include conditions specified as such, or as sequelae, or as due to old or inactive poliomyelitis, without evidence of active disease.

139 Late effects of other infectious and parasitic diseases

Note: This category is to be used to indicate conditions classifiable to categories 001-009, 020-041, 046-136 as the cause of late effects, which are themselves classified elsewhere. The "late effects" include conditions specified as such; they also include sequela of diseases classifiable to the above categories if there is evidence that the disease itself is no longer present.

139.0 Late effects of viral encephalitis
　　Late effects of conditions classifiable to 049.8-049.9, 062-064

139.1 Late effects of trachoma
　　Late effects of conditions classifiable to 076

139.8 Late effects of other and unspecified infectious and parasitic diseases

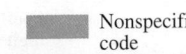 Add 4th or
5th digit　　Nonspecific
code

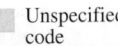 Unspecified
code　　Manifestation
code

2. NEOPLASMS (140-239)

Notes:

1. Content
This chapter contains the following broad groups:

140-195	**Malignant neoplasms, stated or presumed to be primary, of specified sites, except of lymphatic and hematopoietic tissue**
196-198	**Malignant neoplasms, stated or presumed to be secondary, of specified sites**
199	**Malignant neoplasms, without specification of site**
200-208	**Malignant neoplasms, stated or presumed to be primary, of lymphatic and hematopoietic tissue**
210-229	**Benign neoplasms**
230-234	**Carcinoma in situ**
235-238	**Neoplasms of uncertain behavior [see Note, page 92]**
239	**Neoplasms of unspecified nature**

2. Functional activity
All neoplasms are classified in this chapter, whether or not functionally active. An additional code from Chapter 3 may be used, if desired, to identify such functional activity associated with any neoplasm, e.g.:

catecholamine-producing malignant pheochromocytoma of adrenal:
code 194.0, additional code 255.6
basophil adenoma of pituitary with Cushing's syndrome:
code 227.3, additional code 255.0

3. Morphology [Histology]
For those wishing to identify the histological type of neoplasms, a comprehensive coded nomenclature, which comprises the morphology rubrics of the ICD-Oncology, is given on pages 529-542.

4. Malignant neoplasms overlapping site boundaries
Categories 140-195 are for the classification of primary malignant neoplasms according to their point of origin. A malignant neoplasm that overlaps two or more subcategories within a three-digit rubric and whose point of origin cannot be determined should be classified to the subcategory .8 "Other." For example, "carcinoma involving tip and ventral surface of tongue" should be assigned to 141.8. On the other hand, "carcinoma of tip of tongue, extending to involve the ventral surface" should be coded to 141.2, as the point of origin, the tip, is known. Three subcategories (149.8, 159.8, 165.8) have been provided for malignant neoplasms that overlap the boundaries of three-digit rubrics within certain systems. Overlapping malignant neoplasms that cannot be classified as indicated above should be assigned to the appropriate subdivision of category 195 (Malignant neoplasm of other and ill-defined sites).

MALIGNANT NEOPLASM OF LIP, ORAL CAVITY, AND PHARYNX (140-149)

> Excludes: carcinoma in situ (230.0)

140 **Malignant neoplasm of lip**

> Excludes: skin of lip (173.0)

140.0 Upper lip, vermilion border
Upper lip:
NOS
external
lipstick area

140.1 Lower lip, vermilion border
Lower lip:
NOS
external
lipstick area

140.3 Upper lip, inner aspect
Upper lip: Upper lip:
buccal aspect mucosa
frenulum oral aspect

140.4 Lower lip, inner aspect
Lower lip: Lower lip:
buccal aspect mucosa
frenulum oral aspect

	Add 4th or 5th digit		Nonspecific code		Unspecified code		Manifestation code

140.5 Lip, unspecified, inner aspect
Lip, not specified whether upper or lower:
buccal aspect
frenulum
mucosa
oral aspect

140.6 Commissure of lip
Labial commissure

140.8 Other sites of lip
Malignant neoplasm of contiguous or overlapping sites of lip whose point of origin
cannot be determined

140.9 Lip, unspecified, vermilion border
Lip, not specified as upper or lower:
NOS
external
lipstick area

141 Malignant neoplasm of tongue

141.0 Base of tongue
Dorsal surface of base of tongue
Fixed part of tongue NOS

141.1 Dorsal surface of tongue
Anterior two-thirds of tongue, dorsal surface
Dorsal tongue NOS
Midline of tongue

Excludes: *dorsal surface of base of tongue (141.0)*

141.2 Tip and lateral border of tongue

141.3 Ventral surface of tongue
Anterior two-thirds of tongue, ventral surface
Frenulum linguae

141.4 Anterior two-thirds of tongue, part unspecified
Mobile part of tongue NOS

141.5 Junctional zone
Border of tongue at junction of fixed and mobile parts at insertion of anterior tonsillar
pillar

141.6 Lingual tonsil

141.8 Other sites of tongue
Malignant neoplasm of contiguous or overlapping sites of tongue whose point of origin
cannot be determined

141.9 Tongue, unspecified
Tongue NOS

142 Malignant neoplasm of major salivary glands
Includes: salivary ducts

Excludes: *malignant neoplasm of minor salivary glands:*
NOS (145.9)
buccal mucosa (145.0)
soft palate (145.3)
tongue (141.0-141.9)
tonsil, palatine (146.0)

142.0 Parotid gland

142.1 Submandibular gland
Submaxillary gland

142.2 Sublingual gland

142.8 Other major salivary glands
Malignant neoplasm of contiguous or overlapping sites of salivary glands and ducts
whose point of origin cannot be determined

142.9 Salivary gland, unspecified
Salivary gland (major) NOS

● Code new
to this edition
▲ Revision of
existing code
④ ⑤ Fourth or fifth
digit required

143 **Malignant neoplasm of gum**
Includes: alveolar (ridge) mucosa
gingiva (alveolar) (marginal)
interdental papillae

Excludes: *malignant odontogenic neoplasms (170.0-170.1)*

143.0 **Upper gum**

143.1 **Lower gum**

143.8 **Other sites of gum**
Malignant neoplasm of contiguous or overlapping sites of gum whose point of origin cannot be determined

143.9 **Gum, unspecified**

144 **Malignant neoplasm of floor of mouth**

144.0 **Anterior portion**
Anterior to the premolar-canine junction

144.1 **Lateral portion**

144.8 **Other sites of floor of mouth**
Malignant neoplasm of contiguous or overlapping sites of floor of mouth whose point of origin cannot be determined

144.9 **Floor of mouth, part unspecified**

145 **Malignant neoplasm of other and unspecified parts of mouth**

Excludes: *mucosa of lips (140.0-140.9)*

145.0 **Cheek mucosa**
Buccal mucosa   Cheek, inner aspect

145.1 **Vestibule of mouth**
Buccal sulcus (upper) (lower)
Labial sulcus (upper) (lower)

145.2 **Hard palate**

145.3 **Soft palate**

Excludes: *nasopharyngeal [posterior] [superior] surface of soft palate (147.3)*

145.4 **Uvula**

145.5 **Palate, unspecified**
Junction of hard and soft palate
Roof of mouth

145.6 **Retromolar area**

145.8 **Other specified parts of mouth**
Malignant neoplasm of contiguous or overlapping sites of mouth whose point of origin cannot be determined

145.9 **Mouth, unspecified**
Buccal cavity NOS
Minor salivary gland, unspecified site
Oral cavity NOS

146 **Malignant neoplasm of oropharynx**

146.0 **Tonsil**
Tonsil:
NOS
faucial
palatine

Excludes: *lingual tonsil (141.6)*
pharyngeal tonsil (147.1)

146.1 **Tonsillar fossa**

146.2 **Tonsillar pillars (anterior) (posterior)**
Faucial pillar
Glossopalatine fold
Palatoglossal arch
Palatopharyngeal arch

146.3 **Vallecula**
Anterior and medial surface of the pharyngoepiglottic fold

| | Add 4th or 5th digit | | Nonspecific code | | Unspecified code | | Manifestation code |

146.4 Anterior aspect of epiglottis
Epiglottis, free border [margin] Glossoepiglottic fold(s)

Excludes: epiglottis:
  NOS (161.1)
  suprahyoid portion (161.1)

146.5 Junctional region
Junction of the free margin of the epiglottis, the aryepiglottic fold, and the
pharyngoepiglottic fold

146.6 Lateral wall of oropharynx

146.7 Posterior wall of oropharynx

146.8 Other specified sites of oropharynx
Branchial cleft
Malignant neoplasm of contiguous or overlapping sites of oropharynx whose point of
origin cannot be determined

146.9 Oropharynx, unspecified

147 Malignant neoplasm of nasopharynx

147.0 Superior wall
Roof of nasopharynx

147.1 Posterior wall
Adenoid
Pharyngeal tonsil

147.2 Lateral wall
Fossa of Rosenmüller
Opening of auditory tube
Pharyngeal recess

147.3 Anterior wall
Floor of nasopharynx
Nasopharyngeal [posterior] [superior] surface of soft palate
Posterior margin of nasal septum and choanae

147.8 Other specified sites of nasopharynx
Malignant neoplasm of contiguous or overlapping sites of nasopharynx whose point of
origin cannot be determined

147.9 Nasopharynx, unspecified
Nasopharyngeal wall NOS

148 Malignant neoplasm of hypopharynx

148.0 Postcricoid region

148.1 Pyriform sinus
Pyriform fossa

148.2 Aryepiglottic fold, hypopharyngeal aspect
Aryepiglottic fold or interarytenoid fold:
  NOS
  marginal zone

Excludes: aryepiglottic fold or interarytenoid fold, laryngeal aspect (161.1)

148.3 Posterior hypopharyngeal wall

148.8 Other specified sites of hypopharynx
Malignant neoplasm of contiguous or overlapping sites of hypopharynx whose point of
origin cannot be determined

148.9 Hypopharynx, unspecified
Hypopharyngeal wall NOS
Hypopharynx NOS

149 Malignant neoplasm of other and ill-defined sites within the lip, oral cavity, and pharynx

149.0 Pharynx, unspecified

149.1 Waldeyer's ring

149.8 Other
Malignant neoplasms of lip, oral cavity, and pharynx whose point of origin cannot be
assigned to any one of the categories 140-148

Excludes: "book leaf" neoplasm [ventral surface of tongue and floor of mouth] (145.8)

149.9 Ill-defined

● Code new
to this edition
▲ Revision of
existing code
④ ⑤ Fourth or fifth
digit required

MALIGNANT NEOPLASM OF DIGESTIVE ORGANS AND PERITONEUM (150-159)

> *Excludes:* *carcinoma in situ (230.1-230.9)*

150 **Malignant neoplasm of esophagus**

150.0 **Cervical esophagus**

150.1 **Thoracic esophagus**

150.2 **Abdominal esophagus**

> *Excludes:* *adenocarcinoma (151.0)*
> *cardio-esophageal junction (151.0)*

150.3 **Upper third of esophagus**
Proximal third of esophagus

150.4 **Middle third of esophagus**

150.5 **Lower third of esophagus**
Distal third of esophagus

> *Excludes:* *adenocarcinoma (151.0)*
> *cardio-esophageal junction (151.0)*

150.8 **Other specified part**
Malignant neoplasm of contiguous or overlapping sites of esophagus whose point of origin cannot be determined

150.9 **Esophagus, unspecified**

151 **Malignant neoplasm of stomach**

151.0 **Cardia**
Cardiac orifice
Cardio-esophageal junction

> *Excludes:* *squamous cell carcinoma (150.2, 150.5)*

151.1 **Pylorus**
Prepylorus
Pyloric canal

151.2 **Pyloric antrum**
Antrum of stomach NOS

151.3 **Fundus of stomach**

151.4 **Body of stomach**

151.5 **Lesser curvature, unspecified**
Lesser curvature, not classifiable to 151.1-151.4

151.6 **Greater curvature, unspecified**
Greater curvature, not classifiable to 151.0-151.4

151.8 **Other specified sites of stomach**
Anterior wall, not classifiable to 151.0-151.4
Posterior wall, not classifiable to 151.0-151.4
Malignant neoplasm of contiguous or overlapping sites of stomach whose point of origin cannot be determined

151.9 **Stomach, unspecified**
Carcinoma ventriculi
Gastric cancer

152 **Malignant neoplasm of small intestine, including duodenum**

152.0 **Duodenum**

152.1 **Jejunum**

152.2 **Ileum**

> *Excludes:* *ileocecal valve (153.4)*

152.3 **Meckel's diverticulum**

152.8 **Other specified sites of small intestine**
Duodenojejunal junction
Malignant neoplasm of contiguous or overlapping sites of small intestine whose point of origin cannot be determined

152.9 **Small intestine, unspecified**

153 **Malignant neoplasm of colon**

153.0 **Hepatic flexure**

153.1 **Transverse colon**

■ Add 4th or 5th digit   ■ Nonspecific code   ▨ Unspecified code   ■ Manifestation code

153.2 Descending colon
Left colon

153.3 Sigmoid colon
Sigmoid (flexure)

[Excludes:] *rectosigmoid junction (154.0)*

153.4 Cecum
Ileocecal valve

153.5 Appendix

153.6 Ascending colon
Right colon

153.7 Splenic flexure

153.8 Other specified sites of large intestine
Malignant neoplasm of contiguous or overlapping sites of colon whose point of origin cannot be determined

[Excludes:] *ileocecal valve (153.4)*
rectosigmoid junction (154.0)

153.9 Colon, unspecified
Large intestine NOS

154 Malignant neoplasm of rectum, rectosigmoid junction, and anus

154.0 Rectosigmoid junction
Colon with rectum
Rectosigmoid (colon)

154.1 Rectum
Rectal ampulla

154.2 Anal canal
Anal sphincter

[Excludes:] *skin of anus (172.5, 173.5)*

154.3 Anus, unspecified

[Excludes:] *anus:*
margin (172.5, 173.5)
skin (172.5, 173.5)
perianal skin (172.5, 173.5)

154.8 Other
Anorectum
Cloacogenic zone
Malignant neoplasm of contiguous or overlapping sites of rectum, rectosigmoid junction, and anus whose point of origin cannot be determined

155 Malignant neoplasm of liver and intrahepatic bile ducts

155.0 Liver, primary
Carcinoma:
liver, specified as primary
hepatocellular
liver cell
Hepatoblastoma

155.1 Intrahepatic bile ducts
Canaliculi biliferi
Interlobular:
bile ducts
biliary canals
Intrahepatic:
biliary passages
canaliculi
gall duct

[Excludes:] *hepatic duct (156.1)*

155.2 Liver, not specified as primary or secondary

156 Malignant neoplasm of gallbladder and extrahepatic bile ducts

156.0 Gallbladder

156.1 Extrahepatic bile ducts
Biliary duct or passage NOS
Common bile duct
Cystic duct
Hepatic duct
Sphincter of Oddi

156.2 Ampulla of Vater

156.8 Other specified sites of gallbladder and extrahepatic bile ducts
Malignant neoplasm of contiguous or overlapping sites of gallbladder and extrahepatic bile ducts whose point of origin cannot be determined

156.9 Biliary tract, part unspecified
Malignant neoplasm involving both intrahepatic and extrahepatic bile ducts

157 Malignant neoplasm of pancreas

157.0 Head of pancreas

157.1 Body of pancreas

157.2 Tail of pancreas

157.3 Pancreatic duct
Duct of:
  Santorini
  Wirsung

157.4 Islets of Langerhans
Islets of Langerhans, any part of pancreas
Use additional code, if desired, to identify any functional activity

157.8 Other specified sites of pancreas
Ectopic pancreatic tissue
Malignant neoplasm of contiguous or overlapping sites of pancreas whose point of origin cannot be determined

157.9 Pancreas, part unspecified

158 Malignant neoplasm of retroperitoneum and peritoneum

158.0 Retroperitoneum
Periadrenal tissue	Perirenal tissue
Perinephric tissue	Retrocecal tissue

158.8 Specified parts of peritoneum
Cul-de-sac (of Douglas)	Peritoneum:
Mesentery	parietal
Mesocolon	pelvic
Omentum	Rectouterine pouch

Malignant neoplasm of contiguous or overlapping sites of retroperitoneum and peritoneum whose point of origin cannot be determined

158.9 Peritoneum, unspecified

159 Malignant neoplasm of other and ill-defined sites within the digestive organs and peritoneum

159.0 Intestinal tract, part unspecified
Intestine NOS

159.1 Spleen, not elsewhere classified
Angiosarcoma of spleen
Fibrosarcoma of spleen

Excludes: Hodgkin's disease (201.0-201.9)
  lymphosarcoma (200.1)
  reticulosarcoma (200.0)

159.8 Other sites of digestive system and intra-abdominal organs
Malignant neoplasm of digestive organs and peritoneum whose point of origin cannot be assigned to any one of the categories 150-158

Excludes: anus and rectum (154.8)
  cardio-esophageal junction (151.0)
  colon and rectum ORANGE (154.0)

159.9 Ill-defined
Alimentary canal or tract NOS
Gastrointestinal tract NOS

Excludes: abdominal NOS (195.2)
  intra-abdominal NOS (195.2)

	Add 4th or 5th digit		Nonspecific code		Unspecified code		Manifestation code

MALIGNANT NEOPLASM OF RESPIRATORY AND INTRATHORACIC ORGANS (160-165)

[Excludes:] *carcinoma in situ (231.0-231.9)*

160 Malignant neoplasm of nasal cavities, middle ear, and accessory sinuses

160.0 Nasal cavities

Cartilage of nose
Conchae, nasal
Internal nose
Septum of nose
Vestibule of nose

[Excludes:] *nasal bone (170.0)*
nose NOS (195.0)
olfactory bulb (192.0)
posterior margin of septum and choanae (147.3)
skin of nose (172.3, 173.3)
turbinates (170.0)

160.1 Auditory tube, middle ear, and mastoid air cells

Antrum tympanicum
Eustachian tube
Tympanic cavity

[Excludes:] *auditory canal (external) (172.2, 173.2)*
bone of ear (meatus) (170.0)
cartilage of ear (171.0)
ear (external) (skin) (172.2, 173.2)

160.2 Maxillary sinus

Antrum (Highmore) (maxillary)

160.3 Ethmoidal sinus

160.4 Frontal sinus

160.5 Sphenoidal sinus

160.8 Other

Malignant neoplasm of contiguous or overlapping sites of nasal cavities, middle ear, and accessory sinuses whose point of origin cannot be determined

160.9 Accessory sinus, unspecified

161 Malignant neoplasm of larynx

161.0 Glottis

Intrinsic larynx
Laryngeal commissure (anterior) (posterior)
True vocal cord
Vocal cord NOS

161.1 Supraglottis

Aryepiglottic fold or interarytenoid fold, laryngeal aspect
Epiglottis (suprahyoid portion) NOS
Extrinsic larynx
False vocal cords
Posterior (laryngeal) surface of epiglottis
Ventricular bands

[Excludes:] *anterior aspect of epiglottis (146.4)*
aryepiglottic fold or interarytenoid fold:
NOS (148.2)
hypopharyngeal aspect (148.2)
marginal zone (148.2)

161.2 Subglottis

161.3 Laryngeal cartilages

Cartilage:
arytenoid
cricoid

Cartilage:
cuneiform
thyroid

161.8 Other specified sites of larynx

Malignant neoplasm of contiguous or overlapping sites of larynx whose point of origin cannot be determined

161.9 Larynx, unspecified

162 Malignant neoplasm of trachea, bronchus, and lung

162.0 Trachea

Cartilage of trachea
Mucosa of trachea

● Code new to this edition ▲ Revision of existing code ④ ⑤ Fourth or fifth digit required

162.2 Main bronchus
  Carina
  Hilus of lung

162.3 Upper lobe, bronchus or lung

162.4 Middle lobe, bronchus or lung

162.5 Lower lobe, bronchus or lung

162.8 Other parts of bronchus or lung
  Malignant neoplasm of contiguous or overlapping sites of bronchus or lung whose point
    of origin cannot be determined

162.9 Bronchus and lung, unspecified

163 Malignant neoplasm of pleura

163.0 Parietal pleura

163.1 Visceral pleura

163.8 Other specified sites of pleura
  Malignant neoplasm of contiguous or overlapping sites of pleura whose point of origin
    cannot be determined

163.9 Pleura, unspecified

164 Malignant neoplasm of thymus, heart, and mediastinum

164.0 Thymus

164.1 Heart
  Endocardium   Myocardium
  Epicardium   Pericardium

  Excludes: *great vessels (171.4)*

164.2 Anterior mediastinum

164.3 Posterior mediastinum

164.8 Other
  Malignant neoplasm of contiguous or overlapping sites of thymus, heart, and
    mediastinum whose point of origin cannot be determined

164.9 Mediastinum, part unspecified

165 Malignant neoplasm of other and ill-defined sites within the respiratory system and intrathoracic organs

165.0 Upper respiratory trace, part unspecified

165.8 Other
  Malignant neoplasm of respiratory and intrathoracic organs whose point of origin
    cannot be assigned to any one of the categories 160-164

165.9 Ill-defined sites within the respiratory system
  Respiratory tract NOS

  Excludes: *intrathoracic NOS (195.1)*
      thoracic NOS (195.1)

MALIGNANT NEOPLASM OF BONE, CONNECTIVE TISSUE, SKIN, AND BREAST (170-176)

  Excludes: *carcinoma in situ:*
      breast (233.0)
      skin (232.0-232.9)

170 Malignant neoplasm of bone and articular cartilage
  Includes: cartilage (articular) (joint)
       periosteum

  Excludes: *bone marrow NOS (202.9)*
      cartilage:
      ear (171.0)
      eyelid (171.0)
      larynx (161.3)
      nose (160.0)
      synovia (171.0-171.9)

| | Add 4th or 5th digit | | Nonspecific code | | Unspecified code | | Manifestation code |

170.0 Bones of skull and face, except mandible

Bone:
  ethmoid
  frontal
  malar
  nasal
  occipital
  orbital
  parietal

Bone:
  sphenoid
  temporal
  zygomatic
Maxilla (superior)
Turbinate
Upper jaw bone
Vomer

Excludes: *carcinoma, any type except intraosseous or odontogenic:*
  maxilla, maxillary (sinus) (160.2)
  upper jaw bone (143.0)
  jaw bone (lower) (170.1)

170.1 Mandible

Inferior maxilla
Jaw bone NOS

Lower jaw bone

Excludes: *carcinoma, any type except intraosseous or odontogenic:*
  jaw bone NOS (143.9)
  lower (143.1)
  upper jaw bone (170.0)

170.2 Vertebral column, excluding sacrum and coccyx

Spinal column
Spine

Vertebra

Excludes: *sacrum and coccyx (170.6)*

170.3 Ribs, sternum, and clavicle

Costal cartilage
Costovertebral joint

Xiphoid process

170.4 Scapula and long bones of upper limb

Acromion
Bones NOS of upper limb
Humerus

Radius
Ulna

170.5 Short bones of upper limb

Carpal
Cuneiform, wrist
Metacarpal
Navicular, of hand
Phalanges of hand
Pisiform

Scaphoid (of hand)
Semilunar or lunate
Trapezium
Trapezoid
Unciform

170.6 Pelvic bones, sacrum, and coccyx

Coccygeal vertebra
Ilium
Ischium

Pubic bone
Sacral vertebra

170.7 Long bones of lower limb

Bones NOS of lower limb
Femur

Fibula
Tibia

170.8 Short bones of lower limb

Astragalus [talus]
Calcaneus
Cuboid
Cuneiform, ankle
Metatarsal

Navicular (of ankle)
Patella
Phalanges of foot
Tarsal

170.9 Bone and articular cartilage, site unspecified

● Code new
  to this edition

▲ Revision of
  existing code

④ ⑤ Fourth or fifth
    digit required

171 **Malignant neoplasm of connective and other soft tissue**
Includes: blood vessel
bursa
fascia
fat
ligament, except uterine
muscle
peripheral, sympathetic, and parasympathetic nerves and ganglia
synovia
tendon (sheath)

Excludes: *cartilage (of):*
articular (170.0-170.9)
larynx (161.3)
nose (160.0)
connective tissue:
breast (174.0-175.9)
internal organs—code to malignant neoplasm of the site [e.g., leiomyosarcoma
of stomach, 151.9]
heart (164.1)
uterine ligament (183.4)

171.0   Head, face, and neck
Cartilage of:
ear
eyelid

171.2   Upper limb, including shoulder
Arm   Forearm
Finger   Hand

171.3   Lower limb, including hip
Foot   Thigh
Leg   Toe
Popliteal space

171.4   Thorax
Axilla   Great vessels
Diaphragm

Excludes: *heart (164.1)*
mediastinum (164.2-164.9)
thymus (164.0)

171.5   Abdomen
Abdominal wall   Hypochondrium

Excludes: *peritoneum (158.8)*
retroperitoneum (158.0)

171.6   Pelvis
Buttock   Inguinal region
Groin   Perineum

Excludes: *pelvic peritoneum (158.8)*
retroperitoneum (158.0)
uterine ligament, any (183.3-183.5)

171.7   Trunk, unspecified
Back NOS
Flank NOS

171.8   Other specified sites of connective and other soft tissue
Malignant neoplasm of contiguous or overlapping sites of connective tissue whose point
of origin cannot be determined

171.9   Connective and other soft tissue, site unspecified

172 **Malignant melanoma of skin**
Includes: melanocarcinoma
melanoma (skin) NOS

Excludes: *skin of genital organs (184.0-184.9, 187.1-187.9)*
sites other than skin—code to malignant neoplasm of the site

172.0   Lip
Excludes: *vermilion border of lip (140.0-140.1, 140.9)*

172.1   Eyelid, including canthus

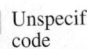

Add 4th or   Nonspecific   Unspecified   Manifestation
5th digit   code   code   code

172.2 Ear and external auditory canal
  Auricle (ear)
  Auricular canal, external
  External [acoustic] meatus
  Pinna

172.3 Other and unspecified parts of face
  Cheek (external)   Forehead
  Chin   Nose, external
  Eyebrow   Temple

172.4 Scalp and neck

172.5 Trunk, except scrotum
  Axilla   Perianal skin
  Breast   Perineum
  Buttock   Umbilicus
  Groin

Excludes:	*anal canal (154.2)*
	anus NOS (154.3)
	scrotum (187.7)

172.6 Upper limb, including shoulder
  Arm   Forearm
  Finger   Hand

172.7 Lower limb, including hip
  Ankle   Leg
  Foot   Popliteal area
  Heel   Thigh
  Knee   Toe

172.8 Other specified sites of skin
  Malignant melanoma of contiguous or overlapping sites of skin whose point of origin
    cannot be determined

172.9 Melanoma of skin, site unspecified

173 Other malignant neoplasm of skin
  Includes: malignant neoplasm of:
       sebaceous glands
       sudoriferous, sudoriparous glands
       sweat glands

  Excludes: *Kaposi's sarcoma (176.0-176.9)*
       malignant melanoma of skin (172.0-172.9)
       skin of genital organs (184.0-184.9, 187.1-187.9)

173.0 Skin of lip

  Excludes: *vermilion border of lip (140.0-140.1, 140.9)*

173.1 Eyelid, including canthus

  Excludes: *cartilage of eyelid (171.0)*

173.2 Skin of ear and external auditory canal
  Auricle (ear)   External meatus
  Auricular canal, external Pinna

  Excludes: *cartilage of ear (171.0)*

173.3 Skin of other and unspecified parts of face
  Cheek, external   Forehead
  Chin   Nose, external
  Eyebrow   Temple

173.4 Scalp and skin of neck

● Code new   ▲ Revision of   ④ ⑤ Fourth or fifth
   to this edition   existing code   digit required

173.5 Skin of trunk, except scrotum

Axillary fold
Perianal skin
Skin of:
  abdominal wall
  anus
  back
  breast

Skin of:
  buttock
  chest wall
  groin
  perineum
Umbilicus

> Excludes: *anal canal (154.2)*
> *anus NOS (154.3)*
> *skin of scrotum (187.7)*

173.6 Skin of upper limb, including shoulder

Arm
Finger

Forearm
Hand

173.7 Skin of lower limb, including hip

Ankle
Foot
Heel
Knee

Leg
Popliteal area
Thigh
Toe

173.8 Other specified sites of skin
Malignant neoplasm of contiguous or overlapping sites of skin whose point of origin cannot be determined

173.9 Skin, site unspecified

174 Malignant neoplasm of female breast
Includes:

breast (female)
connective tissue
soft parts

Paget's disease of:
  breast
  nipple

> Excludes: *skin of breast (172.5, 173.5)*

174.0 Nipple and areola

174.1 Central portion

174.2 Upper-inner quadrant

174.3 Lower-inner quadrant

174.4 Upper-outer quadrant

174.5 Lower-outer quadrant

174.6 Axillary tail

174.8 Other specified sites of female breast

Ectopic sites
Inner breast
Lower breast
Malignant neoplasm of
  contiguous or overlapping
  sites of breast whose point
  of origin cannot be
  determined

Midline of breast
Outer breast
Upper breast

174.9 Breast (female), unspecified

175 Malignant neoplasm of male breast

> Excludes: *skin of breast (172.5, 173.5)*

175.0 Nipple and areola

175.9 Other and unspecified sites of male breast
Ectopic breast tissue, male

176 Kaposi's sarcoma

176.0 Skin

176.1 Soft Tissue
Includes:

blood vessel
connective tissue
fascia

ligament
lymphatic(s) NEC
muscle

> Excludes: *lymph glands and nodes (176.5)*

176.2 Palate

176.3 Gastrointestinal sites

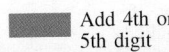

| | Add 4th or 5th digit | | Nonspecific code | | Unspecified code | | Manifestation code |

176.4 **Lung**

176.5 **Lymph nodes**

176.8 **Other specified sites**
Includes: oral cavity NEC

176.9 **Unspecified**
Viscera NOS

MALIGNANT NEOPLASM OF GENITOURINARY ORGANS (179-189)

Excludes: carcinoma in situ (233.1-233.9)

179 **Malignant neoplasm of uterus, part unspecified**

180 **Malignant neoplasm of cervix uteri**
Includes: invasive malignancy [carcinoma]

Excludes: carcinoma in situ (233.1)

180.0 **Endocervix**
Cervical canal NOS   Endocervical gland
Endocervical canal

180.1 **Exocervix**

180.8 **Other specified sites of cervix**
Cervical stump
Squamocolumnar junction of cervix
Malignant neoplasm of contiguous or overlapping sites of cervix uteri whose point of
origin cannot be determined

180.9 **Cervix uteri, unspecified**

181 **Malignant neoplasm of placenta**
Choriocarcinoma NOS   Chorioepithelioma NOS

Excludes: chorioadenoma (destruens) (236.1)
hydatidiform mole (630)
malignant (236.1)
invasive mole (236.1)
male choriocarcinoma NOS (186.0-186.9)

182 **Malignant neoplasm of body of uterus**
Excludes: carcinoma in situ (233.2)

182.0 **Corpus uteri, except isthmus**
Cornu   Fundus
Endometrium   Myometrium

182.1 **Isthmus**
Lower uterine segment

182.8 **Other specified sites of body of uterus**
Malignant neoplasm of contiguous or overlapping sites of body of uterus whose point
of origin cannot be determined
Excludes: uterus NOS (179)

183 **Malignant neoplasm of ovary and other uterine adnexa**
Excludes: Douglas' cul-de-sac (158.8)

183.0 **Ovary**
Use additional code, if desired, to identify any functional activity

183.2 **Fallopian tube**
Oviduct
Uterine tube

183.3 **Broad ligament**
Mesovarium
Parovarian region

183.4 **Parametrium**
Uterine ligament NOS
Uterosacral ligament

183.5 **Round ligament**

183.8 **Other specified sites of uterine adnexa**
Tubo-ovarian
Utero-ovarian
Malignant neoplasm of contiguous or overlapping sites of ovary and other uterine
adnexa whose point of origin cannot be determined

183.9 **Uterine adnexa, unspecified**

● Code new
to this edition
▲ Revision of
existing code
④ ⑤ Fourth or fifth
digit required

184 **Malignant neoplasm of other and unspecified female genital organs**

> Excludes: *carcinoma in situ (233.3)*

184.0 **Vagina**
Gartner's duct   Vaginal vault

184.1 **Labia majora**
Greater vestibular [Bartholin's] gland

184.2 **Labia minora**

184.3 **Clitoris**

184.4 **Vulva, unspecified**
External female genitalia NOS
Pudendum

184.8 **Other specified sites of female genital organs**
Malignant neoplasm of contiguous or overlapping sites of female genital organs whose point of origin cannot be determined

184.9 **Female genital organ, site unspecified**
Female genitourinary tract NOS

185 **Malignant neoplasm of prostate**

> Excludes: *seminal vesicles (187.8)*

186 **Malignant neoplasm of testis**
Use additional code, if desired, to identify any functional activity

186.0 **Undescended testis**
Ectopic testis   Retained testis

186.9 **Other and unspecified testis**
Testis:
  NOS
  descended
  scrotal

187 **Malignant neoplasm of penis and other male genital organs**

187.1 **Prepuce**
Foreskin

187.2 **Glans penis**

187.3 **Body of penis**
Corpus cavernosum

187.4 **Penis, part unspecified**
Skin of penis NOS

187.5 **Epididymis**

187.6 **Spermatic cord**
Vas deferens

187.7 **Scrotum**
Skin of scrotum

187.8 **Other specified sites of male genital organs**
Seminal vesicle
Tunica vaginalis
Malignant neoplasm of contiguous or overlapping sites of penis and other male genital organs whose point of origin cannot be determined

187.9 **Male genital organ, site unspecified**
Male genital organ or tract NOS

188 **Malignant neoplasm of bladder**

> Excludes: *carcinoma in situ (233.7)*

188.0 **Trigone of urinary bladder**

188.1 **Dome of urinary bladder**

188.2 **Lateral wall of urinary bladder**

188.3 **Anterior wall of urinary bladder**

188.4 **Posterior wall of urinary bladder**

188.5 **Bladder neck**
Internal urethral orifice

188.6 **Ureteric orifice**

188.7 **Urachus**

159

Add 4th or 5th digit   Nonspecific code   Unspecified code   Manifestation code

188.8 Other specified sites of bladder
Malignant neoplasm of contiguous or overlapping sites of bladder whose point of origin cannot be determined

188.9 Bladder, part unspecified
Bladder wall NOS

189 Malignant neoplasm of kidney and other and unspecified urinary organs

189.0 Kidney, except pelvis
Kidney NOS   Kidney parenchyma

189.1 Renal pelvis
Renal calyces   Ureteropelvic junction

189.2 Ureter
Excludes: *ureteric orifice of bladder (188.6)*

189.3 Urethra
Excludes: *urethral orifice of bladder (188.5)*

189.4 Paraurethral glands

189.8 Other specified sites of urinary organs
Malignant neoplasm of contiguous or overlapping sites of kidney and other urinary organs whose point of origin cannot be determined

189.9 Urinary organ, site unspecified
Urinary system NOS

MALIGNANT NEOPLASM OF OTHER AND UNSPECIFIED SITES (190-199)

Excludes: *carcinoma in situ (234.0-234.9)*

190 Malignant neoplasm of eye
Excludes: *carcinoma in situ (234.0)*
eyelid (skin) (172.1, 173.1)
cartilage (171.0)
optic nerve (192.0)
orbital bone (170.0)

190.0 Eyeball, except conjunctiva, cornea, retina, and choroid
Ciliary body   Sclera
Crystalline lens   Uveal tract
Iris

190.1 Orbit
Connective tissue of orbit
Extraocular muscle
Retrobulbar
Excludes: *bone of orbit (170.0)*

190.2 Lacrimal gland

190.3 Conjunctiva

190.4 Cornea

190.5 Retina

190.6 Choroid

190.7 Lacrimal duct
Lacrimal sac   Nasolacrimal duct

190.8 Other specified sites of eye
Malignant neoplasm of contiguous or overlapping sites of eye whose point of origin cannot be determined

190.9 Eye, part unspecified

191 Malignant neoplasm of brain
Excludes: *cranial nerves (192.0)*
retrobulbar area (190.1)

191.0 Cerebrum, except lobes and ventricles
Basal ganglia   Globus pallidus
Cerebral cortex   Hypothalamus
Corpus striatum   Thalamus

191.1 Frontal lobe

● Code new
to this edition
▲ Revision of
existing code
④ ⑤ Fourth or fifth
digit required

191.2 Temporal lobe
    Hippocampus   Uncus

191.3 Parietal lobe

191.4 Occipital lobe

191.5 Ventricles
    Choroid plexus   Floor of ventricle

191.6 Cerebellum NOS
    Cerebellopontine angle

191.7 Brain stem
    Cerebral peduncle   Midbrain
    Medulla oblongata   Pons

191.8 Other parts of brain
    Corpus callosum
    Tapetum
    Malignant neoplasm of contiguous or overlapping sites of brain whose point of origin
        cannot be determined

191.9 Brain, unspecified
    Cranial fossa NOS

192 Malignant neoplasm of other and unspecified parts of nervous system
    Excludes: *peripheral, sympathetic, and parasympathetic nerves and ganglia (171.0-171.9)*

192.0 Cranial nerves
    Olfactory bulb

192.1 Cerebral meninges
    Dura (mater)   Meninges NOS
    Falx (cerebelli) (cerebri)   Tentorium

192.2 Spinal cord
    Cauda equina

192.3 Spinal meninges

192.8 Other specified sites of nervous system
    Malignant neoplasm of contiguous or overlapping sites of other parts of nervous system
        whose point of origin cannot be determined

192.9 Nervous system, part unspecified
    Nervous system (central) NOS
    Excludes: *meninges NOS (192.1)*

193 Malignant neoplasm of thyroid gland
    Sipple's syndrome   Thyroglossal duct
Use additional code, if desired, to identify any functional activity

194 Malignant neoplasm of other endocrine glands and related structures
Use additional code, if desired, to identify any functional activity
    Excludes: *islets of Langerhans (157.4)*
             ovary (183.0)
             testis (186.0-186.9)
             thymus (164.0)

194.0 Adrenal gland
    Adrenal cortex   Suprarenal gland
    Adrenal medulla

194.1 Parathyroid gland

194.3 Pituitary gland and craniopharyngeal duct
    Craniobuccal pouch   Rathke's pouch
    Hypophysis   Sella turcica

194.4 Pineal gland

194.5 Carotid body

194.6 Aortic body and other paraganglia
    Coccygeal body   Para-aortic body
    Glomus jugulare

194.8 Other
    Pluriglandular involvement NOS
Note: If the sites of multiple involvements are known, they should be coded separately.

194.9 Endocrine gland, site unspecified

    Add 4th or   Nonspecific   Unspecified   Manifestation
    5th digit   code   code   code

195 Malignant neoplasm of other and ill-defined sites
Includes: malignant neoplasms of contiguous sites, not elsewhere classified, whose point of origin cannot be determined

Excludes: *malignant neoplasm:*
lymphatic and hematopoietic tissue (200.0-208.9)
secondary sites (196.0-198.8)
unspecified site (199.0-199.1)

195.0 Head, face, and neck
Cheek NOS
Jaw NOS
Nose NOS
Supraclavicular region NOS

195.1 Thorax
Axilla
Chest (wall) NOS
Intrathoracic NOS

195.2 Abdomen
Intra-abdominal NOS

195.3 Pelvis
Groin
Inguinal region NOS
Presacral region
Sacrococcygeal region
Sites overlapping systems within pelvis, as:
rectovaginal (septum)
rectovesical (septum)

195.4 Upper limb

195.5 Lower limb

195.8 Other specified sites
Back NOS
Flank NOS
Trunk NOS

196 Secondary and unspecified malignant neoplasm of lymph nodes

Excludes: *any malignant neoplasm of lymph nodes, specified as primary (200.0-202.9)*
Hodgkin's disease (201.0-201.9)
lymphosarcoma (200.1)
reticulosarcoma (200.0)
other forms of lymphoma (202.0-202.9)

196.0 Lymph nodes of head, face, and neck
Cervical
Cervicofacial
Scalene
Supraclavicular

196.1 Intrathoracic lymph nodes
Bronchopulmonary
Intercostal
Mediastinal
Tracheobronchial

196.2 Intra-abdominal lymph nodes
Intestinal
Mesenteric
Retroperitoneal

196.3 Lymph nodes of axilla and upper limb
Brachial
Epitrochlear
Infraclavicular
Pectoral

196.5 Lymph nodes of inguinal region and lower limb
Femoral
Groin
Popliteal
Tibial

196.6 Intrapelvic lymph nodes
Hypogastric
Iliac
Obturator
Parametrial

196.8 Lymph nodes of multiple sites

196.9 Site unspecified
Lymph nodes NOS

197 Secondary malignant neoplasm of respiratory and digestive systems

Excludes: *lymph node metastasis (196.0-196.9)*

197.0 Lung
Bronchus

197.1 Mediastinum

197.2 Pleura

● Code new
to this edition
▲ Revision of
existing code
④ ⑤ Fourth or fifth
digit required

197.3 Other respiratory organs
Trachea

197.4 Small intestine, including duodenum

197.5 Large intestine and rectum

197.6 Retroperitoneum and peritoneum

197.7 Liver, specified as secondary

197.8 Other digestive organs and spleen

198 Secondary malignant neoplasm of other specified sites
[Excludes:] *lymph node metastasis (196.0-196.9)*

198.0 Kidney

198.1 Other urinary organs

198.2 Skin
Skin of breast

198.3 Brain and spinal cord

198.4 Other parts of nervous system
Meninges (cerebral) (spinal)

198.5 Bone and bone marrow

198.6 Ovary

198.7 Adrenal gland
Suprarenal gland

[5] **198.8 Other specified sites**

198.81 Breast
[Excludes:] *skin of breast (198.2)*

198.82 Genital organs

198.89 Other
[Excludes:] *retroperitoneal lymph nodes (196.2)*

199 Malignant neoplasm without specification of site

199.0 Disseminated
Carcinomatosis unspecified site (primary) (secondary)
Generalized:
cancer unspecified site (primary) (secondary)
malignancy unspecified site (primary) (secondary)
Multiple cancer unspecified site (primary) (secondary)

199.1 Other
Cancer unspecified site (primary) (secondary)
Carcinoma unspecified site (primary) (secondary)
Malignancy unspecified site (primary) (secondary)

MALIGNANT NEOPLASM OF LYMPHATIC AND HEMATOPOIETIC TISSUE (200-208)

[Excludes:] *secondary neoplasm of:*
bone marrow (198.5)
spleen (197.8)
secondary and unspecified neoplasm of lymph nodes (196.0-196.9)

The following fifth-digit subclassification is for use with categories 200-202:

0 unspecified site, extranodal and solid organ sites
1 lymph nodes of head, face, and neck
2 intrathoracic lymph nodes
3 intra-abdominal lymph nodes
4 lymph nodes of axilla and upper limb
5 lymph nodes of inguinal region and lower limb
6 intrapelvic lymph nodes
7 spleen
8 lymph nodes of multiple sites

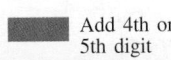

Add 4th or 5th digit | Nonspecific code | Unspecified code | Manifestation code

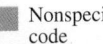

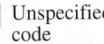

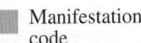

[5] **200 Lymphosarcoma and reticulosarcoma**

[5] **200.0 Reticulosarcoma**

Lymphoma (malignant):
- histiocytic (diffuse):
  - nodular
  - pleomorphic cell type
- reticulum cell type

Reticulum cell sarcoma:
- NOS
- pleomorphic cell type

[5] **200.1 Lymphosarcoma**

Lymphoblastoma (diffuse)

Lymphoma (malignant):
- lymphoblastic (diffuse)
- lymphocytic (cell type) (diffuse)
- lymphosarcoma type

Lymphosarcoma:
- NOS
- diffuse NOS
- lymphoblastic (diffuse)
- lymphocytic (diffuse)
- prolymphocytic

[Excludes:] *lymphosarcoma:*
- *follicular or nodular (202.0)*
- *mixed cell type (200.8)*

lymphosarcoma cell leukemia (207.8)

[5] **200.2 Burkitt's tumor or lymphoma**

Malignant lymphoma, Burkitt's type

[5] **200.8 Other named variants**

Lymphoma (malignant):
- lymphoplasmacytoid type
- mixed lymphocytic-histiocytic (diffuse)

Lymphosarcoma, mixed cell type (diffuse)

Reticulolymphosarcoma (diffuse)

[5] **201 Hodgkin's disease**

[5] **201.0 Hodgkin's paragranuloma**

[5] **201.1 Hodgkin's granuloma**

[5] **201.2 Hodgkin's sarcoma**

[5] **201.4 Lymphocytic-histiocytic predominance**

[5] **201.5 Nodular sclerosis**

Hodgkin's disease, nodular sclerosis:
- NOS
- cellular phase

[5] **201.6 Mixed cellularity**

[5] **201.7 Lymphocytic depletion**

Hodgkin's disease, lymphocytic depletion:
- NOS
- diffuse fibrosis
- reticular type

[5] **201.9 Hodgkin's disease, unspecified**

Hodgkin's:
- disease NOS
- lymphoma NOS

Malignant:
- lymphogranuloma
- lymphogranulomatosis

[5] **202 Other malignant neoplasms of lymphoid and histiocytic tissue**

[5] **202.0 Nodular lymphoma**

Brill-Symmers disease

Lymphoma:
- follicular (giant)
- lymphocytic, nodular

Lymphosarcoma:
- follicular (giant)
- nodular

Reticulosarcoma, follicular or nodular

[5] **202.1 Mycosis fungoides**

[5] **202.2 Sézary's disease**

[5] **202.3 Malignant histiocytosis**

Histiocytic medullary reticulosis

Malignant:
- reticuloendotheliosis
- reticulosis

[5] **202.4 Leukemic reticuloendotheliosis**

Hairy-cell leukemia

[5] **202.5 Letterer-Siwe disease**
Acute:
differentiated progressive histiocytosis
histiocytosis X (progressive)
infantile reticuloendotheliosis
reticulosis of infancy

[Excludes:] *Hand-Schüller-Christian disease (277.8)*
histiocytosis (acute) (chronic) (277.8)
histiocytosis X (chronic) (277.8)

[5] **202.6 Malignant mast cell tumors**
Malignant:
mastocytoma
mastocytosis
Mast cell sarcoma
Systemic tissue mast cell disease

[Excludes:] *mast cell leukemia (207.8)*

[5] **202.8 Other lymphomas**
Lymphoma (malignant):
NOS
diffuse

[Excludes:] *benign lymphoma (229.0)*

[5] **202.9 Other and unspecified malignant neoplasms of lymphoid and histiocytic tissue**
Malignant neoplasm of bone marrow NOS

[5] **203 Multiple myeloma and immunoproliferative neoplasms**
The following fifth-digit subclassification is for use with category 203

0 without mention of remission

1 in remission

[5] **203.0 Multiple myeloma**
Kahler's disease
Myelomatosis

[Excludes:] *solitary myeloma (238.6)*

[5] **203.1 Plasma cell leukemia**
Plasmacytic leukemia

[5] **203.8 Other immunoproliferative neoplasms**

[5] **204 Lymphoid leukemia**
Includes:
leukemia:
lymphatic
lymphoblastic
leukemia:
lymphocytic
lymphogenous

The following fifth-digit subclassification is for use with category 204

0 without mention of remission

1 in remission

[5] **204.0 Acute**

[Excludes:] *acute exacerbation of chronic lymphoid leukemia (204.1)*

[5] **204.1 Chronic**

[5] **204.2 Subacute**

[5] **204.8 Other lymphoid leukemia**
Aleukemic leukemia:
lymphatic
lymphocytic
lymphoid

[5] **204.9 Unspecified lymphoid leukemia**

[5] **205 Myeloid leukemia**
Includes:
leukemia:
granulocytic
myeloblastic
myelocytic
Tmyelogenous
leukemia:
myelomonocytic
myelosclerotic
myelosis

The following fifth-digit subclassification is for use with category 205

0 without mention of remission

1 in remission

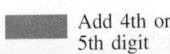

Add 4th or 5th digit | Nonspecific code | Unspecified code | Manifestation code

⑤ **205.0 Acute**
  Acute promyelocytic leukemia
  Excludes: *acute exacerbation of chronic myeloid leukemia (205.1)*

⑤ **205.1 Chronic**
  Eosinophilic leukemia   Neutrophilic leukemia

⑤ **205.2 Subacute**

⑤ **205.3 Myeloid sarcoma**
  Chloroma
  Granulocytic sarcoma

⑤ **205.8 Other myeloid leukemia**
  Aleukemic leukemia:
    granulocytic
    myelogenous
    myeloid
  Aleukemic myelosis

⑤ **205.9 Unspecified myeloid leukemia**

⑤ **206 Monocytic leukemia**
  Includes: leukemia:
        histiocytic
        monoblastic
        monocytoid

  The following fifth-digit subclassification is for use with category 206

    0 without mention of remission

    1 in remission

⑤ **206.0 Acute**
  Excludes: *acute exacerbation of chronic monocytic leukemia (206.1)*

⑤ **206.1 Chronic**

⑤ **206.2 Subacute**

⑤ **206.8 Other monocytic leukemia**
  Aleukemic:
    monocytic leukemia
    monocytoid leukemia

⑤ **206.9 Unspecified monocytic leukemia**

⑤ **207 Other specified leukemia**
  Excludes: *leukemic reticuloendotheliosis (202.4)*
        plasma cell leukemia (203.1)

  The following fifth-digit subclassification is for use with category 207

    0 without mention of remission

    1 in remission

⑤ **207.0 Acute erythremia and erythroleukemia**
  Acute erythremic myelosis   Erythremic myelosis
  Di Guglielmo's disease

⑤ **207.1 Chronic erythremia**
  Heilmeyer-Schöner disease

⑤ **207.2 Megakaryocytic leukemia**
  Megakaryocytic myelosis   Thrombocytic leukemia

⑤ **207.8 Other specified leukemia**
  Lymphosarcoma cell leukemia

⑤ **208 Leukemia of unspecified cell type**
  The following fifth-digit subclassification is for use with category 208

    0 without mention of remission

    1 in remission

⑤ **208.0 Acute**
  Acute leukemia NOS   Stem cell leukemia
  Blast cell leukemia
  Excludes: *acute exacerbation of chronic unspecified leukemia (208.1)*

⑤ **208.1 Chronic**
  Chronic leukemia NOS

● Code new   ▲ Revision of   ④ ⑤ Fourth or fifth
        to this edition   existing code   digit required

[5] **208.2 Subacute**
Subacute leukemia NOS

[5] **208.8 Other leukemia of unspecified cell type**

[5] **208.9 Unspecified leukemia**
Leukemia NOS

BENIGN NEOPLASMS (210-229)

210 Benign neoplasm of lip, oral cavity, and pharynx

[Excludes:] *cyst (of):*
jaw (526.0-526.2, 526.89)
oral soft tissue (528.4)
radicular (522.8)

210.0 Lip
Frenulum labii
Lip (inner aspect) (mucosa) (vermilion border)

[Excludes:] *labial commissure (210.4)*
skin of lip (216.0)

210.1 Tongue
Lingual tonsil

210.2 Major salivary glands
Gland:
parotid
sublingual
submandibular

[Excludes:] *benign neoplasms of minor salivary glands:*
NOS (210.4)
buccal mucosa (210.4)
lips (210.0)
palate (hard) (soft) (210.4)
tongue (210.1)
tonsil, palatine (210.5)

210.3 Floor of mouth

210.4 Other and unspecified parts of mouth
Gingiva
Gum (upper) (lower)
Labial commissure
Oral cavity NOS
Oral mucosa
Palate (hard) (soft)
Uvula

[Excludes:] *benign odontogenic neoplasms of bone (213.0-213.1)*
developmental odontogenic cysts (526.0)
mucosa of lips (210.0)
nasopharyngeal [posterior] [superior] surface of soft palate (210.7)

210.5 Tonsil
Tonsil (faucial) (palatine)

[Excludes:] *lingual tonsil (210.1)*
pharyngeal tonsil (210.7)
tonsillar:
fossa (210.6)
pillars (210.6)

210.6 Other parts of oropharynx
Branchial cleft or vestiges
Epiglottis, anterior aspect
Fauces NOS
Mesopharynx NOS
Tonsillar:
fossa
pillars
Vallecula

[Excludes:] *epiglottis:*
NOS (212.1)
suprahyoid portion (212.1)

210.7 Nasopharynx
Adenoid tissue
Lymphadenoid tissue
Pharyngeal tonsil
Posterior nasal septum

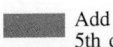

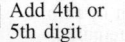

210.8 Hypopharynx
Arytenoid fold
Laryngopharynx

Postcricoid region
Pyriform fossa

210.9 Pharynx, unspecified
Throat NOS

211 **Benign neoplasm of other parts of digestive system**

211.0 Esophagus

211.1 Stomach
Body (stomach)
Cardia (stomach)
Fundus (stomach)

Cardiac orifice
Pylorus

211.2 Duodenum, jejunum, and ileum
Small intestine NOS

Excludes: *ampulla of Vater (211.5)*
ileocecal valve (211.3)

211.3 Colon
Appendix
Cecum

Ileocecal valve
Large intestine NOS

Excludes: *rectosigmoid junction (211.4)*

211.4 Rectum and anal canal
Anal canal or sphincter
Anus NOS

Rectosigmoid junction

Excludes: *anus:*
margin (216.5)
skin (216.5)
perianal skin (216.5)

211.5 Liver and biliary passages
Ampulla of Vater
Common bile duct
Cystic duct

Gallbladder
Hepatic duct
Sphincter of Oddi

211.6 Pancreas, except islets of Langerhans

211.7 Islets of Langerhans
Islet cell tumor

Use additional code, if desired, to identify any functional activity

211.8 Retroperitoneum and peritoneum
Mesentery
Mesocolon

Omentum
Retroperitoneal tissue

211.9 **Other and unspecified site**
Alimentary tract NOS
Digestive system NOS
Gastrointestinal tract NOS

Intestinal tract NOS
Intestine NOS
Spleen, not elsewhere classified

212 **Benign neoplasm of respiratory and intrathoracic organs**

212.0 Nasal cavities, middle ear, and accessory sinuses
Cartilage of nose
Eustachian tube
Nares
Septum of nose

Sinus:
ethmoidal
frontal
maxillary
sphenoidal

Excludes: *auditory canal (external) (216.2)*
bone of:
ear (213.0)
nose [turbinates] (213.0)
cartilage of ear (215.0)
ear (external) (skin) (216.2)
nose NOS (229.8)
skin (216.3)
olfactory bulb (225.1)
polyp of:
accessory sinus (471.8)
ear (385.30-385.35)
nasal cavity (471.0)
posterior margin of septum and choanae (210.7)

● Code new
to this edition

▲ Revision of
existing code

④ ⑤ Fourth or fifth
digit required

212.1 Larynx
Cartilage:
    arytenoid
    cricoid
    cuneiform
    thyroid

Epiglottis (suprahyoid portion) NOS
Glottis
Vocal cords (false) (true)

Excludes: epiglottis, anterior aspect (210.6)
         polyp of vocal cord or larynx (478.4)

212.2 Trachea

212.3 Bronchus and lung
Carina
Hilus of lung

212.4 Pleura

212.5 Mediastinum

212.6 Thymus

212.7 Heart
Excludes: great vessels (215.4)

212.8 Other specified sites

212.9 Site unspecified
Respiratory organ NOS
Upper respiratory tract NOS
Excludes: intrathoracic NOS (229.8)
        thoracic NOS (229.8)

213 Benign neoplasm of bone and articular cartilage
Includes: cartilage (articular) (joint)
         periosteum

Excludes: cartilage of:
      ear (215.0)
      eyelid (215.0)
      larynx (212.1)
      nose (212.0)
      exostosis NOS (726.91)
      synovia (215.0-215.9)

213.0 Bones of skull and face
Excludes: lower jaw bone (213.1)

213.1 Lower jaw bone

213.2 Vertebral column, excluding sacrum and coccyx

213.3 Ribs, sternum, and clavicle

213.4 Scapula and long bones of upper limb

213.5 Short bones of upper limb

213.6 Pelvic bones, sacrum, and coccyx

213.7 Long bones of lower limb

213.8 Short bones of lower limb

213.9 Bone and articular cartilage, site unspecified

214 Lipoma
Includes: angiolipoma
         fibrolipoma
         hibernoma
         lipoma (fetal) (infiltrating) (intramuscular)
         myelolipoma
         myxolipoma

214.0 Skin and subcutaneous tissue of face

214.1 Other skin and subcutaneous tissue

214.2 Intrathoracic organs

214.3 Intra-abdominal organs

214.4 Spermatic cord

214.8 Other specified sites

214.9 Lipoma, unspecified site

Add 4th or   Nonspecific   Unspecified   Manifestation
5th digit   code   code   code

215 **Other benign neoplasm of connective and other soft tissue**
Includes:

blood vessel	peripheral, sympathetic, and parasympathetic nerves
bursa	and ganglia
fascia	synovia
ligament	tendon (sheath)
muscle	

Excludes: *cartilage:*
articular (213.0-213.9)
larynx (212.1)
nose (212.0)
connective tissue of:
breast (217)
internal organ, except lipoma and hemangioma — code to benign neoplasm of the site
lipoma (214.0-214.9)

215.0 Head, face, and neck

215.2 Upper limb, including shoulder

215.3 Lower limb, including hip

215.4 Thorax

Excludes: *heart (212.7)*
mediastinum (212.5)
thymus (212.6)

215.5 Abdomen
Abdominal wall
Hypochondrium

215.6 Pelvis

Buttock	Inguinal region
Groin	Perineum

Excludes: *uterine:*
leiomyoma (218.0-218.9)
ligament, any (221.0)

215.7 Trunk, unspecified
Back NOS
Flank NOS

215.8 Other specified sites

215.9 Site unspecified

216 **Benign neoplasm of skin**
Includes:

blue nevus	pigmented nevus
dermatofibroma	syringoadenoma
hydrocystoma	syringoma

Excludes: *skin of genital organs (221.0-222.9)*

216.0 Skin of lip

Excludes: *vermilion border of lip (210.0)*

216.1 Eyelid, including canthus

Excludes: *cartilage of eyelid (215.0)*

216.2 Ear and external auditory canal

Auricle (ear)	External meatus
Auricular canal, external	Pinna

Excludes: *cartilage of ear (215.0)*

216.3 Skin of other and unspecified parts of face

Cheek, external	Nose, external
Eyebrow	Temple

216.4 Scalp and skin of neck

▲ Revision of
existing code   ④ ⑤ Fourth or fifth
digit required

216.5 Skin of trunk, except scrotum

Axillary fold	Skin of:
Perianal skin	buttock
Skin of:	chest wall
abdominal wall	groin
anus	perineum
back	Umbilicus
breast	

> Excludes: anal canal (211.4)
> anus NOS (211.4)
> skin of scrotum (222.4)

216.6 Skin of upper limb, including shoulder

216.7 Skin of lower limb, including hip

216.8 Other specified sites of skin

216.9 Skin, site unspecified

217 Benign neoplasm of breast
Breast (male) (female)
connective tissue
glandular tissue
soft parts

> Excludes: adenofibrosis (610.2)
> benign cyst of breast (610.0)
> fibrocystic disease (610.1)
> skin of breast (216.5)

218 Uterine leiomyoma
Includes: fibroid (bleeding) (uterine)
uterine:
fibromyoma
myoma

218.0 Submucous leiomyoma of uterus

218.1 Intramural leiomyoma of uterus
Interstitial leiomyoma of uterus

218.2 Subserous leiomyoma of uterus
Subperitoneal leiomyoma of uterus

218.9 Leiomyoma of uterus, unspecified

219 Other benign neoplasm of uterus

219.0 Cervix uteri

219.1 Corpus uteri
Endometrium   Myometrium
Fundus

219.8 Other specified parts of uterus

219.9 Uterus, part unspecified

220 Benign neoplasm of ovary
Use additional code, if desired, to identify any functional activity (256.0-256.1)

> Excludes: cyst:
> corpus albicans (620.2)
> corpus luteum (620.1)
> endometrial (617.1)
> follicular (atretic) (620.0)
> graafian follicle (620.0)
> ovarian NOS (620.2)
> retention (620.2)

221 Benign neoplasm of other female genital organs
Includes: adenomatous polyp
benign teratoma

> Excludes: cyst:
> epoophoron (752.11)
> fimbrial (752.11)
> Gartner's duct (752.11)
> parovarian (752.11)

	Add 4th or 5th digit		Nonspecific code		Unspecified code		Manifestation code

221.0 Fallopian tube and uterine ligaments

Oviduct
Parametrium
Uterine ligament (broad) (round) (uterosacral)
Uterine tube

221.1 Vagina

221.2 Vulva

Clitoris
External female genitalia NOS
Greater vestibular [Bartholin's] gland
Labia (majora) (minora)
Pudendum

[Excludes:] *Bartholin's (duct) (gland) cyst (616.2)*

221.8 Other specified sites of female genital organs

221.9 Female genital organ, site unspecified

Female genitourinary tract NOS

222 Benign neoplasm of male genital organs

222.0 Testis

Use additional code, if desired, to identify any functional activity

222.1 Penis

Corpus cavernosum
Glans penis
Prepuce

222.2 Prostate

[Excludes:] *adenomatous hyperplasia of prostate (600.2)*
prostatic:
adenoma (600.2)
enlargement (600.0)
hypertrophy (600.0)

222.3 Epididymis

222.4 Scrotum

Skin of scrotum

222.8 Other specified sites of male genital organs

Seminal vesicle
Spermatic cord

222.9 Male genital organ, site unspecified

Male genitourinary tract NOS

223 Benign neoplasm of kidney and other urinary organs

223.0 Kidney, except pelvis

Kidney NOS

[Excludes:] *renal:*
calyces (223.1)
pelvis (223.1)

223.1 Renal pelvis

223.2 Ureter

[Excludes:] *ureteric orifice of bladder (223.3)*

223.3 Bladder

[5] **223.8 Other specified sites of urinary organs**

223.81 Urethra

[Excludes:] *urethral orifice of bladder (223.3)*

223.89 Other

Paraurethral glands

223.9 Urinary organ, site unspecified

Urinary system NOS

224 Benign neoplasm of eye

[Excludes:] *cartilage of eyelid (215.0)*
eyelid (skin) (216.1)
optic nerve (225.1)
orbital bone (213.0)

224.0 Eyeball, except conjunctiva, cornea, retina, and choroid

Ciliary body
Iris
Sclera
Uveal tract

224.1 Orbit
> Excludes: bone of orbit (213.0)

224.2 Lacrimal gland

224.3 Conjunctiva

224.4 Cornea

224.5 Retina
> Excludes: hemangioma of retina (228.03)

224.6 Choroid

224.7 Lacrimal duct
Lacrimal sac   Nasolacrimal duct

224.8 Other specified parts of eye

224.9 Eye, part unspecified

225 Benign neoplasm of brain and other parts of nervous system
> Excludes: hemangioma (228.02)
> neurofibromatosis (237.7)
> peripheral, sympathetic, and parasympathetic nerves and ganglia (215.0-215.9)
> retrobulbar (224.1)

225.0 Brain

225.1 Cranial nerves

225.2 Cerebral meninges
Meninges NOS   Meningioma (cerebral)

225.3 Spinal cord
Cauda equina

225.4 Spinal meninges
Spinal meningioma

225.8 Other specified sites of nervous system

225.9 Nervous system, part unspecified
Nervous system (central) NOS
> Excludes: meninges NOS (225.2)

226 Benign neoplasm of thyroid glands
Use additional code, if desired, to identify any functional activity

227 Benign neoplasm of other endocrine glands and related structures
Use additional code, if desired, to identify any functional activity
> Excludes: ovary (220)
> pancreas (211.6)
> testis (222.0)

227.0 Adrenal gland
Suprarenal gland

227.1 Parathyroid gland

227.3 Pituitary gland and craniopharyngeal duct (pouch)
Craniobuccal pouch   Rathke's pouch
Hypophysis   Sella turcica

227.4 Pineal gland
Pineal body

227.5 Carotid body

227.6 Aortic body and other paraganglia
Coccygeal body   Para-aortic body
Glomus jugulare

227.8 Other

227.9 Endocrine gland, site unspecified

| | Add 4th or 5th digit | | Nonspecific code | | Unspecified code | | Manifestation code |

228 Hemangioma and lymphangioma, any site

Includes: angioma (benign) (cavernous) (congenital) NOS
cavernous nevus
glomus tumor
hemangioma (benign) (congenital)

Excludes: *benign neoplasm of spleen, except hemangioma and lymphangioma (211.9)*
glomus jugulare (227.6)
nevus:
NOS (216.0-216.9)
blue or pigmented (216.0-216.9)
vascular (757.32)

⑤ **228.0 Hemangioma, any site**

228.00 Of unspecified site

228.01 Of skin and subcutaneous tissue

228.02 Of intracranial structures

228.03 Of retina

228.04 Of intra-abdominal structures
Peritoneum   Retroperitoneal tissue

228.09 Of other sites
Systemic angiomatosis

228.1 Lymphangioma, any site
Congenital lymphangioma   Lymphatic nevus

229 Benign neoplasm of other and unspecified sites

229.0 Lymph nodes

Excludes: *lymphangioma (228.1)*

229.8 Other specified sites
Intrathoracic NOS   Thoracic NOS

229.9 Site unspecified

CARCINOMA IN SITU (230-234)

Includes: Bowen's disease
erythroplasia
Queyrat's erythroplasia

Excludes: *leukoplakia—see Alphabetic Index*

230 Carcinoma in situ of digestive organs

230.0 Lip, oral cavity, and pharynx
Gingiva   Oropharynx
Hypopharynx   Salivary gland or duct
Mouth [any part]   Tongue
Nasopharynx

Excludes: *aryepiglottic fold or interarytenoid fold, laryngeal aspect (231.0)*
epiglottis:
NOS (231.0)
suprahyoid portion (231.0)
skin of lip (232.0)

230.1 Esophagus

230.2 Stomach
Body of stomach   Cardiac orifice
Cardia of stomach   Pylorus
Fundus of stomach

230.3 Colon
Appendix   Ileocecal valve
Cecum   Large intestine NOS

Excludes: *rectosigmoid junction (230.4)*

230.4 Rectum
Rectosigmoid junction

230.5 Anal canal
Anal sphincter

● Code new
to this edition

▲ Revision of
existing code

④ ⑤ Fourth or fifth
digit required

230.6 Anus, unspecified

Excludes: anus:
    margin (232.5)
    skin (232.5)
    perianal skin (232.5)

230.7 Other and unspecified parts of intestine

| Duodenum | Jejunum |
| Ileum | Small intestine NOS |

Excludes: ampulla of Vater (230.8)

230.8 Liver and biliary system

Ampulla of Vater	Gallbladder
Common bile duct	Hepatic duct
Cystic duct	Sphincter of Oddi

230.9 Other and unspecified digestive organs

| Digestive organ NOS | Pancreas |
| Gastrointestinal tract NOS | Spleen |

231 Carcinoma in situ of respiratory system

231.0 Larynx

Cartilage:	Epiglottis:
arytenoid	NOS
cricoid	posterior surface
cuneiform	suprahyoid portion
thyroid	Vocal cords (false) (true)

Excludes: aryepiglottic fold or interarytenoid fold:
    NOS (230.0)
    hypopharyngeal aspect (230.0)
    marginal zone (230.0)

231.1 Trachea

231.2 Bronchus and lung

| Carina | Hilus of lung |

231.8 Other specified parts of respiratory system

| Accessory sinuses | Nasal cavities |
| Middle ear | Pleura |

Excludes: ear (external) (skin) (232.2)
    nose NOS (234.8)
    skin (232.3)

231.9 Respiratory system, part unspecified

Respiratory organ NOS

232 Carcinoma in situ of skin

Includes: pigment cells

232.0 Skin of lip

Excludes: vermilion border of lip (230.0)

232.1 Eyelid, including canthus

232.2 Ear and external auditory canal

232.3 Skin of other and unspecified parts of face

232.4 Scalp and skin of neck

232.5 Skin of trunk, except scrotum

Anus, margin	Skin of:
Axillary fold	breast
Perianal skin	buttock
Skin of:	chest wall
abdominal wall	groin
anus	perineum
back	Umbilicus

Excludes: anal canal (230.5)
    anus NOS (230.6)
    skin of genital organs (233.3, 233.5-233.6)

232.6 Skin of upper limb, including shoulder

232.7 Skin of lower limb, including hip

232.8 Other specified sites of skin

| Add 4th or 5th digit | Nonspecific code | Unspecified code | Manifestation code |

232.9 Skin, site unspecified

233 Carcinoma in situ of breast and genitourinary system

233.0 Breast

Excludes: *Paget's disease (174.0-174.9)*
skin of breast (232.5)

233.1 Cervix uteri

233.2 Other and unspecified parts of uterus

233.3 Other and unspecified female genital organs

233.4 Prostate

233.5 Penis

233.6 Other and unspecified male genital organs

233.7 Bladder

233.9 Other and unspecified urinary organs

234 Carcinoma in situ of other and unspecified sites

234.0 Eye

Excludes: *cartilage of eyelid (234.8)*
eyelid (skin) (232.1)
optic nerve (234.8)
orbital bone (234.8)

234.8 Other specified sites
Endocrine gland [any]

234.9 Site unspecified
Carcinoma in situ NOS

NEOPLASMS OF UNCERTAIN BEHAVIOR (235-238)

Note: Categories 235-238 classify by site certain histo-morphologically well-defined neoplasms, the subsequent behavior of which cannot be predicted from the present appearance.

235 Neoplasm of uncertain behavior of digestive and respiratory systems

235.0 Major salivary glands
Gland:
parotid
sublingual
submandibular

Excludes: *minor salivary glands (235.1)*

235.1 Lip, oral cavity, and pharynx

Gingiva	Nasopharynx
Hypopharynx	Oropharynx
Minor salivary glands	Tongue
Mouth	

Excludes: *aryepiglottic fold or interarytenoid fold, laryngeal aspect (235.6)*
epiglottis:
NOS (235.6)
suprahyoid portion (235.6)
skin of lip (238.2)

235.2 Stomach, intestines, and rectum

235.3 Liver and biliary passages

Ampulla of Vater	Gallbladder
Bile ducts [any]	Liver

235.4 Retroperitoneum and peritoneum

235.5 Other and unspecified digestive organs

Anal:	Esophagus
canal	Pancreas
sphincter	Spleen
Anus NOS	

Excludes: *anus:*
margin (238.2)
skin (238.2)
perianal skin (238.2)

● Code new
to this edition

▲ Revision of
existing code

④ ⑤ Fourth or fifth
digit required

235.6 Larynx

[Excludes:] *aryepiglottic fold or interarytenoid fold:*
NOS (235.1)
hypopharyngeal aspect (235.1)
marginal zone (235.1)

235.7 Trachea, bronchus, and lung

235.8 Pleura, thymus, and mediastinum

235.9 Other and unspecified respiratory organs
Accessory sinuses
Middle ear
Nasal cavities
Respiratory organ NOS

[Excludes:] *ear (external) (skin) (238.2)*
nose (238.8)
skin (238.2)

236 Neoplasm of uncertain behavior of genitourinary organs

236.0 Uterus

236.1 Placenta
Chorioadenoma (destruens)
Invasive mole
Malignant hydatid(iform) mole

236.2 Ovary
Use additional code, if desired, to identify any functional activity

236.3 Other and unspecified female genital organs

236.4 Testis
Use additional code, if desired, to identify any functional activity

236.5 Prostate

236.6 Other and unspecified male genital organs

236.7 Bladder

[5] **236.9 Other and unspecified urinary organs**

236.90 Urinary organ, unspecified

236.91 Kidney and ureter

236.99 Other

237 Neoplasm of uncertain behavior of endocrine glands and nervous system

237.0 Pituitary gland and craniopharyngeal duct
Use additional code, if desired, to identify any functional activity

237.1 Pineal gland

237.2 Adrenal gland
Suprarenal gland
Use additional code, if desired, to identify any functional activity

237.3 Paraganglia
Aortic body
Carotid body
Coccygeal body
Glomus jugulare

237.4 Other and unspecified endocrine glands
Parathyroid gland
Thyroid gland

237.5 Brain and spinal cord

237.6 Meninges
Meninges:
NOS
cerebral
spinal

[5] **237.7 Neurofibromatosis**
von Recklinghausen's disease

237.70 Neurofibromatosis, unspecified

237.71 Neurofibromatosis, Type I [von Recklinghausen's disease]

237.72 Neurofibromatosis, Type II [acoustic neurofibromatosis]

237.9 Other and unspecified parts of nervous system
Cranial nerves

[Excludes:] *peripheral, sympathetic, and parasympathetic nerves and ganglia (238.1)*

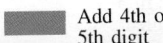

238 **Neoplasm of uncertain behavior of other and unspecified sites and tissues**

238.0 Bone and articular cartilage

Excludes: *cartilage:*
> *ear (238.1)*
> *eyelid (238.1)*
> *larynx (235.6)*
> *nose (235.9)*
> *synovia (238.1)*

238.1 **Connective and other soft tissue**
> Peripheral, sympathetic, and parasympathetic nerves and ganglia

Excludes: *cartilage (of):*
> *articular (238.0)*
> *larynx (235.6)*
> *nose (235.9)*
> *connective tissue of breast (238.3)*

238.2 Skin

Excludes: *anus NOS (235.5)*
> *skin of genital organs (236.3, 236.6)*
> *vermilion border of lip (235.1)*

238.3 Breast

Excludes: *skin of breast (238.2)*

238.4 Polycythemia vera

238.5 Histiocytic and mast cells
> Mast cell tumor NOS
> Mastocytoma NOS

238.6 Plasma cells
> Plasmacytoma NOS
> Solitary myeloma

238.7 **Other lymphatic and hematopoietic tissues**
> Disease:
>> lymphoproliferative (chronic) NOS
>> myeloproliferative (chronic) NOS
> Idiopathic thrombocythemia
> Megakaryocytic myelosclerosis
> Myelodysplastic syndrome
> Myelosclerosis with myeloid metaplasia
> Panmyelosis (acute)

Excludes: *myelofibrosis (289.8)*
> *myelosclerosis NOS (289.8)*
> *myelosis:*
>> *NOS (205.9)*
>> *megakaryocytic (207.2)*

238.8 **Other specified sites**
> Eye
> Heart

Excludes: *eyelid (skin) (238.2)*
> *cartilage (238.1)*

238.9 Site unspecified

NEOPLASMS OF UNSPECIFIED NATURE (239)

239 **Neoplasms of unspecified nature**

Note: Category 239 classifies by site neoplasms of unspecified morphology and behavior. The term "mass," unless otherwise stated, is not to be regarded as a neoplastic growth.
> Includes: "growth" NOS
>> neoplasm NOS
>> new growth NOS
>> tumor NOS

239.0 **Digestive system**

Excludes: *anus:*
> *margin (239.2)*
> *skin (239.2)*
> *perianal skin (239.2)*

239.1 Respiratory system

● Code new
to this edition

▲ Revision of
existing code

④ ⑤ Fourth or fifth
digit required

239.2 Bone, soft tissue, and skin

> *Excludes:* anal canal (239.0)
> anus NOS (239.0)
> bone marrow (202.9)
> cartilage:
>   larynx (239.1)
>   nose (239.1)
> connective tissue of breast (239.3)
> skin of genital organs (239.5)
> vermilion border of lip (239.0)

239.3 Breast

> *Excludes:* skin of breast (239.2)

239.4 Bladder

239.5 Other genitourinary organs

239.6 Brain

> *Excludes:* cerebral meninges (239.7)
> cranial nerves (239.7)

239.7 Endocrine glands and other parts of nervous system

> *Excludes:* peripheral, sympathetic, and parasympathetic nerves and ganglia (239.2)

239.8 Other specified sites

> *Excludes:* eyelids (skin) (239.2)
>   cartilage (239.2)
>   great vessels (239.2)
>   optic nerve (239.7)

239.9 Site unspecified

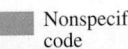

| Add 4th or 5th digit | Nonspecific code | Unspecified code | Manifestation code |

● Code new
to this edition ▲ Revision of
existing code ④ ⑤ Fourth or fifth
digit required

3. ENDOCRINE, NUTRITIONAL AND METABOLIC DISEASES, AND IMMUNITY DISORDERS (240-279)

[Excludes:] *endocrine and metabolic disturbances specific to the fetus and newborn (775.0-775.9)*

Note: All neoplasms, whether functionally active or not, are classified in Chapter 2. Codes in Chapter 3 (i.e., 242.8, 246.0, 251-253, 255-259) may be used, if desired, to identify such functional activity associated with any neoplasm, or by ectopic endocrine tissue.

DISORDERS OF THYROID GLAND (240-246)

240 Simple and unspecified goiter

240.0 Goiter, specified as simple
Any condition classifiable to 240.9, specified as simple

240.9 Goiter, unspecified
Enlargement of thyroid
Goiter or struma:
NOS
diffuse colloid
endemic
Goiter or struma:
hyperplastic
nontoxic (diffuse)
parenchymatous
sporadic

[Excludes:] *congenital (dyshormonogenic) goiter (246.1)*

241 Nontoxic nodular goiter

[Excludes:] *adenoma of thyroid (226)*
cystadenoma of thyroid (226)

241.0 Nontoxic uninodular goiter
Thyroid nodule
Uninodular goiter (nontoxic)

241.1 Nontoxic multinodular goiter
Multinodular goiter (nontoxic)

241.9 Unspecified nontoxic nodular goiter
Adenomatous goiter
Nodular goiter (nontoxic) NOS
Struma nodosa (simplex)

[5] **242 Thyrotoxicosis with or without goiter**

[Excludes:] *neonatal thyrotoxicosis (775.3)*

The following fifth-digit subclassification is for use with category 242:

0 without mention of thyrotoxic crisis or storm

1 with mention of thyrotoxic crisis or storm

[5] **242.0 Toxic diffuse goiter**
Basedow's disease
Exophthalmic or toxic goiter NOS
Graves' disease
Primary thyroid hyperplasia

[5] **242.1 Toxic uninodular goiter**
Thyroid nodule, toxic or with hyperthyroidism
Uninodular goiter, toxic or with hyperthyroidism

[5] **242.2 Toxic multinodular goiter**
Secondary thyroid hyperplasia

[5] **242.3 Toxic nodular goiter, unspecified**
Adenomatous goiter, toxic or with hyperthyroidism
Nodular goiter, toxic or with hyperthyroidism
Struma nodosa, toxic or with hyperthyroidism
Any condition classifiable to 241.9 specified as toxic or with hyperthyroidism

[5] **242.4 Thyrotoxicosis from ectopic thyroid nodule**

[5] **242.8 Thyrotoxicosis of other specified origin**
Overproduction of thyroid-stimulating hormone [TSH]
Thyrotoxicosis:
factitia
from ingestion of excessive thyroid material

Use additional E code to identify cause, if drug-induced

[5] **242.9 Thyrotoxicosis without mention of goiter or other cause**
Hyperthyroidism NOS
Thyrotoxicosis NOS

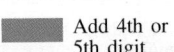

Add 4th or 5th digit | Nonspecific code | Unspecified code | Manifestation code

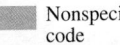

243 Congenital hypothyroidism
Congenital thyroid insufficiency
Cretinism (athyrotic) (endemic)
Use additional code to identify associated mental retardation
[Excludes:] *congenital (dyshormonogenic) goiter (246.1)*

244 Acquired hypothyroidism
Includes: athyroidism (acquired)
hypothyroidism (acquired)
myxedema (adult) (juvenile)
thyroid (gland) insufficiency (acquired)

244.0 Postsurgical hypothyroidism

244.1 Other postablative hypothyroidism
Hypothyroidism following therapy, such as irradiation

244.2 Iodine hypothyroidism
Hypothyroidism resulting from administration or ingestion of iodide
Use additional E code to identify drug

244.3 Other iatrogenic hypothyroidism
Hypothyroidism resulting from:
P-aminosalicylic acid [PAS]
Phenylbutazone
Resorcinol
Iatrogenic hypothyroidism NOS
Use additional E code to identify drug

244.8 Other specified acquired hypothyroidism
Secondary hypothyroidism NEC

244.9 Unspecified hypothyroidism
Hypothyroidism, primary or NOS
Myxedema, primary or NOS

245 Thyroiditis

245.0 Acute thyroiditis
Abscess of thyroid
Thyroiditis:
nonsuppurative, acute
pyogenic
suppurative
Use additional code to identify organism

245.1 Subacute thyroiditis
Thyroiditis:
de Quervain's
giant cell
Thyroiditis:
granulomatous
viral

245.2 Chronic lymphocytic thyroiditis
Hashimoto's disease
Struma lymphomatosa
Thyroiditis:
autoimmune
lymphocytic (chronic)

245.3 Chronic fibrous thyroiditis
Struma fibrosa
Thyroiditis:
invasive (fibrous)
ligneous
Riedel's

245.4 Iatrogenic thyroiditis
Use additional code to identify cause

245.8 Other and unspecified chronic thyroiditis
Chronic thyroiditis:
NOS
nonspecific

245.9 Thyroiditis, unspecified
Thyroiditis NOS

246 Other disorders of thyroid

246.0 Disorders of thyrocalcitonin secretion
Hypersecretion of calcitonin or thyrocalcitonin

● Code new to this edition ▲ Revision of existing code ④ ⑤ Fourth or fifth digit required

246.1 Dyshormonogenic goiter
Congenital (dyshormonogenic) goiter
Goiter due to enzyme defect in synthesis of thyroid hormone
Goitrous cretinism (sporadic)

246.2 Cyst of thyroid
[Excludes:] *cystadenoma of thyroid (226)*

246.3 Hemorrhage and infarction of thyroid

246.8 Other specified disorders of thyroid
Abnormality of thyroid-binding globulin
Atrophy of thyroid
Hyper-TBG-nemia
Hypo-TBG-nemia

246.9 Unspecified disorder of thyroid

DISEASES OF OTHER ENDOCRINE GLANDS (250-259)

[5] **250 Diabetes mellitus**
[Excludes:] *gestational diabetes (648.8)*
hyperglycemia NOS (790.6)
neonatal diabetes mellitus (775.1)
nonclinical diabetes (790.2)

The following fifth-digit subclassification is for use with category 250:

0 type II [non-insulin dependent type] [NIDDM type] [adult-onset type] or unspecified type, not stated as uncontrolled

Fifth-digit 0 is for use with type II, adult-onset diabetic patients, even if the patient requires insulin

1 type I [insulin dependent type] [IDDM] [juvenile type], not stated as uncontrolled

2 type II [non-insulin dependent type] [NIDDM type] [adult-onset type] or unspecified type, uncontrolled

Fifth-digit 2 is for use with type II, adult-onset diabetic patients, even if the patient requires insulin

3 type I [insulin dependent type] [IDDM] [juvenile type], uncontrolled

[5] **250.0 Diabetes mellitus without mention of complication**
Diabetes mellitus without mention of complication or manifestation classifiable to 250.1-250.9
Diabetes (mellitus) NOS

[5] **250.1 Diabetes with ketoacidosis**
Diabetic:
acidosis without mention of coma
ketosis without mention of coma

[5] **250.2 Diabetes with hyperosmolarity**
Hyperosmolar (nonketotic) coma

[5] **250.3 Diabetes with other coma**
Diabetic coma (with ketoacidosis)
Diabetic hypoglycemic coma
Insulin coma NOS

[Excludes:] *diabetes with hyperosmolar coma (250.2)*

[5] **250.4 Diabetes with renal manifestations**
Use additional code to identify manifestation, as:
diabetic:
nephropathy NOS (583.81)
nephrosis (581.81)
intercapillary glomerulosclerosis (581.81)
Kimmelstiel-Wilson syndrome (581.81)

[5] **250.5 Diabetes with ophthalmic manifestations**
Use additional code to identify manifestation, as:
diabetic:
blindness (369.00-369.9)
cataract (366.41)
glaucoma (365.44)
retinal edema (362.83)
retinopathy (362.01-362.02)

[5] **250.6 Diabetes with neurological manifestations**

Use additional code to identify manifestation, as:

diabetic:
- amyotrophy (358.1)
- mononeuropathy (354.0-355.9)
- neurogenic arthropathy (713.5)
- peripheral autonomic neuropathy (337.1)
- polyneuropathy (357.2)

[5] **250.7 Diabetes with peripheral circulatory disorders**

Use additional code to identify manifestation, as:

diabetic:
- gangrene (785.4)
- peripheral angiopathy (443.81)

[5] **250.8 Diabetes with other specified manifestations**

Diabetic hypoglycemia
Hypoglycemic shock

Use additional code to identify manifestation, as:
- any associated ulceration (707.10-707.9)
- diabetic bone changes (731.8)

Use additional E code to identify cause, if drug-induced

[5] **250.9 Diabetes with unspecified complication**

251 Other disorders of pancreatic internal secretion

251.0 Hypoglycemic coma

Iatrogenic hyperinsulinism
Non-diabetic insulin coma

Use additional E code to identify cause, if drug-induced

[*Excludes:*] *hypoglycemic coma in diabetes mellitus (250.3)*

251.1 Other specified hypoglycemia

Use additional E code to identify cause, if drug-induced

Hyperinsulinism:
- NOS
- ectopic
- functional

Hyperplasia of pancreatic islet beta cells NOS

[*Excludes:*] *hypoglycemia in diabetes mellitus (250.8)*
hypoglycemia in infant of diabetic mother (775.0)
hypoglycemic coma (251.0)
neonatal hypoglycemia (775.6)

251.2 Hypoglycemia, unspecified

Hypoglycemia:
- NOS
- reactive
- spontaneous

[*Excludes:*] *hypoglycemia:*
- *with coma (251.0)*
- *in diabetes mellitus (250.8)*
- *leucine-induced (270.3)*

251.3 Postsurgical hypoinsulinemia

Hypoinsulinemia following complete or partial pancreatectomy
Postpancreatectomy hyperglycemia

251.4 Abnormality of secretion of glucagon

Hyperplasia of pancreatic islet alpha cells with glucagon excess

251.5 Abnormality of secretion of gastrin

Hyperplasia of pancreatic alpha cells with gastrin excess
Zollinger-Ellison syndrome

251.8 Other specified disorders of pancreatic internal secretion

251.9 Unspecified disorder of pancreatic internal secretion

Islet cell hyperplasia NOS

● Code new to this edition
▲ Revision of existing code
[4] [5] Fourth or fifth digit required

252 **Disorders of parathyroid gland**

252.0 **Hyperparathyroidism**
Hyperplasia of parathyroid
Osteitis fibrosa cystica generalisata
von Recklinghausen's disease of bone

Excludes: ectopic hyperparathyroidism (259.3)
secondary hyperparathyroidism (of renal origin) (588.8)

252.1 **Hypoparathyroidism**
Parathyroiditis (autoimmune)
Tetany:
parathyroid
parathyroprival

Excludes: pseudohypoparathyroidism (275.4)
pseudo-pseudohypoparathyroidism (275.4)
tetany NOS (781.7)
transitory neonatal hypoparathyroidism (775.4)

252.8 **Other specified disorders of parathyroid gland**
Cyst of parathyroid gland
Hemorrhage of parathyroid gland

252.9 **Unspecified disorder of parathyroid gland**

253 **Disorders of the pituitary gland and its hypothalamic control**
Includes: the listed conditions whether the disorder is in the pituitary or the hypothalamus

Excludes: Cushing's syndrome (255.0)

253.0 **Acromegaly and gigantism**
Overproduction of growth hormone

253.1 **Other and unspecified anterior pituitary hyperfunction**
Forbes-Albright syndrome

Excludes: overproduction of:
ACTH (255.3)
thyroid-stimulating hormone [TSH] (242.8)

253.2 **Panhypopituitarism**
Cachexia, pituitary   Sheehan's syndrome
Necrosis of pituitary   Simmonds' disease
(postpartum)
Pituitary insufficiency NOS

Excludes: iatrogenic hypopituitarism (253.7)

253.3 **Pituitary dwarfism**
Isolated deficiency of (human) growth hormone [HGH]
Lorain-Levi dwarfism

253.4 **Other anterior pituitary disorders**
Isolated or partial deficiency of an anterior pituitary hormone, other than growth
hormone
Prolactin deficiency

253.5 **Diabetes insipidus**
Vasopressin deficiency

Excludes: nephrogenic diabetes insipidus (588.1)

253.6 **Other disorders of neurohypophysis**
Syndrome of inappropriate secretion of antidiuretic hormone [ADH]
Excludes: ectopic antidiuretic hormone secretion (259.3)

253.7 **Iatrogenic pituitary disorders**
Hypopituitarism:
hormone-induced
hypophysectomy-induced
postablative
radiotherapy-induced
Use additional E code to identify cause

253.8 **Other disorders of the pituitary and other syndromes of diencephalohypophyseal**
origin
Abscess of pituitary   Cyst of Rathke's pouch
Adiposogenital dystrophy   Fröhlich's syndrome

Excludes: craniopharyngioma (237.0)

| | Add 4th or 5th digit | | Nonspecific code | | Unspecified code | | Manifestation code |

253.9 **Unspecified**
Dyspituitarism

254 **Diseases of thymus gland**

Excludes: *aplasia or dysplasia with immunodeficiency (279.2)*
hypoplasia with immunodeficiency (279.2)
myasthenia gravis (358.0)

254.0 **Persistent hyperplasia of thymus**
Hypertrophy of thymus

254.1 **Abscess of thymus**

254.8 **Other specified diseases of thymus gland**
Atrophy of thymus
Cyst of thymus

Excludes *thymoma (212.6)*

254.9 **Unspecified disease of thymus gland**

255 **Disorders of adrenal glands**
Includes: the listed conditions whether the basic disorder is in the adrenals or is
pituitary-induced

255.0 **Cushing's syndrome**

Adrenal hyperplasia due to
excess ACTH
Cushing's syndrome:
NOS
iatrogenic
idiopathic
pituitary-dependent

Ectopic ACTH syndrome
Iatrogenic syndrome of excess cortisol
Overproduction of cortisol

Use additional E code to identify cause, if drug-induced

Excludes: *congenital adrenal hyperplasia (255.2)*

255.1 **Hyperaldosteronism**

Aldosteronism (primary)
(secondary)

Bartter's syndrome
Conn's syndrome

255.2 **Adrenogenital disorders**
Adrenogenital syndromes, virilizing or feminizing, whether acquired or associated with
congenital adrenal hyperplasia consequent on inborn enzyme defects in hormone
synthesis
Achard-Thiers syndrome
Congenital adrenal hyperplasia
Female adrenal pseudohermaphroditism
Male:
macrogenitosomia praecox
sexual precocity with adrenal hyperplasia
Virilization (female) (suprarenal)

Excludes: *adrenal hyperplasia due to excess ACTH (255.0)*
isosexual virilization (256.4)

255.3 **Other corticoadrenal overactivity**
Acquired benign adrenal androgenic overactivity
Overproduction of ACTH

255.4 **Corticoadrenal insufficiency**

Addisonian crisis
Addison's disease NOS
Adrenal:
atrophy (autoimmune)
calcification

Adrenal:
crisis
hemorrhage
infarction
insufficiency NOS

Excludes: *tuberculous Addison's disease (017.6)*

255.5 **Other adrenal hypofunction**
Adrenal medullary insufficiency

Excludes: *Waterhouse-Friderichsen syndrome (meningococcal) (036.3)*

255.6 **Medulloadrenal hyperfunction**
Catecholamine secretion by pheochromocytoma

255.8 **Other specified disorders of adrenal glands**
Abnormality of cortisol-binding globulin

255.9 **Unspecified disorder of adrenal glands**

● Code new
to this edition
▲ Revision of
existing code
④ ⑤ Fourth or fifth
digit required

256 Ovarian dysfunction

256.0 Hyperestrogenism

256.1 Other ovarian hyperfunction
Hypersecretion of ovarian androgens

256.2 Postablative ovarian failure
Ovarian failure:
iatrogenic
postirradiation
postsurgical
Use additional code for states associated with artifical menopause (627.4)

Excludes: *asymptomatic age-related (natural) postmenopausal status (V49.81)*
acquired absence of ovary (V45.77)

⑤ **256.3 Other ovarian failure**
Use additional code for states associated with natural menopause (627.2)

Excludes: *asymptomatic age-related (natural) postmenopausal status (V49.81)*

256.31 Premature menopause

256.39 Other ovarian failure
Delayed menarche
Ovarian hypofunction
Primary ovarian failure NOS

256.4 Polycystic ovaries
Isosexual virilization
Stein-Leventhal syndrome

256.8 Other ovarian dysfunction

256.9 Unspecified ovarian dysfunction

257 Testicular dysfunction

257.0 Testicular hyperfunction
Hypersecretion of testicular hormones

257.1 Postablative testicular hypofunction
Testicular hypofunction:
iatrogenic
postirradiation
postsurgical

257.2 Other testicular hypofunction
Defective biosynthesis of testicular androgen
Eunuchoidism:
NOS
hypogonadotropic
Failure:
Leydig's cell, adult
seminiferous tubule, adult
Testicular hypogonadism

Excludes: *azoospermia (606.0)*

257.8 Other testicular dysfunction
Goldberg-Maxwell syndrome
Male pseudohermaphroditism with testicular feminization
Testicular feminization

257.9 Unspecified testicular dysfunction

258 Polyglandular dysfunction and related disorders

258.0 Polyglandular activity in multiple endocrine adenomatosis
Wermer's syndrome

258.1 Other combinations of endocrine dysfunction
Lloyd's syndrome
Schmidt's syndrome

258.8 Other specified polyglandular dysfunction

258.9 Polyglandular dysfunction, unspecified

259 Other endocrine disorders

259.0 Delay in sexual development and puberty, not elsewhere classified
Delayed puberty

 Add 4th or 5th digit   Nonspecific code   Unspecified code   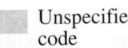 Manifestation code

259.1 Precocious sexual development and puberty, not elsewhere classified
Sexual precocity:
NOS
constitutional
cryptogenic
idiopathic

259.2 Carcinoid syndrome
Hormone secretion by carcinoid tumors

259.3 Ectopic hormone secretion, not elsewhere classified
Ectopic:
antidiuretic hormone secretion [ADH]
hyperparathyroidism

Excludes: *ectopic ACTH syndrome (255.0)*

259.4 Dwarfism, not elsewhere classified
Dwarfism:
NOS
constitutional

Excludes: *dwarfism:*
achondroplastic (756.4)
intrauterine (759.7)
nutritional (263.2)
pituitary (253.3)
renal (588.0)
progeria (259.8)

259.8 Other specified endocrine disorders
Pineal gland dysfunction   Werner's syndrome
Progeria

259.9 Unspecified endocrine disorder
Disturbance: Infantilism NOS
endocrine NOS
hormone NOS

NUTRITIONAL DEFICIENCIES (260-269)

Excludes: *deficiency anemias (280.0-281.9)*

260 Kwashiorkor
Nutritional edema with dyspigmentation of skin and hair

261 Nutritional marasmus
Nutritional atrophy   Severe malnutrition NOS
Severe calorie deficiency

262 Other severe protein-calorie malnutrition
Nutritional edema without mention of dyspigmentation of skin and hair

263 Other and unspecified protein-calorie malnutrition

263.0 Malnutrition of moderate degree

263.1 Malnutrition of mild degree

263.2 Arrested development following protein-calorie malnutrition
Nutritional dwarfism
Physical retardation due to malnutrition

263.8 Other protein-calorie malnutrition

263.9 Unspecified protein-calorie malnutrition
Dystrophy due to malnutrition
Malnutrition (calorie) NOS

Excludes: *nutritional deficiency NOS (269.9)*

264 Vitamin A deficiency

264.0 With conjunctival xerosis

264.1 With conjunctival xerosis and Bitot's spot
Bitot's spot in the young child

264.2 With corneal xerosis

264.3 With corneal ulceration and xerosis

264.4 With keratomalacia

264.5 With night blindness

264.6 With xerophthalmic scars of cornea

● Code new
  to this edition   ▲ Revision of
     existing code   ④ ⑤ Fourth or fifth
     digit required

264.7 Other ocular manifestations of vitamin A deficiency
Xerophthalmia due to vitamin A deficiency

264.8 Other manifestations of vitamin A deficiency
Follicular keratosis due to vitamin A deficiency
Xeroderma due to vitamin A deficiency

264.9 Unspecified vitamin A deficiency
Hypovitaminosis A NOS

265 Thiamine and niacin deficiency states

265.0 Beriberi

265.1 Other and unspecified manifestations of thiamine deficiency
Other vitamin B_1 deficiency states

265.2 Pellagra
Deficiency:
  niacin (-tryptophan)
  nicotinamide
  nicotinic acid
  vitamin PP
Pellagra (alcoholic)

266 Deficiency of B-complex components

266.0 Ariboflavinosis
Riboflavin [vitamin B_2] deficiency

266.1 Vitamin B_6 deficiency
Deficiency: Vitamin B_6 deficiency syndrome
  pyridoxal
  pyridoxamine
  pyridoxine

  Excludes: *vitamin B_6-responsive sideroblastic anemia (285.0)*

266.2 Other B-complex deficiencies
Deficiency:
  cyanocobalamin
  folic acid
  vitamin B_{12}

  Excludes: *combined system disease with anemia (281.0-281.1)*
         deficiency anemias (281.0-281.9)
         subacute degeneration of spinal cord with anemia (281.0-281.1)

266.9 Unspecified vitamin B deficiency

267 Ascorbic acid deficiency
Deficiency of vitamin C   Scurvy

  Excludes: *scorbutic anemia (281.8)*

268 Vitamin D deficiency

  Excludes: *vitamin D-resistant:*
         osteomalacia (275.3)
         rickets (275.3)

268.0 Rickets, active

  Excludes: *celiac rickets (579.0)*
         renal rickets (588.0)

268.1 Rickets, late effect
Any condition specified as due to rickets and stated to be a late effect or sequela of
  rickets
Use additional code to identify the nature of late effect

268.2 Osteomalacia, unspecified

268.9 Unspecified vitamin D deficiency
Avitaminosis D

269 Other nutritional deficiencies

269.0 Deficiency of vitamin K

  Excludes: *deficiency of coagulation factor due to vitamin K deficiency (286.7)*
         vitamin K deficiency of newborn (776.0)

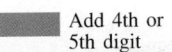

| | Add 4th or 5th digit | | Nonspecific code | | Unspecified code | | Manifestation code |

269.1 **Deficiency of other vitamins**
Deficiency:
    vitamin E
    vitamin P

269.2 **Unspecified vitamin deficiency**
Multiple vitamin deficiency NOS

269.3 **Mineral deficiency, not elsewhere classified**
Deficiency:
    calcium, dietary
    iodine
Excludes: *deficiency:*
    calcium NOS (275.4)
    potassium (276.8)
    sodium (276.1)

269.8 **Other nutritional deficiency**
Excludes: *adult failure to thrive (783.7)*
    failure to thrive in childhood (783.41)
    feeding problems (783.3)
      newborn (779.3)

269.9 **Unspecified nutritional deficiency**

OTHER METABOLIC AND IMMUNITY DISORDERS (270-279)

Use additional code to identify any associated mental retardation

270 **Disorders of amino-acid transport and metabolism**
Excludes: *abnormal findings without manifest disease (790.0-796.9)*
    disorders of purine and pyrimidine metabolism (277.1-277.2)
    gout (274.0-274.9)

270.0 **Disturbances of amino-acid transport**
Cystinosis
Cystinuria
Fanconi (-de Toni) (-Debré) syndrome
Glycinuria (renal)
Hartnup disease

270.1 **Phenylketonuria [PKU]**
Hyperphenylalaninemia

270.2 **Other disturbances of aromatic amino-acid metabolism**

Albinism	Hypertyrosinemia
Alkaptonuria	Indicanuria
Alkaptonuric ochronosis	Kynureninase defects
Disturbances of metabolism	Oasthouse urine disease
of tyrosine and	Ochronosis
tryptophan	Tyrosinosis
Homogentisic acid defects	Tyrosinuria
Hydroxykynureninuria	Waardenburg syndrome

Excludes: *vitamin B$_6$-deficiency syndrome (266.1)*

270.3 **Disturbances of branched-chain amino-acid metabolism**
Disturbances of metabolism of leucine, isoleucine, and valine
Hypervalinemia
Intermittent branched-chain ketonuria
Leucine-induced hypoglycemia
Leucinosis
Maple syrup urine disease

270.4 **Disturbances of sulphur-bearing amino-acid metabolism**
Cystathioninemia
Cystathioninuria
Disturbances of metabolism of methionine, homocystine, and cystathionine
Homocystinuria
Hypermethioninemia
Methioninemia

270.5 **Disturbances of histidine metabolism**

Carnosinemia	Hyperhistidinemia
Histidinemia	Imidazole aminoaciduria

● Code new
to this edition
   ▲ Revision of
existing code
   ④ ⑤ Fourth or fifth
digit required

270.6 Disorders of urea cycle metabolism
Argininosuccinic aciduria
Citrullinemia
Disorders of metabolism of ornithine, citrulline, argininosuccinic acid, arginine, and ammonia
Hyperammonemia
Hyperornithinemia

270.7 Other disturbances of straight-chain amino-acid metabolism
Glucoglycinuria
Glycinemia (with methyl-malonic acidemia)
Hyperglycinemia
Hyperlysinemia
Pipecolic acidemia
Saccharopinuria
Other disturbances of metabolism of glycine, threonine, serine, glutamine, and lysine

270.8 Other specified disorders of amino-acid metabolism
Alaninemia
Ethanolaminuria
Glycoprolinuria
Hydroxyprolinemia
Hyperprolinemia
Iminoacidopathy
Prolinemia
Prolinuria
Sarcosinemia

270.9 Unspecified disorder of amino-acid metabolism

271 Disorders of carbohydrate transport and metabolism
Excludes: *abnormality of secretion of glucagon (251.4)*
diabetes mellitus (250.0-250.9)
hypoglycemia NOS (251.2)
mucopolysaccharidosis (277.5)

271.0 Glycogenosis
Amylopectinosis
Glucose-6-phosphatase deficiency
Glycogen storage disease
McArdle's disease
Pompe's disease
von Gierke's disease

271.1 Galactosemia
Galactose-1-phosphate uridyl transferase deficiency
Galactosuria

271.2 Hereditary fructose intolerance
Essential benign fructosuria
Fructosemia

271.3 Intestinal disaccharidase deficiencies and disaccharide malabsorption
Intolerance or malabsorption (congenital) (of):
glucose-galactose
lactose
sucrose-isomaltose

271.4 Renal glycosuria
Renal diabetes

271.8 Other specified disorders of carbohydrate transport and metabolism
Essential benign pentosuria
Fucosidosis
Glycolic aciduria
Hyperoxaluria (primary)
Mannosidosis
Oxalosis
Xylosuria
Xylulosuria

271.9 Unspecified disorder of carbohydrate transport and metabolism

272 Disorders of lipoid metabolism
Excludes: *localized cerebral lipidoses (330.1)*

272.0 Pure hypercholesterolemia
Familial hypercholesterolemia
Fredrickson Type IIa hyperlipoproteinemia
Hyperbetalipoproteinemia
Hyperlipidemia, Group A
Low-density-lipoid-type [LDL] hyperlipoproteinemia

272.1 Pure hyperglyceridemia
Endogenous hyperglyceridemia
Fredrickson Type IV hyperlipoproteinemia
Hyperlipidemia, Group B
Hyperprebetalipoproteinemia
Hypertriglyceridemia, essential
Very-low-density-lipoid-type [VLDL] hyperlipoproteinemia

Add 4th or 5th digit   Nonspecific code   Unspecified code   Manifestation code

272.2 Mixed hyperlipidemia
  Broad- or floating-betalipoproteinemia
  Fredrickson Type IIb or III hyperlipoproteinemia
  Hypercholesterolemia with endogenous hyperglyceridemia
  Hyperbetalipoproteinemia with prebetalipoproteinemia
  Tubo-eruptive xanthoma
  Xanthoma tuberosum

272.3 Hyperchylomicronemia
  Bürger-Grütz syndrome
  Fredrickson type I or V
    hyperlipoproteinemia

  Hyperlipidemia, Group D
  Mixed hyperglyceridemia

272.4 Other and unspecified hyperlipidemia
  Alpha-lipoproteinemia
  Combined hyperlipidemia

  Hyperlipidemia NOS
  Hyperlipoproteinemia NOS

272.5 Lipoprotein deficiencies
  Abetalipoproteinemia
  Bassen-Kornzweig syndrome
  High-density lipoid deficiency
  Hypoalphalipoproteinemia
  Hypobetalipoproteinemia (familial)

272.6 Lipodystrophy
  Barraquer-Simons disease
  Progressive lipodystrophy
Use additional E code to identify cause, if iatrogenic

Excludes: intestinal lipodystrophy (040.2)

272.7 Lipidoses
  Chemically-induced lipidosis
  Disease:
    Anderson's
    Fabry's
    Gaucher's
    I cell [mucolipidosis I]
    lipoid storage NOS
    Neimann-Pick
    pseudo-Hurler's or
    mucolipidosis III

  Disease:
    triglyceride storage, Type I or II
    Wolman's or triglyceride storage, Type III
  Mucolipidosis II
  Primary familial xanthomatosis

Excludes: cerebral lipidoses (330.1)
    Tay-Sachs disease (330.1)

272.8 Other disorders of lipoid metabolism
  Hoffa's disease or liposynovitis prepatellaris
  Launois-Bensaude's lipomatosis
  Lipoid dermatoarthritis

272.9 Unspecified disorder of lipoid metabolism

273 Disorders of plasma protein metabolism

Excludes: agammaglobulinemia and hypogammaglobulinemia (279.0 -279.2)
    coagulation defects (286.0-286.9)
    hereditary hemolytic anemias (282.0-282.9)

273.0 Polyclonal hypergammaglobulinemia
  Hypergammaglobulinemic purpura:
    benign primary
    Waldenström's

273.1 Monoclonal paraproteinemia
  Benign monoclonal hypergammaglobulinemia [BMH]
  Monoclonal gammopathy:
    NOS
    associated with lymphoplasmacytic dyscrasias
    benign
  Paraproteinemia:
    benign (familial)
    secondary to malignant or inflammatory disease

273.2 Other paraproteinemias
  Cryoglobulinemic:
    purpura
    vasculitis

  Mixed cryoglobulinemia

● Code new
  to this edition
▲ Revision of
  existing code
④ ⑤ Fourth or fifth
  digit required

273.3 Macroglobulinemia
Macroglobulinemia (idiopathic) (primary)
Waldenström's macroglobulinemia

273.8 Other disorders of plasma protein metabolism
Abnormality of transport protein
Bisalbuminemia

273.9 Unspecified disorder of plasma protein metabolism

274 Gout

[Excludes:] *lead gout (984.0-984.9)*

274.0 Gouty arthropathy

[5] **274.1 Gouty nephropathy**

274.10 Gouty nephropathy, unspecified

274.11 Uric acid nephrolithiasis

274.19 Other

[5] **274.8 Gout with other specified manifestations**

274.81 Gouty tophi of ear

274.82 Gouty tophi of other sites
Gouty tophi of heart

274.89 Other
Use additional code to identify manifestations, as:
gouty:
iritis (364.11)
neuritis (357.4)

274.9 Gout, unspecified

275 Disorders of mineral metabolism

[Excludes:] *abnormal findings without manifest disease (790.0-796.9)*

275.0 Disorders of iron metabolism
Bronzed diabetes
Hemochromatosis
Pigmentary cirrhosis (of liver)

[Excludes:] *anemia:*
iron deficiency (280.0-280.9)
sideroblastic (285.0)

275.1 Disorders of copper metabolism
Hepatolenticular degeneration
Wilson's disease

275.2 Disorders of magnesium metabolism
Hypermagnesemia
Hypomagnesemia

275.3 Disorders of phosphorus metabolism
Familial hypophosphatemia
Hypophosphatasia
Vitamin D-resistant:
osteomalacia
rickets

[5] **275.4 Disorders of calcium metabolism**

[Excludes:] *parathyroid disorders (252.0-252.9)*
vitamin D deficiency (268.0-268.9)

275.40 Unspecified disorder of calcium metabolism

275.41 Hypocalcemia

275.42 Hypercalcemia

275.49 Other disorders of calcium metabolism
Nephrocalcinosis
Pseudohypoparathyroidism
Pseudopseudohypoparathyroidism

275.8 Other specified disorders of mineral metabolism

275.9 Unspecified disorder of mineral metabolism

276 Disorders of fluid, electrolyte, and acid-base balance

[Excludes:] *diabetes insipidus (253.5)*
familial periodic paralysis (359.3)

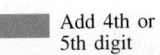

Add 4th or 5th digit — Nonspecific code — Unspecified code — Manifestation code

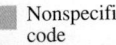

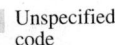

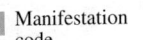

276.0 Hyperosmolality and/or hypernatremia
Sodium [Na] excess
Sodium [Na] overload

276.1 Hyposmolality and/or hyponatremia
Sodium [Na] deficiency

276.2 Acidosis
Acidosis:
NOS
lactic
metabolic
respiratory

[Excludes:] *diabetic acidosis (250.1)*

276.3 Alkalosis
Alkalosis:
NOS
metabolic
respiratory

276.4 Mixed acid-base balance disorder
Hypercapnia with mixed acid-base disorder

276.5 Volume depletion
Dehydration
Depletion of volume of plasma or extracellular fluid
Hypovolemia

[Excludes:] *hypovolemic shock:*
postoperative (998.0)
traumatic (958.4)

276.6 Fluid overload
Fluid retention

[Excludes:] *ascites (789.5)*
localized edema (782.3)

276.7 Hyperpotassemia
Hyperkalemia
Potassium [K]:
excess
intoxication
overload

276.8 Hypopotassemia
Hypokalemia
Potassium [K] deficiency

276.9 Electrolyte and fluid disorders not elsewhere classified
Electrolyte imbalance
Hypochloremia
Hyperchloremia

[Excludes:] *electrolyte imbalance:*
associated with hyperemesis gravidarum (643.1)
complicating labor and delivery (669.0)
following abortion and ectopic or molar pregnancy (634-638 with .4, 639.4)

277 Other and unspecified disorders of metabolism

⑤ **277.0 Cystic fibrosis**
Fibrocystic disease of the pancreas
Mucoviscidosis

277.00 Without mention of meconium ileus
Cystic fibrosis NOS

277.01 With meconium ileus
Meconium:
ileus (of newborn)
obstruction of intestine in mucoviscidosis

● **277.02 With pulmonary manifestations**
Cystic fibrosis with pulmonary exacerbation
Use additional code to identify any infectious organism present, such as:
pseudomonas (041.7)

● **277.03 With gastrointestinal manifestations**

[Excludes:] *with meconium ileus (277.01)*

● **277.09 With other manifestations**

● Code new to this edition
▲ Revision of existing code
④ ⑤ Fourth or fifth digit required

277.1 Disorders of porphyrin metabolism
Hematoporphyria
Hematoporphyrinuria
Hereditary coproporphyria
Porphyria
Porphyrinuria
Protocoproporphyria
Protoporphyria
Pyrroloporphyria

277.2 Other disorders of purine and pyrimidine metabolism
Hypoxanthine-guanine-phosphoribosyltransferase deficiency [HG-PRT deficiency]
Lesch-Nyhan syndrome
Xanthinuria

[Excludes:] *gout (274.0-274.9)*
orotic aciduric anemia (281.4)

277.3 Amyloidosis
Amyloidosis:
NOS
inherited systemic
nephropathic
neuropathic (Portuguese) (Swiss)
secondary
Benign paroxysmal peritonitis
Familial Mediterranean fever
Hereditary cardiac amyloidosis

277.4 Disorders of bilirubin excretion
Hyperbilirubinemia:
congenital
constitutional
Syndrome:
Crigler-Najjar
Dubin-Johnson
Gilbert's
Rotor's

[Excludes:] *hyperbilirubinemias specific to the perinatal period (774.0-774.7)*

277.5 Mucopolysaccharidosis
Gargoylism
Hunter's syndrome
Hurler's syndrome
Lipochondrodystrophy
Maroteaux-Lamy syndrome
Morquio-Brailsford disease
Osteochondrodystrophy
Sanfilippo's syndrome
Scheie's syndrome

277.6 Other deficiencies of circulating enzymes
Alpha 1-antitrypsin deficiency
Hereditary angioedema

277.7 Dysmetabolic syndrome X
Use additional code for associated manifestation, such as:
cardiovascular disease (414.00-414.06)
obesity (278.00-278.01)

277.8 Other specified disorders of metabolism
Hand-Schüller-Christian disease
Histiocytosis (acute) (chronic)
Histiocytosis X (chronic)

[Excludes:] *histiocytosis:*
acute differentiated progressive (202.5)
X, acute (progressive) (202.5)

277.9 Unspecified disorder of metabolism
Enzymopathy NOS

278 Obesity and other hyperalimentation

[Excludes:] *hyperalimentation NOS (783.6)*
poisoning by vitamins NOS (963.5)
polyphagia (783.6)

[5] **278.0 Obesity**

[Excludes:] *adiposogenital dystrophy (253.8)*
obesity of endocrine origin NOS (259.9)

278.00 Obesity, unspecified
Obesity NOS

278.01 Morbid obesity

278.1 Localized adiposity
Fat pad

278.2 Hypervitaminosis A

Add 4th or 5th digit | Nonspecific code | Unspecified code | Manifestation code

278.3 **Hypercarotinemia**

278.4 **Hypervitaminosis D**

278.8 **Other hyperalimentation**

279 **Disorders involving the immune mechanism**

⑤ 279.0 **Deficiency of humoral immunity**

279.00 **Hypogammaglobulinemia, unspecified**
Agammaglobulinemia NOS

279.01 **Selective IgA immunodeficiency**

279.02 **Selective IgM immunodeficiency**

279.03 **Other selective immunoglobulin deficiencies**
Selective deficiency of IgG

279.04 **Congenital hypogammaglobulinemia**
Agammaglobulinemia:
Bruton's type
X-linked

279.05 **Immunodeficiency with increased IgM**
Immunodeficiency with hyper-IgM:
autosomal recessive
X-linked

279.06 **Common variable immunodeficiency**
Dysgammaglobulinemia (acquired) (congenital) (primary)
Hypogammaglobulinemia:
acquired primary
congenital non-sex-linked
sporadic

279.09 **Other**
Transient hypogammaglobulinemia of infancy

⑤ 279.1 **Deficiency of cell-mediated immunity**

279.10 **Immunodeficiency with predominant T-cell defect, unspecified**

279.11 **DiGeorge's syndrome**
Pharyngeal pouch syndrome
Thymic hypoplasia

279.12 **Wiskott-Aldrich syndrome**

279.13 **Nezelof's syndrome**
Cellular immunodeficiency with abnormal immunoglobulin deficiency

279.19 **Other**

Excludes: *ataxia-telangiectasia (334.8)*

279.2 **Combined immunity deficiency** ·
Agammaglobulinemia:
autosomal recessive
Swiss-type
x-linked recessive
Severe combined immunodeficiency [SCID]
Thymic:
alymphoplasia
aplasia or dysplasia with immunodeficiency

Excludes: *thymic hypoplasia (279.11)*

279.3 **Unspecified immunity deficiency**

279.4 **Autoimmune disease, not elsewhere classified**
Autoimmune disease NOS

Excludes: *transplant failure or rejection (996.80-996.89)*

279.8 **Other specified disorders involving the immune mechanism**
Single complement [C_1-C_9] deficiency or dysfunction

279.9 **Unspecified disorder of immune mechanism**

● Code new
to this edition

▲ Revision of
existing code

④ ⑤ Fourth or fifth
digit required

4. DISEASES OF THE BLOOD AND BLOOD-FORMING ORGANS (280-289)

Excludes: anemia complicating pregnancy or the puerperium (648.2)

280 Iron deficiency anemias
Includes: anemia:
    asiderotic
    hypochromic-microcytic
    sideropenic

Excludes: familial microcytic anemia (282.4)

280.0 Secondary to blood loss (chronic)
Normocytic anemia due to blood loss

Excludes: acute posthemorrhagic anemia (285.1)

280.1 Secondary to inadequate dietary iron intake

280.8 Other specified iron deficiency anemias
Paterson-Kelly syndrome
Plummer-Vinson syndrome
Sideropenic dysphagia

280.9 Iron deficiency anemia, unspecified
Anemia:
    achlorhydric
    chlorotic
    idiopathic hypochromic
    iron [Fe] deficiency NOS

281 Other deficiency anemias

281.0 Pernicious anemia
Anemia: Congenital intrinsic factor [Castle's] deficiency
    Addison's
    Biermer's
    congenital pernicious

Excludes: combined system disease without mention of anemia (266.2)
          subacute degeneration of spinal cord without mention of anemia (266.2)

281.1 Other vitamin B_{12} deficiency anemia
Anemia:
    vegan's
    vitamin B_{12} deficiency (dietary)
    due to selective vitamin B_{12} malabsorption with proteinuria
Syndrome:
    Imerslund's
    Imerslund-Gräsbeck

Excludes: combined system disease without mention of anemia (266.2)
          subacute degeneration of spinal cord without mention of anemia (266.2)

281.2 Folate-deficiency anemia
Congenital folate malabsorption
Folate or folic acid deficiency anemia:
    NOS
    dietary
    drug-induced
Goat's milk anemia
Nutritional megaloblastic anemia (of infancy)
Use additional E code, if desired, to identify drug

281.3 Other specified megaloblastic anemias not elsewhere classified
Combined B_{12} and folate-deficiency anemia
Refractory megaloblastic anemia

281.4 Protein-deficiency anemia
Amino-acid-deficiency anemia

281.8 Anemia associated with other specified nutritional deficiency
Scorbutic anemia

281.9 Unspecified deficiency anemia
Anemia: Anemia:
    dimorphic   nutritional NOS
    macrocytic   simple chronic
    megaloblastic NOS

	Add 4th or 5th digit		Nonspecific code		Unspecified code		Manifestation code

282 **Hereditary hemolytic anemias**

282.0 **Hereditary spherocytosis**
Acholuric (familial) jaundice
Congenital hemolytic anemia (spherocytic)
Congenital spherocytosis
Minkowski-Chauffard syndrome
Spherocytosis (familial)

Excludes: *hemolytic anemia of newborn (773.0-773.5)*

282.1 **Hereditary elliptocytosis**
Elliptocytosis (congenital)
Ovalocytosis (congenital) (hereditary)

282.2 **Anemias due to disorders of glutathione metabolism**
Anemia:
6-phosphogluconic dehydrogenase deficiency
enzyme deficiency, drug-induced
erythrocytic glutathione deficiency
glucose-6-phosphate dehydrogenase [G-6-PD] deficiency
glutathione-reductase deficiency
hemolytic nonspherocytic (hereditary), type I
Disorder of pentose phosphate pathway
Favism

282.3 **Other hemolytic anemias due to enzyme deficiency**
Anemia:
hemolytic nonspherocytic (hereditary), type II
hexokinase deficiency
pyruvate kinase [PK] deficiency
triosephosphate isomerase deficiency

282.4 **Thalassemias**
Cooley's anemia
Hereditary leptocytosis
Mediterranean anemia (with other hemoglobinopathy)
Microdrepanocytosis
Sickle-cell thalassemia
Thalassemia (alpha) (beta) (intermedia) (major) (minima) (minor) (mixed) (trait) (with other hemoglobinopathy)
Thalassemia-Hb-S disease

Excludes: *sickle-cell:*
anemia (282.60-282.69)
trait (282.5)

282.5 **Sickle-cell trait**
Hb-AS genotype   Heterozygous:
Hemoglobin S [Hb-S] trait   hemoglobin S
                                    Hb-S

Excludes: *that with other hemoglobinopathy (282.60-282.69)*
that with thalassemia (282.4)

⑤ **282.6** **Sickle-cell anemia**

Excludes: *sickle-cell thalassemia (282.4)*
sickle-cell trait (282.5)

282.60 **Sickle-cell anemia, unspecified**

282.61 **Hb-S disease without mention of crisis**

282.62 **Hb-S disease with mention of crisis**
Sickle-cell crisis NOS

282.63 **Sickle-cell/Hb-C disease**
Hb-S/Hb-C disease

282.69 **Other**
Disease: Disease:
Hb-S/Hb-D   sickle-cell/Hb-D
Hb-S/Hb-E   sickle-cell/Hb-E

● Code new
to this edition
▲ Revision of
existing code
④ ⑤ Fourth or fifth
digit required

282.7 **Other hemoglobinopathies**
Abnormal hemoglobin NOS
Congenital Heinz-body anemia
Disease:
Hb-Bart's
hemoglobin C [Hb-C]
hemoglobin D [Hb-D]
hemoglobin E [Hb-E]
hemoglobin Zurich [Hb-Zurich]
Hemoglobinopathy NOS
Hereditary persistence of fetal hemoglobin [HPFH]
Unstable hemoglobin hemolytic disease

Excludes: *familial polycythemia (289.6)*
hemoglobin M [Hb-M] disease (289.7)
high-oxygen-affinity hemoglobin (289.0)

282.8 **Other specified hereditary hemolytic anemias**
Stomatocytosis

282.9 **Hereditary hemolytic anemia, unspecified**
Hereditary hemolytic anemia NOS

283 **Acquired hemolytic anemias**

283.0 **Autoimmune hemolytic anemias**
Autoimmune hemolytic anemias (cold type) (warm type)
Chronic cold hemagglutinin disease
Cold agglutinin disease or hemoglobinuria
Hemolytic anemia:
cold type (secondary) (symptomatic)
drug-induced
warm type (secondary) (symptomatic)
Use additional E code, if desired, to identify cause, if drug-induced

Excludes: *Evans' syndrome (287.3)*
hemolytic disease of newborn (773.0-773.5)

⑤ **283.1** **Non-autoimmune hemolytic anemias**

283.10 **Non-autoimmune hemolytic anemia, unspecified**

283.11 **Hemolytic-uremic syndrome**

283.19 **Other non-autoimmune hemolytic anemias**
Hemolytic anemia:
mechanical
microangiopathic
toxic
Use additional E code, if desired, to identify cause

283.2 **Hemoglobinuria due to hemolysis from external causes**
Acute intravascular hemolysis
Hemoglobinuria:
from exertion
march
paroxysmal (cold) (nocturnal)
due to other hemolysis
Marchiafava-Micheli syndrome
Use additional E code, if desired, to identify cause

283.9 **Acquired hemolytic anemia, unspecified**
Acquired hemolytic anemia NOS
Chronic idiopathic hemolytic anemia

284 **Aplastic anemia**

284.0 **Constitutional aplastic anemia**
Aplasia, (pure) red cell: Familial hypoplastic anemia
congenital   Fanconi's anemia
of infants   Pancytopenia with malformations
primary
Blackfan-Diamond syndrome

| | Add 4th or 5th digit | | Nonspecific code | | Unspecified code | | Manifestation code |

284.8 **Other specified aplastic anemias**

Aplastic anemia (due to):
chronic systemic disease
drugs
infection
radiation
toxic (paralytic)

Pancytopenia (acquired)
Red cell aplasia (acquired) (adult) (pure) (with
thymoma)

Use additional E code, if desired, to identify cause

284.9 **Aplastic anemia, unspecified**

Anemia:
aplastic (idiopathic) NOS
aregenerative
hypoplastic NOS

Anemia:
nonregenerative
refractory
Medullary hypoplasia

285 **Other and unspecified anemias**

285.0 **Sideroblastic anemia**

Anemia:
hypochromic with iron loading
sideroachrestic
sideroblastic
acquired
congenital
hereditary
primary
refractory
secondary (drug-induced) (due to disease)
sex-linked hypochromic
vitamin B$_6$-responsive
Pyridoxine-responsive (hypochromic) anemia

Use additional E code, if desired, to identify cause, if drug induced

285.1 **Acute posthemorrhagic anemia**

Anemia due to acute blood loss

Excludes: anemia due to chronic blood loss (280.0)
blood loss anemia NOS (280.0)

⑤ **285.2** **Anemia in chronic illness**

285.21 **Anemia in end-stage renal disease**

285.22 **Anemia in neoplastic disease**

285.29 **Anemia of other chronic illness**

285.8 **Other specified anemias**

Anemia:
dyserythropoietic (congenital)
dyshematopoietic (congenital)
leukoerythroblastic
von Jaksch's
Infantile pseudoleukemia

285.9 **Anemia, unspecified**

Anemia:
NOS
essential
normocytic, not due to blood loss
profound
progressive
secondary
Oligocythemia

Excludes: anemia (due to):
blood loss:
acute (285.1)
chronic or unspecified (280.0)
iron deficiency (280.0-280.9)

● Code new
to this edition

▲ Revision of
existing code

④ ⑤ Fourth or fifth
digit required

286 **Coagulation defects**

286.0 **Congenital factor VIII disorder**

Antihemophilic globulin [AHG] deficiency
Factor VIII (functional) deficiency

Hemophilia:
  NOS
  A
  classical
  familial
  hereditary
Subhemophilia

> Excludes: *factor VIII deficiency with vascular defect (286.4)*

286.1 **Congenital factor IX disorder**

Christmas disease
Deficiency:
  factor IX (functional)
  plasma thromboplastin component [PTC]
Hemophilia B

286.2 **Congenital factor XI deficiency**

Hemophilia C
Plasma thromboplastin antecedent [PTA] deficiency
Rosenthal's disease

286.3 **Congenital deficiency of other clotting factors**

Congenital afibrinogenemia
Deficiency:
  AC globulin factor:
    I [fibrinogen]
    II [prothrombin]
    V [labile]
    VII [stable]
    X [Stuart-Prower]
    XII [Hageman]
    XIII [fibrin stabilizing]

Deficiency:
  Laki-Lorand factor
  proaccelerin
Disease:
  Owren's
  Stuart-Prower
Dysfibrinogenemia (congenital)
Dysprothrombinemia (constitutional)
Hypoproconvertinemia
Hypoprothrombinemia (hereditary)
Parahemophilia

286.4 **von Willebrand's disease**

Angiohemophilia (A) (B)
Constitutional thrombopathy
Factor VIII deficiency with vascular defect
Pseudohemophilia type B
Vascular hemophilia
von Willebrand's (-Jürgens') disease

> Excludes: *factor VIII deficiency:*
> *NOS (286.0)*
> *with functional defect (286.0)*
> *hereditary capillary fragility (287.8)*

286.5 **Hemorrhagic disorder due to circulating anticoagulants**

Antithrombinemia
Antithromboplastinemia
Antithromboplastinogenemia
Hyperheparinemia

Increase in:
  anti-VIIIa
  anti-IXa
  anti-Xa
  anti-XIa
  antithrombin
Systemic lupus erythematosus [SLE] inhibitor

Use additional E code, if desired, to identify cause, if drug induced

286.6 **Defibrination syndrome**

Afibrinogenemia, acquired
Consumption coagulopathy
Diffuse or disseminated intravascular coagulation [DIC syndrome]
Fibrinolytic hemorrhage, acquired
Hemorrhagic fibrinogenolysis
Pathologic fibrinolysis
Purpura:
  fibrinolytic
  fulminans

> Excludes: *that complicating:*
> *abortion (634-638 with .1, 639.1)*
> *pregnancy or the puerperium (641.3, 666.3)*
> *disseminated intravascular coagulation in newborn (776.2)*

| Add 4th or 5th digit | Nonspecific code | Unspecified code | Manifestation code |

286.7 Acquired coagulation factor deficiency
Deficiency of coagulation factor due to:
liver disease
vitamin K deficiency
Hypoprothrombinemia, acquired

[Excludes:] *vitamin K deficiency of newborn (776.0)*

Use additional E-code, if desired, to identify cause, if drug induced

286.9 Other and unspecified coagulation defects
Defective coagulation NOS
Deficiency, coagulation factor NOS
Delay, coagulation
Disorder:
coagulation
hemostasis

[Excludes:] *abnormal coagulation profile (790.92)*
hemorrhagic disease of newborn (776.0)
that complicating:
abortion (634-638 with .1, 639.1)
pregnancy or the puerperium (641.3, 666.3)

287 Purpura and other hemorrhagic conditions

[Excludes:] *hemorrhagic thrombocythemia (238.7)*
purpura fulminans (286.6)

287.0 Allergic purpura
Peliosis rheumatica
Purpura:
anaphylactoid
autoimmune
Henoch's
Purpura:
nonthrombocytopenic:
hemorrhagic
idiopathic
rheumatica
Schönlein-Henoch
vascular
Vasculitis, allergic

[Excludes:] *hemorrhagic purpura (287.3)*
purpura annularis telangiectodes (709.1)

287.1 Qualitative platelet defects
Thrombasthenia (hemorrhagic) (hereditary)
Thrombocytasthenia
Thrombocytopathy (dystrophic)
Thrombopathy (Bernard-Soulier)

[Excludes:] *von Willebrand's disease (286.4)*

287.2 Other nonthrombocytopenic purpuras
Purpura:
NOS
senile
simplex

287.3 Primary thrombocytopenia
Evans' syndrome
Megakaryocytic hypoplasia
Purpura, thrombocytopenic
congenital
hereditary
idiopathic
Thrombocytopenia:
congenital
hereditary
primary
Tidal platelet dysgenesis

[Excludes:] *thrombotic thrombocytopenic purpura (446.6)*
transient thrombocytopenia of newborn (776.1)

287.4 Secondary thrombocytopenia
Posttransfusion purpura
Thrombocytopenia (due to):
dilutional
drugs
extracorporeal circulation of blood
massive blood transfusion
platelet alloimmunization

Use additional E code, if desired, to identify cause

[Excludes:] *transient thrombocytopenia of newborn (776.1)*

287.5 **Thrombocytopenia, unspecified**

287.8 **Other specified hemorrhagic conditions**
Capillary fragility (hereditary)
Vascular pseudohemophilia

287.9 **Unspecified hemorrhagic conditions**
Hemorrhagic diathesis (familial)

288 **Diseases of white blood cells**

Excludes: *leukemia (204.0-208.9)*

288.0 **Agranulocytosis**
Infantile genetic agranulo-
cytosis
Kostmann's syndrome
Neutropenia:
NOS
cyclic
Neutropenia:
drug-induced
immune
periodic
toxic
Neutropenic splenomegaly
Use additional E code, if desired, to identify drug or other cause

Excludes: *transitory neonatal neutropenia (776.7)*

288.1 **Functional disorders of polymorphonuclear neutrophils**
Chronic (childhood) granulomatous disease
Congenital dysphagocytosis
Job's syndrome
Lipochrome histiocytosis (familial)
Progressive septic granulomatosis

288.2 **Genetic anomalies of leukocytes**
Anomaly (granulation) (granulocyte) or syndrome:
Alder's (-Reilly)
Chédiak-Steinbrinck (-Higashi)
Jordan's
May-Hegglin
Pelger-Huet
Hereditary:
hypersegmentation
hyposegmentation
leukomelanopathy

288.3 **Eosinophilia**
Eosinophilia
allergic
hereditary
idiopathic
secondary
Eosinophilic leukocytosis

Excludes: *Löffler's syndrome (518.3)*
pulmonary eosinophilia (518.3)

288.8 **Other specified disease of white blood cells**
Leukemoid reaction
lymphocytic
monocytic
myelocytic
Leukocytosis
Lymphocytopenia
Lymphocytosis (symptomatic)
Lymphopenia
Monocytosis (symptomatic)
Plasmacytosis

Excludes: *immunity disorders (279.0-279.9)*

288.9 **Unspecified disease of white blood cells**

Add 4th or
5th digit

Nonspecific
code

Unspecified
code

Manifestation
code

289 **Other diseases of blood and blood-forming organs**

289.0 **Polycythemia, secondary**

High-oxygen-affinity
   hemoglobin
Polycythemia:
   acquired
   benign
   due to:
     fall in plasma volume
     high altitude

Polycythemia:
   emotional
   erythropoietin
   hypoxemic
   nephrogenous
   relative
   spurious
   stress

Excludes: *polycythemia:*
    neonatal (776.4)
    primary (238.4)
    vera (238.4)

289.1 **Chronic lymphadenitis**

Chronic:
   adenitis, any lymph node, except mesenteric
   lymphadenitis, any lymph node, except mesenteric

Excludes: *acute lymphadenitis (683)*
    mesenteric (289.2)
    enlarged glands NOS (785.6)

289.2 **Nonspecific mesenteric lymphadenitis**

Mesenteric lymphadenitis (acute) (chronic)

289.3 **Lymphadenitis, unspecified, except mesenteric**

289.4 **Hypersplenism**

"Big spleen" syndrome
Dyssplenism

Hypersplenia

Excludes: *primary splenic neutropenia (288.0)*

⑤ **289.5** **Other diseases of spleen**

289.50 **Disease of spleen, unspecified**

289.51 **Chronic congestive splenomegaly**

289.59 **Other**

Lien migrans
Perisplenitis
Splenic:
   abscess
   atrophy
   cyst

Splenic:
   fibrosis
   infarction
   rupture, nontraumatic
Splenitis
Wandering spleen

Excludes: *bilharzial splenic fibrosis (120.0-120.9)*
    hepatolienal fibrosis (571.5)
    splenomegaly NOS (789.2)

289.6 **Familial polycythemia**

Familial:
   benign polycythemia
   erythrocytosis

289.7 **Methemoglobinemia**

Congenital NADH [DPNH]-methemoglobin-reductase deficiency
Hemoglobin M [Hb-M] disease
Methemoglobinemia:
   NOS
   acquired (with sulfhemoglobinemia)
   hereditary
   toxic
Stokvis' disease
Sulfhemoglobinemia

Use additional E code, if desired, to identify cause

289.8 **Other specified diseases of blood and blood-forming organs**

Hypergammaglobulinemia
Myelofibrosis
Pseudocholinesterase deficiency

289.9 **Unspecified diseases of blood and blood-forming organs**

Blood dyscrasia NOS
Erythroid hyperplasia

● Code new
  to this edition

▲ Revision of
  existing code

④ ⑤ Fourth or fifth
    digit required

5. MENTAL DISORDERS (290-319)

In the *International Classification of Diseases, 9th Revision* (*ICD-9*), the corresponding Chapter V, "Mental Disorders," includes a glossary which defines the contents of each category. The introduction to Chapter V in *ICD-9* indicates that the glossary is intended so that psychiatrists can make the diagnosis based on the descriptions provided rather than from the category titles. Lay coders are instructed to code whatever diagnosis the physician records.

Chapter 5, "Mental Disorders," in *ICD-9-CM* uses the standard classification format with inclusion and exclusion terms, omitting the glossary as part of the main text.

The mental disorders section of *ICD-9-CM* has been expanded to incorporate additional psychiatric disorders not listed in *ICD-9*. The glossary from *ICD-9* does not contain all these terms. It now appears in Appendix B, pages 543-564 which also contains descriptions and definitions for the terms added in *ICD-9-CM*. Some of these were provided by the American Psychiatric Association's Task Force on Nomenclature and Statistics who are preparing the *Diagnostic and Statistical Manual*, Third Edition (DSM-III), and others from *A Psychiatric Glossary*.

The American Psychiatric Association provided invaluable assistance in modifying Chapter 5 of *ICD-9-CM* to incorporate detail useful to American clinicians and gave permission to use material from the aforementioned sources.

1. **Manual of the *International Statistical Classification of Diseases, Injuries, and Causes of Death*, 9th Revision, World Health Organization, Geneva, Switzerland, 1975.**
2. **American Psychiatric Association, Task Force on Nomenclature and Statistics, Robert L. Spitzer, M.D., Chairman.**
3. ***A Psychiatric Glossary*, Fourth Edition, American Psychiatric Association, Washington, D.C., 1975.**

PSYCHOSES (290-299)

[*Excludes:*] *mental retardation (317-319)*

ORGANIC PSYCHOTIC CONDITIONS (290-294)

Includes: psychotic organic brain syndrome

[*Excludes:*] *nonpsychotic syndromes of organic etiology (310.0-310.9)*
psychoses classifiable to 295-298 and without impairment of orientation, comprehension, calculation, learning capacity, and judgement, but associated with physical disease, injury, or condition affecting the brain [e.g., following childbirth] (295.0-298.8)

[290] Senile and presenile organic psychotic conditions
Code first the associated neurological condition

[*Excludes:*] *dementia not classified as senile, presenile, or arteriosclerotic (294.10-294.11)*
psychoses classifiable to 295-298 occurring in the senium without dementia or delirium (295.0-298.8)
senility with mental changes of nonpsychotic severity (310.1)
transient organic psychotic conditions (293.0-293.9)

290.0 Senile dementia, uncomplicated
Senile dementia:
NOS
simple type

[*Excludes:*] *mild memory disturbances, not amounting to dementia, associated with senile brain disease (310.1)*
senile dementia with:
delirium or confusion (290.3)
delusional [paranoid] features (290.20)
depressive features (290.21)

[5] **290.1 Presenile dementia**
Brain syndrome with presenile brain disease

[*Excludes:*] *arteriosclerotic dementia (290.40-290.43)*
dementia associated with other cerebral conditions (294.10-294.11)

290.10 Presenile dementia, uncomplicated
Presenile dementia:
NOS
simple type

290.11 Presenile dementia with delirium
Presenile dementia with acute confusional state

Add 4th or 5th digit | Nonspecific code | Unspecified code | Manifestation code

290.12 Presenile dementia with delusional features
Presenile dementia, paranoid type

290.13 Presenile dementia with depressive features
Presenile dementia, depressed type

[5] **290.2 Senile dementia with delusional or depressive features**
[Excludes:] *senile dementia:*
NOS (290.0)
with delirium and/or confusion (290.3)

290.20 Senile dementia with delusional features
Senile dementia, paranoid type
Senile psychosis NOS

290.21 Senile dementia with depressive features

290.3 Senile dementia with delirium
Senile dementia with acute confusional state
[Excludes:] *senile:*
dementia NOS (290.0)
psychosis NOS (290.20)

[5] **290.4 Arteriosclerotic dementia**
Multi-infarct dementia or psychosis
Use additional code to identify cerebral atherosclerosis (437.0)
[Excludes:] *suspected cases with no clear evidence of arteriosclerosis (290.9)*

290.40 Arteriosclerotic dementia, uncomplicated
Arteriosclerotic dementia:
NOS
simple type

290.41 Arteriosclerotic dementia with delirium
Arteriosclerotic dementia with acute confusional state

290.42 Arteriosclerotic dementia with delusional features
Arteriosclerotic dementia, paranoid type

290.43 Arteriosclerotic dementia with depressive features
Arteriosclerotic dementia, depressed type

290.8 Other specified senile psychotic conditions
Presbyophrenic psychosis

290.9 Unspecified senile psychotic condition

291 Alcoholic psychoses
[Excludes:] *alcoholism without psychosis (303.0-303.9)*

291.0 Alcohol withdrawal delirium
Alcoholic delirium
Delirium tremens
[Excludes:] *alcohol withdrawal (291.81)*

291.1 Alcohol amnestic syndrome
Alcoholic polyneuritic psychosis
Korsakoff's psychosis, alcoholic
Wernicke-Korsakoff syndrome (alcoholic)

291.2 Other alcoholic dementia
Alcoholic dementia NOS
Alcoholism associated with dementia NOS
Chronic alcoholic brain syndrome

291.3 Alcohol withdrawal hallucinosis
Alcoholic:
hallucinosis (acute)
psychosis with hallucinosis
[Excludes:] *alcohol withdrawal with delirium (291.0)*
schizophrenia (295.0-295.9) and paranoid states (297.0-297.9) taking the form of chronic hallucinosis with clear consciousness in an alcoholic

● Code new to this edition
▲ Revision of existing code
[4] [5] Fourth or fifth digit required

291.4 Idiosyncratic alcohol intoxication
Pathologic:
alcohol intoxication
drunkenness

Excludes: *acute alcohol intoxication (305.0)*
in alcoholism (303.0)
simple drunkenness (305.0)

291.5 Alcoholic jealousy
Alcoholic:
paranoia
psychosis, paranoid type

Excludes: *nonalcoholic paranoid states (297.0-297.9)*
schizophrenia, paranoid type (295.3)

⑤ **291.8 Other specified alcoholic psychosis**

291.81 Alcohol withdrawal
Alcohol:
withdrawal syndrome or symptoms
abstinence syndrome or symptoms

Excludes: *alcohol withdrawal:*
delirium (291.0)
hallucinosis (291.3)
delirium tremens (291.0)

291.89 Other

291.9 Unspecified alcoholic psychosis
Alcoholic:
mania NOS
psychosis NOS
Alcoholism (chronic) with psychosis

292 Drug psychoses
Includes: drug-induced mental disorders
organic brain syndrome associated with consumption of drugs

Use additional code for any associated drug dependence (304.0-304.9)

Use additional E code, if desired, to identify drug

292.0 Drug withdrawal syndrome
Drug:
abstinence syndrome or symptoms
withdrawal syndrome or symptoms

⑤ **292.1 Paranoid and/or hallucinatory states induced by drugs**

292.11 Drug-induced organic delusional syndrome
Paranoid state induced by drugs

292.12 Drug-induced hallucinosis
Hallucinatory state induced by drugs

Excludes: *states following LSD or other hallucinogens, lasting only a few days or less* *["bad trips"] (305.3)*

292.2 Pathological drug intoxication
Drug reaction:
NOS resulting in brief psychotic states
idiosyncratic resulting in brief psychotic states
pathologic resulting in brief psychotic states

Excludes: *expected brief psychotic reactions to hallucinogens ["bad trips"] (305.3)*
physiological side-effects of drugs (e.g., dystonias)

⑤ **292.8 Other specified drug-induced mental disorders**

292.81 Drug-induced delirium

292.82 Drug-induced dementia

292.83 Drug-induced amnestic syndrome

292.84 Drug-induced organic affective syndrome
Depressive state induced by drugs

292.89 Other
Drug-induced organic personality syndrome

292.9 Unspecified drug-induced mental disorder
Organic psychosis NOS due to or associated with drugs

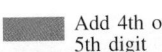

Add 4th or
5th digit   Nonspecific
code   Unspecified
code   Manifestation
code

293 Transient organic psychotic conditions

Includes: transient organic mental disorders not associated with alcohol or drugs

Code first the associated physical or neurological condition

Excludes: *confusional state or delirium superimposed on senile dementia (290.3)*
dementia due to:
alcohol (291.0-291.9)
arteriosclerosis (290.40-290.43)
drugs (292.82)
senility (290.0)

293.0 *Acute delirium*

Acute:
confusional state
infective psychosis
organic reaction
posttraumatic organic
psychosis
psycho-organic syndrome

Acute psychosis associated with endocrine, metabolic, or cerebrovascular disorder
Epileptic:
confusional state
twilight state

293.1 *Subacute delirium*

Subacute:
confusional state
infective psychosis
organic reaction
posttraumatic organic
psychosis

Subacute:
psycho-organic syndrome
psychosis associated with endocrine or metabolic
disorder

⑤ 293.8 *Other specified transient organic mental disorders*

293.81 *Organic delusional syndrome*
Transient organic psychotic condition, paranoid type

293.82 *Organic hallucinosis syndrome*
Transient organic psychotic condition, hallucinatory type

293.83 *Organic affective syndrome*
Transient organic psychotic condition, depressive type

293.84 *Organic anxiety syndrome*

293.89 *Other*

293.9 *Unspecified transient organic mental disorder*

Organic psychosis: Psycho-organic syndrome
infective NOS
posttraumatic NOS
transient NOS

294 Other organic psychotic conditions (chronic)

Includes: organic psychotic brain syndromes (chronic), not elsewhere classified

294.0 Amnestic syndrome

Korsakoff's psychosis or syndrome (nonalcoholic)

Excludes: *alcoholic:*

amnestic syndrome (291.1)
Korsakoff's psychosis (291.1)

⑤ 294.1 *Dementia in conditions classified elsewhere*

Code first any underlying physical condition, as:
dementia in:
Alzheimer's disease (331.0)
cerebral lipidoses (330.1)
epilepsy (345.0-345.9)
general paresis [syphilis] (094.1)
hepatolenticular degeneration (275.1)
Huntington's chorea (333.4)
Jakob-Creutzfeldt disease (046.1)
multiple sclerosis (340)
Pick's disease of the brain (331.1)
polyarteritis nodosa (446.0)
syphilis (094.1)

Excludes: *dementia:*

arteriosclerotic (290.40-290.43)
presenile (290.10-290.13)
senile (290.0)
epileptic psychosis NOS (294.8)

● Code new
to this edition

▲ Revision of
existing code

④ ⑤ Fourth or fifth
digit required

294.10 ***Dementia in conditions classified elsewhere without behavioral disturbance***
Dementia in conditions classified elsewhere NOS

294.11 ***Dementia in conditions classified elsewhere with behavioral disturbance***
Aggressive behavior
Combative behavior
Violent behavior
Wandering off

294.8 Other specified organic brain syndromes (chronic)
Epileptic psychosis NOS
Mixed paranoid and affective organic psychotic states

Use additional code for associated epilepsy (345.0-345.9)

[Excludes:] *mild memory disturbances, not amounting to dementia (310.1)*

294.9 Unspecified organic brain syndrome (chronic)
Organic psychosis (chronic)

OTHER PSYCHOSES (295-299)

Use additional code to identify any associated physical disease, injury, or condition affecting the brain with psychoses classifiable to 295-298

[5] **295 Schizophrenic disorders**
Includes: schizophrenia of the types described in 295.0-295.9 occurring in children

[Excludes:] *childhood type schizophrenia (299.9)*
infantile autism (299.0)

The following fifth-digit subclassification is for use with category 295:

0 unspecified
1 subchronic
2 chronic
3 subchronic with acute exacerbation
4 chronic with acute exacerbation
5 in remission

[5] **295.0 Simple type**
Schizophrenia simplex

[Excludes:] *latent schizophrenia (295.5)*

[5] **295.1 Disorganized type**
Hebephrenia
Hebephrenic type schizophrenia

[5] **295.2 Catatonic type**
Catatonic (schizophrenia):
agitation
excitation
excited type
stupor
withdrawn type

Schizophrenic:
catalepsy
catatonia
flexibilitas cerea

[5] **295.3 Paranoid type**
Paraphrenic schizophrenia

[Excludes:] *involutional paranoid state (297.2)*
paranoia (297.1)
paraphrenia (297.2)

[5] **295.4 Acute schizophrenic episode**
Oneirophrenia
Schizophreniform:
attack
disorder
psychosis, confusional type

[Excludes:] *acute forms of schizophrenia of:*
catatonic type (295.2)
hebephrenic type (295.1)
paranoid type (295.3)
simple type (295.0)
undifferentiated type (295.8)

Add 4th or 5th digit | Nonspecific code | Unspecified code | Manifestation code

⑤ **295.5 Latent schizophrenia**

Latent schizophrenic reaction
Schizophrenia:
borderline
incipient
Schizophrenia:
prepsychotic
prodromal
pseudoneurotic
pseudopsychopathic

[Excludes:] *schizoid personality (301.20-301.22)*

⑤ **295.6 Residual schizophrenia**

Chronic undifferentiated schizophrenia
Restzustand (schizophrenic)
Schizophrenic residual state

⑤ **295.7 Schizo-affective type**

Cyclic schizophrenia
Mixed schizophrenic and affective psychosis
Schizo-affective psychosis
Schizophreniform psychosis, affective type

⑤ **295.8 Other specified types of schizophrenia**

Acute (undifferentiated) schizophrenia
Atypical schizophrenia
Cenesthopathic schizophrenia

[Excludes:] *infantile autism (299.0)*

⑤ **295.9 Unspecified schizophrenia**

Schizophrenia:
NOS
mixed NOS
undifferentiated NOS
Schizophrenic reaction NOS
Schizophreniform psychosis NOS

296 Affective psychoses

Includes: episodic affective disorders

[Excludes:] *neurotic depression (300.4)*
reactive depressive psychosis (298.0)
reactive excitation (298.1)

The following fifth-digit subclassification is for use with categories 296.0-296.6:

0 unspecified
1 mild
2 moderate
3 severe, without mention of psychotic behavior
4 severe, specified as with psychotic behavior
5 in partial or unspecified remission
6 in full remission

⑤ **296.0 Manic disorder, single episode**

Hypomania (mild) NOS, single episode or unspecified
Hypomanic psychosis, single episode or unspecified
Mania (monopolar) NOS, single episode or unspecified
Manic-depressive psychosis or reaction:
hypomanic, single episode or unspecified
manic, single episode or unspecified

[Excludes:] *circular type, if there was a previous attack of depression (296.4)*

⑤ **296.1 Manic disorder, recurrent episode**

Any condition classifiable to 296.0, stated to be recurrent

[Excludes:] *circular type, if there was a previous attack of depression (296.4)*

⑤ **296.2 Major depressive disorder, single episode**

Depressive psychosis, single episode or unspecified
Endogenous depression, single episode or unspecified
Involutional melancholia, single episode or unspecified
Manic-depressive psychosis or reaction, depressed type, single episode or unspecified
Monopolar depression, single episode or unspecified
Psychotic depression, single episode or unspecified

[Excludes:] *circular type, if previous attack was of manic type (296.5)*
depression NOS (311)
reactive depression (neurotic) (300.4)
psychotic (298.0)

[5] **296.3 Major depressive disorder, recurrent episode**
Any condition classifiable to 296.2, stated to be recurrent

[Excludes:] *circular type, if previous attack was of manic type (296.5)*
depression NOS (311)
reactive depression (neurotic) (300.4)
psychotic (298.0)

[5] **296.4 Bipolar affective disorder, manic**
Bipolar disorder, now manic
Manic-depressive psychosis, circular type but currently manic

[Excludes:] *brief compensatory or rebound mood swings (296.99)*

[5] **296.5 Bipolar affective disorder, depressed**
Bipolar disorder, now depressed
Manic-depressive psychosis, circular type but currently depressed

[Excludes:] *brief compensatory or rebound mood swings (296.99)*

[5] **296.6 Bipolar affective disorder, mixed**
Manic-depressive psychosis, circular type, mixed

296.7 Bipolar affective disorder, unspecified
Atypical bipolar affective disorder NOS
Manic-depressive psychosis, circular type, current condition not specified as either manic or depressive

[5] **296.8 Manic-depressive psychosis, other and unspecified**

296.80 Manic-depressive psychosis, unspecified
Manic-depressive:
reaction NOS
syndrome NOS

296.81 Atypical manic disorder

296.82 Atypical depressive disorder

296.89 Other
Manic-depressive psychosis, mixed type

[5] **296.9 Other and unspecified affective psychoses**

[Excludes:] *psychogenic affective psychoses (298.0-298.8)*

296.90 Unspecified affective psychosis
Affective psychosis NOS
Melancholia NOS

296.99 Other specified affective psychoses
Mood swings:
brief compensatory
rebound

297 Paranoid states (Delusional disorders)
Includes: paranoid disorders

[Excludes:] *acute paranoid reaction (298.3)*
alcoholic jealousy or paranoid state (291.5)
paranoid schizophrenia (295.3)

297.0 Paranoid state, simple

297.1 Paranoia
Chronic paranoid psychosis
Sander's disease
Systematized delusions

[Excludes:] *paranoid personality disorder (301.0)*

297.2 Paraphrenia
Involutional paranoid state
Late paraphrenia
Paraphrenia (involutional)

297.3 Shared paranoid disorder
Folie à deux
Induced psychosis or paranoid disorder

297.8 Other specified paranoid states
Paranoia querulans
Sensitiver Beziehungswahn

[Excludes:] *acute paranoid reaction or state (298.3)*
senile paranoid state (290.20)

297.9 Unspecified paranoid state
Paranoid:
disorder NOS
psychosis

Paranoid:
reaction NOS
state NOS

298 Other nonorganic psychoses
Includes: psychotic conditions due to or provoked by:
emotional stress
environmental factors as major part of etiology

298.0 Depressive type psychosis
Psychogenic depressive psychosis
Psychotic reactive depression
Reactive depressive psychosis

[Excludes:] *manic-depressive psychosis, depressed type (296.2-296.3)*
neurotic depression (300.4)
reactive depression NOS (300.4)

298.1 Excitative type psychosis
Acute hysterical psychosis
Psychogenic excitation
Reactive excitation

[Excludes:] *manic-depressive psychosis, manic type (296.0-296.1)*

298.2 Reactive confusion
Psychogenic confusion
Psychogenic twilight state

[Excludes:] *acute confusional state (293.0)*

298.3 Acute paranoid reaction
Acute psychogenic paranoid psychosis
Bouffée délirante

[Excludes:] *paranoid states (297.0-297.9)*

298.4 Psychogenic paranoid psychosis
Protracted reactive paranoid psychosis

298.8 Other and unspecified reactive psychosis
Brief reactive psychosis NOS
Hysterical psychosis
Psychogenic psychosis NOS
Psychogenic stupor

[Excludes:] *acute hysterical psychosis (298.1)*

298.9 Unspecified psychosis
Atypical psychosis
Psychosis NOS

⑤ **299 Psychoses with origin specific to childhood**
Includes: pervasive developmental disorders

[Excludes:] *adult type psychoses occurring in childhood, as:*
affective disorders (296.0-296.9)
manic-depressive disorders (296.0-296.9)
schizophrenia (295.0-295.9)

The following fifth-digit subclassification is for use with category 299:

0 current or active state

1 residual state

⑤ **299.0 Infantile autism**
Childhood autism
Infantile psychosis
Kanner's syndrome

[Excludes:] *disintegrative psychosis (299.1)*
Heller's syndrome (299.1)
schizophrenic syndrome of childhood (299.9)

● Code new to this edition ▲ Revision of existing code ④ ⑤ Fourth or fifth digit required

[5] **299.1 Disintegrative psychosis**
Heller's syndrome

Use additional code to identify any associated neurological disorder

[*Excludes:*] *infantile autism (299.0)*
schizophrenic syndrome of childhood (299.9)

[5] **299.8 Other specified early childhood psychoses**
Atypical childhood psychosis
Borderline psychosis of childhood

[*Excludes:*] *simple stereotypies without psychotic disturbance (307.3)*

[5] **299.9 Unspecified**
Child psychosis NOS
Schizophrenia, childhood type NOS
Schizophrenic syndrome of childhood NOS

[*Excludes:*] *schizophrenia of adult type occurring in childhood (295.0-295.9)*

NEUROTIC DISORDERS, PERSONALITY DISORDERS, AND OTHER NONPSYCHOTIC MENTAL DISORDERS (300-316)

300 Neurotic disorders

[5] **300.0 Anxiety states**

[*Excludes:*] *anxiety in:*
acute stress reaction (308.0)
transient adjustment reaction (309.24)
neurasthenia (300.5)
psychophysiological disorders (306.0-306.9)
separation anxiety (309.21)

300.00 Anxiety state, unspecified
Anxiety:
neurosis
reaction
state (neurotic)
Atypical anxiety disorder

300.01 Panic disorder
Panic:
attack
state

300.02 Generalized anxiety disorder

300.09 Other

[5] **300.1 Hysteria**

[*Excludes:*] *adjustment reaction (309.0-309.9)*
anorexia nervosa (307.1)
gross stress reaction (308.0-308.9)
hysterical personality (301.50-301.59)
psychophysiologic disorders (306.0-306.9)

300.10 Hysteria, unspecified

300.11 Conversion disorder
Astasia-abasia, hysterical
Conversion hysteria or reaction
Hysterical:
blindness
deafness
paralysis

300.12 Psychogenic amnesia
Hysterical amnesia

300.13 Psychogenic fugue
Hysterical fugue

300.14 Multiple personality
Dissociative identity disorder

300.15 Dissociative disorder or reaction, unspecified

300.16 Factitious illness with psychological symptoms
Compensation neurosis
Ganser's syndrome, hysterical

Add 4th or 5th digit | Nonspecific code | Unspecified code | Manifestation code

300.19 **Other and unspecified factitious illness**
Factitious illness (with physical symptoms) NOS

Excludes: *multiple operations or hospital addiction syndrome (301.51)*

⑤ **300.2** **Phobic disorders**

Excludes: *anxiety state not associated with a specific situation or object (300.0-300.09)*
obsessional phobias (300.3)

300.20 **Phobia, unspecified**
Anxiety-hysteria NOS
Phobia NOS

300.21 **Agoraphobia with panic attacks**
Fear of:
open spaces with panic attacks
streets with panic attacks
travel with panic attacks

300.22 **Agoraphobia without mention of panic attacks**
Any condition classifiable to 300.21 without mention of panic attacks

300.23 **Social phobia**
Fear of:
eating in public
public speaking
washing in public

300.29 **Other isolated or simple phobias**
Acrophobia   Claustrophobia
Animal phobias   Fear of crowds

300.3 **Obsessive-compulsive disorders**
Anancastic neurosis   Obsessional phobia [any]
Compulsive neurosis

Excludes: *obsessive-compulsive symptoms occurring in:*
endogenous depression (296.2-296.3)
organic states (e.g., encephalitis)
schizophrenia (295.0-295.9)

300.4 **Neurotic depression**
Anxiety depression   Dysthymic disorder
Depression with anxiety   Neurotic depressive state
Depressive reaction   Reactive depression

Excludes: *adjustment reaction with depressive symptoms (309.0-309.1)*
depression NOS (311)
manic-depressive psychosis, depressed type (296.2-296.3)
reactive depressive psychosis (298.0)

300.5 **Neurasthenia**
Fatigue neurosis   Psychogenic:
Nervous debility   asthenia
                 general fatigue
Use additional code to identify any associated physical disorder

Excludes: *anxiety state (300.00-300.09)*
neurotic depression (300.4)
psychophysiological disorders (306.0-306.9)
specific nonpsychotic mental disorders following organic brain damage
(310.0-310.9)

300.6 **Depersonalization syndrome**
Depersonalization disorder
Derealization (neurotic)
Neurotic state with depersonalization episode

Excludes: *depersonalization associated with:*
anxiety (300.00-300.09)
depression (300.4)
manic-depressive disorder or psychosis (296.0-296.9)
schizophrenia (295.0-295.9)

    ● Code new   ▲ Revision of   ④ ⑤ Fourth or fifth
        to this edition   existing code   digit required

300.7 Hypochondriasis
Body dysmorphic disorder

[Excludes:] *hypochondriasis in:*
hysteria (300.10-300.19)
manic-depressive psychosis, depressed type (296.2-296.3)
neurasthenia (300.5)
obsessional disorder (300.3)
schizophrenia (295.0-295.9)

[5] **300.8 Other neurotic disorders**

300.81 Somatization disorder
Briquet's disorder
Severe somatoform disorder

300.82 Undifferentiated somatoform disorder
Atypical somatoform disorder
Somatoform disorder NOS

300.89 Other
Occupational neurosis, including writers' cramp
Psychasthenia
Psychasthenic neurosis

300.9 Unspecified neurotic disorder
Neurosis NOS
Psychoneurosis NOS

301 Personality disorders
Includes: character neurosis

Use additional code to identify any associated neurosis or psychosis, or physical condition

[Excludes:] *nonpsychotic personality disorder associated with organic brain syndromes (310.0-310.9)*

301.0 Paranoid personality disorder
Fanatic personality
Paranoid personality (disorder)
Paranoid traits

[Excludes:] *acute paranoid reaction (298.3)*
alcoholic paranoia (291.5)
paranoid schizophrenia (295.3)
paranoid states (297.0-297.9)

[5] **301.1 Affective personality disorder**

[Excludes:] *affective psychotic disorders (296.0-296.9)*
neurasthenia (300.5)
neurotic depression (300.4)

301.10 Affective personality disorder, unspecified

301.11 Chronic hypomanic personality disorder
Chronic hypomanic disorder
Hypomanic personality

301.12 Chronic depressive personality disorder
Chronic depressive disorder
Depressive character or personality

301.13 Cyclothymic disorder
Cycloid personality
Cyclothymia
Cyclothymic personality

[5] **301.2 Schizoid personality disorder**

[Excludes:] *schizophrenia (295.0-295.9)*

301.20 Schizoid personality disorder, unspecified

301.21 Introverted personality

301.22 Schizotypal personality

301.3 Explosive personality disorder
Aggressive:
personality
reaction
Aggressiveness
Emotional instability (excessive)
Pathological emotionality
Quarrelsomeness

[Excludes:] *dyssocial personality (301.7)*
hysterical neurosis (300.10-300.19)

301.4 Compulsive personality disorder
Anancastic personality
Obsessional personality

Excludes: *obsessive-compulsive disorder (300.3)*
phobic state (300.20-300.29)

⑤ **301.5 Histrionic personality disorder**

Excludes: *hysterical neurosis (300.10-300.19)*

301.50 Histrionic personality disorder, unspecified
Hysterical personality NOS

301.51 Chronic factitious illness with physical symptoms
Hospital addiction syndrome
Multiple operations syndrome
Munchausen syndrome

301.59 Other histrionic personality disorder
Personality:
emotionally unstable
labile
psychoinfantile

301.6 Dependent personality disorder
Asthenic personality   Passive personality
Inadequate personality

Excludes: *neurasthenia (300.5)*
passive-aggressive personality (301.84)

301.7 Antisocial personality disorder
Amoral personality
Asocial personality
Dyssocial personality
Personality disorder with predominantly sociopathic or asocial manifestation

Excludes: *disturbance of conduct without specifiable personality disorder (312.0-312.9)*
explosive personality (301.3)

⑤ **301.8 Other personality disorders**

301.81 Narcissistic personality

301.82 Avoidant personality

301.83 Borderline personality

301.84 Passive-aggressive personality

301.89 Other
Personality: Personality:
eccentric   masochistic
"haltlose" type   psychoneurotic
immature

Excludes: *psychoinfantile personality (301.59)*

301.9 Unspecified personality disorder
Pathological personality   Psychopathic:
NOS   constitutional state
Personality disorder NOS   personality (disorder)

302 Sexual deviations and disorders

Excludes: *sexual disorder manifest in:*
organic brain syndrome (290.0-294.9, 310.0-310.9)
psychosis (295.0-298.9)

302.0 Ego-dystonic homosexuality
Ego-dystonic lesbianism
Homosexual conflict disorder

Excludes: *homosexual pedophilia (302.2)*

302.1 Zoophilia
Bestiality

302.2 Pedophilia

302.3 Transvestism

Excludes: *trans-sexualism (302.5)*

302.4 Exhibitionism

● Code new   ▲ Revision of   ④ ⑤ Fourth or fifth
to this edition   existing code   digit required

⑤ **302.5 Trans-sexualism**

Excludes: *transvestism (302.3)*

> **302.50 With unspecified sexual history**
>
> **302.51 With asexual history**
>
> **302.52 With homosexual history**
>
> **302.53 With heterosexual history**

302.6 Disorders of psychosexual identity
Feminism in boys
Gender identity disorder of childhood

Excludes: *gender identity disorder in adult (302.85)*
homosexuality (302.0)
trans-sexualism (302.50-302.53)
transvestism (302.3)

⑤ **302.7 Psychosexual dysfunction**

Excludes: *impotence of organic origin (607.84)*
normal transient symptoms from ruptured hymen
transient or occasional failures of erection due to fatigue, anxiety, alcohol, or
drugs

> **302.70 Psychosexual dysfunction, unspecified**
>
> **302.71 With inhibited sexual desire**
>
> **302.72 With inhibited sexual excitement**
> Frigidity
> Impotence
>
> **302.73 With inhibited female orgasm**
>
> **302.74 With inhibited male orgasm**
>
> **302.75 With premature ejaculation**
>
> **302.76 With functional dyspareunia**
> Dyspareunia, psychogenic
>
> **302.79 With other specified psychosexual dysfunctions**

⑤ **302.8 Other specified psychosexual disorders**

> **302.81 Fetishism**
>
> **302.82 Voyeurism**
>
> **302.83 Sexual masochism**
>
> **302.84 Sexual sadism**
>
> **302.85 Gender identity disorder of adolescent or adult life**
>
> **302.89 Other**
> Nymphomania
> Satyriasis

302.9 Unspecified psychosexual disorder
Pathologic sexuality NOS
Sexual deviation NOS

⑤ **303 Alcohol dependence syndrome**
Use additional code to identify any associated condition, as:
alcoholic psychoses (291.0-291.9)
drug dependence (304.0-304.9)
physical complications of alcohol, such as:
cerebral degeneration (331.7)
cirrhosis of liver (571.2)
epilepsy (345.0-345.9)
gastritis (535.3)
hepatitis (571.1)
liver damage NOS (571.3)

Excludes: *drunkenness NOS (305.0)*
The following fifth-digit subclassification is for use with category 303:

> **0 unspecified**
>
> **1 continuous**
>
> **2 episodic**
>
> **3 in remission**

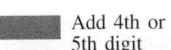

| Add 4th or 5th digit | Nonspecific code | Unspecified code | Manifestation code |

[5] **303.0 Acute alcoholic intoxication**
Acute drunkenness in alcoholism

[5] **303.9 Other and unspecified alcohol dependence**
Chronic alcoholism
Dipsomania

[5] **304 Drug dependence**

[Excludes:] *nondependent abuse of drugs (305.1-305.9)*

The following fifth-digit subclassification is for use with category 304:

0 unspecified
1 continuous
2 episodic
3 in remission

[5] **304.0 Opioid type dependence**
Heroin
Meperidine
Methadone
Morphine
Opium
Opium alkaloids and their derivatives
Synthetics with morphine-like effects

[5] **304.1 Barbiturate and similarly acting sedative or hypnotic dependence**
Barbiturates
Nonbarbiturate sedatives and tranquilizers with a similar effect:
chlordiazepoxide
diazepam
glutethimide
meprobamate
methaqualone

[5] **304.2 Cocaine dependence**
Coca leaves and derivatives

[5] **304.3 Cannabis dependence**
Hashish
Hemp
Marihuana

[5] **304.4 Amphetamine and other psychostimulant dependence**
Methylphenidate
Phenmetrazine

[5] **304.5 Hallucinogen dependence**
Dimethyltryptamine [DMT]
Lysergic acid diethylamide [LSD] and derivatives
Mescaline
Psilocybin

[5] **304.6 Other specified drug dependence**
Absinthe addiction
Glue sniffing

[Excludes:] *tobacco dependence (305.1)*

[5] **304.7 Combinations of opioid type drug with any other**

[5] **304.8 Combinations of drug dependence excluding opioid type drug**

[5] **304.9 Unspecified drug dependence**
Drug addiction NOS
Drug dependence NOS

[5] **305 Nondependent abuse of drugs**

Note: Includes cases where a person, for whom no other diagnosis is possible, has come under medical care because of the maladaptive effect of a drug on which he is not dependent and that he has taken on his own initiative to the detriment of his health or social functioning.

[Excludes:] *alcohol dependence syndrome (303.0-303.9)*
drug dependence (304.0-304.9)
drug withdrawal syndrome (292.0)
poisoning by drugs or medicinal substances (960.0-979.9)

The following fifth-digit subclassification is for use with codes 305.0, 305.2-305.9:

0 unspecified
1 continuous
2 episodic
3 in remission

● Code new to this edition
▲ Revision of existing code
[4] [5] Fourth or fifth digit required

⑤ **305.0 Alcohol abuse**
    Drunkenness NOS   "Hangover" (alcohol)
    Excessive drinking of alcohol NOS   Inebriety NOS

    Excludes: *acute alcohol intoxication in alcoholism (303.0)*
               alcoholic psychoses (291.0-291.9)

305.1 Tobacco use disorder
    Tobacco dependence

    Excludes: *history of tobacco use (V15.82)*

⑤ **305.2 Cannabis abuse**

⑤ **305.3 Hallucinogen abuse**
    Acute intoxication from hallucinogens ["bad trips"]
    LSD reaction

⑤ **305.4 Barbiturate and similarly acting sedative or hypnotic abuse**

⑤ **305.5 Opioid abuse**

⑤ **305.6 Cocaine abuse**

⑤ **305.7 Amphetamine or related acting sympathomimetic abuse**

⑤ **305.8 Antidepressant type abuse**

⑤ **305.9 Other, mixed, or unspecified drug abuse**
    "Laxative habit"
    Misuse of drugs NOS
    Nonprescribed use of drugs or patent medicinals

306 Physiological malfunction arising from mental factors
    Includes: psychogenic:
             physical symptoms not involving tissue damage
             physiological manifestation not involving tissue damage

    Excludes: *hysteria (300.11-300.19)*
             physical symptoms secondary to a psychiatric disorder classified elsewhere
             psychic factors associated with physical conditions involving tissue damage
                classified elsewhere (316)
             specific nonpsychotic mental disorders following organic brain damage
                (310.0-310.9)

306.0 Musculoskeletal
    Psychogenic paralysis   Psychogenic torticollis

    Excludes: *Gilles de la Tourette's syndrome (307.23)*
             paralysis as hysterical or conversion reaction (300.11)
             tics (307.20-307.22)

306.1 Respiratory
    Psychogenic:
        air hunger
        cough
        hiccough
        hyperventilation
        yawning

    Excludes: *psychogenic asthma (316 and 493.9)*

306.2 Cardiovascular
    Cardiac neurosis
    Cardiovascular neurosis
    Neurocirculatory asthenia
    Psychogenic cardiovascular disorder

    Excludes: *psychogenic paroxysmal tachycardia (316 and 427.2)*

306.3 Skin
    Psychogenic pruritus

    Excludes: *psychogenic:*
             alopecia (316 and 704.00)
             dermatitis (316 and 692.9)
             eczema (316 and 691.8 or 692.9)
             urticaria (316 and 708.0-708.9)

■ Add 4th or   ■ Nonspecific   ■ Unspecified   ■ Manifestation
   5th digit   code   code   code

306.4 Gastrointestinal

Aerophagy
Cyclical vomiting, psychogenic
Diarrhea, psychogenic
Nervous gastritis
Psychogenic dyspepsia

[Excludes:] *cyclical vomiting NOS (536.2)*
globus hystericus (300.11)
mucous colitis (316 and 564.9)
psychogenic:
cardiospasm (316 and 530.0)
duodenal ulcer (316 and 532.0-532.9)
gastric ulcer (316 and 531.0-531.9)
peptic ulcer NOS (316 and 533.0-533.9)
vomiting NOS (307.54)

[5] **306.5 Genitourinary**

[Excludes:] *enuresis, psychogenic (307.6)*
frigidity (302.72)
impotence (302.72)
psychogenic dyspareunia (302.76)

306.50 Psychogenic genitourinary malfunction, unspecified

306.51 Psychogenic vaginismus
Functional vaginismus

306.52 Psychogenic dysmenorrhea

306.53 Psychogenic dysuria

306.59 Other

306.6 Endocrine

306.7 Organs of special sense

[Excludes:] *hysterical blindness or deafness (300.11)*
psychophysical visual disturbances (368.16)

306.8 Other specified psychophysiological malfunction

Bruxism
Teeth grinding

306.9 Unspecified psychophysiological malfunction

Psychophysiologic disorder NOS
Psychosomatic disorder NOS

307 Special symptoms or syndromes, not elsewhere classified

Note: This category is intended for use if the psychopathology is manifested by a single specific symptom or group of symptoms which is not part of an organic illness or other mental disorder classifiable elsewhere.

[Excludes:] *those due to mental disorders classified elsewhere*
those of organic origin

307.0 Stammering and stuttering

[Excludes:] *dysphasia (784.5)*
lisping or lalling (307.9)
retarded development of speech (315.31-315.39)

307.1 Anorexia nervosa

[Excludes:] *eating disturbance NOS (307.50)*
feeding problem (783.3)
of nonorganic origin (307.59)
loss of appetite (783.0)
of nonorganic origin (307.59)

[5] **307.2 Tics**

[Excludes:] *nail-biting or thumb-sucking (307.9)*
stereotypies occurring in isolation (307.3)
tics of organic origin (333.3)

307.20 Tic disorder, unspecified

307.21 Transient tic disorder of childhood

307.22 Chronic motor tic disorder

307.23 Gilles de la Tourette's disorder
Motor-verbal tic disorder

307.3 Stereotyped repetitive movements

Body-rocking Spasmus nutans
Head banging Stereotypies NOS

Excludes: tics (307.20-307.23)
of organic origin (333.3)

⑤ **307.4 Specific disorders of sleep of nonorganic origin**

Excludes: narcolepsy (347)
those of unspecified cause (780.50-780.59)

307.40 Nonorganic sleep disorder, unspecified

307.41 Transient disorder of initiating or maintaining sleep
Hyposomnia associated with acute or intermittent emotional reactions or
conflicts
Insomnia associated with acute or intermittent emotional reactions or conflicts
Sleeplessness associated with acute or intermittent emotional reactions or
conflicts

307.42 Persistent disorder of initiating or maintaining sleep
Hyposomnia, insomnia, or sleeplessness associated with:
anxiety
conditioned arousal
depression (major) (minor)
psychosis

307.43 Transient disorder of initiating or maintaining wakefulness
Hypersomnia associated with acute or intermittent emotional reactions or
conflicts

307.44 Persistent disorder of initiating or maintaining wakefulness
Hypersomnia associated with depression (major) (minor)

307.45 Phase-shift disruption of 24-hour sleep-wake cycle
Irregular sleep-wake rhythm, nonorganic origin
Jet lag syndrome
Rapid time-zone change
Shifting sleep-work schedule

307.46 Somnambulism or night terrors

307.47 Other dysfunctions of sleep stages or arousal from sleep
Nightmares: Sleep drunkenness
NOS
REM-sleep type

307.48 Repetitive intrusions of sleep
Repetitive intrusion of sleep with:
atypical polysomnographic features
environmental disturbances
repeated REM-sleep interruptions

307.49 Other
"Short-sleeper"
Subjective insomnia complaint

⑤ **307.5 Other and unspecified disorders of eating**

Excludes: anorexia:
nervosa (307.1)
of unspecified cause (783.0)
overeating, of unspecified cause (783.6)
vomiting:
NOS (787.0)
cyclical (536.2)
psychogenic (306.4)

307.50 Eating disorder, unspecified

307.51 Bulimia
Overeating of nonorganic origin

307.52 Pica
Perverted appetite of nonorganic origin

307.53 Psychogenic rumination
Regurgitation, of nonorganic origin, of food with reswallowing

Excludes: obsessional rumination (300.3)

307.54 Psychogenic vomiting

■ Add 4th or ■ Nonspecific ■ Unspecified ■ Manifestation
5th digit code code code

`307.59` **Other**
Infantile feeding disturbances of nonorganic origin
Loss of appetite of nonorganic origin

307.6 Enuresis
Enuresis (primary) (secondary) of nonorganic origin
Excludes: *enuresis of unspecified cause (788.3)*

307.7 Encopresis
Encopresis (continuous) (discontinuous) of nonorganic origin
Excludes: *encopresis of unspecified cause (787.6)*

⑤ **307.8 Psychalgia**

`307.80` **Psychogenic pain, site unspecified**

`307.81` **Tension headache**
Excludes: *headache:*
NOS (784.0)
migraine (346.0-346.9)

`307.89` **Other**
Psychogenic backache
Excludes: *pains not specifically attributable to a psychological cause (in):*
back (724.5)
joint (719.4)
limb (729.5)
lumbago (724.2)
rheumatic (729.0)

`307.9` **Other and unspecified special symptoms or syndromes, not elsewhere classified**

Hair plucking	Masturbation
Lalling	Nail-biting
Lisping	Thumb-sucking

`308` **Acute reaction to stress**
Includes: catastrophic stress
combat fatigue
gross stress reaction (acute)
transient disorders in response to exceptional physical or mental stress which
usually subside within hours or days
Excludes: *adjustment reaction or disorder (309.0-309.9)*
chronic stress reaction (309.1-309.9)

308.0 Predominant disturbance of emotions
Anxiety as acute reaction to exceptional [gross] stress
Emotional crisis as acute reaction to exceptional [gross] stress
Panic state as acute reaction to exceptional [gross] stress

308.1 Predominant disturbance of consciousness
Fugues as acute reaction to exceptional [gross] stress

308.2 Predominant psychomotor disturbance
Agitation states as acute reaction to exceptional [gross] stress
Stupor as acute reaction to exceptional [gross] stress

`308.3` **Other acute reactions to stress**
Acute situational disturbance
Brief or acute posttraumatic stress disorder
Excludes: *prolonged posttraumatic emotional disturbance (309.81)*

308.4 Mixed disorders as reaction to stress

`308.9` **Unspecified acute reaction to stress**

`309` **Adjustment reaction**
Includes: adjustment disorders
reaction (adjustment) to chronic stress
Excludes: *acute reaction to major stress (308.0-308.9)*
neurotic disorders (300.0-300.9)

● Code new
to this edition
▲ Revision of
existing code
④ ⑤ Fourth or fifth
digit required

309.0 Brief depressive reaction
Adjustment disorder with depressed mood
Grief reaction

[Excludes:] *affective psychoses (296.0-296.9)*
neurotic depression (300.4)
prolonged depressive reaction (309.1)
psychogenic depressive psychosis (298.0)

309.1 Prolonged depressive reaction

[Excludes:] *affective psychoses (296.0-296.9)*
brief depressive reaction (309.0)
neurotic depression (300.4)
psychogenic depressive psychosis (298.0)

[5] **309.2 With predominant disturbance of other emotions**

309.21 Separation anxiety disorder

309.22 Emancipation disorder of adolescence and early adult life

309.23 Specific academic or work inhibition

309.24 Adjustment reaction with anxious mood

309.28 Adjustment reaction with mixed emotional features
Adjustment reaction with anxiety and depression

309.29 Other
Culture shock

309.3 With predominant disturbance of conduct
Conduct disturbance as adjustment reaction
Destructiveness as adjustment reaction

[Excludes:] *destructiveness in child (312.9)*
disturbance of conduct NOS (312.9)
dyssocial behavior without manifest psychiatric disorder (V71.01-V71.02)
personality disorder with predominantly sociopathic or asocial manifestations (301.7)

309.4 With mixed disturbance of emotions and conduct

[5] **309.8 Other specified adjustment reactions**

309.81 Prolonged posttraumatic stress disorder
Chronic posttraumatic stress disorder
Concentration camp syndrome

[Excludes:] *posttraumatic brain syndrome:*
nonpsychotic (310.2)
psychotic (293.0-293.9)

309.82 Adjustment reaction with physical symptoms

309.83 Adjustment reaction with withdrawal
Elective mutism as adjustment reaction
Hospitalism (in children) NOS

309.89 Other

309.9 Unspecified adjustment reaction
Adaptation reaction NOS
Adjustment reaction NOS

310 Specific nonpsychotic mental disorders due to organic brain damage

[Excludes:] *neuroses, personality disorders, or other nonpsychotic conditions occurring in a form similar to that seen with functional disorders but in association with a physical condition (300.0-300.9, 301.0-301.9)*

310.0 Frontal lobe syndrome
Lobotomy syndrome
Postleucotomy syndrome [state]

[Excludes:] *postcontusion syndrome (310.2)*

310.1 Organic personality syndrome
Cognitive or personality change of other type, of nonpsychotic severity
Mild memory disturbance
Organic psychosyndrome of nonpsychotic severity
Presbyophrenia NOS
Senility with mental changes of nonpsychotic severity

310.2 Postconcussion syndrome
Postcontusion syndrome or encephalopathy
Posttraumatic brain syndrome, nonpsychotic
Status postcommotio cerebri

Excludes: *frontal lobe syndrome (310.0)*
postencephalitic syndrome (310.8)
any organic psychotic conditions following head injury (293.0—294.0)

310.8 Other specified nonpsychotic mental disorders following organic brain damage
Postencephalitic syndrome
Other focal (partial) organic psychosyndromes

310.9 Unspecified nonpsychotic mental disorder following organic brain damage

311 Depressive disorder, not elsewhere classified
Depressive disorder NOS
Depressive state NOS
Depression NOS

Excludes: *acute reaction to major stress with depressive symptoms (308.0)*
affective personality disorder (301.10-301.13)
affective psychoses (296.0-296.9)
brief depressive reaction (309.0)
depressive states associated with stressful events (309.0-309.1)
disturbance of emotions specific to childhood and adolescence, with misery and unhappiness (313.1)
mixed adjustment reaction with depressive symptoms (309.4)
neurotic depression (300.4)
prolonged depressive adjustment reaction (309.1)
psychogenic depressive psychosis (298.0)

312 Disturbance of conduct, not elsewhere classified

Excludes: *adjustment reaction with disturbance of conduct (309.3)*
drug dependence (304.0-304.9)
dyssocial behavior without manifest psychiatric disorder (V71.01-V71.02)
personality disorder with predominantly sociopathic or asocial manifestations (301.7)
sexual deviations (302.0-302.9)

The following fifth-digit subclassification is for use with categories 312.0-312.2:

0 unspecified

1 mild

2 moderate

3 severe

⑤ **312.0 Undersocialized conduct disorder, aggressive type**
Aggressive outburst   Unsocialized aggressive disorder
Anger reaction

⑤ **312.1 Undersocialized conduct disorder, unaggressive type**
Childhood truancy,   Solitary stealing
unsocialized   Tantrums

⑤ **312.2 Socialized conduct disorder**
Childhood truancy, socialized
Group delinquency

Excludes: *gang activity without manifest psychiatric disorder (V71.01)*

⑤ **312.3 Disorders of impulse control, not elsewhere classified**

312.30 Impulse control disorder, unspecified

312.31 Pathological gambling

312.32 Kleptomania

312.33 Pyromania

312.34 Intermittent explosive disorder

312.35 Isolated explosive disorder

312.39 Other

312.4 Mixed disturbance of conduct and emotions
Neurotic delinquency

Excludes: *compulsive conduct disorder (312.3)*

⑤ **312.8 Other specified disturbances of conduct, not elsewhere classified**

● Code new   ▲ Revision of   ④ ⑤ Fourth or fifth
   to this edition   existing code   digit required

312.81 Conduct disorder, childhood onset type

312.82 Conduct disorder, adolescent onset type

312.89 Other conduct disorder

312.9 Unspecified disturbance of conduct
Delinquency (juvenile)

313 Disturbance of emotions specific to childhood and adolescence

[Excludes:] *adjustment reaction (309.0-309.9)*
emotional disorder of neurotic type (300.0-300.9)
masturbation, nail-biting, thumb-sucking, and other isolated symptoms (307.0-307.9)

313.0 Overanxious disorder
Anxiety and fearfulness of childhood and adolescence
Overanxious disorder of childhood and adolescence

[Excludes:] *abnormal separation anxiety (309.21)*
anxiety states (300.00-300.09)
hospitalism in children (309.83)
phobic state (300.20-300.29)

313.1 Misery and unhappiness disorder

[Excludes:] *depressive neurosis (300.4)*

[5] **313.2 Sensitivity, shyness, and social withdrawal disorder**

[Excludes:] *infantile autism (299.0)*
schizoid personality (301.20-301.22)
schizophrenia (295.0-295.9)

313.21 Shyness disorder of childhood
Sensitivity reaction of childhood or adolescence

313.22 Introverted disorder of childhood
Social withdrawal of childhood or adolescence
Withdrawal reaction of childhood or adolescence

313.23 Elective mutism

[Excludes:] *elective mutism as adjustment reaction (309.83)*

313.3 Relationship problems
Sibling jealousy

[Excludes:] *relationship problems associated with aggression, destruction, or other forms of conduct disturbance (312.0-312.9)*

[5] **313.8 Other or mixed emotional disturbances of childhood or adolescence**

313.81 Oppositional disorder

313.82 Identity disorder

313.83 Academic underachievement disorder

313.89 Other

313.9 Unspecified emotional disturbance of childhood or adolescence

314 Hyperkinetic syndrome of childhood

[Excludes:] *hyperkinesis as symptom of underlying disorder—code the underlying disorder*

[5] **314.0 Attention deficit disorder**
Adult
Child

314.00 Without mention of hyperactivity
Predominantly inattentive type

314.01 With hyperactivity
Combined type
Overactivity NOS
Predominantly hyperactive/impulsive type
Simple disturbance of attention with overactivity

314.1 Hyperkinesis with developmental delay
Developmental disorder of hyperkinesis

Use additional code to identify any associated neurological disorder

314.2 Hyperkinetic conduct disorder
Hyperkinetic conduct disorder without developmental delay

[Excludes:] *hyperkinesis with significant delays in specific skills (314.1)*

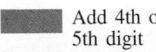

314.8 **Other specified manifestations of hyperkinetic syndrome**

314.9 **Unspecified hyperkinetic syndrome**
Hyperkinetic reaction of childhood or adolescence NOS
Hyperkinetic syndrome NOS

315 **Specific delays in development**
Excludes: *that due to a neurological disorder (320.0-389.9)*

⑤ **315.0** **Specific reading disorder**

315.00 **Reading disorder, unspecified**

315.01 **Alexia**

315.02 **Developmental dyslexia**

315.09 **Other**
Specific spelling difficulty

315.1 **Specific arithmetical disorder**
Dyscalculia

315.2 **Other specific learning difficulties**
Excludes: *specific arithmetical disorder (315.1)*
specific reading disorder (315.00-315.09)

⑤ **315.3** **Developmental speech or language disorder**

315.31 **Developmental language disorder**
Developmental aphasia
Expressive language disorder
Word deafness

Excludes: *acquired aphasia (784.3)*
elective mutism (309.83, 313.0, 313.23)

315.32 **Receptive language disorder (mixed)**
Receptive expressive language disorder

315.39 **Other**
Developmental articulation disorder
Dyslalia

Excludes: *lisping and lalling (307.9)*
stammering and stuttering (307.0)

315.4 **Coordination disorder**
Clumsiness syndrome
Dyspraxia syndrome
Specific motor development disorder

315.5 **Mixed development disorder**

315.8 **Other specified delays in development**

315.9 **Unspecified delay in development**
Developmental disorder NOS

316 **Psychic factors associated with diseases classified elsewhere**
Psychologic factors in physical conditions classified elsewhere
Use additional code to identify the associated physical condition, as:
psychogenic:
asthma (493.9)
dermatitis (692.9)
duodenal ulcer (532.0-532.9)
eczema (691.8, 692.9)
gastric ulcer (531.0-531.9)
mucous colitis (564.9)
paroxysmal tachycardia (427.2)
ulcerative colitis (556)
urticaria (708.0-708.9)
psychosocial dwarfism (259.4)

Excludes: *physical symptoms and physiological malfunctions, not involving tissue damage, of*
mental origin (306.0-306.9)

● Code new
to this edition
▲ Revision of
existing code
④ ⑤ Fourth or fifth
digit required

MENTAL RETARDATION (317-319)

Use additional code(s) to identify any associated psychiatric or physical condition(s)

317 Mild mental retardation
High-grade defect   Mild mental subnormality
IQ 50-70

318 Other specified mental retardation

    318.0 Moderate mental retardation
        IQ 35-49   Moderate mental subnormality

    318.1 Severe mental retardation
        IQ 20-34
        Severe mental subnormality

    318.2 Profound mental retardation
        IQ under 20   Profound mental subnormality

319 Unspecified mental retardation
Mental deficiency NOS   Mental subnormality NOS

 Add 4th or 5th digit   Nonspecific code   Unspecified code   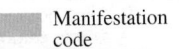 Manifestation code

● Code new
to this edition

▲ Revision of
existing code

④ ⑤ Fourth or fifth
digit required

6. DISEASES OF THE NERVOUS SYSTEM AND SENSE ORGANS (320-389)

INFLAMMATORY DISEASES OF THE CENTRAL NERVOUS SYSTEM (320-326)

320 Bacterial meningitis
Includes:
bacterial:
arachnoiditis
leptomeningitis
meningitis
meningoencephalitis
meningomyelitis
pachymeningitis

320.0 Hemophilus meningitis
Meningitis due to Hemophilus influenzae [H. influenzae]

320.1 Pneumococcal meningitis

320.2 Streptococcal meningitis

320.3 Staphylococcal meningitis

320.7 Meningitis in other bacterial diseases classified elsewhere
Code first underlying disease, as:
actinomycosis (039.8)
listeriosis (027.0)
typhoid fever (002.0)
whooping cough (033.0-033.9)

[*Excludes:*] *meningitis (in):*
epidemic (036.0)
gonococcal (098.82)
meningococcal (036.0)
salmonellosis (003.21)
syphilis:
NOS (094.2)
congenital (090.42)
meningovascular (094.2)
secondary (091.81)
tuberculous (013.0)

[5] **320.8 Meningitis due to other specified bacteria**

320.81 Anaerobic meningitis
Bacteroides (fragilis)
Gram-negative anaerobes

320.82 Meningitis due to Gram-negative bacteria, not elsewhere classified
Aerobacter aerogenes
Escherichia coli [E. coli]
Friedlander bacillus
Klebsiella pneumoniae
Proteus morganii
Pseudomonas

[*Excludes:*] *Gram-negative anaerobes (320.81)*

320.89 Meningitis due to other specified bacteria
Bacillus pyocyaneus

320.9 Meningitis due to unspecified bacterium
Meningitis:
bacterial NOS
purulent NOS
pyogenic NOS
suppurative NOS

321 Meningitis due to other organisms
Includes:
arachnoiditis due to organisms other than bacteria
leptomeningitis due to organisms other than bacteria
meningitis due to organisms other than bacteria
pachymeningitis due to organisms other than bacteria

321.0 Cryptococcal meningitis
Code first underlying disease (117.5)

Add 4th or 5th digit | Nonspecific code | Unspecified code | Manifestation code

321.1 Meningitis in other fungal diseases
Code first underlying disease (110.0-118)

Excludes: meningitis in:
candidiasis (112.83)
coccidioidomycosis (114.2)
histoplasmosis (115.01, 115.11, 115.91)

321.2 Meningitis due to viruses not elsewhere classified
Code first underlying disease, as:
meningitis due to arbovirus (060.0-066.9)

Excludes: meningitis (due to):
abacterial (047.0-047.9)
adenovirus (049.1)
aseptic NOS (047.9)
Coxsackie (virus) (047.0)
ECHO virus (047.1)
enterovirus (047.0-047.9)
herpes simplex virus (054.72)
herpes zoster virus (053.0)
lymphocytic choriomeningitis virus (049.0)
mumps (072.1)
viral NOS (047.9)
meningo-eruptive syndrome (047.1)

321.3 Meningitis due to trypanosomiasis
Code first underlying disease (086.0-086.9)

321.4 Meningitis in sarcoidosis
Code first underlying disease (135)

321.8 Meningitis due to other nonbacterial organisms classified elsewhere
Code first underlying disease

Excludes: leptospiral meningitis (100.81)

322 Meningitis of unspecified cause
Includes:
arachnoiditis with no organism specified as cause
leptomeningitis with no organism specified as cause
meningitis with no organism specified as cause
pachymeningitis with no organism specified as cause

322.0 Nonpyogenic meningitis
Meningitis with clear cerebrospinal fluid

322.1 Eosinophilic meningitis

322.2 Chronic meningitis

322.9 Meningitis, unspecified

323 Encephalitis, myelitis, and encephalomyelitis
Includes: acute disseminated encephalomyelitis
meningoencephalitis, except bacterial
meningomyelitis, except bacterial
myelitis (acute):
ascending
transverse

Excludes: bacterial:
meningoencephalitis (320.0-320.9)
meningomyelitis (320.0-320.9)

● Code new
to this edition

▲ Revision of
existing code

④ ⑤ Fourth or fifth
digit required

323.0 *Encephalitis in viral diseases classified elsewhere*
Code first underlying disease, as:
cat-scratch disease (078.3)
infectious mononucleosis (075)
ornithosis (073.7)

Excludes: *encephalitis (in):*
arthropod-borne viral (062.0-064)
herpes simplex (054.3)
mumps (072.2)
poliomyelitis (045.0-045.9)
rubella (056.01)
slow virus infections of central nervous system (046.0-046.9)
other viral diseases of central nervous system (049.8-049.9)
viral NOS (049.9)

323.1 *Encephalitis in rickettsial diseases classified elsewhere*
Code first underlying disease (080-083.9)

323.2 *Encephalitis in protozoal diseases classified elsewhere*
Code first underlying disease, as:
malaria (084.0-084.9)
trypanosomiasis (086.0-086.9)

323.4 *Other encephalitis due to infection classified elsewhere*
Code first underlying disease

Excludes: *encephalitis (in):*
meningococcal (036.1)
syphilis:
NOS (094.81)
congenital (090.41)
toxoplasmosis (130.0)
tuberculosis (013.6)
meningoencephalitis due to free-living ameba [Naegleria] (136.2)

323.5 Encephalitis following immunization procedures
Encephalitis, postimmunization or postvaccinal
Encephalomyelitis, postimmunization or postvaccinal
Use additional E code, if desired, to identify vaccine

323.6 *Postinfectious encephalitis*
Code first underlying disease

Excludes: *encephalitis:*
postchickenpox (052.0)
postmeasles (055.0)

323.7 *Toxic encephalitis*
Code first underlying cause, as:
carbon tetrachloride (982.1)
hydroxyquinoline derivatives (961.3)
lead (984.0-984.9)
mercury (985.0)
thallium (985.8)

323.8 Other causes of encephalitis

323.9 Unspecified cause of encephalitis

324 Intracranial and intraspinal abscess

324.0 Intracranial abscess

Abscess (embolic):
cerebellar
cerebral

Abscess (embolic) of brain [any part]:
epidural
extradural
otogenic
subdural

Excludes: *tuberculous (013.3)*

324.1 Intraspinal abscess
Abscess (embolic) of spinal cord [any part]:
epidural
extradural
subdural

Excludes: *tuberculous (013.5)*

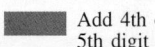 Add 4th or
5th digit

 Nonspecific
code

Unspecified
code

Manifestation
code

324.9 Of unspecified site
Extradural or subdural abscess NOS

325 Phlebitis and thrombophlebitis of intracranial venous sinuses
Embolism
Endophlebitis
Phlebitis, septic or suppurative of cavernous, lateral, or other intracranial or unspecified intracranial venous sinus
Thrombophlebitis of cavernous, lateral, or other intracranial or unspecified intracranial venous sinus
Thrombosis of cavernous, lateral, or other intracranial or unspecified intracranial venous sinus

Excludes: *that specified as:*
> *complicating pregnancy, childbirth, or the puerperium (671.5)*
> *of nonpyogenic origin (437.6)*

326 Late effects of intracranial abscess or pyogenic infection
Note: This category is to be used to indicate conditions whose primary classification is to 320-325 [excluding 320.7, 321.0-321.8, 323.0-323.4, 323.6-323.7] as the cause of late effects, themselves classifiable elsewhere. The "late effects" include conditions specified as such, or as sequelae, which may occur at any time after the resolution of the causal condition.

Use additional code, if desired, to identify condition, as:
hydrocephalus (331.4)
paralysis (342.0-342.9, 344.0-344.9)

HEREDITARY AND DEGENERATIVE DISEASES OF THE CENTRAL NERVOUS SYSTEM (330-337)

Excludes: *hepatolenticular degeneration (275.1)*
> *multiple sclerosis (340)*
> *other demyelinating diseases of central nervous system (341.0-341.9)*

330 Cerebral degenerations usually manifest in childhood
Use additional code, if desired, to identify associated mental retardation

330.0 Leukodystrophy
Krabbe's disease
Pelizaeus-Merzbacher disease
Sulfatide lipidosis
Leukodystrophy:
globoid cell
metachromatic
NOS
sudanophilic

330.1 Cerebral lipidoses
Amaurotic (familial) idiocy
Batten disease
Gangliosidosis
Jansky-Bielschowsky disease
Kufs' disease
Spielmeyer-Vogt disease
Tay-Sachs disease

330.2 *Cerebral degeneration in generalized lipidoses*
Code first underlying disease, as:
Fabry's disease (272.7)
Gaucher's disease (272.7)
Neimann-Pick disease (272.7)
sphingolipidosis (272.7)

330.3 *Cerebral degeneration of childhood in other diseases classified elsewhere*
Code first underlying disease, as:
Hunter's disease (277.5)
mucopolysaccharidosis (277.5)

330.8 Other specified cerebral degenerations in childhood
Alpers' disease or gray-matter degeneration
Infantile necrotizing encephalomyelopathy
Leigh's disease
Subacute necrotizing encephalopathy or encephalomyelopathy

330.9 Unspecified cerebral degeneration in childhood

331 Other cerebral degenerations

331.0 Alzheimer's disease

331.1 Pick's disease

331.2 Senile degeneration of brain
Excludes: *senility NOS (797)*

331.3 Communicating hydrocephalus
Excludes: *congenital hydrocephalus (741.0, 742.3)*

● Code new
to this edition
▲ Revision of
existing code
④ ⑤ Fourth or fifth
digit required

331.4 Obstructive hydrocephalus
Acquired hydrocephalus NOS
[Excludes:] *congenital hydrocephalus (741.0, 742.3)*

331.7 Cerebral degeneration in diseases classified elsewhere
Code first underlying disease, as:
alcoholism (303.0-303.9)
beriberi (265.0)
cerebrovascular disease (430-438)
congenital hydrocephalus (741.0, 742.3)
neoplastic disease (140.0-239.9)
myxedema (244.0-244.9)
vitamin B_{12} deficiency (266.2)
[Excludes:] *cerebral degeneration in:*
Jakob-Creutzfeldt disease (046.1)
progressive multifocal leukoencephalopathy (046.3)
subacute spongiform encephalopathy (046.1)

[5] **331.8 Other cerebral degeneration**

331.81 Reye's syndrome

331.89 Other
Cerebral ataxia

331.9 Cerebral degeneration, unspecified

332 Parkinson's disease

332.0 Paralysis agitans
Parkinsonism or Parkinson's disease:
NOS
idiopathic
primary

332.1 Secondary Parkinsonism
Parkinsonism due to drugs
Use additional E code, if desired, to identify drug, if drug-induced
[Excludes:] *Parkinsonism (in):*
Huntington's disease (333.4)
progressive supranuclear palsy (333.0)
Shy-Drager syndrome (333.0)
syphilitic (094.82)

333 Other extrapyramidal disease and abnormal movement disorders
Includes: other forms of extrapyramidal, basal ganglia, or striatopallidal disease
[Excludes:] *abnormal movements of head NOS (781.0)*

333.0 Other degenerative diseases of the basal ganglia
Atrophy or degeneration:
olivopontocerebellar [Déjérine-Thomas syndrome]
pigmentary pallidal [Hallervorden-Spatz disease]
striatonigral
Parkinsonian syndrome associated with:
idiopathic orthostatic hypotension
symptomatic orthostatic hypotension
Progressive supranuclear ophthalmoplegia
Shy-Drager syndrome

333.1 Essential and other specified forms of tremor
Benign essential tremor
Familial tremor
Use additional E code, if desired, to identify drug, if drug-induced
[Excludes:] *tremor NOS (781.0)*

333.2 Myoclonus
Familial essential myoclonus
Progressive myoclonic epilepsy
Unverricht-Lundborg disease
Use additional E code, if desired, to identify drug, if drug-induced

Add 4th or 5th digit | Nonspecific code | Unspecified code | Manifestation code

333.3 Tics of organic origin
> *Excludes:* *Gilles de la Tourette's syndrome (307.23)*
> *habit spasm (307.22)*
> *tic NOS (307.20)*

Use additional E code, if desired, to identify drug, if drug-induced

333.4 Huntington's chorea

333.5 Other choreas
    Hemiballism(us)
    Paroxysmal choreo-athetosis
> *Excludes:* *Sydenham's or rheumatic chorea (392.0-392.9)*

Use additional E code, if desired, to identify drug, if drug-induced

333.6 Idiopathic torsion dystonia
    Dystonia:
      deformans progressiva
      musculorum deformans
      (Schwalbe-) Ziehen-Oppenheim disease

333.7 Symptomatic torsion dystonia
    Athetoid cerebral palsy [Vogt's disease]
    Double athetosis (syndrome)

Use additional E code, if desired, to identify drug, if drug-induced

⑤ **333.8 Fragments of torsion dystonia**
Use additional E code, if desired, to identify drug, if drug-induced

    333.81 Blepharospasm

    333.82 Orofacial dyskinesia

    333.83 Spasmodic torticollis
> *Excludes:* *torticollis:*
> *NOS (723.5)*
> *hysterical (300.11)*
> *psychogenic (306.0)*

    333.84 Organic writers' cramp
> *Excludes:* *psychogenic (300.89)*

    333.89 Other

⑤ **333.9 Other and unspecified extrapyramidal diseases and abnormal movement disorders**

    333.90 Unspecified extrapyramidal disease and abnormal movement disorder

    333.91 Stiff-man syndrome

    333.92 Neuroleptic malignant syndrome
      Use additional E code to identify drug

    333.93 Benign shuddering attacks

    333.99 Other
      Restless legs

334 Spinocerebellar disease
> *Excludes:* *olivopontocerebellar degeneration (333.0)*
> *peroneal muscular atrophy (356.1)*

334.0 Friedreich's ataxia

334.1 Hereditary spastic paraplegia

334.2 Primary cerebellar degeneration
    Cerebellar ataxia:
      Marie's
      Sanger-Brown
    Dyssynergia cerebellaris myoclonica
    Primary cerebellar degeneration:
      NOS
      hereditary
      sporadic

334.3 Other cerebellar ataxia
    Cerebellar ataxia NOS

Use additional E code, if desired, to identify drug, if drug-induced

● Code new to this edition   ▲ Revision of existing code   ④ ⑤ Fourth or fifth digit required

334.4 Cerebellar ataxia in diseases classified elsewhere
Code first underlying disease, as:
alcoholism (303.0-303.9)
myxedema (244.0-244.9)
neoplastic disease (140.0-239.9)

334.8 Other spinocerebellar diseases
Ataxia-telangiectasia [Louis-Bar syndrome]
Corticostriatal-spinal degeneration

334.9 Spinocerebellar disease, unspecified

335 Anterior horn cell disease

335.0 Werdnig-Hoffmann disease
Infantile spinal muscular atrophy
Progressive muscular atrophy of infancy

[5] **335.1 Spinal muscular atrophy**

335.10 Spinal muscular atrophy, unspecified

335.11 Kugelberg-Welander disease
Spinal muscular atrophy:
familial
juvenile

335.19 Other
Adult spinal muscular atrophy

[5] **335.2 Motor neuron disease**

335.20 Amyotrophic lateral sclerosis
Motor neuron disease (bulbar) (mixed type)

335.21 Progressive muscular atrophy
Duchenne-Aran muscular atrophy
Progressive muscular atrophy (pure)

335.22 Progressive bulbar palsy

335.23 Pseudobulbar palsy

335.24 Primary lateral sclerosis

335.29 Other

335.8 Other anterior horn cell diseases

335.9 Anterior horn cell disease, unspecified

336 Other diseases of spinal cord

336.0 Syringomyelia and syringobulbia

336.1 Vascular myelopathies
Acute infarction of spinal cord (embolic) (nonembolic)
Arterial thrombosis of spinal cord
Edema of spinal cord
Hematomyelia
Subacute necrotic myelopathy

336.2 Subacute combined degeneration of spinal cord in diseases classified elsewhere
Code first underlying disease, as:
pernicious anemia (281.0)
other vitamin B_{12} deficiency anemia (281.1)
vitamin B_{12} deficiency (266.2)

336.3 Myelopathy in other diseases classified elsewhere
Code first underlying disease, as:
myelopathy in neoplastic disease (140.0-239.9)

[*Excludes:*] *myelopathy in:*
intervertebral disc disorder (722.70-722.73)
spondylosis (721.1, 721.41-721.42, 721.91)

336.8 Other myelopathy
Myelopathy:
drug-induced
radiation-induced

Use additional E code, if desired, to identify cause

336.9 Unspecified disease of spinal cord
Cord compression NOS
Myelopathy NOS

[*Excludes:*] *myelitis (323.0-323.9)*
spinal (canal) stenosis (723.0, 724.00-724.09)

Add 4th or 5th digit | Nonspecific code | Unspecified code | Manifestation code

337 Disorders of the autonomic nervous system

Includes: disorders of peripheral autonomic, sympathetic, parasympathetic, or vegetative system

[Excludes:] *familial dysautonomia [Riley-Day syndrome] (742.8)*

337.0 Idiopathic peripheral autonomic neuropathy
Carotid sinus syncope or syndrome
Cervical sympathetic dystrophy or paralysis

337.1 Peripheral autonomic neuropathy in disorders classified elsewhere
Code first underlying disease, as:
amyloidosis (277.3)
diabetes (250.6)

[5] **337.2 Reflex sympathetic dystrophy**

337.20 Reflex sympathetic dystrophy, unspecified

337.21 Reflex sympathetic dystrophy of the upper limb

337.22 Reflex sympathetic dystrophy of the lower limb

337.29 Reflex sympathetic dystrophy of other specified site

337.3 Autonomic dysreflexia
Use additional code to identify the cause, such as:
decubitus ulcer (707.0)
fecal impaction (560.39)
urinary tract infection (599.0)

337.9 Unspecified disorder of autonomic nervous system

OTHER DISORDERS OF THE CENTRAL NERVOUS SYSTEM (340-349)

340 Multiple sclerosis
Disseminated or multiple sclerosis:
NOS
brain stem
cord
generalized

341 Other demyelinating diseases of central nervous system

341.0 Neuromyelitis optica

341.1 Schilder's disease
Baló's concentric sclerosis
Encephalitis periaxialis:
concentrica [Baló's]
diffusa [Schilder's]

341.8 Other demyelinating diseases of central nervous system
Central demyelination of corpus callosum
Central pontine myelinosis
Marchiafava (-Bignami) disease

341.9 Demyelinating disease of central nervous system, unspecified

[5] **342 Hemiplegia and hemiparesis**

[Excludes:] *congenital (343.1)*
hemiplegia due to late effect of cerebrovascular accident (438.20-438.22)
infantile NOS (343.4)

Note: This category is to be used when hemiplegia (complete) (incomplete) is reported without further specification, or is stated to be old or long-standing but of unspecified cause. The category is also for use in multiple coding to identify these types of hemiplegia resulting from any cause.

The following fifth-digits are for use with codes 342.0-342.9

0 affecting unspecified site

1 affecting dominant site

2 affecting nondominant site

[5] **342.0 Flaccid hemiplegia**

[5] **342.1 Spastic hemiplegia**

[5] **342.8 Other specified hemiplegia**

[5] **342.9 Hemiplegia, unspecified**

● Code new to this edition ▲ Revision of existing code [4] [5] Fourth or fifth digit required

343 Infantile cerebral palsy

Includes: cerebral:
- palsy NOS
- spastic infantile paralysis

congenital spastic paralysis (cerebral)
Little's disease
paralysis (spastic) due to birth injury:
- intracranial
- Spinal

[Excludes:] *hereditary cerebral paralysis, such as:*
- *hereditary spastic paraplegia (334.1)*
- *Vogt's disease (333.7)*

spastic paralysis specified as noncongenital or noninfantile (344.0-344.9)

343.0 Diplegic
Congenital diplegia
Congenital paraplegia

343.1 Hemiplegic
Congenital hemiplegia

[Excludes:] *infantile hemiplegia NOS (343.4)*

343.2 Quadriplegic
Tetraplegic

343.3 Monoplegic

343.4 Infantile hemiplegia
Infantile hemiplegia (postnatal) NOS

343.8 Other specified infantile cerebral palsy

343.9 Infantile cerebral palsy, unspecified
Cerebral palsy NOS

344 Other paralytic syndromes

Note: This category is to be used when the listed conditions are reported without further specification or are stated to be old or long-standing but of unspecified cause. The category is also for use in multiple coding to identify these conditions resulting from any cause.

Includes: paralysis (complete) (incomplete), except as classifiable to 342 and 343

[Excludes:] *congenital or infantile cerebral palsy (343.0-343.9)*
hemiplegia (342.0-342.9)
- *congenital or infantile (343.1, 343.4)*

[5] **344.0 Quadriplegia and quadriparesis**

344.00 Quadriplegia, unspecified

344.01 C1-C4, complete

344.02 C1-C4, incomplete

344.03 C5-C7, complete

344.04 C5-C7, incomplete

344.09 Other

344.1 Paraplegia
Paralysis of both lower limbs
Paraplegia (lower)

344.2 Diplegia of upper limbs
Diplegia (upper)
Paralysis of both upper limbs

[5] **344.3 Monoplegia of lower limb**
Paralysis of lower limb

[Excludes:] *monoplegia of lower limb due to late effect of cerebrovascular accident (438.40-438.42)*

344.30 affecting unspecified side

344.31 affecting dominant side

344.32 affecting nondominant side

[5] **344.4 Monoplegia of upper limb**
Paralysis of upper limb

[Excludes:] *monoplegia of upper limb due to late effect of cerebrovascular accident (438.30-438.32)*

344.40 affecting unspecified side

344.41   **affecting dominant side**

344.42   **affecting nondominant side**

344.5 **Unspecified monoplegia**

⑤ **344.6** **Cauda equina syndrome**

344.60   **Without mention of neurogenic bladder**

344.61   **With neurogenic bladder**
Acontractile bladder
Autonomic hyperreflexia of bladder
Cord bladder
Detrusor hyperreflexia

⑤ **344.8** **Other specified paralytic syndromes**

344.81   **Locked-in state**

344.89   **Other specified paralytic syndrome**

344.9 **Paralysis, unspecified**

345 **Epilepsy**

The following fifth-digit subclassification is for use with categories 345.0, 345.1, 345.4-345.9:

0   **without mention of intractable epilepsy**

1   **with intractable epilepsy**

Excludes: *progressive myoclonic epilepsy (333.2)*

⑤ **345.0** **Generalized nonconvulsive epilepsy**

Absences:	Pykno-epilepsy
atonic	Seizures:
typical	akinetic
Minor epilepsy	atonic
Petit mal	

⑤ **345.1** **Generalized convulsive epilepsy**

Epileptic seizures:	Grand mal
clonic	Major epilepsy
myoclonic	
tonic	
tonic-clonic	

Excludes: *convulsions:*
NOS (780.3)
infantile (780.3)
newborn (779.0)
infantile spasms (345.6)

345.2 **Petit mal status**
Epileptic absence status

345.3 **Grand mal status**
Status epilepticus NOS

Excludes: *epilepsia partialis continua (345.7)*
status:
psychomotor (345.7)
temporal lobe (345.7)

⑤ **345.4** **Partial epilepsy, with impairment of consciousness**
Epilepsy:
limbic system
partial:
secondarily generalized
with memory and ideational disturbances
psychomotor
psychosensory
temporal lobe
Epileptic automatism

⑤ **345.5** **Partial epilepsy, without mention of impairment of consciousness**

Epilepsy:	Epilepsy:
Bravais-Jacksonian NOS	sensory-induced
focal (motor) NOS	somatomotor
Jacksonian NOS	somatosensory
motor partial	visceral
partial NOS	visual

   ● Code new
to this edition   ▲ Revision of
existing code   ④ ⑤ Fourth or fifth
digit required

⑤ **345.6 Infantile spasms**
Hypsarrhythmia   Salaam attacks
Lightning spasms

Excludes: salaam tic (781.0)

⑤ **345.7 Epilepsia partialis continua**
Kojevnikov's epilepsy

⑤ **345.8 Other forms of epilepsy**
Epilepsy:
 cursive [running]
 gelastic

⑤ **345.9 Epilepsy, unspecified**
Epileptic convulsions, fits, or seizures NOS

Excludes: convulsive seizure or fit NOS (780.3)

⑤ **346 Migraine**
The following fifth-digit subclassification is for use with category 346:

 0 **without mention of intractable migraine**

 1 **with intractable migraine, so stated**

⑤ **346.0 Classical migraine**
Migraine preceded or accompanied by transient focal neurological phenomena
Migraine with aura

⑤ **346.1 Common migraine**
Atypical migraine   Sick headache

⑤ **346.2 Variants of migraine**

Cluster headache	Migraine:
Histamine cephalgia	lower half
Horton's neuralgia	retinal
Migraine:	Neuralgia:
abdominal	ciliary
basilar	migrainous

⑤ **346.8 Other forms of migraine**
Migraine:
 hemiplegic
 ophthalmoplegic

⑤ **346.9 Migraine, unspecified**

347 Cataplexy and narcolepsy

348 Other conditions of brain

348.0 Cerebral cysts
Arachnoid cyst   Porencephaly, acquired
Porencephalic cyst   Pseudoporencephaly

Excludes: porencephaly (congenital) (742.4)

348.1 Anoxic brain damage

Excludes: that occurring in:
 abortion (634-638 with .7, 639.8)
 ectopic or molar pregnancy (639.8)
 labor or delivery (668.2, 669.4)
 that of newborn (767.0, 768.0-768.9, 772.1-772.2)

Use additional E code, if desired, to identify cause

348.2 Benign intracranial hypertension
Pseudotumor cerebri

Excludes: hypertensive encephalopathy (437.2)

348.3 Encephalopathy, unspecified

348.4 Compression of brain
Compression, brain (stem)
Herniation, brain (stem)
Posterior fossa compression syndrome

348.5 Cerebral edema

	Add 4th or 5th digit		Nonspecific code		Unspecified code		Manifestation code

348.8 **Other conditions of brain**
Cerebral:
calcification
fungus

348.9 **Unspecified condition of brain**

349 **Other and unspecified disorders of the nervous system**

349.0 **Reaction to spinal or lumbar puncture**
Headache following lumbar puncture

349.1 **Nervous system complications from surgically implanted device**
Excludes: immediate postoperative complications (997.00-997.09)
mechanical complications of nervous system device (996.2)

349.2 **Disorders of meninges, not elsewhere classified**
Adhesions, meningeal (cerebral) (spinal)
Cyst, spinal meninges
Meningocele, acquired
Pseudomeningocele, acquired

⑤ **349.8** **Other specified disorders of nervous system**

349.81 **Cerebrospinal fluid rhinorrhea**
Excludes: cerebrospinal fluid otorrhea (388.61)

349.82 **Toxic encephalopathy**
Use additional E code, if desired, to identify cause

349.89 **Other**

349.9 **Unspecified disorders of nervous system**
Disorder of nervous system (central) NOS

DISORDERS OF THE PERIPHERAL NERVOUS SYSTEM (350-359)

Excludes: diseases of:
acoustic [8th] nerve (388.5)
oculomotor [3rd, 4th, 6th] nerves (378.0-378.9)
optic [2nd] nerve (377.0-377.9)
peripheral autonomic nerves (337.0-337.9)
neuralgia NOS or "rheumatic" (729.2)
neuritis NOS or "rheumatic" (729.2)
radiculitis NOS or "rheumatic" (729.2)
peripheral neuritis in pregnancy (646.4)

350 **Trigeminal nerve disorders**
Includes: disorders of 5th cranial nerve

350.1 **Trigeminal neuralgia**
Tic douloureux   Trigeminal neuralgia NOS
Trifacial neuralgia
Excludes: postherpetic (053.12)

350.2 **Atypical face pain**

350.8 **Other specified trigeminal nerve disorders**

350.9 **Trigeminal nerve disorder, unspecified**

351 **Facial nerve disorders**
Includes: disorders of 7th cranial nerve
Excludes: that in newborn (767.5)

351.0 **Bell's palsy**
Facial palsy

351.1 **Geniculate ganglionitis**
Geniculate ganglionitis NOS
Excludes: herpetic (053.11)

351.8 **Other facial nerve disorders**
Facial myokymia   Melkersson's syndrome

351.9 **Facial nerve disorder, unspecified**

352 **Disorders of other cranial nerves**

352.0 **Disorders of olfactory [1st] nerve**

352.1 **Glossopharyngeal neuralgia**

● Code new
to this edition

▲ Revision of
existing code

④ ⑤ Fourth or fifth
digit required

352.2 Other disorders of glossopharyngeal [9th] nerve

352.3 Disorders of pneumogastric [10th] nerve
Disorders of vagal nerve

Excludes: paralysis of vocal cords or larynx (478.30-478.34)

352.4 Disorders of accessory [11th] nerve

352.5 Disorders of hypoglossal [12th] nerve

352.6 Multiple cranial nerve palsies
Collet-Sicard syndrome   Polyneuritis cranialis

352.9 Unspecified disorder of cranial nerves

353 Nerve root and plexus disorders

Excludes: conditions due to:
intervertebral disc disorders (722.0-722.9)
spondylosis (720.0-721.9)
vertebrogenic disorders (723.0-724.9)

353.0 Brachial plexus lesions
Cervical rib syndrome   Thoracic outlet syndrome
Costoclavicular syndrome
Scalenus anticus syndrome

Excludes: brachial neuritis or radiculitis NOS (723.4)
that in newborn (767.6)

353.1 Lumbosacral plexus lesions

353.2 Cervical root lesions, not elsewhere classified

353.3 Thoracic root lesions, not elsewhere classified

353.4 Lumbosacral root lesions, not elsewhere classified

353.5 Neuralgic amyotrophy
Parsonage-Aldren-Turner syndrome

353.6 Phantom limb (syndrome)

353.8 Other nerve root and plexus disorders

353.9 Unspecified nerve root and plexus disorder

354 Mononeuritis of upper limb and mononeuritis multiplex

354.0 Carpal tunnel syndrome
Median nerve entrapment   Partial thenar atrophy

354.1 Other lesion of median nerve
Median nerve neuritis

354.2 Lesion of ulnar nerve
Cubital tunnel syndrome   Tardy ulnar nerve palsy

354.3 Lesion of radial nerve
Acute radial nerve palsy

354.4 Causalgia of upper limb

Excludes: causalgia:
NOS (355.9)
lower limb (355.71)

354.5 Mononeuritis multiplex
Combinations of single conditions classifiable to 354 or 355

354.8 Other mononeuritis of upper limb

354.9 Mononeuritis of upper limb, unspecified

355 Mononeuritis of lower limb and unspecified site

355.0 Lesion of sciatic nerve

Excludes: sciatica NOS (724.3)

355.1 Meralgia paresthetica
Lateral cutaneous femoral nerve of thigh compression or syndrome

355.2 Other lesion of femoral nerve

355.3 Lesion of lateral popliteal nerve
Lesion of common peroneal nerve

355.4 Lesion of medial popliteal nerve

355.5 Tarsal tunnel syndrome

| | Add 4th or 5th digit | | Nonspecific code | | Unspecified code | | Manifestation code |

355.6 Lesion of plantar nerve
Morton's metatarsalgia, neuralgia, or neuroma

⑤ **355.7 Other mononeuritis of lower limb**

355.71 Causalgia of lower limb

Excludes: causalgia:
NOS (355.9)
upper limb (354.4)

355.79 Other mononeuritis of lower limb

355.8 Mononeuritis of lower limb, unspecified

355.9 Mononeuritis of unspecified site
Causalgia NOS

Excludes: causalgia:
lower limb (355.71)
upper limb (354.4)

356 Hereditary and idiopathic peripheral neuropathy

356.0 Hereditary peripheral neuropathy
Déjérine-Sottas disease

356.1 Peroneal muscular atrophy
Charcot-Marie-Tooth disease
Neuropathic muscular atrophy

356.2 Hereditary sensory neuropathy

356.3 Refsum's disease
Heredopathia atactica polyneuritiformis

356.4 Idiopathic progressive polyneuropathy

356.8 Other specified idiopathic peripheral neuropathy
Supranuclear paralysis

356.9 Unspecified

357 Inflammatory and toxic neuropathy

357.0 Acute infective polyneuritis
Guillain-Barré syndrome
Postinfectious polyneuritis

357.1 Polyneuropathy in collagen vascular disease
Code first underlying disease, as:
disseminated lupus erythematosus (710.0)
polyarteritis nodosa (446.0)
rheumatoid arthritis (714.0)

357.2 Polyneuropathy in diabetes
Code first underlying disease (250.6)

357.3 Polyneuropathy in malignant disease
Code first underlying disease (140.0-208.9)

357.4 Polyneuropathy in other diseases classified elsewhere
Code first underlying disease, as:
amyloidosis (277.3)
beriberi (265.0)
deficiency of B vitamins (266.0-266.9)
diphtheria (032.0-032.9)
hypoglycemia (251.2)
pellagra (265.2)
porphyria (277.1)
sarcoidosis (135)
uremia (585)

Excludes: polyneuropathy in:
herpes zoster (053.13)
mumps (072.72)

357.5 Alcoholic polyneuropathy

357.6 Polyneuropathy due to drugs
Use additional E code, if desired, to identify drug

357.7 Polyneuropathy due to other toxic agents
Use additional E code, if desired, to identify toxic agent

● Code new to this edition   ▲ Revision of existing code   ④ ⑤ Fourth or fifth digit required

[5] **357.8 Other**

● **357.81 Chronic inflammatory demyelinating polyneuritis**

● **357.82 Critical illness polyneuropathy**
Acute motor neuropathy

● **357.89 Other inflammatory and toxic neuropathy**

357.9 Unspecified

358 Myoneural disorders

358.0 Myasthenia gravis

358.1 Myasthenic syndromes in diseases classified elsewhere
Amyotrophy from stated cause classified elsewhere
Eaton-Lambert syndrome from stated cause classified elsewhere

Code first underlying disease, as:
botulism (005.1)
diabetes mellitus (250.6)
hypothyroidism (244.0-244.9)
malignant neoplasm (140.0-208.9)
pernicious anemia (281.0)
thyrotoxicosis (242.0-242.9)

358.2 Toxic myoneural disorders
Use additional E code, if desired, to identify toxic agent

358.8 Other specified myoneural disorders

358.9 Myoneural disorders, unspecified

359 Muscular dystrophies and other myopathies
[Excludes:] *idiopathic polymyositis (710.4)*

359.0 Congenital hereditary muscular dystrophy
Benign congenital myopathy
Central core disease
Centronuclear myopathy
Myotubular myopathy
Nemaline body disease

[Excludes:] *arthrogryposis multiplex congenita (754.89)*

359.1 Hereditary progressive muscular dystrophy
Muscular dystrophy:
NOS
distal
Duchenne
Erb's
fascioscapulohumeral
Muscular dystrophy:
Gower's
Landouzy-Déjérine
limb-girdle
ocular
oculopharyngeal

359.2 Myotonic disorders
Dystrophia myotonica
Eulenburg's disease
Myotonia congenita
Paramyotonia congenita
Steinert's disease
Thomsen's disease

359.3 Familial periodic paralysis
Hypokalemic familial periodic paralysis

359.4 Toxic myopathy
Use additional E code, if desired, to identify toxic agent

359.5 Myopathy in endocrine diseases classified elsewhere
Code first underlying disease, as:
Addison's disease (255.4)
Cushing's syndrome (255.0)
hypopituitarism (253.2)
myxedema (244.0-244.9)
thyrotoxicosis (242.0-242.9)

Add 4th or 5th digit | Nonspecific code | Unspecified code | Manifestation code

359.6 Symptomatic inflammatory myopathy in diseases classified elsewhere
Code first underlying disease, as:
amyloidosis (277.3)
disseminated lupus erythematosus (710.0)
malignant neoplasm (140.0-208.9)
polyarteritis nodosa (446.0)
rheumatoid arthritis (714.0)
sarcoidosis (135)
scleroderma (710.1)
Sjögren's disease (710.2)

⑤ **359.8 Other myopathies**

● **359.81 Critical illness myopathy**
Acute necrotizing myopathy
Acute quadriplegic myopathy
Intensive care (ICU) myopathy
Myopathy of critical illness

● **359.89 Other myopathies**

359.9 Myopathy, unspecified

DISORDERS OF THE EYE AND ADNEXA (360-379)

360 Disorders of the globe
Includes: disorders affecting multiple structures of eye

⑤ **360.0 Purulent endophthalmitis**

360.00 Purulent endophthalmitis, unspecified

360.01 Acute endophthalmitis

360.02 Panophthalmitis

360.03 Chronic endophthalmitis

360.04 Vitreous abscess

⑤ **360.1 Other endophthalmitis**

360.11 Sympathetic uveitis

360.12 Panuveitis

360.13 Parasitic endophthalmitis NOS

360.14 Ophthalmia nodosa

360.19 Other
Phacoanaphylactic endophthalmitis

⑤ **360.2 Degenerative disorders of globe**

360.20 Degenerative disorder of globe, unspecified

360.21 Progressive high (degenerative) myopia
Malignant myopia

360.23 Siderosis

360.24 Other metallosis
Chalcosis

360.29 Other

Excludes: xerophthalmia (264.7)

⑤ **360.3 Hypotony of eye**

360.30 Hypotony, unspecified

360.31 Primary hypotony

360.32 Ocular fistula causing hypotony

360.33 Hypotony associated with other ocular disorders

360.34 Flat anterior chamber

⑤ **360.4 Degenerated conditions of globe**

360.40 Degenerated globe or eye, unspecified

360.41 Blind hypotensive eye
Atrophy of globe   Phthisis bulbi

360.42 Blind hypertensive eye
Absolute glaucoma

360.43 Hemophthalmos, except current injury

Excludes: traumatic (871.0-871.9, 921.0-921.9)

● Code new
to this edition

▲ Revision of
existing code

④ ⑤ Fourth or fifth
digit required

360.44 Leucocoria

⑤ **360.5 Retained (old) intraocular foreign body, magnetic**

> Excludes: *current penetrating injury with magnetic foreign body (871.5)*
> *retained (old) foreign body of orbit (376.6)*

360.50 Foreign body, magnetic, intraocular, unspecified

360.51 Foreign body, magnetic, in anterior chamber

360.52 Foreign body, magnetic, in iris or ciliary body

360.53 Foreign body, magnetic, in lens

360.54 Foreign body, magnetic, in vitreous

360.55 Foreign body, magnetic, in posterior wall

360.59 Foreign body, magnetic, in other or multiple sites

⑤ **360.6 Retained (old) intraocular foreign body, nonmagnetic**
Retained (old) foreign body:
  NOS
  nonmagnetic

> Excludes: *current penetrating injury with (nonmagnetic) foreign body (871.6)*
> *retained (old) foreign body in orbit (376.6)*

360.60 Foreign body, intraocular, unspecified

360.61 Foreign body in anterior chamber

360.62 Foreign body in iris or ciliary body

360.63 Foreign body in lens

360.64 Foreign body in vitreous

360.65 Foreign body in posterior wall

360.69 Foreign body in other or multiple sites

⑤ **360.8 Other disorders of globe**

360.81 Luxation of globe

360.89 Other

360.9 Unspecified disorder of globe

361 Retinal detachments and defects

⑤ **361.0 Retinal detachment with retinal defect**
Rhegmatogenous retinal detachment

> Excludes: *detachment of retinal pigment epithelium (362.42-362.43)*
> *retinal detachment (serous) (without defect) (361.2)*

361.00 Retinal detachment with retinal defect, unspecified

361.01 Recent detachment, partial, with single defect

361.02 Recent detachment, partial, with multiple defects

361.03 Recent detachment, partial, with giant tear

361.04 Recent detachment, partial, with retinal dialysis
Dialysis (juvenile) of retina (with detachment)

361.05 Recent detachment, total or subtotal

361.06 Old detachment, partial
Delimited old retinal detachment

361.07 Old detachment, total or subtotal

⑤ **361.1 Retinoschisis and retinal cysts**

> Excludes: *juvenile retinoschisis (362.73)*
> *microcystoid degeneration of retina (362.62)*
> *parasitic cyst of retina (360.13)*

361.10 Retinoschisis, unspecified

361.11 Flat retinoschisis

361.12 Bullous retinoschisis

361.13 Primary retinal cysts

361.14 Secondary retinal cysts

361.19 Other
Pseudocyst of retina

| | Add 4th or 5th digit | | Nonspecific code | | Unspecified code | | Manifestation code |

361.2 Serous retinal detachment
Retinal detachment without retinal defect
[Excludes:] *central serous retinopathy (362.41)*
retinal pigment epithelium detachment (362.42-362.43)

[5] **361.3 Retinal defects without detachment**
[Excludes:] *chorioretinal scars after surgery for detachment (363.30-363.35)*
peripheral retinal degeneration without defect (362.60-362.66)

361.30 Retinal defect, unspecified
Retinal break(s) NOS

361.31 Round hole of retina without detachment

361.32 Horseshoe tear of retina without detachment
Operculum of retina without mention of detachment

361.33 Multiple defects of retina without detachment

[5] **361.8 Other forms of retinal detachment**

361.81 Traction detachment of retina
Traction detachment with vitreoretinal organization

361.89 Other

361.9 Unspecified retinal detachment

362 Other retinal disorders
[Excludes:] *chorioretinal scars (363.30-363.35)*
chorioretinitis (363.0-363.2)

[5] ***362.0 Diabetic retinopathy***
Code first diabetes (250.5)

362.01 Background diabetic retinopathy
Diabetic retinal microaneurysms
Diabetic retinopathy NOS

362.02 Proliferative diabetic retinopathy

[5] **362.1 Other background retinopathy and retinal vascular changes**

362.10 Background retinopathy, unspecified

362.11 Hypertensive retinopathy

362.12 Exudative retinopathy
Coats' syndrome

362.13 Changes in vascular appearance
Vascular sheathing of retina
Use additional code for any associated atherosclerosis (440.8)

362.14 Retinal microaneurysms NOS

362.15 Retinal telangiectasia

362.16 Retinal neovascularization NOS
Neovascularization:
choroidal
subretinal

362.17 Other intraretinal microvascular abnormalities
Retinal varices

362.18 Retinal vasculitis
Eales' disease
Retinal:
arteritis
endarteritis
Retinal:
perivasculitis
phlebitis

[5] **362.2 Other proliferative retinopathy**

362.21 Retrolental fibroplasia

362.29 Other nondiabetic proliferative retinopathy

[5] **362.3 Retinal vascular occlusion**

362.30 Retinal vascular occlusion, unspecified

362.31 Central retinal artery occlusion

362.32 Arterial branch occlusion

● Code new to this edition
▲ Revision of existing code
[4] [5] Fourth or fifth digit required

362.33 Partial arterial occlusion
Hollenhorst plaque   Retinal microembolism

362.34 Transient arterial occlusion
Amaurosis fugax

362.35 Central retinal vein occlusion

362.36 Venous tributary (branch) occlusion

362.37 Venous engorgement
Occlusion:
incipient of retinal vein
partial of retinal vein

[5] **362.4 Separation of retinal layers**

[Excludes:] *retinal detachment (serous) (361.2)*
rhegmatogenous (361.00-361.07)

362.40 Retinal layer separation, unspecified

362.41 Central serous retinopathy

362.42 Serous detachment of retinal pigment epithelium
Exudative detachment of retinal pigment epithelium

362.43 Hemorrhagic detachment of retinal pigment epithelium

[5] **362.5 Degeneration of macula and posterior pole**

[Excludes:] *degeneration of optic disc (377.21-377.24)*
hereditary retinal degeneration [dystrophy] (362.70-362.77)

362.50 Macular degeneration (senile), unspecified

362.51 Nonexudative senile macular degeneration
Senile macular degeneration:
atrophic
dry

362.52 Exudative senile macular degeneration
Kuhnt-Junius degeneration
Senile macular degeneration:
disciform
wet

362.53 Cystoid macular degeneration
Cystoid macular edema

362.54 Macular cyst, hole, or pseudohole

362.55 Toxic maculopathy
Use additional E code, if desired, to identify drug, if drug induced

362.56 Macular puckering
Preretinal fibrosis

362.57 Drusen (degenerative)

[5] **362.6 Peripheral retinal degenerations**

[Excludes:] *hereditary retinal degeneration [dystrophy] (362.70-362.77)*
retinal degeneration with retinal defect (361.00-361.07)

362.60 Peripheral retinal degeneration, unspecified

362.61 Paving stone degeneration

362.62 Microcystoid degeneration
Blessig's cysts   Iwanoff's cysts

362.63 Lattice degeneration
Palisade degeneration of retina

362.64 Senile reticular degeneration

362.65 Secondary pigmentary degeneration
Pseudoretinitis pigmentosa

362.66 Secondary vitreoretinal degenerations

[5] **362.7 Hereditary retinal dystrophies**

362.70 Hereditary retinal dystrophy, unspecified

362.71 Retinal dystrophy in systemic or cerebroretinal lipidoses
Code first underlying disease, as:
cerebroretinal lipidoses (330.1)
systemic lipidoses (272.7)

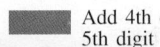

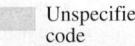

362.72 ***Retinal dystrophy in other systemic disorders and syndromes***
Code first underlying disease, as:
Bassen-Kornzweig syndrome (272.5)
Refsum's disease (356.3)

362.73 Vitreoretinal dystrophies
Juvenile retinoschisis

362.74 Pigmentary retinal dystrophy
Retinal dystrophy, albipunctate
Retinitis pigmentosa

362.75 Other dystrophies primarily involving the sensory retina
Progressive cone (-rod) dystrophy
Stargardt's disease

362.76 Dystrophies primarily involving the retinal pigment epithelium
Fundus flavimaculatus
Vitelliform dystrophy

362.77 Dystrophies primarily involving Bruch's membrane
Dystrophy:
hyaline
pseudoinflammatory foveal
Hereditary drusen

[5] **362.8 Other retinal disorders**
[Excludes:] *chorioretinal inflammations (363.0-363.2)*
chorioretinal scars (363.30-363.35)

362.81 Retinal hemorrhage
Hemorrhage:
preretinal
retinal (deep) (superficial)
subretinal

362.82 Retinal exudates and deposits

362.83 Retinal edema
Retinal:
cotton wool spots
edema (localized) (macular) (peripheral)

362.84 Retinal ischemia

362.85 Retinal nerve fiber bundle defects

362.89 Other retinal disorders

362.9 Unspecified retinal disorder

363 Chorioretinal inflammations, scars, and other disorders of choroid

[5] **363.0 Focal chorioretinitis and focal retinochoroiditis**
[Excludes:] *focal chorioretinitis or retinochoroiditis in:*
histoplasmosis (115.02, 115.12, 115.92)
toxoplasmosis (130.2)
congenital infection (771.2)

363.00 Focal chorioretinitis, unspecified
Focal:
choroiditis or chorioretinitis NOS
retinitis or retinochoroiditis NOS

363.01 Focal choroiditis and chorioretinitis, juxtapapillary

363.03 Focal choroiditis and chorioretinitis of other posterior pole

363.04 Focal choroiditis and chorioretinitis, peripheral

363.05 Focal retinitis and retinochoroiditis, juxtapapillary
Neuroretinitis

363.06 Focal retinitis and retinochoroiditis, macular or paramacular

363.07 Focal retinitis and retinochoroiditis of other posterior pole

363.08 Focal retinitis and retinochoroiditis, peripheral

[5] **363.1 Disseminated chorioretinitis and disseminated retinochoroiditis**
[Excludes:] *disseminated choroiditis or chorioretinitis in secondary syphilis (091.51)*
neurosyphilitic disseminated retinitis or retinochoroiditis (094.83)
retinal (peri)vasculitis (362.18)

363.10 Disseminated chorioretinitis, unspecified
Disseminated:
choroiditis or chorioretinitis NOS
retinitis or retinochoroiditis NOS

363.11 Disseminated choroiditis and chorioretinitis, posterior pole

363.12 Disseminated choroiditis and chorioretinitis, peripheral

363.13 Disseminated choroiditis and chorioretinitis, generalized
Code first any underlying disease, as:
tuberculosis (017.3)

363.14 Disseminated retinitis and retinochoroiditis, metastatic

363.15 Disseminated retinitis and retinochoroiditis, pigment epitheliopathy
Acute posterior multifocal placoid pigment epitheliopathy

[5] **363.2 Other and unspecified forms of chorioretinitis and retinochoroiditis**
[*Excludes:*] *panophthalmitis (360.02)*
sympathetic uveitis (360.11)
uveitis NOS (364.3)

363.20 Chorioretinitis, unspecified
Choroiditis NOS
Retinitis NOS
Uveitis, posterior NOS

363.21 Pars planitis
Posterior cyclitis

363.22 Harada's disease

[5] **363.3 Chorioretinal scars**
Scar (postinflammatory) (postsurgical) (posttraumatic):
choroid
retina

363.30 Chorioretinal scar, unspecified

363.31 Solar retinopathy

363.32 Other macular scars

363.33 Other scars of posterior pole

363.34 Peripheral scars

363.35 Disseminated scars

[5] **363.4 Choroidal degenerations**

363.40 Choroidal degeneration, unspecified
Choroidal sclerosis NOS

363.41 Senile atrophy of choroid

363.42 Diffuse secondary atrophy of choroid

363.43 Angioid streaks of choroid

[5] **363.5 Hereditary choroidal dystrophies**
Hereditary choroidal atrophy:
partial [choriocapillaris]
total [all vessels]

363.50 Hereditary choroidal dystrophy or atrophy, unspecified

363.51 Circumpapillary dystrophy of choroid, partial

363.52 Circumpapillary dystrophy of choroid, total
Helicoid dystrophy of choroid

363.53 Central dystrophy of choroid, partial
Dystrophy, choroidal:
central areolar
circinate

363.54 Central choroidal atrophy, total
Dystrophy, choroidal:
central gyrate
serpiginous

363.55 Choroideremia

363.56 Other diffuse or generalized dystrophy, partial
Diffuse choroidal sclerosis

363.57 Other diffuse or generalized dystrophy, total
Generalized gyrate atrophy, choroid

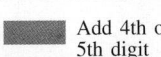

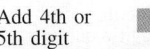

⑤ **363.6 Choroidal hemorrhage and rupture**

    363.61 Choroidal hemorrhage, unspecified

    363.62 Expulsive choroidal hemorrhage

    363.63 Choroidal rupture

⑤ **363.7 Choroidal detachment**

    363.70 Choroidal detachment, unspecified

    363.71 Serous choroidal detachment

    363.72 Hemorrhagic choroidal detachment

363.8 Other disorders of choroid

363.9 Unspecified disorder of choroid

364 Disorders of iris and ciliary body

⑤ **364.0 Acute and subacute iridocyclitis**
Anterior uveitis, acute and subacute
Cyclitis, acute and subacute
Iridocyclitis, acute and subacute
Iritis, acute and subacute

Excludes: *gonococcal (098.41)*
    herpes simplex (054.44)
    herpes zoster (053.22)

    364.00 Acute and subacute iridocyclitis, unspecified

    364.01 Primary iridocyclitis

    364.02 Recurrent iridocyclitis

    364.03 Secondary iridocyclitis, infectious

    364.04 Secondary iridocyclitis, noninfectious
        Aqueous:
          cells
          fibrin
          flare

    364.05 Hypopyon

⑤ **364.1 Chronic iridocyclitis**

Excludes: *posterior cyclitis (363.21)*

    364.10 Chronic iridocyclitis, unspecified

    364.11 Chronic iridocyclitis in diseases classified elsewhere
        Code first underlying disease, as:
          sarcoidosis (135)
          tuberculosis (017.3)

Excludes: *syphilitic iridocyclitis (091.52)*

⑤ **364.2 Certain types of iridocyclitis**

Excludes: *posterior cyclitis (363.21)*
    sympathetic uveitis (360.11)

    364.21 Fuchs' heterochromic cyclitis

    364.22 Glaucomatocyclitic crises

    364.23 Lens-induced iridocyclitis

    364.24 Vogt-Koyanagi syndrome

364.3 Unspecified iridocyclitis
    Uveitis NOS

⑤ **364.4 Vascular disorders of iris and ciliary body**

    364.41 Hyphema
        Hemorrhage of iris or ciliary body

    364.42 Rubeosis iridis
        Neovascularization of iris or ciliary body

⑤ **364.5 Degenerations of iris and ciliary body**

    364.51 Essential or progressive iris atrophy

    364.52 Iridoschisis

  ● Code new
    to this edition
  ▲ Revision of
    existing code
  ④ ⑤ Fourth or fifth
    digit required

364.53 Pigmentary iris degeneration
Acquired heterochromia of iris
Pigment dispersion syndrome of iris
Translucency of iris

364.54 Degeneration of pupillary margin
Atrophy of sphincter of iris
Ectropion of pigment epithelium of iris

364.55 Miotic cysts of pupillary margin

364.56 Degenerative changes of chamber angle

364.57 Degenerative changes of ciliary body

364.59 Other iris atrophy
Iris atrophy (generalized) (sector shaped)

⑤ **364.6 Cysts of iris, ciliary body, and anterior chamber**
Excludes: miotic pupillary cyst (364.55)
parasitic cyst (360.13)

364.60 Idiopathic cysts

364.61 Implantation cysts
Epithelial down-growth, anterior chamber
Implantation cysts (surgical) (traumatic)

364.62 Exudative cysts of iris or anterior chamber

364.63 Primary cyst of pars plana

364.64 Exudative cyst of pars plana

⑤ **364.7 Adhesions and disruptions of iris and ciliary body**
Excludes: flat anterior chamber (360.34)

364.70 Adhesions of iris, unspecified
Synechiae (iris) NOS

364.71 Posterior synechiae

364.72 Anterior synechiae

364.73 Goniosynechiae
Peripheral anterior synechiae

364.74 Pupillary membranes
Iris bombé
Pupillary:
  occlusion
  seclusion

364.75 Pupillary abnormalities
Deformed pupil   Rupture of sphincter, pupil
Ectopic pupil

364.76 Iridodialysis

364.77 Recession of chamber angle

364.8 Other disorders of iris and ciliary body
Prolapse of iris NOS
Excludes: prolapse of iris in recent wound (871.1)

364.9 Unspecified disorder of iris and ciliary body

365 Glaucoma
Excludes: blind hypertensive eye [absolute glaucoma] (360.42)
congenital glaucoma (743.20-743.22)

⑤ **365.0 Borderline glaucoma [glaucoma suspect]**

365.00 Preglaucoma, unspecified

365.01 Open angle with borderline findings
Open angle with:
  borderline intraocular pressure
  cupping of optic discs

365.02 Anatomical narrow angle

365.03 Steroid responders

365.04 Ocular hypertension

Add 4th or 5th digit   Nonspecific code   Unspecified code   Manifestation code

⑤ **365.1 Open-angle glaucoma**

  365.10 Open-angle glaucoma, unspecified
  Wide-angle glaucoma NOS

  365.11 Primary open angle glaucoma
  Chronic simple glaucoma

  365.12 Low tension glaucoma

  365.13 Pigmentary glaucoma

  365.14 Glaucoma of childhood
  Infantile or juvenile glaucoma

  365.15 Residual stage of open angle glaucoma

⑤ **365.2 Primary angle-closure glaucoma**

  365.20 Primary angle-closure glaucoma, unspecified

  365.21 Intermittent angle-closure glaucoma
  Angle-closure glaucoma:
    interval
    subacute

  365.22 Acute angle-closure glaucoma

  365.23 Chronic angle-closure glaucoma

  365.24 Residual stage of angle-closure glaucoma

⑤ **365.3 Corticosteroid-induced glaucoma**

  365.31 Glaucomatous stage

  365.32 Residual stage

⑤ **365.4 Glaucoma associated with congenital anomalies, dystrophies, and systemic syndromes**

  365.41 *Glaucoma associated with chamber angle anomalies*
  Code first associated disorder, as:
    Axenfeld's anomaly (743.44)
    Rieger's anomaly or syndrome (743.44)

  365.42 *Glaucoma associated with anomalies of iris*
  Code first associated disorder, as:
    aniridia (743.45)
    essential iris atrophy (364.51)

  365.43 *Glaucoma associated with other anterior segment anomalies*
  Code first associated disorder, as:
    microcornea (743.41)

  365.44 *Glaucoma associated with systemic syndromes*
  Code first associated disease, as:
    neurofibromatosis (237.7)
    Sturge-Weber (-Dimitri) syndrome (759.6)

⑤ **365.5 Glaucoma associated with disorders of the lens**

  365.51 Phacolytic glaucoma
  Use additional code for associated hypermature cataract (366.18)

  365.52 Pseudoexfoliation glaucoma
  Use additional code for associated pseudoexfoliation of capsule (366.11)

  365.59 Glaucoma associated with other lens disorders
  Use additional code for associated disorder, as:
    dislocation of lens (379.33-379.34)
    spherophakia (743.36)

⑤ **365.6 Glaucoma associated with other ocular disorders**

  365.60 Glaucoma associated with unspecified ocular disorder

  365.61 Glaucoma associated with pupillary block
  Use additional code for associated disorder, as:
    seclusion of pupil [iris bombé] (364.74)

  365.62 Glaucoma associated with ocular inflammations
  Use additional code for associated disorder, as:
    glaucomatocyclitic crises (364.22)
    iridocyclitis (364.0-364.3)

  365.63 Glaucoma associated with vascular disorders
  Use additional code for associated disorder, as:
    central retinal vein occlusion (362.35)
    hyphema (364.41)

● Code new
  to this edition ▲ Revision of
  existing code ④ ⑤ Fourth or fifth
  digit required

365.64 Glaucoma associated with tumors or cysts
Use additional code for associated disorder, as:
benign neoplasm (224.0-224.9)
epithelial down-growth (364.61)
malignant neoplasm (190.0-190.9)

365.65 Glaucoma associated with ocular trauma
Use additional code for associated condition, as:
contusion of globe (921.3)
recession of chamber angle (364.77)

⑤ **365.8 Other specified forms of glaucoma**

365.81 Hypersecretion glaucoma

365.82 Glaucoma with increased episcleral venous pressure

● **365.83 Aqueous misdirection**
Malignant glaucoma

365.89 Other specified glaucoma

365.9 Unspecified glaucoma

366 Cataract
Excludes: congenital cataract (743.30-743.34)

⑤ **366.0 Infantile, juvenile, and presenile cataract**

366.00 Nonsenile cataract, unspecified

366.01 Anterior subcapsular polar cataract

366.02 Posterior subcapsular polar cataract

366.03 Cortical, lamellar, or zonular cataract

366.04 Nuclear cataract

366.09 Other and combined forms of nonsenile cataract

⑤ **366.1 Senile cataract**

366.10 Senile cataract, unspecified

366.11 Pseudoexfoliation of lens capsule

366.12 Incipient cataract
Cataract: Water clefts
coronary
immature NOS
punctate

366.13 Anterior subcapsular polar senile cataract

366.14 Posterior subcapsular polar senile cataract

366.15 Cortical senile cataract

366.16 Nuclear sclerosis
Cataracta brunescens
Nuclear cataract

366.17 Total or mature cataract

366.18 Hypermature cataract
Morgagni cataract

366.19 Other and combined forms of senile cataract

⑤ **366.2 Traumatic cataract**

366.20 Traumatic cataract, unspecified

366.21 Localized traumatic opacities
Vossius' ring

366.22 Total traumatic cataract

366.23 Partially resolved traumatic cataract

⑤ **366.3 Cataract secondary to ocular disorders**

366.30 Cataracts complicata, unspecified

366.31 Glaucomatous flecks (subcapsular)
Code first underlying glaucoma (365.0-365.9)

366.32 Cataract in inflammatory disorders
Code first underlying condition, as:
chronic choroiditis (363.0-363.2)

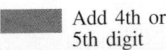 Add 4th or
5th digit

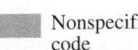 Nonspecific
code

Unspecified
code

Manifestation
code

366.33 *Cataract with neovascularization*
Code first underlying condition, as:
chronic iridocyclitis (364.10)

366.34 *Cataract in degenerative disorders*
Sunflower cataract
Code first underlying condition, as:
chalcosis (360.24)
degenerative myopia (360.21)
pigmentary retinal dystrophy (362.74)

⑤ **366.4 Cataract associated with other disorders**

366.41 *Diabetic cataract*
Code first diabetes (250.5)

366.42 *Tetanic cataract*
Code first underlying disease, as:
calcinosis (275.4)
hypoparathyroidism (252.1)

366.43 *Myotonic cataract*
Code first underlying disorder (359.2)

366.44 *Cataract associated with other syndromes*
Code first underlying condition, as:
craniofacial dysostosis (756.0)
galactosemia (271.1)

366.45 Toxic cataract
Drug-induced cataract
Use additional E code, if desired, to identify drug or other toxic substance

366.46 Cataract associated with radiation and other physical influences
Use additional E code, if desired, to identify cause

⑤ **366.5 After-cataract**

366.50 After-cataract, unspecified
Secondary cataract NOS

366.51 Soemmering's ring

366.52 Other after-cataract, not obscuring vision

366.53 After-cataract, obscuring vision

366.8 Other cataract
Calcification of lens

366.9 Unspecified cataract

367 Disorders of refraction and accommodation

367.0 Hypermetropia
Far-sightedness   Hyperopia

367.1 Myopia
Near-sightedness

⑤ **367.2 Astigmatism**

367.20 Astigmatism, unspecified

367.21 Regular astigmatism

367.22 Irregular astigmatism

⑤ **367.3 Anisometropia and aniseikonia**

367.31 Anisometropia

367.32 Aniseikonia

367.4 Presbyopia

⑤ **367.5 Disorders of accommodation**

367.51 Paresis of accommodation
Cycloplegia

367.52 Total or complete internal ophthalmoplegia

367.53 Spasm of accommodation

⑤ **367.8 Other disorders of refraction and accommodation**

367.81 Transient refractive change

367.89 Other
Drug-induced disorders of refraction and accommodation
Toxic disorders of refraction and accommodation

● Code new
to this edition
▲ Revision of
existing code
④ ⑤ Fourth or fifth
digit required

367.9 Unspecified disorder of refraction and accommodation

368 Visual disturbances

[Excludes:] *electrophysiological disturbances (794.11-794.14)*

[5] **368.0 Amblyopia ex anopsia**

368.00 Amblyopia, unspecified

368.01 Strabismic amblyopia
Suppression amblyopia

368.02 Deprivation amblyopia

368.03 Refractive amblyopia

[5] **368.1 Subjective visual disturbances**

368.10 Subjective visual disturbance, unspecified

368.11 Sudden visual loss

368.12 Transient visual loss
Concentric fading
Scintillating scotoma

368.13 Visual discomfort
Asthenopia
Eye strain
Photophobia

368.14 Visual distortions of shape and size
Macropsia
Metamorphopsia
Micropsia

368.15 Other visual distortions and entoptic phenomena
Photopsia
Refractive:
  diplopia
  polyopia
Visual halos

368.16 Psychophysical visual disturbances
Visual:
  agnosia
  disorientation syndrome
  hallucinations

368.2 Diplopia
Double vision

[5] **368.3 Other disorders of binocular vision**

368.30 Binocular vision disorder, unspecified

368.31 Suppression of binocular vision

368.32 Simultaneous visual perception without fusion

368.33 Fusion with defective stereopsis

368.34 Abnormal retinal correspondence

[5] **368.4 Visual field defects**

368.40 Visual field defect, unspecified

368.41 Scotoma involving central area
Scotoma:
  central
  centrocecal
  paracentral

368.42 Scotoma of blind spot area
Enlarged:
  angioscotoma
  blind spot
Paracecal scotoma

368.43 Sector or arcuate defects
Scotoma:
  arcuate
  Bjerrum
  Seidel

368.44 Other localized visual field defect
Scotoma:
  NOS
  ring
Visual field defect:
  nasal step
  peripheral

368.45 Generalized contraction or constriction

368.46 Homonymous bilateral field defects
Hemianopsia (altitudinal) (homonymous)
Quadrant anopia

368.47 Heteronymous bilateral field defects
Hemianopsia:
binasal
bitemporal

⑤ **368.5 Color vision deficiencies**
Color blindness

368.51 Protan defect
Protanomaly   Protanopia

368.52 Deutan defect
Deuteranomaly   Deuteranopia

368.53 Tritan defect
Tritanomaly   Tritanopia

368.54 Achromatopsia
Monochromatism (cone) (rod)

368.55 Acquired color vision deficiencies

368.59 Other color vision deficiencies

⑤ **368.6 Night blindness**
Nyctalopia

368.60 Night blindness, unspecified

368.61 Congenital night blindness
Hereditary night blindness
Oguchi's disease

368.62 Acquired night blindness

Excludes: *that due to vitamin A deficiency (264.5)*

368.63 Abnormal dark adaptation curve
Abnormal threshold of cones or rods
Delayed adaptation of cones or rods

368.69 Other night blindness

368.8 Other specified visual disturbances
Blurred vision NOS

368.9 Unspecified visual disturbance

369 Blindness and low vision

Note: Visual impairment refers to a functional limitation of the eye (e.g., limited visual acuity or visual field). It should be distinguished from visual disability, indicating a limitation of the abilities of the individual (e.g., limited reading skills, vocational skills), and from visual handicap, indicating a limitation of personal and socioeconomic independence (e.g., limited mobility, limited employability.)

The levels of impairment defined in the table on page 174 are based on the recommendations of the WHO Study Group on Prevention of Blindness (Geneva, November 6-10, 1972; WHO Technical Report Series 518), and of the International Council of Ophthalmology (1976).
Note that definitions of blindness vary in different settings.

For international reporting WHO defines blindness as profound impairment. This definition can be applied to blindness of one eye (369.1, 369.6) and to blindness of the individual (369.0).

For determination of benefits in the U.S.A., the definition of legal blindness as severe impairment is often used. This definition applies to blindness of the individual only.

Excludes: *correctable impaired vision due to refractive errors (367.0-367.9)*

⑤ **369.0 Profound impairment, both eyes**

369.00 Impairment level not further specified
Blindness:
NOS according to WHO definition
both eyes

**369.01 Better eye: total impairment;
lesser eye: total impairment**

● Code new
to this edition

▲ Revision of
existing code

④ ⑤ Fourth or fifth
digit required

369.02 Better eye: near-total impairment; lesser eye: not further specified

369.03 Better eye: near-total impairment; lesser eye: total impairment

369.04 Better eye: near-total impairment; lesser eye: near-total impairment

369.05 Better eye: profound impairment; lesser eye: not further specified

369.06 Better eye: profound impairment; lesser eye: total impairment

369.07 Better eye: profound impairment; lesser eye: near-total impairment

369.08 Better eye: profound impairment; lesser eye: profound impairment

[5] **369.1 Moderate or severe impairment, better eye, profound impairment lesser eye**

369.10 Impairment level not further specified
Blindness, one eye, low vision other eye

369.11 Better eye: severe impairment; lesser eye: blind, not further specified

369.12 Better eye: severe impairment; lesser eye: total impairment

369.13 Better eye: severe impairment; lesser eye: near-total impairment

369.14 Better eye: severe impairment; lesser eye: profound impairment

369.15 Better eye: moderate impairment; lesser eye: blind, not further specified

369.16 Better eye: moderate impairment; lesser eye: total impairment

369.17 Better eye: moderate impairment; lesser eye: near-total impairment

369.18 Better eye: moderate impairment; lesser eye: profound impairment

[5] **369.2 Moderate or severe impairment, both eyes**

369.20 Impairment level not further specified
Low vision, both eyes NOS

369.21 Better eye: severe impairment; lesser eye: not further specified

369.22 Better eye: severe impairment; lesser eye: severe impairment

369.23 Better eye: moderate impairment; lesser eye: not further specified

369.24 Better eye: moderate impairment; lesser eye: severe impairment

369.25 Better eye: moderate impairment; lesser eye: moderate impairment

369.3 Unqualified visual loss, both eyes

[*Excludes:*] *blindness NOS:*
legal [U.S.A. definition] (369.4)
WHO definition (369.00)

369.4 Legal blindness, as defined in U.S.A.
Blindness NOS according to U.S.A. definition

[*Excludes:*] *legal blindness with specification of impairment level (369.01-369.08, 369.11-369.14, 369.21-369.22)*

[5] **369.6 Profound impairment, one eye**

369.60 Impairment level not further specified
Blindness, one eye

369.61 One eye: total impairment; other eye: not specified

369.62 One eye: total impairment; other eye: near-normal vision

369.63 **One eye: total impairment; other eye: normal vision**

369.64 **One eye: near-total impairment; other eye: not specified**

369.65 **One eye: near-total impairment; other eye: near-normal vision**

369.66 **One eye: near-total impairment; other eye: normal vision**

369.67 **One eye: profound impairment; other eye: not specified**

369.68 **One eye: profound impairment; other eye: near-normal vision**

369.69 **One eye: profound impairment; other eye: normal vision**

[5] **369.7** **Moderate or severe impairment, one eye**

369.70 **Impairment level not further specified**
Low vision, one eye

369.71 **One eye: severe impairment; other eye: not specified**

369.72 **One eye: severe impairment; other eye: near-normal vision**

369.73 **One eye: severe impairment; other eye: normal vision**

369.74 **One eye: moderate impairment; other eye: not specified**

Classification "legal"	Classification WHO	LEVELS OF VISUAL IMPAIRMENT Visual Acuity and/or Visual Field Limitation (whichever is worse)	Additional Descriptors which may be encountered
	(NEAR-) NORMAL VISION	**RANGE OF NORMAL VISION** 20/10 0.7; 20/13 0.6; 20/16 0.5; 20/20 0.4; 20/25 0.8	
	(NEAR-) NORMAL VISION	**NEAR-NORMAL VISION** 0.7; 20/30 0.6; 20/40 0.5; 20/50 0.4; 20/60 0.4	
	LOW VISION	**MODERATE VISUAL IMPAIRMENT** 20/70; 20/80 0.25; 20/100 0.20; 20/125 0.16; 20/160 0.12	Moderate low vision
LEGAL BLINDNESS	LOW VISION	**SEVERE VISUAL IMPAIRMENT** 20/200 0.10; 20/250 0.08; 20/320 0.06; 20/400 0.05 Visual Field: 20 degrees or less	Severe low vision, "legal blindness"
LEGAL BLINDNESS	BLINDNESS	**PROFOUND VISUAL IMPAIRMENT** 20/500 0.04; 20/630 0.03; 20/800 0.025; 20/1000 0.02 Count Fingers at: less than 3 m (10ft) Visual Field: 10 degrees or less	Profound low vision, moderate blindness
LEGAL BLINDNESS	BLINDNESS	**NEAR-TOTAL VISUAL IMPAIRMENT** Visual Acuity: less than 0.02 (20/1000) Count Fingers at: 1 m (3 ft) or less Hand Movements: 5m (15ft) or less Light projection, light perception Visual Field: 5 degrees or less	Severe blindness Near-Total blindness
(USA) both eyes	(WHO) one or both eyes	**TOTAL VISUAL IMPAIRMENT** No light perception (NLP)	Total blindness

Visual acuity refers to best achievable acuity with correction
Non-listed Snellen fractions may be classified by converting to the nearest decimal equivalent, e.g., 10/200=0.05, 6/30=0.20
CF (count fingers) without designation of distance, may be classified to profound impairment
HM (hand motion) without designation of distance, may be classified to near-total impairment.
Visual field measurements refer to the largest field diameter for a 1/100 white test object.

369.75 **One eye: moderate impairment; other eye: near-normal vision**

369.76 **One eye: moderate impairment; other eye: normal vision**

369.8 **Unqualified visual loss, one eye**

369.9 **Unspecified visual loss**

● Code new to this edition ▲ Revision of existing code [4] [5] Fourth or fifth digit required

370 Keratitis

[5] **370.0 Corneal ulcer**

[Excludes:] *that due to vitamin A deficiency (264.3)*

370.00 Corneal ulcer, unspecified

370.01 Marginal corneal ulcer

370.02 Ring corneal ulcer

370.03 Central corneal ulcer

370.04 Hypopyon ulcer
Serpiginous ulcer

370.05 Mycotic corneal ulcer

370.06 Perforated corneal ulcer

370.07 Mooren's ulcer

[5] **370.2 Superficial keratitis without conjunctivitis**

[Excludes:] *dendritic [herpes simplex] keratitis (054.42)*

370.20 Superficial keratitis, unspecified

370.21 Punctate keratitis
Thygeson's superficial punctate keratitis

370.22 Macular keratitis
Keratitis:
areolar
nummular
Keratitis:
stellate
striate

370.23 Filamentary keratitis

370.24 Photokeratitis
Snow blindness
Welders' keratitis

[5] **370.3 Certain types of keratoconjunctivitis**

370.31 Phlyctenular keratoconjunctivitis
Phlyctenulosis
Use additional code for any associated tuberculosis (017.3)

370.32 Limbar and corneal involvement in vernal conjunctivitis
Use additional code for vernal conjunctivitis (372.13)

370.33 Keratoconjunctivitis sicca, not specified as Sjögren's

[Excludes:] *Sjögren's syndrome (710.2)*

370.34 Exposure keratoconjunctivitis

370.35 Neurotrophic keratoconjunctivitis

[5] **370.4 Other and unspecified keratoconjunctivitis**

370.40 Keratoconjunctivitis, unspecified
Superficial keratitis with conjunctivitis NOS

370.44 Keratitis or keratoconjunctivitis in exanthema
Code first underlying condition (050.0-052.9)

[Excludes:] *herpes simplex (054.43)*
herpes zoster (053.21)
measles (055.71)

370.49 Other

[Excludes:] *epidemic keratoconjunctivitis (077.1)*

[5] **370.5 Interstitial and deep keratitis**

370.50 Interstitial keratitis, unspecified

370.52 Diffuse interstitial keratitis
Cogan's syndrome

370.54 Sclerosing keratitis

370.55 Corneal abscess

370.59 Other

[Excludes:] *disciform herpes simplex keratitis (054.43)*
syphilitic keratitis (090.3)

[5] **370.6 Corneal neovascularization**

370.60 Corneal neovascularization, unspecified

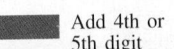

Add 4th or 5th digit | Nonspecific code | Unspecified code | Manifestation code

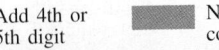

370.61 **Localized vascularization of cornea**

370.62 **Pannus (corneal)**

370.63 **Deep vascularization of cornea**

370.64 **Ghost vessels (corneal)**

370.8 Other forms of keratitis

370.9 Unspecified keratitis

371 Corneal opacity and other disorders of cornea

⑤ **371.0 Corneal scars and opacities**

Excludes: that due to vitamin A deficiency (264.6)

371.00 **Corneal opacity, unspecified**
Corneal scar NOS

371.01 **Minor opacity of cornea**
Corneal nebula

371.02 **Peripheral opacity of cornea**
Corneal macula not interfering with central vision

371.03 **Central opacity of cornea**
Corneal:
leucoma interfering with central vision
macula interfering with central vision

371.04 **Adherent leucoma**

371.05 *Phthisical cornea*
Code first underlying tuberculosis (017.3)

⑤ **371.1 Corneal pigmentations and deposits**

371.10 **Corneal deposit, unspecified**

371.11 **Anterior pigmentations**
Stähli's lines

371.12 **Stromal pigmentations**
Hematocornea

371.13 **Posterior pigmentations**
Krukenberg spindle

371.14 **Kayser-Fleischer ring**

371.15 **Other deposits associated with metabolic disorders**

371.16 **Argentous deposits**

⑤ **371.2 Corneal edema**

371.20 **Corneal edema, unspecified**

371.21 **Idiopathic corneal edema**

371.22 **Secondary corneal edema**

371.23 **Bullous keratopathy**

371.24 **Corneal edema due to wearing of contact lenses**

⑤ **371.3 Changes of corneal membranes**

371.30 **Corneal membrane change, unspecified**

371.31 **Folds and rupture of Bowman's membrane**

371.32 **Folds in Descemet's membrane**

371.33 **Rupture in Descemet's membrane**

⑤ **371.4 Corneal degenerations**

371.40 **Corneal degeneration, unspecified**

371.41 **Senile corneal changes**
Arcus senilis   Hassall-Henle bodies

371.42 **Recurrent erosion of cornea**

Excludes: Mooren's ulcer (370.07)

371.43 **Band-shaped keratopathy**

371.44 **Other calcerous degenerations of cornea**

371.45 **Keratomalacia NOS**

Excludes: that due to vitamin A deficiency (264.4)

● Code new to this edition   ▲ Revision of existing code   ④ ⑤ Fourth or fifth digit required

371.46 Nodular degeneration of cornea
Salzmann's nodular dystrophy

371.48 Peripheral degenerations of cornea
Marginal degeneration of cornea [Terrien's]

371.49 Other
Discrete colliquative keratopathy

[5] **371.5 Hereditary corneal dystrophies**

371.50 Corneal dystrophy, unspecified

371.51 Juvenile epithelial corneal dystrophy

371.52 Other anterior corneal dystrophies
Corneal dystrophy:
microscopic cystic
ring-like

371.53 Granular corneal dystrophy

371.54 Lattice corneal dystrophy

371.55 Macular corneal dystrophy

371.56 Other stromal corneal dystrophies
Crystalline corneal dystrophy

371.57 Endothelial corneal dystrophy
Combined corneal dystrophy
Cornea guttata
Fuchs' endothelial dystrophy

371.58 Other posterior corneal dystrophies
Polymorphous corneal dystrophy

[5] **371.6 Keratoconus**

371.60 Keratoconus, unspecified

371.61 Keratoconus, stable condition

371.62 Keratoconus, acute hydrops

[5] **371.7 Other corneal deformities**

371.70 Corneal deformity, unspecified

371.71 Corneal ectasia

371.72 Descemetocele

371.73 Corneal staphyloma

[5] **371.8 Other corneal disorders**

371.81 Corneal anesthesia and hypoesthesia

371.82 Corneal disorder due to contact lens

[Excludes:] *corneal edema due to contact lens (371.24)*

371.89 Other

371.9 Unspecified corneal disorder

372 Disorders of conjunctiva

[Excludes:] *keratoconjunctivitis (370.3-370.4)*

[5] **372.0 Acute conjunctivitis**

372.00 Acute conjunctivitis, unspecified

372.01 Serous conjunctivitis, except viral

[Excludes:] *viral conjunctivitis NOS (077.9)*

372.02 Acute follicular conjunctivitis
Conjunctival folliculosis NOS

[Excludes:] *conjunctivitis:*
adenoviral (acute follicular) (077.3)
epidemic hemorrhagic (077.4)
inclusion (077.0)
Newcastle (077.8)
epidemic keratoconjunctivitis (077.1)
pharyngoconjunctival fever (077.2)

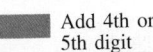

Add 4th or 5th digit | Nonspecific code | Unspecified code | Manifestation code

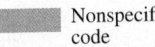

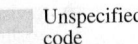

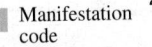

372.03 **Other mucopurulent conjunctivitis**
Catarrhal conjunctivitis

Excludes: *blennorrhea neonatorum (gonococcal) (098.40)*
neonatal conjunctivitis (771.6)
ophthalmia neonatorum NOS (771.6)

372.04 **Pseudomembranous conjunctivitis**
Membranous conjunctivitis

Excludes: *diphtheritic conjunctivitis (032.81)*

372.05 **Acute atopic conjunctivitis**

⑤ **372.1** **Chronic conjunctivitis**

372.10 **Chronic conjunctivitis, unspecified**

372.11 **Simple chronic conjunctivitis**

372.12 **Chronic follicular conjunctivitis**

372.13 **Vernal conjunctivitis**

372.14 **Other chronic allergic conjunctivitis**

372.15 *Parasitic conjunctivitis*
Code first underlying disease, as:
filariasis (125.0-125.9)
mucocutaneous leishmaniasis (085.5)

⑤ **372.2** **Blepharoconjunctivitis**

372.20 **Blepharoconjunctivitis, unspecified**

372.21 **Angular blepharoconjunctivitis**

372.22 **Contact blepharoconjunctivitis**

⑤ **372.3** **Other and unspecified conjunctivitis**

372.30 **Conjunctivitis, unspecified**

372.31 *Rosacea conjunctivitis*
Code first underlying rosacea dermatitis (695.3)

372.33 *Conjunctivitis in mucocutaneous disease*
Code first underlying disease, as:
erythema multiforme (695.1)
Reiter's disease (099.3)

Excludes: *ocular pemphigoid (694.61)*

372.39 **Other**

⑤ **372.4** **Pterygium**

Excludes: *pseudopterygium (372.52)*

372.40 **Pterygium, unspecified**

372.41 **Peripheral pterygium, stationary**

372.42 **Peripheral pterygium, progressive**

372.43 **Central pterygium**

372.44 **Double pterygium**

372.45 **Recurrent pterygium**

⑤ **372.5** **Conjunctival degenerations and deposits**

372.50 **Conjunctival degeneration, unspecified**

372.51 **Pinguecula**

372.52 **Pseudopterygium**

372.53 **Conjunctival xerosis**

Excludes: *conjunctival xerosis due to vitamin A deficiency (264.0, 264.1, 264.7)*

372.54 **Conjunctival concretions**

372.55 **Conjunctival pigmentations**
Conjunctival argyrosis

372.56 **Conjunctival deposits**

⑤ **372.6** **Conjunctival scars**

372.61 **Granuloma of conjunctiva**

372.62 **Localized adhesions and strands of conjunctiva**

● Code new
to this edition
▲ Revision of
existing code
④ ⑤ Fourth or fifth
digit required

372.63 Symblepharon
Extensive adhesions of conjunctiva

372.64 Scarring of conjunctiva
Contraction of eye socket (after enucleation)

[5] **372.7 Conjunctival vascular disorders and cysts**

372.71 Hyperemia of conjunctiva

372.72 Conjunctival hemorrhage
Hyposphagma
Subconjunctival hemorrhage

372.73 Conjunctival edema
Chemosis of conjunctiva
Subconjunctival edema

372.74 Vascular abnormalities of conjunctiva
Aneurysm(ata) of conjunctiva

372.75 Conjunctival cysts

[5] **372.8 Other disorders of conjunctiva**

372.81 Conjunctivochalasis

372.89 Other disorders of conjunctiva

372.9 Unspecified disorder of conjunctiva

373 Inflammation of eyelids

[5] **373.0 Blepharitis**

[Excludes:] *blepharoconjunctivitis (372.20-372.22)*

373.00 Blepharitis, unspecified

373.01 Ulcerative blepharitis

373.02 Squamous blepharitis

[5] **373.1 Hordeolum and other deep inflammation of eyelid**

373.11 Hordeolum externum
Hordeolum NOS
Stye

373.12 Hordeolum internum
Infection of meibomian gland

373.13 Abscess of eyelid
Furuncle of eyelid

373.2 Chalazion
Meibomian (gland) cyst

[Excludes:] *infected meibomian gland (373.12)*

[5] **373.3 Noninfectious dermatoses of eyelid**

373.31 Eczematous dermatitis of eyelid

373.32 Contact and allergic dermatitis of eyelid

373.33 Xeroderma of eyelid

373.34 Discoid lupus erythematosus of eyelid

373.4 Infective dermatitis of eyelid of types resulting in deformity
Code first underlying disease, as:
leprosy (030.0-030.9)
lupus vulgaris (tuberculous) (017.0)
yaws (102.0-102.9)

373.5 Other infective dermatitis of eyelid
Code first underlying disease, as:
actinomycosis (039.3)
impetigo (684)
mycotic dermatitis (110.0-111.9)
vaccinia (051.0)
postvaccination (999.0)

[Excludes:] *herpes:*
simplex (054.41)
zoster (053.20)

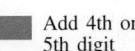

Add 4th or 5th digit | Nonspecific code | Unspecified code | Manifestation code

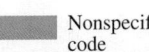

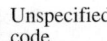

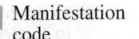

373.6 *Parasitic infestation of eyelid*
Code first underlying disease, as:
leishmaniasis (085.0-085.9)
loiasis (125.2)
onchocerciasis (125.3)
pediculosis (132.0)

373.8 Other inflammations of eyelids

373.9 Unspecified inflammation of eyelid

374 Other disorders of eyelids

[5] **374.0 Entropion and trichiasis of eyelid**

374.00 Entropion, unspecified

374.01 Senile entropion

374.02 Mechanical entropion

374.03 Spastic entropion

374.04 Cicatricial entropion

374.05 Trichiasis without entropion

[5] **374.1 Ectropion**

374.10 Ectropion, unspecified

374.11 Senile ectropion

374.12 Mechanical ectropion

374.13 Spastic ectropion

374.14 Cicatricial ectropion

[5] **374.2 Lagophthalmos**

374.20 Lagophthalmos, unspecified

374.21 Paralytic lagophthalmos

374.22 Mechanical lagophthalmos

374.23 Cicatricial lagophthalmos

[5] **374.3 Ptosis of eyelid**

374.30 Ptosis of eyelid, unspecified

374.31 Paralytic ptosis

374.32 Myogenic ptosis

374.33 Mechanical ptosis

374.34 Blepharochalasis
Pseudoptosis

[5] **374.4 Other disorders affecting eyelid function**

[Excludes:] *blepharoclonus (333.81)*
blepharospasm (333.81)
facial nerve palsy (351.0)
third nerve palsy or paralysis (378.51-378.52)
tic (psychogenic) (307.20-307.23)
organic (333.3)

374.41 Lid retraction or lag

374.43 Abnormal innervation syndrome
Jaw-blinking
Paradoxical facial movements

374.44 Sensory disorders

374.45 Other sensorimotor disorders
Deficient blink reflex

374.46 Blepharophimosis
Ankyloblepharon

[5] **374.5 Degenerative disorders of eyelid and periocular area**

374.50 Degenerative disorder of eyelid, unspecified

374.51 ***Xanthelasma***
Xanthoma (planum) (tuberosum) of eyelid
Code first underlying condition (272.0-272.9)

374.52 Hyperpigmentation of eyelid
Chloasma
Dyspigmentation

● Code new to this edition
▲ Revision of existing code
[4] [5] Fourth or fifth digit required

374.53 **Hypopigmentation of eyelid**
Vitiligo of eyelid

374.54 **Hypertrichosis of eyelid**

374.55 **Hypotrichosis of eyelid**
Madarosis of eyelid

374.56 **Other degenerative disorders of skin affecting eyelid**

[5] **374.8 Other disorders of eyelid**

374.81 **Hemorrhage of eyelid**

[Excludes:] *black eye (921.0)*

374.82 **Edema of eyelid**
Hyperemia of eyelid

374.83 **Elephantiasis of eyelid**

374.84 **Cysts of eyelids**
Sebaceous cyst of eyelid

374.85 **Vascular anomalies of eyelid**

374.86 **Retained foreign body of eyelid**

374.87 **Dermatochalasis**

374.89 **Other disorders of eyelid**

374.9 Unspecified disorder of eyelid

375 Disorders of lacrimal system

[5] **375.0 Dacryoadenitis**

375.00 **Dacryoadenitis, unspecified**

375.01 **Acute dacryoadenitis**

375.02 **Chronic dacryoadenitis**

375.03 **Chronic enlargement of lacrimal gland**

[5] **375.1 Other disorders of lacrimal gland**

375.11 **Dacryops**

375.12 **Other lacrimal cysts and cystic degeneration**

375.13 **Primary lacrimal atrophy**

375.14 **Secondary lacrimal atrophy**

375.15 **Tear film insufficiency, unspecified**
Dry eye syndrome

375.16 **Dislocation of lacrimal gland**

[5] **375.2 Epiphora**

375.20 **Epiphora, unspecified as to cause**

375.21 **Epiphora due to excess lacrimation**

375.22 **Epiphora due to insufficient drainage**

[5] **375.3 Acute and unspecified inflammation of lacrimal passages**

[Excludes:] *neonatal dacryocystitis (771.6)*

375.30 **Dacryocystitis, unspecified**

375.31 **Acute canaliculitis, lacrimal**

375.32 **Acute dacryocystitis**
Acute peridacryocystitis

375.33 **Phlegmonous dacryocystitis**

[5] **375.4 Chronic inflammation of lacrimal passages**

375.41 **Chronic canaliculitis**

375.42 **Chronic dacryocystitis**

375.43 **Lacrimal mucocele**

[5] **375.5 Stenosis and insufficiency of lacrimal passages**

375.51 **Eversion of lacrimal punctum**

375.52 **Stenosis of lacrimal punctum**

375.53 **Stenosis of lacrimal canaliculi**

375.54 **Stenosis of lacrimal sac**

375.55 Obstruction of nasolacrimal duct, neonatal
Excludes: *congenital anomaly of nasolacrimal duct (743.65)*

    375.56 Stenosis of nasolacrimal duct, acquired

    375.57 Dacryolith

⑤ **375.6 Other changes of lacrimal passages**

    375.61 Lacrimal fistula

    375.69 Other

⑤ **375.8 Other disorders of lacrimal system**

    375.81 Granuloma of lacrimal passages

    375.89 Other

375.9 Unspecified disorder of lacrimal system

376 Disorders of the orbit

⑤ **376.0 Acute inflammation of orbit**

    376.00 Acute inflammation of orbit, unspecified

    376.01 Orbital cellulitis
        Abscess of orbit

    376.02 Orbital periostitis

    376.03 Orbital osteomyelitis

    376.04 Tenonitis

⑤ **376.1 Chronic inflammatory disorders of orbit**

    376.10 Chronic inflammation of orbit, unspecified

    376.11 Orbital granuloma
        Pseudotumor (inflammatory) of orbit

    376.12 Orbital myositis

    376.13 *Parasitic infestation of orbit*
        Code first underlying disease, as:
          hydatid infestation of orbit (122.3, 122.6, 122.9)
          myiasis of orbit (134.0)

⑤ **376.2 *Endocrine exophthalmos***
    Code first underlying thyroid disorder (242.0-242.9)

    376.21 *Thyrotoxic exophthalmos*

    376.22 *Exophthalmic ophthalmoplegia*

⑤ **376.3 Other exophthalmic conditions**

    376.30 Exophthalmos, unspecified

    376.31 Constant exophthalmos

    376.32 Orbital hemorrhage

    376.33 Orbital edema or congestion

    376.34 Intermittent exophthalmos

    376.35 Pulsating exophthalmos

    376.36 Lateral displacement of globe

⑤ **376.4 Deformity of orbit**

    376.40 Deformity of orbit, unspecified

    376.41 Hypertelorism of orbit

    376.42 Exostosis of orbit

    376.43 Local deformities due to bone disease

    376.44 Orbital deformities associated with craniofacial deformities

    376.45 Atrophy of orbit

    376.46 Enlargement of orbit

    376.47 Deformity due to trauma or surgery

⑤ **376.5 Enophthalmos**

    376.50 Enophthalmos, unspecified as to cause

    376.51 Enophthalmos due to atrophy of orbital tissue

    376.52 Enophthalmos due to trauma or surgery

● Code new
  to this edition

▲ Revision of
  existing code

④ ⑤ Fourth or fifth
    digit required

376.6 **Retained (old) foreign body following penetrating wound of orbit**
Retrobulbar foreign body

⑤ **376.8** **Other orbital disorders**

376.81 **Orbital cysts**
Encephalocele of orbit

376.82 **Myopathy of extraocular muscles**

376.89 **Other**

376.9 **Unspecified disorder of orbit**

377 **Disorders of optic nerve and visual pathways**

⑤ **377.0** **Papilledema**

377.00 **Papilledema, unspecified**

377.01 **Papilledema associated with increased intracranial pressure**

377.02 **Papilledema associated with decreased ocular pressure**

377.03 **Papilledema associated with retinal disorder**

377.04 **Foster-Kennedy syndrome**

⑤ **377.1** **Optic atrophy**

377.10 **Optic atrophy, unspecified**

377.11 **Primary optic atrophy**

Excludes: *neurosyphilitic optic atrophy (094.84)*

377.12 **Postinflammatory optic atrophy**

377.13 **Optic atrophy associated with retinal dystrophies**

377.14 **Glaucomatous atrophy [cupping] of optic disc**

377.15 **Partial optic atrophy**
Temporal pallor of optic disc

377.16 **Hereditary optic atrophy**
Optic atrophy:
dominant hereditary
Leber's

⑤ **377.2** **Other disorders of optic disc**

377.21 **Drusen of optic disc**

377.22 **Crater-like holes of optic disc**

377.23 **Coloboma of optic disc**

377.24 **Pseudopapilledema**

⑤ **377.3** **Optic neuritis**

Excludes: *meningococcal optic neuritis (036.81)*

377.30 **Optic neuritis, unspecified**

377.31 **Optic papillitis**

377.32 **Retrobulbar neuritis (acute)**

Excludes: *syphilitic retrobulbar neuritis (094.85)*

377.33 **Nutritional optic neuropathy**

377.34 **Toxic optic neuropathy**
Toxic amblyopia

377.39 **Other**

Excludes: *ischemic optic neuropathy (377.41)*

⑤ **377.4** **Other disorders of optic nerve**

377.41 **Ischemic optic neuropathy**

377.42 **Hemorrhage in optic nerve sheaths**

377.49 **Other**
Compression of optic nerve

⑤ **377.5** **Disorders of optic chiasm**

377.51 **Associated with pituitary neoplasms and disorders**

377.52 **Associated with other neoplasms**

377.53 **Associated with vascular disorders**

 Add 4th or
5th digit

Nonspecific
code

Unspecified
code

Manifestation
code

377.54   Associated with inflammatory disorders

⑤ **377.6 Disorders of other visual pathways**

377.61   Associated with neoplasms

377.62   Associated with vascular disorders

377.63   Associated with inflammatory disorders

⑤ **377.7 Disorders of visual cortex**

Excludes: *visual:*

> *agnosia (368.16)*
> *hallucinations (368.16)*
> *halos (368.15)*

377.71   Associated with neoplasms

377.72   Associated with vascular disorders

377.73   Associated with inflammatory disorders

377.75   Cortical blindness

377.9 Unspecified disorder of optic nerve and visual pathways

378 Strabismus and other disorders of binocular eye movements

Excludes: *nystagmus and other irregular eye movements (379.50-379.59)*

⑤ **378.0 Esotropia**

Convergent concomitant strabismus

Excludes: *intermittent esotropia (378.20-378.22)*

378.00   Esotropia, unspecified

378.01   Monocular esotropia

378.02   Monocular esotropia with A pattern

378.03   Monocular esotropia with V pattern

378.04   Monocular esotropia with other noncomitancies
Monocular esotropia with X or Y pattern

378.05   Alternating esotropia

378.06   Alternating esotropia with A pattern

378.07   Alternating esotropia with V pattern

378.08   Alternating esotropia with other noncomitancies
Alternating esotropia with X or Y pattern

⑤ **378.1 Exotropia**

Divergent concomitant strabismus

Excludes: *intermittent exotropia (378.20, 378.23-378.24)*

378.10   Exotropia, unspecified

378.11   Monocular exotropia

378.12   Monocular exotropia with A pattern

378.13   Monocular exotropia with V pattern

378.14   Monocular exotropia with other noncomitancies
Monocular exotropia with X or Y pattern

378.15   Alternating exotropia

378.16   Alternating exotropia with A pattern

378.17   Alternating exotropia with V pattern

378.18   Alternating exotropia with other noncomitancies
Alternating exotropia with X or Y pattern

⑤ **378.2 Intermittent heterotropia**

Excludes: *vertical heterotropia (intermittent) (378.31)*

378.20   Intermittent heterotropia, unspecified
Intermittent:
  esotropia NOS
  exotropia NOS

378.21   Intermittent esotropia, monocular

378.22   Intermittent esotropia, alternating

378.23   Intermittent exotropia, monocular

● Code new
to this edition   ▲ Revision of
existing code   ④ ⑤ Fourth or fifth
digit required

378.24 Intermittent exotropia, alternating

[5] **378.3 Other and unspecified heterotropia**

378.30 Heterotropia, unspecified

378.31 Hypertropia
Vertical heterotropia (constant) (intermittent)

378.32 Hypotropia

378.33 Cyclotropia

378.34 Monofixation syndrome
Microtropia

378.35 Accommodative component in esotropia

[5] **378.4 Heterophoria**

378.40 Heterophoria, unspecified

378.41 Esophoria

378.42 Exophoria

378.43 Vertical heterophoria

378.44 Cyclophoria

378.45 Alternating hyperphoria

[5] **378.5 Paralytic strabismus**

378.50 Paralytic strabismus, unspecified

378.51 Third or oculomotor nerve palsy, partial

378.52 Third or oculomotor nerve palsy, total

378.53 Fourth or trochlear nerve palsy

378.54 Sixth or abducens nerve palsy

378.55 External ophthalmoplegia

378.56 Total ophthalmoplegia

[5] **378.6 Mechanical strabismus**

378.60 Mechanical strabismus, unspecified

378.61 Brown's (tendon) sheath syndrome

378.62 Mechanical strabismus from other musculofascial disorders

378.63 Limited duction associated with other conditions

[5] **378.7 Other specified strabismus**

378.71 Duane's syndrome

378.72 Progressive external ophthalmoplegia

378.73 Strabismus in other neuromuscular disorders

[5] **378.8 Other disorders of binocular eye movements**

[*Excludes:*] *nystagmus (379.50-379.56)*

378.81 Palsy of conjugate gaze

378.82 Spasm of conjugate gaze

378.83 Convergence insufficiency or palsy

378.84 Convergence excess or spasm

378.85 Anomalies of divergence

378.86 Internuclear ophthalmoplegia

378.87 Other dissociated deviation of eye movements
Skew deviation

378.9 Unspecified disorder of eye movements
Ophthalmoplegia NOS   Strabismus NOS

379 Other disorders of eye

[5] **379.0 Scleritis and episcleritis**

[*Excludes:*] *syphilitic episcleritis (095.0)*

379.00 Scleritis, unspecified
Episcleritis NOS

379.01 Episcleritis periodica fugax

379.02 Nodular episcleritis

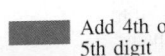

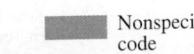

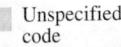

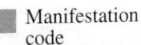

379.03	**Anterior scleritis**	
379.04	**Scleromalacia perforans**	
379.05	**Scleritis with corneal involvement**	
	Scleroperikeratitis	
379.06	**Brawny scleritis**	
379.07	**Posterior scleritis**	
	Sclerotenonitis	
`379.09`	**Other**	
	Scleral abscess	

⑤ **379.1 Other disorders of sclera**

Excludes: blue sclera (743.47)

379.11	**Scleral ectasia**
	Scleral staphyloma NOS
379.12	**Staphyloma posticum**
379.13	**Equatorial staphyloma**
379.14	**Anterior staphyloma, localized**
`379.15`	**Ring staphyloma**
`379.16`	**Other degenerative disorders of sclera**
379.19	**Other**

⑤ **379.2 Disorders of vitreous body**

379.21	**Vitreous degeneration**
	Vitreous:
	cavitation
	detachment
	liquefaction
379.22	**Crystalline deposits in vitreous**
	Asteroid hyalitis Synchysis scintillans
379.23	**Vitreous hemorrhage**
`379.24`	**Other vitreous opacities**
	Vitreous floaters
379.25	**Vitreous membranes and strands**
379.26	**Vitreous prolapse**
`379.29`	**Other disorders of vitreous**

Excludes: vitreous abscess (360.04)

⑤ **379.3 Aphakia and other disorders of lens**

Excludes: after-cataract (366.50-366.53)

379.31	**Aphakia**

Excludes: cataract extraction status (V45.61)

379.32	**Subluxation of lens**
379.33	**Anterior dislocation of lens**
379.34	**Posterior dislocation of lens**
`379.39`	**Other disorders of lens**

⑤ **379.4 Anomalies of pupillary function**

`379.40`	**Abnormal pupillary function, unspecified**
379.41	**Anisocoria**
379.42	**Miosis (persistent), not due to miotics**
379.43	**Mydriasis (persistent) not due to mydriatics**
379.45	**Argyll Robertson pupil, atypical**
	Argyll Robertson phenomenon or pupil, nonsyphilitic

Excludes: Argyll Robertson pupil (syphilitic) (094.89)

379.46	**Tonic pupillary reaction**
	Adie's pupil or syndrome
`379.49`	**Other**
	Hippus
	Pupillary paralysis

● Code new
to this edition

▲ Revision of
existing code

④ ⑤ Fourth or fifth
digit required

[5] **379.5 Nystagmus and other irregular eye movements**

379.50 Nystagmus, unspecified

379.51 Congenital nystagmus

379.52 Latent nystagmus

379.53 Visual deprivation nystagmus

379.54 Nystagmus associated with disorders of the vestibular system

379.55 Dissociated nystagmus

379.56 Other forms of nystagmus

379.57 Deficiencies of saccadic eye movements
Abnormal optokinetic response

379.58 Deficiencies of smooth pursuit movements

379.59 Other irregularities of eye movements
Opsoclonus

379.8 Other specified disorders of eye and adnexa

[5] **379.9 Unspecified disorder of eye and adnexa**

379.90 Disorder of eye, unspecified

379.91 Pain in or around eye

379.92 Swelling or mass of eye

379.93 Redness or discharge of eye

379.99 Other ill-defined disorders of eye

[*Excludes:*] *blurred vision NOS (368.8)*

DISEASES OF THE EAR AND MASTOID PROCESS (380-389)

380 Disorders of external ear

[5] **380.0 Perichondritis of pinna**
Perichondritis of auricle

380.00 Perichondritis of pinna, unspecified

380.01 Acute perichondritis of pinna

380.02 Chronic perichondritis of pinna

[5] **380.1 Infective otitis externa**

380.10 Infective otitis externa, unspecified
Otitis externa (acute):
NOS
circumscribed
diffuse
hemorrhagica
infective NOS

380.11 Acute infection of pinna

[*Excludes:*] *furuncular otitis externa (680.0)*

380.12 Acute swimmers' ear
Beach ear   Tank ear

380.13 Other acute infections of external ear
Code first underlying disease, as:
erysipelas (035)
impetigo (684)
seborrheic dermatitis (690.10-690.18)

[*Excludes:*] *herpes simplex (054.73)*
herpes zoster (053.71)

380.14 Malignant otitis externa

380.15 Chronic mycotic otitis externa
Code first underlying disease, as:
aspergillosis (117.3)
otomycosis NOS (111.9)

[*Excludes:*] *candidal otitis externa (112.82)*

380.16 Other chronic infective otitis externa
Chronic infective otitis externa NOS

[5] **380.2 Other otitis externa**

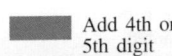

Add 4th or 5th digit   Nonspecific code   Unspecified code   Manifestation code

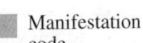

380.21 Cholesteatoma of external ear
Keratosis obturans of external ear (canal)

[Excludes:] *cholesteatoma NOS (385.30-385.35)*
postmastoidectomy (383.32)

380.22 Other acute otitis externa
Acute otitis externa:
- actinic
- chemical
- contact
- eczematoid
- reactive

380.23 Other chronic otitis externa
Chronic otitis externa NOS

[5] **380.3 Noninfectious disorders of pinna**

380.30 Disorder of pinna, unspecified

380.31 Hematoma of auricle or pinna

380.32 Acquired deformities of auricle or pinna

[Excludes:] *cauliflower ear (738.7)*

380.39 Other

[Excludes:] *gouty tophi of ear (274.81)*

380.4 Impacted cerumen
Wax in ear

[5] **380.5 Acquired stenosis of external ear canal**
Collapse of external ear canal

380.50 Acquired stenosis of external ear canal, unspecified as to cause

380.51 Secondary to trauma

380.52 Secondary to surgery

380.53 Secondary to inflammation

[5] **380.8 Other disorders of external ear**

380.81 Exostosis of external ear canal

380.89 Other

380.9 Unspecified disorder of external ear

381 Nonsuppurative otitis media and Eustachian tube disorders

[5] **381.0 Acute nonsuppurative otitis media**
Acute tubotympanic catarrh
Otitis media, acute or subacute:
- catarrhal
- exudative
- transudative
- with effusion

[Excludes:] *otitic barotrauma (993.0)*

381.00 Acute nonsuppurative otitis media, unspecified

381.01 Acute serous otitis media
Acute or subacute secretory otitis media

381.02 Acute mucoid otitis media
Acute or subacute seromucinous otitis media
Blue drum syndrome

381.03 Acute sanguinous otitis media

381.04 Acute allergic serous otitis media

381.05 Acute allergic mucoid otitis media

381.06 Acute allergic sanguinous otitis media

[5] **381.1 Chronic serous otitis media**
Chronic tubotympanic catarrh

381.10 Chronic serous otitis media, simple or unspecified

381.19 Other
Serosanguinous chronic otitis media

● Code new to this edition ▲ Revision of existing code [4] [5] Fourth or fifth digit required

⑤ **381.2 Chronic mucoid otitis media**
Glue ear

Excludes: *adhesive middle ear disease (385.10-385.19)*

381.20 Chronic mucoid otitis media, simple or unspecified

381.29 Other
Mucosanguinous chronic otitis media

381.3 Other and unspecified chronic nonsuppurative otitis media
Otitis media, chronic: Otitis media, chronic:
  allergic   seromucinous
  exudative   transudative
  secretory   with effusion

381.4 Nonsuppurative otitis media, not specified as acute or chronic
Otitis media: Otitis media:
  allergic   secretory
  catarrhal   seromucinous
  exudative   serous
  mucoid   transudative
                 with effusion

⑤ **381.5 Eustachian salpingitis**

381.50 Eustachian salpingitis, unspecified

381.51 Acute Eustachian salpingitis

381.52 Chronic Eustachian salpingitis

⑤ **381.6 Obstruction of Eustachian tube**
Stenosis of Eustachian tube
Stricture of Eustachian tube

381.60 Obstruction of Eustachian tube, unspecified

381.61 Osseous obstruction of Eustachian tube
Obstruction of Eustachian tube from cholesteatoma, polyp, or other osseous lesion

381.62 Intrinsic cartilagenous obstruction of Eustachian tube

381.63 Extrinsic cartilagenous obstruction of Eustachian tube
Compression of Eustachian tube

381.7 Patulous Eustachian tube

⑤ **381.8 Other disorders of Eustachian tube**

381.81 Dysfunction of Eustachian tube

381.89 Other

381.9 Unspecified Eustachian tube disorder

382 Suppurative and unspecified otitis media

⑤ **382.0 Acute suppurative otitis media**
Otitis media, acute:
  necrotizing NOS
  purulent

382.00 Acute suppurative otitis media without spontaneous rupture of ear drum

382.01 Acute suppurative otitis media with spontaneous rupture of ear drum

382.02 Acute suppurative otitis media in diseases classified elsewhere
Code first underlying disease, as:
  influenza (487.8)
  scarlet fever (034.1)

Excludes: *postmeasles otitis (055.2)*

382.1 Chronic tubotympanic suppurative otitis media
Benign chronic suppurative otitis media (with anterior perforation of ear drum)
Chronic tubotympanic disease (with anterior perforation of ear drum)

382.2 Chronic atticoantral suppurative otitis media
Chronic atticoantral disease (with posterior or superior marginal perforation of ear drum)
Persistent mucosal disease (with posterior or superior marginal perforation of ear drum)

382.3 Unspecified chronic suppurative otitis media
Chronic purulent otitis media

Excludes: *tuberculous otitis media (017.4)*

273

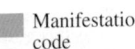

382.4 Unspecified suppurative otitis media
Purulent otitis media NOS

382.9 Unspecified otitis media
Otitis media:
  NOS
  acute NOS
  chronic NOS

383 Mastoiditis and related conditions

⑤ **383.0 Acute mastoiditis**
Abscess of mastoid   Empyema of mastoid

  383.00 Acute mastoiditis without complications

  383.01 Subperiosteal abscess of mastoid

  383.02 Acute mastoiditis with other complications
    Gradenigo's syndrome

383.1 Chronic mastoiditis
Caries of mastoid   Fistula of mastoid

Excludes: *tuberculous mastoiditis (015.6)*

⑤ **383.2 Petrositis**
Coalescing osteitis of petrous bone
Inflammation of petrous bone
Osteomyelitis of petrous bone

  383.20 Petrositis, unspecified

  383.21 Acute petrositis

  383.22 Chronic petrositis

⑤ **383.3 Complications following mastoidectomy**

  383.30 Postmastoidectomy complication, unspecified

  383.31 Mucosal cyst of postmastoidectomy cavity

  383.32 Recurrent cholesteatoma of postmastoidectomy cavity

  383.33 Granulations of postmastoidectomy cavity
    Chronic inflammation of postmastoidectomy cavity

⑤ **383.8 Other disorders of mastoid**

  383.81 Postauricular fistula

  383.89 Other

383.9 Unspecified mastoiditis

384 Other disorders of tympanic membrane

⑤ **384.0 Acute myringitis without mention of otitis media**

  384.00 Acute myringitis, unspecified
    Acute tympanitis NOS

  384.01 Bullous myringitis
    Myringitis bullosa hemorrhagica

  384.09 Other

384.1 Chronic myringitis without mention of otitis media
Chronic tympanitis

⑤ **384.2 Perforation of tympanic membrane**
Perforation of ear drum:
  NOS
  persistent posttraumatic
  postinflammatory

Excludes: *otitis media with perforation of tympanic membrane (382.00-382.9)*
    traumatic perforation [current injury] (872.61)

  384.20 Perforation of tympanic membrane, unspecified

  384.21 Central perforation of tympanic membrane

  384.22 Attic perforation of tympanic membrane
    Pars flaccida

  384.23 Other marginal perforation of tympanic membrane

  384.24 Multiple perforations of tympanic membrane

  384.25 Total perforation of tympanic membrane

● Code new
to this edition
▲ Revision of
existing code
④ ⑤ Fourth or fifth
digit required

⑤ **384.8 Other specified disorders of tympanic membrane**

384.81 Atrophic flaccid tympanic membrane
Healed perforation of ear drum

384.82 Atrophic nonflaccid tympanic membrane

384.9 Unspecified disorder of tympanic membrane

385 Other disorders of middle ear and mastoid

Excludes: mastoiditis (383.0-383.9)

⑤ **385.0 Tympanosclerosis**

385.00 Tympanosclerosis, unspecified as to involvement

385.01 Tympanosclerosis involving tympanic membrane only

385.02 Tympanosclerosis involving tympanic membrane and ear ossicles

385.03 Tympanosclerosis involving tympanic membrane, ear ossicles, and middle ear

385.09 Tympanosclerosis involving other combination of structures

⑤ **385.1 Adhesive middle ear disease**
Adhesive otitis

Otitis media:
chronic adhesive
fibrotic

Excludes: glue ear (381.20-381.29)

385.10 Adhesive middle ear disease, unspecified as to involvement

385.11 Adhesions of drum head to incus

385.12 Adhesions of drum head to stapes

385.13 Adhesions of drum head to promontorium

385.19 Other adhesions and combinations

⑤ **385.2 Other acquired abnormality of ear ossicles**

385.21 Impaired mobility of malleus
Ankylosis of malleus

385.22 Impaired mobility of other ear ossicles
Ankylosis of ear ossicles, except malleus

385.23 Discontinuity or dislocation of ear ossicles

385.24 Partial loss or necrosis of ear ossicles

⑤ **385.3 Cholesteatoma of middle ear and mastoid**
Cholesterosis of (middle) ear
Epidermosis of (middle) ear
Keratosis of (middle) ear
Polyp of (middle) ear

Excludes: cholesteatoma:
external ear canal (380.21)
recurrent of postmastoidectomy cavity (383.32)

385.30 Cholesteatoma, unspecified

385.31 Cholesteatoma of attic

385.32 Cholesteatoma of middle ear

385.33 Cholesteatoma of middle ear and mastoid

385.35 Diffuse cholesteatosis

⑤ **385.8 Other disorders of middle ear and mastoid**

385.82 Cholesterin granuloma

385.83 Retained foreign body of middle ear

385.89 Other

385.9 Unspecified disorder of middle ear and mastoid

386 Vertiginous syndromes and other disorders of vestibular system

Excludes: vertigo NOS (780.4)

⑤ **386.0 Ménière's disease**
Endolymphatic hydrops
Lermoyez's syndrome

Ménière's syndrome or vertigo

386.00 Ménière's disease, unspecified
Ménière's disease (active)

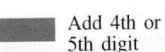 Add 4th or
5th digit

Nonspecific
code

Unspecified
code

Manifestation
code

386.01 **Active Ménière's disease, cochleovestibular**

386.02 **Active Ménière's disease, cochlear**

386.03 **Active Ménière's disease, vestibular**

386.04 **Inactive Ménière's disease**
Ménière's disease in remission

⑤ 386.1 **Other and unspecified peripheral vertigo**

| Excludes: | epidemic vertigo (078.81)

386.10 **Peripheral vertigo, unspecified**

386.11 **Benign paroxysmal positional vertigo**
Benign paroxysmal positional nystagmus

386.12 **Vestibular neuronitis**
Acute (and recurrent) peripheral vestibulopathy

386.19 **Other**
Aural vertigo   Otogenic vertigo

386.2 **Vertigo of central origin**
Central positional nystagmus
Malignant positional vertigo

⑤ 386.3 **Labyrinthitis**

386.30 **Labyrinthitis, unspecified**

386.31 **Serous labyrinthitis**
Diffuse labyrinthitis

386.32 **Circumscribed labyrinthitis**
Focal labyrinthitis

386.33 **Suppurative labyrinthitis**
Purulent labyrinthitis

386.34 **Toxic labyrinthitis**

386.35 **Viral labyrinthitis**

⑤ 386.4 **Labyrinthine fistula**

386.40 **Labyrinthine fistula, unspecified**

386.41 **Round window fistula**

386.42 **Oval window fistula**

386.43 **Semicircular canal fistula**

386.48 **Labyrinthine fistula of combined sites**

⑤ 386.5 **Labyrinthine dysfunction**

386.50 **Labyrinthine dysfunction, unspecified**

386.51 **Hyperactive labyrinth, unilateral**

386.52 **Hyperactive labyrinth, bilateral**

386.53 **Hypoactive labyrinth, unilateral**

386.54 **Hypoactive labyrinth, bilateral**

386.55 **Loss of labyrinthine reactivity, unilateral**

386.56 **Loss of labyrinthine reactivity, bilateral**

386.58 **Other forms and combinations**

386.8 **Other disorders of labyrinth**

386.9 **Unspecified vertiginous syndromes and labyrinthine disorders**

387 **Otosclerosis**
Includes: otospongiosis

387.0 **Otosclerosis involving oval window, nonobliterative**

387.1 **Otosclerosis involving oval window, obliterative**

387.2 **Cochlear otosclerosis**
Otosclerosis involving:
otic capsule
round window

387.8 **Other otosclerosis**

387.9 **Otosclerosis, unspecified**

388 **Other disorders of ear**

● Code new
to this edition
▲ Revision of
existing code
④ ⑤ Fourth or fifth
digit required

[5] **388.0 Degenerative and vascular disorders of ear**

388.00 Degenerative and vascular disorders, unspecified

388.01 Presbyacusis

388.02 Transient ischemic deafness

[5] **388.1 Noise effects on inner ear**

388.10 Noise effects on inner ear, unspecified

388.11 Acoustic trauma (explosive) to ear
Otitic blast injury

388.12 Noise-induced hearing loss

388.2 Sudden hearing loss, unspecified

[5] **388.3 Tinnitus**

388.30 Tinnitus, unspecified

388.31 Subjective tinnitus

388.32 Objective tinnitus

[5] **388.4 Other abnormal auditory perception**

388.40 Abnormal auditory perception, unspecified

388.41 Diplacusis

388.42 Hyperacusis

388.43 Impairment of auditory discrimination

388.44 Recruitment

388.5 Disorders of acoustic nerve
Acoustic neuritis
Degeneration of acoustic or eighth nerve
Disorder of acoustic or eighth nerve

[*Excludes:*] *acoustic neuroma (225.1)*
syphilitic acoustic neuritis (094.86)

[5] **388.6 Otorrhea**

388.60 Otorrhea, unspecified
Discharging ear NOS

388.61 Cerebrospinal fluid otorrhea

[*Excludes:*] *cerebrospinal fluid rhinorrhea (349.81)*

388.69 Other
Otorrhagia

[5] **388.7 Otalgia**

388.70 Otalgia, unspecified
Earache NOS

388.71 Otogenic pain

388.72 Referred pain

388.8 Other disorders of ear

388.9 Unspecified disorder of ear

389 Hearing loss

[5] **389.0 Conductive hearing loss**
Conductive deafness

389.00 Conductive hearing loss, unspecified

389.01 Conductive hearing loss, external ear

389.02 Conductive hearing loss, tympanic membrane

389.03 Conductive hearing loss, middle ear

389.04 Conductive hearing loss, inner ear

389.08 Conductive hearing loss of combined types

[5] **389.1 Sensorineural hearing loss**
Perceptive hearing loss or deafness

[*Excludes:*] *abnormal auditory perception (388.40-388.44)*
psychogenic deafness (306.7)

389.10 Sensorineural hearing loss, unspecified

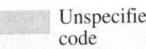

389.11 Sensory hearing loss

389.12 Neural hearing loss

389.14 Central hearing loss

389.18 Sensorineural hearing loss of combined types

389.2 Mixed conductive and sensorineural hearing loss
Deafness or hearing loss of type classifiable to 389.0 with type classifiable to 389.1

389.7 Deaf mutism, not elsewhere classifiable
Deaf, nonspeaking

389.8 Other specified forms of hearing loss

389.9 Unspecified hearing loss
Deafness NOS

● Code new to this edition ▲ Revision of existing code ④ ⑤ Fourth or fifth digit required

7. DISEASES OF THE CIRCULATORY SYSTEM (390-459)

ACUTE RHEUMATIC F

EVER (390-392)

390 Rheumatic fever without mention of heart involvement
Arthritis, rheumatic, acute or subacute
Rheumatic fever (active) (acute)
Rheumatism, articular, acute or subacute

| Excludes: | that with heart involvement (391.0-391.9) |

391 Rheumatic fever with heart involvement

| Excludes: | chronic heart diseases of rheumatic origin (393.0-398.9) unless rheumatic fever is also present or there is evidence of recrudescence or activity of the rheumatic process |

391.0 Acute rheumatic pericarditis
Rheumatic:
  fever (active) (acute) with pericarditis
  pericarditis (acute)
Any condition classifiable to 390 with pericarditis

| Excludes: | that not specified as rheumatic (420.0-420.9) |

391.1 Acute rheumatic endocarditis
Rheumatic:
  endocarditis, acute
  fever (active) (acute) with endocarditis or valvulitis
  valvulitis acute
Any condition classifiable to 390 with endocarditis or valvulitis

391.2 Acute rheumatic myocarditis
Rheumatic fever (active) (acute) with myocarditis
Any condition classifiable to 390 with myocarditis

391.8 Other acute rheumatic heart disease
Rheumatic:
  fever (active) (acute) with other or multiple types of heart involvement
  pancarditis, acute
Any condition classifiable to 390 with other or multiple types of heart involvement

391.9 Acute rheumatic heart disease, unspecified
Rheumatic:
  carditis, acute
  fever (active) (acute) with unspecified type of heart involvement
  heart disease, active or acute
Any condition classifiable to 390 with unspecified type of heart involvement

392 Rheumatic chorea
Includes: Sydenham's chorea

Excludes:	chorea:
	NOS (333.5)
	Huntington's (333.4)

392.0 With heart involvement
Rheumatic chorea with heart involvement of any type classifiable to 391

392.9 Without mention of heart involvement

CHRONIC RHEUMATIC HEART DISEASE (393-398)

393 Chronic rheumatic pericarditis
Adherent pericardium, rheumatic
Chronic rheumatic:
  mediastinopericarditis
  myopericarditis

| Excludes: | pericarditis NOS or not specified as rheumatic (423.0-423.9) |

394 Diseases of mitral valve

| Excludes: | that with aortic valve involvement (396.0-396.9) |

394.0 Mitral stenosis
Mitral (valve):
  obstruction (rheumatic)
  stenosis NOS

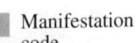

| | Add 4th or 5th digit | | Nonspecific code | | Unspecified code | | Manifestation code |

394.1 Rheumatic mitral insufficiency
    Rheumatic mitral:
        incompetence
        regurgitation

    Excludes: *that not specified as rheumatic (424.0)*

394.2 Mitral stenosis with insufficiency
    Mitral stenosis with incompetence or regurgitation

394.9 Other and unspecified mitral valve diseases
    Mitral (valve):
        disease (chronic)
        failure

395 Diseases of aortic valve

    Excludes: *that not specified as rheumatic (424.1)*
        that with mitral valve involvement (396.0-396.9)

395.0 Rheumatic aortic stenosis
    Rheumatic aortic (valve) obstruction

395.1 Rheumatic aortic insufficiency
    Rheumatic aortic:
        incompetence
        regurgitation

395.2 Rheumatic aortic stenosis with insufficiency
    Rheumatic aortic stenosis with incompetence or regurgitation

395.9 Other and unspecified rheumatic aortic diseases
    Rheumatic aortic (valve) disease

396 Diseases of mitral and aortic valves
    Includes: involvement of both mitral and aortic valves, whether specified as rheumatic or
        not

396.0 Mitral valve stenosis and aortic valve stenosis
    Atypical aortic (valve) stenosis
    Mitral and aortic (valve) obstruction (rheumatic)

396.1 Mitral valve stenosis and aortic valve insufficiency

396.2 Mitral valve insufficiency and aortic valve stenosis

396.3 Mitral valve insufficiency and aortic valve insufficiency
    Mitral and aortic (valve):
        incompetence
        regurgitation

396.8 Multiple involvement of mitral and aortic valves
    Stenosis and insufficiency of mitral or aortic valve with stenosis or insufficiency, or
        both, of the other valve

396.9 Mitral and aortic valve diseases, unspecified

397 Diseases of other endocardial structures

397.0 Diseases of tricuspid valve
    Tricuspid (valve) (rheumatic):
        disease
        insufficiency
        obstruction
        regurgitation
        stenosis

397.1 Rheumatic diseases of pulmonary valve

    Excludes: *that not specified as rheumatic (424.3)*

397.9 Rheumatic diseases of endocardium, valve unspecified
    Rheumatic:
        endocarditis (chronic)
        valvulitis (chronic)

    Excludes: *that not specified as rheumatic (424.90-424.99)*

398 Other rheumatic heart disease

398.0 Rheumatic myocarditis
    Rheumatic degeneration of myocardium

    Excludes: *myocarditis not specified as rheumatic (429.0)*

⑤ **398.9 Other and unspecified rheumatic heart diseases**

● Code new
    to this edition
▲ Revision of
    existing code
④ ⑤ Fourth or fifth
    digit required

398.90 Rheumatic heart disease, unspecified
Rheumatic:
carditis
heart disease NOS

[Excludes:] *carditis not specified as rheumatic (429.89)*
heart disease NOS not specified as rheumatic (429.9)

398.91 Rheumatic heart failure (congestive)
Rheumatic left ventricular failure

398.99 Other

HYPERTENSIVE DISEASE (401-405)

[Excludes:] *that complicating pregnancy, childbirth, or the puerperium (642.0-642.9)*
that involving coronary vessels (410.00-414.9)

401 Essential hypertension
Includes: high blood pressure
hyperpiesia
hyperpiesis
hypertension (arterial) (essential) (primary) (systemic)
hypertensive vascular:
degeneration
disease

[Excludes:] *elevated blood pressure without diagnosis of hypertension (796.2)*
pulmonary hypertension (416.0-416.9)
that involving vessels of:
brain (430-438)
eye (362.11)

401.0 Malignant

401.1 Benign

401.9 Unspecified

402 Hypertensive heart disease
Use additional code to specify type of heart failure (428.0, 428.20-428.23, 428.30-428.33, 428.40-428.43)
Includes: hypertensive:
cardiomegaly
cardiopathy
cardiovascular disease
heart (disease) (failure)
any condition classifiable to 428, 429.0-429.3, 429.8, 429.9 due to hypertension

[5] **402.0 Malignant**

▲ **402.00 Without heart failure**

▲ **402.01 With heart failure**

[5] **402.1 Benign**

▲ **402.10 Without heart failure**

▲ **402.11 With heart failure**

[5] **402.9 Unspecified**

▲ **402.90 Without heart failure**

▲ **402.91 With heart failure**

Add 4th or 5th digit | Nonspecific code | Unspecified code | Manifestation code

[5] **403 Hypertensive renal disease**

The following fifth-digit subclassification is for use with category 403:

- **0 without mention of renal failure**
- **1 with renal failure**

Includes: arteriolar nephritis
arteriosclerosis of:
kidney
renal arterioles
arteriosclerotic nephritis (chronic) (interstitial)
hypertensive:
nephropathy
renal failure
uremia (chronic)
nephrosclerosis
renal sclerosis with hypertension
any condition classifiable to 585, 586, or 587 with any condition classifiable to 401

Excludes: *acute renal failure (584.5-584.9)*
renal disease stated as not due to hypertension
renovascular hypertension (405.0-405.9 with fifth-digit 1)

[5] **403.0 Malignant**

[5] **403.1 Benign**

[5] **403.9 Unspecified**

▲ **404 Hypertensive heart and renal disease**

Use additional code to specify type of heart failure (428.0, 428.20-428.23, 428.30-428.33, 428.40-428.43)

The following fifth-digit subclassification is for use with category 404:

- **0 without mention of heart failure or renal failure**
- **1 with heart failure**
- **2 with renal failure**
- **3 with heart failure and renal failure**

Includes: disease:
cardiornal
cardiovascular renal
any condition classifiable to 402 with any condition classifiable to 403

[5] **404.0 Malignant**

[5] **404.1 Benign**

[5] **404.9 Unspecified**

405 Secondary hypertension

[5] **405.0 Malignant**

405.01 Renovascular

405.09 Other

[5] **405.1 Benign**

405.11 Renovascular

405.19 Other

[5] **405.9 Unspecified**

405.91 Renovascular

405.99 Other

● Code new to this edition ▲ Revision of existing code [4] [5] Fourth or fifth digit required

ISCHEMIC HEART DISEASE (410-414)

Includes: that with mention of hypertension

Use additional code, if desired, to identify presence of hypertension (401.0-405.9)

[5] 410 Acute myocardial infarction

Includes: cardiac infarction
coronary (artery):
embolism
occlusion
rupture
thrombosis
infarction of heart, myocardium, or ventricle
rupture of heart, myocardium, or ventricle
any condition classifiable to 414.1-414.9 specified as acute or with a stated duration of 8 weeks or less

The following fifth-digit subclassification is for use with category 410:

0 episode of care unspecified
Use when the source document does not contain sufficient information for the assignment of fifth digit 1 or 2.

1 initial episode of care
Use fifth digit 1 to designate the first episode of care (regardless of facility site) for a newly diagnosed myocardial infarction. The fifth digit 1 is assigned regardless of the number of times a patient may be transferred during the initial episode of care

2 subsequent episode of care
Use fifth digit 2 to designate an episode of care following the initial episode when the patient is admitted for further observation, evaluation, or treatment for a myocardial infarction that has received initial treatment, but is still less than 8 weeks old.

[5] 410.0 Of anterolateral wall

[5] 410.1 Of other anterior wall
Infarction:
anterior (wall) NOS (with contiguous portion of intraventricular septum)
anteroapical (with contiguous portion of intraventricular septum)
anteroseptal (with contiguous portion of intraventricular septum)

[5] 410.2 Of inferolateral wall

[5] 410.3 Of inferoposterior wall

[5] 410.4 Of other inferior wall
Infarction:
diaphragmatic wall (with contiguous portion of intraventricular septum)
inferior (wall) NOS (with contiguous portion of intraventricular septum)

[5] 410.5 Of other lateral wall
Infarction:
apical-lateral
basal-lateral
Infarction:
high lateral
posterolateral

[5] 410.6 True posterior wall infarction
Infarction:
posterobasal
strictly posterior

[5] 410.7 Subendocardial infarction
Nontransmural infarction

[5] 410.8 Of other specified sites
Infarction of:
atrium
papillary muscle
septum alone

[5] 410.9 Unspecified site
Acute myocardial infarction NOS
Coronary occlusion NOS

411 Other acute and subacute forms of ischemic heart disease

411.0 Postmyocardial infarction syndrome
Dressler's syndrome

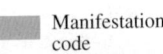

411.1 Intermediate coronary syndrome
  Impending infarction   Preinfarction syndrome
  Preinfarction angina   Unstable angina
  Excludes: *angina (pectoris) (413.9)*
      decubitus (413.0)

⑤ **411.8 Other**

  411.81 Acute coronary occlusion without myocardial infarction
    Acute coronary (artery):
     embolism without or not resulting in myocardial infarction
     obstruction without or not resulting in myocardial infarction
     occlusion without or not resulting in myocardial infarction
     thrombosis without or not resulting in myocardial infarction

  Excludes: *occlusion without infarction due to atherosclerosis (414.00-414.06)*
      obstruction without infarction due to atherosclerosis (414.00-414.06)

  411.89 Other
    Coronary insufficiency (acute)
    Subendocardial ischemia

412 Old myocardial infarction
  Healed myocardial infarction
  Past myocardial infarction diagnosed on ECG [EKG] or other special investigation, but
   currently presenting no symptoms

413 Angina pectoris

 413.0 Angina decubitus
   Nocturnal angina

 413.1 Prinzmetal angina
   Variant angina pectoris

 413.9 Other and unspecified angina pectoris
   Angina: Anginal syndrome
    NOS   Status anginosus
    cardiac   Stenocardia
    of effort   Syncope anginosa
   Excludes: *preinfarction angina (411.1)*

414 Other forms of chronic ischemic heart disease
  Excludes: *arteriosclerotic cardiovascular disease [ASCVD] (429.2)*
      cardiovascular:
       arteriosclerosis or sclerosis (429.2)
       degeneration or disease (429.2)

⑤ **414.0 Coronary atherosclerosis**
   Arteriosclerotic heart disease [ASHD]
   Atherosclerotic heart disease
   Coronary (artery):
    arteriosclerosis
    arteritis or endarteritis
    atheroma
    sclerosis
    stricture

  Excludes: *embolism of graft (996.72)*
      occlusion NOS of graft (996.72)
      thrombus of graft (996.72)

  414.00 Of unspecified type of vessel, native or graft

  414.01 Of native coronary artery

  414.02 Of autologous vein bypass graft

  414.03 Of nonautologous biological bypass graft

  414.04 Of artery bypass graft
    Internal mammary artery

  414.05 Of unspecified type of bypass graft
    Bypass graft NOS

 ● **414.06 Of coronary artery of transplanted heart**

● Code new
to this edition ▲ Revision of
existing code ④ ⑤ Fourth or fifth
digit required

▲ **414.1** **Aneurysm and dissection of heart**

    ▲ **414.10** **Aneurysm of heart (wall)**
        Aneurysm (arteriovenous):
          mural
          ventricular

    ▲ **414.11** **Aneurysm of coronary vessels**
        Aneurysm (arteriovenous) of coronary vessels

    ● **414.12** **Dissection of coronary artery**

    ▲ **414.19** **Other aneurysm of heart**
        Arteriovenous fistula, acquired, of heart

414.8 **Other specified forms of chronic ischemic heart disease**
    Chronic coronary insufficiency
    Ischemia, myocardial (chronic)
    Any condition classifiable to 410 specified as chronic, or presenting with symptoms
        after 8 weeks from date of infarction

    Excludes: *coronary insufficiency (acute) (411.89)*

414.9 **Chronic ischemic heart disease, unspecified**
    Ischemic heart disease NOS

DISEASES OF PULMONARY CIRCULATION (415-417)

415 **Acute pulmonary heart disease**

    415.0 **Acute cor pulmonale**
        Excludes: *cor pulmonale NOS (416.9)*

⑤ **415.1** **Pulmonary embolism and infarction**
    Pulmonary (artery) (vein):
        apoplexy
        embolism
        infarction (hemorrhagic)
        thrombosis

    Excludes: *that complicating:*
        abortion (634-638 with .6, 639.6)
        ectopic or molar pregnancy (639.6)
        pregnancy, childbirth, or the puerperium (673.0-673.8)

        415.11 **Iatrogenic pulmonary embolism and infarction**

        415.19 **Other**

416 **Chronic pulmonary heart disease**

    416.0 **Primary pulmonary hypertension**
        Idiopathic pulmonary arteriosclerosis
        Pulmonary hypertension (essential) (idiopathic) (primary)

    416.1 **Kyphoscoliotic heart disease**

    416.8 **Other chronic pulmonary heart diseases**
        Pulmonary hypertension, secondary

    416.9 **Chronic pulmonary heart disease, unspecified**
        Chronic cardiopulmonary disease
        Cor pulmonale (chronic) NOS

417 **Other diseases of pulmonary circulation**

    417.0 **Arteriovenous fistula of pulmonary vessels**
        Excludes: *congenital arteriovenous fistula (747.3)*

    417.1 **Aneurysm of pulmonary artery**
        Excludes: *congenital aneurysm (747.3)*

    417.8 **Other specified diseases of pulmonary circulation**
        Pulmonary:
          arteritis
          endarteritis
        Rupture of pulmonary vessel
        Stricture of pulmonary vessel

    417.9 **Unspecified disease of pulmonary circulation**

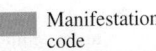

| | Add 4th or 5th digit | | Nonspecific code | | Unspecified code | | Manifestation code |

OTHER FORMS OF HEART DISEASE (420-429)

420 Acute pericarditis

Includes: acute:
mediastinopericarditis
myopericarditis
pericardial effusion
pleuropericarditis
pneumopericarditis

Excludes: *acute rheumatic pericarditis (391.0)*
postmyocardial infarction syndrome [Dressler's] (411.0)

420.0 Acute pericarditis in diseases classified elsewhere
Code first underlying disease, as:
actinomycosis (039.8)
amebiasis (006.8)
nocardiosis (039.8)
tuberculosis (017.9)
uremia (585)

Excludes: *pericarditis (acute) (in):*
Coxsackie (virus) (074.21)
gonococcal (098.83)
histoplasmosis (115.0-115.9 with fifth-digit 3)
meningococcal infection (036.41)
syphilitic (093.81)

⑤ **420.9 Other and unspecified acute pericarditis**

420.90 Acute pericarditis, unspecified
Pericarditis (acute):
NOS
infective NOS
sicca

420.91 Acute idiopathic pericarditis
Pericarditis, acute:
benign
nonspecific
viral

420.99 Other

Pericarditis (acute):	Pericarditis (acute):
pneumococcal	streptococcal
purulent	suppurative
staphylococcal	Pneumopyopericardium
	Pyopericardium

Excludes: *pericarditis in diseases classified elsewhere (420.0)*

421 Acute and subacute endocarditis

421.0 Acute and subacute bacterial endocarditis

Endocarditis (acute) (chronic) (subacute):	Endocarditis (acute) (chronic) (subacute):
bacterial	septic
infective NOS	ulcerative
lenta	vegetative
malignant	Infective aneurysm
purulent	Subacute bacterial endocarditis [SBE]

Use additional code, if desired, to identify infectious organism [e.g., Streptococcus 041.0, Staphylococcus 041.1]

421.1 Acute and subacute infective endocarditis in diseases classified elsewhere
Code first underlying disease, as:
blastomycosis (116.0)
Q fever (083.0)
typhoid (fever) (002.0)

Excludes: *endocarditis (in):*
Coxsackie (virus) (074.22)
gonococcal (098.84)
histoplasmosis (115.0-115.9 with fifth-digit 4)
meningococcal infection (036.42)
monilial (112.81)

● Code new to this edition ▲ Revision of existing code ④ ⑤ Fourth or fifth digit required

421.9 Acute endocarditis, unspecified
Endocarditis, acute or subacute
Myoendocarditis, acute or subacute
Periendocarditis, acute or subacute

[Excludes:] *acute rheumatic endocarditis (391.1)*

422 Acute myocarditis

[Excludes:] *acute rheumatic myocarditis (391.2)*

422.0 Acute myocarditis in diseases classified elsewhere
Code first underlying disease, as:
myocarditis (acute):
influenzal (487.8)
tuberculous (017.9)

[Excludes:] *myocarditis (acute) (due to):*
aseptic, of newborn (074.23)
Coxsackie (virus) (074.23)
diphtheritic (032.82)
meningococcal infection (036.43)
syphilitic (093.82)
toxoplasmosis (130.3)

[5] **422.9 Other and unspecified acute myocarditis**

422.90 Acute myocarditis, unspecified
Acute or subacute (interstitial) myocarditis

422.91 Idiopathic myocarditis
Myocarditis (acute or subacute):
Fiedler's
giant cell
isolated (diffuse) (granulomatous)
nonspecific granulomatous

422.92 Septic myocarditis
Myocarditis, acute or subacute:
pneumococcal
staphylococcal

Use additional code, if desired, to identify infectious organism [e.g., Staphylococcus 041.1]

[Excludes:] *myocarditis, acute or subacute:*
in bacterial diseases classified elsewhere (422.0)
streptococcal (391.2)

422.93 Toxic myocarditis

422.99 Other

423 Other diseases of pericardium

[Excludes:] *that specified as rheumatic (393)*

423.0 Hemopericardium

423.1 Adhesive pericarditis
Adherent pericardium
Fibrosis of pericardium
Milk spots
Pericarditis:
adhesive
obliterative
Soldiers' patches

423.2 Constrictive pericarditis
Concato's disease
Pick's disease of heart (and liver)

423.8 Other specified diseases of pericardium
Calcification of pericardium
Fistula of pericardium

423.9 Unspecified disease of pericardium

424 Other diseases of endocardium

[Excludes:] *bacterial endocarditis (421.0-421.9)*
rheumatic endocarditis (391.1, 394.0-397.9)
syphilitic endocarditis (093.20-093.24)

424.0 Mitral valve disorders
Mitral (valve):
incompetence NOS of specified cause, except rheumatic
insufficiency NOS of specified cause, except rheumatic
regurgitation NOS of specified cause, except rheumatic
[Excludes:] *mitral (valve):*
disease (394.9)
failure (394.9)
stenosis (394.0)
the listed conditions:
specified as rheumatic (394.1)
unspecified as to cause but with mention of:
diseases of aortic valve (396.0-396.9)
mitral stenosis or obstruction (394.2)

424.1 Aortic valve disorders
Aortic (valve):
incompetence NOS of specified cause, except rheumatic
insufficiency NOS of specified cause, except rheumatic
regurgitation NOS of specified cause, except rheumatic
stenosis NOS of specified cause, except rheumatic
[Excludes:] *hypertrophic subaortic stenosis (425.1)*
that specified as rheumatic (395.0-395.9)
that of unspecified cause but with mention of diseases of mitral valve (396.0-396.9)

424.2 Tricuspid valve disorders, specified as nonrheumatic
Tricuspid valve:
incompetence of specified cause, except rheumatic
insufficiency of specified cause, except rheumatic
regurgitation of specified cause, except rheumatic
stenosis of specified cause, except rheumatic
[Excludes:] *rheumatic or of unspecified cause (397.0)*

424.3 Pulmonary valve disorders
Pulmonic:
incompetence NOS
insufficiency NOS
Pulmonic:
regurgitation NOS
stenosis NOS
[Excludes:] *that specified as rheumatic (397.1)*

⑤ **424.9 Endocarditis, valve unspecified**

424.90 Endocarditis, valve unspecified, unspecified cause
Endocarditis (chronic):
NOS
nonbacterial thrombotic
Valvular:
incompetence of unspecified valve, unspecified cause
insufficiency of unspecified valve, unspecified cause
regurgitation of unspecified valve, unspecified cause
stenosis of unspecified valve, unspecified cause
Valvulitis (chronic) of unspecified valve, unspecified cause

424.91 Endocarditis in diseases classified elsewhere
Code first underlying disease, as:
atypical verrucous endocarditis [Libman-Sacks] (710.0)
disseminated lupus erythematosus (710.0)
tuberculosis (017.9)
[Excludes:] *syphilitic (093.20-093.24)*

424.99 Other
Any condition classifiable to 424.90 with specified cause, except rheumatic
[Excludes:] *endocardial fibroelastosis (425.3)*
that specified as rheumatic (397.9)

425 Cardiomyopathy
Includes: myocardiopathy

425.0 Endomyocardial fibrosis

425.1 Hypertrophic obstructive cardiomyopathy
Hypertrophic subaortic stenosis (idiopathic)

● Code new to this edition ▲ Revision of existing code ④ ⑤ Fourth or fifth digit required

425.2 Obscure cardiomyopathy of Africa
Becker's disease
Idiopathic mural endomyocardial disease

425.3 Endocardial fibroelastosis
Elastomyofibrosis

425.4 Other primary cardiomyopathies
Cardiomyopathy:
NOS
congestive
constrictive
familial
hypertrophic
Cardiomyopathy:
idiopathic
nonobstructive
obstructive
restrictive
Cardiovascular collagenosis

425.5 Alcoholic cardiomyopathy

425.7 Nutritional and metabolic cardiomyopathy
Code first underlying disease, as:
amyloidosis (277.3)
beriberi (265.0)
cardiac glycogenosis (271.0)
mucopolysaccharidosis (277.5)
thyrotoxicosis (242.0-242.9)

[*Excludes:*] *gouty tophi of heart (274.82)*

425.8 Cardiomyopathy in other diseases classified elsewhere
Code first underlying disease, as:
Friedreich's ataxia (334.0)
myotonia atrophica (359.2)
progressive muscular dystrophy (359.1)
sarcoidosis (135)

[*Excludes:*] *cardiomyopathy in Chagas' disease (086.0)*

425.9 Secondary cardiomyopathy, unspecified

426 Conduction disorders

426.0 Atrioventricular block, complete
Third degree atrioventricular block

[5] **426.1 Atrioventricular block, other and unspecified**

426.10 Atrioventricular block, unspecified
Atrioventricular [AV] block (incomplete) (partial)

426.11 First degree atrioventricular block
Incomplete atrioventricular block, first degree
Prolonged P-R interval NOS

426.12 Mobitz (type) II atrioventricular block
Incomplete atrioventricular block:
Mobitz (type) II
second degree, Mobitz (type) II

426.13 Other second degree atrioventricular block
Incomplete atrioventricular block:
Mobitz (type) I [Wenckebach's]
second degree:
NOS
Mobitz (type) I
with 2:1 atrioventricular response [block]
Wenckebach's phenomenon

426.2 Left bundle branch hemiblock
Block:
left anterior fascicular
left posterior fascicular

426.3 Other left bundle branch block
Left bundle branch block:
NOS
anterior fascicular with posterior fascicular
complete
main stem

426.4 Right bundle branch block

[5] **426.5 Bundle branch block, other and unspecified**

426.50 Bundle branch block, unspecified

Add 4th or 5th digit | Nonspecific code | Unspecified code | Manifestation code

426.51 **Right bundle branch block and left posterior fascicular block**

426.52 **Right bundle branch block and left anterior fascicular block**

426.53 **Other bilateral bundle branch block**
Bifascicular block NOS
Bilateral bundle branch block NOS
Right bundle branch with left bundle branch block (incomplete) (main stem)

426.54 **Trifascicular block**

426.6 **Other heart block**
Intraventricular block: Sinoatrial block
  NOS   Sinoauricular block
  diffuse
  myofibrillar

426.7 **Anomalous atrioventricular excitation**
Atrioventricular conduction:
  accelerated
  accessory
  pre-excitation
Ventricular pre-excitation
Wolff-Parkinson-White syndrome

⑤ **426.8** **Other specified conduction disorders**

426.81 **Lown-Ganong-Levine syndrome**
Syndrome of short P-R interval, normal QRS complexes, and supraventricular tachycardias

426.89 **Other**
Dissociation:
  atrioventricular [AV]
  interference
  isorhythmic
Nonparoxysmal AV nodal tachycardia

426.9 **Conduction disorder, unspecified**
Heart block NOS
Stokes-Adams syndrome

427 **Cardiac dysrhythmias**
> Excludes: that complicating:
>   abortion (634-638 with .7, 639.8)
>   ectopic or molar pregnancy (639.8)
>   labor or delivery (668.1, 669.4)

427.0 **Paroxysmal supraventricular tachycardia**
Paroxysmal tachycardia:
  atrial [PAT]
  atrioventricular [AV]
  junctional
  nodal

427.1 **Paroxysmal ventricular tachycardia**
Ventricular tachycardia (paroxysmal)

427.2 **Paroxysmal tachycardia, unspecified**
Bouveret-Hoffmann syndrome
Paroxysmal tachycardia:
  NOS
  essential

⑤ **427.3** **Atrial fibrillation and flutter**

427.31 **Atrial fibrillation**

427.32 **Atrial flutter**

⑤ **427.4** **Ventricular fibrillation and flutter**

427.41 **Ventricular fibrillation**

427.42 **Ventricular flutter**

427.5 **Cardiac arrest**
Cardiorespiratory arrest

⑤ **427.6** **Premature beats**

● Code new
to this edition
▲ Revision of
existing code
④ ⑤ Fourth or fifth
digit required

427.60 Premature beats, unspecified
Ectopic beats
Extrasystoles
Extrasystolic arrhythmia
Premature contractions or systoles NOS

427.61 Supraventricular premature beats
Atrial premature beats, contractions, or systoles

427.69 Other
Ventricular premature beats, contractions, or systoles

⑤ **427.8 Other specified cardiac dysrhythmias**

427.81 Sinoatrial node dysfunction
Sinus bradycardia:
persistent
severe
Syndrome:
sick sinus
tachycardia-bradycardia

[Excludes:] *sinus bradycardia NOS (427.89)*

427.89 Other
Rhythm disorder:
coronary sinus
ectopic
nodal
Wandering (atrial) pacemaker

[Excludes:] *carotid sinus syncope (337.0)*
neonatal bradycardia (779.81)
neonatal tachycardia (779.82)
reflex bradycardia (337.0)
tachycardia (785.0)

427.9 Cardiac dysrhythmia, unspecified
Arrhythmia (cardiac) NOS

428 Heart failure

[Excludes:] *following cardiac surgery (429.4)*
rheumatic (398.91)
that complicating:
abortion (634-638 with .7, 639.8)
ectopic or molar pregnancy (639.8)
labor or delivery (668.1, 669.4)

Code, if applicable, heart failure due to hypertension first (402.0-402.9, with fifth-digit 1 or 404.0-404.9 with fifth digit 1 or 3)

▲ **428.0 Congestive heart failure, unspecified**
Congestive heart disease
Right heart failure (secondary to left heart failure)

[Excludes:] *fluid overload NOS (276.6)*

428.1 Left heart failure
Acute edema of lung with heart disease NOS or heart failure
Acute pulmonary edema with heart disease NOS or heart failure
Cardiac asthma
Left ventricular failure

● **428.2 Systolic heart failure**

[Excludes:] *combined systolic and diastolic heart failure (428.40-428.43)*

● **428.20 Unspecified**
● **428.21 Acute**
● **428.22 Chronic**
● **428.23 Acute on chronic**

● **428.3 Diastolic heart failure**

[Excludes:] *combined systolic and diastolic heart failure (428.40-428.43)*

● **428.30 Unspecified**
● **428.31 Acute**
● **428.32 Chronic**
● **428.33 Acute on chronic**

Add 4th or 5th digit | Nonspecific code | Unspecified code | Manifestation code

● **428.4 Combined systolic and diastolic heart failure**

● **428.40 Unspecified**

● **428.41 Acute**

● **428.42 Chronic**

● **428.43 Acute on chronic**

428.9 Heart failure, unspecified

Cardiac failure NOS
Heart failure NOS
Myocardial failure NOS
Weak heart

429 Ill-defined descriptions and complications of heart disease

429.0 Myocarditis, unspecified

Myocarditis:
NOS (with mention of arteriosclerosis)
chronic (interstitial) (with mention of arteriosclerosis)
fibroid (with mention of arteriosclerosis)
senile (with mention of arteriosclerosis)

Use additional code, if desired, to identify presence of arteriosclerosis

[Excludes:] *acute or subacute (422.0-422.9)*
rheumatic (398.0)
acute (391.2)
that due to hypertension (402.0-402.9)

429.1 Myocardial degeneration

Degeneration of heart or myocardium:
fatty (with mention of arteriosclerosis)
mural (with mention of arteriosclerosis)
muscular (with mention of arteriosclerosis)
Myocardial:
degeneration disease (with mention of arteriosclerosis)

Use additional code, if desired, to identify presence of arteriosclerosis

[Excludes:] *that due to hypertension (402.0-402.9)*

429.2 Cardiovascular disease, unspecified

Arteriosclerotic cardiovascular disease [ASCVD]
Cardiovascular arteriosclerosis
Cardiovascular:
degeneration (with mention of arteriosclerosis)
disease (with mention of arteriosclerosis)
sclerosis (with mention of arteriosclerosis)

Use additional code, if desired, to identify presence of arteriosclerosis

[Excludes:] *that due to hypertension (402.0-402.9)*

429.3 Cardiomegaly

Cardiac:
dilatation
hypertrophy
Ventricular dilatation

[Excludes:] *that due to hypertension (402.0-402.9)*

429.4 Functional disturbances following cardiac surgery

Cardiac insufficiency following cardiac surgery or due to prosthesis
Heart failure following cardiac surgery or due to prosthesis
Postcardiotomy syndrome
Postvalvulotomy syndrome

[Excludes:] *cardiac failure in the immediate postoperative period (997.1)*

429.5 Rupture of chordae tendineae

429.6 Rupture of papillary muscle

[5] **429.7 Certain sequelae of myocardial infarction, not elsewhere classified**

Use additional code to identify the associated myocardial infarction:
with onset of 8 weeks or less (410.00-410.92)
with onset of more than 8 weeks (414.8)

[Excludes:] *congenital defects of heart (745, 746)*
coronary aneurysm (414.11)
disorders of papillary muscle (429.6, 429.81)
postmyocardial infarction syndrome (411.0)
rupture of chordae tendineae (429.5)

429.71 Acquired cardiac septal defect

[Excludes:] *acute septal infarction (410.00-410.92)*

429.79 Other
Mural thrombus (atrial) (ventricular), acquired, following myocardial infarction

[5] **429.8 Other ill-defined heart diseases**

429.81 Other disorders of papillary muscle
Papillary muscle:
atrophy
degeneration
dysfunction
Papillary muscle:
incompetence
incoordination
scarring

429.82 Hyperkinetic heart disease

429.89 Other
Carditis

[Excludes:] *that due to hypertension (402.0-402.9)*

429.9 Heart disease, unspecified
Heart disease (organic) NOS
Morbus cordis NOS

[Excludes:] *that due to hypertension (402.0-402.9)*

CEREBROVASCULAR DISEASE (430-438)

Includes: with mention of hypertension (conditions classifiable to 401-405)

Use additional code, if desired, to identify presence of hypertension

[Excludes:] *any condition classifiable to 430-434, 436, 437 occurring during pregnancy, childbirth, or the puerperium, or specified as puerperal (674.0)*
iatrogenic cerebrovascular infarction or hemorrhage (997.02)

430 Subarachnoid hemorrhage
Meningeal hemorrhage
Ruptured:
berry aneurysm
(congenital) cerebral aneurysm NOS

[Excludes:] *syphilitic ruptured cerebral aneurysm (094.87)*

431 Intracerebral hemorrhage
Hemorrhage (of):
basilar
bulbar
cerebellar
cerebral
cerebromeningeal
cortical
internal capsule
Hemorrhage (of):
intrapontine
pontine
subcortical
ventricular
Rupture of blood vessel in brain

432 Other and unspecified intracranial hemorrhage

432.0 Nontraumatic extradural hemorrhage
Nontraumatic epidural hemorrhage

432.1 Subdural hemorrhage
Subdural hematoma, nontraumatic

432.9 Unspecified intracranial hemorrhage
Intracranial hemorrhage NOS

[5] **433 Occlusion and stenosis of precerebral arteries**

The following fifth-digit subclassification is for use with category 433:

0 without mention of cerebral infarction

1 with cerebral infarction

Includes:
embolism of basilar, carotid, and vertebral arteries
narrowing of basilar, carotid, and vertebral arteries
obstruction of basilar, carotid, and vertebral arteries
thrombosis of basilar, carotid, and vertebral arteries

[Excludes:] *insufficiency NOS of precerebral arteries (435.0-435.9)*

[5] **433.0 Basilar artery**

[5] **433.1 Carotid artery**

[5] **433.2 Vertebral artery**

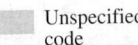

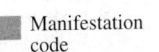

⑤ **433.3** Multiple and bilateral

⑤ **433.8** Other specified precerebral artery

⑤ **433.9** Unspecified precerebral artery
Precerebral artery NOS

⑤ **434** Occlusion of cerebral arteries
The following fifth-digit subclassification is for use with category 434:

    0 without mention of cerebral infarction

    1 with cerebral infarction

⑤ **434.0** Cerebral thrombosis
Thrombosis of cerebral arteries

⑤ **434.1** Cerebral embolism

⑤ **434.9** Cerebral artery occlusion, unspecified

435 Transient cerebral ischemia
Includes: cerebrovascular insufficiency (acute) with transient focal neurological signs and
symptoms
insufficiency of basilar, carotid, and vertebral arteries
spasm of cerebral arteries

Excludes: *acute cerebrovascular insufficiency NOS (437.1)*
that due to any condition classifiable to 433 (433.0-433.9)

435.0 Basilar artery syndrome

435.1 Vertebral artery syndrome

435.2 Subclavian steal syndrome

435.3 Vertebrobasilar artery syndrome

435.8 Other specified transient cerebral ischemias

435.9 Unspecified transient cerebral ischemia
Impending cerebrovascular accident
Intermittent cerebral ischemia
Transient ischemic attack [TIA]

436 Acute, but ill-defined, cerebrovascular disease
Apoplexy, apoplectic: Cerebral seizure
  NOS   Cerebrovascular accident [CVA] NOS
  attack   Stroke
  cerebral
  seizure

Excludes: *any condition classifiable to categories 430-435*
postoperative cerebrovascular accident (997.02)

437 Other and ill-defined cerebrovascular disease

437.0 Cerebral atherosclerosis
Atheroma of cerebral arteries
Cerebral arteriosclerosis

437.1 Other generalized ischemic cerebrovascular disease
Acute cerebrovascular insufficiency NOS
Cerebral ischemia (chronic)

437.2 Hypertensive encephalopathy

437.3 Cerebral aneurysm, nonruptured
Internal carotid artery, intracranial portion
Internal carotid artery NOS

Excludes: *congenital cerebral aneurysm, nonruptured (747.81)*
internal carotid artery, extracranial portion (442.81)

437.4 Cerebral arteritis

437.5 Moyamoya disease

437.6 Nonpyogenic thrombosis of intracranial venous sinus

Excludes: *pyogenic (325)*

437.7 Transient global amnesia

437.8 Other

437.9 Unspecified
Cerebrovascular disease or lesion NOS

● Code new   ▲ Revision of   ④ ⑤ Fourth or fifth
   to this edition   existing code   digit required

438 Late effects of cerebrovascular disease

Note: This category is to be used to indicate conditions in 430-437 as the cause of late effects. The "late effects" include conditions specified as such, as sequelae, which may occur at any time after the onset of the causal condition.

438.0 Cognitive deficits

[5] **438.1 Speech and language deficits**

- **438.10 Speech and language deficit, unspecified**
- **438.11 Aphasia**
- **438.12 Dysphasia**
- **438.19 Other speech and language deficits**

[5] **438.2 Hemiplegia/hemiparesis**

- **438.20 Hemiplegia affecting unspecified side**
- **438.21 Hemiplegia affecting dominant side**
- **438.22 Hemiplegia affecting nondominant side**

[5] **438.3 Monoplegia of upper limb**

- **438.30 Monoplegia of upper limb affecting unspecified side**
- **438.31 Monoplegia of upper limb affecting dominant side**
- **438.32 Monoplegia of upper limb affecting nondominant side**

[5] **438.4 Monoplegia of lower limb**

- **438.40 Monoplegia of lower limb affecting unspecified side**
- **438.41 Monoplegia of lower limb affecting dominant side**
- **438.42 Monoplegia of lower limb affecting nondominant side**

[5] **438.5 Other paralytic syndrome**

Use additional code to identify type of paralytic syndrome, such as:
locked-in state (344.81)
quadriplegia (344.00-344.09)

[*Excludes:*] *late effects of cerebrovascular accident with:*
hemiplegia/hemiparesis (438.20-438.22)
monoplegia of lower limb (438.40-438.42)
monoplegia of upper limb (438.30-438.32)

- **438.50 Other paralytic syndrome affecting unspecified side**
- **438.51 Other paralytic syndrome affecting dominant side**
- **438.52 Other paralytic syndrome affecting nondominant side**
- **438.53 Other paralytic syndrome, bilateral**

● **438.6 Alterations of sensations**

Use additional code to identify the altered sensation

● **438.7 Disturbances of vision**

Use additional code to identify the visual disturbance

[5] **438.8 Other late effects of cerebrovascular disease**

- **438.81 Apraxia**
- **438.82 Dysphagia**
- ● **438.83 Facial weakness**
  Facial droop
- ● **438.84 Ataxia**
- ● **438.85 Vertigo**
- **438.89 Other late effects of cerebrovascular disease**
  Use additional code to identify the late effect

438.9 Unspecified late effects of cerebrovascular disease

Add 4th or 5th digit | Nonspecific code | Unspecified code | Manifestation code

DISEASES OF ARTERIES, ARTERIOLES, AND CAPILLARIES (440-448)

440 **Atherosclerosis**

Includes: arteriolosclerosis
arteriosclerosis (obliterans) (senile)
arteriosclerotic vascular disease
atheroma
degeneration:
arterial
arteriovascular
vascular
endarteritis deformans or obliterans
senile arteritis
senile endarteritis

Excludes: *atheroembolism (445.01-445.89)*
atherosclerosis of bypass graft of the extremities (440.30-440.32)

440.0 **Of aorta**

440.1 **Of renal artery**

Excludes: *atherosclerosis of renal arterioles (403.00-403.91)*

⑤ **440.2** **Of native arteries of the extremities**

Excludes: *atherosclerosis of bypass graft of the extremities (440.30-440.32)*

440.20 **Atherosclerosis of the extremities, unspecified**

440.21 **Atherosclerosis of the extremities with intermittent claudication**

440.22 **Atherosclerosis of the extremities with rest pain**
Includes: any condition classifiable to 440.21

440.23 **Atherosclerosis of the extremities with ulceration**
Includes: any condition classifiable to 440.21 and 440.22
Use additional code for any associated ulceration (707.10-707.9)

440.24 **Atherosclerosis of the extremities with gangrene**
Includes: any condition classifiable to 440.21, 440.22, and 440.23
with ischemic gangrene 785.4

Excludes: *gas gangrene 040.0*

440.29 **Other**

⑤ **440.3** **Of bypass graft of the extremities**

Excludes: *atherosclerosis of native artery of the extremity (440.21-440.24)*
embolism [occlusion NOS] [thrombus]
of graft (996.74)

440.30 **Of unspecified graft**

440.31 **Of autologous vein bypass graft**

440.32 **Of nonautologous biological bypass graft**

440.8 **Of other specified arteries**

Excludes: *basilar (433.0)*
carotid (433.1)
cerebral (437.0)
coronary (414.00-414.06)
mesenteric (557.1)
precerebral (433.0-433.9)
pulmonary (416.0)
vertebral (433.2)

440.9 **Generalized and unspecified atherosclerosis**
Arteriosclerotic vascular disease NOS

Excludes: *arteriosclerotic cardiovascular disease [ASCVD] (429.2)*

441 **Aortic aneurysm and dissection**

Excludes: *syphilitic aortic aneurysm (093.0)*
traumatic aortic aneurysm (901.0, 902.0)

⑤ **441.0** **Dissection of aorta**

441.00 **Unspecified site**

441.01 **Thoracic**

441.02 **Abdominal**

● Code new
to this edition

▲ Revision of
existing code

④ ⑤ Fourth or fifth
digit required

441.03 Thoracoabdominal

441.1 Thoracic aneurysm, ruptured

441.2 Thoracic aneurysm without mention of rupture

441.3 Abdominal aneurysm, ruptured

441.4 Abdominal aneurysm without mention of rupture

441.5 Aortic aneurysm of unspecified site, ruptured
Rupture of aorta NOS

441.6 Thoracoabdominal aneurysm, ruptured

441.7 Thoracoabdominal aneurysm, without mention of rupture

441.9 Aortic aneurysm of unspecified site without mention of rupture
Aneurysm of aorta
Dilatation of aorta
Hyaline necrosis of aorta

442 Other aneurysm
Includes: aneurysm (ruptured) (cirsoid) (false) (varicose)
aneurysmal varix

[Excludes:] *arteriovenous aneurysm or fistula:*
acquired (447.0)
congenital (747.60-747.69)
traumatic (900.0-904.9)

442.0 Of artery of upper extremity

442.1 Of renal artery

442.2 Of iliac artery

442.3 Of artery of lower extremity
Aneurysm:
femoral artery
popliteal artery

[5] **442.8 Of other specified artery**

442.81 Artery of neck
Aneurysm of carotid artery (common) (external) (internal, extracranial portion)

[Excludes:] *internal carotid artery, intracranial portion (437.3)*

442.82 Subclavian artery

442.83 Splenic artery

442.84 Other visceral artery
Aneurysm:
celiac artery
gastroduodenal artery
gastroepiploic artery
hepatic artery
pancreaticoduodenal artery
superior mesenteric artery

442.89 Other
Aneurysm:
mediastinal artery
spinal artery

[Excludes:] *cerebral (nonruptured) (437.3)*
congenital (747.81)
ruptured (430)
coronary (414.11)
heart (414.10)
pulmonary (417.1)

442.9 Of unspecified site

443 Other peripheral vascular disease

443.0 Raynaud's syndrome
Raynaud's:
disease
phenomenon (secondary)

Use additional code, if desired, to identify gangrene (785.4)

443.1 Thromboangiitis obliterans [Buerger's disease]
Presenile gangrene

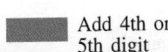

Add 4th or 5th digit | Nonspecific code | Unspecified code | Manifestation code

● **443.2** **Other arterial dissection**

Excludes: *dissection of aorta (441.00-441.03)*
dissection of coronary arteries (414.12)

- ● **443.21** **Dissection of carotid artery**
- ● **443.22** **Dissection of iliac artery**
- ● **443.23** **Dissection of renal artery**
- ● **443.24** **Dissection of vertebral artery**
- ● **443.29** **Dissection of other artery**

⑤ **443.8** **Other specified peripheral vascular diseases**

443.81 ***Peripheral angiopathy in diseases classified elsewhere***
Code first underlying disease, as:
diabetes mellitus (250.7)

443.89 **Other**
Acrocyanosis
Acroparesthesia:
simple [Schultze's type]
vasomotor [Nothnagel's type]
Erythrocyanosis
Erythromelalgia

Excludes: *chilblains (991.5)*
frostbite (991.0-991.3)
immersion foot (991.4)

443.9 **Peripheral vascular disease, unspecified**
Intermittent claudication NOS
Peripheral:
angiopathy NOS
vascular disease NOS
Spasm of artery

Excludes: *atherosclerosis of the arteries of the extremities (440.20-440.22)*
spasm of cerebral artery (435.0-435.9)

444 **Arterial embolism and thrombosis**
Includes: infarction:
embolic
thrombotic
occlusion

Excludes: *atheroembolism (445.01-445.89)*
that complicating:
abortion (634-638 with .6, 639.6)
ectopic or molar pregnancy (639.6)
pregnancy, childbirth, or the puerperium (673.0-673.8)

444.0 **Of abdominal aorta**
Aortic bifurcation syndrome   Leriche's syndrome
Aortoiliac obstruction   Saddle embolus

444.1 **Of thoracic aorta**
Embolism or thrombosis of aorta (thoracic)

⑤ **444.2** **Of arteries of the extremities**

444.21 **Upper extremity**

444.22 **Lower extremity**
Arterial embolism or thrombosis:
femoral
peripheral NOS
popliteal

Excludes: *iliofemoral (444.81)*

⑤ **444.8** **Of other specified artery**

444.81 **Iliac artery**

● Code new
to this edition   ▲ Revision of
existing code   ④ ⑤ Fourth or fifth
digit required

444.89 Other

[xcludes:] *basilar (433.0)*
carotid (433.1)
cerebral (434.0-434.9)
coronary (410.00-410.92)
mesenteric (557.0)
ophthalmic (362.30-362.34)
precerebral (433.0-433.9)
pulmonary (415.19)
renal (593.81)
retinal (362.30-362.34)
vertebral (433.2)

444.9 Of unspecified artery

● **445 Atheroembolism**
Includes: Atherothrombotic microembolism
Cholesterol embolism

● **445.0 Of extremities**

● **445.01 Upper extremity**

● **445.02 Lower extremity**

● **445.8 Of other sites**

● **445.81 Kidney**
Use additional code for any associated kidney failure (584, 585)

● **445.89 Other site**

446 Polyarteritis nodosa and allied conditions

446.0 Polyarteritis nodosa
Disseminated necrotizing periarteritis
Necrotizing angiitis
Panarteritis (nodosa)
Periarteritis (nodosa)

446.1 Acute febrile mucocutaneous lymph node syndrome [MCLS]
Kawasaki disease

[5] **446.2 Hypersensitivity angiitis**
[Excludes:] *antiglomerular basement membrane disease without pulmonary hemorrhage (583.89)*

446.20 Hypersensitivity angiitis, unspecified

446.21 Goodpasture's syndrome
Antiglomerular basement membrane antibody-mediated nephritis with pulmonary hemorrhage
Use additional code, if desired, to identify renal disease (583.81)

446.29 Other specified hypersensitivity angiitis

446.3 Lethal midline granuloma
Malignant granuloma of face

446.4 Wegener's granulomatosis
Necrotizing respiratory granulomatosis
Wegener's syndrome

446.5 Giant cell arteritis
Cranial arteritis
Horton's disease
Temporal arteritis

446.6 Thrombotic microangiopathy
Moschcowitz's syndrome
Thrombotic thrombocytopenic purpura

446.7 Takayasu's disease
Aortic arch arteritis
Pulseless disease

447 Other disorders of arteries and arterioles

447.0 Arteriovenous fistula, acquired
Arteriovenous aneurysm, acquired

[Excludes:] *cerebrovascular (437.3)*
coronary (414.19)
pulmonary (417.0)
surgically created arteriovenous shunt or fistula:
complication (996.1, 996.61-996.62)
status or presence (V45.1)
traumatic (900.0-904.9)

447.1 Stricture of artery

447.2 Rupture of artery
Erosion of artery
Fistula, except arteriovenous of artery
Ulcer of artery

[Excludes:] *traumatic rupture of artery (900.0-904.9)*

447.3 Hyperplasia of renal artery
Fibromuscular hyperplasia of renal artery

447.4 Celiac artery compression syndrome
Celiac axis syndrome
Marable's syndrome

447.5 Necrosis of artery

447.6 Arteritis, unspecified
Aortitis NOS
Endarteritis NOS

[Excludes:] *arteritis, endarteritis:*
aortic arch (446.7)
cerebral (437.4)
coronary (414.00-414.06)
deformans (440.0-440.9)
obliterans (440.0-440.9)
pulmonary (417.8)
senile (440.0-440.9)
polyarteritis NOS (446.0)
syphilitic aortitis (093.1)

447.8 Other specified disorders of arteries and arterioles
Fibromuscular hyperplasia of arteries, except renal

447.9 Unspecified disorders of arteries and arterioles

448 Disease of capillaries

448.0 Hereditary hemorrhagic telangiectasia
Rendu-Osler-Weber disease

448.1 Nevus, non-neoplastic
Nevus:
araneus
senile
Nevus:
spider
stellar

[Excludes:] *neoplastic (216.0-216.9)*
port wine (757.32)
strawberry (757.32)

448.9 Other and unspecified capillary diseases
Capillary:
hemorrhage
hyperpermeability
thrombosis

[Excludes:] *capillary fragility (hereditary) (287.8)*

DISEASES OF VEINS AND LYMPHATICS, AND OTHER DISEASES OF CIRCULATORY SYSTEM (451-459)

451 Phlebitis and thrombophlebitis
Includes: endophlebitis
inflammation, vein
periphlebitis
suppurative phlebitis

Use additional E Code, if desired, to identify drug, if drug-induced

[Excludes:] *that complicating:*
abortion (634-638 with .7, 639.8)
ectopic or molar pregnancy (639.8)
pregnancy, childbirth, or the puerperium (671.0-671.9)
that due to or following:
implant or catheter device (996.61-996.62)
infusion, perfusion, or transfusion (999.2)

451.0 Of superficial vessels of lower extremities
Saphenous vein (greater) (lesser)

⑤ **451.1 Of deep vessels of lower extremities**

● Code new to this edition
▲ Revision of existing code
④ ⑤ Fourth or fifth digit required

451.11 Femoral vein (deep) (superficial)

451.19 Other
Femoropopliteal vein
Popliteal vein
Tibial vein

451.2 Of lower extremities, unspecified

[5] **451.8 Of other sites**

[Excludes:] *intracranial venous sinus (325)*
nonpyogenic (437.6)
portal (vein) (572.1)

451.81 Iliac vein

451.82 Of superficial veins of upper extremities
Antecubital vein
Basilic vein
Cephalic vein

451.83 Of deep veins of upper extremities
Brachial vein
Radial vein
Ulnar vein

451.84 Of upper extremities, unspecified

451.89 Other
Axillary vein
Jugular vein
Subclavian vein
Thrombophlebitis of breast (Mondor's disease)

451.9 Of unspecified site

452 Portal vein thrombosis
Portal (vein) obstruction

[Excludes:] *hepatic vein thrombosis (453.0)*
phlebitis of portal vein (572.1)

453 Other venous embolism and thrombosis

[Excludes:] *that complicating:*
abortion (634-638 with .7, 639.8)
ectopic or molar pregnancy (639.8)
pregnancy, childbirth, or the puerperium (671.0-671.9)
that with inflammation, phlebitis, and thrombophlebitis (451.0-451.9)

453.0 Budd-Chiari syndrome
Hepatic vein thrombosis

453.1 Thrombophlebitis migrans

453.2 Of vena cava

453.3 Of renal vein

453.8 Of other specified veins

[Excludes:] *cerebral (434.0-434.9)*
coronary (410.00-410.92)
intracranial venous sinus (325)
nonpyogenic (437.6)
mesenteric (557.0)
portal (452)
precerebral (433.0-433.9)
pulmonary (415.19)

453.9 Of unspecified site
Embolism of vein
Thrombosis (vein)

454 Varicose veins of lower extremities

[Excludes:] *that complicating pregnancy, childbirth, or the puerperium (671.0)*

454.0 With ulcer
Varicose ulcer (lower extremity, any part)
Varicose veins with ulcer of lower extremity [any part] or of unspecified site
Any condition classifiable to 454.9 with ulcer or specified as ulcerated

454.1 With inflammation
Stasis dermatitis
Varicose veins with inflammation of lower extremity [any part] or of unspecified site
Any condition classifiable to 454.9 with inflammation or specified as inflamed

454.2 With ulcer and inflammation
Varicose veins with ulcer and inflammation of lower extremity [any part] or of
  unspecified site
Any condition classifiable to 454.9 with ulcer and inflammation

● **454.8 With other complications**
Edema
Pain
Swelling

▲ **454.9 Asymptomatic varicose veins**
Phlebectasia of lower extremity [any part] or of unspecified site
Varicose veins NOS
Varicose veins of lower extremity [any part] or of unspecified site
Varix of lower extremity [any part] or of unspecified site

455 Hemorrhoids
Includes: hemorrhoids (anus) (rectum)
           piles
           varicose veins, anus or rectum

| Excludes: | that complicating pregnancy, childbirth or the puerperium (671.8) |

455.0 Internal hemorrhoids without mention of complication

455.1 Internal thrombosed hemorrhoids

455.2 Internal hemorrhoids with other complication
Internal hemorrhoids: Internal hemorrhoids:
  bleeding   strangulated
  prolapsed   ulcerated

455.3 External hemorrhoids without mention of complication

455.4 External thrombosed hemorrhoids

455.5 External hemorrhoids with other complication
External hemorrhoids: External hemorrhoids:
  bleeding   strangulated
  prolapsed   ulcerated

455.6 Unspecified hemorrhoids without mention of complication
Hemorrhoids NOS

455.7 Unspecified thrombosed hemorrhoids
Thrombosed hemorrhoids, unspecified whether internal or external

455.8 Unspecified hemorrhoids with other complication
Hemorrhoids, unspecified whether internal or external:
  bleeding
  prolapsed
  strangulated
  ulcerated

455.9 Residual hemorrhoidal skin tags
Skin tags, anus or rectum

456 Varicose veins of other sites

456.0 Esophageal varices with bleeding

456.1 Esophageal varices without mention of bleeding

⑤ **456.2 Esophageal varices in diseases classified elsewhere**
Code first underlying cause, as:
  cirrhosis of liver (571.0-571.9)
  portal hypertension (572.3)

   456.20 With bleeding

   456.21 Without mention of bleeding

456.3 Sublingual varices

456.4 Scrotal varices
Varicocele

456.5 Pelvic varices
Varices of broad ligament

● Code new   ▲ Revision of   ④ ⑤ Fourth or fifth
  to this edition   existing code   digit required

456.6 Vulval varices
Varices of perineum

Excludes: *that complicating pregnancy, childbirth, or the puerperium (671.1)*

456.8 Varices of other sites
Varicose veins of nasal septum (with ulcer)

Excludes: *placental varices (656.7)*
retinal varices (362.17)
varicose ulcer of unspecified site (454.0)
varicose veins of unspecified site (454.9)

457 Noninfectious disorders of lymphatic channels

457.0 Postmastectomy lymphedema syndrome
Elephantiasis due to mastectomy
Obliteration of lymphatic vessel due to mastectomy

457.1 Other lymphedema
Elephantiasis (nonfilarial) NOS
Lymphangiectasis
Lymphedema:
  acquired (chronic)
  praecox
  secondary
Obliteration, lymphatic vessel

Excludes: *elephantiasis (nonfilarial):*
congenital (757.0)
eyelid (374.83)
vulva (624.8)

457.2 Lymphangitis
Lymphangitis:
  NOS
  chronic
  subacute

Excludes: *acute lymphangitis (682.0-682.9)*

457.8 Other noninfectious disorders of lymphatic channels
Chylocele (nonfilarial)   Lymph node or vessel:
Chylous: fistula
  ascites   infarction
  cyst   rupture

Excludes: *chylocele:*
filarial (125.0-125.9)
tunica vaginalis (nonfilarial) (608.84)

457.9 Unspecified noninfectious disorder of lymphatic channels

458 Hypotension
Includes: hypopiesis

Excludes: *cardiovascular collapse (785.50)*
maternal hypotension syndrome (669.2)
shock (785.50-785.59)
Shy-Drager syndrome (333.0)

458.0 Orthostatic hypotension
Hypotension:
  orthostatic (chronic)
  postural

458.1 Chronic hypotension
Permanent idiopathic hypotension

458.2 Iatrogenic hypotension
Postoperative hypotension

458.8 Other specified hypotension

458.9 Hypotension, unspecified
Hypotension (arterial) NOS

459 Other disorders of circulatory system

| | Add 4th or 5th digit | | Nonspecific code | | Unspecified code | | Manifestation code |

459.0 Hemorrhage, unspecified
Rupture of blood vessel NOS
Spontaneous hemorrhage NEC

Excludes: *hemorrhage:*
gastrointestinal NOS (578.9)
in newborn NOS (772.9)
secondary or recurrent following trauma (958.2)
traumatic rupture of blood vessel (900.0-904.9)

⑤ **459.1 Postphlebitic syndrome**
Chronic venous hypertension due to deep vein thrombosis

Excludes: *chronic venous hyptertension without deep vein thrombosis (459.30-459.39)*

● **459.10 Postphlebetic syndrome without complications**
Asymptomatic postphlebetic syndrome
Postphlebetic syndrome NOS

● **459.11 Postphlebetic syndrome with ulcer**

● **459.12 Postphlebetic syndrome with inflammation**

● **459.13 Postphlebetic syndrome with ulcer and inflammation**

● **459.19 Postphlebetic syndrome with other complication**

459.2 Compression of vein
Stricture of vein
Vena cava syndrome (inferior) (superior)

● **459.3 Chronic venous hypertension (idiopathic)**
Statis edema

Excludes: *chronic venous hypertension due to deep vein thrombosis (459.10-459.19)*
varicose veins (454.0-454.9)

● **459.30 Chronic venous hypertension without complications**
Asymptomatic chronic venous hypertension
Chronic venous hypertension NOS

● **459.31 Chronic venous hypertension with ulcer**

● **459.32 Chronic venous hypertension with inflammation**

● **459.33 Chronic venous hypertension with ulcer and inflammation**

● **459.39 Chronic venous hypertension with other complication**

⑤ **459.8 Other specified disorders of circulatory system**

459.81 Venous (peripheral) insufficiency, unspecified
Chronic venous insufficiency NOS
Use additional code for any associated ulceration (707.10-707.9)

459.89 Other
Collateral circulation (venous), any site
Phlebosclerosis
Venofibrosis

459.9 Unspecified circulatory system disorder

● Code new
to this edition   ▲ Revision of
existing code   ④ ⑤ Fourth or fifth
digit required

8. DISEASES OF THE RESPIRATORY SYSTEM (460-519)

Use additional code, if desired, to identify infectious organism

ACUTE RESPIRATORY INFECTIONS (460-466)

Excludes: *pneumonia and influenza (480.0-487.8)*

460 Acute nasopharyngitis [common cold]

Coryza (acute)	Rhinitis:
Nasal catarrh, acute	acute
Nasopharyngitis:	infective
NOS	
acute	
infective NOS	

Excludes: *nasopharyngitis, chronic (472.2)*
pharyngitis:
acute or unspecified (462)
chronic (472.1)
rhinitis:
allergic (477.0-477.9)
chronic or unspecified (472.0)
sore throat:
acute or unspecified (462)
chronic (472.1)

461 Acute sinusitis

Includes: abscess
empyema acute, of sinus (accessory) (nasal)
infection acute, of sinus (accessory) (nasal)
inflammation acute, of sinus (accessory) (nasal)
suppuration acute, of sinus (accessory) (nasal)

Excludes: *chronic or unspecified sinusitis (473.0-473.9)*

461.0 Maxillary
Acute antritis

461.1 Frontal

461.2 Ethmoidal

461.3 Sphenoidal

461.8 Other acute sinusitis
Acute pansinusitis

461.9 Acute sinusitis, unspecified
Acute sinusitis NOS

462 Acute pharyngitis

Acute sore throat NOS	Pharyngitis (acute):
Pharyngitis (acute):	staphylococcal
NOS	suppurative
gangrenous	ulcerative
infective	Sore throat (viral) NOS
phlegmonous	Viral pharyngitis
pneumococcal	

Excludes: *abscess:*
peritonsillar [quinsy] (475)
pharyngeal NOS (478.29)
retropharyngeal (478.24)
chronic pharyngitis (472.1)
infectious mononucleosis (075)
that specified as (due to):
Coxsackie (virus) (074.0)
gonococcus (098.6)
herpes simplex (054.79)
influenza (487.1)
septic (034.0)
streptococcal (034.0)

Add 4th or 5th digit	Nonspecific code	Unspecified code	Manifestation code

463 Acute tonsillitis

Tonsillitis (acute):	Tonsillitis (acute):
NOS	septic
follicular	staphylococcal
gangrenous	suppurative
infective	ulcerative
pneumococcal	viral

Excludes: *chronic tonsillitis (474.0)*
hypertrophy of tonsils (474.1)
peritonsillar abscess [quinsy] (475)
sore throat:
    acute or NOS (462)
    septic (034.0)
streptococcal tonsillitis (034.0)

464 Acute laryngitis and tracheitis

Excludes: *that associated with influenza (487.1)*
that due to Streptococcus (034.0)

⑤ **464.0 Acute laryngitis**

Laryngitis (acute):	Laryngitis (acute):
NOS	pneumococcal
edematous	septic
Hemophilus influenza	suppurative
[H. influenzae]	ulcerative

Excludes: *chronic laryngitis (476.0-476.1)*
influenzal laryngitis (487.1)

    464.00 Without mention of obstruction

    464.01 With obstruction

⑤ **464.1 Acute tracheitis**
Tracheitis (acute):
NOS
catarrhal
viral

Excludes: *chronic tracheitis (491.8)*

    464.10 Without mention of obstruction

    464.11 With obstruction

⑤ **464.2 Acute laryngotracheitis**
Laryngotracheitis (acute)
Tracheitis (acute) with laryngitis (acute)

Excludes: *chronic laryngotracheitis (476.1)*

    464.20 Without mention of obstruction

    464.21 With obstruction

⑤ **464.3 Acute epiglottitis**
Viral epiglottitis

Excludes: *epiglottitis, chronic (476.1)*

    464.30 Without mention of obstruction

    464.31 With obstruction

  464.4 Croup
Croup syndrome

⑤ **464.5 Supraglottitis, unspecified**

    464.50 Without mention of obstruction

    464.51 With obstruction

465 Acute upper respiratory infections of multiple or unspecified sites

Excludes: *upper respiratory infection due to:*
influenza (487.1)
Streptococcus (034.0)

  465.0 Acute laryngopharyngitis

465.8 Other multiple sites
Multiple URI

● Code new
       to this edition   ▲ Revision of
                               existing code   ④ ⑤ Fourth or fifth
                                                         digit required

465.9 Unspecified site
Acute URI NOS
Upper respiratory infection (acute)

466 Acute bronchitis and bronchiolitis
Includes: that with:
bronchospasm
obstruction

466.0 Acute bronchitis
Bronchitis, acute or subacute:
fibrinous
membranous
pneumococcal
purulent
septic
viral
with tracheitis
Croupous bronchitis
Tracheobronchitis, acute

[*Excludes:*] *acute bronchitis with:*
bronchiectasis (494.1)
chronic obstructive pulmonary disease (491.21)

[5] **466.1 Acute bronchiolitis**
Bronchiolitis (acute)
Capillary pneumonia

466.11 Acute bronchiolitis due to respiratory syncytial virus (RSV)

466.19 Acute bronchiolitis due to other infectious organisms
Use additional code to identify organism

OTHER DISEASES OF THE UPPER RESPIRATORY TRACT (470-478)

470 Deviated nasal septum
Deflected septum (nasal) (acquired)

[*Excludes:*] *congenital (754.0)*

471 Nasal polyps

[*Excludes:*] *adenomatous polyps (212.0)*

471.0 Polyp of nasal cavity
Polyp:
choanal
nasopharyngeal

471.1 Polypoid sinus degeneration
Woakes' syndrome or ethmoiditis

471.8 Other polyp of sinus
Polyp of sinus:
accessory
ethmoidal
Polyp of sinus:
maxillary
sphenoidal

471.9 Unspecified nasal polyp
Nasal polyp NOS

472 Chronic pharyngitis and nasopharyngitis

472.0 Chronic rhinitis
Ozena
Rhinitis:
NOS
atrophic
granulomatous
Rhinitis:
hypertrophic
obstructive
purulent
ulcerative

[*Excludes:*] *allergic rhinitis (477.0-477.9)*

472.1 Chronic pharyngitis
Chronic sore throat
Pharyngitis:
atrophic
granular (chronic)
hypertrophic

472.2 Chronic nasopharyngitis

[*Excludes:*] *acute or unspecified nasopharyngitis (460)*

473 **Chronic sinusitis**
Includes:

abscess (chronic) of sinus (accessory) (nasal)
empyema (chronic) of sinus (accessory) (nasal)
infection (chronic) of sinus (accessory) (nasal)
suppuration (chronic) of sinus (accessory) (nasal)

Excludes: *acute sinusitis (461.0-461.9)*

473.0 Maxillary
Antritis (chronic)

473.1 Frontal

473.2 Ethmoidal

Excludes: *Woakes' ethmoiditis (471.1)*

473.3 Sphenoidal

473.8 **Other chronic sinusitis**
Pansinusitis (chronic)

473.9 Unspecified sinusitis (chronic)
Sinusitis (chronic) NOS

474 **Chronic disease of tonsils and adenoids**

⑤ **474.0 Chronic tonsillitis and adenoiditis**

Excludes: *acute or unspecified tonsillitis (463)*

474.00   Chronic tonsillitis

474.01   Chronic adenoiditis

474.02   Chronic tonsillitis and adenoiditis

⑤ **474.1 Hypertrophy of tonsils and adenoids**
Enlargement of tonsils or adenoids
Hyperplasia of tonsils or adenoids
Hypertrophy of tonsils or adenoids

Excludes: *that with adenoiditis (474.01)*
that with adenoiditis and tonsillitis (474.02)
that with tonsillitis (474.00)

474.10   Tonsils with adenoids

474.11   Tonsils alone

474.12   Adenoids alone

474.2 Adenoid vegetations

474.8 **Other chronic disease of tonsils and adenoids**
Amygdalolith
Calculus, tonsil
Cicatrix of tonsil (and adenoid)
Tonsillar tag
Ulcer, tonsil

474.9 Unspecified chronic disease of tonsils and adenoids
Disease (chronic) of tonsils (and adenoids)

475 Peritonsillar abscess
Abscess of tonsil   Quinsy
Peritonsillar cellulitis

Excludes: *tonsillitis:*
acute or NOS (463)
chronic (474.0)

476 **Chronic laryngitis and laryngotracheitis**

476.0 Chronic laryngitis
Laryngitis:
catarrhal
hypertrophic
Sicca

● Code new
to this edition   ▲ Revision of
existing code   ④ ⑤ Fourth or fifth
digit required

476.1 Chronic laryngotracheitis
Laryngitis, chronic, with tracheitis (chronic)
Tracheitis, chronic, with laryngitis

[Excludes:] *chronic tracheitis (491.8)*
laryngitis and tracheitis, acute or unspecified (464.00-464.51)

477 Allergic rhinitis
Includes: allergic rhinitis (nonseasonal) (seasonal)
hay fever
spasmodic rhinorrhea

[Excludes:] *allergic rhinitis with asthma (bronchial) (493.0)*

477.0 Due to pollen
Pollinosis

477.1 Due to food

477.8 Due to other allergen

477.9 Cause unspecified

478 Other diseases of upper respiratory tract

478.0 Hypertrophy of nasal turbinates

478.1 Other diseases of nasal cavity and sinuses
Abscess of nose (septum)
Necrosis of nose (septum)
Ulcer of nose (septum)
Cyst or mucocele of sinus (nasal)
Rhinolith

[Excludes:] *varicose ulcer of nasal septum (456.8)*

[5] **478.2 Other diseases of pharynx, not elsewhere classified**

478.20 Unspecified disease of pharynx

478.21 Cellulitis of pharynx or nasopharynx

478.22 Parapharyngeal abscess

478.24 Retropharyngeal abscess

478.25 Edema of pharynx or nasopharynx

478.26 Cyst of pharynx or nasopharynx

478.29 Other
Abscess of pharynx or nasopharynx

[Excludes:] *ulcerative pharyngitis (462)*

[5] **478.3 Paralysis of vocal cords or larynx**

478.30 Paralysis, unspecified
Laryngoplegia Paralysis of glottis

478.31 Unilateral, partial

478.32 Unilateral, complete

478.33 Bilateral, partial

478.34 Bilateral, complete

478.4 Polyp of vocal cord or larynx

[Excludes:] *adenomatous polyps (212.1)*

478.5 Other diseases of vocal cords
Abscess of vocal cords
Cellulitis of vocal cords
Granuloma of vocal cords
Leukoplakia of vocal cords
Chorditis (fibrinous) (nodosa) (tuberosa)
Singers' nodes

478.6 Edema of larynx
Edema (of):
glottis
subglottic
supraglottic

[5] **478.7 Other diseases of larynx, not elsewhere classified**

478.70 Unspecified disease of larynx

Add 4th or 5th digit | Nonspecific code | Unspecified code | Manifestation code

478.71 **Cellulitis and perichondritis of larynx**

478.74 **Stenosis of larynx**

478.75 **Laryngeal spasm**
Laryngismus (stridulus)

478.79 **Other**
Abscess of larynx
Necrosis of larynx
Obstruction of larynx
Pachyderma of larynx
Ulcer of larynx

Excludes: *ulcerative laryngitis (464.00-464.01)*

478.8 **Upper respiratory tract hypersensitivity reaction, site unspecified**

Excludes: *hypersensitivity reaction of lower respiratory tract, as:*
extrinsic allergic alveolitis (495.0-495.9)
pneumoconiosis (500-505)

478.9 **Other and unspecified diseases of upper respiratory tract**
Abscess of trachea
Cicatrix of trachea

PNEUMONIA AND INFLUENZA (480-487)

Excludes: *pneumonia:*
allergic or eosinophilic (518.3)
aspiration:
NOS (507.0)
newborn (770.1)
solids and liquids (507.0-507.8)
congenital (770.0)
lipoid (507.1)
passive (514)
rheumatic (390)

480 **Viral pneumonia**

480.0 **Pneumonia due to adenovirus**

480.1 **Pneumonia due to respiratory syncytial virus**

480.2 **Pneumonia due to parainfluenza virus**

480.8 **Pneumonia due to other virus not elsewhere classified**

Excludes: *congenital rubella pneumonitis (771.0)*
influenza with pneumonia, any form (487.0)
pneumonia complicating viral diseases classified elsewhere (484.1-484.8)

480.9 **Viral pneumonia, unspecified**

481 **Pneumococcal pneumonia [Streptococcus pneumoniae pneumonia]**
Lobar pneumonia, organism unspecified

482 **Other bacterial pneumonia**

482.0 **Pneumonia due to Klebsiella pneumoniae**

482.1 **Pneumonia due to Pseudomonas**

482.2 **Pneumonia due to Hemophilus influenzae [H. influenzae]**

⑤ 482.3 **Pneumonia due to Streptococcus**

Excludes: *Streptococcus pneumoniae pneumonia (481)*

482.30 **Streptococcus, unspecified**

482.31 **Group A**

482.32 **Group B**

482.39 **Other Streptococcus**

⑤ 482.4 **Pneumonia due to Staphylococcus**

482.40 **Pneumonia due to Staphylococcus, unspecified**

482.41 **Pneumonia due to Staphylococcus aureus**

482.49 **Other Staphylococcus pneumonia**

⑤ 482.8 **Pneumonia due to other specified bacteria**

Excludes: *pneumonia complicating infectious disease classified elsewhere (484.1-484.8)*

● Code new
to this edition

▲ Revision of
existing code

④ ⑤ Fourth or fifth
digit required

482.81 Anaerobes
Bacteroides (melaninogenicus)
Gram-negative anaerobes

482.82 Escherichia coli [E. coli]

482.83 Other gram-negative bacteria
Gram-negative pneumonia NOS
Proteus
Serratia marcescens

Excludes: Gram-negative anaerobes (482.81)
Legionnaires' disease (482.84)

482.84 Legionnaires' disease

482.89 Other specified bacteria

482.9 Bacterial pneumonia unspecified

483 Pneumonia due to other specified organism

483.0 Mycoplasma pneumoniae
Eaton's agent
Pleuropneumonia-like organism [PPLO]

483.1 Chlamydia

483.8 Other specified organism

484 Pneumonia in infectious diseases classified elsewhere

Excludes: influenza with pneumonia, any form (487.0)

484.1 Pneumonia in cytomegalic inclusion disease
Code first underlying disease (078.5)

484.3 Pneumonia in whooping cough
Code first underlying disease (033.0-033.9)

484.5 Pneumonia in anthrax
Code first underlying disease (022.1)

484.6 Pneumonia in aspergillosis
Code first underlying disease (117.3)

484.7 Pneumonia in other systemic mycoses
Code first underlying disease

Excludes: pneumonia in:
candidiasis (112.4)
coccidioidomycosis (114.0)
histoplasmosis (115.0-115.9 with fifth-digit 5)

484.8 Pneumonia in other infectious diseases classified elsewhere
Code first underlying disease, as:
Q fever (083.0)
typhoid fever (002.0)

Excludes: pneumonia in:
actinomycosis (039.1)
measles (055.1)
nocardiosis (039.1)
ornithosis (073.0)
Pneumocystis carinii (136.3)
salmonellosis (003.22)
toxoplasmosis (130.4)
tuberculosis (011.6)
tularemia (021.2)
varicella (052.1)

485 Bronchopneumonia, organism unspecified

Bronchopneumonia:
hemorrhagic
terminal
Pleurobronchopneumonia

Pneumonia:
lobular
segmental

Excludes: bronchiolitis (acute) (466.11-466.19)
chronic (491.8)
lipoid pneumonia (507.1)

Add 4th or 5th digit	Nonspecific code	Unspecified code	Manifestation code

486 Pneumonia, organism unspecified

Excludes: hypostatic or passive pneumonia (514)
   influenza with pneumonia, any form (487.0)
   inhalation or aspiration pneumonia due to foreign materials (507.0-507.8)
   pneumonitis due to fumes and vapors (506.0)

487 Influenza

Excludes: Hemophilus influenzae [H. influenzae]:
   infection NOS (041.5)
   laryngitis (464.00-464.01)
   meningitis (320.0)
   pneumonia (482.2)

487.0 With pneumonia
Influenza with pneumonia, any form
Influenzal:
   bronchopneumonia
   pneumonia

487.1 With other respiratory manifestations
Influenza NOS
Influenzal:
   laryngitis
   pharyngitis
   respiratory infection (upper) (acute)

487.8 With other manifestations
Encephalopathy due to influenza
Influenza with involvement of gastrointestinal tract

Excludes: "intestinal flu" [viral gastroenteritis] (008.8)

CHRONIC OBSTRUCTIVE PULMONARY DISEASE AND ALLIED CONDITIONS (490-496)

490 Bronchitis, not specified as acute or chronic
Bronchitis NOS: Tracheobronchitis NOS
   catarrhal
   with tracheitis NOS

Excludes: bronchitis:
   allergic NOS (493.9)
   asthmatic NOS (493.9)
   due to fumes and vapors (506.0)

491 Chronic bronchitis

Excludes: chronic obstructive asthma (493.2)

491.0 Simple chronic bronchitis
Catarrhal bronchitis, chronic
Smokers' cough

491.1 Mucopurulent chronic bronchitis
Bronchitis (chronic) (recurrent):
   fetid
   mucopurulent
   purulent

⑤ 491.2 Obstructive chronic bronchitis
Bronchitis: Bronchitis with:
   emphysematous   chronic airway obstruction
   obstructive (chronic) (diffuse)   emphysema

Excludes: asthmatic bronchitis (acute) NOS (493.9)
   chronic obstructive asthma (493.2)

491.20 Without mention of acute exacerbation
Emphysema with chronic bronchitis

491.21 With acute exacerbation
Acute bronchitis with chronic obstructive pulmonary disease [COPD]
Acute and chronic obstructive bronchitis
Acute exacerbation of chronic obstructive pulmonary disease [COPD]
Emphysema with both acute and chronic bronchitis

Excludes: chronic obstructive asthma with acute exacerbation (493.22)

● Code new   ▲ Revision of   ④ ⑤ Fourth or fifth
   to this edition   existing code   digit required

491.8 Other chronic bronchitis
Chronic:
- tracheitis
- tracheobronchitis

491.9 Unspecified chronic bronchitis

492 Emphysema

492.0 Emphysematous bleb
Giant bullous emphysema
Ruptured emphysematous bleb
Tension pneumatocele
Vanishing lung

492.8 Other emphysema
Emphysema (lung or pulmonary):
- NOS
- centriacinar
- centrilobular
- obstructive
- panacinar

Emphysema (lung or pulmonary):
- panlobular
- unilateral
- vesicular

MacLeod's syndrome
Swyer-James syndrome
Unilateral hyperlucent lung

[Excludes:] *emphysema:*
- *compensatory (518.2)*
- *due to fumes and vapors (506.4)*
- *interstitial (518.1)*
  - *newborn (770.2)*
- *mediastinal (518.1)*
- *surgical (subcutaneous) (998.81)*
- *traumatic (958.7)*
- *with chronic bronchitis (491.20)*
- *with both acute and chronic bronchitis (491.21)*

[5] 493 Asthma

[Excludes:] *wheezing NOS (786.07)*

The following fifth-digit subclassification is for use with category 493:

0 without mention of status asthmaticus or acute exacerbation or unspecified

1 with status asthmaticus

2 with acute exacerbation

[5] **493.0 extrinsic asthma**
Asthma:
- allergic with stated cause
- atopic
- childhood
- hay
- platinum

Hay fever with asthma

[Excludes:] *asthma:*
- *allergic NOS (493.9)*
- *detergent (507.8)*
- *miners' (500)*
- *wood (495.8)*

[5] **493.1 Intrinsic asthma**
Late-onset asthma

[5] **493.2 Chronic obstructive asthma**
Asthma with chronic obstructive pulmonary disease [COPD]
Chronic asthmatic bronchitis

[Excludes:] *chronic obstructive bronchitis (491.2)*
acute bronchitis (466.0)

[5] **493.9 Asthma, unspecified**
Asthma (bronchial) (allergic NOS)
Bronchitis:
- allergic
- asthmatic

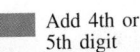

Add 4th or 5th digit | Nonspecific code | Unspecified code | Manifestation code

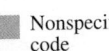

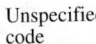

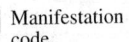

494 Bronchiectasis
  Bronchiectasis (fusiform) (postinfectious) (recurrent)
  Bronchiolectasis

  > Excludes: congenital (748.61)
  > tuberculous bronchiectasis (current disease) (011.5)

  494.0 Bronchiectasis without acute exacerbation

  494.1 Bronchiectasis with acute exacerbation
    Acute bronchitis with bronchiectasis

495 Extrinsic allergic alveolitis
  Includes: allergic alveolitis and pneumonitis due to inhaled organic dust particles of fungal, thermophilic actinomycete, or other origin

  495.0 Farmers' lung

  495.1 Bagassosis

  495.2 Bird-fanciers' lung
    Budgerigar-fanciers' disease or lung
    Pigeon-fanciers' disease or lung

  495.3 Suberosis
    Cork-handlers' disease or lung

  495.4 Malt workers' lung
    Alveolitis due to Aspergillus clavatus

  495.5 Mushroom workers' lung

  495.6 Maple bark-strippers' lung
    Alveolitis due to Cryptostroma corticale

  495.7 "Ventilation" pneumonitis
    Allergic alveolitis due to fungal, thermophilic actinomycete, and other organisms growing in ventilation [air conditioning] systems

  495.8 Other specified allergic alveolitis and pneumonitis
    Cheese-washers' lung   Pituitary snuff-takers' disease
    Coffee workers' lung   Sequoiosis or red-cedar asthma
    Fish-meal workers' lung   Wood asthma
    Furriers' lung
    Grain-handlers' disease or lung

  495.9 Unspecified allergic alveolitis and pneumonitis
    Alveolitis, allergic (extrinsic)
    Hypersensitivity pneumonitis

496 Chronic airway obstruction, not elsewhere classified
  Note: This code is not to be used with any code from categories 491-493
    Chronic:
    nonspecific lung disease
    obstructive lung disease
    obstructive pulmonary disease [COPD] NOS

  > Excludes: chronic obstructive lung disease [COPD] specified (as) (with):
  > allergic alveolitis (495.0-495.9)
  > asthma (493.2)
  > bronchiectasis (494.0-494.1)
  > bronchitis (491.20-491.21)
  > with emphysema (491.20-491.21)
  > emphysema (492.0-492.8)

PNEUMOCONIOSES AND OTHER LUNG DISEASES DUE TO EXTERNAL AGENTS (500-508)

500 Coal workers' pneumoconiosis
  Anthracosilicosis   Coal workers' lung
  Anthracosis   Miner's asthma
  Black lung disease

501 Asbestosis

502 Pneumoconiosis due to other silica or silicates
  Pneumoconiosis due to talc
  Silicotic fibrosis (massive) of lung
  Silicosis (simple) (complicated)

● Code new to this edition   ▲ Revision of existing code   ④ ⑤ Fourth or fifth digit required

503 **Pneumoconiosis due to other inorganic dust**
    Aluminosis (of lung)   Graphite fibrosis (of lung)
    Bauxite fibrosis (of lung)   Siderosis
    Berylliosis   Stannosis

504 **Pneumonopathy due to inhalation of other dust**
    Byssinosis   Flax-dressers' disease
    Cannabinosis

       | Excludes: | *allergic alveolitis (495.0-495.9)*
                asbestosis (501)
                bagassosis (495.1)
                farmers' lung (495.0)

505 **Pneumoconiosis, unspecified**

506 **Respiratory conditions due to chemical fumes and vapors**
Use additional E code, if desired, to identify cause

    506.0 **Bronchitis and pneumonitis due to fumes and vapors**
        Chemical bronchitis (acute)

    506.1 **Acute pulmonary edema due to fumes and vapors**
        Chemical pulmonary edema (acute)

       | Excludes: | *acute pulmonary edema NOS (518.4)*
                  chronic or unspecified pulmonary edema (514)

    506.2 **Upper respiratory inflammation due to fumes and vapors**

    506.3 **Other acute and subacute respiratory conditions due to fumes and vapors**

    506.4 **Chronic respiratory conditions due to fumes and vapors**
        Emphysema (diffuse) (chronic) due to inhalation of chemical fumes and vapors
        Obliterative bronchiolitis (chronic) (subacute) due to inhalation of chemical fumes and vapors
        Pulmonary fibrosis (chronic) due to inhalation of chemical fumes and vapors

    506.9 **Unspecified respiratory conditions due to fumes and vapors**
        Silo-fillers' disease

507 **Pneumonitis due to solids and liquids**

       | Excludes: | *fetal aspiration pneumonitis (770.1)*

    507.0 **Due to inhalation of food or vomitus**
        Aspiration pneumonia (due to):
          NOS
          food (regurgitated)
          gastric secretions
          milk
          saliva
          vomitus

    507.1 **Due to inhalation of oils and essences**
        Lipoid pneumonia (exogenous)

       | Excludes: | *endogenous lipoid pneumonia (516.8)*

    507.8 **Due to other solids and liquids**
        Detergent asthma

508 **Respiratory conditions due to other and unspecified external agents**
Use additional E code, if desired, to identify cause

    508.0 **Acute pulmonary manifestations due to radiation**
        Radiation pneumonitis

    508.1 **Chronic and other pulmonary manifestations due to radiation**
        Fibrosis of lung following radiation

    508.8 **Respiratory conditions due to other specified external agents**

    508.9 **Respiratory conditions due to unspecified external agent**

OTHER DISEASES OF RESPIRATORY SYSTEM (510-519)

510 **Empyema**
Use additional code, if desired, to identify infectious organism (041.0-041.9)

       | Excludes: | *abscess of lung (513.0)*

315

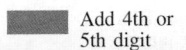 Add 4th or
5th digit

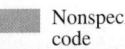 Nonspecific
code

Unspecified
code

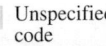 Manifestation
code

510.0 With fistula

Fistula:
  bronchocutaneous
  bronchopleural
  hepatopleural

Fistula:
  mediastinal
  pleural
  thoracic

Any condition classifiable to 510.9 with fistula

510.9 Without mention of fistula

Abscess:
  pleura
  thorax
Empyema (chest) (lung)
  (pleura)
Fibrinopurulent pleurisy

Pleurisy:
  purulent
  septic
  seropurulent
  suppurative
Pyopneumothorax
Pyothorax

511 Pleurisy

Excludes: malignant pleural effusion (197.2)
  pleurisy with mention of tuberculosis, current disease (012.0)

511.0 Without mention of effusion or current tuberculosis

Adhesion, lung or pleura
Calcification of pleura
Pleurisy (acute) (sterile):
  diaphragmatic
  fibrinous
  interlobar

Pleurisy:
  NOS
  pneumococcal
  staphylococcal
  streptococcal
Thickening of pleura

511.1 With effusion, with mention of a bacterial cause other than tuberculosis

Pleurisy with effusion (exudative) (serous):
  pneumococcal
  staphylococcal
  streptococcal
  other specified nontuberculous bacterial cause

511.8 Other specified forms of effusion, except tuberculous

Encysted pleurisy
Hemopneumothorax
Hemothorax

Hydropneumothorax
Hydrothorax

Excludes: traumatic (860.2-860.5, 862.29, 862.39)

511.9 Unspecified pleural effusion

Pleural effusion NOS
Pleurisy:
  exudative
  serofibrinous

Pleurisy:
  serous
  with effusion NOS

512 Pneumothorax

512.0 Spontaneous tension pneumothorax

512.1 Iatrogenic pneumothorax

Postoperative pneumothorax

512.8 Other spontaneous pneumothorax

Pneumothorax:
  NOS
  acute
  chronic

Excludes: pneumothorax:
  congenital (770.2)
  traumatic (860.0-860.1, 860.4-860.5)
  tuberculous, current disease (011.7)

513 Abscess of lung and mediastinum

513.0 Abscess of lung

Abscess (multiple) of lung
Gangrenous or necrotic pneumonia
Pulmonary gangrene or necrosis

513.1 Abscess of mediastinum

● Code new
  to this edition

▲ Revision of
  existing code

④ ⑤ Fourth or fifth
  digit required

514 Pulmonary congestion and hypostasis
Hypostatic:
  bronchopneumonia
  pneumonia
Passive pneumonia
Pulmonary congestion (chronic) (passive)
Pulmonary edema:
  NOS
  chronic

> Excludes: *acute pulmonary edema:*
>   *NOS (518.4)*
>   *with mention of heart disease or failure (428.1)*

515 Postinflammatory pulmonary fibrosis
Cirrhosis of lung, chronic or unspecified
Fibrosis of lung (atrophic) (confluent) (massive) (perialveolar) (peribronchial), chronic or unspecified
Induration of lung, chronic or unspecified

516 Other alveolar and parietoalveolar pneumonopathy

516.0 Pulmonary alveolar proteinosis

516.1 Idiopathic pulmonary hemosiderosis
Essential brown induration of lung
Code first underlying disease (275.0)

516.2 Pulmonary alveolar microlithiasis

516.3 Idiopathic fibrosing alveolitis
Alveolar capillary block
Diffuse (idiopathic) (interstitial) pulmonary fibrosis
Hamman-Rich syndrome

516.8 Other specified alveolar and parietoalveolar pneumonopathies
Endogenous lipoid pneumonia
Interstitial pneumonia (desquamative) (lymphoid)

> Excludes: *lipoid pneumonia, exogenous or unspecified (507.1)*

516.9 Unspecified alveolar and parietoalveolar pneumonopathy

517 Lung involvement in conditions classified elsewhere

> Excludes: *rheumatoid lung (714.81)*

517.1 Rheumatic pneumonia
Code first underlying disease (390)

517.2 Lung involvement in systemic sclerosis
Code first underlying disease (710.1)

517.8 Lung involvement in other diseases classified elsewhere
Code first underlying disease, as:
  amyloidosis (277.3)
  polymyositis (710.4)
  sarcoidosis (135)
  Sjögren's disease (710.2)
  systemic lupus erythematosus (710.0)

> Excludes: *syphilis (095.1)*

518 Other diseases of lung

518.0 Pulmonary collapse
Atelectasis
Collapse of lung
Middle lobe syndrome

> Excludes: *atelectasis:*
>   *congenital (partial) (770.5)*
>   *primary (770.4)*
>   *tuberculous, current disease (011.8)*

518.1 Interstitial emphysema
Mediastinal emphysema

> Excludes: *surgical (subcutaneous) emphysema (998.81)*
>   *that in fetus or newborn (770.2)*
>   *traumatic emphysema (958.7)*

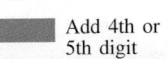

| | Add 4th or 5th digit | | Nonspecific code | | Unspecified code | | Manifestation code |

518.2 Compensatory emphysema

518.3 Pulmonary eosinophilia
Eosinophilic asthma
Löffler's syndrome
Pneumonia:
allergic
eosinophilic
Tropical eosinophilia

518.4 Acute edema of lung, unspecified
Acute pulmonary edema NOS
Pulmonary edema, postoperative

[Excludes:] *pulmonary edema:*
acute, with mention of heart disease or failure (428.1)
chronic or unspecified (514)
due to external agents (506.0-508.9)

518.5 Pulmonary insufficiency following trauma and surgery
Adult respiratory distress syndrome
Pulmonary insufficiency following:
shock
surgery
trauma
Shock lung

[Excludes:] *adult respiratory distress syndrome associated with other conditions (518.82)*
pneumonia:
aspiration (507.0)
hypostatic (514)
respiratory failure in other conditions (518.81, 518.83-518.84)

518.6 Allergic bronchopulmonary aspergillosis

⑤ **518.8 Other diseases of lung**

518.81 Acute respiratory failure
Respiratory failure NOS

[Excludes:] *acute and chronic respiratory failure (518.84)*
acute respiratory distress (518.82)
chronic respiratory failure (518.83)
respiratory arrest (799.1)
respiratory failure, newborn (770.84)

518.82 Other pulmonary insufficiency, not elsewhere classified
Acute respiratory distress
Acute respiratory insufficiency
Adult respiratory distress syndrome NEC

[Excludes:] *adult respiratory distress syndrome associated with trauma and surgery (518.5)*
pulmonary insufficiency following trauma and surgery (518.5)
respiratory distress:
NOS (786.09)
newborn (770.89)
syndrome, newborn (769)
shock lung (518.5)

518.83 Chronic respiratory failure

518.84 Acute and chronic respiratory failure
Acute or chronic respiratory failure

518.89 Other diseases of lung, not elsewhere classified
Broncholithiasis
Calcification of lung
Lung disease NOS
Pulmolithiasis

519 Other diseases of respiratory system

⑤ **519.0 Tracheostomy complications**

519.00 Tracheostomy complication, unspecified

519.01 Infection of tracheostomy
Use additional code to identify type of infection, such as:
abscess or cellulitis of neck (682.1)
septicemia (038.0-038.9)
Use additional code to identify organism (041.00-041.9)

519.02 Mechanical complication of tracheostomy
Tracheal stenosis due to tracheostomy

● Code new to this edition
▲ Revision of existing code
④ ⑤ Fourth or fifth digit required

519.09 **Other tracheostomy complications**
Hemorrhage due to tracheostomy
Tracheoesophageal fistula due to tracheostomy

519.1 **Other diseases of trachea and bronchus, not elsewhere classified**
Calcification of bronchus or trachea
Stenosis of bronchus or trachea
Ulcer of bronchus or trachea

519.2 **Mediastinitis**

519.3 **Other diseases of mediastinum, not elsewhere classified**
Fibrosis of mediastinum
Hernia of mediastinum
Retraction of mediastinum

519.4 **Disorders of diaphragm**
Diaphragmitis
Paralysis of diaphragm
Relaxation of diaphragm

Excludes: *congenital defect of diaphragm (756.6)*
diaphragmatic hernia (551-553 with .3)
congenital (756.6)

519.8 **Other diseases of respiratory system, not elsewhere classified**

519.9 **Unspecified disease of respiratory system**
Respiratory disease (chronic) NOS

Add 4th or
5th digit
Nonspecific
code
Unspecified
code
Manifestation
code

● Code new
to this edition

▲ Revision of
existing code

④ ⑤ Fourth or fifth
digit required

9. DISEASES OF THE DIGESTIVE SYSTEM (520-579)

DISEASES OF ORAL CAVITY, SALIVARY GLANDS, AND JAWS (520-529)

`520` **Disorders of tooth development and eruption**

520.0 Anodontia
Absence of teeth (complete) (congenital) (partial)
Hypodontia
Oligodontia

Excludes: *acquired absence of teeth (525.10-525.19)*

520.1 Supernumerary teeth
Distomolar
Fourth molar
Mesiodens
Paramolar
Supplemental teeth

Excludes: *supernumerary roots (520.2)*

520.2 Abnormalities of size and form
Concrescence of teeth
Fusion of teeth
Gemination of teeth
Dens evaginatus of teeth
Dens in dente of teeth
Dens invaginatus of teeth
Enamel pearls of teeth
Macrodontia
Microdontia
Peg-shaped [conical] teeth
Supernumerary roots
Taurodontism
Tuberculum paramolare

Excludes: *that due to congenital syphilis (090.5)*
tuberculum Carabelli, which is regarded as a normal variation

520.3 Mottled teeth
Dental fluorosis
Mottling of enamel
Nonfluoride enamel opacities

520.4 Disturbances of tooth formation
Aplasia and hypoplasia of cementum
Dilaceration of tooth
Enamel hypoplasia (neonatal) (postnatal) (prenatal)
Horner's teeth
Hypocalcification of teeth
Regional odontodysplasia
Turner's tooth

Excludes: *Hutchinson's teeth and mulberry molars in congenital syphilis (090.5)*
mottled teeth (520.3)

520.5 Hereditary disturbances in tooth structure, not elsewhere classified
Amelogenesis imperfecta
Dentinogenesis imperfecta
Odontogenesis imperfecta
Dentinal dysplasia
Shell teeth

520.6 Disturbances of tooth eruption
Teeth:
  embedded
  impacted
  natal
  neonatal
  primary [deciduous]:
    persistent
    shedding, premature
Tooth eruption:
  late
  obstructed
  premature

Excludes: *exfoliation of teeth (attributable to disease of surrounding tissues) (525.0-525.19)*
impacted or embedded teeth with abnormal position of such teeth or adjacent teeth (524.3)

520.7 Teething syndrome

`520.8` **Other specified disorders of tooth development and eruption**
Color changes during tooth formation
Pre-eruptive color changes

Excludes: *posteruptive color changes (521.7)*

`520.9` **Unspecified disorder of tooth development and eruption**

Add 4th or 5th digit

Nonspecific code

Unspecified code

Manifestation code

521 Diseases of hard tissues of teeth

⑤ **521.0 Dental caries**

521.00 Dental caries, unspecified

521.01 Dental caries limited to enamel
Initial caries
White spot lesion

521.02 Dental caries extending into dentine

521.03 Dental caries extending into pulp

521.04 Arrested dental caries

521.05 Odontoclasia
Infantile melanodontia
Melanodontoclasia

[*Excludes:*] *internal and external resorption of teeth (521.4)*

521.09 Other dental caries

521.1 Excessive attrition
Approximal wear
Occlusal wear

521.2 Abrasion
Abrasion:
dentifrice of teeth
habitual of teeth
occupational of teeth
ritual of teeth
traditional of teeth
Wedge defect NOS of teeth

521.3 Erosion
Erosion of teeth:
NOS
due to:
medicine
persistent vomiting
Erosion of teeth:
idiopathic
occupational

521.4 Pathological resorption
Internal granuloma of pulp
Resorption of tooth or root (external) (internal)

521.5 Hypercementosis
Cementation hyperplasia

521.6 Ankylosis of teeth

521.7 Posteruptive color changes
Staining [discoloration] of teeth:
NOS
due to:
drugs
metals
pulpal bleeding

[*Excludes:*] *accretions [deposits] on teeth (523.6)*
pre-eruptive color changes (520.8)

521.8 Other specified diseases of hard tissues of teeth
Irradiated enamel
Sensitive dentin

521.9 Unspecified disease of hard tissues of teeth

522 Diseases of pulp and periapical tissues

522.0 Pulpitis
Pulpal:
abscess
polyp
Pulpitis:
acute
chronic (hyperplastic) (ulcerative)
suppurative

522.1 Necrosis of the pulp
Pulp gangrene

522.2 Pulp degeneration
Denticles   Pulp stones
  Pulp calcifications

522.3 Abnormal hard tissue formation in pulp
Secondary or irregular dentin

522.4 Acute apical periodontitis of pulpal origin

522.5 Periapical abscess without sinus
Abscess:
  dental
  dentoalveolar

> *Excludes:* *periapical abscess with sinus (522.7)*

522.6 Chronic apical periodontitis
Apical or periapical granuloma
Apical periodontitis NOS

522.7 Periapical abscess with sinus
Fistula:
  alveolar process
  dental

522.8 Radicular cyst
Cyst:
  apical (periodontal)
  periapical
  radiculodental
  residual radicular

> *Excludes:* *lateral developmental or lateral periodontal cyst (526.0)*

522.9 **Other and unspecified diseases of pulp and periapical tissues**

523 **Gingival and periodontal diseases**

523.0 Acute gingivitis

> *Excludes:* *acute necrotizing ulcerative gingivitis (101)*
> *herpetic gingivostomatitis (054.2)*

523.1 Chronic gingivitis
Gingivitis (chronic):   Gingivitis (chronic):
  NOS   simple marginal
  desquamative   ulcerative
  hyperplastic   Gingivostomatitis

> *Excludes:* *herpetic gingivostomatitis (054.2)*

523.2 Gingival recession
Gingival recession (generalized) (localized) (postinfective) (postoperative)

523.3 Acute periodontitis
Acute: Paradontal abscess
  pericementitis   Periodontal abscess
  pericoronitis

> *Excludes:* *acute apical periodontitis (522.4)*
> *periapical abscess (522.5, 522.7)*

523.4 Chronic periodontitis
Alveolar pyorrhea   Periodontitis:
Chronic pericoronitis   NOS
Pericementitis (chronic)   complex
                               simplex

> *Excludes:* *chronic apical periodontitis (522.6)*

523.5 Periodontosis

523.6 Accretions on teeth
Dental calculus: Deposits on teeth:
  subgingival   betel
  supragingival   materia alba
                               soft
                               tartar
                               tobacco

Add 4th or   Nonspecific   Unspecified   Manifestation
5th digit   code   code   code

523.8 Other specified periodontal diseases

Giant cell:
- epulis
- peripheral granuloma

Gingival:
- cysts
- enlargement NOS
- fibromatosis

Gingival polyp
Periodontal lesions due to traumatic occlusion
Peripheral giant cell granuloma

[Excludes:] *leukoplakia of gingiva (528.6)*

523.9 Unspecified gingival and periodontal disease

524 Dentofacial anomalies, including malocclusion

[5] **524.0 Major anomalies of jaw size**

[Excludes:] *hemifacial atrophy or hypertrophy (754.0)*
unilateral condylar hyperplasia or hypoplasia of mandible (526.89)

524.00 Unspecified anomaly

524.01 Maxillary hyperplasia

524.02 Mandibular hyperplasia

524.03 Maxillary hypoplasia

524.04 Mandibular hypoplasia

524.05 Macrogenia

524.06 Microgenia

524.09 Other specified anomaly

[5] **524.1 Anomalies of relationship of jaw to cranial base**

524.10 Unspecified anomaly
prognathism
retrognathism

524.11 Maxillary asymmetry

524.12 Other jaw asymmetry

524.19 Other specified anomaly

524.2 Anomalies of dental arch relationship

Crossbite (anterior) (posterior)
Disto-occlusion
Mesio-occlusion
Midline deviation
Open bite (anterior) (posterior)
Overbite (excessive)
- deep
- horizontal
- vertical

Overjet
Posterior lingual occlusion of mandibular teeth
Soft tissue impingement

[Excludes:] *hemifacial atrophy or hypertrophy (754.0)*
unilateral condylar hyperplasia or hypoplasia of mandible (526.89)

524.3 Anomalies of tooth position

Crowding of tooth, teeth
Diastema of tooth, teeth
Displacement of tooth, teeth
Rotation of tooth, teeth
Spacing, abnormal of tooth, teeth
Transposition of tooth, teeth
Impacted or embedded teeth with abnormal position of such teeth or adjacent teeth

524.4 Malocclusion, unspecified

524.5 Dentofacial functional abnormalities

Abnormal jaw closure
Malocclusion due to:
- abnormal swallowing
- mouth breathing
- tongue, lip, or finger habits

[5] **524.6 Temporomandibular joint disorders**

[Excludes:] *current temporomandibular joint:*
- *dislocation (830.0-830.1)*
- *strain (848.1)*

524.60 Temporomandibular joint disorders, unspecified
Temporomandibular joint-pain-dysfunction syndrome [TMJ]

524.61 **Adhesions and ankylosis (bony or fibrous)**

524.62 **Arthralgia of temporomandibular joint**

524.63 **Articular disc disorder (reducing or non-reducing)**

524.69 **Other specified temporomandibular joint disorders**

[5] 524.7 **Dental alveolar anomalies**

524.70 **Unspecified alveolar anomaly**

524.71 **Alveolar maxillary hyperplasia**

524.72 **Alveolar mandibular hyperplasia**

524.73 **Alveolar maxillary hypoplasia**

524.74 **Alveolar mandibular hypoplasia**

524.79 **Other specified alveolar anomaly**

524.8 **Other specified dentofacial anomalies**

524.9 **Unspecified dentofacial anomalies**

525 **Other diseases and conditions of the teeth and supporting structures**

525.0 **Exfoliation of teeth due to systemic causes**

[5] 525.1 **Loss of teeth due to trauma, extraction, or periodontal disease**

525.10 **Acquired absence of teeth, unspecified**
Edentulism
Tooth extraction status, NOS

525.11 **Loss of teeth due to trauma**

525.12 **Loss of teeth due to periodontal disease**

525.13 **Loss of teeth due to caries**

525.19 **Other loss of teeth**

525.2 **Atrophy of edentulous alveolar ridge**

525.3 **Retained dental root**

525.8 **Other specified disorders of the teeth and supporting structures**
Enlargement of alveolar ridge NOS
Irregular alveolar process

525.9 **Unspecified disorder of the teeth and supporting structures**

526 **Diseases of the jaws**

526.0 **Developmental odontogenic cysts**
Cyst:
dentigerous
eruption
follicular
lateral developmental
Cyst:
lateral periodontal
primordial
Keratocyst

[Excludes:] *radicular cyst (522.8)*

526.1 **Fissural cysts of jaw**
Cyst:
globulomaxillary
incisor canal
median anterior maxillary
median palatal
nasopalatine
palatine of papilla

[Excludes:] *cysts of oral soft tissues (528.4)*

526.2 **Other cysts of jaws**
Cyst of jaw:
NOS
aneurysmal
Cyst of jaw:
hemorrhagic
traumatic

526.3 **Central giant cell (reparative) granuloma**

[Excludes:] *peripheral giant cell granuloma (523.8)*

Add 4th or 5th digit | Nonspecific code | Unspecified code | Manifestation code

526.4 Inflammatory conditions
Abscess
Osteitis
Osteomyelitis (neonatal) } of jaw (acute) (chronic) (suppurative)
Periostitis
Sequestrum of jaw bone

Excludes: alveolar osteitis (526.5)

526.5 Alveolitis of jaw
Alveolar osteitis
Dry socket

⑤ **526.8 Other specified diseases of the jaws**

526.81 Exostosis of jaw
Torus mandibularis
Torus palatinus

526.89 Other
Cherubism
Fibrous dysplasia } of jaw(s)
Latent bone cyst
Osteoradionecrosis of jaw(s)
Unilateral condylar hyperplasia or hypoplasia of mandible

526.9 Unspecified disease of the jaws

527 Diseases of the salivary glands

527.0 Atrophy

527.1 Hypertrophy

527.2 Sialoadenitis
Parotitis: Sialoangitis
  NOS   Sialodochitis
  allergic
  toxic

Excludes: epidemic or infectious parotitis (072.0-072.9)
            uveoparotid fever (135)

527.3 Abscess

527.4 Fistula

Excludes: congenital fistula of salivary glands (750.24)

527.5 Sialolithiasis
Calculus
Stone } of salivary gland or duct
Sialodocholithiasis

527.6 Mucocele
Mucous:
  extravasation cyst of salivary gland
  retention cyst of salivary gland
  Ranula

527.7 Disturbance of salivary secretion
Hyposecretion   Sialorrhea
Ptyalism   Xerostomia

527.8 Other specified diseases of the salivary glands
Benign lymphoepithelial lesion of salivary gland
Sialectasia
Sialosis
Stenosis
Stricture } of salivary duct

527.9 Unspecified disease of the salivary glands

● Code new   ▲ Revision of   ④ ⑤ Fourth or fifth
  to this edition   existing code   digit required

528 Diseases of the oral soft tissues, excluding lesions specific for gingiva and tongue

528.0 Stomatitis

Stomatitis:
NOS
ulcerative

Vesicular stomatitis

Excludes: *stomatitis:*

acute necrotizing ulcerative (101)
aphthous (528.2)
gangrenous (528.1)
herpetic (054.2)
Vincent's (101)

528.1 Cancrum oris

Gangrenous stomatitis

Noma

528.2 Oral aphthae

Aphthous stomatitis
Canker sore
Periadenitis mucosa necrotica recurrens

Recurrent aphthous ulcer
Stomatitis herpetiformis

Excludes: *herpetic stomatitis (054.2)*

528.3 Cellulitis and abscess

Cellulitis of mouth (floor)
Ludwig's angina
Oral fistula

Excludes: *abscess of tongue (529.0)*

cellulitis or abscess of lip (528.5)
fistula (of):
dental (522.7)
lip (528.5)
gingivitis (523.0-523.1)

528.4 Cysts

Dermoid cyst of mouth
Epidermoid cyst of mouth
Epstein's pearl of mouth
Lymphoepithelial cyst of mouth
Nasoalveolar cyst of mouth
Nasolabial cyst of mouth

Excludes: *cyst:*

gingiva (523.8)
tongue (529.8)

528.5 Diseases of lips

Abscess of lip(s)
Cellulitis of lip(s)
Fistula of lip(s)
Hypertrophy of lip(s)

Cheilitis:
NOS
angular
Cheilodynia
Cheilosis

Excludes: *actinic cheilitis (692.79)*

congenital fistula of lip (750.25)
leukoplakia of lips (528.6)

528.6 Leukoplakia of oral mucosa, including tongue

Leukokeratosis of oral mucosa
Leukoplakia of:
gingiva
lips
tongue

Excludes: *carcinoma in situ (230.0, 232.0)*

leukokeratosis nicotina palati (528.7)

528.7 Other disturbances of oral epithelium, including tongue

Erythroplakia of mouth or tongue
Focal epithelial hyperplasia of mouth or tongue
Leukoedema of mouth or tongue
Leukokeratosis nicotina palati of mouth or tongue

Excludes: *carcinoma in situ (230.0, 232.0)*

leukokeratosis NOS (702)

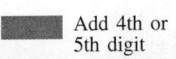

| Add 4th or 5th digit | Nonspecific code | Unspecified code | Manifestation code |

528.8 Oral submucosal fibrosis, including of tongue

528.9 Other and unspecified diseases of the oral soft tissues
Cheek and lip biting
Denture sore mouth
Denture stomatitis
Melanoplakia
Papillary hyperplasia of palate
Eosinophilic granuloma of oral mucosa
Irritative hyperplasia of oral mucosa
Pyogenic granuloma of oral mucosa
Ulcer (traumatic) of oral mucosa

529 Diseases and other conditions of the tongue

529.0 Glossitis
Abscess of tongue
Ulceration (traumatic) of tongue

Excludes: glossitis:
  benign migratory (529.1)
  Hunter's (529.4)
  median rhomboid (529.2)
  Moeller's (529.4)

529.1 Geographic tongue
Benign migratory glossitis
Glossitis areata exfoliativa

529.2 Median rhomboid glossitis

529.3 Hypertrophy of tongue papillae
Black hairy tongue
Coated tongue
Hypertrophy of foliate papillae
Lingua villosa nigra

529.4 Atrophy of tongue papillae
Bald tongue
Glazed tongue
Glossitis:
  Hunter's
  Moeller's

Glossodynia exfoliativa
Smooth atrophic tongue

529.5 Plicated tongue
Fissured tongue
Furrowed tongue
Scrotal tongue

Excludes: fissure of tongue, congenital (750.13)

529.6 Glossodynia
Glossopyrosis   Painful tongue

Excludes: glossodynia exfoliativa (529.4)

529.8 Other specified conditions of the tongue
Atrophy (of) tongue
Crenated (of) tongue
Enlargement (of) tongue
Hypertrophy (of) tongue
Glossocele (of) tongue
Glossoptosis (of) tongue

Excludes: erythroplasia of tongue (528.7)
  leukoplakia of tongue (528.6)
  macroglossia (congenital) (750.15)
  microglossia (congenital) (750.16)
  oral submucosal fibrosis (528.8)

529.9 Unspecified condition of the tongue

DISEASES OF ESOPHAGUS, STOMACH, AND DUODENUM (530-537)

530 Diseases of esophagus

Excludes: esophageal varices (456.0-456.2)

● Code new
to this edition

▲ Revision of
existing code

④ ⑤ Fourth or fifth
digit required

530.0 Achalasia and cardiospasm
Achalasia (of cardia)
Aperistalsis of esophagus
Megaesophagus
Excludes: *congenital cardiospasm (750.7)*

[5] **530.1 Esophagitis**
Abscess of esophagus
Esophagitis:
NOS
chemical
peptic
Esophagitis:
postoperative
regurgitant

Use additional E code, if desired, to identify cause, if induced by chemical
Excludes: *tuberculous esophagitis (017.8)*

530.10 Esophagitis, unspecified

530.11 Reflux esophagitis

530.12 Acute esophagitis

530.19 Other esophagitis

530.2 Ulcer of esophagus
Ulcer of esophagus
fungal
peptic
Ulcer of esophagus due to ingestion of:
aspirin
chemicals
medicines

Use additional E code, if desired, to identify cause, if induced by chemical or drug

530.3 Stricture and stenosis of esophagus
Compression of esophagus
Obstruction of esophagus
Excludes: *congenital stricture of esophagus (750.3)*

530.4 Perforation of esophagus
Rupture of esophagus
Excludes: *traumatic perforation of esophagus (862.22, 862.32, 874.4-874.5)*

530.5 Dyskinesia of esophagus
Corkscrew esophagus
Curling esophagus
Esophagospasm
Spasm of esophagus
Excludes: *cardiospasm (530.0)*

530.6 Diverticulum of esophagus, acquired
Diverticulum, acquired:
epiphrenic
pharyngoesophageal
pulsion
subdiaphragmatic
traction
Zenker's (hypopharyngeal)
Esophageal pouch, acquired
Esophagocele, acquired
Excludes: *congenital diverticulum of esophagus (750.4)*

530.7 Gastroesophageal laceration-hemorrhage syndrome
Mallory-Weiss syndrome

[5] **530.8 Other specified disorders of esophagus**

530.81 Esophageal reflux
Gastroesophageal reflux
Excludes: *reflux esophagitis (530.11)*

530.82 Esophageal hemorrhage
Excludes: *hemorrhage due to esophageal varices (456.0-456.2)*

530.83 Esophageal leukoplakia

530.84 Tracheoesophageal fistula
Excludes: *congenital tracheoesophageal fistula (750.3)*

530.89 Other
Excludes: *Paterson-Kelly syndrome (280.8)*

530.9 Unspecified disorder of esophagus

[5] **531 Gastric ulcer**

Includes: ulcer (peptic):
  prepyloric
  pylorus
  stomach

Use additional E code, if desired, to identify drug, if drug-induced

[Excludes:] *peptic ulcer NOS (533.0-533.9)*

The following fifth-digit subclassification is for use with category 531:

0 without mention of obstruction

1 with obstruction

[5] **531.0 Acute with hemorrhage**

[5] **531.1 Acute with perforation**

[5] **531.2 Acute with hemorrhage and perforation**

[5] **531.3 Acute without mention of hemorrhage or perforation**

[5] **531.4 Chronic or unspecified with hemorrhage**

[5] **531.5 Chronic or unspecified with perforation**

[5] **531.6 Chronic or unspecified with hemorrhage and perforation**

[5] **531.7 Chronic without mention of hemorrhage or perforation**

[5] **531.9 Unspecified as acute or chronic, without mention of hemorrhage or perforation**

[5] **532 Duodenal ulcer**

Includes: erosion (acute) of duodenum
  ulcer (peptic):
    duodenum
    postpyloric

Use additional E code, if desired, to identify drug, if drug-induced

[Excludes:] *peptic ulcer NOS (533.0-533.9)*

The following fifth-digit subclassification is for use with category 532:

0 without mention of obstruction

1 with obstruction

[5] **532.0 Acute with hemorrhage**

[5] **532.1 Acute with perforation**

[5] **532.2 Acute with hemorrhage and perforation**

[5] **532.3 Acute without mention of hemorrhage or perforation**

[5] **532.4 Chronic or unspecified with hemorrhage**

[5] **532.5 Chronic or unspecified with perforation**

[5] **532.6 Chronic or unspecified with hemorrhage and perforation**

[5] **532.7 Chronic without mention of hemorrhage or perforation**

[5] **532.9 Unspecified as acute or chronic, without mention of hemorrhage or perforation**

[5] **533 Peptic ulcer, site unspecified**

Includes: gastroduodenal ulcer NOS
  peptic ulcer NOS
  stress ulcer NOS

Use additional E code, if desired, to identify drug, if drug-induced

[Excludes:] *peptic ulcer:*
  duodenal (532.0-532.9)
  gastric (531.0-531.9)

The following fifth-digit subclassification is for use with category 533:

0 without mention of obstruction

1 with obstruction

[5] **533.0 Acute with hemorrhage**

[5] **533.1 Acute with perforation**

[5] **533.2 Acute with hemorrhage and perforation**

[5] **533.3 Acute without mention of hemorrhage and perforation**

[5] **533.4 Chronic or unspecified with hemorrhage**

[5] **533.5 Chronic or unspecified with perforation**

[5] **533.6 Chronic or unspecified with hemorrhage and perforation**

[5] **533.7 Chronic without mention of hemorrhage or perforation**

[5] **533.9 Unspecified as acute or chronic, without mention of hemorrhage or perforation**

[5] **534 Gastrojejunal ulcer**

Includes: ulcer (peptic) or erosion:
- anastomotic
- gastrocolic
- gastrointestinal
- gastrojejunal
- jejunal
- marginal
- stomal

[Excludes:] *primary ulcer of small intestine (569.82)*

The following fifth-digit subclassification is for use with category 534:

0 without mention of obstruction

1 with obstruction

[5] **534.0 Acute with hemorrhage**

[5] **534.1 Acute with perforation**

[5] **534.2 Acute with hemorrhage and perforation**

[5] **534.3 Acute without mention of hemorrhage or perforation**

[5] **534.4 Chronic or unspecified with hemorrhage**

[5] **534.5 Chronic or unspecified with perforation**

[5] **534.6 Chronic or unspecified with hemorrhage and perforation**

[5] **534.7 Chronic without mention of hemorrhage or perforation**

[5] **534.9 Unspecified as acute or chronic, without mention of hemorrhage or perforation**

[5] **535 Gastritis and duodenitis**

The following fifth-digit subclassification is for use with category 535

0 without mention of hemorrhage

1 with hemorrhage

[5] **535.0 Acute gastritis**

[5] **535.1 Atrophic gastritis**

Gastritis:
- atrophic-hyperplastic
- chronic (atrophic)

[5] **535.2 Gastric mucosal hypertrophy**

Hypertrophic gastritis

[5] **535.3 Alcoholic gastritis**

[5] **535.4 Other specified gastritis**

Gastritis:
- allergic
- bile induced
- irritant

Gastritis:
- superficial
- toxic

[5] **535.5 Unspecified gastritis and gastroduodenitis**

[5] **535.6 Duodenitis**

536 Disorders of function of stomach

[Excludes:] *functional disorders of stomach specified as psychogenic (306.4)*

536.0 Achlorhydria

536.1 Acute dilatation of stomach

Acute distention of stomach

536.2 Persistent vomiting

Habit vomiting
Persistent vomiting [not of pregnancy]
Uncontrollable vomiting

[Excludes:] *excessive vomiting in pregnancy (643.0-643.9)*
vomiting NOS (787.0)

536.3 Gastroparesis

[5] **536.4 Gastrostomy complications**

536.40 Gastrostomy complications, unspecified

536.41 Infection of gastrostomy
Use additional code to specify type of infection, such as:
abscess or cellulitis of abdomen (682.2)
septicemia (038.0-038.9)
Use additional code to identify organism (041.00-041.9)

536.42 Mechanical complication of gastrostomy

536.49 Other gastrostomy complications

536.8 Dyspepsia and other specified disorders of function of stomach
Achylia gastrica
Hourglass contraction of stomach
Hyperacidity
Hyperchlorhydria
Hypochlorhydria
Indigestion

[Excludes:] *achlorhydria (536.0)*
heartburn (787.1)

536.9 Unspecified functional disorder of stomach
Functional gastrointestinal:
disorder
disturbance
irritation

537 Other disorders of stomach and duodenum

537.0 Acquired hypertrophic pyloric stenosis
Constriction of pylorus, acquired or adult
Obstruction of pylorus, acquired or adult
Stricture of pylorus, acquired or adult

[Excludes:] *congenital or infantile pyloric stenosis (750.5)*

537.1 Gastric diverticulum

[Excludes:] *congenital diverticulum of stomach (750.7)*

537.2 Chronic duodenal ileus

537.3 Other obstruction of duodenum
Cicatrix of duodenum
Stenosis of duodenum
Stricture of duodenum
Volvulus of duodenum

[Excludes:] *congenital obstruction of duodenum (751.1)*

537.4 Fistula of stomach or duodenum
Gastrocolic fistula
Gastrojejunocolic fistula

537.5 Gastroptosis

537.6 Hourglass stricture or stenosis of stomach
Cascade stomach

[Excludes:] *congenital hourglass stomach (750.7)*
hourglass contraction of stomach (536.8)

[5] **537.8 Other specified disorders of stomach and duodenum**

537.81 Pylorospasm

[Excludes:] *congenital pylorospasm (750.5)*

537.82 Angiodysplasia of stomach and duodenum without mention of hemorrhage

537.83 Angiodysplasia of stomach and duodenum with hemorrhage

● **537.84 Dieulafoy lesion (hemorrhagic) of stomach and duodenum**

537.89 Other
Gastric or duodenal:
prolapse
rupture
Intestinal metaplasia of gastric mucosa
Passive congestion of stomach

[Excludes:] *diverticula of duodenum (562.00-562.01)*
gastrointestinal hemorrhage (578.0-578.9)

537.9 Unspecified disorder of stomach and duodenum

● Code new to this edition ▲ Revision of existing code [4] [5] Fourth or fifth digit required

APPENDICITIS (540-543)

540 Acute appendicitis

540.0 With generalized peritonitis
Appendicitis (acute):
fulminating with: perforation peritonitis (generalized) rupture
gangrenous with: perforation peritonitis (generalized) rupture
obstructive with: perforation peritonitis (generalized) rupture
Cecitis (acute) with: perforation peritonitis (generalized) rupture
Rupture of appendix with: perforation peritonitis (generalized) rupture

[*Excludes:*] *acute appendicitis with peritoneal abscess (540.1)*

540.1 With peritoneal abscess
Abscess of appendix
With generalized peritonitis

540.9 Without mention of peritonitis
Acute:
appendicitis:
fulminating without mention of perforation, peritonitis, or rupture
gangrenous without mention of perforation, peritonitis, or rupture
inflamed without mention of perforation, peritonitis, or rupture
obstructive without mention of perforation, peritonitis, or rupture
cecitis without mention of perforation, peritonitis, or rupture

541 Appendicitis, unqualified

542 Other appendicitis
Appendicitis:
chronic
recurrent
Appendicitis:
relapsing
subacute

[*Excludes:*] *hyperplasia (lymphoid) of appendix (543.0)*

543 Other diseases of appendix

543.0 Hyperplasia of appendix (lymphoid)

543.9 Other and unspecified diseases of appendix
Appendicular or appendiceal:
colic
concretion
fistula
Diverticulum of appendix
Fecalith of appendix
Intussusception of appendix
Mucocele of appendix
Stercolith of appendix

HERNIA OF ABDOMINAL CAVITY (550-553)

Includes: hernia:
acquired
congenital, except diaphragmatic or hiatal

[5] **550 Inguinal hernia**
Includes: bubonocele
inguinal hernia (direct) (double) (indirect) (oblique) (sliding)
scrotal hernia

The following fifth-digit subclassification is for use with category 550:

0 unilateral or unspecified (not specified as recurrent)
Unilateral NOS

1 unilateral or unspecified, recurrent

2 bilateral (not specified as recurrent)
Bilateral NOS

3 bilateral, recurrent

[5] **550.0 Inguinal hernia, with gangrene**
Inguinal hernia with gangrene (and obstruction)

[5] **550.1 Inguinal hernia, with obstruction, without mention of gangrene**
Inguinal hernia with mention of incarceration, irreducibility, or strangulation

[5] **550.9 Inguinal hernia, without mention of obstruction or gangrene**
Inguinal hernia NOS

551 Other hernia of abdominal cavity, with gangrene
Includes: that with gangrene (and obstruction)

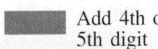

[5] **551.0 Femoral hernia with gangrene**

551.00 Unilateral or unspecified (not specified as recurrent)
Femoral hernia NOS with gangrene

551.01 Unilateral or unspecified, recurrent

551.02 Bilateral (not specified as recurrent)

551.03 Bilateral, recurrent

551.1 Umbilical hernia with gangrene
Parumbilical hernia specified as gangrenous

[5] **551.2 Ventral hernia with gangrene**

551.20 Ventral, unspecified, with gangrene

551.21 Incisional, with gangrene
Postoperative hernia, specified as gangrenous
Recurrent ventral hernia, specified as gangrenous

551.29 Other
Epigastric hernia specified as gangrenous

551.3 Diaphragmatic hernia with gangrene
Hiatal hernia (esophageal) (sliding), specified as gangrenous
Paraesophageal hernia, specified as gangrenous
Thoracic stomach, specified as gangrenous

[*Excludes:*] *congenital diaphragmatic hernia (756.6)*

551.8 Hernia of other specified sites, with gangrene
Any condition classifiable to 553.8 if specified as gangrenous

551.9 Hernia of unspecified site, with gangrene
Any condition classifiable to 553.9 if specified as gangrenous

552 Other hernia of abdominal cavity, with obstruction, but without mention of gangrene

[*Excludes:*] *that with mention of gangrene (551.0-551.9)*

[5] **552.0 Femoral hernia with obstruction**
Femoral hernia specified as incarcerated, irreducible, strangulated, or causing obstruction

552.00 Unilateral or unspecified (not specified as recurrent)

552.01 Unilateral or unspecified, recurrent

552.02 Bilateral (not specified as recurrent)

552.03 Bilateral, recurrent

552.1 Umbilical hernia with obstruction
Parumbilical hernia specified as incarcerated, irreducible, strangulated, or causing obstruction

[5] **552.2 Ventral hernia with obstruction**
Ventral hernia specified as incarcerated, irreducible, strangulated, or causing obstruction

552.20 Ventral, unspecified, with obstruction

552.21 Incisional, with obstruction
Postoperative hernia, specified as incarcerated, irreducible, strangulated, or causing obstruction
Recurrent ventral hernia, specified as incarcerated, irreducible, strangulated, or causing obstruction

552.29 Other
Epigastric hernia specified as incarcerated, irreducible, strangulated, or causing obstruction

552.3 Diaphragmatic hernia with obstruction
Hiatal hernia (esophageal) (sliding), specified as incarcerated, irreducible, strangulated, or causing obstruction
Paraesophageal hernia, specified as incarcerated, irreducible, strangulated, or causing obstruction
Thoracic stomach, specified as incarcerated, irreducible, strangulated, or causing obstruction

[*Excludes:*] *congenital diaphragmatic hernia (756.6)*

552.8 Hernia of other specified sites, with obstruction
Any condition classifiable to 553.8 if specified as incarcerated, irreducible, strangulated, or causing obstruction

552.9 Hernia of unspecified site, with obstruction
Any condition classifiable to 553.9 if specified as incarcerated, irreducible, strangulated, or causing obstruction

553 Other hernia of abdominal cavity without mention of obstruction or gangrene

[*Excludes:*] *the listed conditions with mention of:*
gangrene (and obstruction) (551.0-551.9)
obstruction (552.0-552.9)

[5] **553.0 Femoral hernia**

553.00 Unilateral or unspecified (not specified as recurrent)
Femoral hernia NOS

553.01 Unilateral or unspecified, recurrent

553.02 Bilateral (not specified as recurrent)

553.03 Bilateral, recurrent

553.1 Umbilical hernia
Parumbilical hernia

[5] **553.2 Ventral hernia**

553.20 Ventral, unspecified

553.21 Incisional
Hernia:
postoperative
recurrent, ventral

553.29 Other
Hernia:
epigastric
spigelian

553.3 Diaphragmatic hernia
Hernia:
hiatal (esophageal) (sliding)
paraesophageal
Thoracic stomach

[*Excludes:*] *congenital:*
diaphragmatic hernia (756.6)
hiatal hernia (750.6)
esophagocele (530.6)

553.8 Hernia of other specified sites
Hernia:
ischiatic
ischiorectal
lumbar
obturator
pudendal
Hernia:
retroperitoneal
sciatic
Other abdominal hernia of specified site

[*Excludes:*] *vaginal enterocele (618.6)*

553.9 Hernia of unspecified site
Enterocele
Epiplocele
Hernia:
NOS
interstitial
Hernia:
intestinal
intra-abdominal
Rupture (nontraumatic)
Sarcoepiplocele

NONINFECTIOUS ENTERITIS AND COLITIS (555-558)

555 Regional enteritis
Includes: Crohn's disease
Granulomatous enteritis

[*Excludes:*] *ulcerative colitis (556)*

555.0 Small intestine
Ileitis:
regional
segmental
terminal
Regional enteritis or Crohn's disease of:
duodenum
ileum
jejunum

555.1 Large intestine
Colitis:
granulomatous
regional
transmural
Regional enteritis or Crohn's disease of:
colon
large bowel
rectum

555.2 Small intestine with large intestine
Regional ileocolitis

555.9 Unspecified site
Crohn's disease NOS
Regional enteritis NOS

556 Ulcerative colitis

556.0 Ulcerative (chronic) enterocolitis

556.1 Ulcerative (chronic) ileocolitis

556.2 Ulcerative (chronic) proctitis

556.3 Ulcerative (chronic) proctosigmoiditis

556.4 Pseudopolyposis of colon

556.5 Left-sided ulcerative (chronic) colitis

556.6 Universal ulcerative (chronic) colitis
Pancolitis

556.8 Other ulcerative colitis

556.9 Ulcerative colitis, unspecified
Ulcerative enteritis NOS

557 Vascular insufficiency of intestine

> Excludes: *necrotizing enterocolitis of the newborn (777.5)*

557.0 Acute vascular insufficiency of intestine
Acute:
  hemorrhagic enterocolitis
  ischemic colitis, enteritis, or enterocolitis
  massive necrosis of intestine
Bowel infarction
Embolism of mesenteric artery
Fulminant enterocolitis
Hemorrhagic necrosis of intestine
Infarction of appendices epiploicae
Intestinal gangrene
Intestinal infarction (acute) (agnogenic) (hemorrhagic) (nonocclusive)
Mesenteric infarction (embolic) (thrombotic)
Necrosis of intestine
Terminal hemorrhagic enteropathy
Thrombosis of mesenteric artery

557.1 Chronic vascular insufficiency of intestine
Angina, abdominal
Chronic ischemic colitis, enteritis, or enterocolitis
Ischemic stricture of intestine
Mesenteric:
  angina
  artery syndrome (superior)
  vascular insufficiency

557.9 Unspecified vascular insufficiency of intestine
Alimentary pain due to vascular insufficiency
Ischemic colitis, enteritis, or enterocolitis NOS

558 Other and unspecified noninfectious gastroenteritis and colitis

> Excludes: *infectious:*
>   *colitis, enteritis, or gastroenteritis (009.0-009.1)*
>   *diarrhea (009.2-009.3)*

558.1 Gastroenteritis and colitis due to radiation
Radiation enterocolitis

558.2 Toxic gastroenteritis and colitis
Use additional E code, if desired, to identify cause

558.3 Allergic gastroenteritis and colitis

558.9 Other and unspecified noninfectious gastroenteritis and colitis
Colitis NOS, dietetic, or noninfectious
Enteritis NOS, dietetic, or noninfectious
Gastroenteritis NOS, dietetic, or noninfectious
Ileitis NOS, dietetic, or noninfectious
Jejunitis NOS, dietetic, or noninfectious
Sigmoiditis NOS, dietetic, or noninfectious

● Code new
  to this edition
▲ Revision of
  existing code
④ ⑤ Fourth or fifth
  digit required

OTHER DISEASES OF INTESTINES AND PERITONEUM (560-569)

560 Intestinal obstruction without mention of hernia

[Excludes:] *duodenum (537.2-537.3)*
inguinal hernia with obstruction (550.1)
intestinal obstruction complicating hernia (552.0-552.9)
mesenteric:
embolism (557.0)
infarction (557.0)
thrombosis (557.0)
neonatal intestinal obstruction (277.01, 777.1-777.2, 777.4)

560.0 Intussusception
Intussusception (colon) (intestine) (rectum)
Invagination of intestine or colon

[Excludes:] *intussusception of appendix (543.9)*

560.1 Paralytic ileus
Adynamic ileus
Ileus (of intestine) (of bowel) (of colon)
Paralysis of intestine or colon

[Excludes:] *gallstone ileus (560.31)*

560.2 Volvulus
Knotting of intestine, bowel, or colon
Strangulation of intestine, bowel, or colon
Torsion of intestine, bowel, or colon
Twist of intestine, bowel, or colon

[5] **560.3 Impaction of intestine**

560.30 Impaction of intestine, unspecified
Impaction of colon

560.31 Gallstone ileus
Obstruction of intestine by gallstone

560.39 Other
Concretion of intestine
Enterolith
Fecal impaction

[5] **560.8 Other specified intestinal obstruction**

560.81 Intestinal or peritoneal adhesions with obstruction (postoperative) (postinfection)

[Excludes:] *adhesions without obstruction (568.0)*

560.89 Other
Mural thickening causing obstruction

[Excludes:] *ischemic stricture of intestine (557.1)*

560.9 Unspecified intestinal obstruction
Enterostenosis
Obstruction of intestine or colon
Occlusion of intestine or colon
Stenosis of intestine or colon
Stricture of intestine or colon

[Excludes:] *congenital stricture or stenosis of intestine (751.1-751.2)*

562 Diverticula of intestine
Use additional code, if desired, to identify any associated:
peritonitis (567.0-567.9)

[Excludes:] *congenital diverticulum of colon (751.5)*
diverticulum of appendix (543.9)
Meckel's diverticulum (751.0)

[5] **562.0 Small intestine**

562.00 Diverticulosis of small intestine (without mention of hemorrhage)
Diverticulosis:
duodenum without mention of diverticulitis
ileum without mention of diverticulitis
jejunum without mention of diverticulitis

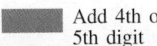

562.01 Diverticulitis of small intestine (without mention of hemorrhage)
Diverticulitis (with diverticulosis):
  duodenum
  ileum
  jejunum
  small intestine

562.02 Diverticulosis of small intestine with hemorrhage

562.03 Diverticulitis of small intestine with hemorrhage

⑤ **562.1 Colon**

562.10 Diverticulosis of colon (without mention of hemorrhage)
Diverticulosis:
  NOS without mention of diverticulitis
  intestine (large) without mention of diverticulitis
Diverticular disease (colon) without mention of diverticulitis

562.11 Diverticulitis of colon (without mention of hemorrhage)
Diverticulitis (with diverticulosis):
  NOS
  colon
  intestine (large)

562.12 Diverticulosis of colon with hemorrhage

562.13 Diverticulitis of colon with hemorrhage

564 **Functional digestive disorders, not elsewhere classified**
Excludes: functional disorders of stomach (536.0-536.9)
  those specified as psychogenic (306.4)

⑤ **564.0 Constipation**

564.00 Constipation, unspecified

564.01 Slow transit constipation

564.02 Outlet dysfunction constipation

564.09 Other constipation

564.1 Irritable bowel syndrome
Irritable colon   Spastic colon

564.2 Postgastric surgery syndromes
Dumping syndrome   Postgastrectomy syndrome
Jejunal syndrome   Postvagotomy syndrome
Excludes: malnutrition following gastrointestinal surgery (579.3)
  postgastrojejunostomy ulcer (534.0-534.9)

564.3 Vomiting following gastrointestinal surgery
Vomiting (bilious) following gastrointestinal surgery

564.4 Other postoperative functional disorders
Diarrhea following gastrointestinal surgery
Excludes: colostomy and enterostomy complications (569.60-569.69)

564.5 Functional diarrhea
Excludes: diarrhea:
  NOS (787.91)
  psychogenic (306.4)

564.6 Anal spasm
Proctalgia fugax

564.7 Megacolon, other than Hirschsprung's
Dilatation of colon
Excludes: megacolon:
  congenital [Hirschsprung's] (751.3)
  toxic (556)

⑤ **564.8 Other specified functional disorders of intestine**
Excludes: malabsorption (579.0-579.9)

564.81 Neurogenic bowel

564.89 Other functional disorders of intestine
Atony of colon

564.9 Unspecified functional disorder of intestine

● Code new   ▲ Revision of   ④ ⑤ Fourth or fifth
  to this edition   existing code   digit required

565 **Anal fissure and fistula**

565.0 **Anal fissure**
Tear of anus, nontraumatic

Excludes: traumatic *(863.89, 863.99)*

565.1 **Anal fistula**
Fistula:
anorectal
rectal
rectum to skin

Excludes: fistula of rectum to internal organs—see Alphabetic Index
ischiorectal fistula (566)
rectovaginal fistula (619.1)

566 **Abscess of anal and rectal regions**

Abscess:
ischiorectal
perianal
perirectal

Cellulitis:
anal
perirectal
rectal
Ischiorectal fistula

567 **Peritonitis**

Excludes: peritonitis:
benign paroxysmal (277.3)
pelvic, female (614.5, 614.7)
periodic familial (277.3)
puerperal (670)
with or following:
abortion (634-638 with .0, 639.0)
appendicitis (540.0-540.1)
ectopic or molar pregnancy (639.0)

567.0 *Peritonitis in infectious diseases classified elsewhere*
Code first underlying disease

Excludes: peritonitis:
gonococcal (098.86)
syphilitic (095.2)
tuberculous (014.0)

567.1 **Pneumococcal peritonitis**

567.2 **Other suppurative peritonitis**

Abscess (of):
abdominopelvic
mesenteric
omentum
peritoneum
retrocecal
retroperitoneal
subdiaphragmatic

Abscess (of):
subhepatic
subphrenic
Peritonitis (acute):
general
pelvic, male
subphrenic
suppurative

567.8 **Other specified peritonitis**
Chronic proliferative peritonitis
Fat necrosis of peritoneum
Mesenteric saponification
Peritonitis due to:
bile
urine

567.9 **Unspecified peritonitis**
Peritonitis:
NOS
of unspecified cause

Add 4th or
5th digit

Nonspecific
code

Unspecified
code

Manifestation
code

568 Other disorders of peritoneum

568.0 Peritoneal adhesions (postoperative) (postinfection)

Adhesions (of):
- abdominal (wall)
- diaphragm
- intestine
- male pelvis

Adhesions (of):
- mesenteric
- omentum
- stomach

Adhesive bands

[Excludes:] *adhesions:*
pelvic, female (614.6)
with obstruction:
duodenum (537.3)
intestine (560.81)

[5] **568.8 Other specified disorders of peritoneum**

568.81 Hemoperitoneum (nontraumatic)

568.82 Peritoneal effusion (chronic)

[Excludes:] *ascites NOS (789.5)*

568.89 Other

Peritoneal:
- cyst
- granuloma

568.9 Unspecified disorder of peritoneum

569 Other disorders of intestine

569.0 Anal and rectal polyp

Anal and rectal polyp NOS

[Excludes:] *adenomatous anal and rectal polyp (211.4)*

569.1 Rectal prolapse

Procidentia:
- anus (sphincter)
- rectum (sphincter)

Proctoptosis

Prolapse:
- anal canal
- rectal mucosa

[Excludes:] *prolapsed hemorrhoids (455.2, 455.5)*

569.2 Stenosis of rectum and anus

Stricture of anus (sphincter)

569.3 Hemorrhage of rectum and anus

[Excludes:] *gastrointestinal bleeding NOS (578.9)*
melena (578.1)

[5] **569.4 Other specified disorders of rectum and anus**

569.41 Ulcer of anus and rectum

Solitary ulcer of anus (sphincter) or rectum (sphincter)
Stercoral ulcer of anus (sphincter) or rectum (sphincter)

569.42 Anal or rectal pain

569.49 Other

Granuloma of rectum (sphincter)
Rupture of rectum (sphincter)
Hypertrophy of anal papillae
Proctitis NOS

[Excludes:] *fistula of rectum to:*
internal organs—see Alphabetic Index
skin (565.1)
hemorrhoids (455.0-455.9)
incontinence of sphincter ani (787.6)

569.5 Abscess of intestine

[Excludes:] *appendiceal abscess (540.1)*

[5] **569.6 Colostomy and enterostomy complications**

569.60 Colostomy and enterostomy complication, unspecified

● Code new to this edition ▲ Revision of existing code [4] [5] Fourth or fifth digit required

569.61 Infection of colostomy or enterostomy
Use additional code to specify type of infection, such as:
abscess or cellulitis of abdomen (682.2)
septicemia (038.0-038.9)
Use additional code to identify organism (041.00-041.9)

569.62 Mechanical complication of colostomy and enterostomy
Malfunction of colostomy and enterostomy

569.69 **Other complication**
Fistula
Hernia
Prolapse

⑤ **569.8 Other specified disorders of intestine**

569.81 Fistula of intestine, excluding rectum and anus
Fistula: Fistula:
abdominal wall   enteroenteric
enterocolic   ileorectal

Excludes: *fistula of intestine to internal organs —see Alphabetic Index*
persistent postoperative fistula (998.6)

569.82 Ulceration of intestine
Primary ulcer of intestine
Ulceration of colon

Excludes: *that with perforation (569.83)*

569.83 Perforation of intestine

569.84 Angiodysplasia of intestine (without mention of hemorrhage)

569.85 Angiodysplasia of intestine with hemorrhage

● **569.86 Dieulafoy lesion (hemorrhagic of intestine)**

569.89 **Other**
Enteroptosis
Granuloma of intestine
Prolapse of intestine
Pericolitis
Perisigmoiditis
Visceroptosis

Excludes: *gangrene of intestine, mesentery, or omentum (557.0)*
hemorrhage of intestine NOS (578.9)
obstruction of intestine (560.0-560.9)

569.9 **Unspecified disorder of intestine**

OTHER DISEASES OF DIGESTIVE SYSTEM (570-579)

570 Acute and subacute necrosis of liver
Acute hepatic failure
Acute or subacute hepatitis, not specified as infective
Necrosis of liver (acute) (diffuse) (massive) (subacute)
Parenchymatous degeneration of liver
Yellow atrophy (liver) (acute) (subacute)

Excludes: *icterus gravis of newborn (773.0-773.2)*
serum hepatitis (070.2-070.3)
that with:
abortion (634-638 with .7, 639.8)
ectopic or molar pregnancy (639.8)
pregnancy, childbirth, or the puerperium (646.7)
viral hepatitis (070.0-070.9)

571 **Chronic liver disease and cirrhosis**

571.0 Alcoholic fatty liver

571.1 Acute alcoholic hepatitis
Acute alcoholic liver disease

571.2 Alcoholic cirrhosis of liver
Florid cirrhosis
Laennec's cirrhosis (alcoholic)

571.3 **Alcoholic liver damage, unspecified**

341

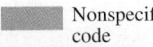 Add 4th or
5th digit

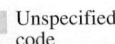 Nonspecific
code

Unspecified
code

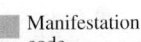 Manifestation
code

⑤ **571.4 Chronic hepatitis**

> *Excludes:* viral hepatitis (acute) (chronic) (070.0-070.9)

> **571.40** **Chronic hepatitis, unspecified**
>
> **571.41** **Chronic persistent hepatitis**
>
> **571.49** **Other**
> Chronic hepatitis:
> active
> aggressive
> Recurrent hepatitis

571.5 Cirrhosis of liver without mention of alcohol
Cirrhosis of liver: Cirrhosis of liver:
 NOS   posthepatitic
 cryptogenic   postnecrotic
 macronodular   Healed yellow atrophy (liver)
 micronodular   Portal cirrhosis

571.6 Biliary cirrhosis
Chronic nonsuppurative destructive cholangitis
Cirrhosis:
 cholangitic
 cholestatic

571.8 Other chronic nonalcoholic liver disease
Chronic yellow atrophy (liver)
Fatty liver, without mention of alcohol

571.9 Unspecified chronic liver disease without mention of alcohol

572 Liver abscess and sequelae of chronic liver disease

572.0 Abscess of liver

> *Excludes:* amebic liver abscess (006.3)

572.1 Portal pyemia
Phlebitis of portal vein   Pylephlebitis
Portal thrombophlebitis   Pylethrombophlebitis

572.2 Hepatic coma
Hepatic encephalopathy
Hepatocerebral intoxication
Portal-systemic encephalopathy

572.3 Portal hypertension

572.4 Hepatorenal syndrome

> *Excludes:* that following delivery (674.8)

572.8 Other sequelae of chronic liver disease

573 Other disorders of liver

> *Excludes:* amyloid or lardaceous degeneration of liver (277.3)
>   congenital cystic disease of liver (751.62)
>   glycogen infiltration of liver (271.0)
>   hepatomegaly NOS (789.1)
>   portal vein obstruction (452)

573.0 Chronic passive congestion of liver

573.1 Hepatitis in viral diseases classified elsewhere
Code first underlying disease as:
 Coxsackie virus disease (074.8)
 cytomegalic inclusion virus disease (078.5)
 infectious mononucleosis (075)

> *Excludes:* hepatitis (in):
>   mumps (072.71)
>   viral (070.0-070.9)
>   yellow fever (060.0-060.9)

● Code new   ▲ Revision of   ④ ⑤ Fourth or fifth
     to this edition   existing code   digit required

573.2 ***Hepatitis in other infectious diseases classified elsewhere***
Code first underlying disease, as:
malaria (084.9)

[Excludes:] *hepatitis in:*
late syphilis (095.3)
secondary syphilis (091.62)
toxoplasmosis (130.5)

573.3 Hepatitis, unspecified
Toxic (noninfectious) hepatitis

Use additional E code, if desired, to identify cause

573.4 Hepatic infarction

573.8 Other specified disorders of liver
Hepatoptosis

573.9 Unspecified disorder of liver

[5] **574 Cholelithiasis**

The following fifth-digit subclassification is for use with category 574:

0 without mention of obstruction

1 with obstruction

[5] **574.0 Calculus of gallbladder with acute cholecystitis**
Biliary calculus with acute cholecystitis
Calculus of cystic duct with acute cholecystitis
Cholelithiasis with acute cholecystitis
Any condition classifiable to 574.2 with acute cholecystitis

[5] **574.1 Calculus of gallbladder with other cholecystitis**
Biliary calculus with cholecystitis
Calculus of cystic duct with cholecystitis
Cholelithiasis with cholecystitis
Cholecystitis with cholelithiasis NOS
Any condition classifiable to 574.2 with cholecystitis (chronic)

[5] **574.2 Calculus of gallbladder without mention of cholecystitis**
Biliary:
calculus NOS
colic NOS
Calculus of cystic duct
Cholelithiasis NOS
Colic (recurrent) of gallbladder
Gallstone (impacted)

[5] **574.3 Calculus of bile duct with acute cholecystitis**
Calculus of bile duct [any] with acute cholecystitis
Choledocholithiasis with acute cholecystitis
Any condition classifiable to 574.5 with acute cholecystitis

[5] **574.4 Calculus of bile duct with other cholecystitis**
Calculus of bile duct [any] with cholecystitis (chronic)
Choledocholithiasis with cholecystitis (chronic)
Any condition classifiable to 574.5 with cholecystitis (chronic)

[5] **574.5 Calculus of bile duct without mention of cholecystitis**
Calculus of:
bile duct [any]
common duct
hepatic duct
Choledocholithiasis
Hepatic:
colic (recurrent)
lithiasis

[5] **574.6 Calculus of gallbladder and bile duct with acute cholecystitis**
Any condition classifiable to 574.0 and 574.3

[5] **574.7 Calculus of gallbladder and bile duct with other cholecystitis**
Any condition classifiable to 574.1 and 574.4

[5] **574.8 Calculus of gallbladder and bile duct with acute and chronic cholecystitis**
Any condition classifiable to 574.6 and 574.7

[5] **574.9 Calculus of gallbladder and bile duct without cholecystitis**
Any condition classifiable to 574.2 and 574.5

575 **Other disorders of gallbladder**

575.0 **Acute cholecystitis**
Abscess of gallbladder without mention of calculus
Angiocholecystitis without mention of calculus
Cholecystitis: without mention of calculus
emphysematous (acute) without mention of calculus
gangrenous without mention of calculus
suppurative without mention of calculus
Empyema of gallbladder without mention of calculus
Gangrene of gallbladder without mention of calculus

Excludes: *that with:*

acute and chronic cholecystitis (575.12)
choledocholithiasis (574.3)
choledocholithiasis and cholelithiasis (574.6)
cholelithiasis (574.0)

⑤ **575.1** **Other cholecystitis**
Cholecystitis:
NOS without mention of calculus
chronic without mention of calculus

Excludes: *that with:*

choledocholithiasis (574.4)
choledocholithiasis and cholelithiasis (574.8)
cholelithiasis (574.1)

575.10 **Cholecystitis, unspecified**
Cholecystitis NOS

575.11 **Chronic cholecystitis**

575.12 **Acute and chronic cholecystits**

575.2 **Obstruction of gallbladder**
Occlusion of cystic duct or gallbladder without mention of calculus
Stenosis of cystic duct or gallbladder without mention of calculus
Stricture of cystic duct or gallbladder without mention of calculus

Excludes: *that with calculus (574.0-574.2 with fifth-digit 1)*

575.3 **Hydrops of gallbladder**
Mucocele of gallbladder

575.4 **Perforation of gallbladder**
Rupture of cystic duct or gallbladder

575.5 **Fistula of gallbladder**
Fistula:
cholecystoduodenal
cholecystoenteric

575.6 **Cholesterolosis of gallbladder**
Strawberry gallbladder

575.8 **Other specified disorders of gallbladder**
Adhesions (of) cystic duct or gallbladder
Atrophy (of) cystic duct or gallbladder
Cyst (of) cystic duct or gallbladder
Hypertrophy (of) cystic duct or gallbladder
Nonfunctioning (of) cystic duct or gallbladder
Ulcer (of) cystic duct or gallbladder
Biliary dyskinesia (of) cystic duct or gallbladder

Excludes: *nonvisualization of gallbladder (793.3)*
Hartmann's pouch of intestine (V44.3)

575.9 **Unspecified disorder of gallbladder**

576 **Other disorders of biliary tract**

Excludes: *that involving the:*
cystic duct (575.0-575.9)
gallbladder (575.0-575.9)

576.0 **Postcholecystectomy syndrome**

● Code new
to this edition
▲ Revision of
existing code
④ ⑤ Fourth or fifth
digit required

576.1 Cholangitis

Cholangitis:
  NOS
  acute
  ascending
  chronic
  primary

Cholangitis:
  recurrent
  sclerosing
  secondary
  stenosing
  suppurative

576.2 Obstruction of bile duct
Occlusion of bile duct, except cystic duct, without mention of calculus
Stenosis of bile duct, except cystic duct, without mention of calculus
Stricture of bile duct, except cystic duct, without mention of calculus

Excludes: *congenital (751.61)*
  that with calculus (574.3-574.5 with fifth-digit 1)

576.3 Perforation of bile duct
Rupture of bile duct, except cystic duct

576.4 Fistula of bile duct
Choledochoduodenal fistula

576.5 Spasm of sphincter of Oddi

576.8 Other specified disorders of biliary tract
Adhesions of bile duct [any]
Atrophy of bile duct [any]
Cyst of bile duct [any]
Hypertrophy of bile duct [any]
Stasis of bile duct [any]
Ulcer of bile duct [any]

Excludes: *congenital choledochal cyst (751.69)*

576.9 Unspecified disorder of biliary tract

577 Diseases of pancreas

577.0 Acute pancreatitis
Abscess of pancreas
Necrosis of pancreas:
  acute
  infective

Pancreatitis:
  NOS
  acute (recurrent)
  apoplectic
  hemorrhagic
  subacute
  suppurative

Excludes: *mumps pancreatitis (072.3)*

577.1 Chronic pancreatitis
Chronic pancreatitis:
  NOS
  infectious
  interstitial

Pancreatitis:
  painless
  recurrent
  relapsing

577.2 Cyst and pseudocyst of pancreas

577.8 Other specified diseases of pancreas
Atrophy of pancreas
Calculus of pancreas
Cirrhosis of pancreas
Fibrosis of pancreas

Pancreatic:
  infantilism
  necrosis:
    NOS
    aseptic
    fat
Pancreatolithiasis

Excludes: *fibrocystic disease of pancreas (277.00-277.09)*
  islet cell tumor of pancreas (211.7)
  pancreatic steatorrhea (579.4)

577.9 Unspecified disease of pancreas

Add 4th or
5th digit

Nonspecific
code

Unspecified
code

Manifestation
code

578 **Gastrointestinal hemorrhage**

Excludes: *that with mention of :*

angiodysplasia of stomach and duodenum (537.83)
angiodysplasia of intestine (569.85)
diverticulitis, intestine:
    large (562.13)
    small (562.03)
diverticulosis, intestine:
    large (562.12)
    small (562.02)
gastritis and duodenitis (535.0-535.6)
ulcer:
    duodenal (532.0-532.9)
    gastric (531.0-531.9)
    gastrojejunal (534.0-534.9)
    peptic (533.0-533.9)

578.0 **Hematemesis**
Vomiting of blood

578.1 **Blood in stool**
Melena

Excludes: *occult blood (792.1)*

578.9 **Hemorrhage of gastrointestinal tract, unspecified**
Gastric hemorrhage   Intestinal hemorrhage

579 **Intestinal malabsorption**

579.0 **Celiac disease**
Celiac: Gee (-Herter) disease
    crisis   Gluten enteropathy
    infantilism   Idiopathic steatorrhea
    rickets   Nontropical sprue

579.1 **Tropical sprue**
Sprue: Tropical steatorrhea
    NOS
    tropical

579.2 **Blind loop syndrome**
Postoperative blind loop syndrome

579.3 **Other and unspecified postsurgical nonabsorption**
Hypoglycemia following gastrointestinal surgery
Malnutrition following gastrointestinal surgery

579.4 **Pancreatic steatorrhea**

579.8 **Other specified intestinal malabsorption**
Enteropathy: Steatorrhea (chronic)
    exudative
    protein-losing

579.9 **Unspecified intestinal malabsorption**
Malabsorption syndrome NOS

● Code new   ▲ Revision of   ④ ⑤ Fourth or fifth
  to this edition   existing code   digit required

chapter

10. DISEASES OF THE GENITOURINARY SYSTEM (580-629)

NEPHRITIS, NEPHROTIC SYNDROME, AND NEPHROSIS (580-589) section

[Excludes:] *hypertensive renal disease (403.00-403.91)*

580 Acute glomerulonephritis category
Includes: acute nephritis

580.0 With lesion of proliferative glomerulonephritis
Acute (diffuse) proliferative glomerulonephritis
Acute poststreptococcal glomerulonephritis

580.4 With lesion of rapidly progressive glomerulonephritis
Acute nephritis with lesion of necrotizing glomerulitis

⑤ **580.8 With other specified pathological lesion in kidney** – subcategory

580.81 Acute glomerulonephritis in diseases classified elsewhere subclassification.
Code first underlying disease, as:
infectious hepatitis (070.0-070.9)
mumps (072.79)
subacute bacterial endocarditis (421.0)
typhoid fever (002.0)

580.89 Other
Glomerulonephritis, acute, with lesion of:
exudative nephritis
interstitial (diffuse) (focal) nephritis

580.9 Acute glomerulonephritis with unspecified pathological lesion in kidney
Glomerulonephritis:
NOS specified as acute
hemorrhagic specified as acute
Nephritis specified as acute
Nephropathy specified as acute

581 Nephrotic syndrome

581.0 With lesion of proliferative glomerulonephritis

581.1 With lesion of membranous glomerulonephritis
Epimembranous nephritis
Idiopathic membranous glomerular disease
Nephrotic syndrome with lesion of:
focal glomerulosclerosis
sclerosing membranous glomerulonephritis
segmental hyalinosis

581.2 With lesion of membranoproliferative glomerulonephritis
Nephrotic syndrome with lesion (of):
endothelial glomerulonephritis
hypocomplementemic persistent glomerulonephritis
lobular glomerulonephritis
mesangiocapillary glomerulonephritis
mixed membranous and proliferative glomerulonephritis

581.3 With lesion of minimal change glomerulonephritis
Foot process disease
Lipoid nephrosis
Minimal change:
glomerular disease
glomerulitis
nephrotic syndrome

⑤ **581.8 With other specified pathological lesion in kidney**

581.81 Nephrotic syndrome in diseases classified elsewhere
Code first underlying disease, as:
amyloidosis (277.3)
diabetes mellitus (250.4)
malaria (084.9)
polyarteritis (446.0)
systemic lupus erythematosus (710.0)

[Excludes:] *nephrosis in epidemic hemorrhagic fever (078.6)*

581.89 Other
Glomerulonephritis with edema and lesion of:
exudative nephritis
interstitial (diffuse) (focal) nephritis

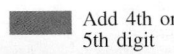

Add 4th or 5th digit | Nonspecific code | Unspecified code | Manifestation code

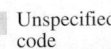

581.9 Nephrotic syndrome with unspecified pathological lesion in kidney
Glomerulonephritis with edema NOS
Nephritis:
nephrotic NOS
with edema NOS
Nephrosis NOS
Renal disease with edema NOS

582 Chronic glomerulonephritis
Includes: chronic nephritis

582.0 With lesion of proliferative glomerulonephritis
Chronic (diffuse) proliferative glomerulonephritis

582.1 With lesion of membranous glomerulonephritis
Chronic glomerulonephritis:
membranous
sclerosing
Focal glomerulosclerosis
Segmental hyalinosis

582.2 With lesion of membranoproliferative glomerulonephritis
Chronic glomerulonephritis:
endothelial
hypocomplementemic persistent
lobular
membranoproliferative
mesangiocapillary
mixed membranous and proliferative

582.4 With lesion of rapidly progressive glomerulonephritis
Chronic nephritis with lesion of necrotizing glomerulitis

[5] **582.8 With other specified pathological lesion in kidney**

582.81 Chronic glomerulonephritis in diseases classified elsewhere
Code first underlying disease, as:
amyloidosis (277.3)
systemic lupus erythematosus (710.0)

582.89 Other
Chronic glomerulonephritis with lesion of:
exudative nephritis
interstitial (diffuse) (focal) nephritis

582.9 Chronic glomerulonephritis with unspecified pathological lesion in kidney
Glomerulonephritis:
NOS specified as chronic
hemorrhagic specified as chronic
Nephritis specified as chronic
Nephropathy specified as chronic

583 Nephritis and nephropathy, not specified as acute or chronic
Includes: "renal disease" so stated, not specified as acute or chronic but with stated pathology or cause

583.0 With lesion of proliferative glomerulonephritis
Proliferative:
glomerulonephritis (diffuse) NOS
nephritis NOS
nephropathy NOS

583.1 With lesion of membranous glomerulonephritis
Membranous:
glomerulonephritis NOS
nephritis NOS
Membranous nephropathy NOS

583.2 With lesion of membranoproliferative glomerulonephritis
Membranoproliferative:
glomerulonephritis NOS
nephritis NOS
nephropathy NOS
Nephritis NOS, with lesion of:
hypocomplementemic persistent glomerulonephritis
lobular glomerulonephritis
mesangiocapillary glomerulonephritis
mixed membranous and proliferative glomerulonephritis

● Code new to this edition ▲ Revision of existing code [4] [5] Fourth or fifth digit required

583.4 With lesion of rapidly progressive glomerulonephritis
Necrotizing or rapidly progressive:
glomerulitis NOS
glomerulonephritis NOS
nephritis NOS
nephropathy NOS
Nephritis, unspecified, with lesion of necrotizing glomerulitis

583.6 With lesion of renal cortical necrosis
Nephritis NOS with (renal) cortical necrosis
Nephropathy NOS with (renal) cortical necrosis
Renal cortical necrosis NOS

583.7 With lesion of renal medullary necrosis
Nephritis NOS with (renal) medullary [papillary] necrosis
Nephropathy NOS with (renal) medullary [papillary] necrosis

[5] **583.8 With other specified pathological lesion in kidney**

583.81 Nephritis and nephropathy, not specified as acute or chronic, in diseases classified elsewhere
Code first underlying disease, as:
amyloidosis (277.3)
diabetes mellitus (250.4)
gonococcal infection (098.19)
Goodpasture's syndrome (446.21)
systemic lupus erythematosus (710.0)
tuberculosis (016.0)

[Excludes:] *gouty nephropathy (274.10)*
syphilitic nephritis (095.4)

583.89 Other
Glomerulitis with lesion of: exudative nephritis and interstitial nephritis
Glomerulonephritis with lesion of: exudative nephritis and interstitial nephritis
Nephritis with lesion of: exudative nephritis and interstitial nephritis
Nephropathy with lesion of: exudative nephritis and interstitial nephritis
Renal disease with lesion of: exudative nephritis and interstitial nephritis

583.9 With unspecified pathological lesion in kidney
Glomerulitis NOS
Glomerulonephritis NOS
Nephritis NOS
Nephropathy NOS

[Excludes:] *nephropathy complicating pregnancy, labor, or the puerperium (642.0-642.9, 646.2)*
renal disease NOS with no stated cause (593.9)

584 Acute renal failure

[Excludes:] *following labor and delivery (669.3)*
posttraumatic (958.5)
that complicating:
abortion (634-638 with .3, 639.3)
ectopic or molar pregnancy (639.3)

584.5 With lesion of tubular necrosis
Lower nephron nephrosis
Renal failure with (acute) tubular necrosis
Tubular necrosis:
NOS
acute

584.6 With lesion of renal cortical necrosis

584.7 With lesion of renal medullary [papillary] necrosis
Necrotizing renal papillitis

584.8 With other specified pathological lesion in kidney

584.9 Acute renal failure, unspecified

Add 4th or 5th digit | Nonspecific code | Unspecified code | Manifestation code

585 Chronic renal failure
Chronic uremia

Use additional code, if desired, to identify manifestation as:
uremic:
  neuropathy (357.4)
  pericarditis (420.0)

Excludes: *that with any condition classifiable to 401 (403.0-403.9 with fifth-digit 1)*

586 Renal failure, unspecified
Uremia NOS

Excludes: *following labor and delivery (669.3)*
    posttraumatic renal failure (958.5)
    that complicating:
      abortion (634-638 with .3, 639.3)
      ectopic or molar pregnancy (639.3)
    uremia:
      extrarenal (788.9)
      prenal (788.9)
    with any condition classifiable to 401 (403.0-403.9 with fifth-digit 1)

587 Renal sclerosis, unspecified
Atrophy of kidney   Renal:
Contracted kidney   cirrhosis
                        fibrosis

Excludes: *nephrosclerosis (arteriolar) (arteriosclerotic) (403.00-403.92)*
    with hypertension (403.00-403.92)

588 Disorders resulting from impaired renal function

588.0 Renal osteodystrophy
Azotemic osteodystrophy   Renal:
Phosphate-losing tubular   dwarfism
    disorders   infantilism
                        rickets

588.1 Nephrogenic diabetes insipidus
Excludes: *diabetes insipidus NOS (253.5)*

588.8 Other specified disorders resulting from impaired renal function
Hypokalemic nephropathy
Secondary hyperparathyroidism (of renal origin)
Excludes: *secondary hypertension (405.0-405.9)*

588.9 Unspecified disorder resulting from impaired renal function

589 Small kidney of unknown cause

589.0 Unilateral small kidney

589.1 Bilateral small kidneys

589.9 Small kidney, unspecified

OTHER DISEASES OF URINARY SYSTEM (590-599)

590 Infections of kidney
Use additional code, if desired, to identify organism, such as Escherichia coli [E. coli] (041.4)

⑤ **590.0 Chronic pyelonephritis**
Chronic pyelitis   Chronic pyonephrosis
Code, if applicable, any causal condition first

    590.00 Without lesion of renal medullary necrosis

    590.01 With lesion of renal medullary necrosis

⑤ **590.1 Acute pyelonephritis**
Acute pyelitis   Acute pyonephrosis

    590.10 Without lesion of renal medullary necrosis

    590.11 With lesion of renal medullary necrosis

● Code new
   to this edition
▲ Revision of
   existing code
④ ⑤ Fourth or fifth
     digit required

590.2 Renal and perinephric abscess
    Abscess: Carbuncle of kidney
      kidney
      nephritic
      perirenal

590.3 Pyeloureteritis cystica
    Infection of renal pelvis and ureter
    Ureteritis cystica

⑤ **590.8 Other pyelonephritis or pyonephrosis, not specified as acute or chronic**

    590.80 Pyelonephritis, unspecified
        Pyelitis NOS   Pyelonephritis NOS

    590.81 *Pyelitis or pyelonephritis in diseases classified elsewhere*
        Code first underlying disease, as:
        tuberculosis (016.0)

590.9 Infection of kidney, unspecified
    Excludes: *urinary tract infection NOS (599.0)*

591 Hydronephrosis
    Hydrocalycosis   Hydroureteronephrosis
    Hydronephrosis
    Excludes: *congenital hydronephrosis (753.29)*
          hydroureter (593.5)

592 Calculus of kidney and ureter
    Excludes: *nephrocalcinosis (275.4)*

592.0 Calculus of kidney
    Nephrolithiasis NOS   Staghorn calculus
    Renal calculus or stone   Stone in kidney
    Excludes: *uric acid nephrolithiasis (274.11)*

592.1 Calculus of ureter
    Ureteric stone   Ureterolithiasis

592.9 Urinary calculus, unspecified

593 Other disorders of kidney and ureter

593.0 Nephroptosis
    Floating kidney   Mobile kidney

593.1 Hypertrophy of kidney

593.2 Cyst of kidney, acquired
    Cyst (multiple) (solitary) of kidney, not congenital
    Peripelvic (lymphatic) cyst
    Excludes: *calyceal or pyelogenic cyst of kidney (591)*
          congenital cyst of kidney (753.1)
          polycystic (disease of) kidney (753.1)

593.3 Stricture or kinking of ureter
    Angulation of ureter (postoperative)
    Constriction of ureter (postoperative)
    Stricture of pelviureteric junction

593.4 Other ureteric obstruction
    Idiopathic retroperitoneal fibrosis
    Occlusion NOS of ureter
    Excludes: *that due to calculus (592.1)*

593.5 Hydroureter
    Excludes: *congenital hydroureter (753.22)*
          hydroureteronephrosis (591)

593.6 Postural proteinuria
    Benign postural proteinuria
    Orthostatic proteinuria
    Excludes: *proteinuria NOS (791.0)*

	Add 4th or 5th digit		Nonspecific code		Unspecified code		Manifestation code

⑤ **593.7** **Vesicoureteral reflux**

 593.70 **Unspecified or without reflux nephropathy**

 593.71 **With reflux nephropathy, unilateral**

 593.72 **With reflux nephropathy, bilateral**

 593.73 **With reflux nephropathy NOS**

⑤ **593.8** **Other specified disorders of kidney and ureter**

 593.81 **Vascular disorders of kidney**
Renal (artery):   Renal infarction
 embolism
 hemorrhage
 thrombosis

 593.82 **Ureteral fistula**
Intestinoureteral fistula

 Excludes: fistula between ureter and female genital tract (619.0)

 593.89 **Other**
Adhesions, kidney or   Polyp of ureter
 ureter   Pyelectasia
Periureteritis   Ureterocele

 Excludes: tuberculosis of ureter (016.2)
 ureteritis cystica (590.3)

 593.9 **Unspecified disorder of kidney and ureter**
Renal disease NOS
Salt-losing nephritis or syndrome

 Excludes: cystic kidney disease (753.1)
 nephropathy, so stated (583.0-583.9)
 renal disease:
 acute (580.0-580.9)
 arising in pregnancy or the puerperium (642.1-642.2, 642.4-642.7, 646.2)
 chronic (582.0-582.9)
 not specified as acute or chronic, but with stated pathology or cause
 (583.0-583.9)

594 **Calculus of lower urinary tract**

 594.0 **Calculus in diverticulum of bladder**

 594.1 **Other calculus in bladder**
Urinary bladder stone

 Excludes: staghorn calculus (592.0)

 594.2 **Calculus in urethra**

 594.8 **Other lower urinary tract calculus**

 594.9 **Calculus of lower urinary tract, unspecified**

 Excludes: calculus of urinary tract NOS (592.9)

595 **Cystitis**

 Excludes: prostatocystitis (601.3)
Use additional code, if desired, to identify organism, such as Escherichia coli [E. coli] (041.4)

 595.0 **Acute cystitis**

 Excludes: trigonitis (595.3)

 595.1 **Chronic interstitial cystitis**
Hunner's ulcer   Submucous cystitis
Panmural fibrosis of bladder

 595.2 **Other chronic cystitis**
Chronic cystitis NOS   Subacute cystitis

 Excludes: trigonitis (595.3)

 595.3 **Trigonitis**
Follicular cystitis
Trigonitis (acute) (chronic)
Urethrotrigonitis

● Code new   ▲ Revision of   ④ ⑤ Fourth or fifth
 to this edition   existing code   digit required

595.4 Cystitis in diseases classified elsewhere

Code first underlying disease, as:
actinomycosis (039.8)
amebiasis (006.8)
bilharziasis (120.0-120.9)
Echinococcus infestation (122.3, 122.6)

[Excludes:] *cystitis:*
diphtheritic (032.84)
gonococcal (098.11, 098.31)
monilial (112.2)
trichomonal (131.09)
tuberculous (016.1)

[5] **595.8 Other specified types of cystitis**

595.81 Cystitis cystica

595.82 Irradiation cystitis
Use additional E code, if desired, to identify cause

595.89 Other
Abscess of bladder
Cystitis:
bullous
emphysematous
glandularis

595.9 Cystitis, unspecified

596 Other disorders of bladder
Use additional code, if desired, to identify urinary incontinence (625.6, 788.30-788.39)

596.0 Bladder neck obstruction
Contracture (acquired) of bladder neck or vesicourethral orifice
Obstruction (acquired) of bladder neck or vesicourethral orifice
Stenosis (acquired) of bladder neck or vesicourethral orifice

[Excludes:] *congenital (753.6)*

596.1 Intestinovesical fistula
Fistula:
enterovesical
vesicocolic
Fistula:
vesicoenteric
vesicorectal

596.2 Vesical fistula, not elsewhere classified
Fistula:
bladder NOS
urethrovesical
Fistula:
vesicocutaneous
vesicoperineal

[Excludes:] *fistula between bladder and female genital tract (619.0)*

596.3 Diverticulum of bladder
Diverticulitis of bladder
Diverticulum (acquired) (false) of bladder

[Excludes:] *that with calculus in diverticulum of bladder (594.0)*

596.4 Atony of bladder
High compliance bladder, of bladder
Hypotonicity of bladder
Inertia of bladder

[Excludes:] *neurogenic bladder (596.54)*

[5] **596.5 Other functional disorders of bladder**

[Excludes:] *cauda equina syndrome*
with neurogenic bladder (344.61)

596.51 Hypertonicity of bladder
Hyperactivity
Overactive bladder

596.52 Low bladder compliance

596.53 Paralysis of bladder

596.54 Neurogenic bladder NOS

596.55 Detrusor sphincter dyssynergia

596.59 Other functional disorder of bladder
Detrusor instability

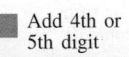

Add 4th or 5th digit
Nonspecific code
Unspecified code
Manifestation code

596.6 Rupture of bladder, nontraumatic

596.7 Hemorrhage into bladder wall
Hyperemia of bladder

Excludes: *acute hemorrhagic cystitis (595.0)*

596.8 Other specified disorders of bladder

Bladder:
  calcified
  contracted

Bladder:
  hemorrhage
  hypertrophy

Excludes: *cystocele, female (618.0, 618.2-618.4)*
  hernia or prolapse of bladder, female (618.0, 618.2-618.4)

596.9 Unspecified disorder of bladder

597 Urethritis, not sexually transmitted, and urethral syndrome

Excludes: *nonspecific urethritis, so stated (099.4)*

597.0 Urethral abscess

Abscess of:
  bulbourethral gland
  Cowper's gland
  Littré's gland

Abscess:
  periurethral
  urethral (gland)
Periurethral cellulitis

Excludes: *urethral caruncle (599.3)*

⑤ **597.8 Other urethritis**

  597.80 Urethritis, unspecified

  597.81 Urethral syndrome NOS

  597.89 Other

Adenitis, Skene's
  glands
Cowperitis

Meatitis, urethral
Ulcer, urethra (meatus)
Verumontanitis

Excludes: *trichomonal (131.02)*

598 Urethral stricture
Includes: pinhole meatus
  stricture of urinary meatus

Excludes: *congenital stricture of urethra and urinary meatus (753.6)*
Use additional code to identify urinary incontinence (625.6, 788.30-788.39)

⑤ **598.0 Urethral stricture due to infection**

  598.00 Due to unspecified infection

  598.01 Due to infective diseases classified elsewhere
    Code first underlying disease, as:
    gonococcal infection (098.2)
    schistosomiasis (120.0-120.9)
    syphilis (095.8)

598.1 Traumatic urethral stricture
Stricture of urethra:
  late effect of injury
  postobstetric

Excludes: *postoperative following surgery on genitourinary tract (598.2)*

598.2 Postoperative urethral stricture
Postcatheterization stricture of urethra

598.8 Other specified causes of urethral stricture

598.9 Urethral stricture, unspecified

599 Other disorders of urethra and urinary tract

599.0 Urinary tract infection, site not specified
Pyuria

Excludes: *candidiasis of urinary tract (112.2)*
  urinary tract infection of newborn (771.82)

Use additional code to identify organism, such as Escherichia coli [E. coli] (041.4)

● Code new
  to this edition
▲ Revision of
  existing code
④ ⑤ Fourth or fifth
  digit required

599.1 Urethral fistula
Fistula:
urethroperineal
urethrorectal
Urinary fistula NOS

[Excludes:] *fistula:*
urethroscrotal (608.89)
urethrovaginal (619.0)
urethrovesicovaginal (619.0)

599.2 Urethral diverticulum

599.3 Urethral caruncle
Polyp of urethra

599.4 Urethral false passage

599.5 Prolapsed urethral mucosa
Prolapse of urethra
Urethrocele

[Excludes:] *urethrocele, female (618.0, 618.2-618.4)*

599.6 Urinary obstruction, unspecified
Obstructive uropathy NOS
Urinary (tract) obstruction NOS

[Excludes:] *obstructive nephropathy NOS (593.89)*

Use additional code, if desired, to identify urinary incontinence (625.6, 788.30-788.39)

599.7 Hematuria
Hematuria (benign) (essential)

[Excludes:] *hemoglobinuria (791.2)*

[5] **599.8 Other specified disorders of urethra and urinary tract**

[Excludes:] *symptoms and other conditions classifiable to 788.0-788.9, 791.0-791.9*

Use additional code, if desired, to identify urinary incontinence (625.6, 788.30-788.39)

599.81 Urethral hypermobility

599.82 Intrinsic (urethral) sphincter deficiency [ISD]

599.83 Urethral instability

599.84 Other specified disorders of urethra
Rupture of urethra (nontraumatic)
Urethral:
cyst
granuloma

599.89 Other specified disorders of urinary tract

599.9 Unspecified disorder of urethra and urinary tract

DISEASES OF MALE GENITAL ORGANS (600-608)

600 Hyperplasia of prostate

Use additional code, if desired, to identify urinary incontinence (788.30-788.39)

600.0 Hypertrophy (benign) of prostate
Benign prostatic hypertrophy
Enlargement of prostate
Smooth enlarged prostate
Soft enlarged prostate

600.1 Nodular prostate
Hard, firm prostate
Multinodular prostate

[Excludes:] *malignant neoplasm of prostate (185)*

600.2 Benign localized hyperplasia of prostate
Adenofibromatous hypertrophy of prostate
Adenoma of prostate
Fibroadenoma of prostate
Fibroma of prostate
Myoma of prostate
Polyp of prostate

[Excludes:] *benign neoplasms of prostate (222.2)*
hypertrophy of prostate (600.0)
malignant neoplasm of prostate (185)

600.3 Cyst of prostate

600.9 Hyperplasia of prostate, unspecified
Median bar
Prostatic obstruction NOS

601 Inflammatory diseases of prostate
Use additional code, if desired, to identify organism, such as Staphylococcus (041.1), or Streptococcus (041.0)

601.0 Acute prostatitis

601.1 Chronic prostatitis

601.2 Abscess of prostate

601.3 Prostatocystitis

601.4 Prostatitis in diseases classified elsewhere
Code first underlying disease, as:
actinomycosis (039.8)
blastomycosis (116.0)
syphilis (095.8)
tuberculosis (016.5)

[*Excludes:*] *prostatitis:*
gonococcal (098.12, 098.32)
monilial (112.2)
trichomonal (131.03)

601.8 Other specified inflammatory diseases of prostate
Prostatitis:
cavitary
diverticular
granulomatous

601.9 Prostatitis, unspecified
Prostatitis NOS

602 Other disorders of prostate

602.0 Calculus of prostate
Prostatic stone

602.1 Congestion or hemorrhage of prostate

602.2 Atrophy of prostate

602.3 Dysplasia of prostate
Prostatic intraepithelial neoplasia I (PIN I)
Prostatic intraepithelial neoplasia II (PIN II)

[*Excludes:*] *Prostatic intraepithelial neoplasia III (PIN III) (233.4)*

602.8 Other specified disorders of prostate
Fistula of prostate
Infarction of prostate
Stricture of prostate
Periprostatic adhesions

602.9 Unspecified disorder of prostate

603 Hydrocele
Includes: hydrocele of spermatic cord, testis, or tunica vaginalis
[*Excludes:*] *congenital (778.6)*

603.0 Encysted hydrocele

603.1 Infected hydrocele
Use additional code, if desired, to identify organism

603.8 Other specified types of hydrocele

603.9 Hydrocele, unspecified

604 Orchitis and epididymitis
Use additional code, if desired, to identify organism, such as Escherichia coli [E. coli] (041.4), Staphylococcus (041.1), or Streptococcus (041.0)

604.0 Orchitis, epididymitis, and epididymo-orchitis, with abscess
Abscess of epididymis or testis

[5] **604.9 Other orchitis, epididymitis, and epididymo-orchitis, without mention of abscess**

604.90 Orchitis and epididymitis, unspecified

● Code new to this edition
▲ Revision of existing code
[4] [5] Fourth or fifth digit required

604.91 ***Orchitis and epididymitis in diseases classified elsewhere***
Code first underlying disease, as:
diphtheria (032.89)
filariasis (125.0-125.9)
syphilis (095.8)

[Excludes:] *orchitis:*
gonococcal (098.13, 098.33)
mumps (072.0)
tuberculous (016.5)
tuberculous epididymitis (016.4)

604.99 Other

605 Redundant prepuce and phimosis
Adherent prepuce
Paraphimosis
Phimosis (congenital)
Tight foreskin

606 Infertility, male

606.0 Azoospermia
Absolute infertility
Infertility due to:
germinal (cell) aplasia
spermatogenic arrest (complete)

606.1 Oligospermia
Infertility due to:
germinal cell desquamation
hypospermatogenesis
incomplete spermatogenic arrest

606.8 Infertility due to extratesticular causes
Infertility due to:
drug therapy
infection
obstruction of efferent ducts
radiation
systemic disease

606.9 Male infertility, unspecified

607 Disorders of penis
[Excludes:] *phimosis (605)*

607.0 Leukoplakia of penis
Kraurosis of penis

[Excludes:] *carcinoma in situ of penis (233.5)*
erythroplasia of Queyrat (233.5)

607.1 Balanoposthitis
Balanitis

Use additional code, if desired, to identify organism

607.2 Other inflammatory disorders of penis
Abscess of corpus cavernosum or penis
Boil of corpus cavernosum or penis
Carbuncle of corpus cavernosum or penis
Cellulitis of corpus cavernosum or penis
Cavernitis (penis) of corpus cavernosum or penis

Use additional code, if desired, to identify organism

[Excludes:] *herpetic infection (054.13)*

607.3 Priapism
Painful erection

[5] **607.8 Other specified disorders of penis**

607.81 Balanitis xerotica obliterans
Induratio penis plastica

607.82 Vascular disorders of penis
Embolism of corpus cavernosum or penis
Hematoma (nontraumatic) of corpus cavernosum or penis
Hemorrhage of corpus cavernosum or penis
Thrombosis of corpus cavernosum or penis

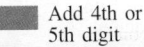

Add 4th or 5th digit | Nonspecific code | Unspecified code | Manifestation code

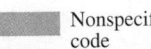

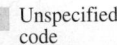

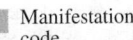

607.83 Edema of penis

607.84 Impotence of organic origin

[Excludes:] *nonorganic or unspecified (302.72)*

607.89 Other

Atrophy of corpus cavernosum or penis
Fibrosis of corpus cavernosum or penis
Hypertrophy of corpus cavernosum or penis
Ulcer (chronic) of corpus cavernosum or penis

607.9 Unspecified disorder of penis

608 Other disorders of male genital organs

608.0 Seminal vesiculitis

Abscess of seminal vesicle
Cellulitis of seminal vesicle
Vesiculitis (seminal)

Use additional code, if desired, to identify organism

[Excludes:] *gonococcal infection (098.14, 098.34)*

608.1 Spermatocele

608.2 Torsion of testis

Torsion of:
epididymis
spermatic cord
testicle

608.3 Atrophy of testis

608.4 Other inflammatory disorders of male genital organs

Abscess of scrotum, spermatic cord, testis [except abscess], tunica vaginalis, or vas deferens
Boil of scrotum, spermatic cord, testis [except abscess], tunica vaginalis, or vas deferens
Carbuncle of scrotum, spermatic cord, testis [except abscess], tunica vaginalis, or vas deferens
Cellulitis of scrotum, spermatic cord, testis [except abscess], tunica vaginalis, or vas deferens
Vasitis of scrotum, spermatic cord, testis [except abscess], tunica vaginalis, or vas deferens

Use additional code, if desired, to identify organism

[Excludes:] *abscess of testis (604.0)*

[5] **608.8 Other specified disorders of male genital organs**

608.81 Disorders of male genital organs in diseases classified elsewhere

Code first underlying disease, as:
filariasis (125.0-125.9)
tuberculosis (016.5)

608.82 Hematospermia

608.83 Vascular disorders

Hematoma (nontraumatic) of seminal vesicle, spermatic cord, testis, scrotum, tunica vaginalis, or vas deferens
Hemorrhage of seminal vesicle, spermatic cord, testis, scrotum, tunica vaginalis, or vas deferens
Thrombosis of seminal vesicle, spermatic cord, testis, scrotum, tunica vaginalis, or vas deferens
Hematocele NOS, male

608.84 Chylocele of tunica vaginalis

608.85 Stricture

Stricture of spermatic cord
Stricture of tunica vaginalis
Stricture of vas deferens

608.86 Edema

608.87 Retrograde ejaculation

608.89 Other

Atrophy of seminal vesicle, spermatic cord, testis, scrotum, tunica vaginalis, or vas deferens
Fibrosis of seminal vesicle, spermatic cord, testis, scrotum, tunica vaginalis, or vas deferens
Hypertrophy of seminal vesicle, spermatic cord, testis, scrotum, tunica vaginalis, or vas deferens
Ulcer of seminal vesicle, spermatic cord, testis, scrotum, tunica vaginalis, or vas deferens

[Excludes:] *atrophy of testis (608.3)*

608.9 Unspecified disorder of male genital organs

● Code new to this edition
▲ Revision of existing code
[4] [5] Fourth or fifth digit required

DISORDERS OF BREAST (610-611)

610 Benign mammary dysplasias

610.0 Solitary cyst of breast
Cyst (solitary) of breast

610.1 Diffuse cystic mastopathy
Chronic cystic mastitis
Cystic breast
Fibrocystic disease of breast

610.2 Fibroadenosis of breast
Fibroadenosis of breast:
- NOS
- chronic
- cystic

Fibroadenosis of breast:
- diffuse
- periodic
- segmental

610.3 Fibrosclerosis of breast

610.4 Mammary duct ectasia
Comedomastitis
Dust ectasia
Mastitis:
- periductal
- plasma cell

610.8 Other specified benign mammary dysplasias
Mazoplasia
Sebaceous cyst of breast

610.9 Benign mammary dysplasia, unspecified

611 Other disorders of breast
[Excludes:] *that associated with lactation or the puerperium (675.0-676.9)*

611.0 Inflammatory disease of breast
Abscess (acute) (chronic) (nonpuerperal) of:
- areola
- breast

Mammillary fistula
Mastitis (acute) (subacute) (nonpuerperal):
- NOS
- infective
- retromammary
- submammary

[Excludes:] *carbuncle of breast (680.2)*
chronic cystic mastitis (610.1)
neonatal infective mastitis (771.5)
thrombophlebitis of breast [Mondor's disease] (451.89)

611.1 Hypertrophy of breast
Gynecomastia
Hypertrophy of breast:
- NOS
- massive pubertal

611.2 Fissure of nipple

611.3 Fat necrosis of breast
Fat necrosis (segmental) of breast

611.4 Atrophy of breast

611.5 Galactocele

611.6 Galactorrhea not associated with childbirth

[5] **611.7 Signs and symptoms in breast**

611.71 Mastodynia
Pain in breast

611.72 Lump or mass in breast

611.79 Other
Induration of breast
Inversion of nipple
Nipple discharge
Retraction of nipple

611.8 Other specified disorders of breast
Hematoma (nontraumatic) of breast
Infarction of breast
Occlusion of breast duct
Subinvolution of breast (postlactational) (postpartum)

611.9 Unspecified breast disorder

INFLAMMATORY DISEASE OF FEMALE PELVIC ORGANS (614-616)

Use additional code, if desired, to identify organism, such as Staphylococcus (041.1), or Streptococcus (041.0)

Excludes: that associated with pregnancy, abortion, childbirth, or the puerperium (630-676.9)

614 **Inflammatory disease of ovary, fallopian tube, pelvic cellular tissue, and peritoneum**

Excludes: endometritis (615.0-615.9)
major infection following delivery (670)
that complicating:
abortion (634-638 with .0, 639.0)
ectopic or molar pregnancy (639.0)
pregnancy or labor (646.6)

614.0 **Acute salpingitis and oophoritis**
Any condition classifiable to 614.2, specified as acute or subacute

614.1 **Chronic salpingitis and oophoritis**
Hydrosalpinx
Salpingitis:
follicularis
isthmica nodosa
Any condition classifiable to 614.2, specified as chronic

614.2 **Salpingitis and oophoritis not specified as acute, subacute, or chronic**
Abscess (of):   Perisalpingitis
  fallopian tube   Pyosalpinx
  ovary   Salpingitis
  tubo-ovarian   Salpingo-oophoritisRTubo-ovarian inflammatory disease
Oophoritis
Perioophoritis

Excludes: gonococcal infection (chronic) (098.37)
acute (098.17)
tuberculous (016.6)

614.3 **Acute parametritis and pelvic cellulitis**
Acute inflammatory pelvic disease
Any condition classifiable to 614.4, specified as acute

614.4 **Chronic or unspecified parametritis and pelvic cellulitis**
Abscess (of):
  broad ligament, chronic or NOS
  parametrium, chronic or NOS
  pelvis, female, chronic or NOS
  pouch of Douglas, chronic or NOS
Chronic inflammatory pelvic disease
Pelvic cellulitis, female

Excludes: tuberculous (016.7)

614.5 **Acute or unspecified pelvic peritonitis, female**

614.6 **Pelvic peritoneal adhesions, female (postoperative) (postinfection)**
Adhesions:
  peritubal
  tubo-ovarian

Use additional code, if desired, to identify any associated infertility (628.2)

614.7 **Other chronic pelvic peritonitis, female**
Excludes: tuberculous (016.7)

614.8 **Other specified inflammatory disease of female pelvic organs and tissues**

614.9 **Unspecified inflammatory disease of female pelvic organs and tissues**
Pelvic infection or inflammation, female NOS
Pelvic inflammatory disease [PID]

● Code new   ▲ Revision of   ④ ⑤ Fourth or fifth
  to this edition   existing code   digit required

615 Inflammatory diseases of uterus, except cervix

[Excludes:] *following delivery (670)*
hyperplastic endometritis (621.3)
that complicating:
abortion (634-638 with .0, 639.0)
ectopic or molar pregnancy (639.0)
pregnancy or labor (646.6)

615.0 Acute
Any condition classifiable to 615.9, specified as acute or subacute

615.1 Chronic
Any condition classifiable to 615.9, specified as chronic

615.9 Unspecified inflammatory disease of uterus
Endometritis
Endomyometritis
Metritis
Myometritis
Perimetritis
Pyometra
Uterine abscess

616 Inflammatory disease of cervix, vagina, and vulva

[Excludes:] *that complicating:*
abortion (634-638 with .0, 639.0)
ectopic or molar pregnancy (639.0)
pregnancy, childbirth, or the puerperium (646.6)

616.0 Cervicitis and endocervicitis
Cervicitis with or without mention of erosion or ectropion
Endocervicitis with or without mention of erosion or ectropion
Nabothian (gland) cyst or follicle

[Excludes:] *erosion or ectropion without mention of cervicitis (622.0)*

[5] **616.1 Vaginitis and vulvovaginitis**

616.10 Vaginitis and vulvovaginitis, unspecified
Vaginitis:
NOS
postirradiation
Vulvitis NOS
Vulvovaginitis NOS

Use additional code, if desired, to identify organism, such as Escherichia coli [E. coli] (041.4), Staphylococcus (041.1), or Streptococcus (041.0)

[Excludes:] *noninfective leukorrhea (623.5)*
postmenopausal or senile vaginitis (627.3)

616.11 Vaginitis and vulvovaginitis in diseases classified elsewhere
Code first underlying disease, as:
pinworm vaginitis (127.4)

[Excludes:] *herpetic vulvovaginitis (054.11)*
monilial vulvovaginitis (112.1)
trichomonal vaginitis or vulvovaginitis (131.01)

616.2 Cyst of Bartholin's gland
Bartholin's duct cyst

616.3 Abscess of Bartholin's gland
Vulvovaginal gland abscess

616.4 Other abscess of vulva
Abscess of vulva
Carbuncle of vulva
Furuncle of vulva

[5] **616.5 Ulceration of vulva**

616.50 Ulceration of vulva, unspecified
Ulcer NOS of vulva

616.51 Ulceration of vulva in diseases classified elsewhere
Code first underlying disease, as:
Behçet's syndrome (136.1)
tuberculosis (016.7)

[Excludes:] *vulvar ulcer (in):*
gonococcal (098.0)
herpes simplex (054.12)
syphilitic (091.0)

616.8 Other specified inflammatory diseases of cervix, vagina, and vulva
Caruncle, vagina or labium
Ulcer, vagina

Excludes: *noninflammatory disorders of:*
cervix (622.0-622.9)
vagina (623.0-623.9)
vulva (624.0-624.9)

616.9 Unspecified inflammatory disease of cervix, vagina, and vulva

OTHER DISORDERS OF FEMALE GENITAL TRACT (617-629)

617 Endometriosis

617.0 Endometriosis of uterus
Adenomyosis

Endometriosis:
cervix
internal
myometrium

Excludes: *stromal endometriosis (236.0)*

617.1 Endometriosis of ovary
Chocolate cyst of ovary
Endometrial cystoma of ovary

617.2 Endometriosis of fallopian tube

617.3 Endometriosis of pelvic peritoneum
Endometriosis:
broad ligament
cul-de-sac (Douglas')

Endometriosis:
parametrium
round ligament

617.4 Endometriosis of rectovaginal septum and vagina

617.5 Endometriosis of intestine
Endometriosis:
appendix
colon
rectum

617.6 Endometriosis in scar of skin

617.8 Endometriosis of other specified sites
Endometriosis:
bladder
lung

Endometriosis:
umbilicus
vulva

617.9 Endometriosis, site unspecified

618 Genital prolapse
Use additional code, if desired, to identify urinary incontinence (625.6, 788.31, 788.33-788.39)
Excludes: *that complicating pregnancy, labor, or delivery (654.4)*

618.0 Prolapse of vaginal walls without mention of uterine prolapse
Cystocele without mention of uterine prolapse
Cystourethrocele without mention of uterine prolapse
Proctocele, female without mention of uterine prolapse
Rectocele without mention of uterine prolapse
Urethrocele, female without mention of uterine prolapse
Vaginal prolapse without mention of uterine prolapse

Excludes: *that with uterine prolapse (618.2-618.4)*
enterocele (618.6)
vaginal vault prolapse following hysterectomy (618.5)

618.1 Uterine prolapse without mention of vaginal wall prolapse
Descensus uteri
Uterine prolapse:
NOS
complete

Uterine prolapse:
first degree
second degree
third degree

Excludes: *that with mention of cystocele, urethrocele, or rectocele (618.2-618.4)*

618.2 Uterovaginal prolapse, incomplete

618.3 Uterovaginal prolapse, complete

618.4 Uterovaginal prolapse, unspecified

618.5 Prolapse of vaginal vault after hysterectomy

● Code new
to this edition

▲ Revision of
existing code

④ ⑤ Fourth or fifth
digit required

618.6 Vaginal enterocele, congenital or acquired
Pelvic enterocele, congenital or acquired

618.7 Old laceration of muscles of pelvic floor

618.8 Other specified genital prolapse
Incompetence or weakening of pelvic fundus
Relaxation of vaginal outlet or pelvis

618.9 Unspecified genital prolapse

619 Fistula involving female genital tract
Excludes: *vesicorectal and intestinovesical fistula (596.1)*

619.0 Urinary-genital tract fistula, female

Fistula:
cervicovesical
ureterovaginal
urethrovaginal
urethrovesicovaginal

Fistula:
uteroureteric
uterovesical
vesicocervicovaginal
vesicovaginal

619.1 Digestive-genital tract fistula, female

Fistula:
intestinouterine
intestinovaginal
rectovaginal

Fistula:
rectovulval
sigmoidovaginal
uterorectal

619.2 Genital tract-skin fistula, female
Fistula:
uterus to abdominal wall
vaginoperineal

619.8 Other specified fistulas involving female genital tract

Fistula:
cervix
cul-de-sac (Douglas')

Fistula:
uterus
vagina

619.9 Unspecified fistula involving female genital tract

620 Noninflammatory disorders of ovary, fallopian tube, and broad ligament
Excludes: *hydrosalpinx (614.1)*

620.0 Follicular cyst of ovary
Cyst of graafian follicle

620.1 Corpus luteum cyst or hematoma
Corpus luteum hemorrhage or rupture
Lutein cyst

620.2 Other and unspecified ovarian cyst
Cyst:
NOS of ovary
corpus albicans of ovary
retention NOS of ovary
serous of ovary
theca-lutein of ovary
Simple cystoma of ovary

Excludes: *cystadenoma (benign) (serous) (220)*
developmental cysts (752.0)
neoplastic cysts (220)
polycystic ovaries (256.4)
Stein-Leventhal syndrome (256.4)

620.3 Acquired atrophy of ovary and fallopian tube
Senile involution of ovary

620.4 Prolapse or hernia of ovary and fallopian tube
Displacement of ovary and fallopian tube
Salpingocele

620.5 Torsion of ovary, ovarian pedicle, or fallopian tube
Torsion:
accessory tube
hydatid of Morgagni

620.6 Broad ligament laceration syndrome
Masters-Allen syndrome

620.7 Hematoma of broad ligament
Hematocele, broad ligament

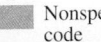 Add 4th or 5th digit   Nonspecific code   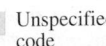 Unspecified code   Manifestation code

620.8 **Other noninflammatory disorders of ovary, fallopian tube, and broad ligament**
Cyst of broad ligament or fallopian tube
Polyp of broad ligament or fallopian tube
Infarction of ovary or fallopian tube
Rupture of ovary or fallopian tube
Hematosalpinx

Excludes: *hematosalpinx in ectopic pregnancy (639.2)*
peritubal adhesions (614.6)
torsion of ovary, ovarian pedicle, or fallopian tube (620.5)

620.9 **Unspecified noninflammatory disorder of ovary, fallopian tube, and broad ligament**

621 **Disorders of uterus, not elsewhere classified**

621.0 **Polyp of corpus uteri**
Polyp:
endometrium
uterus NOS

Excludes: *cervical polyp NOS (622.7)*

621.1 **Chronic subinvolution of uterus**
Excludes: *puerperal (674.8)*

621.2 **Hypertrophy of uterus**
Bulky or enlarged uterus

Excludes: *puerperal (674.8)*

621.3 **Endometrial cystic hyperplasia**
Hyperplasia (adenomatous) (cystic) (glandular) of endometrium
Hyperplastic endometritis

621.4 **Hematometra**
Hemometra

Excludes: *that in congenital anomaly (752.2-752.3)*

621.5 **Intrauterine synechiae**
Adhesions of uterus   Band(s) of uterus

621.6 **Malposition of uterus**
Anteversion of uterus
Retroflexion of uterus
Retroversion of uterus

Excludes: *malposition complicating pregnancy, labor, or delivery (654.3-654.4)*
prolapse of uterus (618.1-618.4)

621.7 **Chronic inversion of uterus**
Excludes: *current obstetrical trauma (665.2)*
prolapse of uterus (618.1-618.4)

621.8 **Other specified disorders of uterus, not elsewhere classified**
Atrophy, acquired of uterus
Cyst of uterus
Fibrosis NOS of uterus
Old laceration (postpartum) of uterus
Ulcer of uterus

Excludes: *bilharzial fibrosis (120.0-120.9)*
endometriosis (617.0)
fistulas (619.0-619.8)
inflammatory diseases (615.0-615.9)

621.9 **Unspecified disorder of uterus**

622 **Noninflammatory disorders of cervix**
Excludes: *abnormality of cervix complicating pregnancy, labor, or delivery (654.5-654.6)*
fistula (619.0-619.8)

622.0 **Erosion and ectropion of cervix**
Eversion of cervix
Ulcer of cervix

Excludes: *that in chronic cervicitis (616.0)*

● Code new
to this edition   ▲ Revision of
existing code   ④ ⑤ Fourth or fifth
digit required

622.1 Dysplasia of cervix (uteri)
Anaplasia of cervix
Cervical atypism
Cervical intraepithelial neoplasia I (CIN I)
Cervical intraepithelial neoplasia II (CIN II)
High grade squamous intraepithelial dysplasia (HGSIL)
Low grade squamous intraepithelial dysplasia (LGSIL)

| Excludes: | carcinoma in situ of cervix (233.1)
cervical intraepithelial neoplasia III [CIN III] (233.1) |

622.2 Leukoplakia of cervix (uteri)

| Excludes: | carcinoma in situ of cervix (233.1) |

622.3 Old laceration of cervix
Adhesions of cervix
Band(s) of cervix
Cicatrix (postpartum) of cervix

| Excludes: | current obstetrical trauma (665.3) |

622.4 Stricture and stenosis of cervix
Atresia (acquired) of cervix
Contracture of cervix
Occlusion of cervix
Pinpoint os uteri of cervix

| Excludes: | congenital (752.49)
that complicating labor (654.6) |

622.5 Incompetence of cervix

| Excludes: | complicating pregnancy (654.5)
that affecting fetus or newborn (761.0) |

622.6 Hypertrophic elongation of cervix

622.7 Mucous polyp of cervix
Polyp NOS of cervix

| Excludes: | adenomatous polyp of cervix (219.0) |

622.8 Other specified noninflammatory disorders of cervix
Atrophy (senile) of cervix
Cyst of cervix
Fibrosis of cervix
Hemorrhage of cervix

| Excludes: | endometriosis (617.0)
fistula (619.0-619.8)
inflammatory diseases (616.0) |

622.9 Unspecified noninflammatory disorder of cervix

623 Noninflammatory disorders of vagina

| Excludes: | abnormality of vagina complicating pregnancy, labor, or delivery (654.7)
congenital absence of vagina (752.49)
congenital diaphragm or bands (752.49)
fistulas involving vagina (619.0-619.8) |

623.0 Dysplasia of vagina

| Excludes: | carcinoma in situ of vagina (233.3) |

623.1 Leukoplakia of vagina

623.2 Stricture or atresia of vagina
Adhesions (postoperative) (postradiation) of vagina
Occlusion of vagina
Stenosis, vagina

Use additional E code, if desired, to identify any external cause

| Excludes: | congenital atresia or stricture (752.49) |

623.3 Tight hymenal ring
Rigid hymen acquired or congenital
Tight hymenal ring acquired or congenital
Tight introitus acquired or congenital

| Excludes: | imperforate hymen (752.42) |

| | Add 4th or 5th digit | | Nonspecific code | | Unspecified code | | Manifestation code |

623.4 Old vaginal laceration

[Excludes:] *old laceration involving muscles of pelvic floor (618.7)*

623.5 Leukorrhea, not specified as infective

Leukorrhea NOS of vagina
Vaginal discharge NOS

[Excludes:] *trichomonal (131.00)*

623.6 Vaginal hematoma

[Excludes:] *current obstetrical trauma (665.7)*

623.7 Polyp of vagina

623.8 Other specified noninflammatory disorders of vagina

Cyst of vagina
Hemorrhage of vagina

623.9 Unspecified noninflammatory disorder of vagina

624 Noninflammatory disorders of vulva and perineum

[Excludes:] *abnormality of vulva and perineum complicating pregnancy, labor, or delivery (654.8)*
condyloma acuminatum (078.1)
fistulas involving:
perineum—see Alphabetic Index
vulva (619.0-619.8)
vulval varices (456.6)
vulvar involvement in skin conditions (690-709.9)

624.0 Dystrophy of vulva

Kraurosis of vulva
Leukoplakia of vulva

[Excludes:] *carcinoma in situ of vulva (233.3)*

624.1 Atrophy of vulva

624.2 Hypertrophy of clitoris

[Excludes:] *that in endocrine disorders (255.2, 256.1)*

624.3 Hypertrophy of labia

Hypertrophy of vulva NOS

624.4 Old laceration or scarring of vulva

624.5 Hematoma of vulva

[Excludes:] *that complicating delivery (664.5)*

624.6 Polyp of labia and vulva

624.8 Other specified noninflammatory disorders of vulva and perineum

Cyst of vulva
Edema of vulva
Stricture of vulva

624.9 Unspecified noninflammatory disorder of vulva and perineum

625 Pain and other symptoms associated with female genital organs

625.0 Dyspareunia

[Excludes:] *psychogenic dyspareunia (302.76)*

625.1 Vaginismus

Colpospasm
Vulvismus

[Excludes:] *psychogenic vaginismus (306.51)*

625.2 Mittelschmerz

Intermenstrual pain
Ovulation pain

625.3 Dysmenorrhea

Painful menstruation

[Excludes:] *psychogenic dysmenorrhea (306.52)*

625.4 Premenstrual tension syndromes

Menstrual:
migraine
molimen
Premenstrual syndrome
Premenstrual tension NOS

● Code new to this edition ▲ Revision of existing code ④ ⑤ Fourth or fifth digit required

625.5 Pelvic congestion syndrome
Congestion-fibrosis syndrome
Taylor's syndrome

625.6 Stress incontinence, female
Excludes: mixed incontinence (788.33)
stress incontinence, male (788.32)

625.8 Other specified symptoms associated with female genital organs

625.9 Unspecified symptom associated with female genital organs

626 Disorders of menstruation and other abnormal bleeding from female genital tract
Excludes: menopausal and premenopausal bleeding (627.0)
pain and other symptoms associated with menstrual cycle (625.2-625.4)
postmenopausal bleeding (627.1)

626.0 Absence of menstruation
Amenorrhea (primary) (secondary)

626.1 Scanty or infrequent menstruation
Hypomenorrhea   Oligomenorrhea

626.2 Excessive or frequent menstruation
Heavy periods   Menorrhagia
Menometrorrhagia   Polymenorrhea
Excludes: premenopausal (627.0)
that in puberty (626.3)

626.3 Puberty bleeding
Excessive bleeding associated with onset of menstrual periods
Pubertal menorrhagia

626.4 Irregular menstrual cycle
Irregular:
bleeding NOS
menstruation
periods

626.5 Ovulation bleeding
Regular intermenstrual bleeding

626.6 Metrorrhagia
Bleeding unrelated to menstrual cycle
Irregular intermenstrual bleeding

626.7 Postcoital bleeding

626.8 Other
Dysfunctional or functional uterine hemorrhage NOS
Menstruation:
retained
suppression of

626.9 Unspecified

627 Menopausal and postmenopausal disorders
Excludes: asymptomatic age-related (natural) postmenopausal status (V49.81)

627.0 Premenopausal menorrhagia
Excessive bleeding   Menorrhagia:
associated   climacteric
with onset of menopause   menopausal
preclimacteric

627.1 Postmenopausal bleeding

▲ **627.2 Symptomatic menopausal or female climacteric states**
Symptoms, such as flushing, sleeplessness, headache, lack of concentration, associated with the menopause

627.3 Postmenopausal atrophic vaginitis
Senile (atrophic) vaginitis

▲ **627.4 Symptomatic states associated with artificial menopause**
Postartificial menopause syndromes
Any condition classifiable to 627.1, 627.2, or 627.3 which follows induced menopause

627.8 Other specified menopausal and postmenopausal disorders
Excludes: premature menopause NOS (256.31)

627.9 Unspecified menopausal and postmenopausal disorder

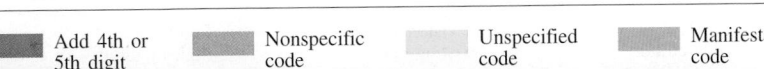

| | Add 4th or 5th digit | | Nonspecific code | | Unspecified code | | Manifestation code |

628 **Infertility, female**
Includes: primary and secondary sterility

628.0 **Associated with anovulation**
Anovulatory cycle
Use additional code for any associated Stein-Leventhal syndrome (256.4)

628.1 *Of pituitary-hypothalamic origin*
Code first underlying cause, as:
adiposogenital dystrophy (253.8)
anterior pituitary disorder (253.0-253.4)

628.2 **Of tubal origin**
Infertility associated with congenital anomaly of tube
Tubal:
block
occlusion
stenosis
Use additional code for any associated peritubal adhesions (614.6)

628.3 **Of uterine origin**
Infertility associated with congenital anomaly of uterus
Nonimplantation
Use additional code for any associated tuberculous endometritis (016.7)

628.4 **Of cervical or vaginal origin**
Infertility associated with:
anomaly of cervical mucus
congenital structural anomaly
dysmucorrhea

628.8 **Of other specified origin**

628.9 **Of unspecified origin**

629 **Other disorders of female genital organs**

629.0 **Hematocele, female, not elsewhere classified**
Excludes: *hematocele or hematoma:*
broad ligament (620.7)
fallopian tube (620.8)
that associated with ectopic pregnancy (633.00-633.91)
uterus (621.4)
vagina (623.6)
vulva (624.5)

629.1 **Hydrocele, canal of Nuck**
Cyst of canal of Nuck (acquired)
Excludes: *congenital (752.41)*

629.8 **Other specified disorders of female genital organs**

629.9 **Unspecified disorder of female genital organs**
Habitual aborter without current pregnancy

● Code new
to this edition
▲ Revision of
existing code
④ ⑤ Fourth or fifth
digit required

11. COMPLICATIONS OF PREGNANCY, CHILDBIRTH, AND THE PUERPERIUM (630-677)

ECTOPIC AND MOLAR PREGNANCY (630-633)

Use additional code from category 639 to identify any complications

630 Hydatidiform mole
Trophoblastic disease NOS
Vesicular mole

[*Excludes:*] *chorioadenoma (destruens) (236.1)*
chorionepithelioma (181)
malignant hydatidiform mole (236.1)

631 Other abnormal product of conception
Blighted ovum
Mole:
NOS
carneous
Mole:
fleshy
stone

632 Missed abortion
Early fetal death before completion of 22 weeks' gestation with retention of dead fetus
Retained products of conception, not following spontaneous or induced abortion or delivery

[*Excludes:*] *failed induced abortion (638.0-638.9)*
fetal death (intrauterine) (late) (656.4)
missed delivery (656.4)
that with abnormal product of conception (630, 631)

633 Ectopic pregnancy
Includes: ruptured ectopic pregnancy

[5] **633.0 Abdominal pregnancy**
Intraperitoneal pregnancy

● **633.00 Abdominal pregnancy without intrauterine pregnancy**

● **633.01 Abdominal pregnancy with intrauterine pregnancy**

[5] **633.1 Tubal pregnancy**
Fallopian pregnancy
Rupture of (fallopian) tube due to pregnancy
Tubal abortion

● **633.10 Tubal pregnancy without intrauterine pregnancy**

● **633.11 Tubal pregnancy with intrauterine pregnancy**

[5] **633.2 Ovarian pregnancy**

● **633.20 Ovarian pregnancy without intrauterine pregnancy**

● **633.21 Ovarian pregnancy with intrauterine pregnancy**

[5] **633.8 Other ectopic pregnancy**
Pregnancy:
cervical
combined
cornual
Pregnancy:
intraligamentous
mesometric
mural

● **633.80 Other ectopic pregnancy without intrauterine pregnancy**

● **633.81 Other ectopic pregnancy with intrauterine pregnancy**

[5] **633.9 Unspecified ectopic pregnancy**

● **633.90 Unspecified ectopic pregnancy without intrauterine pregnancy**

● **633.91 Unspecified ectopic pregnancy with intrauterine pregnancy**

OTHER PREGNANCY WITH ABORTIVE OUTCOME (634-639)

Note: Use the following fifth-digit subclassification with categories 634-637:

0 Unspecified

1 Incomplete

2 Complete

The following fourth-digit subdivisions are for use with categories 634-638:

.0 Complicated by genital tract and pelvic infection
Endometritis
Salpingo-oophoritis
Sepsis NOS
Septicemia NOS
Any condition classifiable to 639.0, with condition classifiable to 634-638

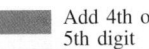

Add 4th or 5th digit | Nonspecific code | Unspecified code | Manifestation code

[Excludes:] *urinary tract infection (634-638 with .7)*

.1 Complicated by delayed or excessive hemorrhage
Afibrinogenemia
Defibrination syndrome
Intravascular hemolysis
Any condition classifiable to 639.1, with condition classifiable to 634-638

.2 Complicated by damage to pelvic organs and tissues
Laceration, perforation, or tear of:
bladder
uterus
Any condition classifiable to 639.2, with condition classifiable to 634-638

.3 Complicated by renal failure
Oliguria
Uremia
Any condition classifiable to 639.3, with condition classifiable to 634-638

.4 Complicated by metabolic disorder
Electrolyte imbalance with conditions classifiable to 634-638

.5 Complicated by shock
Circulatory collapse
Shock (postoperative) (septic)
Any condition classifiable to 639.5, with condition classifiable to 634-638

.6 Complicated by embolism
Embolism:
NOS
amniotic fluid
pulmonary
Any condition classifiable to 639.6, with condition classifiable to 634-638

.7 With other specified complications
Cardiac arrest or failure
Urinary tract infection
Any condition classifiable to 639.8, with condition classifiable to 634-638

.8 With unspecified complication

.9 Without mention of complication

[5] 634 Abortion
Includes: miscarriage
spontaneous abortion

- [5] **634.0 Complicated by genital tract and pelvic infection**
- [5] **634.1 Complicated by delayed or excessive hemorrhage**
- [5] **634.2 Complicated by damage to pelvic organs or tissues**
- [5] **634.3 Complicated by renal failure**
- [5] **634.4 Complicated by metabolic disorder**
- [5] **634.5 Complicated by shock**
- [5] **634.6 Complicated by embolism**
- [5] **634.7 With other specified complications**
- [5] **634.8 With unspecified complication**
- [5] **634.9 Without mention of complication**

[5] 635 Legally induced abortion
Includes: abortion or termination of pregnancy:
elective
legal
therapeutic

[Excludes:] *menstrual extraction or regulation (V25.3)*

- [5] **635.0 Complicated by genital tract and pelvic infection**
- [5] **635.1 Complicated by delayed or excessive hemorrhage**
- [5] **635.2 Complicated by damage to pelvic organs or tissues**
- [5] **635.3 Complicated by renal failure**
- [5] **635.4 Complicated by metabolic disorder**
- [5] **635.5 Complicated by shock**
- [5] **635.6 Complicated by embolism**
- [5] **635.7 With other specified complications**

[5] **635.8 With unspecified complication**

[5] **635.9 Without mention of complication**

[5] **636 Illegally induced abortion**

Includes: abortion:
criminal
illegal
self-induced

[5] **636.0 Complicated by genital tract and pelvic infection**

[5] **636.1 Complicated by delayed or excessive hemorrhage**

[5] **636.2 Complicated by damage to pelvic organs or tissues**

[5] **636.3 Complicated by renal failure**

[5] **636.4 Complicated by metabolic disorder**

[5] **636.5 Complicated by shock**

[5] **636.6 Complicated by embolism**

[5] **636.7 With other specified complications**

[5] **636.8 With unspecified complication**

[5] **636.9 Without mention of complication**

[5] **637 Unspecified abortion**

Includes: abortion NOS
retained products of conception following abortion, not classifiable elsewhere

[5] **637.0 Complicated by genital tract and pelvic infection**

[5] **637.1 Complicated by delayed or excessive hemorrhage**

[5] **637.2 Complicated by damage to pelvic organs or tissues**

[5] **637.3 Complicated by renal failure**

[5] **637.4 Complicated by metabolic disorder**

[5] **637.5 Complicated by shock**

[5] **637.6 Complicated by embolism**

[5] **637.7 With other specified complications**

[5] **637.8 With unspecified complication**

[5] **637.9 Without mention of complication**

638 Failed attempted abortion

Includes: failure of attempted induction of (legal) abortion

[Excludes:] incomplete abortion (634.0-637.9)

638.0 Complicated by genital tract and pelvic infection

638.1 Complicated by delayed or excessive hemorrhage

638.2 Complicated by damage to pelvic organs or tissues

638.3 Complicated by renal failure

638.4 Complicated by metabolic disorder

638.5 Complicated by shock

638.6 Complicated by embolism

638.7 With other specified complications

638.8 With unspecified complication

638.9 Without mention of complication

639 Complications following abortion and ectopic and molar pregnancies

Note: This category is provided for use when it is required to classify separately the complications classifiable to the fourth-digit level in categories 634-638; for example:

a) when the complication itself was responsible for an episode of medical care, the abortion, ectopic or molar pregnancy itself having been dealt with at a previous episode

b) when these conditions are immediate complications of ectopic or molar pregnancies classifiable to 630-633 where they cannot be identified at fourth-digit level.

639.0 Genital tract and pelvic infection
Endometritis following conditions classifiable to 630-638
Parametritis following conditions classifiable to 630-638
Pelvic peritonitis following conditions classifiable to 630-638
Salpingitis following conditions classifiable to 630-638
Salpingo-oophoritis following conditions classifiable to 630-638
Sepsis NOS following conditions classifiable to 630-638
Septicemia NOS following conditions classifiable to 630-638

| Excludes: | urinary tract infection (639.8) |

639.1 Delayed or excessive hemorrhage
Afibrinogenemia following conditions classifiable to 630-638
Defibrination syndrome following conditions classifiable to 630-638
Intravascular hemolysis following conditions classifiable to 630-638

639.2 Damage to pelvic organs and tissues
Laceration, perforation, or tear of:
bladder following conditions classifiable to 630-638
bowel following conditions classifiable to 630-638
broad ligament following conditions classifiable to 630-638
cervix following conditions classifiable to 630-638
periurethral tissue following conditions classifiable to 630-638
uterus following conditions classifiable to 630-638
vagina following conditions classifiable to 630-638

639.3 Renal failure
Oliguria following conditions classifiable to 630-638
Renal: following conditions classifiable to 630-638
failure (acute) following conditions classifiable to 630-638
shutdown following conditions classifiable to 630-638
tubular necrosis following conditions classifiable to 630-638
Uremia following conditions classifiable to 630-638

639.4 Metabolic disorders
Electrolyte imbalance following conditions classifiable to 630-638

639.5 Shock
Circulatory collapse following conditions classifiable to 630-638
Shock (postoperative) (septic) following conditions classifiable to 630-638

639.6 Embolism
Embolism NOS following conditions classifiable to 630-638
Embolism, air following conditions classifiable to 630-638
Embolism, amniotic fluid following conditions classifiable to 630-638
Embolism, blood-clot following conditions classifiable to 630-638
Embolism, fat following conditions classifiable to 630-638
Embolism, pulmonary following conditions classifiable to 630-638
Embolism, pyemic following conditions classifiable to 630-638
Embolism, septic following conditions classifiable to 630-638
Embolism, soap following conditions classifiable to 630-638

639.8 Other specified complications following abortion or ectopic and molar pregnancy
Acute yellow atrophy or necrosis of liver following conditions classifiable to 630-638
Cardiac arrest or failure following conditions classifiable to 630-638
Cerebral anoxia following conditions classifiable to 630-638
Urinary tract infection following conditions classifiable to 630-638

639.9 Unspecified complication following abortion or ectopic and molar pregnancy
Complication(s) not further specified following conditions classifiable to 630-638

COMPLICATIONS MAINLY RELATED TO PREGNANCY (640-648)

Includes: listed conditions even if it arose or was present during labor, delivery, or puerperium

The following fifth-digit subclassification is for use with categories 640-648 to denote the current episode of care:

0 unspecified as to episode of care or not applicable

1 delivered, with or without mention of antepartum condition
Antepartum condition with delivery
Delivery NOS (with mention of antepartum complication during current episode of care)
Intrapartum obstetric condition (with mention of antepartum complication during current episode of care)
Pregnancy, delivered (with mention of antepartum complication during current episode of care)

2 delivered, with mention of postpartum complication
Delivery with mention of puerperal complication during current episode of care

● Code new
　to this edition
▲ Revision of
　existing code
④ ⑤ Fourth or fifth
　　digit required

3 antepartum condition or complication
Antepartum obstetric condition, not delivered during the current episode of care

4 postpartum condition or complication
Postpartum or puerperal obstetric condition or complication following delivery that occurred:
during previous episode of care
outside hospital, with subsequent admission for observation or care

[5] **640 Hemorrhage in early pregnancy**
Includes: hemorrhage before completion of 22 weeks' gestation

[5] **640.0 Threatened abortion**
[0,1,3]

[5] **640.8 Other specified hemorrhage in early pregnancy**
[0,1,3]

[5] **640.9 Unspecified hemorrhage in early pregnancy**
[0,1,3]

[5] **641 Antepartum hemorrhage, abruptio placentae, and placenta previa**

[5] **641.0 Placenta previa without hemorrhage**
[0,1,3] Low implantation of placenta
Placenta previa noted:
during pregnancy without hemorrhage
before labor (and delivered by cesarean delivery) without hemorrhage

[5] **641.1 Hemorrhage from placenta previa**
[0,1,3] Low-lying placenta NOS or with hemorrhage (intrapartum)
Placenta previa NOS or with hemorrhage (intrapartum)
incomplete NOS or with hemorrhage (intrapartum)
marginal NOS or with hemorrhage (intrapartum)
partial NOS or with hemorrhage (intrapartum)
total NOS or with hemorrhage (intrapartum)

[*Excludes:*] *hemorrhage from vasa previa (663.5)*

[5] **641.2 Premature separation of placenta**
[0,1,3] Ablatio placentae
Abruptio placentae
Accidental antepartum hemorrhage
Couvelaire uterus
Detachment of placenta (premature)
Premature separation of normally implanted placenta

[5] **641.3 Antepartum hemorrhage associated with coagulation defects**
[0,1,3] Antepartum or intrapartum hemorrhage associated with:
afibrinogenemia
hyperfibrinolysis
hypofibrinogenemia

[5] **641.8 Other antepartum hemorrhage**
[0,1,3] Antepartum or intrapartum hemorrhage associated with:
trauma
uterine leiomyoma

[5] **641.9 Unspecified antepartum hemorrhage**
[0,1,3] Hemorrhage antepartum NOS
Hemorrhage intrapartum NOS
Hemorrhage of pregnancy NOS

[5] **642 Hypertension complicating pregnancy, childbirth, and the puerperium**

[5] **642.0 Benign essential hypertension complicating pregnancy, childbirth, and the puerperium**
[0-4] Hypertension:
benign essential specified as complicating, or as a reason for obstetric care during pregnancy, childbirth, or the puerperium
chronic NOS specified as complicating, or as a reason for obstetric care during pregnancy, childbirth, or the puerperium
essential specified as complicating, or as a reason for obstetric care during pregnancy, childbirth, or the puerperium
pre-existing NOS specified as complicating, or as a reason for obstetric care during pregnancy, childbirth, or the puerperium

[5] **642.1 Hypertension secondary to renal disease, complicating pregnancy, childbirth, and the puerperium**
[0-4] Hypertension secondary to renal disease, specified as complicating, or as a reason for obstetric care during pregnancy, childbirth, or the puerperium

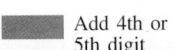

[5] **642.2 Other pre-existing hypertension complicating pregnancy, childbirth, and the puerperium**
[0-4] Hypertensive:
heart and renal disease specified as complicating, as a reason for obstetric care during pregnancy, childbirth, or the puerperium
heart disease specified as complicating, as a reason for obstetric care during pregnancy, childbirth, or the puerperium
renal disease specified as complicating, as a reason for obstetric care during pregnancy, childbirth, or the puerperium
Malignant hypertension specified as complicating, as a reason for obstetric care during pregnancy, childbirth, or the puerperium

[5] **642.3 Transient hypertension of pregnancy**
[0-4] Gestational hypertension
Transient hypertension, so described, in pregnancy, childbirth, or the puerperium

[5] **642.4 Mild or unspecified pre-eclampsia**
[0-4] Hypertension in pregnancy, childbirth, or the puerperium, not specified as pre-existing, with either albuminuria or edema, or both; mild or unspecified
Pre-eclampsia:
NOS
mild
Toxemia (pre-eclamptic):
NOS
mild

[Excludes:] *albuminuria in pregnancy, without mention of hypertension (646.2)*
edema in pregnancy, without mention of hypertension (646.1)

[5] **642.5 Severe pre-eclampsia**
[0-4] Hypertension in pregnancy, childbirth, or the puerperium, not specified as pre-existing, with either albuminuria or edema, or both; specified as severe
Pre-eclampsia, severe
Toxemia (pre-eclamptic), severe

[5] **642.6 Eclampsia**
[0-4] Toxemia:
eclamptic
with convulsions

[5] **642.7 Pre-eclampsia or eclampsia superimposed on pre-existing hypertension**
[0-4] Conditions classifiable to 642.4-642.6, with conditions classifiable to 642.0-642.2

[5] **642.9 Unspecified hypertension complicating pregnancy, childbirth, or the puerperium**
[0-4] Hypertension NOS, without mention of albuminuria or edema, complicating pregnancy, childbirth, or the puerperium

[5] **643 Excessive vomiting in pregnancy**
Includes:
hyperemesis arising during pregnancy
vomiting:
persistent, arising during pregnancy
vicious, arising during pregnancy
hyperemesis gravidarum

[5] **643.0 Mild hyperemesis gravidarum**
[0,1,3] Hyperemesis gravidarum, mild or unspecified, starting before the end of the 22nd week of gestation

[5] **643.1 Hyperemesis gravidarum with metabolic disturbance**
[0,1,3] Hyperemesis gravidarum, starting before the end of the 22nd week of gestation, with metabolic disturbance, such as:
carbohydrate depletion
dehydration
electrolyte imbalance

[5] **643.2 Late vomiting of pregnancy**
[0,1,3] Excessive vomiting starting after 22 completed weeks of gestation

[5] **643.8 Other vomiting complicating pregnancy**
[0,1,3] Vomiting due to organic disease or other cause, specified as complicating pregnancy, or as a reason for obstetric care during pregnancy
Use additional code, if desired, to specify cause

[5] **643.9 Unspecified vomiting of pregnancy**
[0,1,3] Vomiting as a reason for care during pregnancy, length of gestation unspecified

[5] **644 Early or threatened labor**

[5] **644.0 Threatened premature labor**
[0,3] Premature labor after 22 weeks, but before 37 completed weeks of gestation without delivery

[Excludes:] *that occurring before 22 completed weeks of gestation (640.0)*

● Code new to this edition ▲ Revision of existing code [4] [5] Fourth or fifth digit required

[5] **644.1 Other threatened labor**
[0,3] False labor:
NOS without delivery
after 37 completed weeks of gestation without delivery
Threatened labor NOS without delivery

[5] **644.2 Early onset of delivery**
[0,1] Onset (spontaneous) of delivery before 37 completed weeks of gestation
Premature labor with onset of delivery before 37 completed weeks of gestation

[5] **645 Late pregnancy**

[5] **645.1 Post term pregnancy**
[0,1,3] Pregnancy over 40 completed weeks to 42 completed weeks gestation

[5] **645.2 Prolonged pregnancy**
[0,1,3] Pregnancy which has advanced beyond 42 completed weeks gestation

[5] **646 Other complications of pregnancy, not elsewhere classified**
Use additional code(s) to further specify complication

[5] **646.0 Papyraceous fetus**
[0,1,3]

[5] **646.1 Edema or excessive weight gain in pregnancy, without mention of hypertension**
[0-4] Gestational edema
Maternal obesity syndrome

[Excludes:] *that with mention of hypertension (642.0-642.9)*

[5] **646.2 Unspecified renal disease in pregnancy, without mention of hypertension**
[0-4] Albuminuria in pregnancy or the puerperium, without mention of hypertension
Nephropathy NOS in pregnancy or the puerperium, without mention of hypertension
Renal disease NOS in pregnancy or the puerperium, without mention of hypertension
Uremia in pregnancy or the puerperium, without mention of hypertension
Gestational proteinuria in pregnancy or the puerperium, without mention of hypertension

[Excludes:] *that with mention of hypertension (642.0-642.9)*

[5] **646.3 Habitual aborter**
[0,1,3]

[Excludes:] *with current abortion (634.0-634.9)*
without current pregnancy (629.9)

[5] **646.4 Peripheral neuritis in pregnancy**
[0-4]

[5] **646.5 Asymptomatic bacteriuria in pregnancy**
[0-4]

[5] **646.6 Infections of genitourinary tract in pregnancy**
[0-4] Conditions classifiable to 590, 595, 597, 599.0, 616 complicating pregnancy, childbirth, or the puerperium
Conditions classifiable to 614.0-614.5, 617.7-614.9, 615

[Excludes:] *major puerperal infection (670)*

[5] **646.7 Liver disorders in pregnancy**
[0,1,3] Acute yellow atrophy of liver (obstetric) (true) of pregnancy
Icterus gravis of pregnancy
Necrosis of liver of pregnancy

[Excludes:] *hepatorenal syndrome following delivery (674.8)*
viral hepatitis (647.6)

[5] **646.8 Other specified complications of pregnancy**
[0-4] Fatigue during pregnancy
Herpes gestationis
Insufficient weight gain of pregnancy
Uterine size-date discrepancy

[5] **646.9 Unspecified complication of pregnancy**
[0,1,3]

[5] **647 Infectious and parasitic conditions in the mother classifiable elsewhere, but complicating pregnancy, childbirth, or the puerperium**
Includes: the listed conditions when complicating the pregnant state, aggravated by the pregnancy, or when a main reason for obstetric care

[Excludes:] *those conditions in the mother known or suspected to have affected the fetus (655.0-655.9)*

Use additional code(s) to further specify complication

Add 4th or 5th digit | Nonspecific code | Unspecified code | Manifestation code

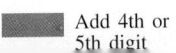

[5] **647.0 Syphilis**
[0-4] Conditions classifiable to 090-097

[5] **647.1 Gonorrhea**
[0-4] Conditions classifiable to 098

[5] **647.2 Other venereal diseases**
[0-4] Conditions classifiable to 099

[5] **647.3 Tuberculosis**
[0-4] Conditions classifiable to 010-018

[5] **647.4 Malaria**
[0-4] Conditions classifiable to 084

[5] **647.5 Rubella**
[0-4] Conditions classifiable to 056

[5] **647.6 Other viral diseases**
[0-4] Conditions classifiable to 042 and 050-079, except 056

[5] **647.8 Other specified infectious and parasitic diseases**
[0-4]

[5] **647.9 Unspecified infection or infestation**
[0-4]

[5] **648 Other current conditions in the mother classifiable elsewhere, but complicating pregnancy, childbirth, or the puerperium**

Includes: the listed conditions when complicating the pregnant state, aggravated by the pregnancy, or when a main reason for obstetric care

[Excludes:] *those conditions in the mother known or suspected to have affected the fetus (655.0-655.9)*

Use additional code(s) to identify the condition

[5] **648.0 Diabetes mellitus**
[0-4] Conditions classifiable to 250

[Excludes:] *gestational diabetes (648.8)*

[5] **648.1 Thyroid dysfunction**
[0-4] Conditions classifiable to 240-246

[5] **648.2 Anemia**
[0-4] Conditions classifiable to 280-285

[5] **648.3 Drug dependence**
[0-4] Conditions classifiable to 304

[5] **648.4 Mental disorders**
[0-4] Conditions classifiable to 290-303, 305-316, 317-319

[5] **648.5 Congenital cardiovascular disorders**
[0-4] Conditions classifiable to 745-747

[5] **648.6 Other cardiovascular diseases**
[0-4] Conditions classifiable to 390-398, 410-429

[Excludes:] *cerebrovascular disorders in the puerperium (674.0)*
venous complications (671.0-671.9)

[5] **648.7 Bone and joint disorders of back, pelvis, and lower limbs**
[0-4] Conditions classifiable to 720-724, and those classifiable to 711-719 or 725-738, specified as affecting the lower limbs

[5] **648.8 Abnormal glucose tolerance**
[0-4] Conditions classifiable to 790.2
Gestational diabetes

[5] **648.9 Other current conditions classifiable elsewhere**
[0-4] Conditions classifiable to 440-459
Nutritional deficiencies [conditions classifiable to 260-269]

● Code new to this edition ▲ Revision of existing code [4] [5] Fourth or fifth digit required

NORMAL DELIVERY, AND OTHER INDICATIONS FOR CARE IN PREGNANCY, LABOR, AND DELIVERY (650-659)

650 Normal delivery

Delivery requiring minimal or no assistance, with or without episiotomy, without fetal manipulation [e.g., rotation version] or instrumentation [forceps] of spontaneous, cephalic, vaginal, full-term, single, live born infant. This code is for use as a single diagnosis code and is not to be used with any other code in the range 630-676.

[Excludes:] *breech delivery (assisted) (spontaneous) NOS (652.2)*
delivery by vacuum extractor, forceps, cesarean section, or breech extraction, without specified complication (669.5-669.7)

Use additional code to indicate outcome of delivery (V27.0)

The following fifth-digit subclassification is for use with categories 651-659 to denote the current episode of care:

- **0 unspecified as to episode of care or not applicable**
- **1 delivered, with or without mention of antepartum condition**
- **2 delivered, with mention of postpartum complication**
- **3 antepartum condition or complication**
- **4 postpartum condition or complication**

[5] **651 Multiple gestation**

[5] **651.0 Twin pregnancy**
[0,1,3]

[5] **651.1 Triplet pregnancy**
[0,1,3]

[5] **651.2 Quadruplet pregnancy**
[0,1,3]

[5] **651.3 Twin pregnancy with fetal loss and retention of one fetus**
[0,1,3]

[5] **651.4 Triplet pregnancy with fetal loss and retention of one or more fetus(es)**
[0,1,3]

[5] **651.5 Quadruplet pregnancy with fetal loss and retention of one or more fetus(es)**
[0,1,3]

[5] **651.6 Other multiple pregnancy with fetal loss and retention of one or more fetus(es)**
[0,1,3]

[5] **651.8 Other specified multiple gestation**
[0,1,3]

[5] **651.9 Unspecified multiple gestation**
[0,1,3]

[5] **652 Malposition and malpresentation of fetus**
Code first any associated obstructed labor (660.0)

[5] **652.0 Unstable lie**
[0,1,3]

[5] **652.1 Breech or other malpresentation successfully converted to cephalic presentation**
[0,1,3] Cephalic version NOS

[5] **652.2 Breech presentation without mention of version**
[0,1,3] Breech delivery (assisted) (spontaneous) NOS
Buttocks presentation
Complete breech
Frank breech

[Excludes:] *footling presentation (652.8)*
incomplete breech (652.8)

[5] **652.3 Transverse or oblique presentation**
[0,1,3] Oblique lie — Transverse lie

[Excludes:] *transverse arrest of fetal head (660.3)*

[5] **652.4 Face or brow presentation**
[0,1,3] Mentum presentation

[5] **652.5 High head at term**
[0,1,3] Failure of head to enter pelvic brim

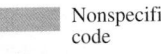

Add 4th or 5th digit — Nonspecific code — Unspecified code — Manifestation code

⑤ **652.6 Multiple gestation with malpresentation of one fetus or more**
[0,1,3]

⑤ **652.7 Prolapsed arm**
[0,1,3]

⑤ **652.8 Other specified malposition or malpresentation**
[0,1,3]   Compound presentation

⑤ **652.9 Unspecified malposition or malpresentation**
[0,1,3]

⑤ **653 Disproportion**
Code first any associated obstructed labor (660.1)

⑤ **653.0 Major abnormality of bony pelvis, not further specified**
[0,1,3]   Pelvic deformity NOS

⑤ **653.1 Generally contracted pelvis**
[0,1,3]   Contracted pelvis NOS

⑤ **653.2 Inlet contraction of pelvis**
[0,1,3]   Inlet contraction (pelvis)

⑤ **653.3 Outlet contraction of pelvis**
[0,1,3]   Outlet contraction (pelvis)

⑤ **653.4 Fetopelvic disproportion**
[0,1,3]   Cephalopelvic disproportion NOS
Disproportion of mixed maternal and fetal origin, with normally formed fetus

⑤ **653.5 Unusually large fetus causing disproportion**
[0,1,3]   Disproportion of fetal origin with normally formed fetus
Fetal disproportion NOS

Excludes: *that when the reason for medical care was concern for the fetus (656.6)*

⑤ **653.6 Hydrocephalic fetus causing disproportion**
[0,1,3]

Excludes: *that when the reason for medical care was concern for the fetus (655.0)*

⑤ **653.7 Other fetal abnormality causing disproportion**
[0,1,3]   Conjoined twins   Fetal myelomeningocele
Fetal ascites   Fetal sacral teratoma
Fetal hydrops   Fetal tumor

⑤ **653.8 Disproportion of other origin**
[0,1,3]

Excludes: *shoulder (girdle) dystocia (660.4)*

⑤ **653.9 Unspecified disproportion**
[0,1,3]

⑤ **654 Abnormality of organs and soft tissues of pelvis**
Includes: the listed conditions during pregnancy, childbirth, or the puerperium
Code first any associated obstructed labor (660.2)

⑤ **654.0 Congenital abnormalities of uterus**
[0-4]   Double uterus   Uterus bicornis

⑤ **654.1 Tumors of body of uterus**
[0-4]   Uterine fibroids

⑤ **654.2 Previous cesarean delivery NOS**
[0,1,3]   Uterine scar from previous cesarean delivery

⑤ **654.3 Retroverted and incarcerated gravid uterus**
[0-4]

⑤ **654.4 Other abnormalities in shape or position of gravid uterus and of neighboring structures**
[0-4]   Cystocele   Prolapse of gravid uterus
Pelvic floor repair   Rectocele
Pendulous abdomen   Rigid pelvic floor

⑤ **654.5 Cervical incompetence**
[0-4]   Presence of Shirodkar suture with or without mention of cervical incompetence

⑤ **654.6 Other congenital or acquired abnormality of cervix**
[0-4]   Cicatricial cervix   Stenosis or stricture of cervix
Polyp of cervix   Tumor of cervix
Previous surgery to cervix
Rigid cervix (uteri)

● Code new
to this edition   ▲ Revision of
existing code   ④ ⑤ Fourth or fifth
digit required

[5] **654.7 Congenital or acquired abnormality of vagina**
[0-4]
Previous surgery to vagina
Septate vagina
Stenosis of vagina (acquired) (congenital)
Stricture of vagina
Tumor of vagina

[5] **654.8 Congenital or acquired abnormality of vulva**
[0-4]
Fibrosis of perineum
Persistent hymen
Previous surgery to perineum or vulva
Rigid perineum
Tumor of vulva

[Excludes:] *varicose veins of vulva (671.1)*

[5] **654.9 Other and unspecified**
[0-4]
Uterine scar NEC

[5] **655 Known or suspected fetal abnormality affecting management of mother**
Includes: the listed conditions in the fetus as a reason for observation or obstetrical care of the mother, or for termination of pregnancy

[5] **655.0 Central nervous system malformation in fetus**
[0,1,3]
Fetal or suspected fetal:
- anencephaly
- hydrocephalus
- spina bifida (with myelomeningocele)

[5] **655.1 Chromosomal abnormality in fetus**
[0,1,3]

[5] **655.2 Hereditary disease in family possibly affecting fetus**
[0,1,3]

[5] **655.3 Suspected damage to fetus from viral disease in the mother**
[0,1,3]
Suspected damage to fetus from maternal rubella

[5] **655.4 Suspected damage to fetus from other disease in the mother**
[0,1,3]
Suspected damage to fetus from maternal:
- alcohol addiction
- listeriosis
- toxoplasmosis

[5] **655.5 Suspected damage to fetus from drugs**
[0,1,3]

[5] **655.6 Suspected damage to fetus from radiation**
[0,1,3]

[5] **655.7 Decreased fetal movements**
[0,1,3]

[5] **655.8 Other known or suspected fetal abnormality, not elsewhere classified**
[0,1,3]
Suspected damage to fetus from:
- environmental toxins
- intrauterine contraceptive device

[5] **655.9 Unspecified**
[0,1,3]

[5] **656 Other fetal and placental problems affecting management of mother**

[5] **656.0 Fetal-maternal hemorrhage**
[0,1,3]
Leakage (microscopic) of fetal blood into maternal circulation

[5] **656.1 Rhesus isoimmunization**
[0,1,3]
Anti-D [Rh] antibodies
Rh incompatibility

[5] **656.2 Isoimmunization from other and unspecified blood-group incompatibility**
[0,1,3]
ABO isoimmunization

[5] **656.3 Fetal distress**
[0,1,3]
Fetal metabolic acidemia

[Excludes:] *abnormal fetal acid-base balance (656.8)*
abnormality in fetal heart rate or rhythm (659.7)
fetal bradycardia (659.7)
fetal tachycardia (659.7)
meconium in liquor (656.8)

Add 4th or 5th digit | Nonspecific code | Unspecified code | Manifestation code

[5] **656.4 Intrauterine death**
[0,1,3] Fetal death:
NOS
after completion of 22 weeks' gestation
late
Missed delivery
[Excludes:] *missed abortion (632)*

[5] **656.5 Poor fetal growth**
[0,1,3] "Light-for-dates"
"Placental insufficiency"
"Small-for-dates"

[5] **656.6 Excessive fetal growth**
[0,1,3] "Large-for-dates"

[5] **656.7 Other placental conditions**
[0,1,3] Abnormal placenta
Placental infarct
[Excludes:] *placental polyp (674.4)*
placentitis (658.4)

[5] **656.8 Other specified fetal and placental problems**
[0,1,3] Abnormal acid-base balance
Intrauterine acidosis
Lithopedian
Meconium in liquor

[5] **656.9 Unspecified fetal and placental problem**
[0,1,3]

[5] **657 Polyhydramnios**
[0,1,3] Hydramnios
Use 0 as fourth-digit for this category

[5] **658 Other problems associated with amniotic cavity and membranes**
[Excludes:] *amniotic fluid embolism (673.1)*

[5] **658.0 Oligohydramnios**
[0,1,3] Oligohydramnios without mention of rupture of membranes

[5] **658.1 Premature rupture of membranes**
[0,1,3] Rupture of amniotic sac less than 24 hours prior to the onset of labor

[5] **658.2 Delayed delivery after spontaneous or unspecified rupture of membranes**
[0,1,3] Prolonged rupture of membranes NOS
Rupture of amniotic sac 24 hours or more prior to the onset of labor

[5] **658.3 Delayed delivery after artificial rupture of membranes**
[0,1,3]

[5] **658.4 Infection of amniotic cavity**
[0,1,3] Amnionitis
Chorioamnionitis
Membranitis
Placentitis

[5] **658.8 Other**
[0,1,3] Amnion nodosum
Amniotic cyst

[5] **658.9 Unspecified**
[0,1,3]

[5] **659 Other indications for care or intervention related to labor and delivery, not elsewhere classified**

[5] **659.0 Failed mechanical induction**
[0,1,3] Failure of induction of labor by surgical or other instrumental methods

[5] **659.1 Failed medical or unspecified induction**
[0,1,3] Failed induction NOS
Failure of induction of labor by medical methods, such as oxytocic drugs

[5] **659.2 Maternal pyrexia during labor, unspecified**
[0,1,3]

[5] **659.3 Generalized infection during labor**
[0,1,3] Septicemia during labor

[5] **659.4 Grand multiparity**
[0,1,3]
[Excludes:] *supervision only, in pregnancy (V23.3)*
without current pregnancy (V61.5)

● Code new to this edition
▲ Revision of existing code
[4] [5] Fourth or fifth digit required

⑤ **659.5 Elderly primigravida**
[0,1,3]   First pregnancy in a woman who will be 35 years of age or older at expected date of delivery

> Excludes: *supervision only, in pregnancy (V23.81)*

⑤ **659.6 Elderly multigravida**
[0,1,3]   Second or more pregnancy in a woman who will be 35 years of age or older at expected date of delivery

> Excludes: *elderly primigravida 659.5*
> *supervision only, in pregnancy (V23.82)*

⑤ **659.7 Abnormality in fetal heart rate or rhythm**
[0,1,3]   Depressed fetal heart tones
Fetal:
  bradycardia
  tachycardia
Fetal heart rate decelerations
Non-reassuring fetal heart rate or rhythm

⑤ **659.8 Other specified indications for care or intervention related to labor and delivery**
[0,1,3]   Pregnancy in female less than 16 years old at expected date of delivery
Very young maternal age

⑤ **659.9 Unspecified indication for care or intervention related to labor and delivery**
[0,1,3]

COMPLICATIONS OCCURRING MAINLY IN THE COURSE OF LABOR AND DELIVERY (660-669)

The following fifth-digit subclassification is for use with categories 660-669 to denote the current episode of care:

0   unspecified as to episode of care or not applicable

1   delivered, with or without mention of antepartum condition

2   delivered, with mention of postpartum complication

3   antepartum condition or complication

4   postpartum condition or complication

⑤ **660** **Obstructed labor**

⑤ **660.0 Obstruction caused by malposition of fetus at onset of labor**
[0,1,3]   Any condition classifiable to 652, causing obstruction during labor
Use additional code from 652.0-652.9, if desired, to identify condition

⑤ **660.1 Obstruction by bony pelvis**
[0,1,3]   Any condition classifiable to 653, causing obstruction during labor
Use additional code from 653.0-653.9, if desired, to identify condition

⑤ **660.2 Obstruction by abnormal pelvic soft tissues**
[0,1,3]   Prolapse of anterior lip of cervix
Any condition classifiable to 654, causing obstruction during labor
Use additional code from 654.0-654.9, if desired, to identify condition

⑤ **660.3 Deep transverse arrest and persistent occipitoposterior position**
[0,1,3]

⑤ **660.4 Shoulder (girdle) dystocia**
[0,1,3]   Impacted shoulders

⑤ **660.5 Locked twins**
[0,1,3]

⑤ **660.6 Failed trial of labor, unspecified**
[0,1,3]   Failed trial of labor, without mention of condition or suspected condition

⑤ **660.7 Failed forceps or vacuum extractor, unspecified**
[0,1,3]   Application of ventouse or forceps, without mention of condition

⑤ **660.8 Other causes of obstructed labor**
[0,1,3]

⑤ **660.9 Unspecified obstructed labor**
[0,1,3]   Dystocia:
  NOS
  fetal NOS
  maternal NOS

381

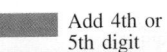 Add 4th or 5th digit   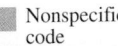 Nonspecific code   Unspecified code   Manifestation code

[5] **661 Abnormality of forces of labor**

[5] **661.0 Primary uterine inertia**
[0,1,3]
Failure of cervical dilation
Hypotonic uterine dysfunction, primary
Prolonged latent phase of labor

[5] **661.1 Secondary uterine inertia**
[0,1,3]
Arrested active phase of labor
Hypotonic uterine dysfunction, secondary

[5] **661.2 Other and unspecified uterine inertia**
[0,1,3]
Desultory labor
Irregular labor
Poor contractions
Slow slope active phase of labor

[5] **661.3 Precipitate labor**
[0,1,3]

[5] **661.4 Hypertonic, incoordinate, or prolonged uterine contractions**
[0,1,3]
Cervical spasm
Contraction ring (dystocia)
Dyscoordinate labor
Hourglass contraction of uterus
Hypertonic uterine dysfunction
Incoordinate uterine action
Retraction ring (Bandl's) (pathological)
Tetanic contractions
Uterine dystocia NOS
Uterine spasm

[5] **661.9 Unspecified abnormality of labor**
[0,1,3]

[5] **662 Long labor**

[5] **662.0 Prolonged first stage**
[0,1,3]

[5] **662.1 Prolonged labor, unspecified**
[0,1,3]

[5] **662.2 Prolonged second stage**
[0,1,3]

[5] **662.3 Delayed delivery of second twin, triplet, etc.**
[0,1,3]

[5] **663 Umbilical cord complications**

[5] **663.0 Prolapse of cord**
[0,1,3]
Presentation of cord

[5] **663.1 Cord around neck, with compression**
[0,1,3]
Cord tightly around neck

[5] **663.2 Other and unspecified cord entanglement, with compression**
[0,1,3]
Entanglement of cords of twins in mono-amniotic sac
Knot in cord (with compression)

[5] **663.3 Other and unspecified cord entanglement, without mention of compression**
[0,1,3]

[5] **663.4 Short cord**
[0,1,3]

[5] **663.5 Vasa previa**
[0,1,3]

[5] **663.6 Vascular lesions of cord**
[0,1,3]
Bruising of cord
Hematoma of cord
Thrombosis of vessels of cord

[5] **663.8 Other umbilical cord complications**
[0,1,3]
Velamentous insertion of umbilical cord

[5] **663.9 Unspecified umbilical cord complication**
[0,1,3]

[5] **664 Trauma to perineum and vulva during delivery**
Includes: damage from instruments
that from extension of episiotomy

⑤ **664.0 First-degree perineal laceration**
[0,1,4]   Perineal laceration, rupture, or tear involving:
      fourchette
      hymen
      labia
      skin
      vagina
      vulva

⑤ **664.1 Second-degree perineal laceration**
[0,1,4]   Perineal laceration, rupture, or tear (following episiotomy) involving:
      pelvic floor
      perineal muscles
      vaginal muscles

   | Excludes: | that involving anal sphincter (664.2) |

⑤ **664.2 Third-degree perineal laceration**
[0,1,4]   Perineal laceration, rupture, or tear (following episiotomy) involving:
      anal sphincter
      rectovaginal septum
      sphincter NOS

   | Excludes: | that with anal or rectal mucosal laceration (664.3) |

⑤ **664.3 Fourth-degree perineal laceration**
[0,1,4]   Perineal laceration, rupture, or tear as classifiable to 664.2 and involving also:
      anal mucosa
      rectal mucosa

⑤ **664.4 Unspecified perineal laceration**
[0,1,4]   Central laceration

⑤ **664.5 Vulval and perineal hematoma**
[0,1,4]

⑤ **664.8 Other specified trauma to perineum and vulva**
[0,1,4]

⑤ **664.9 Unspecified trauma to perineum and vulva**
[0,1,4]

⑤ **665 Other obstetrical trauma**
      Includes: damage from instruments

⑤ **665.0 Rupture of uterus before onset of labor**
[0,1,3]

⑤ **665.1 Rupture of uterus during labor**
[0,1]   Rupture of uterus NOS

⑤ **665.2 Inversion of uterus**
[0,2,4]

⑤ **665.3 Laceration of cervix**
[0,1,4]

⑤ **665.4 High vaginal laceration**
[0,1,4]   Laceration of vaginal wall or sulcus without mention of perineal laceration

⑤ **665.5 Other injury to pelvic organs**
[0,1,4]   Injury to:
      bladder
      urethra

⑤ **665.6 Damage to pelvic joints and ligaments**
[0,1,4]   Avulsion of inner symphyseal cartilage
      Damage to coccyx
      Separation of symphysis (pubis)

⑤ **665.7 Pelvic hematoma**
[0,1,2,4]   Hematoma of vagina

⑤ **665.8 Other specified obstetrical trauma**
[0-4]

⑤ **665.9 Unspecified obstetrical trauma**
[0-4]

⑤ **666 Postpartum hemorrhage**

⑤ **666.0 Third-stage hemorrhage**
[0,2,4]   Hemorrhage associated with retained, trapped, or adherent placenta
      Retained placenta NOS

383

| ▨ | Add 4th or 5th digit | ▨ | Nonspecific code | ▨ | Unspecified code | ▨ | Manifestation code |

[5] **666.1 Other immediate postpartum hemorrhage**
[0,2,4] Atony of uterus
Hemorrhage within the first 24 hours following delivery of placenta
Postpartum hemorrhage (atonic) NOS

[5] **666.2 Delayed and secondary postpartum hemorrhage**
[0,2,4] Hemorrhage:
after the first 24 hours following delivery
associated with retained portions of placenta or membranes
Postpartum hemorrhage specified as delayed or secondary
Retained products of conception NOS, following delivery

[5] **666.3 Postpartum coagulation defects**
[0,2,4] Postpartum afibrinogenemia
Postpartum fibrinolysis

[5] **667 Retained placenta or membranes, without hemorrhage**

[5] **667.0 Retained placenta without hemorrhage**
[0,2,4] Placenta accreta without hemorrhage
Retained placenta:
NOS without hemorrhage
total without hemorrhage

[5] **667.1 Retained portions of placenta or membranes, without hemorrhage**
[0,2,4] Retained products of conception following delivery, without hemorrhage

[5] **668 Complications of the administration of anesthetic or other sedation in labor and delivery**
Includes: complications arising from the administration of a general or local anesthetic, analgesic, or other sedation in labor and delivery

[Excludes:] *reaction to spinal or lumbar puncture (349.0)*
spinal headache (349.0)

Use additional code(s) to further specify complication

[5] **668.0 Pulmonary complications**
[0-4] Inhalation [aspiration] of stomach contents or secretions following anesthesia or other sedation in labor or delivery
Mendelson's syndrome following anesthesia or other sedation in labor or delivery
Pressure collapse of lung following anesthesia or other sedation in labor or delivery

[5] **668.1 Cardiac complications**
[0-4] Cardiac arrest or failure following anesthesia or other sedation in labor and delivery

[5] **668.2 Central nervous system complications**
[0-4] Cerebral anoxia following anesthesia or other sedation in labor and delivery

[5] **668.8 Other complications of anesthesia or other sedation in labor and delivery**
[0-4]

[5] **668.9 Unspecified complication of anesthesia and other sedation**
[0-4]

[5] **669 Other complications of labor and delivery, not elsewhere classified**

[5] **669.0 Maternal distress**
[0-4] Metabolic disturbance in labor and delivery

[5] **669.1 Shock during or following labor and delivery**
[0-4] Obstetric shock

[5] **669.2 Maternal hypotension syndrome**
[0-4]

[5] **669.3 Acute renal failure following labor and delivery**
[0,2,4]

[5] **669.4 Other complications of obstetrical surgery and procedures**
[0-4] Cardiac:
arrest following cesarean or other obstetrical surgery or procedure, including delivery NOS
failure following cesarean or other obstetrical surgery or procedure, including delivery NOS
Cerebral anoxia following cesarean or other obstetrical surgery or procedure, including delivery NOS

[Excludes:] *complications of obstetrical surgical wounds (674.1-674.3)*

[5] **669.5 Forceps or vacuum extractor delivery without mention of indication**
[0,1] Delivery by ventouse, without mention of indication

[5] **669.6 Breech extraction, without mention of indication**
[0,1]

[Excludes:] *breech delivery NOS (652.2)*

[5] **669.7 Cesarean delivery, without mention of indication**
[0,1]

[5] **669.8 Other complications of labor and delivery**
[0-4]

[5] **669.9 Unspecified complication of labor and delivery**
[0-4]

COMPLICATIONS OF THE PUERPERIUM (670-677)

Note: Categories 671 and 673-676 include the listed conditions even if they occur during pregnancy or childbirth.

The following fifth-digit subclassification is for use with categories 670-676 to denote the current episode of care:

0 unspecified as to episode of care or not applicable
1 delivered, with or without mention of antepartum condition
2 delivered, with mention of postpartum complication
3 antepartum condition or complication
4 postpartum condition or complication

[5] **670 Major puerperal infection**
[0,2,4]
Puerperal:
  endometritis
  fever (septic)
  pelvic:
    cellulitis
    sepsis
Puerperal:
  peritonitis
  pyemia
  salpingitis
  septicemia

Use 0 as fourth-digit for this category

[Excludes:] *infection following abortion (639.0)*
minor genital tract infection following delivery (646.6)
puerperal pyrexia NOS (672)
puerperal fever NOS (672)
puerperal pyrexia of unknown origin (672)
urinary tract infection following delivery (646.6)

[5] **671 Venous complications in pregnancy and the puerperium**

[5] **671.0 Varicose veins of legs**
[0-4] Varicose veins NOS

[5] **671.1 Varicose veins of vulva and perineum**
[0-4]

[5] **671.2 Superficial thrombophlebitis**
[0-4] Thrombophlebitis (superficial)

[5] **671.3 Deep phlebothrombosis, antepartum**
[0,1,3] Deep-vein thrombosis, antepartum

[5] **671.4 Deep phlebothrombosis, postpartum**
[0,2,4] Deep-vein thrombosis, postpartum
Pelvic thrombophlebitis, postpartum
Phlegmasia alba dolens (puerperal)

[5] **671.5 Other phlebitis and thrombosis**
[0-4] Cerebral venous thrombosis
Thrombosis of intracranial venous sinus

[5] **671.8 Other venous complications**
[0-4] Hemorrhoids

[5] **671.9 Unspecified venous complication**
[0-4] Phlebitis NOS
Thrombosis NOS

[5] **672 Pyrexia of unknown origin during the puerperium**
[0,2,4] Puerperal fever NOS
Postpartum fever NOS

Use 0 as fourth-digit for this category

[5] **673 Obstetrical pulmonary embolism**
Includes: pulmonary emboli in pregnancy, childbirth, or the puerperium, or specified as puerperal

[Excludes:] *embolism following abortion (639.6)*

[5] **673.0 Obstetrical air embolism**
[0-4]

[5] **673.1 Amniotic fluid embolism**
[0-4]

[5] **673.2 Obstetrical blood-clot embolism**
[0-4] Puerperal pulmonary embolism NOS

[5] **673.3 Obstetrical pyemic and septic embolism**
[0-4]

[5] **673.8 Other pulmonary embolism**
[0-4] Fat embolism

[5] **674 Other and unspecified complications of the puerperium, not elsewhere classified**

[5] **674.0 Cerebrovascular disorders in the puerperium**
[0-4] Any condition classifiable to 430-434, 436-437 occurring during pregnancy, childbirth, or the puerperium, or specified as puerperal

[Excludes:] *intracranial venous sinus thrombosis (671.5)*

[5] **674.1 Disruption of cesarean wound**
[0,2,4] Dehiscence or disruption of uterine wound

[Excludes:] *uterine rupture before onset of labor (665.0)*
uterine rupture during labor (665.1)

[5] **674.2 Disruption of perineal wound**
[0,2,4] Breakdown of perineum
Disruption of wound of:
episiotomy
perineal laceration
Secondary perineal tear

[5] **674.3 Other complications of obstetrical surgical wounds**
[0,2,4] Hematoma of cesarean section or perineal wound
Hemorrhage of cesarean section or perineal wound
Infection of cesarean section or perineal wound

[Excludes:] *damage from instruments in delivery (664.0-665.9)*

[5] **674.4 Placental polyp**
[0,2,4]

[5] **674.8 Other**
[0,2,4] Hepatorenal syndrome, following delivery
Postpartum:
cardiomyopathy
subinvolution of uterus
uterine hypertrophy

[5] **674.9 Unspecified**
[0,2,4] Sudden death of unknown cause during the puerperium

[5] **675 Infections of the breast and nipple associated with childbirth**
Includes: the listed conditions during pregnancy, childbirth, or the puerperium

[5] **675.0 Infections of nipple**
[0-4] Abscess of nipple

[5] **675.1 Abscess of breast**
[0-4] Abscess:
mammary
subareolar
submammary
Mastitis:
purulent
retromammary
submammary

[5] **675.2 Nonpurulent mastitis**
[0-4] Lymphangitis of breast
Mastitis:
NOS
interstitial
parenchymatous

[5] **675.8 Other specified infections of the breast and nipple**
[0-4]

[5] **675.9 Unspecified infection of the breast and nipple**
[0-4]

[5] **676 Other disorders of the breast associated with childbirth and disorders of lactation**
Includes: the listed conditions during pregnancy, the puerperium, or lactation

[5] **676.0 Retracted nipple**
[0-4]

[5] **676.1 Cracked nipple**
[0-4] Fissure of nipple

[5] **676.2 Engorgement of breasts**
[0-4]

[5] **676.3 Other and unspecified disorder of breast**
[0-4]

[5] **676.4 Failure of lactation**
[0-4] Agalactia

[5] **676.5 Suppressed lactation**
[0-4]

[5] **676.6 Galactorrhea**
[0-4]

[*Excludes:*] *galactorrhea not associated with childbirth (611.6)*

[5] **676.8 Other disorders of lactation**
[0-4] Galactocele

[5] **676.9 Unspecified disorder of lactation**
[0-4]

677 Late effect of complication of pregnancy, childbirth, and the puerperium

Note: This category is to be used to indicate conditions in 632-648.9 and 651-676.9 as the cause of the late effect, themselves classifiable elsewhere. The "late effects" include conditions specified as such, or as sequelae, which may occur at any time after the puerperium.

Code first any sequelae

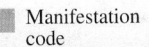

● Code new
to this edition

▲ Revision of
existing code

④ ⑤ Fourth or fifth
digit required

12. DISEASES OF THE SKIN AND SUBCUTANEOUS TISSUE (680-709)

INFECTIONS OF SKIN AND SUBCUTANEOUS TISSUE (680-686)

[Excludes:] *certain infections of skin classified under "Infectious and Parasitic Diseases," such as:*
erysipelas (035)
erysipeloid of Rosenbach (027.1)
herpes:
simplex (054.0-054.9)
zoster (053.0-053.9)
molluscum contagiosum (078.0)
viral warts (078.1)

680 Carbuncle and furuncle
Includes: boil
furunculosis

680.0 Face
Ear [any part]
Face [any part, except eye]
Nose (septum)
Temple (region)

[Excludes:] *eyelid (373.13)*
lacrimal apparatus (375.31)
orbit (376.01)

680.1 Neck

680.2 Trunk
Abdominal wall
Back [any part, except buttocks]
Breast
Chest wall
Flank
Groin
Pectoral region
Perineum
Umbilicus

[Excludes:] *buttocks (680.5)*
external genital organs:
female (616.4)
male (607.2, 608.4)

680.3 Upper arm and forearm
Arm [any part, except hand]
Axilla
Shoulder

680.4 Hand
Finger [any]
Thumb
Wrist

680.5 Buttock
Anus
Gluteal region

680.6 Leg, except foot
Ankle
Hip
Knee
Thigh

680.7 Foot
Heel
Toe

680.8 Other specified sites
Head [any part, except face]
Scalp

[Excludes:] *external genital organs:*
female (616.4)
male (607.2, 608.4)

680.9 Unspecified site
Boil NOS
Carbuncle NOS
Furuncle NOS

681 Cellulitis and abscess of finger and toe
Includes: that with lymphangitis

Use additional code, if desired, to identify organism, such as Staphylococcus (041.1)

[5] **681.0 Finger**

681.00 Cellulitis and abscess, unspecified

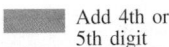

Add 4th or 5th digit — Nonspecific code — Unspecified code — Manifestation code

681.01 Felon
Pulp abscess
Whitlow

[Excludes:] *herpetic whitlow (054.6)*

681.02 Onychia and paronychia of finger
Panaritium of finger
Perionychia of finger

⑤ **681.1 Toe**

681.10 Cellulitis and abscess, unspecified

681.11 Onychia and paronychia of toe
Panaritium of toe
Perionychia of toe

681.9 Cellulitis and abscess of unspecified digit
Infection of nail NOS

682 Other cellulitis and abscess
Includes:
abscess (acute) (with lymphangitis) except of finger or toe
cellulitis (diffuse) (with lymphangitis) except of finger or toe
lymphangitis, acute (with lymphangitis) except of finger or toe

Use additional code, if desired, to identify organism, such as Staphylococcus (041.1)

[Excludes:] *lymphangitis (chronic) (subacute) (457.2)*

682.0 Face
Cheek, external
Chin
Forehead
Nose, external
Submandibular
Temple (region)

[Excludes:] *ear [any part] (380.10-380.16)*
eyelid (373.13)
lacrimal apparatus (375.31)
lip (528.5)
mouth (528.3)
nose (internal) (478.1)
orbit (376.01)

682.1 Neck

682.2 Trunk
Abdominal wall
Back [any part, except buttock]
Chest wall
Flank
Groin
Pectoral region
Perineum
Umbilicus, except newborn

[Excludes:] *anal and rectal regions (566)*
breast:
NOS (611.0)
puerperal (675.1)
external genital organs:
female (616.3-616.4)
male (604.0, 607.2, 608.4)
umbilicus, newborn (771.4)

682.3 Upper arm and forearm
Arm [any part, except hand]
Axilla
Shoulder

[Excludes:] *hand (682.4)*

682.4 Hand, except fingers and thumb
Wrist

[Excludes:] *finger and thumb (681.00-681.02)*

682.5 Buttock
Gluteal region

[Excludes:] *anal and rectal regions (566)*

682.6 Leg, except foot
Ankle
Hip
Knee
Thigh

● Code new to this edition
▲ Revision of existing code
④ ⑤ Fourth or fifth digit required

682.7 Foot, except toes
Heel

Excludes: toe (681.10-681.11)

682.8 Other specified sites
Head [except face]   Scalp

Excludes: face (682.0)

682.9 Unspecified site
Abscess NOS   Lymphangitis, acute NOS
Cellulitis NOS

Excludes: lymphangitis NOS (457.2)

683 Acute lymphadenitis
Abscess (acute), lymph gland or node, except mesenteric
Adenitis, acute, lymph gland or node, except mesenteric
Lymphadenitis, acute, lymph gland or node, except mesenteric

Use additional code, if desired, to identify organism, such as Staphylococcus (041.1)

Excludes: enlarged glands NOS (785.6)

lymphadenitis:
chronic or subacute, except mesenteric (289.1)
mesenteric (acute) (chronic) (subacute) (289.2)
unspecified (289.3)

684 Impetigo
Impetiginization of other dermatoses
Impetigo (contagiosa) [any site] [any organism]:
bullous
circinate
neonatorum
simplex
Pemphigus neonatorum

Excludes: impetigo herpetiformis (694.3)

685 Pilonidal cyst
Includes:
fistula, coccygeal or pilonidal
sinus, coccygeal or pilonidal

685.0 With abscess

685.1 Without mention of abscess

686 Other local infections of skin and subcutaneous tissue
Use additional code, if desired, to identify any infectious organism (041.0-041.8)

⑤ **686.0 Pyoderma**
Dermatitis:
purulent
septic
suppurative

686.00 Pyoderma, unspecified

686.01 Pyoderma gangrenosum

686.09 Other pyoderma

686.1 Pyogenic granuloma
Granuloma:
septic
suppurative
telangiectaticum

Excludes: pyogenic granuloma of oral mucosa (528.9)

686.8 Other specified local infections of skin and subcutaneous tissue
Bacterid (pustular)   Ecthyma
Dermatitis vegetans   Perlèche

Excludes: dermatitis infectiosa eczematoides (690.8)
panniculitis (729.30-729.39)

686.9 Unspecified local infection of skin and subcutaneous tissue
Fistula of skin NOS   Skin infection NOS

Excludes: fistula to skin from internal organs—see Alphabetic Index

| Add 4th or 5th digit | Nonspecific code | Unspecified code | Manifestation code |

OTHER INFLAMMATORY CONDITIONS OF SKIN AND SUBCUTANEOUS TISSUE (690-698)

[Excludes:] *panniculitis (729.30-729.39)*

690 Erythematosquamous dermatosis

[Excludes:] *eczematous dermatitis of eyelid (373.31)*
parakeratosis variegata (696.2)
psoriasis (696.0-696.1)
seborrheic keratosis (702.11-702.19)

[5] **690.1 Seborrheic dermatitis**

690.10 Seborrheic dermatitis, unspecified
Seborrheic dermatitis NOS

690.11 Seborrhea capitis
Cradle cap

690.12 Seborrheic infantile dermatitis

690.18 Other seborrheic dermatitis

690.8 Other erythematosquamous dermatosis

691 Atopic dermatitis and related conditions

691.0 Diaper or napkin rash
Ammonia dermatitis
Diaper or napkin:
- dermatitis
- erythema
- rash

Psoriasiform napkin eruption

691.8 Other atopic dermatitis and related conditions
Atopic dermatitis
Besnier's prurigo
Eczema:
- atopic
- flexural
- intrinsic (allergic)

Neurodermatitis:
- atopic
- diffuse (of Brocq)

692 Contact dermatitis and other eczema
Includes:
dermatitis:
- NOS
- contact
- occupational
- venenata

eczema (acute) (chronic):
- NOS
- allergic
- erythematous
- occupational

[Excludes:] *allergy NOS (995.3)*
contact dermatitis of eyelids (373.32)
dermatitis due to substances taken internally (693.0-693.9)
eczema of external ear (380.22)
perioral dermatitis (695.3)
urticarial reactions (708.0-708.9, 995.1)

692.0 Due to detergents

692.1 Due to oils and greases

692.2 Due to solvents
Dermatitis due to solvents of:
- chlorocompound group
- cyclohexane group
- ester group
- glycol group
- hydrocarbon group
- ketone group

692.3 Due to drugs and medicines in contact with skin
Dermatitis (allergic) (contact) due to:
arnica
fungicides
iodine
keratolytics
mercurials
neomycin
pediculocides
phenols
scabicides
any drug applied to skin
Dermatitis medicamentosa due to drug applied to skin

Use additional E code, if desired, to identify drug

[Excludes:] *allergy NOS due to drugs (995.2)*
dermatitis due to ingested drugs (693.0)
dermatitis medicamentosa NOS (693.0)

692.4 Due to other chemical products
Dermatitis due to:
acids
adhesive plaster
alkalis
caustics
dichromate
insecticide
nylon
plastic
rubber

692.5 Due to food in contact with skin
Dermatitis, contact, due to:
cereals
fish
flour
fruit
meat
milk

[Excludes:] *dermatitis due to:*
dyes (692.89)
ingested foods (693.1)
preservatives (692.89)

692.6 Due to plants [except food]
Dermatitis due to:
lacquer tree [Rhus verniciflua]
poison ivy [Rhus toxicodendron]
poison oak [Rhus diversiloba]
poison sumac [Rhus venenata]
poison vine [Rhus radicans]
primrose [Primula]
ragweed [Senecio jacobae]
other plants in contact with the skin

[Excludes:] *allergy NOS due to pollen (477.0)*
nettle rash (708.8)

[5] **692.7 Due to solar radiation**

[Excludes:] *sunburn due to other ultraviolet radiation exposure (692.82)*

692.70 Unspecified dermatitis due to sun

692.71 Sunburn
First degree sunburn
Sunburn NOS

692.72 Acute dermatitis due to solar radiation
Berloque dermatitis
Photoallergic response
Phototoxic response
Polymorphus light eruption
Acute solar skin damage NOS

[Excludes:] *sunburn (692.71, 692.76-692.77)*

Use additional E code, if desired, to identify drug, if drug induced

692.73 Actinic reticuloid and actinic granuloma

692.74 Other chronic dermatitis due to solar radiation
solar elastosis
chronic solar skin damage NOS

[Excludes:] *actinic [solar] keratosis (702.0)*

Add 4th or 5th digit | Nonspecific code | Unspecified code | Manifestation code

692.75 Disseminated superficial actinic porokeratosis (DSAP)

692.76 Sunburn of second degree

692.77 Sunburn of third degree

692.79 Other dermatitis due to solar radiation
Hydroa aestivale
Photodermatitis due to sun
Photosensitiveness due to sun
Solar skin damage NOS

⑤ **692.8 Due to other specified agents**

692.81 Dermatitis due to cosmetics

692.82 Dermatitis due to other radiation
Infrared rays
Light, except from sun
Radiation NOS
Ultraviolet rays, except from sun
X-rays
Tanning bed

[Excludes:] *that due to solar radiation (692.70-692.79)*

692.83 Dermatitis due to metals
jewelry

692.89 Other
Dermatitis due to:
cold weather
dyes
furs
hot weather
preservatives

[Excludes:] *allergy NOS due to animal hair, dander (animal), or dust (477.8)*
sunburn (692.71, 692.76-692.77)

692.9 Unspecified cause
Dermatitis:
NOS
contact NOS
venenata NOS
Eczema NOS

693 Dermatitis due to substances taken internally

[Excludes:] *adverse effect NOS of drugs and medicines (995.2)*
allergy NOS (995.3)
contact dermatitis (692.0-692.9)
urticarial reactions (708.0-708.9, 995.1)

693.0 Due to drugs and medicines
Dermatitis medicamentosa NOS

Use additional E code, if desired, to identify drug

[Excludes:] *that due to drugs in contact with skin (692.3)*

693.1 Due to food

693.8 Due to other specified substances taken internally

693.9 Due to unspecified substance taken internally

[Excludes:] *dermatitis NOS (692.9)*

694 Bullous dermatoses

694.0 Dermatitis herpetiformis
Dermatosis herpetiformis
Duhring's disease
Hydroa herpetiformis

[Excludes:] *herpes gestationis (646.8)*
dermatitis herpetiformis:
juvenile (694.2)
senile (694.5)

694.1 Subcorneal pustular dermatosis
Sneddon-Wilkinson disease or syndrome

694.2 Juvenile dermatitis herpetiformis
Juvenile pemphigoid

694.3 Impetigo herpetiformis

694.4 Pemphigus

Pemphigus:
- NOS
- erythematosus
- foliaceus

Pemphigus:
- malignant
- vegetans
- vulgaris

[Excludes:] *pemphigus neonatorum (684)*

694.5 Pemphigoid

Benign pemphigus NOS
Bullous pemphigoid
Herpes circinatus bullosus
Senile dermatitis herpetiformis

[5] **694.6 Benign mucous membrane pemphigoid**

Cicatricial pemphigoid
Mucosynechial atrophic bullous dermatitis

694.60 Without mention of ocular involvement

694.61 With ocular involvement

Ocular pemphigus

694.8 Other specified bullous dermatoses

[Excludes:] *herpes gestationis (646.8)*

694.9 Unspecified bullous dermatoses

695 Erythematous conditions

695.0 Toxic erythema

Erythema venenatum

695.1 Erythema multiforme

Erythema iris
Herpes iris
Lyell's syndrome
Scalded skin syndrome
Stevens-Johnson syndrome
Toxic epidermal necrolysis

695.2 Erythema nodosum

[Excludes:] *tuberculous erythema nodosum (017.1)*

695.3 Rosacea

Acne:
- erythematosa
- rosacea

Perioral dermatitis
Rhinophyma

695.4 Lupus erythematosus

Lupus:
- erythematodes (discoid)
- erythematosus (discoid), not disseminated

[Excludes:] *lupus (vulgaris) NOS (017.0)*
systemic [disseminated] lupus erythematosus (710.0)

[5] **695.8 Other specified erythematous conditions**

695.81 Ritter's disease

Dermatitis exfoliativa neonatorum

695.89 Other

Erythema intertrigo
Intertrigo
Pityriasis rubra (Hebra)

[Excludes:] *mycotic intertrigo (111.0-111.9)*

695.9 Unspecified erythematous condition

Erythema NOS
Erythroderma (secondary)

696 Psoriasis and similar disorders

696.0 Psoriatic arthropathy

696.1 Other psoriasis

Acrodermatitis continua
Dermatitis repens
Psoriasis:
- NOS
- any type, except arthropathic

[Excludes:] *psoriatic arthropathy (696.0)*

Add 4th or 5th digit | Nonspecific code | Unspecified code | Manifestation code

696.2 Parapsoriasis
Parakeratosis variegata
Parapsoriasis lichenoides chronica
Pityriasis lichenoides et varioliformis

696.3 Pityriasis rosea
Pityriasis circinata (et maculata)

696.4 Pityriasis rubra pilaris
Devergie's disease
Lichen ruber acuminatus

Excludes: *pityriasis rubra (Hebra) (695.89)*

696.5 Other and unspecified pityriasis
Pityriasis:
NOS
alba
streptogenes

Excludes: *pityriasis simplex (690.18)*
pityriasis versicolor (111.0)

696.8 Other

697 Lichen

Excludes: *lichen:*

obtusus corneus (698.3)
pilaris (congenital) (757.39)
ruber acuminatus (696.4)
sclerosus et atrophicus (701.0)
scrofulosus (017.0)
simplex chronicus (698.3)
spinulosus (congenital) (757.39)
urticatus (698.2)

697.0 Lichen planus
Lichen:
planopilaris
ruber planus

697.1 Lichen nitidus
Pinkus' disease

697.8 Other lichen, not elsewhere classified
Lichen:
ruber moniliforme
striata

697.9 Lichen, unspecified

698 Pruritus and related conditions

Excludes: *pruritus specified as psychogenic (306.3)*

698.0 Pruritus ani
Perianal itch

698.1 Pruritus of genital organs

698.2 Prurigo
Lichen urticatus   Urticaria papulosa (Hebra)
Prurigo:
NOS
Hebra's
mitis
simplex

Excludes: *prurigo nodularis (698.3)*

698.3 Lichenification and lichen simplex chronicus
Hyde's disease
Neurodermatitis (circumscripta) (local)
Prurigo nodularis

Excludes: *neurodermatitis, diffuse (of Brocq) (691.8)*

698.4 Dermatitis factitia [artefacta]
Dermatitis ficta
Neurotic excoriation
Use additional code, if desired, to identify any associated mental disorder

---

● Code new   ▲ Revision of   ④ ⑤ Fourth or fifth
to this edition   existing code   digit required

698.8 **Other specified pruritic conditions**
    Pruritus: Winter itch
      hiemalis
      senilis

698.9 **Unspecified pruritic disorder**
    Itch NOS   Pruritus NOS

OTHER DISEASES OF SKIN AND SUBCUTANEOUS TISSUE (700-709)

Excludes: *conditions confined to eyelids (373.0-374.9)*
                  congenital conditions of skin, hair, and nails (757.0-757.9)

700 **Corns and callosities**
    Callus   Clavus

701 **Other hypertrophic and atrophic conditions of skin**

Excludes: *dermatomyositis (710.3)*
                  hereditary edema of legs (757.0)
                  scleroderma (generalized) (710.1)

701.0 **Circumscribed scleroderma**
    Addison's keloid
    Dermatosclerosis, localized
    Lichen sclerosus et atrophicus
    Morphea
    Scleroderma, circumscribed or localized

701.1 **Keratoderma, acquired**
    Acquired:
      ichthyosis
      keratoderma palmaris et plantaris
    Elastosis perforans serpiginosa
    Hyperkeratosis:
      NOS
      follicularis in cutem penetrans
      palmoplantaris climacterica
    Keratoderma:
      climactericum
      tylodes, progressive
    Keratosis (blennorrhagica)

Excludes: *Darier's disease [keratosis follicularis] (congenital) (757.39)*
                  keratosis:
                    arsenical (692.4)
                    gonococcal (098.81)

701.2 **Acquired acanthosis nigricans**
    Keratosis nigricans

701.3 **Striae atrophicae**
    Atrophic spots of skin
    Atrophoderma maculatum
    Atrophy blanche (of Milian)
    Degenerative colloid atrophy
    Senile degenerative atrophy
    Striae distensae

701.4 **Keloid scar**
    Cheloid   Keloid
    Hypertrophic scar

701.5 **Other abnormal granulation tissue**
    Excessive granulation

701.8 **Other specified hypertrophic and atrophic conditions of skin**
    Acrodermatitis atrophicans chronica
    Atrophia cutis senilis
    Atrophoderma neuriticum
    Confluent and reticulate papillomatosis
    Cutis laxa senilis
    Elastosis senilis
    Folliculitis ulerythematosa reticulata
    Gougerot-Carteaud syndrome or disease

701.9 **Unspecified hypertrophic and atrophic conditions of skin**
    Atrophoderma

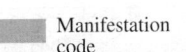

Add 4th or   Nonspecific   Unspecified   Manifestation
5th digit   code   code   code

702 Other dermatoses

[Excludes:] *carcinoma in situ (232.0-232.9)*

702.0 Actinic keratosis

⑤ **702.1 Seborrheic keratosis**

702.11 Inflamed seborrheic keratosis

702.19 Other seborrheic keratosis
Seborrheic keratosis NOS

702.8 Other specified dermatoses

703 Diseases of nail

[Excludes:] *congenital anomalies (757.5)*
onychia and paronychia (681.02, 681.11)

703.0 Ingrowing nail
Ingrowing nail with infection
Unguis incarnatus

[Excludes:] *infection, nail NOS (681.9)*

703.8 Other specified diseases of nail
Dystrophia unguium
Hypertrophy of nail
Koilonychia
Leukonychia (punctata) (striata)
Onychauxis
Onychogryposis
Onycholysis

703.9 Unspecified disease of nail

704 Diseases of hair and hair follicles

[Excludes:] *congenital anomalies (757.4)*

⑤ **704.0 Alopecia**

[Excludes:] *madarosis (374.55)*
syphilitic alopecia (091.82)

704.00 Alopecia, unspecified
Baldness
Loss of hair

704.01 Alopecia areata
Ophiasis

704.02 Telogen effluvim

704.09 Other
Folliculitis decalvans
Hypotrichosis:
NOS
postinfectional NOS
Pseudopelade

704.1 Hirsutism
Hypertrichosis:
NOS
lanuginosa, acquired
Polytrichia

[Excludes:] *hypertrichosis of eyelid (374.54)*

704.2 Abnormalities of the hair
Atrophic hair
Clastothrix
Fragilitas crinium
Trichiasis:
NOS
cicatrical
Trichorrhexis (nodosa)

[Excludes:] *trichiasis of eyelid (374.05)*

704.3 Variations in hair color
Canities (premature)
Grayness, hair (premature)
Heterochromia of hair
Poliosis:
NOS
circumscripta, acquired

● Code new to this edition
▲ Revision of existing code
④ ⑤ Fourth or fifth digit required

704.8 Other specified diseases of hair and hair follicles

Folliculitis:
- NOS
- abscedens et suffodiens
- pustular

Perifolliculitis:
- NOS
- capitis abscedens et suffodiens
- scalp

Sycosis:
- NOS
- barbae [not parasitic]
- lupoid
- vulgaris

704.9 Unspecified disease of hair and hair follicles

705 Disorders of sweat glands

705.0 Anhidrosis

Hypohidrosis
Oligohidrosis

705.1 Prickly heat

Heat rash
Miliaria rubra (tropicalis)
Sudamina

[5] **705.8 Other specified disorders of sweat glands**

705.81 Dyshidrosis

Cheiropompholyx
Pompholyx

705.82 Fox-Fordyce disease

705.83 Hidradenitis

Hidradenitis suppurativa

705.89 Other

Bromhidrosis
Chromhidrosis
Granulosis rubra nasi
Urhidrosis

[Excludes:] *hidrocystoma (216.0-216.9)*
hyperhidrosis (780.8)

705.9 Unspecified disorder of sweat glands

Disorder of sweat glands NOS

706 Diseases of sebaceous glands

706.0 Acne varioliformis

Acne:
- frontalis
- necrotica

706.1 Other acne

Acne:
- NOS
- conglobata
- cystic
- pustular
- vulgaris

Blackhead
Comedo

[Excludes:] *acne rosacea (695.3)*

706.2 Sebaceous cyst

Atheroma, skin
Keratin cyst
Wen

706.3 Seborrhea

[Excludes:] *seborrhea:*
- *capitis (690.11)*
- *sicca (690.18)*

seborrheic dermatitis (690.11)
seborrheic keratosis (702.11-702.19)

706.8 Other specified diseases of sebaceous glands

Asteatosis (cutis)
Xerosis cutis

706.9 Unspecified disease of sebaceous glands

707 Chronic ulcer of skin

Includes: non-infected sinus of skin
non-healing ulcer

[Excludes:] *specific infections classified under "Infectious and Parasitic Diseases" (001.0-136.9)*
varicose ulcer (454.0, 454.2)

707.0 Decubitus ulcer
Bed sore
Decubitus ulcer [any site]
Plaster ulcer
Pressure ulcer

[5] **707.1 Ulcer of lower limbs, except decubitus**
Ulcer, chronic, neurogenic, of lower limb
Ulcer, chronic, trophic, of lower limb

Code, if applicable, any causal condition first:
atherosclerosis of the extremities with ulceration (440.23)
Chronic venous hypertension with ulcer (459.31)
Chronic venous hypertension with ulcer and inflammation (459.33)
diabetes mellitus (250.80-250.83)
Postphlebetic syndrome with ulcer (459.11)
Postphlebetic syndrome with ulcer and inflammation (459.13)

707.10 Ulcer of lower limb, unspecified

707.11 Ulcer of thigh

707.12 Ulcer of calf

707.13 Ulcer of ankle

707.14 Ulcer of heel and midfoot
Plantar surface of midfoot

707.15 Ulcer of other part of foot
Toes

707.19 Ulcer of other part of lower limb

707.8 Chronic ulcer of other specified sites
Ulcer, chronic:
neurogenic of other specified sites
trophic of other specified sites

707.9 Chronic ulcer of unspecified site
Chronic ulcer NOS
Trophic ulcer NOS
Tropical ulcer NOS
Ulcer of skin NOS

708 Urticaria

[*Excludes:*] *edema:*
angioneurotic (995.1)
Quincke's (995.1)
hereditary angioedema (277.6)
urticaria:
giant (995.1)
papulosa (Hebra) (698.2)
pigmentosa (juvenile) (congenital) (757.33)

708.0 Allergic urticaria

708.1 Idiopathic urticaria

708.2 Urticaria due to cold and heat
Thermal urticaria

708.3 Dermatographic urticaria
Dermatographia
Factitial urticaria

708.4 Vibratory urticaria

708.5 Cholinergic urticaria

708.8 Other specified urticaria
Nettle rash
Urticaria:
chronic
recurrent periodic

708.9 Urticaria, unspecified
Hives NOS

709 Other disorders of skin and subcutaneous tissue

[5] **709.0 Dyschromia**

[*Excludes:*] *albinism (270.2)*
pigmented nevus (216.0-216.9)
that of eyelid (374.52-374.53)

709.00 Dyschromia, unspecified

709.01 Vitiligo

709.09 Other

● Code new to this edition
▲ Revision of existing code
[4] [5] Fourth or fifth digit required

709.1 Vascular disorders of skin
    Angioma serpiginosum
    Purpura (primary) annularis telangiectodes

709.2 Scar conditions and fibrosis of skin
    Adherent scar (skin)
    Cicatrix
    Disfigurement (due to scar)
    Fibrosis, skin NOS
    Scar NOS

    | Excludes: | *keloid scar (701.4)*

709.3 Degenerative skin disorders

Calcinosis:	Degeneration, skin
circumscripta	Deposits, skin
cutis	Senile dermatosis NOS
Colloid milium	Subcutaneous calcification

709.4 Foreign body granuloma of skin and subcutaneous tissue

    | Excludes: | *residual foreign body without granuloma of skin and subcutaneous tissue (729.6)*
    that of muscle (728.82)

709.8 Other specified disorders of skin
    Epithelial hyperplasia   Vesicular eruption
    Menstrual dermatosis

709.9 Unspecified disorder of skin and subcutaneous tissue
    Dermatosis NOS

Add 4th or 5th digit	Nonspecific code	Unspecified code	Manifestation code

● Code new
  to this edition

▲ Revision of
  existing code

④ ⑤ Fourth or fifth
  digit required

13. DISEASES OF THE MUSCULOSKELETAL SYSTEM AND CONNECTIVE TISSUE (710-739)

The following fifth-digit subclassification is for use with categories 711-712, 715-716, 718-719, and 730:

0 **site unspecified**

1 **shoulder region**
Acromioclavicular joint(s)
Glenohumeral joint(s)
Sternoclavicular joint(s)
Clavicle joint(s)
Scapula joint(s)

2 **upper arm**
Elbow joint   Humerus

3 **forearm**
Radius   Wrist joint
Ulna

4 **hand**
Carpus   Phalanges [fingers]
Metacarpus

5 **pelvic region and thigh**
Buttock   Hip (joint)
Femur

6 **lower leg**
Fibula   Patella
Knee joint   Tibia

7 **ankle and foot**
Ankle joint   Phalanges, foot
Digits [toes]   Tarsus
Metatarsus   Other joints in foot

8 **other specified sites**
Head   Skull
Neck   Trunk
Ribs   Vertebral column

9 **multiple sites**

ARTHROPATHIES AND RELATED DISORDERS (710-719)

Excludes: disorders of spine (720.0-724.9)

710 **Diffuse diseases of connective tissue**
Includes: all collagen diseases whose effects are not mainly confined to a single system

Excludes: those affecting mainly the cardiovascular system, i.e., polyarteritis nodosa and allied conditions (446.0-446.7)

710.0 **Systemic lupus erythematosus**
Disseminated lupus erythematosus
Libman-Sacks disease

Use additional code, if desired, to identify manifestation, as:
endocarditis (424.91)
nephritis (583.81)
chronic (582.81)
nephrotic syndrome (581.81)

Excludes: lupus erythematosus (discoid) NOS (695.4)

710.1 **Systemic sclerosis**
Acrosclerosis
CRST syndrome
Progressive systemic sclerosis
Scleroderma

Use additional code, if desired, to identify manifestation, as:
lung involvement (517.8)
myopathy (359.6)

Excludes: circumscribed scleroderma (701.0)

710.2 **Sicca syndrome**
Keratoconjunctivitis sicca
Sjögren's disease

403

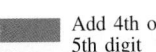 Add 4th or 5th digit   Nonspecific code   Unspecified code   Manifestation code

710.3 Dermatomyositis
Poikilodermatomyositis
Polymyositis with skin involvement

710.4 Polymyositis

710.5 Eosinophilia myalgia syndrome
Toxic oil syndrome

Use additional E code, if desired, to identify drug, if drug induced

710.8 Other specified diffuse diseases of connective tissue
Multifocal fibrosclerosis (idiopathic) NEC
Systemic fibrosclerosing syndrome

710.9 Unspecified diffuse connective tissue disease
Collagen disease NOS

⑤ **711 Arthropathy associated with infections**
Includes:
arthritis associated with conditions classifiable below
arthropathy associated with conditions classifiable below
polyarthritis associated with conditions classifiable below
polyarthropathy associated with conditions classifiable below

[Excludes:] *rheumatic fever (390)*

The following fifth-digit subclassification is for use with category 711; valid digits are in [brackets] under each code. For definitions, see the beginning of this chapter:

0 site unspecified
1 shoulder region
2 upper arm
3 forearm
4 hand
5 pelvic region and thigh
6 lower leg
7 ankle and foot
8 other specified sites
9 multiple sites

⑤ **711.0 Pyogenic arthritis**
[0-9] Arthritis or polyarthritis (due to):
coliform [Escherichia coli]
Hemophilus influenzae [H. influenzae]
pneumococcal
Pseudomonas
staphylococcal
streptococcal
Pyarthrosis

Use additional code, if desired, to identify infectious organism (041.0-041.8)

⑤ ***711.1 Arthropathy associated with Reiter's disease and nonspecific urethritis***
[0-9] *Code first underlying disease, as:*
nonspecific urethritis (099.4)
Reiter's disease (099.3)

⑤ ***711.2 Arthropathy in Behçet's syndrome***
[0-9] *Code first underlying disease (136.1)*

⑤ ***711.3 Postdysenteric arthropathy***
[0-9] *Code first underlying disease, as:*
dysentery (009.0)
enteritis, infectious (008.0-009.3)
paratyphoid fever (002.1-002.9)
typhoid fever (002.0)

[Excludes:] *salmonella arthritis (003.23)*

● Code new to this edition ▲ Revision of existing code ④ ⑤ Fourth or fifth digit required

⑤ **711.4** *Arthropathy associated with other bacterial diseases*
[0-9] *Code first underlying disease, as:*
diseases classifiable to 010-040, 090-099, except as in 711.1, 711.3, and 713.5
leprosy (030.0-030.9)
tuberculosis (015.0-015.9)

Excludes: *gonococcal arthritis (098.50)*
meningococcal arthritis (036.82)

⑤ **711.5** *Arthropathy associated with other viral diseases*
[0-9] *Code first underlying disease, as:*
diseases classifiable to 045-049, 050-079, 480, 487
O'nyong nyong (066.3)

Excludes: *that due to rubella (056.71)*

⑤ **711.6** *Arthropathy associated with mycoses*
[0-9] *Code first underlying disease (110.0-118)*

⑤ **711.7** *Arthropathy associated with helminthiasis*
[0-9] *Code first underlying disease, as:*
filariasis (125.0-125.9)

⑤ **711.8** *Arthropathy associated with other infectious and parasitic diseases*
[0-9] *Code first underlying disease, as:*
diseases classifiable to 080-088, 100-104, 130-136

Excludes: *arthropathy associated with sarcoidosis (713.7)*

⑤ **711.9** **Unspecified infective arthritis**
[0-9] Infective arthritis or polyarthritis (acute) (chronic) (subacute) NOS

⑤ **712** **Crystal arthropathies**
Includes: crystal-induced arthritis and synovitis

Excludes: *gouty arthropathy (274.0)*

The following fifth-digit subclassification is for use with category 712; valid digits are in [brackets] under each code. See beginning of this chapter for definitions:

0 **site unspecified**

1 **shoulder region**

2 **upper arm**

3 **forearm**

4 **hand**

5 **pelvic region and thigh**

6 **lower leg**

7 **ankle and foot**

8 **other specified sites**

9 **multiple sites**

⑤ **712.1** *Chondrocalcinosis due to dicalcium phosphate crystals*
[0-9] Chondrocalcinosis due to dicalcium phosphate crystals (with other crystals)
Code first underlying disease (275.4)

⑤ **712.2** *Chondrocalcinosis due to pyrophosphate crystals*
[0-9] *Code first underlying disease (275.4)*

⑤ **712.3** *Chondrocalcinosis, unspecified*
[0-9] *Code first underlying disease (275.4)*

⑤ **712.8** **Other specified crystal arthropathies**
[0-9]

⑤ **712.9** **Unspecified crystal arthropathy**
[0-9]

| | Add 4th or 5th digit | | Nonspecific code | | Unspecified code | | Manifestation code |

713 **Arthropathy associated with other disorders classified elsewhere**
Includes:
> arthritis associated with conditions classifiable below
> arthropathy associated with conditions classifiable below
> polyarthritis associated with conditions classifiable below
> polyarthropathy associated with conditions classifiable below

713.0 *Arthropathy associated with other endocrine and metabolic disorders*
Code first underlying disease, as:
acromegaly (253.0)
hemochromatosis (275.0)
hyperparathyroidism (252.0)
hypogammaglobulinemia (279.00-279.09)
hypothyroidism (243-244.9)
lipoid metabolism disorder (272.0-272.9)
ochronosis (270.2)

Excludes: *arthropathy associated with:*
> *amyloidosis (713.7)*
> *crystal deposition disorders, except gout (712.1-712.9)*
> *diabetic neuropathy (713.5)*
> *gouty arthropathy (274.0)*

713.1 *Arthropathy associated with gastrointestinal conditions other than infections*
Code first underlying disease, as:
regional enteritis (555.0-555.9)
ulcerative colitis (556)

713.2 *Arthropathy associated with hematological disorders*
Code first underlying disease, as:
hemoglobinopathy (282.4-282.7)
hemophilia (286.0-286.2)
leukemia (204.0-208.9)
malignant reticulosis (202.3)
multiple myelomatosis (203.0)

Excludes: *arthropathy associated with Henoch-Schönlein purpura (713.6)*

713.3 *Arthropathy associated with dermatological disorders*
Code first underlying disease, as:
erythema multiforme (695.1)
erythema nodosum (695.2)

Excludes: *psoriatic arthropathy (696.0)*

713.4 *Arthropathy associated with respiratory disorders*
Code first underlying disease, as:
diseases classifiable to 490-519

Excludes: *arthropathy associated with respiratory infections (711.0, 711.4-711.8)*

713.5 *Arthropathy associated with neurological disorders*
Charcot's arthropathy associated with diseases classifiable elsewhere
Neuropathic arthritis associated with diseases classifiable elsewhere
Code first underlying disease, as:
neuropathic joint disease [Charcot's joints]:
NOS (094.0)
diabetic (250.6)
syringomyelic (336.0)
tabetic [syphilitic] (094.0)

713.6 *Arthropathy associated with hypersensitivity reaction*
Code first underlying disease, as:
Henoch (-Schönlein) purpura (287.0)
serum sickness (999.5)

Excludes: *allergic arthritis NOS (716.2)*

713.7 *Other general diseases with articular involvement*
Code first underlying disease, as:
amyloidosis (277.3)
familial Mediterranean fever (277.3)
sarcoidosis (135)

● Code new
   to this edition
▲ Revision of
   existing code
④ ⑤ Fourth or fifth
   digit required

713.8 ***Arthropathy associated with other conditions classifiable elsewhere***
Code first underlying disease, as:
conditions classifiable elsewhere except as in 711.1-711.8, 712, and 713.0-713.7

714 Rheumatoid arthritis and other inflammatory polyarthropathies

[*Excludes:*] *rheumatic fever (390)*
rheumatoid arthritis of spine NOS (720.0)

714.0 Rheumatoid arthritis
Arthritis or polyarthritis:
atrophic
rheumatic (chronic)

Use additional code, if desired, to identify manifestation, as:
myopathy (359.6)
polyneuropathy (357.1)

[*Excludes:*] *juvenile rheumatoid arthritis NOS (714.30)*

714.1 Felty's syndrome
Rheumatoid arthritis with splenoadenomegaly and leukopenia

714.2 Other rheumatoid arthritis with visceral or systemic involvement
Rheumatoid carditis

[5] **714.3 Juvenile chronic polyarthritis**

714.30 Polyarticular juvenile rheumatoid arthritis, chronic or unspecified
Juvenile rheumatoid arthritis NOS
Still's disease

714.31 Polyarticular juvenile rheumatoid arthritis, acute

714.32 Pauciarticular juvenile rheumatoid arthritis

714.33 Monoarticular juvenile rheumatoid arthritis

714.4 Chronic postrheumatic arthropathy
Chronic rheumatoid nodular fibrositis
Jaccoud's syndrome

[5] **714.8 Other specified inflammatory polyarthropathies**

714.81 Rheumatoid lung
Caplan's syndrome
Diffuse interstitial rheumatoid disease of lung
Fibrosing alveolitis, rheumatoid

714.89 Other

714.9 Unspecified inflammatory polyarthropathy
Inflammatory polyarthropathy or polyarthritis NOS

[*Excludes:*] *polyarthropathy NOS (716.5)*

[5] 715 Osteoarthrosis and allied disorders

Note: Localized, in the subcategories below, includes bilateral involvement of the same site.
Includes: arthritis or polyarthritis:
degenerative
hypertrophic
degenerative joint disease
osteoarthritis

[*Excludes:*] *Marie-Strümpell spondylitis (720.0)*
osteoarthrosis [osteoarthritis] of spine (721.0-721.9)

The following fifth-digit subclassification is for use with category 715; valid digits are in [brackets] under each code. See beginning of this chapter for definitions:

0 site unspecified
1 shoulder region
2 upper arm
3 forearm
4 hand
5 pelvic region and thigh
6 lower leg
7 ankle and foot
8 other specified sites
9 multiple sites

[5] **715.0 Osteoarthrosis, generalized**
[0,4,9] Degenerative joint disease, involving multiple joints
Primary generalized hypertrophic osteoarthrosis

[5] **715.1 Osteoarthrosis, localized, primary**
[0-8] Localized osteoarthropathy, idiopathic

[5] **715.2 Osteoarthrosis, localized, secondary**
[0-8] Coxae malum senilis

[5] **715.3 Osteoarthrosis, localized, not specified whether primary or secondary**
[0-8] Otto's pelvis

[5] **715.8 Osteoarthrosis involving, or with mention of more than one site, but not specified as generalized**
[0,9]

[5] **715.9 Osteoarthrosis, unspecified whether generalized or localized**
[0-8]

[5] **716 Other and unspecified arthropathies**

[Excludes:] *cricoarytenoid arthropathy (478.79)*

The following fifth-digit subclassification is for use with category 716; valid digits are in [brackets] under each code. See beginning of this chapter for definitions:

0 site unspecified
1 shoulder region
2 upper arm
3 forearm
4 hand
5 pelvic region and thigh
6 lower leg
7 ankle and foot
8 other specified sites
9 multiple sites

[5] **716.0 Kaschin-Beck disease**
[0-9] Endemic polyarthritis

[5] **716.1 Traumatic arthropathy**
[0-9]

[5] **716.2 Allergic arthritis**
[0-9]

[Excludes:] *arthritis associated with Henoch-Schönlein purpura or serum sickness (713.6)*

[5] **716.3 Climacteric arthritis**
[0-9] Menopausal arthritis

[5] **716.4 Transient arthropathy**
[0-9]

[Excludes:] *palindromic rheumatism (719.3)*

[5] **716.5 Unspecified polyarthropathy or polyarthritis**
[0-9]

[5] **716.6 Unspecified monoarthritis**
[0-8] Coxitis

[5] **716.8 Other specified arthropathy**
[0-9]

[5] **716.9 Arthropathy, unspecified**
[0-9] Arthritis (acute) (chronic) (subacute)
Arthropathy (acute) (chronic) (subacute)
Articular rheumatism (chronic)
Inflammation of joint NOS

717 Internal derangement of knee
Includes:
degeneration of articular cartilage or meniscus of knee
rupture, old, of articular cartilage or meniscus of knee
tear, old, of articular cartilage or meniscus of knee

[Excludes:] *acute derangement of knee (836.0-836.6)*
ankylosis (718.5)
contracture (718.4)
current injury (836.0-836.6)
deformity (736.4-736.6)
recurrent dislocation (718.3)

717.0 Old bucket handle tear of medial meniscus
Old bucket handle tear of unspecified cartilage

717.1 Derangement of anterior horn of medial meniscus

717.2 Derangement of posterior horn of medial meniscus

717.3 Other and unspecified derangement of medial meniscus
Degeneration of internal semilunar cartilage

[5] **717.4 Derangement of lateral meniscus**

717.40 Derangement of lateral meniscus, unspecified

717.41 Bucket handle tear of lateral meniscus

717.42 Derangement of anterior horn of lateral meniscus

717.43 Derangement of posterior horn of lateral meniscus

717.49 Other

717.5 Derangement of meniscus, not elsewhere classified
Congenital discoid meniscus
Cyst of semilunar cartilage
Derangement of semilunar cartilage NOS

717.6 Loose body in knee
Joint mice, knee
Rice bodies, knee (joint)

717.7 Chondromalacia of patella
Chondromalacia patellae
Degeneration [softening] of articular cartilage of patella

[5] **717.8 Other internal derangement of knee**

717.81 Old disruption of lateral collateral ligament

717.82 Old disruption of medial collateral ligament

717.83 Old disruption of anterior cruciate ligament

717.84 Old disruption of posterior cruciate ligament

717.85 Old disruption of other ligaments of knee
Capsular ligament of knee

717.89 Other
Old disruption of ligaments of knee NOS

717.9 Unspecified internal derangement of knee
Derangement NOS of knee

[5] **718 Other derangement of joint**

[Excludes:] *current injury (830.0-848.9)*
jaw (524.6)

The following fifth-digit subclassification is for use with category 718; valid digits are in [brackets] under each code. See beginning of this chapter for definitions:

0 site unspecified
1 shoulder region
2 upper arm
3 forearm
4 hand
5 pelvic region and thigh
6 lower leg
7 ankle and foot

8 **other specified sites**

9 **multiple sites**

⑤ **718.0 Articular cartilage disorder**
[0-5, 7-9] Meniscus:
disorder
rupture, old
tear, old
Old rupture of ligament(s) of joint NOS

[Excludes:] *articular cartilage disorder:*
in ochronosis (270.2)
knee (717.0-717.9)
chondrocalcinosis (275.4)
metastatic calcification (275.4)

⑤ **718.1 Loose body in joint**
[0-5, 7-9] Joint mice

[Excludes:] *knee (717.6)*

⑤ **718.2 Pathological dislocation**
[0-9] Dislocation or displacement of joint, not recurrent and not current injury
Spontaneous dislocation (joint)

⑤ **718.3 Recurrent dislocation of joint**
[0-9]

⑤ **718.4 Contracture of joint**
[0-9]

⑤ **718.5 Ankylosis of joint**
[0-9] Ankylosis of joint (fibrous) (osseous)

[Excludes:] *spine (724.9)*
stiffness of joint without mention of ankylosis (719.5)

⑤ **718.6 Unspecified intrapelvic protrusion of acetabulum**
[0, 5] Protrusio acetabuli, unspecified

⑤ **718.7 Developmental dislocation of joint**
[0-9]

[Excludes:] *congenital dislocation of joint (754.0-755.8)*
traumatic dislocation of joint (830-839)

⑤ **718.8 Other joint derangement, not elsewhere classified**
[0-9] Flail joint (paralytic) Instability of joint

[Excludes:] *deformities classifiable to 736 (736.0-736.9)*

⑤ **718.9 Unspecified derangement of joint**
[0-5, 7-9]

[Excludes:] *knee (717.9)*

⑤ **719 Other and unspecified disorders of joint**

[Excludes:] *jaw (524.6)*

The following fifth-digit subclassification is for use with category 719; valid digits are in [brackets] under each code. See beginning of this chapter for definitions:

0 **site unspecified**

1 **shoulder region**

2 **upper arm**

3 **forearm**

4 **hand**

5 **pelvic region and thigh**

6 **lower leg**

7 **ankle and foot**

8 **other specified sites**

9 **multiple sites**

⑤ **719.0 Effusion of joint**
[0-9] Hydrarthrosis
Swelling of joint, with or without pain

[Excludes:] *intermittent hydrarthrosis (719.3)*

⑤ **719.1 Hemarthrosis**
[0-9]
> Excludes: *current injury (840.0-848.9)*

⑤ **719.2 Villonodular synovitis**
[0-9]

⑤ **719.3 Palindromic rheumatism**
[0-9]   Hench-Rosenberg syndrome
        Intermittent hydrarthrosis

⑤ **719.4 Pain in joint**
[0-9]   Arthralgia

⑤ **719.5 Stiffness of joint, not elsewhere classified**
[0-9]

⑤ **719.6 Other symptoms referable to joint**
[0-9]   Joint crepitus   Snapping hip

⑤ **719.7 Difficulty in walking**
[0, 5-9]
> Excludes: *abnormality of gait (781.2)*

⑤ **719.8 Other specified disorders of joint**
[0-9]   Calcification of joint   Fistula of joint
> Excludes: *temporomandibular joint-pain-dysfunction syndrome [Costen's syndrome] (524.6)*

⑤ **719.9 Unspecified disorder of joint**
[0-9]

DORSOPATHIES (720-724)

> Excludes: *curvature of spine (737.0-737.9)*
> *osteochondrosis of spine (juvenile) (732.0)*
> *adult (732.8)*

720 **Ankylosing spondylitis and other inflammatory spondylopathies**

720.0 Ankylosing spondylitis
        Rheumatoid arthritis of spine NOS
        Spondylitis:
          Marie-Strümpell
          rheumatoid

720.1 Spinal enthesopathy
        Disorder of peripheral ligamentous or muscular attachments of spine
        Romanus lesion

720.2 Sacroiliitis, not elsewhere classified
        Inflammation of sacroiliac joint NOS

⑤ **720.8 Other inflammatory spondylopathies**

> **720.81** *Inflammatory spondylopathies in diseases classified elsewhere*
> *Code first underlying disease, as:*
> tuberculosis (015.0)

> **720.89** **Other**

720.9 Unspecified inflammatory spondylopathy
        Spondylitis NOS

721 **Spondylosis and allied disorders**

721.0 Cervical spondylosis without myelopathy
        Cervical or cervicodorsal:
          arthritis
          osteoarthritis
          spondylarthritis

721.1 Cervical spondylosis with myelopathy
        Anterior spinal artery compression syndrome
        Spondylogenic compression of cervical spinal cord
        Vertebral artery compression syndrome

Add 4th or 5th digit	Nonspecific code	Unspecified code	Manifestation code

721.2 Thoracic spondylosis without myelopathy
Thoracic:
arthritis
osteoarthritis
spondylarthritis

721.3 Lumbosacral spondylosis without myelopathy
Lumbar or lumbosacral:
arthritis
osteoarthritis
spondylarthritis

⑤ **721.4 Thoracic or lumbar spondylosis with myelopathy**

    721.41 Thoracic region
Spondylogenic compression of thoracic spinal cord

    721.42 Lumbar region
Spondylogenic compression of lumbar spinal cord

721.5 Kissing spine
Baastrup's syndrome

721.6 Ankylosing vertebral hyperostosis

721.7 Traumatic spondylopathy
Kümmell's disease or spondylitis

721.8 Other allied disorders of spine

⑤ **721.9 Spondylosis of unspecified site**

    721.90 Without mention of myelopathy
Spinal:
arthritis (deformans) (degenerative) (hypertrophic)
osteoarthritis NOS
Spondylarthrosis NOS

    721.91 With myelopathy
Spondylogenic compression of spinal cord NOS

722 Intervertebral disc disorders

722.0 Displacement of cervical intervertebral disc without myelopathy
Neuritis (brachial) or radiculitis due to displacement or rupture of cervical intervertebral disc
Any condition classifiable to 722.2 of the cervical or cervicothoracic intervertebral disc

⑤ **722.1 Displacement of thoracic or lumbar intervertebral disc without myelopathy**

    722.10 Lumbar intervertebral disc without myelopathy
Lumbago or sciatica due to displacement of intervertebral disc
Neuritis or radiculitis due to displacement or rupture of lumbar intervertebral disc
Any condition classifiable to 722.2 of the lumbar or lumbosacral intervertebral disc

    722.11 Thoracic intervertebral disc without myelopathy
Any condition classifiable to 722.2 of thoracic intervertebral disc

722.2 Displacement of intervertebral disc, site unspecified, without myelopathy
Discogenic syndrome NOS
Herniation of nucleus pulposus NOS
Intervertebral disc NOS:
extrusion
prolapse
protrusion
rupture
Neuritis or radiculitis due to displacement or rupture of intervertebral disc

⑤ **722.3 Schmorl's nodes**

    722.30 Unspecified region

    722.31 Thoracic region

    722.32 Lumbar region

    722.39 Other

722.4 Degeneration of cervical intervertebral disc
Degeneration of cervicothoracic intervertebral disc

⑤ **722.5 Degeneration of thoracic or lumbar intervertebral disc**

    722.51 Thoracic or thoracolumbar intervertebral disc

    722.52 Lumbar or lumbosacral intervertebral disc

● Code new
   to this edition
▲ Revision of
   existing code
④ ⑤ Fourth or fifth
     digit required

722.6 Degeneration of intervertebral disc, site unspecified
Degenerative disc disease NOS
Narrowing of intervertebral disc or space NOS

[5] **722.7 Intervertebral disc disorder with myelopathy**

722.70 Unspecified region

722.71 Cervical region

722.72 Thoracic region

722.73 Lumbar region

[5] **722.8 Postlaminectomy syndrome**

722.80 Unspecified region

722.81 Cervical region

722.82 Thoracic region

722.83 Lumbar region

[5] **722.9 Other and unspecified disc disorder**
Calcification of intervertebral cartilage or disc
Discitis

722.90 Unspecified region

722.91 Cervical region

722.92 Thoracic region

722.93 Lumbar region

723 Other disorders of cervical region

[*Excludes:*] *conditions due to:*
intervertebral disc disorders (722.0-722.9)
spondylosis (721.0-721.9)

723.0 Spinal stenosis in cervical region

723.1 Cervicalgia
Pain in neck

723.2 Cervicocranial syndrome
Barré-Liéou syndrome
Posterior cervical sympathetic syndrome

723.3 Cervicobrachial syndrome (diffuse)

723.4 Brachial neuritis or radiculitis NOS
Cervical radiculitis
Radicular syndrome of upper limbs

723.5 Torticollis, unspecified
Contracture of neck

[*Excludes:*] *congenital (754.1)*
due to birth injury (767.8)
hysterical (300.11)
ocular torticollis (781.93)
psychogenic (306.0)
spasmodic (333.83)
traumatic, current (847.0)

723.6 Panniculitis specified as affecting neck

723.7 Ossification of posterior longitudinal ligament in cervical region

723.8 Other syndromes affecting cervical region
Cervical syndrome NEC
Klippel's disease
Occipital neuralgia

723.9 Unspecified musculoskeletal disorders and symptoms referable to neck
Cervical (region) disorder NOS

724 Other and unspecified disorders of back

[*Excludes:*] *collapsed vertebra (code to cause, e.g., osteoporosis, 733.00-733.09)*
conditions due to:
intervertebral disc disorders (722.0-722.9)
spondylosis (721.0-721.9)

[5] **724.0 Spinal stenosis, other than cervical**

724.00 Spinal stenosis, unspecified region

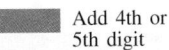

Add 4th or 5th digit | Nonspecific code | Unspecified code | Manifestation code

724.01 **Thoracic region**

724.02 **Lumbar region**

724.09 **Other**

724.1 **Pain in thoracic spine**

724.2 **Lumbago**
Low back pain   Lumbalgia
Low back syndrome

724.3 **Sciatica**
Neuralgia or neuritis of sciatic nerve
Excludes: *specified lesion of sciatic nerve (355.0)*

724.4 **Thoracic or lumbosacral neuritis or radiculitis, unspecified**
Radicular syndrome of lower limbs

724.5 **Backache, unspecified**
Vertebrogenic (pain) syndrome NOS

724.6 **Disorders of sacrum**
Ankylosis, lumbosacral or sacroiliac (joint)
Instability, lumbosacral or sacroiliac (joint)

⑤ **724.7** **Disorders of coccyx**

724.70 **Unspecified disorder of coccyx**

724.71 **Hypermobility of coccyx**

724.79 **Other**
Coccygodynia

724.8 **Other symptoms referable to back**
Ossification of posterior longitudinal ligament NOS
Panniculitis specified as sacral or affecting back

724.9 **Other unspecified back disorders**
Ankylosis of spine NOS
Compression of spinal nerve root NEC
Spinal disorder NOS
Excludes: *sacroiliitis (720.2)*

RHEUMATISM, EXCLUDING THE BACK (725-729)

Includes: disorders of muscles and tendons and their attachments, and of other soft tissues

725 **Polymyalgia rheumatica**

726 **Peripheral enthesopathies and allied syndromes**
Note: Enthesopathies are disorders of peripheral ligamentous or muscular attachments.
Excludes: *spinal enthesopathy (720.1)*

726.0 **Adhesive capsulitis of shoulder**

⑤ **726.1** **Rotator cuff syndrome of shoulder and allied disorders**

726.10 **Disorders of bursae and tendons in shoulder region, unspecified**
Rotator cuff syndrome NOS
Supraspinatus syndrome NOS

726.11 **Calcifying tendinitis of shoulder**

726.12 **Bicipital tenosynovitis**

726.19 **Other specified disorders**
Excludes: *complete rupture of rotator cuff, nontraumatic (727.61)*

726.2 **Other affections of shoulder region, not elsewhere classified**
Periarthritis of shoulder
Scapulohumeral fibrositis

⑤ **726.3** **Enthesopathy of elbow region**

726.30 **Enthesopathy of elbow, unspecified**

726.31 **Medial epicondylitis**

726.32 **Lateral epicondylitis**
Epicondylitis NOS   Tennis elbow
Golfers' elbow

726.33 **Olecranon bursitis**
Bursitis of elbow

● Code new to this edition   ▲ Revision of existing code   ④ ⑤ Fourth or fifth digit required

726.39 Other

726.4 Enthesopathy of wrist and carpus
Bursitis of hand or wrist
Periarthritis of wrist

726.5 Enthesopathy of hip region
Bursitis of hip
Gluteal tendinitis
Iliac crest spur
Psoas tendinitis
Trochanteric tendinitis

[5] **726.6 Enthesopathy of knee**

726.60 Enthesopathy of knee, unspecified
Bursitis of knee NOS

726.61 Pes anserinus tendinitis or bursitis

726.62 Tibial collateral ligament bursitis
Pellegrini-Stieda syndrome

726.63 Fibular collateral ligament bursitis

726.64 Patellar tendinitis

726.65 Prepatellar bursitis

726.69 Other
Bursitis:
infrapatellar
subpatellar

[5] **726.7 Enthesopathy of ankle and tarsus**

726.70 Enthesopathy of ankle and tarsus, unspecified
Metatarsalgia NOS

[*Excludes:*] *Morton's metatarsalgia (355.6)*

726.71 Achilles bursitis or tendinitis

726.72 Tibialis tendinitis
Tibialis (anterior) (posterior) tendinitis

726.73 Calcaneal spur

726.79 Other
Peroneal tendinitis

726.8 Other peripheral enthesopathies

[5] **726.9 Unspecified enthesopathy**

726.90 Enthesopathy of unspecified site
Capsulitis NOS
Periarthritis NOS
Tendinitis NOS

726.91 Exostosis of unspecified site
Bone spur NOS

727 Other disorders of synovium, tendon, and bursa

[5] **727.0 Synovitis and tenosynovitis**

727.00 Synovitis and tenosynovitis, unspecified
Synovitis NOS
Tenosynovitis NOS

727.01 Synovitis and tenosynovitis in diseases classified elsewhere
Code first underlying disease, as:
tuberculosis (015.0-015.9)

[*Excludes:*] *crystal-induced (275.4)*
gonococcal (098.51)
gouty (274.0)
syphilitic (095.7)

727.02 Giant cell tumor of tendon sheath

727.03 Trigger finger (acquired)

727.04 Radial styloid tenosynovitis
de Quervain's disease

727.05 Other tenosynovitis of hand and wrist

727.06 Tenosynovitis of foot and ankle

727.09 Other

727.1 Bunion

Add 4th or 5th digit | Nonspecific code | Unspecified code | Manifestation code

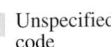

727.2 **Specific bursitides often of occupational origin**

Beat:
   elbow
   hand
   knee

Chronic crepitant synovitis of wrist
Miners':
   elbow
   knee

727.3 **Other bursitis**
Bursitis NOS

Excludes: *bursitis:*
        gonococcal (098.52)
        subacromial (726.19)
        subcoracoid (726.19)
        subdeltoid (726.19)
        syphilitic (095.7)
        "frozen shoulder" (726.0)

⑤ **727.4** **Ganglion and cyst of synovium, tendon, and bursa**

   727.40 **Synovial cyst, unspecified**

Excludes: *that of popliteal space (727.51)*

   727.41 **Ganglion of joint**

   727.42 **Ganglion of tendon sheath**

   727.43 **Ganglion, unspecified**

   727.49 **Other**
      Cyst of bursa

⑤ **727.5** **Rupture of synovium**

   727.50 **Rupture of synovium, unspecified**

   727.51 **Synovial cyst of popliteal space**
      Baker's cyst (knee)

   727.59 **Other**

⑤ **727.6** **Rupture of tendon, nontraumatic**

   727.60 **Nontraumatic rupture of unspecified tendon**

   727.61 **Complete rupture of rotator cuff**

   727.62 **Tendons of biceps (long head)**

   727.63 **Extensor tendons of hand and wrist**

   727.64 **Flexor tendons of hand and wrist**

   727.65 **Quadriceps tendon**

   727.66 **Patellar tendon**

   727.67 **Achilles tendon**

   727.68 **Other tendons of foot and ankle**

   727.69 **Other**

⑤ **727.8** **Other disorders of synovium, tendon, and bursa**

   727.81 **Contracture of tendon (sheath)**
      Short Achilles tendon (acquired)

   727.82 **Calcium deposits in tendon and bursa**
      Calcification of tendon NOS
      Calcific tendinitis NOS

Excludes: *peripheral ligamentous or muscular attachments (726.0-726.9)*

   727.83 **Plica syndrome**
      Plica knee

   727.89 **Other**
      Abscess of bursa or tendon

Excludes: *xanthomatosis localized to tendons (272.7)*

  727.9 **Unspecified disorder of synovium, tendon, and bursa**

728 **Disorders of muscle, ligament, and fascia**

Excludes: *enthesopathies (726.0-726.9)*
      muscular dystrophies (359.0-359.1)
      myoneural disorders (358.0-358.9)
      myopathies (359.2-359.9)
      old disruption of ligaments of knee (717.81-717.89)

  ● Code new   ▲ Revision of   ④ ⑤ Fourth or fifth
      to this edition   existing code   digit required

728.0 Infective myositis
Myositis:
purulent
suppurative

[Excludes:] *myositis:*
epidemic (074.1)
interstitial (728.81)
syphilitic (095.6)
tropical (040.81)

5 **728.1 Muscular calcification and ossification**

728.10 Calcification and ossification, unspecified
Massive calcification (paraplegic)

728.11 Progressive myositis ossificans

728.12 Traumatic myositis ossificans
Myositis ossificans (circumscripta)

728.13 Postoperative heterotopic calcification

728.19 Other
Polymyositis ossificans

728.2 Muscular wasting and disuse atrophy, not elsewhere classified
Amyotrophia NOS
Myofibrosis

[Excludes:] *neuralgic amyotrophy (353.5)*
progressive muscular atrophy (335.0-335.9)

728.3 Other specific muscle disorders
Arthrogryposis
Immobility syndrome (paraplegic)

[Excludes:] *arthrogryposis multiplex congenita (754.89)*
stiff-man syndrome (333.91)

728.4 Laxity of ligament

728.5 Hypermobility syndrome

728.6 Contracture of palmar fascia
Dupuytren's contracture

5 **728.7 Other fibromatoses**

728.71 Plantar fascial fibromatosis
Contracture of plantar fascia
Plantar fasciitis (traumatic)

728.79 Other
Garrod's or knuckle pads
Nodular fasciitis
Pseudosarcomatous fibromatosis (proliferative) (subcutaneous)

5 **728.8 Other disorders of muscle, ligament, and fascia**

728.81 Interstitial myositis

728.82 Foreign body granuloma of muscle
Talc granuloma of muscle

728.83 Rupture of muscle, nontraumatic

728.84 Diastasis of muscle
Diastasis recti (abdomen)

[Excludes:] *diastasis recti complicating pregnancy, labor, and delivery (665.8)*

728.85 Spasm of muscle

728.86 Necrotizing fasciitis
Use additional code to identify:
infectious organism (041.00 - 041.89)
gangrene (785.4), if applicable

728.89 Other
Eosinophilic fasciitis
Use additional E code, if desired, to identify drug, if drug induced

728.9 Unspecified disorder of muscle, ligament, and fascia

Add 4th or 5th digit | Nonspecific code | Unspecified code | Manifestation code

729 **Other disorders of soft tissues**

Excludes: *acroparesthesia (443.89)*
carpal tunnel syndrome (354.0)
disorders of the back (720.0-724.9)
entrapment syndromes (354.0-355.9)
palindromic rheumatism (719.3)
periarthritis (726.0-726.9)
psychogenic rheumatism (306.0)

729.0 **Rheumatism, unspecified and fibrositis**

729.1 **Myalgia and myositis, unspecified**
Fibromyositis NOS

729.2 **Neuralgia, neuritis, and radiculitis, unspecified**

Excludes: *brachial radiculitis (723.4)*
cervical radiculitis (723.4)
lumbosacral radiculitis (724.4)
mononeuritis (354.0-355.9)
radiculitis due to intervertebral disc involvement (722.0-722.2, 722.7)
sciatica (724.3)

⑤ **729.3** **Panniculitis, unspecified**

729.30 **Panniculitis, unspecified site**
Weber-Christian disease

729.31 **Hypertrophy of fat pad, knee**
Hypertrophy of infrapatellar fat pad

729.39 **Other site**

Excludes: *panniculitis specified as (affecting):*
back (724.8)
neck (723.6)
sacral (724.8)

729.4 **Fasciitis, unspecified**

Excludes: *necrotizing fasciitis (728.86)*
nodular fasciitis (728.79)

729.5 **Pain in limb**

729.6 **Residual foreign body in soft tissue**

Excludes: *foreign body granuloma:*
muscle (728.82)
skin and subcutaneous tissue (709.4)

⑤ **729.8** **Other musculoskeletal symptoms referable to limbs**

729.81 **Swelling of limb**

729.82 **Cramp**

729.89 **Other**

Excludes: *abnormality of gait (781.2)*
tetany (781.7)
transient paralysis of limb (781.4)

729.9 **Other and unspecified disorders of soft tissue**
Polyalgia

OSTEOPATHIES, CHONDROPATHIES, AND ACQUIRED MUSCULOSKELETAL DEFORMITIES (730-739)

⑤ **730** **Osteomyelitis, periostitis, and other infections involving bone**

Excludes: *jaw (526.4-526.5)*
petrous bone (383.2)

Use additional code, if desired, to identify organism, such as Staphylococcus (041.1)

The following fifth-digit subclassification is for use with category 730; valid digits are in [brackets] under each code. See beginning of this chapter for definitions:

0 **site unspecified**

1 **shoulder region**

2 **upper arm**

3 **forearm**

● Code new
to this edition

▲ Revision of
existing code

④ ⑤ Fourth or fifth
digit required

4 **hand**
5 **pelvic region and thigh**
6 **lower leg**
7 **ankle and foot**
8 **other specified sites**
9 **multiple sites**

[5] **730.0 Acute osteomyelitis**
[0-9] Abscess of any bone except accessory sinus, jaw, or mastoid
Acute or subacute osteomyelitis, with or without mention of periostitis

[5] **730.1 Chronic osteomyelitis**
[0-9] Brodie's abscess
Chronic or old osteomyelitis, with or without mention of periostitis
Sequestrum of bone
Sclerosing osteomyelitis of Garré

[*Excludes:*] *aseptic necrosis of bone (733.40-733.49)*

[5] **730.2 Unspecified osteomyelitis**
[0-9] Osteitis or osteomyelitis NOS, with or without mention of periostitis

[5] **730.3 Periostitis without mention of osteomyelitis**
[0-9] Abscess of periosteum without mention of osteomyelitis
Periostosis without mention of osteomyelitis

[*Excludes:*] *that in secondary syphilis (091.61)*

[5] ***730.7 Osteopathy resulting from poliomyelitis***
[0-9] *Code first underlying disease (045.0-045.9)*

[5] ***730.8 Other infections involving bone in diseases classified elsewhere***
[0-9] *Code first underlying disease, as:*
tuberculosis (015.0-015.9)
typhoid fever (002.0)

[*Excludes:*] *syphilis of bone NOS (095.5)*

[5] **730.9 Unspecified infection of bone**
[0-9]

731 Osteitis deformans and osteopathies associated with other disorders classified elsewhere

731.0 Osteitis deformans without mention of bone tumor
Paget's disease of bone

731.1 Osteitis deformans in diseases classified elsewhere
Code first underlying disease, as:
malignant neoplasm of bone (170.0-170.9)

731.2 Hypertrophic pulmonary osteoarthropathy
Bamberger-Marie disease

731.8 Other bone involvement in diseases classified elsewhere
Code first underlying disease, as:
diabetes mellitus (250.8)
Use additional code to specify bone condition, such as:
acute osteomyelitis (730.00-730.09)

732 Osteochondropathies

732.0 Juvenile osteochondrosis of spine
Juvenile osteochondrosis (of):
marginal or vertebral epiphysis (of Scheuermann)
spine NOS
Vertebral epiphysitis

[*Excludes:*] *adolescent postural kyphosis (737.0)*

732.1 Juvenile osteochondrosis of hip and pelvis
Coxa plana
Ischiopubic synchondrosis (of van Neck)
Osteochondrosis (juvenile) of:
acetabulum
head of femur (of Legg-Calvé-Perthes)
iliac crest (of Buchanan)
symphysis pubis (of Pierson)
Pseudocoxalgia

Add 4th or 5th digit | Nonspecific code | Unspecified code | Manifestation code

732.2 Nontraumatic slipped upper femoral epiphysis
Slipped upper femoral epiphysis NOS

732.3 Juvenile osteochondrosis of upper extremity
Osteochondrosis (juvenile) of:
  capitulum of humerus (of Panner)
  carpal lunate (of Kienbock)
  hand NOS
  head of humerus (of Haas)
  heads of metacarpals (of Mauclaire)
  lower ulna (of Burns)
  radial head (of Brailsford)
  upper extremity NOS

732.4 Juvenile osteochondrosis of lower extremity, excluding foot
Osteochondrosis (juvenile) of:
  lower extremity NOS
  primary patellar center (of Köhler)
  proximal tibia (of Blount)
  secondary patellar center (of Sinding-Larsen)
  tibial tubercle (of Osgood-Schlatter)
Tibia vara

732.5 Juvenile osteochondrosis of foot
Calcaneal apophysitis
Epiphysitis, os calcis
Osteochondrosis (juvenile) of:
  astragalus (of Diaz)
  calcaneum (of Sever)
  foot NOS
  metatarsal
    second (of Freiberg)
    fifth (of Iselin)
  os tibiale externum (Haglund)
  tarsal navicular (of Köhler)

732.6 Other juvenile osteochondrosis
Apophysitis specified as juvenile, of other site, or site NOS
Epiphysitis specified as juvenile, of other site, or site NOS
Osteochondritis specified as juvenile, of other site, or site NOS
Osteochondrosis specified as juvenile, of other site, or site NOS

732.7 Osteochondritis dissecans

732.8 Other specified forms of osteochondropathy
Adult osteochondrosis of spine

732.9 Unspecified osteochondropathy
Apophysitis NOS, not specified as adult or juvenile, of unspecified site
Epiphysitis NOS, not specified as adult or juvenile, of unspecified site
Osteochondritis NOS, not specified as adult or juvenile, of unspecified site
Osteochondrosis NOS, not specified as adult or juvenile, of unspecified site

733 Other disorders of bone and cartilage
Excludes: *bone spur (726.91)*
      cartilage of, or loose body in, joint (717.0-717.9, 718.0-718.9)
      giant cell granuloma of jaw (526.3)
      osteitis fibrosa cystica generalisata (252.0)
      osteomalacia (268.2)
      polyostotic fibrous dysplasia of bone (756.54)
      prognathism, retrognathism (524.1)
      xanthomatosis localized to bone (272.7)

⑤ **733.0 Osteoporosis**

  733.00 Osteoporosis, unspecified
  Wedging of vertebra NOS

  733.01 Senile osteoporosis
  Postmenopausal osteoporosis

  733.02 Idiopathic osteoporosis

  733.03 Disuse osteoporosis

  733.09 Other
  Drug-induced osteoporosis
  Use additional E code, if desired, to identify drug

● Code new
  to this edition
▲ Revision of
  existing code
④ ⑤ Fourth or fifth
  digit required

[5] **733.1 Pathologic fracture**
Spontaneous fracture

[Excludes:] *traumatic fracture (800-829)*
stress fracture (733.93-733.95)

733.10 Pathologic fracture, unspecified site

733.11 Pathologic fracture of humerus

733.12 Pathologic fracture of distal radius and ulna
Wrist NOS

733.13 Pathologic fracture of vertebrae
Collapse of vertebra NOS

733.14 Pathologic fracture of neck of femur
Femur NOS
Hip NOS

733.15 Pathologic fracture of other specified part of femur

733.16 Pathologic fracture of tibia or fibula
Ankle NOS

733.19 Pathologic fracture of other specified site

[5] **733.2 Cyst of bone**

733.20 Cyst of bone (localized), unspecified

733.21 Solitary bone cyst
Unicameral bone cyst

733.22 Aneurysmal bone cyst

733.29 Other
Fibrous dysplasia (monostotic)

[Excludes:] *cyst of jaw (526.0-526.2, 526.89)*
osteitis fibrosa cystica (252.0)
polyostotic fibrous dysplasia of bone (756.54)

733.3 Hyperostosis of skull
Hyperostosis interna frontalis
Leontiasis ossium

[5] **733.4 Aseptic necrosis of bone**

[Excludes:] *osteochondropathies (732.0-732.9)*

733.40 Aseptic necrosis of bone, site unspecified

733.41 Head of humerus

733.42 Head and neck of femur
Femur NOS

[Excludes:] *Legg-Calvé-Perthes disease (732.1)*

733.43 Medial femoral condyle

733.44 Talus

733.49 Other

733.5 Osteitis condensans
Piriform sclerosis of ilium

733.6 Tietze's disease
Costochondral junction syndrome
Costochondritis

733.7 Algoneurodystrophy
Disuse atrophy of bone
Sudeck's atrophy

[5] **733.8 Malunion and nonunion of fracture**

733.81 Malunion of fracture

733.82 Nonunion of fracture
Pseudoarthrosis (bone)

[5] **733.9 Other and unspecified disorders of bone and cartilage**

733.90 Disorder of bone and cartilage, unspecified

733.91 Arrest of bone development or growth
Epiphyseal arrest

Add 4th or 5th digit | Nonspecific code | Unspecified code | Manifestation code

733.92 Chondromalacia
Chondromalacia:
NOS
localized, except patella
systemic
tibial plateau

Excludes: chondromalacia of patella (717.7)

733.93 Stress fracture of tibia or fibula
Stress reaction of tibia or fibula

733.94 Stress fracture of the metatarsals
Stress reaction of metatarsals

733.95 Stress fracture of other bone
Stress reaction of other bone

733.99 Other
Diaphysitis   Relapsing polychondritis
Hypertrophy of bone

734 Flat foot
Pes planus (acquired)
Talipes planus (acquired)

Excludes: congenital (754.61)
rigid flat foot (754.61)
spastic (everted) flat foot (754.61)

735 Acquired deformities of toe

Excludes: congenital (754.60-754.69, 755.65-755.66)

735.0 Hallux valgus (acquired)

735.1 Hallux varus (acquired)

735.2 Hallux rigidus

735.3 Hallux malleus

735.4 Other hammer toe (acquired)

735.5 Claw toe (acquired)

735.8 Other acquired deformities of toe

735.9 Unspecified acquired deformity of toe

736 Other acquired deformities of limbs

Excludes: congenital (754.3-755.9)

⑤ **736.0 Acquired deformities of forearm, excluding fingers**

736.00 Unspecified deformity
Deformity of elbow, forearm, hand, or wrist (acquired) NOS

736.01 Cubitus valgus (acquired)

736.02 Cubitus varus (acquired)

736.03 Valgus deformity of wrist (acquired)

736.04 Varus deformity of wrist (acquired)

736.05 Wrist drop (acquired)

736.06 Claw hand (acquired)

736.07 Club hand, acquired

736.09 Other

736.1 Mallet finger

⑤ **736.2 Other acquired deformities of finger**

736.20 Unspecified deformity
Deformity of finger (acquired) NOS

736.21 Boutonniere deformity

736.22 Swan-neck deformity

736.29 Other

Excludes: trigger finger (727.03)

⑤ **736.3 Acquired deformities of hip**

● Code new
to this edition

▲ Revision of
existing code

④ ⑤ Fourth or fifth
digit required

736.30 Unspecified deformity
Deformity of hip (acquired) NOS

736.31 Coxa valga (acquired)

736.32 Coxa vara (acquired)

736.39 Other

5 **736.4 Genu valgum or varum (acquired)**

736.41 Genu valgum (acquired)

736.42 Genu varum (acquired)

736.5 Genu recurvatum (acquired)

736.6 Other acquired deformities of knee
Deformity of knee (acquired) NOS

5 **736.7 Other acquired deformities of ankle and foot**

[Excludes:] *deformities of toe (acquired) (735.0-735.9)*
pes planus (acquired) (734)

736.70 Unspecified deformity of ankle and foot, acquired

736.71 Acquired equinovarus deformity
Clubfoot, acquired

[Excludes:] *clubfoot not specified as acquired (754.5-754.7)*

736.72 Equinus deformity of foot, acquired

736.73 Cavus deformity of foot

[Excludes:] *that with claw foot (736.74)*

736.74 Claw foot, acquired

736.75 Cavovarus deformity of foot, acquired

736.76 Other calcaneus deformity

736.79 Other
Acquired:
pes not elsewhere classified
talipes not elsewhere classified

5 **736.8 Acquired deformities of other parts of limbs**

736.81 Unequal leg length (acquired)

736.89 Other
Deformity (acquired):
arm or leg, not elsewhere classified
shoulder

736.9 Acquired deformity of limb, site unspecified

737 Curvature of spine

[Excludes:] *congenital (754.2)*

737.0 Adolescent postural kyphosis

[Excludes:] *osteochondrosis of spine (juvenile) (732.0)*
adult (732.8)

5 **737.1 Kyphosis (acquired)**

737.10 Kyphosis (acquired) (postural)

737.11 Kyphosis due to radiation

737.12 Kyphosis, postlaminectomy

737.19 Other

[Excludes:] *that associated with conditions classifiable elsewhere (737.41)*

5 **737.2 Lordosis (acquired)**

737.20 Lordosis (acquired) (postural)

737.21 Lordosis, postlaminectomy

737.22 Other postsurgical lordosis

737.29 Other

[Excludes:] *that associated with conditions classifiable elsewhere (737.42)*

⑤ **737.3 Kyphoscoliosis and scoliosis**

    737.30 Scoliosis [and kyphoscoliosis], idiopathic

    737.31 Resolving infantile idiopathic scoliosis

    737.32 Progressive infantile idiopathic scoliosis

    737.33 Scoliosis due to radiation

    737.34 Thoracogenic scoliosis

    737.39 Other

    Excludes: that associated with conditions classifiable elsewhere (737.43)
               that in kyphoscoliotic heart disease (416.1)

⑤ **737.4 *Curvature of spine associated with other conditions***

    Code first associated condition, as:
      Charcot-Marie-Tooth disease (356.1)
      mucopolysaccharidosis (277.5)
      neurofibromatosis (237.7)
      osteitis deformans (731.0)
      osteitis fibrosa cystica (252.0)
      osteoporosis (733.00-733.09)
      poliomyelitis (138)
      tuberculosis [Pott's curvature] (015.0)

    737.40 Curvature of spine, unspecified

    737.41 Kyphosis

    737.42 Lordosis

    737.43 Scoliosis

737.8 Other curvatures of spine

737.9 Unspecified curvature of spine
    Curvature of spine (acquired) (idiopathic) NOS
    Hunchback, acquired

    Excludes: deformity of spine NOS (738.5)

738 Other acquired deformity

    Excludes: congenital (754.0-756.9, 758.0-759.9)
               dentofacial anomalies (524.0-524.9)

738.0 Acquired deformity of nose
    Deformity of nose (acquired)
    Overdevelopment of nasal bones

    Excludes: deflected or deviated nasal septum (470)

⑤ **738.1 Other acquired deformity of head**

    738.10 Unspecified deformity

    738.11 Zygomatic hyperplasia

    738.12 Zygomatic hypoplasia

    738.19 Other specified deformity

738.2 Acquired deformity of neck

738.3 Acquired deformity of chest and rib
    Deformity: Pectus:
      chest (acquired)   carinatum, acquired
      rib (acquired)   excavatum, acquired

738.4 Acquired spondylolisthesis
    Degenerative spondylolisthesis
    Spondylolysis, acquired

    Excludes: congenital (756.12)

738.5 Other acquired deformity of back or spine
    Deformity of spine NOS

    Excludes: curvature of spine (737.0-737.9)

738.6 Acquired deformity of pelvis
    Pelvic obliquity

    Excludes: intrapelvic protrusion of acetabulum (718.6)
               that in relation to labor and delivery (653.0-653.4, 653.8-653.9)

738.7 Cauliflower ear

● Code new   ▲ Revision of   ④ ⑤ Fourth or fifth
   to this edition   existing code   digit required

738.8 **Acquired deformity of other specified site**
Deformity of clavicle

738.9 **Acquired deformity of unspecified site**

739 **Nonallopathic lesions, not elsewhere classified**
Includes: segmental dysfunction
somatic dysfunction

739.0 **Head region**
Occipitocervical region

739.1 **Cervical region**
Cervicothoracic region

739.2 **Thoracic region**
Thoracolumbar region

739.3 **Lumbar region**
Lumbosacral region

739.4 **Sacral region**
Sacrococcygeal region   Sacroiliac region

739.5 **Pelvic region**
Hip region   Pubic region

739.6 **Lower extremities**

739.7 **Upper extremities**
Acromioclavicular region   Sternoclavicular region

739.8 **Rib cage**
Costochondral region   Sternochondral region
Costovertebral region

739.9 **Abdomen and other**

Add 4th or 5th digit   Nonspecific code   Unspecified code   Manifestation code

● Code new
to this edition

▲ Revision of
existing code

④ ⑤ Fourth or fifth
digit required

14. CONGENITAL ANOMALIES (740-759)

740 **Anencephalus and similar anomalies**

740.0 **Anencephalus**
Acrania
Amyelencephalus
Hemianencephaly
Hemicephaly

740.1 **Craniorachischisis**

740.2 **Iniencephaly**

⑤ **741** **Spina bifida**

Excludes: *spina bifida occulta (756.17)*

The following fifth-digit subclassification is for use with category 741:

0 **unspecified region**

1 **cervical region**

2 **dorsal [thoracic] region**

3 **lumbar region**

⑤ **741.0** **With hydrocephalus**
Arnold-Chiari syndrome, type II
Any condition classifiable to 741.9 with any condition classifiable to 742.3
Chiari malformation, type II

⑤ **741.9** **Without mention of hydrocephalus**
Hydromeningocele (spinal)
Hydromyelocele
Meningocele (spinal)
Meningomyelocele
Myelocele
Myelocystocele
Rachischisis
Spina bifida (aperta)
Syringomyelocele

742 **Other congenital anomalies of nervous system**

742.0 **Encephalocele**
Encephalocystocele
Encephalomyelocele
Hydroencephalocele
Hydromeningocele, cranial
Meningocele, cerebral
Meningoencephalocele

742.1 **Microcephalus**
Hydromicrocephaly
Micrencephaly

742.2 **Reduction deformities of brain**
Absence of part of brain
Agenesis of part of brain
Aplasia of part of brain
Hypoplasia of part of brain
Agyria
Arhinencephaly
Holoprosencephaly
Microgyria

742.3 **Congenital hydrocephalus**
Aqueduct of Sylvius:
anomaly
obstruction, congenital
stenosis
Atresia of foramina of Magendie and Luschka
Hydrocephalus in newborn

Excludes: *hydrocephalus:*
acquired (331.3-331.4)
due to congenital toxoplasmosis (771.2)
with any condition classifiable to 741.9 (741.0)

742.4 **Other specified anomalies of brain**
Congenital cerebral cyst
Macroencephaly
Macrogyria
Megalencephaly
Multiple anomalies of brain NOS
Porencephaly
Ulegyria

⑤ **742.5** **Other specified anomalies of spinal cord**

742.51 **Diastematomyelia**

742.53 **Hydromyelia**
Hydrorhachis

■ Add 4th or
5th digit
■ Nonspecific
code
■ Unspecified
code
■ Manifestation
code

742.59 **Other**
Amyelia
Atelomyelia
Congenital anomaly of spinal meninges
Defective development of cauda equina
Hypoplasia of spinal cord
Myelatelia
Myelodysplasia

742.8 **Other specified anomalies of nervous system**
Agenesis of nerve
Displacement of brachial
plexus
Familial dysautonomia

Jaw-winking syndrome
Marcus-Gunn syndrome
Riley-Day syndrome

Excludes: *neurofibromatosis (237.7)*

742.9 **Unspecified anomaly of brain, spinal cord, and nervous system**
Anomaly of brain, nervous system, and spinal cord
Congenital:
disease of brain, nervous system, and spinal cord
lesion of brain, nervous system, and spinal cord
Deformity of brain, nervous system, and spinal cord

743 **Congenital anomalies of eye**

⑤ **743.0** **Anophthalmos**

743.00 **Clinical anophthalmos, unspecified**
Agenesis of eye
Congenital absence of eye
Anophthalmos NOS

743.03 **Cystic eyeball, congenital**

743.06 **Cryptophthalmos**

⑤ **743.1** **Microphthalmos**
Dysplasia of eye
Hypoplasia of eye
Rudimentary eye, of eye

743.10 **Microphthalmos, unspecified**

743.11 **Simple microphthalmos**

743.12 **Microphthalmos associated with other anomalies of eye and adnexa**

⑤ **743.2** **Buphthalmos**
Glaucoma:
congenital
newborn

Hydrophthalmos

Excludes: *glaucoma of childhood (365.14)*
traumatic glaucoma due to birth injury (767.8)

743.20 **Buphthalmos, unspecified**

743.21 **Simple buphthalmos**

743.22 **Buphthalmos associated with other ocular anomalies**
Keratoglobus, congenital, associated with buphthalmos
Megalocornea associated with buphthalmos

⑤ **743.3** **Congenital cataract and lens anomalies**
Excludes: *infantile cataract (366.00-366.09)*

743.30 **Congenital cataract, unspecified**

743.31 **Capsular and subcapsular cataract**

743.32 **Cortical and zonular cataract**

743.33 **Nuclear cataract**

743.34 **Total and subtotal cataract, congenital**

743.35 **Congenital aphakia**
Congenital absence of lens

743.36 **Anomalies of lens shape**
Microphakia
Spherophakia

743.37 **Congenital ectopic lens**

743.39 **Other**

● Code new
to this edition

▲ Revision of
existing code

④ ⑤ Fourth or fifth
digit required

[5] **743.4 Coloboma and other anomalies of anterior segment**

743.41 Anomalies of corneal size and shape
Microcornea

[Excludes:] *that associated with buphthalmos (743.22)*

743.42 Corneal opacities, interfering with vision, congenital

743.43 Other corneal opacities, congenital

743.44 Specified anomalies of anterior chamber, chamber angle, and related structures
Anomaly:
  Axenfeld's
  Peters'
  Rieger's

743.45 Aniridia

743.46 Other specified anomalies of iris and ciliary body
Anisocoria, congenital
Atresia of pupil
Coloboma of iris
Corectopia

743.47 Specified anomalies of sclera

743.48 Multiple and combined anomalies of anterior segment

743.49 Other

[5] **743.5 Congenital anomalies of posterior segment**

743.51 Vitreous anomalies
Congenital vitreous opacity

743.52 Fundus coloboma

743.53 Chorioretinal degeneration, congenital

743.54 Congenital folds and cysts of posterior segment

743.55 Congenital macular changes

743.56 Other retinal changes, congenital

743.57 Specified anomalies of optic disc
Coloboma of optic disc (congenital)

743.58 Vascular anomalies
Congenital retinal aneurysm

743.59 Other

[5] **743.6 Congenital anomalies of eyelids, lacrimal system, and orbit**

743.61 Congenital ptosis

743.62 Congenital deformities of eyelids
Ablepharon
Absence of eyelid
Accessory eyelid
Congenital:
  ectropion
  entropion

743.63 Other specified congenital anomalies of eyelid
Absence, agenesis, of cilia

743.64 Specified congenital anomalies of lacrimal gland

743.65 Specified congenital anomalies of lacrimal passages
Absence, agenesis of:
  lacrimal apparatus
  punctum lacrimale
Accessory lacrimal canal

743.66 Specified congenital anomalies of orbit

743.69 Other
Accessory eye muscles

743.8 Other specified anomalies of eye

[Excludes:] *congenital nystagmus (379.51)*
ocular albinism (270.2)
retinitis pigmentosa (362.74)

■ Add 4th or 5th digit
■ Nonspecific code
■ Unspecified code
■ Manifestation code

743.9 Unspecified anomaly of eye
Congenital:
anomaly NOS of eye [any part]
deformity NOS of eye [any part]

744 Congenital anomalies of ear, face, and neck

Excludes: anomaly of:
cervical spine (754.2, 756.10-756.19)
larynx (748.2-748.3)
nose (748.0-748.1)
parathyroid gland (759.2)
thyroid gland (759.2)
cleft lip (749.10-749.25)

⑤ **744.0 Anomalies of ear causing impairment of hearing**

Excludes: congenital deafness without mention of cause (389.0-389.9)

744.00 Unspecified anomaly of ear with impairment of hearing

744.01 Absence of external ear
Absence of:
auditory canal (external)
auricle (ear) (with stenosis or atresia of auditory canal)

744.02 Other anomalies of external ear with impairment of hearing
Atresia or stricture of auditory canal (external)

744.03 Anomaly of middle ear, except ossicles
Atresia or stricture of osseous meatus (ear)

744.04 Anomalies of ear ossicles
Fusion of ear ossicles

744.05 Anomalies of inner ear
Congenital anomaly of:
membranous labyrinth
organ of Corti

744.09 Other
Absence of ear, congenital

744.1 Accessory auricle
Accessory tragus   Supernumerary:
Polyotia   ear
Preauricular appendage   lobule

⑤ **744.2 Other specified anomalies of ear**

Excludes: that with impairment of hearing (744.00-744.09)

744.21 Absence of ear lobe, congenital

744.22 Macrotia

744.23 Microtia

744.24 Specified anomalies of Eustachian tube
Absence of Eustachian tube

744.29 Other
Bat ear   Prominence of auricle
Darwin's tubercle   Ridge ear
Pointed ear

Excludes: preauricular sinus (744.46)

744.3 Unspecified anomaly of ear
Congenital:
anomaly NOS of ear, not elsewhere classified
deformity NOS of ear, not elsewhere classified

⑤ **744.4 Branchial cleft cyst or fistula; preauricular sinus**

744.41 Branchial cleft sinus or fistula
Branchial:
sinus (external) (internal)
vestige

744.42 Branchial cleft cyst

744.43 Cervical auricle

744.46 Preauricular sinus or fistula

744.47 Preauricular cyst

● Code new   ▲ Revision of   ④ ⑤ Fourth or fifth
to this edition   existing code   digit required

744.49 Other
Fistula (of):
auricle, congenital
cervicoaural

744.5 Webbing of neck
Pterygium colli

[5] **744.8 Other specified anomalies of face and neck**

744.81 Macrocheilia
Hypertrophy of lip, congenital

744.82 Microcheilia

744.83 Macrostomia

744.84 Microstomia

744.89 Other

[Excludes:] *congenital fistula of lip (750.25)*
musculoskeletal anomalies (754.0-754.1, 756.0)

744.9 Unspecified anomalies of face and neck
Congenital:
anomaly NOS of face [any part] or neck [any part]
deformity NOS of face [any part] or neck [any part]

745 Bulbus cordis anomalies and anomalies of cardiac septal closure

745.0 Common truncus
Absent septum between aorta and pulmonary artery
Communication (abnormal) between aorta and pulmonary artery
Aortic septal defect
Common aortopulmonary trunk
Persistent truncus arteriosus

[5] **745.1 Transposition of great vessels**

745.10 Complete transposition of great vessels
Transposition of great vessels:
NOS
classical

745.11 Double outlet right ventricle
Dextratransposition of aorta
Incomplete transposition of great vessels
Origin of both great vessels from right ventricle
Taussig-Bing syndrome or defect

745.12 Corrected transposition of great vessels

745.19 Other

745.2 Tetralogy of Fallot
Fallot's pentalogy
Ventricular septal defect with pulmonary stenosis or atresia, dextraposition of aorta, and hypertrophy of right ventricle

[Excludes:] *Fallot's triad (746.09)*

745.3 Common ventricle
Cor triloculare biatriatum
Single ventricle

745.4 Ventricular septal defect
Eisenmenger's defect or complex
Gerbode defect
Interventricular septal defect
Left ventricular-right atrial communication
Roger's disease

[Excludes:] *common atrioventricular canal type (745.69)*
single ventricle (745.3)

745.5 Ostium secundum type atrial septal defect
Defect:
atrium secundum
fossa ovalis
Lutembacher's syndrome
Patent or persistent:
foramen ovale
ostium secundum

[5] **745.6 Endocardial cushion defects**

745.60 Endocardial cushion defect, unspecified type

745.61 Ostium primum defect
Persistent ostium primum

745.69 Other
Absence of atrial septum
Atrioventricular canal type ventricular septal defect
Common atrioventricular canal
Common atrium

745.7 Cor biloculare
Absence of atrial and ventricular septa

745.8 Other

745.9 Unspecified defect of septal closure
Septal defect NOS

746 Other congenital anomalies of heart
Excludes: endocardial fibroelastosis (425.3)

⑤ **746.0 Anomalies of pulmonary valve**
Excludes: infundibular or subvalvular pulmonic stenosis (746.83)
tetralogy of Fallot (745.2)

746.00 Pulmonary valve anomaly, unspecified

746.01 Atresia, congenital
Congenital absence of pulmonary valve

746.02 Stenosis, congenital

746.09 Other
Congenital insufficiency of pulmonary valve
Fallot's triad or trilogy

746.1 Tricuspid atresia and stenosis, congenital
Absence of tricuspid valve

746.2 Ebstein's anomaly

746.3 Congenital stenosis of aortic valve
Congenital aortic stenosis
Excludes: congenital:
subaortic stenosis (746.81)
supravalvular aortic stenosis (747.22)

746.4 Congenital insufficiency of aortic valve
Bicuspid aortic valve
Congenital aortic insufficiency

746.5 Congenital mitral stenosis
Fused commissure of mitral valve
Parachute deformity of mitral valve
Supernumerary cusps of mitral valve

746.6 Congenital mitral insufficiency

746.7 Hypoplastic left heart syndrome
Atresia, or marked hypoplasia, of aortic orifice or valve, with hypoplasia of ascending
aorta and defective development of left ventricle (with mitral valve atresia)

⑤ **746.8 Other specified anomalies of heart**

746.81 Subaortic stenosis

746.82 Cor triatriatum

746.83 Infundibular pulmonic stenosis
Subvalvular pulmonic stenosis

746.84 Obstructive anomalies of heart, not elsewhere classified
Uhl's disease

746.85 Coronary artery anomaly
Anomalous origin or communication of coronary artery
Arteriovenous malformation of coronary artery
Coronary artery:
absence
arising from aorta or pulmonary trunk
single

746.86 Congenital heart block
Complete or incomplete atrioventricular [AV] block

● Code new
  to this edition

▲ Revision of
  existing code

④ ⑤ Fourth or fifth
  digit required

746.87 Malposition of heart and cardiac apex
Abdominal heart
Dextrocardia
Ectopia cordis
Levocardia (isolated)
Mesocardia

[Excludes:] *dextrocardia with complete transposition of viscera (759.3)*

746.89 Other
Atresia of cardiac vein
Hypoplasia of cardiac vein
Congenital:
 cardiomegaly
 diverticulum, left ventricle
 pericardial defect

746.9 Unspecified anomaly of heart
Congenital:
 anomaly of heart NOS
 heart disease NOS

747 Other congenital anomalies of circulatory system

747.0 Patent ductus arteriosus
Patent ductus Botalli
Persistent ductus arteriosus

[5] **747.1 Coarctation of aorta**

747.10 Coarctation of aorta (preductal) (postductal)
Hypoplasia of aortic arch

747.11 Interruption of aortic arch

[5] **747.2 Other anomalies of aorta**

747.20 Anomaly of aorta, unspecified

747.21 Anomalies of aortic arch
Anomalous origin, right subclavian artery
Dextraposition of aorta
Double aortic arch
Kommerell's diverticulum
Overriding aorta
Persistent:
 convolutions, aortic arch
 right aortic arch
Vascular ring

[Excludes:] *hypoplasia of aortic arch (747.10)*

747.22 Atresia and stenosis of aorta
Absence of aorta
Aplasia of aorta
Hypoplasia of aorta
Stricture of aorta
Supra (valvular)-aortic stenosis

[Excludes:] *congenital aortic (valvular) stenosis or stricture, so stated (746.3)*
hypoplasia of aorta in hypoplastic left heart syndrome (746.7)

747.29 Other
Aneurysm of sinus of Valsalva
Congenital:
 aneurysm of aorta
 dilation of aorta

747.3 Anomalies of pulmonary artery
Agenesis of pulmonary artery
Anomaly of pulmonary artery
Atresia of pulmonary artery
Coarctation of pulmonary artery
Hypoplasia of pulmonary artery
Stenosis of pulmonary artery
Pulmonary arteriovenous aneurysm

[5] **747.4 Anomalies of great veins**

747.40 Anomaly of great veins, unspecified
Anomaly NOS of:
 pulmonary veins
 vena cava

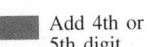

Add 4th or 5th digit | Nonspecific code | Unspecified code | Manifestation code

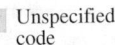

747.41 Total anomalous pulmonary venous connection
Total anomalous pulmonary venous return [TAPVR]:
subdiaphragmatic
supradiaphragmatic

747.42 Partial anomalous pulmonary venous connection
Partial anomalous pulmonary venous return

747.49 Other anomalies of great veins
Absence of vena cava (inferior) (superior)
Congenital stenosis of vena cava (inferior) (superior)
Persistent:
left posterior cardinal vein
left superior vena cava
Scimitar syndrome
Transposition of pulmonary veins NOS

747.5 Absence or hypoplasia of umbilical artery
Single umbilical artery

[5] **747.6 Other anomalies of peripheral vascular system**
Absence of artery or vein, not elsewhere classified
Anomaly of artery or vein, not elsewhere classified
Atresia of artery or vein, not elsewhere classified
Arteriovenous aneurysm (peripheral)
Arteriovenous malformation of the peripheral vascular system
Congenital:
aneurysm (peripheral)
phlebectasia
stricture, artery
varix
Multiple renal arteries

[Excludes:] *anomalies of:*
cerebral vessels (747.81)
pulmonary artery (747.3)
congenital retinal aneurysm (743.58)
hemangioma (228.00-228.09)
lymphangioma (228.1)

747.60 Anomaly of the peripheral vascular system, unspecified site

747.61 Gastrointestinal vessel anomaly

747.62 Renal vessel anomaly

747.63 Upper limb vessel anomaly

747.64 Lower limb vessel anomaly

747.69 Anomalies of other specified sites of peripheral vascular system

[5] **747.8 Other specified anomalies of circulatory system**

747.81 Anomalies of cerebrovascular system
Arteriovenous malformation of brain
Cerebral arteriovenous aneurysm, congenital
Congenital anomalies of cerebral vessels

[Excludes:] *ruptured cerebral (arteriovenous) aneurysm (430)*

747.82 Spinal vessel anomaly
Arteriovenous malformation of spinal vessel

● **747.83 Persistent fetal circulation**
Persistent pulmonary hypertension
Primary pulmonary hypertension of newborn

747.89 Other
Aneurysm, congenital, specified site not elsewhere classified

[Excludes:] *congenital aneurysm:*
coronary (746.85)
peripheral (747.6)
pulmonary (747.3)
retinal (743.58)

747.9 Unspecified anomaly of circulatory system

748 Congenital anomalies of respiratory system

[Excludes:] *congenital defect of diaphragm (756.6)*

748.0 Choanal atresia
Atresia of nares (anterior) (posterior)
Congenital stenosis of nares (anterior) (posterior)

748.1 Other anomalies of nose
Absent nose
Accessory nose
Cleft nose
Deformity of wall of nasal sinus
Congenital:
deformity of nose
notching of tip of nose
perforation of wall of nasal sinus

[Excludes:] *congenital deviation of nasal septum (754.0)*

748.2 Web of larynx
Web of larynx:
NOS
glottic
subglottic

748.3 Other anomalies of larynx, trachea, and bronchus
Absence or agenesis of:
bronchus
larynx
trachea
Anomaly (of):
cricoid cartilage
epiglottis
thyroid cartilage
tracheal cartilage
Atresia (of):
epiglottis
glottis
larynx
trachea
Cleft thyroid, cartilage, congenital
Congenital:
dilation, trachea
stenosis:
larynx
trachea
tracheocele
Diverticulum:
bronchus
trachea
Fissure of epiglottis
Laryngocele
Posterior cleft of cricoid cartilage (congenital)
Rudimentary tracheal bronchus
Stridor, laryngeal, congenital

748.4 Congenital cystic lung
Disease, lung:
cystic, congenital
polycystic, congenital
Honeycomb lung, congenital

[Excludes:] *acquired or unspecified cystic lung (518.89)*

748.5 Agenesis, hypoplasia, and dysplasia of lung
Absence of lung (fissures) (lobe)
Aplasia of lung
Hypoplasia of lung (lobe)
Sequestration of lung

[5] **748.6 Other anomalies of lung**

748.60 Anomaly of lung, unspecified

748.61 Congenital bronchiectasis

748.69 Other
Accessory lung (lobe)
Azygos lobe (fissure), lung

748.8 Other specified anomalies of respiratory system
Abnormal communication between pericardial and pleural sacs
Anomaly, pleural folds
Atresia of nasopharynx
Congenital cyst of mediastinum

748.9 Unspecified anomaly of respiratory system
Anomaly of respiratory system NOS

749 Cleft palate and cleft lip

[5] **749.0 Cleft palate**

749.00 Cleft palate, unspecified

749.01 Unilateral, complete

749.02 Unilateral, incomplete
Cleft uvula

749.03 Bilateral, complete

749.04 Bilateral, incomplete

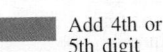

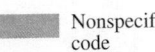

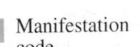

⑤ **749.1 Cleft lip**

Cheiloschisis
Congenital fissure of lip
Harelip
Labium leporinum

749.10 Cleft lip, unspecified

749.11 Unilateral, complete

749.12 Unilateral, incomplete

749.13 Bilateral, complete

749.14 Bilateral, incomplete

⑤ **749.2 Cleft palate with cleft lip**

Cheilopalatoschisis

749.20 Cleft palate with cleft lip, unspecified

749.21 Unilateral, complete

749.22 Unilateral, incomplete

749.23 Bilateral, complete

749.24 Bilateral, incomplete

749.25 Other combinations

750 Other congenital anomalies of upper alimentary tract

[Excludes:] *dentofacial anomalies (524.0-524.9)*

750.0 Tongue tie

Ankyloglossia

⑤ **750.1 Other anomalies of tongue**

750.10 Anomaly of tongue, unspecified

750.11 Aglossia

750.12 Congenital adhesions of tongue

750.13 Fissure of tongue

Bifid tongue
Double tongue

750.15 Macroglossia

Congenital hypertrophy of tongue

750.16 Microglossia

Hypoplasia of tongue

750.19 Other

⑤ **750.2 Other specified anomalies of mouth and pharynx**

750.21 Absence of salivary gland

750.22 Accessory salivary gland

750.23 Atresia, salivary duct

Imperforate salivary duct

750.24 Congenital fistula of salivary gland

750.25 Congenital fistula of lip

Congenital (mucus) lip pits

750.26 Other specified anomalies of mouth

Absence of uvula

750.27 Diverticulum of pharynx

Pharyngeal pouch

750.29 Other specified anomalies of pharynx

Imperforate pharynx

750.3 Tracheoesophageal fistula, esophageal atresia and stenosis

Absent esophagus
Atresia of esophagus
Congenital:
  esophageal ring
  stenosis of esophagus
  stricture of esophagus
Congenital fistula:
  esophagobronchial
  esophagotracheal
Imperforate esophagus
Webbed esophagus

750.4 Other specified anomalies of esophagus
Dilatation, congenital (of) esophagus
Displacement, congenital (of) esophagus
Diverticulum (of) esophagus
Duplication (of) esophagus
Giant (of) esophagus
Esophageal pouch (of) esophagus

Excludes: *congenital hiatus hernia (750.6)*

750.5 Congenital hypertrophic pyloric stenosis
Congenital or infantile:
constriction of pylorus
hypertrophy of pylorus
spasm of pylorus
stenosis of pylorus
stricture of pylorus

750.6 Congenital hiatus hernia
Displacement of cardia through esophageal hiatus

Excludes: *congenital diaphragmatic hernia (756.6)*

750.7 Other specified anomalies of stomach
Congenital: Duplication of stomach
  cardiospasm   Megalogastria
  hourglass stomach   Microgastria
Displacement of stomach   Transposition of stomach
Diverticulum of stomach,
  congenital

750.8 Other specified anomalies of upper alimentary tract

750.9 Unspecified anomaly of upper alimentary tract
Congenital:
anomaly NOS of upper alimentary tract [any part, except tongue]
deformity NOS of upper alimentary tract [any part, except tongue]

751 Other congenital anomalies of digestive system

751.0 Meckel's diverticulum
Meckel's diverticulum (displaced) (hypertrophic)
Persistent:
omphalomesenteric duct
vitelline duct

751.1 Atresia and stenosis of small intestine
Atresia of:
duodenum
ileum
intestine NOS
Congenital:
absence of small intestine or intestine NOS
obstruction of small intestine or intestine NOS
stenosis of small intestine or intestine NOS
stricture of small intestine or intestine NOS
Imperforate jejunum

751.2 Atresia and stenosis of large intestine, rectum, and anal canal
Absence: Congenital or infantile:
  anus (congenital)   obstruction of large intestine
  appendix, congenital   occlusion of anus
  large intestine, congenital   stricture of anus
  rectum   Imperforate:
Atresia of: anus
  anus   rectum
  colon   Stricture of rectum, congenital
  rectum

751.3 Hirschsprung's disease and other congenital functional disorders of colon
Aganglionosis   Congenital megacolon
Congenital dilation of colon   Macrocolon

Add 4th or 5th digit   Nonspecific code   Unspecified code   Manifestation code

751.4 Anomalies of intestinal fixation

Congenital adhesions:
  omental, anomalous
  peritoneal
Jackson's membrane
Malrotation of colon

Rotation of cecum or colon:
  failure of
  incomplete
  insufficient
Universal mesentery

751.5 Other anomalies of intestine

Congenital diverticulum,
  colon
Dolichocolon
Duplication of:
  anus
  appendix
  cecum
  intestine
Ectopic anus

Megaloappendix
Megaloduodenum
Microcolon
Persistent cloaca
Transposition of:
  appendix
  colon
  intestine

⑤ **751.6 Anomalies of gallbladder, bile ducts, and liver**

751.60 Unspecified anomaly of gallbladder, bile ducts, and liver

751.61 Biliary atresia
  Congenital:
    absence of bile duct (common) or passage
    hypoplasia of bile duct (common) or passage
    obstruction of bile duct (common) or passage
    stricture of bile duct (common) or passage

751.62 Congenital cystic disease of liver
  Congenital polycystic disease of liver
  Fibrocystic disease of liver

751.69 Other anomalies of gallbladder, bile ducts, and liver

Absence of:
  gallbladder,
    congenital
  liver (lobe)
Accessory:
  hepatic ducts
  liver
Congenital:
  choledochal cyst
  hepatomegaly

Duplication of:
  biliary duct
  cystic duct
  gallbladder
  liver
Floating:
  gallbladder
  liver
Intrahepatic gallbladder

751.7 Anomalies of pancreas

Absence of pancreas
Agenesis of pancreas
Hypoplasia of pancreas
Accessory pancreas

Annular pancreas
Ectopic pancreatic tissue
Pancreatic heterotopia

Excludes: *diabetes mellitus:*
          congenital (250.0-250.9)
          neonatal (775.1)
        fibrocystic disease of pancreas (277.00-277.09)

751.8 Other specified anomalies of digestive system
  Absence (complete) (partial) of alimentary tract NOS
  Duplication of digestive organs NOS
  Malposition, congenital, of digestive organs NOS

Excludes: *congenital diaphragmatic hernia (756.6)*
          congenital hiatus hernia (750.6)

751.9 Unspecified anomaly of digestive system
  Congenital:
    anomaly NOS of digestive system NOS
    deformity NOS of digestive system NOS

752 Congenital anomalies of genital organs

Excludes: *syndromes associated with anomalies in the number and form of chromosomes*
          (758.0-758.9)
          testicular feminization syndrome (257.8)

● Code new   ▲ Revision of   ④ ⑤ Fourth or fifth
        to this edition   existing code   digit required

752.0 Anomalies of ovaries
Absence, congenital (of) ovary
Accessory (of) ovary
Ectopic (of) ovary
Streak (of) ovary

[5] **752.1 Anomalies of fallopian tubes and broad ligaments**

752.10 Unspecified anomaly of fallopian tubes and broad ligaments

752.11 Embryonic cyst of fallopian tubes and broad ligaments
Cyst:
- epoophoron
- fimbrial

Cyst:
- Gartner's duct
- parovarian

752.19 Other
Absence (of) fallopian tube or broad ligament
Accessory (of) fallopian tube or broad ligament
Atresia (of) fallopian tube or broad ligament

752.2 Doubling of uterus
Didelphic uterus
Doubling of uterus [any degree] (associated with doubling of cervix and vagina)

752.3 Other anomalies of uterus
Absence, congenital of uterus
Agenesis of uterus
Aplasia of uterus
Bicornuate uterus
Uterus unicornis
Uterus with only one functioning horn

[5] **752.4 Anomalies of cervix, vagina, and external female genitalia**

752.40 Unspecified anomaly of cervix, vagina, and external female genitalia

752.41 Embryonic cyst of cervix, vagina, and external female genitalia
Cyst of:
- canal of Nuck, congenital
- vagina, embryonal
- vulva, congenital

752.42 Imperforate hymen

752.49 Other anomalies of cervix, vagina, and external female genitalia
Absence of cervix, clitoris, vagina, or vulva
Agenesis of cervix, clitoris, vagina, or vulva
Congenital stenosis or stricture of:
- cervical canal
- vagina

[*Excludes:*] *double vagina associated with total duplication (752.2)*

[5] **752.5 Undescended and retractile testicle**

752.51 Undescended testis
Cryptorchism
Ectopic testis

752.52 Retractile testis

[5] **752.6 Hypospadias and epispadias and other penile anomalies**

752.61 Hypospadias

752.62 Epispadias
Anaspadias

752.63 Congenital chordee

752.64 Micropenis

752.65 Hidden penis

752.69 Other penile anomalies

Add 4th or 5th digit | Nonspecific code | Unspecified code | Manifestation code

752.7 Indeterminate sex and pseudohermaphroditism
Gynandrism
Hermaphroditism
Ovotestis
Pseudohermaphroditism (male) (female)
Pure gonadal dysgenesis

[Excludes:] *pseudohermaphroditism:*
female, with adrenocortical disorder (255.2)
male, with gonadal disorder (257.8)
with specified chromosomal anomaly (758.0-758.9)
testicular feminization syndrome (257.8)

752.8 Other specified anomalies of genital organs
Absence of:
prostate
spermatic cord
vas deferens
Anorchism
Aplasia (congenital) of:
prostate
round ligament
testicle
Atresia of:
ejaculatory duct
vas deferens
Fusion of testes
Hypoplasia of testis
Monorchism
Polyorchism

[Excludes:] *congenital hydrocele (778.6)*
penile anomalies (752.61-752.69)
phimosis or paraphimosis (605)

752.9 Unspecified anomaly of genital organs
Congenital:
anomaly NOS of genital organ, not elsewhere classified
deformity NOS of genital organ, not elsewhere classified

753 Congenital anomalies of urinary system

753.0 Renal agenesis and dysgenesis
Atrophy of kidney:
congenital
infantile
Congenital absence of kidney(s)
Hypoplasia of kidney(s)

⑤ **753.1 Cystic kidney disease**
[Excludes:] *acquired cyst of kidney (593.2)*

753.10 Cystic kidney disease, unspecified

753.11 Congenital single renal cyst

753.12 Polycystic kidney, unspecified type

753.13 Polycystic kidney, autosomal dominant

753.14 Polycystic kidney, autosomal recessive

753.15 Renal dysplasia

753.16 Medullary cystic kidney
Nephronopthisis

753.17 Medullary sponge kidney

753.19 Other specified cystic kidney disease
Multicystic kidney

⑤ **753.2 Obstructive defects of renal pelvis and ureter**

753.20 Unspecified obstructive defect of renal pelvis and ureter

753.21 Congenital obstruction of ureteropelvic junction

753.22 Congenital obstruction of ureterovesical junction
Adynamic ureter
Congenital hydroureter

753.23 Congenital ureterocele

753.29 Other

753.3 Other specified anomalies of kidney

Accessory kidney
Congenital:
  calculus of kidney
  displaced kidney
Discoid kidney
Double kidney with double pelvis
Ectopic kidney
Fusion of kidneys
Giant kidney
Horseshoe kidney
Hyperplasia of kidney
Lobulation of kidney
Malrotation of kidney
Trifid kidney (pelvis)

753.4 Other specified anomalies of ureter

Absent ureter
Accessory ureter
Deviation of ureter
Displaced ureteric orifice
Double ureter
Ectopic ureter
Implantation, anomalous of ureter

753.5 Exstrophy of urinary bladder

Ectopia vesicae
Extroversion of bladder

753.6 Atresia and stenosis of urethra and bladder neck

Congenital obstruction:
  bladder neck
  urethra
Congenital stricture of:
  urethra (valvular)
  urinary meatus
  vesicourethral orifice
Imperforate urinary meatus
Impervious urethra
Urethral valve formation

753.7 Anomalies of urachus

Cyst (of) urachus
Fistula (of) urachus
Patent (of) urachus
Persistent umbilical sinus

753.8 Other specified anomalies of bladder and urethra

Absence, congenital of:
  bladder
  urethra
Accessory:
  bladder
  urethra
Congenital:
  diverticulum of bladder
  hernia of bladder
Congenital urethrorectal fistula
Congenital prolapse of:
  bladder (mucosa)
  urethra
Double:
  urethra
  urinary meatus

753.9 Unspecified anomaly of urinary system

Congenital:
  anomaly NOS of urinary system [any part, except urachus]
  deformity NOS of urinary system [any part, except urachus]

754 Certain congenital musculoskeletal deformities

Includes: nonteratogenic deformities which are considered to be due to intrauterine malposition and pressure

754.0 Of skull, face, and jaw

Asymmetry of face
Compression facies
Depressions in skull
Deviation of nasal septum, congenital
Dolichocephaly
Plagiocephaly
Potter's facies
Squashed or bent nose, congenital

[Excludes:] *dentofacial anomalies (524.0-524.9)*
syphilitic saddle nose (090.5)

754.1 Of sternocleidomastoid muscle

Congenital sternomastoid torticollis
Congenital wryneck
Contracture of sternocleidomastoid (muscle)
Sternomastoid tumor

754.2 Of spine

Congenital postural:
  lordosis
  scoliosis

[5] **754.3 Congenital dislocation of hip**

754.30 Congenital dislocation of hip, unilateral
Congenital dislocation of hip NOS

754.31 Congenital dislocation of hip, bilateral

754.32 Congenital subluxation of hip, unilateral
Congenital flexion deformity, hip or thigh
Predislocation status of hip at birth
Preluxation of hip, congenital

754.33 Congenital subluxation of hip, bilateral

754.35 Congenital dislocation of one hip with subluxation of other hip

⑤ **754.4 Congenital genu recurvatum and bowing of long bones of leg**

754.40 Genu recurvatum

754.41 Congenital dislocation of knee (with genu recurvatum)

754.42 Congenital bowing of femur

754.43 Congenital bowing of tibia and fibula

754.44 Congenital bowing of unspecified long bones of leg

⑤ **754.5 Varus deformities of feet**

[Excludes:] *acquired (736.71, 736.75, 736.79)*

754.50 Talipes varus
Congenital varus deformity of foot, unspecified
Pes varus

754.51 Talipes equinovarus
Equinovarus (congenital)

754.52 Metatarsus primus varus

754.53 Metatarsus varus

754.59 Other
Talipes calcaneovarus

⑤ **754.6 Valgus deformities of feet**

[Excludes:] *valgus deformity of foot (acquired) (736.79)*

754.60 Talipes valgus
Congenital valgus deformity of foot, unspecified

754.61 Congenital pes planus
Congenital rocker bottom flat foot
Flat foot, congenital

[Excludes:] *pes planus (acquired) (734)*

754.62 Talipes calcaneovalgus

754.69 Other
Talipes:
equinovalgus
planovalgus

⑤ **754.7 Other deformities of feet**

[Excludes:] *acquired (736.70-736.79)*

754.70 Talipes, unspecified
Congenital deformity of foot NOS

754.71 Talipes cavus
Cavus foot (congenital)

754.79 Other
Asymmetric talipes
Talipes:
calcaneus
equinus

⑤ **754.8 Other specified nonteratogenic anomalies**

754.81 Pectus excavatum
Congenital funnel chest

754.82 Pectus carinatum
Congenital pigeon chest [breast]

754.89 Other
Club hand (congenital)
Congenital:
deformity of chest wall
dislocation of elbow
Generalized flexion contractures of lower limb joints, congenital
Spade-like hand (congenital)

● Code new to this edition ▲ Revision of existing code ④ ⑤ Fourth or fifth digit required

755 Other congenital anomalies of limbs
[*Excludes:*] *those deformities classifiable to 754.0-754.8*

[5] **755.0 Polydactyly**

755.00 Polydactyly, unspecified digits
Supernumerary digits

755.01 Of fingers
Accessory fingers

755.02 Of toes
Accessory toes

[5] **755.1 Syndactyly**
Symphalangy
Webbing of digits

755.10 Of multiple and unspecified sites

755.11 Of fingers without fusion of bone

755.12 Of fingers with fusion of bone

755.13 Of toes without fusion of bone

755.14 Of toes with fusion of bone

[5] **755.2 Reduction deformities of upper limb**

755.20 Unspecified reduction deformity of upper limb
Ectromelia NOS of upper limb
Hemimelia NOS of upper limb
Shortening of arm, congenital

755.21 Transverse deficiency of upper limb
Amelia of upper limb
Congenital absence of:
  fingers, all (complete or partial)
  forearm, including hand and fingers
  upper limb, complete
Congenital amputation of upper limb
Transverse hemimelia of upper limb

755.22 Longitudinal deficiency of upper limb, not elsewhere classified
Phocomelia NOS of upper limb
Rudimentary arm

755.23 Longitudinal deficiency, combined, involving humerus, radius, and ulna (complete or incomplete)
Congenital absence of arm and forearm (complete or incomplete) with or without metacarpal deficiency and/or phalangeal deficiency, incomplete
Phocomelia, complete, of upper limb

755.24 Longitudinal deficiency, humeral, complete or partial (with or without distal deficiencies, incomplete)
Congenital absence of humerus (with or without absence of some [but not all] distal elements)
Proximal phocomelia of upper limb

755.25 Longitudinal deficiency, radioulnar, complete or partial (with or without distal deficiencies, incomplete)
Congenital absence of radius and ulna (with or without absence of some [but not all] distal elements)
Distal phocomelia of upper limb

755.26 Longitudinal deficiency, radial, complete or partial (with or without distal deficiencies, incomplete)
Agenesis of radius
Congenital absence of radius (with or without absence of some [but not all] distal elements)

755.27 Longitudinal deficiency, ulnar, complete or partial (with or without distal deficiencies, incomplete)
Agenesis of ulna
Congenital absence of ulna (with or without absence of some [but not all] distal elements)

755.28 Longitudinal deficiency, carpals or metacarpals, complete or partial (with or without incomplete phalangeal deficiency)

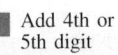

Add 4th or 5th digit | Nonspecific code | Unspecified code | Manifestation code

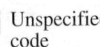

755.29 Longitudinal deficiency, phalanges, complete or partial
Absence of finger, congenital
Aphalangia of upper limb, terminal, complete or partial

> *Excludes:* terminal deficiency of all five digits (755.21)
> transverse deficiency of phalanges (755.21)

⑤ **755.3 Reduction deformities of lower limb**

755.30 Unspecified reduction deformity of lower limb
Ectromelia NOS of lower limb
Hemimelia NOS of lower limb
Shortening of leg, congenital

755.31 Transverse deficiency of lower limb
Amelia of lower limb
Congenital absence of:
  foot
  leg, including foot and toes
  lower limb, complete
  toes, all, complete
Transverse hemimelia of lower limb

755.32 Longitudinal deficiency of lower limb, not elsewhere classified
Phocomelia NOS of lower limb

755.33 Longitudinal deficiency, combined, involving femur, tibia, and fibula (complete or incomplete)
Congenital absence of thigh and (lower) leg (complete or incomplete) with or without metacarpal deficiency and/or phalangeal deficiency, incomplete
Phocomelia, complete, of lower limb

755.34 Longitudinal deficiency, femoral, complete or partial (with or without distal deficiencies, incomplete)
Congenital absence of femur (with or without absence of some [but not all] distal elements)
Proximal phocomelia of lower limb

755.35 Longitudinal deficiency, tibiofibular, complete or partial (with or without distal deficiencies, incomplete)
Congenital absence of tibia and fibula (with or without absence of some [but not all] distal elements)
Distal phocomelia of lower limb

755.36 Longitudinal deficiency, tibia, complete or partial (with or without distal deficiencies, incomplete)
Agenesis of tibia
Congenital absence of tibia (with or without absence of some [but not all] distal elements)

755.37 Longitudinal deficiency, fibular, complete or partial (with or without distal deficiencies, incomplete)
Agenesis of fibula
Congenital absence of fibula (with or without absence of some [but not all] distal elements)

755.38 Longitudinal deficiency, tarsals or metatarsals, complete or partial (with or without incomplete phalangeal deficiency)

755.39 Longitudinal deficiency, phalanges, complete or partial
Absence of toe, congenital
Aphalangia of lower limb, terminal, complete or partial

> *Excludes:* terminal deficiency of all five digits (755.31)
> transverse deficiency of phalanges (755.31)

755.4 Reduction deformities, unspecified limb
Absence, congenital (complete or partial) of limb NOS
Amelia of unspecified limb
Ectromelia of unspecified limb
Hemimelia of unspecified limb
Phocomelia of unspecified limb

⑤ **755.5 Other anomalies of upper limb, including shoulder girdle**

755.50 Unspecified anomaly of upper limb

755.51 Congenital deformity of clavicle

755.52 Congenital elevation of scapula
Sprengel's deformity

755.53 Radioulnar synostosis

● Code new
to this edition

▲ Revision of
existing code

④ ⑤ Fourth or fifth
digit required

755.54 **Madelung's deformity**

755.55 **Acrocephalosyndactyly**
Apert's syndrome

755.56 **Accessory carpal bones**

755.57 **Macrodactylia (fingers)**

755.58 **Cleft hand, congenital**
Lobster-claw hand

755.59 **Other**
Cleidocranial dysostosis
Cubitus:
valgus, congenital
varus, congenital

Excludes: *club hand (congenital) (754.89)*
congenital dislocation of elbow (754.89)

⑤ **755.6 Other anomalies of lower limb, including pelvic girdle**

755.60 **Unspecified anomaly of lower limb**

755.61 **Coxa valga, congenital**

755.62 **Coxa vara, congenital**

755.63 **Other congenital deformity of hip (joint)**
Congenital anteversion of femur (neck)

Excludes: *congenital dislocation of hip (754.30-754.35)*

755.64 **Congenital deformity of knee (joint)**
Congenital:
absence of patella
genu valgum [knock-knee]
genu varum [bowleg]
Rudimentary patella

755.65 **Macrodactylia of toes**

755.66 **Other anomalies of toes**
Congenital:
hallux valgus
hallux varus
hammer toe

755.67 **Anomalies of foot, not elsewhere classified**
Astragaloscaphoid synostosis
Calcaneonavicular bar
Coalition of calcaneus
Talonavicular synostosis
Tarsal coalitions

755.69 **Other**
Congenital:
angulation of tibia
deformity (of):
ankle (joint)
sacroiliac (joint)
fusion of sacroiliac joint

755.8 Other specified anomalies of unspecified limb

755.9 Unspecified anomaly of unspecified limb
Congenital:
anomaly NOS of unspecified limb
deformity NOS of unspecified limb

Excludes: *reduction deformity of unspecified limb (755.4)*

756 Other congenital musculoskeletal anomalies
Excludes: *those deformities classifiable to 754.0-754.8*

▬	Add 4th or 5th digit	▬ Nonspecific code	▬ Unspecified code	▬ Manifestation code

756.0 Anomalies of skull and face bones

Absence of skull bones	Imperfect fusion of skull
Acrocephaly	Oxycephaly
Congenital deformity of	Platybasia
forehead	Premature closure of cranial sutures
Craniosynostosis	Tower skull
Crouzon's disease	Trigonocephaly
Hypertelorism	

Excludes: *acrocephalosyndactyly [Apert's syndrome] (755.55)*
dentofacial anomalies (524.0-524.9)
skull defects associated with brain anomalies, such as:
anencephalus (740.0)
encephalocele (742.0)
hydrocephalus (742.3)
microcephalus (742.1)

⑤ **756.1 Anomalies of spine**

756.10 Anomaly of spine, unspecified

756.11 Spondylolysis, lumbosacral region
Prespondylolisthesis (lumbosacral)

756.12 Spondylolisthesis

756.13 Absence of vertebra, congenital

756.14 Hemivertebra

756.15 Fusion of spine [vertebra], congenital

756.16 Klippel-Feil syndrome

756.17 Spina bifida occulta

Excludes: *spina bifida (aperta) (741.0-741.9)*

756.19 Other
Platyspondylia
Supernumerary vertebra

756.2 Cervical rib
Supernumerary rib in the cervical region

756.3 Other anomalies of ribs and sternum

Congenital absence of:	Congenital:
rib	fissure of sternum
sternum	fusion of ribs
	Sternum bifidum

Excludes: *nonteratogenic deformity of chest wall (754.81-754.89)*

756.4 Chondrodystrophy

Achondroplasia	Dyschondroplasia
Chondrodystrophia (fetalis)	Enchondromatosis
	Ollier's disease

Excludes: *lipochondrodystrophy [Hurler's syndrome] (277.5)*
Morquio's disease (277.5)

⑤ **756.5 Osteodystrophies**

756.50 Osteodystrophy, unspecified

756.51 Osteogenesis imperfecta
Fragilitas ossium
Osteopsathyrosis

756.52 Osteopetrosis

756.53 Osteopoikilosis

756.54 Polyostotic fibrous dysplasia of bone

756.55 Chondroectodermal dysplasia
Ellis-van Creveld syndrome

756.56 Multiple epiphyseal dysplasia

756.59 Other
Albright (-McCune)-Sternberg syndrome

● Code new
to this edition

▲ Revision of
existing code

④ ⑤ Fourth or fifth
digit required

756.6 Anomalies of diaphragm
Absence of diaphragm
Congenital hernia:
diaphragmatic
foramen of Morgagni
Eventration of diaphragm
[Excludes:] *congenital hiatus hernia (750.6)*

[5] **756.7 Anomalies of abdominal wall**
Omphalocele
Exomphalos
Gastroschisis
Prune belly (syndrome)

756.70 Anomaly of abdominal wall, unspecified

756.71 Prune belly syndrome
Eagle-Barrett syndrome
Prolapse of bladder mucosa

756.79 Other congenital anomalies of abdominal wall
Exomphalos
Gastroschisis
Omphalocele

[Excludes:] *umbilical hernia (551-553 with .1)*

[5] **756.8 Other specified anomalies of muscle, tendon, fascia, and connective tissue**

756.81 Absence of muscle and tendon
Absence of muscle (pectoral)

756.82 Accessory muscle

756.83 Ehlers-Danlos syndrome

756.89 Other
Amyotrophia congenita
Congenital shortening of tendon

756.9 Other and unspecified anomalies of musculoskeletal system
Congenital:
anomaly NOS of musculoskeletal system, not elsewhere classified
deformity NOS of musculoskeletal system, not elsewhere classified

757 Congenital anomalies of the integument
Includes: anomalies of skin, subcutaneous tissue, hair, nails, and breast
[Excludes:] *hemangioma (228.00-228.09)*
pigmented nevus (216.0-216.9)

757.0 Hereditary edema of legs
Congenital lymphedema
Hereditary trophedema
Milroy's disease

757.1 Ichthyosis congenita
Congenital ichthyosis
Harlequin fetus
Ichthyosiform erythroderma

757.2 Dermatoglyphic anomalies
Abnormal palmar creases

[5] **757.3 Other specified anomalies of skin**

757.31 Congenital ectodermal dysplasia

757.32 Vascular hamartomas
Birthmarks
Port-wine stain
Strawberry nevus

757.33 Congenital pigmentary anomalies of skin
Congenital poikiloderma
Urticaria pigmentosa
Xeroderma pigmentosum

[Excludes:] *albinism (270.2)*

757.39 **Other**
Accessory skin tags, congenital
Congenital scar
Epidermolysis bullosa
Keratoderma (congenital)

Excludes: pilonidal cyst (685.0-685.1)

757.4 **Specified anomalies of hair**
Congenital:
alopecia
atrichosis
beaded hair
Congenital:
hypertrichosis
monilethrix
Persistent lanugo

757.5 **Specified anomalies of nails**
Anonychia
Congenital:
clubnail
koilonychia
Congenital:
leukonychia
onychauxis
pachyonychia

757.6 **Specified anomalies of breast**
Absent breast or nipple
Accessory breast or nipple
Supernumerary breast or nipple
Hypoplasia of breast

Excludes: absence of pectoral muscle (756.81)

757.8 **Other specified anomalies of the integument**

757.9 **Unspecified anomaly of the integument**
Congenital:
anomaly NOS of integument
deformity NOS of integument

758 **Chromosomal anomalies**
Includes: syndromes associated with anomalies in the number and form of chromosomes

758.0 **Down's syndrome**
Mongolism
Translocation Down's
syndrome
Trisomy:
21 or 22
G

758.1 **Patau's syndrome**
Trisomy:
13
D_1

758.2 **Edwards' syndrome**
Trisomy:
18
E_3

758.3 **Autosomal deletion syndromes**
Antimongolism syndrome   Cri-du-chat syndrome

758.4 **Balanced autosomal translocation in normal individual**

758.5 **Other conditions due to autosomal anomalies**
Accessory autosomes NEC

758.6 **Gonadal dysgenesis**
Ovarian dysgenesis   XO syndrome
Turner's syndrome

Excludes: pure gonadal dysgenesis (752.7)

758.7 **Klinefelter's syndrome**
XXY syndrome

⑤ **758.8** **Other conditions due to chromosome anomalies**

758.81 **Other conditions due to sex chromosome anomalies**

758.89 **Other**

758.9 **Conditions due to anomaly of unspecified chromosome**

759 **Other and unspecified congenital anomalies**

759.0 **Anomalies of spleen**
Aberrant spleen
Absent spleen
Accessory spleen
Congenital splenomegaly
Ectopic spleen
Lobulation of spleen

● Code new
to this edition

▲ Revision of
existing code

④ ⑤ Fourth or fifth
digit required

759.1 Anomalies of adrenal gland
Aberrant adrenal gland
Absent adrenal gland
Accessory adrenal gland

[Excludes:] *adrenogenital disorders (255.2)*
congenital disorders of steroid metabolism (255.2)

759.2 Anomalies of other endocrine glands
Absent parathyroid gland
Accessory thyroid gland
Persistent thyroglossal or thyrolingual duct
Thyroglossal (duct) cyst

[Excludes:] *congenital:*
goiter (246.1)
hypothyroidism (243)

759.3 Situs inversus
Situs inversus or transversus:
abdominalis
thoracis
Transposition of viscera:
abdominal
thoracic

[Excludes:] *dextrocardia without mention of complete transposition (746.87)*

759.4 Conjoined twins
Craniopagus
Dicephalus
Pygopagus
Thoracopagus
Xiphopagus

759.5 Tuberous sclerosis
Bourneville's disease
Epiloia

759.6 Other hamartoses, not elsewhere classified
Syndrome:
Peutz-Jeghers
Sturge-Weber (-Dimitri)
von Hippel-Lindau

[Excludes:] *neurofibromatosis (237.7)*

759.7 Multiple congenital anomalies, so described
Congenital:
anomaly, multiple NOS
deformity, multiple NOS

[5] **759.8 Other specified anomalies**

759.81 Prader-Willi syndrome

759.82 Marfan syndrome

759.83 Fragile X syndrome

759.89 Other
Congenital malformation syndromes affecting multiple systems, not elsewhere classified
Laurence-Moon-Biedl syndrome

759.9 Congenital anomaly, unspecified

● Code new
to this edition

▲ Revision of
existing code

④ ⑤ Fourth or fifth
digit required

15. CERTAIN CONDITIONS ORIGINATING IN THE PERINATAL PERIOD (760-779)

Includes: conditions which have their origin in the perinatal period even though death or morbidity occurs later

Use additional code(s) to further specify condition

MATERNAL CAUSES OF PERINATAL MORBIDITY AND MORTALITY (760-763)

760 Fetus or newborn affected by maternal conditions which may be unrelated to present pregnancy

Includes: the listed maternal conditions only when specified as a cause of mortality or morbidity of the fetus or newborn

[Excludes:] *maternal endocrine and metabolic disorders affecting fetus or newborn (775.0-775.9)*

760.0 Maternal hypertensive disorders
Fetus or newborn affected by maternal conditions classifiable to 642

760.1 Maternal renal and urinary tract diseases
Fetus or newborn affected by maternal conditions classifiable to 580-599

760.2 Maternal infections
Fetus or newborn affected by maternal infectious disease classifiable to 001-136 and 487, but fetus or newborn not manifesting that disease

[Excludes:] *congenital infectious diseases (771.0-771.8)*
maternal genital tract and other localized infections (760.8)

760.3 Other chronic maternal circulatory and respiratory diseases
Fetus or newborn affected by chronic maternal conditions classifiable to 390-459, 490-519, 745-748

760.4 Maternal nutritional disorders
Fetus or newborn affected by:
maternal disorders classifiable to 260-269
maternal malnutrition NOS

[Excludes:] *fetal malnutrition (764.10-764.29)*

760.5 Maternal injury
Fetus or newborn affected by maternal conditions classifiable to 800-995

760.6 Surgical operation on mother

[Excludes:] *cesarean section for present delivery (763.4)*
damage to placenta from amniocentesis, cesarean section, or surgical induction (762.1)
previous surgery to uterus or pelvic organs (763.89)

[5] **760.7 Noxious influences affecting fetus via placenta or breast milk**
Fetus or newborn affected by noxious substance transmitted via placenta or breast milk

[Excludes:] *anesthetic and analgesic drugs administered during labor and delivery (763.5)*
drug withdrawal syndrome in newborn (779.5)

760.70 Unspecified noxious substance
Fetus or newborn affected by:
Drug NEC

760.71 Alcohol
Fetal alcohol syndrome

760.72 Narcotics

760.73 Hallucinogenic agents

760.74 Anti-infectives
Antibiotics

760.75 Cocaine

760.76 Diethylstilbestrol (DES)

760.79 Other
Fetus or newborn affected by:
immune sera transmitted via placenta or breast milk
medicinal agents NEC transmitted via placenta or breast milk
toxic substance NEC transmitted via placenta or breast milk

760.8 Other specified maternal conditions affecting fetus or newborn
Maternal genital tract and other localized infection affecting fetus or newborn, but fetus or newborn not manifesting that disease

[Excludes:] *maternal urinary tract infection affecting fetus or newborn (760.1)*

Add 4th or 5th digit | Nonspecific code | Unspecified code | Manifestation code

760.9 Unspecified maternal condition affecting fetus or newborn

761 Fetus or newborn affected by maternal complications of pregnancy

Includes: the listed maternal conditions only when specified as a cause of mortality or morbidity of the fetus or newborn

761.0 Incompetent cervix

761.1 Premature rupture of membranes

761.2 Oligohydramnios

[Excludes:] *that due to premature rupture of membranes (761.1)*

761.3 Polyhydramnios

Hydramnios (acute) (chronic)

761.4 Ectopic pregnancy

Pregnancy:
abdominal
intraperitoneal
tubal

761.5 Multiple pregnancy

Triplet (pregnancy)
Twin (pregnancy)

761.6 Maternal death

761.7 Malpresentation before labor

Breech presentation before labor
External version before labor
Oblique lie before labor
Transverse lie before labor
Unstable lie before labor

761.8 Other specified maternal complications of pregnancy affecting fetus or newborn

Spontaneous abortion, fetus

761.9 Unspecified maternal complication of pregnancy affecting fetus or newborn

762 Fetus or newborn affected by complications of placenta, cord, and membranes

Includes: the listed maternal conditions only when specified as a cause of mortality or morbidity in the fetus or newborn

762.0 Placenta previa

762.1 Other forms of placental separation and hemorrhage

Abruptio placentae
Antepartum hemorrhage
Damage to placenta from amniocentesis, cesarean section, or surgical induction
Maternal blood loss
Premature separation of placenta
Rupture of marginal sinus

762.2 Other and unspecified morphological and functional abnormalities of placenta

Placental:
dysfunction
infarction
insufficiency

762.3 Placental transfusion syndromes

Placental and cord abnormality resulting in twin-to-twin or other transplacental transfusion

Use additional code, if desired, to indicate resultant condition in fetus or newborn:
fetal blood loss (772.0)
polycythemia neonatorum (776.4)

762.4 Prolapsed cord

Cord presentation

762.5 Other compression of umbilical cord

Cord around neck
Entanglement of cord
Knot in cord
Torsion of cord

762.6 Other and unspecified conditions of umbilical cord

Short cord
Thrombosis of umbilical cord
Varices of umbilical cord
Velamentous insertion of umbilical cord
Vasa previa or umbilical cord

[Excludes:] *infection of umbilical cord (771.4)*
single umbilical artery (747.5)

● Code new to this edition
▲ Revision of existing code
④ ⑤ Fourth or fifth digit required

762.7 Chorioamnionitis
Amnionitis
Membranitis
Placentitis

762.8 Other specified abnormalities of chorion and amnion

762.9 Unspecified abnormality of chorion and amnion

763 Fetus or newborn affected by other complications of labor and delivery
Includes: the listed conditions only when specified as a cause of mortality or morbidity in the fetus or newborn

763.0 Breech delivery and extraction

763.1 Other malpresentation, malposition, and disproportion during labor and delivery
Fetus or newborn affected by:
abnormality of bony pelvis
contracted pelvis
persistent occipitoposterior position
shoulder presentation
transverse lie
conditions classifiable to 652, 653, and 660

763.2 Forceps delivery
Fetus or newborn affected by forceps extraction

763.3 Delivery by vacuum extractor

763.4 Cesarean delivery
[Excludes:] *placental separation or hemorrhage from cesarean section (762.1)*

763.5 Maternal anesthesia and analgesia
Reactions and intoxications from maternal opiates and tranquilizers during labor and delivery
[Excludes:] *drug withdrawal syndrome in newborn (779.5)*

763.6 Precipitate delivery
Rapid second stage

763.7 Abnormal uterine contractions
Fetus or newborn affected by:
contraction ring
hypertonic labor
hypotonic uterine dysfunction
uterine inertia or dysfunction
conditions classifiable to 661, except 661.3

[5] **763.8 Other specified complications of labor and delivery affecting fetus or newborn**

763.81 Abnormality in fetal heart rate or rhythm before the onset of labor

763.82 Abnormality in fetal heart rate or rhythm during labor

763.83 Abnormality in fetal heart rate or rhythm, unspecified as to time of onset

763.89 Other specified complications of labor and delivery affecting fetus or newborn
Fetus or newborn affected by:
abnormality of maternal soft tissues
destructive operation on live fetus to facilitate delivery
induction of labor (medical)
previous surgery to uterus or pelvic organs
other conditions classifiable to 650-669
other procedures used in labor and delivery

763.9 Unspecified complication of labor and delivery affecting fetus or newborn

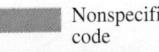

OTHER CONDITIONS ORIGINATING IN THE PERINATAL PERIOD (764-779)

The following fifth-digit subclassification is for use with categories 764 and codes 765.0 and 765.1 to denote birthweight:

0 unspecified [weight]
1 less than 500 grams
2 500-749 grams
3 750-999 grams
4 1,000- 1,249 grams
5 1,250-1,499 grams
6 1,500-1,749 grams
7 1,750-1,999 grams
8 2,000-2,499 grams
9 2,500 grams and over

[5] **764 Slow fetal growth and fetal malnutrition**

[5] **764.0 "Light-for-dates" without mention of fetal malnutrition**
Infants underweight for gestational age
"Small-for-dates"

[5] **764.1 "Light-for-dates" with signs of fetal malnutrition**
Infants "light-for-dates" classifiable to 764.0, who in addition show signs of fetal malnutrition, such as dry peeling skin and loss of subcutaneous tissue

[5] **764.2 Fetal malnutrition without mention of "light-for-dates"**
Infants, not underweight for gestational age, showing signs of fetal malnutrition, such as dry peeling skin and loss of subcutaneous tissue
Intrauterine malnutrition

[5] **764.9 Fetal growth retardation, unspecified**
Intrauterine growth retardation

▲ **765 Disorders relating to short gestation and low birthweight**
Includes: the listed conditions, without further specification, as causes of mortality, morbidity, or additional care, in fetus or newborn

[5] **765.0 Extreme immaturity**
Note: Usually implies a birthweight of less than 1000 grams
Use additional code for weeks of gestation (765.20-765.29)

[5] **765.1 Other preterm infants**
Note: Usually implies a birthweight of 1000-2499 grams
Prematurity NOS
Prematurity or small size, not classifiable to 765.0 or as "light-for-dates" in 764
Use additional code for weeks of gestation (765.20-765.29)

● **765.2 Weeks of gestation**

● **765.20 Unspecified weeks of gestation**
● **765.21 Less than 24 completed weeks of gestation**
● **765.22 24 completed weeks of gestation**
● **765.23 25-26 completed weeks of gestation**
● **765.24 27-28 completed weeks of gestation**
● **765.25 29-30 completed weeks of gestation**
● **765.26 31-32 completed weeks of gestation**
● **765.27 33-34 completed weeks of gestation**
● **765.28 35-36 completed weeks of gestation**
● **765.29 37 or more completed weeks of gestation**

766 Disorders relating to long gestation and high birthweight
Includes: the listed conditions, without further specification, as causes of mortality, morbidity, or additional care, in fetus or newborn

766.0 Exceptionally large baby
Note: Usually implies a birthweight of 4500 grams or more.

766.1 Other "heavy-for-dates" infants
Other fetus or infant "heavy-" or "large-for-dates" regardless of period of gestation

766.2 Post-term infant, not "heavy-for-dates"
Fetus or infant with gestation period of 294 days or more [42 or more completed weeks], not "heavy-" or "large-for-dates"
Postmaturity NOS

767 Birth trauma

767.0 Subdural and cerebral hemorrhage
Subdural and cerebral hemorrhage, whether described as due to birth trauma or to intrapartum anoxia or hypoxia
Subdural hematoma (localized)
Tentorial tear

Use additional code, if desired, to identify cause

Excludes: *intraventricular hemorrhage (772.10-772.14)*
subarachnoid hemorrhage (772.2)

767.1 Injuries to scalp
Caput succedaneum
Cephalhematoma
Chignon (from vacuum extraction)
Massive epicranial subaponeurotic hemorrhage

767.2 Fracture of clavicle

767.3 Other injuries to skeleton
Fracture of:
long bones
skull

Excludes: *congenital dislocation of hip (754.30-754.35)*
fracture of spine, congenital (767.4)

767.4 Injury to spine and spinal cord
Dislocation of spine or spinal cord due to birth trauma
Fracture of spine or spinal cord due to birth trauma
Laceration of spine or spinal cord due to birth trauma
Rupture of spine or spinal cord due to birth trauma

767.5 Facial nerve injury
Facial palsy

767.6 Injury to brachial plexus
Palsy or paralysis:
brachial
Erb (-Duchenne)
Klumpke (-Déjérine)

767.7 Other cranial and peripheral nerve injuries
Phrenic nerve paralysis

767.8 Other specified birth trauma

Eye damage	Rupture of:
Hematoma of:	liver
liver (subcapsular)	spleen
testes	Scalpel wound
vulva	Traumatic glaucoma

Excludes: *hemorrhage classifiable to 772.0-772.9*

767.9 Birth trauma, unspecified
Birth injury NOS

768 Intrauterine hypoxia and birth asphyxia
Use only when associated with newborn morbidity classifiable elsewhere

768.0 Fetal death from asphyxia or anoxia before onset of labor or at unspecified time

768.1 Fetal death from asphyxia or anoxia during labor

768.2 Fetal distress before onset of labor, in liveborn infant
Fetal metabolic acidemia before onset of labor, in liveborn infant

768.3 Fetal distress first noted during labor, in liveborn infant
Fetal metabolic acidemia first noted during labor, in liveborn infant

768.4 Fetal distress, unspecified as to time of onset, in liveborn infant
Fetal metabolic acidemia unspecified as to time of onset, in liveborn infant

768.5 Severe birth asphyxia
Birth asphyxia with neurologic involvement

768.6 Mild or moderate birth asphyxia
Other specified birth asphyxia (without mention of neurologic involvement)

	Add 4th or 5th digit		Nonspecific code		Unspecified code		Manifestation code

768.9 Unspecified birth asphyxia in liveborn infant
Anoxia NOS, in liveborn infant
Asphyxia NOS, in liveborn infant
Hypoxia NOS, in liveborn infant

769 Respiratory distress syndrome
Cardiorespiratory distress syndrome of newborn
Hyaline membrane disease (pulmonary)
Idiopathic respiratory distress syndrome [IRDS or RDS] of newborn
Pulmonary hypoperfusion syndrome

Excludes: transient tachypnea of newborn (770.6)

770 Other respiratory conditions of fetus and newborn

770.0 Congenital pneumonia
Infective pneumonia acquired prenatally

Excludes: pneumonia from infection acquired after birth (480.0-486)

770.1 Meconium aspiration syndrome
Aspiration of contents of birth canal NOS
Meconium aspiration below vocal cords
Pneumonitis:
    fetal aspiration
    meconium

770.2 Interstitial emphysema and related conditions
Pneumomediastinum originating in the perinatal period
Pneumopericardium originating in the perinatal period
Pneumothorax originating in the perinatal period

770.3 Pulmonary hemorrhage
Hemorrhage:
    alveolar (lung) originating in the perinatal period
    intra-alveolar (lung) originating in the perinatal period
    massive pulmonary originating in the perinatal period

770.4 Primary atelectasis
Pulmonary immaturity NOS

770.5 Other and unspecified atelectasis
Atelectasis:
    NOS, originating in the perinatal period
    partial, originating in the perinatal period
    secondary, originating in the perinatal period
Pulmonary collapse, originating in the perinatal period

770.6 Transitory tachypnea of newborn
Idiopathic tachypnea of newborn
Wet lung syndrome

Excludes: respiratory distress syndrome (769)

770.7 Chronic respiratory disease arising in the perinatal period
Bronchopulmonary dysplasia
Interstitial pulmonary fibrosis of prematurity
Wilson-Mikity syndrome

⑤ **770.8 Other respiratory problems after birth**

● **770.81 Primary apnea of newborn**
Apneic spells of newborn NOS
Essential apnea of newborn
Sleep apnea of newborn

● **770.82 Other apnea of newborn**
Obstructure apnea of newborn

● **770.83 Cyanotic attacks of newborn**

● **770.84 Respiratory failure of newborn**
Excludes: respiratory distress syndrom (769)

● **770.89 Other respiratory problems after birth**

770.9 Unspecified respiratory condition of fetus and newborn

● Code new
to this edition
▲ Revision of
existing code
④ ⑤ Fourth or fifth
digit required

771 Infections specific to the perinatal period
Includes: infections acquired before or during birth or via the umbilicus

[Excludes:] *congenital pneumonia (770.0)*
congenital syphilis (090.0-090.9)
maternal infectious disease as a cause of mortality or morbidity in fetus or newborn, but fetus or newborn not manifesting the disease (760.2)
ophthalmia neonatorum due to gonococcus (098.40)
other infections not specifically classified to this category

771.0 Congenital rubella
Congenital rubella pneumonitis

771.1 Congenital cytomegalovirus infection
Congenital cytomegalic inclusion disease

771.2 Other congenital infections
Congenital:
- herpes simplex
- listeriosis
- malaria

Congenital:
- toxoplasmosis
- tuberculosis

771.3 Tetanus neonatorum
Tetanus omphalitis

[Excludes:] *hypocalcemic tetany (775.4)*

771.4 Omphalitis of the newborn
Infection:
- navel cord
- umbilical stump

[Excludes:] *tetanus omphalitis (771.3)*

771.5 Neonatal infective mastitis

[Excludes:] *noninfective neonatal mastitis (778.7)*

771.6 Neonatal conjunctivitis and dacryocystitis
Ophthalmia neonatorum NOS

[Excludes:] *ophthalmia neonatorum due to gonococcus (098.40)*

771.7 Neonatal Candida infection
Neonatal moniliasis
Thrush in newborn

[5] **771.8 Other infection specific to the perinatal period**
Use additional code to identify organism

● **771.81 Septicemia [sepsis] of newborn**

● **771.82 Urinary tract infection of newborn**

● **771.83 Bacteremia of newborn**

● **771.89 Other infections specific to the perinatal period**
Intra-amniotic infection of fetus NOS
Infection of newborn NOS

772 Fetal and neonatal hemorrhage

[Excludes:] *hematological disorders of fetus and newborn (776.0-776.9)*

772.0 Fetal blood loss
Fetal blood loss from:
- cut end of co-twin's cord
- placenta
- ruptured cord
- vasa previa

Fetal exsanguination
Fetal hemorrhage into:
- co-twin
- mother's circulation

[5] **772.1 Intraventricular hemorrhage**
Intraventricular hemorrhage from any perinatal cause

772.10 Unspecified grade

772.11 Grade I
Bleeding into germinal matrix

772.12 Grade II
Bleeding into ventricle

772.13 Grade III
Bleeding with enlargement of ventricle

Add 4th or 5th digit | Nonspecific code | Unspecified code | Manifestation code

772.14 Grade IV
Bleeding into cerebral cortex

772.2 Subarachnoid hemorrhage
Subarachnoid hemorrhage from any perinatal cause

Excludes: subdural and cerebral hemorrhage (767.0)

772.3 Umbilical hemorrhage after birth
Slipped umbilical ligature

772.4 Gastrointestinal hemorrhage

Excludes: swallowed maternal blood (777.3)

772.5 Adrenal hemorrhage

772.6 Cutaneous hemorrhage
Bruising in fetus or newborn
Ecchymoses in fetus or newborn
Petechiae in fetus or newborn
Superficial hematoma in fetus or newborn

772.8 Other specified hemorrhage of fetus or newborn

Excludes: hemorrhagic disease of newborn (776.0)
    pulmonary hemorrhage (770.3)

772.9 Unspecified hemorrhage of newborn

773 Hemolytic disease of fetus or newborn, due to isoimmunization

773.0 Hemolytic disease due to Rh isoimmunization
Anemia due to RH antibodies, isoimmunization, or maternal/fetal incompatibility
Erythroblastosis (fetalis) due to RH antibodies, isoimmunization, or maternal/fetal
    incompatibility
Hemolytic disease (fetus) (newborn) due to RH antibodies, isoimmunization, or
    maternal/fetal incompatibility
Jaundice due to RH antibodies, isoimmunization, or maternal/fetal incompatibility
Rh hemolytic disease
Rh isoimmunization

773.1 Hemolytic disease due to ABO isoimmunization
ABO hemolytic disease
ABO isoimmunization
Anemia due to ABO antibodies, isoimmunization, or maternal/fetal incompatibility
Erythroblastosis (fetalis) due to ABO antibodies, isoimmunization, or maternal/fetal
    incompatibility
Hemolytic disease (fetus) (newborn) due to ABO antibodies, isoimmunization, or
    maternal/fetal incompatibility
Jaundice due to ABO antibodies, isoimmunization, or maternal/fetal incompatibility

773.2 Hemolytic disease due to other and unspecified isoimmunization
Erythroblastosis (fetalis) (neonatorum) NOS
Hemolytic disease (fetus) (newborn) NOS
Jaundice or anemia due to other and unspecified blood-group incompatibility

773.3 Hydrops fetalis due to isoimmunization
Use additional code, if desired, to identify type of isoimmunization (773.0-773.2)

773.4 Kernicterus due to isoimmunization
Use additional code, if desired, to identify type of isoimmunization (773.0-773.2)

773.5 Late anemia due to isoimmunization

774 Other perinatal jaundice

774.0 *Perinatal jaundice from hereditary hemolytic anemias*
Code first underlying disease (282.0-282.9)

774.1 Perinatal jaundice from other excessive hemolysis
Fetal or neonatal jaundice from:
    bruising
    drugs or toxins transmitted from mother
    infection
    polycythemia
    swallowed maternal blood
Use additional code, if desired, to identify cause

Excludes: jaundice due to isoimmunization (773.0-773.2)

774.2 Neonatal jaundice associated with preterm delivery
Hyperbilirubinemia of prematurity
Jaundice due to delayed conjugation associated with preterm delivery

● Code new   ▲ Revision of   ④ ⑤ Fourth or fifth
  to this edition   existing code   digit required

⑤ **774.3** **Neonatal jaundice due to delayed conjugation from other causes**

    774.30   **Neonatal jaundice due to delayed conjugation, cause unspecified**

    774.31   *Neonatal jaundice due to delayed conjugation in diseases classified elsewhere*
        Code first underlying diseases, as:
          congenital hypothyroidism (243)
          Crigler-Najjar syndrome (277.4)
          Gilbert's syndrome (277.4)

    774.39   **Other**
        Jaundice due to delayed conjugation from causes, such as:
        breast milk inhibitors
        delayed development of conjugating system

774.4 **Perinatal jaundice due to hepatocellular damage**
    Fetal or neonatal hepatitis
    Giant cell hepatitis
    Inspissated bile syndrome

774.5 *Perinatal jaundice from other causes*
    Code first underlying cause, as:
        congenital obstruction of bile duct (751.61)
        galactosemia (271.1)
        mucoviscidosis (277.00-277.09)

774.6 **Unspecified fetal and neonatal jaundice**
    Icterus neonatorum
    Neonatal hyperbilirubinemia (transient)
    Physiologic jaundice NOS in newborn

    Excludes: *that in preterm infants (774.2)*

774.7 **Kernicterus not due to isoimmunization**
    Bilirubin encephalopathy
    Kernicterus of newborn NOS

    Excludes: *kernicterus due to isoimmunization (773.4)*

775 **Endocrine and metabolic disturbances specific to the fetus and newborn**
    Includes: transitory endocrine and metabolic disturbances caused by the infant's response to
               maternal endocrine and metabolic factors, its removal from them, or its adjustment
               to extrauterine existence

775.0 **Syndrome of "infant of a diabetic mother"**
    Maternal diabetes mellitus affecting fetus or newborn (with hypoglycemia)

775.1 **Neonatal diabetes mellitus**
    Diabetes mellitus syndrome in newborn infant

775.2 **Neonatal myasthenia gravis**

775.3 **Neonatal thyrotoxicosis**
    Neonatal hyperthyroidism (transient)

775.4 **Hypocalcemia and hypomagnesemia of newborn**
    Cow's milk hypocalcemia
    Hypocalcemic tetany, neonatal
    Neonatal hypoparathyroidism
    Phosphate-loading hypocalcemia

775.5 **Other transitory neonatal electrolyte disturbances**
    Dehydration, neonatal

775.6 **Neonatal hypoglycemia**

    Excludes: *infant of mother with diabetes mellitus (775.0)*

775.7 **Late metabolic acidosis of newborn**

775.8 **Other transitory neonatal endocrine and metabolic disturbances**
    Amino-acid metabolic disorders described as transitory

775.9 **Unspecified endocrine and metabolic disturbances specific to the fetus and newborn**

776 **Hematological disorders of fetus and newborn**
    Includes: disorders specific to the fetus or newborn

    776.0 **Hemorrhagic disease of newborn**
        Hemorrhagic diathesis of newborn
        Vitamin K deficiency of newborn

        Excludes: *fetal or neonatal hemorrhage (772.0-772.9)*

▓	Add 4th or 5th digit	▓	Nonspecific code	▓	Unspecified code	▓ Manifestation code

776.1 Transient neonatal thrombocytopenia
Neonatal thrombocytopenia due to:
exchange transfusion
idiopathic maternal thrombocytopenia
isoimmunization

776.2 Disseminated intravascular coagulation in newborn

776.3 Other transient neonatal disorders of coagulation
Transient coagulation defect, newborn

776.4 Polycythemia neonatorum
Plethora of newborn
Polycythemia due to:
donor twin transfusion
maternal-fetal transfusion

776.5 Congenital anemia
Anemia following fetal blood loss

Excludes: anemia due to isoimmunization (773.0-773.2, 773.5)
hereditary hemolytic anemias (282.0-282.9)

776.6 Anemia of prematurity

776.7 Transient neonatal neutropenia
Isoimmune neutropenia
Maternal transfer neutropenia

Excludes: congenital neutropenia (nontransient) (288.0)

776.8 Other specified transient hematological disorders

776.9 Unspecified hematological disorder specific to fetus or newborn

777 Perinatal disorders of digestive system
Includes: disorders specific to the fetus and newborn

Excludes: intestinal obstruction classifiable to 560.0-560.9

777.1 Meconium obstruction
Congenital fecaliths
Delayed passage of meconium
Meconium ileus NOS
Meconium plug syndrome

Excludes: meconium ileus in cystic fibrosis (277.01)

777.2 Intestinal obstruction due to inspissated milk

777.3 Hematemesis and melena due to swallowed maternal blood
Swallowed blood syndrome in newborn

Excludes: that not due to swallowed maternal blood (772.4)

777.4 Transitory ileus of newborn

Excludes: Hirschsprung's disease (751.3)

777.5 Necrotizing enterocolitis in fetus or newborn
Pseudomembranous enterocolitis in newborn

777.6 Perinatal intestinal perforation
Meconium peritonitis

777.8 Other specified perinatal disorders of digestive system

777.9 Unspecified perinatal disorder of digestive system

778 Conditions involving the integument and temperature regulation of fetus and newborn

778.0 Hydrops fetalis not due to isoimmunization
Idiopathic hydrops

Excludes: hydrops fetalis due to isoimmunization (773.3)

778.1 Sclerema neonatorum
Subcutaneous fat necrosis

778.2 Cold injury syndrome of newborn

778.3 Other hypothermia of newborn

778.4 Other disturbances of temperature regulation of newborn
Dehydration fever in newborn
Environmentally-induced pyrexia
Hyperthermia in newborn
Transitory fever of newborn

● Code new
to this edition

▲ Revision of
existing code

④ ⑤ Fourth or fifth
digit required

778.5 Other and unspecified edema of newborn
Edema neonatorum

778.6 Congenital hydrocele
Congenital hydrocele of tunica vaginalis

778.7 Breast engorgement in newborn
Noninfective mastitis of newborn

[Excludes:] *infective mastitis of newborn (771.5)*

778.8 Other specified conditions involving the integument of fetus and newborn
Urticaria neonatorum

[Excludes:] *impetigo neonatorum (684)*
pemphigus neonatorum (684)

778.9 Unspecified condition involving the integument and temperature regulation of fetus and newborn

779 Other and ill-defined conditions originating in the perinatal period

779.0 Convulsions in newborn
Fits in newborn
Seizures in newborn

779.1 Other and unspecified cerebral irritability in newborn

779.2 Cerebral depression, coma, and other abnormal cerebral signs
CNS dysfunction in newborn NOS

779.3 Feeding problems in newborn
Regurgitation of food in newborn
Slow feeding in newborn
Vomiting in newborn

779.4 Drug reactions and intoxications specific to newborn
Gray syndrome from chloramphenicol administration in newborn

[Excludes:] *fetal alcohol syndrome (760.71)*
reactions and intoxications from maternal opiates and tranquilizers (763.5)

779.5 Drug withdrawal syndrome in newborn
Drug withdrawal syndrome in infant of dependent mother

[Excludes:] *fetal alcohol syndrome (760.71)*

779.6 Termination of pregnancy (fetus)
Fetus death due to:
induced abortion
termination of pregnancy

[Excludes:] *spontaneous abortion (fetus) (761.8)*

779.7 Periventricular leukomalacia

[5] **779.8 Other specified conditions originating in the perinatal period**

● **779.81 Neonatal bradycardia**

[Excludes:] *abnormality in fetal heart rate or rhythm complicating labor and delivery (763.81-763.83)*
bradycardia due to birth asphyxia (768.5-768.9)

● **779.82 Neonatal tachycardia**

[Excludes:] *abnormality in fetal heart rate or rhythm complicating labor and delivery (763.81-763.83)*

● **779.89 Other specified conditions originating in the perinatal period**

779.9 Unspecified condition originating in the perinatal period
Congenital debility NOS
Stillbirth NEC

16. SYMPTOMS, SIGNS, AND ILL-DEFINED CONDITIONS (780-799)

This section includes symptoms, signs, abnormal results of laboratory or other investigative procedures, and ill-defined conditions regarding which no diagnosis classifiable elsewhere is recorded.

Signs and symptoms that point rather definitely to a given diagnosis are assigned to some category in the preceding part of the classification. In general, categories 780-796 include the more ill-defined conditions and symptoms that point with perhaps equal suspicion to two or more diseases or to two or more systems of the body, and without the necessary study of the case to make a final diagnosis. Practically all categories in this group could be designated as "not otherwise specified," or as "unknown etiology," or as "transient." The Alphabetic Index should be consulted to determine which symptoms and signs are to be allocated here and which to more specific sections of the classification; the residual subcategories numbered .9 are provided for other relevant symptoms which cannot be allocated elsewhere in the classification.

The conditions and signs or symptoms included in categories 780-796 consist of: (a) cases for which no more specific diagnosis can be made even after all facts bearing on the case have been investigated; (b) signs or symptoms existing at the time of initial encounter that proved to be transient and whose causes could not be determined; (c) provisional diagnoses in a patient who failed to return for further investigation or care; (d) cases referred elsewhere for investigation or treatment before the diagnosis was made; (e) cases in which a more precise diagnosis was not available for any other reason; (f) certain symptoms which represent important problems in medical care and which it might be desired to classify in addition to a known cause.

SYMPTOMS (780-789)

780 General symptoms

[5] **780.0 Alteration of consciousness**

[Excludes:] *coma:*
diabetic (250.2-250.3)
hepatic (572.2)
originating in the perinatal period (779.2)

780.01 Coma

780.02 Transient alteration of awareness

780.03 Persistent vegetative state

780.09 Other
Drowsiness
Semicoma
Unconsciousness
Somnolence
Stupor

780.1 Hallucinations
Hallucinations:
NOS
auditory
gustatory
olfactory
tactile

[Excludes:] *those associated with mental disorders, as functional psychoses (295.0-298.9)*
organic brain syndromes (290.0-294.9, 310.0-310.9)
visual hallucinations (368.16)

780.2 Syncope and collapse
Blackout
Fainting
(Near) (Pre) syncope
Vasovagal attack

[Excludes:] *carotid sinus syncope (337.0)*
heat syncope (992.1)
neurocirculatory asthenia (306.2)
orthostatic hypotension (458.0)
shock NOS (785.50)

[5] **780.3 Convulsions**

[Excludes:] *convulsions:*
epileptic (345.10-345.91)
in newborn (779.0)

780.31 Febrile convulsions
Febrile seizure

780.39 Other convulsions
Convulsive disorder NOS
Fit NOS
Seizure NOS

780.4 Dizziness and giddiness
Light-headedness   Vertigo NOS

Excludes: *Ménière's disease and other specified vertiginous syndromes (386.0-386.9)*

⑤ **780.5 Sleep disturbances**

Excludes: *that of nonorganic origin (307.40-307.49)*

 780.50 Sleep disturbance, unspecified

 780.51 Insomnia with sleep apnea

 780.52 Other insomnia
   Insomnia NOS

 780.53 Hypersomnia with sleep apnea

 780.54 Other hypersomnia
   Hypersomnia NOS

 780.55 Disruptions of 24-hour sleep-wake cycle
   Inversion of sleep rhythm
   Irregular sleep-wake rhythm NOS
   Non-24-hour sleep-wake rhythm

 780.56 Dysfunctions associated with sleep stages or arousal from sleep

 780.57 Other and unspecified sleep apnea

 780.59 Other

780.6 Fever
Chills with fever   Hyperpyrexia NOS
Fever NOS   Pyrexia NOS
Fever of unknown origin   Pyrexia of unknown origin
 (FUO)

Excludes: *pyrexia of unknown origin (during):*
   in newborn (778.4)
   labor (659.2)
   the puerperium (672)

⑤ **780.7 Malaise and fatigue**

Excludes: *debility, unspecified (799.3)*

  fatigue (during):
   combat (308.0-308.9)
   heat (992.6)
   pregnancy (646.8)
  neurasthenia (300.5)
  senile asthenia (797.5)

 780.71 Chronic fatigue syndrome

 780.79 Other malaise and fatigue
   Asthenia NOS
   Lethargy
   Postviral (asthenic) syndrome
   Tiredness

780.8 Hyperhidrosis
Diaphoresis
Excessive sweating

⑤ **780.9 Other general symptoms**

Excludes: *hypothermia:*
   NOS (accidental) (991.6)
   due to anesthesia (995.89)
   of newborn (778.2-778.3)
   memory disturbance as part of a pattern of mental disorder

 ● **780.91 Fussy infant (baby)**

 ● **780.92 Excessive crying of infant (baby)**

 ● **780.99 Other general symptoms**
   Amnesia (retrograde)
   Chill(s) NOS
   Generalized pain
   Hypothermia, not associated with low environmental temperature

● Code new
 to this edition

▲ Revision of
 existing code

④ ⑤ Fourth or fifth
  digit required

781 Symptoms involving nervous and musculoskeletal systems

[Excludes:] *depression NOS (311)*
disorders specifically relating to:
back (724.0-724.9)
hearing (388.0-389.9)
joint (718.0-719.9)
limb (729.0-729.9)
neck (723.0-723.9)
vision (368.0-369.9)
pain in limb (729.5)

781.0 Abnormal involuntary movements
Abnormal head movements
Fasciculation
Spasms NOS
Tremor NOS

[Excludes:] *abnormal reflex (796.1)*
chorea NOS (333.5)
infantile spasms (345.60-345.61)
spastic paralysis (342.1, 343.0-344.9)
specified movement disorders classifiable to 333 (333.0-333.9)
that of nonorganic origin (307.2-307.3)

781.1 Disturbances of sensation of smell and taste
Anosmia
Parageusia
Parosmia

781.2 Abnormality of gait
Gait:
ataxic
paralytic
Gait:
spastic
staggering

[Excludes:] *ataxia:*
NOS (781.3)
locomotor (progressive) (094.0)
difficulty in walking (719.7)

781.3 Lack of coordination
Ataxia NOS
Muscular incoordination

[Excludes:] *ataxic gait (781.2)*
cerebellar ataxia (334.0-334.9)
difficulty in walking (719.7)
vertigo NOS (780.4)

781.4 Transient paralysis of limb
Monoplegia, transient NOS

[Excludes:] *paralysis (342.0-344.9)*

781.5 Clubbing of fingers

781.6 Meningismus
Dupré's syndrome
Meningism

781.7 Tetany
Carpopedal spasm

[Excludes:] *tetanus neonatorum (771.3)*
tetany:
hysterical (300.11)
newborn (hypocalcemic) (775.4)
parathyroid (252.1)
psychogenic (306.0)

781.8 Neurologic neglect syndrome
Asomatognosia
Hemi-akinesia
Hemi-inattention
Hemispatial neglect
Left-sided neglect
Sensory extinction
Sensory neglect
Visuospatial neglect

[5] **781.9 Other symptoms involving nervous and musculoskeletal systems**

781.91 Loss of height

[Excludes:] *osteoporosis (733.00-733.09)*

781.92 Abnormal posture

● **781.93 Ocular torticollis**

781.99 Other symptoms involving nervous and musculoskeletal systems

782 Symptoms involving skin and other integumentary tissue

[Excludes:] *symptoms relating to breast (611.71-611.79)*

782.0 Disturbance of skin sensation

Anesthesia of skin
Burning or prickling sensation
Hyperesthesia
Hypoesthesia
Numbness
Paresthesia
Tingling

782.1 Rash and other nonspecific skin eruption

Exanthem

[Excludes:] *vesicular eruption (709.8)*

782.2 Localized superficial swelling, mass, or lump

Subcutaneous nodules

[Excludes:] *localized adiposity (278.1)*

782.3 Edema

Anasarca
Dropsy
Localized edema NOS

[Excludes:] *ascites (789.5)*
edema of:
newborn NOS (778.5)
pregnancy (642.0-642.9, 646.1)
fluid retention (276.6)
hydrops fetalis (773.3, 778.0)
hydrothorax (511.8)
nutritional edema (260, 262)

782.4 Jaundice, unspecified, not of newborn

Cholemia NOS
Icterus NOS

[Excludes:] *jaundice in newborn (774.0-774.7)*
due to isoimmunization (773.0-773.2, 773.4)

782.5 Cyanosis

[Excludes:] *newborn (770.83)*

[5] **782.6 Pallor and flushing**

782.61 Pallor

782.62 Flushing

Excessive blushing

782.7 Spontaneous ecchymoses

Petechiae

[Excludes:] *ecchymosis in fetus or newborn (772.6)*
purpura (287.0-287.9)

782.8 Changes in skin texture

Induration of skin
Thickening of skin

782.9 Other symptoms involving skin and integumentary tissues

783 Symptoms concerning nutrition, metabolism, and development

783.0 Anorexia

Loss of appetite

[Excludes:] *anorexia nervosa (307.1)*
loss of appetite of nonorganic origin (307.59)

783.1 Abnormal weight gain

[Excludes:] *excessive weight gain in pregnancy (646.1)*
obesity (278.00)
morbid (278.01)

[5] **783.2 Abnormal loss of weight and underweight**

783.21 Loss of weight

783.22 Underweight

783.3 Feeding difficulties and mismanagement
Feeding problem (elderly) (infant)

Excludes: *feeding disturbance or problems:*
in newborn (779.3)
of nonorganic origin (307.50-307.59)

⑤ **783.4 Lack of expected normal physiological development in childhood**

Excludes: *delay in sexual development and puberty (259.0)*
gonadal dysgenesis (758.6)
pituitary dwarfism (253.3)
slow fetal growth and fetal malnutrition (764.00-764.99)
specific delays in mental development (315.0-315.9)

783.40 Lack of normal physiological development, unspecified
Inadequate development
Lack of development

783.41 Failure to thrive
Failure to gain weight

783.42 Delayed milestones
Late talker
Late walker

783.43 Short stature
Growth failure
Growth retardation
Lack of growth
Physical retardation

783.5 Polydipsia
Excessive thirst

783.6 Polyphagia
Excessive eating
Hyperalimentation NOS

Excludes: *disorders of eating of nonorganic origin (307.50-307.59)*

783.7 Adult failure to thrive

783.9 Other symptoms concerning nutrition, metabolism, and development
Hypometabolism

Excludes: *abnormal basal metabolic rate (794.7)*
dehydration (276.5)
other disorders of fluid, electrolyte, and acid-base balance (276.0-276.9)

784 Symptoms involving head and neck

Excludes: *encephalopathy NOS (348.3)*
specific symptoms involving neck classifiable to 723 (723.0-723.9)

784.0 Headache
Facial pain   Pain in head NOS

Excludes: *atypical face pain (350.2)*
migraine (346.0-346.9)
tension headache (307.81)

784.1 Throat pain

Excludes: *dysphagia (787.2)*
neck pain (723.1)
sore throat (462)
chronic (472.1)

784.2 Swelling, mass, or lump in head and neck
Space-occupying lesion, intracranial NOS

784.3 Aphasia

Excludes: *developmental aphasia (315.31)*

⑤ **784.4 Voice disturbance**

784.40 Voice disturbance, unspecified

784.41 Aphonia
Loss of voice

Add 4th or 5th digit	Nonspecific code	Unspecified code	Manifestation code

784.49 Other
Change in voice
Dysphonia
Hoarseness
Hypernasality
Hyponasality

784.5 Other speech disturbance
Dysarthria
Dysphasia
Slurred speech

Excludes: *stammering and stuttering (307.0)*
that of nonorganic origin (307.0, 307.9)

⑤ **784.6 Other symbolic dysfunction**

Excludes: *developmental learning delays (315.0-315.9)*

784.60 Symbolic dysfunction, unspecified

784.61 Alexia and dyslexia
Alexia (with agraphia)

784.69 Other
Acalculia
Agnosia
Agraphia NOS
Apraxia

784.7 Epistaxis
Hemorrhage from nose
Nosebleed

784.8 Hemorrhage from throat

Excludes: *hemoptysis (786.3)*

784.9 Other symptoms involving head and neck
Choking sensation
Halitosis
Mouth breathing
Sneezing

785 Symptoms involving cardiovascular system

Excludes: *heart failure NOS (428.9)*

785.0 Tachycardia, unspecified
Rapid heart beat

Excludes: *neonatal tachycardia (779.82)*
paroxysmal tachycardia (427.0-427.2)

785.1 Palpitations
Awareness of heart beat

Excludes: *specified dysrhythmias (427.0-427.9)*

785.2 Undiagnosed cardiac murmurs
Heart murmur NOS

785.3 Other abnormal heart sounds
Cardiac dullness, increased or decreased
Friction fremitus, cardiac
Precordial friction

785.4 Gangrene
Gangrenous cellulitis
Gangrene NOS
Gangrene spreading cutaneous
Phagedena

Code first any associated underlying condition, as:
diabetes (250.7)
Raynaud's syndrome (443.0)

Excludes: *gangrene of certain sites—see Alphabetic Index*
gangrene with atherosclerosis of the extremities (440.24)
gas gangrene (040.0)

⑤ **785.5 Shock without mention of trauma**

785.50 Shock, unspecified
Failure of peripheral circulation

785.51 Cardiogenic shock

● Code new
to this edition
▲ Revision of
existing code
④ ⑤ Fourth or fifth
digit required

785.59 Other

Shock:
- endotoxic
- gram-negative

Shock:
- hypovolemic
- septic

[Excludes:] *shock (due to):*
- *anesthetic (995.4)*
- *anaphylactic (995.0)*
  - *due to serum (999.4)*
- *electric (994.8)*
- *following abortion (639.5)*
- *lightning (994.0)*
- *obstetrical (669.1)*
- *postoperative (998.0)*
- *traumatic (958.4)*

785.6 Enlargement of lymph nodes

Lymphadenopathy

"Swollen glands"

[Excludes:] *lymphadenitis (chronic) (289.1-289.3)*
- *acute (683)*

785.9 Other symptoms involving cardiovascular system

Bruit (arterial)

Weak pulse

786 Symptoms involving respiratory system and other chest symptoms

⑤ 786.0 Dyspnea and respiratory abnormalities

786.00 Respiratory abnormality, unspecified

786.01 Hyperventilation

[Excludes:] *hyperventilation, psychogenic (306.1)*

786.02 Orthopnea

786.03 Apnea

[Excludes:] *apnea of newborn (770.81, 770.82)*
sleep apnea (780.51, 780.53, 780.57)

786.04 Cheyne-Stokes respiration

786.05 Shortness of breath

786.06 Tachypnea

[Excludes:] *transitory tachypnea of newborn (770.6)*

786.07 Wheezing

[Excludes:] *asthma (493.00-493.92)*

786.09 Other

Respiratory:
- distress
- insufficiency

[Excludes:] *respiratory distress:*
- *following trauma and surgery (518.5)*
- *newborn (770.89)*
- *syndrome (newborn) (769)*
  - *adult (518.5)*

respiratory failure (518.81, 518.83-518.84)
- *newborn (770.84)*

786.1 Stridor

[Excludes:] *congenital laryngeal stridor (748.3)*

786.2 Cough

[Excludes:] *cough:*
- *psychogenic (306.1)*
- *smokers' (491.0)*
- *with hemorrhage (786.3)*

786.3 Hemoptysis

Cough with hemorrhage

Pulmonary hemorrhage NOS

[Excludes:] *pulmonary hemorrhage of newborn (770.3)*

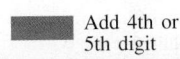

Add 4th or 5th digit | Nonspecific code | Unspecified code | Manifestation code

786.4 Abnormal sputum
Abnormal:
amount of sputum
color of sputum
odor of sputum
Excessive sputum

[5] **786.5 Chest pain**

786.50 Chest pain, unspecified

786.51 Precordial pain

786.52 Painful respiration
Pain:
anterior chest wall
pleuritic
Pleurodynia

[Excludes:] *epidemic pleurodynia (074.1)*

786.59 Other
Discomfort in chest
Pressure in chest
Tightness in chest

[Excludes:] *pain in breast (611.71)*

786.6 Swelling, mass, or lump in chest

[Excludes:] *lump in breast (611.72)*

786.7 Abnormal chest sounds
Abnormal percussion, chest
Friction sounds, chest
Rales
Tympany, chest

[Excludes:] *wheezing (786.07)*

786.8 Hiccough

[Excludes:] *psychogenic hiccough (306.1)*

786.9 Other symptoms involving respiratory system and chest
Breath-holding spell

787 Symptoms involving digestive system

[Excludes:] *constipation (564.00-564.09)*
pylorospasm (537.81)
congenital (750.5)

[5] **787.0 Nausea and vomiting**
Emesis

[Excludes:] *hematemesis NOS (578.0)*
vomiting:
bilious, following gastrointestinal surgery (564.3)
cyclical (536.2)
psychogenic (306.4)
excessive, in pregnancy (643.0-643.9)
habit (536.2)
of newborn (779.3)
psychogenic NOS (307.54)

787.01 Nausea with vomiting

787.02 Nausea alone

787.03 Vomiting alone

787.1 Heartburn
Pyrosis
Waterbrash

[Excludes:] *dyspepsia or indigestion (536.8)*

787.2 Dysphagia
Difficulty in swallowing

787.3 Flatulence, eructation, and gas pain
Abdominal distention (gaseous)
Bloating
Tympanites (abdominal) (intestinal)

[Excludes:] *aerophagy (306.4)*

● Code new to this edition ▲ Revision of existing code [4] [5] Fourth or fifth digit required

787.4 Visible peristalsis
Hyperperistalsis

787.5 Abnormal bowel sounds
Absent bowel sounds
Hyperactive bowel sounds

787.6 Incontinence of feces
Encopresis NOS
Incontinence of sphincter ani

[Excludes:] *that of nonorganic origin (307.7)*

787.7 Abnormal feces
Bulky stools

[Excludes:] *abnormal stool content (792.1)*
melena:
NOS (578.1)
newborn (772.4, 777.3)

[5] **787.9 Other symptoms involving digestive system**

[Excludes:] *gastrointestinal hemorrhage (578.0-578.9)*
intestinal obstruction (560.0-560.9)
specific functional digestive disorders:
esophagus (530.0-530.9)
stomach and duodenum (536.0-536.9)
those not elsewhere classified (564.00-564.9)

787.91 Diarrhea
Diarrhea NOS

787.99 Other
Change in bowel habits
Tenesmus (rectal)

788 Symptoms involving urinary system

[Excludes:] *hematuria (599.7)*
nonspecific findings on examination of the urine (791.0-791.9)
small kidney of unknown cause (589.0-589.9)
uremia NOS (586)

788.0 Renal colic
Colic (recurrent) of:
kidney
ureter

788.1 Dysuria
Painful urination
Strangury

[5] **788.2 Retention of urine**

788.20 Retention of urine, unspecified

788.21 Incomplete bladder emptying

788.29 Other specified retention of urine

[5] **788.3 Incontinence of urine**

[Excludes:] *that of nonorganic origin (307.6)*

Code, if applicable, any causal condition first, such as:
congenital ureterocele (753.23)
genital prolapse (618.0-618.9)

788.30 Urinary incontinence, unspecified
Enuresis NOS

788.31 Urge incontinence

788.32 Stress incontinence, male

[Excludes:] *stress incontinence (female) (625.6)*

788.33 Mixed incontinence (male) (female)
Urge and stress

788.34 Incontinence without sensory awareness

788.35 Post-void dribbling

788.36 Nocturnal enuresis

788.37 Continuous leakage

Add 4th or 5th digit | Nonspecific code | Unspecified code | Manifestation code

788.39 **Other urinary incontinence**

⑤ **788.4** **Frequency of urination and polyuria**

788.41 **Urinary frequency**
Frequency of micturition

788.42 **Polyuria**

788.43 **Nocturia**

788.5 **Oliguria and anuria**
Deficient secretion of urine
Suppression of urinary secretion

Excludes: *that complicating:*
abortion (634-638 with .3, 639.3)
ectopic or molar pregnancy (639.3)
pregnancy, childbirth, or the puerperium (642.0-642.9, 646.2)

⑤ **788.6** **Other abnormality of urination**

788.61 **Splitting of urinary stream**
Intermittent urinary stream

788.62 **Slowing of urinary stream**
Weak stream

788.69 **Other**

788.7 **Urethral discharge**
Penile discharge   Urethrorrhea

788.8 **Extravasation of urine**

788.9 **Other symptoms involving urinary system**
Extrarenal uremia
Vesical:
pain
tenesmus

789 **Other symptoms involving abdomen and pelvis**
The following fifth-digit subclassification is to be used for codes 789.0, 789.3, 789.4, 789.6

0 **unspecified site**

1 **right upper quadrant**

2 **left upper quadrant**

3 **right lower quadrant**

4 **left lower quadrant**

5 **periumbilic**

6 **epigastric**

7 **generalized**

9 **other specified site**
multiple sites

Excludes: *symptoms referable to genital organs:*
female (625.0-625.9)
male (607.0-608.9)
psychogenic (302.70-302.79)

⑤ **789.0** **Abdominal pain**
Colic:
NOS
infantile
Cramps, abdominal

Excludes: *renal colic (788.0)*

789.1 **Hepatomegaly**
Enlargement of liver

789.2 **Splenomegaly**
Enlargement of spleen

⑤ **789.3** **Abdominal or pelvic swelling, mass, or lump**
Diffuse or generalized swelling or mass:
abdominal NOS
umbilical

Excludes: *abdominal distention (gaseous) (787.3)*
ascites (789.5)

● Code new
to this edition

▲ Revision of
existing code

④ ⑤ Fourth or fifth
digit required

[5] **789.4 Abdominal rigidity**

789.5 Ascites
Fluid in peritoneal cavity

[5] **789.6 Abdominal tenderness**
Rebound tenderness

789.9 Other symptoms involving abdomen and pelvis
Umbilical:
bleeding
discharge

NONSPECIFIC ABNORMAL FINDINGS (790-796)

790 Nonspecific findings on examination of blood

[Excludes:] *abnormality of:*
platelets (287.0-287.9)
thrombocytes (287.0-287.9)
white blood cells (288.0-288.9)

[5] **790.0 Abnormality of red blood cells**

[Excludes:] *anemia:*
congenital (776.5)
newborn, due to isoimmunization (773.0-773.2, 773.5)
of premature infant (776.6)
other specified types (280.0-285.9)
hemoglobin disorders (282.5-282.7)
polycythemia:
familial (289.6)
neonatorum (776.4)
secondary (289.0)
vera (238.4)

790.01 Precipitous drop in hematocrit
Drop in hematocrit

790.09 Other abnormality of red blood cells
Abnormal red cell morphology NOS
Abnormal red cell volume NOS
Anisocytosis
Poikilocytosis

790.1 Elevated sedimentation rate

790.2 Abnormal glucose tolerance test

[Excludes:] *that complicating pregnancy, childbirth, or the puerperium (648.8)*

790.3 Excessive blood level of alcohol
Elevated blood-alcohol

790.4 Nonspecific elevation of levels of transaminase or lactic acid dehydrogenase [LDH]

790.5 Other nonspecific abnormal serum enzyme levels
Abnormal serum level of:
acid phosphatase
alkaline phosphatase
Abnormal serum level of:
amylase
lipase

[Excludes:] *deficiency of circulating enzymes (277.6)*

790.6 Other abnormal blood chemistry
Abnormal blood level of:
cobalt
copper
iron
lithium
Abnormal blood level of:
magnesium
mineral
zinc

[Excludes:] *abnormality of electrolyte or acid-base balance (276.0-276.9)*
hypoglycemia NOS (251.2)
specific finding indicating abnormality of:
amino-acid transport and metabolism (270.0-270.9)
carbohydrate transport and metabolism (271.0-271.9)
lipid metabolism (272.0-272.9)
uremia NOS (586)

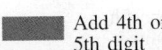

790.7 Bacteremia

> Excludes: *bacteremia of newborn (771.83)*
> > *septicemia (038)*

Use additional code, if desired, to identify organism (041)

790.8 Viremia, unspecified

⑤ **790.9 Other nonspecific findings on examination of blood**

> **790.91 Abnormal arterial blood gases**

> **790.92 Abnormal coagulation profile**
> > Abnormal or prolonged:
> > > bleeding time
> > > coagulation time
> > > partial thromboplastin time [PTT]
> > > prothrombin time [PT]

> Excludes: *coagulation (hemorrhagic) disorders (286.0-286.9)*

> **790.93 Elevated prostate specific antigen (PSA)**
> **790.94 Euthyroid sick syndrome**
> **790.99 Other**

791 Nonspecific findings on examination of urine

> Excludes: *hematuria NOS (599.7)*
> > *specific findings indicating abnormality of:*
> > > *amino-acid transport and metabolism (270.0-270.9)*
> > > *carbohydrate transport and metabolism (271.0-271.9)*

791.0 Proteinuria
  Albuminuria   Bence-Jones proteinuria

> Excludes: *postural proteinuria (593.6)*
> > *that arising during pregnancy or the puerperium (642.0-642.9, 646.2)*

791.1 Chyluria

> Excludes: *filarial (125.0-125.9)*

791.2 Hemoglobinuria

791.3 Myoglobinuria

791.4 Biliuria

791.5 Glycosuria

> Excludes: *renal glycosuria (271.4)*

791.6 Acetonuria
  Ketonuria

791.7 Other cells and casts in urine

791.9 Other nonspecific findings on examination of urine
  Crystalluria
  Elevated urine levels of:
    17-ketosteroids
    catecholamines
    indolacetic acid
    vanillylmandelic acid [VMA]
  Melanuria

792 Nonspecific abnormal findings in other body substances

> Excludes: *that in chromosomal analysis (795.2)*

792.0 Cerebrospinal fluid

792.1 Stool contents
  Abnormal stool color
  Fat in stool   Occult blood
  Mucus in stool   Pus in stool

> Excludes: *blood in stool [melena] (578.1)*
> > *newborn (772.4, 777.3)*

792.2 Semen
  Abnormal spermatozoa

> Excludes: *azoospermia (606.0)*
> > *oligospermia (606.1)*

● Code new   ▲ Revision of   ④ ⑤ Fourth or fifth
     to this edition   existing code   digit required

792.3 Amniotic fluid

792.4 Saliva

[Excludes:] *that in chromosomal analysis (795.2)*

792.5 Cloudy (hemodialysis) (peritoneal) dialysis effluent

792.9 Other nonspecific abnormal findings in body substances

Peritoneal fluid
Pleural fluid
Synovial fluid
Vaginal fluids

793 Nonspecific abnormal findings on radiological and other examinations of body structure

Includes: nonspecific abnormal findings of:
thermography
ultrasound examination [echogram]
x-ray examination

[Excludes:] *abnormal results of function studies and radioisotope scans (794.0-794.9)*

793.0 Skull and head

[Excludes:] *nonspecific abnormal echoencephalogram (794.01)*

793.1 Lung field

Coin lesion of lung
Shadow of lung

793.2 Other intrathoracic organ

Abnormal:
echocardiogram
heart shadow
ultrasound cardiogram
Mediastinal shift

793.3 Biliary tract

Nonvisualization of gallbladder

793.4 Gastrointestinal tract

793.5 Genitourinary organs

Filling defect:
bladder
kidney
ureter

793.6 Abdominal area, including retroperitoneum

793.7 Musculoskeletal system

[5] **793.8 Breast**

793.80 Abnormal mammogram, unspecified

793.81 Mammographic microcalcification

793.89 Other abnormal findings on radiological examination of breast

793.9 Other

Abnormal:
placental finding by x-ray or ultrasound method
radiological findings in skin and subcutaneous tissue

[Excludes:] *abnormal finding by radioisotope localization of placenta (794.9)*

794 Nonspecific abnormal results of function studies

Includes: radioisotope:
scans
uptake studies
scintiphotography

[5] **794.0 Brain and central nervous system**

794.00 Abnormal function study, unspecified

794.01 Abnormal echoencephalogram

794.02 Abnormal electroencephalogram [EEG]

794.09 Other

Abnormal brain scan

[5] **794.1 Peripheral nervous system and special senses**

794.10 Abnormal response to nerve stimulation, unspecified

794.11 Abnormal retinal function studies

Abnormal electroretinogram [ERG]

794.12 Abnormal electro-oculogram [EOG]

Add 4th or 5th digit | Nonspecific code | Unspecified code | Manifestation code

794.13 Abnormal visually evoked potential

794.14 Abnormal oculomotor studies

794.15 Abnormal auditory function studies

794.16 Abnormal vestibular function studies

794.17 Abnormal electromyogram [EMG]
> Excludes: *that of eye (794.14)*

794.19 Other

794.2 Pulmonary
Abnormal lung scan
Reduced:
  ventilatory capacity
  vital capacity

⑤ **794.3 Cardiovascular**

794.30 Abnormal function study, unspecified

794.31 Abnormal electrocardiogram [ECG] [EKG]

794.39 Other
Abnormal:
  ballistocardiogram
  phonocardiogram
  vectorcardiogram

794.4 Kidney
Abnormal renal function test

794.5 Thyroid
Abnormal thyroid:
  scan
  uptake

794.6 Other endocrine function study

794.7 Basal metabolism
Abnormal basal metabolic rate [BMR]

794.8 Liver
Abnormal liver scan

794.9 Other
Bladder
Pancreas
Placenta
Spleen

795 Nonspecific abnormal histological and immunological findings
> Excludes: *nonspecific abnormalities of red blood cells (790.01-790.09)*

⑤ **795.0 Nonspecific abnormal Papanicolaou smear of cervix**
> Excludes: *carcinoma in-situ of cervix (233.1)*
> *cervical intraepithelial neoplasia I (CIN I) (622.1)*
> *cervical intraepithelial neoplasia II (CINN II) (622.1)*
> *cervical intraepithelial neoplasia III (CIN III) (233.1)*
> *dysplasia of cervix (uteri) (622.1)*
> *high grade squamous intraepithelial dysplasia (HGSIL) (622.1)*
> *low grade squamous intraepithelial dysplasia (LGSIL) (622.1)*

● **795.00 Nonspecific abnormal Papanicolaou smear of cervix, unspecified**

● **795.01 Atypical squamous cell changes of undetermined significance favor benign (ASCUS favor benign)**
Atypical glandular cell changes of undetermined significance favor benign (AGCUS favor benign)

● **795.02 Atypical squamous cell changes of undetermined significance favor dysplasia (ASCUS favor dysplasia)**
Atypical glandular cell changes of undetermined significance favor dysplasia (AGCUS favor dysplasia)

● **795.09 Other nonspecific abnormal Papanicolaou smear of cervix**
Benign cellular changes
Unsatisfactory smear

795.1 Nonspecific abnormal Papanicolaou smear of other site

● Code new
to this edition

▲ Revision of
existing code

④ ⑤ Fourth or fifth
digit required

795.2 Nonspecific abnormal findings on chromosomal analysis
Abnormal karyotype

[5] **795.3 Nonspecific positive culture findings**
Positive culture findings in:
nose
sputum
throat
wound

[Excludes:] *that of:*
blood (790.7-790.8)
urine (791.9)

● **795.31 Nonspecific positive findings for anthrax**
Positive findings by nasal swab

● **795.39 Other nonspecific positive culture findings**

795.4 Other nonspecific abnormal histological findings

795.5 Nonspecific reaction to tuberculin skin test without active tuberculosis
Abnormal result of Mantoux test
PPD positive
Tuberculin (skin test):
positive
reactor

795.6 False positive serological test for syphilis
False positive Wassermann reaction

[5] **795.7 Other nonspecific immunological findings**

[Excludes:] *isoimmunization, in pregnancy (656.1-656.2)*
affecting fetus or newborn (773.0-773.2)

795.71 Nonspecific serologic evidence of human immunodeficiency virus [HIV]
Inconclusive human immunodeficiency virus [HIV] test (adult) (infant)

Note: This code is ONLY to be used when a test finding is reported as nonspecific. Asymptomatic positive findings are coded to V08. If any HIV infection symptom or condition is present, see code 042. Negative findings are not coded.

[Excludes:] *acquired immunodeficiency syndrome [AIDS] (042)*
asymptomatic human immunodeficiency virus, [HIV] infection status (V08)
HIV infection, symptomatic (042)
human immunodeficiency virus [HIV] disease (042)
positive (status) NOS (V08)

795.79 Other and unspecified nonspecific immunological findings
Raised antibody titer
Raised level of immunoglobulins

796 Other nonspecific abnormal findings

796.0 Nonspecific abnormal toxicological findings
Abnormal levels of heavy metals or drugs in blood, urine, or other tissue

[Excludes:] *excessive blood level of alcohol (790.3)*

796.1 Abnormal reflex

796.2 Elevated blood pressure reading without diagnosis of hypertension

Note: This category is to be used to record an episode of elevated blood pressure in a patient in whom no formal diagnosis of hypertension has been made, or as an incidental finding.

796.3 Nonspecific low blood pressure reading

796.4 Other abnormal clinical findings

796.5 Abnormal finding on antenatal screening

796.9 Other

ILL-DEFINED AND UNKNOWN CAUSES OF MORBIDITY AND MORTALITY (797-799)

797 Senility without mention of psychosis
Old age
Senescence
Senile asthenia
Senile debility
Senile exhaustion

[Excludes:] *senile psychoses (290.0-290.9)*

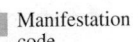

798 **Sudden death, cause unknown**

798.0 Sudden infant death syndrome
Cot death
Crib death
Sudden death of nonspecific cause in infancy

798.1 Instantaneous death

798.2 Death occurring in less than 24 hours from onset of symptoms, not otherwise explained
Death known not to be violent or instantaneous, for which no cause could be discovered
Died without sign of disease

798.9 Unattended death
Death in circumstances where the body of the deceased was found and no cause could be discovered
Found dead

799 **Other ill-defined and unknown causes of morbidity and mortality**

799.0 Asphyxia
Excludes: *asphyxia (due to):*
  carbon monoxide (986)
  inhalation of food or foreign body (932-934.9)
  newborn (768.0-768.9)
  traumatic (994.7)

799.1 Respiratory arrest
Cardiorespiratory failure
Excludes: *cardiac arrest (427.5)*
  failure of peripheral circulation (785.50)
  respiratory distress:
    NOS (786.09)
    acute (518.82)
    following trauma and surgery (518.5)
    newborn (770.89)
    syndrome (newborn) (769)
      adult (following trauma and surgery) (518.5)
      other (518.82)
  respiratory failure (518.81, 518.83-518.84)
    newborn (770.84)
  respiratory insufficiency (786.09)
    acute (518.82)

799.2 Nervousness
"Nerves"

799.3 Debility, unspecified
Excludes: *asthenia (780.79)*
  nervous debility (300.5)
  neurasthenia (300.5)
  senile asthenia (797)

799.4 Cachexia
Wasting disease
Excludes: *nutritional marasmus (261)*

799.8 Other ill-defined conditions

799.9 Other unknown and unspecified cause
Undiagnosed disease, not specified as to site or system involved
Unknown cause of morbidity or mortality

● Code new
to this edition

▲ Revision of
existing code

④ ⑤ Fourth or fifth
digit required

17. INJURY AND POISONING (800-999)

Use E code(s) to identify the cause and intent of the injury or poisoning (E800-E999)

Note:

1. The principle of multiple coding of injuries should be followed wherever possible. Combination categories for multiple injuries are provided for use when there is insufficient detail as to the nature of the individual conditions, or for primary tabulation purposes when it is more convenient to record a single code; otherwise, the component injuries should be coded separately.

   Where multiple sites of injury are specified in the titles, the word "with" indicates involvement of both sites, and the word "and" indicates involvement of either or both sites. The word "finger" includes thumb.
2. Categories for "late effect" of injuries are to be found at 905-909.

FRACTURES (800-829)

[Excludes:] malunion (733.81)
nonunion (733.82)
pathologic or spontaneous fracture (733.10-733.19)
stress fractures (733.93-733.95)

The terms "condyle," "coronoid process," "ramus," and "symphysis" indicate the portion of the bone fractured, not the name of the bone involved.

The descriptions "closed" and "open" used in the fourth-digit subdivisions include the following terms:

closed (with or without delayed healing):
comminuted
depressed
elevated
fissured
fracture NOS
greenstick
impacted
linear
simple
slipped epiphysis
spiral

open (with or without delayed healing):
compound
infected
missile
puncture
with foreign body

A fracture not indicated as closed or open should be classified as closed.

FRACTURE OF SKULL (800-804)

The following fifth-digit subclassification is for use with the appropriate codes in categories 800, 801, 803, and 804:

0 unspecified state of consciousness
1 with no loss of consciousness
2 with brief [less than one hour] loss of consciousness
3 with moderate [1-24 hours] loss of consciousness and return to pre-existing conscious level
4 with prolonged [more than 24 hours] loss of consciousness and return to pre-existing conscious level
5 with prolonged [more than 24 hours] loss of consciousness, without return to pre-existing conscious level
Use fifth-digit 5 to designate when a patient is unconscious and dies before regaining consciousness, regardless of the duration of the loss of consciousness
6 with loss of consciousness of unspecified duration
9 with concussion, unspecified

[5] **800 Fracture of vault of skull**
Includes: frontal bone
parietal bone

[5] **800.0 Closed without mention of intracranial injury**
[5] **800.1 Closed with cerebral laceration and contusion**
[5] **800.2 Closed with subarachnoid, subdural, and extradural hemorrhage**
[5] **800.3 Closed with other and unspecified intracranial hemorrhage**
[5] **800.4 Closed with intracranial injury of other and unspecified nature**
[5] **800.5 Open without mention of intracranial injury**
[5] **800.6 Open with cerebral laceration and contusion**
[5] **800.7 Open with subarachnoid, subdural, and extradural hemorrhage**

Add 4th or 5th digit | Nonspecific code | Unspecified code | Medicare secondary payer (MSP) alert

[5] **800.8 Open with other and unspecified intracranial hemorrhage**

[5] **800.9 Open with intracranial injury of other and unspecified nature**

[5] **801 Fracture of base of skull**

Includes:

fossa:
  anterior
  middle
  posterior
occiput bone
orbital roof
sinus:
  ethmoid
  frontal
sphenoid bone
temporal bone

[5] **801.0 Closed without mention of intracranial injury**

[5] **801.1 Closed with cerebral laceration and contusion**

[5] **801.2 Closed with subarachnoid, subdural, and extradural hemorrhage**

[5] **801.3 Closed with other and unspecified intracranial hemorrhage**

[5] **801.4 Closed with intracranial injury of other and unspecified nature**

[5] **801.5 Open without mention of intracranial injury**

[5] **801.6 Open with cerebral laceration and contusion**

[5] **801.7 Open with subarachnoid, subdural, and extradural hemorrhage**

[5] **801.8 Open with other and unspecified intracranial hemorrhage**

[5] **801.9 Open with intracranial injury of other and unspecified nature**

802 Fracture of face bones

802.0 Nasal bones, closed

802.1 Nasal bones, open

[5] **802.2 Mandible, closed**

Inferior maxilla
Lower jaw (bone)

802.20 Unspecified site

802.21 Condylar process

802.22 Subcondylar

802.23 Coronoid process

802.24 Ramus, unspecified

802.25 Angle of jaw

802.26 Symphysis of body

802.27 Alveolar border of body

802.28 Body, other and unspecified

802.29 Multiple sites

[5] **802.3 Mandible, open**

802.30 Unspecified site

802.31 Condylar process

802.32 Subcondylar

802.33 Coronoid process

802.34 Ramus, unspecified

802.35 Angle of jaw

802.36 Symphysis of body

802.37 Alveolar border of body

802.38 Body, other and unspecified

802.39 Multiple sites

802.4 Malar and maxillary bones, closed

Superior maxilla
Upper jaw (bone)
Zygoma
Zygomatic arch

802.5 Malar and maxillary bones, open

802.6 Orbital floor (blow-out), closed

802.7 Orbital floor (blow-out), open

802.8 Other facial bones, closed
Alveolus
Orbit:
    NOS
    part other than roof or floor
Palate

Excludes: orbital:
        floor (802.6)
        roof (801.0-801.9)

802.9 Other facial bones, open

⑤ **803 Other and unqualified skull fractures**
Includes: skull NOS
            skull multiple NOS

⑤ **803.0 Closed without mention of intracranial injury**

⑤ **803.1 Closed with cerebral laceration and contusion**

⑤ **803.2 Closed with subarachnoid, subdural, and extradural hemorrhage**

⑤ **803.3 Closed with other and unspecified intracranial hemorrhage**

⑤ **803.4 Closed with intracranial injury of other and unspecified nature**

⑤ **803.5 Open without mention of intracranial injury**

⑤ **803.6 Open with cerebral laceration and contusion**

⑤ **803.7 Open with subarachnoid, subdural, and extradural hemorrhage**

⑤ **803.8 Open with other and unspecified intracranial hemorrhage**

⑤ **803.9 Open with intracranial injury of other and unspecified nature**

⑤ **804 Multiple fractures involving skull or face with other bones**

⑤ **804.0 Closed without mention of intracranial injury**

⑤ **804.1 Closed with cerebral laceration and contusion**

⑤ **804.2 Closed with subarachnoid, subdural, and extradural hemorrhage**

⑤ **804.3 Closed with other and unspecified intracranial hemorrhage**

⑤ **804.4 Closed with intracranial injury of other and unspecified nature**

⑤ **804.5 Open without mention of intracranial injury**

⑤ **804.6 Open with cerebral laceration and contusion**

⑤ **804.7 Open with subarachnoid, subdural, and extradural hemorrhage**

⑤ **804.8 Open with other and unspecified intracranial hemorrhage**

⑤ **804.9 Open with intracranial injury of other and unspecified nature**

FRACTURE OF NECK AND TRUNK (805-809)

805 Fracture of vertebral column without mention of spinal cord injury
Includes:

neural arch	transverse process
spine	vertebra
spinous process	

The following fifth-digit subclassification is for use with codes 805.0-805.1:

0 cervical vertebra, unspecified level

1 first cervical vertebra

2 second cervical vertebra

3 third cervical vertebra

4 fourth cervical vertebra

5 fifth cervical vertebra

6 sixth cervical vertebra

7 seventh cervical vertebra

8 multiple cervical vertebrae

⑤ **805.0 Cervical, closed**
Atlas   Axis

⑤ **805.1 Cervical, open**

805.2 Dorsal [thoracic], closed

805.3 Dorsal [thoracic], open

Add 4th or 5th digit	Nonspecific code	Unspecified code	Medicare secondary payer (MSP) alert

805.4 Lumbar, closed

805.5 Lumbar, open

805.6 Sacrum and coccyx, closed

805.7 Sacrum and coccyx, open

805.8 Unspecified, closed

805.9 Unspecified, open

806 Fracture of vertebral column with spinal cord injury

Includes: any condition classifiable to 805 with:
  complete or incomplete transverse lesion (of cord)
  hematomyelia
  injury to:
    cauda equina
    nerve
  paralysis
  paraplegia
  quadriplegia
  spinal concussion

⑤ **806.0** Cervical, closed

806.00 C_1-C_4 level with unspecified spinal cord injury
Cervical region NOS with spinal cord injury NOS

806.01 C_1-C_4 level with complete lesion of cord

806.02 C_1-C_4 level with anterior cord syndrome

806.03 C_1-C_4 level with central cord syndrome

806.04 C_1-C_4 level with other specified spinal cord injury
C_1-C_4 level with:
  incomplete spinal cord lesion NOS
  posterior cord syndrome

806.05 C_5-C_7 level with unspecified spinal cord injury

806.06 C_5-C_7 level with complete lesion of cord

806.07 C_5-C_7 level with anterior cord syndrome

806.08 C_5-C_7 level with central cord syndrome

806.09 C_5-C_7 level with other specified spinal cord injury
C_5-C_7 level with:
  incomplete spinal cord lesion NOS
  posterior cord syndrome

⑤ **806.1** Cervical, open

806.10 C_1-C_4 level with unspecified spinal cord injury

806.11 C_1-C_4 level with complete lesion of cord

806.12 C_1-C_4 level with anterior cord syndrome

806.13 C_1-C_4 level with central cord syndrome

806.14 C_1-C_4 level with other specified spinal cord injury
C_1-C_4 level with:
  incomplete spinal cord lesion NOS
  posterior cord syndrome

806.15 C_5-C_7 level with unspecified spinal cord injury

806.16 C_5-C_7 level with complete lesion of cord

806.17 C_5-C_7 level with anterior cord syndrome

806.18 C_5-C_7 level with central cord syndrome

806.19 C_5-C_7 level with other specified spinal cord injury
C_5-C_7 level with:
  incomplete spinal cord lesion NOS
  posterior cord syndrome

⑤ **806.2** Dorsal [thoracic], closed

806.20 T_1-T_6 level with unspecified spinal cord injury
Thoracic region NOS with spinal cord injury NOS

806.21 T_1-T_6 level with complete lesion of cord

806.22 T_1-T_6 level with anterior cord syndrome

806.23 T_1-T_6 level with central cord syndrome

● Code new
to this edition

▲ Revision of
existing code

④ ⑤ Fourth or fifth
digit required

806.24 **T_1-T_6 level with other specified spinal cord injury**
T_1-T_6 level with:
incomplete spinal cord lesion NOS
posterior cord syndrome

806.25 **T_7-T_{12} level with unspecified spinal cord injury**

806.26 **T_7-T_{12} level with complete lesion of cord**

806.27 **T_7-T_{12} level with anterior cord syndrome**

806.28 **T_7-T_{12} level with central cord syndrome**

806.29 **T_7-T_{12} level with other specified spinal cord injury**
T_7-T_{12} level with:
incomplete spinal cord lesion NOS
posterior cord syndrome

[5] **806.3 Dorsal [thoracic], open**

806.30 **T_1-T_6 level with unspecified spinal cord injury**

806.31 **T_1-T_6 level with complete lesion of cord**

806.32 **T_1-T_6 level with anterior cord syndrome**

806.33 **T_1-T_6 level with central cord syndrome**

806.34 **T_1-T_6 level with other specified spinal cord injury**
T_1-T_6 level with:
incomplete spinal cord lesion NOS
posterior cord syndrome

806.35 **T_7-T_{12} level with unspecified spinal cord injury**

806.36 **T_7-T_{12} level with complete lesion of cord**

806.37 **T_7-T_{12} level with anterior cord syndrome**

806.38 **T_7-T_{12} level with central cord syndrome**

806.39 **T_7-T_{12} level with other specified spinal cord injury**
T_7-T_{12} level with:
incomplete spinal cord lesion NOS
posterior cord syndrome

806.4 **Lumbar, closed**

806.5 **Lumbar, open**

[5] **806.6 Sacrum and coccyx, closed**

806.60 **With unspecified spinal cord injury**

806.61 **With complete cauda equina lesion**

806.62 **With other cauda equina injury**

806.69 **With other spinal cord injury**

[5] **806.7 Sacrum and coccyx, open**

806.70 **With unspecified spinal cord injury**

806.71 **With complete cauda equina lesion**

806.72 **With other cauda equina injury**

806.79 **With other spinal cord injury**

806.8 **Unspecified, closed**

806.9 **Unspecified, open**

807 Fracture of rib(s), sternum, larynx, and trachea

The following fifth-digit subclassification is for use with codes 807.0-807.1:

- **0 rib(s), unspecified**
- **1 one rib**
- **2 two ribs**
- **3 three ribs**
- **4 four ribs**
- **5 five ribs**
- **6 six ribs**
- **7 seven ribs**
- **8 eight or more ribs**
- **9 multiple ribs, unspecified**

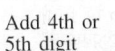

Add 4th or 5th digit | Nonspecific code | Unspecified code | Medicare secondary payer (MSP) alert

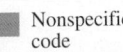

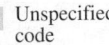

⑤ **807.0 Rib(s), closed**

⑤ **807.1 Rib(s), open**

807.2 Sternum, closed

807.3 Sternum, open

807.4 Flail chest

807.5 Larynx and trachea, closed
Hyoid bone
Thyroid cartilage
Trachea

807.6 Larynx and trachea, open

808 Fracture of pelvis

808.0 Acetabulum, closed

808.1 Acetabulum, open

808.2 Pubis, closed

808.3 Pubis, open

⑤ **808.4 Other specified part, closed**

808.41 Ilium

808.42 Ischium

808.43 Multiple pelvic fractures with disruption of pelvic circle

808.49 Other
Innominate bone
Pelvic rim

⑤ **808.5 Other specified part, open**

808.51 Ilium

808.52 Ischium

808.53 Multiple pelvic fractures with disruption of pelvic circle

808.59 Other

808.8 Unspecified, closed

808.9 Unspecified, open

809 Ill-defined fractures of bones of trunk
Includes: bones of trunk with other bones except those of skull and face
multiple bones of trunk

[Excludes:] *multiple fractures of:*
pelvic bones alone (808.0-808.9)
ribs alone (807.0-807.1, 807.4)
ribs or sternum with limb bones (819.0-819.1, 828.0-828.1)
skull or face with other bones (804.0-804.9)

809.0 Fracture of bones of trunk, closed

809.1 Fracture of bones of trunk, open

FRACTURE OF UPPER LIMB (810-819)

⑤ **810 Fracture of clavicle**
Includes: collar bone
interligamentous part of clavicle

The following fifth-digit subclassification is for use with category 810:

0 unspecified part
Clavicle NOS

1 sternal end of clavicle

2 shaft of clavicle

3 acromial end of clavicle

⑤ **810.0 Closed**

⑤ **810.1 Open**

⑤ **811 Fracture of scapula**
Includes: shoulder blade

The following fifth-digit subclassification is for use with category 811:

0 unspecified part

1 acromial process
Acromion (process)

continued

● Code new to this edition ▲ Revision of existing code ④ ⑤ Fourth or fifth digit required

        2   coracoid process

        3   glenoid cavity and neck of scapula

        9   other
                Scapula body

⑤ **811.0** Closed

⑤ **811.1** Open

812 Fracture of humerus

⑤ **812.0** Upper end, closed

    812.00 **Upper end, unspecified part**
        Proximal end
        Shoulder

    812.01 **Surgical neck**
        Neck of humerus NOS

    812.02 **Anatomical neck**

    812.03 **Greater tuberosity**

    812.09 **Other**
        Head   Upper epiphysis

⑤ **812.1** Upper end, open

    812.10 **Upper end, unspecified part**

    812.11 **Surgical neck**

    812.12 **Anatomical neck**

    812.13 **Greater tuberosity**

    812.19 **Other**

⑤ **812.2** Shaft or unspecified part, closed

    812.20 **Unspecified part of humerus**
        Humerus NOS   Upper arm NOS

    812.21 **Shaft of humerus**

⑤ **812.3** Shaft or unspecified part, open

    812.30 **Unspecified part of humerus**

    812.31 **Shaft of humerus**

⑤ **812.4** Lower end, closed
        Distal end of humerus   Elbow

    812.40 **Lower end, unspecified part**

    812.41 **Supracondylar fracture of humerus**

    812.42 **Lateral condyle**
        External condyle

    812.43 **Medial condyle**
        Internal epicondyle

    812.44 **Condyle(s), unspecified**
        Articular process NOS
        Lower epiphysis NOS

    812.49 **Other**
        Multiple fractures of lower end
        Trochlea

⑤ **812.5** Lower end, open

    812.50 **Lower end, unspecified part**

    812.51 **Supracondylar fracture of humerus**

    812.52 **Lateral condyle**

    812.53 **Medial condyle**

    812.54 **Condyle(s), unspecified**

    812.59 **Other**

813 Fracture of radius and ulna

⑤ **813.0** Upper end, closed
        Proximal end

    813.00 **Upper end of forearm, unspecified**

    813.01 **Olecranon process of ulna**

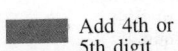 Add 4th or 5th digit	Nonspecific code	Unspecified code	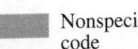 Medicare secondary payer (MSP) alert

813.02 Coronoid process of ulna

813.03 Monteggia's fracture

813.04 Other and unspecified fractures of proximal end of ulna (alone)
Multiple fractures of ulna, upper end

813.05 Head of radius

813.06 Neck of radius

813.07 Other and unspecified fractures of proximal end of radius (alone)
Multiple fractures of radius, upper end

813.08 Radius with ulna, upper end [any part]

⑤ **813.1 Upper end, open**

813.10 Upper end of forearm, unspecified

813.11 Olecranon process of ulna

813.12 Coronoid process of ulna

813.13 Monteggia's fracture

813.14 Other and unspecified fractures of proximal end of ulna (alone)

813.15 Head of radius

813.16 Neck of radius

813.17 Other and unspecified fractures of proximal end of radius (alone)

813.18 Radius with ulna, upper end [any part]

⑤ **813.2 Shaft, closed**

813.20 Shaft, unspecified

813.21 Radius (alone)

813.22 Ulna (alone)

813.23 Radius with ulna

⑤ **813.3 Shaft, open**

813.30 Shaft, unspecified

813.31 Radius (alone)

813.32 Ulna (alone)

813.33 Radius with ulna

⑤ **813.4 Lower end, closed**
Distal end

813.40 Lower end of forearm, unspecified

813.41 Colles' fracture
Smith's fracture

813.42 Other fractures of distal end of radius (alone)
Dupuytren's fracture, radius
Radius, lower end

813.43 Distal end of ulna (alone)

Ulna:	Ulna:
head	lower epiphysis
lower end	styloid process

813.44 Radius with ulna, lower end

● **813.45 Torus fracture of radius**

⑤ **813.5 Lower end, open**

813.50 Lower end of forearm, unspecified

813.51 Colles' fracture

813.52 Other fractures of distal end of radius (alone)

813.53 Distal end of ulna (alone)

813.54 Radius with ulna, lower end

⑤ **813.8 Unspecified part, closed**

813.80 Forearm, unspecified

813.81 Radius (alone)

813.82 Ulna (alone)

813.83 Radius with ulna

● Code new to this edition ▲ Revision of existing code ④ ⑤ Fourth or fifth digit required

[5] **813.9 Unspecified part, open**

- **813.90 Forearm, unspecified**
- **813.91 Radius (alone)**
- **813.92 Ulna (alone)**
- **813.93 Radius with ulna**

[5] **814 Fracture of carpal bone(s)**

The following fifth-digit subclassification is for use with category 814:

- **0 carpal bone, unspecified**
  Wrist NOS
- **1 navicular [scaphoid] of wrist**
- **2 lunate [semilunar] bone of wrist**
- **3 triquetral [cuneiform] bone of wrist**
- **4 pisiform**
- **5 trapezium bone [larger multangular]**
- **6 trapezoid bone [smaller multangular]**
- **7 capitate bone [os magnum]**
- **8 hamate [unciform] bone**
- **9 other**

[5] **814.0 Closed**

[5] **814.1 Open**

[5] **815 Fracture of metacarpal bone(s)**

Includes: hand [except finger]
metacarpus

The following fifth-digit subclassification is for use with category 815:

- **0 metacarpal bone(s), site unspecified**
- **1 base of thumb [first] metacarpal**
  Bennett's fracture
- **2 base of other metacarpal bone(s)**
- **3 shaft of metacarpal bone(s)**
- **4 neck of metacarpal bone(s)**
- **9 multiple sites of metacarpus**

[5] **815.0 Closed**

[5] **815.1 Open**

[5] **816 Fracture of one or more phalanges of hand**

Includes: finger(s)
thumb

The following fifth-digit subclassification is for use with category 816:

- **0 phalanx or phalanges, unspecified**
- **1 middle or proximal phalanx or phalanges**
- **2 distal phalanx or phalanges**
- **3 multiple sites**

[5] **816.0 Closed**

[5] **816.1 Open**

817 Multiple fractures of hand bones

Includes: metacarpal bone(s) with phalanx or phalanges of same hand

817.0 Closed

817.1 Open

818 Ill-defined fractures of upper limb

Includes: arm NOS
multiple bones of same upper limb

[*Excludes:*] *multiple fractures of:*
metacarpal bone(s) with phalanx or phalanges (817.0-817.1)
phalanges of hand alone (816.0-816.1)
radius with ulna (813.0-813.9)

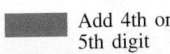

818.0 **Closed**

818.1 **Open**

819 **Multiple fractures involving both upper limbs, and upper limb with rib(s) and sternum**
Includes: arm(s) with rib(s) or sternum
both arms [any bones]

819.0 **Closed**

819.1 **Open**

FRACTURE OF LOWER LIMB (820-829)

820 **Fracture of neck of femur**

⑤ 820.0 **Transcervical fracture, closed**

820.00 **Intracapsular section, unspecified**

820.01 **Epiphysis (separation) (upper)**
Transepiphyseal

820.02 **Midcervical section**
Transcervical NOS

820.03 **Base of neck**
Cervicotrochanteric section

820.09 **Other**
Head of femur
Subcapital

⑤ 820.1 **Transcervical fracture, open**

820.10 **Intracapsular section, unspecified**

820.11 **Epiphysis (separation) (upper)**

820.12 **Midcervical section**

820.13 **Base of neck**

820.19 **Other**

⑤ 820.2 **Pertrochanteric fracture, closed**

820.20 **Trochanteric section, unspecified**
Trochanter:
NOS
greater
lesser

820.21 **Intertrochanteric section**

820.22 **Subtrochanteric section**

⑤ 820.3 **Pertrochanteric fracture, open**

820.30 **Trochanteric section, unspecified**

820.31 **Intertrochanteric section**

820.32 **Subtrochanteric section**

820.8 **Unspecified part of neck of femur, closed**
Hip NOS   Neck of femur NOS

820.9 **Unspecified part of neck of femur, open**

821 **Fracture of other and unspecified parts of femur**

⑤ 821.0 **Shaft or unspecified part, closed**

821.00 **Unspecified part of femur**
Thigh   Upper leg

Excludes: hip NOS (820.8)

821.01 **Shaft**

⑤ 821.1 **Shaft or unspecified part, open**

821.10 **Unspecified part of femur**

821.11 **Shaft**

⑤ 821.2 **Lower end, closed**
Distal end

821.20 **Lower end, unspecified part**

821.21 **Condyle, femoral**

821.22 **Epiphysis, lower (separation)**

● Code new
to this edition

▲ Revision of
existing code

④ ⑤ Fourth or fifth
digit required

821.23 Supracondylar fracture of femur

821.29 Other
Multiple fractures of lower end

[5] **821.3 Lower end, open**

821.30 Lower end, unspecified part

821.31 Condyle, femoral

821.32 Epiphysis, lower (separation)

821.33 Supracondylar fracture of femur

821.39 Other

822 Fracture of patella

822.0 Closed

822.1 Open

[5] **823 Fracture of tibia and fibula**

[Excludes:] *Dupuytren's fracture (824.4-824.5)*
ankle (824.4-824.5)
radius (813.42, 813.52)
Pott's fracture (824.4-824.5)
that involving ankle (824.0-824.9)

The following fifth-digit subclassification is for use with category 823:

0 tibia alone

1 fibula alone

2 fibula with tibia

[5] **823.0 Upper end, closed**
Head
Proximal end
Tibia:
condyles
tuberosity

[5] **823.1 Upper end, open**

[5] **823.2 Shaft, closed**

[5] **823.3 Shaft, open**

● **823.4 Torus fracture**

[5] **823.8 Unspecified part, closed**
Lower leg NOS

[5] **823.9 Unspecified part, open**

824 Fracture of ankle

824.0 Medial malleolus, closed
Tibia involving:
ankle
malleolus

824.1 Medial malleolus, open

824.2 Lateral malleolus, closed
Fibula involving:
ankle
malleolus

824.3 Lateral malleolus, open

824.4 Bimalleolar, closed
Dupuytren's fracture, fibula
Pott's fracture

824.5 Bimalleolar, open

824.6 Trimalleolar, closed
Lateral and medial malleolus with anterior or posterior lip of tibia

824.7 Trimalleolar, open

824.8 Unspecified, closed
Ankle NOS

824.9 Unspecified, open

825 Fracture of one or more tarsal and metatarsal bones

825.0 Fracture of calcaneus, closed
Heel bone
Os calcis

Add 4th or 5th digit | Nonspecific code | Unspecified code | Medicare secondary payer (MSP) alert

825.1 Fracture of calcaneus, open

⑤ **825.2 Fracture of other tarsal and metatarsal bones, closed**

> **825.20 Unspecified bone(s) of foot [except toes]**
> Instep

> **825.21 Astragalus**
> Talus

> **825.22 Navicular [scaphoid], foot**

> **825.23 Cuboid**

> **825.24 Cuneiform, foot**

> **825.25 Metatarsal bone(s)**

> **825.29 Other**
> Tarsal with metatarsal bone(s) only

> Excludes: calcaneus (825.0)

⑤ **825.3 Fracture of other tarsal and metatarsal bones, open**

> **825.30 Unspecified bone(s) of foot [except toes]**

> **825.31 Astragalus**

> **825.32 Navicular [scaphoid], foot**

> **825.33 Cuboid**

> **825.34 Cuneiform, foot**

> **825.35 Metatarsal bone(s)**

> **825.39 Other**

826 Fracture of one or more phalanges of foot
Includes: toe(s)

826.0 Closed

826.1 Open

827 Other, multiple, and ill-defined fractures of lower limb
Includes: leg NOS
multiple bones of same lower limb

> Excludes: multiple fractures of:
> ankle bones alone (824.4-824.9)
> phalanges of foot alone (826.0-826.1)
> tarsal with metatarsal bones (825.29, 825.39)
> tibia with fibula (823.0-823.9 with fifth-digit 2)

827.0 Closed

827.1 Open

828 Multiple fractures involving both lower limbs, lower with upper limb, and lower limb(s) with rib(s) and sternum
Includes: arm(s) with leg(s) [any bones]
both legs [any bones]
leg(s) with rib(s) or sternum

828.0 Closed

828.1 Open

829 Fracture of unspecified bones

829.0 Unspecified bone, closed

829.1 Unspecified bone, open

● Code new
to this edition

▲ Revision of
existing code

④ ⑤ Fourth or fifth
digit required

DISLOCATION (830-839)

Includes: displacement
subluxation

[Excludes:] *congenital dislocation (754.0-755.8)*
pathological dislocation (718.2)
recurrent dislocation (718.3)

The descriptions "closed" and "open", used in the fourth-digit subdivisions, include the following terms:

closed:	open:
complete	compound
dislocation NOS	infected
partial	with foreign body
simple	
uncomplicated	

A dislocation not indicated as closed or open should be classified as closed.

830 Dislocation of jaw
Includes: jaw (cartilage) (meniscus)
mandible
maxilla (inferior)
temporomandibular (joint)

830.0 Closed dislocation

830.1 Open dislocation

[5] **831 Dislocation of shoulder**

[Excludes:] *sternoclavicular joint (839.61, 839.71)*
sternum (839.61, 839.71)

The following fifth-digit subclassification is for use with category 831:

0 shoulder, unspecified
Humerus NOS

1 anterior dislocation of humerus

2 posterior dislocation of humerus

3 inferior dislocation of humerus

4 acromioclavicular (joint)
Clavicle

9 other
Scapula

[5] **831.0 Closed dislocation**

[5] **831.1 Open dislocation**

[5] **832 Dislocation of elbow**

The following fifth-digit subclassification is for use with category 832:

0 elbow unspecified

1 anterior dislocation of elbow

2 posterior dislocation of elbow

3 medial dislocation of elbow

4 lateral dislocation of elbow

9 other

[5] **832.0 Closed dislocation**

[5] **832.1 Open dislocation**

[5] **833 Dislocation of wrist**

The following fifth-digit subclassification is for use with category 833:

0 wrist, unspecified part
Carpal (bone)
Radius, distal end

1 radioulnar (joint), distal

2 radiocarpal (joint)

3 midcarpal (joint)

4 carpometacarpal (joint)

5 metacarpal (bone), proximal end

Add 4th or 5th digit | Nonspecific code | Unspecified code | Medicare secondary payer (MSP) alert

9 other
Ulna, distal end

⑤ **833.0 Closed dislocation**

⑤ **833.1 Open dislocation**

⑤ **834 Dislocation of finger**
Includes: finger(s)
phalanx of hand
thumb

The following fifth-digit subclassification is for use with category 834:

0 finger, unspecified part

1 metacarpophalangeal (joint)
Metacarpal (bone), distal end

2 interphalangeal (joint), hand

⑤ **834.0 Closed dislocation**

⑤ **834.1 Open dislocation**

⑤ **835 Dislocation of hip**

The following fifth-digit subclassification is for use with category 835:

0 dislocation of hip, unspecified

1 posterior dislocation

2 obturator dislocation

3 other anterior dislocation

⑤ **835.0 Closed dislocation**

⑤ **835.1 Open dislocation**

836 Dislocation of knee

[*Excludes:*] *dislocation of knee:*
old or pathological (718.2)
recurrent (718.3)
internal derangement of knee joint (717.0-717.5, 717.8-717.9)
old tear of cartilage or meniscus of knee (717.0-717.5, 717.8-717.9)

836.0 Tear of medial cartilage or meniscus of knee, current
Bucket handle tear:
NOS, current injury
medial meniscus, current injury

836.1 Tear of lateral cartilage or meniscus of knee, current

836.2 Other tear of cartilage or meniscus of knee, current
Tear of:
cartilage (semilunar), current injury, not specified as medial or lateral
meniscus, current injury, not specified as medial or lateral

836.3 Dislocation of patella, closed

836.4 Dislocation of patella, open

⑤ **836.5 Other dislocation of knee, closed**

836.50 Dislocation of knee, unspecified

836.51 Anterior dislocation of tibia, proximal end
Posterior dislocation of femur, distal end

836.52 Posterior dislocation of tibia, proximal end
Anterior dislocation of femur, distal end

836.53 Medial dislocation of tibia, proximal end

836.54 Lateral dislocation of tibia, proximal end

836.59 Other

⑤ **836.6 Other dislocation of knee, open**

836.60 Dislocation of knee, unspecified

836.61 Anterior dislocation of tibia, proximal end

836.62 Posterior dislocation of tibia, proximal end

836.63 Medial dislocation of tibia, proximal end

836.64 Lateral dislocation of tibia, proximal end

836.69 Other

● Code new to this edition ▲ Revision of existing code ④ ⑤ Fourth or fifth digit required

837 Dislocation of ankle

Includes:

astragalus	navicular, foot
fibula, distal end	scaphoid, foot
	tibia, distal end

837.0 Closed dislocation

837.1 Open dislocation

[5] **838 Dislocation of foot**

The following fifth-digit subclassification is for use with category 838:

0 foot, unspecified

1 tarsal (bone), joint unspecified

2 midtarsal (joint)

3 tarsometatarsal (joint)

4 metatarsal (bone), joint unspecified

5 metatarsophalangeal (joint)

6 interphalangeal (joint), foot

9 other

Phalanx of foot — Toe(s)

[5] **838.0 Closed dislocation**

[5] **838.1 Open dislocation**

839 Other, multiple, and ill-defined dislocations

[5] **839.0 Cervical vertebra, closed**

Cervical spine — Neck

839.00 Cervical vertebra, unspecified

839.01 First cervical vertebra

839.02 Second cervical vertebra

839.03 Third cervical vertebra

839.04 Fourth cervical vertebra

839.05 Fifth cervical vertebra

839.06 Sixth cervical vertebra

839.07 Seventh cervical vertebra

839.08 Multiple cervical vertebrae

[5] **839.1 Cervical vertebra, open**

839.10 Cervical vertebra, unspecified

839.11 First cervical vertebra

839.12 Second cervical vertebra

839.13 Third cervical vertebra

839.14 Fourth cervical vertebra

839.15 Fifth cervical vertebra

839.16 Sixth cervical vertebra

839.17 Seventh cervical vertebra

839.18 Multiple cervical vertebrae

[5] **839.2 Thoracic and lumbar vertebra, closed**

839.20 Lumbar vertebra

839.21 Thoracic vertebra

Dorsal [thoracic] vertebra

[5] **839.3 Thoracic and lumbar vertebra, open**

839.30 Lumbar vertebra

839.31 Thoracic vertebra

[5] **839.4 Other vertebra, closed**

839.40 Vertebra, unspecified site

Spine NOS

839.41 Coccyx

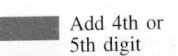

839.42 **Sacrum**
Sacroiliac (joint)

`839.49` **Other**

⑤ **839.5 Other vertebra, open**

`839.50` **Vertebra, unspecified site**

839.51 **Coccyx**

839.52 **Sacrum**

`839.59` **Other**

⑤ **839.6 Other location, closed**

839.61 **Sternum**
Sternoclavicular joint

`839.69` **Other**
Pelvis

⑤ **839.7 Other location, open**

`839.71` **Sternum**

`839.79` **Other**

`839.8` **Multiple and ill-defined, closed**
Arm
Back
Hand
Multiple locations, except fingers or toes alone
Other ill-defined locations
Unspecified location

`839.9` **Multiple and ill-defined, open**

SPRAINS AND STRAINS OF JOINTS AND ADJACENT MUSCLES (840-848)

Includes:

avulsion of: joint capsule, ligament, muscle, tendon
hemarthrosis of: joint capsule, ligament, muscle, tendon
laceration of: joint capsule, ligament, muscle, tendon
rupture of: joint capsule, ligament, muscle, tendon
sprain of: joint capsule, ligament, muscle, tendon
strain of: joint capsule, ligament, muscle, tendon
tear of: joint capsule, ligament, muscle, tendon

Excludes: *laceration of tendon in open wounds (880-884 and 890-894 with .2)*

`840` **Sprains and strains of shoulder and upper arm**

840.0 **Acromioclavicular (joint) (ligament)**

840.1 **Coracoclavicular (ligament)**

840.2 **Coracohumeral (ligament)**

840.3 **Infraspinatus (muscle) (tendon)**

840.4 **Rotator cuff (capsule)**

Excludes: *complete rupture of rotator cuff, nontraumatic (727.61)*

840.5 **Subscapularis (muscle)**

840.6 **Supraspinatus (muscle) (tendon)**

840.7 **Superior glenoid labrum lesion**
SLAP lesion

`840.8` **Other specified sites of shoulder and upper arm**

`840.9` **Unspecified site of shoulder and upper arm**
Arm NOS   Shoulder NOS

`841` **Sprains and strains of elbow and forearm**

841.0 **Radial collateral ligament**

841.1 **Ulnar collateral ligament**

841.2 **Radiohumeral (joint)**

841.3 **Ulnohumeral (joint)**

`841.8` **Other specified sites of elbow and forearm**

`841.9` **Unspecified site of elbow and forearm**
Elbow NOS

● Code new
to this edition

▲ Revision of
existing code

④ ⑤ Fourth or fifth
digit required

842 Sprains and strains of wrist and hand

[5] **842.0 Wrist**

- **842.00 Unspecified site**
- **842.01 Carpal (joint)**
- **842.02 Radiocarpal (joint) (ligament)**
- **842.09 Other**
  Radioulnar joint, distal

[5] **842.1 Hand**

- **842.10 Unspecified site**
- **842.11 Carpometacarpal (joint)**
- **842.12 Metacarpophalangeal (joint)**
- **842.13 Interphalangeal (joint)**
- **842.19 Other**
  Midcarpal (joint)

843 Sprains and strains of hip and thigh

- **843.0 Iliofemoral (ligament)**
- **843.1 Ischiocapsular (ligament)**
- **843.8 Other specified sites of hip and thigh**
- **843.9 Unspecified site of hip and thigh**
  Hip NOS
  Thigh NOS

844 Sprains and strains of knee and leg

- **844.0 Lateral collateral ligament of knee**
- **844.1 Medial collateral ligament of knee**
- **844.2 Cruciate ligament of knee**
- **844.3 Tibiofibular (joint) (ligament), superior**
- **844.8 Other specified sites of knee and leg**
- **844.9 Unspecified site of knee and leg**
  Knee NOS
  Leg NOS

845 Sprains and strains of ankle and foot

[5] **845.0 Ankle**

- **845.00 Unspecified site**
- **845.01 Deltoid (ligament), ankle**
  Internal collateral (ligament), ankle
- **845.02 Calcaneofibular (ligament)**
- **845.03 Tibiofibular (ligament), distal**
- **845.09 Other**
  Achilles tendon

[5] **845.1 Foot**

- **845.10 Unspecified site**
- **845.11 Tarsometatarsal (joint) (ligament)**
- **845.12 Metatarsophalangeal (joint)**
- **845.13 Interphalangeal (joint), toe**
- **845.19 Other**

846 Sprains and strains of sacroiliac region

- **846.0 Lumbosacral (joint) (ligament)**
- **846.1 Sacroiliac ligament**
- **846.2 Sacrospinatus (ligament)**
- **846.3 Sacrotuberous (ligament)**
- **846.8 Other specified sites of sacroiliac region**
- **846.9 Unspecified site of sacroiliac region**

847 Sprains and strains of other and unspecified parts of back

[*Excludes:*] *lumbosacral (846.0)*

Add 4th or 5th digit | Nonspecific code | Unspecified code | Medicare secondary payer (MSP) alert

847.0 Neck
Anterior longitudinal (ligament), cervical
Atlanto-axial (joints)
Atlanto-occipital (joints)
Whiplash injury

[Excludes:] *neck injury NOS (959.0)*
thyroid region (848.2)

847.1 Thoracic

847.2 Lumbar

847.3 Sacrum
Sacrococcygeal (ligament)

847.4 Coccyx

847.9 Unspecified site of back
Back NOS

848 Other and ill-defined sprains and strains

848.0 Septal cartilage of nose

848.1 Jaw
Temporomandibular (joint) (ligament)

848.2 Thyroid region
Cricoarytenoid (joint) (ligament)
Cricothyroid (joint) (ligament)
Thyroid cartilage

848.3 Ribs
Chondrocostal (joint) without mention of injury to sternum
Costal cartilage without mention of injury to sternum

[5] **848.4 Sternum**

848.40 Unspecified site

848.41 Sternoclavicular (joint) (ligament)

848.42 Chondrosternal (joint)

848.49 Other
Xiphoid cartilage

848.5 Pelvis
Symphysis pubis

[Excludes:] *that in childbirth (665.6)*

848.8 Other specified sites of sprains and strains

848.9 Unspecified site of sprain and strain

INTRACRANIAL INJURY, EXCLUDING THOSE WITH SKULL FRACTURE (850-854)

[Excludes:] *intracranial injury with skull fracture (800-801 and 803-804, except .0 and .5)*
open wound of head without intracranial injury (870.0-873.9)
skull fracture alone (800-801 and 803-804 with .0, .5)

The description "with open intracranial wound," used in the fourth-digit subdivisions, includes those specified as open or with mention of infection or foreign body.

The following fifth-digit subclassification is for use with categories 851-854:

0 unspecified state of consciousness

1 with no loss of consciousness

2 with brief [less than one hour] loss of consciousness

3 with moderate [1-24 hours] loss of consciousness

4 with prolonged [more than 24 hours] loss of consciousness and return to pre-existing conscious level

5 with prolonged [more than 24 hours] loss of consciousness, without return to pre-existing conscious level

Use fifth-digit 5 to designate when a patient is unconscious and dies before regaining consciousness, regardless of the duration of the loss of consciousness

6 with loss of consciousness of unspecified duration

9 with concussion, unspecified

850 Concussion
Includes: commotio cerebri
[Excludes:] *concussion with:*
cerebral laceration or contusion (851.0-851.9)
cerebral hemorrhage (852-853)
head injury NOS (959.01)

850.0 With no loss of consciousness
Concussion with mental confusion or disorientation, without loss of consciousness

850.1 With brief loss of consciousness
Loss of consciousness for less than one hour

850.2 With moderate loss of consciousness
Loss of consciousness for 1-24 hours

850.3 With prolonged loss of consciousness and return to pre-existing conscious level
Loss of consciousness for more than 24 hours with complete recovery

850.4 With prolonged loss of consciousness, without return to pre-existing conscious level

850.5 With loss of consciousness of unspecified duration

850.9 Concussion, unspecified

[5] **851 Cerebral laceration and contusion**

[5] **851.0 Cortex (cerebral) contusion without mention of open intracranial wound**

[5] **851.1 Cortex (cerebral) contusion with open intracranial wound**

[5] **851.2 Cortex (cerebral) laceration without mention of open intracranial wound**

[5] **851.3 Cortex (cerebral) laceration with open intracranial wound**

[5] **851.4 Cerebellar or brain stem contusion without mention of open intracranial wound**

[5] **851.5 Cerebellar or brain stem contusion with open intracranial wound**

[5] **851.6 Cerebellar or brain stem laceration without mention of open intracranial wound**

[5] **851.7 Cerebellar or brain stem laceration with open intracranial wound**

[5] **851.8 Other and unspecified cerebral laceration and contusion, without mention of open intracranial wound**
Brain (membrane) NOS

[5] **851.9 Other and unspecified cerebral laceration and contusion, with open intracranial wound**

[5] **852 Subarachnoid, subdural, and extradural hemorrhage, following injury**
[Excludes:] *Cerebral contusion or laceration (with hemorrhage) (851.0-851.9)*

[5] **852.0 Subarachnoid hemorrhage following injury without mention of open intracranial wound**
Middle meningeal hemorrhage following injury

[5] **852.1 Subarachnoid hemorrhage following injury with open intracranial wound**

[5] **852.2 Subdural hemorrhage following injury without mention of open intracranial wound**

[5] **852.3 Subdural hemorrhage following injury with open intracranial wound**

[5] **852.4 Extradural hemorrhage following injury without mention of open intracranial wound**
Epidural hematoma following injury

[5] **852.5 Extradural hemorrhage following injury with open intracranial wound**

[5] **853 Other and unspecified intracranial hemorrhage following injury**

[5] **853.0 Without mention of open intracranial wound**
Cerebral compression due to injury
Intracranial hematoma following injury
Traumatic cerebral hemorrhage

[5] **853.1 With open intracranial wound**

[5] **854 Intracranial injury of other and unspecified nature**
Includes: brain injury NOS
cavernous sinus
intracranial injury
[Excludes:] *any condition classifiable to 850-853*
head injury NOS (959.01)

[5] **854.0 Without mention of open intracranial wound**

[5] **854.1 With open intracranial wound**

Add 4th or 5th digit | Nonspecific code | Unspecified code | Medicare secondary payer (MSP) alert

INTERNAL INJURY OF THORAX, ABDOMEN, AND PELVIS (860-869)

Includes:

blast injuries of internal organs
blunt trauma of internal organs
bruise of internal organs
concussion injuries (except cerebral) of internal organs
crushing of internal organs
hematoma of internal organs
laceration of internal organs
puncture of internal organs
tear of internal organs
traumatic rupture of internal organs

[Excludes:] *concussion NOS (850.0-850.9)*
flail chest (807.4)
foreign body entering through orifice (930.0-939.9)
injury to blood vessels (901.0-902.9)

The description "with open wound," used in the fourth-digit subdivisions, includes those with mention of infection or foreign body.

860 Traumatic pneumothorax and hemothorax

860.0 Pneumothorax without mention of open wound into thorax

860.1 Pneumothorax with open wound into thorax

860.2 Hemothorax without mention of open wound into thorax

860.3 Hemothorax with open wound into thorax

860.4 Pneumohemothorax without mention of open wound into thorax

860.5 Pneumohemothorax with open wound into thorax

861 Injury to heart and lung

[Excludes:] *injury to blood vessels of thorax (901.0-901.9)*

[5] **861.0 Heart, without mention of open wound into thorax**

861.00 Unspecified injury

861.01 Contusion

Cardiac contusion
Myocardial contusion

861.02 Laceration without penetration of heart chambers

861.03 Laceration with penetration of heart chambers

[5] **861.1 Heart, with open wound into thorax**

861.10 Unspecified injury

861.11 Contusion

861.12 Laceration without penetration of heart chambers

861.13 Laceration with penetration of heart chambers

[5] **861.2 Lung, without mention of open wound into thorax**

861.20 Unspecified injury

861.21 Contusion

861.22 Laceration

[5] **861.3 Lung, with open wound into thorax**

861.30 Unspecified injury

861.31 Contusion

861.32 Laceration

862 Injury to other and unspecified intrathoracic organs

[Excludes:] *injury to blood vessels of thorax (901.0-901.9)*

862.0 Diaphragm, without mention of open wound into cavity

862.1 Diaphragm, with open wound into cavity

[5] **862.2 Other specified intrathoracic organs, without mention of open wound into cavity**

862.21 Bronchus

862.22 Esophagus

862.29 Other

Pleura
Thymus gland

● Code new to this edition
▲ Revision of existing code
[4] [5] Fourth or fifth digit required

⑤ **862.3** Other specified intrathoracic organs, with open wound into cavity

    862.31 Bronchus

    862.32 Esophagus

    862.39 Other

862.8 Multiple and unspecified intrathoracic organs, without mention of open wound into cavity
    Crushed chest
    Multiple intrathoracic organs

862.9 Multiple and unspecified intrathoracic organs, with open wound into cavity

863 Injury to gastrointestinal tract

    Excludes: *anal sphincter laceration during delivery (664.2)*
            bile duct (868.0-868.1 with fifth-digit 2)
            gallbladder (868.0-868.1 with fifth-digit 2)

863.0 Stomach, without mention of open wound into cavity

863.1 Stomach, with open wound into cavity

⑤ **863.2** Small intestine, without mention of open wound into cavity

    863.20 Small intestine, unspecified site

    863.21 Duodenum

    863.29 Other

⑤ **863.3** Small intestine, with open wound into cavity

    863.30 Small intestine, unspecified site

    863.31 Duodenum

    863.39 Other

⑤ **863.4** Colon or rectum, without mention of open wound into cavity

    863.40 Colon, unspecified site

    863.41 Ascending [right] colon

    863.42 Transverse colon

    863.43 Descending [left] colon

    863.44 Sigmoid colon

    863.45 Rectum

    863.46 Multiple sites in colon and rectum

    863.49 Other

⑤ **863.5** Colon or rectum, with open wound into cavity

    863.50 Colon, unspecified site

    863.51 Ascending [right] colon

    863.52 Transverse colon

    863.53 Descending [left] colon

    863.54 Sigmoid colon

    863.55 Rectum

    863.56 Multiple sites in colon and rectum

    863.59 Other

⑤ **863.8** Other and unspecified gastrointestinal sites, without mention of open wound into cavity

    863.80 Gastrointestinal tract, unspecified site

    863.81 Pancreas, head

    863.82 Pancreas, body

    863.83 Pancreas, tail

    863.84 Pancreas, multiple and unspecified sites

    863.85 Appendix

    863.89 Other
        Intestine NOS

⑤ **863.9** Other and unspecified gastrointestinal sites, with open wound into cavity

    863.90 Gastrointestinal tract, unspecified site

| | Add 4th or 5th digit | | Nonspecific code | | Unspecified code | | Medicare secondary payer (MSP) alert |

863.91	**Pancreas, head**
863.92	**Pancreas, body**
863.93	**Pancreas, tail**
863.94	**Pancreas, multiple and unspecified sites**
863.95	**Appendix**
863.99	**Other**

⑤ **864** **Injury to liver**

The following fifth-digit subclassification is for use with category 864:

  0   **unspecified injury**

  1   **hematoma and contusion**

  2   **laceration, minor**
      Laceration involving capsule only, or without significant involvement of hepatic parenchyma [i.e., less than 1 cm deep]

  3   **laceration, moderate**
      Laceration involving parenchyma but without major disruption of parenchyma [i.e., less than 10 cm long and less than 3 cm deep]

  4   **laceration, major**
      Laceration with significant disruption of hepatic parenchyma [i.e., 10 cm long and 3 cm deep]
      Multiple moderate lacerations, with or without hematoma
      Stellate lacerations of liver

  5   **laceration, unspecified**

  9   **other**

⑤ **864.0** **Without mention of open wound into cavity**

⑤ **864.1** **With open wound into cavity**

⑤ **865** **Injury to spleen**

The following fifth-digit subclassification is for use with category 865:

  0   **unspecified injury**

  1   **hematoma without rupture of capsule**

  2   **capsular tears, without major disruption of parenchyma**

  3   **laceration extending into parenchyma**

  4   **massive parenchymal disruption**

  9   **other**

⑤ **865.0** **Without mention of open wound into cavity**

⑤ **865.1** **With open wound into cavity**

⑤ **866** **Injury to kidney**

The following fifth-digit subclassification is for use with category 866:

  0   **unspecified injury**

  1   **hematoma without rupture of capsule**

  2   **laceration**

  3   **complete disruption of kidney parenchyma**

⑤ **866.0** **Without mention of open wound into cavity**

⑤ **866.1** **With open wound into cavity**

867 **Injury to pelvic organs**

    Excludes: *injury during delivery (664.0-665.9)*

867.0 **Bladder and urethra, without mention of open wound into cavity**

867.1 **Bladder and urethra, with open wound into cavity**

867.2 **Ureter, without mention of open wound into cavity**

867.3 **Ureter, with open wound into cavity**

867.4 **Uterus, without mention of open wound into cavity**

867.5 **Uterus, with open wound into cavity**

867.6 **Other specified pelvic organs, without mention of open wound into cavity**

Fallopian tube	Seminal vesicle
Ovary	Vas deferens
Prostate	

   ● Code new to this edition   ▲ Revision of existing code   ④ ⑤ Fourth or fifth digit required

867.7 Other specified pelvic organs, with open wound into cavity

867.8 Unspecified pelvic organs, without mention of open wound into cavity

867.9 Unspecified pelvic organ, with open wound into cavity

5 **868 Injury to other intra-abdominal organs**

The following fifth-digit subclassification is for use with category 868:

0 unspecified intra-abdominal organ
1 adrenal gland
2 bile duct and gallbladder
3 peritoneum
4 retroperitoneum
9 other and multiple intra-abdominal organs

5 **868.0 Without mention of open wound into cavity**

5 **868.1 With open wound into cavity**

869 Internal injury to unspecified or ill-defined organs

Includes: internal injury NOS
multiple internal injury NOS

869.0 Without mention of open wound into cavity

869.1 With open wound into cavity

OPEN WOUND (870-897)

Includes:

animal bite
avulsion
cut
laceration
puncture wound
traumatic amputation

[Excludes:] *burn (940.0-949.5)*
crushing (925-929.9)
puncture of internal organs (860.0-869.1)
superficial injury (910.0-919.9)
that incidental to:
dislocation (830.0-839.9)
fracture (800.0-829.1)
internal injury (860.0-869.1)
intracranial injury (851.0-854.1)

Note: The description "complicated" used in the fourth-digit subdivisions includes those with mention of delayed healing, delayed treatment, foreign body, or infection.

Use additional code to identify infection.

OPEN WOUND OF HEAD, NECK, AND TRUNK (870-879)

870 Open wound of ocular adnexa

870.0 Laceration of skin of eyelid and periocular area

870.1 Laceration of eyelid, full-thickness, not involving lacrimal passages

870.2 Laceration of eyelid involving lacrimal passages

870.3 Penetrating wound of orbit, without mention of foreign body

870.4 Penetrating wound of orbit with foreign body

[Excludes:] *retained (old) foreign body in orbit (376.6)*

870.8 Other specified open wounds of ocular adnexa

870.9 Unspecified open wound of ocular adnexa

871 Open wound of eyeball

[Excludes:] *2nd cranial nerve [optic] injury (950.0-950.9)*
3rd cranial nerve [oculomotor] injury (951.0)

871.0 Ocular laceration without prolapse of intraocular tissue

871.1 Ocular laceration with prolapse or exposure of intraocular tissue

871.2 Rupture of eye with partial loss of intraocular tissue

871.3 Avulsion of eye

Traumatic enucleation

871.4 Unspecified laceration of eye

Add 4th or 5th digit | Nonspecific code | Unspecified code | Medicare secondary payer (MSP) alert

871.5 Penetration of eyeball with magnetic foreign body

> *Excludes:* retained (old) magnetic foreign body in globe (360.50-360.59)

871.6 Penetration of eyeball with (nonmagnetic) foreign body

> *Excludes:* retained (old) (nonmagnetic) foreign body in globe (360.60-360.69)

871.7 Unspecified ocular penetration

871.9 Unspecified open wound of eyeball

872 Open wound of ear

⑤ **872.0 External ear, without mention of complication**

872.00 External ear, unspecified site

872.01 Auricle, ear
Pinna

872.02 Auditory canal

⑤ **872.1 External ear, complicated**

872.10 External ear, unspecified site

872.11 Auricle, ear

872.12 Auditory canal

⑤ **872.6 Other specified parts of ear, without mention of complication**

872.61 Ear drum
Drumhead   Tympanic membrane

872.62 Ossicles

872.63 Eustachian tube

872.64 Cochlea

872.69 Other and multiple sites

⑤ **872.7 Other specified parts of ear, complicated**

872.71 Ear drum

872.72 Ossicles

872.73 Eustachian tube

872.74 Cochlea

872.79 Other and multiple sites

872.8 Ear, part unspecified, without mention of complication
Ear NOS

872.9 Ear, part unspecified, complicated

873 Other open wound of head

873.0 Scalp, without mention of complication

873.1 Scalp, complicated

⑤ **873.2 Nose, without mention of complication**

873.20 Nose, unspecified site

873.21 Nasal septum

873.22 Nasal cavity

873.23 Nasal sinus

873.29 Multiple sites

⑤ **873.3 Nose, complicated**

873.30 Nose, unspecified site

873.31 Nasal septum

873.32 Nasal cavity

873.33 Nasal sinus

873.39 Multiple sites

⑤ **873.4 Face, without mention of complication**

873.40 Face, unspecified site

873.41 Cheek

873.42 Forehead
Eyebrow

873.43 Lip

● Code new to this edition   ▲ Revision of existing code   ④ ⑤ Fourth or fifth digit required

873.44 Jaw

873.49 Other and multiple sites

[5] **873.5 Face, complicated**

873.50 Face, unspecified site

873.51 Cheek

873.52 Forehead

873.53 Lip

873.54 Jaw

873.59 Other and multiple sites

[5] **873.6 Internal structures of mouth, without mention of complication**

873.60 Mouth, unspecified site

873.61 Buccal mucosa

873.62 Gum (alveolar process)

873.63 Tooth (broken)

873.64 Tongue and floor of mouth

873.65 Palate

873.69 Other and multiple sites

[5] **873.7 Internal structures of mouth, complicated**

873.70 Mouth, unspecified site

873.71 Buccal mucosa

873.72 Gum (alveolar process)

873.73 Tooth (broken)

873.74 Tongue and floor of mouth

873.75 Palate

873.79 Other and multiple sites

873.8 Other and unspecified open wound of head without mention of complication
Head NOS

873.9 Other and unspecified open wound of head, complicated

874 Open wound of neck

[5] **874.0 Larynx and trachea, without mention of complication**

874.00 Larynx with trachea

874.01 Larynx

874.02 Trachea

[5] **874.1 Larynx and trachea, complicated**

874.10 Larynx with trachea

874.11 Larynx

874.12 Trachea

874.2 Thyroid gland, without mention of complication

874.3 Thyroid gland, complicated

874.4 Pharynx, without mention of complication
Cervical esophagus

874.5 Pharynx, complicated

874.8 Other and unspecified parts, without mention of complication
Nape of neck
Supraclavicular region
Throat NOS

874.9 Other and unspecified parts, complicated

875 Open wound of chest (wall)

[Excludes:] *open wound into thoracic cavity (860.0-862.9)*
traumatic pneumothorax and hemothorax (860.1, 860.3, 860.5)

875.0 Without mention of complication

875.1 Complicated

Add 4th or 5th digit | Nonspecific code | Unspecified code | Medicare secondary payer (MSP) alert

876 Open wound of back
Includes: loin / lumbar region
[Excludes:] *open wound into thoracic cavity (860.0-862.9)*
traumatic pneumothorax and hemothorax (860.1, 860.3, 860.5)

876.0 Without mention of complication

876.1 Complicated

877 Open wound of buttock
Includes: sacroiliac region

877.0 Without mention of complication

877.1 Complicated

878 Open wound of genital organs (external), including traumatic amputation
[Excludes:] *injury during delivery (664.0-665.9)*
internal genital organs (867.0-867.9)

878.0 Penis, without mention of complication

878.1 Penis, complicated

878.2 Scrotum and testes, without mention of complication

878.3 Scrotum and testes, complicated

878.4 Vulva, without mention of complication
Labium (majus) (minus)

878.5 Vulva, complicated

878.6 Vagina, without mention of complication

878.7 Vagina, complicated

878.8 Other and unspecified parts, without mention of complication

878.9 Other and unspecified parts, complicated

879 Open wound of other and unspecified sites, except limbs

879.0 Breast, without mention of complication

879.1 Breast, complicated

879.2 Abdominal wall, anterior, without mention of complication
Abdominal wall NOS
Epigastric region
Hypogastric region
Pubic region
Umbilical region

879.3 Abdominal wall, anterior, complicated

879.4 Abdominal wall, lateral, without mention of complication
Flank
Groin
Hypochondrium
Iliac (region)
Inguinal region

879.5 Abdominal wall, lateral, complicated

879.6 Other and unspecified parts of trunk, without mention of complication
Pelvic region
Perineum
Trunk NOS

879.7 Other and unspecified parts of trunk, complicated

879.8 Open wound(s) (multiple) of unspecified site(s) without mention of complication
Multiple open wounds NOS
Open wound NOS

879.9 Open wound(s) (multiple) of unspecified site(s), complicated

OPEN WOUND OF UPPER LIMB (880-887)

⑤ **880 Open wound of shoulder and upper arm**
The following fifth-digit subclassification is for use with category 880:
0 shoulder region
1 scapular region
2 axillary region
3 upper arm
9 multiple sites

⑤ **880.0 Without mention of complication**

⑤ **880.1 Complicated**

● Code new to this edition ▲ Revision of existing code ④ ⑤ Fourth or fifth digit required

[5] **880.2 With tendon involvement**

[5] **881 Open wound of elbow, forearm, and wrist**

The following fifth-digit subclassification is for use with category 881:

0 forearm

1 elbow

2 wrist

[5] **881.0 Without mention of complication**

[5] **881.1 Complicated**

[5] **881.2 With tendon involvement**

882 Open wound of hand except finger(s) alone

882.0 Without mention of complication

882.1 Complicated

882.2 With tendon involvement

883 Open wound of finger(s)

Includes: fingernail thumb (nail)

883.0 Without mention of complication

883.1 Complicated

883.2 With tendon involvement

884 Multiple and unspecified open wound of upper limb

Includes: arm NOS
multiple sites of one upper limb
upper limb NOS

884.0 Without mention of complication

884.1 Complicated

884.2 With tendon involvement

885 Traumatic amputation of thumb (complete) (partial)

Includes: thumb(s) (with finger(s) of either hand)

885.0 Without mention of complication

885.1 Complicated

886 Traumatic amputation of other finger(s) (complete) (partial)

Includes: finger(s) of one or both hands, without mention of thumb(s)

886.0 Without mention of complication

886.1 Complicated

887 Traumatic amputation of arm and hand (complete) (partial)

887.0 Unilateral, below elbow, without mention of complication

887.1 Unilateral, below elbow, complicated

887.2 Unilateral, at or above elbow, without mention of complication

887.3 Unilateral, at or above elbow, complicated

887.4 Unilateral, level not specified, without mention of complication

887.5 Unilateral, level not specified, complicated

887.6 Bilateral [any level], without mention of complication

One hand and other arm

887.7 Bilateral [any level], complicated

OPEN WOUND OF LOWER LIMB (890-897)

890 Open wound of hip and thigh

890.0 Without mention of complication

890.1 Complicated

890.2 With tendon involvement

891 Open wound of knee, leg [except thigh], and ankle

Includes: leg NOS
multiple sites of leg, except thigh

[Excludes:] *that of thigh (890.0-890.2)*
with multiple sites of lower limb (894.0-894.2)

891.0 Without mention of complication

Add 4th or 5th digit | Nonspecific code | Unspecified code | Medicare secondary payer (MSP) alert

891.1 Complicated

891.2 With tendon involvement

892 Open wound of foot except toe(s) alone
Includes: heel

892.0 Without mention of complication

892.1 Complicated

892.2 With tendon involvement

893 Open wound of toe(s)
Includes: toenail

893.0 Without mention of complication

893.1 Complicated

893.2 With tendon involvement

894 Multiple and unspecified open wound of lower limb
Includes: lower limb NOS
multiple sites of one lower limb, with thigh

894.0 Without mention of complication

894.1 Complicated

894.2 With tendon involvement

895 Traumatic amputation of toe(s) (complete) (partial)
Includes: toe(s) of one or both feet

895.0 Without mention of complication

895.1 Complicated

896 Traumatic amputation of foot (complete) (partial)

896.0 Unilateral, without mention of complication

896.1 Unilateral, complicated

896.2 Bilateral, without mention of complication
[Excludes:] *one foot and other leg (897.6-897.7)*

896.3 Bilateral, complicated

897 Traumatic amputation of leg(s) (complete) (partial)

897.0 Unilateral, below knee, without mention of complication

897.1 Unilateral, below knee, complicated

897.2 Unilateral, at or above knee, without mention of complication

897.3 Unilateral, at or above knee, complicated

897.4 Unilateral, level not specified, without mention of complication

897.5 Unilateral, level not specified, complicated

897.6 Bilateral [any level], without mention of complication
One foot and other leg

897.7 Bilateral [any level], complicated

INJURY TO BLOOD VESSELS (900-904)

Includes:
arterial hematoma of blood vessel, secondary to other injuries e.g., fracture or open wound
avulsion of blood vessel, secondary to other injuries e.g., fracture or open wound
cut of blood vessel, secondary to other injuries e.g., fracture or open wound
laceration of blood vessel, secondary to other injuries e.g., fracture or open wound
rupture of blood vessel, secondary to other injuries e.g., fracture or open wound
traumatic aneurysm or fistula (arteriovenous) of blood vessel, secondary to other injuries e.g., fracture or open wound

[Excludes:] *accidental puncture or laceration during medical procedure (998.2)*
intracranial hemorrhage following injury (851.0-854.1)

900 Injury to blood vessels of head and neck

[5] **900.0 Carotid artery**

900.00 Carotid artery, unspecified

900.01 Common carotid artery

900.02 External carotid artery

900.03 Internal carotid artery

900.1 Internal jugular vein

⑤ **900.8** Other specified blood vessels of head and neck

    900.81 External jugular vein
        Jugular vein NOS

    900.82 Multiple blood vessels of head and neck

    900.89 Other

900.9 Unspecified blood vessel of head and neck

901 Injury to blood vessels of thorax

    Excludes: traumatic hemothorax (860.2-860.5)

901.0 Thoracic aorta

901.1 Innominate and subclavian arteries

901.2 Superior vena cava

901.3 Innominate and subclavian veins

⑤ **901.4** Pulmonary blood vessels

    901.40 Pulmonary vessel(s), unspecified

    901.41 Pulmonary artery

    901.42 Pulmonary vein

⑤ **901.8** Other specified blood vessels of thorax

    901.81 Intercostal artery or vein

    901.82 Internal mammary artery or vein

    901.83 Multiple blood vessels of thorax

    901.89 Other
        Azygos vein   Hemiazygos vein

901.9 Unspecified blood vessel of thorax

902 Injury to blood vessels of abdomen and pelvis

902.0 Abdominal aorta

⑤ **902.1** Inferior vena cava

    902.10 Inferior vena cava, unspecified

    902.11 Hepatic veins

    902.19 Other

⑤ **902.2** Celiac and mesenteric arteries

    902.20 Celiac and mesenteric arteries, unspecified

    902.21 Gastric artery

    902.22 Hepatic artery

    902.23 Splenic artery

    902.24 Other specified branches of celiac axis

    902.25 Superior mesenteric artery (trunk)

    902.26 Primary branches of superior mesenteric artery
        Ileo-colic artery

    902.27 Inferior mesenteric artery

    902.29 Other

⑤ **902.3** Portal and splenic veins

    902.31 Superior mesenteric vein and primary subdivisions
        Ileo-colic vein

    902.32 Inferior mesenteric vein

    902.33 Portal vein

    902.34 Splenic vein

    902.39 Other
        Cystic vein   Gastric vein

⑤ **902.4** Renal blood vessels

    902.40 Renal vessel(s), unspecified

    902.41 Renal artery

    902.42 Renal vein

▨ Add 4th or 5th digit	▨ Nonspecific code	▨ Unspecified code	▨ Medicare secondary payer (MSP) alert

902.49	Other
	Suprarenal arteries

⑤ 902.5 Iliac blood vessels

902.50	Iliac vessel(s), unspecified
902.51	Hypogastric artery
902.52	Hypogastric vein
902.53	Iliac artery
902.54	Iliac vein
902.55	Uterine artery
902.56	Uterine vein
902.59	Other

⑤ 902.8 Other specified blood vessels of abdomen and pelvis

902.81	Ovarian artery
902.82	Ovarian vein
902.87	Multiple blood vessels of abdomen and pelvis
902.89	Other

902.9 Unspecified blood vessel of abdomen and pelvis

903 Injury to blood vessels of upper extremity

⑤ 903.0 Axillary blood vessels

903.00	Axillary vessel(s), unspecified
903.01	Axillary artery
903.02	Axillary vein

903.1 Brachial blood vessels

903.2 Radial blood vessels

903.3 Ulnar blood vessels

903.4 Palmar artery

903.5 Digital blood vessels

903.8 Other specified blood vessels of upper extremity
Multiple blood vessels of upper extremity

903.9 Unspecified blood vessel of upper extremity

904 Injury to blood vessels of lower extremity and unspecified sites

904.0 Common femoral artery
Femoral artery above profunda origin

904.1 Superficial femoral artery

904.2 Femoral veins

904.3 Saphenous veins
Saphenous vein (greater) (lesser)

⑤ 904.4 Popliteal blood vessels

904.40	Popliteal vessel(s), unspecified
904.41	Popliteal artery
904.42	Popliteal vein

⑤ 904.5 Tibial blood vessels

904.50	Tibial vessel(s), unspecified
904.51	Anterior tibial artery
904.52	Anterior tibial vein
904.53	Posterior tibial artery
904.54	Posterior tibial vein

904.6 Deep plantar blood vessels

904.7 Other specified blood vessels of lower extremity
Multiple blood vessels of lower extremity

904.8 Unspecified blood vessel of lower extremity

904.9 Unspecified site
Injury to blood vessel NOS

● Code new
to this edition

▲ Revision of
existing code

④ ⑤ Fourth or fifth
digit required

LATE EFFECTS OF INJURIES, POISONINGS, TOXIC EFFECTS, AND OTHER EXTERNAL CAUSES (905-909)

Note: These categories are to be used to indicate conditions classifiable to 800-999 as the cause of late effects, which are themselves classified elsewhere. The "late effects" include those specified as such, or as sequelae, which may occur at any time after the acute injury.

905 **Late effects of musculoskeletal and connective tissue injuries**

905.0 **Late effect of fracture of skull and face bones**
Late effect of injury classifiable to 800-804

905.1 **Late effect of fracture of spine and trunk without mention of spinal cord lesion**
Late effect of injury classifiable to 805, 807-809

905.2 **Late effect of fracture of upper extremities**
Late effect of injury classifiable to 810-819

905.3 **Late effect of fracture of neck of femur**
Late effect of injury classifiable to 820

905.4 **Late effect of fracture of lower extremities**
Late effect of injury classifiable to 821-827

905.5 **Late effect of fracture of multiple and unspecified bones**
Late effect of injury classifiable to 828-829

905.6 **Late effect of dislocation**
Late effect of injury classifiable to 830-839

905.7 **Late effect of sprain and strain without mention of tendon injury**
Late effect of injury classifiable to 840-848, except tendon injury

905.8 **Late effect of tendon injury**
Late effect of tendon injury due to:
open wound [injury classifiable to 880-884 with .2, 890-894 with .2]
sprain and strain [injury classifiable to 840-848]

905.9 **Late effect of traumatic amputation**
Late effect of injury classifiable to 885-887, 895-897

> Excludes: late amputation stump complication (997.60-997.69)

906 **Late effects of injuries to skin and subcutaneous tissues**

906.0 **Late effect of open wound of head, neck, and trunk**
Late effect of injury classifiable to 870-879

906.1 **Late effect of open wound of extremities without mention of tendon injury**
Late effect of injury classifiable to 880-884, 890-894 except .2

906.2 **Late effect of superficial injury**
Late effect of injury classifiable to 910-919

906.3 **Late effect of contusion**
Late effect of injury classifiable to 920-924

906.4 **Late effect of crushing**
Late effect of injury classifiable to 925-929

906.5 **Late effect of burn of eye, face, head, and neck**
Late effect of injury classifiable to 940-941

906.6 **Late effect of burn of wrist and hand**
Late effect of injury classifiable to 944

906.7 **Late effect of burn of other extremities**
Late effect of injury classifiable to 943 or 945

906.8 **Late effect of burns of other specified sites**
Late effect of injury classifiable to 942, 946-947

906.9 **Late effect of burn of unspecified site**
Late effect of injury classifiable to 948-949

907 **Late effects of injuries to the nervous system**

907.0 **Late effect of intracranial injury without mention of skull fracture**
Late effect of injury classifiable to 850-854

907.1 **Late effect of injury to cranial nerve**
Late effect of injury classifiable to 950-951

907.2 **Late effect of spinal cord injury**
Late effect of injury classifiable to 806, 952

907.3 **Late effect of injury to nerve root(s), spinal plexus(es), and other nerves of trunk**
Late effect of injury classifiable to 953-954

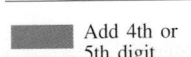

| | Add 4th or 5th digit | | Nonspecific code | | Unspecified code | | Medicare secondary payer (MSP) alert |

907.4 Late effect of injury to peripheral nerve of shoulder girdle and upper limb
Late effect of injury classifiable to 955

907.5 Late effect of injury to peripheral nerve of pelvic girdle and lower limb
Late effect of injury classifiable to 956

907.9 Late effect of injury to other and unspecified nerve
Late effect of injury classifiable to 957

908 Late effects of other and unspecified injuries

908.0 Late effect of internal injury to chest
Late effect of injury classifiable to 860-862

908.1 Late effect of internal injury to intra-abdominal organs
Late effect of injury classifiable to 863-866, 868

908.2 Late effect of internal injury to other internal organs
Late effect of injury classifiable to 867 or 869

908.3 Late effect of injury to blood vessel of head, neck, and extremities
Late effect of injury classifiable to 900, 903-904

908.4 Late effect of injury to blood vessel of thorax, abdomen, and pelvis
Late effect of injury classifiable to 901-902

908.5 Late effect of foreign body in orifice
Late effect of injury classifiable to 930-939

908.6 Late effect of certain complications of trauma
Late effect of complications classifiable to 958

908.9 Late effect of unspecified injury
Late effect of injury classifiable to 959

909 Late effects of other and unspecified external causes

909.0 Late effect of poisoning due to drug, medicinal or biological substance
Late effect of conditions classifiable to 960-979

> Excludes: *late effect of adverse effect of drug, medicinal or biological substance (909.5)*

909.1 Late effect of toxic effects of nonmedical substances
Late effect of conditions classifiable to 980-989

909.2 Late effect of radiation
Late effect of conditions classifiable to 990

909.3 Late effect of complications of surgical and medical care
Late effect of conditions classifiable to 996-999

909.4 Late effect of certain other external causes
Late effect of conditions classifiable to 991-994

909.5 Late effect of adverse effect of drug, medicinal or biological substance

> Excludes: *late effect of poisoning due to drug, medicinal or biological substance (909.0)*

909.9 Late effect of other and unspecified external causes

SUPERFICIAL INJURY (910-919)

> Excludes: *burn (blisters) (940.0-949.5)*
> *contusion (920-924.9)*
> *foreign body:*
> *granuloma (728.82)*
> *inadvertently left in operative wound (998.4)*
> *residual, in soft tissue (729.6)*
> *insect bite, venomous (989.5)*
> *open wound with incidental foreign body (870.0-897.7)*

910 Superficial injury of face, neck, and scalp except eye
Includes:

cheek	lip
ear	nose
gum	throat

> Excludes: *eye and adnexa (918.0-918.9)*

910.0 Abrasion or friction burn without mention of infection

910.1 Abrasion or friction burn, infected

910.2 Blister without mention of infection

910.3 Blister, infected

910.4 Insect bite, nonvenomous, without mention of infection

● Code new
to this edition
▲ Revision of
existing code
④ ⑤ Fourth or fifth
digit required

910.5 Insect bite, nonvenomous, infected

910.6 Superficial foreign body (splinter) without major open wound and without mention of infection

910.7 Superficial foreign body (splinter) without major open wound, infected

910.8 Other and unspecified superficial injury of face, neck, and scalp without mention of infection

910.9 Other and unspecified superficial injury of face, neck, and scalp, infected

911 Superficial injury of trunk

Includes:

abdominal wall	interscapular region
anus	labium (majus) (minus)
back	penis
breast	perineum
buttock	scrotum
chest wall	testis
flank	vagina
groin	vulva

Excludes: hip (916.0-916.9)
scapular region (912.0-912.9)

911.0 Abrasion or friction burn without mention of infection

911.1 Abrasion or friction burn, infected

911.2 Blister without mention of infection

911.3 Blister, infected

911.4 Insect bite, nonvenomous, without mention of infection

911.5 Insect bite, nonvenomous, infected

911.6 Superficial foreign body (splinter) without major open wound and without mention of infection

911.7 Superficial foreign body (splinter) without major open wound, infected

911.8 Other and unspecified superficial injury of trunk without mention of infection

911.9 Other and unspecified superficial injury of trunk, infected

912 Superficial injury of shoulder and upper arm

Includes: axilla   scapular region

912.0 Abrasion or friction burn without mention of infection

912.1 Abrasion or friction burn, infected

912.2 Blister without mention of infection

912.3 Blister, infected

912.4 Insect bite, nonvenomous, without mention of infection

912.5 Insect bite, nonvenomous, infected

912.6 Superficial foreign body (splinter) without major open wound and without mention of infection

912.7 Superficial foreign body (splinter) without major open wound, infected

912.8 Other and unspecified superficial injury of shoulder and upper arm without mention of infection

912.9 Other and unspecified superficial injury of shoulder and upper arm, infected

913 Superficial injury of elbow, forearm, and wrist

913.0 Abrasion or friction burn without mention of infection

913.1 Abrasion or friction burn, infected

913.2 Blister without mention of infection

913.3 Blister, infected

913.4 Insect bite, nonvenomous, without mention of infection

913.5 Insect bite, nonvenomous, infected

913.6 Superficial foreign body (splinter) without major open wound and without mention of infection

913.7 Superficial foreign body (splinter) without major open wound, infected

913.8 Other and unspecified superficial injury of elbow, forearm, and wrist without mention of infection

913.9 Other and unspecified superficial injury of elbow, forearm, and wrist, infected

914 Superficial injury of hand(s) except finger(s) alone

    914.0 Abrasion or friction burn without mention of infection

    914.1 Abrasion or friction burn, infected

    914.2 Blister without mention of infection

    914.3 Blister, infected

    914.4 Insect bite, nonvenomous, without mention of infection

    914.5 Insect bite, nonvenomous, infected

    914.6 Superficial foreign body (splinter) without major open wound and without mention of infection

    914.7 Superficial foreign body (splinter) without major open wound, infected

    914.8 Other and unspecified superficial injury of hand without mention of infection

    914.9 Other and unspecified superficial injury of hand, infected

915 Superficial injury of finger(s)

    Includes: fingernail   thumb (nail)

    915.0 Abrasion or friction burn without mention of infection

    915.1 Abrasion or friction burn, infected

    915.2 Blister without mention of infection

    915.3 Blister, infected

    915.4 Insect bite, nonvenomous, without mention of infection

    915.5 Insect bite, nonvenomous, infected

    915.6 Superficial foreign body (splinter) without major open wound and without mention of infection

    915.7 Superficial foreign body (splinter) without major open wound, infected

    915.8 Other and unspecified superficial injury of fingers without mention of infection

    915.9 Other and unspecified superficial injury of fingers, infected

916 Superficial injury of hip, thigh, leg, and ankle

    916.0 Abrasion or friction burn without mention of infection

    916.1 Abrasion or friction burn, infected

    916.2 Blister without mention of infection

    916.3 Blister, infected

    916.4 Insect bite, nonvenomous, without mention of infection

    916.5 Insect bite, nonvenomous, infected

    916.6 Superficial foreign body (splinter) without major open wound and without mention of infection

    916.7 Superficial foreign body (splinter) without major open wound, infected

    916.8 Other and unspecified superficial injury of hip, thigh, leg, and ankle without mention of infection

    916.9 Other and unspecified superficial injury of hip, thigh, leg, and ankle, infected

917 Superficial injury of foot and toe(s)

    Includes: heel   toenail

    917.0 Abrasion or friction burn without mention of infection

    917.1 Abrasion or friction burn, infected

    917.2 Blister without mention of infection

    917.3 Blister, infected

    917.4 Insect bite, nonvenomous, without mention of infection

    917.5 Insect bite, nonvenomous, infected

    917.6 Superficial foreign body (splinter) without major open wound and without mention of infection

    917.7 Superficial foreign body (splinter) without major open wound, infected

    917.8 Other and unspecified superficial injury of foot and toes without mention of infection

    917.9 Other and unspecified superficial injury of foot and toes, infected

    ● Code new   ▲ Revision of   ④ ⑤ Fourth or fifth

        to this edition   existing code   digit required

918 **Superficial injury of eye and adnexa**

> *Excludes:* burn (940.0-940.9)
>> foreign body on external eye (930.0-930.9)

918.0 Eyelids and periocular area
Abrasion   Superficial foreign body (splinter)
Insect bite

918.1 Cornea
Corneal abrasion   Superficial laceration

> *Excludes:* corneal injury due to contact lens (371.82)

918.2 Conjunctiva

918.9 Other and unspecified superficial injuries of eye
Eye (ball) NOS

919 **Superficial injury of other, multiple, and unspecified sites**

> *Excludes:* multiple sites classifiable to the same three-digit category (910.0-918.9)

919.0 Abrasion or friction burn without mention of infection

919.1 Abrasion or friction burn, infected

919.2 Blister without mention of infection

919.3 Blister, infected

919.4 Insect bite, nonvenomous, without mention of infection

919.5 Insect bite, nonvenomous, infected

919.6 Superficial foreign body (splinter) without major open wound and without mention of infection

919.7 Superficial foreign body (splinter) without major open wound, infected

919.8 Other and unspecified superficial injury without mention of infection

919.9 Other and unspecified superficial injury, infected

CONTUSION WITH INTACT SKIN SURFACE (920-924)

Includes: bruise without fracture or open wound
hematoma without fracture or open wound

> *Excludes:* concussion (850.0-850.9)
>> hemarthrosis (840.0-848.9)
>> internal organs (860.0-869.1)
>> that incidental to:
>>> crushing injury (925-929.9)
>>> dislocation (830.0-839.9)
>>> fracture (800.0-829.1)
>>> internal injury (860.0-869.1)
>>> intracranial injury (850.0-854.1)
>>> nerve injury (950.0-957.9)
>>> open wound (870.0-897.7)

920 **Contusion of face, scalp, and neck except eye(s)**
Cheek   Mandibular joint area
Ear (auricle)   Nose
Gum   Throat
Lip

921 **Contusion of eye and adnexa**

921.0 Black eye, not otherwise specified

921.1 Contusion of eyelids and periocular area

921.2 Contusion of orbital tissues

921.3 Contusion of eyeball

921.9 Unspecified contusion of eye
Injury of eye NOS

922 **Contusion of trunk**

922.0 Breast

922.1 Chest wall

922.2 Abdominal wall
Flank   Groin

Add 4th or   Nonspecific   Unspecified   Medicare secondary
5th digit   code   code   payer (MSP) alert

⑤ **922.3 Back**

> Excludes: *scapular region (923.01)*

922.31 Back

> Excludes: *interscapular region (922.33)*

922.32 Buttock

922.33 Interscapular region

922.4 Genital organs
Labium (majus) (minus)   Testis
Penis   Vagina
Perineum   Vulva
Scrotum

922.8 Multiple sites of trunk

922.9 Unspecified part
Trunk NOS

923 Contusion of upper limb

⑤ **923.0 Shoulder and upper arm**

923.00 Shoulder region

923.01 Scapular region

923.02 Axillary region

923.03 Upper arm

923.09 Multiple sites

⑤ **923.1 Elbow and forearm**

923.10 Forearm

923.11 Elbow

⑤ **923.2 Wrist and hand(s), except finger(s) alone**

923.20 Hand(s)

923.21 Wrist

923.3 Finger
Fingernail   Thumb (nail)

923.8 Multiple sites of upper limb

923.9 Unspecified part of upper limb
Arm NOS

924 Contusion of lower limb and of other and unspecified sites

⑤ **924.0 Hip and thigh**

924.00 Thigh

924.01 Hip

⑤ **924.1 Knee and lower leg**

924.10 Lower leg

924.11 Knee

⑤ **924.2 Ankle and foot, excluding toe(s)**

924.20 Foot
Heel

924.21 Ankle

924.3 Toe
Toenail

924.4 Multiple sites of lower limb

924.5 Unspecified part of lower limb
Leg NOS

924.8 Multiple sites, not elsewhere classified

924.9 Unspecified site

● Code new   ▲ Revision of   ④ ⑤ Fourth or fifth
           to this edition   existing code   digit required

CRUSHING INJURY (925-929)

[Excludes:] *concussion (850.0-850.9)*
fractures (800-829)
internal organs (860.0-869.1)
that incidental to:
internal injury (860.0-869.1)
intracranial injury (850.0-854.1)

925 Crushing injury of face, scalp, and neck
Cheek
Ear
Larynx
Pharynx
Throat

925.1 Crushing injury of face and scalp
Cheek
Ear

925.2 Crushing injury of neck
Larynx
Pharynx
Throat

926 Crushing injury of trunk
[Excludes:] *crush injury of internal organs (860.0-869.1)*

926.0 External genitalia
Labium (majus) (minus)
Penis
Scrotum
Testis
Vulva

[5] **926.1 Other specified sites**

926.11 Back

926.12 Buttock

926.19 Other
Breast

[Excludes:] *crushing of chest (860.0-862.9)*

926.8 Multiple sites of trunk

926.9 Unspecified site
Trunk NOS

927 Crushing injury of upper limb

[5] **927.0 Shoulder and upper arm**

927.00 Shoulder region

927.01 Scapular region

927.02 Axillary region

927.03 Upper arm

927.09 Multiple sites

[5] **927.1 Elbow and forearm**

927.10 Forearm

927.11 Elbow

[5] **927.2 Wrist and hand(s), except finger(s) alone**

927.20 Hand(s)

927.21 Wrist

927.3 Finger(s)

927.8 Multiple sites of upper limb

927.9 Unspecified site
Arm NOS

928 Crushing injury of lower limb

[5] **928.0 Hip and thigh**

928.00 Thigh

928.01 Hip

[5] **928.1 Knee and lower leg**

928.10 Lower leg

928.11 Knee

[5] **928.2 Ankle and foot, excluding toe(s) alone**

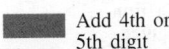

928.20 Foot
Heel

928.21 Ankle

928.3 Toe(s)

928.8 Multiple sites of lower limb

928.9 Unspecified site
Leg NOS

929 Crushing injury of multiple and unspecified sites
[Excludes:] *multiple internal injury NOS (869.0-869.1)*

929.0 Multiple sites, not elsewhere classified

929.9 Unspecified site

EFFECTS OF FOREIGN BODY ENTERING THROUGH ORIFICE (930-939)

[Excludes:] *foreign body:*
granuloma (728.82)
inadvertently left in operative wound (998.4, 998.7)
in open wound (800-839, 851-897)
residual, in soft tissues (729.6)
superficial without major open wound (910-919 with .6 or .7)

930 Foreign body on external eye
[Excludes:] *foreign body in penetrating wound of:*
eyeball (871.5-871.6)
retained (old) (360.5-360.6)
ocular adnexa (870.4)
retained (old) (376.6)

930.0 Corneal foreign body

930.1 Foreign body in conjunctival sac

930.2 Foreign body in lacrimal punctum

930.8 Other and combined sites

930.9 Unspecified site
External eye NOS

931 Foreign body in ear
Auditory canal
Auricle

932 Foreign body in nose
Nasal sinus
Nostril

933 Foreign body in pharynx and larynx

933.0 Pharynx
Nasopharynx
Throat NOS

933.1 Larynx
Asphyxia due to foreign body
Choking due to:
food (regurgitated)
phlegm

934 Foreign body in trachea, bronchus, and lung

934.0 Trachea

934.1 Main bronchus

934.8 Other specified parts
Bronchioles
Lung

934.9 Respiratory tree, unspecified
Inhalation of liquid or vomitus, lower respiratory tract NOS

935 Foreign body in mouth, esophagus, and stomach

935.0 Mouth

935.1 Esophagus

935.2 Stomach

936 Foreign body in intestine and colon

937 Foreign body in anus and rectum
Rectosigmoid (junction)

938 Foreign body in digestive system, unspecified
Alimentary tract NOS
Swallowed foreign body

● Code new to this edition
▲ Revision of existing code
④ ⑤ Fourth or fifth digit required

939 Foreign body in genitourinary tract

939.0 Bladder and urethra

939.1 Uterus, any part

[Excludes:] *intrauterine contraceptive device:*
complications from (996.32, 996.65)
presence of (V45.51)

939.2 Vulva and vagina

939.3 Penis

939.9 Unspecified site

BURNS (940-949)

Includes: burns from:
electrical heating appliance
electricity
flame
hot object
lightning
radiation
chemical burns (external) (internal)
scalds

[Excludes:] *friction burns (910-919 with .0, .1)*
sunburn (692.71, 692.76-692.77)

940 Burn confined to eye and adnexa

940.0 Chemical burn of eyelids and periocular area

940.1 Other burns of eyelids and periocular area

940.2 Alkaline chemical burn of cornea and conjunctival sac

940.3 Acid chemical burn of cornea and conjunctival sac

940.4 Other burn of cornea and conjunctival sac

940.5 Burn with resulting rupture and destruction of eyeball

940.9 Unspecified burn of eye and adnexa

[5] **941 Burn of face, head, and neck**

[Excludes:] *mouth (947.0)*

The following fifth-digit subclassification is for use with category 941:

0 face and head, unspecified site
1 ear [any part]
2 eye (with other parts of face, head, and neck)
3 lip(s)
4 chin
5 nose (septum)
6 scalp [any part]
Temple (region)
7 forehead and cheek
8 neck
9 multiple sites [except with eye] of face, head, and neck

[5] **941.0 Unspecified degree**

[5] **941.1 Erythema [first degree]**

[5] **941.2 Blisters, epidermal loss [second degree]**

[5] **941.3 Full-thickness skin loss [third degree NOS]**

[5] **941.4 Deep necrosis of underlying tissues [deep third degree] without mention of loss of a body part**

[5] **941.5 Deep necrosis of underlying tissues [deep third degree] with loss of a body part**

[5] **942 Burn of trunk**

[Excludes:] *scapular region (943.0-943.5 with fifth-digit 6)*

The following fifth-digit subclassification is for use with category 942:

0 trunk, unspecified site
1 breast

Add 4th or 5th digit | Nonspecific code | Unspecified code | Medicare secondary payer (MSP) alert

2 **chest wall, excluding breast and nipple**

3 **abdominal wall**
Flank   Groin

4 **back [any part]**
Buttock   Interscapular region

5 **genitalia**
Labium (majus) (minus)   Scrotum
Penis   Testis
Perineum   Vulva

9 **other and multiple sites of trunk**

⑤ **942.0** **Unspecified degree**

⑤ **942.1** **Erythema [first degree]**

⑤ **942.2** **Blisters, epidermal loss [second degree]**

⑤ **942.3** **Full-thickness skin loss [third degree NOS]**

⑤ **942.4** **Deep necrosis of underlying tissues [deep third degree] without mention of loss of a body part**

⑤ **942.5** **Deep necrosis of underlying tissues [deep third degree] with loss of a body part**

⑤ **943** **Burn of upper limb, except wrist and hand**
The following fifth-digit subclassification is for use with category 943:

0 **upper limb, unspecified site**

1 **forearm**

2 **elbow**

3 **upper arm**

4 **axilla**

5 **shoulder**

6 **scapular region**

9 **multiple sites of upper limb, except wrist and hand**

⑤ **943.0** **Unspecified degree**

⑤ **943.1** **Erythema [first degree]**

⑤ **943.2** **Blisters, epidermal loss [second degree]**

⑤ **943.3** **Full-thickness skin loss [third degree NOS]**

⑤ **943.4** **Deep necrosis of underlying tissues [deep third degree] without mention of loss of a body part**

⑤ **943.5** **Deep necrosis of underlying tissues [deep third degree] with loss of a body part**

⑤ **944** **Burn of wrist(s) and hand(s)**
The following fifth-digit subclassification is for use with category 944:

0 **hand, unspecified site**

1 **single digit [finger (nail)] other than thumb**

2 **thumb (nail)**

3 **two or more digits, not including thumb**

4 **two or more digits including thumb**

5 **palm**

6 **back of hand**

7 **wrist**

8 **multiple sites of wrist(s) and hand(s)**

⑤ **944.0** **Unspecified degree**

⑤ **944.1** **Erythema [first degree]**

⑤ **944.2** **Blisters, epidermal loss [second degree]**

⑤ **944.3** **Full-thickness skin loss [third degree NOS]**

⑤ **944.4** **Deep necrosis of underlying tissues [deep third degree] without mention of loss of a body part**

⑤ **944.5** **Deep necrosis of underlying tissues [deep third degree] with loss of a body part**

● Code new
to this edition

▲ Revision of
existing code

④ ⑤ Fourth or fifth
digit required

⑤ **945** **Burn of lower limb(s)**

The following fifth-digit subclassification is for use with category 945:

0 **lower limb [leg], unspecified site**

1 **toe(s) (nail)**

2 **foot**

3 **ankle**

4 **lower leg**

5 **knee**

6 **thigh [any part]**

9 **multiple sites of lower limb(s)**

⑤ **945.0** **Unspecified degree**

⑤ **945.1** **Erythema [first degree]**

⑤ **945.2** **Blisters, epidermal loss [second degree]**

⑤ **945.3** **Full-thickness skin loss [third degree NOS]**

⑤ **945.4** **Deep necrosis of underlying tissues [deep third degree] without mention of loss of a body part**

⑤ **945.5** **Deep necrosis of underlying tissues [deep third degree] with loss of a body part**

946 **Burns of multiple specified sites**

Includes: burns of sites classifiable to more than one three-digit category in 940-945

Excludes: *multiple burns NOS (949.0-949.5)*

946.0 **Unspecified degree**

946.1 **Erythema [first degree]**

946.2 **Blisters, epidermal loss [second degree]**

946.3 **Full-thickness skin loss [third degree NOS]**

946.4 **Deep necrosis of underlying tissues [deep third degree] without mention of loss of a body part**

946.5 **Deep necrosis of underlying tissues [deep third degree] with loss of a body part**

947 **Burn of internal organs**

Includes: burns from chemical agents (ingested)

947.0 **Mouth and pharynx**
Gum   Tongue

947.1 **Larynx, trachea, and lung**

947.2 **Esophagus**

947.3 **Gastrointestinal tract**
Colon   Small intestine
Rectum   Stomach

947.4 **Vagina and uterus**

947.8 **Other specified sites**

947.9 **Unspecified site**

⑤ **948** **Burns classified according to extent of body surface involved**

Excludes: *sunburn (692.71, 692.76-692.77)*

Note: This category is to be used when the site of the burn is unspecified, or with categories 940-947 when the site is specified.

The following fifth-digit subclassification is for use with category 948 to indicate the percent of *body surface* with *third degree burn*; valid digits are in [brackets] under each code:

0 **less than 10 percent or unspecified**

1 **10-19%**

2 **20-29%**

3 **30-39%**

4 **40-49%**

5 **50-59%**

6 **60-69%**

| | Add 4th or 5th digit | | Nonspecific code | | Unspecified code | | Medicare secondary payer (MSP) alert |

      7   70-79%

      8   80-89%

      9   90% or more of body surface

⑤ **948.0 Burn [any degree] involving less than 10 percent of body surface**
[0]

⑤ **948.1 10-19 percent of body surface**
[0-1]

⑤ **948.2 20-29 percent of body surface**
[0-2]

⑤ **948.3 30-39 percent of body surface**
[0-3]

⑤ **948.4 40-49 percent of body surface**
[0-4]

⑤ **948.5 50-59 percent of body surface**
[0-5]

⑤ **948.6 60-69 percent of body surface**
[0-6]

⑤ **948.7 70-79 percent of body surface**
[0-7]

⑤ **948.8 80-89 percent of body surface**
[0-8]

⑤ **948.9 90 percent or more of body surface**
[0-9]

949 Burn, unspecified
    Includes: burn NOS
                multiple burns NOS

      Excludes: *burn of unspecified site but with statement of the extent of body surface involved*
              (948.0-948.9)

    949.0 Unspecified degree

    949.1 Erythema [first degree]

    949.2 Blisters, epidermal loss [second degree]

    949.3 Full-thickness skin loss [third degree NOS]

    **949.4 Deep necrosis of underlying tissues [deep third degree] without mention of loss of a
           body part**

    949.5 Deep necrosis of underlying tissues [deep third degree] with loss of a body part

INJURY TO NERVES AND SPINAL CORD (950-957)

    Includes:
                division of nerve (with open wound)
                lesion in continuity (with open wound)
                traumatic neuroma (with open wound)
                traumatic transient paralysis (with open wound)

      Excludes: *accidental puncture or laceration during medical procedure (998.2)*

950 Injury to optic nerve and pathways

    950.0 Optic nerve injury
           Second cranial nerve

    950.1 Injury to optic chiasm

    950.2 Injury to optic pathways

    950.3 Injury to visual cortex

    950.9 Unspecified
           Traumatic blindness NOS

951 Injury to other cranial nerve(s)

    951.0 Injury to oculomotor nerve
           Third cranial nerve

    951.1 Injury to trochlear nerve
           Fourth cranial nerve

    951.2 Injury to trigeminal nerve
           Fifth cranial nerve

    ● Code new
      to this edition
        ▲ Revision of
          existing code
      ④ ⑤ Fourth or fifth
           digit required

951.3 Injury to abducens nerve
Sixth cranial nerve

951.4 Injury to facial nerve
Seventh cranial nerve

951.5 Injury to acoustic nerve
Auditory nerve
Eighth cranial nerve
Traumatic deafness NOS

951.6 Injury to accessory nerve
Eleventh cranial nerve

951.7 Injury to hypoglossal nerve
Twelfth cranial nerve

951.8 Injury to other specified cranial nerves
Glossopharyngeal [9th cranial] nerve
Olfactory [1st cranial] nerve
Pneumogastric [10th cranial] nerve
Traumatic anosmia NOS
Vagus [10th cranial] nerve

951.9 Injury to unspecified cranial nerve

952 Spinal cord injury without evidence of spinal bone injury

[5] **952.0 Cervical**

952.00 C_1-C_4 level with unspecified spinal cord injury
Spinal cord injury, cervical region NOS

952.01 C_1-C_4 level with complete lesion of spinal cord

952.02 C_1-C_4 level with anterior cord syndrome

952.03 C_1-C_4 level with central cord syndrome

952.04 C_1-C_4 level with other specified spinal cord injury
Incomplete spinal cord lesion at C_1-C_4 level:
NOS
with posterior cord syndrome

952.05 C_5-C_7 level with unspecified spinal cord injury

952.06 C_5-C_7 level with complete lesion of spinal cord

952.07 C_5-C_7 level with anterior cord syndrome

952.08 C_5-C_7 level with central cord syndrome

952.09 C_5-C_7 level with other specified spinal cord injury
Incomplete spinal cord lesion at C_5-C_7 level:
NOS
with posterior cord syndrome

[5] **952.1 Dorsal [thoracic]**

952.10 T_1-T_6 level with unspecified spinal cord injury
Spinal cord injury, thoracic region NOS

952.11 T_1-T_6 level with complete lesion of spinal cord

952.12 T_1-T_6 level with anterior cord syndrome

952.13 T_1-T_6 level with central cord syndrome

952.14 T_1-T_6 level with other specified spinal cord injury
Incomplete spinal cord lesion at T_1-T_6 level:
NOS
with posterior cord syndrome

952.15 T_7-T_{12} level with unspecified spinal cord injury

952.16 T_7-T_{12} level with complete lesion of spinal cord

952.17 T_7-T_{12} level with anterior cord syndrome

952.18 T_7-T_{12} level with central cord syndrome

952.19 T_7-T_{12} level with other specified spinal cord injury
Incomplete spinal cord lesion at T_7-T_{12} level:
NOS
with posterior cord syndrome

952.2 Lumbar

952.3 Sacral

952.4 Cauda equina

952.8 Multiple sites of spinal cord

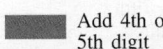

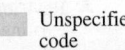

952.9 Unspecified site of spinal cord

953 Injury to nerve roots and spinal plexus

953.0 Cervical root

953.1 Dorsal root

953.2 Lumbar root

953.3 Sacral root

953.4 Brachial plexus

953.5 Lumbosacral plexus

953.8 Multiple sites

953.9 Unspecified site

954 Injury to other nerve(s) of trunk, excluding shoulder and pelvic girdles

954.0 Cervical sympathetic

954.1 Other sympathetic
Celiac ganglion or plexus   Splanchnic nerve(s)
Inferior mesenteric plexus   Stellate ganglion

954.8 Other specified nerve(s) of trunk

954.9 Unspecified nerve of trunk

955 Injury to peripheral nerve(s) of shoulder girdle and upper limb

955.0 Axillary nerve

955.1 Median nerve

955.2 Ulnar nerve

955.3 Radial nerve

955.4 Musculocutaneous nerve

955.5 Cutaneous sensory nerve, upper limb

955.6 Digital nerve

955.7 Other specified nerve(s) of shoulder girdle and upper limb

955.8 Multiple nerves of shoulder girdle and upper limb

955.9 Unspecified nerve of shoulder girdle and upper limb

956 Injury to peripheral nerve(s) of pelvic girdle and lower limb

956.0 Sciatic nerve

956.1 Femoral nerve

956.2 Posterior tibial nerve

956.3 Peroneal nerve

956.4 Cutaneous sensory nerve, lower limb

956.5 Other specified nerve(s) of pelvic girdle and lower limb

956.8 Multiple nerves of pelvic girdle and lower limb

956.9 Unspecified nerve of pelvic girdle and lower limb

957 Injury to other and unspecified nerves

957.0 Superficial nerves of head and neck

957.1 Other specified nerve(s)

957.8 Multiple nerves in several parts
Multiple nerve injury NOS

957.9 Unspecified site
Nerve injury NOS

CERTAIN TRAUMATIC COMPLICATIONS AND UNSPECIFIED INJURIES (958-959)

958 Certain early complications of trauma

Excludes: *adult respiratory distress syndrome (518.5)*
flail chest (807.4)
shock lung (518.5)
that occurring during or following medical procedures (996.0-999.9)

● Code new
to this edition   ▲ Revision of
existing code   ④ ⑤ Fourth or fifth
digit required

958.0 Air embolism
   Pneumathemia

> *Excludes:* *that complicating:*
>> *abortion (634-638 with .6, 639.6)*
>> *ectopic or molar pregnancy (639.6)*
>> *pregnancy, childbirth, or the puerperium (673.0)*

958.1 Fat embolism

> *Excludes:* *that complicating:*
>> *abortion (634-638 with .6, 639.6)*
>> *pregnancy, childbirth, or the puerperium (673.8)*

958.2 Secondary and recurrent hemorrhage

958.3 Posttraumatic wound infection, not elsewhere classified

> *Excludes:* *infected open wounds—code to complicated open wound of site*

958.4 Traumatic shock
   Shock (immediate) (delayed) following injury

> *Excludes:* *shock:*
>> *anaphylactic (995.0)*
>>> *due to serum (999.4)*
>> *anesthetic (995.4)*
>> *electric (994.8)*
>> *following abortion (639.5)*
>> *lightning (994.0)*
>> *nontraumatic NOS (785.50)*
>> *obstetric (669.1)*
>> *postoperative (998.0)*

958.5 Traumatic anuria
   Crush syndrome
   Renal failure following crushing

> *Excludes:* *that due to a medical procedure (997.5)*

958.6 Volkmann's ischemic contracture
   Posttraumatic muscle contracture

958.7 Traumatic subcutaneous emphysema

> *Excludes:* *subcutaneous emphysema resulting from a procedure (998.81)*

958.8 Other early complications of trauma

959 Injury, other and unspecified
   Includes: injury NOS

> *Excludes:* *injury NOS of:*
>> *blood vessels (900.0-904.9)*
>> *eye (921.0-921.9)*
>> *internal organs (860.0-869.1)*
>> *intracranial sites (854.0-854.1)*
>> *nerves (950.0-951.9, 953.0-957.9)*
>> *spinal cord (952.0-952.9)*

⑤ **959.0 Head, face and neck**

Cheek	Mouth
Ear	Nose
Eyebrow	Throat
Lip	

959.01 Head injury, unspecified

> *Excludes:* *concussion (850.1-850.9)*
>> *with head injury NOS (850.1-850.9)*
>> *head injury NOS with loss of consciousness (850.1-850.5)*
>> *specified intracranial injuries (850.0-854.1)*

959.09 Injury of face and neck

▅ Add 4th or 5th digit	▅ Nonspecific code	▅ Unspecified code	▅ Medicare secondary payer (MSP) alert

959.1 Trunk

Abdominal wall	External genital organs
Back	Flank
Breast	Groin
Buttock	Interscapular region
Chest wall	Perineum

Excludes: scapular region (959.2)

959.2 Shoulder and upper arm

Axilla	Scapular region

959.3 Elbow, forearm, and wrist

959.4 Hand, except finger

959.5 Finger

Fingernail	Thumb (nail)

959.6 Hip and thigh
Upper leg

959.7 Knee, leg, ankle, and foot

959.8 Other specified sites, including multiple

Excludes: multiple sites classifiable to the same four-digit category (959.0-959.7)

959.9 Unspecified site

POISONING BY DRUGS, MEDICINAL AND BIOLOGICAL SUBSTANCES (960-979)

Includes: overdose of these substances
wrong substances given or taken in error

Excludes: adverse effects ["hypersensitivity," "reaction," etc.] of correct substance properly
administered. Such cases are to be classified according to the nature of the
adverse effect, such as:
adverse effect NOS (995.2)
allergic lymphadenitis (289.3)
aspirin gastritis (535.4)
blood disorders (280.0-289.9)
dermatitis:
contact (692.0-692.9)
due to ingestion (693.0-693.9)
nephropathy (583.9)
[The drug giving rise to the adverse effect may be identified by use of
categories E930-E949]
drug dependence (304.0-304.9)
drug reaction and poisoning affecting the newborn (760.0-779.9)
nondependent abuse of drugs (305.0-305.9)
pathological drug intoxication (292.2)

Use additional code to specify the effects of the poisoning

960 Poisoning by antibiotics

Excludes: antibiotics:
ear, nose, and throat (976.6)
eye (976.5)
local (976.0)

960.0 Penicillins

Ampicillin	Cloxacillin
Carbenicillin	Penicillin G

960.1 Antifungal antibiotics

Amphotericin B	Nystatin
Griseofulvin	Trichomycin

Excludes: preparations intended for topical use (976.0-976.9)

960.2 Chloramphenicol group

Chloramphenicol	Thiamphenicol

960.3 Erythromycin and other macrolides

Oleandomycin	Spiramycin

960.4 Tetracycline group

Doxycycline	Oxytetracycline
Minocycline	

● Code new to this edition	▲ Revision of existing code	④ ⑤ Fourth or fifth digit required

960.5 Cephalosporin group
Cephalexin
Cephaloglycin
Cephaloridine
Cephalothin

960.6 Antimycobacterial antibiotics
Cycloserine
Kanamycin
Rifampin
Streptomycin

960.7 Antineoplastic antibiotics
Actinomycin such as:
    Cactinomycin
    Dactinomycin
Bleomycin
Daunorubicin
Mitomycin

960.8 Other specified antibiotics

960.9 Unspecified antibiotic

961 Poisoning by other anti-infectives

Excludes: anti-infectives:
        ear, nose, and throat (976.6)
        eye (976.5)
        local (976.0)

961.0 Sulfonamides
Sulfadiazine
Sulfafurazole
Sulfamethoxazole

961.1 Arsenical anti-infectives

961.2 Heavy metal anti-infectives
Compounds of:
    antimony
    bismuth
Compounds of:
    lead
    mercury

Excludes: mercurial diuretics (974.0)

961.3 Quinoline and hydroxyquinoline derivatives
Chiniofon
Diiodohydroxyquin

Excludes: antimalarial drugs (961.4)

961.4 Antimalarials and drugs acting on other blood protozoa
Chloroquine
Cycloguanil
Primaquine
Proguanil [chloroguanide]
Pyrimethamine
Quinine

961.5 Other antiprotozoal drugs
Emetine

961.6 Anthelmintics
Hexylresorcinol
Piperazine
Thiabendazole

961.7 Antiviral drugs
Methisazone

Excludes: amantadine (966.4)
        cytarabine (963.1)
        idoxuridine (976.5)

961.8 Other antimycobacterial drugs
Ethambutol
Ethionamide
Isoniazid
Para-aminosalicylic acid derivatives
Sulfones

961.9 Other and unspecified anti-infectives
Flucytosine
Nitrofuran derivatives

962 Poisoning by hormones and synthetic substitutes

Excludes: oxytocic hormones (975.0)

962.0 Adrenal cortical steroids
Cortisone derivatives
Desoxycorticosterone derivatives
Fluorinated corticosteroids

962.1 Androgens and anabolic congeners
Methandriol
Nandrolone
Oxymetholone
Testosterone

| | Add 4th or 5th digit | | Nonspecific code | | Unspecified code | | Medicare secondary payer (MSP) alert |

962.2 Ovarian hormones and synthetic substitutes
Contraceptives, oral
Estrogens
Estrogens and progestogens, combined
Progestogens

962.3 Insulins and antidiabetic agents
Acetohexamide
Biguanide derivatives, oral
Chlorpropamide
Glucagon
Insulin
Phenformin
Sulfonylurea derivatives, oral
Tolbutamide

962.4 Anterior pituitary hormones
Corticotropin
Gonadotropin
Somatotropin [growth hormone]

962.5 Posterior pituitary hormones
Vasopressin

Excludes: *oxytocic hormones (975.0)*

962.6 Parathyroid and parathyroid derivatives

962.7 Thyroid and thyroid derivatives
Dextrothyroxin
Levothyroxine sodium
Liothyronine
Thyroglobulin

962.8 Antithyroid agents
Iodides
Thiouracil
Thiourea

962.9 Other and unspecified hormones and synthetic substitutes

963 Poisoning by primarily systemic agents

963.0 Antiallergic and antiemetic drugs
Antihistamines
Chlorpheniramine
Diphenhydramine
Diphenylpyraline
Thonzylamine
Tripelennamine

Excludes: *phenothiazine-based tranquilizers (969.1)*

963.1 Antineoplastic and immunosuppressive drugs
Azathioprine
Busulfan
Chlorambucil
Cyclophosphamide
Cytarabine
Fluorouracil
Mercaptopurine
thio-TEPA

Excludes: *antineoplastic antibiotics (960.7)*

963.2 Acidifying agents

963.3 Alkalizing agents

963.4 Enzymes, not elsewhere classified
Penicillinase

963.5 Vitamins, not elsewhere classified
Vitamin A
Vitamin D

Excludes: *nicotinic acid (972.2)*
          vitamin K (964.3)

963.8 Other specified systemic agents
Heavy metal antagonists

963.9 Unspecified systemic agent

964 Poisoning by agents primarily affecting blood constituents

964.0 Iron and its compounds
Ferric salts
Ferrous sulfate and other ferrous salts

964.1 Liver preparations and other antianemic agents
Folic acid

964.2 Anticoagulants
Coumarin
Heparin
Phenindione
Warfarin sodium

964.3 Vitamin K [phytonadione]

● Code new to this edition   ▲ Revision of existing code   ④ ⑤ Fourth or fifth digit required

964.4 Fibrinolysis-affecting drugs
Aminocaproic acid
Streptodornase
Streptokinase
Urokinase

964.5 Anticoagulant antagonists and other coagulants
Hexadimethrine
Protamine sulfate

964.6 Gamma globulin

964.7 Natural blood and blood products
Blood plasma
Human fibrinogen
Packed red cells
Whole blood

[Excludes:] *transfusion reactions (999.4-999.8)*

964.8 Other specified agents affecting blood constituents
Macromolecular blood substitutes
Plasma expanders

964.9 Unspecified agent affecting blood constituents

965 Poisoning by analgesics, antipyretics, and antirheumatics

[Excludes:] *drug dependence (304.0-304.9)*
nondependent abuse (305.0-305.9)

[5] **965.0 Opiates and related narcotics**

965.00 Opium (alkaloids), unspecified

965.01 Heroin
Diacetylmorphine

965.02 Methadone

965.09 Other
Codeine [methylmorphine]
Meperidine [pethidine]
Morphine

965.1 Salicylates
Acetylsalicylic acid [aspirin]
Salicylic acid salts

965.4 Aromatic analgesics, not elsewhere classified
Acetanilid
Paracetamol [acetaminophen]
Phenacetin [acetophenetidin]

965.5 Pyrazole derivatives
Aminophenazone [aminopyrine]
Phenylbutazone

[5] **965.6 Antirheumatics [antiphlogistics]**

[Excludes:] *salicylates (965.1)*
steroids (962.0-962.9)

965.61 Propionic acid derivatives
Fenoprofen
Flurbiprofen
Ibuprofen
Ketoprofen
Naproxen
Oxaprozin

965.69 Other antirheumatics
Gold salts
Indomethacin

965.7 Other non-narcotic analgesics
Pyrabital

965.8 Other specified analgesics and antipyretics
Pentazocine

965.9 Unspecified analgesic and antipyretic

966 Poisoning by anticonvulsants and anti-Parkinsonism drugs

966.0 Oxazolidine derivatives
Paramethadione
Trimethadione

966.1 Hydantoin derivatives
Phenytoin

966.2 Succinimides
Ethosuximide
Phensuximide

966.3 Other and unspecified anticonvulsants
Primidone

[Excludes:] *barbiturates (967.0)*
sulfonamides (961.0)

966.4 Anti-Parkinsonism drugs
Amantadine
Ethopropazine [profenamine]
Levodopa [L-dopa]

967 Poisoning by sedatives and hypnotics

[Excludes:] *drug dependence (304.0-304.9)*
nondependent abuse (305.0-305.9)

967.0 Barbiturates
Amobarbital [amylobarbitone]
Barbital [barbitone]
Butabarbital [butabarbitone]
Pentobarbital [pentobarbitone]
Phenobarbital [phenobarbitone]
Secobarbital [quinalbarbitone]

[Excludes:] *thiobarbiturate anesthetics (968.3)*

967.1 Chloral hydrate group

967.2 Paraldehyde

967.3 Bromine compounds
Bromide
Carbromal (derivatives)

967.4 Methaqualone compounds

967.5 Glutethimide group

967.6 Mixed sedatives, not elsewhere classified

967.8 Other sedatives and hypnotics

967.9 Unspecified sedative or hypnotic
Sleeping:
drug NOS
pill NOS
tablet NOS

968 Poisoning by other central nervous system depressants and anesthetics

[Excludes:] *drug dependence (304.0-304.9)*
nondependent abuse (305.0-305.9)

968.0 Central nervous system muscle-tone depressants
Chlorphenesin (carbamate)
Mephenesin
Methocarbamol

968.1 Halothane

968.2 Other gaseous anesthetics
Ether
Halogenated hydrocarbon derivatives, except halothane
Nitrous oxide

968.3 Intravenous anesthetics

[Excludes:] *Methohexital [methohexitone]*
Thiobarbiturates, such as thiopental sodium

968.4 Other and unspecified general anesthetics

968.5 Surface [topical] and infiltration anesthetics
Cocaine
Lidocaine [lignocaine]
Procaine
Tetracaine

968.6 Peripheral nerve and plexus-blocking anesthetics

968.7 Spinal anesthetics

968.9 Other and unspecified local anesthetics

969 Poisoning by psychotropic agents

[Excludes:] *drug dependence (304.0-304.9)*
nondependent abuse (305.0-305.9)

● Code new to this edition ▲ Revision of existing code ④ ⑤ Fourth or fifth digit required

969.0 Antidepressants
　　Amitriptyline　　　　Monoamine oxidase [MAO] inhibitors
　　Imipramine

969.1 Phenothiazine-based tranquilizers
　　Chlorpromazine　　　Prochlorperazine
　　Fluphenazine　　　　Promazine

969.2 Butyrophenone-based tranquilizers
　　Haloperidol　　　　　Trifluperidol
　　Spiperone

969.3 Other antipsychotics, neuroleptics, and major tranquilizers

969.4 Benzodiazepine-based tranquilizers
　　Chlordiazepoxide　　Lorazepam
　　Diazepam　　　　　Medazepam
　　Flurazepam　　　　　Nitrazepam

969.5 Other tranquilizers
　　Hydroxyzine　　　　Meprobamate

969.6 Psychodysleptics [hallucinogens]
　　Cannabis (derivatives)　Mescaline
　　Lysergide [LSD]　　　Psilocin
　　Marihuana (derivatives)　Psilocybin

969.7 Psychostimulants
　　Amphetamine　　　　Caffeine

　　Excludes: *central appetite depressants (977.0)*

969.8 Other specified psychotropic agents

969.9 Unspecified psychotropic agent

970 Poisoning by central nervous system stimulants

970.0 Analeptics
　　Lobeline　　　　　　Nikethamide

970.1 Opiate antagonists
　　Levallorphan　　　　Naloxone
　　Nalorphine

970.8 Other specified central nervous system stimulants

970.9 Unspecified central nervous system stimulant

971 Poisoning by drugs primarily affecting the autonomic nervous system

971.0 Parasympathomimetics [cholinergics]
　　Acetylcholine　　　　Pilocarpine
　　Anticholinesterase:
　　　organophosphorus
　　　reversible

971.1 Parasympatholytics [anticholinergics and antimuscarinics] and spasmolytics
　　Atropine　　　　　　Hyoscine [scopolamine]
　　Homatropine　　　　Quaternary ammonium derivatives

　　Excludes: *papaverine (972.5)*

971.2 Sympathomimetics [adrenergics]
　　Epinephrine [adrenalin]
　　Levarterenol [noradrenalin]

971.3 Sympatholytics [antiadrenergics]
　　Phenoxybenzamine　　Tolazoline hydrochloride

971.9 Unspecified drug primarily affecting autonomic nervous system

972 Poisoning by agents primarily affecting the cardiovascular system

972.0 Cardiac rhythm regulators
　　Practolol　　　　　　Propranolol
　　Procainamide　　　　Quinidine

　　Excludes: *lidocaine (968.5)*

972.1 Cardiotonic glycosides and drugs of similar action
　　Digitalis glycosides　　Strophanthins
　　Digoxin

972.2 Antilipemic and antiarteriosclerotic drugs
　　Clofibrate
　　Nicotinic acid derivatives

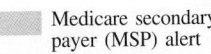

　Add 4th or　　Nonspecific　　Unspecified　　Medicare secondary
　5th digit　　　code　　　　code　　　　payer (MSP) alert

972.3 Ganglion-blocking agents
Pentamethonium bromide

972.4 Coronary vasodilators
Dipyridamole   Nitrites
Nitrates [nitroglycerin]

972.5 Other vasodilators
Cyclandelate   Papaverine
Diazoxide

Excludes: nicotinic acid (972.2)

972.6 Other antihypertensive agents
Clonidine   Rauwolfia alkaloids
Guanethidine   Reserpine

972.7 Antivaricose drugs, including sclerosing agents
Sodium morrhuate   Zinc salts

972.8 Capillary-active drugs
Adrenochrome derivatives
Metaraminol

972.9 Other and unspecified agents primarily affecting the cardiovascular system

973 Poisoning by agents primarily affecting the gastrointestinal system

973.0 Antacids and antigastric secretion drugs
Aluminum hydroxide   Magnesium trisilicate

973.1 Irritant cathartics
Bisacodyl   Phenolphthalein
Castor oil

973.2 Emollient cathartics
Dioctyl sulfosuccinates

973.3 Other cathartics, including intestinal atonia drugs
Magnesium sulfate

973.4 Digestants
Pancreatin   Pepsin
Papain

973.5 Antidiarrheal drugs
Kaolin   Pectin

Excludes: anti-infectives (960.0-961.9)

973.6 Emetics

973.8 Other specified agents primarily affecting the gastrointestinal system

973.9 Unspecified agent primarily affecting the gastrointestinal system

974 Poisoning by water, mineral, and uric acid metabolism drugs

974.0 Mercurial diuretics
Chlormerodrin   Mersalyl
Mercaptomerin

974.1 Purine derivative diuretics
Theobromine   Theophylline

Excludes: aminophylline [theophylline ethylenediamine] (975.7)
         caffeine (969.7)

974.2 Carbonic acid anhydrase inhibitors
Acetazolamide

974.3 Saluretics
Benzothiadiazines   Chlorothiazide group

974.4 Other diuretics
Ethacrynic acid   Furosemide

974.5 Electrolytic, caloric, and water-balance agents

974.6 Other mineral salts, not elsewhere classified

974.7 Uric acid metabolism drugs
Allopurinol   Probenecid
Colchicine

975 Poisoning by agents primarily acting on the smooth and skeletal muscles and respiratory system

975.0 Oxytocic agents
    Ergot alkaloids   Prostaglandins
    Oxytocin

975.1 Smooth muscle relaxants
    Adiphenine
    Metaproterenol [orciprenaline]
    Excludes: papaverine (972.5)

975.2 Skeletal muscle relaxants

975.3 Other and unspecified drugs acting on muscles

975.4 Antitussives
    Dextromethorphan   Pipazethate

975.5 Expectorants
    Acetylcysteine   Terpin hydrate
    Guaifenesin

975.6 Anti-common cold drugs

975.7 Antiasthmatics
    Aminophylline [theophylline ethylenediamine]

975.8 Other and unspecified respiratory drugs

976 Poisoning by agents primarily affecting skin and mucous membrane, ophthalmological, otorhinolaryngological, and dental drugs

976.0 Local anti-infectives and anti-inflammatory drugs

976.1 Antipruritics

976.2 Local astringents and local detergents

976.3 Emollients, demulcents, and protectants

976.4 Keratolytics, keratoplastics, other hair treatment drugs and preparations

976.5 Eye anti-infectives and other eye drugs
    Idoxuridine

976.6 Anti-infectives and other drugs and preparations for ear, nose, and throat

976.7 Dental drugs topically applied
    Excludes: anti-infectives (976.0)
             local anesthetics (968.5)

976.8 Other agents primarily affecting skin and mucous membrane
    Spermicides [vaginal contraceptives]

976.9 Unspecified agent primarily affecting skin and mucous membrane

977 Poisoning by other and unspecified drugs and medicinal substances

977.0 Dietetics
    Central appetite depressants

977.1 Lipotropic drugs

977.2 Antidotes and chelating agents, not elsewhere classified

977.3 Alcohol deterrents

977.4 Pharmaceutical excipients
    Pharmaceutical adjuncts

977.8 Other specified drugs and medicinal substances
    Contrast media used for diagnostic x-ray procedures
    Diagnostic agents and kits

977.9 Unspecified drug or medicinal substance

978 Poisoning by bacterial vaccines

978.0 BCG

978.1 Typhoid and paratyphoid

978.2 Cholera

978.3 Plague

978.4 Tetanus

978.5 Diphtheria

978.6 Pertussis vaccine, including combinations with a pertussis component

978.8 Other and unspecified bacterial vaccines

978.9 Mixed bacterial vaccines, except combinations with a pertussis component

| | Add 4th or 5th digit | | Nonspecific code | | Unspecified code | | Medicare secondary payer (MSP) alert |

979 Poisoning by other vaccines and biological substances

Excludes: gamma globulin (964.6)

979.0 Smallpox vaccine

979.1 Rabies vaccine

979.2 Typhus vaccine

979.3 Yellow fever vaccine

979.4 Measles vaccine

979.5 Poliomyelitis vaccine

979.6 Other and unspecified viral and rickettsial vaccines
Mumps vaccine

979.7 Mixed viral-rickettsial and bacterial vaccines, except combinations with a pertussis component

Excludes: combinations with a pertussis component (978.6)

979.9 Other and unspecified vaccines and biological substances

TOXIC EFFECTS OF SUBSTANCES CHIEFLY NONMEDICINAL AS TO SOURCE (980-989)

Excludes: burns from chemical agents (ingested) (947.0-947.9)
localized toxic effects indexed elsewhere (001.0-799.9)
respiratory conditions due to external agents (506.0-508.9)

Use additional code to specify the nature of the toxic effect

980 Toxic effect of alcohol

980.0 Ethyl alcohol
Denatured alcohol
Ethanol
Grain alcohol
Use additional code to identify any associated:
acute alcohol intoxication (305.0)
in alcoholism (303.0)
drunkenness (simple) (305.0)
pathological (291.4)

980.1 Methyl alcohol
Methanol   Wood alcohol

980.2 Isopropyl alcohol
Dimethyl carbinol   Rubbing alcohol
Isopropanol

980.3 Fusel oil
Alcohol:
amyl
butyl
propyl

980.8 Other specified alcohols

980.9 Unspecified alcohol

981 Toxic effect of petroleum products
Benzine   Petroleum:
Gasoline   ether
Kerosene   naphtha
Paraffin wax   spirit

982 Toxic effect of solvents other than petroleum-based

982.0 Benzene and homologues

982.1 Carbon tetrachloride

982.2 Carbon disulfide
Carbon bisulfide

982.3 Other chlorinated hydrocarbon solvents
Tetrachloroethylene   Trichloroethylene

Excludes: chlorinated hydrocarbon preparations other than solvents (989.2)

982.4 Nitroglycol

982.8 Other nonpetroleum-based solvents
Acetone

● Code new
to this edition   ▲ Revision of
existing code   ④ ⑤ Fourth or fifth
digit required

983 **Toxic effect of corrosive aromatics, acids, and caustic alkalis**

983.0 **Corrosive aromatics**
Carbolic acid or phenol   Cresol

983.1 **Acids**
Acid:
hydrochloric
nitric
sulfuric

983.2 **Caustic alkalis**
Lye   Sodium hydroxide
Potassium hydroxide

983.9 **Caustic, unspecified**

984 **Toxic effect of lead and its compounds (including fumes)**
Includes: that from all sources except medicinal substances

984.0 **Inorganic lead compounds**
Lead dioxide   Lead salts

984.1 **Organic lead compounds**
Lead acetate   Tetraethyl lead

984.8 **Other lead compounds**

984.9 **Unspecified lead compound**

985 **Toxic effect of other metals**
Includes: that from all sources except medicinal substances

985.0 **Mercury and its compounds**
Minamata disease

985.1 **Arsenic and its compounds**

985.2 **Manganese and its compounds**

985.3 **Beryllium and its compounds**

985.4 **Antimony and its compounds**

985.5 **Cadmium and its compounds**

985.6 **Chromium**

985.8 **Other specified metals**
Brass fumes   Iron compounds
Copper salts   Nickel compounds

985.9 **Unspecified metal**

986 **Toxic effect of carbon monoxide**
Carbon monoxide from any source

987 **Toxic effect of other gases, fumes, or vapors**

987.0 **Liquefied petroleum gases**
Butane   Propane

987.1 **Other hydrocarbon gas**

987.2 **Nitrogen oxides**
Nitrogen dioxide   Nitrous fumes

987.3 **Sulfur dioxide**

987.4 **Freon**
Dichloromonofluoromethane

987.5 **Lacrimogenic gas**
Bromobenzyl cyanide   Ethyliodoacetate
Chloroacetophenone

987.6 **Chlorine gas**

987.7 **Hydrocyanic acid gas**

987.8 **Other specified gases, fumes, or vapors**
Phosgene   Polyester fumes

987.9 **Unspecified gas, fume, or vapor**

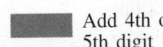 Add 4th or 5th digit   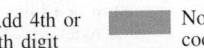 Nonspecific code   Unspecified code   Medicare secondary payer (MSP) alert

988 Toxic effect of noxious substances eaten as food

[Excludes:] *allergic reaction to food, such as:*
gastroenteritis (558.3)
rash (692.5, 693.1)
food poisoning (bacterial) (005.0-005.9)
toxic effects of food contaminants, such as:
aflatoxin and other mycotoxin (989.7)
mercury (985.0)

988.0 Fish and shellfish

988.1 Mushrooms

988.2 Berries and other plants

988.8 Other specified noxious substances eaten as food

988.9 Unspecified noxious substance eaten as food

989 Toxic effect of other substances, chiefly nonmedicinal as to source

989.0 Hydrocyanic acid and cyanides
Potassium cyanide
Sodium cyanide

[Excludes:] *gas and fumes (987.7)*

989.1 Strychnine and salts

989.2 Chlorinated hydrocarbons
Aldrin
Chlordane
DDT
Dieldrin

[Excludes:] *chlorinated hydrocarbon solvents (982.0-982.3)*

989.3 Organophosphate and carbamate
Carbaryl
Dichlorvos
Malathion
Parathion
Phorate
Phosdrin

989.4 Other pesticides, not elsewhere classified
Mixtures of insecticides

989.5 Venom
Bites of venomous snakes, lizards, and spiders
Tick paralysis

989.6 Soaps and detergents

989.7 Aflatoxin and other mycotoxin [food contaminants]

⑤ **989.8 Other substances, chiefly nonmedicinal as to source**

989.81 Asbestos

[Excludes:] *asbestosis (501)*
exposure to asbestos (V15.84)

989.82 Latex

989.83 Silicone

[Excludes:] *silicone used in medical devices, implants and grafts (996.00-996.79)*

989.84 Tobacco

989.89 Other

989.9 Unspecified substance, chiefly nonmedicinal as to source

OTHER AND UNSPECIFIED EFFECTS OF EXTERNAL CAUSES (990-995)

990 Effects of radiation, unspecified
Complication of phototherapy
Complication of radiation therapy
Radiation sickness

[Excludes:] *specified adverse effects of radiation*
Such conditions are to be classified according to the nature of the adverse effect, as:
burns (940.0-949.5)
dermatitis (692.7-692.8)
leukemia (204.0-208.9)
pneumonia (508.0)
sunburn (692.71, 692.76-692.77)
[The type of radiation giving rise to the adverse effect may be identified by use of the E codes.]

● Code new to this edition ▲ Revision of existing code ④ ⑤ Fourth or fifth digit required

991 **Effects of reduced temperature**

991.0 **Frostbite of face**

991.1 **Frostbite of hand**

991.2 **Frostbite of foot**

991.3 **Frostbite of other and unspecified sites**

991.4 **Immersion foot**
Trench foot

991.5 **Chilblains**
Erythema pernio   Perniosis

991.6 **Hypothermia**
Hypothermia (accidental)

Excludes: hypothermia following anesthesia (995.89)
hypothermia not associated with low environmental temperature (780.99)

991.8 **Other specified effects of reduced temperature**

991.9 **Unspecified effect of reduced temperature**
Effects of freezing or excessive cold NOS

992 **Effects of heat and light**

Excludes: burns (940.0-949.5)
diseases of sweat glands due to heat (705.0-705.9)
malignant hyperpyrexia following anesthesia (995.86)
sunburn (692.71, 692.76-692.77)

992.0 **Heat stroke and sunstroke**
Heat apoplexy   Siriasis
Heat pyrexia   Thermoplegia
Ictus solaris

992.1 **Heat syncope**
Heat collapse

992.2 **Heat cramps**

992.3 **Heat exhaustion, anhydrotic**
Heat prostration due to water depletion

Excludes: that associated with salt depletion (992.4)

992.4 **Heat exhaustion due to salt depletion**
Heat prostration due to salt (and water) depletion

992.5 **Heat exhaustion, unspecified**
Heat prostration NOS

992.6 **Heat fatigue, transient**

992.7 **Heat edema**

992.8 **Other specified heat effects**

992.9 **Unspecified**

993 **Effects of air pressure**

993.0 **Barotrauma, otitic**
Aero-otitis media
Effects of high altitude on ears

993.1 **Barotrauma, sinus**
Aerosinusitis
Effects of high altitude on sinuses

993.2 **Other and unspecified effects of high altitude**
Alpine sickness   Hypobaropathy
Andes disease   Mountain sickness
Anoxia due to high altitude

993.3 **Caisson disease**
Bends   Decompression sickness
Compressed-air disease   Divers' palsy or paralysis

993.4 **Effects of air pressure caused by explosion**

993.8 **Other specified effects of air pressure**

993.9 **Unspecified effect of air pressure**

994 **Effects of other external causes**

Excludes: certain adverse effects not elsewhere classified (995.0-995.8)

| | Add 4th or 5th digit | | Nonspecific code | | Unspecified code | | Medicare secondary payer (MSP) alert |

994.0 Effects of lightning
Shock from lightning
Struck by lightning NOS

[Excludes:] *burns (940.0-949.5)*

994.1 Drowning and nonfatal submersion
Bathing cramp
Immersion

994.2 Effects of hunger
Deprivation of food
Starvation

994.3 Effects of thirst
Deprivation of water

994.4 Exhaustion due to exposure

994.5 Exhaustion due to excessive exertion
Overexertion

994.6 Motion sickness
Air sickness
Seasickness
Travel sickness

994.7 Asphyxiation and strangulation
Suffocation (by):
- bedclothes
- cave-in
- constriction
- mechanical

Suffocation (by):
- plastic bag
- pressure
- strangulation

[Excludes:] *asphyxia from:*
- *carbon monoxide (986)*
- *inhalation of food or foreign body (932-934.9)*
- *other gases, fumes, and vapors (987.0-987.9)*

994.8 Electrocution and nonfatal effects of electric current
Shock from electric current

[Excludes:] *electric burns (940.0-949.5)*

994.9 Other effects of external causes
Effects of:
- abnormal gravitational [G] forces or states
- weightlessness

995 Certain adverse effects not elsewhere classified

[Excludes:] *complications of surgical and medical care (996.0-999.9)*

995.0 Other anaphylactic shock
Allergic shock NOS or due to adverse effect of correct medicinal substance properly administered
Anaphylactic reaction NOS or due to adverse effect of correct medicinal substance properly administered
Anaphylaxis NOS or due to adverse effect of correct medicinal substance properly administered

[Excludes:] *anaphylactic reaction to serum (999.4)*
anaphylactic shock due to adverse food reaction (995.60-995.69)

Use additional E code, if desired, to identify external cause, such as:
adverse effects of correct medicinal substance properly administered (E930-E949)

995.1 Angioneurotic edema
Giant urticaria

[Excludes:] *Urticaria:*
- *due to serum (999.5)*
- *other specified (698.2, 708.0-708.9, 757.33)*

995.2 Unspecified adverse effect of drug, medicinal and biological substance
Adverse effect due to correct medicinal substance properly administered
Allergic reaction due to correct medicinal substance properly administered
Hypersensitivity due to correct medicinal substance properly administered
Idiosyncrasy due to correct medicinal substance properly administered
Drug:
- hypersensitivity NOS
- reaction NOS

[Excludes:] *pathological drug intoxication (292.2)*

● Code new to this edition ▲ Revision of existing code ④ ⑤ Fourth or fifth digit required

995.3 Allergy, unspecified
Allergic reaction NOS
Hypersensitivity NOS
Idiosyncrasy NOS

[Excludes:] *allergic reaction NOS to correct medicinal substance properly administered (995.2)*
specific types of allergic reaction, such as:
allergic diarrhea (558.3)
dermatitis (691.0-693.9)
hay fever (477.0-477.9)

995.4 Shock due to anesthesia
Shock due to anesthesia in which the correct substance was properly administered

[Excludes:] *complications of anesthesia in labor or delivery (668.0-668.9)*
overdose or wrong substance given (968.0-969.9)
postoperative shock NOS (998.0)
specified adverse effects of anesthesia classified elsewhere, such as:
anoxic brain damage (348.1)
hepatitis (070.0-070.9), etc.
unspecified adverse effect of anesthesia (995.2)

[5] **995.5 Child maltreatment syndrome**
Use additional code(s), if applicable, to identify any associated injuries
Use additional E code to identify:
nature of abuse (E960-E968)
perpetrator (E967.0-E967.9)

995.50 Child abuse, unspecified

995.51 Child emotional/psychological abuse

995.52 Child neglect (nutritional)

995.53 Child sexual abuse

995.54 Child physical abuse
Battered baby or child syndrome

[Excludes:] *Shaken infant syndrome (995.55)*

995.55 Shaken infant syndrome
Use additional code(s) to identify any associated injuries

995.59 Other child abuse and neglect
Multiple forms of abuse

[5] **995.6 Anaphylactic shock due to adverse food reaction**
Anaphylactic shock due to nonpoisonous foods

995.60 Due to unspecified food

995.61 Due to peanuts

995.62 Due to crustaceans

995.63 Due to fruits and vegetables

995.64 Due to tree nuts and seeds

995.65 Due to fish

995.66 Due to food additives

995.67 Due to milk products

995.68 Due to eggs

995.69 Due to other specified food

995.7 Other adverse food reactions, not elsewhere classified
Use additional code to identify the type of reaction, such as:
hives (708.0)
wheezing (786.07)

[Excludes:] *anaphylactic shock due to adverse food reaction (995.60-995.69)*
asthma (493.0, 493.9)
dermatitis due to food (693.1)
in contact with the skin (692.5)
gastroenteritis and colitis due to food (558.3)
rhinitis due to food (477.1)

[5] **995.8 Other specified adverse effects, not elsewhere classified**

Add 4th or 5th digit — Nonspecific code — Unspecified code — Medicare secondary payer (MSP) alert

995.80 **Adult maltreatment, unspecified**
Abused person NOS
Use additional code to identify:
any associated injury
perpetrator (E967.0-E967.9)

995.81 **Adult physical abuse**
Battered:
person syndrome NEC
man
spouse
woman
Use additional code to identify:
any associated injury
nature of abuse (E960-E968)
perpetrator (E967.0-E967.9)

995.82 **Adult emotional/psychological abuse**
Use additional E code to identify perpetrator (E967.0-E967.9)

995.83 **Adult sexual abuse**
Use additional code to identify:
any associated injury
perpetrator (E967.0-E967.9)

995.84 **Adult neglect (nutritional)**
Use additional code to identify:
intent of neglect (E904.0, E968.4)
perpetrator (E967.0-967.9)

995.85 **Other adult abuse and neglect**
Multiple forms of abuse and neglect
Use additional code to identify:
any associated injury
intent of neglect (E904.0, E968.4)
nature of abuse (E960-E968)
perpetrator (E967.0-E967.9)

995.86 **Malignant hyperthermia**
Malignant hyperpyrexia due to anesthesia

995.89 **Other**
Hypothermia due to anesthesia

● **995.9** **Systemic inflammatory response syndrome (SIRS)**

● **995.90** **Systemic inflammatory response syndrome, unspecified**
SIRS NOS

● **995.91** **Systemic inflammatory response syndrome due to infectious process without organ dysfunction**

● **995.92** **Systemic inflammatory response syndrome due to infectious process with organ dysfunction**
Severe sepsis
Use addition code to specify organ dysfunction, such as:
encephalopathy (348.3)
heart failure (428.0-428.9)
kidney failure (584.5-584.9, 585, 586)

● **995.93** **Systemic inflammatory response syndrome due to non-infectious process without organ dysfunction**

● **995.94** **Systemic inflammatory response syndrome due to non-infectious process with organ dysfunction**
Use addition code to specify organ dysfunction, such as:
encephalopathy (348.3)
heart failure (428.0-428.9)
kidney failure (584.5-584.9, 585, 586)

● Code new
to this edition

▲ Revision of
existing code

④ ⑤ Fourth or fifth
digit required

COMPLICATIONS OF SURGICAL AND MEDICAL CARE, NOT ELSEWHERE CLASSIFIED (996-999)

[Excludes:] *adverse effects of medicinal agents (001.0-799.9, 995.0-995.8)*
burns from local applications and irradiation (940.0-949.5)
complications of:
conditions for which the procedure was performed
surgical procedures during abortion, labor, and delivery (630-676.9)
poisoning and toxic effects of drugs and chemicals (960.0-989.9)
postoperative conditions in which no complications are present, such as:
artificial opening status (V44.0-V44.9)
closure of external stoma (V55.0-V55.9)
fitting of prosthetic device (V52.0-V52.9)
specified complications classified elsewhere
anesthetic shock (995.4)
electrolyte imbalance (276.0-276.9)
postlaminectomy syndrome (772.80-722.83)
postmastectomy lymphedema syndrome (457.0)
postoperative psychosis (293.0-293.9)
any other condition classified elsewhere in the Alphabetic Index when described as due to a procedure

996 Complications peculiar to certain specified procedures

Includes: complications, not elsewhere classified, in the use of artificial substitutes [e.g., Dacron, metal, Silastic, Teflon] or natural sources [e.g., bone] involving:
anastomosis (internal)
graft (bypass) (patch)
implant
internal device:
catheter
electronic
fixation
prosthetic
reimplant
transplant

[Excludes:] *accidental puncture or laceration during procedure (998.2)*
complications of internal anastomosis of:
gastrointestinal tract (997.4)
urinary tract (997.5)
other specified complications classified elsewhere, such as:
hemolytic anemia (283.1)
functional cardiac disturbances (429.4)
serum hepatitis (070.2-070.3)

[5] **996.0 Mechanical complication of cardiac device, implant, and graft**

Breakdown (mechanical)
Displacement
Leakage
Obstruction, mechanical
Perforation
Protrusion

996.00 Unspecified device, implant, and graft

996.01 Due to cardiac pacemaker (electrode)

996.02 Due to heart valve prosthesis

996.03 Due to coronary bypass graft

[Excludes:] *atherosclerosis of graft (414.02, 414.03)*
embolism [occlusion NOS] [thrombus] of graft (996.72)

996.04 Due to automatic implantable cardiac defibrillator

996.09 Other

Add 4th or 5th digit | Nonspecific code | Unspecified code | Medicare secondary payer (MSP) alert

996.1 Mechanical complication of other vascular device, implant, and graft
Mechanical complications involving:
aortic (bifurcation) graft (replacement)
arteriovenous:
dialysis catheter
fistula surgically created
shunt surgicall created
balloon (counterpulsation) device, intra-aortic
carotid artery bypass graft
femoral-popliteal bypass graft
umbrella device, vena cava

[Excludes:] *atherosclerosis of biological graft (440.30-440.32)*
embolism [occlusion NOS] [thrombus] of (biological) (synthetic) graft (996.74)
peritoneal dialysis catheter (996.56)

996.2 Mechanical complication of nervous system device, implant, and graft
Mechanical complications involving:
dorsal column stimulator
electrodes implanted in brain [brain "pacemaker"]
peripheral nerve graft
ventricular (communicating) shunt

[5] **996.3 Mechanical complication of genitourinary device, implant, and graft**

996.30 Unspecified device, implant, and graft

996.31 Due to urethral [indwelling] catheter

996.32 Due to intrauterine contraceptive device

996.39 Other
Cystostomy catheter
Prosthetic reconstruction of vas deferens
Repair (graft) of ureter without mention of resection

[Excludes:] *complications due to:*
external stoma of urinary tract (997.5)
internal anastomosis of urinary tract (997.5)

996.4 Mechanical complication of internal orthopedic device, implant, and graft
Mechanical complications involving:
external (fixation) device utilizing internal screw(s), pin(s) or other methods of fixation
grafts of bone, cartilage, muscle, or tendon
internal (fixation) device such as nail, plate, rod, etc.

[Excludes:] *complications of external orthopedic device, such as:*
pressure ulcer due to cast (707.0)

[5] **996.5 Mechanical complication of other specified prosthetic device, implant, and graft**
Mechanical complications involving:
prosthetic implant in:
bile duct
breast
chin
orbit of eye
nonabsorbable surgical material NOS
other graft, implant, and internal device, not elsewhere classified

996.51 Due to corneal graft

996.52 Due to graft of other tissue, not elsewhere classified
Skin graft failure or rejection

[Excludes:] *failure of artificial skin graft (996.55)*
failure of decellularized allodermis (996.55)
sloughing of temporary skin allografts or xenografts (pigskin)—omit code

996.53 Due to ocular lens prosthesis

[Excludes:] *contact lenses—code to condition*

996.54 Due to breast prosthesis
Breast capsule (prosthesis)
Mammary implant

● Code new to this edition ▲ Revision of existing code [4] [5] Fourth or fifth digit required

996.55 Due to artificial skin graft and decellularized allodermis

Dislodgement	Displacement
Failure	Non-adherence
Poor incorporation	Shearing

996.56 Due to peritoneal dialysis catheter

[Excludes:] *mechanical complication of arteriovenous dialysis catheter (996.1)*

996.59 Due to other implant and internal device, not elsewhere classified

Nonabsorbable surgical material NOS
Prosthetic implant in:
  bile duct
  chin
  orbit of eye

[5] **996.6 Infection and inflammatory reaction due to internal prosthetic device, implant, and graft**

Infection (causing obstruction) due to (presence of) any device, implant and graft classifiable to 996.0-996.5

Inflammation due to (presence of) any device, implant and graft classifiable to 996.0-996.5

Use additional code to identify specified infections

996.60 Due to unspecified device, implant, and graft

996.61 Due to cardiac device, implant, and graft

Cardiac pacemaker or defibrillator:
  electrode(s), lead(s)
  pulse generator
  subcutaneous pocket
Coronary artery bypass graft
Heart valve prosthesis

996.62 Due to other vascular device, implant, and graft

Arterial graft
Arteriovenous fistula or shunt
Infusion pump
Vascular catheter (arterial) (dialysis) (venous)

996.63 Due to nervous system device, implant, and graft

Electrodes implanted in brain
Peripheral nerve graft
Spinal canal catheter
Ventricular (communicating) shunt (catheter)

996.64 Due to indwelling urinary catheter

Use additional code to identify specified infections, such as:
  Cystitis (595.0-595.9)
  Sepsis (038.0-038.9)

996.65 Due to other genitourinary device, implant, and graft

Intrauterine contraceptive device

996.66 Due to internal joint prosthesis

996.67 Due to other internal orthopedic device, implant, and graft

Bone growth stimulator (electrode)
Internal fixation device (pin) (rod) (screw)

996.68 Due to peritoneal dialysis catheter

Exit-site infection or inflammation

996.69 Due to other internal prosthetic device, implant, and graft

Breast prosthesis
Ocular lens prosthesis
Prosthetic orbital implant

[5] **996.7 Other complications of internal (biological) (synthetic) prosthetic device, implant, and graft**

Complication NOS due to (presence of) any device, implant, and graft classifiable to 996.0-996.5
occlusion NOS due to (presence of) any device, implant, and graft classifiable to 996.0-996.5
Embolism due to (presence of) any device, implant, and graft classifiable to 996.0-996.5
Fibrosis due to (presence of) any device, implant, and graft classifiable to 996.0-996.5
Hemorrhage due to (presence of) any device, implant, and graft classifiable to 996.0-996.5
Pain due to (presence of) any device, implant, and graft classifiable to 996.0-996.5
Stenosis due to (presence of) any device, implant, and graft classifiable to 996.0-996.5
Thrombus due to (presence of) any device, implant, and graft classifiable to 996.0-996.5

[Excludes:] *transplant rejection (996.8)*

996.70 Due to unspecified device, implant, and graft

996.71 Due to heart valve prosthesis

996.72 Due to other cardiac device, implant, and graft
Cardiac pacemaker or defibrillator:
electrode(s), lead(s)
subcutaneous pocket
Coronary artery bypass (graft)

[Excludes:] *occlusion due to atherosclerosis (414.02-414.06)*

996.73 Due to renal dialysis device, implant, and graft

996.74 Due to other vascular device, implant, and graft

[Excludes:] *occlusion of biological graft due to atherosclerosis (440.30-440.32)*

996.75 Due to nervous system device, implant, and graft

996.76 Due to genitourinary device, implant, and graft

996.77 Due to internal joint prosthesis

996.78 Due to other internal orthopedic device, implant, and graft

996.79 Due to other internal prosthetic device, implant, and graft

[5] **996.8 Complications of transplanted organ**

Use additional code, if desired, to identify nature of complication, such as:
Cytomegalovirus (CMV) infection (078.5)
Transplant failure or rejection

996.80 Transplanted organ, unspecified

996.81 Kidney

996.82 Liver

996.83 Heart

996.84 Lung

996.85 Bone Marrow
Graft-versus-host disease (acute) (chronic)

996.86 Pancreas

996.87 Intestine

996.89 Other specified transplanted organ

[5] **996.9 Complications of reattached extremity or body part**

996.90 Unspecified extremity

996.91 Forearm

996.92 Hand

996.93 Finger(s)

996.94 Upper extremity, other and unspecified

996.95 Foot and toe(s)

996.96 Lower extremity, other and unspecified

996.99 Other specified body part

997 Complications affecting specified body systems, not elsewhere classified
Use additional code to identify complication

[Excludes:] *the listed conditions when specified as:*
causing shock (998.0)
complications of:
anesthesia:
adverse effect (001.0-799.9, 995.0-995.8)
in labor or delivery (668.0-668.9)
poisoning (968.0-969.9)
implanted device or graft (996.0-996.9)
obstetrical procedures (669.0-669.4)
reattached extremity (996.90-996.96)
transplanted organ (996.80-996.89)

[5] **997.0 Nervous system complications**

997.00 Nervous system complication, unspecified

997.01 Central nervous system complication
Anoxic brain damage
Cerebral hypoxia

[Excludes:] *cerebrovascular hemorrhage or infarction (997.02)*

997.02 Iatrogenic cerebrovascular infarction or hemorrhage
Postoperative stroke

997.09 Other nervous system complications

997.1 Cardiac complications
Cardiac arrest during or resulting from a procedure
Cardiac insufficiency during or resulting from a procedure
Cardiorespiratory failure during or resulting from a procedure
Heart failure during or resulting from a procedure

[Excludes:] *the listed conditions as long-term effects of cardiac surgery or due to the presence of cardiac prosthetic device (429.4)*

997.2 Peripheral vascular complications
Phlebitis or thrombophlebitis during or resulting from a procedure

[Excludes:] *the listed conditions due to:*
implant or catheter device (996.62)
infusion, perfusion, or transfusion (999.2)
complications affecting blood vessels (997.71-997.79)

997.3 Respiratory complications
Mendelson's syndrome resulting from a procedure
Pneumonia (aspiration) resulting from a procedure

[Excludes:] *iatrogenic [postoperative] pneumothorax (512.1)*
iatrogenic pulmonary embolism (415.11)
Mendelson's syndrome in labor and delivery (668.0)
specified complications classified elsewhere, such as:
adult respiratory distress syndrome (518.5)
pulmonary edema, postoperative (518.4)
respiratory insufficiency, acute, postoperative (518.5)
shock lung (518.5)
tracheostomy complications (519.00-519.09)

997.4 Digestive system complications
>
> Complications of intestinal (internal) anastomosis and bypass, not elsewhere classified, except that involving urinary tract
> Hepatic failure specified as due to a procedure
> Hepatorenal syndrome specified as due to a procedure
> Intestinal obstruction NOS specified as due to a procedure

| Excludes: | *specified gastrointestinal complications classified elsewhere, such as:* |

> *blind loop syndrome (579.2)*
> *colostomy or enterostomy complications (569.60-569.69)*
> *gastrostomy complications (536.40-536.49)*
> *gastrojejunal ulcer (534.0-534.9)*
> *infection of external stoma (569.61)*
> *pelvic peritoneal adhesions, female (614.6)*
> *peritoneal adhesions (568.0)*
> *peritoneal adhesions with obstruction (560.81)*
> *postcholecystectomy syndrome (576.0)*
> *postgastric surgery syndromes (564.2)*

997.5 Urinary complications
>
> Complications of:
> external stoma of urinary tract
> internal anastomosis and bypass of urinary tract, including that involving intestinal tract
> Oliguria or anuria specified as due to procedure
> Renal:
> failure (acute) specified as due to procedure
> insufficiency (acute) specified as due to procedure
> Tubular necrosis (acute) specified as due to procedure

| Excludes: | *specified complications classified elsewhere, such as:* |

> *postoperative stricture of:*
> *ureter (593.3)*
> *urethra (598.2)*

⑤ **997.6 Amputation stump complication**

| Excludes: | *admission for treatment for a current traumatic amputation; code to complicated traumatic amputation* |
> *phantom limb (syndrome) (353.6)*

> **997.60** **Unspecified complication**
>
> **997.61** **Neuroma of amputation stump**
>
> **997.62** **Infection (chronic)**

Use additional code to identify the organism

> **997.69** **Other**

⑤ **997.7** **Vascular complications of other vessels**

| Excludes: | *peripheral vascular complications (997.2)* |

> **997.71** **Vascular complications of mesenteric artery**
>
> **997.72** **Vascular complications of renal artery**
>
> **997.79** **Vascular complications of other vessels**

⑤ **997.9 Complications affecting other specified body systems, not elsewhere classified**

| Excludes: | *specified complications classified elsewhere, such as:* |

> *broad ligament laceration syndrome (620.6)*
> *postartificial menopause syndrome (627.4)*
> *postoperative stricture of vagina (623.2)*

> **997.91** **Hypertension**

| Excludes: | *essential hypertension (401.0-401.9)* |

> **997.99** **Other**
> Vitreous touch syndrome

998 **Other complications of procedures, NEC**

● Code new
to this edition

▲ Revision of
existing code

④ ⑤ Fourth or fifth
digit required

998.0 Postoperative shock
Collapse NOS during or resulting from a surgical procedure
Shock (endotoxic) (hypovolemic) (septic) during or resulting from a surgical procedure

[Excludes:] *shock:*
anaphylactic due to serum (999.4)
anesthetic (995.4)
electric (994.8)
following abortion (639.5)
obstetric (669.1)
traumatic (958.4)

[5] **998.1 Hemorrhage or hematoma or seroma complicating a procedure**

[Excludes:] *hemorrhage due to implanted device or graft (996.70-996.79)*
hemorrhage, hematoma or seroma complicating cesarean section or puerperal perineal wound (674.3)

998.11 Hemorrhage complicating a procedure

998.12 Hematoma complicating a procedure

998.13 Seroma complicating a procedure

998.2 Accidental puncture or laceration during a procedure
Accidental perforation by catheter or other instrument during a procedure on:
blood vessel
nerve
organ

[Excludes:] *iatrogenic [postoperative] pneumothorax (512.1)*
puncture or laceration caused by implanted device intentionally left in operation wound (996.0-996.5)
specified complications classified elsewhere, such as:
broad ligament laceration syndrome (620.6)
trauma from instruments during delivery (664.0-665.9)

[5] **998.3 Disruption of operation wound**
Dehiscence of operation wound
Rupture of operation wound

[Excludes:] *disruption of:*
cesarean wound (674.1)
perineal wound, puerperal (674.2)

● **998.31 Disruption of internal operation wound**

● **998.32 Disruption of external operation wound**
Disruption of operation wound NOS

998.4 Foreign body accidentally left during a procedure
Adhesions due to foreign body accidentally left in operative wound or body cavity during a procedure
Obstruction due to foreign body accidentally left in operative wound or body cavity during a procedure
Perforation due to foreign body accidentally left in operative wound or body cavity during a procedure

[Excludes:] *obstruction or perforation caused by implanted device intentionally left in body (996.0-996.5)*

[5] **998.5 Postoperative infection**

[Excludes:] *infection due to:*
implanted device (996.60-996.69)
infusion, perfusion, or transfusion (999.3)
postoperative obstetrical wound infection (674.3)

998.51 Infected postoperative seroma
Use additional code to identify organism

998.59 Other postoperative infection
Abscess: postoperative
intra-abdominal postoperative
stitch postoperative
subphrenic postoperative
wound postoperative
Septicemia postoperative
Use additional code to identify infection

998.6 Persistent postoperative fistula

998.7 **Acute reaction to foreign substance accidentally left during a procedure**
Peritonitis:
aseptic
chemical

⑤ **998.8** **Other specified complications of procedures, not elsewhere classified**

998.81 **Emphysema (subcutaneous) (surgical) resulting from a procedure**

998.82 **Cataract fragments in eye following cataract surgery**

998.83 **Non-healing surgical wound**

998.89 **Other specified complications**

998.9 **Unspecified complication of procedure, not elsewhere classified**
Postoperative complication NOS

Excludes: *complication NOS of obstetrical surgery or procedure (669.4)*

999 **Complications of medical care, not elsewhere classified**
Includes: complications, not elsewhere classified, of:
dialysis (hemodialysis) (peritoneal) (renal)
extracorporeal circulation
hyperalimentation therapy
immunization
infusion
inhalation therapy
injection
inoculation
perfusion
transfusion
vaccination
ventilation therapy

Excludes: *specified complications classified elsewhere such as:*
complications of implanted device (996.0-996.9)
contact dermatitis due to drugs (692.3)
dementia dialysis (294.8)
transient (293.9)
dialysis disequilibrium syndrome (276.0-276.9)
poisoning and toxic effects of drugs and chemicals (960.0-989.9)
postvaccinal encephalitis (323.5)
water and electrolyte imbalance (276.0-276.9)

999.0 **Generalized vaccinia**

999.1 **Air embolism**
Air embolism to any site following infusion, perfusion, or transfusion

Excludes: *embolism specified as:*
complicating:
abortion (634-638 with .6, 639.6)
ectopic or molar pregnancy (639.6)
pregnancy, childbirth, or the puerperium (673.0)
due to implanted device (996.7)
traumatic (958.0)

999.2 **Other vascular complications**
Phlebitis following infusion, perfusion, or transfusion
Thromboembolism following infusion, perfusion, or transfusion
Thrombophlebitis following infusion, perfusion, or transfusion

Excludes: *the listed conditions when specified as:*
due to implanted device (996.61-996.62, 996.72-996.74)
postoperative NOS (997.2, 997.71-997.79)

999.3 **Other infection**
Infection following infusion, injection, transfusion, or vaccination
Sepsis following infusion, injection, transfusion, or vaccination
Septicemia following infusion, injection, transfusion, or vaccination

Excludes: *the listed conditions when specified as:*
due to implanted device (996.60-996.69)
postoperative NOS (998.51-998.59)

● Code new   ▲ Revision of   ④ ⑤ Fourth or fifth
      to this edition   existing code   digit required

999.4 Anaphylactic shock due to serum

Excludes: shock:
    allergic NOS (995.0)
    anaphylactic:
      NOS (995.0)
      due to drugs and chemicals (995.0)

999.5 Other serum reaction

Intoxication by serum   Serum sickness
Protein sickness   Urticaria due to serum
Serum rash

Excludes: serum hepatitis (070.2-070.3)

999.6 ABO incompatibility reaction

Incompatible blood transfusion
Reaction to blood group incompatibility in infusion or transfusion

999.7 Rh incompatibility reaction

Reactions due to Rh factor in infusion or transfusion

999.8 Other transfusion reaction

Septic shock due to transfusion
Transfusion reaction NOS

Excludes: postoperative shock (998.0)

999.9 Other and unspecified complications of medical care, not elsewhere classified

Complications, not elsewhere classified, of:
  electroshock therapy
  inhalation therapy
  ultrasound therapy
  ventilation therapy
Unspecified misadventure of medical care

Excludes: unspecified complication of:
    phototherapy (990)
    radiation therapy (990)

Add 4th or   Nonspecific   Unspecified   Medicare secondary
5th digit   code   code   payer (MSP) alert

SUPPLEMENTARY CLASSIFICATION OF FACTORS INFLUENCING HEALTH STATUS AND CONTACT WITH HEALTH SERVICES (V01-V82)

This classification is provided to deal with occasions when circumstances other than a disease or injury classifiable to categories 001-999 (the main part of ICD)are recorded as “diagnoses” or “problems.” This can arise mainly in three ways:

a) When a person who is not currently sick encounters the health services for some specific purpose, such as to act as a donor of an organ or tissue, to receive prophylactic vaccination, or to discuss a problem which is in itself not a disease or injury. This will be a fairly rare occurrence among hospital inpatients, but will be relatively more common among hospital outpatients and patients of family practitioners, health clinics, etc.

b) When a person with a known disease or injury, whether it is current or resolving, encounters the health care system for a specific treatment of that disease or injury (e.g., dialysis for renal disease; chemotherapy for malignancy; cast change).

c) When some circumstance or problem is present which influences the person’s health status but is not in itself a current illness or injury. Such factors may be elicited during population surveys, when the person may or may not be currently sick, or be recorded as an additional factor to be borne in mind when the person is receiving care for some current illness or injury classifiable to categories 001-999.

In the latter circumstances the V code should be used only as a supplementary code and should not be the one selected for use in primary, single cause tabulations. Examples of these circumstances are a personal history of certain diseases, or a person with an artificial heart valve in situ.

PERSONS WITH POTENTIAL HEALTH HAZARDS RELATED TO COMMUNICABLE DISEASES (V01-V06)

[Excludes:] *family history of infectious and parasitic diseases (V18.8)*
personal history of infectious and parasitic diseases (V12.0)

V01 Contact with or exposure to communicable diseases

V01.0 Cholera
Conditions classifiable to 001

V01.1 Tuberculosis
Conditions classifiable to 010-018

V01.2 Poliomyelitis
Conditions classifiable to 045

V01.3 Smallpox
Conditions classifiable to 050

V01.4 Rubella
Conditions classifiable to 056

V01.5 Rabies
Conditions classifiable to 071

V01.6 Venereal diseases
Conditions classifiable to 090-099

V01.7 Other viral diseases
Conditions classifiable to 042-078 and V08, except as above

[5] **V01.8 Other communicable diseases**
Conditions classifiable to 001-136, except as above

● **V01.81 Anthrax**

● **V01.89 Other communicable diseases**

V01.9 Unspecified communicable disease

V02 Carrier or suspected carrier of infectious diseases

V02.0 Cholera

V02.1 Typhoid

V02.2 Amebiasis

V02.3 Other gastrointestinal pathogens

V02.4 Diphtheria

[5] **V02.5 Other specified bacterial diseases**

V02.51 Group B streptococcus

V02.52 Other streptococcus

V02.59 Other specified bacterial diseases
Meningococcal
Staphylococcal

Add 4th or 5th digit | Nonspecific code | Unspecified code | Manifestation code

⑤ **V02.6 Viral hepatitis**
Hepatitis Australian-antigen [HAA] [SH] carrier
Serum hepatitis carrier

V02.60 Viral hepatitis carrier, unspecified

V02.61 Hepatitis B carrier

V02.62 Hepatitis C carrier

V02.69 Other viral hepatitis carrier

V02.7 Gonorrhea

V02.8 Other venereal diseases

V02.9 Other specified infectious organism

V03 Need for prophylactic vaccination and inoculation against bacterial diseases
Excludes: vaccination not carried out because of contraindication (V64.0)
vaccines against combinations of diseases (V06.0-V06.9)

V03.0 Cholera alone

V03.1 Typhoid-paratyphoid alone [TAB]

V03.2 Tuberculosis [BCG]

V03.3 Plague

V03.4 Tularemia

V03.5 Diphtheria alone

V03.6 Pertussis alone

V03.7 Tetanus toxoid alone

⑤ **V03.8 Other specified vaccinations against single bacterial diseases**

V03.81 Hemophilus influenza, type B [Hib]

V03.82 Streptococcus pneumoniae [pneumococcus]

V03.89 Other specified vaccination

V03.9 Unspecified single bacterial disease

V04 Need for prophylactic vaccination and inoculation against certain viral diseases
Excludes: vaccines against combinations of diseases (V06.0-V06.9)

V04.0 Poliomyelitis

V04.1 Smallpox

V04.2 Measles alone

V04.3 Rubella alone

V04.4 Yellow fever

V04.5 Rabies

V04.6 Mumps alone

V04.7 Common cold

V04.8 Influenza

V05 Need for other prophylactic vaccination and inoculation against single diseases
Excludes: vaccines against combinations of diseases (V06.0-V06.9)

V05.0 Arthropod-borne viral encephalitis

V05.1 Other arthropod-borne viral diseases

V05.2 Leishmaniasis

V05.3 Viral hepatitis

V05.4 Varicella
Chickenpox

V05.8 Other specified disease

V05.9 Unspecified single disease

V06 Need for prophylactic vaccination and inoculation against combinations of diseases
Note: Use additional single vaccination codes from categories V03-V05 to identify any vaccinations not included in a combination code.

V06.0 Cholera with typhoid-paratyphoid [cholera + TAB]

V06.1 Diphtheria-tetanus-pertussis, combined [DTP]

V06.2 Diphtheria-tetanus-pertussis with typhoid-paratyphoid [DTP + TAB]

● Code new
to this edition
▲ Revision of
existing code
④ ⑤ Fourth or fifth
digit required

V06.3 Diphtheria-tetanus-pertussis with poliomyelitis [DTP + polio]

V06.4 Measles-mumps-rubella [MMR]

V06.5 Tetanus-diphtheria [Td]

V06.6 Streptococcus pneumoniae [pneumococcus] and influenza

V06.8 Other combinations

[Excludes:] *multiple single vaccination codes (V03.0-V05.9)*

V06.9 Unspecified combined vaccine

PERSONS WITH NEED FOR ISOLATION, OTHER POTENTIAL HEALTH HAZARDS AND PROPHYLACTIC MEASURES (V07-V09)

V07 Need for isolation and other prophylactic measures

[Excludes:] *prophylactic organ removal (V50.41-V50.49)*

V07.0 Isolation

Admission to protect the individual from his surroundings or for isolation of individual after contact with infectious diseases

V07.1 Desensitization to allergens

V07.2 Prophylactic immunotherapy

Administration of:
- antivenin
- immune sera [gamma globulin]
- RhoGAM
- tetanus antitoxin

[5] **V07.3 Other prophylactic chemotherapy**

V07.31 Prophylactic fluoride administration

V07.39 Other prophylactic chemotherapy

[Excludes:] *maintenance chemotherapy following disease (V58.1)*

V07.4 Postmenopausal hormone replacement therapy

V07.8 Other specified prophylactic measure

V07.9 Unspecified prophylactic measure

V08 Asymptomatic human immunodeficiency virus [HIV] infection status

HIV positive NOS

Note: This code is ONLY to be used when NO HIV infection symptoms or conditions are present. If any HIV infection symptoms or conditions are present, see code 042.

[Excludes:] *AIDS (042)*
human immunodeficiency virus [HIV] disease (042)
exposure to HIV (V01.7)
nonspecific serologic evidence of HIV (795.71)
symptomatic human immunodeficiency virus [HIV] infection (042)

V09 Infection with drug-resistant microorganisms

Note: This category is intended for use as an additional code for infectious conditions classified elsewhere to indicate the presence of drug-resistance of the infectious organism.

V09.0 Infection with microorganisms resistant to penicillins

V09.1 Infection with microorganisms resistant to cephalosporins and other B-lactam antibiotics

V09.2 Infection with microorganisms resistant to macrolides

V09.3 Infection with microorganisms resistant to tetracyclines

V09.4 Infection with microorganisms resistant to aminoglycosides

V09.5 Infection with microorganisms resistant to quinolones and fluoroquinolones

V09.50 Without mention of resistance to multiple quinolones and fluoroquinolones

V09.51 With resistance to multiple quinolones and fluoroquinolones

V09.6 Infection with microorganisms resistant to sulfonamides

[5] **V09.7 Infection with microorganisms resistant to other specified antimycobacterial agents**

[Excludes:] *Amikacin (V09.4)*
Kanamycin (V09.4)
Streptomycin [SM] (V09.4)

V09.70 Without mention of resistance to multiple antimycobacterial agents

V09.71 With resistance to multiple antimycobacterial agents

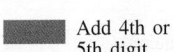

⑤ **V09.8 Infection with microorganisms resistant to other specified drugs**

    V09.80 Without mention of resistance to multiple drugs

    V09.81 With resistance to multiple drugs

⑤ **V09.9 Infection with drug-resistant microorganisms, unspecified**
    Drug resistance NOS

    V09.90 Without mention of multiple drug resistance

    V09.91 With multiple drug resistance
      Multiple drug resistance NOS

PERSONS WITH POTENTIAL HEALTH HAZARDS RELATED TO PERSONAL AND FAMILY HISTORY (V10-V19)

    Excludes: *obstetric patients where the possibility that the fetus might be affected is the reason for observation or management during pregnancy (655.0-655.9)*

V10 **Personal history of malignant neoplasm**

⑤ **V10.0 Gastrointestinal tract**
    History of conditions classifiable to 140-159

    V10.00 Gastrointestinal tract, unspecified

    V10.01 Tongue

    V10.02 Other and unspecified oral cavity and pharynx

    V10.03 Esophagus

    V10.04 Stomach

    V10.05 Large intestine

    V10.06 Rectum, rectosigmoid junction, and anus

    V10.07 Liver

    V10.09 Other

⑤ **V10.1 Trachea, bronchus, and lung**
    History of conditions classifiable to 162

    V10.11 Bronchus and lung

    V10.12 Trachea

⑤ **V10.2 Other respiratory and intrathoracic organs**
    History of conditions classifiable to 160, 161, 163-165

    V10.20 Respiratory organ, unspecified

    V10.21 Larynx

    V10.22 Nasal cavities, middle ear, and accessory sinuses

    V10.29 Other

V10.3 Breast
    History of conditions classifiable to 174 and 175

⑤ **V10.4 Genital organs**
    History of conditions classifiable to 179-187

    V10.40 Female genital organ, unspecified

    V10.41 Cervix uteri

    V10.42 Other parts of uterus

    V10.43 Ovary

    V10.44 Other female genital organs

    V10.45 Male genital organ, unspecified

    V10.46 Prostate

    V10.47 Testis

    V10.48 Epididymis

    V10.49 Other male genital organs

⑤ **V10.5 Urinary organs**
    History of conditions classifiable to 188 and 189

    V10.50 Urinary organ, unspecified

    V10.51 Bladder

● Code new
to this edition
    ▲ Revision of
existing code
    ④ ⑤ Fourth or fifth
digit required

V10.52 Kidney

> *Excludes:* renal pelvis (V10.53)

V10.53 Renal pelvis

V10.59 Other

⑤ **V10.6 Leukemia**
Conditions classifiable to 204-208

> *Excludes:* leukemia in remission (204-208)

V10.60 Leukemia, unspecified

V10.61 Lymphoid leukemia

V10.62 Myeloid leukemia

V10.63 Monocytic leukemia

V10.69 Other

⑤ **V10.7 Other lymphatic and hematopoietic neoplasms**
Conditions classifiable to 200-203

> *Excludes:* listed conditions in 200-203 in remission

V10.71 Lymphosarcoma and reticulosarcoma

V10.72 Hodgkin's disease

V10.79 Other

⑤ **V10.8 Personal history of malignant neoplasm of other sites**
History of conditions classifiable to 170-173, 190-195

V10.81 Bone

V10.82 Malignant melanoma of skin

V10.83 Other malignant neoplasm of skin

V10.84 Eye

V10.85 Brain

V10.86 Other parts of nervous system

> *Excludes:* peripheral, sympathetic, and parasympathetic nerves (V10.89)

V10.87 Thyroid

V10.88 Other endocrine glands and related structures

V10.89 Other

V10.9 Unspecified personal history of malignant neoplasm

V11 Personal history of mental disorder

V11.0 Schizophrenia

> *Excludes:* that in remission (295.0-295.9 with fifth-digit 5)

V11.1 Affective disorders
Personal history of manic-depressive psychosis

> *Excludes:* that in remission (296.0-296.6 with fifth-digit 5, 6)

V11.2 Neurosis

V11.3 Alcoholism

V11.8 Other mental disorders

V11.9 Unspecified mental disorder

V12 Personal history of certain other diseases

⑤ **V12.0 Infectious and parasitic diseases**

V12.00 Unspecified infectious and parasitic disease

V12.01 Tuberculosis

V12.02 Poliomyelitis

V12.03 Malaria

V12.09 Other

V12.1 Nutritional deficiency

V12.2 Endocrine, metabolic, and immunity disorders

> *Excludes:* history of allergy (V14.0-V14.9, V15.01-V15.09)

| | Add 4th or 5th digit | | Nonspecific code | | Unspecified code | | Manifestation code |

V12.3 Diseases of blood and blood-forming organs

⑤ **V12.4 Disorders of nervous system and sense organs**

V12.40 Unspecified disorder of nervous system and sense organs

V12.41 Benign neoplasm of the brain

V12.49 Other disorders of nervous system and sense organs

⑤ **V12.5 Diseases of circulatory system**

Excludes: *old myocardial infarction (412)*
postmyocardial infarction syndrome (411.0)

V12.50 Unspecified circulatory disease

V12.51 Venous thrombosis and embolism
Pulmonary embolism

V12.52 Thrombophlebitis

V12.59 Other

Note: Assign code V12.59 (and not a code from category 438) as an additional code for history of cerebrovascular disease when no neurologic deficits are present.

V12.6 Diseases of respiratory system

⑤ **V12.7 Diseases of digestive system**

V12.70 Unspecified digestive disease

V12.71 Peptic ulcer disease

V12.72 Colonic polyps

V12.79 Other

V13 Personal history of other diseases

⑤ **V13.0 Disorders of urinary system**

V13.00 Unspecified urinary disorder

V13.01 Urinary calculi

V13.09 Other

V13.1 Trophoblastic disease

Excludes: *supervision during a current pregnancy (V23.1)*

⑤ **V13.2 Other genital system and obstetric disorders**

Excludes: *supervision during a current pregnancy of a woman with poor obstetric history*
(V23.0-V23.9)
habitual aborter (646.3)
without current history (629.9)

● **V13.21 Personal history of pre-term labor**

Excludes: *current pregnancy with history of pre-term labor (V23.41)*

● **V13.29 Other genital system and obstetric disorders**

V13.3 Diseases of skin and subcutaneous tissue

V13.4 Arthritis

V13.5 Other musculoskeletal disorders

⑤ **V13.6 Congenital malformations**

V13.61 Hypospadias

V13.69 Other congenital malformations

V13.7 Perinatal problems

Excludes: *low birth weight status (V21.30-V21.35)*

V13.8 Other specified diseases

V13.9 Unspecified disease

V14 Personal history of allergy to medicinal agents

V14.0 Penicillin

V14.1 Other antibiotic agent

V14.2 Sulfonamides

V14.3 Other anti-infective agent

V14.4 Anesthetic agent

V14.5 Narcotic agent

● Code new
to this edition

▲ Revision of
existing code

④ ⑤ Fourth or fifth
digit required

V14.6 **Analgesic agent**

V14.7 **Serum or vaccine**

V14.8 **Other specified medicinal agents**

V14.9 **Unspecified medicinal agent**

V15 **Other personal history presenting hazards to health**

⑤ V15.0 **Allergy, other than to medicinal agents**

> Excludes: *allergy to food substance used as base for medicinal agent (V14.0-V14.9)*

V15.01 **Allergy to peanuts**

V15.02 **Allergy to milk products**

> Excludes: *lactose intolerance (271.3)*

V15.03 **Allergy to eggs**

V15.04 **Allergy to seafood**
Seafood (octopus) (squid) ink
Shellfish

V15.05 **Allergy to other foods**
Food additives
Nuts other than peanuts

V15.06 **Allergy to insects**
Bugs
Insect bites and stings
Spiders

V15.07 **Allergy to latex**
Latex sensitivity

V15.08 **Allergy to radiographic dye**
Contrast media used for diagnostic x-ray procedures

V15.09 **Other allergy, other than to medicinal agents**

V15.1 **Surgery to heart and great vessels**

> Excludes: *replacement by transplant or other means (V42.1-V42.2, V43.2-V43.4)*

V15.2 **Surgery to other major organs**

> Excludes: *replacement by transplant or other means (V42.0-V43.8)*

V15.3 **Irradiation**
Previous exposure to therapeutic or other ionizing radiation

⑤ V15.4 **Psychological trauma**

> Excludes: *history of condition classifiable to 290-316 (V11.0-V11.9)*

V15.41 **History of physical abuse**
Rape

V15.42 **History of emotional abuse**
Neglect

V15.49 **Other**

V15.5 **Injury**

V15.6 **Poisoning**

V15.7 **Contraception**

> Excludes: *current contraceptive management (V25.0-V25.4)*
> *presence of intrauterine contraceptive device as incidental finding (V45.5)*

⑤ V15.8 **Other specified personal history presenting hazards to health**

V15.81 **Noncompliance with medical treatment**

V15.82 **History of tobacco use**

> Excludes: *tobacco dependence (305.1)*

V15.84 **Exposure to asbestos**

V15.85 **Exposure to potentially hazardous body fluids**

V15.86 **Exposure to lead**

V15.89 **Other**

V15.9 **Unspecified personal history presenting hazards to health**

V16 **Family history of malignant neoplasm**

| | Add 4th or 5th digit | | Nonspecific code | | Unspecified code | | Manifestation code |

V16.0 Gastrointestinal tract
Family history of condition classifiable to 140-159

V16.1 Trachea, bronchus, and lung
Family history of condition classifiable to 162

V16.2 Other respiratory and intrathoracic organs
Family history of condition classifiable to 160-161, 163-165

V16.3 Breast
Family history of condition classifiable to 174

⑤ **V16.4 Genital organs**
Family history of condition classifiable to 179-187

   V16.40 Genital organ, unspecified

   V16.41 Ovary

   V16.42 Prostate

   V16.43 Testis

   V16.49 Other

⑤ **V16.5 Urinary organs**
Family history of condition classifiable to 189

   V16.51 Kidney

   V16.59 Other

V16.6 Leukemia
Family history of condition classifiable to 204-208

V16.7 Other lymphatic and hematopoietic neoplasms
Family history of condition classifiable to 200-203

V16.8 Other specified malignant neoplasm
Family history of other condition classifiable to 140-199

V16.9 Unspecified malignant neoplasm

V17 Family history of certain chronic disabling diseases

V17.0 Psychiatric condition

   Excludes: family history of mental retardation (V18.4)

V17.1 Stroke (cerebrovascular)

V17.2 Other neurological diseases
Epilepsy   Huntington's chorea

V17.3 Ischemic heart disease

V17.4 Other cardiovascular diseases

V17.5 Asthma

V17.6 Other chronic respiratory conditions

V17.7 Arthritis

V17.8 Other musculoskeletal diseases

V18 Family history of certain other specific conditions

V18.0 Diabetes mellitus

V18.1 Other endocrine and metabolic diseases

V18.2 Anemia

V18.3 Other blood disorders

V18.4 Mental retardation

V18.5 Digestive disorders

⑤ **V18.6 Kidney diseases**

   V18.61 Polycystic kidney

   V18.69 Other kidney diseases

V18.7 Other genitourinary diseases

V18.8 Infectious and parasitic diseases

V19 Family history of other conditions

V19.0 Blindness or visual loss

V19.1 Other eye disorders

V19.2 Deafness or hearing loss

   ● Code new
to this edition   ▲ Revision of
existing code   ④ ⑤ Fourth or fifth
digit required

V19.3 Other ear disorders

V19.4 Skin conditions

V19.5 Congenital anomalies

V19.6 Allergic disorders

V19.7 Consanguinity

V19.8 Other condition

PERSONS ENCOUNTERING HEALTH SERVICES IN CIRCUMSTANCES RELATED TO REPRODUCTION AND DEVELOPMENT (V20-V29)

V20 Health supervision of infant or child

V20.0 Foundling

V20.1 Other healthy infant or child receiving care
Medical or nursing care supervision of healthy infant in cases of:
maternal illness, physical or psychiatric
socioeconomic adverse condition at home
too many children at home preventing or interfering with normal care

V20.2 Routine infant or child health check
Developmental testing of infant or child
Immunizations appropriate for age
Routine vision and hearing testing

[Excludes:] *special screening for developmental handicaps (V79.3)*

Use additional code(s) to identify:
Special screening examination(s) performed (V73.0-V82.9)

V21 Constitutional states in development

V21.0 Period of rapid growth in childhood

V21.1 Puberty

V21.2 Other adolescence

[5] **V21.3 Low birth weight status**

[Excludes:] *history of perinatal problems (V13.7)*

V21.30 Low birth weight status, unspecified

V21.31 Low birth weight status, less than 500 grams

V21.32 Low birth weight status, 500-999 grams

V21.33 Low birth weight status, 1000-1499 grams

V21.34 Low birth weight status, 1500-1999 grams

V21.35 Low birth weight status, 2000-2500 grams

V21.8 Other specified constitutional states in development

V21.9 Unspecified constitutional state in development

V22 Normal pregnancy

[Excludes:] *pregnancy examination or test, pregnancy unconfirmed (V72.4)*

V22.0 Supervision of normal first pregnancy

V22.1 Supervision of other normal pregnancy

V22.2 Pregnant state, incidental
Pregnant state NOS

V23 Supervision of high-risk pregnancy

V23.0 Pregnancy with history of infertility

V23.1 Pregnancy with history of trophoblastic disease
Pregnancy with history of:
hydatidiform mole
vesicular mole

[Excludes:] *that without current pregnancy (V13.1)*

V23.2 Pregnancy with history of abortion
Pregnancy with history of conditions classifiable to 634-638

[Excludes:] *habitual aborter:*
care during pregnancy (646.3)
that without current pregnancy (629.9)

V23.3 Grand multiparity

Excludes: *care in relation to labor and delivery (659.4)*
that without current pregnancy (V61.5)

⑤ **V23.4 Pregnancy with other poor obstetric history**
Pregnancy with history of other conditions classifiable to 630-676

● **V23.41 Pregnancy with history of pre-term labor**
● **V23.49 Pregnancy with other poor obstetric history**

V23.5 Pregnancy with other poor reproductive history
Pregnancy with history of stillbirth or neonatal death

V23.7 Insufficient prenatal care
History of little or no prenatal care

⑤ **V23.8 Other high-risk pregnancy**

V23.81 Elderly primigravida
First pregnancy in a woman who will be 35 years of age or older at expected
date of delivery

Excludes: *elderly primigravida complicating pregnancy (659.5)*

V23.82 Elderly multigravida
Second or more pregnancy in a woman who will be 35 years of age or older
at expected date of delivery

Excludes: *elderly multigravida complicating pregnancy (659.6)*

V23.83 Young primigravida
First pregnancy in a female less than 16 years old at expected date of delivery

Excludes: *young primigravida complicating pregnancy (659.8)*

V23.84 Young multigravida
Second or more pregnancy in a female less than 16 years old at expected date
of delivery

Excludes: *young multigravida complicating pregnancy (659.8)*

V23.89 Other high-risk pregnancy

V23.9 Unspecified high-risk pregnancy

V24 Postpartum care and examination

V24.0 Immediately after delivery
Care and observation in uncomplicated cases

V24.1 Lactating mother
Supervision of lactation

V24.2 Routine postpartum follow-up

V25 Encounter for contraceptive management

⑤ **V25.0 General counseling and advice**

V25.01 Prescription of oral contraceptives

V25.02 Initiation of other contraceptive measures
Fitting of diaphragm
Prescription of foams, creams, or other agents

V25.09 Other
Family planning advice

V25.1 Insertion of intrauterine contraceptive device

V25.2 Sterilization
Admission for interruption of fallopian tubes or vas deferens

V25.3 Menstrual extraction
Menstrual regulation

⑤ **V25.4 Surveillance of previously prescribed contraceptive methods**
Checking, reinsertion, or removal of contraceptive device
Repeat prescription for contraceptive method
Routine examination in connection with contraceptive maintenance

Excludes: *presence of intrauterine contraceptive device as incidental finding (V45.5)*

V25.40 Contraceptive surveillance, unspecified

V25.41 Contraceptive pill

V25.42 Intrauterine contraceptive device
Checking, reinsertion, or removal of intrauterine device

● Code new
to this edition
▲ Revision of
existing code
④ ⑤ Fourth or fifth
digit required

V25.43 Implantable subdermal contraceptive

V25.49 Other contraceptive method

V25.5 Insertion of implantable subdermal contraceptive

V25.8 Other specified contraceptive management
Postvasectomy sperm count
[Excludes:] *sperm count following sterilization reversal (V26.22)*
sperm count for fertility testing (V26.21)

V25.9 Unspecified contraceptive management

V26 Procreative management

V26.0 Tuboplasty or vasoplasty after previous sterilization

V26.1 Artificial insemination

[5] **V26.2 Investigation and testing**
[Excludes:] *postvasectomy sperm count (V25.8)*

V26.21 Fertility testing
Fallopian insufflation
Sperm count for fertility testing
[Excludes:] *Genetic counseling and testing (V26.3)*

V26.22 Aftercare following sterilization reversal
Fallopian insufflation following sterilization reversal
Sperm count following sterilization reversal

V26.29 Other investigation and testing

V26.3 Genetic counseling and testing
[Excludes:] *fertility testing (V26.21)*

V26.4 General counseling and advice

[5] **V26.5 Sterilization status**

V26.51 Tubal ligation status
[Excludes:] *infertility not due to previous tubal ligation (628.0-628.9)*

V26.52 Vasectomy status

V26.8 Other specified procreative management

V26.9 Unspecified procreative management

V27 Outcome of delivery
Note: This category is intended for the coding of the outcome of delivery on the mother's record.

V27.0 Single liveborn

V27.1 Single stillborn

V27.2 Twins, both liveborn

V27.3 Twins, one liveborn and one stillborn

V27.4 Twins, both stillborn

V27.5 Other multiple birth, all liveborn

V27.6 Other multiple birth, some liveborn

V27.7 Other multiple birth, all stillborn

V27.9 Unspecified outcome of delivery
Single birth, outcome to infant unspecified
Multiple birth, outcome to infant unspecified

V28 Antenatal screening
[Excludes:] *abnormal findings on screening—code to findings*
routine prenatal care (V22.0-V23.9)

V28.0 Screening for chromosomal anomalies by amniocentesis

V28.1 Screening for raised alpha-fetoprotein levels in amniotic fluid

V28.2 Other screening based on amniocentesis

V28.3 Screening for malformation using ultrasonics

V28.4 Screening for fetal growth retardation using ultrasonics

V28.5 Screening for isoimmunization

V28.6 Screening for Streptococcus B

Add 4th or 5th digit | Nonspecific code | Unspecified code | Manifestation code

V28.8 Other specified antenatal screening

V28.9 Unspecified antenatal screening

V29 Observation and evaluation of newborns for suspected condition not found

Note: This category is to be used for newborns, within the neonatal period, (the first 28 days of life) who are suspected of having an abnormal condition resulting from exposure from the mother or the birth process, but without signs or symptoms, and, which after examination and observation, is found not to exist.

V29.0 Observation for suspected infectious condition

V29.1 Observation for suspected neurological condition

V29.2 Observation for suspected respiratory condition

V29.3 Observation for suspected genetic or metabolic condition

V29.8 Observation for other specified suspected condition

V29.9 Observation for unspecified suspected condition

LIVEBORN INFANTS ACCORDING TO TYPE OF BIRTH (V30-V39)

Note: These categories are intended for the coding of liveborn infants who are consuming health care [e.g., crib or bassinet occupancy].

The following fourth-digit subdivisions are for use with categories V30-V39:

.0 **Born in hospital**

.1 **Born before admission to hospital**

.2 **Born outside hospital and not hospitalized**

The following two fifth-digits are for use with the fourth-digit .0, Born in hospital:

0 delivered without mention of cesarean delivery

1 delivered by cesarean delivery

④ **V30 Single liveborn**

④ **V31 Twin, mate liveborn**

④ **V32 Twin, mate stillborn**

④ **V33 Twin, unspecified**

④ **V34 Other multiple, mates all liveborn**

④ **V35 Other multiple, mates all stillborn**

④ **V36 Other multiple, mates live- and stillborn**

④ **V37 Other multiple, unspecified**

④ **V39 Unspecified**

PERSONS WITH A CONDITION INFLUENCING THEIR HEALTH STATUS (V40-V49)

Note: These categories are intended for use when these conditions are recorded as "diagnoses" or "problems."

V40 Mental and behavioral problems

V40.0 Problems with learning

V40.1 Problems with communication [including speech]

V40.2 Other mental problems

V40.3 Other behavioral problems

V40.9 Unspecified mental or behavioral problem

V41 Problems with special senses and other special functions

V41.0 Problems with sight

V41.1 Other eye problems

V41.2 Problems with hearing

V41.3 Other ear problems

V41.4 Problems with voice production

V41.5 Problems with smell and taste

V41.6 Problems with swallowing and mastication

V41.7 Problems with sexual function

Excludes: marital problems (V61.10)

psychosexual disorders (302.0-302.9)

V41.8 Other problems with special functions

● Code new
to this edition
▲ Revision of
existing code
④ ⑤ Fourth or fifth
digit required

V41.9 Unspecified problem with special function

V42 Organ or tissue replaced by transplant
Includes: homologous or heterologous (animal) (human) transplant organ status

V42.0 Kidney

V42.1 Heart

V42.2 Heart valve

V42.3 Skin

V42.4 Bone

V42.5 Cornea

V42.6 Lung

V42.7 Liver

⑤ **V42.8 Other specified organ or tissue**

      V42.81 Bone marrow

      V42.82 Peripheral stem cells

      V42.83 Pancreas

      V42.84 Intestines

      V42.89 Other

V42.9 Unspecified organ or tissue

V43 Organ or tissue replaced by other means
Includes: replacement of organ by:
      artificial device
      mechanical device
      prosthesis

    Excludes: *cardiac pacemaker in situ (V45.01)*
           fitting and adjustment of prosthetic device (V52.0-V52.9)
           renal dialysis status (V45.1)

V43.0 Eye globe

V43.1 Lens
    Pseudophakos

V43.2 Heart

V43.3 Heart valve

V43.4 Blood vessel

V43.5 Bladder

⑤ **V43.6 Joint**

      V43.60 Unspecified joint

      V43.61 Shoulder

      V43.62 Elbow

      V43.63 Wrist

      V43.64 Hip

      V43.65 Knee

      V43.66 Ankle

      V43.69 Other

V43.7 Limb

⑤ **V43.8 Other organ or tissue**

      V43.81 Larynx

      V43.82 Breast

      V43.83 Artificial skin

      V43.89 Other

V44 Artificial opening status

    Excludes: *artificial openings requiring attention or management (V55.0-V55.9)*

V44.0 Tracheostomy

V44.1 Gastrostomy

V44.2 Ileostomy

V44.3 Colostomy

	Add 4th or 5th digit		Nonspecific code		Unspecified code		Manifestation code

V44.4 Other artificial opening of gastrointestinal tract

⑤ **V44.5 Cystostomy**

V44.50 Cystostomy, unspecified

V44.51 Cutaneous-vesicostomy

V44.52 Appendico-vesicostomy

V44.59 Other cystostomy

V44.6 Other artificial opening of urinary tract
Nephrostomy
Ureterostomy
Urethrostomy

V44.7 Artificial vagina

V44.8 Other artificial opening status

V44.9 Unspecified artificial opening status

V45 Other postsurgical states

[Excludes:] *aftercare management (V51-V58.9)*
malfunction or other complication—code to condition

⑤ **V45.0 Cardiac device in situ**

V45.00 Unspecified cardiac device

V45.01 Cardiac pacemaker

V45.02 Automatic implantable cardiac defibrillator

V45.09 Other specified cardiac device
Carotid sinus pacemaker in situ

V45.1 Renal dialysis status
Patient requiring intermittent renal dialysis
Presence of arterial-venous shunt (for dialysis)

[Excludes:] *admission for dialysis treatment, or session (V56.0)*

V45.2 Presence of cerebrospinal fluid drainage device
Cerebral ventricle (communicating) shunt, valve, or device in situ

[Excludes:] *malfunction (996.2)*

V45.3 Intestinal bypass or anastomosis status

V45.4 Arthrodesis status

⑤ **V45.5 Presence of contraceptive device**

[Excludes:] *checking, reinsertion, or removal of device (V25.42)*
complication from device (996.32)
insertion of device (V25.1)

V45.51 Intrauterine contraceptive device

V45.52 Subdermal contraceptive implant

V45.59 Other

⑤ **V45.6 States following surgery of eye and adnexa**
Cataract extraction state following eye surgery
Filtering bleb state following eye surgery
Surgical eyelid adhesion state following eye surgery

[Excludes:] *aphakia (379.31)*
artificial eye globe (V43.0)

V45.61 Cataract extraction status

Use additional code for associated artificial lens status (V43.1)

V45.69 Other states following surgery of eye and adnexa

⑤ **V45.7 Acquired absence of organ**

V45.71 Acquired absence of breast

V45.72 Acquired absence of intestine (large) (small)

V45.73 Acquired absence of kidney

V45.74 Other parts of urinary tract
Bladder

V45.75 Stomach

V45.76 Lung

● Code new to this edition ▲ Revision of existing code ④ ⑤ Fourth or fifth digit required

V45.77 **Genital organs**

V45.78 **Eye**

V45.79 **Other acquired absence of organ**

⑤ V45.8 **Other postsurgical status**

V45.81 **Aortocoronary bypass status**

V45.82 **Percutaneous transluminal coronary angioplasty status**

V45.83 **Breast implant removal status**

V45.84 **Dental restoration status**
Dental crowns status
Dental fillings status

V45.89 **Other**
Presence of neuropacemaker or other electronic device

Excludes: *artificial heart valve in situ (V43.3)*
vascular prosthesis in situ (V43.4)

V46 Other dependence on machines

V46.0 **Aspirator**

V46.1 **Respirator**
Iron lung

● V46.2 **Supplemental oxygen**
Long-term oxygen therapy

V46.8 **Other enabling machines**
Hyperbaric chamber
Possum [Patient-Operated-Selector-Mechanism]

Excludes: *cardiac pacemaker (V45.0)*
kidney dialysis machine (V45.1)

V46.9 **Unspecified machine dependence**

V47 Other problems with internal organs

V47.0 **Deficiencies of internal organs**

V47.1 **Mechanical and motor problems with internal organs**

V47.2 **Other cardiorespiratory problems**
Cardiovascular exercise intolerance with pain (with):
at rest
less than ordinary activity
ordinary activity

V47.3 **Other digestive problems**

V47.4 **Other urinary problems**

V47.5 **Other genital problems**

V47.9 **Unspecified**

V48 Problems with head, neck, and trunk

V48.0 **Deficiencies of head**

Excludes: *deficiencies of ears, eyelids, and nose (V48.8)*

V48.1 **Deficiencies of neck and trunk**

V48.2 **Mechanical and motor problems with head**

V48.3 **Mechanical and motor problems with neck and trunk**

V48.4 **Sensory problem with head**

V48.5 **Sensory problem with neck and trunk**

V48.6 **Disfigurements of head**

V48.7 **Disfigurements of neck and trunk**

V48.8 **Other problems with head, neck, and trunk**

V48.9 **Unspecified problem with head, neck, or trunk**

V49 Other conditions influencing health status

V49.0 **Deficiencies of limbs**

V49.1 **Mechanical problems with limbs**

V49.2 **Motor problems with limbs**

V49.3 **Sensory problems with limbs**

| | Add 4th or 5th digit | | Nonspecific code | | Unspecified code | | Manifestation code |

V49.4 **Disfigurements of limbs**

V49.5 **Other problems of limbs**

⑤ **V49.6 Upper limb amputation status**

    V49.60 **Unspecified level**

    V49.61 **Thumb**

    V49.62 **Other finger(s)**

    V49.63 **Hand**

    V49.64 **Wrist**
        Disarticulation of wrist

    V49.65 **Below elbow**

    V49.66 **Above elbow**
        Disarticulation of elbow

    V49.67 **Shoulder**
        Disarticulation of shoulder

⑤ **V49.7 Lower limb amputation status**

    V49.70 **Unspecified level**

    V49.71 **Great toe**

    V49.72 **Other toe(s)**

    V49.73 **Foot**

    V49.74 **Ankle**
        Disarticulation of ankle

    V49.75 **Below knee**

    V49.76 **Above knee**
        Disarticulation of knee

    V49.77 **Hip**
        Disarticulation of hip

⑤ **V49.8 Other specified conditions influencing health status**

    ▲ V49.81 **Asymptomatic postmenopausal status (age-related) (natural)**

    Excludes: *menopausal and premenopausal disorders (627.0-627.9)*
              postsurgical menopause (256.2)
              premature menopause (256.31)
              symptomatic menopause (627.0-627.9)

    V49.82 **Dental sealant status**

    V49.89 **Other specified conditions influencing health status**

V49.9 **Unspecified**

PERSONS ENCOUNTERING HEALTH SERVICES FOR SPECIFIC PROCEDURES AND AFTERCARE (V50-V59)

Note: Categories V51-V58 are intended for use to indicate a reason for care in patients who may have already been treated for some disease or injury not now present, but who are receiving care to consolidate the treatment, to deal with residual states, or to prevent recurrence.

Excludes: *follow-up examination for medical surveillance following treatment (V67.0-V67.9)*

V50 Elective surgery for purposes other than remedying health states

V50.0 **Hair transplant**

V50.1 **Other plastic surgery for unacceptable cosmetic appearance**
    Breast augmentation or reduction
    Face-lift

Excludes: *plastic surgery following healed injury or operation (V51)*

V50.2 **Routine or ritual circumcision**
    Circumcision in the absence of significant medical indication

V50.3 **Ear piercing**

⑤ V50.4 **Prophylactic organ removal**

    Excludes: *organ donations (V59.0-V59.9)*
              therapeutic organ removal—code to condition

    V50.41 **Breast**

● Code new to this edition   ▲ Revision of existing code   ④ ⑤ Fourth or fifth digit required

V50.42 Ovary

V50.49 Other

V50.8 Other

V50.9 Unspecified

V51 Aftercare involving the use of plastic surgery
Plastic surgery following healed injury or operation

[Excludes:] *cosmetic plastic surgery (V50.1)*
plastic surgery as treatment for current injury—code to condition
repair of scarred tissue—code to scar

V52 Fitting and adjustment of prosthetic device and implant
Includes: removal of device

[Excludes:] *malfunction or complication of prosthetic device (996.0-996.7)*
status only, without need for care (V43.0-V43.8)

V52.0 Artificial arm (complete) (partial)

V52.1 Artificial leg (complete) (partial)

V52.2 Artificial eye

V52.3 Dental prosthetic device

V52.4 Breast prosthesis and implant

[Excludes:] *admission for implant insertion (V50.1)*

V52.8 Other specified prosthetic device

V52.9 Unspecified prosthetic device

V53 Fitting and adjustment of other device
Includes: removal of device
replacement of device

[Excludes:] *status only, without need for care (V45.0-V45.8)*

[5] **V53.0 Devices related to nervous system and special senses**

V53.01 Fitting and adjustment of cerebral ventricular (communicating) shunt

V53.02 Neuropacemaker (brain) (peripheral nerve) (spinal cord)

V53.09 Fitting and adjustment of other devices related to nervous system and special senses
Auditory substitution device
Visual substitution device

V53.1 Spectacles and contact lenses

V53.2 Hearing aid

[5] **V53.3 Cardiac device**
Reprogramming

V53.31 Cardiac pacemaker

[Excludes:] *mechanical complication of cardiac pacemaker (996.01)*

V53.32 Automatic implantable cardiac defibrillator

V53.39 Other cardiac device

V53.4 Orthodontic devices

V53.5 Other intestinal appliance

[Excludes:] *colostomy (V55.3)*
ileostomy (V55.2)
other artificial opening of digestive tract (V55.4)

V53.6 Urinary devices
Urinary catheter

[Excludes:] *cystostomy (V55.5)*
nephrostomy (V55.6)
ureterostomy (V55.6)
urethrostomy (V55.6)

V53.7 Orthopedic devices
Orthopedic:
brace
cast

Orthopedic:
corset
shoes

[Excludes:] *other orthopedic aftercare (V54)*

V53.8 **Wheelchair**

V53.9 Other and unspecified device

V54 Other orthopedic aftercare

> *Excludes:* fitting and adjustment of orthopedic devices (V53.7)
> malfunction of internal orthopedic device (996.4)
> other complication of nonmechanical nature (996.60-996.79)

V54.0 **Aftercare involving removal of fracture plate or other internal fixation device**

Removal of: Removal of:
 pins   rods
 plates   screws

> *Excludes:* removal of external fixation device (V54.89)

● **V54.1** **Aftercare for healing traumatic fracture**

   ● **V54.10** Aftercare for healing traumatic fracture of arm, unspecified
   ● V54.11 Aftercare for healing traumatic fracture of upper arm
   ● V54.12 Aftercare for healing traumatic fracture of lower arm
   ● V54.13 Aftercare for healing traumatic fracture of hip
   ● **V54.14** Aftercare for healing traumatic fracture of leg, unspecified
   ● V54.15 Aftercare for healing traumatic fracture of upper leg

> *Excludes:* aftercare for healing traumatic fracture of hip (V54.13)

   ● V54.16 Aftercare for healing traumatic fracture of lower leg
   ● V54.17 Aftercare for healing traumatic fracture of vertebrae
   ● **V54.19** Aftercare for healing traumatic fracture of other bone

● **V54.2** Aftercare for healing pathologic fracture

   ● **V54.20** Aftercare for healing pathologic fracture of arm, unspecified
   ● V54.21 Aftercare for healing pathologic fracture of upper arm
   ● V54.22 Aftercare for healing pathologic fracture of lower arm
   ● V54.23 Aftercare for healing pathologic fracture of hip
   ● **V54.24** Aftercare for healing pathologic fracture of leg, unspecified
   ● V54.25 Aftercare for healing pathologic fracture of upper leg

> *Excludes:* aftercare for healing pathologic fracture of hip (V54.23)

   ● V54.26 Aftercare for healing pathologic fracture of lower leg
   ● V54.27 Aftercare for healing pathologic fracture of vertebrae
   ● **V54.29** Aftercare for healing pathologic fracture of other bone

⑤ V54.8 **Other orthopedic aftercare**

   ● V54.81 **Aftercare following joint replacement**
Use additional code to identify joint replacement site (V43.60-V43.69)

   ● **V54.89** **Other orthopedic aftercare**
          Aftercare for healing fracture NOS

V54.9 **Unspecified orthopedic aftercare**

V55 Attention to artificial openings

Includes: adjustment or repositioning of catheter
           closure
           passage of sounds or bougies
           reforming
           removal or replacement of catheter
           toilet or cleansing

> *Excludes:* complications of external stoma (519.00-519.09, 569.60-569.69, 997.4, 997.5)
> status only, without need for care (V44.0-V44.9)

V55.0 **Tracheostomy**

V55.1 **Gastrostomy**

V55.2 **Ileostomy**

V55.3 **Colostomy**

V55.4 Other artificial opening of digestive tract

V55.5 **Cystostomy**

● Code new   ▲ Revision of   ④ ⑤ Fourth or fifth
           to this edition   existing code   digit required

V55.6 Other artificial opening of urinary tract
Nephrostomy
Urethrostomy
Ureterostomy

V55.7 Artificial vagina

V55.8 Other specified artificial opening

V55.9 Unspecified artificial opening

V56 Encounter for dialysis and dialysis catheter care
Use additional code to identify the associated condition

[Excludes:] *dialysis preparation—code to condition*

V56.0 Extracorporeal dialysis
Dialysis (renal) NOS

[Excludes:] *dialysis status (V45.1)*

V56.1 Fitting and adjustment of extracorporeal dialysis catheter
Removal or replacement of catheter
Toilet or cleansing

Use additional code for any concurrent extracorporeal dialysis (V56.0)

V56.2 Fitting and adjustment of peritoneal dialysis catheter
Use additional code for any concurrent peritoneal dialysis (V56.8)

[5] **V56.3 Encounter for adequacy testing for dialysis**

V56.31 Encounter for adequacy testing for hemodialysis

V56.32 Encounter for adequacy testing for peritoneal dialysis
Peritoneal equilibration test

V56.8 Other dialysis
Peritoneal dialysis

V57 Care involving use of rehabilitation procedures
Use additional code to identify underlying condition

V57.0 Breathing exercises

V57.1 Other physical therapy
Therapeutic and remedial exercises, except breathing

[5] **V57.2 Occupational therapy and vocational rehabilitation**

V57.21 Encounter for occupational therapy

V57.22 Encounter for vocational therapy

V57.3 Speech therapy

V57.4 Orthoptic training

[5] **V57.8 Other specified rehabilitation procedure**

V57.81 Orthotic training
Gait training in the use of artificial limbs

V57.89 Other
Multiple training or therapy

V57.9 Unspecified rehabilitation procedure

V58 Encounter for other and unspecified procedures and aftercare

[Excludes:] *convalescence and palliative care (V66)*

V58.0 Radiotherapy
Encounter or admission for radiotherapy

[Excludes:] *encounter for radioactive implant—code to condition*
radioactive iodine therapy—code to condition

V58.1 Chemotherapy
Encounter or admission for chemotherapy

[Excludes:] *prophylactic chemotherapy against disease which has never been present (V03.0-V07.9)*

V58.2 Blood transfusion, without reported diagnosis

V58.3 Attention to surgical dressings and sutures
Change of dressings
Removal of sutures

⑤ **V58.4 Other aftercare following surgery**

Note: Codes from this subcategory should be used in conjunction with other aftercare codes to fully identify the reason for the aftercare encounter

Excludes: *aftercare following sterilization reversal surgery (V26.22)*
attention to artificial openings (V55.0-V55.9)
orthopedic aftercare (V54.0-V54.9)

V58.41 Encounter for planned postoperative wound closure

Excludes: *disruption of operative wound (998.3)*

● **V58.42 Aftercare following surgery for neoplasm**
Conditions classifiable to 140-239

● **V58.43 Aftercare following surgery for injury and trauma**
Conditions classifiable to 800-999

Excludes: *aftercare for healing traumatic fracture (V54.10-V54.19)*

V58.49 Other specified aftercare following surgery

V58.5 Orthodontics

Excludes: *fitting and adjustment of orthodontic device (V53.4)*

⑤ **V58.6 Long-term (current) drug use**

Excludes: *drug abuse (305.00-305.93)*
drug dependence (304.00-304.93)

V58.61 Long-term (current) use of anticoagulants

V58.62 Long-term (current) use of antibiotics

V58.69 Long-term (current) use of other medications
High-risk medications

● **V58.7 Aftercare following surgery to specified body systems, not elsewhere classified**

Note: Codes from this subcategory should be used in conjunction with other aftercare codes to fully identify the reason for the aftercare encounter

● **V58.71 Aftercare following surgery of the sense organs, NEC**
Conditions classifiable to 360-379, 380-389

● **V58.72 Aftercare following surgery of the nervous system, NEC**
Conditions classifiable to 320-359

Excludes: *aftercare following surgery of the sense organs, NEC (V58.71)*

● **V58.73 Aftercare following surgery of the circulatory system, NEC**
Conditions classifiable to 390-459

● **V58.74 Aftercare following surgery of the respiratory system, NEC**
Conditions classifiable to 460-519

● **V58.75 Aftercare following suregery of the teeth, oral cavity and digestive system, NEC**
Conditions classifiable to 520-579

● **V58.76 Aftercare following surgery of the genitourinary system, NEC**
Conditions classifiable to 580-629

Excludes: *aftercare following sterilization reversal (V26.22)*

● **V58.77 Aftercare following surgery of the skin and subcutaneous tissue, NEC**
Conditions classifiable to 680-709

● **V58.78 Aftercare following surgery of the musculoskeletal system, NEC**
Conditions classifiable to 710-739

⑤ **V58.8 Other specified procedures and aftercare**

V58.81 Fitting and adjustment of vascular catheter
Removal or replacement of catheter
Toilet or cleansing

Excludes: *complication of renal dialysis catheter (996.73)*
complication of vascular catheter (996.74)
dialysis preparation — code to condition
encounter for dialysis (V56.0-V56.8)
fitting and adjustment of dialysis catheter (V56.1)

● Code new to this edition   ▲ Revision of existing code   ④ ⑤ Fourth or fifth digit required

V58.82 Fitting and adjustment of non-vascular catheter NEC
Removal or replacement of catheter
Toilet or cleansing

Excludes: *fitting and adjustment of peritoneal dialysis catheter (V56.2)*
fitting and adjustment of urinary catheter (V53.6)

V58.83 Encounter for therapeutic drug monitoring
Use additional code for any associated long-term (current) drug use (V58.61-V58.69)

Excludes: *blood-drug testing for medicolegal reasons (V70.4)*

V58.89 Other specified aftercare

V58.9 Unspecified aftercare

V59 Donors

Excludes: *examination of potential donor (V70.8)*
self-donation of organ or tissue—code to condition

⑤ **V59.0 Blood**

V59.01 Whole blood

V59.02 Stem cells

V59.09 Other

V59.1 Skin

V59.2 Bone

V59.3 Bone marrow

V59.4 Kidney

V59.5 Cornea

V59.6 Liver

V59.8 Other specified organ or tissue

V59.9 Unspecified organ or tissue

PERSONS ENCOUNTERING HEALTH SERVICES IN OTHER CIRCUMSTANCES (V60-V69)

V60 Housing, household, and economic circumstances

V60.0 Lack of housing

Hobos	Transients
Social migrants	Vagabonds
Tramps	

V60.1 Inadequate housing
Lack of heating
Restriction of space
Technical defects in home preventing adequate care

V60.2 Inadequate material resources

Economic problem	Poverty NOS

V60.3 Person living alone

V60.4 No other household member able to render care
Person requiring care (has) (is):
family member too handicapped, ill, or otherwise unsuited to render care
partner temporarily away from home
temporarily away from usual place of abode

Excludes: *holiday relief care (V60.5)*

V60.5 Holiday relief care
Provision of health care facilities to a person normally cared for at home, to enable
relatives to take a vacation

V60.6 Person living in residential institution
Boarding school resident

V60.8 Other specified housing or economic circumstances

V60.9 Unspecified housing or economic circumstance

V61 Other family circumstances
Includes: when these circumstances or fear of them, affecting the person directly involved
or others, are mentioned as the reason, justified or not, for seeking or receiving
medical advice or care

V61.0 Family disruption

Divorce	Estrangement

	Add 4th or 5th digit		Nonspecific code		Unspecified code		Manifestation code

⑤ **V61.1 Counseling for marital and partner problems**

Excludes: *problems related to:*
> *psychosexual disorders (302.0-302.9)*
> *sexual function (V41.7)*

> **V61.10 Counseling for marital and partner problems, unspecified**
> Marital conflict
> Partner conflict

> **V61.11 Counseling for victim of spousal and partner abuse**

Excludes: *encounter for treatment of current injuries due to abuse (995.80-995.85)*

> **V61.12 Counseling for perpetrator of spousal and partner abuse**

⑤ **V61.2 Parent-child problems**

> **V61.20 Counseling for parent-child problem, unspecified**
> Concern about behavior of child
> Parent-child conflict

> **V61.21 Counseling for victim of child abuse**
> Child battering
> Child neglect

Excludes: *current injuries due to abuse (995.50-995.59)*

> **V61.22 Counseling for perpetrator of parental child abuse**

Excludes: *counseling for non-parental abuser (V62.83)*

> **V61.29 Other**
> Problem concerning adopted or foster child

V61.3 Problems with aged parents or in-laws

⑤ **V61.4 Health problems within family**

> **V61.41 Alcoholism in family**

> **V61.49 Other**
> Care of sick or handicapped person in family or household
> Presence of sick or handicapped person in family or household

V61.5 Multiparity

V61.6 Illegitimacy or illegitimate pregnancy

V61.7 Other unwanted pregnancy

V61.8 Other specified family circumstances
> Problems with family members NEC

V61.9 Unspecified family circumstance

V62 Other psychosocial circumstances
> Includes: those circumstances or fear of them, affecting the person directly involved or others, mentioned as the reason, justified or not, for seeking or receiving medical advice or care

Excludes: *previous psychological trauma (V15.41-V15.49)*

V62.0 Unemployment

Excludes: *circumstances when main problem is economic inadequacy or poverty (V60.2)*

V62.1 Adverse effects of work environment

V62.2 Other occupational circumstances or maladjustment
> Career choice problem
> Dissatisfaction with employment

V62.3 Educational circumstances
> Dissatisfaction with school environment
> Educational handicap

V62.4 Social maladjustment
Cultural deprivation	Social:
Political, religious, or sex	isolation
discrimination	persecution

V62.5 Legal circumstances
Imprisonment	Litigation
Legal investigation	Prosecution

V62.6 Refusal of treatment for reasons of religion or conscience

⑤ **V62.8 Other psychological or physical stress, not elsewhere classified**

● Code new
to this edition
▲ Revision of
existing code
④ ⑤ Fourth or fifth
digit required

V62.81 Interpersonal problems, not elsewhere classified

V62.82 Bereavement, uncomplicated

[Excludes:] *bereavement as adjustment reaction (309.0)*

V62.83 Counseling for perpetrator of physical/sexual abuse

[Excludes:] *counseling for perpetrator of parental child abuse (V61.22)*
counseling for perpetrator of spousal and partner abuse (V61.12)

V62.89 Other
Life circumstance problems
Phase of life problems

V62.9 Unspecified psychosocial circumstance

V63 Unavailability of other medical facilities for care

V63.0 Residence remote from hospital or other health care facility

V63.1 Medical services in home not available

[Excludes:] *no other household member able to render care (V60.4)*

V63.2 Person awaiting admission to adequate facility elsewhere

V63.8 Other specified reasons for unavailability of medical facilities
Person on waiting list undergoing social agency investigation

V63.9 Unspecified reason for unavailability of medical facilities

V64 Persons encountering health services for specific procedures, not carried out

V64.0 Vaccination not carried out because of contraindication

V64.1 Surgical or other procedure not carried out because of contraindication

V64.2 Surgical or other procedure not carried out because of patient's decision

V64.3 Procedure not carried out for other reasons

V64.4 Laparoscopic surgical procedure converted to open procedure

V65 Other persons seeking consultation without complaint or sickness

V65.0 Healthy person accompanying sick person
Boarder

V65.1 Person consulting on behalf of another person
Advice or treatment for nonattending third party

[Excludes:] *concern (normal) about sick person in family (V61.41-V61.49)*

V65.2 Person feigning illness
Malingerer
Peregrinating patient

V65.3 Dietary surveillance and counseling
Dietary surveillance and counseling (in):
NOS
colitis
diabetes mellitus
food allergies or intolerance
gastritis
hypercholesterolemia
hypoglycemia
obesity

[5] **V65.4 Other counseling, not elsewhere classified**
Health:
advice
education
instruction

[Excludes:] *counseling (for):*
contraception (V25.40-V25.49)
genetic (V26.3)
on behalf of third party (V65.1)
procreative management (V26.4)

V65.40 Counseling NOS

V65.41 Exercise counseling

V65.42 Counseling on substance use and abuse

V65.43 Counseling on injury prevention

V65.44 Human immunodeficiency virus [HIV] counseling

Add 4th or 5th digit | Nonspecific code | Unspecified code | Manifestation code

V65.45 Counseling on other sexually transmitted diseases

V65.49 Other specified counseling

V65.5 Person with feared complaint in whom no diagnosis was made
Feared condition not demonstrated
Problem was normal state
"Worried well"

V65.8 Other reasons for seeking consultation
[Excludes:] *specified symptoms*

V65.9 Unspecified reason for consultation

V66 Convalescence and palliative care

V66.0 Following surgery

V66.1 Following radiotherapy

V66.2 Following chemotherapy

V66.3 Following psychotherapy and other treatment for mental disorder

V66.4 Following treatment of fracture

V66.5 Following other treatment

V66.6 Following combined treatment

V66.7 Encounter for palliative care
End-of-life care
Hospice care
Terminal care

Code first underlying disease

V66.9 Unspecified convalescence

V67 Follow-up examination
Includes: surveillance only following completed treatment
[Excludes:] *surveillance of contraception (V25.40-V25.49)*

⑤ **V67.0 Following surgery**

V67.00 Following surgery, unspecified

V67.01 Follow-up vaginal pap smear
Vaginal pap smear, status-post hysterectomy for malignant condition
Use additional code to identify:
acquired absence of uterus (V45.77)
personal history of malignant neoplasm (V10.40-V10.44)
[Excludes:] *vaginal pap smear status-post hysterectomy for non-malignant condition (V76.47)*

V67.09 Following other surgery
[Excludes:] *sperm count following sterilization reversal (V26.22)*
sperm count for fertility testing (V26.21)

V67.1 Following radiotherapy

V67.2 Following chemotherapy
Cancer chemotherapy follow-up

V67.3 Following psychotherapy and other treatment for mental disorder

V67.4 Following treatment of healed fracture
[Excludes:] *current (healing) fracture aftercare (V54.0-V54.9)*

⑤ **V67.5 Following other treatment**

V67.51 Following completed treatment with high-risk medication, NEC
[Excludes:] *long-term (current) drug use (V58.61-V58.69)*

V67.59 Other

V67.6 Following combined treatment

V67.9 Unspecified follow-up examination

V68 Encounters for administrative purposes

V68.0 Issue of medical certificates
Issue of medical certificate of: cause of death
fitness
incapacity
[Excludes:] *encounter for general medical examination (V70.0-V70.9)*

● Code new to this edition ▲ Revision of existing code ④ ⑤ Fourth or fifth digit required

V68.1 Issue of repeat prescriptions
Issue of repeat prescription for: appliance
glasses
medications

Excludes: *repeat prescription for contraceptives (V25.41-V25.49)*

V68.2 Request for expert evidence

⑤ **V68.8 Other specified administrative purpose**

    V68.81 Referral of patient without examination or treatment

    V68.89 Other

V68.9 Unspecified administrative purpose

V69 Problems related to lifestyle

V69.0 Lack of physical exercise

V69.1 Inappropriate diet and eating habits

Excludes: *anorexia nervosa (307.1)*
bulimia (783.6)
malnutrition and other nutritional deficiencies (260-269.9)
other and unspecified eating disorders (307.50-307.59)

V69.2 High-risk sexual behavior

V69.3 Gambling and betting

Excludes: *pathological gambling (312.31)*

V69.8 Other problems related to lifestyle
Self-damaging behavior

V69.9 Problem related to lifestyle, unspecified

PERSONS WITHOUT REPORTED DIAGNOSIS ENCOUNTERED DURING EXAMINATION AND INVESTIGATION OF INDIVIDUALS AND POPULATIONS (V70-V83)

Note: Nonspecific abnormal findings disclosed at the time of these examinations are classifiable to categories 790-796.

V70 General medical examination
Use additional code(s) to identify any special screening examination(s) performed (V73.0-V82.9)

V70.0 Routine general medical examination at a health care facility
Health checkup

Excludes: *health checkup of infant or child (V20.2)*

V70.1 General psychiatric examination, requested by the authority

V70.2 General psychiatric examination, other and unspecified

V70.3 Other medical examination for administrative purposes
General medical examination for:
admission to old age home   marriage
adoption   prison
camp   school admission
driving license   sports competition
immigration and naturalization
insurance certification

Excludes: *attendance for issue of medical certificates (V68.0)*
pre-employment screening (V70.5)

V70.4 Examination for medicolegal reasons
Blood-alcohol tests
Blood-drug tests
Paternity testing

Excludes: *examination and observation following:*
accidents (V71.3, V71.4)
assault (V71.6)
rape (V71.5)

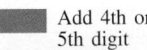 Add 4th or
5th digit

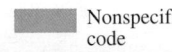 Nonspecific
code

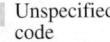 Unspecified
code

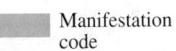 Manifestation
code

V70.5 Health examination of defined subpopulations

Armed forces personnel
Inhabitants of institutions
Occupational health
   examinations
Pre-employment screening

Preschool children
Prisoners
Prostitutes
Refugees
School children
Students

V70.6 Health examination in population surveys

Excludes: *special screening (V73.0-V82.9)*

V70.7 Examination of participant in clinical trial
Examination of participant or control in clinical research

V70.8 Other specified general medical examinations
Examination of potential donor of organ or tissue

V70.9 Unspecified general medical examination

V71 Observation and evaluation for suspected conditions not found

Note: This category is to be used when persons without a diagnosis are suspected of having an
abnormal condition, without signs or symptoms, which requires study, but after
examination and observation, is found not to exist. This category is also for use for
administrative and legal observation status.

⑤ **V71.0 Observation for suspected mental condition**

V71.01 Adult antisocial behavior
Dyssocial behavior or gang activity in adult without manifest psychiatric
disorder

V71.02 Childhood or adolescent antisocial behavior
Dyssocial behavior or gang activity in child or adolescent without manifest
psychiatric disorder

V71.09 Other suspected mental condition

V71.1 Observation for suspected malignant neoplasm

V71.2 Observation for suspected tuberculosis

V71.3 Observation following accident at work

V71.4 Observation following other accident
Examination of individual involved in motor vehicle traffic accident

V71.5 Observation following alleged rape or seduction
Examination of victim or culprit

V71.6 Observation following other inflicted injury
Examination of victim or culprit

V71.7 Observation for suspected cardiovascular disease

▲ **V71.8 Observation and evaluation for other specified suspected conditions**

V71.81 Abuse and neglect

Excludes: *adult abuse and neglect (995.80-995.85)*
child abuse and neglect (995.50-995.59)

● **V71.82 Observation and evaluation for suspected exposure to anthrax**

● **V71.83 Observation and evaluation for suspected exposure to other biological agent**

V71.89 Other specified suspected conditions

V71.9 Observation for unspecified suspected condition

V72 Special investigations and examinations
Includes: routine examination of specific system

Excludes: *general medical examination (V70.0-V70.4)*
general screening examination of defined population groups (V70.5, V70.6, V70.7)
routine examination of infant or child (V20.2)

Use additional code(s) to identify any special screening examination(s) performed (V73.0-V82.9)

V72.0 Examination of eyes and vision

V72.1 Examination of ears and hearing

V72.2 Dental examination

● Code new
to this edition   ▲ Revision of
existing code   ④ ⑤ Fourth or fifth
digit required

V72.3 Gynecological examination
Papanicolaou cervical smear as part of general gynecological examination
Pelvic examination (annual) (periodic)

Use additional code to identify routine vaginal Papanicolaou smear (V76.47)

[Excludes:] *cervical Papanicolaou smear without general gynecological examination (V76.2)*
routine examination in contraceptive management (V25.40-V25.49)

V72.4 Pregnancy examination or test, pregnancy unconfirmed
Possible pregnancy, not (yet) confirmed

[Excludes:] *pregnancy examination with immediate confirmation (V22.0-V22.1)*

V72.5 Radiological examination, not elsewhere classified
Routine chest x-ray

[Excludes:] *examination for suspected tuberculosis (V71.2)*

V72.6 Laboratory examination

[Excludes:] *that for suspected disorder (V71.0-V71.9)*

V72.7 Diagnostic skin and sensitization tests
Allergy tests
Skin tests for hypersensitivity

[Excludes:] *diagnostic skin tests for bacterial diseases (V74.0-V74.9)*

[5] **V72.8 Other specified examinations**

V72.81 Pre-operative cardiovascular examination

V72.82 Pre-operative respiratory examination

V72.83 Other specified pre-operative examination

V72.84 Pre-operative examination, unspecified

V72.85 Other specified examination

V72.9 Unspecified examination

V73 Special screening examination for viral and chlamydial diseases

V73.0 Poliomyelitis

V73.1 Smallpox

V73.2 Measles

V73.3 Rubella

V73.4 Yellow fever

V73.5 Other arthropod-borne viral diseases
Dengue fever
Hemorrhagic fever
Viral encephalitis:
mosquito-borne
tick-borne

V73.6 Trachoma

[5] **V73.8 Other specified viral and chlamydial diseases**

V73.88 Other specified chlamydial diseases

V73.89 Other specified viral diseases

[5] **V73.9 Unspecified viral and chlamydial disease**

V73.98 Unspecified chlamydial disease

V73.99 Unspecified viral disease

V74 Special screening examination for bacterial and spirochetal diseases
Includes: diagnostic skin tests for these diseases

V74.0 Cholera

V74.1 Pulmonary tuberculosis

V74.2 Leprosy [Hansen's disease]

V74.3 Diphtheria

V74.4 Bacterial conjunctivitis

V74.5 Venereal disease

V74.6 Yaws

V74.8 Other specified bacterial and spirochetal diseases
Brucellosis
Leptospirosis
Plague
Tetanus
Whooping cough

Add 4th or 5th digit | Nonspecific code | Unspecified code | Manifestation code

V74.9 **Unspecified bacterial and spirochetal disease**

V75 **Special screening examination for other infectious diseases**

V75.0 **Rickettsial diseases**

V75.1 **Malaria**

V75.2 **Leishmaniasis**

V75.3 **Trypanosomiasis**
Chagas' disease   Sleeping sickness

V75.4 **Mycotic infections**

V75.5 **Schistosomiasis**

V75.6 **Filariasis**

V75.7 **Intestinal helminthiasis**

V75.8 **Other specified parasitic infections**

V75.9 **Unspecified infectious disease**

V76 **Special screening for malignant neoplasms**

V76.0 **Respiratory organs**

⑤ V76.1 **Breast**

V76.10 **Breast screening, unspecified**

V76.11 **Screening mammogram for high-risk patient**

V76.12 **Other screening mammogram**

V76.19 **Other screening breast examination**

V76.2 **Cervix**
Routine cervical Papanicolaou smear

Excludes: *that as part of a general gynecological examination (V72.3)*

V76.3 **Bladder**

⑤ V76.4 **Other sites**

V76.41 **Rectum**

V76.42 **Oral cavity**

V76.43 **Skin**

V76.44 **Prostate**

V76.45 **Testis**

V76.46 **Ovary**

V76.47 **Vagina**
Vaginal pap smear status-post hysterectomy for non-malignant condition
Use additional code to identify acquired absence of uterus (V45.77)

Excludes: *vaginal pap smear status-post hysterectomy for malignant condition (V67.01)*

V76.49 **Other sites**

⑤ V76.5 **Intestine**

V76.50 **Intestine, unspecified**

V76.51 **Colon**

Excludes: *rectum (V76.41)*

V76.52 **Small intestine**

⑤ V76.8 **Other neoplasm**

V76.81 **Nervous system**

V76.89 **Other neoplasm**

V76.9 **Unspecified**

V77 **Special screening for endocrine, nutritional, metabolic, and immunity disorders**

V77.0 **Thyroid disorders**

V77.1 **Diabetes mellitus**

V77.2 **Malnutrition**

V77.3 **Phenylketonuria [PKU]**

V77.4 **Galactosemia**

V77.5 **Gout**

● Code new
to this edition   ▲ Revision of
existing code   ④ ⑤ Fourth or fifth
digit required

V77.6 Cystic fibrosis
Screening for mucoviscidosis

V77.7 Other inborn errors of metabolism

V77.8 Obesity

⑤ **V77.9 Other and unspecified endocrine, nutritional, metabolic, and immunity disorders**

    V77.91 Screening for lipoid disorders
        Screening cholesterol level
        Screening for hypercholesterolemia
        Screening for hyperlipidemia

    V77.99 Other and unspecified endocrine, nutritional, metabolic, and immunity disorders

V78 Special screening for disorders of blood and blood-forming organs

V78.0 Iron deficiency anemia

V78.1 Other and unspecified deficiency anemia

V78.2 Sickle-cell disease or trait

V78.3 Other hemoglobinopathies

V78.8 Other disorders of blood and blood-forming organs

V78.9 Unspecified disorder of blood and blood-forming organs

V79 Special screening for mental disorders and developmental handicaps

V79.0 Depression

V79.1 Alcoholism

V79.2 Mental retardation

V79.3 Developmental handicaps in early childhood

V79.8 Other specified mental disorders and developmental handicaps

V79.9 Unspecified mental disorder and developmental handicap

V80 Special screening for neurological, eye, and ear diseases

V80.0 Neurological conditions

V80.1 Glaucoma

V80.2 Other eye conditions
Screening for:
    cataract
    congenital anomaly of eye
    senile macular lesions

    Excludes: *general vision examination (V72.0)*

V80.3 Ear diseases
    Excludes: *general hearing examination (V72.1)*

V81 Special screening for cardiovascular, respiratory, and genitourinary diseases

V81.0 Ischemic heart disease

V81.1 Hypertension

V81.2 Other and unspecified cardiovascular conditions

V81.3 Chronic bronchitis and emphysema

V81.4 Other and unspecified respiratory conditions
    Excludes: *screening for:*
        lung neoplasm (V76.0)
        pulmonary tuberculosis (V74.1)

V81.5 Nephropathy
Screening for asymptomatic bacteriuria

V81.6 Other and unspecified genitourinary conditions

V82 Special screening for other conditions

V82.0 Skin conditions

V82.1 Rheumatoid arthritis

V82.2 Other rheumatic disorders

V82.3 Congenital dislocation of hip

	Add 4th or 5th digit		Nonspecific code		Unspecified code		Manifestation code

V82.4 Maternal postnatal screening for chromosomal anomalies

> *Excludes:* *antenatal screening by amniocentesis (V28.0)*

V82.5 Chemical poisoning and other contamination
Screening for:
heavy metal poisoning
ingestion of radioactive substance
poisoning from contaminated water supply
radiation exposure

V82.6 Multiphasic screening

⑤ **V82.8 Other specified conditions**

V82.81 Osteoporosis
Use additional code to identify:
postmenopausal hormone replacement therapy status (V07.4)
postmenopausal (natural) status (V49.81)

V82.89 Other specified conditions

V82.9 Unspecified condition

V83 Genetic carrier status

⑤ **V83.0 Hemophilia A carrier**

V83.01 Asymptomatic hemophilia A carrier

V83.02 Symptomatic hemophilia A carrier

● **V83.8 Other genetic carrier status**

● **V83.81 Cystic fibrosis gene carrier**

● **V83.89 Other genetic carrier status**

● Code new
to this edition

▲ Revision of
existing code

④ ⑤ Fourth or fifth
digit required

SUPPLEMENTARY CLASSIFICATION OF EXTERNAL CAUSES OF INJURY AND POISONING (E800-E999)

This section is provided to permit the classification of environmental events, circumstances, and conditions as the cause of injury, poisoning, and other adverse effects. Where a code from this section is applicable, it is intended that it shall be used in addition to a code from one of the main chapters of *ICD-9-CM*, indicating the nature of the condition. Certain other conditions which may be stated to be due to external causes are classified in Chapters 1 to 16 of *ICD-9-CM*. For these, the "E" code classification should be used for more detailed analysis.

Machinery accidents [other than those connected with transport] are classifiable to category E919, in which the fourth-digit allows a broad classification of the type of machinery involved. If a more detailed classification of type of machinery is required, it is suggested that the "Classification of Industrial Accidents according to Agency," prepared by the International Labor Office, be used in addition. This is reproduced on page 571, for optional use.

Categories for "late effects" of accidents and other external causes are to be found at E929, E959, E969, E977, E989, and E999.

Definitions and examples related to transport accidents

(a) A **transport accident** (E800-E848) is any accident involving a device designed primarily for, or being used at the time primarily for, conveying persons or goods from one place to another.

Includes: accidents involving:
    aircraft and spacecraft (E840-E845)
    watercraft (E830-E838)
    motor vehicle (E810-E825)
    railway (E800-E807)
    other road vehicles (E826-E829)

In classifying accidents which involve more than one kind of transport, the above order of precedence of transport accidents should be used.

Accidents involving agriculture and construction machines, such as tractors, cranes, and bulldozers, are regarded as transport accidents only when these vehicles are under their own power on a highway [otherwise the vehicles are regarded as machinery]. Vehicles which can travel on land or water, such as hovercraft and other amphibious vehicles, are regarded as watercraft when on the water, as motor vehicles when on the highway, and as off-road motor vehicles when on land, but off the highway.

Excludes: *accidents:*
    in sports which involve the use of transport but where the transport vehicle itself was not involved in the accident
    involving vehicles which are part of industrial equipment used entirely on industrial premises
    occurring during transportation but unrelated to the hazards associated with the means of transportation [e.g., injuries received in a fight on board ship; transport vehicle involved in a cataclysm such as an earthquake]
    to persons engaged in the maintenance or repair of transport equipment or vehicle not in motion, unless injured by another vehicle in motion

(b) A **railway accident** is a transport accident involving a railway train or other railway vehicle operated on rails, whether in motion or not.

Excludes: *accidents:*
    in repair shops
    in roundhouse or on turntable
    on railway premises but not involving a train or other railway vehicle

(c) A **railway train** or **railway vehicle** is any device with or without cars coupled to it, designed for traffic on a railway.

Includes: interurban:
    electric car (operated chiefly on its own right-of-way, not open to other traffic)
    streetcar (operated chiefly on its own right-of-way, not open to other traffic)
    railway train, any power [diesel] [electric] [steam]
    funicular
    monorail or two-rail
    subterranean or elevated
    other vehicle designed to run on a railway track

Excludes: *interurban electric cars [streetcars] specified to be operating on a right-of-way that forms part of the public street or highway [definition (n)]*

(d) A **railway** or **railroad** is a right-of-way designed for traffic on rails, which is used by carriages or wagons transporting passengers or freight, and by other rolling stock, and which is not open to other public vehicular traffic.

	Add 4th or 5th digit		Nonspecific code		Unspecified code		Manifestation code

(e) A **motor vehicle accident** is a transport accident involving a motor vehicle. It is defined as a motor vehicle traffic accident or as a motor vehicle nontraffic accident according to whether the accident occurs on a public highway or elsewhere.

> Excludes: *injury or damage due to cataclysm*
>
> *injury or damage while a motor vehicle, not under its own power, is being loaded on, or unloaded from, another conveyance*

(f) A **motor vehicle traffic accident** is any motor vehicle accident occurring on a public highway [i.e., originating, terminating, or involving a vehicle partially on the highway]. A motor vehicle accident is assumed to have occurred on the highway unless another place is specified, except in the case of accidents involving only off-road motor vehicles which are classified as nontraffic accidents unless the contrary is stated.

(g) A **motor vehicle nontraffic accident** is any motor vehicle accident which occurs entirely in any place other than a public highway.

(h) A **public highway [trafficway]** or **street** is the entire width between property lines [or other boundary lines] of every way or place, of which any part is open to the use of the public for purposes of vehicular traffic as a matter of right or custom. A roadway is that part of the public highway designed, improved, and ordinarily used, for vehicular travel.

Includes: approaches (public) to:
  docks
  public building
  station

> Excludes: *driveway (private)*
>
> *parking lot*
> *ramp*
> *roads in:*
> *airfield*
> *farm*
> *industrial premises*
> *mine*
> *private grounds*
> *quarry*

(i) A **motor vehicle** is any mechanically or electrically powered device, not operated on rails, upon which any person or property may be transported or drawn upon a highway. Any object such as a trailer, coaster, sled, or wagon being towed by a motor vehicle is considered a part of the motor vehicle.

Includes: automobile [any type]
  bus
  construction machinery, farm and industrial machinery, steam roller, tractor, army tank, highway grader, or similar vehicle on wheels or treads, while in transport under own power
  fire engine (motorized)
  motorcycle
  motorized bicycle [moped] or scooter
  trolley bus not operating on rails
  truck
  van

> Excludes: *devices used solely to move persons or materials within the confines of a building and its premises, such as:*
> *building elevator*
> *coal car in mine*
> *electric baggage or mail truck used solely within a railroad station*
> *electric truck used solely within an industrial plant*
> *moving overhead crane*

(j) A **motorcycle** is a two-wheeled motor vehicle having one or two riding saddles and sometimes having a third wheel for the support of a sidecar. The sidecar is considered part of the motorcycle.

Includes: motorized:
  bicycle [moped]
  scooter
  tricycle

(k) An **off-road motor vehicle** is a motor vehicle of special design, to enable it to negotiate rough or soft terrain or snow. Examples of special design are high construction, special wheels and tires, driven by treads, or support on a cushion of air.

Includes: all terrain vehicle [ATV]
  army tank
  hovercraft, on land or swamp
  snowmobile

● Code new
to this edition   ▲ Revision of
existing code   ④ ⑤ Fourth or fifth
digit required

(l) A **driver** of a motor vehicle is the occupant of the motor vehicle operating it or intending to operate it. A **motorcyclist** is the driver of a motorcycle. Other authorized occupants of a motor vehicle are **passengers.**

(m) An **other road vehicle** is any device, except a motor vehicle, in, on, or by which any person or property may be transported on a highway.

Includes: animal carrying a person or goods
animal-drawn vehicle
animal harnessed to conveyance
bicycle [pedal cycle]
streetcar
tricycle (pedal)

Excludes: *pedestrian conveyance [definition (q)]*

(n) A **streetcar** is a device designed and used primarily for transporting persons within a municipality, running on rails, usually subject to normal traffic control signals, and operated principally on a right-of-way that forms part of the traffic way. A trailer being towed by a streetcar is considered a part of the streetcar.

Includes: interurban or intraurban electric or streetcar, when specified to be operating on a street or public highway
tram (car)
trolley (car)

(o) A **pedal cycle** is any road transport vehicle operated solely by pedals.

Includes: bicycle
pedal cycle
tricycle

Excludes: *motorized bicycle [definition (i)]*

(p) A **pedal cyclist** is any person riding on a pedal cycle or in a sidecar attached to such a vehicle.

(q) A **pedestrian conveyance** is any human powered device by which a pedestrian may move other than by walking or by which a walking person may move another pedestrian.

Includes:

baby carriage	roller skates
coaster wagon	scooter
ice skates	skateboard
perambulator	skis
pushcart	sled
pushchair	wheelchair

(r) A **pedestrian** is any person involved in an accident who was not at the time of the accident riding in or on a motor vehicle, railroad train, streetcar, animal-drawn or other vehicle, or on a bicycle or animal.

Includes: person:
changing tire of vehicle
in or operating a pedestrian conveyance
making adjustment to motor of vehicle
on foot

(s) A **watercraft** is any device for transporting passengers or goods on the water.

(t) A **small boat** is any watercraft propelled by paddle, oars, or small motor, with a passenger capacity of less than ten.

Includes:

boat NOS	rowboat
canoe	rowing shell
coble	scull
dinghy	skiff
punt	small motorboat
raft	

Excludes: *barge*
lifeboat (used after abandoning ship)
raft (anchored) being used as diving platform
yacht

(u) An **aircraft** is any device for transporting passengers or goods in the air.

Includes: airplane [any type]
balloon
bomber
dirigible
glider (hang)
military aircraft
parachute

� Add 4th or 5th digit	▪ Nonspecific code	▫ Unspecified code	▪ Manifestation code

(v) A **commercial transport aircraft** is any device for collective passenger or freight transportation by air, whether run on commercial lines for profit or by government authorities, with the exception of military craft.

RAILWAY ACCIDENTS (E800-E807)

Note: For definitions of railway accident and related terms see definitions (a) to (d).

Excludes: *accidents involving railway train and:*
  aircraft (E840.0-E845.9)
  motor vehicle (E810.0-E825.9)
  watercraft (E830.0-E838.9)

The following fourth-digit subdivisions are for use with categories E800-E807 to identify the injured person:

.0 Railway employee
  Any person who by virtue of his employment in connection with a railway, whether by the railway company or not, is at increased risk of involvement in a railway accident, such as:
  catering staff of train
  driver
  guard
  porter
  postal staff on train
  railway fireman
  shunter
  sleeping car attendant

.1 Passenger on railway
  Any authorized person traveling on a train, except a railway employee.

Excludes: *intending passenger waiting at station (.8)*
  unauthorized rider on railway vehicle (.8)

.2 Pedestrian
  See definition (r)

.3 Pedal cyclist
  See definition (p)

.8 Other specified person
  Intending passenger or bystander waiting at station
  Unauthorized rider on railway vehicle

.9 Unspecified person

④ **E800 Railway accident involving collision with rolling stock**
  Includes: collision between railway trains or railway vehicles, any kind
  collision NOS on railway
  derailment with antecedent collision with rolling stock or NOS

④ **E801 Railway accident involving collision with other object**
  Includes: collision of railway train with:
  buffers
  fallen tree on railway
  gates
  platform
  rock on railway
  streetcar
  other nonmotor vehicle
  other object

  Excludes: *collision with:*
  aircraft (E840.0-E842.9)
  motor vehicle (E810.0-E810.9, E820.0-E822.9)

④ **E802 Railway accident involving derailment without antecedent collision**

④ **E803 Railway accident involving explosion, fire, or burning**
  Excludes: *explosion or fire, with antecedent derailment (E802.0-E802.9)*
  explosion or fire, with mention of antecedent collision (E800.0-E801.9)

④ **E804 Fall in, on, or from railway train**
  Includes: fall while alighting from or boarding railway train
  Excludes: *fall related to collision, derailment, or explosion of railway train (E800.0-E803.9)*

● Code new
  to this edition   ▲ Revision of
  existing code   ④ ⑤ Fourth or fifth
  digit required

④ **E805** **Hit by rolling stock**
　　Includes:

　　　　　　crushed by railway train or part
　　　　　　injured by railway train or part
　　　　　　killed by railway train or part
　　　　　　knocked down by railway train or part
　　　　　　run over by railway train or part

　　　Excludes: pedestrian hit by object set in motion by railway train (E806.0-E806.9)

④ **E806** **Other specified railway accident**
　　Includes:　hit by object falling in railway train
　　　　　　injured by door or window on railway train
　　　　　　nonmotor road vehicle or pedestrian hit by object set in motion by railway train
　　　　　　railway train hit by falling:
　　　　　　　earth NOS
　　　　　　　rock
　　　　　　　tree
　　　　　　　other object

　　　Excludes: railway accident due to cataclysm (E908-E909)

④ **E807** **Railway accident of unspecified nature**
　　Includes:

　　　　　　found dead on railway right-of-way NOS
　　　　　　injured on railway right-of-way NOS
　　　　　　railway accident NOS

MOTOR VEHICLE TRAFFIC ACCIDENTS (E810-E819)

Note: For definitions of motor vehicle traffic accident, and related terms, see definitions (e) to (k).

　　Excludes: accidents involving motor vehicle and aircraft (E840.0-E845.9)

The following fourth-digit subdivisions are for use with categories E810-E819 to identify the injured person:

　.0 Driver of motor vehicle other than motorcycle
　　　See definition (l)

　.1 Passenger in motor vehicle other than motorcycle
　　　See definition (l)

　.2 Motorcyclist
　　　See definition (l)

　.3 Passenger on motorcycle
　　　See definition (l)

　.4 Occupant of streetcar

　.5 Rider of animal; occupant of animal-drawn vehicle

　.6 Pedal cyclist
　　　See definition (p)

　.7 Pedestrian
　　　See definition (r)

　.8 Other specified person
　　　Occupant of vehicle other than above
　　　Person in railway train involved in accident
　　　Unauthorized rider of motor vehicle

　.9 Unspecified person

④ **E810** **Motor vehicle traffic accident involving collision with train**

　　　Excludes: motor vehicle collision with object set in motion by railway train (E815.0-E815.9)
　　　　　　railway train hit by object set in motion by motor vehicle (E818.0-E818.9)

④ **E811** **Motor vehicle traffic accident involving re-entrant collision with another motor vehicle**
　　Includes:　collision between motor vehicle which accidentally leaves the roadway then
　　　　　　re-enters the same roadway, or the opposite roadway on a divided highway,
　　　　　　and another motor vehicle

　　　Excludes: collision on the same roadway when none of the motor vehicles involved have left
　　　　　　and re-entered the roadway (E812.0-E812.9)

④ **E812** **Other motor vehicle traffic accident involving collision with motor vehicle**
　　Includes:　collision with another motor vehicle parked, stopped, stalled, disabled, or
　　　　　　abandoned on the highway
　　　　　　motor vehicle collision NOS

　　　Excludes: collision with object set in motion by another motor vehicle (E815.0-E815.9)
　　　　　　re-entrant collision with another motor vehicle (E811.0-E811.9)

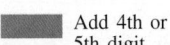 Add 4th or 5th digit　　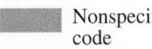 Nonspecific code　　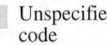 Unspecified code　　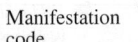 Manifestation code

④ **E813** **Motor vehicle traffic accident involving collision with other vehicle**
  Includes: collision between motor vehicle, any kind, and:
      other road (nonmotor transport) vehicle, such as:
        animal carrying a person
        animal-drawn vehicle
        pedal cycle
        streetcar

  Excludes: *collision with:*
        object set in motion by nonmotor road vehicle (E815.0-E815.9)
        pedestrian (E814.0-E814.9)
        nonmotor road vehicle hit by object set in motion by motor vehicle
          (E818.0-E818.9)

④ **E814** **Motor vehicle traffic accident involving collision with pedestrian**
  Includes: collision between motor vehicle, any kind, and pedestrian
      pedestrian dragged, hit, or run over by motor vehicle, any kind

  Excludes: *pedestrian hit by object set in motion by motor vehicle (E818.0-E818.9)*

④ **E815** **Other motor vehicle traffic accident involving collision on the highway**
  Includes: collision (due to loss of control) (on highway) between motor vehicle, any kind, and:
      abutment (bridge) (overpass)
      animal (herded) (unattended)
      fallen stone, traffic sign, tree, utility pole
      guard rail or boundary fence
      interhighway divider
      landslide (not moving)
      object set in motion by railway train or road vehicle (motor) (nonmotor)
      object thrown in front of motor vehicle
      safety island
      temporary traffic sign or marker
      wall of cut made for road
      other object, fixed, movable, or moving

  Excludes: *collision with:*
        any object off the highway (resulting from loss of control) (E816.0-E816.9)
        any object which normally would have been off the highway and is not stated to
          have been on it (E816.0-E816.9)
        motor vehicle parked, stopped, stalled, disabled, or abandoned on highway
          (E812.0-E812.9)
        moving landslide (E909)
      motor vehicle hit by object:
        set in motion by railway train or road vehicle (motor) (nonmotor)
          (E818.0-E818.9)
        thrown into or on vehicle (E818.0-E818.9)

④ **E816** **Motor vehicle traffic accident due to loss of control, without collision on the highway**
  Includes: motor vehicle:
      failing to make curve and colliding with object off the highway, overturning, or
        stopping abruptly off the highway
      going out of control (due to):
        blowout and colliding with object off the highway, overturning, or stopping
          abruptly off the highway
        burst tire and colliding with object off the highway, overturning, or stopping
          abruptly off the highway
        driver falling asleep and colliding with object off the highway, or overturning,
          stopping abruptly off the highway
        driver inattention and colliding with object off the highway, or overturning,
          stopping abruptly off the highway
        excessive speed and colliding with object off the highway, or overturning,
          stopping abruptly off the highway
        failure of mechanical part and colliding with object off the highway,
          overturning, or stopping abruptly off the highway

  Excludes: *collision on highway following loss of control (E810.0-E815.9)*
      loss of control of motor vehicle following collision on the highway
        (E810.0-E815.9)

④ **E817** **Noncollision motor vehicle traffic accident while boarding or alighting**
  Includes:
        fall down stairs of motor bus while boarding or alighting
        fall from car in street while boarding or alighting
        injured by moving part of the vehicle while boarding or alighting
        trapped by door of motor bus while boarding or alighting

● Code new   ▲ Revision of   ④ ⑤ Fourth or fifth
      to this edition   existing code   digit required

④ **E818** **Other noncollision motor vehicle traffic accident**
　　　Includes:
　　　　　　　accidental poisoning from exhaust gas generated by motor vehicle while in motion
　　　　　　　breakage of any part of motor vehicle while in motion
　　　　　　　explosion of any part of motor vehicle while in motion
　　　　　　　fall, jump, or being accidentally pushed from motor vehicle while in motion
　　　　　　　fire starting in motor vehicle while in motion
　　　　　　　hit by object thrown into or on motor vehicle while in motion
　　　　　　　injured by being thrown against some part of, or object in motor vehicle while in
　　　　　　　　　motion
　　　　　　　injury from moving part of motor vehicle while in motion
　　　　　　　object falling in or on motor vehicle while in motion
　　　　　　　object thrown on motor vehicle while in motion
　　　　　　　collision of railway train or road vehicle except motor vehicle, with object set in
　　　　　　　　　motion by motor vehicle
　　　　　　　motor vehicle hit by object set in motion by railway train or road vehicle (motor)
　　　　　　　　　(nonmotor)
　　　　　　　pedestrian, railway train, or road vehicle (motor) (nonmotor) hit by object set in
　　　　　　　　　motion by motor vehicle

　　　Excludes: *collision between motor vehicle and:*
　　　　　　　object set in motion by railway train or road vehicle (motor) (nonmotor)
　　　　　　　　(E815.0-E815.9)
　　　　　　　object thrown towards the motor vehicle (E815.0-E815.9)
　　　　　　　person overcome by carbon monoxide generated by stationary motor vehicle off
　　　　　　　　the roadway with motor running (E868.2)

④ **E819** **Motor vehicle traffic accident of unspecified nature**
　　　Includes:
　　　　　　　motor vehicle traffic accident NOS
　　　　　　　traffic accident NOS

MOTOR VEHICLE NONTRAFFIC ACCIDENTS (E820-E825)

　　　Note: For definitions of motor vehicle nontraffic accident and related terms see definitions (a) to
　　　　　(k).
　　　Includes: accidents involving motor vehicles being used in recreational or sporting activities
　　　　　　　off
　　　　　　　　the highway
　　　　　　　collision and noncollision motor vehicle accidents occurring entirely off the
　　　　　　　　highway

　　　Excludes: *accidents involving motor vehicle and:*
　　　　　　　aircraft (E840.0-E845.9)
　　　　　　　watercraft (E830.0-E838.9)
　　　　　　　accidents, not on the public highway, involving agricultural and construction
　　　　　　　　machinery but not involving another motor vehicle (E919.0, E919.2, E919.7)

　　　The following fourth-digit subdivisions are for use with categories E820-E825 to identify the
　　　　　injured person:

　　.0 **Driver of motor vehicle other than motorcycle**
　　　　See definition (l)

　　.1 **Passenger in motor vehicle other than motorcycle**
　　　　See definition (l)

　　.2 **Motorcyclist**
　　　　See definition (l)

　　.3 **Passenger on motorcycle**
　　　　See definition (l)

　　.4 **Occupant of streetcar**

　　.5 **Rider of animal; occupant of animal-drawn vehicle**

　　.6 **Pedal cyclist**
　　　　See definition (p)

　　.7 **Pedestrian**
　　　　See definition (r)

　　.8 **Other specified person**
　　　　Occupant of vehicle other than above
　　　　Person on railway train involved in accident
　　　　Unauthorized rider of motor vehicle

　　.9 **Unspecified person**

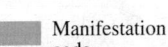

Add 4th or　　Nonspecific　　Unspecified　　Manifestation
5th digit　　　code　　　　　code　　　　code

④ **E820** **Nontraffic accident involving motor-driven snow vehicle**
Includes:

        breakage of part of motor-driven snow vehicle (not on public highway)
        fall from motor-driven snow vehicle (not on public highway)
        hit by motor-driven snow vehicle (not on public highway)
        overturning of motor-driven snow vehicle (not on public highway)
        run over or dragged by motor-driven snow vehicle (not on public highway)
        collision of motor-driven snow vehicle with:
          animal (being ridden) (-drawn vehicle)
          another off-road motor vehicle
          other motor vehicle, not on public highway
          railway train
          other object, fixed or movable
        injury caused by rough landing of motor-driven snow vehicle (after leaving ground on rough terrain)

Excludes: *accident on the public highway involving motor driven snow vehicle (E810.0-E819.9)*

④ **E821** **Nontraffic accident involving other off-road motor vehicle**
Includes:

        breakage of part of off-road motor vehicle, except snow vehicle (not on public highway)
        fall from off-road motor vehicle, except snow vehicle (not on public highway)
        hit by off-road motor vehicle, except snow vehicle (not on public highway)
        overturning of off-road motor vehicle, except snow vehicle (not on public highway)
        run over or dragged by off-road motor vehicle, except snow vehicle (not on public highway)
        thrown against some part of or object in off-road motor vehicle, except snow vehicle (not on public highway)
        collision with:
          animal (being ridden) (-drawn vehicle)
          another off-road motor vehicle, except snow vehicle
          other motor vehicle, not on public highway
          other object, fixed or movable

Excludes: *accident on public highway involving off-road motor vehicle (E810.0-E819.9)*

        collision between motor driven snow vehicle and other off-road motor vehicle (E820.0-E820.9)

        hovercraft accident on water (E830.0-E838.9)

④ **E822** **Other motor vehicle nontraffic accident involving collision with moving object**
Includes: collision, not on public highway, between motor vehicle, except off-road motor vehicle and:
        animal
        nonmotor vehicle
        other motor vehicle, except off-road motor vehicle
        pedestrian
        railway train
        other moving object

Excludes: *collision with:*

        motor-driven snow vehicle (E820.0-E820.9)
        other off-road motor vehicle (E821.0-E821.9)

④ **E823** **Other motor vehicle nontraffic accident involving collision with stationary object**
Includes: collision, not on public highway, between motor vehicle, except off-road motor vehicle, and any object, fixed or movable, but not in motion

④ **E824** **Other motor vehicle nontraffic accident while boarding and alighting**
Includes:

        fall while boarding or alighting from motor vehicle, except off-road motor vehicle, not on public highway
        injury from moving part of motor vehicle while boarding or alighting from motor vehicle, except off-road motor vehicle, not on public highway
        trapped by door of motor vehicle while boarding or alighting from motor vehicle, except off-road motor vehicle, not on public highway

● Code new to this edition   ▲ Revision of existing code   ④ ⑤ Fourth or fifth digit required

④ **E825** **Other motor vehicle nontraffic accident of other and unspecified nature**

    Includes:

        accidental poisoning from carbon monoxide generated by motor vehicle while in motion, not on public highway

        breakage of any part of motor vehicle while in motion, not on public highway

        explosion of any part of motor vehicle while in motion, not on public highway

        fall, jump, or being accidentally pushed from motor vehicle while in motion, not on public highway

        fire starting in motor vehicle while in motion, not on public highway

        hit by object thrown into, towards, or on motor vehicle while in motion, not on public highway

        injured by being thrown against some part of, or object in motor vehicle while in motion, not on public highway

        injury from moving part of motor vehicle while in motion, not on public highway

        object falling in or on motor vehicle while in motion, not on public highway

        motor vehicle nontraffic accident NOS

    Excludes: *fall from or in stationary motor vehicle (E884.9, E885.9)*

        overcome by carbon monoxide or exhaust gas generated by stationary motor vehicle off the roadway with motor running (E868.2)

        struck by falling object from or in stationary motor vehicle (E916)

OTHER ROAD VEHICLE ACCIDENTS (E826-E829)

    Note: Other road vehicle accidents are transport accidents involving road vehicles other than motor vehicles. For definitions of other road vehicle and related terms see definitions (m) to (o).

    Includes: accidents involving other road vehicles being used in recreational or sporting activities

    Excludes: *collision of other road vehicle [any] with:*

        aircraft (E840.0-E845.9)

        motor vehicle (E813.0-E813.9, E820.0-E822.9)

        railway train (E801.0-E801.9)

    The following fourth-digit subdivisions are for use with categories E826-E829 to identify the injured person:

    .0 Pedestrian

        See definition (r)

    .1 Pedal cyclist

        See definition (p)

    .2 Rider of animal

    .3 Occupant of animal-drawn vehicle

    .4 Occupant of streetcar

    .8 Other specified person

    .9 Unspecified person

④ **E826** **Pedal cycle accident**

    [0-9]

    Includes: breakage of any part of pedal cycle

        collision between pedal cycle and:

            animal (being ridden) (herded) (unattended)

            another pedal cycle

            nonmotor road vehicle, any

            pedestrian

            other object, fixed, movable, or moving, not set in motion by motor vehicle, railway train, or aircraft

        entanglement in wheel of pedal cycle

        fall from pedal cycle

        hit by object falling or thrown on the pedal cycle

        pedal cycle accident NOS

        pedal cycle overturned

④ **E827** **Animal-drawn vehicle accident**

[0,2-4,8,9]

Includes: breakage of any part of vehicle
collision between animal-drawn vehicle and:
  animal (being ridden) (herded) (unattended)
  nonmotor road vehicle, except pedal cycle
  pedestrian, pedestrian conveyance, or pedestrian vehicle
  other object, fixed, movable, or moving, not set in motion by motor vehicle,
    railway train, or aircraft
fall from animal-drawn vehicle
knocked down by animal-drawn vehicle
overturning of animal-drawn vehicle
run over by animal-drawn vehicle
thrown from animal-drawn vehicle

Excludes: *collision of animal-drawn vehicle with pedal cycle (E826.0-E826.9)*

④ **E828** **Accident involving animal being ridden**

[0,2,4,8,9]

Includes: collision between animal being ridden and:
  another animal
  nonmotor road vehicle, except pedal cycle, and animal-drawn vehicle
  pedestrian, pedestrian conveyance, or pedestrian vehicle
  other object, fixed, movable, or moving, not set in motion by motor vehicle,
    railway train, or aircraft
fall from animal being ridden
knocked down by animal being ridden
thrown from animal being ridden
trampled by animal being ridden
ridden animal stumbled and fell

Excludes: *collision of animal being ridden with:*
  animal-drawn vehicle (E827.0-E827.9)
  pedal cycle (E826.0-E826.9)

④ **E829** **Other road vehicle accidents**

[0,4,8,9]

Includes:
accident while boarding or alighting from streetcar nonmotor road vehicle not
  classifiable to E826-E828
blow from object in streetcar nonmotor road vehicle not classifiable to E826-E828
breakage of any part of streetcar nonmotor road vehicle not classifiable to
  E826-E828
caught in door of streetcar nonmotor road vehicle not classifiable to E826-E828
derailment of streetcar nonmotor road vehicle not classifiable to E826-E828
fall in, on, or from streetcar nonmotor road vehicle not classifiable to E826-E828
fire in streetcar nonmotor road vehicle not classifiable to E826-E828
collision between streetcar or nonmotor road vehicle, except as in E826-E828, and:
  animal (not being ridden)
  another nonmotor road vehicle not classifiable to E826-E828
  pedestrian
  other object, fixed, movable, or moving, not set in motion by motor vehicle,
    railway train, or aircraft
nonmotor road vehicle accident NOS
streetcar accident NOS

Excludes: *collision with:*
  animal being ridden (E828.0-E828.9)
  animal-drawn vehicle (E827.0-E827.9)
  pedal cycle (E826.0-E826.9)

WATER TRANSPORT ACCIDENTS (E830-E838)

Note: For definitions of water transport accident and related terms see definitions (a), (s), and (t).

Includes: watercraft accidents in the course of recreational activities

Excludes: *accidents involving both aircraft, including objects set in motion by aircraft, and*
  watercraft (E840.0-E845.9)

The following fourth-digit subdivisions are for use with categories E830-E838 to identify the
  injured person:

.0 Occupant of small boat, unpowered

.1 Occupant of small boat, powered
See definition (t)

● Code new
to this edition

▲ Revision of
existing code

④ ⑤ Fourth or fifth
digit required

Excludes: water skier (.4)

.2 Occupant of other watercraft—crew
Persons:
engaged in operation of watercraft
providing passenger services [cabin attendants, ship's physician, catering personnel]
working on ship during voyage in other capacity [musician in band, operators of
shops and beauty parlors]

.3 Occupant of other watercraft—other than crew
Passenger
Occupant of lifeboat, other than crew, after abandoning ship

.4 Water skier

.5 Swimmer

.6 Dockers, stevedores
Longshoreman employed on the dock in loading and unloading ships

.8 Other specified person
Immigration and custom officials on board ship
Person:
accompanying passenger or member of crew
visiting boat
Pilot (guiding ship into port)

.9 Unspecified person

④ **E830 Accident to watercraft causing submersion**
Includes: submersion and drowning due to:
boat overturning
boat submerging
falling or jumping from burning ship
falling or jumping from crushed watercraft
ship sinking
other accident to watercraft

④ **E831 Accident to watercraft causing other injury**
Includes: any injury, except submersion and drowning, as a result of an accident to
watercraft
burned while ship on fire
crushed between ships in collision
crushed by lifeboat after abandoning ship
fall due to collision or other accident to watercraft
hit by falling object due to accident to watercraft
injured in watercraft accident involving collision
struck by boat or part thereof after fall or jump from damaged boat

Excludes: burns from localized fire or explosion on board ship (E837.0-E837.9)

④ **E832 Other accidental submersion or drowning in water transport accident**
Includes: submersion or drowning as a result of an accident other than accident to the
watercraft, such as:
fall:
from gangplank
from ship
overboard
thrown overboard by motion of ship
washed overboard

Excludes: submersion or drowning of swimmer or diver who voluntarily jumps from boat not
involved in an accident (E910.0-E910.9)

④ **E833 Fall on stairs or ladders in water transport**
Excludes: fall due to accident to watercraft (E831.0-E831.9)

④ **E834 Other fall from one level to another in water transport**
Excludes: fall due to accident to watercraft (E831.0-E831.9)

④ **E835 Other and unspecified fall in water transport**
Excludes: fall due to accident to watercraft (E831.0-E831.9)

Add 4th or   Nonspecific   Unspecified   Manifestation
5th digit   code   code   code

[4] **E836 Machinery accident in water transport**
Includes: injuries in water transport caused by:
deck machinery
engine room machinery
galley machinery
laundry machinery
loading machinery

[4] **E837 Explosion, fire, or burning in watercraft**
Includes: explosion of boiler on steamship
localized fire on ship

[Excludes:] *burning ship (due to collision or explosion) resulting in:*
submersion or drowning (E830.0-E830.9)
other injury (E831.0-E831.9)

[4] **E838 Other and unspecified water transport accident**
Includes: accidental poisoning by gases or fumes on ship
atomic power plant malfunction in watercraft
crushed between ship and stationary object [wharf]
crushed between ships without accident to watercraft
crushed by falling object on ship or while loading or unloading
hit by boat while water skiing
struck by boat or part thereof (after fall from boat)
watercraft accident NOS

AIR AND SPACE TRANSPORT ACCIDENTS (E840-E845)

Note: For definition of aircraft and related terms see definitions (u) and (v).

The following fourth-digit subdivisions are for use with categories E840-E845 to identify the injured person:

.0 Occupant of spacecraft

.1 Occupant of military aircraft, any
Crew in military aircraft [air force] [army] [national guard] [navy]
Passenger (civilian) (military) in military aircraft [air force] [army] [national guard] [navy]
Troops in military aircraft [air force] [army] [national guard] [navy]

[Excludes:] *occupants of aircraft operated under jurisdiction of police departments (.5)*
parachutist (.7)

.2 Crew of commercial aircraft (powered) in surface to surface transport

.3 Other occupant of commercial aircraft (powered) in surface to surface transport
Flight personnel:
not part of crew
on familiarization flight
Passenger on aircraft (powered) NOS

.4 Occupant of commercial aircraft (powered) in surface to air transport
Occupant [crew] [passenger] of aircraft (powered) engaged in activities, such as:
aerial spraying (crops) (fire retardants)
air drops of emergency supplies
air drops of parachutists, except from military craft
crop dusting
lowering of construction material [bridge or telephone pole]
sky writing

.5 Occupant of other powered aircraft
Occupant [crew] [passenger] of aircraft [powered] engaged in activities, such as:
aerobatic flying
aircraft racing
rescue operation
storm surveillance
traffic surveillance
Occupant of private plane NOS

.6 Occupant of unpowered aircraft, except parachutist
Occupant of aircraft classifiable to E842

.7 Parachutist (military) (other)
Person making voluntary descent

[Excludes:] *person making descent after accident to aircraft (.1-.6)*

.8 Ground crew, airline employee
Persons employed at airfields (civil) (military) or launching pads, not occupants of aircraft

.9 Other person

④ **E840 Accident to powered aircraft at takeoff or landing**
Includes:
collision of aircraft with any object, fixed, movable, or moving while taking off or landing
crash while taking off or landing
explosion on aircraft while taking off or landing
fire on aircraft while taking off or landing
forced landing while taking off or landing

④ **E841 Accident to powered aircraft, other and unspecified**
Includes: aircraft accident NOS
aircraft crash or wreck NOS
any accident to powered aircraft while in transit or when not specified whether in transit, taking off, or landing
collision of aircraft with another aircraft, bird, or any object, while in transit
explosion on aircraft while in transit
fire on aircraft while in transit

④ **E842 Accident to unpowered aircraft**
[6-9]
Includes: any accident, except collision with powered aircraft, to:
balloon
glider
hang glider
kite carrying a person
hit by object falling from unpowered aircraft

④ **E843 Fall in, on, or from aircraft**
[0-9]
Includes: accident in boarding or alighting from aircraft, any kind
fall in, on, or from aircraft [any kind], while in transit, taking off, or landing, except when as a result of an accident to aircraft

④ **E844 Other specified air transport accidents**
[0-9]
Includes:
hit by:
aircraft without accident to aircraft
object falling from aircraft without accident to aircraft
injury by or from:
machinery on aircraft without accident to aircraft
rotating propeller without accident to aircraft
voluntary parachute descent without accident to aircraft
poisoning by carbon monoxide from aircraft while in transit without accident to aircraft
sucked into jet without accident to aircraft
any accident involving other transport vehicle (motor) (nonmotor) due to being hit by object set in motion by aircraft (powered)

Excludes: *air sickness (E903)*
effects of:
high altitude (E902.0-E902.1)
pressure change (E902.0-E902.1)
injury in parachute descent due to accident to aircraft (840.0-E842.9)

④ **E845 Accident involving spacecraft**
[0,8,9]
Includes: launching pad accident
Excludes: *effects of weightlessness in spacecraft (E928.0)*

	Add 4th or 5th digit		Nonspecific code		Unspecified code		Manifestation code

VEHICLE ACCIDENTS NOT ELSEWHERE CLASSIFIABLE (E846-E848)

E846 Accidents involving powered vehicles used solely within the buildings and premises of industrial or commercial establishment

Accident to, on, or involving:
- battery powered airport passenger vehicle
- battery powered trucks (baggage) (mail)
- coal car in mine
- logging car
- self propelled truck, industrial
- station baggage truck (powered)
- tram, truck, or tub (powered) in mine or quarry

Breakage of any part of vehicle

Collision with:
- pedestrian
- other vehicle or object within premises

Explosion of powered vehicle, industrial or commercial

Fall from powered vehicle, industrial or commercial

Overturning of powered vehicle, industrial or commercial

Struck by powered vehicle, industrial or commercial

[Excludes:] *accidental poisoning by exhaust gas from vehicle not elsewhere classifiable (E868.2)*
injury by crane, lift (fork), or elevator (E919.2)

E847 Accidents involving cable cars not running on rails

Accident to, on, or involving:
- cable car, not on rails
- ski chair-lift
- ski-lift with gondola
- téléférique

Breakage of cable

Caught or dragged by cable car, not on rails

Fall or jump from cable car, not on rails

Object thrown from or in cable car, not on rails

E848 Accidents involving other vehicles, not elsewhere classifiable

Accident to, on, or involving:
- ice yacht
- land yacht
- nonmotor, nonroad vehicle NOS

E849 Place of occurrence

The following category is for use to denote the place where the injury or poisoning occurred.

E849.0 Home

Apartment
Boarding house
Farm house
Home premises
House (residential)
Noninstitutional place of residence
Private:
- *driveway*
- *garage*
- *garden*
- *home*
- *walk*

Swimming pool in private house or garden
Yard of home

[Excludes:] *home under construction but not yet occupied (E849.3)*
institutional place of residence (E849.7)

E849.1 Farm

Farm:
- *buildings*
- *land under cultivation*

[Excludes:] *farm house and home premises of farm (E849.0)*

E849.2 Mine and quarry

Gravel pit
Sand pit
Tunnel under construction

● Code new to this edition ▲ Revision of existing code ④ ⑤ Fourth or fifth digit required

E849.3 **Industrial place and premises**

Building under
  construction
Dockyard
Dry dock
Factory
  building
  premises
Garage (place of work)

Industrial yard
Loading platform (factory) (store)
Plant, industrial
Railway yard
Shop (place of work)
Warehouse
Workhouse

E849.4 **Place for recreation and sport**

Amusement park
Baseball field
Basketball court
Beach resort
Cricket ground
Fives court
Football field
Golf course
Gymnasium
Hockey field
Holiday camp
Ice palace
Lake resort
Mountain resort
Playground, including
  school playground

Public park
Racecourse
Resort NOS
Riding school
Rifle range
Seashore resort
Skating rink
Sports ground
Sports palace
Stadium
Swimming pool, public
Tennis court
Vacation resort

Excludes: that in private house or garden (E849.0)

E849.5 **Street and highway**

E849.6 **Public building**

Building (including adjacent grounds) used by the general public or by a particular
  group of the public, such as:

airport
bank
café
casino
church
cinema
clubhouse
courthouse
dance hall
garage building (for car storage)
hotel
market (grocery or other commodity)
movie house
music hall

nightclub
office
office building
opera house
post office
public hall
radio broadcasting station
restaurant
school (state) (public) (private)
shop, commercial
station (bus) (railway)
store
theater

Excludes: home garage (E849.0)
      industrial building or workplace (E849.3)

E849.7 **Residential institution**

Children's home
Dormitory
Hospital
Jail

Old people's home
Orphanage
Prison
Reform school

E849.8 **Other specified places**

Beach NOS
Canal
Caravan site NOS
Derelict house
Desert
Dock
Forest
Harbor
Hill
Lake NOS
Mountain
Parking lot
Parking place

Pond or pool (natural)
Prairie
Public place NOS
Railway line
Reservoir
River
Sea
Seashore NOS
Stream
Swamp
Trailer court
Woods

E849.9 **Unspecified place**

	Add 4th or 5th digit		Nonspecific code		Unspecified code		Manifestation code

ACCIDENTAL POISONING BY DRUGS, MEDICINAL SUBSTANCES, AND BIOLOGICALS (E850-E858)

Includes: accidental overdose of drug, wrong drug given or taken in error, and drug taken inadvertently

accidents in the use of drugs and biologicals in medical and surgical procedures

Excludes: *administration with suicidal or homicidal intent or intent to harm, or in circumstances classifiable to E980-E989 (E950.0-E950.5, E962.0, E980.0-E980.5)*

correct drug properly administered in therapeutic or prophylactic dosage, as the cause of adverse effect (E930.0-E949.9)

See Alphabetic Index for more complete list of specific drugs to be classified under the fourth-digit subdivisions. The American Hospital Formulary numbers can be used to classify new drugs listed by the American Hospital Formulary Service (AHFS). See appendix C.

E850 **Accidental poisoning by analgesics, antipyretics, and antirheumatics**

  E850.0 **Heroin**
      Diacetylmorphine

  E850.1 **Methadone**

  E850.2 **Other opiates and related narcotics**
      Codeine [methylmorphine]   Morphine
      Meperidine [pethidine]   Opium (alkaloids)

  E850.3 **Salicylates**
      Acetylsalicylic acid [aspirin]
      Amino derivatives of salicylic acid
      Salicylic acid salts

  E850.4 **Aromatic analgesics, not elsewhere classified**
      Acetanilid
      Paracetamol [acetaminophen]
      Phenacetin [acetophenetidin]

  E850.5 **Pyrazole derivatives**
      Aminophenazone [amidopyrine]
      Phenylbutazone

  E850.6 **Antirheumatics [antiphlogistics]**
      Gold salts   Indomethacin
    Excludes: *salicylates (E850.3)*
        steroids (E858.0)

  E850.7 **Other non-narcotic analgesics**
      Pyrabital

  E850.8 **Other specified analgesics and antipyretics**
      Pentazocine

  E850.9 **Unspecified analgesic or antipyretic**

E851 **Accidental poisoning by barbiturates**
    Amobarbital [amylobarbitone]
    Barbital [barbitone]
    Butabarbital [butabarbitone]
    Pentobarbital [pentobarbitone]
    Phenobarbital [phenobarbitone]
    Secobarbital [quinalbarbitone]
    Excludes: *thiobarbiturates (E855.1)*

E852 **Accidental poisoning by other sedatives and hypnotics**

  E852.0 **Chloral hydrate group**

  E852.1 **Paraldehyde**

  E852.2 **Bromine compounds**
      Bromides   Carbromal (derivatives)

  E852.3 **Methaqualone compounds**

  E852.4 **Glutethimide group**

  E852.5 **Mixed sedatives, not elsewhere classified**

  E852.8 **Other specified sedatives and hypnotics**

● Code new
  to this edition
▲ Revision of
  existing code
④ ⑤ Fourth or fifth
    digit required

E852.9 **Unspecified sedative or hypnotic**
Sleeping:
drug NOS
pill NOS
tablet NOS

E853 **Accidental poisoning by tranquilizers**

E853.0 **Phenothiazine-based tranquilizers**
Chlorpromazine   Prochlorperazine
Fluphenazine   Promazine

E853.1 **Butyrophenone-based tranquilizers**
Haloperidol   Trifluperidol
Spiperone

E853.2 **Benzodiazepine-based tranquilizers**
Chlordiazepoxide   Lorazepam
Diazepam   Medazepam
Flurazepam   Nitrazepam

E853.8 **Other specified tranquilizers**
Hydroxyzine   Meprobamate

E853.9 **Unspecified tranquilizer**

E854 **Accidental poisoning by other psychotropic agents**

E854.0 **Antidepressants**
Amitriptyline   Monoamine oxidase [MAO] inhibitors
Imipramine

E854.1 **Psychodysleptics [hallucinogens]**
Cannabis derivatives   Mescaline
Lysergide [LSD]   Psilocin
Marihuana (derivatives) Psilocybin

E854.2 **Psychostimulants**
Amphetamine   Caffeine

Excludes: *central appetite depressants (E858.8)*

E854.3 **Central nervous system stimulants**
Analeptics   Opiate antagonists

E854.8 **Other psychotropic agents**

E855 **Accidental poisoning by other drugs acting on central and autonomic nervous system**

E855.0 **Anticonvulsant and anti-Parkinsonism drugs**
Amantadine
Hydantoin derivatives
Levodopa [L-dopa]
Oxazolidine derivatives [paramethadione] [trimethadione]
Succinimides

E855.1 **Other central nervous system depressants**
Ether   Intravenous anesthetics
Gaseous anesthetics   Thiobarbiturates, such as thiopental sodium
Halogenated hydrocarbon
   derivatives

E855.2 **Local anesthetics**
Cocaine   Procaine
Lidocaine [lignocaine] Tetracaine

E855.3 **Parasympathomimetics [cholinergics]**
Acetylcholine   Pilocarpine
Anticholinesterase:
   organophosphorus
   reversible

E855.4 **Parasympatholytics [anticholinergics and antimuscarinics] and spasmolytics**
Atropine   Hyoscine [scopolamine]
Homatropine   Quaternary ammonium derivatives

E855.5 **Sympathomimetics [adrenergics]**
Epinephrine [adrenalin]
Levarterenol [noradrenalin]

E855.6 **Sympatholytics [antiadrenergics]**
Phenoxybenzamine   Tolazoline hydrochloride

E855.8 **Other specified drugs acting on central and autonomic nervous systems**

| | Add 4th or 5th digit | | Nonspecific code | | Unspecified code | | Manifestation code |

E855.9 Unspecified drug acting on central and autonomic nervous systems

E856 Accidental poisoning by antibiotics

E857 Accidental poisoning by other anti-infectives

E858 Accidental poisoning by other drugs

E858.0 Hormones and synthetic substitutes

E858.1 Primarily systemic agents

E858.2 Agents primarily affecting blood constituents

E858.3 Agents primarily affecting cardiovascular system

E858.4 Agents primarily affecting gastrointestinal system

E858.5 Water, mineral, and uric acid metabolism drugs

E858.6 Agents primarily acting on the smooth and skeletal muscles and respiratory system

E858.7 Agents primarily affecting skin and mucous membrane, ophthalmological, otorhinolaryngological, and dental drugs

E858.8 Other specified drugs
Central appetite depressants

E858.9 Unspecified drug

ACCIDENTAL POISONING BY OTHER SOLID AND LIQUID SUBSTANCES, GASES, AND VAPORS (E860-E869)

Note: Categories in this section are intended primarily to indicate the external cause of poisoning states classifiable to 980-989. They may also be used to indicate external causes of localized effects classifiable to 001-799.

E860 Accidental poisoning by alcohol, not elsewhere classified

E860.0 Alcoholic beverages
Alcohol in preparations intended for consumption

E860.1 Other and unspecified ethyl alcohol and its products
Denatured alcohol
Ethanol NOS
Grain alcohol NOS
Methylated spirit

E860.2 Methyl alcohol
Methanol
Wood alcohol

E860.3 Isopropyl alcohol
Dimethyl carbinol
Isopropanol
Rubbing alcohol substitute
Secondary propyl alcohol

E860.4 Fusel oil
Alcohol:
amyl
butyl
propyl

E860.8 Other specified alcohols

E860.9 Unspecified alcohol

E861 Accidental poisoning by cleansing and polishing agents, disinfectants, paints, and varnishes

E861.0 Synthetic detergents and shampoos

E861.1 Soap products

E861.2 Polishes

E861.3 Other cleansing and polishing agents
Scouring powders

E861.4 Disinfectants
Household and other disinfectants not ordinarily used on the person

[Excludes:] *carbolic acid or phenol (E864.0)*

E861.5 Lead paints

E861.6 Other paints and varnishes
Lacquers
Oil colors
Paints, other than lead
White washes

E861.9 Unspecified

● Code new to this edition ▲ Revision of existing code ④ ⑤ Fourth or fifth digit required

E862 **Accidental poisoning by petroleum products, other solvents and their vapors, not elsewhere classified**

E862.0 **Petroleum solvents**
Petroleum:
ether
benzine
naphtha

E862.1 **Petroleum fuels and cleaners**
Antiknock additives to petroleum fuels
Gas oils
Gasoline or petrol
Kerosene

Excludes: kerosene insecticides (E863.4)

E862.2 **Lubricating oils**

E862.3 **Petroleum solids**
Paraffin wax

E862.4 **Other specified solvents**
Benzene

E862.9 **Unspecified solvent**

E863 **Accidental poisoning by agricultural and horticultural chemical and pharmaceutical preparations other than plant foods and fertilizers**

Excludes: plant foods and fertilizers (E866.5)

E863.0 **Insecticides of organochlorine compounds**
Benzene hexachloride   Dieldrin
Chlordane   Endrine
DDT   Toxaphene

E863.1 **Insecticides of organophosphorus compounds**
Demeton   Parathion
Diazinon   Phenylsulphthion
Dichlorvos   Phorate
Malathion   Phosdrin
Methyl parathion

E863.2 **Carbamates**
Aldicarb   Propoxur
Carbaryl

E863.3 **Mixtures of insecticides**

E863.4 **Other and unspecified insecticides**
Kerosene insecticides

E863.5 **Herbicides**
2, 4-Dichlorophenoxyacetic acid [2, 4-D]
2, 4, 5-Trichlorophenoxyacetic acid [2, 4, 5-T]
Chlorates
Diquat
Mixtures of plant food and fertilizers with herbicides
Paraquat

E863.6 **Fungicides**
Organic mercurials (used in seed dressing)
Pentachlorophenols

E863.7 **Rodenticides**
Fluoroacetates   Warfarin
Squill and derivatives   Zinc phosphide
Thallium

E863.8 **Fumigants**
Cyanides   Phosphine
Methyl bromide

E863.9 **Other and unspecified**

E864 **Accidental poisoning by corrosives and caustics, not elsewhere classified**

Excludes: those as components of disinfectants (E861.4)

E864.0 **Corrosive aromatics**
Carbolic acid or phenol

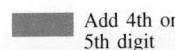 Add 4th or
5th digit

Nonspecific
code

Unspecified
code

Manifestation
code

E864.1 Acids
Acid:
  hydrochloric
  nitric
  sulfuric

E864.2 Caustic alkalis
Lye

E864.3 Other specified corrosives and caustics

E864.4 Unspecified corrosives and caustics

E865 Accidental poisoning from poisonous foodstuffs and poisonous plants
Includes: any meat, fish, or shellfish
plants, berries, and fungi eaten as, or in mistake for, food, or by a child

Excludes: *anaphylactic shock due to adverse food reaction (995.6)*
food poisoning (bacterial) (005.0-005.9)
poisoning and toxic reactions to venomous plants (E905.6-E905.7)

E865.0 Meat

E865.1 Shellfish

E865.2 Other fish

E865.3 Berries and seeds

E865.4 Other specified plants

E865.5 Mushrooms and other fungi

E865.8 Other specified foods

E865.9 Unspecified foodstuff or poisonous plant

E866 Accidental poisoning by other and unspecified solid and liquid substances

Excludes: *these substances as a component of:*
medicines (E850.0-E858.9)
paints (E861.5-E861.6)
pesticides (E863.0-E863.9)
petroleum fuels (E862.1)

E866.0 Lead and its compounds and fumes

E866.1 Mercury and its compounds and fumes

E866.2 Antimony and its compounds and fumes

E866.3 Arsenic and its compounds and fumes

E866.4 Other metals and their compounds and fumes
Beryllium (compounds)   Iron (compounds)
Brass fumes   Manganese (compounds)
Cadmium (compounds)   Nickel (compounds)
Copper salts   Thallium (compounds)

E866.5 Plant foods and fertilizers

Excludes: *mixtures with herbicides (E863.5)*

E866.6 Glues and adhesives

E866.7 Cosmetics

E866.8 Other specified solid or liquid substances

E866.9 Unspecified solid or liquid substance

E867 Accidental poisoning by gas distributed by pipeline
Carbon monoxide from incomplete combustion of piped gas
Coal gas NOS
Liquefied petroleum gas distributed through pipes (pure or mixed with air)
Piped gas (natural) (manufactured)

E868 Accidental poisoning by other utility gas and other carbon monoxide

E868.0 Liquefied petroleum gas distributed in mobile containers
Butane or carbon monoxide from incomplete combustion of these gases
Liquefied hydrocarbon gas NOS or carbon monoxide from incomplete combustion of
  these gases
Propane or carbon monoxide from incomplete combustion of these gases

● Code new   ▲ Revision of   ④ ⑤ Fourth or fifth
     to this edition   existing code   digit required

E868.1 **Other and unspecified utility gas**
Acetylene or or carbon monoxide from incomplete combustion of this gases
Gas NOS used for lighting, heating, cooking, or carbon monoxide from incomplete combustion of this gases
Water gas or carbon monoxide from incomplete combustion of this gases

E868.2 **Motor vehicle exhaust gas**
Exhaust gas from:
farm tractor, not in transit
gas engine
motor pump
motor vehicle, not in transit
any type of combustion engine not in watercraft

Excludes: *poisoning by carbon monoxide from:*
aircraft while in transit (E844.0-E844.9)
motor vehicle while in transit (E818.0-E818.9)
watercraft whether or not in transit (E838.0-E838.9)

E868.3 **Carbon monoxide from incomplete combustion of other domestic fuels**
Carbon monoxide from incomplete combustion of:
coal in domestic stove or fireplace
coke in domestic stove or fireplace
kerosene in domestic stove or fireplace
wood in domestic stove or fireplace

Excludes: *carbon monoxide from smoke and fumes due to conflagration (E890.0-E893.9)*

E868.8 **Carbon monoxide from other sources**
Carbon monoxide from:
blast furnace gas
incomplete combustion of fuels in industrial use
kiln vapor

E868.9 **Unspecified carbon monoxide**

E869 **Accidental poisoning by other gases and vapors**

Excludes: *effects of gases used as anesthetics (E855.1, E938.2)*
fumes from heavy metals (E866.0-E866.4)
smoke and fumes due to conflagration or explosion (E890.0-E899)

E869.0 **Nitrogen oxides**

E869.1 **Sulfur dioxide**

E869.2 **Freon**

E869.3 **Lacrimogenic gas [tear gas]**
Bromobenzyl cyanide   Ethyliodoacetate
Chloroacetophenone

E869.4 **Second-hand tobacco smoke**

E869.8 **Other specified gases and vapors**
Chlorine   Hydrocyanic acid gas

E869.9 **Unspecified gases and vapors**

MISADVENTURES TO PATIENTS DURING SURGICAL AND MEDICAL CARE (E870-E876)

Excludes: *accidental overdose of drug and wrong drug given in error (E850.0-E858.9)*
surgical and medical procedures as the cause of abnormal reaction by the patient,
without mention of misadventure at the time of procedure (E878.0-E879.9)

E870 **Accidental cut, puncture, perforation, or hemorrhage during medical care**

E870.0 **Surgical operation**

E870.1 **Infusion or transfusion**

E870.2 **Kidney dialysis or other perfusion**

E870.3 **Injection or vaccination**

E870.4 **Endoscopic examination**

E870.5 **Aspiration of fluid or tissue, puncture, and catheterization**
Abdominal paracentesis   Lumbar puncture
Aspirating needle biopsy   Thoracentesis
Blood sampling

Excludes: *heart catheterization (E870.6)*

Add 4th or 5th digit   Nonspecific code   Unspecified code   Manifestation code

E870.6 Heart catheterization

E870.7 Administration of enema

E870.8 Other specified medical care

E870.9 Unspecified medical care

E871 Foreign object left in body during procedure

E871.0 Surgical operation

E871.1 Infusion or transfusion

E871.2 Kidney dialysis or other perfusion

E871.3 Injection or vaccination

E871.4 Endoscopic examination

E871.5 Aspiration of fluid or tissue, puncture, and catheterization

Abdominal paracentesis   Lumbar puncture
Aspiration needle biopsy   Thoracentesis
Blood sampling

Excludes: *heart catheterization (E871.6)*

E871.6 Heart catheterization

E871.7 Removal of catheter or packing

E871.8 Other specified procedures

E871.9 Unspecified procedure

E872 Failure of sterile precautions during procedure

E872.0 Surgical operation

E872.1 Infusion or transfusion

E872.2 Kidney dialysis and other perfusion

E872.3 Injection or vaccination

E872.4 Endoscopic examination

E872.5 Aspiration of fluid or tissue, puncture, and catheterization

Abdominal paracentesis   Lumbar puncture
Aspirating needle biopsy   Thoracentesis
Blood sampling

Excludes: *heart catheterization (E872.6)*

E872.6 Heart catheterization

E872.8 Other specified procedures

E872.9 Unspecified procedure

E873 Failure in dosage

Excludes: *accidental overdose of drug, medicinal or biological substance (E850.0-E858.9)*

E873.0 Excessive amount of blood or other fluid during transfusion or infusion

E873.1 Incorrect dilution of fluid during infusion

E873.2 Overdose of radiation in therapy

E873.3 Inadvertent exposure of patient to radiation during medical care

E873.4 Failure in dosage in electroshock or insulin-shock therapy

E873.5 Inappropriate [too hot or too cold] temperature in local application and packing

E873.6 Nonadministration of necessary drug or medicinal substance

E873.8 Other specified failure in dosage

E873.9 Unspecified failure in dosage

E874 Mechanical failure of instrument or apparatus during procedure

E874.0 Surgical operation

E874.1 Infusion and transfusion

Air in system

E874.2 Kidney dialysis and other perfusion

E874.3 Endoscopic examination

● Code new
to this edition

▲ Revision of
existing code

④ ⑤ Fourth or fifth
digit required

E874.4 **Aspiration of fluid or tissue, puncture, and catheterization**
  Abdominal paracentesis   Lumbar puncture
  Aspirating needle biopsy   Thoracentesis
  Blood sampling

  Excludes: heart catheterization (E874.5)

E874.5 **Heart catheterization**

E874.8 **Other specified procedures**

E874.9 **Unspecified procedure**

E875 **Contaminated or infected blood, other fluid, drug, or biological substance**
  Includes: presence of:
        bacterial pyrogens
        endotoxin-producing bacteria
        serum hepatitis-producing agent

E875.0 **Contaminated substance transfused or infused**

E875.1 **Contaminated substance injected or used for vaccination**

E875.2 **Contaminated drug or biological substance administered by other means**

E875.8 **Other**

E875.9 **Unspecified**

E876 **Other and unspecified misadventures during medical care**

E876.0 **Mismatched blood in transfusion**

E876.1 **Wrong fluid in infusion**

E876.2 **Failure in suture and ligature during surgical operation**

E876.3 **Endotracheal tube wrongly placed during anesthetic procedure**

E876.4 **Failure to introduce or to remove other tube or instrument**

  Excludes: foreign object left in body during procedure (E871.0-E871.9)

E876.5 **Performance of inappropriate operation**

E876.8 **Other specified misadventures during medical care**
  Performance of inappropriate treatment NEC

E876.9 **Unspecified misadventure during medical care**

SURGICAL AND MEDICAL PROCEDURES AS THE CAUSE OF ABNORMAL REACTION OF PATIENT OR LATER COMPLICATION, WITHOUT MENTION OF MISADVENTURE AT THE TIME OF PROCEDURE (E878-E879)

  Includes: procedures as the cause of abnormal reaction, such as:
        displacement or malfunction of prosthetic device
        hepatorenal failure, postoperative
        malfunction of external stoma
        postoperative intestinal obstruction
        rejection of transplanted organ

  Excludes: anesthetic management properly carried out as the cause of adverse effect
        (E937.0-E938.9)
        infusion and transfusion, without mention of misadventure in the technique of
        procedure (E930.0-E949.9)

E878 **Surgical operation and other surgical procedures as the cause of abnormal reaction of patient, or of later complication, without mention of misadventure at the time of operation**

E878.0 **Surgical operation with transplant of whole organ**
  Transplantation of:
  heart
  kidney
  liver

E878.1 **Surgical operation with implant of artificial internal device**
  Cardiac pacemaker   Heart valve prosthesis
  Electrodes implanted in brain   Internal orthopedic device

E878.2 **Surgical operation with anastomosis, bypass, or graft, with natural or artificial tissues used as implant**
  Anastomosis: Graft of blood vessel, tendon, or skin
  arteriovenous
  gastrojejunal

  Excludes: external stoma (E878.3)

  Add 4th or   Nonspecific   Unspecified   Manifestation
  5th digit   code   code   code

E878.3 Surgical operation with formation of external stoma
Colostomy
Cystostomy
Duodenostomy
Gastrostomy
Ureterostomy

E878.4 Other restorative surgery

E878.5 Amputation of limb(s)

E878.6 Removal of other organ (partial) (total)

E878.8 Other specified surgical operations and procedures

E878.9 Unspecified surgical operations and procedures

E879 Other procedures, without mention of misadventure at the time of procedure, as the cause of abnormal reaction of patient, or of later complication

E879.0 Cardiac catheterization

E879.1 Kidney dialysis

E879.2 Radiological procedure and radiotherapy

[Excludes:] *radio-opaque dyes for diagnostic x-ray procedures (E947.8)*

E879.3 Shock therapy
Electroshock therapy
Insulin-shock therapy

E879.4 Aspiration of fluid
Lumbar puncture
Thoracentesis

E879.5 Insertion of gastric or duodenal sound

E879.6 Urinary catheterization

E879.7 Blood sampling

E879.8 Other specified procedures
Blood transfusion

E879.9 Unspecified procedure

ACCIDENTAL FALLS (E880-E888)

[Excludes:] *falls (in or from):*
burning building (E890.8, E891.8)
into fire (E890.0-E899)
into water (with submersion or drowning) (E910.0-E910.9)
machinery (in operation) (E919.0-E919.9)
on edged, pointed, or sharp object (E920.0-E920.9)
transport vehicle (E800.0-E845.9)
vehicle not elsewhere classifiable (E846-E848)

E880 Fall on or from stairs or steps

E880.0 Escalator

E880.1 Fall on or from sidewalk curb

[Excludes:] *fall from moving sidewalk (E885.9)*

E880.9 Other stairs or steps

E881 Fall on or from ladders or scaffolding

E881.0 Fall from ladder

E881.1 Fall from scaffolding

E882 Fall from or out of building or other structure
Fall from:
balcony
bridge
building
flagpole
tower
Fall from:
turret
viaduct
wall
window
Fall through roof

[Excludes:] *collapse of a building or structure (E916)*
fall or jump from burning building (E890.8, E891.8)

● Code new to this edition ▲ Revision of existing code ④ ⑤ Fourth or fifth digit required

E883 **Fall into hole or other opening in surface**
Includes:

fall into:	fall into:
cavity	shaft
dock	swimming pool
hole	tank
pit	well
quarry	

Excludes: *fall into water NOS (E910.9)*
that resulting in drowning or submersion without mention of injury (E910.0-E910.9)

E883.0 **Accident from diving or jumping into water [swimming pool]**
Strike or hit:
against bottom when jumping or diving into water
wall or board of swimming pool
water surface

Excludes: *diving with insufficient air supply (E913.2)*
effects of air pressure from diving (E902.2)

E883.1 **Accidental fall into well**

E883.2 **Accidental fall into storm drain or manhole**

E883.9 **Fall into other hole or other opening in surface**

E884 **Other fall from one level to another**

E884.0 **Fall from playground equipment**
Excludes: *recreational machinery (E919.8)*

E884.1 **Fall from cliff**

E884.2 **Fall from chair**

E884.3 **Fall from wheelchair**

E884.4 **Fall from bed**

E884.5 **Fall from other furniture**

E884.6 **Fall from commode**
Toilet

E884.9 **Other fall from one level to another**

Fall from:	Fall from:
embankment	stationary vehicle
haystack	tree

E885 **Fall on same level from slipping, tripping, or stumbling**

● **E885.0** **Fall from (nonmotorized) scooter**

E885.1 **Fall from roller skates**
In-line skates

E885.2 **Fall from skateboard**

E885.3 **Fall from skis**

E885.4 **Fall from snowboard**

E885.9 **Fall from other slipping, tripping or stumbling**
Fall on moving sidewalk

E886 **Fall on same level from collision, pushing, or shoving, by or with other person**
Excludes: *crushed or pushed by a crowd or human stampede (E917.1, E917.6)*

E886.0 **In sports**
Tackles in sports
Excludes: *kicked, stepped on, struck by object, in sports (E917.0, E917.5)*

E886.9 **Other and unspecified**
Fall from collision of pedestrian (conveyance) with another pedestrian (conveyance)

E887 **Fracture, cause unspecified**

E888 **Other and unspecified fall**
Accidental fall NOS
Fall on same level NOS

E888.0 **Fall resulting in striking against sharp object**
Use additional external cause code to identify object (E920)

E888.1 **Fall resulting in striking against other object**

Add 4th or 5th digit	Nonspecific code	Unspecified code	Manifestation code

E888.8   **Other fall**

E888.9   **Unspecified fall**
Fall NOS

ACCIDENTS CAUSED BY FIRE AND FLAMES (E890-E899)

Includes: asphyxia or poisoning due to conflagration or ignition
burning by fire
secondary fires resulting from explosion

Excludes: *arson (E968.0)*

fire in or on:
machinery (in operation) (E919.0-E919.9)
transport vehicle other than stationary vehicle (E800.0-E845.9)
vehicle not elsewhere classifiable (E846-E848)

E890   **Conflagration in private dwelling**
Includes: conflagration in:
apartment
boarding house
camping place
caravan
farmhouse
house
lodging house
mobile home
private garage
rooming house
tenement
conflagration originating from sources classifiable to E893-E898 in the above
buildings

E890.0   **Explosion caused by conflagration**

E890.1   **Fumes from combustion of polyvinylchloride [PVC] and similar material in conflagration**

E890.2   **Other smoke and fumes from conflagration**
Carbon monoxide from conflagration in private building
Fumes NOS from conflagration in private building
Smoke NOS from conflagration in private building

E890.3   **Burning caused by conflagration**

E890.8   **Other accident resulting from conflagration**
Collapse of burning private building
Fall from burning private building
Hit by object falling from burning private building
Jump from burning private building

E890.9   **Unspecified accident resulting from conflagration in private dwelling**

E891   **Conflagration in other and unspecified building or structure**
Conflagration in:
barn
church
convalescent and other
residential home
dormitory of educational
institution
factory

Conflagration in:
farm outbuildings
hospital
hotel
school
store
theater

Conflagration originating from sources classifiable to E893-E898, in the above buildings

E891.0   **Explosion caused by conflagration**

E891.1   **Fumes from combustion of polyvinylchloride [PVC] and similar material in conflagration**

E891.2   **Other smoke and fumes from conflagration**
Carbon monoxide from conflagration in building or structure
Fumes NOS from conflagration in building or structure
Smoke NOS from conflagration in building or structure

E891.3   **Burning caused by conflagration**

● Code new
to this edition

▲ Revision of
existing code

④ ⑤ Fourth or fifth
digit required

E891.8 **Other accident resulting from conflagration**
Collapse of burning building or structure
Fall from burning building or structure
Hit by object falling from burning building or structure
Jump from burning building or structure

E891.9 **Unspecified accident resulting from conflagration of other and unspecified building or structure**

E892 **Conflagration not in building or structure**
Fire (uncontrolled) (in) (of):
forest
grass
hay
lumber
mine
prairie
transport vehicle [any], except while in transit
tunnel

E893 **Accident caused by ignition of clothing**

Excludes: *ignition of clothing:*
from highly inflammable material (E894)
with conflagration (E890.0-E892)

E893.0 **From controlled fire in private dwelling**
Ignition of clothing from:
normal fire (charcoal) (coal) (electric) (gas) (wood) in:
brazier in private dwelling (as listed in E890)
fireplace in private dwelling (as listed in E890)
furnace in private dwelling (as listed in E890)
stove in private dwelling (as listed in E890)

E893.1 **From controlled fire in other building or structure**
Ignition of clothing from:
normal fire (charcoal) (coal) (electric) (gas) (wood) in:
brazier in other building or structure (as listed in E891)
fireplace in other building or structure (as listed in E891)
furnace in other building or structure (as listed in E891)
stove in other building or structure (as listed in E891)

E893.2 **From controlled fire not in building or structure**
Ignition of clothing from:
bonfire (controlled)
brazier fire (controlled), not in building or structure
trash fire (controlled)

Excludes: *conflagration not in building (E892)*
trash fire out of control (E892)

E893.8 **From other specified sources**
Ignition of clothing from:
blowlamp
blowtorch
burning bedspread
candle
cigar
Ignition of clothing from:
cigarette
lighter
matches
pipe
welding torch

E893.9 **Unspecified source**
Ignition of clothing (from controlled fire NOS) (in building NOS) NOS

Add 4th or
5th digit
Nonspecific
code
Unspecified
code
Manifestation
code

E894 Ignition of highly inflammable material
Ignition of:
benzine (with ignition of clothing)
gasoline (with ignition of clothing)
fat (with ignition of clothing)
kerosene (with ignition of clothing)
paraffin (with ignition of clothing)
petrol (with ignition of clothing)

Excludes: *ignition of highly inflammable material with:*
conflagration (E890.0-E892)
explosion (E923.0-E923.9)

E895 Accident caused by controlled fire in private dwelling
Burning by (flame of) normal fire (charcoal) (coal) (electric) (gas) (wood) in:
brazier in private dwelling (as listed in E890)
fireplace in private dwelling (as listed in E890)
furnace in private dwelling (as listed in E890)
stove in private dwelling (as listed in E890)

Excludes: *burning by hot objects not producing fire or flames (E924.0-E924.9)*
ignition of clothing from these sources (E893.0)
poisoning by carbon monoxide from incomplete combustion of fuel (E867-E868.9)
that with conflagration (E890.0-E890.9)

E896 Accident caused by controlled fire in other and unspecified building or structure
Burning by (flame of) normal fire (charcoal) (coal) (electric) (gas) (wood) in:
brazier in other building or structure (as listed in E891)
fireplace in other building or structure (as listed in E891)
furnace in other building or structure (as listed in E891)
stove in other building or structure (as listed in E891)

Excludes: *burning by hot objects not producing fire or flames (E924.0-E924.9)*
ignition of clothing from these sources (E893.1)
poisoning by carbon monoxide from incomplete combustion of fuel (E867-E868.9)
that with conflagration (E891.0-E891.9)

E897 Accident caused by controlled fire not in building or structure
Burns from flame of:
bonfire (controlled)
brazier fire (controlled), not in building or structure
trash fire (controlled)

Excludes: *ignition of clothing from these sources (E893.2)*
trash fire out of control (E892)
that with conflagration (E892)

E898 Accident caused by other specified fire and flames

Excludes: *conflagration (E890.0-E892)*
that with ignition of:
clothing (E893.0-E893.9)
highly inflammable material (E894)

E898.0 Burning bedclothes
Bed set on fire NOS

E898.1 Other

Burning by:	Burning by:
blowlamp	lamp
blowtorch	lighter
candle	matches
cigar	pipe
cigarette	welding torch
fire in room NOS	

E899 Accident caused by unspecified fire
Burning NOS

● Code new
to this edition

▲ Revision of
existing code

④ ⑤ Fourth or fifth
digit required

ACCIDENTS DUE TO NATURAL AND ENVIRONMENTAL FACTORS (E900-E909)

E900 **Excessive heat**

E900.0 **Due to weather conditions**
Excessive heat as the external cause of:
ictus solaris
siriasis
sunstroke

E900.1 **Of man-made origin**

Heat (in):
boiler room
drying room
factory
furnace room

Heat (in):
generated in transport vehicle
kitchen

E900.9 **Of unspecified origin**

E901 **Excessive cold**

E901.0 **Due to weather conditions**
Excessive cold as the cause of:
chilblains NOS
immersion foot

E901.1 **Of man-made origin**
Contact with or inhalation of:
dry ice
liquid air
liquid hydrogen
liquid nitrogen
Prolonged exposure in:
deep freeze unit
refrigerator

E901.8 **Other specified origin**

E901.9 **Of unspecified origin**

E902 **High and low air pressure and changes in air pressure**

E902.0 **Residence or prolonged visit at high altitude**
Residence or prolonged visit at high altitude as the cause of:
Acosta syndrome
Alpine sickness
altitude sickness
Andes disease
anoxia, hypoxia
barotitis, barodontalgia, barosinusitis, otitic barotrauma
hypobarism, hypobaropathy
mountain sickness
range disease

E902.1 **In aircraft**
Sudden change in air pressure in aircraft during ascent or descent as the cause of:
aeroneurosis
aviators' disease

E902.2 **Due to diving**
High air pressure from rapid descent in water as the cause of: caisson disease, divers' disease, divers' palsy or paralysis
Reduction in atmospheric pressure while surfacing from deep water diving as the cause of: caisson disease, divers' disease, divers' palsy or paralysis

E902.8 **Due to other specified causes**
Reduction in atmospheric pressure while surfacing from underground

E902.9 **Unspecified cause**

E903 **Travel and motion**

E904 **Hunger, thirst, exposure, and neglect**

Excludes:	any condition resulting from homicidal intent (E968.0-E968.9)
	hunger, thirst, and exposure resulting from accidents connected with transport (E800.0-E848)

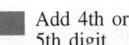 Add 4th or 5th digit   Nonspecific code   Unspecified code   Manifestation code

E904.0 Abandonment or neglect of infants and helpless persons
Exposure to weather conditions resulting from abandonment or neglect
Hunger or thirst resulting from abandonment or neglect
Desertion of newborn
Inattention at or after birth
Lack of care (helpless person) (infant)

[Excludes:] *criminal [purposeful] neglect (E968.4)*

E904.1 Lack of food
Lack of food as the cause of:
- inanition
- insufficient nourishment
- starvation

[Excludes:] *hunger resulting from abandonment or neglect (E904.0)*

E904.2 Lack of water
Lack of water as the cause of:
- dehydration
- inanition

[Excludes:] *dehydration due to acute fluid loss (276.5)*

E904.3 Exposure (to weather conditions), not elsewhere classifiable
Exposure NOS
Humidity
Struck by hailstones

[Excludes:] *struck by lightning (E907)*

E904.9 Privation, unqualified
Destitution

E905 Venomous animals and plants as the cause of poisoning and toxic reactions
Includes: chemical released by animal
insects
release of venom through fangs, hairs, spines, tentacles, and other venom apparatus

[Excludes:] *eating of poisonous animals or plants (E865.0-E865.9)*

E905.0 Venomous snakes and lizards
Cobra
Copperhead snake
Coral snake
Fer de lance
Gila monster
Krait
Mamba
Rattlesnake
Sea snake
Snake (venomous)
Viper
Water moccasin

[Excludes:] *bites of snakes and lizards known to be nonvenomous (E906.2)*

E905.1 Venomous spiders
Black widow spider
Brown spider
Tarantula (venomous)

E905.2 Scorpion

E905.3 Hornets, wasps, and bees
Yellow jacket

E905.4 Centipede and venomous millipede (tropical)

E905.5 Other venomous arthropods
Sting of:
- ant
- caterpillar

E905.6 Venomous marine animals and plants
Puncture by sea urchin spine
Sting of:
- coral
- jelly fish

Sting of:
- nematocysts
- sea anemone
- sea cucumber
- other marine animal or plant

[Excludes:] *bites and other injuries caused by nonvenomous marine animal (E906.2-E906.8)*
bite of sea snake (venomous) (E905.0)

E905.7 **Poisoning and toxic reactions caused by other plants**
Injection of poisons or toxins into or through skin by plant thorns, spines, or other mechanisms

Excludes: puncture wound NOS by plant thorns or spines (E920.8)

E905.8 **Other specified**

E905.9 **Unspecified**
Sting NOS   Venomous bite NOS

E906 **Other injury caused by animals**

Excludes: poisoning and toxic reactions caused by venomous animals and insects
(E905.0-E905.9)
road vehicle accident involving animals (E827.0-E828.9)
tripping or falling over an animal (E885.9)

E906.0 **Dog bite**

E906.1 **Rat bite**

E906.2 **Bite of nonvenomous snakes and lizards**

E906.3 **Bite of other animal except arthropod**
Cats   Rodents, except rats
Moray eel   Shark

E906.4 **Bite of nonvenomous arthropod**
Insect bite NOS

E906.5 **Bite by unspecified animal**
Animal bite NOS

E906.8 **Other specified injury caused by animal**
Butted by animal
Fallen on by horse or other animal, not being ridden
Gored by animal
Implantation of quills of porcupine
Pecked by bird
Run over by animal, not being ridden
Stepped on by animal, not being ridden

Excludes: injury by animal being ridden (E828.0-E828.9)

E906.9 **Unspecified injury caused by animal**

E907 **Lightning**

Excludes: injury from:
fall of tree or other object caused by lightning (E916)
fire caused by lightning (E890.0-E892)

E908 **Cataclysmic storms, and floods resulting from storms**

Excludes: collapse of dam or man-made structure causing flood (E909.3)

E908.0 **Hurricane**
Storm surge
"Tidal wave" caused by storm action
Typhoon

E908.1 **Tornado**
Cyclone
Twisters

E908.2 **Floods**
Torrential rainfall
Flash flood

Excludes: collapse of dam or man-made structure causing flood (909.3)

E908.3 **Blizzard (snow) (ice)**

E908.4 **Dust storm**

E908.8 **Other cataclysmic storms**

E908.9 **Unspecified cataclysmic storms, and floods resulting from storms**
Storm NOS

E909 **Cataclysmic earth surface movements and eruptions**

Excludes: "tidal wave" caused by storm action (E908.0)
transport accident involving collision with avalanche or landslide not in motion
(E800.0-E848)

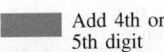

| | Add 4th or 5th digit | | Nonspecific code | | Unspecified code | | Manifestation code |

E909.0	**Earthquakes**
E909.1	**Volcanic eruptions**
	Burns from lava
	Ash inhalation
E909.2	**Avalanche, landslide, or mudslide**
E909.3	**Collapse of dam or man-made structure**
E909.4	**Tidal wave caused by earthquake**
	Tidal wave NOS
	Tsunami

> *Excludes:* *tidal wave caused by tropical storm (E908.0)*

E909.8	**Other cataclysmic earth surface movements and eruptions**
E909.9	**Unspecified cataclysmic earth surface movements and eruptions**

ACCIDENTS CAUSED BY SUBMERSION, SUFFOCATION, AND FOREIGN BODIES (E910-E915)

E910 **Accidental drowning and submersion**
    Includes: immersion
                swimmers' cramp

> *Excludes:* *diving accident (NOS) (resulting in injury except drowning) (E883.0)*
> *diving with insufficient air supply (E913.2)*
> *drowning and submersion due to:*
>   *cataclysm (E908-E909)*
>   *machinery accident (E919.0-E919.9)*
>   *transport accident (E800.0-E845.9)*
> *effect of high and low air pressure (E902.2)*
> *injury from striking against objects while in running water (E917.2)*

E910.0 **While water-skiing**
    Fall from water skis with submersion or drowning

> *Excludes:* *accident to water-skier involving a watercraft and resulting in submersion or*
>   *other injury (E830.4, E831.4)*

E910.1 **While engaged in other sport or recreational activity with diving equipment**
    Scuba diving NOS
    Skin diving NOS
    Underwater spear fishing NOS

E910.2 **While engaged in other sport or recreational activity without diving equipment**
    Fishing or hunting, except from boat or with diving equipment
    Ice skating
    Playing in water
    Surfboarding
    Swimming NOS
    Voluntarily jumping from boat, not involved in accident, for swim NOS
    Wading in water

> *Excludes:* *jumping into water to rescue another person (E910.3)*

E910.3 **While swimming or diving for purposes other than recreation or sport**
    Marine salvage (with diving equipment)
    Pearl diving (with diving equipment)
    Placement of fishing nets (with diving equipment)
    Rescue (attempt) of another person (with diving equipment)
    Underwater construction or repairs (with diving equipment)

E910.4 **In bathtub**

E910.8 **Other accidental drowning or submersion**
    Drowning in:
      quenching tank
      swimming pool

E910.9 **Unspecified accidental drowning or submersion**
    Accidental fall into water NOS
    Drowning NOS

● Code new to this edition   ▲ Revision of existing code   ④ ⑤ Fourth or fifth digit required

E911   Inhalation and ingestion of food causing obstruction of respiratory tract or suffocation
Aspiration and inhalation of food [any] (into respiratory tract) NOS
Asphyxia by food [including bone, seed in food, regurgitated food]
Choked on food [including bone, seed in food, regurgitated food]
Suffocation by food [including bone, seed in food, regurgitated food]
Compression of trachea by food lodged in esophagus
Interruption of respiration by food lodged in esophagus
Obstruction of respiration by food lodged in esophagus
Obstruction of pharynx by food (bolus)

Excludes: *injury, except asphyxia and obstruction of respiratory passage, caused by food*
(E915)
obstruction of esophagus by food without mention of asphyxia or obstruction of
respiratory passage (E915)

E912   Inhalation and ingestion of other object causing obstruction of respiratory tract or suffocation
Aspiration and inhalation of foreign body except food (into respiratory tract) NOS
Foreign object [bean] [marble] in nose
Obstruction of pharynx by foreign body
Compression by foreign body in esophagus
Interruption of respiration by foreign body in esophagus
Obstruction of respiration by foreign body in esophagus

Excludes: *injury, except asphyxia and obstruction of respiratory passage, caused by foreign*
body (E915)
obstruction of esophagus by foreign body without mention of asphyxia or
obstruction in respiratory passage (E915)

E913   Accidental mechanical suffocation

Excludes: *mechanical suffocation from or by:*
accidental inhalation or ingestion of:
food (E911)
foreign object (E912)
cataclysm (E908-E909)
explosion (E921.0-E921.9, E923.0-E923.9)
machinery accident (E919.0-E919.9)

E913.0   In bed or cradle

Excludes: *suffocation by plastic bag (E913.1)*

E913.1   By plastic bag

E913.2   Due to lack of air (in closed place)
Accidentally closed up in refrigerator or other airtight enclosed space
Diving with insufficient air supply

Excludes: *suffocation by plastic bag (E913.1)*

E913.3   By falling earth or other substance
Cave-in NOS

Excludes: *cave-in caused by cataclysmic earth surface movements and eruptions (E909)*
struck by cave-in without asphyxiation or suffocation (E916)

E913.8   Other specified means
Accidental hanging, except in bed or cradle

E913.9   Unspecified means
Asphyxia, mechanical NOS
Strangulation NOS
Suffocation NOS

E914   Foreign body accidentally entering eye and adnexa

Excludes: *corrosive liquid (E924.1)*

E915   Foreign body accidentally entering other orifice

Excludes: *aspiration and inhalation of foreign body, any, (into respiratory tract) NOS*
(E911-E912)

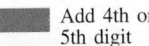 Add 4th or
5th digit

 Nonspecific
code

Unspecified
code

Manifestation
code

OTHER ACCIDENTS (E916-E928)

E916 Struck accidentally by falling object

Collapse of building, except on fire   Object falling from machine, not in operation
Falling rock   Object falling from stationary vehicle
Falling snowslide NOS
Falling stone
Falling tree

Code first: collapse of building on fire (E890.0-E891.9)
        falling object in:
           cataclysm (E908-E909)
           machinery accidents (E919.0-E919.9)
           transport accidents (E800.0-E845.9)
           vehicle accidents not elsewhere classifiable (E846-E848)
        object set in motion by explosion (E921.0-E921.9, E923.0-E923.9)
        object set in motion by firearm (E922.0-E922.9)
        projected object (E917.0-E917.9)

E917 Striking against or struck accidentally by objects or persons

Includes:

    bumping into or against object (moving) (projected) (stationary), pedestrian conveyance, or person

    colliding with object (moving) (projected) (stationary), pedestrian conveyance, or person

    kicking against object (moving) (projected) (stationary), pedestrian conveyance, or person

    stepping on object (moving) (projected) (stationary), pedestrian conveyance, or person

    struck by object (moving) (projected) (stationary), pedestrian conveyance, or person

Excludes: *fall from collision with another person, except when caused by a crowd (E886.0-E886.9)*
    fall from stumbling over object (E885.9)
    fall resulting in striking against object (E888.0, E888.1)
    injury caused by:
        assault (E960.0-E960.1, E967.0-E967.9)
        cutting or piercing instrument (E920.0-E920.9)
        explosion (E921.0-E921.9, E923.0-E923.9)
        firearm (E922.0-E922.9)
        machinery (E919.0-E919.9)
        transport vehicle (E800.0-E845.9)
        vehicle not elsewhere classifiable (E846-E848)

E917.0 In sports without subsequent fall
Kicked or stepped on during game (football) (rugby)
Struck by hit or thrown ball
Struck by hockey stick or puck

E917.1 Caused by a crowd, by collective fear or panic without subsequent fall
Crushed by crown or human stampede
Pushed by crown or human stampede
Stepped on by crown or human stampede

E917.2 In running water without subsequent fall

Excludes: *drowning or submersion (E910.0-E910.9)*
    that in sports (E917.0, E917.5)

E917.3 Furniture without subsequent fall

Excludes: *fall from furniture (E884.2, E884.4-E884.5)*

E917.4 Other stationary object without subsequent fall
Bath tub
Fence
Lamp-post

E917.5 Object in sports with subsequent fall
Knocked down while boxing

E917.6 Caused by a crowd, by collective fear or panic with subsequent fall

E917.7 Furniture with subsequent fall

Excludes: *fall from furniture (E884.2, E884.4-E884.5)*

E917.8 Other stationary object with subsequent fall
Bath tub
Fence
Lamp-post

● Code new to this edition   ▲ Revision of existing code   ④ ⑤ Fourth or fifth digit required

E917.9   Other striking against with or without subsequent fall

E918   Caught accidentally in or between objects
Caught, crushed, jammed, or pinched in or between moving or stationary objects, such as:
escalator
folding object
hand tools, appliances, or implements
sliding door and door frame
under packing crate
washing machine wringer

Excludes: *injury caused by:*
> *cutting or piercing instrument (E920.0-E920.9)*
> *machinery (E919.0-E919.9)*
> *transport vehicle (E800.0-E845.9)*
> *vehicle not elsewhere classifiable (E846-E848)*
> *struck accidentally by:*
> *falling object (E916)*
> *object (moving) (projected) (E917.0-E917.9)*

E919   Accidents caused by machinery
Includes:
> burned by machinery (accident)
> caught in (moving parts of) machinery (accident)
> collapse of machinery (accident)
> crushed by machinery (accident)
> cut or pierced by machinery (accident)
> drowning or submersion caused by machinery (accident)
> explosion of, on, in machinery (accident)
> fall from or into moving part of machinery (accident)
> fire starting in or on machinery (accident)
> mechanical suffocation caused by machinery (accident)
> object falling from, on, in motion by machinery (accident)
> overturning of machinery (accident)
> pinned under machinery (accident)
> run over by machinery (accident)
> struck by machinery (accident)
> thrown from machinery (accident)
> caught between machinery and other object
> machinery accident NOS

Excludes: *accidents involving machinery, not in operation (E884.9, E916-E918)*
> *injury caused by:*
> *electric current in connection with machinery (E925.0-E925.9)*
> *escalator (E880.0, E918)*
> *explosion of pressure vessel in connection with machinery (E921.0-E921.9)*
> *moving sidewalk (E885.9)*
> *powered hand tools, appliances, and implements (E916-E918, E920.0-E921.9,*
> *E923.0-E926.9)*
> *transport vehicle accidents involving machinery (E800.0-E848.9)*
> *poisoning by carbon monoxide generated by machine (E868.8)*

E919.0   Agriculture machines

Animal-powered	Farm tractor
agricultural machine	Harvester
Combine	Hay mower or rake
Derrick, hay	Reaper
Farm machinery NOS	Thresher

Excludes: *that in transport under own power on the highway (E810.0-E819.9)*
> *that being towed by another vehicle on the highway (E810.0-E819.9,*
> *E827.0-E827.9, E829.0-E829.9)*
> *that involved in accident classifiable to E820-E829 (E820.0-E829.9)*

E919.1   Mining and earth-drilling machinery

Bore or drill (land)	Shaft lift
(seabed)	Under-cutter
Shaft hoist	

Excludes: *coal car, tram, truck, and tub in mine (E846)*

Add 4th or 5th digit	Nonspecific code	Unspecified code	Manifestation code

E919.2 Lifting machines and appliances
Chain hoist except in agricultural or mining operations
Crane except in agricultural or mining operations
Derrick except in agricultural or mining operations
Elevator (building) (grain) except in agricultural or mining operations
Forklift truck except in agricultural or mining operations
Lift except in agricultural or mining operations
Pulley block except in agricultural or mining operations
Winch except in agricultural or mining operations

[Excludes:] *that being towed by another vehicle on the highway (E810.0-E819.9, E827.0-E827.9, E829.0-E829.9)*
that in transport under own power on the highway (E810.0-E819.9)
that involved in accident classifiable to E820-E829 (E820.0-E829.9)

E919.3 Metalworking machines
Abrasive wheel
Forging machine
Lathe
Mechanical shears
Metal:
drilling machine
milling machine
power press
rolling-mill
sawing machine

E919.4 Woodworking and forming machines
Band saw
Bench saw
Circular saw
Molding machine
Overhead plane
Powered saw
Radial saw
Sander

[Excludes:] *hand saw (E920.1)*

E919.5 Prime movers, except electrical motors
Gas turbine
Internal combustion engine
Steam engine
Water driven turbine

[Excludes:] *that being towed by other vehicle on the highway (E810.0-E819.9, E827.0-E827.9, E829.0-E829.9)*
that in transport under own power on the highway (E810.0-E819.9)

E919.6 Transmission machinery
Transmission:
belt
cable
chain
gear
Transmission:
pinion
pulley
shaft

E919.7 Earth moving, scraping, and other excavating machines
Bulldozer
Road scraper
Steam shovel

[Excludes:] *that being towed by other vehicle on the highway (E810.0-E819.9, E827.0-E827.9, E829.0-E829.9)*
that in transport under own power on the highway (E810.0-E819.9)

E919.8 Other specified machinery
Machines for manufacture of:
clothing
foodstuffs and beverages
paper
Printing machine
Recreational machinery
Spinning, weaving, and textile machines

E919.9 Unspecified machinery

E920 Accidents caused by cutting and piercing instruments or objects
Includes: accidental injury (by) object:
edged
pointed
sharp

E920.0 Powered lawn mower

E920.1 **Other powered hand tools**
Any powered hand tool [compressed air] [electric] [explosive cartridge] [hydraulic power], such as:

drill	rivet gun
hand saw	snow blower
hedge clipper	staple gun

Excludes: *band saw (E919.4)*
bench saw (E919.4)

E920.2 **Powered household appliances and implements**

Blender	Electric:
Electric:	knife
beater or mixer	sewing machine
can opener	Garbage disposal appliance
fan	

E920.3 **Knives, swords, and daggers**

E920.4 **Other hand tools and implements**

Axe	Paper cutter
Can opener NOS	Pitchfork
Chisel	Rake
Fork	Scissors
Hand saw	Screwdriver
Hoe	Sewing machine, not powered
Ice pick	Shovel
Needle (sewing)	

E920.5 **Hypodermic needle**
Contaminated needle
Needle stick

E920.8 **Other specified cutting and piercing instruments or objects**

Arrow	Nail
Broken glass	Plant thorn
Dart	Splinter
Edge of stiff paper	Tin can lid
Lathe turnings	

Excludes: *animal spines or quills (E906.8)*
flying glass due to explosion (E921.0-E923.9)

E920.9 **Unspecified cutting and piercing instrument or object**

E921 **Accident caused by explosion of pressure vessel**
Includes: accidental explosion of pressure vessels, whether or not part of machinery

Excludes: *explosion of pressure vessel on transport vehicle (E800.0-E845.9)*

E921.0 **Boilers**

E921.1 **Gas cylinders**
Air tank   Pressure gas tank

E921.8 **Other specified pressure vessels**
Aerosol can   Pressure cooker
Automobile tire

E921.9 **Unspecified pressure vessel**

E922 **Accident caused by firearm and air gun missile**

E922.0 **Handgun**
Pistol   Revolver

Excludes: *Verey pistol (E922.8)*

E922.1 **Shotgun (automatic)**

E922.2 **Hunting rifle**

E922.3 **Military firearms**
Army rifle   Machine gun

E922.4 **Air gun**
BB gun   Pellet gun

● **E922.5** **Paintball gun**

E922.8 **Other specified firearm missile**
Verey pistol [flare]

E922.9 **Unspecified firearm missile**
Gunshot wound NOS   Shot NOS

	Add 4th or 5th digit		Nonspecific code		Unspecified code		Manifestation code

E923 Accident caused by explosive material

Includes: flash burns and other injuries resulting from explosion of explosive material
ignition of highly explosive material with explosion

[Excludes:] *explosion:*
in or on machinery (E919.0-E919.9)
on any transport vehicle, except stationary motor vehicle (E800.0-E848)
with conflagration (E890.0, E891.0, E892)
secondary fires resulting from explosion (E890.0-E899)

E923.0 Fireworks

E923.1 Blasting materials

Blasting cap
Detonator
Dynamite
Explosive [any] used in blasting operations

E923.2 Explosive gases

Acetylene
Butane
Coal gas
Explosion in mine NOS
Fire damp
Gasoline fumes
Methane
Propane

E923.8 Other explosive materials

Bomb
Explosive missile
Grenade
Mine
Shell
Torpedo
Explosion in munitions:
dump
factory

E923.9 Unspecified explosive material

Explosion NOS

E924 Accident caused by hot substance or object, caustic or corrosive material, and steam

[Excludes:] *burning NOS (E899)*
chemical burn resulting from swallowing a corrosive substance (E860.0-E864.4)
fire caused by these substances and objects (E890.0-E894)
radiation burns (E926.0-E926.9)
therapeutic misadventures (E870.0-E876.9)

E924.0 Hot liquids and vapors, including steam

Burning or scalding by:
boiling water
hot or boiling liquids not primarily caustic or corrosive
liquid metal
steam
other hot vapor

[Excludes:] *hot (boiling) tap water (E924.2)*

E924.1 Caustic and corrosive substances

Burning by:
acid [any kind]
ammonia
caustic oven cleaner or other substance
corrosive substance
lye
vitriol

E924.2 Hot (boiling) tap water

E924.8 Other

Burning by:
heat from electric heating appliance
hot object NOS
light bulb
steam pipe

E924.9 Unspecified

● Code new to this edition ▲ Revision of existing code ④ ⑤ Fourth or fifth digit required

E925   Accident caused by electric current
Includes: electric current from exposed wire, faulty appliance, high voltage cable, live rail, or open electric socket as the cause of:

burn	electrocution
cardiac fibrillation	puncture wound
convulsion	respiratory paralysis
electric shock	

Excludes: *burn by heat from electrical appliance (E924.8)*
lightning (E907)

E925.0   Domestic wiring and appliances

E925.1   Electric power generating plants, distribution stations, transmission lines
Broken power line

E925.2   Industrial wiring, appliances, and electrical machinery

Conductors	Electrical equipment and machinery
Control apparatus	Transformers

E925.8   Other electric current

Wiring and appliances in or on:	Wiring and appliances in or on:
farm [not farmhouse]	residential institutions
outdoors	schools
public building	

E925.9   Unspecified electric current
Burns or other injury from electric current NOS
Electric shock NOS
Electrocution NOS

E926   Exposure to radiation
Excludes: *abnormal reaction to or complication of treatment without mention of misadventure (E879.2)*
atomic power plant malfunction in water transport (E838.0-E838.9)
misadventure to patient in surgical and medical procedures (E873.2-E873.3)
use of radiation in war operations (E996-E997.9)

E926.0   Radiofrequency radiation
Overexposure to:
microwave radiation from: high-powered radio and television transmitters, industrial radiofrequency induction heaters, or radar installations
radar radiation from: high-powered radio and television transmitters, industrial radiofrequency induction heaters, or radar installations
radiofrequency from: high-powered radio and television transmitters, industrial radiofrequency induction heaters, or radar installations
radiofrequency radiation [any] from: high-powered radio and television transmitters, industrial radiofrequency induction heaters, or radar installations

E926.1   Infra-red heaters and lamps
Exposure to infra-red radiation from heaters and lamps as the cause of:
blistering
burning
charring
inflammatory change

Excludes: *physical contact with heater or lamp (E924.8)*

E926.2   Visible and ultraviolet light sources

Arc lamps	Oxygas welding torch
Black light sources	Sun rays
Electrical welding arc	Tanning bed

Excludes: *excessive heat from these sources (E900.1-E900.9)*

E926.3   X-rays and other electromagnetic ionizing radiation

Gamma rays	X-rays (hard) (soft)

E926.4   Lasers

E926.5   Radioactive isotopes

Radiobiologicals	Radiopharmaceuticals

E926.8   Other specified radiation
Artificially accelerated beams of ionized particles generated by:
betatrons
synchrotrons

E926.9   Unspecified radiation
Radiation NOS

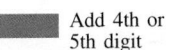 Add 4th or 5th digit

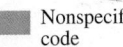 Nonspecific code

Unspecified code

Manifestation code

E927 Overexertion and strenuous movements
  Excessive physical exercise
  Overexertion (from):
    lifting
    pulling
    pushing
  Strenuous movements in:
    recreational activities
    other activities

E928 Other and unspecified environmental and accidental causes

  E928.0 Prolonged stay in weightless environment
    Weightlessness in spacecraft (simulator)

  E928.1 Exposure to noise
    Noise (pollution)
    Sound waves
    Supersonic waves

  E928.2 Vibration

  E928.3 Human bite

  E928.8 Other

  E928.9 Unspecified accident
    Accident NOS
    Blow NOS
    Casualty (not due to war), stated as accidentally inflicted, but not otherwise specified
    Decapitation, stated as accidentally inflicted, but not otherwise specified
    Injury [any part of body, or unspecified], stated as accidentally inflicted, but not
      otherwise specified
    Killed, stated as accidentally inflicted, but not otherwise specified
    Knocked down, stated as accidentally inflicted, but not otherwise specified
    Mangled, stated as accidentally inflicted, but not otherwise specified
    Wound, stated as accidentally inflicted, but not otherwise specified

  Excludes: *fracture, cause unspecified (E887)*
        injuries undetermined whether accidentally or purposely inflicted (E980.0-E989)

LATE EFFECTS OF ACCIDENTAL INJURY (E929)

  Note: This category is to be used to indicate accidental injury as the cause of death or disability
      from late effects, which are themselves classifiable elsewhere. The "late effects" include
      conditions reported as such or as sequelae which may occur at any time after the acute
      injury.

E929 Late effects of accidental injury
  Excludes: *late effects of:*
        surgical and medical procedures (E870.0-E879.9)
        therapeutic use of drugs and medicines (E930.0-E949.9)

  E929.0 Late effects of motor vehicle accident
    Late effects of accidents classifiable to E810-E825

  E929.1 Late effects of other transport accident
    Late effects of accidents classifiable to E800-E807, E826-E838, E840-E848

  E929.2 Late effects of accidental poisoning
    Late effects of accidents classifiable to E850-E858, E860-E869

  E929.3 Late effects of accidental fall
    Late effects of accidents classifiable to E880-E888

  E929.4 Late effects of accident caused by fire
    Late effects of accidents classifiable to E890-E899

  E929.5 Late effects of accident due to natural and environmental factors
    Late effects of accidents classifiable to E900-E909

  E929.8 Late effects of other accidents
    Late effects of accidents classifiable to E910-E928.8

  E929.9 Late effects of unspecified accident
    Late effects of accidents classifiable to E928.9

● Code new
  to this edition
▲ Revision of
  existing code
④ ⑤ Fourth or fifth
  digit required

DRUGS, MEDICINAL AND BIOLOGICAL SUBSTANCES CAUSING ADVERSE EFFECTS IN THERAPEUTIC USE (E930-E949)

Includes: correct drug properly administered in therapeutic or prophylactic dosage, as the cause of any adverse effect including allergic or hypersensitivity reactions

Excludes: *accidental overdose of drug and wrong drug given or taken in error (E850.0-E858.9)*

accidents in the technique of administration of drug or biological substance, such as accidental puncture during injection, or contamination of drug (E870.0-E876.9)

administration with suicidal or homicidal intent or intent to harm, or in circumstances classifiable to E980-E989 (E950.0-E950.5, E962.0, E980.0-E980.5)

See Alphabetic Index for more complete list of specific drugs to be classified under the fourth-digit subdivisions. The American Hospital Formulary numbers can be used to classify new drugs listed by the American Hospital Formulary Service (AHFS). See appendix C.

E930 Antibiotics

Excludes: *that used as eye, ear, nose, and throat [ENT], and local anti-infectives (E946.0-E946.9)*

E930.0 Penicillins
Natural
Synthetic
Semisynthetic, such as:
  ampicillin

Semisynthetic, such as:
  cloxacillin
  nafcillin
  oxacillin

E930.1 Antifungal antibiotics
Amphotericin B
Griseofulvin

Hachimycin [trichomycin]
Nystatin

E930.2 Chloramphenicol group
Chloramphenicol

Thiamphenicol

E930.3 Erythromycin and other macrolides
Oleandomycin

Spiramycin

E930.4 Tetracycline group
Doxycycline
Minocycline

Oxytetracycline

E930.5 Cephalosporin group
Cephalexin
Cephaloglycin

Cephaloridine
Cephalothin

E930.6 Antimycobacterial antibiotics
Cycloserine
Kanamycin

Rifampin
Streptomycin

E930.7 Antineoplastic antibiotics
Actinomycins, such as:
  Cactinomycin
  Dactinomycin

Bleomycin
Daunorubicin
Mitomycin

Excludes: *other antineoplastic drugs (E933.1)*

E930.8 Other specified antibiotics

E930.9 Unspecified antibiotic

E931 Other anti-infectives

Excludes: *ENT, and local anti-infectives (E946.0-E946.9)*

E931.0 Sulfonamides
Sulfadiazine
Sulfafurazole

Sulfamethoxazole

E931.1 Arsenical anti-infectives

E931.2 Heavy metal anti-infectives
Compounds of:
  antimony
  bismuth

Compounds of:
  lead
  mercury

Excludes: *mercurial diuretics (E944.0)*

E931.3 Quinoline and hydroxyquinoline derivatives
Chiniofon

Diiodohydroxyquin

Excludes: *antimalarial drugs (E931.4)*

| | Add 4th or 5th digit | | Nonspecific code | | Unspecified code | | Manifestation code |

E931.4 Antimalarials and drugs acting on other blood protozoa
Chloroquine phosphate   Proguanil [chloroguanide]
Cycloguanil   Pyrimethamine
Primaquine   Quinine (sulphate)

E931.5 Other antiprotozoal drugs
Emetine

E931.6 Anthelmintics
Hexylresorcinol   Piperazine
Male fern oleoresin   Thiabendazole

E931.7 Antiviral drugs
Methisazone

Excludes: *amantadine (E936.4)*
         cytarabine (E933.1)
         idoxuridine (E946.5)

E931.8 Other antimycobacterial drugs
Ethambutol   Para-aminosalicylic acid derivatives
Ethionamide   Sulfones
Isoniazid

E931.9 Other and unspecified anti-infectives
Flucytosine   Nitrofuran derivatives

E932 Hormones and synthetic substitutes

E932.0 Adrenal cortical steroids
Cortisone derivatives
Desoxycorticosterone derivatives
Fluorinated corticosteroids

E932.1 Androgens and anabolic congeners
Nandrolone phenpropionate
Oxymetholone
Testosterone and preparations

E932.2 Ovarian hormones and synthetic substitutes
Contraceptives, oral
Estrogens
Estrogens and progestogens combined
Progestogens

E932.3 Insulins and antidiabetic agents
Acetohexamide   Insulin
Biguanide derivatives, oral   Phenformin
Chlorpropamide   Sulfonylurea derivatives, oral
Glucagon   Tolbutamide

Excludes: *adverse effect of insulin administered for shock therapy (E879.3)*

E932.4 Anterior pituitary hormones
Corticotropin   Somatotropin [growth hormone]
Gonadotropin

E932.5 Posterior pituitary hormones
Vasopressin

Excludes: *oxytocic agents (E945.0)*

E932.6 Parathyroid and parathyroid derivatives

E932.7 Thyroid and thyroid derivatives
Dextrothyroxine   Liothyronine
Levothyroxine sodium   Thyroglobulin

E932.8 Antithyroid agents
Iodides   Thiourea
Thiouracil

E932.9 Other and unspecified hormones and synthetic substitutes

E933 Primarily systemic agents

E933.0 Antiallergic and antiemetic drugs
Antihistamines   Diphenylpyraline
Chlorpheniramine   Thonzylamine
Diphenhydramine   Tripelennamine

Excludes: *phenothiazine-based tranquilizers (E939.1)*

● Code new to this edition   ▲ Revision of existing code   ④ ⑤ Fourth or fifth digit required

E933.1 Antineoplastic and immunosuppressive drugs
 Azathioprine   Mechlorethamine hydrochloride
 Busulfan   Mercaptopurine
 Chlorambucil   Triethylenethiophosphoramide [thio-TEPA]
 Cyclophosphamide
 Cytarabine
 Fluorouracil

 Excludes: antineoplastic antibiotics (E930.7)

E933.2 Acidifying agents

E933.3 Alkalizing agents

E933.4 Enzymes, not elsewhere classified
 Penicillinase

E933.5 Vitamins, not elsewhere classified
 Vitamin A   Vitamin D

 Excludes: nicotinic acid (E942.2)
      vitamin K (E934.3)

E933.8 Other systemic agents, not elsewhere classified
 Heavy metal antagonists

E933.9 Unspecified systemic agent

E934 Agents primarily affecting blood constituents

E934.0 Iron and its compounds
 Ferric salts
 Ferrous sulphate and other ferrous salts

E934.1 Liver preparations and other antianemic agents
 Folic acid

E934.2 Anticoagulants
 Coumarin   Prothrombin synthesis inhibitor
 Heparin   Warfarin sodium
 Phenindione

E934.3 Vitamin K [phytonadione]

E934.4 Fibrinolysis-affecting drugs
 Aminocaproic acid   Streptokinase
 Streptodornase   Urokinase

E934.5 Anticoagulant antagonists and other coagulants
 Hexadimethrine bromide   Protamine sulfate

E934.6 Gamma globulin

E934.7 Natural blood and blood products
 Blood plasma   Packed red cells
 Human fibrinogen   Whole blood

E934.8 Other agents affecting blood constituents
 Macromolecular blood substitutes

E934.9 Unspecified agent affecting blood constituents

E935 Analgesics, antipyretics, and antirheumatics

E935.0 Heroin
 Diacetylmorphine

E935.1 Methadone

E935.2 Other opiates and related narcotics
 Codeine [methylmorphine]   Opium (alkaloids)
 Morphine   Meperidine [pethidine]

E935.3 Salicylates
 Acetylsalicylic acid [aspirin]
 Amino derivatives of salicylic acid
 Salicylic acid salts

E935.4 Aromatic analgesics, not elsewhere classified
 Acetanilid
 Paracetamol [acetaminophen]
 Phenacetin [acetophenetidin]

E935.5 Pyrazole derivatives
 Aminophenazone [aminopyrine]
 Phenylbutazone

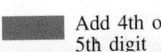

Add 4th or   Nonspecific   Unspecified   Manifestation
5th digit   code   code   code

E935.6 Antirheumatics [antiphlogistics]
    Gold salts   Indomethacin
   Excludes: salicylates (E935.3)
             steroids (E932.0)

E935.7 Other non-narcotic analgesics
    Pyrabital

E935.8 Other specified analgesics and antipyretics
    Pentazocine

E935.9 Unspecified analgesic and antipyretic

E936 Anticonvulsants and anti-Parkinsonism drugs

E936.0 Oxazolidine derivatives
    Paramethadione   Trimethadione

E936.1 Hydantoin derivatives
    Phenytoin

E936.2 Succinimides
    Ethosuximide   Phensuximide

E936.3 Other and unspecified anticonvulsants
    Beclamide   Primidone

E936.4 Anti-Parkinsonism drugs
    Amantadine
    Ethopropazine [profenamine]
    Levodopa [L-dopa]

E937 Sedatives and hypnotics

E937.0 Barbiturates
    Amobarbital [amylobarbitone]
    Barbital [barbitone]
    Butabarbital [butabarbitone]
    Pentobarbital [pentobarbitone]
    Phenobarbital [phenobarbitone]
    Secobarbital [quinalbarbitone]
   Excludes: thiobarbiturates (E938.3)

E937.1 Chloral hydrate group

E937.2 Paraldehyde

E937.3 Bromine compounds
    Bromide   Carbromal (derivatives)

E937.4 Methaqualone compounds

E937.5 Glutethimide group

E937.6 Mixed sedatives, not elsewhere classified

E937.8 Other sedatives and hypnotics

E937.9 Unspecified
    Sleeping:
      drug NOS
      pill NOS
      tablet NOS

E938 Other central nervous system depressants and anesthetics

E938.0 Central nervous system muscle-tone depressants
    Chlorphenesin (carbamate)   Methocarbamol
    Mephenesin

E938.1 Halothane

E938.2 Other gaseous anesthetics
    Ether
    Halogenated hydrocarbon derivatives, except halothane
    Nitrous oxide

E938.3 Intravenous anesthetics
    Ketamine   Thiobarbiturates, such as thiopental sodium
    Methohexital
    [methohexitone]

E938.4 Other and unspecified general anesthetics

● Code new to this edition   ▲ Revision of existing code   ④ ⑤ Fourth or fifth digit required

E938.5 Surface and infiltration anesthetics
    Cocaine   Procaine
    Lidocaine [lignocaine]   Tetracaine

E938.6 Peripheral nerve- and plexus-blocking anesthetics

E938.7 Spinal anesthetics

E938.9 Other and unspecified local anesthetics

E939 Psychotropic agents

E939.0 Antidepressants
    Amitriptyline   Monoamine oxidase [MAO] inhibitors
    Imipramine

E939.1 Phenothiazine-based tranquilizers
    Chlorpromazine   Prochlorperazine
    Fluphenazine   Promazine
    Phenothiazine

E939.2 Butyrophenone-based tranquilizers
    Haloperidol   Trifluperidol
    Spiperone

E939.3 Other antipsychotics, neuroleptics, and major tranquilizers

E939.4 Benzodiazepine-based tranquilizers
    Chlordiazepoxide   Lorazepam
    Diazepam   Medazepam
    Flurazepam   Nitrazepam

E939.5 Other tranquilizers
    Hydroxyzine   Meprobamate

E939.6 Psychodysleptics [hallucinogens]
    Cannabis (derivatives)   Mescaline
    Lysergide [LSD]   Psilocin
    Marihuana (derivatives) Psilocybin

E939.7 Psychostimulants
    Amphetamine   Caffeine
    Excludes: central appetite depressants (E947.0)

E939.8 Other psychotropic agents

E939.9 Unspecified psychotropic agent

E940 Central nervous system stimulants

E940.0 Analeptics
    Lobeline   Nikethamide

E940.1 Opiate antagonists
    Levallorphan   Naloxone
    Nalorphine

E940.8 Other specified central nervous system stimulants

E940.9 Unspecified central nervous system stimulant

E941 Drugs primarily affecting the autonomic nervous system

E941.0 Parasympathomimetics [cholinergics]
    Acetylcholine   Pilocarpine
    Anticholinesterase:
     organophosphorus
     reversible

E941.1 Parasympatholytics [anticholinergics and antimuscarinics] and spasmolytics
    Atropine   Hyoscine [scopolamine]
    Homatropine   Quaternary ammonium derivatives
    Excludes: papaverine (E942.5)

E941.2 Sympathomimetics [adrenergics]
    Epinephrine [adrenalin]
    Levarterenol [noradrenalin]

E941.3 Sympatholytics [antiadrenergics]
    Phenoxybenzamine   Tolazoline hydrochloride

E941.9 Unspecified drug primarily affecting the autonomic nervous system

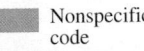 Add 4th or 5th digit
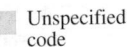 Nonspecific code
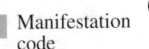 Unspecified code
Manifestation code

E942 **Agents primarily affecting the cardiovascular system**

E942.0 **Cardiac rhythm regulators**
Practolol
Procainamide
Propranolol
Quinidine

E942.1 **Cardiotonic glycosides and drugs of similar action**
Digitalis glycosides
Digoxin
Strophanthins

E942.2 **Antilipemic and antiarteriosclerotic drugs**
Cholestyramine
Clofibrate
Nicotinic acid derivatives
Sitosterols

Excludes: *dextrothyroxine (E932.7)*

E942.3 **Ganglion-blocking agents**
Pentamethonium bromide

E942.4 **Coronary vasodilators**
Dipyridamole
Nitrates [nitroglycerin]
Nitrites
Prenylamine

E942.5 **Other vasodilators**
Cyclandelate
Diazoxide
Hydralazine
Papaverine

E942.6 **Other antihypertensive agents**
Clonidine
Guanethidine
Rauwolfia alkaloids
Reserpine

E942.7 **Antivaricose drugs, including sclerosing agents**
Monoethanolamine
Zinc salts

E942.8 **Capillary-active drugs**
Adrenochrome derivatives
Bioflavonoids
Metaraminol

E942.9 **Other and unspecified agents primarily affecting the cardiovascular system**

E943 **Agents primarily affecting gastrointestinal system**

E943.0 **Antacids and antigastric secretion drugs**
Aluminum hydroxide
Magnesium trisilicate

E943.1 **Irritant cathartics**
Bisacodyl
Castor oil
Phenolphthalein

E943.2 **Emollient cathartics**
Sodium dioctyl sulfosuccinate

E943.3 **Other cathartics, including intestinal atonia drugs**
Magnesium sulfate

E943.4 **Digestants**
Pancreatin
Papain
Pepsin

E943.5 **Antidiarrheal drugs**
Bismuth subcarbonate
Kaolin
Pectin

Excludes: *anti-infectives (E930.0-E931.9)*

E943.6 **Emetics**

E943.8 **Other specified agents primarily affecting the gastrointestinal system**

E943.9 **Unspecified agent primarily affecting the gastrointestinal system**

E944 **Water, mineral, and uric acid metabolism drugs**

E944.0 **Mercurial diuretics**
Chlormerodrin
Mercaptomerin
Mercurophylline
Mersalyl

E944.1 **Purine derivative diuretics**
Theobromine
Theophylline

Excludes: *aminophylline [theophylline ethylenediamine] (E945.7)*

E944.2 **Carbonic acid anhydrase inhibitors**
Acetazolamide

E944.3 **Saluretics**
Benzothiadiazides
Chlorothiazide group

● Code new
to this edition

▲ Revision of
existing code

④ ⑤ Fourth or fifth
digit required

E944.4 **Other diuretics**
    Ethacrynic acid   Furosemide

E944.5 **Electrolytic, caloric, and water-balance agents**

E944.6 **Other mineral salts, not elsewhere classified**

E944.7 **Uric acid metabolism drugs**
    Cinchophen and congeners   Phenoquin
    Colchicine   Probenecid

E945 **Agents primarily acting on the smooth and skeletal muscles and respiratory system**

E945.0 **Oxytocic agents**
    Ergot alkaloids   Prostaglandins

E945.1 **Smooth muscle relaxants**
    Adiphenine
    Metaproterenol [orciprenaline]
    Excludes: papaverine (E942.5)

E945.2 **Skeletal muscle relaxants**
    Alcuronium chloride   Suxamethonium chloride

E945.3 **Other and unspecified drugs acting on muscles**

E945.4 **Antitussives**
    Dextromethorphan   Pipazethate hydrochloride

E945.5 **Expectorants**
    Acetylcysteine   Ipecacuanha
    Cocillana   Terpin hydrate
    Guaifenesin [glyceryl guaiacolate]

E945.6 **Anti-common cold drugs**

E945.7 **Antiasthmatics**
    Aminophylline [theophylline ethylenediamine]

E945.8 **Other and unspecified respiratory drugs**

E946 **Agents primarily affecting skin and mucous membrane, ophthalmological, otorhinolaryngological, and dental drugs**

E946.0 **Local anti-infectives and anti-inflammatory drugs**

E946.1 **Antipruritics**

E946.2 **Local astringents and local detergents**

E946.3 **Emollients, demulcents, and protectants**

E946.4 **Keratolytics, keratoplastics, other hair treatment drugs and preparations**

E946.5 **Eye anti-infectives and other eye drugs**
    Idoxuridine

E946.6 **Anti-infectives and other drugs and preparations for ear, nose, and throat**

E946.7 **Dental drugs topically applied**

E946.8 **Other agents primarily affecting skin and mucous membrane**
    Spermicides

E946.9 **Unspecified agent primarily affecting skin and mucous membrane**

E947 **Other and unspecified drugs and medicinal substances**

E947.0 **Dietetics**

E947.1 **Lipotropic drugs**

E947.2 **Antidotes and chelating agents, not elsewhere classified**

E947.3 **Alcohol deterrents**

E947.4 **Pharmaceutical excipients**

E947.8 **Other drugs and medicinal substances**
    Contrast media used for diagnostic x-ray procedures
    Diagnostic agents and kits

E947.9 **Unspecified drug or medicinal substance**

E948 **Bacterial vaccines**

E948.0 **BCG vaccine**

E948.1 **Typhoid and paratyphoid**

E948.2 **Cholera**

E948.3 **Plague**

E948.4 **Tetanus**

Add 4th or 5th digit   Nonspecific code   Unspecified code   Manifestation code

E948.5 Diphtheria

E948.6 Pertussis vaccine, including combinations with a pertussis component

E948.8 Other and unspecified bacterial vaccines

E948.9 Mixed bacterial vaccines, except combinations with a pertussis component

E949 Other vaccines and biological substances

[Excludes:] *gamma globulin (E934.6)*

E949.0 Smallpox vaccine

E949.1 Rabies vaccine

E949.2 Typhus vaccine

E949.3 Yellow fever vaccine

E949.4 Measles vaccine

E949.5 Poliomyelitis vaccine

E949.6 Other and unspecified viral and rickettsial vaccines

Mumps vaccine

E949.7 Mixed viral-rickettsial and bacterial vaccines, except combinations with a pertussis component

[Excludes:] *combinations with a pertussis component (E948.6)*

E949.9 Other and unspecified vaccines and biological substances

SUICIDE AND SELF-INFLICTED INJURY (E950-E959)

Includes: injuries in suicide and attempted suicide
self-inflicted injuries specified as intentional

E950 Suicide and self-inflicted poisoning by solid or liquid substances

E950.0 Analgesics, antipyretics, and antirheumatics

E950.1 Barbiturates

E950.2 Other sedatives and hypnotics

E950.3 Tranquilizers and other psychotropic agents

E950.4 Other specified drugs and medicinal substances

E950.5 Unspecified drug or medicinal substances

E950.6 Agricultural and horticultural chemical and pharmaceutical preparations other than plant foods and fertilizers

E950.7 Corrosive and caustic substances

Suicide and self-inflicted poisoning by substances classifiable to E864

E950.8 Arsenic and its compounds

E950.9 Other and unspecified solid and liquid substances

E951 Suicide and self-inflicted poisoning by gases in domestic use

E951.0 Gas distributed by pipeline

E951.1 Liquefied petroleum gas distributed in mobile containers

E951.8 Other utility gas

E952 Suicide and self-inflicted poisoning by other gases and vapors

E952.0 Motor vehicle exhaust gas

E952.1 Other carbon monoxide

E952.8 Other specified gases and vapors

E952.9 Unspecified gases and vapors

E953 Suicide and self-inflicted injury by hanging, strangulation, and suffocation

E953.0 Hanging

E953.1 Suffocation by plastic bag

E953.8 Other specified means

E953.9 Unspecified means

E954 Suicide and self-inflicted injury by submersion [drowning]

E955 Suicide and self-inflicted injury by firearms, air guns and explosives

E955.0 Handgun

E955.1 Shotgun

● Code new to this edition ▲ Revision of existing code ④ ⑤ Fourth or fifth digit required

 E955.2 **Hunting rifle**

 E955.3 **Military firearms**

 E955.4 **Other and unspecified firearm**
   Gunshot NOS   Shot NOS

 E955.5 **Explosives**

 E955.6 **Air gun**
   BB gun   Pellet gun

● E955.7 **Paintball gun**

 E955.9 **Unspecified**

E956 **Suicide and self-inflicted injury by cutting and piercing instrument**

E957 **Suicide and self-inflicted injuries by jumping from high place**

 E957.0 **Residential premises**

 E957.1 **Other man-made structures**

 E957.2 **Natural sites**

 E957.9 **Unspecified**

E958 **Suicide and self-inflicted injury by other and unspecified means**

 E958.0 **Jumping or lying before moving object**

 E958.1 **Burns, fire**

 E958.2 **Scald**

 E958.3 **Extremes of cold**

 E958.4 **Electrocution**

 E958.5 **Crashing of motor vehicle**

 E958.6 **Crashing of aircraft**

 E958.7 **Caustic substances, except poisoning**
   Excludes: *poisoning by caustic substance (E950.7)*

 E958.8 **Other specified means**

 E958.9 **Unspecified means**

E959 **Late effects of self-inflicted injury**
  Note: This category is to be used to indicate circumstances classifiable to E950-E958 as the
  cause of death or disability from late effects, which are themselves classifiable elsewhere.
  The "late effects" include conditions reported as such or as sequelae which may occur at
  any time after the attempted suicide or self-inflicted injury.

HOMICIDE AND INJURY PURPOSELY INFLICTED BY OTHER PERSONS (E960-E969)

  Includes: injuries inflicted by another person with intent to injure or kill, by any means

  Excludes: *injuries due to:*
     legal intervention (E970-E978)
     operations of war (E990-E999)
     terrorism (E979)

E960 **Fight, brawl, rape**

 E960.0 **Unarmed fight or brawl**
   Beatings NOS
   Brawl or fight with hands, fists, feet
   Injured or killed in fight NOS

  Excludes: *homicidal:*
     injury by weapons (E965.0-E966, E969)
     strangulation (E963)
     submersion (E964)

 E960.1 **Rape**

E961 **Assault by corrosive or caustic substance, except poisoning**
  Injury or death purposely caused by corrosive or caustic substance, such as:
   acid [any]
   corrosive substance
   vitriol

  Excludes: *burns from hot liquid (E968.3)*
     chemical burns from swallowing a corrosive substance (E962.0-E962.9)

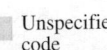

| | Add 4th or
5th digit | | Nonspecific
code | | Unspecified
code | | Manifestation
code |

E962 **Assault by poisoning**

E962.0 **Drugs and medicinal substances**
Homicidal poisoning by any drug or medicinal substance

E962.1 **Other solid and liquid substances**

E962.2 **Other gases and vapors**

E962.9 **Unspecified poisoning**

E963 **Assault by hanging and strangulation**
Homicidal (attempt):
garrotting or ligature
hanging
strangulation
suffocation

E964 **Assault by submersion [drowning]**

E965 **Assault by firearms and explosives**

E965.0 **Handgun**
Pistol   Revolver

E965.1 **Shotgun**

E965.2 **Hunting rifle**

E965.3 **Military firearms**

E965.4 **Other and unspecified firearm**

E965.5 **Antipersonnel bomb**

E965.6 **Gasoline bomb**

E965.7 **Letter bomb**

E965.8 **Other specified explosive**
Bomb NOS (placed in) car
Bomb NOS (placed in) house
Dynamite

E965.9 **Unspecified explosive**

E966 **Assault by cutting and piercing instrument**
Assassination (attempt), homicide (attempt) by any instrument classifiable under E920
Homicidal cut, any part of the body
Homicidal puncture, any part of the body
Homicidal stab, any part of the body
Stabbed, any part of the body

E967 **Perpetrator of child and adult abuse**
Note: selection of the correct perpetrator code is based on the relationship between the perpetrator and the victim

E967.0 **By father, stepfather or boyfriend**
Male partner of child's parent or guardian

E967.1 **By other specified person**

E967.2 **By mother, stepmother or girlfriend**
Female partner of child's parent or guardian

E967.3 **By spouse or partner**
Abuse of spouse or partner by ex-spouse or ex-partner

E967.4 **By child**

E967.5 **By sibling**

E967.6 **By grandparent**

E967.7 **By other relative**

E967.8 **By non-related caregiver**

E967.9 **By unspecified person**

E968 **Assault by other and unspecified means**

E968.0 **Fire**
Arson   Homicidal burns NOS

Excludes: *burns from hot liquid (E968.3)*

E968.1 **Pushing from a high place**

E968.2 **Striking by blunt or thrown object**

● Code new
to this edition   ▲ Revision of
existing code   ④ ⑤ Fourth or fifth
digit required

E968.3 **Hot liquid**
Homicidal burns by scalding

E968.4 **Criminal neglect**
Abandonment of child, infant, or other helpless person with intent to injure or kill

E968.5 **Transport vehicle**
Being struck by other vehicle or run down with intent to injure
Pushed in front of, thrown from, or dragged by moving vehicle with intent to injure

E968.6 **Air gun**
BB gun
Pellet gun

E968.7 **Human bite**

E968.8 **Other specified means**

E968.9 **Unspecified means**
Assassination (attempt) NOS   Manslaughter (nonaccidental)
Homicidal (attempt):   Murder (attempt) NOS
    injury NOS   Violence, non-accidental
    wound NOS

E969 Late effects of injury purposely inflicted by other person
Note: This category is to be used to indicate circumstances classifiable to E960-E968 as the
cause of death or disability from late effects, which are themselves classifiable elsewhere.
The "late effects" include conditions reported as such, or as sequelae which may occur at
any time after the acute injury.

LEGAL INTERVENTION (E970-E978)

Includes: injuries inflicted by the police or other law-enforcing agents, including military on
duty, in the course of arresting or attempting to arrest lawbreakers, suppressing
disturbances, maintaining order, and other legal action
legal execution

Excludes: *injuries caused by civil insurrections (E990.0-E999)*

E970 Injury due to legal intervention by firearms
Gunshot wound   Injury by:
Injury by: rifle pellet or rubber bullet
    machine gun   shot NOS
    revolver

E971 Injury due to legal intervention by explosives
Injury by:
    dynamite
    explosive shell
    grenade
    mortar bomb

E972 Injury due to legal intervention by gas
Asphyxiation by gas
Injury by tear gas
Poisoning by gas

E973 Injury due to legal intervention by blunt object
Hit, struck by:
    baton (nightstick)
    blunt object
    stave

E974 Injury due to legal intervention by cutting and piercing instrument
Cut   Incised wound
Injured by bayonet   Stab wound

E975 Injury due to legal intervention by other specified means
Blow
Manhandling

E976 Injury due to legal intervention by unspecified means

E977 Late effects of injuries due to legal intervention
Note: This category is to be used to indicate circumstances classifiable to E970-E976 as the
cause of death or disability from late effects, which are themselves classifiable elsewhere.
The "late effects" include conditions reported as such, or as sequelae which may occur at
any time after the acute injury due to legal intervention.

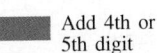 Add 4th or
5th digit

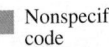 Nonspecific
code

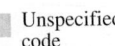 Unspecified
code

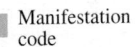 Manifestation
code

E978 Legal execution

All executions performed at the behest of the judiciary or ruling authority [whether permanent or temporary] as:

asphyxiation by gas
beheading, decapitation
  (by guillotine)
capital punishment
electrocution

hanging
poisoning
shooting
other specified means

TERRORISM (E979)

● **E979** **Terrorism**

Injuries resulting from the unlawful use of force or violence against persons or property to intimidate or coerce a Government, the civilian population, or any segment thereof, in furtherance of political or social objective

● **E979.0** **Terrorism involving explosion of marine weapons**
Depth-charge
Marine mine
Mine NOS, at sea or in harbor
Sea-based artillery shell
Torpedo
Underwater blast

● **E979.1** **Terrorism involving destruction of aircraft**
Aircraft used as a weapon
Aircraft:
  burned
  exploded
  shot down
Crushed by falling aircraft

● **E979.2** **Terrorism involving other explosions and fragments**
Antipersonnel bomb
  (fragments)
Blast NOS
Explosion (of):
  artillery shell
  breech-block
  cannon block
  mortar bomb
  munitions being used in
    terrorism NOS

Fragments from:
  artillery shell
  bomb
  grenade
  guided missile
  land-mine
  rocket
  shell
  shrapnel
Mine NOS

● **E979.3** **Terrorism involving fires, conflagration and hot substances**
Burning building or structure:
  collapse of
  fall from
  hit by falling object in
  jump from
Conflagration NOS
Fire (causing):
  asphyxia
  burns
  NOS
  other injury
Melting of fittings and furniture in burning
Petrol bomb
Smouldering building or structure

● **E979.4** **Terrorism involving firearms**
Bullet:
  carbine
  machine gun
  pistol
  rifle
  rubber (rifle)
Pellets (shotgun)

● Code new
  to this edition

▲ Revision of
  existing code

④ ⑤ Fourth or fifth
    digit required

● **E979.5** **Terrorism involving nuclear weapons**
    Blast effects
    Exposure to ionizing radiation from nuclear weapon
    Fireball effects
    Heat from nuclear weapon
    Other direct and secondary effects of nuclear weapons

● **E979.6** **Terrorism involving biological weapons**
    Anthrax
    Cholera
    Smallpox

● **E979.7** **Terrorism involving chemical weapons**
    Gases, fumes, chemicals
    Hydrogen cyanide
    Phosgene
    Sarin

● **E979.8** **Terrorism involving other means**
    Drowning and submersion
    Lasers
    Piercing or stabbing instruments
    Terrorism NOS

● **E979.9** **Terrorism, secondary effects**
    Note: This code is for use to identify conditions occuring subsequent to a terrorist attack not
        those that are due to the intial terrorist act

      | Excludes: | *late effect of terrorist attack (E999.1)*

INJURY UNDETERMINED WHETHER ACCIDENTALLY OR PURPOSELY INFLICTED (E980-E989)

    Note: Categories E980-E989 are for use when it is unspecified or it cannot be determined
        whether the injuries are accidental (unintentional), suicide (attempted), or assault.

E980 **Poisoning by solid or liquid substances, undetermined whether accidentally or purposely inflicted**

    E980.0 **Analgesics, antipyretics, and antirheumatics**

    E980.1 **Barbiturates**

    E980.2 **Other sedatives and hypnotics**

    E980.3 **Tranquilizers and other psychotropic agents**

    E980.4 **Other specified drugs and medicinal substances**

    E980.5 **Unspecified drug or medicinal substance**

    E980.6 **Corrosive and caustic substances**
        Poisoning, undetermined whether accidental or purposeful, by substances classifiable
        to E864

    E980.7 **Agricultural and horticultural chemical and pharmaceutical preparations other than plant foods and fertilizers**

    E980.8 **Arsenic and its compounds**

    E980.9 **Other and unspecified solid and liquid substances**

E981 **Poisoning by gases in domestic use, undetermined whether accidentally or purposely inflicted**

    E981.0 **Gas distributed by pipeline**

    E981.1 **Liquefied petroleum gas distributed in mobile containers**

    E981.8 **Other utility gas**

E982 **Poisoning by other gases, undetermined whether accidentally or purposely inflicted**

    E982.0 **Motor vehicle exhaust gas**

    E982.1 **Other carbon monoxide**

    E982.8 **Other specified gases and vapors**

    E982.9 **Unspecified gases and vapors**

E983 **Hanging, strangulation, or suffocation, undetermined whether accidentally or purposely inflicted**

    E983.0 **Hanging**

    E983.1 **Suffocation by plastic bag**

    E983.8 **Other specified means**

    E983.9 **Unspecified means**

| ■ | Add 4th or 5th digit | ■ | Nonspecific code | ■ | Unspecified code | ■ | Manifestation code |

E984 Submersion [drowning], undetermined whether accidentally or purposely inflicted

E985 Injury by firearms, air guns and explosives, undetermined whether accidentally or purposely inflicted

E985.0 Handgun

E985.1 Shotgun

E985.2 Hunting rifle

E985.3 Military firearms

E985.4 Other and unspecified firearm

E985.5 Explosives

E985.6 Air gun
BB gun
Pellet gun

● **E985.7 Paintball gun**

E986 Injury by cutting and piercing instruments, undetermined whether accidentally or purposely inflicted

E987 Falling from high place, undetermined whether accidentally or purposely inflicted

E987.0 Residential premises

E987.1 Other man-made structures

E987.2 Natural sites

E987.9 Unspecified site

E988 Injury by other and unspecified means, undetermined whether accidentally or purposely inflicted

E988.0 Jumping or lying before moving object

E988.1 Burns, fire

E988.2 Scald

E988.3 Extremes of cold

E988.4 Electrocution

E988.5 Crashing of motor vehicle

E988.6 Crashing of aircraft

E988.7 Caustic substances, except poisoning

E988.8 Other specified means

E988.9 Unspecified means

E989 Late effects of injury, undetermined whether accidentally or purposely inflicted

Note: This category is to be used to indicate circumstances classifiable to E980-E988 as the cause of death or disability from late effects, which are themselves classifiable elsewhere. The "late effects" include conditions reported as such or as sequelae which may occur at any time after the acute injury, undetermined whether accidentally or purposely inflicted.

INJURY RESULTING FROM OPERATIONS OF WAR (E990-E999)

Includes: injuries to military personnel and civilians caused by war and civil insurrections and occurring during the time of war and insurrection

[Excludes:] *accidents during training of military personnel, manufacture of war material and transport, unless attributable to enemy action*

E990 Injury due to war operations by fires and conflagrations

Includes: asphyxia, burns, or other injury originating from fire caused by a fire-producing device or indirectly by any conventional weapon

E990.0 From gasoline bomb

E990.9 From other and unspecified source

E991 Injury due to war operations by bullets and fragments

E991.0 Rubber bullets (rifle)

E991.1 Pellets (rifle)

● Code new to this edition ▲ Revision of existing code ④ ⑤ Fourth or fifth digit required

E991.2   Other bullets
>   Bullet [any, except rubber bullets and pellets]
>   carbine
>   machine gun
>   pistol
>   rifle
>   shotgun

E991.3   Antipersonnel bomb (fragments)

E991.9   Other and unspecified fragments
>   Fragments from: Fragments from:
>   artillery shell   land mine
>   bombs, except antipersonnel   rockets
>   grenade   shell
>   guided missile   Shrapnel

E992   Injury due to war operations by explosion of marine weapons
>   Depth charge   Sea-based artillery shell
>   Marine mines   Torpedo
>   Mine NOS, at sea or in harbor   Underwater blast

E993   Injury due to war operations by other explosion
>   Accidental explosion of munitions   Explosion of:
>   being used in war   artillery shell
>   Accidental explosion of own weapons   breech block
>   Air blast NOS   cannon block
>   Blast NOS   mortar bomb
>   Explosion NOS   Injury by weapon burst

E994   Injury due to war operations by destruction of aircraft
>   Airplane: Crushed by falling airplane
>   burned
>   exploded
>   shot down

E995   Injury due to war operations by other and unspecified forms of conventional warfare
>   Battle wounds   Drowned in war operations
>   Bayonet injury

E996   Injury due to war operations by nuclear weapons
>   Blast effects
>   Exposure to ionizing radiation from nuclear weapons
>   Fireball effects
>   Heat
>   Other direct and secondary effects of nuclear weapons

E997   Injury due to war operations by other forms of unconventional warfare

E997.0   Lasers

E997.1   Biological warfare

E997.2   Gases, fumes, and chemicals

E997.8   Other specified forms of unconventional warfare

E997.9   Unspecified form of unconventional warfare

E998   Injury due to war operations but occurring after cessation of hostilities
>   Injuries due to operations of war but occurring after cessation of hostilities by any means classifiable under E990-E997
>   Injuries by explosion of bombs or mines placed in the course of operations of war, if the explosion occurred after cessation of hostilities

▲ **E999   Late effect of injury due to war operations and terrorism**
>   Note: This category is to be used to indicate circumstances classifiable to E979, E990-E998 as the cause of death or disability from late effects, which are themselves classifiable elsewhere. The "late effects" include conditions reported as such or as sequelae which may occur at any time after the acute injury, resulting from operations of war or terrorism.

● **E999.0   Late effect of injury due to war operations**

● **E999.1   Late effect of injury due to terrorism**

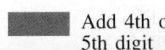

| | Add 4th or 5th digit | | Nonspecific code | | Unspecified code | | Manifestation code |

● Code new
to this edition

▲ Revision of
existing code

④ ⑤ Fourth or fifth
digit required

MORPHOLOGY OF NEOPLASMS

The World Health Organization has published an adaptation of the International Classification of Diseases for oncology (ICD-O). It contains a coded nomenclature for the morphology of neoplasms, which is reproduced here for those who wish to use it in conjunction with Chapter 2 of the *International Classification of Diseases, 9th Revision, Clinical Modification.*

The morphology code numbers consist of five digits; the first four identify the histological type of the neoplasm and the fifth indicates its behavior. The one-digit behavior code is as follows:

/0 Benign

/1 Uncertain whether benign or malignant
    Borderline malignancy

/2 Carcinoma in situ
    Intraepithelial
    Noninfiltrating
    Noninvasive

/3 Malignant, primary site

/6 Malignant, metastatic site
    Secondary site

/9 Malignant, uncertain whether primary or metastatic site

In the nomenclature below, the morphology code numbers include the behavior code appropriate to the histological type of neoplasm, but this behavior code should be changed if other reported information makes this necessary. For example, "chordoma (M9370/3)" is assumed to be malignant; the term "benign chordoma" should be coded M9370/0. Similarly, "superficial spreading adenocarcinoma (M8143/3)" described as "noninvasive" should be coded M8143/2 and "melanoma (M8720/3)" described as "secondary" should be coded M8720/6.

The following table shows the correspondence between the morphology code and the different sections of Chapter 2:

Morphology code Histology/Behavior			ICD-9-CM Chapter 2
Any	0	210-229	Benign neoplasms
M8000-M8004	1	239	Neoplasms of unspecified nature
M8010+	1	235-238	Neoplasms of uncertain behavior
Any	2	230-234	Carcinoma in situ
Any	3	140-195 200-208	Malignant neoplasms, stated or presumed to be primary
Any	6	196-198	Malignant neoplasms, stated or presumed to be secondary

The ICD-O behavior digit /9 is inapplicable in an ICD context, since all malignant neoplasms are presumed to be primary (/3) or secondary (/6) according to other information on the medical record.

Only the first-listed term of the full ICD-O morphology nomenclature appears against each code number in the list below. The ICD-9-CM Alphabetical Index (Volume 2), however, includes all the ICD-O synonyms as well as a number of other morphological names still likely to be encountered on medical records but omitted from ICD-O as outdated or otherwise undesirable.

A coding difficulty sometimes arises where a morphological diagnosis contains two qualifying adjectives that have different code numbers. An example is "transitional cell epidermoid carcinoma." "Transitional cell carcinoma NOS" is M8120/3 and "epidermoid carcinoma NOS" is M8070/3. In such circumstances, the higher number (M8120/3 in this example) should be used, as it is usually more specific.

CODED NOMENCLATURE FOR MORPHOLOGY OF NEOPLASMS

M800   **Neoplasms NOS**
M8000/0   *Neoplasm, benign*
M8000/1   *Neoplasm, uncertain whether benign or malignant*
M8000/3   *Neoplasm, malignant*
M8000/6   *Neoplasm, metastatic*
M8000/9   *Neoplasm, malignant, uncertain whether primary or metastatic*
M8001/0   *Tumor cells, benign*
M8001/1   *Tumor cells, uncertain whether benign or malignant*
M8001/3   *Tumor cells, malignant*
M8002/3   *Malignant tumor, small cell type*
M8003/3   *Malignant tumor, giant cell type*
M8004/3   *Malignant tumor, fusiform cell type*

M801-M804 Epithelial neoplasms NOS
M8010/0   *Epithelial tumor, benign*
M8010/2   *Carcinoma in situ NOS*
M8010/3   *Carcinoma NOS*
M8010/6   *Carcinoma, metastatic NOS*
M8010/9   *Carcinomatosis*
M8011/0   *Epithelioma, benign*
M8011/3   *Epithelioma, malignant*
M8012/3   *Large cell carcinoma NOS*
M8020/3   *Carcinoma, undifferentiated type NOS*
M8021/3   *Carcinoma, anaplastic type NOS*
M8022/3   *Pleomorphic carcinoma*
M8030/3   *Giant cell and spindle cell carcinoma*
M8031/3   *Giant cell carcinoma*
M8032/3   *Spindle cell carcinoma*
M8033/3   *Pseudosarcomatous carcinoma*
M8034/3   *Polygonal cell carcinoma*
M8035/3   *Spheroidal cell carcinoma*
M8040/1   *Tumorlet*
M8041/3   *Small cell carcinoma NOS*
M8042/3   *Oat cell carcinoma*
M8043/3   *Small cell carcinoma, fusiform cell type*

M805-M808 Papillary and squamous cell neoplasms
M8050/0   *Papilloma NOS (except Papilloma of urinary bladder M8120/1)*
M8050/2   *Papillary carcinoma in situ*
M8050/3   *Papillary carcinoma NOS*
M8051/0   *Verrucous papilloma*
M8051/3   *Verrucous carcinoma NOS*
M8052/0   *Squamous cell papilloma*
M8052/3   *Papillary squamous cell carcinoma*
M8053/0   *Inverted papilloma*
M8060/0   *Papillomatosis NOS*
M8070/2   *Squamous cell carcinoma in situ NOS*
M8070/3   *Squamous cell carcinoma NOS*
M8070/6   *Squamous cell carcinoma, metastatic NOS*
M8071/3   *Squamous cell carcinoma, keratinizing type NOS*
M8072/3   *Squamous cell carcinoma, large cell, nonkeratinizing type*
M8073/3   *Squamous cell carcinoma, small cell, nonkeratinizing type*
M8074/3   *Squamous cell carcinoma, spindle cell type*
M8075/3   *Adenoid squamous cell carcinoma*
M8076/2   *Squamous cell carcinoma in situ with questionable stromal invasion*
M8076/3   *Squamous cell carcinoma, microinvasive*
M8080/2   *Queyrat's erythroplasia*
M8081/2   *Bowen's disease*
M8082/3   *Lymphoepithelial carcinoma*

M809-M811 Basal cell neoplasms
M8090/1   *Basal cell tumor*
M8090/3   *Basal cell carcinoma NOS*
M8091/3   *Multicentric basal cell carcinoma*
M8092/3   *Basal cell carcinoma, morphea type*
M8093/3   *Basal cell carcinoma, fibroepithelial type*
M8094/3   *Basosquamous carcinoma*
M8095/3   *Metatypical carcinoma*
             Intraepidermal epithelioma of Jadassohn
             Trichoepithelioma
             Trichofolliculoma

M8102/0	*Tricholemmoma*
M8110/0	*Pilomatrixoma*

M812-M813 Transitional cell papillomas and carcinomas

M8120/0	*Transitional cell papilloma NOS*
M8120/1	*Urothelial papilloma*
M8120/2	*Transitional cell carcinoma in situ*
M8120/3	*Transitional cell carcinoma NOS*
M8121/0	*Schneiderian papilloma*
M8121/1	*Transitional cell papilloma, inverted type*
M8121/3	*Schneiderian carcinoma*
M8122/3	*Transitional cell carcinoma, spindle cell type*
M8123/3	*Basaloid carcinoma*
M8124/3	*Cloacogenic carcinoma*
M8130/3	*Papillary transitional cell carcinoma*

M814-M838 Adenomas and adenocarcinomas

M8140/0	*Adenoma NOS*
M8140/1	*Bronchial adenoma NOS*
M8140/2	*Adenocarcinoma in situ*
M8140/3	*Adenocarcinoma NOS*
M8140/6	*Adenocarcinoma, metastatic NOS*
M8141/3	*Scirrhous adenocarcinoma*
M8142/3	*Linitis plastica*
M8143/3	*Superficial spreading adenocarcinoma*
M8144/3	*Adenocarcinoma, intestinal type*
M8145/3	*Carcinoma, diffuse type*
M8146/0	*Monomorphic adenoma*
M8147/0	*Basal cell adenoma*
M8150/0	*Islet cell adenoma*
M8150/3	*Islet cell carcinoma*
M8151/0	*Insulinoma NOS*
M8151/3	*Insulinoma, malignant*
M8152/0	*Glucagonoma NOS*
M8152/3	*Glucagonoma, malignant*
M8153/1	*Gastrinoma NOS*
M8153/3	*Gastrinoma, malignant*
M8154/3	*Mixed islet cell and exocrine adenocarcinoma*
M8160/0	*Bile duct adenoma*
M8160/3	*Cholangiocarcinoma*
M8161/0	*Bile duct cystadenoma*
M8161/3	*Bile duct cystadenocarcinoma*
M8170/0	*Liver cell adenoma*
M8170/3	*Hepatocellular carcinoma NOS*
M8180/0	*Hepatocholangioma, benign*
M8180/3	*Combined hepatocellular carcinoma and cholangiocarcinoma*
M8190/0	*Trabecular adenoma*
M8190/3	*Trabecular adenocarcinoma*
M8191/0	*Embryonal adenoma*
M8200/0	*Eccrine dermal cylindroma*
M8200/3	*Adenoid cystic carcinoma*
M8201/3	*Cribriform carcinoma*
M8210/0	*Adenomatous polyp NOS*
M8210/3	*Adenocarcinoma in adenomatous polyp*
M8211/0	*Tubular adenoma NOS*
M8211/3	*Tubular adenocarcinoma*
M8220/0	*Adenomatous polyposis coli*
M8220/3	*Adenocarcinoma in adenomatous polyposis coli*
M8221/0	*Multiple adenomatous polyps*
M8230/3	*Solid carcinoma NOS*
M8231/3	*Carcinoma simplex*
M8240/1	*Carcinoid tumor NOS*
M8240/3	*Carcinoid tumor, malignant*
M8241/1	*Carcinoid tumor, argentaffin NOS*
M8241/3	*Carcinoid tumor, argentaffin, malignant*
M8242/1	*Carcinoid tumor, nonargentaffin NOS*
M8242/3	*Carcinoid tumor, nonargentaffin, malignant*
M8243/3	*Mucocarcinoid tumor, malignant*
M8244/3	*Composite carcinoid*
M8250/1	*Pulmonary adenomatosis*
M8250/3	*Bronchiolo-alveolar adenocarcinoma*
M8251/0	*Alveolar adenoma*

M8251/3	*Alveolar adenocarcinoma*
M8260/0	*Papillary adenoma NOS*
M8260/3	*Papillary adenocarcinoma NOS*
M8261/1	*Villous adenoma NOS*
M8261/3	*Adenocarcinoma in villous adenoma*
M8262/3	*Villous adenocarcinoma*
M8263/0	*Tubulovillous adenoma*
M8270/0	*Chromophobe adenoma*
M8270/3	*Chromophobe carcinoma*
M8280/0	*Acidophil adenoma*
M8280/3	*Acidophil carcinoma*
M8281/0	*Mixed acidophil-basophil adenoma*
M8281/3	*Mixed acidophil-basophil carcinoma*
M8290/0	*Oxyphilic adenoma*
M8290/3	*Oxyphilic adenocarcinoma*
M8300/0	*Basophil adenoma*
M8300/3	*Basophil carcinoma*
M8310/0	*Clear cell adenoma*
M8310/3	*Clear cell adenocarcinoma NOS*
M8311/1	*Hypernephroid tumor*
M8312/3	*Renal cell carcinoma*
M8313/0	*Clear cell adenofibroma*
M8320/3	*Granular cell carcinoma*
M8321/0	*Chief cell adenoma*
M8322/0	*Water-clear cell adenoma*
M8322/3	*Water-clear cell adenocarcinoma*
M8323/0	*Mixed cell adenoma*
M8323/3	*Mixed cell adenocarcinoma*
M8324/0	*Lipoadenoma*
M8330/0	*Follicular adenoma*
M8330/3	*Follicular adenocarcinoma NOS*
M8331/3	*Follicular adenocarcinoma, well differentiated type*
M8332/3	*Follicular adenocarcinoma, trabecular type*
M8333/0	*Microfollicular adenoma*
M8334/0	*Macrofollicular adenoma*
M8340/3	*Papillary and follicular adenocarcinoma*
M8350/3	*Nonencapsulated sclerosing carcinoma*
M8360/1	*Multiple endocrine adenomas*
M8361/1	*Juxtaglomerular tumor*
M8370/0	*Adrenal cortical adenoma NOS*
M8370/3	*Adrenal cortical carcinoma*
M8371/0	*Adrenal cortical adenoma, compact cell type*
M8372/0	*Adrenal cortical adenoma, heavily pigmented variant*
M8373/0	*Adrenal cortical adenoma, clear cell type*
M8374/0	*Adrenal cortical adenoma, glomerulosa cell type*
M8375/0	*Adrenal cortical adenoma, mixed cell type*
M8380/0	*Endometrioid adenoma NOS*
M8380/1	*Endometrioid adenoma, borderline malignancy*
M8380/3	*Endometrioid carcinoma*
M8381/0	*Endometrioid adenofibroma NOS*
M8381/1	*Endometrioid adenofibroma, borderline malignancy*
M8381/3	*Endometrioid adenofibroma, malignant*

M839-M842 Adnexal and skin appendage neoplasms

M8390/0	*Skin appendage adenoma*
M8390/3	*Skin appendage carcinoma*
M8400/0	*Sweat gland adenoma*
M8400/1	*Sweat gland tumor NOS*
M8400/3	*Sweat gland adenocarcinoma*
M8401/0	*Apocrine adenoma*
M8401/3	*Apocrine adenocarcinoma*
M8402/0	*Eccrine acrospiroma*
M8403/0	*Eccrine spiradenoma*
M8404/0	*Hidrocystoma*
M8405/0	*Papillary hydradenoma*
M8406/0	*Papillary syringadenoma*
M8407/0	*Syringoma NOS*
M8410/0	*Sebaceous adenoma*
M8410/3	*Sebaceous adenocarcinoma*
M8420/0	*Ceruminous adenoma*
M8420/3	*Ceruminous adenocarcinoma*

M843   **Mucoepidermoid neoplasms**
M8430/1   *Mucoepidermoid tumor*
M8430/3   *Mucoepidermoid carcinoma*

M844-M849 **Cystic, mucinous, and serous neoplasms**
M8440/0   *Cystadenoma NOS*
M8440/3   *Cystadenocarcinoma NOS*
M8441/0   *Serous cystadenoma NOS*
M8441/1   *Serous cystadenoma, borderline malignancy*
M8441/3   *Serous cystadenocarcinoma NOS*
M8450/0   *Papillary cystadenoma NOS*
M8450/1   *Papillary cystadenoma, borderline malignancy*
M8450/3   *Papillary cystadenocarcinoma NOS*
M8460/0   *Papillary serous cystadenoma NOS*
M8460/1   *Papillary serous cystadenoma, borderline malignancy*
M8460/3   *Papillary serous cystadenocarcinoma*
M8461/0   *Serous surface papilloma NOS*
M8461/1   *Serous surface papilloma, borderline malignancy*
M8461/3   *Serous surface papillary carcinoma*
M8470/0   *Mucinous cystadenoma NOS*
M8470/1   *Mucinous cystadenoma, borderline malignancy*
M8470/3   *Mucinous cystadenocarcinoma NOS*
M8471/0   *Papillary mucinous cystadenoma NOS*
M8471/1   *Papillary mucinous cystadenoma, borderline malignancy*
M8471/3   *Papillary mucinous cystadenocarcinoma*
M8480/0   *Mucinous adenoma*
M8480/3   *Mucinous adenocarcinoma*
M8480/6   *Pseudomyxoma peritonei*
M8481/3   *Mucin-producing adenocarcinoma*
M8490/3   *Signet ring cell carcinoma*
M8490/6   *Metastatic signet ring cell carcinoma*

M850-M854 **Ductal, lobular, and medullary neoplasms**
M8500/2   *Intraductal carcinoma, noninfiltrating NOS*
M8500/3   *Infiltrating duct carcinoma*
M8501/2   *Comedocarcinoma, noninfiltrating*
M8501/3   *Comedocarcinoma NOS*
M8502/3   *Juvenile carcinoma of the breast*
M8503/0   *Intraductal papilloma*
M8503/2   *Noninfiltrating intraductal papillary adenocarcinoma*
M8504/0   *Intracystic papillary adenoma*
M8504/2   *Noninfiltrating intracystic carcinoma*
M8505/0   *Intraductal papillomatosis NOS*
M8506/0   *Subareolar duct papillomatosis*
M8510/3   *Medullary carcinoma NOS*
M8511/3   *Medullary carcinoma with amyloid stroma*
M8512/3   *Medullary carcinoma with lymphoid stroma*
M8520/2   *Lobular carcinoma in situ*
M8520/3   *Lobular carcinoma NOS*
M8521/3   *Infiltrating ductular carcinoma*
M8530/3   *Inflammatory carcinoma*
M8540/3   *Paget's disease, mammary*
M8541/3   *Paget's disease and infiltrating duct carcinoma of breast*
M8542/3   *Paget's disease, extramammary (except Paget's disease of bone)*

M855   **Acinar cell neoplasms**
M8550/0   *Acinar cell adenoma*
M8550/1   *Acinar cell tumor*
M8550/3   *Acinar cell carcinoma*

M856-M858 **Complex epithelial neoplasms**
M8560/3   *Adenosquamous carcinoma*
M8561/0   *Adenolymphoma*
M8570/3   *Adenocarcinoma with squamous metaplasia*
M8571/3   *Adenocarcinoma with cartilaginous and osseous metaplasia*
M8572/3   *Adenocarcinoma with spindle cell metaplasia*
M8573/3   *Adenocarcinoma with apocrine metaplasia*
M8580/0   *Thymoma, benign*
M8580/3   *Thymoma, malignant*

M859-M867 **Specialized gonadal neoplasms**
M8590/1   *Sex cord-stromal tumor*
M8600/0   *Thecoma NOS*
M8600/3   *Theca cell carcinoma*

M8610/0	*Luteoma NOS*
M8620/1	*Granulosa cell tumor NOS*
M8620/3	*Granulosa cell tumor, malignant*
M8621/1	*Granulosa cell-theca cell tumor*
M8630/0	*Androblastoma, benign*
M8630/1	*Androblastoma NOS*
M8630/3	*Androblastoma, malignant*
M8631/0	*Sertoli-Leydig cell tumor*
M8632/1	*Gynandroblastoma*
M8640/0	*Tubular androblastoma NOS*
M8640/3	*Sertoli cell carcinoma*
M8641/0	*Tubular androblastoma with lipid storage*
M8650/0	*Leydig cell tumor, benign*
M8650/1	*Leydig cell tumor NOS*
M8650/3	*Leydig cell tumor, malignant*
M8660/0	*Hilar cell tumor*
M8670/0	*Lipid cell tumor of ovary*
M8671/0	*Adrenal rest tumor*

M868-M871 Paragangliomas and glomus tumors

M8680/1	*Paraganglioma NOS*
M8680/3	*Paraganglioma, malignant*
M8681/1	*Sympathetic paraganglioma*
M8682/1	*Parasympathetic paraganglioma*
M8690/1	*Glomus jugulare tumor*
M8691/1	*Aortic body tumor*
M8692/1	*Carotid body tumor*
M8693/1	*Extra-adrenal paraganglioma NOS*
M8693/3	*Extra-adrenal paraganglioma, malignant*
M8700/0	*Pheochromocytoma NOS*
M8700/3	*Pheochromocytoma, malignant*
M8710/3	*Glomangiosarcoma*
M8711/0	*Glomus tumor*
M8712/0	*Glomangioma*

M872-M879 Nevi and melanomas

M8720/0	*Pigmented nevus NOS*
M8720/3	*Malignant melanoma NOS*
M8721/3	*Nodular melanoma*
M8722/0	*Balloon cell nevus*
M8722/3	*Balloon cell melanoma*
M8723/0	*Halo nevus*
M8724/0	*Fibrous papule of the nose*
M8725/0	*Neuronevus*
M8726/0	*Magnocellular nevus*
M8730/0	*Nonpigmented nevus*
M8730/3	*Amelanotic melanoma*
M8740/0	*Junctional nevus*
M8740/3	*Malignant melanoma in junctional nevus*
M8741/2	*Precancerous melanosis NOS*
M8741/3	*Malignant melanoma in precancerous melanosis*
M8742/2	*Hutchinson's melanotic freckle*
M8742/3	*Malignant melanoma in Hutchinson's melanotic freckle*
M8743/3	*Superficial spreading melanoma*
M8750/0	*Intradermal nevus*
M8760/0	*Compound nevus*
M8761/1	*Giant pigmented nevus*
M8761/3	*Malignant melanoma in giant pigmented nevus*
M8770/0	*Epithelioid and spindle cell nevus*
M8771/3	*Epithelioid cell melanoma*
M8772/3	*Spindle cell melanoma NOS*
M8773/3	*Spindle cell melanoma, type A*
M8774/3	*Spindle cell melanoma, type B*
M8775/3	*Mixed epithelioid and spindle cell melanoma*
M8780/0	*Blue nevus NOS*
M8780/3	*Blue nevus, malignant*
M8790/0	*Cellular blue nevus*

M880 Soft tissue tumors and sarcomas NOS

M8800/0	*Soft tissue tumor, benign*
M8800/3	*Sarcoma NOS*
M8800/9	*Sarcomatosis NOS*
M8801/3	*Spindle cell sarcoma*

M8802/3	*Giant cell sarcoma (except of bone M9250/3)*
M8803/3	*Small cell sarcoma*
M8804/3	*Epithelioid cell sarcoma*

M881-M883 Fibromatous neoplasms

M8810/0	*Fibroma NOS*
M8810/3	*Fibrosarcoma NOS*
M8811/0	*Fibromyxoma*
M8811/3	*Fibromyxosarcoma*
M8812/0	*Periosteal fibroma*
M8812/3	*Periosteal fibrosarcoma*
M8813/0	*Fascial fibroma*
M8813/3	*Fascial fibrosarcoma*
M8814/3	*Infantile fibrosarcoma*
M8820/0	*Elastofibroma*
M8821/1	*Aggressive fibromatosis*
M8822/1	*Abdominal fibromatosis*
M8823/1	*Desmoplastic fibroma*
M8830/0	*Fibrous histiocytoma NOS*
M8830/1	*Atypical fibrous histiocytoma*
M8830/3	*Fibrous histiocytoma, malignant*
M8831/0	*Fibroxanthoma NOS*
M8831/1	*Atypical fibroxanthoma*
M8831/3	*Fibroxanthoma, malignant*
M8832/0	*Dermatofibroma NOS*
M8832/1	*Dermatofibroma protuberans*
M8832/3	*Dermatofibrosarcoma NOS*

M884 Myxomatous neoplasms

M8840/0	*Myxoma NOS*
M8840/3	*Myxosarcoma*

M885-M888 Lipomatous neoplasms

M8850/0	*Lipoma NOS*
M8850/3	*Liposarcoma NOS*
M8851/0	*Fibrolipoma*
M8851/3	*Liposarcoma, well differentiated type*
M8852/0	*Fibromyxolipoma*
M8852/3	*Myxoid liposarcoma*
M8853/3	*Round cell liposarcoma*
M8854/3	*Pleomorphic liposarcoma*
M8855/3	*Mixed type liposarcoma*
M8856/0	*Intramuscular lipoma*
M8857/0	*Spindle cell lipoma*
M8860/0	*Angiomyolipoma*
M8860/3	*Angiomyoliposarcoma*
M8861/0	*Angiolipoma NOS*
M8861/1	*Angiolipoma, infiltrating*
M8870/0	*Myelolipoma*
M8880/0	*Hibernoma*
M8881/0	*Lipoblastomatosis*

M889-M892 Myomatous neoplasms

M8890/0	*Leiomyoma NOS*
M8890/1	*Intravascular leiomyomatosis*
M8890/3	*Leiomyosarcoma NOS*
M8891/1	*Epithelioid leiomyoma*
M8891/3	*Epithelioid leiomyosarcoma*
M8892/1	*Cellular leiomyoma*
M8893/0	*Bizarre leiomyoma*
M8894/0	*Angiomyoma*
M8894/3	*Angiomyosarcoma*
M8895/0	*Myoma*
M8895/3	*Myosarcoma*
M8900/0	*Rhabdomyoma NOS*
M8900/3	*Rhabdomyosarcoma NOS*
M8901/3	*Pleomorphic rhabdomyosarcoma*
M8902/3	*Mixed type rhabdomyosarcoma*
M8903/0	*Fetal rhabdomyoma*
M8904/0	*Adult rhabdomyoma*
M8910/3	*Embryonal rhabdomyosarcoma*
M8920/3	*Alveolar rhabdomyosarcoma*

M893-M899 Complex mixed and stromal neoplasms

M8930/3	*Endometrial stromal sarcoma*
M8931/1	*Endolymphatic stromal myosis*
M8932/0	*Adenomyoma*
M8940/0	*Pleomorphic adenoma*
M8940/3	*Mixed tumor, malignant NOS*
M8950/3	*Mullerian mixed tumor*
M8951/3	*Mesodermal mixed tumor*
M8960/1	*Mesoblastic nephroma*
M8960/3	*Nephroblastoma NOS*
M8961/3	*Epithelial nephroblastoma*
M8962/3	*Mesenchymal nephroblastoma*
M8970/3	*Hepatoblastoma*
M8980/3	*Carcinosarcoma NOS*
M8981/3	*Carcinosarcoma, embryonal type*
M8982/0	*Myoepithelioma*
M8990/0	*Mesenchymoma, benign*
M8990/1	*Mesenchymoma, NOS*
M8990/3	*Mesenchymoma, malignant*
M8991/3	*Embryonal sarcoma*

M900-M903 Fibroepithelial neoplasms

M9000/0	*Brenner tumor NOS*
M9000/1	*Brenner tumor, borderline malignancy*
M9000/3	*Brenner tumor, malignant*
M9010/0	*Fibroadenoma NOS*
M9011/0	*Intracanalicular fibroadenoma NOS*
M9012/0	*Pericanalicular fibroadenoma*
M9013/0	*Adenofibroma NOS*
M9014/0	*Serous adenofibroma*
M9015/0	*Mucinous adenofibroma*
M9020/0	*Cellular intracanalicular fibroadenoma*
M9020/1	*Cystosarcoma phyllodes NOS*
M9020/3	*Cystosarcoma phyllodes, malignant*
M9030/0	*Juvenile fibroadenoma*

M904 Synovial neoplasms

M9040/0	*Synovioma, benign*
M9040/3	*Synovial sarcoma NOS*
M9041/3	*Synovial sarcoma, spindle cell type*
M9042/3	*Synovial sarcoma, epithelioid cell type*
M9043/3	*Synovial sarcoma, biphasic type*
M9044/3	*Clear cell sarcoma of tendons and aponeuroses*

M905 Mesothelial neoplasms

M9050/0	*Mesothelioma, benign*
M9050/3	*Mesothelioma, malignant*
M9051/0	*Fibrous mesothelioma, benign*
M9051/3	*Fibrous mesothelioma, malignant*
M9052/0	*Epithelioid mesothelioma, benign*
M9052/3	*Epithelioid mesothelioma, malignant*
M9053/0	*Mesothelioma, biphasic type, benign*
M9053/3	*Mesothelioma, biphasic type, malignant*
M9054/0	*Adenomatoid tumor NOS*

M906-M909 Germ cell neoplasms

M9060/3	*Dysgerminoma*
M9061/3	*Seminoma NOS*
M9062/3	*Seminoma, anaplastic type*
M9063/3	*Spermatocytic seminoma*
M9064/3	*Germinoma*
M9070/3	*Embryonal carcinoma NOS*
M9071/3	*Endodermal sinus tumor*
M9072/3	*Polyembryoma*
M9073/1	*Gonadoblastoma*
M9080/0	*Teratoma, benign*
M9080/1	*Teratoma NOS*
M9080/3	*Teratoma, malignant NOS*
M9081/3	*Teratocarcinoma*
M9082/3	*Malignant teratoma, undifferentiated type*
M9083/3	*Malignant teratoma, intermediate type*
M9084/0	*Dermoid cyst*
M9084/3	*Dermoid cyst with malignant transformation*

M9090/0	*Struma ovarii NOS*
M9090/3	*Struma ovarii, malignant*
M9091/1	*Strumal carcinoid*

M910   **Trophoblastic neoplasms**

M9100/0	*Hydatidiform mole NOS*
M9100/1	*Invasive hydatidiform mole*
M9100/3	*Choriocarcinoma*
M9101/3	*Choriocarcinoma combined with teratoma*
M9102/3	*Malignant teratoma, trophoblastic*

M911   **Mesonephromas**

M9110/0	*Mesonephroma, benign*
M9110/1	*Mesonephric tumor*
M9110/3	*Mesonephroma, malignant*
M9111/1	*Endosalpingioma*

M912-M916   **Blood vessel tumors**

M9120/0	*Hemangioma NOS*
M9120/3	*Hemangiosarcoma*
M9121/0	*Cavernous hemangioma*
M9122/0	*Venous hemangioma*
M9123/0	*Racemose hemangioma*
M9124/3	*Kupffer cell sarcoma*
M9130/0	*Hemangioendothelioma, benign*
M9130/1	*Hemangioendothelioma NOS*
M9130/3	*Hemangioendothelioma, malignant*
M9131/0	*Capillary hemangioma*
M9132/0	*Intramuscular hemangioma*
M9140/3	*Kaposi's sarcoma*
M9141/0	*Angiokeratoma*
M9142/0	*Verrucous keratotic hemangioma*
M9150/0	*Hemangiopericytoma, benign*
M9150/1	*Hemangiopericytoma NOS*
M9150/3	*Hemangiopericytoma, malignant*
M9160/0	*Angiofibroma NOS*
M9161/1	*Hemangioblastoma*

M917   **Lymphatic vessel tumors**

M9170/0	*Lymphangioma NOS*
M9170/3	*Lymphangiosarcoma*
M9171/0	*Capillary lymphangioma*
M9172/0	*Cavernous lymphangioma*
M9173/0	*Cystic lymphangioma*
M9174/0	*Lymphangiomyoma*
M9174/1	*Lymphangiomyomatosis*
M9175/0	*Hemolymphangioma*

M918-M920   **Osteomas and osteosarcomas**

M9180/0	*Osteoma NOS*
M9180/3	*Osteosarcoma NOS*
M9181/3	*Chondroblastic osteosarcoma*
M9182/3	*Fibroblastic osteosarcoma*
M9183/3	*Telangiectatic osteosarcoma*
M9184/3	*Osteosarcoma in Paget's disease of bone*
M9190/3	*Juxtacortical osteosarcoma*
M9191/0	*Osteoid osteoma NOS*
M9200/0	*Osteoblastoma*

M921-M924   **Chondromatous neoplasms**

M9210/0	*Osteochondroma*
M9210/1	*Osteochondromatosis NOS*
M9220/0	*Chondroma NOS*
M9220/1	*Chondromatosis NOS*
M9220/3	*Chondrosarcoma NOS*
M9221/0	*Juxtacortical chondroma*
M9221/3	*Juxtacortical chondrosarcoma*
M9230/0	*Chondroblastoma NOS*
M9230/3	*Chondroblastoma, malignant*
M9240/3	*Mesenchymal chondrosarcoma*
M9241/0	*Chondromyxoid fibroma*

M925   **Giant cell tumors**

M9250/1	*Giant cell tumor of bone NOS*
M9250/3	*Giant cell tumor of bone, malignant*

M9251/1	Giant cell tumor of soft parts NOS
M9251/3	Malignant giant cell tumor of soft parts

M926   **Miscellaneous bone tumors**

M9260/3	Ewing's sarcoma
M9261/3	Adamantinoma of long bones
M9262/0	Ossifying fibroma

M927-M934   **Odontogenic tumors**

M9270/0	Odontogenic tumor, benign
M9270/1	Odontogenic tumor NOS
M9270/3	Odontogenic tumor, malignant
M9271/0	Dentinoma
M9272/0	Cementoma NOS
M9273/0	Cementoblastoma, benign
M9274/0	Cementifying fibroma
M9275/0	Gigantiform cementoma
M9280/0	Odontoma NOS
M9281/0	Compound odontoma
M9282/0	Complex odontoma
M9290/0	Ameloblastic fibro-odontoma
M9290/3	Ameloblastic odontosarcoma
M9300/0	Adenomatoid odontogenic tumor
M9301/0	Calcifying odontogenic cyst
M9310/0	Ameloblastoma NOS
M9310/3	Ameloblastoma, malignant
M9311/0	Odontoameloblastoma
M9312/0	Squamous odontogenic tumor
M9320/0	Odontogenic myxoma
M9321/0	Odontogenic fibroma NOS
M9330/0	Ameloblastic fibroma
M9330/3	Ameloblastic fibrosarcoma
M9340/0	Calcifying epithelial odontogenic tumor

M935-M937   **Miscellaneous tumors**

M9350/1	Craniopharyngioma
M9360/1	Pinealoma
M9361/1	Pineocytoma
M9362/3	Pineoblastoma
M9363/0	Melanotic neuroectodermal tumor
M9370/3	Chordoma

M938-M948   **Gliomas**

M9380/3	Glioma, malignant
M9381/3	Gliomatosis cerebri
M9382/3	Mixed glioma
M9383/1	Subependymal glioma
M9384/1	Subependymal giant cell astrocytoma
M9390/0	Choroid plexus papilloma NOS
M9390/3	Choroid plexus papilloma, malignant
M9391/3	Ependymoma NOS
M9392/3	Ependymoma, anaplastic type
M9393/1	Papillary ependymoma
M9394/1	Myxopapillary ependymoma
M9400/3	Astrocytoma NOS
M9401/3	Astrocytoma, anaplastic type
M9410/3	Protoplasmic astrocytoma
M9411/3	Gemistocytic astrocytoma
M9420/3	Fibrillary astrocytoma
M9421/3	Pilocytic astrocytoma
M9422/3	Spongioblastoma NOS
M9423/3	Spongioblastoma polare
M9430/3	Astroblastoma
M9440/3	Glioblastoma NOS
M9441/3	Giant cell glioblastoma
M9442/3	Glioblastoma with sarcomatous component
M9443/3	Primitive polar spongioblastoma
M9450/3	Oligodendroglioma NOS
M9451/3	Oligodendroglioma, anaplastic type
M9460/3	Oligodendroblastoma
M9470/3	Medulloblastoma NOS
M9471/3	Desmoplastic medulloblastoma
M9472/3	Medullomyoblastoma

M9480/3	*Cerebellar sarcoma NOS*
M9481/3	*Monstrocellular sarcoma*

M949-M952 Neuroepitheliomatous neoplasms

M9490/0	*Ganglioneuroma*
M9490/3	*Ganglioneuroblastoma*
M9491/0	*Ganglioneuromatosis*
M9500/3	*Neuroblastoma NOS*
M9501/3	*Medulloepithelioma NOS*
M9502/3	*Teratoid medulloepithelioma*
M9503/3	*Neuroepithelioma NOS*
M9504/3	*Spongioneuroblastoma*
M9505/1	*Ganglioglioma*
M9506/0	*Neurocytoma*
M9507/0	*Pacinian tumor*
M9510/3	*Retinoblastoma NOS*
M9511/3	*Retinoblastoma, differentiated type*
M9512/3	*Retinoblastoma, undifferentiated type*
M9520/3	*Olfactory neurogenic tumor*
M9521/3	*Esthesioneurocytoma*
M9522/3	*Esthesioneuroblastoma*
M9523/3	*Esthesioneuroepithelioma*

M953   **Meningiomas**

M9530/0	*Meningioma NOS*
M9530/1	*Meningiomatosis NOS*
M9530/3	*Meningioma, malignant*
M9531/0	*Meningotheliomatous meningioma*
M9532/0	*Fibrous meningioma*
M9533/0	*Psammomatous meningioma*
M9534/0	*Angiomatous meningioma*
M9535/0	*Hemangioblastic meningioma*
M9536/0	*Hemangiopericytic meningioma*
M9537/0	*Transitional meningioma*
M9538/1	*Papillary meningioma*
M9539/3	*Meningeal sarcomatosis*

M954-M957 Nerve sheath tumor

M9540/0	*Neurofibroma NOS*
M9540/1	*Neurofibromatosis NOS*
M9540/3	*Neurofibrosarcoma*
M9541/0	*Melanotic neurofibroma*
M9550/0	*Plexiform neurofibroma*
M9560/0	*Neurilemmoma NOS*
M9560/1	*Neurinomatosis*
M9560/3	*Neurilemmoma, malignant*
M9570/0	*Neuroma NOS*

M958   **Granular cell tumors and alveolar soft part sarcoma**

M9580/0	*Granular cell tumor NOS*
M9580/3	*Granular cell tumor, malignant*
M9581/3	*Alveolar soft part sarcoma*

M959-M963 Lymphomas, NOS or diffuse

M9590/0	*Lymphomatous tumor, benign*
M9590/3	*Malignant lymphoma NOS*
M9591/3	*Malignant lymphoma, non Hodgkin's type*
M9600/3	*Malignant lymphoma, undifferentiated cell type NOS*
M9601/3	*Malignant lymphoma, stem cell type*
M9602/3	*Malignant lymphoma, convoluted cell type NOS*
M9610/3	*Lymphosarcoma NOS*
M9611/3	*Malignant lymphoma, lymphoplasmacytoid type*
M9612/3	*Malignant lymphoma, immunoblastic type*
M9613/3	*Malignant lymphoma, mixed lymphocytic-histiocytic NOS*
M9614/3	*Malignant lymphoma, centroblastic-centrocytic, diffuse*
M9615/3	*Malignant lymphoma, follicular center cell NOS*
M9620/3	*Malignant lymphoma, lymphocytic, well differentiated NOS*
M9621/3	*Malignant lymphoma, lymphocytic, intermediate differentiation NOS*
M9622/3	*Malignant lymphoma, centrocytic*
M9623/3	*Malignant lymphoma, follicular center cell, cleaved NOS*
M9630/3	*Malignant lymphoma, lymphocytic, poorly differentiated NOS*
M9631/3	*Prolymphocytic lymphosarcoma*
M9632/3	*Malignant lymphoma, centroblastic type NOS*
M9633/3	*Malignant lymphoma, follicular center cell, noncleaved NOS*

M964   **Reticulosarcomas**
M9640/3   *Reticulosarcoma NOS*
M9641/3   *Reticulosarcoma, pleomorphic cell type*
M9642/3   *Reticulosarcoma, nodular*

M965-M966 Hodgkin's disease
M9650/3   *Hodgkin's disease NOS*
M9651/3   *Hodgkin's disease, lymphocytic predominance*
M9652/3   *Hodgkin's disease, mixed cellularity*
M9653/3   *Hodgkin's disease, lymphocytic depletion NOS*
M9654/3   *Hodgkin's disease, lymphocytic depletion, diffuse fibrosis*
M9655/3   *Hodgkin's disease, lymphocytic depletion, reticular type*
M9656/3   *Hodgkin's disease, nodular sclerosis NOS*
M9657/3   *Hodgkin's disease, nodular sclerosis, cellular phase*
M9660/3   *Hodgkin's paragranuloma*
M9661/3   *Hodgkin's granuloma*
M9662/3   *Hodgkin's sarcoma*

M969   **Lymphomas, nodular or follicular**
M9690/3   *Malignant lymphoma, nodular NOS*
M9691/3   *Malignant lymphoma, mixed lymphocytic-histiocytic, nodular*
M9692/3   *Malignant lymphoma, centroblastic-centrocytic, follicular*
M9693/3   *Malignant lymphoma, lymphocytic, well differentiated, nodular*
M9694/3   *Malignant lymphoma, lymphocytic, intermediate differentiation, nodular*
M9695/3   *Malignant lymphoma, follicular center cell, cleaved, follicular*
M9696/3   *Malignant lymphoma, lymphocytic, poorly differentiated, nodular*
M9697/3   *Malignant lymphoma, centroblastic type, follicular*
M9698/3   *Malignant lymphoma, follicular center cell, noncleaved, follicular*

M970   **Mycosis fungoides**
M9700/3   *Mycosis fungoides*
M9701/3   *Sezary's disease*

M971-M972 Miscellaneous reticuloendothelial neoplasms
M9710/3   *Microglioma*
M9720/3   *Malignant histiocytosis*
M9721/3   *Histiocytic medullary reticulosis*
M9722/3   *Letterer-Siwe's disease*

M973   **Plasma cell tumors**
M9730/3   *Plasma cell myeloma*
M9731/0   *Plasma cell tumor, benign*
M9731/1   *Plasmacytoma NOS*
M9731/3   *Plasma cell tumor, malignant*

M974   **Mast cell tumors**
M9740/1   *Mastocytoma NOS*
M9740/3   *Mast cell sarcoma*
M9741/3   *Malignant mastocytosis*

M975   **Burkitt's tumor**
M9750/3   *Burkitt's tumor*

M980-M994 Leukemias

M980   **Leukemias NOS**
M9800/3   *Leukemia NOS*
M9801/3   *Acute leukemia NOS*
M9802/3   *Subacute leukemia NOS*
M9803/3   *Chronic leukemia NOS*
M9804/3   *Aleukemic leukemia NOS*

M981   **Compound leukemias**
M9810/3   *Compound leukemia*

M982   **Lymphoid leukemias**
M9820/3   *Lymphoid leukemia NOS*
M9821/3   *Acute lymphoid leukemia*
M9822/3   *Subacute lymphoid leukemia*
M9823/3   *Chronic lymphoid leukemia*
M9824/3   *Aleukemic lymphoid leukemia*
M9825/3   *Prolymphocytic leukemia*

M983   **Plasma cell leukemias**
M9830/3   *Plasma cell leukemia*

M984   **Erythroleukemias**
M9840/3   *Erythroleukemia*
M9841/3   *Acute erythremia*

M9842/3	*Chronic erythremia*
M985	**Lymphosarcoma cell leukemias**
M9850/3	*Lymphosarcoma cell leukemia*
M986	**Myeloid leukemias**
M9860/3	*Myeloid leukemia NOS*
M9861/3	*Acute myeloid leukemia*
M9862/3	*Subacute myeloid leukemia*
M9863/3	*Chronic myeloid leukemia*
M9864/3	*Aleukemic myeloid leukemia*
M9865/3	*Neutrophilic leukemia*
M9866/3	*Acute promyelocytic leukemia*
M987	**Basophilic leukemias**
M9870/3	*Basophilic leukemia*
M988	**Eosinophilic leukemias**
M9880/3	*Eosinophilic leukemia*
M989	**Monocytic leukemias**
M9890/3	*Monocytic leukemia NOS*
M9891/3	*Acute monocytic leukemia*
M9892/3	*Subacute monocytic leukemia*
M9893/3	*Chronic monocytic leukemia*
M9894/3	*Aleukemic monocytic leukemia*
M990-M994	**Miscellaneous leukemias**
M9900/3	*Mast cell leukemia*
M9910/3	*Megakaryocytic leukemia*
M9920/3	*Megakaryocytic myelosis*
M9930/3	*Myeloid sarcoma*
M9940/3	*Hairy cell leukemia*
M995-M997	**Miscellaneous myeloproliferative and lymphoproliferative disorders**
M9950/1	*Polycythemia vera*
M9951/1	*Acute panmyelosis*
M9960/1	*Chronic myeloproliferative disease*
M9961/1	*Myelosclerosis with myeloid metaplasia*
M9962/1	*Idiopathic thrombocythemia*
M9970/1	*Chronic lymphoproliferative disease*

GLOSSARY OF MENTAL DISORDERS

The psychiatric terms which appear in Chapter 5, "Mental Disorders," are listed here in alphabetic sequence. Many of the glossary descriptions originally appeared in the section on Mental Disorders in the *International Classification of Diseases, 9th Revision,*[1] and others are included to define the psychiatric conditions added to *ICD-9-CM.* The additional definitions are based on material furnished by the American Psychiatric Association's Task Force on Nomenclature and Statistics[2] and from *A Psychiatric Glossary.*[3] In a few instances definitions were obtained from *Dorland's Illustrated Medical Dictionary*[4] *and from Stedman's Medical Dictionary, Illustrated.*[5]

1. Manual of the *International Classification of Diseases, Injuries, and Causes of Death,* 9th Revision. World Health Organization, Geneva, Switzerland, 1975.
2. American Psychiatric Association, Task Force on Nomenclature and Statistics, Robert L. Spitzer, Chairman.
3. *A Psychiatric Glossary,* Fourth Edition, American Psychiatric Association, Washington, D.C., 1975.
4. *Dorland's Illustrated Medical Dictionary,* Twenty-fifth Edition, W.B. Saunders Company, Philadelphia, 1974.
5. *Stedman's Medical Dictionary,* Illustrated, Twenty-third Edition, Williams and Wilkins, Baltimore, 1976.

Academic underachievement disorder: Failure to achieve in most school tasks despite adequate intellectual capacity, a supportive and encouraging social environment, and apparent effort. The failure occurs in the absence of a demonstrable specific learning disability and is caused by emotional conflict not clearly associated with any other mental disorder.[2]

Adaptation reaction—*see* Adjustment reaction

Adjustment reaction or disorder: Mild or transient disorders lasting longer than acute stress reactions which occur in individuals of any age without any apparent pre-existing mental disorder. Such disorders are often relatively circumscribed or situation-specific, are generally reversible, and usually last only a few months. They are usually closely related in time and content to stresses such as bereavement, migration, or other experiences. Reactions to major stress that last longer than a few days are also included. In children such disorders are associated with no significant distortion of development.[1]

    conduct disturbance: Mild or transient disorders in which the main disturbance predominantly involves a disturbance of conduct (e.g., an adolescent grief reaction resulting in aggressive or antisocial disorder).[1]

    depressive reaction: States of depression, not specifiable as manic-depressive, psychotic, or neurotic.[1]

        brief: Generally transient, in which the depressive symptoms are usually closely related in time and content to some stressful event.[1]

        prolonged: Generally long-lasting, usually developing in association with prolonged exposure to a stressful situation.[1]

    emotional disturbance: An adjustment disorder in which the main symptoms are emotional in type (e.g., anxiety, fear, worry) but not specifically depressive.[1]

    mixed conduct and emotional disturbance: An adjustment reaction in which both emotional disturbance and disturbance of conduct are prominent features.[1]

Affective psychoses: Mental disorders, usually recurrent, in which there is a severe disturbance of mood (mostly compounded of depression and anxiety but also manifested as elation, and excitement) which is accompanied by one or more of the following: delusions, perplexity, disturbed attitude to self, disorder of perception and behavior; these are all in keeping with the individual's prevailing mood (as are hallucinations when they occur). There is a strong tendency to suicide. For practical reasons, mild disorders of mood may also be included here if the symptoms match closely the descriptions given; this applies particularly to mild hypomania.[1]

    bipolar: A manic-depressive psychosis which has appeared in both the depressive and manic form, either alternating or separated by an interval of normality.[1]

        atypical: An episode of affective psychosis with some, but not all, of the features of the one form of the disorder in individuals who have had a previous episode of the other form of the disorder.[2]

        depressed: A manic-depressive psychosis, circular type, in which the depressive form is currently present.[1]

        manic: A manic-depressive psychosis, circular type, in which the manic form is currently present.[1]

        mixed: A manic-depressive psychosis, circular type, in which both manic and depressive symptoms are present at the same time.[1]

    depressed type: A manic-depressive psychosis in which there is a widespread depressed mood of gloom and wretchedness with some degree of anxiety. There is often reduced activity but there may be restlessness and agitation. There is marked tendency to recurrence; in a few cases this may be at regular intervals.[1]

atypical: An affective depressive disorder that cannot be classified as a manic-depressive psychosis, depressed type, or chronic depressive personality disorder, or as an adjustment disorder.[2]

manic type: A manic-depressive psychosis characterized by states of elation or excitement out of keeping with the individual's circumstances and varying from enhanced liveliness (hypomania) to violent, almost uncontrollable, excitement. Aggression and anger, flight of ideas, distractibility, impaired judgement, and grandiose ideas are common.[1]

mixed type: Manic-depressive psychosis syndromes corresponding to both the manic and depressed types, but which for other reasons cannot be classified more specifically.[1]

Aggressive personality—*see* Personality disorder, explosive type

Agoraphobia—*see* agoraphobia under Phobia

Alcohol dependence syndrome: A state, psychic and usually also physical, resulting from taking alcohol, characterized by behavioral and other responses that always include a compulsion to take alcohol on a continuous or periodic basis in order to experience its psychic effects, and sometimes to avoid the discomfort of its absence; tolerance may or may not be present. A person may be dependent on alcohol and other drugs; if so, also record the diagnosis of drug dependence to identify the agent. If alcohol dependence is associated with alcoholic psychosis or with physical complications, *both* diagnoses should be recorded.[1]

Alcohol intoxication

acute: A psychic and physical state resulting from alcohol ingestion characterized by slurred speech, unsteady gait, poor coordination, flushed facies, nystagmus, sluggish reflexes, fetor alcoholica, loud speech, emotional instability (e.g., jollity followed by lugubriousness), excessive conviviality, loquacity, and poorly inhibited sexual and aggressive behavior.[2]

idiosyncratic: Acute psychotic episodes induced by relatively small amounts of alcohol. These are regarded as individual idiosyncratic reactions to alcohol, not due to excessive consumption and without conspicuous neurological signs of intoxication.[1]

pathological—*see* Alcohol intoxication, idiosyncratic

Alcoholic psychoses: Organic psychotic states due mainly to excessive consumption of alcohol; defects of nutrition are thought to play an important role.[1]

alcohol abstinence syndrome—*see* alcohol withdrawal syndrome below

alcohol amnestic syndrome: A syndrome of prominent and lasting reduction of memory span, including striking loss of recent memory, disordered time appreciation and confabulation, occurring in alcoholics as the sequel to an acute alcoholic psychosis (especially delirium tremens) or, more rarely, in the course of chronic alcoholism. It is usually accompanied by peripheral neuritis and may be associated with Wernicke's encephalopathy.[1]

alcohol withdrawal delirium [delirium tremens]: Acute or subacute organic psychotic states in alcoholics, characterized by clouded consciousness, disorientation, fear, illusions, delusions, hallucinations of any kind, notably visual and tactile, and restlessness, tremor and sometimes fever.[1]

alcohol withdrawal hallucinosis: A psychosis usually of less than six months' duration, with slight or no clouding of consciousness and much anxious restlessness in which auditory hallucinations, mostly of voices uttering insults and threats, predominate.[1]

alcohol withdrawal syndrome: Tremor of hands, tongue, and eyelids following cessation of prolonged heavy drinking of alcohol. Nausea and vomiting, dry mouth, headache, heavy perspiration, fitful sleep, acute anxiety attacks, mood depression, feelings of guilt and remorse, and irritability are associated features.[2]

alcohol delirium—*see* alcohol withdrawal delirium above

alcoholic dementia: Nonhallucinatory dementias occurring in association with alcoholism, but not characterized by the features of either alcohol withdrawal delirium [delirium tremens] or alcohol amnestic syndrome [Korsakoff's alcoholic psychosis].[1]

alcoholic hallucinosis—*see* alcohol withdrawal hallucinosis above

alcoholic jealousy: Chronic paranoid psychosis characterized by delusional jealousy and associated with alcoholism.[1]

alcoholic paranoia—*see* Alcoholic jealousy

alcoholic polyneuritic psychosis—*see* alcohol amnestic syndrome above

Alcoholism

acute—*see* Alcohol intoxication, acute

chronic—*see* Alcohol dependence syndrome

Alexia: Loss of a previously possessed reading facility that cannot be explained by defective visual acuity.[3]

Amnesia, psychogenic: A form of dissociative hysteria in which there is a temporary disturbance in the ability to recall important personal information which has already been registered and stored in memory. The sudden onset of this disturbance in the absence of an underlying organic mental disorder, and the extent of the disturbance being too great to be explained by ordinary forgetfulness, are the essential features.[2]

Amnestic syndrome: A syndrome of prominent and lasting reduction of memory span, including striking loss of recent memory, disordered time appreciation, and confabulation. The commonest causes are chronic alcoholism [alcohol amnestic syndrome; Korsakoff's alcoholic psychosis], chronic barbiturate dependence, and malnutrition. An amnestic syndrome may be the predominating disturbance in the early states of presenile and senile dementia, arteriosclerotic dementia, and in encephalitis and other inflammatory and degenerative diseases in which there is particular bilateral involvement of the temporal lobes, and certain temporal lobe tumors.[2]

alcoholic—*see* alcohol amnestic syndrome under Alcoholic psychoses

Amoral personality—*see* Personality disorder, antisocial type

Anancastic [anankastic] neurosis—*see* Neurotic disorder, obsessive-compulsive

Anancastic [anankastic] personality—*see* Personality disorder, compulsive type

Anorexia nervosa: A disorder in which the main features are persistent active refusal to eat and marked loss of weight. The level of activity and alertness is characteristically high in relation to the degree of emaciation. Typically the disorder begins in teenage girls but it may sometimes begin before puberty and rarely it occurs in males. Amenorrhea is usual and there may be a variety of other physiological changes including slow pulse and respiration, low body temperature, and dependent edema. Unusual eating habits and attitudes toward food are typical and sometimes starvation follows or alternates with periods of overeating. The accompanying psychiatric symptoms are diverse.[1]

Anxiety hysteria—*see* phobia under Neurotic disorders

Anxiety state (neurotic): Apprehension, tension, or uneasiness that stems from the anticipation of danger, the source of which is largely unknown or unrecognized.[3]

atypical: An anxiety disorder that does not fulfill the criteria of generalized or panic attack anxiety. An example might be an individual with a single morbid fear.[2]

generalized: A disorder of at least six months' duration in which the predominant feature is limited to diffuse and persistent anxiety without the specific symptoms that characterize phobic disorders, panic disorder, or obsessive-compulsive disorder.[2]

panic attack: An episodic and often chronic, recurrent disorder in which the predominant features are anxiety attacks and nervousness. The anxiety attacks are manifested by discrete periods of sudden onset of intense apprehension, fearfulness, or terror often associated with feelings of impending doom.[2]

Aphasia, developmental: A delay in the production of spoken language. Rarely, there is also a developmental delay in the comprehension of speech sounds.[1]

Arteriosclerotic dementia: Dementia attributable, because of physical signs (on examination of the central nervous system), to degenerative arterial disease of the brain. Symptoms suggesting a focal lesion in the brain are common. There may be a fluctuating or patchy intellectual defect with insight, and an intermittent course is common. Clinical differentiation from senile or presenile dementia, which may coexist with it, may be very difficult or impossible. The diagnosis of cerebral atherosclerosis should also be recorded.[1]

Asocial personality—*see* Personality disorder, antisocial type

Astasia-abasia, hysterical: A form of conversion hysteria in which the individual is unable to stand or walk although the legs are otherwise under control.[4]

Asthenia, psychogenic—*see* neurasthenia under Neurotic disorders

Asthenic personality—*see* Personality disorder, dependent type

Attention deficit disorder—*see* attention deficit disorder under Hyperkinetic syndrome of childhood.

Autism, infantile: A syndrome present from birth or beginning almost invariably in the first 30 months. Responses to auditory and sometimes to visual stimuli are abnormal, and there are usually severe problems in the understanding of spoken language. Speech is delayed and, if it develops, is characterized by echolalia, the reversal of pronouns, immature grammatical structure, and inability to use abstract terms. There is generally an impairment in the social use of both verbal and gestural language. Problems in social relationships are most severe before the age of five years and include an impairment in the development of eye-to-eye gaze, social attachments, and cooperative play. Ritualistic behavior is usual and may include abnormal routines, resistance to change, attachment to odd objects and stereotyped patterns of play. The capacity for abstract or symbolic thought and for imaginative play is diminished. Intelligence ranges from severely subnormal to normal or above. Performance is usually better on tasks involving rote memory or visuospatial skills than on those requiring symbolic or linguistic skills.[1]

Avoidant personality—*see* Personality disorder, avoidant type

"Bad trips": Acute intoxication from hallucinogen abuse, manifested by hallucinatory states lasting only a few days or less.[1]

Barbiturate abuse: Cases where an individual has taken the drug to the detriment of his health or social functioning, in doses above or for periods beyond those normally regarded as therapeutic.[1]

Bestiality—*see* Zoophilia

Bipolar disorder—*see* Affective psychosis, bipolar

   atypical—*see* Affective psychosis, bipolar, atypical

Body-rocking—*see* Stereotyped repetitive movements

Borderline personality—*see* Personality disorder, borderline type

Borderline psychosis of childhood—*see* Psychosis, atypical childhood

Borderline schizophrenia—*see* Schizophrenia, latent

Bouffée délirante—*see* Paranoid reaction, acute

Briquet's disorder—*see* somatization disorder under Neurotic disorders

Bulimia: An episodic pattern of overeating [binge eating] accompanied by an awareness of the disordered eating pattern with a fear of not being able to stop eating voluntarily. Depressive moods and self-deprecating thoughts follow the episodes of binge eating.[2]

Catalepsy schizophrenia—*see* Schizophrenia, catatonic type

Catastrophic stress—*see* Gross stress reaction

Catatonia (schizophrenic)—*see* Schizophrenia, catatonic type

Character neurosis—*see* Personality disorders

Childhood autism—*see* Autism, infantile

Childhood type schizophrenia—*see* Psychosis, child

Chronic alcoholic brain syndrome—*see* alcoholic dementia under Alcoholic psychoses

Clay-eating—*see* Pica

Clumsiness syndrome—*see* coordination disorder under Developmental delay disorders, specific

Combat fatigue—*see* Posttraumatic disorder, acute

Compensation neurosis—*see* compensation neurosis under Neurotic disorders

Compulsive conduct disorder—*see* impulse control disorders under Conduct disorders

Compulsive neurosis—*see* Neurotic disorder, obsessive-compulsive

Compulsive personality—*see* Personality disorder, compulsive type

Concentration camp syndrome—*see* Posttraumatic stress disorder, prolonged

Conduct disorders: Disorders mainly involving aggressive and destructive behavior and disorders involving delinquency. It should be used for abnormal behavior, in individuals of any age, which gives rise to social disapproval but which is not part of any other psychiatric condition. Minor emotional disturbances may also be present. To be included, the behavior, as judged by its frequency, severity, and type of associations with other symptoms, must be abnormal in its context. Disturbances of conduct are distinguished from an adjustment reaction by a longer duration and by a lack of close relationship in time and content to some stress. They differ from a personality disorder by the absence of deeply ingrained maladaptive patterns of behavior present from adolescence or earlier.[1]

   impulse control disorders: A failure to resist an impulse, drive, or temptation to perform some action which is harmful to the individual or to others. The impulse may or may not be consciously resisted, and the act may or may not be premeditated or planned. Prior to committing the act, there is an increasing sense of tension, and at the time of committing the act, there is an experience of either pleasure, gratification, or release. Immediately following the act, there may or may not be genuine regret, self-reproach, or guilt.[2] *See also* Intermittent explosive disorder, Isolated explosive disorder, Kleptomania, Pathological gambling, and Pyromania.

   mixed disturbance of conduct and emotions: A disorder characterized by features of undersocialized and socialized disturbance of conduct, but in which there is also considerable emotional disturbance as shown, for example, by anxiety, misery, or obsessive manifestations.[1]

   socialized conduct disorder: Conduct disorders in individuals who have acquired the values or behavior of a delinquent peer group to whom they are loyal and with whom they characteristically steal, play truant, and stay out late at night. There may also be sexual promiscuity.[1]

   undersocialized conduct disturbance

      aggressive type: A disorder characterized by a persistent pattern of disrespect for the feelings and well-being of others (bullying, physical aggression, cruel behavior, hostility, verbal abusiveness, impudence, defiance, negativism), aggressive antisocial behavior (destructiveness, stealing, persistent lying, frequent truancy, and vandalism), and failure to develop close and stable relationships with others.[2]

unaggressive type: A disorder in which there is a lack of concern for the rights and feelings of others to a degree which indicates a failure to establish a normal degree of affection, empathy, or bond with others. There are two patterns of behavior found. In one, the child is fearful and timid, lacking self-assertiveness, resorts to self-protective and manipulative lying, indulges in whining demandingness and temper tantrums, feels rejected and unfairly treated, and is mistrustful of others. In the other pattern of the disorder, the child approaches others strictly for his own gains and acts exclusively because of exploitative and extractive goals. The child lies brazenly and steals, appearing to feel no guilt, and forms no social bonds to other individuals.[2]

Confusion, psychogenic—*see* Psychosis, reactive confusion

Confusion, reactive—*see* Psychosis, reactive confusion

Confusional state

    acute—*see* Delirium, acute

    epileptic—*see* Delirium, acute

    subacute—*see* Delirium, subacute

Conversion hysteria—*see* hysteria, conversion type under Neurotic disorders

Coordination disorder—*see* coordination disorder under Developmental delay disorders, specific

Culture shock: A form of stress reaction associated with an individual's assimilation into a new culture which is vastly different from that in which he was raised.[5]

Cyclic schizophrenia—*see* Schizophrenia, schizo-affective type

Cyclothymic personality or disorder—*see* Personality disorder, cyclothymic type

Delirium: Transient organic psychotic conditions with a short course in which there is a rapidly developing onset of disorganization of higher mental processes manifested by some degree of impairment of information processing, impaired or abnormal attention, perception, memory, and thinking. Clouded consciousness, confusion, disorientation, delusions, illusions, and often vivid hallucinations predominate in the clinical picture.[1,2]

    acute: short-lived states, lasting hours or days, of the above type.[1]

    subacute: states of the above type in which the symptoms, usually less florid, last for several weeks or longer, during which they may show marked fluctuations in intensity.[1]

Delirium tremens—*see* alcohol withdrawal delirium under Alcoholic psychoses

Delusions, systematized—*see* Paranoia

Dementia: A decrement in intellectual functioning of sufficient severity to interfere with occupational or social performance, or both. There is impairment of memory and abstract thinking, the ability to learn new skills, problem solving, and judgment. There is often also personality change or impairment in impulse control. Dementia in organic psychoses may be of a chronic or progressive nature, which if untreated are usually irreversible and terminal.[1,2]

    alcoholic—*see* alcoholic dementia under Alcoholic psychoses

    arteriosclerotic—*see* Arteriosclerotic dementia

    multi-infarct—*see* Arteriosclerotic dementia

    presenile—*see* Presenile dementia

    repeated infarct—*see* Arteriosclerotic dementia

    senile—*see* Senile dementia

Depersonalization syndrome—*see* depersonalization syndrome under Neurotic disorders

Depression: States of depression, usually of moderate but occasionally of marked intensity, which have no specifically manic-depressive or other psychotic depressive features, and which do not appear to be associated with stressful events or other features specified under neurotic depression.[1]

    anxiety—*see* depression under Neurotic disorders

    endogenous—*see* Affective psychosis, depressed type

    monopolar—*see* Affective psychosis, depressed type

    neurotic—*see* depression under Neurotic disorders

    psychotic—*see* Affective psychosis, depressed type

    psychotic reactive—*see* Psychosis, depressive

    reactive—*see* depression under Neurotic disorders

    reactive psychotic—*see* Psychosis, depressive

Depressive personality or character—*see* Personality disorder, chronic depressive type

Depressive reaction—*see* depressive reaction under Adjustment reaction

Depressive psychosis—*see* Affective psychosis, depressed type

Derealization (neurotic)—*see* depersonalization syndrome under Neurotic disorders

Developmental delay disorders, specific: A group of disorders in which a specific delay in development is the main feature. For many the delay is not explicable in terms of general intellectual retardation or of inadequate schooling. In each case development is related to biological maturation, but it is also influenced by nonbiological factors. A diagnosis of a specific developmental delay carries no etiological implications. A diagnosis of specific delay in development should not be made if it is due to a known neurological disorder.[1]

    arithmetical disorder: Disorders in which the main feature is a serious impairment in the development of arithmetical skills.[1]

    articulation disorder: A delay in the development of normal word-sound production resulting in defects of articulation. Omissions or substitutions of consonants are most frequent.[1]

    coordination disorder: Disorders in which the main feature is a serious impairment in the development of motor coordination which is not explicable in terms of general intellectual retardation. The clumsiness is commonly associated with perceptual difficulties.[1]

    mixed development disorder: A delay in the development of one specific skill (e.g., reading, arithmetic, speech, or coordination) is frequently associated with lesser delays in other skills. When this occurs the diagnosis should be made according to the skill most seriously impaired. The mixed category should be used only where the mixture of delayed skills is such that no one skill is preponderantly affected.[1]

    motor retardation—*see* coordination disorder above

    reading disorder or retardation: Disorders in which the main feature is a serious impairment in the development of reading or spelling skills which is not explicable in terms of general intellectual retardation or of inadequate schooling. Speech or language difficulties, impaired right-left differentiation, perceptuo-motor problems, and coding difficulties are frequently associated. Similar problems are often present in other members of the family. Adverse psychosocial factors may be present.[1]

    speech or language disorder: Disorders in which the main feature is a serious impairment in the development of speech or language (syntax or semantic) which is not explicable in terms of general intellectual retardation. Most commonly there is a delay in the development of normal word-sound production resulting in defects of articulation. Omissions or substitutions of consonants are most frequent. There may also be a delay in the production of spoken language. Rarely, there is also a developmental delay in the comprehension of sounds. Includes cases in which delay is largely due to environmental privation.[1]

Dipsomania—*see* Alcohol dependence syndrome

Disorganized schizophrenia—*see* Schizophrenia, disorganized type

Dissociative hysteria—*see* hysteria, dissociative type under Neurotic disorders

Drug abuse: Includes cases where an individual, for whom no other diagnosis is possible, has come under medical care because of the maladaptive effect of a drug on which he is not dependent (*see* Drug dependence) and that he has taken on his own initiative to the detriment of his health or social functioning. When drug abuse is secondary to a psychiatric disorder, record the disorder as an additional diagnosis.[1]

Drug dependence: A state, psychic and sometimes also physical, resulting from taking a drug, characterized by behavioral and other responses that always include a compulsion to take a drug on a continuous or periodic basis in order to experience its psychic effects, and sometimes to avoid the discomfort of its absence. Tolerance may or may not be present. A person may be dependent on more than one drug.[1]

Drug psychoses: Organic mental syndromes which are due to consumption of drugs (notably amphetamines, barbiturates, and opiate and LSD groups) and solvents. Some of the syndromes in this group are not as severe as most conditions labeled "psychotic," but they are included here for practical reasons. The drug should be identified, and also a diagnosis of drug dependence should be recorded, if present.[1]

    drug-induced hallucinosis: Hallucinatory states of more than a few days, but not more than a few months' duration, associated with large or prolonged intake of drugs, notably of the amphetamine and LSD groups. Auditory hallucinations usually predominate and there may be anxiety or restlessness. States following LSD or other hallucinogens lasting only a few days or less ["bad trips"] are not included.[1]

    drug-induced organic delusional syndrome: Paranoid states of more than a few days, but not more than a few months' duration, associated with large or prolonged intake of drugs, notably of the amphetamine and LSD groups.[1]

    drug withdrawal syndrome: States associated with drug withdrawal ranging from severe, as specified for alcohol withdrawal delirium [delirium tremens], to less severe states characterized by one or more symptoms such as convulsions, tremor, anxiety, restlessness, gastrointestinal and muscular complaints, and mild disorientation and memory disturbance.[1]

Drunkenness:

    acute—*see* Alcohol intoxication, acute

    pathologic—*see* Alcohol intoxication, idiosyncratic

    simple: A state of inebriation due to alcohol consumption without conspicuous neurological signs of intoxication.[2]

    sleep: An inability to fully arouse from the sleep state characterized by failure to attain full consciousness after arousal.[2]

Dyscalculia—*see* arithmetical disorder under Developmental delay disorders, specific

Dyslalia—*see* articulation disorder under Developmental delay disorders, specific

Dyslexia, developmental: A disorder in which the main feature is a serious impairment of reading skills which is not explicable in terms of general intellectual retardation or of inadequate schooling. Word-blindness and strephosymbolia (tendency to reverse letters and words in reading) are included.[1,3]

Dysmenorrhea, psychogenic: Painful menstruation due to disturbance of psychic control.[4]

Dyspareunia, functional—*see* functional dyspareunia under Psychosexual dysfunctions

Dyspraxia syndrome—*see* coordination disorder under Developmental delay disorders, specific

Dyssocial personality—*see* Personality disorder, antisocial type

Dysuria, psychogenic: Difficulty in passing urine due to psychic factors.[4]

Eating disorders: A group of disorders characterized by a conspicuous disturbance in eating behavior.[2] *See also* Bulimia, Pica, and Rumination, psychogenic.

Eccentric personality—*see* Personality disorder, eccentric type

Elective mutism: A pervasive and persistent refusal to speak in situations not attributable to a mental disorder. In some cases the behavior may manifest a form of withdrawal reaction to a specific stressful situation, or as a predominant feature in children exhibiting shyness or social withdrawal disorders.[2]

Emancipation disorder: An adjustment reaction in adolescents or young adults in which there is symptomatic expression (e.g., difficulty in making independent decisions, increased dependence on parental advice, adoption of values deliberately oppositional to parents) of a conflict over independence following the recent assumption of a status in which the individual is more independent of parental control or supervision.[2]

Emotional disturbances specific to childhood and adolescence: Less well-differentiated emotional disorders characteristic of the childhood period. When the emotional disorder takes the form of a neurosis, the appropriate diagnosis should be made. These disorders differ from adjustment reactions in terms of longer duration and by the lack of close relationship in time and content to some stress.[1] *See also* Academic underachievement disorder, Elective mutism, Identity disorder, Introverted disorder of childhood, Misery and unhappiness disorder, Oppositional disorder, Overanxious disorder, and Shyness disorder of childhood.

Encopresis: A disorder in which the main manifestation is the persistent voluntary or involuntary passage of formed stools of normal or near-normal consistency into places not intended for that purpose in the individual's own sociocultural setting. Sometimes the child has failed to gain bowel control, and sometimes he has gained control but then later again became encopretic. There may be a variety of associated psychiatric symptoms and there may be smearing of feces. The condition would not usually be diagnosed under the age of four years.[1]

Endogenous depression—*see* Affective psychosis, depressed type

Enuresis: A disorder in which the main manifestation is a persistent involuntary voiding of urine by day or night which is considered abnormal for the age of the individual. Sometimes the child will have failed to gain bladder control and in other cases he will have gained control and then lost it. Episodic or fluctuating enuresis should be included. The disorder would not usually be diagnosed under the age of four years.[1]

Epileptic confusional or twilight state—*see* Delirium, acute

Excitation

    catatonic—*see* Schizophrenia, catatonic type

    psychogenic—*see* Psychosis, excitative type

    reactive—*see* Psychosis, excitative type

Exhaustion delirium—*see* Stress reaction, acute

Exhibitionism: Sexual deviation in which the main sexual pleasure and gratification is derived from exposure of the genitals to a person of the opposite sex.[1]

Explosive personality disorder—*see* Personality disorder, explosive type

Factitious illness: A form of hysterical neurosis in which there are physical or psychological symptoms that are not real, genuine, or natural, which are produced by the individual and are under his voluntary control.[2]

physical symptom type: The presentation of physical symptoms that may be total fabrication, self-inflicted, an exaggeration or exacerbation of a pre-existing physical condition, or any combination or variation of these.[2]

psychological symptom type: The voluntary production of symptoms suggestive of a mental disorder. Behavior may mimic psychosis or, rather, the individual's idea of psychosis.[2]

Fanatic personality—*see* Personality disorder, paranoid type

Fatigue neurosis—*see* neurasthenia under Neurotic disorders

Feeble-minded—*see* Mental retardation, mild

Fetishism: A sexual deviation in which nonliving objects are utilized as a preferred or exclusive method of stimulating erotic arousal.[2]

Finger-flicking—*see* Stereotyped repetitive movements

Folie à deux—*see* Shared paranoid disorder

Frigidity: A psychosexual dysfunction in which there is partial or complete failure to attain or maintain the lubrication-swelling response of sexual excitement until completion of the sexual act.[2]

Frontal lobe syndrome: Changes in behavior following damage to the frontal areas of the brain or following interference with the connections of those areas. There is a general diminution of self-control, foresight, creativity, and spontaneity, which may be manifest as increased irritability, selfishness, restlessness and lack of concern for others. Conscientiousness and powers of concentration are often diminished, but measurable deterioration of intellect or memory is not necessarily present. The overall picture is often one of emotional dullness, lack of drive, and slowness; but, particularly in persons previously with energetic, restless, or aggressive characteristics, there may be a change towards impulsiveness, boastfulness, temper outbursts, silly fatuous humor, and the development of unrealistic ambitions; the direction of change usually depends upon the previous personality. A considerable degree of recovery is possible and may continue over the course of several years.[1]

Fugue, psychogenic: A form of dissociative hysteria characterized by an episode of wandering with inability to recall one's prior identity. Both onset and recovery are rapid. Following recovery there is no recollection of events which took place during the fugue state.[2]

Ganser's syndrome (hysterical): A form of factitious illness in which the patient voluntarily produces symptoms suggestive of a mental disorder.[2]

Gender identity disorder—*see* gender identity disorder under Psychosexual identity disorders

Gilles de la Tourette's disorder or syndrome—*see* Gilles de la Tourette's disorder under Tics

Grief reaction—*see* depressive reaction, brief under Adjustment reaction

Gross stress reaction—*see* Stress reaction, acute

Group delinquency—*see* socialized conduct disorder under Conduct disorders

Habit spasm—*see* chronic motor tic disorder under Tics

Hangover (alcohol)—*see* Drunkenness, simple

Head-banging—*see* Stereotyped repetitive movements

Hebephrenia—*see* Schizophrenia, disorganized type

Heller's syndrome—*see* Psychosis, disintegrative

High grade defect—*see* Mental retardation, mild

Homosexuality: Exclusive or predominant sexual attraction for persons of the same sex with or without physical relationship. Record homosexuality as a diagnosis whether or not it is considered as a mental disorder.[1]

Hospital addiction syndrome—*see* Munchausen syndrome

Hospital hoboes—*see* Munchausen syndrome

Hospitalism: A mild or transient adjustment reaction characterized by withdrawal seen in hospitalized patients. In young children this may be manifested by elective mutism.[1]

Hyperkinetic syndrome of childhood: Disorders in which the essential features are short attention-span and distractibility. In early childhood the most striking symptom is disinhibited, poorly organized and poorly regulated extreme overactivity but in adolescence this may be replaced by underactivity. Impulsiveness, marked mood fluctuations, and aggression are also common symptoms. Delays in the development of specific skills are often present and disturbed, poor relationships are common. If the hyperkinesis is symptomatic of an underlying disorder, the diagnosis of the underlying disorder is recorded instead.[1]

attention deficit disorder: Cases of hyperkinetic syndrome in which short attention span, distractibility, and overactivity are the main manifestations without significant disturbance of conduct or delay in specific skills.[1]

hyperkinesis with developmental delay: Cases in which the hyperkinetic syndrome is associated with speech delay, clumsiness, reading difficulties, or other delays of specific skills.[1]

hyperkinetic conduct disorder: Cases in which the hyperkinetic syndrome is associated with marked conduct disturbance but not developmental delay.[1]

Hypersomnia: A disorder of initiating arousal from sleep or maintaining wakefulness.

persistent: Chronic difficulty in initiating arousal from sleep or maintaining wakefulness associated with major or minor depressive mental disorders.[2]

transient: Episodes of difficulty in arousal from sleep or maintaining wakefulness associated with acute or intermittent emotional reactions or conflicts.[2]

Hypochondriasis—*see* hypochondriasis under Neurotic disorders

Hypomania—*see* Affective psychosis, manic type

Hypomanic personality—*see* Personality disorder, chronic hypomanic type

Hyposomnia—*see* Insomnia

Hysteria—*see* hysteria under Neurotic disorders

anxiety—*see* phobia under Neurotic disorders

psychosis—*see* Psychosis, reactive

acute—*see* Psychosis, excitative type

Hysterical personality—*see* Personality disorder, histrionic type

Identity disorder: An emotional disorder caused by distress over the inability to reconcile aspects of the self into a relatively coherent and acceptable sense of self, not secondary to another mental disorder. The disturbance is manifested by intense subjective distress regarding uncertainty about a variety of issues relating to identity, including long-term goals, career choice, friendship patterns, values, and loyalties.[2]

Idiocy—*see* Mental retardation, profound

Imbecile—*see* Mental retardation, moderate

Impotence: A psychosexual dysfunction in which there is partial or complete failure to attain or maintain erection until completion of the sexual act.[2]

Impulse control disorder—*see* impulse control disorders under Conduct disorders

Inadequate personality—*see* Personality disorder, dependent type

Induced paranoid disorder—*see* Shared paranoid disorder

Inebriety—*see* Drunkenness, simple

Infantile autism—*see* Autism, infantile

Insomnia: A disorder of initiating or maintaining sleep.[2]

persistent: A chronic state of sleeplessness associated with chronic anxiety, major or minor depressive disorders, or psychoses.[2]

transient: Episodes of sleeplessness associated with acute or intermittent emotional reactions or conflicts.[2]

Intermittent explosive disorder: Recurrent episodes of sudden and significant loss of control of aggressive impulses, not accounted for by any other mental disorder, which results in serious assault or destruction of property. The magnitude of the behavior during an episode is grossly out of proportion to any psychosocial stressors which may have played a role in eliciting the episode of lack of control. Following each episode there is genuine regret or self-reproach at the consequences of the action and the inability to control the aggressive impulse.[2]

Introverted disorder of childhood: An emotional disturbance in children chiefly manifested by a lack of interest in social relationships and indifference to social praise or criticism.[2]

Introverted personality—*see* Personality disorder, introverted type

Involutional melancholia—*see* Affective psychosis, depressed type

Involutional paranoid state—*see* Paraphrenia

Isolated explosive disorder: A disorder of impulse control in which there is a single discrete episode characterized by failure to resist an impulse which leads to a single, violent externally- directed act, which has a catastrophic impact on others, and for which the available information does not justify the diagnosis of another mental disorder.[2]

Isolated phobia—*see* simple phobia under Phobia

Jet lag syndrome: A phase-shift disruption of the 24-hour sleep-wake cycle due to rapid time-zone changes experienced in long-distance travel.[2]

Kanner's syndrome—*see* Autism, infantile

Kleptomania: A disorder of impulse control characterized by a recurrent failure to resist impulses to steal objects not for immediate use or their monetary value. An increasing sense of tension is experienced prior to committing the act, with an intense experience of gratification at the time of committing the theft.[2]

Korsakoff's psychosis:

    alcoholic—*see* alcohol amnestic syndrome under Alcoholic psychoses

    nonalcoholic—*see* Amnestic syndrome

Latent schizophrenia—*see* Schizophrenia, latent

Lesbianism—*see* Homosexuality

Lobotomy syndrome—*see* Frontal lobe syndrome

LSD reaction: Acute intoxication from hallucinogen abuse, manifested by hallucinatory states lasting only a few days or less.[1]

Major depressive disorder—*see* Affective psychosis, depressed type

Malingering: A clinical picture in which the predominant feature is the presentation of fake or grossly exaggerated physical or psychiatric illness apparently under voluntary control. In contrast to factitious illness, the symptoms produced in malingering are in pursuit of a goal which, when known, is recognizable and obviously understandable in light of knowledge of the individual's circumstances. Examples of understandable goals include, but are not limited to, becoming a "patient" in order to avoid conscription or military duty, avoid work, obtain financial compensation, evade criminal prosecution, and obtain drugs.[2]

Mania (monopolar)—*see* Affective psychosis, manic type

Manic-depressive psychosis

    circular type—*see* Affective psychosis, bipolar

    depressed type—*see* Affective psychosis, depressed type

    manic type—*see* Affective psychosis, manic type

    mixed type—*see* Affective psychosis, mixed type

Manic disorder—*see* Affective psychosis, manic type

    atypical—*see* Affective psychosis, manic type, atypical

Masochistic personality—*see* Personality disorder, masochistic type

Melancholia—*see* Affective psychoses

    involutional—*see* Affective psychosis, depressed type

Mental retardation: A condition of arrested or incomplete development of mind which is especially characterized by subnormality of intelligence. The coding should be made on the individual's *current* level of functioning *without regard to its nature* or causation, such as psychosis, cultural deprivation, Down's syndrome, etc. Where there is a specific cognitive handicap—such as in speech—the diagnosis of mental retardation should be based on assessments of cognition *outside the area of specific handicap.* The assessment of intellectual level should be based on whatever information is available, including clinical evidence, adaptive behavior, and psychometric findings. The IQ levels given are based on a test with a mean of 100 and a standard deviation of 15, such as the Wechsler scales. They are provided only as a guide and should not be applied rigidly. Mental retardation often involves psychiatric disturbances and may often develop as a result of some physical disease or injury. In these cases, an additional diagnosis should be recorded to identify any associated condition, psychiatric or physical.[1]

    mild mental retardation: IQ criteria 50-70. Individuals with this level of retardation are usually educable. During the pre-school period they can develop social and communication skills, have minimal retardation in sensorimotor areas, and often are not distinguished from normal children until a later age. During the school age period they can learn academic skills up to approximately the sixth-grade level. During the adult years, they can usually achieve social and vocational skills adequate for minimum self-support, but may need guidance and assistance when under social or economic stress.[2]

    moderate mental retardation: IQ criteria 35-49. Individuals with this level of retardation are usually trainable. During the pre-school period they can talk or learn to communicate. They have poor social awareness and fair motor development. During the school age period they can profit from training in social and occupational skills, but they are unlikely to progress beyond the second-grade level in academic subjects. During their adult years they may achieve self-maintenance in unskilled or semi-skilled work under sheltered conditions. They need supervision and guidance when under mild social or economic stress.[2]

    severe mental retardation: IQ criteria 20-34. Individuals with this level of retardation evidence poor motor development, minimal speech, and are generally unable to profit from training and self-help during the pre-school period. During the school age period they can talk or learn to communicate, can be trained in elementary health habits, and may profit from systematic habit training. During the adult years they may contribute partially to self-maintenance under complete supervision.[2]

profound mental retardation: IQ criteria under 20. Individuals with this level of retardation evidence minimal capacity for sensorimotor functioning and need nursing care during the pre-school period. During the school age period some further motor development may occur, and they may respond to minimal or limited training in self-help. During the adult years some motor and speech development may occur, and they may achieve very limited self-care and need nursing care.[2]

Merycism—*see* Rumination, psychogenic

Minimal brain dysfunction [MBD]—*see* Hyperkinetic syndrome of childhood

Misery and unhappiness disorder: An emotional disorder characteristic of childhood in which the main symptoms involve misery and unhappiness. There may also be eating and sleep disturbances.[1]

Mood swings (brief compensatory) (rebound): Mild disorders of mood (depression and anxiety or elation and excitement, occurring alternatingly or episodically) seen in affective psychosis.[1]

Motor tic disorders—*see* Tics

Motor-verbal tic disorder—*see* Gilles de la Tourette's disorder under Tics

Multi-infarct dementia or psychosis—*see* Arteriosclerotic dementia

Multiple operations syndrome—*see* Munchausen syndrome

Multiple personality: A form of dissociative hysteria in which there is the domination of the individual at any one time by one of two or more distinct personalities. Each personality is a full-integrated and complex unit with memories, behavior patterns, and social friendships which determine the nature of the individual's acts when uppermost in consciousness.[2]

Munchausen syndrome: A chronic form of factitious illness in which the individual demonstrates a plausible presentation of voluntarily produced physical symptomatology of such a degree that he is able to obtain and sustain multiple hospitalizations.[2]

Narcissistic personality—*see* Personality disorder, narcissistic type

Nervous debility—*see* neurasthenia under Neurotic disorders

Neurasthenia—*see* neurasthenia under Neurotic disorders

Neurotic delinquency—*see* mixed disturbance of conduct and emotions under Conduct disorders

Neurotic disorders: Neurotic disorders are mental disorders without any demonstrable organic basis in which the individual may have considerable insight and has unimpaired reality testing, in that he usually does not confuse his morbid subjective experiences and fantasies with external reality. Behavior may be greatly affected although usually remaining within socially acceptable limits, but personality is not disorganized. The principal manifestations include excessive anxiety, hysterical symptoms, phobias, obsessional and compulsive symptoms, and depression.[1]

    anxiety states: Various combinations of physical and mental manifestations of anxiety, not attributable to real danger and occurring either in attacks [*see* Anxiety state, panic attacks] or as a persisting state [*see* Anxiety state, generalized]. The anxiety is usually diffuse and may extend to panic. Other neurotic features such as obsessional or hysterical symptoms may be present but do not dominate the clinical picture.[1]

    compensation neurosis: Certain unconscious neurotic reactions in which features of secondary gain, such as a situational or financial advantage, are prominent.[3]

    depersonalization: A neurotic disorder with an unpleasant state of disturbed perception in which external objects or parts of one's own body are experienced as changed in their quality, unreal, remote, or automatized. The patient is aware of the subjective nature of the change he experiences. If depersonalization occurs as a feature of anxiety, schizophrenia, or other mental disorder, the condition is classified according to the major psychiatric disorder.[1]

    depression: A neurotic disorder characterized by disproportionate depression which has usually recognizably ensued on a distressing experience; it does not include among its features delusions or hallucinations, and there is often preoccupation with the psychic trauma which preceded the illness, e.g., loss of a cherished person or possession. Anxiety is also frequently present and mixed states of anxiety and depression should be included here. The distinction between depressive neurosis and psychosis should be made not only upon the degree of depression but also on the presence or absence of other neurotic and psychotic characteristics, and upon the degree of disturbance of the individual's behavior.[1]

    hypochondriasis: A neurotic disorder in which the conspicuous features are excessive concern with one's health in general or the integrity and functioning of some part of one's body, or less frequently, one's mind. It is usually associated with anxiety and depression. It may occur as a feature of some other severe mental disorder (e.g., manic-depressive psychosis, depressed type, schizophrenia, hysteria) and in that case should be classified according to the corresponding major disorder.[1]

    hysteria: A neurotic mental disorder in which motives, of which the patient seems unaware, produce either a restriction of the field of consciousness or disturbances of motor or sensory function which may seem to have psychological advantage or symbolic value.[1] There are three subtypes:

conversion type: The chief or only symptoms of the hysterical neurosis consist of psychogenic disturbance of function in some part of the body, e.g., paralysis, tremor, blindness, deafness, seizures.[1]

dissociative type: The most prominent feature of the hysterical neurosis is a narrowing of the field of consciousness which seems to serve an unconscious purpose and is commonly accompanied or followed by a selective amnesia. There may be dramatic but essentially superficial changes of personality [multiple personality], or sometimes the patient enters into a wandering state [fugue].[1]

factitious illness: Physical or psychological symptoms that are not real, genuine, or natural, which are produced by the individual and are under his voluntary control.[2]

neurasthenia: A neurotic disorder characterized by fatigue, irritability, headache, depression, insomnia, difficulty in concentration, and lack of capacity for enjoyment [anhedonia]. It may follow or accompany an infection or exhaustion, or arise from continued emotional stress. If neurasthenia is associated with a physical disorder, the latter should also be recorded as a diagnosis.[1]

obsessive-compulsive: States in which the outstanding symptom is a feeling of subjective compulsion, which must be resisted, to carry out some action, to dwell on an idea, to recall an experience, or to ruminate on an abstract topic. Unwanted thoughts which intrude, the insistency of words or ideas, ruminations or trains of thought are perceived by the individual to be inappropriate or nonsensical. The obsessional urge or idea is recognized as alien to the personality but as coming from within the self. Obsessional actions may be quasi-ritual performances designed to relieve anxiety, e.g., washing the hands to cope with contamination. Attempts to dispel the unwelcome thought or urges may lead to a severe inner struggle, with intense anxiety.[1]

occupational: A neurosis characterized by a functional disorder of a group of muscles used chiefly in one's occupation, marked by the occurrence of spasm, paresis, or incoordination on attempt to repeat the habitual movements (e.g., writers' cramp).[5]

phobic disorders: Neurotic states with abnormally intense dread of certain objects or specific situations which would not normally have that effect. If the anxiety tends to spread from a specified situation or object to a wider range of circumstances, it becomes akin to or identical with anxiety state and should be classified as such.[1] *See also* Phobia.

somatization disorder: A chronic, but fluctuating, neurotic disorder which begins early in life and is characterized by recurrent and multiple somatic complaints for which medical attention is sought but which are not apparently due to any physical illness. Complaints are presented in a dramatic, vague, or exaggerated way, or are part of a complicated medical history in which often many specific diagnoses have allegedly been made by other physicians. Complaints invariably refer to many organ systems (headache, fatigue, palpitations, fainting, nausea and vomiting, abdominal pains, bowel trouble, allergies, menstrual and sexual difficulties), and the individual frequently receives medical care from a number of physicians, sometimes simultaneously.[2]

Neurosis—*see* Neurotic disorders

Nightmares: Anxiety attacks occurring in dreams during REM sleep.[2]

Night terrors: A pathology of arousal from stage 4 sleep in which the individual experiences excessive terror and extreme panic (screaming, verbalizations), symptoms of autonomic activity, confusion, and poor recall for event.[2]

Nymphomania: Abnormal and excessive need or desire in the woman for sexual intercourse.[3]

Obsessional personality—*see* Personality disorder, compulsive type

Occupational neurosis—*see* Neurotic disorder, occupational

Oneirophrenia—*see* Schizophrenia, acute episode

Oppositional disorder of childhood or adolescence: A disorder characterized by pervasive opposition to all in authority regardless of self-interest, a continuous argumentativeness, and an unwillingness to respond to reasonable persuasion, not accounted for by a conduct disorder, adjustment disorder, or a psychosis of childhood. The oppositional behavior in this disorder is evoked by any demand, rule, suggestion, request, or admonishment placed on the individual.[2]

Organic affective syndrome: A clinical picture in which the predominating symptoms closely resemble those seen in either the depressive or manic affective disorders, occurring in the presence of evidence or history of a specific organic factor which is etiologically related to the disturbance, such as head trauma, endocranial tumors, and exocranial tumors secreting neurotoxic diatheses (e.g., pancreatic carcinoma). Excessive use of steroids, Cushing's syndrome, and other endocrine disorders may lead to an organic affective syndrome.[2]

Organic personality syndrome: Chronic, mild states of memory disturbance and intellectual deterioration, of nonpsychotic nature, often accompanied by increased irritability, querulousness, lassitude, and complaints of physical weakness. These states are often associated with old age, and may precede more severe states due to brain damage classifiable under senile or presenile dementia, dementia associated with other chronic organic psychotic brain syndromes, or delirium, delusions, hallucinosis, and depression in transient organic psychotic conditions.[1]

Organic psychosyndrome, focal (partial): A nonpsychotic organic mental disorder resembling the postconcussion syndrome associated with localized diseases of the brain or surrounding tissues.[1]

Organic psychotic conditions: Syndromes in which there is impairment of orientation, memory, comprehension, calculation, learning capacity, and judgment. These are the essential features but there may also be shallowness or lability of affect, or a more persistent disturbance of mood, lowering of ethical standards and exaggeration or emergence of personality traits, and diminished capacity for independent decision.[1] See also Alcohol psychoses, Arteriosclerotic dementia, Drug psychoses, Presenile dementia, and Senile dementia.

    mixed paranoid and affective: Organic psychosis in which depressive and paranoid symptoms are the main features.[1]

    transient: States characterized by clouded consciousness, confusion, disorientation, illusions, and often vivid hallucinations. They are usually due to some intra- or extracerebral toxic, infectious, metabolic or other systemic disturbance and are generally reversible. Depressive and paranoid symptoms may also be present but are not the main feature. The diagnosis of the associated physical or neurological condition should also be recorded.[1]

        acute delirium: Short-lived states, lasting hours or days, of the above type.[1]

        subacute delirium: States of the above type in which the symptoms, usually less florid, last for several weeks or longer during which they may show marked fluctuations in intensity.[1]

Organic reaction—*see* Organic psychotic conditions, transient

Overanxious disorder: An ill-defined emotional disorder characteristic of childhood in which the main symptoms involve anxiety and fearfulness.[1]

Panic disorder—*see* panic attack under Anxiety state

Paranoia: A rare chronic psychosis in which logically constructed systematized delusions have developed gradually without concomitant hallucinations or the schizophrenic type of disordered thinking. The delusions are mostly of grandeur (the paranoiac prophet or inventor), persecution, or somatic abnormality.[1]

    alcoholic—*see* alcoholic jealousy under Alcoholic psychoses

    querulans: A paranoid state which, though in many ways akin to schizophrenic or affective states, differs from other paranoid states and psychogenic paranoid psychosis.[1]

    senile—*see* Paraphrenia

Paranoid personality—*see* Personality disorder, paranoid type

Paranoid reaction, acute: Paranoid states apparently provoked by some emotional stress. The stress is often misconstrued as an attack or threat. Such states are particularly prone to occur in prisoners or as acute reactions to a strange and threatening environment, e.g., in immigrants.[1]

Paranoid schizophrenia—*see* Schizophrenia, paranoid type

Paranoid state

    involutional—*see* Paraphrenia

    senile—*see* Paraphrenia

    simple: A psychosis, acute or chronic, not classifiable as schizophrenia or affective psychosis, in which delusions, especially of being influenced, persecuted, or treated in some special way, are the main symptoms. The delusions are of a fairly fixed, elaborate, and systematized kind.[1]

Paranoid traits—*see* Personality disorder, paranoid type

Paraphilia—*see* Sexual deviations

Paraphrenia: Paranoid psychosis in which there are conspicuous hallucinations, often in several modalities. Affective symptoms and disordered thinking, if present, do not dominate the clinical picture, and the personality is well preserved.[1]

Paraphrenic schizophrenia—*see* Schizophrenia, paranoid type

Passive-aggressive personality — *see* Personality disorder, passive- aggressive type

Passive personality—*see* Personality disorder, dependent type

Pathological

    alcohol intoxication—*see* Alcohol intoxication, idiosyncratic

    drug intoxication: Individual idiosyncratic reactions to comparatively small quantities of a drug, which take the form of acute, brief psychotic states of any type.[1]

    drunkenness—*see* Alcohol intoxication, idiosyncratic

    gambling: A disorder of impulse control characterized by a chronic and progressive preoccupation with gambling and urge to gamble, with subsequent gambling behavior that compromises, disrupts, or damages personal, family, and vocational pursuits.[2]

    personality—*see* Personality disorder

Pedophilia: Sexual deviations in which an adult engages in sexual activity with a child of the same or opposite sex.[1]

Peregrinating patient—*see* Malingering

Personality disorders: Deeply ingrained maladaptive patterns of behavior generally recognizable by the time of adolescence or earlier and continuing throughout most of adult life, although often becoming less obvious in middle or old age. The personality is abnormal either in the balance of its components, their quality and expression, or in its total aspect. Because of this deviation or psychopathy the patient suffers or others have to suffer, and there is an adverse effect upon the individual or on society. It includes what is sometimes called psychopathic personality, but if this is determined primarily by malfunctioning of the brain, it should be classified as one of the nonpsychotic organic brain syndromes. When the patient exhibits an anomaly of personality directly related to his neurosis or psychosis, e.g., schizoid personality and schizophrenia or anancastic personality and obsessive compulsive neurosis, the relevant neurosis or psychosis which is in evidence should be diagnosed in addition.[1]

affective type: A chronic personality disorder characterized by lifelong predominance of a pronounced mood. The illness does not have a clear onset, and there may be intermittent periods of disturbed mood separated by periods of normal mood.[1]

anancastic [anankastic] type—*see* Personality disorder, compulsive type

antisocial type: A personality disorder characterized by disregard for social obligations, lack of feeling for others, and impetuous violence or callous unconcern. There is a gross disparity between behavior and the prevailing social norms. Behavior is not readily modifiable by experience, including punishment. People with this personality are often affectively cold, and may be abnormally aggressive or irresponsible. Their tolerance to frustration is low; they blame others or offer plausible rationalizations for the behavior which brings them into conflict with society.[1]

asthenic type—*see* Personality disorder, dependent type

avoidant type: Individuals with this disorder exhibit excessive social inhibitions and shyness, a tendency to withdraw from opportunities for developing close relationships, and a fearful expectation that they will be belittled and humiliated. Desires for affection and acceptance are strong, but they are unwilling to enter relationships unless given unusually strong guarantees that they will be uncritically accepted. Therefore, they have few close relationships and suffer from feelings of loneliness and isolation.[2]

borderline type: Individuals with this disorder are characterized by instability in a variety of areas, including interpersonal relationships, behavior, mood, and self image. Interpersonal relationships are often intense and unstable with marked shifts of attitude over time. Frequently there is impulsive and unpredictable behavior which is potentially physically self-damaging. There may be problems tolerating being alone, and chronic feelings of emptiness or boredom.[2]

chronic depressive type: An affective personality disorder characterized by lifelong predominance of a chronic nonpsychotic disturbance involving either intermittent or sustained periods of depressed mood (marked by worry, pessimism, low output of energy, and a sense of futility).[2]

chronic hypomanic type: An affective personality disorder characterized by lifelong predominance of a chronic nonpsychotic disturbance involving either intermittent or sustained periods of abnormally elevated mood (unshakable optimism and an enhanced zest for life and activity).[2]

compulsive type: A personality disorder characterized by feelings of personal insecurity, doubt, and incompleteness leading to excessive conscientiousness, checking, stubbornness, and caution. There may be insistent and unwelcome thoughts or impulses which do not attain the severity of an obsessional neurosis. There is perfectionism and meticulous accuracy and a need to check repeatedly in an attempt to ensure this. Rigidity and excessive doubt may be conspicuous.[1]

cyclothymic type: A chronic nonpsychotic disturbance involving depressed and elevated mood, lasting at least two years, separated by periods of normal mood.[2]

dependent type: A personality disorder characterized by passive compliance with the wishes of elders and others and a weak inadequate response to the demands of daily life. Lack of vigor may show itself in the intellectual or emotional spheres; there is little capacity for enjoyment.[1]

eccentric type: A personality disorder characterized by oddities of behavior which do not conform to the clinical syndromes of personality disorders described elsewhere.[2]

explosive type: A personality disorder characterized by instability of mood with liability to intemperate outbursts of anger, hate, violence, or affection. Aggression may be expressed in words or in physical violence. The outbursts cannot readily be controlled by the affected persons, who are not otherwise prone to antisocial behavior.[1]

histrionic type: A personality disorder characterized by shallow, labile affectivity, dependence on others, craving for appreciation and attention, suggestibility, and theatricality. There is often sexual immaturity, e.g., frigidity and over-responsiveness to stimuli. Under stress hysterical symptoms [neurosis] may develop.[1]

hysterical type—*see* Personality disorder, histrionic type

inadequate type—*see* Personality disorder, dependent type

introverted type: A form of schizoid personality in which the essential features are a profound defect in the ability to form social relationships and to respond to the usual forms of social reinforcements. Such patients are characteristically "loners" who do not appear distressed by their social distance and are not interested in greater social involvements.[2]

masochistic type: A personality disorder in which the individual appears to arrange life situations so as to be defeated and humiliated.[2]

narcissistic type: A personality disorder in which interpersonal difficulties are caused by an inflated sense of self-worth, and indifference to the welfare of others. Achievement deficits and social irresponsibilities are justified and sustained by a boastful arrogance, expansive fantasies, facile rationalization, and frank prevarication.[2]

paranoid type: A personality disorder in which there is excessive sensitiveness to setbacks or to what are taken to be humiliations and rebuffs, a tendency to distort experience by misconstruing the neutral or friendly actions of others as hostile or contemptuous, and a combative and tenacious sense of personal rights. There may be a proneness to jealousy or excessive self-importance. Such persons may feel helplessly humiliated and put upon; others, likewise excessively sensitive, are aggressive and insistent. In all cases there is excessive self-reference.[1]

passive-aggressive type: A personality disorder characterized by aggressive behavior manifested in passive ways, such as obstructionism, pouting, procrastination, intentional inefficiency, or stubbornness. The *aggression* often arises from resentment at failing to find gratification in a relationship with an individual or institution upon which the individual is overdependent.[3]

passive type—*see* Personality disorder, dependent type

schizoid type: A personality disorder in which there is withdrawal from affectional, social, and other contacts with autistic preference for fantasy and introspective reserve. Behavior may be slightly eccentric or indicate avoidance of competitive situations. Apparent coolness and detachment may mask an incapacity to express feeling.

schizotypal type: A form of schizoid personality in which individuals with this disorder manifest various oddities of thinking, perception, communication, and behavior. The disturbance in thinking may be expressed as magical thinking, ideas of reference, or paranoid ideation. Perceptual disturbances may include recurrent illusions and derealization [depersonalization]. Frequently, but not invariably, the behavioral manifestations include social isolation and constricted or inappropriate affect which interferes with rapport in face-to-face interaction without any of the frank psychotic features which characterize schizophrenia.[2]

Phobia: Neurotic states with abnormally intense dread of certain objects or specific situations which would not normally have that effect. If the anxiety tends to spread from a specified situation or object to a wider range of circumstances, it becomes akin to or identical with anxiety state, and should be classified as such.[1]

acrophobia: Fear of heights[3]

agoraphobia: fear of leaving the familiar setting of the home, and is almost always preceded by a phase during which there are recurrent panic attacks. Because of the anticipatory fear of helplessness when having a panic attack, the patient is reluctant or refuses to be alone, travel or walk alone, or to be in situations where there is no ready access to help, such as in crowds, closed or open spaces, or crowded stores.[2]

ailurophobia: Fear of cats[3]

algophobia: Fear of pain[3]

claustrophobia: Fear of closed spaces[3]

isolated phobia—*see* simple phobia below

mysophobia: Fear of dirt or germs[3]

obsessional—*see* Neurotic disorder, obsessive-compulsive

panphobia: Fear of everything[3]

simple phobia: Fear of a discrete object or situation which is neither fear of leaving the familiar setting of the home [agoraphobia], or of being observed by others in certain situations [social phobia]. Examples of simple phobia are fear of animals, acrophobia, and claustrophobia.

social phobia: Fear of situations in which the subject is exposed to possible scrutiny by others, and the possibility exists that he may act in a fashion that will be considered shameful. The most common social phobias are fears of public speaking, blushing, eating in public, writing in front of others, or using public lavatories.[2]

xenophobia: Fear of strangers[3]

Pica: Perverted appetite of nonorganic origin in which there is persistent eating of non-nutritional substances. Typically, infants ingest paint, plaster, string, hair, or cloth. Older children may have access to animal droppings, sand, bugs, leaves, or pebbles. In the adult, eating of starch or clay-earth has been observed.[2]

Postconcussion syndrome: States occurring after generalized contusion of the brain, in which the symptom picture may resemble that of the frontal lobe syndrome or that of any of the neurotic disorders, but in which in addition, headache, giddiness, fatigue, insomnia, and a subjective feeling of impaired intellectual ability are usually prominent. Mood may fluctuate, and quite ordinary stress may produce exaggerated fear and apprehension. There may be marked intolerance of mental and physical exertion, undue sensitivity to noise, and hypochondriacal preoccupation. The symptoms are more common in persons who have previously suffered from neurotic or personality disorders, or when there is a possibility of compensation. This syndrome is particularly associated with the closed type of head injury when signs of localized brain damage are slight or absent, but it may also occur in other conditions.[1]

Postcontusion syndrome or encephalopathy—*see* Postconcussion syndrome

Postencephalitic syndrome: A nonpsychotic organic mental disorder resembling the postconcussion syndrome associated with central nervous system infections.[1]

Postleucotomy syndrome—*see* Frontal lobe syndrome

Posttraumatic brain syndrome, nonpsychotic—*see* Postconcussion syndrome

Posttraumatic organic psychosis—*see* Organic psychotic conditions, transient

Posttraumatic stress disorder: The development of characteristic symptoms (re-experiencing the traumatic event, numbing of responsiveness to or involvement with the external world, and a variety of other autonomic, dysphoric, or cognitive symptoms) after experiencing a psychologically traumatic event or events outside the normal range of human experience (e.g., rape or assault, military combat, natural catastrophes such as flood or earthquake, or other disaster, such as airplane crash, fires, bombings).[2]

> **acute:** Brief, episodic, or recurrent disorders lasting less than six months' duration after the onset of trauma.[2]

> **prolonged:** Chronic disorders of the above type lasting six months or more following the trauma.[2]

Premature ejaculation—*see* premature ejaculation under Psychosexual dysfunction.

Prepsychotic schizophrenia—*see* Schizophrenia, latent

Presbyophrenia—*see* Organic personality syndrome

Presenile dementia: Dementia occuring usually before the age of 65 in patients with the relatively rare forms of diffuse or lobar cerebral atrophy. The associated neurological condition (e.g., Alzheimer's disease, Pick's disease, Jakob-Creutzfeldt disease) should also be recorded as a diagnosis.[1]

Prodromal schizophrenia—*see* Schizophrenia, latent

Pseudoneurotic schizophrenia—*see* Schizophrenia, latent

Psychalgia: Pains of mental origin, e.g., headache or backache, for which a more precise medical or psychiatric diagnosis cannot be made.[1]

Psychasthenia: A functional neurosis marked by stages of pathological fear or anxiety, obsessions, fixed ideas, tics, feelings of inadequacy, self-accusation, and peculiar feelings of strangeness, unreality, and depersonalization.[4]

Psychic shock: A sudden disturbance of mental equilibrium produced by strong emotion in response to physical or mental stress.[4]

Psychic factors associated with physical diseases: Mental disturbances or psychic factors of any type thought to have played a major part in the etiology of physical conditions, usually involving tissue damage, classified elsewhere. The mental disturbance is usually mild and nonspecific, and the psychic factors (worry, fear, conflict, etc.) may be present without any overt psychiatric disorder. Examples of these conditions are asthma, dermatitis, eczema, duodenal ulcer, ulcerative colitis, and urticaria, specified as due to psychogenic factors.
Use an additional diagnosis to identify the physical condition. In the rare instance that an overt psychiatric disorder is thought to have caused the physical condition, the psychiatric diagnosis should be recorded in addition.[1]

Psychoneurosis—*see* Neurotic disorders

Psycho-organic syndrome—*see* Organic psychotic conditions, transient

Psychopathic constitutional state—*see* Personality disorders

Psychopathic personality—*see* Personality disorders

Psychophysiological disorders: A variety of physical symptoms or types of physiological malfunctions of mental origin, not involving tissue damage, and usually mediated through the autonomic nervous system. The disorders are classified according to the body system involved. If the physical symptom is secondary to a psychiatric disorder classifiable elsewhere, the physical symptom is not classified as a psychophysiological disorder. If tissue damage is involved, then the diagnosis is classified as a *Psychic factor associated with diseases classified elsewhere.*[1]

Psychosexual dysfunctions: A group of disorders in which there is recurrent and persistent dysfunction encountered during sexual activity. The dysfunction may be lifelong or acquired, generalized or situational, and total or partial.[2]

functional dyspareunia: Recurrent and persistent genital pain associated with coitus.[2]

functional vaginismus: A history of recurrent and persistent involuntary spasm of the musculature of the outer one-third of the vagina that interferes with sexual activity.[2]

inhibited female orgasm: Recurrent and persistent inhibition of the female orgasm as manifested by a delay or absence of orgasm following a normal sexual excitement phase during sexual activity.[2]

inhibited male orgasm: Recurrent and persistent inhibition of the male orgasm as manifested by a delay or absence of either the emission or ejaculation phases, or more usually, both following an adequate phase of sexual excitement.[2]

inhibited sexual desire: Persistent inhibition of desire for engaging in a particular form of sexual activity.[2]

inhibited sexual excitement: Recurrent and persistent inhibition of sexual excitement during sexual activity, manifested either by partial or complete failure to attain or maintain erection until completion of the sexual act [impotence], or partial or complete failure to attain or maintain the lubrication-swelling response of sexual excitement until completion of the sexual act [frigidity].[2]

premature ejaculation: Ejaculation occurs before the individual wishes it, because of recurrent and persistent absence of reasonable voluntary control of ejaculation and orgasm during sexual activity.[2]

Psychosexual gender identity disorders: Behavior occurring in preadolescents of immature psychosexuality, or in adults, in which there is an incongruence between the individual's anatomic sex and gender identity.[2]

gender identity disorder: In children or in adults a condition in which the individual would prefer to be of the other sex, and strongly prefers the clothes, toys, activities, and companionship of the other sex. Cross-dressing is intermittent, although it may be frequent. In children the commonest form is feminism in boys.[2]

trans-sexualism: A psychosexual identity disorder centered around fixed beliefs that the overt bodily sex is wrong. The resulting behavior is directed towards either changing the sexual organs by operation, or completely concealing the bodily sex by adopting both the dress and behavior of the opposite sex.[1]

Psychosomatic disorders—*see* Psychophysiological disorders

Psychosis: Mental disorders in which impairment of mental function has developed to a degree that interferes grossly with insight, ability to meet some ordinary demands of life or to maintain adequate contact with reality. It is not an exact or well defined term. Mental retardation is excluded.[1]

affective—*see* Affective psychoses

alcoholic—*see* Alcoholic psychoses

atypical childhood: A variety of atypical infantile psychoses which may show some, but not all, of the features of infantile autism. Symptoms may include stereotyped repetitive movements, hyperkinesis, self-injury, retarded speech development, echolalia, and impaired social relationships. Such disorders may occur in children of any level of intelligence but are particularly common in those with mental retardation.[1]

borderline, of childhood—*see* Psychosis, atypical childhood

child: A group of disorders in children, characterized by distortions in the timing, rate, and sequence of many psychological functions involving language development and social relations in which the severe qualitative abnormalities are not normal for any stage of development.[2] See also Autism, infantile, Psychosis, disintegrative, Psychosis, atypical childhood.

depressive—*see* Affective psychosis, depressed type

depressive type: A depressive psychosis which can be similar in its symptoms to manic-depressive psychosis, depressed type but is apparently provoked by saddening stress such as a bereavement, or a severe disappointment or frustration. There may be less diurnal variation of symptoms than in manic-depressive psychosis, depressed type, and the delusions are more often understandable in the context of the life experiences. There is usually a serious disturbance of behavior, e.g., major suicidal attempt.[1]

disintegrative: A disorder in which normal or near-normal development for the first few years is followed by a loss of social skills and of speech, together with a severe disorder of emotions, behavior, and relationships. Usually this loss of speech and of social competence takes place over a period of a few months and is accompanied by the emergence of overactivity and of stereotypies. In most cases there is intellectual impairment, but this is not a necessary part of the disorder. The condition may follow overt brain disease, such as measles encephalitis, but it may also occur in the absence of any known organic brain disease or damage. Any associated neurological disorder should also be recorded.[1]

epileptic: An organic psychotic condition associated with epilepsy.[1]

excitative type: An affective psychosis similar in its symptoms to manic-depressive psychosis, manic type, but apparently provoked by emotional stress.[1]

hypomanic—*see* Affective psychosis, manic type

hysterical—*see* Psychosis, reactive

    acute—*see* Psychosis, excitative type

induced—*see* Shared paranoid disorder

infantile—*see* Autism, infantile

infective—*see* Organic psychotic conditions, transient

Korsakoff's:

    alcoholic—*see* alcohol amnestic syndrome under Alcoholic psychoses

    nonalcoholic—*see* Amnestic syndrome

manic-depressive—*see* Affective psychoses

multi-infarct—*see* Arteriosclerotic dementia

paranoid

    chronic—*see* Paranoia

    protracted reactive—*see* Psychosis, paranoid, psychogenic

    psychogenic: Psychogenic or reactive paranoid psychosis of any type which is more protracted than the reactions described under paranoid reaction, acute.[1]
    acute—*see* Paranoid reaction, acute

postpartum—*see* Psychosis, puerperal

psychogenic—*see* Psychosis, reactive

    depressive—*see* Psychosis, depressive type

puerperal: Any psychosis occurring within a fixed period (approximately 90 days) after childbirth.[3] The diagnosis should be classified according to the predominant symptoms or characteristics, such as schizophrenia, affective psychosis, paranoid states, or other specified psychosis.

reactive: A psychotic condition which is largely or entirely attributable to a recent life experience. This diagnosis is not used for the wider range of psychoses in which environmental factors play some, but not the *major,* part in etiology.[1]

    brief: A florid psychosis of at least a few hours' duration but lasting no more than two weeks, with sudden onset immediately following a severe environmental stress and eventually terminating in complete recovery to the pre-psychotic state.[2]

    confusion: Mental disorders with clouded consciousness, disorientation (though less marked than in organic confusion), and diminished accessibility often accompanied by excessive activity and apparently provoked by emotional stress.[1]

    depressive—*see* Psychosis, depressive type

schizo-affective—*see* Schizophrenia, schizo-affective type

schizophrenic—*see* Schizophrenia

schizophreniform—*see* Schizophrenia

    affective type—*See* Schizophrenia, schizo-affective type

    confusional type—*see* Schizophrenia, acute episode

senile—*see* Senile dementia, delusional type

Pyromania: A disorder of impulse control characterized by a recurrent failure to resist impulses to set fires without regard for the consequences, or with deliberate destructive intent. Invariably there is intense fascination with the setting of fires, seeing fires burn, and a satisfaction with the resultant destruction.[2]

Relationship problems of childhood: Emotional disorders characteristic of childhood in which the main symptoms involve relationship problems.[1]

Repeated infarct dementia—*see* Arteriosclerotic dementia

Residual schizophrenia—*.see* Schizophrenia, residual type

Restzustand (schizophrenia)—*see* Schizophrenia, residual type

Rumination:

    obsessional: The constant preoccupation with certain thoughts, with inability to dismiss them from the mind.[4] *see* Neurotic disorder, obsessive-compulsive.

    psychogenic: In children the regurgitation of food, with failure to thrive or weight loss developing after a period of normal functioning. Food is brought up without nausea, retching, or disgust. The food is then ejected from the mouth, or chewed and reswallowed.[2]

Sander's disease—*see* Paranoia

Satyriasis: Pathologic or exaggerated sexual desire or excitement in the man.[3]

Schizoid personality disorder—*see* Personality disorder, schizoid type

Schizophrenia: A group of psychoses in which there is a fundamental disturbance of personality, a characteristic distortion of thinking, often a sense of being controlled by alien forces, delusions which may be bizarre, disturbed perception, abnormal affect out of keeping with the real situation, and autism. Nevertheless, clear consciousness and intellectual capacity are usually maintained. The disturbance of personality involves its most basic functions which give the normal person his feeling of individuality, uniqueness, and self-direction. The most intimate thoughts, feelings, and acts are often felt to be known to or shared by others and explanatory delusions may develop, to the effect that natural or supernatural forces are at work to influence the schizophrenic person's thoughts and actions in ways that are often bizarre. He may see himself as the pivot of all that happens. Hallucinations, especially of hearing, are common and may comment on the patient or address him. Perception is frequently disturbed in other ways; there may be perplexity, irrelevant features may become all-important and accompanied by passivity feeling, may lead the patient to believe that everyday objects and situations possess a special, usually sinister, meaning intended for him. In the characteristic schizophrenic disturbance of thinking, peripheral and irrelevant features of a total concept, which are inhibited in normal directed mental activity, are brought to the forefront and utilized in place of the elements relevant and appropriate to the situation. Thus, thinking becomes vague, elliptical and obscure, and its expression in speech sometimes incomprehensible. Breaks and interpolations in the flow of consecutive thought are frequent, and the patient may be convinced that his thoughts are being withdrawn by some outside agency. Mood may be shallow, capricious, or incongruous. Ambivalence and disturbance of volition may appear as inertia, negativism, or stupor. Catatonia may be present. The diagnosis "schizophrenia" should not be made unless there is, or has been evident during the same illness, characteristic disturbance of thought, perception, mood, conduct, or personality—preferably in at least two of these areas. The diagnosis should not be restricted to conditions running a protracted, deteriorating, or chronic course. In addition to making the diagnosis on the criteria just given, effort should be made to specify one of the following subtypes of schizophrenia, according to the predominant symptoms.[1]

acute (undifferentiated): Schizophrenia of florid nature which cannot be classified as simple, catatonic, hebephrenic, paranoid, or any other types.[1]

acute episode: Schizophrenic disorders, other than simple, hebephrenic, catatonic, and paranoid, in which there is a dream-like state with slight clouding of consciousness and perplexity. External things, people, and events may become charged with personal significance for the patient. There may be ideas of reference and emotional turmoil. In many such cases remission occurs within a few weeks or months, even without treatment.[1]

atypical—*see* Schizophrenia, acute (undifferentiated)

borderline—*see* Schizophrenia, latent

catatonic type: Includes as an essential feature prominent psychomotor disturbances often alternating between extremes such as hyperkinesis and stupor, or automatic obedience and negativism. Constrained attitudes may be maintained for long periods: if the patient's limbs are put in some unnatural position they may be held there for some time after the external force has been removed. Severe excitement may be a striking feature of the condition. Depressive or hypomanic concomitants may be present.[1]

cenesthopathic—*see* Schizophrenia, acute (undifferentiated)

childhood type—*see* Psychosis, child

chronic undifferentiated—*see* Schizophrenia, residual

cyclic—*see* Schizophrenia, schizo-affective type

disorganized type: A form of schizophrenia in which affective changes are prominent, delusions and hallucinations fleeting and fragmentary, behavior irresponsible and unpredictable, and mannerisms common. The mood is shallow and inappropriate, accompanied by giggling or self-satisfied, self—absorbed smiling, or by a lofty manner, grimaces, mannerisms, pranks, hypochondriacal complaints, and reiterated phrases. Thought is disorganized. There is a tendency to remain solitary, and behavior seems empty of purpose and feeling. This form of schizophrenia usually starts between the ages of 15 and 25 years.[1]

hebephrenic type:—*see* Schizophrenia, disorganized type

latent: It has not been possible to produce a generally acceptable description for this condition. It is not recommended for general use, but a description is provided for those who believe it to be useful: a condition of eccentric or inconsequent behavior and anomalies of affect which give the impression of schizophrenia though no definite and characteristic schizophrenic anomalies, present or past, have been manifest.[1]

paranoid type: The form of schizophrenia in which relatively stable delusions, which may be accompanied by hallucinations, dominate the clinical picture. The delusions are frequently of persecution, but may take other forms (for example, of jealousy, exalted birth, Messianic mission, or bodily change). Hallucinations and erratic behavior may occur; in some cases conduct is seriously disturbed from the outset, thought disorder may be gross, and affective flattening with fragmentary delusions and hallucinations may develop.[1]

prepsychotic—*see* Schizophrenia, latent

prodromal—*see* Schizophrenia, latent

pseudoneurotic—*see* Schizophrenia, latent

residual: A chronic form of schizophrenia in which the symptoms that persist from the acute phase have mostly lost their sharpness. Emotional response is blunted and thought disorder, even when gross, does not prevent the accomplishment of routine work.[1]

schizo-affective type: A psychosis in which pronounced manic or depressive features are intermingled with schizophrenic features and which tends towards remission without permanent defect, but which is prone to recur. The diagnosis should be made only when both the affective and schizophrenic symptoms are pronounced.[1]

simple type: A psychosis in which there is insidious development of oddities of conduct, inability to meet the demands of society, and decline in total performance. Delusions and hallucinations are not in evidence and the condition is less obviously psychotic than are the hebephrenic, catatonic, and paranoid types of schizophrenia. With increasing social impoverishment vagrancy may ensue and the patient becomes self-absorbed, idle, and aimless. Because the schizophrenic symptoms are not clear-cut, diagnosis of this form should be made sparingly, if at all.[1]

simplex—*see* Schizophrenia, simple type

Schizophrenic syndrome of childhood—*see* Psychosis, child

Schizophreniform

attack—*see* Schizophrenia, acute episode

disorder—*see* Schizophrenia, acute episode

psychosis—*see* Schizophrenia

affective type—*see* Schizophrenia, schizo-affective type

confusional type—*see* Schizophrenia, acute episode

Schizotypal personality—Dementia occurring usually after the age of 65 in which any cerebral pathology other than that of senile atrophic change can be reasonably excluded.[1]

delirium: Senile dementia with a superimposed reversible episode of acute confusional state.[1]

delusional type: A type of senile dementia characterized by development in advanced old age, progressive in nature, in which delusions, varying from simple poorly formed paranoid delusions to highly formed paranoid delusional states, and hallucinations are also present.[1,2]

depressed type: A type of senile dementia characterized by development in advanced old age, progressive in nature, in which depressive features, ranging from mild to severe forms of manic-depressive affective psychosis, are also present. Disturbance of the sleep-waking cycle and preoccupation with dead people are often particularly prominent.[1,2]

paranoid type—*see* Senile dementia, delusional type

simple type—*see* Senile dementia

Sensitiver Beziehungswahn: A paranoid state which, though in many ways akin to schizophrenic or affective states, differs from paranoia, simple paranoid state, shared paranoid disorder, or psychogenic psychosis.[1]

Sensitivity reaction of childhood or adolescence—*see* Shyness disorder of childhood

Separation anxiety disorder: A clinical disorder in children in which the predominant disturbance is exaggerated distress at separation from parents, home, or other familial surroundings. When separation is instituted, the child may experience anxiety to the point of panic. In adults a similar disorder is seen in agoraphobic reactions.[2]

Sexual deviations: Abnormal sexual inclinations or behavior which are part of a referral problem. The limits and features of normal sexual behavior have not been stated absolutely in different societies and cultures, but are broadly such as serve approved social and biological purposes. The sexual activity of affected persons is directed primarily either towards people not of the opposite sex, or towards sexual acts not associated with coitus normally, or towards coitus performed under abnormal circumstances. If the anomalous behavior becomes manifest only during psychosis or other mental illness the condition should be classified under the major illness. It is common for more than one anomaly to occur together in the same individual; in that case the predominant deviation is classified. It is preferable not to diagnose sexual deviation in individuals who perform deviant sexual acts when normal sexual outlets are not available to them.[1] *see also* exhibitionism, Fetishism, Homosexuality, Nymphomania, Pedophilia, Satyriasis, Sexual masochism, Sexual sadism, Transvestism, Voyeurism, and Zoophilia.

Gender identity disorder and trans-sexualism are considered to be psychosexual gender identity disorders and are not included here.

Sexual masochism: A sexual deviation in which sexual arousal and pleasure is produced in an individual by his own physical or psychological suffering, and in which there are insistent and persistent fantasies wherein sexual excitement is produced as a result of suffering.[2]

Sexual sadism: A sexual deviation in which physical or psychological suffering inflicted on another person is utilized as a method of stimulating erotic excitement and orgasm, and in which there are insistent and persistent fantasies wherein sexual excitement is produced as a result of suffering inflicted on the partner.[2]

Shared paranoid disorder: Mainly delusional psychosis, usually chronic and often without florid features, which appears to have developed as a result of a close, if not dependent, relationship with another person who already has an established similar psychosis. The delusions are at least partly shared. The rare cases in which several persons are affected should also be included here.[1]

Shifting sleep-work schedule: A sleep disorder in which the phase- shift disruption of the 24-hour sleep-wake cycle occurs due to rapid changes in the individual's work schedule.[2]

Short sleeper: Individuals who typically need only 4-6 hours of sleep within the 24-hour cycle.[2]

Shyness disorder of childhood: A persistent and excessive shrinking from familiarity or contact with all strangers of sufficient severity as to interfere with peer functioning, yet there are warm and satisfying relationships with family members. A critical feature of this disorder is that the avoidant behavior with strangers persists even after prolonged exposure or contact.[2]

Sibling jealousy or rivalry: An emotional disorder related to competition between siblings for the love of a parent or for other recognition or gain.[3]

Simple phobia—*see* simple phobia under Phobia

Situational disturbance, acute—*see* Stress reaction, acute

Social phobia—*see* social phobia under Phobia

Social withdrawal of childhood—*see* Introverted disorder of childhood

Socialized conduct disorder—*see* socialized conduct disorder under Conduct disorders

Somatization disorder—*see* somatization disorder under Neurotic disorders

Somatoform disorder, atypical—*see* hypochondriasis under Neurotic disorders

Spasmus nutans—*see* Stereotyped repetitive movements

Specific academic or work inhibition: An adjustment reaction in which a specific academic or work inhibition occurs in an individual whose intellectual capacity, skills, and previous academic or work performance have been at least adequate, and in which the inhibition occurs despite apparent effort and is not due to any other mental disorder.[2]

Stammering—*see* Stuttering

Starch-eating—*see* Pica

Status postcommotio cerebri—*see* Postconcussion syndrome

Stereotyped repetitive movements: Disorders in which voluntary repetitive stereotyped movements, which are not due to any psychiatric or neurological condition, constitute the main feature. Includes head-banging, spasmus nutans, rocking, twirling, finger-flicking mannerisms, and eye poking. Such movements are particularly common in cases of mental retardation with sensory impairment or with environmental monotony.[1]

Stereotypies—*see* Stereotyped repetitive movements

Stress reaction

> **acute**: Acute transient disorders of any severity and nature of emotions, consciousness, and psychomotor states (singly or in combination) which occur in individuals, without any apparent pre-existing mental disorder, in response to exceptional physical or mental stress, such as natural catastrophe or battle, and which usually subside within hours or days.[1]

> **chronic**—*see* Adjustment reaction

Stupor

> **catatonic**—*see* Schizophrenia, catatonic type

> **psychogenic**—*see* Psychosis, reactive

Stuttering: Disorders in the rhythm of speech, in which the individual knows precisely what he wishes to say, but at the time is unable to say it because of an involuntary, repetitive prolongation or cessation of a sound.[1]

Subjective insomnia complaint: a complaint of insomnia made by the individual, which has not been investigated or proven.[2]

Systematized delusions—*see* Paranoia

Tension headache: Headache of mental origin for which a more precise medical or psychiatric diagnosis cannot be made.[1]

Tics: Disorders of no known organic origin in which the outstanding feature consists of quick, involuntary, apparently purposeless, and frequently repeated movements which are not due to any neurological condition. Any part of the body may be involved but the face is most frequently affected. Only one form of tic may be present, or there may be a combination of tics which are carried out simultaneously, alternatively, or consecutively.[1]

> **chronic motor tic disorder:** A tic disorder starting in childhood and persisting into adult life. The tic is limited to no more than three motor areas, and rarely has a verbal component.[2]

Gilles de la Tourette's disorder [motor-verbal tic disorder]: a rare disorder occurring in individuals of any level of intelligence in which facial tics and tic-like throat noises become more marked and more generalized, and in which later whole words or short sentences (often with obscene content) are ejaculated spasmodically and involuntarily. There is some overlap with other varieties of tic.[1]

transient tic disorder of childhood: Facial or other tics beginning in childhood, but limited to one year in duration.[2]

Tobacco use disorder: Cases in which tobacco is used to the detriment of a person's health or social functioning or in which there is tobacco dependence. Dependence is included here rather than under drug dependence because tobacco differs from other drugs of dependence in its psychotoxic effects.[1]

Tranquilizer abuse: Cases where an individual has taken the drug to the detriment of his health or social functioning, in doses above or for periods beyond those normally regarded as therapeutic.[1]

Transient organic psychotic condition—*see* Organic psychotic conditions, transient

Trans-sexualism—*see* trans-sexualism under Psychosexual identity disorders

Transvestism: Sexual deviation in which there is recurrent and persistent dressing in clothes of the opposite sex, and initially in the early stage of the illness, for the purpose of sexual arousal.[2]

Twilight state

confusional—*see* Delirium, acute

psychogenic—*see* Psychosis, reactive confusion

Undersocialized conduct disorder—*see* undersocialized conduct disorder under Conduct disorders

Unsocialized aggressive disorder—*see* undersocialized conduct disorder, aggressive type under Conduct disorders

Vaginismus, functional—*see* functional vaginismus under Psychosexual dysfunctions

Vorbeireden: The symptom of the approximate answer or talking past the point, seen in the Ganser syndrome, a form of factitious illness.[2]

Voyeurism: A sexual deviation in which the individual repetitively seeks out situations in which he engages in looking at unsuspecting women who are either naked, in the act of disrobing, or engaging in sexual activity. The act of looking is accompanied by sexual excitement, frequently with orgasm. In its severe form, the act of peeping constitutes the preferred or exclusive sexual activity of the individual.[2]

Wernicke-Korsakoff syndrome—*see* alcohol amnestic syndrome under Alcoholic psychoses

Withdrawal reaction of childhood or adolescence—*see* Introverted disorder of childhood

Word-deafness: A developmental delay in the comprehension of speech sounds.[1]

Zoophilia: Sexual or anal intercourse with animals.[1]

1. Manual of the *International Classification of Diseases, Injuries, and Causes of Death.* 9th Revision. World Health Organization, Geneva, Switzerland, 1975.
2. American Psychiatric Association, Task Force on Nomenclature and Statistics, Robert L. Spitzer, Chairman.
3. *A Psychiatric Glossary*, Fourth Edition, American Psychiatric Association, Washington, D.C., 1975.
4. *Dorland's Illustrated Medical Dictionary.* Twenty-fifth Edition, W. B. Saunders Company, Philadelphia, 1974.
5. *Stedman's Medical Dictionary. Illustrated,* Twenty-third Edition, Williams and Wilkins, Baltimore, 1976.

CLASSIFICATION OF DRUGS BY AMERICAN HOSPITAL FORMULARY SERVICE LIST NUMBER AND THEIR ICD-9-CM EQUIVALENTS

The coding of adverse effects of drugs is keyed to the continually revised Hospital Formulary of the American Hospital Formulary Service (AHFS) published under the direction of the American Society of Hospital Pharmacists.

The following section gives the ICD-9-CM diagnosis code for each AHFS list.

	AHFS* LIST	ICD-9-CM Diagnosis Code
4:00	**ANTIHISTAMINE DRUGS**	963.0
8:00	**ANTI-INFECTIVE AGENTS**	
8:04	Amebacides	961.5
	hydroxyquinoline derivatives	961.3
	arsenical anti-infectives	961.1
8:08	Anthelmintics	961.6
	quinoline derivatives	961.3
8:12.04	Antifungal Antibiotics	960.1
	nonantibiotics	961.9
8:12.06	Cephalosporins	960.5
8:12.08	Chloramphenicol	960.2
8:12.12	The Erythromycins	960.3
8:12.16	The Penicillins	960.0
8:12.20	The Streptomycins	960.6
8:12.24	The Tetracyclines	960.4
8:12.28	Other Antibiotics	960.8
	antimycobacterial antibiotics	960.6
	macrolides	960.3
8:16	Antituberculars	961.8
	antibiotics	960.6
8:18	Antivirals	961.7
8:20	Plasmodicides (antimalarials)	961.4
8:24	Sulfonamides	961.0
8:26	The Sulfones	961.8
8:28	Treponemicides	961.2
8:32	Trichomonacides	961.5
	hydroxyquinoline derivatives	961.3
	nitrofuran derivatives	961.9
8:36	Urinary Germicides	961.9
	quinoline derivatives	961.3
8:40	Other Anti-Infectives	961.9
10:00	**ANTINEOPLASTIC AGENTS**	963.1
	antibiotics	960.7
	progestogens	962.2
12:00	**AUTONOMIC DRUGS**	
12:04	Parasympathomimetic (Cholinergic) Agents	971.0
12:08	Parasympatholytic (Cholinergic Blocking) Agents	971.1
12:12	Sympathomimetic (Adrenergic) Agents	971.2
12:16	Sympatholytic (Adrenergic Blocking) Agents	971.3
12:20	Skeletal Muscle Relaxants	975.2
	central nervous system muscle-tone depressants	968.0

	AHFS* LIST	ICD-9-CM Diagnosis Code
16:00	**BLOOD DERIVATIVES**	964.7
20:00	**BLOOD FORMATION AND COAGULATION**	
20:04	Antianemia Drugs	964.1
20:04.04	Iron Preparations	964.0
20:04.08	Liver and Stomach Preparations	964.1
20:12.04	Anticoagulants	964.2
20:12.08	Antiheparin agents	964.5
20:12.12	Coagulants	964.5
20:12.16	Hemostatics	964.5
	capillary-active drugs	972.8
	fibrinolysis-affecting agents	964.4
	natural products	964.7
24:00	**CARDIOVASCULAR DRUGS**	
24:04	Cardiac Drugs	972.9
	cardiotonic agents	972.1
	rhythm regulators	972.0
24:06	Antilipemic Agents	972.2
	thyroid derivatives	962.7
24:08	Hypotensive Agents	972.6
	adrenergic blocking agents	971.3
	ganglion-blocking agents	972.3
	vasodilators	972.5
24:12	Vasodilating Agents	972.5
	coronary	972.4
	nicotinic acid derivatives	972.2
24:16	Sclerosing Agents	972.7
28:00	**CENTRAL NERVOUS SYSTEM DRUGS**	
28:04	General Anesthetics	968.4
	gaseous anesthetics	968.2
	halothane	968.1
	intravenous anesthetics	968.3
28:08	Analgesics and Antipyretics	965.9
	antirheumatics	965.6
	aromatic analgesics	965.4
	non-narcotics NEC	965.7
	opium alkaloids	965.00
	heroin	965.01
	methadone	965.02
	specified type NEC	965.09
	pyrazole derivatives	965.5
	salicylates	965.1
	specified type NEC	965.8
28:10	Narcotic Antagonists	970.1
28:12	Anticonvulsants	966.3
	barbiturates	967.0
	benzodiazepine-based tranquilizers	969.4
	bromides	967.3
	hydantoin derivatives	966.1
	oxazolidine derivative	966.0
	succinimides	966.2
28:16.04	Antidepressants	969.0
28:16.08	Tranquilizers	969.5
	benzodiazepine-based	969.4
	butyrophenone-based	969.2
	major NEC	969.3
	phenothiazine-based	969.1

	AHFS* LIST	ICD-9-CM Diagnosis Code
28:16.12	Other Psychotherapeutic Agents	969.8
28:20	Respiratory and Cerebral Stimulants	970.9
	analeptics	970.0
	anorexigenic agents	977.0
	psychostimulants	969.7
	specified type NEC	970.8
28:24	Sedatives and Hypnotics	967.9
	barbiturates	967.0
	benzodiazepine-based tranquilizers	969.4
	chloral hydrate group	967.1
	glutethamide group	967.5
	intravenous anesthetics	968.3
	methaqualone	967.4
	paraldehyde	967.2
	phenothiazine-based tranquilizers	969.1
	specified type NEC	967.8
	thiobarbiturates	968.3
	tranquilizer NEC	969.5
36:00	**DIAGNOSTIC AGENTS**	977.8
40:00	**ELECTROLYTE, CALORIC, AND WATER BALANCE AGENTS NEC**	974.5
40:04	Acidifying Agents	963.2
40:08	Alkalinizing Agents	963.3
40:10	Ammonia Detoxicants	974.5
40:12	Replacement Solutions NEC	974.5
	plasma volume expanders	964.8
40:16	Sodium-Removing Resins	974.5
40:18	Potassium-Removing Resins	974.5
40:20	Caloric Agents	974.5
40:24	Salt and Sugar Substitutes	974.5
40:28	Diuretics NEC	974.4
	carbonic acid anhydrase inhibitors	974.2
	mercurials	974.0
	purine derivatives	974.1
	saluretics	974.3
40:36	Irrigating Solutions	974.5
40:40	Uricosuric Agents	974.7
44:00	**ENZYMES NEC**	963.4
	fibrinolysis-affecting agents	964.4
	gastric agents	973.4
48:00	**EXPECTORANTS AND COUGH PREPARATIONS**	
	antihistamine agents	963.0
	antitussives	975.4
	codeine derivatives	965.09
	expectorants	975.5
	narcotic agents NEC	965.09
52:00	**EYE, EAR, NOSE, AND THROAT PREPARATIONS**	
52:04	Anti-Infectives	
	ENT	976.6
	ophthalmic	976.5
52:04.04	Antibiotics	
	ENT	976.6
	ophthalmic	976.5

AHFS* LIST	ICD-9-CM Diagnosis Code
52:04.06 Antivirals	
ENT	976.6
ophthalmic	976.5
52:04.08 Sulfonamides	
ENT	976.6
ophthalmic	976.5
52:04.12 Miscellaneous Anti-Infectives	
ENT	976.6
ophthalmic	976.5
52:08 Anti-Inflammatory Agents	
ENT	976.6
ophthalmic	976.5
52:10 Carbonic Anhydrase Inhibitors	974.2
52:12 Contact Lens Solutions	976.5
52:16 Local Anesthetics	968.5
52:20 Miotics	971.0
52:24 Mydriatics	
adrenergics	971.2
anticholinergics	971.1
antimuscarinics	971.1
parasympatholytics	971.1
spasmolytics	971.1
sympathomimetics	971.2
52:28 Mouth Washes and Gargles	976.6
52:32 Vasoconstrictors	971.2
52:36 Unclassified Agents	
ENT	976.6
ophthalmic	976.5
56:00 **GASTROINTESTINAL DRUGS**	
56:04 Antacids and Absorbants	973.0
56:08 Anti-Diarrhea Agents	973.5
56:10 Antiflatulents	973.8
56:12 Cathartics NEC	973.3
emollients	973.2
irritants	973.1
56:16 Digestants	973.4
56:20 Emetics and Antiemetics	
antiemetics	963.0
emetics	973.6
56:24 Lipotropic Agents	977.1
60:00 **GOLD COMPOUNDS**	965.6
64:00 **HEAVY METAL ANTAGONISTS**	963.8
68:00 **HORMONES AND SYNTHETIC SUBSTITUTES**	
68:04 Adrenals	962.0
68:08 Androgens	962.1
68:12 Contraceptives	962.2
68:16 Estrogens	962.2
68:18 Gonadotropins	962.4
68:20 Insulins and Antidiabetic Agents	962.3
68:20.08 Insulins	962.3
68:24 Parathyroid	962.6

* American Hospital Formulary Service

AHFS* LIST	ICD-9-CM Diagnosis Code
68:28 Pituitary	
anterior	962.4
posterior	962.5
68:32 Progestogens	962.2
68:34 Other Corpus Luteum Hormones	962.2
68:36 Thyroid and Antithyroid	
antithyroid	962.8
thyroid	962.7
72:00 **LOCAL ANESTHETICS NEC**	968.9
topical (surface) agents	968.5
infiltrating agents (intradermal) (subcutaneous) (submucosal)	968.5
nerve blocking agents (peripheral) (plexus)(regional)	968.6
spinal	968.7
76:00 **OXYTOCICS**	975.0
78:00 **RADIOACTIVE AGENTS**	990
80:00 **SERUMS, TOXOIDS, AND VACCINES**	
80:04 Serums	979.9
immune globulin (gamma) (human)	964.6
80:08 Toxoids NEC	978.8
diphtheria	978.5
and tetanus	978.9
with pertussis component	978.6
tetanus	978.4
and diphtheria	978.9
with pertussis component	978.6
80:12 Vaccines NEC	979.9
bacterial NEC	978.8
with	
other bacterial component	978.9
pertussis component	978.6
viral and rickettsial component	979.7
rickettsial NEC	979.6
with	
bacterial component	979.7
pertussis component	978.6
viral component	979.7
viral NEC	979.6
with	
bacterial component	979.7
pertussis component	978.6
rickettsial component	979.7
84:00 **SKIN AND MUCOUS MEMBRANE PREPARATIONS**	
84:04 Anti-Infectives	976.0
84:04.04 Antibiotics	976.0
84:04.08 Fungicides	976.0
84:04.12 Scabicides and Pediculicides	976.0
84:04.16 Miscellaneous Local Anti-Infectives	976.0
84:06 Anti-Inflammatory Agents	976.0
84:08 Antipruritics and Local Anesthetics	
antipruritics	976.1
local anesthetics	968.5
84:12 Astringents	976.2
84:16 Cell Stimulants and Proliferants	976.8
84:20 Detergents	976.2

	AHFS* LIST	ICD-9-CM Diagnosis Code
84:24	Emollients, Demulcents, and Protectants	976.3
84:28	Keratolytic Agents	976.4
84:32	Keratoplastic Agents	976.4
84:36	Miscellaneous Agents	976.8
86:00	**SPASMOLYTIC AGENTS**	975.1
	antiasthmatics	975.7
	papaverine	972.5
	theophyllin	974.1
88:00	**VITAMINS**	
88:04	Vitamin A	963.5
88:08	Vitamin B Complex	963.5
	hematopoietic vitamin	964.1
	nicotinic acid derivatives	972.2
88:12	Vitamin C	963.5
88:16	Vitamin D	963.5
88:20	Vitamin E	963.5
88:24	Vitamin K Activity	964.3
88:28	Multivitamin Preparations	963.5
92:00	**UNCLASSIFIED THERAPEUTIC AGENTS**	977.8

* American Hospital Formulary Service

CLASSIFICATION OF INDUSTRIAL ACCIDENTS ACCORDING TO AGENCY

Annex B to the Resolution concerning Statistics of Employment Injuries adopted by the Tenth International Conference of Labor Statisticians on 12 October 1962

1 MACHINES

11 Prime-Movers, except Electrical Motors
111 Steam engines
112 Internal combustion engines
119 Others

12 Transmission Machinery
121 Transmission shafts
122 Transmission belts, cables, pulleys, pinions, chains, gears
129 Others

13 Metalworking Machines
131 Power presses
132 Lathes
133 Milling machines
134 Abrasive wheels
135 Mechanical shears
136 Forging machines
137 Rolling-mills
139 Others

14 Wood and Assimilated Machines
141 Circular saws
142 Other saws
143 Molding machines
144 Overhand planes
149 Others

15 Agricultural Machines
151 Reapers (including combine reapers)
152 Threshers
159 Others

16 Mining Machinery
161 Under-cutters
169 Others

19 Other Machines Not Elsewhere Classified
191 Earth-moving machines, excavating and scraping machines, except means of transport
192 Spinning, weaving and other textile machines
193 Machines for the manufacture of foodstuffs and beverages
194 Machines for the manufacture of paper
195 Printing machines
199 Others

2 MEANS OF TRANSPORT AND LIFTING EQUIPMENT

21 Lifting Machines and Appliances
211 Cranes
212 Lifts and elevators
213 Winches
214 Pulley blocks
219 Others

22 Means of Rail Transport
221 Inter-urban railways
222 Rail transport in mines, tunnels, quarries, industrial establishments, docks, etc.
229 Others

23 Other Wheeled Means of Transport, Excluding Rail Transport
231 Tractors
232 Lorries
233 Trucks
234 Motor vehicles, not elsewhere classified
235 Animal-drawn vehicles

2 MEANS OF TRANSPORT AND LIFTING EQUIPMENT *continued*

236 Hand-drawn vehicles
239 Others

24 Means of Air Transport

25 Means of Water Transport
251 Motorized means of water transport
252 Non-motorized means of water transport

26 Other Means of Transport
261 Cable-cars
262 Mechanical conveyors, except cable-cars
269 Others

3 OTHER EQUIPMENT

31 Pressure Vessels
311 Boilers
312 Pressurized containers
313 Pressurized piping and accessories
314 Gas cylinders
315 Caissons, diving equipment
319 Others

32 Furnaces, Ovens, Kilns
321 Blast furnaces
322 Refining furnaces
323 Other furnaces
324 Kilns
325 Ovens

33 Refrigerating Plants

34 Electrical Installations, Including Electric Motors, but Excluding Electric Hand Tools
341 Rotating machines
342 Conductors
343 Transformers
344 Control apparatus
349 Others

35 Electric Hand Tools

36 Tools, Implements, and Appliances, Except Electric Hand Tools
361 Power-driven hand tools, except electric hand tools
362 Hand tools, not power-driven
369 Others

37 Ladders, Mobile Ramps

38 Scaffolding

39 Other Equipment, Not Elsewhere Classified

4 MATERIALS, SUBSTANCES AND RADIATIONS

41 Explosives

42 Dusts, Gases, Liquids and Chemicals, Excluding Explosives
421 Dusts
422 Gases, vapors, fumes
423 Liquids, not elsewhere classified
424 Chemicals, not elsewhere classified

43 Flying Fragments

44 Radiations
441 Ionizing radiations
449 Others

49 Other Materials and Substances Not Elsewhere Classified

5 WORKING ENVIRONMENT

51 Outdoor
511 Weather

5 WORKING ENVIRONMENT *continued*

512 Traffic and working surfaces
513 Water
519 Others

52 Indoor

521 Floors
522 Confined quarters
523 Stairs
524 Other traffic and working surfaces
525 Floor openings and wall openings
526 Environmental factors (lighting, ventilation, temperature, noise, etc.)
529 Others

53 Underground

531 Roofs and faces of mine roads and tunnels, etc.
532 Floors of mine roads and tunnels, etc.
533 Working-faces of mines, tunnels, etc.
534 Mine shafts
535 Fire
536 Water
539 Others

6 OTHER AGENCIES, NOT ELSEWHERE CLASSIFIED

61 Animals

611 Live animals
612 Animals products

69 Other Agencies, Not Elsewhere Classified

7 AGENCIES NOT CLASSIFIED FOR LACK OF SUFFICIENT DATA

LIST OF THREE-DIGIT CATEGORIES

1. INFECTIOUS AND PARASITIC DISEASES

Intestinal infectious diseases (001-009)
- 001 Cholera
- 002 Typhoid and paratyphoid fevers
- 003 Other salmonella infections
- 004 Shigellosis
- 005 Other food poisoning (bacterial)
- 006 Amebiasis
- 007 Other protozoal intestinal diseases
- 008 Intestinal infections due to other organisms
- 009 Ill-defined intestinal infections

Tuberculosis (010-018)
- 010 Primary tuberculous infection
- 011 Pulmonary tuberculosis
- 012 Other respiratory tuberculosis
- 013 Tuberculosis of meninges and central nervous system
- 014 Tuberculosis of intestines, peritoneum, and mesenteric glands
- 015 Tuberculosis of bones and joints
- 016 Tuberculosis of genitourinary system
- 017 Tuberculosis of other organs
- 018 Miliary tuberculosis

Zoonotic bacterial diseases (020-027)
- 020 Plague
- 021 Tularemia
- 022 Anthrax
- 023 Brucellosis
- 024 Glanders
- 025 Melioidosis
- 026 Rat-bite fever
- 027 Other zoonotic bacterial diseases

Other bacterial diseases (030-041)
- 030 Leprosy
- 031 Diseases due to other mycobacteria
- 032 Diphtheria
- 033 Whooping cough
- 034 Streptococcal sore throat and scarlet fever
- 035 Erysipelas
- 036 Meningococcal infection
- 037 Tetanus
- 038 Septicemia
- 039 Actinomycotic infections
- 040 Other bacterial diseases
- 041 Bacterial infection in conditions classified elsewhere and of unspecified site

Human immunodeficiency virus (042)
- 042 Human immunodeficiency virus [HIV] disease

Poliomyelitis and other non-arthropod-borne viral diseases of central nervous system (045-049)
- 045 Acute poliomyelitis
- 046 Slow virus infection of central nervous system
- 047 Meningitis due to enterovirus
- 048 Other enterovirus diseases of central nervous system
- 049 Other non-arthropod-borne viral diseases of central nervous system

Viral diseases accompanied by exanthem (050-057)
- 050 Smallpox
- 051 Cowpox and paravaccinia
- 052 Chickenpox
- 053 Herpes zoster
- 054 Herpes simplex
- 055 Measles
- 056 Rubella
- 057 Other viral exanthemata

1. INFECTIOUS AND PARASITIC DISEASES *continued*

Arthropod-borne viral diseases (060-066)
060 Yellow fever
061 Dengue
062 Mosquito-borne viral encephalitis
063 Tick-borne viral encephalitis
064 Viral encephalitis transmitted by other and unspecified arthropods
065 Arthropod-borne hemorrhagic fever
066 Other arthropod-borne viral diseases

Other diseases due to viruses and Chlamydiae (070-079)
070 Viral hepatitis
071 Rabies
072 Mumps
073 Ornithosis
074 Specific diseases due to Coxsackie virus
075 Infectious mononucleosis
076 Trachoma
077 Other diseases of conjunctiva due to viruses and Chlamydiae
078 Other diseases due to viruses and Chlamydiae
079 Viral and Chlamydial infection in conditions classified elsewhere and of unspecified site

Rickettsioses and other arthropod-borne diseases (080-088)
080 Louse-borne [epidemic] typhus
081 Other typhus
082 Tick-borne rickettsioses
083 Other rickettsioses
084 Malaria
085 Leishmaniasis
086 Trypanosomiasis
087 Relapsing fever
088 Other arthropod-borne diseases

Syphilis and other venereal diseases (090-099)
090 Congenital syphilis
091 Early syphilis, symptomatic
092 Early syphilis, latent
093 Cardiovascular syphilis
094 Neurosyphilis
095 Other forms of late syphilis, with symptoms
096 Late syphilis, latent
097 Other and unspecified syphilis
098 Gonococcal infections
099 Other venereal diseases

Other spirochetal diseases (100-104)
100 Leptospirosis
101 Vincent's angina
102 Yaws
103 Pinta
104 Other spirochetal infection

Mycoses (110-118)
110 Dermatophytosis
111 Dermatomycosis, other and unspecified
112 Candidiasis
114 Coccidioidomycosis
115 Histoplasmosis
116 Blastomycotic infection
117 Other mycoses
118 Opportunistic mycoses

Helminthiases (120-129)
120 Schistosomiasis [bilharziasis]
121 Other trematode infections
122 Echinococcosis
123 Other cestode infection
124 Trichinosis

1. INFECTIOUS AND PARASITIC DISEASES *continued*

    125   Filarial infection and dracontiasis
    126   Ancylostomiasis and necatoriasis
    127   Other intestinal helminthiases
    128   Other and unspecified helminthiases
    129   Intestinal parasitism, unspecified

Other infectious and parasitic diseases (130-136)

    130   Toxoplasmosis
    131   Trichomoniasis
    132   Pediculosis and phthirus infestation
    133   Acariasis
    134   Other infestation
    135   Sarcoidosis
    136   Other and unspecified infectious and parasitic diseases

Late effects of infectious and parasitic diseases (137-139)

    137   Late effects of tuberculosis
    138   Late effects of acute poliomyelitis
    139   Late effects of other infectious and parasitic diseases

2. NEOPLASMS

Malignant neoplasm of lip, oral cavity, and pharynx (140-149)

    140   Malignant neoplasm of lip
    141   Malignant neoplasm of tongue
    142   Malignant neoplasm of major salivary glands
    143   Malignant neoplasm of gum
    144   Malignant neoplasm of floor of mouth
    145   Malignant neoplasm of other and unspecified parts of mouth
    146   Malignant neoplasm of oropharynx
    147   Malignant neoplasm of nasopharynx
    148   Malignant neoplasm of hypopharynx
    149   Malignant neoplasm of other and ill-defined sites within the lip, oral cavity, and pharynx

Malignant neoplasm of digestive organs and peritoneum (150-159)

    150   Malignant neoplasm of esophagus
    151   Malignant neoplasm of stomach
    152   Malignant neoplasm of small intestine, including duodenum
    153   Malignant neoplasm of colon
    154   Malignant neoplasm of rectum, rectosigmoid junction, and anus
    155   Malignant neoplasm of liver and intrahepatic bile ducts
    156   Malignant neoplasm of gallbladder and extrahepatic bile ducts
    157   Malignant neoplasm of pancreas
    158   Malignant neoplasm of retroperitoneum and peritoneum
    159   Malignant neoplasm of other and ill-defined sites within the digestive organs and peritoneum

Malignant neoplasm of respiratory and intrathoracic organs (160-165)

    160   Malignant neoplasm of nasal cavities, middle ear, and accessory sinuses
    161   Malignant neoplasm of larynx
    162   Malignant neoplasm of trachea, bronchus, and lung
    163   Malignant neoplasm of pleura
    164   Malignant neoplasm of thymus, heart, and mediastinum
    165   Malignant neoplasm of other and ill-defined sites within the respiratory system and intrathoracic organs

Malignant neoplasm of bone, connective tissue, skin, and breast (170-176)

    170   Malignant neoplasm of bone and articular cartilage
    171   Malignant neoplasm of connective and other soft tissue
    172   Malignant melanoma of skin
    173   Other malignant neoplasm of skin
    174   Malignant neoplasm of female breast
    175   Malignant neoplasm of male breast
    176   Kaposi's sarcoma

Malignant neoplasm of genitourinary organs (179-189)

    179   Malignant neoplasm of uterus, part unspecified
    180   Malignant neoplasm of cervix uteri

2. NEOPLASMS *continued*

181   Malignant neoplasm of placenta
182   Malignant neoplasm of body of uterus
183   Malignant neoplasm of ovary and other uterine adnexa
184   Malignant neoplasm of other and unspecified female genital organs
185   Malignant neoplasm of prostate
186   Malignant neoplasm of testis
187   Malignant neoplasm of penis and other male genital organs
188   Malignant neoplasm of bladder
189   Malignant neoplasm of kidney and other and unspecified urinary organs

Malignant neoplasm of other and unspecified sites (190-199)

190   Malignant neoplasm of eye
191   Malignant neoplasm of brain
192   Malignant neoplasm of other and unspecified parts of nervous system
193   Malignant neoplasm of thyroid gland
194   Malignant neoplasm of other endocrine glands and related structures
195   Malignant neoplasm of other and ill-defined sites
196   Secondary and unspecified malignant neoplasm of lymph nodes
197   Secondary malignant neoplasm of respiratory and digestive systems
198   Secondary malignant neoplasm of other specified sites
199   Malignant neoplasm without specification of site

Malignant neoplasm of lymphatic and hematopoietic tissue (200-208)

200   Lymphosarcoma and reticulosarcoma
201   Hodgkin's disease
202   Other malignant neoplasm of lymphoid and histiocytic tissue
203   Multiple myeloma and immunoproliferative neoplasms
204   Lymphoid leukemia
205   Myeloid leukemia
206   Monocytic leukemia
207   Other specified leukemia
208   Leukemia of unspecified cell type

Benign neoplasms (210-229)

210   Benign neoplasm of lip, oral cavity, and pharynx
211   Benign neoplasm of other parts of digestive system
212   Benign neoplasm of respiratory and intrathoracic organs
213   Benign neoplasm of bone and articular cartilage
214   Lipoma
215   Other benign neoplasm of connective and other soft tissue
216   Benign neoplasm of skin
217   Benign neoplasm of breast
218   Uterine leiomyoma
219   Other benign neoplasm of uterus
220   Benign neoplasm of ovary
221   Benign neoplasm of other female genital organs
222   Benign neoplasm of male genital organs
223   Benign neoplasm of kidney and other urinary organs
224   Benign neoplasm of eye
225   Benign neoplasm of brain and other parts of nervous system
226   Benign neoplasm of thyroid gland
227   Benign neoplasm of other endocrine glands and related structures
228   Hemangioma and lymphangioma, any site
229   Benign neoplasm of other and unspecified sites

Carcinoma in situ (230-234)

230   Carcinoma in situ of digestive organs
231   Carcinoma in situ of respiratory system
232   Carcinoma in situ of skin
233   Carcinoma in situ of breast and genitourinary system
234   Carcinoma in situ of other and unspecified sites

Neoplasms of uncertain behavior (235-238)

235   Neoplasm of uncertain behavior of digestive and respiratory systems
236   Neoplasm of uncertain behavior of genitourinary organs
237   Neoplasm of uncertain behavior of endocrine glands and nervous system
238   Neoplasm of uncertain behavior of other and unspecified sites and tissues

2. NEOPLASMS *continued*

Neoplasm of unspecified nature (239)
- 239   Neoplasm of unspecified nature

3. ENDOCRINE, NUTRITIONAL AND METABOLIC DISEASES, AND IMMUNITY DISORDERS

Disorders of thyroid gland (240-246)
- 240   Simple and unspecified goiter
- 241   Nontoxic nodular goiter
- 242   Thyrotoxicosis with or without goiter
- 243   Congenital hypothyroidism
- 244   Acquired hypothyroidism
- 245   Thyroiditis
- 246   Other disorders of thyroid

Diseases of other endocrine glands (250-259)
- 250   Diabetes mellitus
- 251   Other disorders of pancreatic internal secretion
- 252   Disorders of parathyroid gland
- 253   Disorders of the pituitary gland and its hypothalamic control
- 254   Diseases of thymus gland
- 255   Disorders of adrenal glands
- 256   Ovarian dysfunction
- 257   Testicular dysfunction
- 258   Polyglandular dysfunction and related disorders
- 259   Other endocrine disorders

Nutritional deficiencies (260-269)
- 260   Kwashiorkor
- 261   Nutritional marasmus
- 262   Other severe protein-calorie malnutrition
- 263   Other and unspecified protein-calorie malnutrition
- 264   Vitamin A deficiency
- 265   Thiamine and niacin deficiency states
- 266   Deficiency of B-complex components
- 267   Ascorbic acid deficiency
- 268   Vitamin D deficiency
- 269   Other nutritional deficiencies

Other metabolic disorders and immunity disorders (270-279)
- 270   Disorders of amino-acid transport and metabolism
- 271   Disorders of carbohydrate transport and metabolism
- 272   Disorders of lipoid metabolism
- 273   Disorders of plasma protein metabolism
- 274   Gout
- 275   Disorders of mineral metabolism
- 276   Disorders of fluid, electrolyte, and acid-base balance
- 277   Other and unspecified disorders of metabolism
- 278   Obesity and other hyperalimentation
- 279   Disorders involving the immune mechanism

4. DISEASES OF THE BLOOD AND BLOOD-FORMING ORGANS

Diseases of blood and blood-forming organs (280-289)
- 280   Iron deficiency anemias
- 281   Other deficiency anemias
- 282   Hereditary hemolytic anemias
- 283   Acquired hemolytic anemias
- 284   Aplastic anemia
- 285   Other and unspecified anemias
- 286   Coagulation defects
- 287   Purpura and other hemorrhagic conditions
- 288   Diseases of white blood cells
- 289   Other diseases of blood and blood-forming organs

5. MENTAL DISORDERS

Organic psychotic conditions (290-294)
- 290 Senile and presenile organic psychotic conditions
- 291 Alcoholic psychoses
- 292 Drug psychoses
- 293 Transient organic psychotic conditions
- 294 Other organic psychotic conditions (chronic)

Other psychoses (295-299)
- 295 Schizophrenic psychoses
- 296 Affective psychoses
- 297 Paranoid states (Delusional disorders)
- 298 Other nonorganic psychoses
- 299 Psychoses with origin specific to childhood

Neurotic disorders, personality disorders, and other nonpsychotic mental disorders (300-316)
- 300 Neurotic disorders
- 301 Personality disorders
- 302 Sexual deviations and disorders
- 303 Alcohol dependence syndrome
- 304 Drug dependence
- 305 Nondependent abuse of drugs
- 306 Physiological malfunction arising from mental factors
- 307 Special symptoms or syndromes, not elsewhere classified
- 308 Acute reaction to stress
- 309 Adjustment reaction
- 310 Specific nonpsychotic mental disorders due to organic brain damage
- 311 Depressive disorder, not elsewhere classified
- 312 Disturbance of conduct, not elsewhere classified
- 313 Disturbance of emotions specific to childhood and adolescence
- 314 Hyperkinetic syndrome of childhood
- 315 Specific delays in development
- 316 Psychic factors associated with diseases classified elsewhere

Mental retardation (317-319)
- 317 Mild mental retardation
- 318 Other specified mental retardation
- 319 Unspecified mental retardation

6. DISEASES OF THE NERVOUS SYSTEM AND SENSE ORGANS

Inflammatory diseases of the central nervous system (320-326)
- 320 Bacterial meningitis
- 321 Meningitis due to other organisms
- 322 Meningitis of unspecified cause
- 323 Encephalitis, myelitis, and encephalomyelitis
- 324 Intracranial and intraspinal abscess
- 325 Phlebitis and thrombophlebitis of intracranial venous sinuses
- 326 Late effects of intracranial abscess or pyogenic infection

Hereditary and degenerative diseases of the central nervous system (330-337)
- 330 Cerebral degenerations usually manifest in childhood
- 331 Other cerebral degenerations
- 332 Parkinson's disease
- 333 Other extrapyramidal disease and abnormal movement disorders
- 334 Spinocerebellar disease
- 335 Anterior horn cell disease
- 336 Other diseases of spinal cord
- 337 Disorders of the autonomic nervous system

Other disorders of the central nervous system (340-349)
- 340 Multiple sclerosis
- 341 Other demyelinating diseases of central nervous system
- 342 Hemiplegia and hemiparesis
- 343 Infantile cerebral palsy
- 344 Other paralytic syndromes
- 345 Epilepsy
- 346 Migraine
- 347 Cataplexy and narcolepsy

6. DISEASES OF THE NERVOUS SYSTEM AND SENSE ORGANS *continued*

348   Other conditions of brain
349   Other and unspecified disorders of the nervous system

Disorders of the peripheral nervous system (350-359)

350   Trigeminal nerve disorders
351   Facial nerve disorders
352   Disorders of other cranial nerves
353   Nerve root and plexus disorders
354   Mononeuritis of upper limb and mononeuritis multiplex
355   Mononeuritis of lower limb and unspecified site
356   Hereditary and idiopathic peripheral neuropathy
357   Inflammatory and toxic neuropathy
358   Myoneural disorders
359   Muscular dystrophies and other myopathies

Disorders of the eye and adnexa (360-379)

360   Disorders of the globe
361   Retinal detachments and defects
362   Other retinal disorders
363   Chorioretinal inflammations and scars and other disorders of choroid
364   Disorders of iris and ciliary body
365   Glaucoma
366   Cataract
367   Disorders of refraction and accommodation
368   Visual disturbances
369   Blindness and low vision
370   Keratitis
371   Corneal opacity and other disorders of cornea
372   Disorders of conjunctiva
373   Inflammation of eyelids
374   Other disorders of eyelids
375   Disorders of lacrimal system
376   Disorders of the orbit
377   Disorders of optic nerve and visual pathways
378   Strabismus and other disorders of binocular eye movements
379   Other disorders of eye

Diseases of the ear and mastoid process (380-389)

380   Disorders of external ear
381   Nonsuppurative otitis media and Eustachian tube disorders
382   Suppurative and unspecified otitis media
383   Mastoiditis and related conditions
384   Other disorders of tympanic membrane
385   Other disorders of middle ear and mastoid
386   Vertiginous syndromes and other disorders of vestibular system
387   Otosclerosis
388   Other disorders of ear
389   Hearing loss

7. DISEASES OF THE CIRCULATORY SYSTEM

Acute rheumatic fever (390-392)

390   Rheumatic fever without mention of heart involvement
391   Rheumatic fever with heart involvement
392   Rheumatic chorea

Chronic rheumatic heart disease (393-398)

393   Chronic rheumatic pericarditis
394   Diseases of mitral valve
395   Diseases of aortic valve
396   Diseases of mitral and aortic valves
397   Diseases of other endocardial structures
398   Other rheumatic heart disease

Hypertensive disease (401-405)

401   Essential hypertension
402   Hypertensive heart disease
403   Hypertensive renal disease

7. DISEASES OF THE CIRCULATORY SYSTEM *continued*

    404   Hypertensive heart and renal disease
    405   Secondary hypertension

Ischemic heart disease (410-414)
    410   Acute myocardial infarction
    411   Other acute and subacute form of ischemic heart disease
    412   Old myocardial infarction
    413   Angina pectoris
    414   Other forms of chronic ischemic heart disease

Diseases of pulmonary circulation (415-417)
    415   Acute pulmonary heart disease
    416   Chronic pulmonary heart disease
    417   Other diseases of pulmonary circulation

Other forms of heart disease (420-429)
    420   Acute pericarditis
    421   Acute and subacute endocarditis
    422   Acute myocarditis
    423   Other diseases of pericardium
    424   Other diseases of endocardium
    425   Cardiomyopathy
    426   Conduction disorders
    427   Cardiac dysrhythmias
    428   Heart failure
    429   Ill-defined descriptions and complications of heart disease

Cerebrovascular disease (430-438)
    430   Subarachnoid hemorrhage
    431   Intracerebral hemorrhage
    432   Other and unspecified intracranial hemorrhage
    433   Occlusion and stenosis of precerebral arteries
    434   Occlusion of cerebral arteries
    435   Transient cerebral ischemia
    436   Acute but ill-defined cerebrovascular disease
    437   Other and ill-defined cerebrovascular disease
    438   Late effects of cerebrovascular disease

Diseases of arteries, arterioles, and capillaries (440-448)
    440   Atherosclerosis
    441   Aortic aneurysm and dissection
    442   Other aneurysm
    443   Other peripheral vascular disease
    444   Arterial embolism and thrombosis
    445   Atheroembolism
    446   Polyarteritis nodosa and allied conditions
    447   Other disorders of arteries and arterioles
    448   Diseases of capillaries

Diseases of veins and lymphatics, and other diseases of circulatory system (451-459)
    451   Phlebitis and thrombophlebitis
    452   Portal vein thrombosis
    453   Other venous embolism and thrombosis
    454   Varicose veins of lower extremities
    455   Hemorrhoids
    456   Varicose veins of other sites
    457   Noninfective disorders of lymphatic channels
    458   Hypotension
    459   Other disorders of circulatory system

8. DISEASES OF THE RESPIRATORY SYSTEM

Acute respiratory infections (460-466)
    460   Acute nasopharyngitis [common cold]
    461   Acute sinusitis
    462   Acute pharyngitis
    463   Acute tonsillitis
    464   Acute laryngitis and tracheitis

8. DISEASES OF THE RESPIRATORY SYSTEM *continued*

465   Acute upper respiratory infections of multiple or unspecified sites
466   Acute bronchitis and bronchiolitis

Other diseases of upper respiratory tract (470-478)

470   Deviated nasal septum
471   Nasal polyps
472   Chronic pharyngitis and nasopharyngitis
473   Chronic sinusitis
474   Chronic disease of tonsils and adenoids
475   Peritonsillar abscess
476   Chronic laryngitis and laryngotracheitis
477   Allergic rhinitis
478   Other diseases of upper respiratory tract

Pneumonia and influenza (480-487)

480   Viral pneumonia
481   Pneumococcal pneumonia [Streptococcus pneumoniae pneumonia]
482   Other bacterial pneumonia
483   Pneumonia due to other specified organism
484   Pneumonia in infectious diseases classified elsewhere
485   Bronchopneumonia, organism unspecified
486   Pneumonia, organism unspecified
487   Influenza

Chronic obstructive pulmonary disease and allied conditions (490-496)

490   Bronchitis, not specified as acute or chronic
491   Chronic bronchitis
492   Emphysema
493   Asthma
494   Bronchiectasis
495   Extrinsic allergic alveolitis
496   Chronic airway obstruction, not elsewhere classified

Pneumoconioses and other lung diseases due to external agents (500-508)

500   Coalworkers' pneumoconiosis
501   Asbestosis
502   Pneumoconiosis due to other silica or silicates
503   Pneumoconiosis due to other inorganic dust
504   Pneumopathy due to inhalation of other dust
505   Pneumoconiosis, unspecified
506   Respiratory conditions due to chemical fumes and vapors
507   Pneumonitis due to solids and liquids
508   Respiratory conditions due to other and unspecified external agents

Other diseases of respiratory system (510-519)

510   Empyema
511   Pleurisy
512   Pneumothorax
513   Abscess of lung and mediastinum
514   Pulmonary congestion and hypostasis
515   Postinflammatory pulmonary fibrosis
516   Other alveolar and parietoalveolar pneumopathy
517   Lung involvement in conditions classified elsewhere
518   Other diseases of lung
519   Other diseases of respiratory system

9. DISEASES OF THE DIGESTIVE SYSTEM

Diseases of oral cavity, salivary glands, and jaws (520-529)

520   Disorders of tooth development and eruption
521   Diseases of hard tissues of teeth
522   Diseases of pulp and periapical tissues
523   Gingival and periodontal diseases
524   Dentofacial anomalies, including malocclusion
525   Other diseases and conditions of the teeth and supporting structures
526   Diseases of the jaws
527   Diseases of the salivary glands
528   Diseases of the oral soft tissues, excluding lesions specific for gingiva and tongue
529   Diseases and other conditions of the tongue

9. DISEASES OF THE DIGESTIVE SYSTEM *continued*

Diseases of esophagus, stomach, and duodenum (530-537)

530   Diseases of esophagus
531   Gastric ulcer
532   Duodenal ulcer
533   Peptic ulcer, site unspecified
534   Gastrojejunal ulcer
535   Gastritis and duodenitis
536   Disorders of function of stomach
537   Other disorders of stomach and duodenum

Appendicitis (540-543)

540   Acute appendicitis
541   Appendicitis, unqualified
542   Other appendicitis
543   Other diseases of appendix

Hernia of abdominal cavity (550-553)

550   Inguinal hernia
551   Other hernia of abdominal cavity, with gangrene
552   Other hernia of abdominal cavity, with obstruction, but without mention of gangrene
553   Other hernia of abdominal cavity without mention of obstruction or gangrene

Noninfectious enteritis and colitis (555-558)

555   Regional enteritis
556   Ulcerative colitis
557   Vascular insufficiency of intestine
558   Other and unspecified noninfectious gastroenteritis and colitis

Other diseases of intestines and peritoneum (560-569)

560   Intestinal obstruction without mention of hernia
562   Diverticula of intestine
564   Functional digestive disorders, not elsewhere classified
565   Anal fissure and fistula
566   Abscess of anal and rectal regions
567   Peritonitis
568   Other disorders of peritoneum
569   Other disorders of intestine

Other diseases of digestive system (570-579)

570   Acute and subacute necrosis of liver
571   Chronic liver disease and cirrhosis
572   Liver abscess and sequelae of chronic liver disease
573   Other disorders of liver
574   Cholelithiasis
575   Other disorders of gallbladder
576   Other disorders of biliary tract
577   Diseases of pancreas
578   Gastrointestinal hemorrhage
579   Intestinal malabsorption

10. DISEASES OF THE GENITOURINARY SYSTEM

Nephritis, nephrotic syndrome, and nephrosis (580-589)

580   Acute glomerulonephritis
581   Nephrotic syndrome
582   Chronic glomerulonephritis
583   Nephritis and nephropathy, not specified as acute or chronic
584   Acute renal failure
585   Chronic renal failure
586   Renal failure, unspecified
587   Renal sclerosis, unspecified
588   Disorders resulting from impaired renal function
589   Small kidney of unknown cause

Other diseases of urinary system (590-599)

590   Infections of kidney
591   Hydronephrosis
592   Calculus of kidney and ureter
593   Other disorders of kidney and ureter

10. DISEASES OF THE GENITOURINARY SYSTEM *continued*

594 Calculus of lower urinary tract
595 Cystitis
596 Other disorders of bladder
597 Urethritis, not sexually transmitted, and urethral syndrome
598 Urethral stricture
599 Other disorders of urethra and urinary tract

Diseases of male genital organs (600-608)
600 Hyperplasia of prostate
601 Inflammatory diseases of prostate
602 Other disorders of prostate
603 Hydrocele
604 Orchitis and epididymitis
605 Redundant prepuce and phimosis
606 Infertility, male
607 Disorders of penis
608 Other disorders of male genital organs

Disorders of breast (610-611)
610 Benign mammary dysplasias
611 Other disorders of breast

Inflammatory disease of female pelvic organs (614-616)
614 Inflammatory disease of ovary, fallopian tube, pelvic cellular tissue, and peritoneum
615 Inflammatory diseases of uterus, except cervix
616 Inflammatory disease of cervix, vagina, and vulva

Other disorders of female genital tract (617-629)
617 Endometriosis
618 Genital prolapse
619 Fistula involving female genital tract
620 Noninflammatory disorders of ovary, fallopian tube, and broad ligament
621 Disorders of uterus, not elsewhere classified
622 Noninflammatory disorders of cervix
623 Noninflammatory disorders of vagina
624 Noninflammatory disorders of vulva and perineum
625 Pain and other symptoms associated with female genital organs
626 Disorders of menstruation and other abnormal bleeding from female genital tract
627 Menopausal and postmenopausal disorders
628 Infertility, female
629 Other disorders of female genital organs

11. COMPLICATIONS OF PREGNANCY, CHILDBIRTH AND THE PUERPERIUM

Ectopic and molar pregnancy (630-633)
630 Hydatidiform mole
631 Other abnormal product of conception
632 Missed abortion
633 Ectopic pregnancy

Other pregnancy with abortive outcome (634-639)
634 Abortion
635 Legally induced abortion
636 Illegally induced abortion
637 Unspecified abortion
638 Failed attempted abortion
639 Complications following abortion and ectopic and molar pregnancies

Complications mainly related to pregnancy (640-648)
640 Hemorrhage in early pregnancy
641 Antepartum hemorrhage, abruptio placentae, and placenta previa
642 Hypertension complicating pregnancy, childbirth, and the puerperium
643 Excessive vomiting in pregnancy
644 Early or threatened labor
645 Late pregnancy
646 Other complications of pregnancy, not elsewhere classified
647 Infective and parasitic conditions in the mother classifiable elsewhere but complicating pregnancy, childbirth, and the puerperium
648 Other current conditions in the mother classifiable elsewhere but complicating pregnancy, childbirth, and the puerperium

11. COMPLICATIONS OF PREGNANCY, CHILDBIRTH AND THE PUERPERIUM *continued*

Normal delivery, and other indications for care in pregnancy, labor, and delivery (650-659)

- 650 Normal delivery
- 651 Multiple gestation
- 652 Malposition and malpresentation of fetus
- 653 Disproportion
- 654 Abnormality of organs and soft tissues of pelvis
- 655 Known or suspected fetal abnormality affecting management of mother
- 656 Other fetal and placental problems affecting management of mother
- 657 Polyhydramnios
- 658 Other problems associated with amniotic cavity and membranes
- 659 Other indications for care or intervention related to labor and delivery and not elsewhere classified

Complications occurring mainly in the course of labor and delivery (660-669)

- 660 Obstructed labor
- 661 Abnormality of forces of labor
- 662 Long labor
- 663 Umbilical cord complications
- 664 Trauma to perineum and vulva during delivery
- 665 Other obstetrical trauma
- 666 Postpartum hemorrhage
- 667 Retained placenta or membranes, without hemorrhage
- 668 Complications of the administration of anesthetic or other sedation in labor and delivery
- 669 Other complications of labor and delivery, not elsewhere classified

Complications of the puerperium (670-677)

- 670 Major puerperal infection
- 671 Venous complications in pregnancy and the puerperium
- 672 Pyrexia of unknown origin during the puerperium
- 673 Obstetrical pulmonary embolism
- 674 Other and unspecified complications of the puerperium, not elsewhere classified
- 675 Infections of the breast and nipple associated with childbirth
- 676 Other disorders of the breast associated with childbirth, and disorders of lactation
- 677 Late effect of complication of pregnancy, childbirth, and the puerperium

12. DISEASES OF THE SKIN AND SUBCUTANEOUS TISSUE

Infections of skin and subcutaneous tissue (680-686)

- 680 Carbuncle and furuncle
- 681 Cellulitis and abscess of finger and toe
- 682 Other cellulitis and abscess
- 683 Acute lymphadenitis
- 684 Impetigo
- 685 Pilonidal cyst
- 686 Other local infections of skin and subcutaneous tissue

Other inflammatory conditions of skin and subcutaneous tissue (690-698)

- 690 Erythematosquamous dermatosis
- 691 Atopic dermatitis and related conditions
- 692 Contact dermatitis and other eczema
- 693 Dermatitis due to substances taken internally
- 694 Bullous dermatoses
- 695 Erythematous conditions
- 696 Psoriasis and similar disorders
- 697 Lichen
- 698 Pruritus and related conditions

Other diseases of skin and subcutaneous tissue (700-709)

- 700 Corns and callosities
- 701 Other hypertrophic and atrophic conditions of skin
- 702 Other dermatoses
- 703 Diseases of nail
- 704 Diseases of hair and hair follicles
- 705 Disorders of sweat glands
- 706 Diseases of sebaceous glands
- 707 Chronic ulcer of skin

12. DISEASES OF THE SKIN AND SUBCUTANEOUS TISSUE *continued*

708 Urticaria
709 Other disorders of skin and subcutaneous tissue

13. DISEASES OF THE MUSCULOSKELETAL SYSTEM AND CONNECTIVE TISSUE

Arthropathies and related disorders (710-719)

710 Diffuse diseases of connective tissue
711 Arthropathy associated with infections
712 Crystal arthropathies
713 Arthropathy associated with other disorders classified elsewhere
714 Rheumatoid arthritis and other inflammatory polyarthropathies
715 Osteoarthrosis and allied disorders
716 Other and unspecified arthropathies
717 Internal derangement of knee
718 Other derangement of joint
719 Other and unspecified disorder of joint

Dorsopathies (720-724)

720 Ankylosing spondylitis and other inflammatory spondylopathies
721 Spondylosis and allied disorders
722 Intervertebral disc disorders
723 Other disorders of cervical region
724 Other and unspecified disorders of back

Rheumatism, excluding the back (725-729)

725 Polymyalgia rheumatica
726 Peripheral enthesopathies and allied syndromes
727 Other disorders of synovium, tendon, and bursa
728 Disorders of muscle, ligament, and fascia
729 Other disorders of soft tissues

Osteopathies, chondropathies, and acquired musculoskeletal deformities (730-739)

730 Osteomyelitis, periostitis, and other infections involving bone
731 Osteitis deformans and osteopathies associated with other disorders classified elsewhere
732 Osteochondropathies
733 Other disorders of bone and cartilage
734 Flat foot
735 Acquired deformities of toe
736 Other acquired deformities of limbs
737 Curvature of spine
738 Other acquired deformity
739 Nonallopathic lesions, not elsewhere classified

14. CONGENITAL ANOMALIES

740 Anencephalus and similar anomalies
741 Spina bifida
742 Other congenital anomalies of nervous system
743 Congenital anomalies of eye
744 Congenital anomalies of ear, face, and neck
745 Bulbus cordis anomalies and anomalies of cardiac septal closure
746 Other congenital anomalies of heart
747 Other congenital anomalies of circulatory system
748 Congenital anomalies of respiratory system
749 Cleft palate and cleft lip
750 Other congenital anomalies of upper alimentary tract
751 Other congenital anomalies of digestive system
752 Congenital anomalies of genital organs
753 Congenital anomalies of urinary system
754 Certain congenital musculoskeletal deformities
755 Other congenital anomalies of limbs
756 Other congenital musculoskeletal anomalies
757 Congenital anomalies of the integument
758 Chromosomal anomalies
759 Other and unspecified congenital anomalies

15. CERTAIN CONDITIONS ORIGINATING IN THE PERINATAL PERIOD

Maternal causes of perinatal morbidity and mortality (760-763)

760 Fetus or newborn affected by maternal conditions which may be unrelated to present pregnancy
761 Fetus or newborn affected by maternal complications of pregnancy
762 Fetus or newborn affected by complications of placenta, cord, and membranes
763 Fetus or newborn affected by other complications of labor and delivery

Other conditions originating in the perinatal period (764-779)

764 Slow fetal growth and fetal malnutrition
765 Disorders relating to short gestation and low birthweight
766 Disorders relating to long gestation and high birthweight
767 Birth trauma
768 Intrauterine hypoxia and birth asphyxia
769 Respiratory distress syndrome
770 Other respiratory conditions of fetus and newborn
771 Infections specific to the perinatal period
772 Fetal and neonatal hemorrhage
773 Hemolytic disease of fetus or newborn, due to isoimmunization
774 Other perinatal jaundice
775 Endocrine and metabolic disturbances specific to the fetus and newborn
776 Hematological disorders of fetus and newborn
777 Perinatal disorders of digestive system
778 Conditions involving the integument and temperature regulation of fetus and newborn
779 Other and ill-defined conditions originating in the perinatal period

16. SYMPTOMS, SIGNS, AND ILL-DEFINED CONDITIONS

Symptoms (780-789)

780 General symptoms
781 Symptoms involving nervous and musculoskeletal systems
782 Symptoms involving skin and other integumentary tissue
783 Symptoms concerning nutrition, metabolism, and development
784 Symptoms involving head and neck
785 Symptoms involving cardiovascular system
786 Symptoms involving respiratory system and other chest symptoms
787 Symptoms involving digestive system
788 Symptoms involving urinary system
789 Other symptoms involving abdomen and pelvis

Nonspecific abnormal findings (790-796)

790 Nonspecific findings on examination of blood
791 Nonspecific findings on examination of urine
792 Nonspecific abnormal findings in other body substances
793 Nonspecific abnormal findings on radiological and other examination of body structure
794 Nonspecific abnormal results of function studies
795 Nonspecific abnormal histological and immunological findings
796 Other nonspecific abnormal findings

Ill-defined and unknown causes of morbidity and mortality (797-799)

797 Senility without mention of psychosis
798 Sudden death, cause unknown
799 Other ill-defined and unknown causes of morbidity and mortality

17. INJURY AND POISONING

Fracture of skull (800-804)

800 Fracture of vault of skull
801 Fracture of base of skull
802 Fracture of face bones
803 Other and unqualified skull fractures
804 Multiple fractures involving skull or face with other bones

Fracture of neck and trunk (805-809)

805 Fracture of vertebral column without mention of spinal cord injury
806 Fracture of vertebral column with spinal cord injury
807 Fracture of rib(s), sternum, larynx, and trachea
808 Fracture of pelvis
809 Ill-defined fractures of bones of trunk

17. INJURY AND POISONING *continued*

Fracture of upper limb (810-819)

810 Fracture of clavicle
811 Fracture of scapula
812 Fracture of humerus
813 Fracture of radius and ulna
814 Fracture of carpal bone(s)
815 Fracture of metacarpal bone(s)
816 Fracture of one or more phalanges of hand
817 Multiple fractures of hand bones
818 Ill-defined fractures of upper limb
819 Multiple fractures involving both upper limbs, and upper limb with rib(s) and sternum

Fracture of lower limb (820-829)

820 Fracture of neck of femur
821 Fracture of other and unspecified parts of femur
822 Fracture of patella
823 Fracture of tibia and fibula
824 Fracture of ankle
825 Fracture of one or more tarsal and metatarsal bones
826 Fracture of one or more phalanges of foot
827 Other, multiple, and ill-defined fractures of lower limb
828 Multiple fractures involving both lower limbs, lower with upper limb, and lower
        limb(s) with rib(s) and sternum
829 Fracture of unspecified bones

Dislocation (830-839)

830 Dislocation of jaw
831 Dislocation of shoulder
832 Dislocation of elbow
833 Dislocation of wrist
834 Dislocation of finger
835 Dislocation of hip
836 Dislocation of knee
837 Dislocation of ankle
838 Dislocation of foot
839 Other, multiple, and ill-defined dislocations

Sprains and strains of joints and adjacent muscles (840-848)

840 Sprains and strains of shoulder and upper arm
841 Sprains and strains of elbow and forearm
842 Sprains and strains of wrist and hand
843 Sprains and strains of hip and thigh
844 Sprains and strains of knee and leg
845 Sprains and strains of ankle and foot
846 Sprains and strains of sacroiliac region
847 Sprains and strains of other and unspecified parts of back
848 Other and ill-defined sprains and strains

Intracranial injury, excluding those with skull fracture (850-854)

850 Concussion
851 Cerebral laceration and contusion
852 Subarachnoid, subdural, and extradural hemorrhage, following injury
853 Other and unspecified intracranial hemorrhage following injury
854 Intracranial injury of other and unspecified nature

Internal injury of thorax, abdomen, and pelvis (860-869)

860 Traumatic pneumothorax and hemothorax
861 Injury to heart and lung
862 Injury to other and unspecified intrathoracic organs
863 Injury to gastrointestinal tract
864 Injury to liver
865 Injury to spleen
866 Injury to kidney
867 Injury to pelvic organs
868 Injury to other intra-abdominal organs
869 Internal injury to unspecified or ill-defined organs

17. INJURY AND POISONING continued

Open wound of head, neck, and trunk (870-879)

870 Open wound of ocular adnexa
871 Open wound of eyeball
872 Open wound of ear
873 Other open wound of head
874 Open wound of neck
875 Open wound of chest (wall)
876 Open wound of back
877 Open wound of buttock
878 Open wound of genital organs (external), including traumatic amputation
879 Open wound of other and unspecified sites, except limbs

Open wound of upper limb (880-887)

880 Open wound of shoulder and upper arm
881 Open wound of elbow, forearm, and wrist
882 Open wound of hand except finger(s) alone
883 Open wound of finger(s)
884 Multiple and unspecified open wound of upper limb
885 Traumatic amputation of thumb (complete) (partial)
886 Traumatic amputation of other finger(s) (complete) (partial)
887 Traumatic amputation of arm and hand (complete) (partial)

Open wound of lower limb (890-897)

890 Open wound of hip and thigh
891 Open wound of knee, leg [except thigh], and ankle
892 Open wound of foot except toe(s) alone
893 Open wound of toe(s)
894 Multiple and unspecified open wound of lower limb
895 Traumatic amputation of toe(s) (complete) (partial)
896 Traumatic amputation of foot (complete) (partial)
897 Traumatic amputation of leg(s) (complete) (partial)

Injury to blood vessels (900-904)

900 Injury to blood vessels of head and neck
901 Injury to blood vessels of thorax
902 Injury to blood vessels of abdomen and pelvis
903 Injury to blood vessels of upper extremity
904 Injury to blood vessels of lower extremity and unspecified sites

Late effects of injuries, poisonings, toxic effects, and other external causes (905-909)

905 Late effects of musculoskeletal and connective tissue injuries
906 Late effects of injuries to skin and subcutaneous tissues
907 Late effects of injuries to the nervous system
908 Late effects of other and unspecified injuries
909 Late effects of other and unspecified external causes

Superficial injury (910-919)

910 Superficial injury of face, neck, and scalp except eye
911 Superficial injury of trunk
912 Superficial injury of shoulder and upper arm
913 Superficial injury of elbow, forearm, and wrist
914 Superficial injury of hand(s) except finger(s) alone
915 Superficial injury of finger(s)
916 Superficial injury of hip, thigh, leg, and ankle
917 Superficial injury of foot and toe(s)
918 Superficial injury of eye and adnexa
919 Superficial injury of other, multiple, and unspecified sites

Contusion with intact skin surface (920-924)

920 Contusion of face, scalp, and neck except eye(s)
921 Contusion of eye and adnexa
922 Contusion of trunk
923 Contusion of upper limb
924 Contusion of lower limb and of other and unspecified sites

Crushing injury (925-929)

925 Crushing injury of face, scalp, and neck
926 Crushing injury of trunk
927 Crushing injury of upper limb

17. INJURY AND POISONING *continued*

928   Crushing injury of lower limb
929   Crushing injury of multiple and unspecified sites

Effects of foreign body entering through orifice (930-939)

930   Foreign body on external eye
931   Foreign body in ear
932   Foreign body in nose
933   Foreign body in pharynx and larynx
934   Foreign body in trachea, bronchus, and lung
935   Foreign body in mouth, esophagus, and stomach
936   Foreign body in intestine and colon
937   Foreign body in anus and rectum
938   Foreign body in digestive system, unspecified
939   Foreign body in genitourinary tract

Burns (940-949)

940   Burn confined to eye and adnexa
941   Burn of face, head, and neck
942   Burn of trunk
943   Burn of upper limb, except wrist and hand
944   Burn of wrist(s) and hand(s)
945   Burn of lower limb(s)
946   Burns of multiple specified sites
947   Burn of internal organs
948   Burns classified according to extent of body surface involved
949   Burn, unspecified

Injury to nerves and spinal cord (950-957)

950   Injury to optic nerve and pathways
951   Injury to other cranial nerve(s)
952   Spinal cord injury without evidence of spinal bone injury
953   Injury to nerve roots and spinal plexus
954   Injury to other nerve(s) of trunk excluding shoulder and pelvic girdles
955   Injury to peripheral nerve(s) of shoulder girdle and upper limb
956   Injury to peripheral nerve(s) of pelvic girdle and lower limb
957   Injury to other and unspecified nerves

Certain traumatic complications and unspecified injuries (958-959)

958   Certain early complications of trauma
959   Injury, other and unspecified

Poisoning by drugs, medicinal and biological substances (960-979)

960   Poisoning by antibiotics
961   Poisoning by other anti-infectives
962   Poisoning by hormones and synthetic substitutes
963   Poisoning by primarily systemic agents
964   Poisoning by agents primarily affecting blood constituents
965   Poisoning by analgesics, antipyretics, and antirheumatics
966   Poisoning by anticonvulsants and anti-Parkinsonism drugs
967   Poisoning by sedatives and hypnotics
968   Poisoning by other central nervous system depressants and anesthetics
969   Poisoning by psychotropic agents
970   Poisoning by central nervous system stimulants
971   Poisoning by drugs primarily affecting the autonomic nervous system
972   Poisoning by agents primarily affecting the cardiovascular system
973   Poisoning by agents primarily affecting the gastrointestinal system
974   Poisoning by water, mineral, and uric acid metabolism drugs
975   Poisoning by agents primarily acting on the smooth and skeletal muscles and respiratory system
976   Poisoning by agents primarily affecting skin and mucous membrane, ophthalmological, otorhinolaryngological, and dental drugs
977   Poisoning by other and unspecified drugs and medicinals
978   Poisoning by bacterial vaccines
979   Poisoning by other vaccines and biological substances

Toxic effects of substances chiefly nonmedicinal as to source (980-989)

980   Toxic effect of alcohol
981   Toxic effect of petroleum products
982   Toxic effect of solvents other than petroleum-based

17. INJURY AND POISONING *continued*

983 Toxic effect of corrosive aromatics, acids, and caustic alkalis
984 Toxic effect of lead and its compounds (including fumes)
985 Toxic effect of other metals
986 Toxic effect of carbon monoxide
987 Toxic effect of other gases, fumes, or vapors
988 Toxic effect of noxious substances eaten as food
989 Toxic effect of other substances, chiefly nonmedicinal as to source

Other and unspecified effects of external causes (990-995)

990 Effects of radiation, unspecified
991 Effects of reduced temperature
992 Effects of heat and light
993 Effects of air pressure
994 Effects of other external causes
995 Certain adverse effects, not elsewhere classified

Complications of surgical and medical care, not elsewhere classified (996-999)

996 Complications peculiar to certain specified procedures
997 Complications affecting specified body systems, not elsewhere classified
998 Other complications of procedures, not elsewhere classified
999 Complications of medical care, not elsewhere classified

SUPPLEMENTARY CLASSIFICATION OF FACTORS INFLUENCING HEALTH STATUS AND CONTACT WITH HEALTH SERVICES

Persons with potential health hazards related to communicable diseases (V01-V06)

V01 Contact with or exposure to communicable diseases
V02 Carrier or suspected carrier of infectious diseases
V03 Need for prophylactic vaccination and inoculation against bacterial diseases
V04 Need for prophylactic vaccination and inoculation against certain viral diseases
V05 Need for other prophylactic vaccination and inoculation against single diseases
V06 Need for prophylactic vaccination and inoculation against combinations of diseases

Persons with need for isolation, other potential health hazards and prophylactic measures (V07-V09)

V07 Need for isolation and other prophylactic measures
V08 Asymptomatic human immunodeficiency virus (HIV) infection status
V09 Infection with drug-resistant microorganisms

Persons with potential health hazards related to personal and family history (V10-V19)

V10 Personal history of malignant neoplasm
V11 Personal history of mental disorder
V12 Personal history of certain other diseases
V13 Personal history of other diseases
V14 Personal history of allergy to medicinal agents
V15 Other personal history presenting hazards to health
V16 Family history of malignant neoplasm
V17 Family history of certain chronic disabling diseases
V18 Family history of certain other specific conditions
V19 Family history of other conditions

Persons encountering health services in circumstances related to reproduction and development (V20-V29)

V20 Health supervision of infant or child
V21 Constitutional states in development
V22 Normal pregnancy
V23 Supervision of high-risk pregnancy
V24 Postpartum care and examination
V25 Encounter for contraceptive management
V26 Procreative management
V27 Outcome of delivery
V28 Antenatal screening
V29 Observation and evaluation of newborns and infants for suspected condition not found

Liveborn infants according to type of birth (V30-V39)

V30 Single liveborn
V31 Twin, mate liveborn
V32 Twin, mate stillborn
V33 Twin, unspecified
V34 Other multiple, mates all liveborn

SUPPLEMENTARY CLASSIFICATION...HEALTH STATUS/HEALTH SERVICES *continued*

     V35 Other multiple, mates all stillborn
     V36 Other multiple, mates live- and stillborn
     V37 Other multiple, unspecified
     V39 Unspecified

Persons with a condition influencing their health status (V40-V49)

     V40 Mental and behavioral problems
     V41 Problems with special senses and other special functions
     V42 Organ or tissue replaced by transplant
     V43 Organ or tissue replaced by other means
     V44 Artificial opening status
     V45 Other postsurgical states
     V46 Other dependence on machines
     V47 Other problems with internal organs
     V48 Problems with head, neck, and trunk
     V49 Other conditions influencing health status

Persons encountering health services for specific procedures and aftercare (V50-V59)

     V50 Elective surgery for purposes other than remedying health states
     V51 Aftercare involving the use of plastic surgery
     V52 Fitting and adjustment of prosthetic device and implant
     V53 Fitting and adjustment of other device
     V54 Other orthopedic aftercare
     V55 Attention to artificial openings
     V56 Encounter for dialysis and dialysis catheter care
     V57 Care involving use of rehabilitation procedures
     V58 Encounter for other and unspecified procedures and aftercare
     V59 Donors

Persons encountering health services in other circumstances (V60-V69)

     V60 Housing, household, and economic circumstances
     V61 Other family circumstances
     V62 Other psychosocial circumstances
     V63 Unavailability of other medical facilities for care
     V64 Persons encountering health services for specific procedures, not carried out
     V65 Other persons seeking consultation without complaint or sickness
     V66 Convalescence and palliative care
     V67 Follow-up examination
     V68 Encounters for administrative purposes
     V69 Problems related to lifestyle

Persons without reported diagnosis encountered during examination and investigation of individuals and populations (V70-V82)

     V70 General medical examination
     V71 Observation and evaluation for suspected conditions not found
     V72 Special investigations and examinations
     V73 Special screening examination for viral and chlamydial diseases
     V74 Special screening examination for bacterial and spirochetal diseases
     V75 Special screening examination for other infectious diseases
     V76 Special screening for malignant neoplasms
     V77 Special screening for endocrine, nutritional, metabolic, and immunity disorders
     V78 Special screening for disorders of blood and blood-forming organs
     V79 Special screening for mental disorders and developmental handicaps
     V80 Special screening for neurological, eye, and ear diseases
     V81 Special screening for cardiovascular, respiratory, and genitourinary diseases
     V82 Special screening for other conditions
     V83 Genetic carrier status

SUPPLEMENTARY CLASSIFICATION OF EXTERNAL CAUSES OF INJURY AND POISONING

Railway accidents (E800-E807)

     E800 Railway accident involving collision with rolling stock
     E801 Railway accident involving collision with other object
     E802 Railway accident involving derailment without antecedent collision
     E803 Railway accident involving explosion, fire, or burning
     E804 Fall in, on, or from railway train
     E805 Hit by rolling stock

SUPPLEMENTARY CLASSIFICATION...INJURY AND POISONING *continued*

E806 Other specified railway accident
E807 Railway accident of unspecified nature

Motor vehicle traffic accidents (E810-E819)

E810 Motor vehicle traffic accident involving collision with train
E811 Motor vehicle traffic accident involving re-entrant collision with another motor vehicle
E812 Other motor vehicle traffic accident involving collision with another motor vehicle
E813 Motor vehicle traffic accident involving collision with other vehicle
E814 Motor vehicle traffic accident involving collision with pedestrian
E815 Other motor vehicle traffic accident involving collision on the highway
E816 Motor vehicle traffic accident due to loss of control, without collision on the highway
E817 Noncollision motor vehicle traffic accident while boarding or alighting
E818 Other noncollision motor vehicle traffic accident
E819 Motor vehicle traffic accident of unspecified nature

Motor vehicle nontraffic accidents (E820-E825)

E820 Nontraffic accident involving motor-driven snow vehicle
E821 Nontraffic accident involving other off-road motor vehicle
E822 Other motor vehicle nontraffic accident involving collision with moving object
E823 Other motor vehicle nontraffic accident involving collision with stationary object
E824 Other motor vehicle nontraffic accident while boarding and alighting
E825 Other motor vehicle nontraffic accident of other and unspecified nature

Other road vehicle accidents (E826-E829)

E826 Pedal cycle accident
E827 Animal-drawn vehicle accident
E828 Accident involving animal being ridden
E829 Other road vehicle accidents

Water transport accidents (E830-E838)

E830 Accident to watercraft causing submersion
E831 Accident to watercraft causing other injury
E832 Other accidental submersion or drowning in water transport accident
E833 Fall on stairs or ladders in water transport
E834 Other fall from one level to another in water transport
E835 Other and unspecified fall in water transport
E836 Machinery accident in water transport
E837 Explosion, fire, or burning in watercraft
E838 Other and unspecified water transport accident

Air and space transport accidents (E840-E845)

E840 Accident to powered aircraft at takeoff or landing
E841 Accident to powered aircraft, other and unspecified
E842 Accident to unpowered aircraft
E843 Fall in, on, or from aircraft
E844 Other specified air transport accidents
E845 Accident involving spacecraft

Vehicle accidents, not elsewhere classifiable (E846-E849)

E846 Accidents involving powered vehicles used solely within the buildings and premises
of an industrial or commercial establishment
E847 Accidents involving cable cars not running on rails
E848 Accidents involving other vehicles, not elsewhere classifiable
E849 Place of occurrence

Accidental poisoning by drugs, medicinal substances, and biologicals (E850-E858)

E850 Accidental poisoning by analgesics, antipyretics, and antirheumatics
E851 Accidental poisoning by barbiturates
E852 Accidental poisoning by other sedatives and hypnotics
E853 Accidental poisoning by tranquilizers
E854 Accidental poisoning by other psychotropic agents
E855 Accidental poisoning by other drugs acting on central and autonomic nervous systems
E856 Accidental poisoning by antibiotics
E857 Accidental poisoning by other anti-infectives
E858 Accidental poisoning by other drugs

Accidental poisoning by other solid and liquid substances, gases, and vapors (E860-E869)

E860 Accidental poisoning by alcohol, not elsewhere classified
E861 Accidental poisoning by cleansing and polishing agents, disinfectants, paints, and
varnishes

SUPPLEMENTARY CLASSIFICATION...INJURY AND POISONING *continued*

E862 Accidental poisoning by petroleum products, other solvents and their vapors, not elsewhere classified

E863 Accidental poisoning by agricultural and horticultural chemical and pharmaceutical preparations other than plant foods and fertilizers

E864 Accidental poisoning by corrosives and caustics, not elsewhere classified

E865 Accidental poisoning from poisonous foodstuffs and poisonous plants

E866 Accidental poisoning by other and unspecified solid and liquid substances

E867 Accidental poisoning by gas distributed by pipeline

E868 Accidental poisoning by other utility gas and other carbon monoxide

E869 Accidental poisoning by other gases and vapors

Misadventures to patients during surgical and medical care (E870-E876)

E870 Accidental cut, puncture, perforation, or hemorrhage during medical care

E871 Foreign object left in body during procedure

E872 Failure of sterile precautions during procedure

E873 Failure in dosage

E874 Mechanical failure of instrument or apparatus during procedure

E875 Contaminated or infected blood, other fluid, drug, or biological substance

E876 Other and unspecified misadventures during medical care

Surgical and medical procedures as the cause of abnormal reaction of patient or later complication, without mention of misadventure at the time of procedure (E878-E879)

E878 Surgical operation and other surgical procedures as the cause of abnormal reaction of patient, or of later complication, without mention of misadventure at the time of operation

E879 Other procedures, without mention of misadventure at the time of procedure, as the cause of abnormal reaction of patient, or of later complication

Accidental falls (E880-E888)

E880 Fall on or from stairs or steps

E881 Fall on or from ladders or scaffolding

E882 Fall from or out of building or other structure

E883 Fall into hole or other opening in surface

E884 Other fall from one level to another

E885 Fall on same level from slipping, tripping, or stumbling

E886 Fall on same level from collision, pushing or shoving, by or with other person

E887 Fracture, cause unspecified

E888 Other and unspecified fall

Accidents caused by fire and flames (E890-E899)

E890 Conflagration in private dwelling

E891 Conflagration in other and unspecified building or structure

E892 Conflagration not in building or structure

E893 Accident caused by ignition of clothing

E894 Ignition of highly inflammable material

E895 Accident caused by controlled fire in private dwelling

E896 Accident caused by controlled fire in other and unspecified building or structure

E897 Accident caused by controlled fire not in building or structure

E898 Accident caused by other specified fire and flames

E899 Accident caused by unspecified fire

Accidents due to natural and environmental factors (E900-E909)

E900 Excessive heat

E901 Excessive cold

E902 High and low air pressure and changes in air pressure

E903 Travel and motion

E904 Hunger, thirst, exposure, and neglect

E905 Venomous animals and plants as the cause of poisoning and toxic reactions

E906 Other injury caused by animals

E907 Lightning

E908 Cataclysmic storms, and floods resulting from storms

E909 Cataclysmic earth surface movements and eruptions

Accidents caused by submersion, suffocation, and foreign bodies (E910-E915)

E910 Accidental drowning and submersion

E911 Inhalation and ingestion of food causing obstruction of respiratory tract or suffocation

E912 Inhalation and ingestion of other object causing obstruction of respiratory tract or suffocation

E913 Accidental mechanical suffocation

SUPPLEMENTARY CLASSIFICATION...INJURY AND POISONING *continued*

  E914 Foreign body accidentally entering eye and adnexa
  E915 Foreign body accidentally entering other orifice

Other accidents (E916-E928)
  E916 Struck accidentally by falling object
  E917 Striking against or struck accidentally by objects or persons
  E918 Caught accidentally in or between objects
  E919 Accidents caused by machinery
  E920 Accidents caused by cutting and piercing instruments or objects
  E921 Accident caused by explosion of pressure vessel
  E922 Accident caused by firearm and air gun missile
  E923 Accident caused by explosive material
  E924 Accident caused by hot substance or object, caustic or corrosive material, and steam
  E925 Accident caused by electric current
  E926 Exposure to radiation
  E927 Overexertion and strenuous movements
  E928 Other and unspecified environmental and accidental causes

Late effects of accidental injury (E929)
  E929 Late effects of accidental injury

Drugs, medicinal and biological substances causing adverse effects in therapeutic use (E930-E949)
  E930 Antibiotics
  E931 Other anti-infectives
  E932 Hormones and synthetic substitutes
  E933 Primarily systemic agents
  E934 Agents primarily affecting blood constituents
  E935 Analgesics, antipyretics, and antirheumatics
  E936 Anticonvulsants and anti-Parkinsonism drugs
  E937 Sedatives and hypnotics
  E938 Other central nervous system depressants and anesthetics
  E939 Psychotropic agents
  E940 Central nervous system stimulants
  E941 Drugs primarily affecting the autonomic nervous system
  E942 Agents primarily affecting the cardiovascular system
  E943 Agents primarily affecting gastrointestinal system
  E944 Water, mineral, and uric acid metabolism drugs
  E945 Agents primarily acting on the smooth and skeletal muscles and respiratory system
  E946 Agents primarily affecting skin and mucous membrane, ophthalmological,
    otorhinolaryngological, and dental drugs
  E947 Other and unspecified drugs and medicinal substances
  E948 Bacterial vaccines
  E949 Other vaccines and biological substances

Suicide and self-inflicted injury (E950-E959)
  E950 Suicide and self-inflicted poisoning by solid or liquid substances
  E951 Suicide and self-inflicted poisoning by gases in domestic use
  E952 Suicide and self-inflicted poisoning by other gases and vapors
  E953 Suicide and self inflicted injury by hanging, strangulation, and suffocation
  E954 Suicide and self-inflicted injury by submersion [drowning]
  E955 Suicide and self-inflicted injury by firearms, air guns and explosives
  E956 Suicide and self-inflicted injury by cutting and piercing instruments
  E957 Suicide and self-inflicted injuries by jumping from high place
  E958 Suicide and self-inflicted injury by other and unspecified means
  E959 Late effects of self-inflicted injury

Homicide and injury purposely inflicted by other persons (E960-E969)
  E960 Fight, brawl, and rape
  E961 Assault by corrosive or caustic substance, except poisoning
  E962 Assault by poisoning
  E963 Assault by hanging and strangulation
  E964 Assault by submersion [drowning]
  E965 Assault by firearms and explosives
  E966 Assault by cutting and piercing instrument
  E967 Perpetrator of child and adult abuse
  E968 Assault by other and unspecified means
  E969 Late effects of injury purposely inflicted by other person

SUPPLEMENTARY CLASSIFICATION...INJURY AND POISONING *continued*

Legal intervention (E970-E978)

E970 Injury due to legal intervention by firearms
E971 Injury due to legal intervention by explosives
E972 Injury due to legal intervention by gas
E973 Injury due to legal intervention by blunt object
E974 Injury due to legal intervention by cutting and piercing instruments
E975 Injury due to legal intervention by other specified means
E976 Injury due to legal intervention by unspecified means
E977 Late effects of injuries due to legal intervention
E978 Legal execution
E979 Terrorism

Injury undetermined whether accidentally or purposely inflicted (E980-E989)

E980 Poisoning by solid or liquid substances, undetermined whether accidentally or
    purposely inflicted
E981 Poisoning by gases in domestic use, undetermined whether accidentally or purposely
    inflicted
E982 Poisoning by other gases, undetermined whether accidentally or purposely inflicted
E983 Hanging, strangulation, or suffocation, undetermined whether accidentally or
    purposely inflicted
E984 Submersion [drowning], undetermined whether accidentally or purposely inflicted
E985 Injury by firearms, air guns and explosives, undetermined whether accidentally or
    purposely inflicted
E986 Injury by cutting and piercing instruments, undetermined whether accidentally or
    purposely inflicted
E987 Falling from high place, undetermined whether accidentally or purposely inflicted
E988 Injury by other and unspecified means, undetermined whether accidentally or
    purposely inflicted
E989 Late effects of injury, undetermined whether accidentally or purposely inflicted

Injury resulting from operations of war (E990-E999)

E990 Injury due to war operations by fires and conflagrations
E991 Injury due to war operations by bullets and fragments
E992 Injury due to war operations by explosion of marine weapons
E993 Injury due to war operations by other explosion
E994 Injury due to war operations by destruction of aircraft
E995 Injury due to war operations by other and unspecified forms of conventional warfare
E996 Injury due to war operations by nuclear weapons
E997 Injury due to war operations by other forms of unconventional warfare
E998 Injury due to war operations but occurring after cessation of hostilities
E999 Late effects of injury due to war operations and terrorism

DISEASES: ALPHABETIC INDEX
VOLUME 2

A

AAV (disease) (illness) (infection)—*see* Human immunodeficiency virus (disease) (illness) (infection)
Abactio —*see* Abortion, induced
Abactus venter —*see* Abortion, induced
Abarognosis 781.99
Abasia (-astasia) 307.9
  atactica 781.3
  choreic 781.3
  hysterical 300.11
  paroxysmal trepidant 781.3
  spastic 781.3
  trembling 781.3
  trepidans 781.3
Abderhalden-Kaufmann-Lignac syndrome (cystinosis) 270.0
Abdomen, abdominal —*see also* condition
  accordion 306.4
  acute 789.0
  angina 557.1
  burst 868.00
  convulsive equivalent (*see also* Epilepsy) 345.5
  heart 746.87
  muscle deficiency syndrome 756.79
  obstipum 756.79
Abdominalgia 789.0
  periodic 277.3
Abduction contracture, hip or other joint —*see* Contraction, joint
Abercrombie's syndrome (amyloid degeneration) 277.3
Aberrant (congenital)—*see also* Malposition, congenital
  adrenal gland 759.1
  blood vessel NEC 747.60
    arteriovenous NEC 747.60
    cerebrovascular 747.81
    gastrointestinal 747.61
    lower limb 747.64
    renal 747.62
    spinal 747.82
    upper limb 747.63
  breast 757.6
  endocrine gland NEC 759.2
  gastrointestinal vessel (peripheral) 747.61
  hepatic duct 751.69
  lower limb vessel (peripheral) 747.64
  pancreas 751.7
  parathyroid gland 759.2
  peripheral vascular vessel NEC 747.60
  pituitary gland (pharyngeal) 759.2
  renal blood vessel 747.62
  sebaceous glands, mucous membrane, mouth 750.26
  spinal vessel 747.82
  spleen 759.0
  testis (descent) 752.51
  thymus gland 759.2
  thyroid gland 759.2
  upper limb vessel (peripheral) 747.63
Aberratio
  lactis 757.6
  testis 752.51
Aberration —*see also* Anomaly
  chromosome—*see* Anomaly, chromosome(s)
  distantial 368.9
  mental (*see also* Disorder, mental, nonpsychotic) 300.9

Abetalipoproteinemia 272.5
Abionarce 780.79
Abiotrophy 799.8
Ablatio
  placentae—*see* Placenta, ablatio
  retinae (*see also* Detachment, retina) 361.9
Ablation
  pituitary (gland) (with hypofunction) 253.7
  placenta—*see* Placenta, ablatio
  uterus 621.8
Ablepharia, ablepharon, ablephary 743.62
Ablepsia —*see* Blindness
Ablepsy —*see* Blindness
Ablutomania 300.3
Abnormal, abnormality, abnormalities —*see also* Anomaly
  acid-base balance 276.4
    fetus or newborn—*see* Distress, fetal
  adaptation curve, dark 368.63
  alveolar ridge 525.9
  amnion 658.9
    affecting fetus or newborn 762.9
  anatomical relationship NEC 759.9
  apertures, congenital, diaphragm 756.6
  auditory perception NEC 388.40
  autosomes NEC 758.5
    13 758.1
    18 758.2
    21 or 22 758.0
    D_1 758.1
    E_3 758.2
    G 758.0
  ballistocardiogram 794.39
  basal metabolic rate (BMR) 794.7
  biosynthesis, testicular androgen 257.2
  blood level (of)
    cobalt 790.6
    copper 790.6
    iron 790.6
    lithium 790.6
    magnesium 790.6
    mineral 790.6
    zinc 790.6
  blood pressure
    elevated (without diagnosis of hypertension) 796.2
    low (*see also* Hypotension) 458.9
      reading (incidental) (isolated) (nonspecific) 796.3
  bowel sounds 787.5
  breathing behavior—*see* Respiration
  caloric test 794.19
  cervix (acquired) NEC 622.9
    congenital 752.40
    in pregnancy or childbirth 654.6
      causing obstructed labor 660.2
        affecting fetus or newborn 763.1
  chemistry, blood NEC 790.6
  chest sounds 786.7
  chorion 658.9
    affecting fetus or newborn 762.9
  chromosomal NEC 758.89
    analysis, nonspecific result 795.2
    autosomes (*see also* Abnormal, autosomes NEC) 758.5
    fetal, (suspected) affecting management of pregnancy 655.1
    sex 758.81

Abnormal, abnormality . . .—*continued*
narrowness, eyelid 743.62
optokinetic response 379.57
organs or tissues of pelvis NEC
  in pregnancy or childbirth 654.9
    affecting fetus or newborn 763.89
    causing obstructed labor 660.2
      affecting fetus or newborn 763.1
origin—*see* Malposition, congenital
palmar creases 757.2
Papanicolaou (smear)
  cervix 795.00
    atypical squamous cell changes of
      undetermined significance
      favor benign (ASCUS favor benign)
        795.01
      favor dysplasia (ASCUS favor dysplasia)
        795.02
    nonspecific finding NEC 795.09
  other site 795.1
parturition
  affecting fetus or newborn 763.9
  mother—*see* Delivery, complicated
pelvis (bony)—*see* Deformity, pelvis
percussion, chest 786.7
periods (grossly) (see also Menstruation) 626.9
phonocardiogram 794.39
placenta—*see* Placenta, abnormal
plantar reflex 796.1
plasma protein—*see* Deficiency, plasma, protein
pleural folds 748.8
position—*see also* Malposition
  gravid uterus 654.4
    causing obstructed labor 660.2
      affecting fetus or newborn 763.1
posture NEC 781.92
presentation (fetus)—*see* Presentation, fetus,
  abnormal
product of conception NEC 631
puberty—*see* Puberty
pulmonary
  artery 747.3
  function, newborn 770.89
  test results 794.2
  ventilation, newborn 770.89
    hyperventilation 786.01
pulsations in neck 785.1
pupil reflexes 379.40
quality of milk 676.8
radiological examination 793.9
  abdomen NEC 793.6
  biliary tract 793.3
  breast 793.89
    mammogram NOS 793.80
    mammographic microcalcification 793.81
  gastrointestinal tract 793.4
  genitourinary organs 793.5
  head 793.0
  intrathoracic organ NEC 793.2
  lung (field) 793.1
  musculoskeletal system 793.7
  retroperitoneum 793.6
  skin and subcutaneous tissue 793.9
  skull 793.0
red blood cells 790.09
  morphology 790.09
  volume 790.09
reflex NEC 796.1
renal function test 794.4
respiration signs—*see* Respiration
response to nerve stimulation 794.10

Abnormal, abnormality . . .—*continued*
retinal correspondence 368.34
rhythm, heart—*see also* Arrhythmia fetus—*see*
  Distress, fetal
saliva 792.4
scan
  brain 794.09
  kidney 794.4
  liver 794.8
  lung 794.2
  thyroid 794.5
secretion
  gastrin 251.5
  glucagon 251.4
semen 792.2
serum level (of)
  acid phosphatase 790.5
  alkaline phosphatase 790.5
  amylase 790.5
  enzymes NEC 790.5
  lipase 790.5
shape
  cornea 743.41
  gallbladder 751.69
  gravid uterus 654.4
    affecting fetus or newborn 763.89
    causing obstructed labor 660.2
      affecting fetus or newborn 763.1
  head (see also Anomaly, skull) 756.0
  organ or site, congenital NEC—*see* Distortion
sinus venosus 747.40
size
  fetus, complicating delivery 653.5
    causing obstructed labor 660.1
  gallbladder 751.69
  head (*see also* Anomaly, skull) 756.0
  organ or site, congenital NEC—*see* Distortion
  teeth 520.2
skin and appendages, congenital NEC 757.9
soft parts of pelvis—*see* Abnormal, organs or
  tissues of pelvis
spermatozoa 792.2
sputum (amount) (color) (excessive) (odor)
  (purulent) 786.4
stool NEC 787.7
  bloody 578.1
    occult 792.1
  bulky 787.7
  color (dark) (light) 792.1
  content (fat) (mucus) (pus) 792.1
  occult blood 792.1
synchondrosis 756.9
test results without manifest disease—*see*
  Findings, abnormal
thebesian valve 746.9
thermography—*see* Findings, abnormal,
  structure
threshold, cones or rods (eye) 368.63
thyroid-binding globulin 246.8
thyroid product 246.8
toxicology (findings) NEC 796.0
tracheal cartilage (congenital) 748.3
transport protein 273.8
ultrasound results—*see* Findings, abnormal,
  structure
umbilical cord
  affecting fetus or newborn 762.6
  complicating delivery 663.9
  specified NEC 663.8
union
  cricoid cartilage and thyroid cartilage 748.3

Abnormal, abnormality . . .—*continued*
  larynx and trachea 748.3
    thyroid cartilage and hyoid bone 748.3
  urination NEC 788.69
    psychogenic 306.53
    stream
      intermittent 788.61
      slowing 788.62
      splitting 788.61
      weak 788.62
  urine (constituents) NEC 791.9
  uterine hemorrhage (*see also* Hemorrhage,
      uterus) 626.9
    climacteric 627.0
    postmenopausal 627.1
  vagina (acquired) (congenital)
    in pregnancy or childbirth 654.7
      affecting fetus or newborn 763.89
      causing obstructed labor 660.2
        affecting fetus or newborn 763.1
  vascular sounds 785.9
  vectorcardiogram 794.39
  visually evoked potential (VEP) 794.13
  vulva (acquired) (congenital)
    in pregnancy or childbirth 654.8
      affecting fetus or newborn 763.89
      causing obstructed labor 660.2
        affecting fetus or newborn 763.1
  weight
    gain 783.1
      of pregnancy 646.1
        with hypertension—see Toxemia, of
          pregnancy
    loss 783.21
  x-ray examination—*see* Abnormal, radiological
      examination
Abnormally formed uterus —*see* Anomaly,
    uterus
Abnormity (any organ or part)—*see* Anomaly
ABO
  hemolytic disease 773.1
  incompatibility reaction 999.6
Abocclusion 524.2
Abolition, language 784.69
Aborter, habitual or recurrent NEC
  without current pregnancy 629.9
  current abortion (*see also* Abortion,
      spontaneous) 634.9
    affecting fetus or newborn 761.8
  observation in current pregnancy 646.3
Abortion (complete) (incomplete) (inevitable)
    (with retained products of conception) 637.9

> *Note—Use the following fifth-digit*
> *subclassification with categories 634-637:*
>
> 0 *unspecified*
> 1 *incomplete*
> 2 *complete*

  with
    complication(s) (any) following previous
        abortion—*see* category 639
    damage to pelvic organ (laceration) (rupture)
        (tear) 637.2
    embolism (air) (amniotic fluid) (blood clot)
        (pulmonary) (pyemic) (septic) (soap) 637.6
    genital tract and pelvic infection 637.0
    hemorrhage, delayed or excessive 637.1
    metabolic disorder 637.4
    renal failure (acute) 637.3
    sepsis (genital tract) (pelvic organ) 637.0

Abortion—*continued*
    urinary tract 637.7
    shock (postoperative) (septic) 637.5
    specified complication NEC 637.7
    toxemia 637.3
    unspecified complication(s) 637.8
    urinary tract infection 637.7
  accidental—*see* Abortion, spontaneous
  artificial—*see* Abortion, induced
  attempted (failed)—*see* Abortion, failed
  criminal—*see* Abortion, illegal
  early—*see* Abortion, spontaneous
  elective—*see* Abortion, legal
  failed (legal) 638.9
    with
      damage to pelvic organ (laceration)
          (rupture) (tear) 638.2
      embolism (air) (amniotic fluid) (blood clot)
          (pulmonary) (pyemic) (septic) (soap)
          638.6
      genital tract and pelvic infection 638.0
      hemorrhage, delayed or excessive 638.1
      metabolic disorder 638.4
      renal failure (acute) 638.3
      sepsis (genital tract) (pelvic organ) 638.0
        urinary tract 638.7
      shock (postoperative) (septic) 638.5
      specified complication NEC 638.7
      toxemia 638.3
      unspecified complication(s) 638.8
      urinary tract infection 638.7
  fetal indication—*see* Abortion, legal
  fetus 779.6
  following threatened abortion—*see* Abortion,
      by type
  habitual or recurrent (care during pregnancy)
      646.3
    with current abortion (*see also* Abortion,
        spontaneous) 634.9
      affecting fetus or newborn 761.8
    without current pregnancy 629.9
  homicidal—*see* Abortion, illegal
  illegal 636.9
    with
      damage to pelvic organ (laceration)
          (rupture) (tear) 636.2
      embolism (air) (amniotic fluid) (blood clot)
          (pulmonary) (pyemic) (septic) (soap)
          636.6
      genital tract and pelvic infection 636.0
      hemorrhage, delayed or excessive 636.1
      metabolic disorder 636.4
      renal failure 636.3
      sepsis (genital tract) (pelvic organ) 636.0
        urinary tract 636.7
      shock (postoperative) (septic) 636.5
      specified complication NEC 636.7
      toxemia 636.3
      unspecified complication(s) 636.8
      urinary tract infection 636.7
    fetus 779.6
  induced 637.9
    illegal—*see* Abortion, illegal
    legal indications—*see* Abortion, legal
    medical indications—*see* Abortion, legal
    therapeutic—*see* Abortion, legal
  late—*see* Abortion, spontaneous
  legal (legal indication) (medical indication)
      (under medical supervision) 635.9

Abscess—*continued*
  bladder (wall) 595.89
    amebic 006.8
  bone (subperiosteal) (*see also* Osteomyelitis) 730.0
    accessory sinus (chronic) (*see also* Sinusitis) 473.9
    acute 730.0
    chronic or old 730.1
    jaw (lower) (upper) 526.4
    mastoid—*see* Mastoiditis, acute
    petrous (*see also* Petrositis) 383.20
    spinal (tuberculous) (*see also* Tuberculosis) 015.0 *[730.88]*
      nontuberculous 730.08
  bowel 569.5
  brain (any part) 324.0
    amebic (with liver or lung abscess) 006.5
    cystic 324.0
    late effect—*see* category 326
    otogenic 324.0
    tuberculous (*see also* Tuberculosis) 013.3
  breast (acute) (chronic) (nonpuerperal) 611.0
    newborn 771.5
    puerperal, postpartum 675.1
    tuberculous (*see also* Tuberculosis) 017.9
  broad ligament (chronic) (*see also* Disease, pelvis, inflammatory) 614.4
    acute 614.3
  Brodie's (chronic) (localized) (*see also* Osteomyelitis) 730.1
  bronchus 519.1
  buccal cavity 528.3
  bulbourethral gland 597.0
  bursa 727.89
    pharyngeal 478.29
  buttock 682.5
  canaliculus, breast 611.0
  canthus 372.20
  cartilage 733.99
  cecum 569.5
    with appendicitis 540.1
  cerebellum, cerebellar 324.0
    late effect—*see* category 326
  cerebral (embolic) 324.0
    late effect—*see* category 326
  cervical (neck region) 682.1
    lymph gland or node 683
    stump (*see also* Cervicitis) 616.0
  cervix (stump) (uteri) (*see also* Cervicitis) 616.0
  cheek, external 682.0
    inner 528.3
  chest 510.9
    with fistula 510.0
    wall 682.2
  chin 682.0
  choroid 363.00
  ciliary body 364.3
  circumtonsillar 475
  cold (tuberculous)—*see also* Tuberculosis, abscess
    articular—*see* Tuberculosis, joint
  colon (wall) 569.5
  colostomy or enterostomy 569.6
  conjunctiva 372.00
  connective tissue NEC 682.9
  cornea 370.55
    with ulcer 370.00
  corpus
    cavernosum 607.2
    luteum (*see also* Salpingo-oophoritis) 614.2

Abscess—*continued*
  Cowper's gland 597.0
  cranium 324.0
  cul-de-sac (Douglas') (posterior) (*see also* Disease, pelvis, inflammatory) 614.4
    acute 614.3
  dental 522.5
    with sinus (alveolar) 522.7
  dentoalveolar 522.5
    with sinus (alveolar) 522.7
  diaphragm, diaphragmatic—*see* Abscess, peritoneum
  digit NEC 681.9
  Douglas' cul-de-sac or pouch (*see also* Disease, pelvis, inflammatory) 614.4
    acute 614.3
  Dubois' 090.5
  ductless gland 259.8
  ear
    acute 382.00
    external 380.10
    inner 386.30
    middle—*see* Otitis media
  elbow 682.3
  endamebic—*see* Abscess, amebic
  entamebic—*see* Abscess, amebic
  enterostomy 569.6
  epididymis 604.0
  epidural 324.9
    brain 324.0
    late effect—*see* category 326
    spinal cord 324.1
  epiglottis 478.79
  epiploon, epiploic—*see* Abscess, peritoneum
  erysipelatous (*see also* Erysipelas) 035
  esophagus 530.19
  ethmoid (bone) (chronic) (sinus) (*see also* Sinusitis, ethmoidal) 473.2
  external auditory canal 380.10
  extradural 324.9
    brain 324.0
    late effect—*see* category 326
    spinal cord 324.1
  extraperitoneal—*see* Abscess, peritoneum
  eye 360.00
  eyelid 373.13
  face (any part, except eye) 682.0
  fallopian tube (*see also* Salpingo-oophoritis) 614.2
  fascia 728.89
  fauces 478.29
  fecal 569.5
  femoral (region) 682.6
  filaria, filarial (*see also* Infestation, filarial) 125.9
  finger (any) (intrathecal) (periosteal) (subcutaneous) (subcuticular) 681.00
  fistulous NEC 682.9
  flank 682.2
  foot (except toe) 682.7
  forearm 682.3
  forehead 682.0
  frontal (sinus) (chronic) (*see also* Sinusitis, frontal) 473.1
  gallbladder (*see also* Cholecystitis, acute) 575.0
  gastric 535.0
  genital organ or tract NEC
    female 616.9
      with
        abortion—*see* Abortion, by type, with sepsis

Abscess—*continued*
  ectopic pregnancy (*see also* categories
    633.0-633.9) 639.0
  molar pregnancy (*see also* categories
    630-632) 639.0
  following
    abortion 639.0
    ectopic or molar pregnancy 639.0
  puerperal, postpartum, childbirth 670
  male 608.4
  genitourinary system, tuberculous (*see also*
    Tuberculosis) 016.9
  gingival 523.3
  gland, glandular (lymph) (acute) NEC 683
  glottis 478.79
  gluteal (region) 682.5
  gonorrheal NEC (*see also* Gonococcus) 098.0
  groin 682.2
  gum 523.3
  hand (except finger or thumb) 682.4
  head (except face) 682.8
  heart 429.89
  heel 682.7
  helminthic (*see also* Infestation, by specific
    parasite) 128.9
  hepatic 572.0
    amebic (*see also* Abscess, liver, amebic) 006.3
    duct 576.8
  hip 682.6
    tuberculous (active) (*see also* Tuberculosis)
      015.1
  ileocecal 540.1
  ileostomy (bud) 569.6
  iliac (region) 682.2
    fossa 540.1
  iliopsoas (tuberculous) (*see also* Tuberculosis)
    015.0 *[730.88]*
    nontuberculous 728.89
  infraclavicular (fossa) 682.3
  inguinal (region) 682.2
    lymph gland or node 683
  intersphincteric (anus) 566
  intestine, intestinal 569.5
    rectal 566
  intra-abdominal (*see also* Abscess, peritoneum)
    567.2
    postoperative 998.59
  intracranial 324.0
    late effect—*see* category 326
  intramammary—*see* Abscess, breast
  intramastoid (*see also* Mastoiditis, acute) 383.00
  intraorbital 376.01
  intraperitoneal—*see* Abscess, peritoneum
  intraspinal 324.1
    late effect—*see* category 326
  intratonsillar 475
  iris 364.3
  ischiorectal 566
  jaw (bone) (lower) (upper) 526.4
    skin 682.0
  joint (*see also* Arthritis, pyogenic) 711.0
    vertebral (tuberculous) (*see also* Tuberculosis)
      015.0 *[730.88]*
    nontuberculous 724.8
  kidney 590.2
    with
      abortion—*see* Abortion, by type, with
        urinary tract infection
      calculus 592.0
      ectopic pregnancy (*see also* categories
        633.0-633.9) 639.8

Abscess—*continued*
  molar pregnancy (*see also* categories
    630-632) 639.8
  complicating pregnancy or puerperium 646.6
    affecting fetus or newborn 760.1
  following
    abortion 639.8
    ectopic or molar pregnancy 639.8
  knee 682.6
    joint 711.06
    tuberculous (active) (*see also* Tuberculosis)
      015.2
  labium (majus) (minus) 616.4
    complicating pregnancy, childbirth, or
      puerperium 646.6
  lacrimal (passages) (sac) (*see also*
    Dacryocystitis) 375.30
    caruncle 375.30
    gland (*see also* Dacryoadenitis) 375.00
  lacunar 597.0
  larynx 478.79
  lateral (alveolar) 522.5
    with sinus 522.7
  leg, except foot 682.6
  lens 360.00
  lid 373.13
  lingual 529.0
    tonsil 475
  lip 528.5
  Littre's gland 597.0
  liver 572.0
    amebic 006.3
      with
        brain abscess (and lung abscess) 006.5
        lung abscess 006.4
      due to Entamoeba histolytica 006.3
    dysenteric (*see also* Abscess, liver, amebic)
      006.3
    pyogenic 572.0
    tropical (*see also* Abscess, liver, amebic) 006.3
  loin (region) 682.2
  lumbar (tuberculous) (*see also* Tuberculosis)
    015.0 *[730.88]*
    nontuberculous 682.2
  lung (miliary) (putrid) 513.0
    amebic (with liver abscess) 006.4
      with brain abscess 006.5
  lymph, lymphatic, gland or node (acute) 683
    any site, except mesenteric 683
    mesentery 289.2
  lymphangitic, acute—*see* Cellulitis
  malar 526.4
  mammary gland—*see* Abscess, breast
  marginal (anus) 566
  mastoid (process) (*see also* Mastoiditis, acute)
    383.00
    subperiosteal 383.01
  maxilla, maxillary 526.4
    molar (tooth) 522.5
      with sinus 522.7
    premolar 522.5
    sinus (chronic) (*see also* Sinusitis, maxillary)
      473.0
  mediastinum 513.1
  meibomian gland 373.12
  meninges (*see also* Meningitis) 320.9
  mesentery, mesenteric—*see* Abscess,
    peritoneum
  mesosalpinx (*see also* Salpingo-oophoritis)
    614.2
  milk 675.1

Abscess—*continued*
  Monro's (psoriasis) 696.1
  mons pubis 682.2
  mouth (floor) 528.3
  multiple sites NEC 682.9
  mural 682.2
  muscle 728.89
  myocardium 422.92
  nabothian (follicle) (*see also* Cervicitis) 616.0
  nail (chronic) (with lymphangitis) 681.9
    finger 681.02
    toe 681.11
  nasal (fossa) (septum) 478.1
    sinus (chronic) (*see also* Sinusitis) 473.9
  nasopharyngeal 478.29
  nates 682.5
  navel 682.2
    newborn NEC 771.4
  neck (region) 682.1
    lymph gland or node 683
  nephritic (*see also* Abscess, kidney) 590.2
  nipple 611.0
    puerperal, postpartum 675.0
  nose (septum) 478.1
    external 682.0
  omentum—*see* Abscess, peritoneum
  operative wound 998.59
  orbit, orbital 376.01
  ossifluent—*see* Abscess, bone
  ovary, ovarian (corpus luteum) (*see also*
      Salpingo-oophoritis) 614.2
  oviduct (*see also* Salpingo-oophoritis) 614.2
  palate (soft) 528.3
    hard 526.4
  palmar (space) 682.4
  pancreas (duct) 577.0
  paradental 523.3
  parafrenal 607.2
  parametric, parametrium (chronic) (*see also*
      Disease, pelvis, inflammatory) 614.4
    acute 614.3
  paranephric 590.2
  parapancreatic 577.0
  parapharyngeal 478.22
  pararectal 566
  parasinus (*see also* Sinusitis) 473.9
  parauterine (*see also* Disease, pelvis,
      inflammatory) 614.4
    acute 614.3
  paravaginal (*see also* Vaginitis) 616.10
  parietal region 682.8
  parodontal 523.3
  parotid (duct) (gland) 527.3
    region 528.3
  parumbilical 682.2
    newborn 771.4
  pectoral (region) 682.2
  pelvirectal— *see* Abscess, peritoneum
  pelvis, pelvic
    female (chronic) (*see also* Disease, pelvis,
        inflammatory) 614.4
      acute 614.3
    male, peritoneal (cellular tissue)—*see*
        Abscess, peritoneum
    tuberculous (*see also* Tuberculosis) 016.9
  penis 607.2
    gonococcal (acute) 098.0
      chronic or duration of 2 months or over
          098.2
  perianal 566
  periapical 522.5

Abscess—*continued*
    with sinus (alveolar) 522.7
  periappendiceal 540.1
  pericardial 420.99
  pericecal 540.1
  pericemental 523.3
  pericholecystic (*see also* Cholecystitis, acute)
      575.0
  pericoronal 523.3
  peridental 523.3
  perigastric 535.0
  perimetric (*see also* Disease, pelvis,
      inflammatory) 614.4
    acute 614.3
  perinephric, perinephritic (*see also* Abscess,
      kidney) 590.2
  perineum, perineal (superficial) 682.2
    deep (with urethral involvement) 597.0
    urethra 597.0
  periodontal (parietal) 523.3
    apical 522.5
  periosteum, periosteal (*see also* Periostitis) 730.3
    with osteomyelitis (*see also* Osteomyelitis)
        730.2
      acute or subacute 730.0
      chronic or old 730.1
  peripleuritic 510.9
    with fistula 510.0
  periproctic 566
  periprostatic 601.2
  perirectal (staphylococcal) 566
  perirenal (tissue) (*see also* Abscess, kidney)
      590.2
  perisinuous (nose) (*see also* Sinusitis) 473.9
  peritoneum, peritoneal (perforated) (ruptured)
      567.2
    with
      abortion—*see* Abortion, by type, with sepsis
      appendicitis 540.1
      ectopic pregnancy (*see also* categories
          633.0-633.9) 639.0
      molar pregnancy (*see also* categories
          630-632) 639.0
    following
      abortion 639.0
      ectopic or molar pregnancy 639.0
    pelvic, female (*see also* Disease, pelvis,
        inflammatory) 614.4
      acute 614.3
    postoperative 998.59
    puerperal, postpartum, childbirth 670
    tuberculous (*see also* Tuberculosis) 014.0
  peritonsillar 475
  perityphlic 540.1
  periureteral 593.89
  periurethral 597.0
    gonococcal (acute) 098.0
      chronic or duration of 2 months or over
          098.2
  periuterine (*see also* Disease, pelvis,
      inflammatory) 614.4
    acute 614.3
  perivesical 595.89
  pernicious NEC 682.9
  petrous bone—*see* Petrositis
  phagedenic NEC 682.9
    chancroid 099.0
  pharynx, pharyngeal (lateral) 478.29
  phlegmonous NEC 682.9
  pilonidal 685.0
  pituitary (gland) 253.8

Abscess—*continued*
  pleura 510.9
    with fistula 510.0
  popliteal 682.6
  postanal 566
  postcecal 540.1
  postlaryngeal 478.79
  postnasal 478.1
  postpharyngeal 478.24
  posttonsillar 475
  posttyphoid 002.0
  Pott's (*see also* Tuberculosis) 015.0 *[730.88]*
  pouch of Douglas (chronic) (*see also* Disease,
    pelvis, inflammatory) 614.4
  premammary—*see* Abscess, breast
  prepatellar 682.6
  prostate (*see also* Prostatitis) 601.2
    gonococcal (acute) 098.12
      chronic or duration of 2 months or over
        098.32
  psoas (tuberculous) (*see also* Tuberculosis)
    015.0 *[730.88]*
    nontuberculous 728.89
  pterygopalatine fossa 682.8
  pubis 682.2
  puerperal—Puerperal, abscess, by site
  pulmonary—*see* Abscess, lung
  pulp, pulpal (dental) 522.0
    finger 681.01
    toe 681.10
  pyemic—*see* Septicemia
  pyloric valve 535.0
  rectovaginal septum 569.5
  rectovesical 595.89
  rectum 566
  regional NEC 682.9
  renal (*see also* Abscess, kidney) 590.2
  retina 363.00
  retrobulbar 376.01
  retrocecal—*see* Abscess, peritoneum
  retrolaryngeal 478.79
  retromammary—*see* Abscess, breast
  retroperineal 682.2
  retroperitoneal—*see* Abscess, peritoneum
  retropharyngeal 478.24
    tuberculous (*see also* Tuberculosis) 012.8
  retrorectal 566
  retrouterine (*see also* Disease, pelvis,
    inflammatory) 614.4
    acute 614.3
  retrovesical 595.89
  root, tooth 522.5
    with sinus (alveolar) 522.7
  round ligament (*see also* Disease, pelvis,
    inflammatory) 614.4
    acute 614.3
  rupture (spontaneous) NEC 682.9
  sacrum (tuberculous) (*see also* Tuberculosis)
    015.0 *[730.88]*
    nontuberculous 730.08
  salivary duct or gland 527.3
  scalp (any part) 682.8
  scapular 730.01
  sclera 379.09
  scrofulous (*see also* Tuberculosis) 017.2
  scrotum 608.4
  seminal vesicle 608.0
    amebic 006.8
  septal, dental 522.5
    with sinus (alveolar) 522.7
  septum (nasal) 478.1

Abscess—*continued*
  serous (*see also* Periostitis) 730.3
  shoulder 682.3
  side 682.2
  sigmoid 569.5
  sinus (accessory) (chronic) (nasal) (*see also*
    Sinusitis) 473.9
    intracranial venous (any) 324.0
    late effect—*see* category 326
  Skene's duct or gland 597.0
  skin NEC 682.9
    tuberculous (primary) (*see also* Tuberculosis)
      017.0
  sloughing NEC 682.9
  specified site NEC 682.8
    amebic 006.8
  spermatic cord 608.4
  sphenoidal (sinus) (*see also* Sinusitis,
    sphenoidal) 473.3
  spinal
    cord (any part) (staphylococcal) 324.1
      tuberculous (*see also* Tuberculosis) 013.5
    epidural 324.1
  spine (column) (tuberculous) (*see also*
    Tuberculosis) 015.0 *[730.88]*
    nontuberculous 730.08
  spleen 289.59
    amebic 006.8
  staphylococcal NEC 682.9
  stitch 998.59
  stomach (wall) 535.0
  strumous (tuberculous) (*see also* Tuberculosis)
    017.2
  subarachnoid 324.9
    brain 324.0
    cerebral 324.0
    late effect—*see* category 326
    spinal cord 324.1
  subareolar—*see also* Abscess, breast
    puerperal, postpartum 675.1
  subcecal 540.1
  subcutaneous NEC 682.9
  subdiaphragmatic—*see* Abscess, peritoneum
  subdorsal 682.2
  subdural 324.9
    brain 324.0
    late effect—*see* category 326
    spinal cord 324.1
  subgaleal 682.8
  subhepatic—*see* Abscess, peritoneum
  sublingual 528.3
    gland 527.3
  submammary—*see* Abscess, breast
  submandibular (region) (space) (triangle) 682.0
    gland 527.3
  submaxillary (region) 682.0
    gland 527.3
  submental (pyogenic) 682.0
    gland 527.3
  subpectoral 682.2
  subperiosteal—*see* Abscess, bone
  subperitoneal—*see* Abscess, peritoneum
  subphrenic—*see also* Abscess, peritoneum
    postoperative 998.59
  subscapular 682.2
  subungual 681.9
  suburethral 597.0
  sudoriparous 705.89
  suppurative NEC 682.9
  supraclavicular (fossa) 682.3
  suprahepatic—*see* Abscess, peritoneum

Abscess—*continued*
  suprapelvic (*see also* Disease, pelvis,
    inflammatory) 614.4
    acute 614.3
  suprapubic 682.2
  suprarenal (capsule) (gland) 255.8
  sweat gland 705.89
  syphilitic 095.8
  teeth, tooth (root) 522.5
    with sinus (alveolar) 522.7
    supporting structures NEC 523.3
  temple 682.0
  temporal region 682.0
  temporosphenoidal 324.0
    late effect—*see* category 326
  tendon (sheath) 727.89
  testicle—*see* Orchitis
  thecal 728.89
  thigh (acquired) 682.6
  thorax 510.9
    with fistula 510.0
  throat 478.29
  thumb (intrathecal) (periosteal) (subcutaneous)
    (subcuticular) 681.00
  thymus (gland) 254.1
  thyroid (gland) 245.0
  toe (any) (intrathecal) (periosteal)
    (subcutaneous) (subcuticular) 681.10
  tongue (staphylococcal) 529.0
  tonsil(s) (lingual) 475
  tonsillopharyngeal 475
  tooth, teeth (root) 522.5
    with sinus (alveolar) 522.7
    supporting structure NEC 523.3
  trachea 478.9
  trunk 682.2
  tubal (*see also* Salpingo-oophoritis) 614.2
  tuberculous—*see* Tuberculosis, abscess
  tubo-ovarian (*see also* Salpingo-oophoritis)
    614.2
  tunica vaginalis 608.4
  umbilicus NEC 682.2
    newborn 771.4
  upper arm 682.3
  upper respiratory 478.9
  urachus 682.2
  urethra (gland) 597.0
  urinary 597.0
  uterus, uterine (wall) (*see also* Endometritis)
    615.9
    ligament (*see also* Disease, pelvis,
      inflammatory) 614.4
      acute 614.3
    neck (*see also* Cervicitis) 616.0
  uvula 528.3
  vagina (wall) (*see also* Vaginitis) 616.10
  vaginorectal (*see also* Vaginitis) 616.10
  vas deferens 608.4
  vermiform appendix 540.1
  vertebra (column) (tuberculous) (*see also*
    Tuberculosis) 015.0 *[730.88]*
    nontuberculous 730.0
  vesical 595.89
  vesicouterine pouch (*see also* Disease, pelvis,
    inflammatory) 614.4
  vitreous (humor) (pneumococcal) 360.04
  vocal cord 478.5
  von Bezold's 383.01
  vulva 616.4
    complicating pregnancy, childbirth, or
      puerperium 646.6

Abscess—*continued*
  vulvovaginal gland (*see also* Vaginitis) 616.3
  web-space 682.4
  wrist 682.4
Absence (organ or part) (complete or partial)
  acoustic nerve 742.8
  adrenal (gland) (congenital) 759.1
    acquired V45.79
  albumin (blood) 273.8
  alimentary tract (complete) (congenital) (partial)
    751.8
    lower 751.5
    upper 750.8
  alpha-fucosidase 271.8
  alveolar process (acquired) 525.8
    congenital 750.26
  anus, anal (canal) (congenital) 751.2
  aorta (congenital) 747.22
  aortic valve (congenital) 746.89
  appendix, congenital 751.2
  arm (acquired) V49.60
    above elbow V49.66
    below elbow V49.65
    congenital (*see also* Deformity, reduction,
      upper limb) 755.20
      lower—*see* Absence, forearm, congenital
      upper (complete) (partial) (with absence of
        distal elements, incomplete) 755.24
        with
          complete absence of distal elements
            755.21
          forearm (incomplete) 755.23
  artery (congenital) (peripheral) NEC (*see also*
    Anomaly, peripheral vascular system)
    747.60
    brain 747.81
    cerebral 747.81
    coronary 746.85
    pulmonary 747.3
    umbilical 747.5
  atrial septum 745.69
  auditory canal (congenital) (external) 744.01
  auricle (ear) (with stenosis or atresia of auditory
    canal), congenital 744.01
  bile, biliary duct (common) or passage
    (congenital) 751.61
  bladder (acquired) V45.74
    congenital 753.8
  bone (congenital) NEC 756.9
    marrow 284.9
      acquired (secondary) 284.8
      congenital 284.0
      hereditary 284.0
      idiopathic 284.9
    skull 756.0
  bowel sounds 787.5
  brain 740.0
    specified part 742.2
  breast(s) (acquired) V45.71
    congenital 757.6
  broad ligament (congenital) 752.19
  bronchus (congenital) 748.3
  calvarium, calvaria (skull) 756.0
  canaliculus lacrimalis, congenital 743.65
  carpal(s) (congenital) (complete) (partial) (with
    absence of distal elements, incomplete) (*see
    also* Deformity, reduction, upper limb)
    755.28
    with complete absence of distal elements
      755.21
  cartilage 756.9

Absence—*continued*
    caudal spine 756.13
    cecum (acquired) (postoperative)
        (posttraumatic) V45.72
        congenital 751.2
    cementum 520.4
    cerebellum (congenital) (vermis) 742.2
    cervix (acquired) (uteri) V45.77
        congenital 752.49
    chin, congenital 744.89
    cilia (congenital) 743.63
        acquired 374.89
    circulatory system, part NEC 747.89
    clavicle 755.51
    clitoris (congenital) 752.49
    coccyx, congenital 756.13
    cold sense (see also Disturbance, sensation)
        782.0
    colon (acquired) (postoperative) V45.72
        congenital 751.2
    congenital
        lumen—see Atresia
        organ or site NEC—*see* Agenesis
        septum—*see* Imperfect, closure
    corpus callosum (congenital) 742.2
    cricoid cartilage 748.3
    diaphragm (congenital) (with hernia) 756.6
        with obstruction 756.6
    digestive organ(s) or tract, congenital
        (complete) (partial) 751.8
        acquired V45.79
        lower 751.5
        upper 750.8
    ductus arteriosus 747.89
    duodenum (acquired) (postoperative) V45.72
        congenital 751.1
    ear, congenital 744.09
        acquired V45.79
        auricle 744.01
        external 744.01
        inner 744.05
        lobe, lobule 744.21
        middle, except ossicles 744.03
            ossicles 744.04
        ossicles 744.04
    ejaculatory duct (congenital) 752.8
    endocrine gland NEC (congenital) 759.2
    epididymis (congenital) 752.8
        acquired V45.77
    epiglottis, congenital 748.3
    epileptic (atonic) (typical) (*see also* Epilepsy)
        345.0
    erythrocyte 284.9
    erythropoiesis 284.9
        congenital 284.0
    esophagus (congenital) 750.3
    Eustachian tube (congenital) 744.24
    extremity (acquired)
        congenital (*see also* Deformity, reduction)
            755.4
        lower V49.70
        upper V49.60
    extrinsic muscle, eye 743.69
    eye (acquired) V45.78
        adnexa (congenital) 743.69
        congenital 743.00
        muscle (congenital) 743.69
    eyelid (fold), congenital 743.62
        acquired 374.89
    face
        bones NEC 756.0

Absence—*continued*
    specified part NEC 744.89
    fallopian tube(s) (acquired) V45.77
        congenital 752.19
    femur, congenital (complete) (partial) (with
        absence of distal elements, incomplete) (*see
        also* Deformity, reduction, lower limb)
        755.34
        with
            complete absence of distal elements 755.31
            tibia and fibula (incomplete) 755.33
    fibrin 790.92
        fibrinogen (congenital) 286.3
        acquired 286.6
    fibula, congenital (complete) (partial) (with
        absence of distal elements, incomplete) (*see
        also* Deformity, reduction, lower limb)
        755.37
        with
            complete absence of distal elements 755.31
            tibia 755.35
                with
                    complete absence of distal elements
                        755.31
                    femur (incomplete) 755.33
                        with complete absence of distal
                            elements 755.31
    finger (acquired) V49.62
        congenital (complete) (partial) (*see also*
            Deformity, reduction, upper limb) 755.29
            meaning all fingers (complete) (partial)
                755.21
            transverse 755.21
    fissures of lungs (congenital) 748.5
    foot (acquired) V49.73
        congenital (complete) 755.31
    forearm (acquired) V49.65
        congenital (complete) (partial) (with absence
            of distal elements, incomplete) (*see also*
            Deformity, reduction, upper limb) 755.25
            with
                complete absence of distal elements (hand
                    and fingers) 755.21
                humerus (incomplete) 755.23
    fovea centralis 743.55
    fucosidase 271.8
    gallbladder (acquired) V45.79
        congenital 751.69
    gamma globulin (blood) 279.00
    genital organs
        acquired V45.77
        congenital
            female 752.8
                external 752.49
                internal NEC 752.8
            male 752.8
                penis 752.69
    genitourinary organs, congenital NEC 752.8
    glottis 748.3
    gonadal, congenital NEC 758.6
    hair (congenital) 757.4
        acquired—*see* Alopecia
    hand (acquired) V49.63
        congenital (complete) (*see also* Deformity,
            reduction, upper limb) 755.21
    heart (congenital) 759.89
        acquired—*see* Status, organ replacement
    heat sense (*see also* Disturbance, sensation)
        782.0

Absence—*continued*

humerus, congenital (complete) (partial) (with absence of distal elements, incomplete) (*see also* Deformity, reduction, upper limb) 755.24
with
complete absence of distal elements 755.21
radius and ulna (incomplete) 755.23
hymen (congenital) 752.49
ileum (acquired) (postoperative) (posttraumatic) V45.72
congenital 751.1
immunoglobulin, isolated NEC 279.03
IgA 279.01
IgG 279.03
IgM 279.02
incus (acquired) 385.24
congenital 744.04
internal ear (congenital) 744.05
intestine (acquired) (small) V45.72
congenital 751.1
large 751.2
large V45.72
congenital 751.2
iris (congenital) 743.45
jaw—*see* Absence, mandible
jejunum (acquired) V45.72
congenital 751.1
joint, congenital NEC 755.8
kidney(s) (acquired) V45.73
congenital 753.0
labium (congenital) (majus) (minus) 752.49
labyrinth, membranous 744.05
lacrimal apparatus (congenital) 743.65
larynx (congenital) 748.3
leg (acquired) V49.70
above knee V49.76
below knee V49.75
congenital (partial) (unilateral) (*see also* Deformity, reduction, lower limb) 755.31
lower (complete) (partial) (with absence of distal elements, incomplete) 755.35
with
complete absence of distal elements (foot and toes) 755.31
thigh (incomplete) 755.33
with complete absence of distal elements 755.31
upper—*see* Absence, femur
lens (congenital) 743.35
acquired 379.31
ligament, broad (congenital) 752.19
limb (acquired)
congenital (complete) (partial) (*see also* Deformity, reduction) 755.4
lower 755.30
complete 755.31
incomplete 755.32
longitudinal—*see* Deficiency, lower limb, longitudinal
transverse 755.31
upper 755.20
complete 755.21
incomplete 755.22
longitudinal—*see* Deficiency, upper limb, longitudinal
transverse 755.21
lower NEC V49.70
upper NEC V49.60
lip 750.26
liver (congenital) (lobe) 751.69

Absence—*continued*

lumbar (congenital) (vertebra) 756.13
isthmus 756.11
pars articularis 756.11
lumen—*see* Atresia
lung (bilateral) (congenital) (fissure) (lobe) (unilateral) 748.5
acquired (any part) V45.76
mandible (congenital) 524.09
maxilla (congenital) 524.09
menstruation 626.0
metacarpal(s), congenital (complete) (partial) (with absence of distal elements, incomplete) (*see also* Deformity, reduction, upper limb) 755.28
with all fingers, complete 755.21
metatarsal(s), congenital (complete) (partial) (with absence of distal elements, incomplete) (*see also* Deformity, reduction, lower limb) 755.38
with complete absence of distal elements 755.31
muscle (congenital) (pectoral) 756.81
ocular 743.69
musculoskeletal system (congenital) NEC 756.9
nail(s) (congenital) 757.5
neck, part 744.89
nerve 742.8
nervous system, part NEC 742.8
neutrophil 288.0
nipple (congenital) 757.6
nose (congenital) 748.1
acquired 738.0
nuclear 742.8
ocular muscle (congenital) 743.69
organ
of Corti (congenital) 744.05
or site
acquired V45.79
congenital NEC 759.89
osseous meatus (ear) 744.03
ovary (acquired) V45.77
congenital 752.0
oviduct (acquired) V45.77
congenital 752.19
pancreas (congenital) 751.7
acquired (postoperative) (posttraumatic) V45.79
parathyroid gland (congenital) 759.2
parotid gland(s) (congenital) 750.21
patella, congenital 755.64
pelvic girdle (congenital) 755.69
penis (congenital) 752.69
acquired V45.77
pericardium (congenital) 746.89
perineal body (congenital) 756.81
phalange(s), congenital 755.4
lower limb (complete) (intercalary) (partial) (terminal) (*see also* Deformity, reduction, lower limb) 755.39
meaning all toes (complete) (partial) 755.31
transverse 755.31
upper limb (complete) (intercalary) (partial) (terminal) (*see also* Deformity, reduction, upper limb) 755.29
meaning all digits (complete) (partial) 755.21
transverse 755.21
pituitary gland (congenital) 759.2
postoperative—*see* Absence, by site, acquired
prostate (congenital) 752.8

Absence—*continued*
  acquired V45.77
  pulmonary
    artery 747.3
    trunk 747.3
    valve (congenital) 746.01
    vein 747.49
  punctum lacrimale (congenital) 743.65
  radius, congenital (complete) (partial) (with
    absence of distal elements, incomplete)
    755.26
    with
      complete absence of distal elements 755.21
      ulna 755.25
        with
          complete absence of distal elements
            755.21
          humerus (incomplete) 755.23
  ray, congenital 755.4
    lower limb (complete) (partial) (*see also*
      Deformity, reduction, lower limb) 755.38
      meaning all rays 755.31
      transverse 755.31
    upper limb (complete) (partial) (*see also*
      Deformity, reduction, upper limb) 755.28
      meaning all rays 755.21
      transverse 755.21
  rectum (congenital) 751.2
    acquired V45.79
  red cell 284.9
    acquired (secondary) 284.8
    congenital 284.0
    hereditary 284.0
    idiopathic 284.9
  respiratory organ (congenital) NEC 748.9
  rib (acquired) 738.3
    congenital 756.3
  roof of orbit (congenital) 742.0
  round ligament (congenital) 752.8
  sacrum, congenital 756.13
  salivary gland(s) (congenital) 750.21
  scapula 755.59
  scrotum, congenital 752.8
  seminal tract or duct (congenital) 752.8
    acquired V45.77
  septum (congenital)—*see also* Imperfect,
    closure, septum
    atrial 745.69
      and ventricular 745.7
    between aorta and pulmonary artery 745.0
    ventricular 745.3
      and atrial 745.7
  sex chromosomes 758.81
  shoulder girdle, congenital (complete) (partial)
    755.59
  skin (congenital) 757.39
  skull bone 756.0
    with
      anencephalus 740.0
      encephalocele 742.0
      hydrocephalus 742.3
        with spina bifida (*see also* Spina bifida)
          741.0
      microcephalus 742.1
  spermatic cord (congenital) 752.8
  spinal cord 742.59
  spine, congenital 756.13
  spleen (congenital) 759.0
    acquired V45.79
  sternum, congenital 756.3

Absence—*continued*
  stomach (acquired) (partial) (postoperative)
    V45.75
    congenital 750.7
    with postgastric surgery syndrome 564.2
  submaxillary gland(s) (congenital) 750.21
  superior vena cava (congenital) 747.49
  tarsal(s), congenital (complete) (partial) (with
    absence of distal elements, incomplete) (*see
    also* Deformity, reduction, lower limb)
    755.38
  teeth, tooth (congenital) 520.0
    with abnormal spacing 524.3
    acquired 525.10
      due to
        caries 525.13
        extraction 525.10
        periodontal disease 525.12
        trauma 525.11
      with malocclusion 524.3
  tendon (congenital) 756.81
  testis (congenital) 752.8
    acquired V45.77
  thigh (acquired) 736.89
  thumb (acquired) V49.61
    congenital 755.29
  thymus gland (congenital) 759.2
  thyroid (gland) (surgical) 246.8
    with hypothyroidism 244.0
    cartilage, congenital 748.3
    congenital 243
  tibia, congenital (complete) (partial) (with
    absence of distal elements, incomplete) (*see
    also* Deformity, reduction, lower limb)
    755.36
    with
      complete absence of distal elements 755.31
      fibula 755.35
        with
          complete absence of distal elements
            755.31
      femur (incomplete) 755.33
        with complete absence of distal
          elements 755.31
  toe (acquired) V49.72
    congenital (complete) (partial) 755.39
      meaning all toes 755.31
      transverse 755.31
    great V49.71
  tongue (congenital) 750.11
  tooth, teeth, (congenital) 520.0
    with abnormal spacing 524.3
    acquired 525.10
      due to
        caries 525.13
        extraction 525.10
        periodontal disease 525.12
        trauma 525.11
      with malocclusion 524.3
  trachea (cartilage) (congenital) (rings) 748.3
  transverse aortic arch (congenital) 747.21
  tricuspid valve 746.1
  ulna, congenital (complete) (partial) (with
    absence of distal elements, incomplete) (*see
    also* Deformity, reduction, upper limb)
    755.27
    with
      complete absence of distal elements 755.21
      radius 755.25
        with

*Note—Use the following fifth-digit
subclassification with the following codes:
305.0, 305.2-305.9:*

0 unspecified
1 continuous
2 episodic
3 in remission

Abuse—*continued*
  mixed 305.9
  morphine type 305.5
  opioid type 305.5
  phencyclidine (PCP) 305.9
  specified NEC 305.9
  tranquilizers 305.4
  spouse 995.80
  tobacco 305.1
Acalcerosis 275.40
Acalcicosis 275.40
Acalculia 784.69
  developmental 315.1
Acanthocheilonemiasis 125.4
Acanthocytosis 272.5
Acanthokeratodermia 701.1
Acantholysis 701.8
  bullosa 757.39
Acanthoma (benign) (M8070/0)—*see also*
  Neoplasm, by site, benign
  malignant (M8070/3)—*see* Neoplasm, by site,
    malignant
Acanthosis (acquired) (nigricans) 701.2
  adult 701.2
  benign (congenital) 757.39
  congenital 757.39
  glycogenic
    esophagus 530.8
  juvenile 701.2
  tongue 529.8
Acanthrocytosis 272.5
Acapnia 276.3
Acarbia 276.2
Acardia 759.89
Acardiacus amorphus 759.89
Acardiotrophia 429.1
Acardius 759.89
Acariasis 133.9
  sarcoptic 133.0
Acaridiasis 133.9
Acarinosis 133.9
Acariosis 133.9
Acarodermatitis 133.9
  urticarioides 133.9
Acarophobia 300.29
Acatalasemia 277.8
Acatalasia 277.8
Acatamathesia 784.69
Acataphasia 784.5
Acathisia 781.0
  due to drugs 333.99
Acceleration, accelerated
  atrioventricular conduction 426.7
  idioventricular rhythm 427.89
Accessory (congenital)
  adrenal gland 759.1
  anus 751.5
  appendix 751.5
  atrioventricular conduction 426.7
  auditory ossicles 744.04
  auricle (ear) 744.1
  autosome(s) NEC 758.5
    21 or 22 758.0
  biliary duct or passage 751.69
  bladder 753.8
  blood vessels (peripheral) (congenital) NEC
    (*see also* Anomaly, peripheral vascular
    system) 747.60
    cerebral 747.81
    coronary 746.85
  bone NEC 756.9

Accessory—*continued*
  foot 755.67
  breast tissue, axilla 757.6
  carpal bones 755.56
  cecum 751.5
  cervix 752.49
  chromosome(s) NEC 758.5
    13-15 758.1
    16-18 758.2
    21 or 22 758.0
    autosome(s) NEC 758.5
    D_1 758.1
    E_3 758.2
    G 758.0
    sex 758.81
  coronary artery 746.85
  cusp(s), heart valve NEC 746.89
    pulmonary 746.09
  cystic duct 751.69
  digits 755.00
  ear (auricle) (lobe) 744.1
  endocrine gland NEC 759.2
  external os 752.49
  eyelid 743.62
  eye muscle 743.69
  face bone(s) 756.0
  fallopian tube (fimbria) (ostium) 752.19
  fingers 755.01
  foreskin 605
  frontonasal process 756.0
  gallbladder 751.69
  genital organ(s)
    female 752.8
      external 752.49
      internal NEC 752.8
    male NEC 752.8
      penis 752.69
  genitourinary organs NEC 752.8
  heart 746.89
    valve NEC 746.89
      pulmonary 746.09
  hepatic ducts 751.69
  hymen 752.49
  intestine (large) (small) 751.5
  kidney 753.3
  lacrimal canal 743.65
  leaflet, heart valve NEC 746.89
    pulmonary 746.09
  ligament, broad 752.19
  liver (duct) 751.69
  lobule (ear) 744.1
  lung (lobe) 748.69
  muscle 756.82
  navicular of carpus 755.56
  nervous system, part NEC 742.8
  nipple 757.6
  nose 748.1
  organ or site NEC—*see* Anomaly, specified
    type NEC
  ovary 752.0
  oviduct 752.19
  pancreas 751.7
  parathyroid gland 759.2
  parotid gland (and duct) 750.22
  pituitary gland 759.2
  placental lobe—*see* Placenta, abnormal
  preauricular appendage 744.1
  prepuce 605
  renal arteries (multiple) 747.62
  rib 756.3
    cervical 756.2

Acidemia 276.2
　arginosuccinic 270.6
　fetal
　　affecting management of pregnancy 656.3
　　before onset of labor, in liveborn infant 768.2
　　during labor, in liveborn infant 768.3
　　intrauterine—*see* Distress, fetal 656.3
　　unspecified as to time of onset, in liveborn
　　　infant 768.4
　pipecolic 270.7
Acidity, gastric (high) (low) 536.8
　psychogenic 306.4
Acidocytopenia 288.0
Acidocytosis 288.3
Acidopenia 288.0
Acidosis 276.2
　diabetic 250.1
　fetal, affecting newborn 768.9
　fetal, affecting management of pregnancy 656.8
　kidney tubular 588.8
　lactic 276.2
　metabolic NEC 276.2
　　with respiratory acidosis 276.4
　　late, of newborn 775.7
　renal
　　hyperchloremic 588.8
　　tubular (distal) (proximal) 588.8
　respiratory 276.2
　　complicated by
　　　metabolic acidosis 276.4
　　　metabolic alkalosis 276.4
Aciduria 791.9
　arginosuccinic 270.6
　beta-aminoisobutyric (BAIB) 277.2
　glycolic 271.8
　methylmalonic 270.3
　　with glycinemia 270.7
　organic 270.9
　orotic (congenital) (hereditary) (pyrimidine
　　deficiency) 281.4
Acladiosis 111.8
　skin 111.8
Aclasis
　diaphyseal 756.4
　tarsoepiphyseal 756.59
Acleistocardia 745.5
Aclusion 524.4
Acmesthesia 782.0
Acne (pustular) (vulgaris) 706.1
　agminata (*see also* Tuberculosis) 017.0
　artificialis 706.1
　atrophica 706.0
　cachecticorum (Hebra) 706.1
　conglobata 706.1
　conjunctiva 706.1
　cystic 706.1
　decalvans 704.09
　erythematosa 695.3
　eyelid 706.1
　frontalis 706.0
　indurata 706.1
　keloid 706.1
　lupoid 706.0
　necrotic, necrotica 706.0
　　miliaris 704.8
　nodular 706.1
　occupational 706.1
　papulosa 706.1
　rodens 706.0
　rosacea 695.3
　scorbutica 267

Acne—*continued*
　scrofulosorum (Bazin) (*see also* Tuberculosis)
　　017.0
　summer 692.72
　tropical 706.1
　varioliformis 706.0
Acneiform drug eruptions 692.3
Acnitis (primary) (*see also* Tuberculosis) 017.0
Acomia 704.00
Acontractile bladder 344.61
Aconuresis (*see also* Incontinence) 788.30
Acosta's disease 993.2
Acousma 780.1
Acoustic —*see* condition
Acousticophobia 300.29
Acquired —*see* condition
Acquired immunodeficiency syndrome —*see*
　　Human immunodeficiency virus (disease)
　　(illness) (infection)
Acragnosis 781.99
Acrania (monster) 740.0
Acroagnosis 781.99
Acroasphyxia, chronic 443.89
Acrobrachycephaly 756.0
Acrobystiolith 608.89
Acrobystitis 607.2
Acrocephalopolysyndactyly 755.55
Acrocephalosyndactyly 755.55
Acrocephaly 756.0
Acrochondrohyperplasia 759.82
Acrocyanosis 443.89
　newborn 770.83
Acrodermatitis 686.8
　atrophicans (chronica) 701.8
　continua (Hallopeau) 696.1
　enteropathica 686.8
　Hallopeau's 696.1
　perstans 696.1
　pustulosa continua 696.1
　recalcitrant pustular 696.1
Acrodynia 985.0
Acrodysplasia 755.55
Acrohyperhidrosis 780.8
Acrokeratosis verruciformis 757.39
Acromastitis 611.0
Acromegaly, acromegalia (skin) 253.0
Acromelalgia 443.89
Acromicria, acromikria 756.59
Acronyx 703.0
Acropachy, thyroid (*see also* Thyrotoxicosis)
　　242.9
Acropachyderma 757.39
Acroparesthesia 443.89
　simple (Schultz's type) 443.89
　vasomotor (Nothnagel's type) 443.89
Acropathy thyroid (*see also* Thyrotoxicosis)
　　242.9
Acrophobia 300.29
Acroposthitis 607.2
Acroscleriasis (*see also* Scleroderma) 710.1
Acroscleroderma (*see also* Scleroderma) 710.1
Acrosclerosis (*see also* Scleroderma) 710.1
Acrosphacelus 785.4
Acrosphenosyndactylia 755.55
Acrospiroma, eccrine (M8402/0)—*see*
　　Neoplasm, skin, benign
Acrostealgia 732.9
Acrosyndactyly (*see also* Syndactylism) 755.10
Acrotrophodynia 991.4

Actinic —*see also* condition
  cheilitis (due to sun) 692.72
    chronic NEC 692.74
    due to radiation, except from sun 692.82
  conjunctivitis 370.24
  dermatitis (due to sun) (*see also* Dermatitis,
    actinic) 692.70
  due to
    roentgen rays or radioactive substance
      692.82
    ultraviolet radiation, except from sun 692.82
    sun NEC 692.70
  elastosis solare 692.74
  granuloma 692.73
  keratitis 370.24
  ophthalmia 370.24
  reticuloid 692.73
Actinobacillosis, general 027.8
Actinobacillus
  lignieresii 027.8
  mallei 024
  muris 026.1
Actinocutitis NEC (*see also* Dermatitis, actinic)
  692.70
Actinodermatitis NEC (*see also* Dermatitis,
  actinic) 692.70
Actinomyces
  israelii (infection)—*see* Actinomycosis
  muris-ratti (infection) 026.1
Actinomycosis actinomycotic 039.9
  with
    pneumonia 039.1
  abdominal 039.2
  cervicofacial 039.3
  cutaneous 039.0
  pulmonary 039.1
  specified site NEC 039.8
  thoracic 039.1
Actinoneuritis 357.89
Action, heart
  disorder 427.9
    postoperative 997.1
  irregular 427.9
    postoperative 997.1
  psychogenic 306.2
Active —*see* condition
Activity decrease, functional 780.99
Acute —*see also* condition
  abdomen NEC 789.0
  gallbladder (*see also* Cholecystitis, acute) 575.0
Acyanoblepsia 368.53
Acyanopsia 368.53
Acystia 753.8
Acystinervia —*see* Neurogenic, bladder
Acystineuria —*see* Neurogenic, bladder
Adactylia, adactyly (congenital) 755.4
  lower limb (complete) (intercalary) (partial)
    (terminal) (*see also* Deformity, reduction,
    lower limb) 755.39
Adactylia, adactyly—*continued*
  meaning all digits (complete) (partial) 755.31
    transverse (complete) (partial) 755.31
  upper limb (complete) (intercalary) (partial)
    (terminal) (*see also* Deformity, reduction,
    upper limb) 755.29
    meaning all digits (complete) (partial) 755.21
    transverse (complete) (partial) 755.21
Adair-Dighton syndrome (brittle bones and blue
  sclera, deafness) 756.51
Adamantinoblastoma (M9310/0)—*see*
  Ameloblastoma
Adamantinoma (M9310/0)—*see* Ameloblastoma

Adamantoblastoma (M9310/0)—*see*
  Ameloblastoma
Adams-Stokes (-Morgagni) disease or syndrome
  (syncope with heart block) 426.9
Adaptation reaction (*see also* Reaction,
  adjustment) 309.9
Addiction —*see also* Dependence
  absinthe 304.6
  alcoholic (ethyl) (methyl) (wood) 303.9
    complicating pregnancy, childbirth, or
      puerperium 648.4
      affecting fetus or newborn 760.71
    suspected damage to fetus affecting
      management of pregnancy 655.4
  drug (*see also* Dependence) 304.9
  ethyl alcohol 303.9
  heroin 304.0
  hospital 301.51
  methyl alcohol 303.9
  methylated spirit 303.9
  morphine (-like substances) 304.0
  nicotine 305.1
  opium 304.0
  tobacco 305.1
  wine 303.9
Addison's
  anemia (pernicious) 281.0
  disease (bronze) (primary adrenal insufficiency)
    255.4
    tuberculous (*see also* Tuberculosis) 017.6
  keloid (morphea) 701.0
  melanoderma (adrenal cortical hypofunction)
    255.4
Addison-Biermer anemia (pernicious) 281.0
Addison-Gull disease —*see* Xanthoma
Addisonian crisis or melanosis (acute
  adrenocortical insufficiency) 255.4
Additional —*see also* Accessory
  chromosome(s) 758.5
    13-15 758.1
    16-18 758.2
    21 758.0
    autosome(s) NEC 758.5
    sex 758.81
Adduction contracture, hip or other joint
  —*see* Contraction, joint
Adenasthenia gastrica 536.0
Aden fever 061
Adenitis (*see also* Lymphadenitis) 289.3
  acute, unspecified site 683
    epidemic infectious 075
  axillary 289.3
    acute 683
    chronic or subacute 289.1
  Bartholin's gland 616.8
  bulbourethral gland (*see also* Urethritis) 597.89
  cervical 289.3
    acute 683
    chronic or subacute 289.1
  chancroid (Ducrey's bacillus) 099.0
  chronic (any lymph node, except mesenteric)
    289.1
    mesenteric 289.2
  Cowper's gland (*see also* Urethritis) 597.89
  epidemic, acute 075
  gangrenous 683
  gonorrheal NEC 098.89
  groin 289.3
    acute 683
    chronic or subacute 289.1
  infectious 075

Note—The list of adjectival modifiers below is not exhaustive. A description of adenocarcinoma that does not appear in this list should be coded in the same manner as carcinoma with that description. Thus, "mixed acidophil-basophil adenocarcinoma," should be coded in the same manner as "mixed acidophil-basophil carcinoma," which appears in the list under "Carcinoma."

Except where otherwise indicated, the morphological varieties of adenocarcinoma in the list below should be coded by site as for "Neoplasm, malignant."

Adenocarcinoma—*continued*
  in situ (M8140/2)—*see* Neoplasm, by site, in
    situ
  intestinal type (M8144/3)
    specified site—*see* Neoplasm, by site,
      malignant
    unspecified site 151.9
  intraductal (noninfiltrating) (M8500/2)
    papillary (M8503/2)
      specified site—*see* Neoplasm, by site, in situ
      unspecified site 233.0
    specified site—*see* Neoplasm, by site, in situ
    unspecified site 233.0
  islet cell (M8150/3)
    and exocrine, mixed (M8154/3)
      specified site—*see* Neoplasm, by site,
        malignant
      unspecified site 157.9
    pancreas 157.4
    specified site NEC—*see* Neoplasm, by site,
      malignant
    unspecified site 157.4
  lobular (M8520/3)
    specified site—*see* Neoplasm, by site,
      malignant
    unspecified site 174.9
  medullary (M8510/3)
  mesonephric (M9110/3)
  mixed cell (M8323/3)
  mucinous (M8480/3)
  mucin-producing (M8481/3)
  mucoid (M8480/3)—*see also* Neoplasm, by
    site, malignant
    cell (M8300/3)
      specified site—*see* Neoplasm, by site,
        malignant
      unspecified site 194.3
  nonencapsulated sclerosing (M8350/3) 193
  oncocytic (M8290/3)
  oxyphilic (M8290/3)
  papillary (M8260/3)
    and follicular (M8340/3) 193
    intraductal (noninfiltrating) (M8503/2)
      specified site—*see* Neoplasm, by site, in situ
      unspecified site 233.0
    serous (M8460/3)
      specified site—*see* Neoplasm, by site,
        malignant
      unspecified site 183.0
  papillocystic (M8450/3)
    specified site—*see* Neoplasm, by site,
      malignant
    unspecified site 183.0
  pseudomucinous (M8470/3)
    specified site—*see* Neoplasm, by site,
      malignant
    unspecified site 183.0
  renal cell (M8312/3) 189.0
  sebaceous (M8410/3)
  serous (M8441/3)—*see also* Neoplasm, by site,
    malignant
    papillary
      specified site—*see* Neoplasm, by site,
        malignant
      unspecified site 183.0
  signet ring cell (M8490/3)
  superficial spreading (M8143/3)
  sweat gland (M8400/3)—*see* Neoplasm, skin,
    malignant
  trabecular (M8190/3)
  tubular (M8211/3)

Adenocarcinoma—*continued*
  villous (M8262/3)
  water-clear cell (M8322/3) 194.1
Adenofibroma (M9013/0)
  clear cell (M8313/0)—*see* Neoplasm, by site,
    benign
  endometrioid (M8381/0) 220
    borderline malignancy (M8381/1) 236.2
    malignant (M8381/3) 183.0
  mucinous (M9015/0)
    specified site—*see* Neoplasm, by site, benign
    unspecified site 220
  prostate 600.2
  serous (M9014/0)
    specified site—*see* Neoplasm, by site, benign
    unspecified site 220
  specified site—*see* Neoplasm, by site, benign
  unspecified site 220
Adenofibrosis
  breast 610.2
  endometrioid 617.0
Adenoiditis 474.01
  acute 463
  chronic 474.01
    with chronic tonsillitis 474.02
Adenoids (congenital) (of nasal fossa) 474.9
  hypertrophy 474.12
  vegetations 474.2
Adenolipomatosis (symmetrical) 272.8
Adenolymphoma (M8561/0)
  specified site—*see* Neoplasm, by site, benign
  unspecified 210.2
Adenoma (sessile) (M8140/0)—*see also*
    Neoplasm, by site, benign

---

*Note—Except where otherwise indicated, the
morphological varieties of adenoma in the list
below should be coded by site as for
"Neoplasm, benign."*

---

  acidophil (M8280/0)
    specified site—*see* Neoplasm, by site, benign
    unspecified site 227.3
  acinar (cell) (M8550/0)
  acinic cell (M8550/0)
  adrenal (cortex) (cortical) (functioning)
      (M8370/0) 227.0
    clear cell type (M8373/0) 227.0
    compact cell type (M8371/0) 227.0
    glomerulosa cell type (M8374/0) 227.0
    heavily pigmented variant (M8372/0) 227.0
    mixed cell type (M8375/0) 227.0
  alpha cell (M8152/0)
    pancreas 211.7
    specified site NEC—*see* Neoplasm, by site,
      benign
    unspecified site 211.7
  alveolar (M8251/0)
  apocrine (M8401/0)
    breast 217
    specified site NEC—*see* Neoplasm, skin,
      benign
    unspecified site 216.9
  basal cell (M8147/0)
  basophil (M8300/0)
    specified site—*see* Neoplasm, by site, benign
    unspecified site 227.3
  beta cell (M8151/0)
    pancreas 211.7
    specified site NEC—*see* Neoplasm, by site,
      benign
    unspecified site 211.7

Adenoma—*continued*
bile duct (M8160/0) 211.5
black (M8372/0) 227.0
bronchial (M8140/1) 235.7
  carcinoid type (M8240/3)—*see* Neoplasm,
    lung, malignant
  cylindroid type (M8200/3)—*see* Neoplasm,
    lung, malignant
ceruminous (M8420/0) 216.2
chief cell (M8321/0) 227.1
chromophobe (M8270/0)
  (specified site—*see* Neoplasm, by site, benign
  unspecified site 227.3
clear cell (M8310/0)
colloid (M8334/0)
  specified site—*see* Neoplasm, by site, benign
  unspecified site 226
cylindroid type, bronchus (M8200/3)—*see*
    Neoplasm, lung, malignant
duct (M8503/0)
embryonal (M8191/0)
endocrine, multiple (M8360/1)
  single specified site—*see* Neoplasm, by site,
    uncertain behavior
  two or more specified sites 237.4
  unspecified site 237.4
endometrioid (M8380/0)—*see also* Neoplasm,
    by site, benign
  borderline malignancy (M8380/1)—*see*
    Neoplasm, by site, uncertain behavior
eosinophil (M8280/0)
  specified site—*see* Neoplasm, by site, benign
  unspecified site 227.3
fetal (M8333/0)
  specified site—*see* Neoplasm, by site, benign
  unspecified site 226
follicular (M8330/0)
  specified site—*see* Neoplasm, by site, benign
  unspecified site 226
hepatocellular (M8170/0) 211.5
Hürthle cell (M8290/0) 226
intracystic papillary (M8504/0)
islet cell (functioning) (M8150/0)
  pancreas 211.7
  specified site NEC—*see* Neoplasm, by site,
    benign
  unspecified site 211.7
liver cell (M8170/0) 211.5
macrofollicular (M8334/0)
  specified site NEC—*see* Neoplasm, by site,
    benign
  unspecified site 226
malignant, malignum (M8140/3)—*see*
    Neoplasm, by site, malignant
mesonephric (M9110/0)
microfollicular (M8333/0)
  specified site—*see* Neoplasm, by site, benign
  unspecified site 226
mixed cell (M8323/0)
monomorphic (M8146/0)
mucinous (M8480/0)
mucoid cell (M8300/0)
  specified site—*see* Neoplasm, by site, benign
  unspecified site 227.3
multiple endocrine (M8360/1)
  single specified site—*see* Neoplasm, by site,
    uncertain behavior
  two or more specified sites 237.4
  unspecified site 237.4
nipple (M8506/0) 217
oncocytic (M8290/0)

Adenoma—*continued*
oxyphilic (M8290/0)
papillary (M8260/0)—*see also* Neoplasm, by
    site, benign
  intracystic (M8504/0)
papillotubular (M8263/0)
Pick's tubular (M8640/0)
  specified site—*see* Neoplasm, by site, benign
  unspecified site
    female 220
    male 222.0
pleomorphic (M8940/0)
polypoid (M8210/0)
prostate (benign) 600.2
rete cell 222.0
sebaceous, sebaceum (gland) (senile)
  (M8410/0)—*see also* Neoplasm, skin,
    benign
  disseminata 759.5
Sertoli cell (M8640/0)
  specified site—*see* Neoplasm, by site, benign
  unspecified site
    female 220
    male 222.0
skin appendage (M8390/0)—*see* Neoplasm,
    skin, benign
sudoriferous gland (M8400/0)—*see* Neoplasm,
    skin, benign
sweat gland or duct (M8400/0)—*see* Neoplasm,
    skin, benign
testicular (M8640/0)
  specified site—*see* Neoplasm, by site, benign
  unspecified site
    female 220
    male 222.0
thyroid 226
trabecular (M8190/0)
tubular (M8211/0)—*see also* Neoplasm, by site,
    benign
  papillary (M8460/3)
  Pick's (M8640/0)
    specified site—*see* Neoplasm, by site,
      benign
    unspecified site
      female 220
      male 222.0
tubulovillous (M8263/0)
villoglandular (M8263/0)
villous (M8261/1)—*see* Neoplasm, by site,
    uncertain behavior
water-clear cell (M8322/0) 227.1
wolffian duct (M9110/0)
Adenomatosis (M8220/0)
endocrine (multiple) (M8360/1)
  single specified site—*see* Neoplasm, by site,
    uncertain behavior
  two or more specified sites 237.4
  unspecified site 237.4
erosive of nipple (M8506/0) 217
pluriendocrine—*see* Adenomatosis, endocrine
pulmonary (M8250/1) 235.7
  malignant (M8250/3)—*see* Neoplasm, lung,
    malignant
  specified site—*see* Neoplasm, by site, benign
  unspecified site 211.3
Adenomatous
cyst, thyroid (gland)—*see* Goiter, nodular
goiter (nontoxic) (*see also* Goiter, nodular)
    241.9
  toxic or with hyperthyroidism 242.3

Adenomyoma (M8932/0)—*see also* Neoplasm,
by site, benign
prostate 600.2
Adenomyometritis 617.0
Adenomyosis (uterus) (internal) 617.0
Adenopathy (lymph gland) 785.6
inguinal 785.6
mediastinal 785.6
mesentery 785.6
syphilitic (secondary) 091.4
tracheobronchial 785.6
tuberculous (*see also* Tuberculosis) 012.1
primary, progressive 010.8
tuberculous (*see also* Tuberculosis, lymph
gland) 017.2
tracheobronchial 012.1
primary, progressive 010.8
Adenopharyngitis 462
Adenophlegmon 683
Adenosalpingitis 614.1
Adenosarcoma (M8960/3) 189.0
Adenosclerosis 289.3
Adenosis
breast (sclerosing) 610.2
vagina, congenital 752.49
Adentia (complete) (partial) (*see also* Absence,
teeth) 520.0
Adherent
labium (minus) 624.4
pericardium (nonrheumatic) 423.1
rheumatic 393
placenta 667.0
with hemorrhage 666.0
prepuce 605
scar (skin) NEC 709.2
tendon in scar 709.2
**Adhesion(s), adhesive (postinfectional)(postop-
erative)**
abdominal (wall) (*see also* Adhesions,
peritoneum) 568.0
amnion to fetus 658.8
affecting fetus or newborn 762.8
appendix 543.9
arachnoiditis—*see* Meningitis
auditory tube (Eustachian) 381.89
bands—*see also* Adhesions, peritoneum
cervix 622.3
uterus 621.5
bile duct (any) 576.8
bladder (sphincter) 596.8
bowel (*see also* Adhesions, peritoneum) 568.0
cardiac 423.1
rheumatic 398.99
cecum (*see also* Adhesions, peritoneum) 568.0
cervicovaginal 622.3
congenital 752.49
postpartal 674.8
old 622.3
cervix 622.3
clitoris 624.4
colon (*see also* Adhesions, peritoneum) 568.0
common duct 576.8
congenital—*see also* Anomaly, specified type
NEC
fingers (*see also* Syndactylism, fingers) 755.11
labium (majus) (minus) 752.49
omental, anomalous 751.4
ovary 752.0
peritoneal 751.4
toes (*see also* Syndactylism, toes) 755.13
tongue (to gum or roof of mouth) 750.12

Adhesion(s)—*continued*
conjunctiva (acquired) (localized) 372.62
congenital 743.63
extensive 372.63
cornea—*see* Opacity, cornea
cystic duct 575.8
diaphragm (*see also* Adhesions, peritoneum)
568.0
due to foreign body—*see* Foreign body
duodenum (*see also* Adhesions, peritoneum)
568.0
with obstruction 537.3
ear, middle—*see* Adhesions, middle ear
epididymis 608.89
epidural—*see* Adhesions, meninges
epiglottis 478.79
Eustachian tube 381.89
eyelid 374.46
postoperative 997.99
surgically created V45.69
gallbladder (*see also* Disease, gallbladder) 575.8
globe 360.89
heart 423.1
rheumatic 398.99
ileocecal (coil) (*see also* Adhesions,
peritoneum) 568.0
ileum (*see also* Adhesions, peritoneum) 568.0
intestine (postoperative) (*see also* Adhesions,
peritoneum) 568.0
with obstruction 560.81
with hernia—*see also* Hernia, by site, with
obstruction
gangrenous—*see* Hernia, by site, with
gangrene
intra-abdominal (*see also* Adhesions,
peritoneum) 568.0
iris 364.70
to corneal graft 996.79
joint (*see also* Ankylosis) 718.5
kidney 593.89
labium (majus) (minus), congenital 752.49
liver 572.8
lung 511.0
mediastinum 519.3
meninges 349.2
cerebral (any) 349.2
congenital 742.4
congenital 742.8
spinal (any) 349.2
congenital 742.59
tuberculous (cerebral) (spinal) (*see also*
Tuberculosis, meninges) 013.0
mesenteric (*see also* Adhesions, peritoneum)
568.0
middle ear (fibrous) 385.10
drum head 385.19
to
incus 385.11
promontorium 385.13
stapes 385.12
specified NEC 385.19
nasal (septum) (to turbinates) 478.1
nerve NEC 355.9
spinal 355.9
root 724.9
cervical NEC 723.4
lumbar NEC 724.4
lumbosacral 724.4
thoracic 724.4
ocular muscle 378.60

Adhesion—*continued*
  omentum (*see also* Adhesions, peritoneum)
    568.0
  organ or site, congenital NEC—*see* Anomaly,
    specified type NEC
  ovary 614.6
    congenital (to cecum, kidney, or omentum)
      752.0
  parauterine 614.6
  parovarian 614.6
  pelvic (peritoneal)
    female 614.6
    male (*see also* Adhesions, peritoneum) 568.0
    postpartal (old) 614.6
    tuberculous (*see also* Tuberculosis) 016.9
  penis to scrotum (congenital) 752.69
  periappendiceal (*see also* Adhesions,
    peritoneum) 568.0
  pericardium (nonrheumatic) 423.1
    rheumatic 393
    tuberculous (*see also* Tuberculosis) 017.9
      [420.0]
  pericholecystic 575.8
  perigastric (*see also* Adhesions, peritoneum)
    568.0
  periovarian 614.6
  periprostatic 602.8
  perirectal (*see also* Adhesions, peritoneum)
    568.0
  perirenal 593.89
  peritoneum, peritoneal (fibrous) (postoperative)
    568.0
    with obstruction (intestinal) 560.81
      with hernia—*see also* Hernia, by site, with
        obstruction
        gangrenous—*see* Hernia, by site, with
          gangrene
    duodenum 537.3
    congenital 751.4
    female, (postoperative) (postinfective) 614.6
    pelvic, female 614.6
    pelvic, male 568.0
    postpartal, pelvic 614.6
    to uterus 614.6
  peritubal 614.6
  periureteral 593.89
  periuterine 621.5
  perivesical 596.8
  perivesicular (seminal vesicle) 608.89
  pleura, pleuritic 511.0
    tuberculous (*see also* Tuberculosis, pleura)
      012.0
  pleuropericardial 511.0
  postoperative (gastrointestinal tract) (*See also*
    Adhesions, peritoneum) 568.0
    eyelid 997.99
      surgically created V45.69
    urethra 598.2
  postpartal, old 624.4
  preputial, prepuce 605
  pulmonary 511.0
  pylorus (*see also* Adhesions, peritoneum) 568.0
  Rosenmüller's fossa 478.29
  sciatic nerve 355.0
  seminal vesicle 608.89
  shoulder (joint) 726.0
  sigmoid flexure (*see also* Adhesions,
    peritoneum) 568.0
  spermatic cord (acquired) 608.89
    congenital 752.8
  spinal canal 349.2

Adhesion—*continued*
  nerve 355.9
    root 724.9
      cervical NEC 723.4
      lumbar NEC 724.4
      lumbosacral 724.4
      thoracic 724.4
  stomach (*see also* Adhesions, peritoneum) 568.0
  subscapular 726.2
  tendonitis 726.90
    shoulder 726.0
  testicle 608.89
  tongue (congenital) (to gum or roof of mouth)
    750.12
    acquired 529.8
  trachea 519.1
  tubo-ovarian 614.6
  tunica vaginalis 608.89
  ureter 593.89
  uterus 621.5
    to abdominal wall 614.6
      in pregnancy or childbirth 654.4
        affecting fetus or newborn 763.89
  vagina (chronic) (postoperative) (postradiation)
    623.2
  vaginitis (congenital) 752.49
  vesical 596.8
  vitreous 379.29
Adie (-Holmes) syndrome (tonic pupillary
  reaction) 379.46
Adiponecrosis neonatorum 778.1
Adiposa dolorosa 272.8
Adiposalgia 272.8
Adiposis 278.0
  cerebralis 253.8
  dolorosa 272.8
  tuberosa simplex 272.8
Adiposity 278.0
  heart (*see also* Degeneration, myocardial) 429.1
  localized 278.1
Adiposogenital dystrophy 253.8
Adjustment
  prosthesis or other device—*see* Fitting of
  reaction—*see* Reaction, adjustment
Administration, prophylactic
  antibiotics V07.39
  antitoxin, any V07.2
  antivenin V07.2
  chemotherapeutic agent NEC V07.39
  chemotherapy NEC V07.39
  diphtheria antitoxin V07.2
  fluoride V07.31
  gamma globulin V07.2
  immune sera (gamma globulin) V07.2
  passive immunization agent V07.2
  RhoGAM V07.2
Admission (encounter)
  as organ donor—*see* Donor
  by mistake V68.9
  for
    adequacy testing (for)
      hemodialysis V56.31
      peritoneal dialysis V56.32
    adjustment (of)
      artificial
        arm (complete) (partial) V52.0
        eye V52.2
        leg (complete) (partial) V52.1
      brain neuropacemaker V53.02
      breast
        implant V50.1

Admission—*continued*
    prosthesis V52.4
    cardiac device V53.39
      defibrillator, automatic implantable V53.32
      pacemaker V53.31
        carotid sinus V53.39
    catheter
      non-vascular V58.82
      vascular V58.81
    cerebral ventricle (communicating) shunt V53.01
    colostomy belt V53.5
    contact lenses V53.1
    cystostomy device V53.6
    dental prosthesis V52.3
    device NEC V53.9
      abdominal V53.5
      cardiac V53.39
        defibrillator, automatic implantable V53.32
        pacemaker V53.31
          carotid sinus V53.39
      cerebral ventricle (communicating) shunt V53.01
      intrauterine contraceptive V25.1
      nervous system V53.09
      orthodontic V53.4
      prosthetic V52.9
        breast V52.4
        dental V52.3
        eye V52.2
        specified type NEC V52.8
      special senses V53.09
      substitution
        auditory V53.09
        nervous system V53.09
        visual V53.09
      urinary V53.6
    dialysis catheter
      extracorporeal V56.1
      peritoneal V56.2
    diaphragm (contraceptive) V25.02
    hearing aid V53.2
    ileostomy device V53.5
    intestinal appliance or device NEC V53.5
    intrauterine contraceptive device V25.1
    neuropacemaker (brain) (peripheral nerve) (spinal cord) V53.02
    orthodontic device V53.4
    orthopedic (device) V53.7
      brace V53.7
      cast V53.7
      shoes V53.7
    pacemaker
      brain V53.02
      cardiac V53.31
      carotid sinus V53.39
      peripheral nerve V53.02
      spinal cord V53.02
    prosthesis V52.9
      arm (complete) (partial) V52.0
      breast V52.4
      dental V52.3
      eye V52.2
      leg (complete) (partial) V52.1
      specified type NEC V52.8
    spectacles V53.1
    wheelchair V53.8
    adoption referral or proceedings V68.89
    aftercare (*see also* Aftercare) V58.9
      cardiac pacemaker V53.31

Admission—*continued*
    chemotherapy V58.1
    dialysis
      extracorporeal (renal) V56.0
      peritoneal V56.8
      renal V56.0
    fracture (*see also* Aftercare, fracture) V54.9
    medical NEC V58.89
    orthopedic V54.9
      specified care NEC V54.89
      specified type NEC V54.8
    pacemaker device
      brain V53.02
      cardiac V53.31
      carotid sinus V53.39
      nervous system V53.02
      spinal cord V53.02
    postoperative NEC V58.49
      wound closure, planned V58.41
    postpartum
      immediately after delivery V24.0
      routine follow-up V24.2
    postradiation V58.0
    radiation therapy V58.0
    removal of
      non-vascular catheter V58.82
      vascular catheter V58.81
    specified NEC V58.89
      removal of vascular catheter V58.81
    surgical NEC V58.49
      wound closure, planned V58.41
    artificial insemination V26.1
    attention to artificial opening (of) V55.9
      artificial vagina V55.7
      colostomy V55.3
      cystostomy V55.5
      enterostomy V55.4
      gastrostomy V55.1
      ileostomy V55.2
      jejunostomy V55.4
      nephrostomy V55.6
      specified site NEC V55.8
        intestinal tract V55.4
        urinary tract V55.6
      tracheostomy V55.0
      ureterostomy V55.6
      urethrostomy V55.6
    battery replacement
      cardiac pacemaker V53.31
    boarding V65.0
    breast
      augmentation or reduction V50.1
      removal, prophylactic V50.41
    change of
      cardiac pacemaker (battery) V53.31
      carotid sinus pacemaker V53.39
      catheter in artificial opening—*see* Attention to, artificial, opening
      dressing V58.3
      fixation device
        external V54.89
        internal V54.0
      Kirschner wire V54.89
      neuropacemaker device (brain) (peripheral nerve) (spinal cord) V53.02
      pacemaker device
        brain V53.02
        cardiac V53.31
        carotid sinus V53.39
        nervous system V53.02
      plaster cast V54.89

Admission—*continued*
  splint, external V54.89
  Steinmann pin V54.89
  surgical dressing V58.3
  traction device V54.89
 checkup only V70.0
 chemotherapy V58.1
 circumcision, ritual or routine (in absence of
    medical indication) V50.2
 clinical research investigation (control)
    (normal comparison) (participant) V70.7
 closure of artificial opening—*see* Attention to,
    artificial, opening
 contraceptive
  counseling V25.09
  management V25.9
   specified type NEC V25.8
 convalescence following V66.9
  chemotherapy V66.2
  psychotherapy V66.3
  radiotherapy V66.1
  surgery V66.0
  treatment (for) V66.5
   combined V66.6
   fracture V66.4
   mental disorder NEC V66.3
   specified condition NEC V66.5
 cosmetic surgery NEC V50.1
  following healed injury or operation V51
 counseling (*see also* Counseling) V65.40
  without complaint or sickness V65.49
  contraceptive management V25.09
  dietary V65.3
  exercise V65.41
  for
   nonattending third party V65.1
   victim of abuse
    child V61.21
    partner or spouse V61.11
  genetic V26.3
  gonorrhea V65.45
  HIV V65.44
  human immunodeficiency virus V65.44
  injury prevention V65.43
  procreative management V26.4
  sexually transmitted disease NEC V65.45
   HIV V65.44
  specified reason NEC V65.49
  substance use and abuse V65.42
  syphilis V65.45
  victim of abuse
   child V61.21
   partner or spouse V61.11
 desensitization to allergens V07.1
 dialysis V56.0
  catheter
   fitting and adjustment
    extracorporeal V56.1
    peritoneal V56.2
   removal or replacement
    extracorporeal V56.1
    peritoneal V56.2
  extracorporeal (renal) V56.0
  peritoneal V56.8
  renal V56.0
 dietary surveillance and counseling V65.3
 drug monitoring, therapeutic V58.83
 ear piercing V50.3
 elective surgery V50.9
  breast
   augmentation or reduction V50.1

Admission—*continued*
  removal, prophylactic V50.41
 circumcision, ritual or routine (in absence of
    medical indication) V50.2
 cosmetic NEC V50.1
  following healed injury or operation V51
 ear piercing V50.3
 face-lift V50.1
 hair transplant V50.0
 plastic
  cosmetic NEC V50.1
  following healed injury or operation V51
 prophylactic organ removal V50.49
  breast V50.41
  ovary V50.42
 repair of scarred tissue (following healed
    injury or operation) V51
 specified type NEC V50.8
 end-of-life care V66.7
 examination (*see also* Examination) V70.9
  administrative purpose NEC V70.3
  adoption V70.3
  allergy V72.7
  at health care facility V70.0
  athletic team V70.3
  camp V70.3
  cardiovascular, preoperative V72.81
  clinical research investigation (control)
    (participant) V70.7
  dental V72.2
  developmental testing (child) (infant) V20.2
  donor (potential) V70.8
  driver's license V70.3
  ear V72.1
  employment V70.5
  eye V72.0
  follow-up (routine)—*see* Examination,
    follow-up
  for admission to
   old age home V70.3
   school V70.3
  general V70.9
   specified reason NEC V70.8
  gynecological V72.3
  health supervision (child) (infant) V20.2
  hearing V72.1
  immigration V70.3
  insurance certification V70.3
  laboratory V72.6
  marriage license V70.3
  medical (general) (*see also* Examination,
    medical) V70.9
  medicolegal reasons V70.4
  naturalization V70.3
  pelvic (annual) (periodic) V72.3
  postpartum checkup V24.2
  pregnancy (possible) (unconfirmed) V72.4
  preoperative V72.84
   cardiovascular V72.81
   respiratory V72.82
   specified NEC V72.83
  prison V70.3
  psychiatric (general) V70.2
   requested by authority V70.1
  radiological NEC V72.5
  respiratory, preoperative V72.82
  school V70.3
  screening—*see* Screening
  skin hypersensitivity V72.7
  specified type NEC V72.85
  sport competition V70.3

Admission—*continued*
    vision V72.0
    well baby and child care V20.2
    exercise therapy V57.1
    face-lift, cosmetic reason V50.1
    fitting (of)
        artificial
            arm (complete) (partial) V52.0
            eye V52.2
            leg (complete) (partial) V52.1
        biliary drainage tube V58.82
        brain neuropacemaker V53.02
        breast V52.4
            implant V50.1
            prosthesis V52.4
        cardiac pacemaker V53.31
        catheter
            non-vascular V58.82
            vascular V58.81
        cerebral ventricle (communicating) shunt
            V53.01
        chest tube V58.82
        colostomy belt V53.5
        contact lenses V53.1
        cystostomy device V53.6
        dental prosthesis V52.3
        device NEC V53.9
            abdominal V53.5
            cerebral ventricle (communicating) shunt
                V53.01
            intrauterine contraceptive V25.1
            nervous system V53.09
            orthodontic V53.4
            prosthetic V52.9
                breast V52.4
                dental V52.3
                eye V52.2
            special senses V53.09
            substitution
                auditory V53.09
                nervous system V53.09
                visual V53.09
        diaphragm (contraceptive) V25.02
        fistula (sinus tract) drainage tube V58.82
        hearing aid V53.2
        ileostomy device V53.5
        intestinal appliance or device NEC V53.5
        intrauterine contraceptive device V25.1
        neuropacemaker (brain) (peripheral nerve)
            (spinal cord) V53.02
        orthodontic device V53.4
        orthopedic (device) V53.7
            brace V53.7
            cast V53.7
            shoes V53.7
        pacemaker
            brain V53.02
            cardiac V53.31
            carotid sinus V53.39
            spinal cord V53.02
        pleural drainage tube V58.82
        prosthesis V52.9
            arm (complete) (partial) V52.0
            breast V52.4
            dental V52.3
            eye V52.2
            leg (complete) (partial) V52.1
            specified type NEC V52.8
        spectacles V53.1
        wheelchair V53.8

Admission—*continued*
    follow-up examination (routine) (following)
        V67.9
        cancer chemotherapy V67.2
        chemotherapy V67.2
        high-risk medication NEC V67.51
        injury NEC V67.59
        psychiatric V67.3
        psychotherapy V67.3
        radiotherapy V67.1
        specified surgery NEC V67.09
        surgery V67.00
            vaginal pap smear V67.01
        treatment (for) V67.9
            combined V67.6
            fracture V67.4
            involving high-risk medication NEC
                V67.51
            mental disorder V67.3
            specified NEC V67.59
    hair transplant, for cosmetic reason V50.0
    health advice, education, or instruction V65.4
    hospice care V66.7
    insertion (of)
        subdermal implantable contraceptive V25.5
    intrauterine device
        insertion V25.1
        management V25.42
    investigation to determine further disposition
        V63.8
    isolation V07.0
    issue of
        medical certificate NEC V68.0
        repeat prescription NEC V68.1
            contraceptive device NEC V25.49
    kidney dialysis V56.0
    mental health evaluation V70.2
        requested by authority V70.1
    nonmedical reason NEC V68.89
    nursing care evaluation V63.8
    observation (without need for further medical
        care) (*see also* Observation) V71.9
        accident V71.4
        alleged rape or seduction V71.5
        criminal assault V71.6
        following accident V71.4
            at work V71.3
        foreign body ingestion V71.89
        growth and development variations,
            childhood V21.0
        inflicted injury NEC V71.6
        ingestion of deleterious agent or foreign
            body V71.89
        injury V71.6
        malignant neoplasm V71.1
        mental disorder V71.09
        newborn—*see* Observation, suspected
            condition, newborn
        rape V71.5
        specified NEC V71.89
        suspected disorder V71.9
            abuse V71.81
            accident V71.4
                at work V71.3
            benign neoplasm V71.89
            cardiovascular V71.7
            exposure
                anthrax V71.82
                biological agent NEC V71.83
            heart V71.7
            inflicted injury NEC V71.6

Admission—*continued*

malignant neoplasm V71.1
mental NEC V71.09
neglect V71.81
specified condition NEC V71.89
tuberculosis V71.2
tuberculosis V71.2
occupational therapy V57.21
organ transplant, donor—*see* Donor
ovary, ovarian removal, prophylactic V50.42
palliative care V66.7
Papanicolaou smear
cervix V76.2
for suspected malignant neoplasm V76.2
no disease found V71.1
routine, as part of gynecological
examination V72.3
vaginal V76.47
following hysterectomy for malignant
condition V67.01
passage of sounds or bougie in artificial
opening—*see* Attention to, artificial,
opening
paternity testing V70.4
peritoneal dialysis V56.8
physical therapy NEC V57.1
plastic surgery
cosmetic NEC V50.1
following healed injury or operation V51
postmenopausal hormone replacement therapy
V07.4
postpartum observation
immediately after delivery V24.0
routine follow-up V24.2
poststerilization (for restoration) V26.0
procreative management V26.9
specified type NEC V26.8
prophylactic
administration of
antibiotics V07.39
antitoxin, any V07.2
antivenin V07.2
chemotherapeutic agent NEC V07.39
chemotherapy NEC V07.39
diphtheria antitoxin V07.2
fluoride V07.31
gamma globulin V07.2
immune sera (gamma globulin) V07.2
RhoGAM V07.2
tetanus antitoxin V07.2
breathing exercises V57.0
chemotherapy NEC V07.39
fluoride V07.31
measure V07.9
specified type NEC V07.8
organ removal V50.49
breast V50.41
ovary V50.42
psychiatric examination (general) V70.2
requested by authority V70.1
radiation management V58.0
radiotherapy V58.0
reforming of artificial opening—*see* Attention
to, artificial, opening
rehabilitation V57.9
multiple types V57.89
occupational V57.21
orthoptic V57.4
orthotic V57.81
physical NEC V57.1
specified type NEC V57.89

Admission—*continued*

speech V57.3
vocational V57.22
removal of
cardiac pacemaker V53.31
cast (plaster) V54.89
catheter from artificial opening—*see*
Attention to, artificial, opening
cerebral ventricle (communicating) shunt
V53.01
cystostomy catheter V55.5
device
cerebral ventricle (communicating) shunt
V53.01
fixation
external V54.89
internal V54.0
intrauterine contraceptive V25.42
traction, external V54.89
dressing V58.3
fixation device
external V54.89
internal V54.0
intrauterine contraceptive device V25.42
Kirschner wire V54.89
neuropacemaker (brain) (peripheral nerve)
(spinal cord) V53.02
orthopedic fixation device
external V54.89
internal V54.0
pacemaker device
brain V53.02
cardiac V53.31
carotid sinus V53.39
nervous system V53.02
plaster cast V54.89
plate (fracture) V54.0
rod V54.0
screw (fracture) V54.0
splint, traction V54.89
Steinmann pin V54.89
subdermal implantable contraceptive V25.43
surgical dressing V58.3
sutures V58.3
traction device, external V54.89
ureteral stent V53.6
repair of scarred tissue (following healed
injury or operation) V51
reprogramming of cardiac pacemaker V53.31
restoration of organ continuity
(poststerilization) (tuboplasty)
(vasoplasty) V26.0
sensitivity test—*see also* Test, skin
allergy NEC V72.7
bacterial disease NEC V74.9
Dick V74.8
Kveim V82.89
Mantoux V74.1
mycotic infection NEC V75.4
parasitic disease NEC V75.8
Schick V74.3
Schultz-Charlton V74.8
social service (agency) referral or evaluation
V63.8
speech therapy V57.3
sterilization V25.2
suspected disorder (ruled out) (without need
for further care)—*see* Observation
terminal care V66.7
tests only—*see* Test
therapeutic drug monitoring V58.83

Admission—*continued*

therapy

blood transfusion, without reported diagnosis V58.2

breathing exercises V57.0

chemotherapy V58.1

prophylactic NEC V07.39

fluoride V07.31

dialysis (intermittent) (treatment)

extracorporeal V56.0

peritoneal V56.8

renal V56.0

specified type NEC V56.8

exercise (remedial) NEC V57.1

breathing V57.0

long-term (current) drug use NEC V58.69

antibiotics V58.62

anticoagulant V58.61

occupational V57.21

orthoptic V57.4

physical NEC V57.1

radiation V58.0

speech V57.3

vocational V57.22

toilet or cleaning

of artificial opening — *see* Attention to, artificial, opening

of non-vascular catheter V58.82

of vascular catheter V58.81

tubal ligation V25.2

tuboplasty for previous sterilization V26.0

vaccination, prophylactic (against)

arthropod-borne virus, viral NEC V05.1

disease NEC V05.1

encephalitis V05.0

Bacille Calmette Guérin (BCG) V03.2

BCG V03.2

chickenpox V05.4

cholera alone V03.0

with typhoid-paratyphoid (cholera + TAB) V06.0

common cold V04.7

dengue V05.1

diphtheria alone V03.5

diphtheria-tetanus [Td] without pertussis V06.5

diphtheria-tetanus-pertussis (DTP) V06.1

with

poliomyelitis (DTP + polio) V06.3

typhoid-paratyphoid (DTP + TAB) V06.2

disease (single) NEC V05.9

bacterial NEC V03.9

specified type NEC V03.89

combinations NEC V06.9

specified type NEC V06.8

specified type NEC V05.8

encephalitis, viral, arthropod-borne V05.0

Hemophilus influenzae, type B [Hib] V03.81

hepatitis, viral V05.3

immune sera (gamma globulin) V07.2

influenza V04.8

with

Streptococcus pneumoniae [pneumococcus] V06.6

Leishmaniasis V05.2

measles alone V04.2

measles-mumps-rubella (MMR) V06.4

mumps alone V04.6

with measles and rubella (MMR) V06.4

not done because of contraindication V64.0

Admission—*continued*

pertussis alone V03.6

plague V03.3

pneumonia V03.82

poliomyelitis V04.0

with diphtheria-tetanus-pertussis (DTP + polio) V06.3

rabies V04.5

rubella alone V04.3

with measles and mumps (MMR) V06.4

smallpox V04.1

specified type NEC V05.8

Streptococcus pneumoniae [pneumococcus] V03.82

with

influenza V06.6

tetanus toxoid alone V03.7

with diphtheria [Td] V06.5

and pertussis (DTP) V06.1

tuberculosis (BCG) V03.2

tularemia V03.4

typhoid alone V03.1

with diphtheria-tetanus-pertussis (TAB + DTP) V06.2

typhoid-paratyphoid alone (TAB) V03.1

typhus V05.8

varicella V05.4

viral encephalitis, arthropod-borne V05.0

viral hepatitis V05.3

yellow fever V04.4

vasectomy V25.2

vasoplasty for previous sterilization V26.0

vision examination V72.0

vocational therapy V57.22

waiting period for admission to other facility V63.2

undergoing social agency investigation V63.8

well baby and child care V20.2

x-ray of chest

for suspected tuberculosis V71.2

routine V72.5

Adnexitis (suppurative) (*see also* Salpingo-oophoritis) 614.2

Adolescence NEC V21.2

Adoption

agency referral V68.89

examination V70.3

held for V68.89

Adrenal gland —*see* condition

Adrenalism 255.9

tuberculous (*see also* Tuberculosis) 017.6

Adrenalitis, adrenitis 255.8

meningococcal hemorrhagic 036.3

Adrenarche, precocious 259.1

Adrenocortical syndrome 255.2

Adrenogenital syndrome (acquired) (congenital) 255.2

iatrogenic, fetus or newborn 760.79

Adventitious bursa —*see* Bursitis

Adynamia (episodica) (hereditary) (periodic) 359.3

Adynamic

ileus or intestine (see also ileus) 560.1

ureter 753.22

Aeration lung imperfect, newborn 770.5

Aerobullosis 993.3

Aerocele —*see* Embolism, air

Aerodermectasia

subcutaneous (traumatic) 958.7

surgical 998.81

surgical 998.81

Aerodontalgia 993.2
Aeroembolism 993.3
Aerogenes capsulatus infection (*see also*
   Gangrene, gas) 040.0
Aero-otitis media 993.0
Aerophagy, aerophagia 306.4
   psychogenic 306.4
Aerosinusitis 993.1
Aerotitis 993.0
Affection, affections —*see also* Disease
   sacroiliac (joint), old 724.6
   shoulder region NEC 726.2
Afibrinogenemia 286.3
   acquired 286.6
   congenital 286.3
   postpartum 666.3
African
   sleeping sickness 086.5
   tick fever 087.1
   trypanosomiasis 086.5
      Gambian 086.3
      Rhodesian 086.4
Aftercare V58.9
   artificial openings—*see* Attention to, artificial,
      opening
   blood transfusion without reported diagnosis
      V58.2
   breathing exercise V57.0
   cardiac device V53.39
      defibrillator, automatic implantable V53.32
      pacemaker V53.31
         carotid sinus V53.39
   carotid sinus pacemaker V53.39
   cerebral ventricle (communicating) shunt
      V53.01
   chemotherapy session (adjunctive)
      (maintenance) V58.1
   defibrillator, automatic implantable cardiac
      V53.32
   exercise (remedial) (therapeutic) V57.1
      breathing V57.0
   extracorporeal dialysis (intermittent) (treatment)
      V56.0
   following surgery NEC V58.49
      for
         injury V58.43
         neoplasm V58.42
         trauma V58.43
      joint replacement V54.81
      of
         circulatory system V58.73
         digestive system V58.75
         genital organs V58.76
         genitourinary system V58.76
         musculoskeletal system V58.78
         nervous system V58.72
         oral cavity V58.75
         respiratory system V58.74
         sense organs V58.71
         skin V58.77
         subcutaneous tissue V58.77
         teeth V58.75
         urinary system V58.76
      wound closure, planned V58.41
   fracture V54.9
      healing V54.89
         pathologic
            arm V54.20
               lower V54.22
               upper V54.21
            hip V54.23

Aftercare—*continued*
      leg V54.24
         lower V54.26
         upper V54.25
      specified site NEC V54.29
      vertebrae V54.27
      traumatic
         arm V54.10
            lower V54.12
            upper V54.11
         hip V54.13
         leg V54.14
            lower V54.16
            upper V54.15
         specified site NEC V54.19
         vertebrae V54.17
   removal of
      external fixation device V54.89
      internal fixation device V54.0
      specified care NEC V54.89
   gait training V57.1
      for use of artificial limb(s) V57.81
   involving
      dialysis (intermittent) (treatment)
         extracorporeal V56.0
         peritoneal V56.8
         renal V56.0
      gait training V57.1
         for use of artificial limb(s) V57.81
      orthoptic training V57.4
      orthotic training V57.81
      radiotherapy session V58.0
      removal of
         dressings V58.3
         fixation device
            external V54.89
            internal V54.0
         fracture plate V54.0
         pins V54.0
         plaster cast V54.89
         rods V54.0
         screws V54.0
         surgical dressings V58.3
         sutures V58.3
         traction device, external V54.89
   neuropacemaker (brain) (peripheral nerve)
      (spinal cord) V53.02
   occupational therapy V57.21
   orthodontic V58.5
   orthopedic V54.9
      change of external fixation or traction device
         V54.89
      following joint replacement V54.81
      removal of fixation device
         external V54.89
         internal V54.0
      specified care NEC V54.89
   orthoptic training V57.4
   orthotic training V57.81
   pacemaker
      brain V53.02
      cardiac V53.31
      carotid sinus V53.39
      peripheral nerve V53.02
      spinal cord V53.02
   peritoneal dialysis (intermittent) (treatment)
      V56.8
   physical therapy NEC V57.1
      breathing exercises V57.0
   radiotherapy session V58.0
   rehabilitation procedure V57.9

Aftercare—*continued*
  breathing exercises V57.0
  multiple types V57.89
  occupational V57.21
  orthoptic V57.4
  orthotic V57.81
  physical therapy NEC V57.1
  remedial exercises V57.1
  specified type NEC V57.89
  speech V57.3
  therapeutic exercises V57.1
  vocational V57.22
  renal dialysis (intermittent) (treatment) V56.0
  specified type NEC V58.89
    removal of non-vascular catheter V58.82
    removal of vascular catheter V58.81
  speech therapy V57.3
  vocational rehabilitation V57.22
After-cataract 366.50
  obscuring vision 366.53
  specified type, not obscuring vision 366.52
Agalactia 676.4
Agammaglobulinemia 279.00
  with lymphopenia 279.2
  acquired (primary) (secondary) 279.06
  Bruton's X-linked 279.04
  infantile sex-linked (Bruton's) (congenital)
    279.04
  Swiss-type 279.2
Aganglionosis (bowel) (colon) 751.3
AGCUS (atypical glandular cell changes of un-
    determined significance)
  favor benign 795.01
  favor dysplasia 795.02
Age (old) (*see also* Senile) 797
Agenesis —*see also* Absence, by site, congenital
  acoustic nerve 742.8
  adrenal (gland) 759.1
  alimentary tract (complete) (partial) NEC 751.8
    lower 751.2
    upper 750.8
  anus, anal (canal) 751.2
  aorta 747.22
  appendix 751.2
  arm (complete) (partial) (*see also* Deformity,
    reduction, upper limb) 755.20
  artery (peripheral) NEC (*see also* Anomaly,
    peripheral vascular system) 747.60
    brain 747.81
    coronary 746.85
    pulmonary 747.3
    umbilical 747.5
  auditory (canal) (external) 744.01
  auricle (ear) 744.01
  bile, biliary duct or passage 751.61
  bone NEC 756.9
  brain 740.0
    specified part 742.2
  breast 757.6
  bronchus 748.3
  canaliculus lacrimalis 743.65
  carpus NEC (*see also* Deformity, reduction,
    upper limb) 755.28
  cartilage 756.9
  cecum 751.2
  cerebellum 742.2
  cervix 752.49
  chin 744.89
  cilia 743.63
  circulatory system, part NEC 747.89

Agenesis—*continued*
  clavicle 755.51
  clitoris 752.49
  coccyx 756.13
  colon 751.2
  corpus callosum 742.2
  cricoid cartilage 748.3
  diaphragm (with hernia) 756.6
  digestive organ(s) or tract (complete) (partial)
    NEC 751.8
    lower 751.2
    upper 750.8
  ductus arteriosus 747.89
  duodenum 751.1
  ear NEC 744.09
    auricle 744.01
    lobe 744.21
  ejaculatory duct 752.8
  endocrine (gland) NEC 759.2
  epiglottis 748.3
  esophagus 750.3
  Eustachian tube 744.24
  extrinsic muscle, eye 743.69
  eye 743.00
    adnexa 743.69
  eyelid (fold) 743.62
  face
    bones NEC 756.0
    specified part NEC 744.89
  fallopian tube 752.19
  femur NEC (*see also* Absence, femur,
    congenital) 755.34
  fibula NEC (*see also* Absence, fibula,
    congenital) 755.37
  finger NEC (*see also* Absence, finger,
    congenital) 755.29
  foot (complete) (*see also* Deformity, reduction,
    lower limb) 755.31
  gallbladder 751.69
  gastric 750.8
  genitalia, genital (organ)
    female 752.8
      external 752.49
      internal NEC 752.8
    male 752.8
      penis 752.69
  glottis 748.3
  gonadal 758.6
  hair 757.4
  hand (complete) (*see also* Deformity, reduction,
    upper limb) 755.21
  heart 746.89
    valve NEC 746.89
      aortic 746.89
      mitral 746.89
      pulmonary 746.01
  hepatic 751.69
  humerus NEC (*see also* Absence, humerus,
    congenital) 755.24
  hymen 752.49
  ileum 751.1
  incus 744.04
  intestine (small) 751.1
    large 751.2
  iris (dilator fibers) 743.45
  jaw 524.09
  jejunum 751.1
  kidney(s) (partial) (unilateral) 753.0
  labium (majus) (minus) 752.49
  labyrinth, membranous 744.05
  lacrimal apparatus (congenital) 743.65

Agenesis—*continued*
  larynx 748.3
  leg NEC (*see also* Deformity, reduction, lower
    limb) 755.30
  lens 743.35
  limb (complete) (partial) (*see also* Deformity,
    reduction) 755.4
    lower NEC 755.30
    upper 755.20
  lip 750.26
  liver 751.69
  lung (bilateral) (fissures) (lobe) (unilateral)
    748.5
  mandible 524.09
  maxilla 524.09
  metacarpus NEC 755.28
  metatarsus NEC 755.38
  muscle (any) 756.81
  musculoskeletal system NEC 756.9
  nail(s) 757.5
  neck, part 744.89
  nerve 742.8
  nervous system, part NEC 742.8
  nipple 757.6
  nose 748.1
  nuclear 742.8
  organ
    of Corti 744.05
    or site not listed—*see* Anomaly, specified
      type NEC
  osseous meatus (ear) 744.03
  ovary 752.0
  oviduct 752.19
  pancreas 751.7
  parathyroid (gland) 759.2
  patella 755.64
  pelvic girdle (complete) (partial) 755.69
  penis 752.69
  pericardium 746.89
  perineal body 756.81
  pituitary (gland) 759.2
  prostate 752.8
  pulmonary
    artery 747.3
    trunk 747.3
    vein 747.49
  punctum lacrimale 743.65
  radioulnar NEC (*see also* Absence, forearm,
    congenital) 755.25
  radius NEC (*see also* Absence, radius,
    congenital) 755.26
  rectum 751.2
  renal 753.0
  respiratory organ NEC 748.9
  rib 756.3
  roof of orbit 742.0
  round ligament 752.8
  sacrum 756.13
  salivary gland 750.21
  scapula 755.59
  scrotum 752.8
  seminal duct or tract 752.8
  septum
    atrial 745.69
    between aorta and pulmonary artery 745.0
    ventricular 745.3
  shoulder girdle (complete) (partial) 755.59
  skull (bone) 756.0
    with
      anencephalus 740.0
      encephalocele 742.0

Agenesis—*continued*
  hydrocephalus 742.3
    with spina bifida (*see also* Spina bifida)
      741.0
  microcephalus 742.1
  spermatic cord 752.8
  spinal cord 742.59
  spine 756.13
    lumbar 756.13
      isthmus 756.11
      pars articularis 756.11
  spleen 759.0
  sternum 756.3
  stomach 750.7
  tarsus NEC 755.38
  tendon 756.81
  testicular 752.8
  testis 752.8
  thymus (gland) 759.2
  thyroid (gland) 243
    cartilage 748.3
  tibia NEC (*see also* Absence, tibia, congenital)
    755.36
  tibiofibular NEC 755.35
  toe (complete) (partial) (*see also* Absence, toe,
    congenital) 755.39
  tongue 750.11
  trachea (cartilage) 748.3
  ulna NEC (*see also* Absence, ulna, congenital)
    755.27
  ureter 753.4
  urethra 753.8
  urinary tract NEC 753.8
  uterus 752.3
  uvula 750.26
  vagina 752.49
  vas deferens 752.8
  vein(s) (peripheral) NEC (*see also* Anomaly,
    peripheral vascular system) 747.60
    brain 747.81
    great 747.49
    portal 747.49
    pulmonary 747.49
  vena cava (inferior) (superior) 747.49
  vermis of cerebellum 742.2
  vertebra 756.13
    lumbar 756.13
      isthmus 756.11
      pars articularis 756.11
  vulva 752.49
Ageusia (*see also* Disturbance, sensation) 781.1
Aggressiveness 301.3
Aggressive outburst (*see also* Disturbance,
  conduct) 312.0
  in children and adolescents 313.9
Aging skin 701.8
Agitated —*see* condition
Agitation 307.9
  catatonic (*see also* Schizophrenia) 295.2
Aglossia (congenital) 750.11
Aglycogenosis 271.0
Agnail (finger) (with lymphangitis) 681.02
Agnosia (body image) (tactile) 784.69
  verbal 784.69
    auditory 784.69
      secondary to organic lesion 784.69
    developmental 315.8
    secondary to organic lesion 784.69
    visual 784.69
      developmental 315.8
      secondary to organic lesion 784.69

Agnosia—*continued*
  visual 368.16
    developmental 315.31
Agoraphobia 300.22
  with panic attacks 300.21
Agrammatism 784.69
Agranulocytopenia 288.0
Agranulocytosis (angina) (chronic) (cyclical)
  (genetic) (infantile) (periodic) (pernicious)
  288.0
Agraphia (absolute) 784.69
  with alexia 784.61
  developmental 315.39
Agrypnia (*see also* Insomnia) 780.52
Ague (*see also* Malaria) 084.6
  brass-founders' 985.8
  dumb 084.6
  tertian 084.1
Agyria 742.2
Ahumada-del Castillo syndrome (nonpuerperal
  galactorrhea and amenorrhea) 253.1
AIDS 042
AIDS-associated retrovirus (disease) (illness)
  042
  infection—*see* Human immunodeficiency virus,
    infection
AIDS-associated virus (disease) (illness) 042
  infection—*see* Human immunodeficiency virus,
    infection
AIDS-like disease (illness) (syndrome) 042
AIDS-related complex 042
AIDS-related conditions 042
AIDS-related virus (disease) (illness) 042
  infection—*see* Human immunodeficiency virus,
    infection
AIDS virus (disease) (illness) 042
  infection—*see* Human immunodeficiency virus,
    infection
Ailment, heart —*see* Disease, heart
Ailurophobia 300.29
Ainhum (disease) 136.0
Air
  anterior mediastinum 518.1
  compressed, disease 993.3
  embolism (any site) (artery) (cerebral) 958.0
    with
      abortion—*see* Abortion, by type, with
        embolism
      ectopic pregnancy (*see also* categories
        633.0-633.9) 639.6
      molar pregnancy (*see also* categories
        630-632) 639.6
    due to implanted device—*see* Complications,
      due to (presence of) any device, implant,
      or graft classified to 996.0-996.5 NEC
    following
      abortion 639.6
      ectopic or molar pregnancy 639.6
      infusion, perfusion, or transfusion 999.1
    in pregnancy, childbirth, or puerperium 673.0
    traumatic 958.0
  hunger 786.09
    psychogenic 306.1
  leak (lung) (pulmonary) (thorax) 512.8
    iatrogenic 512.1
    postoperative 512.1
  rarefied, effects of—*see* Effect, adverse, high
    altitude
  sickness 994.6
Airplane sickness 994.6
Akathisia, acathisia 781.0
  due to drugs 333.99

Akinesia algeria 352.6
Akiyami 100.89
Akureyri disease (epidemic neuromyasthenia)
  049.8
Alacrima (congenital) 743.65
Alactasia (hereditary) 271.3
Alalia 784.3
  developmental 315.31
    receptive-expressive 315.32
  secondary to organic lesion 784.3
Alaninemia 270.8
Alastrim 050.1
Albarrán's disease (colibacilluria) 791.9
Albers-Schönberg's disease (marble bones)
  756.52
Albert's disease 726.71
Albinism, albino (choroid) (cutaneous) (eye)
  (generalized) (isolated) (ocular)
  (oculocutaneous) (partial) 270.2
Albinismus 270.2
Albright (-Martin) (-Bantam) disease
  (pseudohypoparathyroidism) 275.49
Albright (-McCune) (-Sternberg) syndrome
  (osteitis fibrosa disseminata) 756.59
Albuminous —*see* condition
Albuminuria, albuminuric (acute) (chronic)
  (subacute) 791.0
  Bence-Jones 791.0
  cardiac 785.9
  complicating pregnancy, childbirth, or
    puerperium 646.2
    with hypertension—*see* Toxemia, of
      pregnancy
    affecting fetus or newborn 760.1
  cyclic 593.6
  gestational 646.2
  gravidarum 646.2
    with hypertension—*see* Toxemia, of
      pregnancy
    affecting fetus or newborn 760.1
  heart 785.9
  idiopathic 593.6
  orthostatic 593.6
  postural 593.6
  pre-eclamptic (mild) 642.4
    affecting fetus or newborn 760.0
    severe 642.5
      affecting fetus or newborn 760.0
  recurrent physiologic 593.6
  scarlatinal 034.1
Albumosuria 791.0
  Bence-Jones 791.0
  myelopathic (M9730/3) 203.0
Alcaptonuria 270.2
Alcohol, alcoholic
  abstinence 291.81
  acute intoxication 305.0
    with dependence 303.0
  addiction (*see also* Alcoholism) 303.9
    maternal
      with suspected fetal damage affecting
        management of pregnancy 655.4
      affecting fetus or newborn 760.71
  amnestic disorder, persisting 291.1
  anxiety 291.89
  brain syndrome, chronic 291.2
  cardiopathy 425.5
  chronic (*see also* Alcoholism) 303.9
  cirrhosis (liver) 571.2
  delirium 291.0
    acute 291.0

Alcohol, alcoholic—*continued*
  chronic 291.1
    tremens 291.0
    withdrawal 291.0
  dementia NEC 291.2
  deterioration 291.2
  drunkenness (simple) 305.0
  hallucinosis (acute) 291.3
  insanity 291.9
  intoxication (acute) 305.0
    with dependence 303.0
    pathological 291.4
  jealousy 291.5
  Korsakoff's, Korsakov's, Korsakow's 291.1
  liver NEC 571.3
    acute 571.1
    chronic 571.2
  mania (acute) (chronic) 291.9
  mood 291.89
  paranoia 291.5
  paranoid (type) psychosis 291.5
  pellagra 265.2
  poisoning, accidental (acute) NEC 980.9
    specified type of alcohol—*see* Table of drugs
      and chemicals
  psychosis (*see also* Psychosis, alcoholic) 291.9
    Korsakoff's, Korsakov's, Korsakow's 291.1
    polyneuritic 291.1
      with
        delusions 291.5
        hallucinations 291.3
  withdrawal symptoms, syndrome NEC 291.81
    delirium 291.0
    hallucinosis 291.3
Alcoholism 303.9

> *Note—Use the following fifth-digit*
> *subclassification with category 303:*
>
> *0 unspecified*
> *1 continuous*
> *2 episodic*
> *3 in remission*

  with psychosis (*see also* Psychosis, alcoholic)
    291.9
  acute 303.0
  chronic 303.9
    with psychosis 291.9
  complicating pregnancy, childbirth, or
    puerperium 648.4
    affecting fetus or newborn 760.71
  history V11.3
  Korsakoff's, Korsakov's, Korsakow's 291.1
  suspected damage to fetus affecting
    management of pregnancy 655.4
Alder's anomaly or syndrome (leukocyte
  granulation anomaly) 288.2
Alder-Reilly anomaly (leukocyte granulation)
  288.2
Aldosteronism (primary) (secondary) 255.1
  congenital 255.1
Aldosteronoma (M8370/1) 237.2
Aldrich (-Wiskott) syndrome
  (eczema-thrombocytopenia) 279.12
Aleppo boil 085.1
Aleukemic —*see* condition

Aleukia
  congenital 288.0
  hemorrhagica 284.9
    acquired (secondary) 284.8
    congenital 284.0
    idiopathic 284.9
  splenica 289.4
Alexia (congenital) (developmental) 315.01
  secondary to organic lesion 784.61
Algoneurodystrophy 733.7
Algophobia 300.29
Alibert's disease (mycosis fungoides) (M9700/3)
  202.1
Alibert-Bazin disease (M9700/3) 202.1
Alice in Wonderland syndrome 293.89
Alienation, mental (*see also* Psychosis) 298.9
Alkalemia 276.3
Alkalosis 276.3
  metabolic 276.3
    with respiratory acidosis 276.4
  respiratory 276.3
Alkaptonuria 270.2
Allen-Masters syndrome 620.6
Allergic bronchopulmonary aspergillosis 518.6
Allergy, allergic (reaction) 995.3
  air-borne substance (*see also* Fever, hay) 477.9
    specified allergen NEC 477.8
  alveolitis (extrinsic) 495.9
    due to
      Aspergillus clavatus 495.4
      cryptostroma corticale 495.6
      organisms (fungal, thermophilic
        actinomycete, other) growing in
        ventilation (air conditioning systems)
        495.7
    specified type NEC 495.8
  anaphylactic shock 999.4
    due to
      food—*see* Anaphylactic shock, due to, food
  angioneurotic edema 995.1
  animal (dander) (epidermal) (hair) 477.8
  arthritis (*see also* Arthritis, allergic) 716.2
  asthma—*see* Asthma
  bee sting (anaphylactic shock) 989.5
  biological—*see* Allergy, drug
  bronchial asthma—*see* Asthma
  conjunctivitis (eczematous) 372.14
  dander (animal) 477.8
  dandruff 477.8
  dermatitis (venenata)—*see* Dermatitis
  diathesis V15.09
  drug, medicinal substance, and biological (any)
    (correct medicinal substance properly
    administered) (external) (internal) 995.2
    wrong substance given or taken NEC 977.9
      specified drug or substance—*see* Table of
        drugs and chemicals
  dust (house) (stock) 477.8
  eczema—*see* Eczema
  endophthalmitis 360.19
  epidermal (animal) 477.8
  feathers 477.8
  food (any) (ingested) 693.1
    atopic 691.8
    in contact with skin 692.5
  gastritis 535.4
  gastroenteritis 558.3
  gastrointestinal 558.3
  grain 477.0
  grass (pollen) 477.0
    asthma (*see also* Asthma) 493.0

Allergy, allergic—*continued*
  hay fever 477.0
  hair (animal) 477.8
  hay fever (grass) (pollen) (ragweed) (tree) (*see also* Fever, hay) 477.9
  history (of) V15.09
    to
      eggs V15.03
      food additives V15.05
      insect bite V15.06
      latex V15.07
      milk products V15.02
      nuts V15.05
        peanuts V15.01
      radiographic dye V15.08
      seafood V15.04
      specified food NEC V15.05
      spider bite V15.06
  horse serum—*see* Allergy, serum
  inhalant 477.9
    dust 477.8
    pollen 477.0
    specified allergen other than pollen 477.8
  kapok 477.8
  medicine—*see* Allergy, drug
  migraine 346.2
  pannus 370.62
  pneumonia 518.3
  pollen (any) (hay fever) 477.0
    asthma (*see also* Asthma) 493.0
  primrose 477.0
  primula 477.0
  purpura 287.0
  ragweed (pollen) (Senecio jacobae) 477.0
    asthma (*see also* Asthma) 493.0
    hay fever 477.0
  respiratory (*see also* Allergy, inhalant) 477.9
    due to
      drug—*see* Allergy, drug
      food—*see* Allergy, food
  rhinitis (*see also* Fever, hay) 477.9
    due to food 477.1
  rose 477.0
  Senecio jacobae 477.0
  serum (prophylactic) (therapeutic) 999.5
    anaphylactic shock 999.4
  shock (anaphylactic)
    due to
      adverse effect of correct medicinal
        substance properly administered 995.0
      food—*see* Anaphylactic shock, due to, food
    from serum or immunization 999.5
      anaphylactic 999.4
  sinusitis (*see also* Fever, hay) 477.9
  skin reaction 692.9
    specified substance—*see* Dermatitis, due to
  tree (any) (hay fever) (pollen) 477.0
    asthma (*see also* Asthma) 493.0
  upper respiratory (*see also* Fever, hay) 477.9
  urethritis 597.89
  urticaria 708.0
  vaccine—*see* Allergy, serum
Allescheriosis 117.6
Alligator skin disease (ichthyosis congenita) 757.1
  acquired 701.1
Allocheiria, allochiria (*see also* Disturbance, sensation) 782.0
Almeida's disease (Brazilian blastomycosis) 116.1

Alopecia (atrophicans) (pregnancy) (premature) (senile) 704.00
  adnata 757.4
  areata 704.01
  (celsi 704.01
  cicatrisata 704.09
  circumscripta 704.01
  congenital, congenitalis 757.4
  disseminata 704.01
  effluvium (telogen) 704.02
  febrile 704.09
  generalisata 704.09
  hereditaria 704.09
  marginalis 704.01
  mucinosa 704.09
  postinfectional 704.09
  seborrheica 704.09
  specific 091.82
  syphilitic (secondary) 091.82
  telogen effluvium 704.02
  totalis 704.09
  toxica 704.09
  universalis 704.09
  x-ray 704.09
Alper's disease 330.8
Alpha-lipoproteinemia 272.4
Alpha thalassemia 282.4
Alphos 696.1
Alpine sickness 993.2
Alport's syndrome (hereditary hematuria-nephropathy-deafness) 759.89
Alteration (of), altered
  awareness 780.09
    transient 780.02
  consciousness 780.09
    persistent vegetative state 780.03
    transient 780.02
  mental status 780.99
Alternaria (infection) 118
Alternating —*see* condition
Altitude, high (effects)—*see* Effect, adverse, high altitude
Aluminosis (of lung) 503
Alvarez syndrome (transient cerebral ischemia) 435.9
Alveolar capillary block syndrome 516.3
Alveolitis
  allergic (extrinsic) 495.9
    due to organisms (fungal, thermophilic actinomycete, other) growing in ventilation (air conditioning systems) 495.7
    specified type NEC 495.8
  due to
    Aspergillus clavatus 495.4
    Cryptostroma corticale 495.6
  fibrosing (chronic) (cryptogenic) (lung) 516.3
    idiopathic 516.3
    rheumatoid 714.81
  jaw 526.5
  sicca dolorosa 526.5
Alveolus, alveolar —*see* condition
Alymphocytosis (pure) 279.2
Alymphoplasia, thymic 279.2
Alzheimer's
  dementia (senile)
    with behavioral disturbance 331.0 *[294.11]*
    without behavioral disturbance 331.0 *[294.10]*
  disease or sclerosis 331.0
    with dementia—*see* Alzheimer's, dementia
Amastia (*see also* Absence, breast) 611.8

Amaurosis (acquired) (congenital) (*see also* Blindness) 369.00
  fugax 362.34
  hysterical 300.11
  Leber's (congenital) 362.76
  tobacco 377.34
  uremic—*see* Uremia
Amaurotic familial idiocy (infantile) (juvenile) (late) 330.1
Ambisexual 752.7
Amblyopia (acquired) (congenital) (partial) 368.00
  color 368.59
    acquired 368.55
  deprivation 368.02
  ex anopsia 368.00
  hysterical 300.11
  nocturnal 368.60
    vitamin A deficiency 264.5
  refractive 368.03
  strabismic 368.01
  suppression 368.01
  tobacco 377.34
  toxic NEC 377.34
  uremic—*see* Uremia
Ameba, amebic (histolytica)–*see also* Amebiasis
  abscess 006.3
    bladder 006.8
    brain (with liver and lung abscess) 006.5
    liver 006.3
      with
        brain abscess (and lung abscess) 006.5
        lung abscess 006.4
      lung (with liver abscess) 006.4
        with brain abscess 006.5
    seminal vesicle 006.8
    spleen 006.8
  carrier (suspected of) V02.2
  meningoencephalitis
    due to Naegleria (gruberi) 136.2
    primary 136.2
Amebiasis NEC 006.9
  with
    brain abscess (with liver or lung abscess) 006.5
    liver abscess (without mention of brain or lung abscess) 006.3
    lung abscess (with liver abscess) 006.4
      with brain abscess 006.5
  acute 006.0
  bladder 006.8
  chronic 006.1
  cutaneous 006.6
  cutis 006.6
  due to organism other than Entamoeba histolytica 007.8
  hepatic (*see also* Abscess, liver, amebic) 006.3
  nondysenteric 006.2
  seminal vesicle 006.8
  specified
    organism NEC 007.8
    site NEC 006.8
Ameboma 006.8
Amelia 755.4
  lower limb 755.31
  upper limb 755.21
Ameloblastoma (M9310/0) 213.1
  jaw (bone) (lower) 213.1
    upper 213.0
  long bones (M9261/3)—*see* Neoplasm, bone, malignant

Ameloblastoma—*continued*
  malignant (M9310/3) 170.1
    jaw (bone) (lower) 170.1
      upper 170.0
  mandible 213.1
  tibial (M9261/3) 170.7
Amelogenesis imperfecta 520.5
  nonhereditaria (segmentalis) 520.4
Amenorrhea (primary) (secondary) 626.0
  due to ovarian dysfunction 256.8
  hyperhormonal 256.8
Amentia (*see also* Retardation, mental) 319
  Meynert's (nonalcoholic) 294.0
    alcoholic 291.1
  nevoid 759.6
American
  leishmaniasis 085.5
  mountain tick fever 066.1
  trypanosomiasis—*see* Trypanosomiasis, American
Ametropia (*see also* Disorder, accommodation) 367.9
Amianthosis 501
Amimia 784.69
Amino acid
  deficiency 270.9
    anemia 281.4
  metabolic disorder (*see also* Disorder, amino acid) 270.9
Aminoaciduria 270.9
  imidazole 270.5
Amnesia (retrograde) 780.99
  auditory 784.69
    developmental 315.31
    secondary to organic lesion 784.69
  hysterical or dissociative type 300.12
  psychogenic 300.12
  transient global 437.7
Amnestic (confabulatory) syndrome 294.0
  alcohol-induced 291.1
  drug-induced 292.83
  posttraumatic 294.0
Amniocentesis screening (for) V28.2
  alphafetoprotein level, raised V28.1
  chromosomal anomalies V28.0
Amnion, amniotic —*see also* condition
  nodosum 658.8
Amnionitis (complicating pregnancy) 658.4
  affecting fetus or newborn 762.7
Amoral trends 301.7
Amotio retinae (*see also* Detachment, retina) 361.9
Ampulla
  lower esophagus 530.89
  phrenic 530.89
Amputation
  any part of fetus, to facilitate delivery 763.89
  cervix (supravaginal) (uteri) 622.8
    in pregnancy or childbirth 654.6
      affecting fetus or newborn 763.89
  clitoris—*see* Wound, open, clitoris
  congenital
    lower limb 755.31
    upper limb 755.21
  neuroma (traumatic)—*see also* Injury, nerve, by site
    surgical complications (late) 997.61
  penis—*see* Amputation, traumatic, penis
  status (without complication)—*see* Absence, by site, acquired
  stump (surgical)(posttraumatic)

Amputation—*continued*
  abnormal, painful, or with complication (late)
      997.60
  healed or old NEC —*see also* Absence, by
      site, acquired
      lower V49.70
      upper V49.60
  traumatic (complete) (partial)

---

*Note—"Complicated" includes traumatic
amputation with delayed healing, delayed
treatment, foreign body, or infection.*

---

  arm 887.4
    at or above elbow 887.2
      complicated 887.3
    below elbow 887.0
      complicated 887.1
    both (bilateral) (any level(s)) 887.6
      complicated 887.7
    complicated 887.5
  finger(s) (one or both hands) 886.0
    with thumb(s) 885.0
      complicated 885.1
    complicated 886.1
  foot (except toe(s) only) 896.0
    and other leg 897.6
      complicated 897.7
    both (bilateral) 896.2
      complicated 896.3
    complicated 896.1
    toe(s) only (one or both feet) 895.0
      complicated 895.1
  genital organ(s) (external) NEC 878.8
    complicated 878.9
  hand (except finger(s) only) 887.0
    and other arm 887.6
      complicated 887.7
    both (bilateral) 887.6
      complicated 887.7
    complicated 887.1
    finger(s) (one or both hands) 886.0
      with thumb(s) 885.0
        complicated 885.1
      complicated 886.1
    thumb(s) (with fingers of either hand) 885.0
      complicated 885.1
  head 874.9
  late effect—*see* Late, effects (of), amputation
  leg 897.4
    and other foot 897.6
      complicated 897.7
    at or above knee 897.2
      complicated 897.3
    below knee 897.0
      complicated 897.1
    both (bilateral) 897.6
      complicated 897.7
    complicated 897.5
  lower limb(s) except toe(s)—*see* Amputation,
      traumatic, leg
  nose—*see* Wound, open, nose
  penis 878.0
    complicated 878.1
  sites other than limbs—*see* Wound, open, by
      site
  thumb(s) (with finger(s) of either hand) 885.0
    complicated 885.1
  toe(s) (one or both feet) 895.0
    complicated 895.1
  upper limb(s)—*see* Amputation, traumatic,
      arm

Amputee (bilateral) (old) —*see also* Absence, by
    site, acquired V49.70
Amusia 784.69
  developmental 315.39
  secondary to organic lesion 784.69
Amyelencephalus 740.0
Amyelia 742.59
Amygdalitis— *see* Tonsillitis
Amygdalolith 474.8
Amyloid disease or degeneration 277.3
  heart 277.3 *[425.7]*
Amyloidosis (familial) (general) (generalized)
    (genetic) (primary) (secondary) 277.3
  with lung involvement 277.3 *[517.8]*
  heart 277.3 *[425.7]*
  nephropathic 277.3 *[583.81]*
  neuropathic (Portuguese) (Swiss) 277.3 *[357.4]*
  pulmonary 277.3 *[517.8]*
  systemic, inherited 277.3
Amylopectinosis (brancher enzyme deficiency)
    271.0
Amylophagia 307.52
Amyoplasia, congenita 756.89
Amyotonia 728.2
  congenita 358.8
Amyotrophia, amyotrophy, amyotrophic 728.2
  congenita 756.89
  diabetic 250.6 *[358.1]*
  lateral sclerosis (syndrome) 335.20
  neuralgic 353.5
  sclerosis (lateral) 335.20
  spinal progressive 335.21
Anacidity
  gastric 536.0
  psychogenic 306.4
Anaerosis of newborn 768.9
Analbuminemia 273.8
Analgesia (*see also* Anesthesia) 782.0
Analphalipoproteinemia 272.5
Anaphylactic shock or reaction (correct
    substance properly administered) 995.0
  due to
    food 995.60
      additives 995.66
      crustaceans 995.62
      eggs 995.68
      fish 995.65
      fruits 995.63
      milk products 995.67
      nuts (tree) 995.64
      peanuts 995.61
      seeds 995.64
      specified NEC 995.69
      tree nuts 995.64
      vegetables 995.63
    immunization 999.4
    overdose or wrong substance given or taken
        977.9
      specified drug—*see* Table of drugs and
          chemicals
    following sting(s) 989.5
    purpura 287.0
    serum 999.4
Anaphylactoid shock or reaction —*see*
    Anaphylactic shock
Anaphylaxis —*see* Anaphylactic shock
Anaplasia, cervix 622.1
Anarthria 784.5
Anarthritic rheumatoid disease 446.5

Anasarca 782.3
cardiac (*see also* Failure, heart) 428.0
fetus or newborn 778.0
lung 514
nutritional 262
pulmonary 514
renal (*see also* Nephrosis) 581.9
Anaspadias 752.62
Anastomosis
aneurysmal—*see* Aneurysm
arteriovenous, congenital NEC (*see also*
Anomaly, arteriovenous) 747.60
ruptured, of brain (*see also* Hemorrhage,
subarachnoid) 430
intestinal 569.89
complicated NEC 997.4
involving urinary tract 997.5
retinal and choroidal vessels 743.58
acquired 362.17
Anatomical narrow angle (glaucoma) 365.02
Ancylostoma (infection) (infestation) 126.9
americanus 126.1
braziliense 126.2
caninum 126.8
ceylanicum 126.3
duodenale 126.0
Necator americanus 126.1
Ancylostomiasis (intestinal) 126.9
Ancylostoma
americanus 126.1
caninum 126.8
ceylanicum 126.3
duodenale 126.0
braziliense 126.2
Necator americanus 126.1
Anders' disease or syndrome (adiposis tuberosa
simplex) 272.8
Andersen's glycogen storage disease 271.0
Anderson's disease 272.7
Andes disease 993.2
Andrews' disease (bacterid) 686.8
Androblastoma (M8630/1)
benign (M8630/0)
specified site—*see* Neoplasm, by site, benign
unspecified site
female 220
male 222.0
malignant (M8630/3)
specified site—*see* Neoplasm, by site,
malignant
unspecified site
female 183.0
male 186.9
specified site—*see* Neoplasm, by site, uncertain
behavior
tubular (M8640/0)
with lipid storage (M8641/0)
specified site—*see* Neoplasm, by site,
benign
unspecified site
female 220
male 222.0
specified site—*see* Neoplasm, by site, benign
unspecified site
female 220
male 222.0
unspecified site
female 236.2
male 236.4

Android pelvis 755.69
with disproportion (fetopelvic) 653.3
affecting fetus or newborn 763.1
causing obstructed labor 660.1
affecting fetus or newborn 763.1
Anectasis, pulmonary (newborn or fetus) 770.5
Anemia 285.9
in
chronic illness NEC 285.29
end-stage renal disease 285.21
neoplastic disease 285.22
of chronic illness NEC 285.29
with
disorder of
anaerobic glycolysis 282.3
pentose phosphate pathway 282.2
koilonychia 280.9
6-phosphogluconic dehydrogenase deficiency
282.2
achlorhydric 280.9
achrestic 281.8
Addison's (pernicious) 281.0
Addison-Biermer (pernicious) 281.0
agranulocytic 288.0
amino acid deficiency 281.4
aplastic 284.9
acquired (secondary) 284.8
congenital 284.0
constitutional 284.0
due to
chronic systemic disease 284.8
drugs 284.8
infection 284.8
radiation 284.8
idiopathic 284.9
myxedema 244.9
of or complicating pregnancy 648.2
red cell (acquired) (pure) (with thymoma)
284.8
congenital 284.0
specified type NEC 284.8
toxic (paralytic) 284.8
aregenerative 284.9
congenital 284.0
asiderotic 280.9
atypical (primary) 285.9
autohemolysis of Selwyn and Dacie (type I)
282.2
autoimmune hemolytic 283.0
Baghdad Spring 282.2
Balantidium coli 007.0
Biermer's (pernicious) 281.0
blood loss (chronic) 280.0
acute 285.1
bothriocephalus 123.4
brickmakers' (*see also* Ancylostomiasis) 126.9
cerebral 437.8
childhood 285.9
chlorotic 280.9
chronica congenita aregenerativa 284.0
chronic simple 281.9
combined system disease NEC 281.0 *[336.2]*
due to dietary deficiency 281.1 *[336.2]*
complicating pregnancy or childbirth 648.2
congenital (following fetal blood loss) 776.5
aplastic 284.0
due to isoimmunization NEC 773.2
Heinz-body 282.7
hereditary hemolytic NEC 282.9
nonspherocytic
Type I 282.2

Anemia—*continued*
  myelopathic 285.8
  myelophthisic (normocytic) 285.8
  newborn (*see also* Disease, hemolytic) 773.2
    due to isoimmunization (*see also* Disease,
      hemolytic) 773.2
    late, due to isoimmunization 773.5
    posthemorrhagic 776.5
  nonregenerative 284.9
  nonspherocytic hemolytic—*see* Anemia,
    hemolytic, nonspherocytic
  normocytic (infectional) (not due to blood loss)
    285.9
    due to blood loss (chronic) 280.0
      acute 285.1
    myelophthisic 284.8
  nutritional (deficiency) 281.9
    with
      poor iron absorption 280.9
      specified deficiency NEC 281.8
    due to inadequate dietary iron intake 280.1
    megaloblastic (of infancy) 281.2
  of childhood (*see also* Thalassemia) 282.4
  of or complicating pregnancy 648.2
    affecting fetus or newborn 760.8
  of prematurity 776.6
  orotic aciduric (congenital) (hereditary) 281.4
  osteosclerotic 289.8
  ovalocytosis (hereditary) (*see also*
    Elliptocytosis) 282.1
  paludal (*see also* Malaria) 084.6
  pentose phosphate pathway deficiency 282.2
  pernicious (combined system disease)
      (congenital) (dorsolateral spinal
      degeneration) (juvenile) (myelopathy)
      (neuropathy) (posterior sclerosis) (primary)
      (progressive) (spleen) 281.0
    of or complicating pregnancy 648.2
  pleochromic 285.9
    of sprue 281.8
  portal 285.8
  posthemorrhagic (chronic) 280.0
    acute 285.1
    newborn 776.5
  pressure 285.9
  primary 285.9
  profound 285.9
  progressive 285.9
    malignant 281.0
    pernicious 281.0
  protein-deficiency 281.4
  pseudoleukemica infantum 285.8
  puerperal 648.2
  pure red cell 284.8
    congenital 284.0
  pyridoxine-responsive (hypochromic) 285.0
  pyruvate kinase (PK) deficiency 282.3
  refractoria sideroblastica 285.0
  refractory (primary) 284.9
    with hemochromatosis 285.0
    megaloblastic 281.3
    sideroblastic 285.0
    sideropenic 280.9
  Rietti-Greppi-Micheli (thalassemia minor) 282.4
  scorbutic 281.8
  secondary (to) 285.9
    blood loss (chronic) 280.0
      acute 285.1
    hemorrhage 280.0
      acute 285.1
    inadequate dietary iron intake 280.1

Anemia—*continued*
  semiplastic 284.9
  septic 285.9
  sickle-cell (*see also* Disease, sickle-cell) 282.60
  sideroachrestic 285.0
  sideroblastic (acquired) (any type) (congenital)
      (drug-induced) (due to disease) (hereditary)
      (primary) (refractory) (secondary)
      (sex-linked hypochromic) (vitamin B_6
      responsive) 285.0
  sideropenic (refractory) 280.9
    due to blood loss (chronic) 280.0
      acute 285.1
  simple chronic 281.9
  specified type NEC 285.8
  spherocytic (hereditary) (*see also*
    Spherocytosis) 282.0
  splenic 285.8
    familial (Gaucher's) 272.7
  splenomegalic 285.8
  stomatocytosis 282.8
  syphilitic 095.8
  target cell (oval) 282.4
  thalassemia 282.4
  thrombocytopenic (*see also* Thrombocytopenia)
    287.5
  toxic 284.8
  triosephosphate isomerase deficiency 282.3
  tropical, macrocytic 281.2
  tuberculous (*see also* Tuberculosis) 017.9
  vegan's 281.1
  vitamin
    B_6-responsive 285.0
    B_{12} deficiency (dietary) 281.1
      pernicious 281.0
  von Jaksch's (pseudoleukemia infantum) 285.8
  Witts' (achlorhydric anemia) 280.9
  Zuelzer (-Ogden) (nutritional megaloblastic
    anemia) 281.2
Anencephalus, anencephaly 740.0
  fetal, affecting management of pregnancy 655.0
Anergasia (*see also* Psychosis, organic) 294.9
  senile 290.0
Anesthesia, anesthetic 782.0
  complication or reaction NEC 995.2
    due to
      correct substance properly administered
        995.2
      overdose or wrong substance given 968.4
        specified anesthetic—*see* Table of drugs
          and chemicals
  cornea 371.81
  death from
    correct substance properly administered 995.4
    during delivery 668.9
    overdose or wrong substance given 968.4
      specified anesthetic—*see* Table of drugs
        and chemicals
  eye 371.81
  functional 300.11
  hyperesthetic, thalamic 348.8
  hysterical 300.11
  local skin lesion 782.0
  olfactory 781.1
  sexual (psychogenic) 302.72
  shock
    due to
      correct substance properly administered
        995.4
      overdose or wrong substance given 968.4

Anesthesia, anesthetic—*continued*
    specified anesthetic—*see* Table of drugs
      and chemicals
  skin 782.0
  tactile 782.0
  testicular 608.9
  thermal 782.0
Anetoderma (maculosum) 701.3
Aneuploidy NEC 758.5
Aneurin deficiency 265.1
Aneurysm (anastomotic) (artery) (cirsoid)
    (diffuse) (false) (fusiform) (multiple)
    (ruptured) (saccular) (varicose) 442.9
  abdominal (aorta) 441.4
    ruptured 441.3
    syphilitic 093.0
  aorta, aortic (nonsyphilitic) 441.9
    abdominal 441.4
      dissecting 441.02
      ruptured 441.3
      syphilitic 093.0
    arch 441.2
      ruptured 441.1
    arteriosclerotic NEC 441.9
      ruptured 441.5
    ascending 441.2
      ruptured 441.1
    congenital 747.29
    descending 441.9
      abdominal 441.4
        ruptured 441.3
      ruptured 441.5
      thoracic 441.2
        ruptured 441.1
    dissecting 441.00
      abdominal 441.02
      thoracic 441.01
      thoracoabdominal 441.03
    due to coarctation (aorta) 747.10
    ruptured 441.5
    sinus, right 747.29
    syphilitic 093.0
    thoracoabdominal 441.7
      ruptured 441.6
    thorax, thoracic (arch) (nonsyphilitic) 441.2
      dissecting 441.01
      ruptured 441.1
      syphilitic 093.0
    transverse 441.2
      ruptured 441.1
    valve (heart) (*see also* Endocarditis, aortic)
      424.1
  arteriosclerotic NEC 442.9
    cerebral 437.3
      ruptured (*see also* Hemorrhage,
        subarachnoid) 430
  arteriovenous (congenital) (peripheral) NEC
    (*see also* Anomaly, arteriovenous) 747.60
    acquired NEC 447.0
      brain 437.3
        ruptured (*see also* Hemorrhage,
          subarachnoid) 430
      coronary 414.11
      pulmonary 417.0
    brain (cerebral) 747.81
      ruptured (*see also* Hemorrhage,
        subarachnoid) 430
    coronary 746.85
    pulmonary 747.3
    retina 743.58
    specified site NEC 747.89

Aneurysm—*continued*
  acquired 447.0
  traumatic (*see also* Injury, blood vessel, by
    site) 904.9
  basal—*see* Aneurysm, brain
  berry (congenital) (ruptured) (*see also*
    Hemorrhage, subarachnoid) 430
  brain 437.3
    arteriosclerotic 437.3
      ruptured (*see also* Hemorrhage,
        subarachnoid) 430
    arteriovenous 747.81
      acquired 437.3
        ruptured (*see also* Hemorrhage,
          subarachnoid) 430
      ruptured (*see also* Hemorrhage,
        subarachnoid) 430
    berry (congenital) (ruptured) (*see also*
      Hemorrhage, subarachnoid) 430
    congenital 747.81
      ruptured (*see also* Hemorrhage,
        subarachnoid) 430
    meninges 437.3
      ruptured (*see also* Hemorrhage,
        subarachnoid) 430
    miliary (congenital) (ruptured) (*see also*
      Hemorrhage, subarachnoid) 430
    mycotic 421.0
      ruptured (*see also* Hemorrhage,
        subarachnoid) 430
    nonruptured 437.3
    ruptured (*see also* Hemorrhage, subarachnoid)
      430
    syphilitic 094.87
    syphilitic (hemorrhage) 094.87
    traumatic—*see* Injury, intracranial
  cardiac (false) (*see also* Aneurysm, heart)
    414.10
  carotid artery (common) (external) 442.81
    internal (intracranial portion) 437.3
      extracranial portion 442.81
      ruptured into brain (*see also* Hemorrhage,
        subarachnoid) 430
      syphilitic 093.89
        intracranial 094.87
  cavernous sinus (*see also* Aneurysm, brain)
    437.3
    arteriovenous 747.81
      ruptured (*see also* Hemorrhage,
        subarachnoid) 430
    congenital 747.81
      ruptured (*see also* Hemorrhage,
        subarachnoid) 430
  celiac 442.84
  central nervous system, syphilitic 094.89
  cerebral—*see* Aneurysm, brain
  chest—*see* Aneurysm, thorax
  circle of Willis (*see also* Aneurysm, brain) 437.3
    congenital 747.81
      ruptured (*see also* Hemorrhage,
        subarachnoid) 430
    ruptured (*see also* Hemorrhage, subarachnoid)
      430
  common iliac artery 442.2
  congenital (peripheral) NEC 747.60
    brain 747.81
      ruptured (*see also* Hemorrhage,
        subarachnoid) 430
    cerebral—*see* Aneurysm, brain, congenital
    coronary 746.85
    gastrointestinal 747.61

Aneurysm—*continued*
  lower limb 747.64
  pulmonary 747.3
  renal 747.62
  retina 743.58
  specified site NEC 747.89
  spinal 747.82
  upper limb 747.63
conjunctiva 372.74
conus arteriosus (*see also* Aneurysm, heart)
  414.10
coronary (arteriosclerotic) (artery) (vein) (*see
  also* Aneurysm, heart) 414.11
  arteriovenous 746.85
  congenital 746.85
  syphilitic 093.89
cylindrical 441.9
  ruptured 441.5
  syphilitic 093.9
dissecting 442.9
  aorta 441.00
    abdominal 441.02
    thoracic 441.01
    thoracoabdominal 441.03
  syphilitic 093.9
ductus arteriosus 747.0
embolic—*see* Embolism, artery
endocardial, infective (any valve) 421.0
femoral 442.3
gastroduodenal 442.84
gastroepiploic 442.84
heart (chronic or with a stated duration of over 8
  weeks) (infectional) (wall) 414.10
  acute or with a stated duration of 8 weeks or
    less (*see also* Infarct, myocardium) 410.9
  congenital 746.89
  valve—*see* Endocarditis
hepatic 442.84
iliac (common) 442.2
infective (any valve) 421.0
innominate (nonsyphilitic) 442.89
  syphilitic 093.89
interauricular septum (*see also* Aneurysm,
  heart) 414.10
interventricular septum (*see also* Aneurysm,
  heart) 414.10
intracranial—*see* Aneurysm, brain
intrathoracic (nonsyphilitic) 441.2
  ruptured 441.1
  syphilitic 093.0
jugular vein 453.8
lower extremity 442.3
lung (pulmonary artery) 417.1
malignant 093.9
mediastinal (nonsyphilitic) 442.89
  syphilitic 093.89
miliary (congenital) (ruptured) (*see also*
  Hemorrhage, subarachnoid) 430
mitral (heart) (valve) 424.0
mural (arteriovenous) (heart) (*see also*
  Aneurysm, heart) 414.10
mycotic, any site 421.0
  ruptured, brain (*see also* Hemorrhage,
    subarachnoid) 430
myocardium (*see also* Aneurysm, heart) 414.10
neck 442.81
pancreaticoduodenal 442.84
patent ductus arteriosus 747.0
peripheral NEC 442.89
  congenital NEC (*see also* Aneurysm,
    congenital) 747.60

Aneurysm—*continued*
  popliteal 442.3
  pulmonary 417.1
    arteriovenous 747.3
    acquired 417.0
    syphilitic 093.89
    valve (heart) (*see also* Endocarditis,
      pulmonary) 424.3
  racemose 442.9
    congenital (peripheral) NEC 747.60
  radial 442.0
  Rasmussen's (*see also* Tuberculosis) 011.2
  renal 442.1
  retinal (acquired) 362.17
    congenital 743.58
    diabetic 250.5 *[362.01]*
  sinus, aortic (of Valsalva) 747.29
  specified site NEC 442.89
  spinal (cord) 442.89
    congenital 747.82
    syphilitic (hemorrhage) 094.89
  spleen, splenic 442.83
  subclavian 442.82
    syphilitic 093.89
  superior mesenteric 442.84
  syphilitic 093.9
    aorta 093.0
    central nervous system 094.89
    congenital 090.5
    spine, spinal 094.89
  thoracoabdominal 441.7
    ruptured 441.6
  thorax, thoracic (arch) (nonsyphilitic) 441.2
    dissecting 441.01
    ruptured 441.1
    syphilitic 093.0
  traumatic (complication) (early)—*see* Injury,
    blood vessel, by site
  tricuspid (heart) (valve)—*see* Endocarditis,
    tricuspid
  ulnar 442.0
  upper extremity 442.0
  valve, valvular—*see* Endocarditis
  venous 456.8
    congenital NEC (*see also* Aneurysm,
      congenital) 747.60
  ventricle (arteriovenous) (*see also* Aneurysm,
    heart) 414.10
  visceral artery NEC 442.84
Angiectasis 459.89
Angiectopia 459.9
Angiitis 447.6
  allergic granulomatous 446.4
  hypersensitivity 446.20
    Goodpasture's syndrome 446.21
    specified NEC 446.29
  necrotizing 446.0
  Wegener's (necrotizing respiratory
    granulomatosis) 446.4
Angina (attack) (cardiac) (chest) (effort) (heart)
  (pectoris) (syndrome) (vasomotor) 413.9
  abdominal 557.1
  agranulocytic 288.0
  aphthous 074.0
  catarrhal 462
  crescendo 411.1
  croupous 464.4
  cruris 443.9
    due to atherosclerosis NEC (*see also*
      Arteriosclerosis, extremities) 440.20
  decubitus 413.0

Angioscotoma, enlarged 368.42
Angiospasm 443.9
  brachial plexus 353.0
  cerebral 435.9
  cervical plexus 353.2
  nerve
    arm 354.9
      axillary 353.0
      median 354.1
      ulnar 354.2
    autonomic (*see also* Neuropathy, peripheral,
      autonomic) 337.9
    axillary 353.0
    leg 355.8
      plantar 355.6
    lower extremity—*see* Angiospasm, nerve, leg
    median 354.1
    peripheral NEC 355.9
    spinal NEC 355.9
    sympathetic (*see also* Neuropathy, peripheral,
      autonomic) 337.9
    ulnar 354.2
    upper extremity—*see* Angiospasm, nerve, arm
  peripheral NEC 443.9
  traumatic 443.9
    foot 443.9
    leg 443.9
  vessel 443.9
Angiospastic disease or edema 443.9
Anguillulosis 127.2
Angulation
  cecum (*see also* Obstruction, intestine) 560.9
  coccyx (acquired) 738.6
    congenital 756.19
  femur (acquired) 736.39
    congenital 755.69
  intestine (large) (small) (*see also* Obstruction,
    intestine) 560.9
  sacrum (acquired) 738.5
    congenital 756.19
  sigmoid (flexure) (*see also* Obstruction,
    intestine) 560.9
  spine (*see also* Curvature, spine) 737.9
  tibia (acquired) 736.89
    congenital 755.69
  ureter 593.3
  wrist (acquired) 736.09
    congenital 755.59
Angulus infectiosus 686.8
Anhedonia 302.72
Anhidrosis (lid) (neurogenic) (thermogenic)
  705.0
Anhydration 276.5
  with
    hypernatremia 276.0
    hyponatremia 276.1
Anhydremia 276.5
  with
    hypernatremia 276.0
    hyponatremia 276.1
Anidrosis 705.0
Aniridia (congenital) 743.45
Anisakiasis (infection) (infestation) 127.1
Anisakis larva infestation 127.1
Aniseikonia 367.32
Anisocoria (pupil) 379.41
  congenital 743.46
Anisocytosis 790.09
Anisometropia (congenital) 367.31
Ankle —*see* condition

Ankyloblepharon (acquired) (eyelid) 374.46
  filiforme (adnatum) (congenital) 743.62
  total 743.62
Ankylodactly (*see also* Syndactylism) 755.10
Ankyloglossia 750.0
Ankylosis (fibrous) (osseous) 718.50
  ankle 718.57
  any joint, produced by surgical fusion V45.4
  cricoarytenoid (cartilage) (joint) (larynx) 478.79
  dental 521.6
  ear ossicle NEC 385.22
    malleus 385.21
  elbow 718.52
  finger 718.54
  hip 718.55
  incostapedial joint (infectional) 385.22
  joint, produced by surgical fusion NEC V45.4
  knee 718.56
  lumbosacral (joint) 724.6
  malleus 385.21
  multiple sites 718.59
  postoperative (status) V45.4
  sacroiliac (joint) 724.6
  shoulder 718.51
  specified site NEC 718.58
  spine NEC 724.9
  surgical V45.4
  teeth, tooth (hard tissues) 521.6
  temporomandibular joint 524.61
  wrist 718.53
Ankylostoma— *see* Ancylostoma
Ankylostomiasis (intestinal)—*see*
  Ancylostomiasis
Ankylurethria (*see also* Stricture, urethra) 598.9
Annular —*see also* condition
  detachment, cervix 622.8
  organ or site, congenital NEC—*see* Distortion
  pancreas (congenital) 751.7
Anodontia (complete) (partial) (vera) 520.0
  with abnormal spacing 524.3
  acquired 525.10
    causing malocclusion 524.3
    due to
      caries 525.13
      extraction 525.10
      periodontal disease 525.12
      trauma 525.11
Anomaly, anomalous (congenital) (unspecified
  type) 759.9
  abdomen 759.9
  abdominal wall 756.70
  acoustic nerve 742.9
  adrenal (gland) 759.1
  Alder (-Reilly) (leukocyte granulation) 288.2
  alimentary tract 751.9
    lower 751.5
    specified type NEC 751.8
    upper (any part, except tongue) 750.9
      tongue 750.10
        specified type NEC 750.19
  alveolar ridge (process) 525.8
  ankle (joint) 755.69
  anus, anal (canal) 751.5
  aorta, aortic 747.20
    arch 747.21
    coarctation (postductal) (preductal) 747.10
    cusp or valve NEC 746.9
    septum 745.0
    specified type NEC 747.29
  aorticopulmonary septum 745.0
  apertures, diaphragm 756.6

Anomaly, anomalous—*continued*
  appendix 751.5
  aqueduct of Sylvius 742.3
    with spina bifida (*see also* Spina bifida) 741.0
  arm 755.50
    reduction (*see also* Deformity, reduction,
      upper limb) 755.20
  arteriovenous (congenital) (peripheral) NEC
    747.60
    brain 747.81
    cerebral 747.81
    coronary 746.85
    gastrointestinal 747.61
    lower limb 747.64
    renal 747.62
    specified site NEC 747.69
    spinal 747.82
    upper limb 747.63
  artery (*see also* Anomaly, peripheral vascular
      system) NEC 747.60
    brain 747.81
    cerebral 747.81
    coronary 746.85
    eye 743.9
    pulmonary 747.3
    renal 747.62
    retina 743.9
    umbilical 747.5
  arytenoepiglottic folds 748.3
  atrial
    bands 746.9
    folds 746.9
    septa 745.5
  atrioventricular
    canal 745.69
    common 745.69
    conduction 426.7
    excitation 426.7
    septum 745.4
  atrium—*see* Anomaly, atrial
  auditory canal 744.3
    specified type NEC 744.29
      with hearing impairment 744.02
  auricle
    ear 744.3
      causing impairment of hearing 744.02
    heart 746.9
      septum 745.5
  autosomes, autosomal NEC 758.5
  Axenfeld's 743.44
  back 759.9
  band
    atrial 746.9
    heart 746.9
    ventricular 746.9
  Bartholin's duct 750.9
  biliary duct or passage 751.60
    atresia 751.61
  bladder (neck) (sphincter) (trigone) 753.9
    specified type NEC 753.8
  blood vessel 747.9
    artery—*see* Anomaly, artery
    peripheral vascular—*see* Anomaly, peripheral
      vascular system
    vein—*see* Anomaly, vein
  bone NEC 756.9
    ankle 755.69
    arm 755.50
    chest 756.3
    cranium 756.0
    face 756.0

Anomaly, anomalous— *continued*
  finger 755.50
  foot 755.67
  forearm 755.50
  frontal 756.0
  head 756.0
  hip 755.63
  leg 755.60
  lumbosacral 756.10
  nose 748.1
  pelvic girdle 755.60
  rachitic 756.4
  rib 756.3
  shoulder girdle 755.50
  skull 756.0
    with
      anencephalus 740.0
      encephalocele 742.0
      hydrocephalus 742.3
        with spina bifida (*see also* Spina bifida)
          741.0
      microcephalus 742.1
  toe 755.66
  brain 742.9
    multiple 742.4
    reduction 742.2
    specified type NEC 742.4
    vessel 747.81
  branchial cleft NEC 744.49
    cyst 744.42
    fistula 744.41
    persistent 744.41
    sinus (external) (internal) 744.41
  breast 757.9
  broad ligament 752.10
    specified type NEC 752.19
  bronchus 748.3
  bulbar septum 745.0
  bulbus cordis 745.9
    persistent (in left ventricle) 745.8
  bursa 756.9
  canal of Nuck 752.9
  canthus 743.9
  capillary NEC (*see also* Anomaly, peripheral
      vascular system) 747.60
  cardiac 746.9
    septal closure 745.9
      acquired 429.71
    valve NEC 746.9
      pulmonary 746.00
      specified type NEC 746.89
  cardiovascular system 746.9
    complicating pregnancy, childbirth, or
      puerperium 648.5
  carpus 755.50
  cartilage, trachea 748.3
  cartilaginous 756.9
  caruncle, lacrimal, lachrymal 743.9
  cascade stomach 750.7
  cauda equina 742.59
  cecum 751.5
  cerebral—*see also* Anomaly, brain
    vessels 747.81
  cerebrovascular system 747.81
  cervix (uterus) 752.40
    with doubling of vagina and uterus 752.2
    in pregnancy or childbirth 654.6
      affecting fetus or newborn 763.89
      causing obstructed labor 660.2
        affecting fetus or newborn 763.1

Anomaly, anomalous—*continued*
   Chédiak-Higashi (-Steinbrinck) (congenital
      gigantism of peroxidase granules) 288.2
   cheek 744.9
   chest (wall) 756.3
   chin 744.9
      specified type NEC 744.89
   chordae tendineae 746.9
   choroid 743.9
      plexus 742.9
   chromosomes, chromosomal 758.9
      13 (13-15) 758.1
      18 (16-18) 758.2
      21 or 22 758.0
      autosomes NEC (*see also* Abnormality,
         autosomes) 758.5
         deletion 758.3
      Christchurch 758.3
      D₁ 758.1
      E₃ 758.2
      G 758.0
      mitochondrial 758.9
      mosaics 758.89
      sex 758.81
         complement, XO 758.6
         complement, XXX 758.81
         complement, XYY 758.81
         gonadal dysgenesis 758.6
         Klinefelter's 758.7
         Turner's 758.6
      trisomy 21 758.0
   cilia 743.9
   circulatory system 747.9
      specified type NEC 747.89
   clavicle 755.51
   clitoris 752.40
   coccyx 756.10
   colon 751.5
   common duct 751.60
   communication
      coronary artery 746.85
      left ventricle with right atrium 745.4
   concha (ear) 744.3
   connection
      renal vessels with kidney 747.62
      total pulmonary venous 747.41
   connective tissue 756.9
      specified type NEC 756.89
   cornea 743.9
      shape 743.41
      size 743.41
      specified type NEC 743.49
   coronary
      artery 746.85
      vein 746.89
   cranium—*see* Anomaly, skull
   cricoid cartilage 748.3
   cushion, endocardial 745.60
      specified type NEC 745.69
   cystic duct 751.60
   dental arch relationship 524.2
   dentition 520.6
   dentofacial NEC 524.9
      functional 524.5
      specified type NEC 524.8
   dermatoglyphic 757.2
   Descemet's membrane 743.9
      specified type NEC 743.49
   development
      cervix 752.40
      vagina 752.40

Anomaly, anomalous— *continued*
   vulva 752.40
   diaphragm, diaphragmatic (apertures) NEC
      756.6
   digestive organ(s) or system 751.9
      lower 751.5
      specified type NEC 751.8
      upper 750.9
   distribution, coronary artery 746.85
   ductus
      arteriosus 747.0
      Botalli 747.0
   duodenum 751.5
   dura 742.9
      brain 742.4
      spinal cord 742.59
   ear 744.3
      causing impairment of hearing 744.00
         specified type NEC 744.09
      external 744.3
         causing impairment of hearing 744.02
         specified type NEC 744.29
      inner (causing impairment of hearing) 744.05
      middle, except ossicles (causing impairment
         of hearing) 744.03
         ossicles 744.04
      ossicles 744.04
      prominent auricle 744.29
      specified type NEC 744.29
         with hearing impairment 744.09
   Ebstein's (heart) 746.2
      tricuspid valve 746.2
   ectodermal 757.9
   Eisenmenger's (ventricular septal defect) 745.4
   ejaculatory duct 752.9
      specified type NEC 752.8
   elbow (joint) 755.50
   endocardial cushion 745.60
      specified type NEC 745.69
   endocrine gland NEC 759.2
   epididymis 752.9
   epiglottis 748.3
   esophagus 750.9
      specified type NEC 750.4
   Eustachian tube 744.3
      specified type NEC 744.24
   eye (any part) 743.9
      adnexa 743.9
         specified type NEC 743.69
      anophthalmos 743.00
      anterior
         chamber and related structures 743.9
            angle 743.9
               specified type NEC 743.44
            specified type NEC 743.44
         segment 743.9
            combined 743.48
            multiple 743.48
            specified type NEC 743.49
      cataract (*see also* Cataract) 743.30
      glaucoma (*see also* Buphthalmia) 743.20
      lid 743.9
         specified type NEC 743.63
      microphthalmos (*see also* Microphthalmos)
         743.10
      posterior segment 743.9
         specified type NEC 743.59
         vascular 743.58
         vitreous 743.9
            specified type NEC 743.51
      ptosis (eyelid) 743.61

Anomaly, anomalous—*continued*
  retina 743.9
    specified type NEC 743.59
  sclera 743.9
    specified type NEC 743.47
    specified type NEC 743.8
  eyebrow 744.89
  eyelid 743.9
    specified type NEC 743.63
  face (any part) 744.9
    bone(s) 756.0
    specified type NEC 744.89
  fallopian tube 752.10
    specified type NEC 752.19
  fascia 756.9
    specified type NEC 756.89
  femur 755.60
  fibula 755.60
  finger 755.50
    supernumerary 755.01
    webbed (*see also* Syndactylism, fingers) 755.11
  fixation, intestine 751.4
  flexion (joint) 755.9
    hip or thigh (*see also* Dislocation, hip, congenital) 754.30
  folds, heart 746.9
  foot 755.67
  foramen
    Botalli 745.5
    ovale 745.5
  forearm 755.50
  forehead (*see also* Anomaly, skull) 756.0
  form, teeth 520.2
  fovea centralis 743.9
  frontal bone (*see also* Anomaly, skull) 756.0
  gallbladder 751.60
  Gartner's duct 752.11
  gastrointestinal tract 751.9
    specified type NEC 751.8
    vessel 747.61
  genitalia, genital organ(s) or system
    female 752.9
      external 752.40
        specified type NEC 752.49
      internal NEC 752.9
    male (external and internal) 752.9
      epispadias 752.62
      hidden penis 752.65
      hydrocele, congenital 778.6
      hypospadias 752.61
      micropenis 752.64
      testis, undescended 752.51
        retractile 752.52
    specified type NEC 752.8
  genitourinary NEC 752.9
  Gerbode 745.4
  globe (eye) 743.9
  glottis 748.3
  granulation or granulocyte, genetic 288.2
    constitutional 288.2
    leukocyte 288.2
  gum 750.9
  gyri 742.9
  hair 757.9
    specified type NEC 757.4
  hand 755.50
  hard tissue formation in pulp 522.3
  head (*see also* Anomaly, skull) 756.0
  heart 746.9
    auricle 746.9

Anomaly, anomalous—*continued*
    bands 746.9
    fibroelastosis cordis 425.3
    folds 746.9
    malposition 746.87
    maternal, affecting fetus or newborn 760.3
    obstructive NEC 746.84
    patent ductus arteriosus (Botalli) 747.0
    septum 745.9
      acquired 429.71
      aortic 745.0
      aorticopulmonary 745.0
      atrial 745.5
      auricular 745.5
      between aorta and pulmonary artery 745.0
      endocardial cushion type 745.60
        specified type NEC 745.69
      interatrial 745.5
      interventricular 745.4
        with pulmonary stenosis or atresia, dextraposition of aorta, and hypertrophy of right ventricle 745.2
        acquired 429.71
        specified type NEC 745.8
      ventricular 745.4
        with pulmonary stenosis or atresia, dextraposition of aorta, and hypertrophy of right ventricle 745.2
        acquired 429.71
    specified type NEC 746.89
    tetralogy of Fallot 745.2
    valve NEC 746.9
      aortic 746.9
        atresia 746.89
        bicuspid valve 746.4
        insufficiency 746.4
        specified type NEC 746.89
        stenosis 746.3
          subaortic 746.81
          supravalvular 747.22
      mitral 746.9
        atresia 746.89
        insufficiency 746.6
        specified type NEC 746.89
        stenosis 746.5
      pulmonary 746.00
        atresia 746.01
        insufficiency 746.09
        stenosis 746.02
          infundibular 746.83
          subvalvular 746.83
      tricuspid 746.9
        atresia 746.1
        stenosis 746.1
    ventricle 746.9
  heel 755.67
  Hegglin's 288.2
  hemianencephaly 740.0
  hemicephaly 740.0
  hemicrania 740.0
  hepatic duct 751.60
  hip (joint) 755.63
  hourglass
    bladder 753.8
    gallbladder 751.69
    stomach 750.7
  humerus 755.50
  hymen 752.40
  hypersegmentation of neutrophils, hereditary 288.2
  hypophyseal 759.2

Anomaly, anomalous—*continued*
  ileocecal (coil) (valve) 751.5
  ileum (intestine) 751.5
  ilium 755.60
  integument 757.9
    specified type NEC 757.8
  intervertebral cartilage or disc 756.10
  intestine (large) (small) 751.5
    fixational type 751.4
  iris 743.9
    specified type NEC 743.46
  ischium 755.60
  jaw NEC 524.9
    closure 524.5
    size NEC 524.00
    specified type NEC 524.8
  jaw-cranial base relationship 524.10
    specified NEC 524.19
  jejunum 751.5
  joint 755.9
    hip
      dislocation (*see also* Dislocation, hip,
        congenital) 754.30
      predislocation (*see also* Subluxation,
        congenital, hip) 754.32
      preluxation (*see also* Subluxation,
        congenital, hip) 754.32
      subluxation (*see also* Subluxation,
        congenital, hip) 754.32
    lumbosacral 756.10
      spondylolisthesis 756.12
      spondylosis 756.11
    multiple arthrogryposis 754.89
    sacroiliac 755.69
  Jordan's 288.2
  kidney(s) (calyx) (pelvis) 753.9
    vessel 747.62
  Klippel-Feil (brevicollis) 756.16
  knee (joint) 755.64
  labium (majus) (minus) 752.40
  labyrinth, membranous (causing impairment of
    hearing) 744.05
  lacrimal
    apparatus, duct or passage 743.9
      specified type NEC 743.65
    gland 743.9
      specified type NEC 743.64
  Langdon Down (mongolism) 758.0
  larynx, laryngeal (muscle) 748.3
    web, webbed 748.2
  leg (lower) (upper) 755.60
    reduction NEC (*see also* Deformity,
      reduction, lower limb) 755.30
  lens 743.9
    shape 743.36
    specified type NEC 743.39
  leukocytes, genetic 288.2
    granulation (constitutional) 288.2
  lid (fold) 743.9
  ligament 756.9
    broad 752.10
    round 752.9
  limb, except reduction deformity 755.9
    lower 755.60
      reduction deformity (*see also* Deformity,
        reduction, lower limb) 755.30
      specified type NEC 755.69
    upper 755.50
      reduction deformity (*see also* Deformity,
        reduction, upper limb) 755.20
      specified type NEC 755.59

Anomaly, anomalous—*continued*
  lip 750.9
    harelip (*see also* Cleft, lip) 749.10
    specified type NEC 750.26
  liver (duct) 751.60
    atresia 751.69
  lower extremity 755.60
    vessel 747.64
  lumbosacral (joint) (region) 756.10
  lung (fissure) (lobe) NEC 748.60
    agenesis 748.5
    specified type NEC 748.69
  lymphatic system 759.9
  Madelung's (radius) 755.54
  mandible 524.9
    size NEC 524.00
  maxilla 524.9
    size NEC 524.00
  May (-Hegglin) 288.2
  meatus urinarius 753.9
    specified type NEC 753.8
  meningeal bands or folds, constriction of 742.8
  meninges 742.9
    brain 742.4
    spinal 742.59
  meningocele (*see also* Spina bifida) 741.9
  mesentery 751.9
  metacarpus 755.50
  metatarsus 755.67
  middle ear, except ossicles (causing impairment
    of hearing) 744.03
    ossicles 744.04
  mitral (leaflets) (valve) 746.9
    atresia 746.89
    insufficiency 746.6
    specified type NEC 746.89
    stenosis 746.5
  mouth 750.9
    specified type NEC 750.26
  multiple NEC 759.7
    specified type NEC 759.89
  muscle 756.9
    eye 743.9
      specified type NEC 743.69
    specified type NEC 756.89
  musculoskeletal system, except limbs 756.9
    specified type NEC 756.9
  nail 757.9
    specified type NEC 757.5
  narrowness, eyelid 743.62
  nasal sinus or septum 748.1
  neck (any part) 744.9
    specified type NEC 744.89
  nerve 742.9
    acoustic 742.9
      specified type NEC 742.8
    optic 742.9
      specified type NEC 742.8
    specified type NEC 742.8
  nervous system NEC 742.9
    brain 742.9
      specified type NEC 742.4
    specified type NEC 742.8
  neurological 742.9
  nipple 757.9
  nonteratogenic NEC 754.89
  nose, nasal (bone) (cartilage) (septum) (sinus)
    748.1
  ocular muscle 743.9
  omphalomesenteric duct 751.0
  opening, pulmonary veins 747.49

Anomaly, anomalous—*continued*
  optic
    disc 743.9
      specified type NEC 743.57
    nerve 742.9
  opticociliary vessels 743.9
  orbit (eye) 743.9
    specified type NEC 743.66
  organ
    of Corti (causing impairment of hearing)
      744.05
    or site 759.9
      specified type NEC 759.89
  origin
    both great arteries from same ventricle 745.11
    coronary artery 746.85
    innominate artery 747.69
    left coronary artery from pulmonary artery
      746.85
    pulmonary artery 747.3
    renal vessels 747.62
    subclavian artery (left) (right) 747.21
  osseous meatus (ear) 744.03
  ovary 752.0
  oviduct 752.10
  palate (hard) (soft) 750.9
    cleft (*see also* Cleft, palate) 749.00
  pancreas (duct) 751.7
  papillary muscles 746.9
  parathyroid gland 759.2
  paraurethral ducts 753.9
  parotid (gland) 750.9
  patella 755.64
  Pelger-Huët (hereditary hyposegmentation)
    288.2
  pelvic girdle 755.60
    specified type NEC 755.69
  pelvis (bony) 755.60
    complicating delivery 653.0
    rachitic 268.1
      fetal 756.4
  penis (glans) 752.69
  pericardium 746.89
  peripheral vascular system NEC 747.60
    gastrointestinal 747.61
    lower limb 747.64
    renal 747.62
    specified site NEC 747.69
    spinal 747.82
    upper limb 747.63
  Peter's 743.44
  pharynx 750.9
    branchial cleft 744.41
    specified type NEC 750.29
  Pierre Robin 756.0
  pigmentation NEC 709.00
    congenital 757.33
  pituitary (gland) 759.2
  pleural folds 748.8
  portal vein 747.40
  position tooth, teeth 524.3
  preauricular sinus 744.46
  prepuce 752.9
  prostate 752.9
  pulmonary 748.60
    artery 747.3
    circulation 747.3
    specified type NEC 748.69
    valve 746.00
      atresia 746.01
      insufficiency 746.09

Anomaly, anomalous—*continued*
    specified type NEC 746.09
    stenosis 746.02
      infundibular 746.83
      subvalvular 746.83
  vein 747.40
  venous
    connection 747.49
      partial 747.42
      total 747.41
    return 747.49
      partial 747.42
      total (TAPVR) (complete)
        (subdiaphragmatic)
        (supradiaphragmatic) 747.41
  pupil 743.9
  pylorus 750.9
    hypertrophy 750.5
    stenosis 750.5
  rachitic, fetal 756.4
  radius 755.50
  rectovaginal (septum) 752.40
  rectum 751.5
  refraction 367.9
  renal 753.9
    vessel 747.62
  respiratory system 748.9
    specified type NEC 748.8
  rib 756.3
    cervical 756.2
  Rieger's 743.44
  rings, trachea 748.3
  rotation—*see also* Malrotation
    hip or thigh (*see also* Subluxation, congenital,
      hip) 754.32
  round ligament 752.9
  sacroiliac (joint) 755.69
  sacrum 756.10
  saddle
    back 754.2
    nose 754.0
      syphilitic 090.5
  salivary gland or duct 750.9
    specified type NEC 750.26
  scapula 755.50
  sclera 743.9
    specified type NEC 743.47
  scrotum 752.9
  sebaceous gland 757.9
  seminal duct or tract 752.9
  sense organs 742.9
    specified type NEC 742.8
  septum
    heart—*see* Anomaly, heart, septum
    nasal 748.1
  sex chromosomes NEC (*see also* Anomaly,
    chromosomes) 758.81
  shoulder (girdle) (joint) 755.50
    specified type NEC 755.59
  sigmoid (flexure) 751.5
  sinus of Valsalva 747.29
  site NEC 759.9
  skeleton generalized NEC 756.50
  skin (appendage) 757.9
    specified type NEC 757.39
  skull (bone) 756.0
    with
      anencephalus 740.0
      encephalocele 742.0
      hydrocephalus 742.3

Anomaly, anomalous—*continued*
 with spina bifida (*see also* Spina bifida)
  741.0
 microcephalus 742.1
specified type NEC
 adrenal (gland) 759.1
 alimentary tract (complete) (partial) 751.8
  lower 751.5
  upper 750.8
 ankle 755.69
 anus, anal (canal) 751.5
 aorta, aortic 747.29
  arch 747.21
 appendix 751.5
 arm 755.59
 artery (peripheral) NEC (*see also* Anomaly,
  peripheral vascular system) 747.60
  brain 747.81
  coronary 746.85
  eye 743.58
  pulmonary 747.3
  retinal 743.58
  umbilical 747.5
 auditory canal 744.29
  causing impairment of hearing 744.02
 bile duct or passage 751.69
 bladder 753.8
  neck 753.8
 bone(s) 756.9
  arm 755.59
  face 756.0
  leg 755.69
  pelvic girdle 755.69
  shoulder girdle 755.59
  skull 756.0
   with
    anencephalus 740.0
    encephalocele 742.0
    hydrocephalus 742.3
     with spina bifida (*see also* Spina
      bifida) 741.0
    microcephalus 742.1
 brain 742.4
 breast 757.6
 broad ligament 752.19
 bronchus 748.3
 canal of Nuck 752.8
 cardiac septal closure 745.8
 carpus 755.59
 cartilaginous 756.9
 cecum 751.5
 cervix 752.49
 chest (wall) 756.3
 chin 744.89
 ciliary body 743.46
 circulatory system 747.89
 clavicle 755.51
 clitoris 752.49
 coccyx 756.19
 colon 751.5
 common duct 751.69
 connective tissue 756.89
 cricoid cartilage 748.3
 cystic duct 751.69
 diaphragm 756.6
 digestive organ(s) or tract 751.8
  lower 751.5
  upper 750.8
 duodenum 751.5
 ear 744.29
  auricle 744.29

Anomaly, anomalous—*continued*
 causing impairment of hearing 744.02
 causing impairment of hearing 744.09
 inner (causing impairment of hearing)
  744.05
 middle, except ossicles 744.03
  ossicles 744.04
 ejaculatory duct 752.8
 endocrine 759.2
 epiglottis 748.3
 esophagus 750.4
 Eustachian tube 744.24
 eye 743.8
  lid 743.63
  muscle 743.69
 face 744.89
  bone(s) 756.0
 fallopian tube 752.19
 fascia 756.89
 femur 755.69
 fibula 755.69
 finger 755.59
 foot 755.67
 fovea centralis 743.55
 gallbladder 751.69
 Gartner's duct 752.8
 gastrointestinal tract 751.8
 genitalia, genital organ(s)
  female 752.8
   external 752.49
   internal NEC 752.8
  male 752.8
   penis 752.69
 genitourinary tract NEC 752.8
 glottis 748.3
 hair 757.4
 hand 755.59
 heart 746.89
  valve NEC 746.89
  pulmonary 746.09
 hepatic duct 751.69
 hydatid of Morgagni 752.8
 hymen 752.49
 integument 757.8
 intestine (large) (small) 751.5
  fixational type 751.4
 iris 743.46
 jejunum 751.5
 joint 755.8
 kidney 753.3
 knee 755.64
 labium (majus) (minus) 752.49
 labyrinth, membranous 744.05
 larynx 748.3
 leg 755.69
 lens 743.39
 limb, except reduction deformity 755.8
  lower 755.69
   reduction deformity (*see also* Deformity,
    reduction, lower limb) 755.30
  upper 755.59
   reduction deformity (*see also* Deformity,
    reduction, upper limb) 755.20
 lip 750.26
 liver 751.69
 lung (fissure) (lobe) 748.69
 meatus urinarius 753.8
 metacarpus 755.59
 mouth 750.26
 muscle 756.89
  eye 743.69

Anomaly, anomalous—*continued*
  musculoskeletal system, except limbs 756.9
  nail 757.5
  neck 744.89
  nerve 742.8
    acoustic 742.8
    optic 742.8
  nervous system 742.8
  nipple 757.6
  nose 748.1
  organ NEC 759.89
    of Corti 744.05
  osseous meatus (ear) 744.03
  ovary 752.0
  oviduct 752.19
  pancreas 751.7
  parathyroid 759.2
  patella 755.64
  pelvic girdle 755.69
  penis 752.69
  pericardium 746.89
  peripheral vascular system NEC (*see also*
    Anomaly, peripheral vascular system)
    747.60
  pharynx 750.29
  pituitary 759.2
  prostate 752.8
  radius 755.59
  rectum 751.5
  respiratory system 748.8
  rib 756.3
  round ligament 752.8
  sacrum 756.19
  salivary duct or gland 750.26
  scapula 755.59
  sclera 743.47
  scrotum 752.8
  seminal duct or tract 752.8
  shoulder girdle 755.59
  site NEC 759.89
  skin 757.39
  skull (bone(s)) 756.0
    with
      anencephalus 740.0
      encephalocele 742.0
      hydrocephalus 742.3
        with spina bifida (*see also* Spina bifida)
        741.0
      microcephalus 742.1
  specified organ or site NEC 759.89
  spermatic cord 752.8
  spinal cord 742.59
  spine 756.19
  spleen 759.0
  sternum 756.3
  stomach 750.7
  tarsus 755.67
  tendon 756.89
  testis 752.8
  thorax (wall) 756.3
  thymus 759.2
  thyroid (gland) 759.2
    cartilage 748.3
  tibia 755.69
  toe 755.66
  tongue 750.19
  trachea (cartilage) 748.3
  ulna 755.59
  urachus 753.7
  ureter 753.4
    obstructive 753.29

Anomaly, anomalous—*continued*
  urethra 753.8
    obstructive 753.6
  urinary tract 753.8
  uterus 752.3
  uvula 750.26
  vagina 752.49
  vascular NEC (*see also* Anomaly, peripheral
    vascular system) 747.60
    brain 747.81
  vas deferens 752.8
  vein(s) (peripheral) NEC (*see also* Anomaly,
    peripheral vascular system) 747.60
    brain 747.81
    great 747.49
    portal 747.49
    pulmonary 747.49
  vena cava (inferior) (superior) 747.49
  vertebra 756.19
  vulva 752.49
  spermatic cord 752.9
  spine, spinal 756.10
    column 756.10
    cord 742.9
      meningocele (*see also* Spina bifida) 741.9
      specified type NEC 742.59
      spina bifida (*see also* Spina bifida) 741.9
      vessel 747.82
    meninges 742.59
    nerve root 742.9
  spleen 759.0
  Sprengel's 755.52
  sternum 756.3
  stomach 750.9
    specified type NEC 750.7
  submaxillary gland 750.9
  superior vena cava 747.40
  talipes—*see* Talipes
  tarsus 755.67
    with complete absence of distal elements
    755.31
  teeth, tooth NEC 520.9
    position 524.3
    spacing 524.3
  tendon 756.9
    specified type NEC 756.89
  termination
    coronary artery 746.85
  testis 752.9
  thebesian valve 746.9
  thigh 755.60
    flexion (*see also* Subluxation, congenital, hip)
    754.32
  thorax (wall) 756.3
  throat 750.9
  thumb 755.50
    supernumerary 755.01
  thymus gland 759.2
  thyroid (gland) 759.2
    cartilage 748.3
  tibia 755.60
    saber 090.5
  toe 755.66
    supernumerary 755.02
    webbed (*see also* Syndactylism, toes) 755.13
  tongue 750.10
    specified type NEC 750.19
  trachea, tracheal 748.3
    cartilage 748.3
    rings 748.3
  tragus 744.3

Anomaly, anomalous—*continued*
transverse aortic arch 747.21
trichromata 368.59
trichromatopsia 368.59
tricuspid (leaflet) (valve) 746.9
  atresia 746.1
  Ebstein's 746.2
  specified type NEC 746.89
  stenosis 746.1
trunk 759.9
Uhl's (hypoplasia of myocardium, right
  ventricle) 746.84
ulna 755.50
umbilicus 759.9
  artery 747.5
union, trachea with larynx 748.3
unspecified site 759.9
upper extremity 755.50
  vessel 747.63
urachus 753.7
  specified type NEC 753.7
ureter 753.9
  obstructive 753.20
  specified type NEC 753.4
    obstructive 753.29
urethra (valve) 753.9
  obstructive 753.6
  specified type NEC 753.8
urinary tract or system (any part, except
  urachus) 753.9
  specified type NEC 753.8
  urachus 753.7
uterus 752.3
  with only one functioning horn 752.3
  in pregnancy or childbirth 654.0
    affecting fetus or newborn 763.89
    causing obstructed labor 660.2
      affecting fetus or newborn 763.1
uvula 750.9
vagina 752.40
valleculae 748.3
valve (heart) NEC 746.9
  formation, ureter 753.29
  pulmonary 746.00
  specified type NEC 746.89
vascular NEC (*see also* Anomaly, peripheral
  vascular system) 747.60
  ring 747.21
vas deferens 752.9
vein(s) (peripheral) NEC (*see also* Anomaly,
  peripheral vascular system) 747.60
  brain 747.81
  cerebral 747.81
  coronary 746.89
  great 747.40
    specified type NEC 747.49
  portal 747.40
  pulmonary 747.40
  retina 743.9
vena cava (inferior) (superior) 747.40
venous return (pulmonary) 747.49
  partial 747.42
  total 747.41
ventricle, ventricular (heart) 746.9
  bands 746.9
  folds 746.9
  septa 745.4
vertebra 756.10
vesicourethral orifice 753.9
vessels NEC (*see also* Anomaly, peripheral
  vascular system) 747.60

Anomaly, anomalous—*continued*
  optic papilla 743.9
  vitelline duct 751.0
  vitreous humor 743.9
    specified type NEC 743.51
  vulva 752.40
  wrist (joint) 755.50
Anomia 784.69
Anonychia 757.5
  acquired 703.8
Anophthalmos, anophthalmus (clinical)
  (congenital) (globe) 743.00
  acquired V45.78
Anopsia (altitudinal) (quadrant) 368.46
Anorchia 752.8
Anorchism, anorchidism 752.8
Anorexia 783.0
  hysterical 300.11
  nervosa 307.1
Anosmia (*see also* Disturbance, sensation) 781.1
  hysterical 300.11
  postinfectional 478.9
  psychogenic 306.7
  traumatic 951.8
Anosognosia 780.99
Anosphrasia 781.1
Anosteoplasia 756.50
Anotia 744.09
Anovulatory cycle 628.0
Anoxemia 799.0
  newborn 768.9
Anoxia 799.0
  altitude 993.2
  cerebral 348.1
    with
      abortion—*see* Abortion, by type,
        with specified complication NEC
      ectopic pregnancy (*see also* categories
        633.0-633.9) 639.8
      molar pregnancy (*see also* categories
        630-632) 639.8
    complicating
      delivery (cesarean) (instrumental) 669.4
      ectopic or molar pregnancy 639.8
      obstetric anesthesia or sedation 668.2
    during or resulting from a procedure 997.01
    following
      abortion 639.8
      ectopic or molar pregnancy 639.8
    newborn (*see also* Distress, fetal, liveborn
      infant) 768.9
  due to drowning 994.1
  fetal, affecting newborn 768.9
  heart—*see* Insufficiency, coronary
  high altitude 993.2
  intrauterine
    fetal death (before onset of labor) 768.0
      during labor 768.1
    liveborn infant—*see* Distress, fetal, liveborn
      infant
  myocardial—*see* Insufficiency, coronary
  newborn 768.9
    mild or moderate 768.6
    severe 768.5
  pathological 799.0
Anteflexion —*see* Anteversion
Antenatal
  care, normal pregnancy V22.1
    first V22.0
  screening (for) V28.9
    based on amniocentesis NEC V28.2

Antenatal—*continued*
   chromosomal anomalies V28.0
    raised alphafetoprotein levels V28.1
   chromosomal anomalies V28.0
   fetal growth retardation using ultrasonics
    V28.4
   isoimmunization V28.5
   malformations using ultrasonics V28.3
   raised alphafetoprotein levels in amniotic fluid
    V28.1
   specified condition NEC V28.8
   Streptococcus B V28.6
Antepartum —*see* condition
Anterior —*see also* condition
   spinal artery compression syndrome 721.1
Antero-occlusion 524.2
Anteversion
   cervix (*see also* Anteversion, uterus) 621.6
   femur (neck), congenital 755.63
   uterus, uterine (cervix) (postinfectional)
    (postpartal, old) 621.6
   congenital 752.3
   in pregnancy or childbirth 654.4
    affecting fetus or newborn 763.89
    causing obstructed labor 660.2
     affecting fetus or newborn 763.1
Anthracosilicosis (occupational) 500
Anthracosis (lung) (occupational) 500
   lingua 529.3
Anthrax 022.9
   with pneumonia 022.1 *[484.5]*
   colitis 022.2
   cutaneous 022.0
   gastrointestinal 022.2
   intestinal 022.2
   pulmonary 022.1
   respiratory 022.1
   septicemia 022.3—
   specified manifestation NEC 022.8
Anthropoid pelvis 755.69
   with disproportion (fetopelvic) 653.2
    affecting fetus or newborn 763.1
    causing obstructed labor 660.1
     affecting fetus or newborn 763.1
Anthropophobia 300.29
Antibioma, breast 611.0
Antibodies
   maternal (blood group) (*see also*
    Incompatibility) 656.2
   anti-D, cord blood 656.1
    fetus or newborn 773.0
Antibody deficiency syndrome
   agammaglobulinemic 279.00
   congenital 279.04
   hypogammaglobulinemic 279.00
Anticoagulant, circulating (*see also* Circulating
   anticoagulants) 286.5
Antimongolism syndrome 758.3
Antimonial cholera 985.4
Antisocial personality 301.7
Antithrombinemia (*see also* Circulating
   anticoagulants) 286.5
Antithromboplastinemia (*see also* Circulating
   anticoagulants) 286.5
Antithromboplastinogenemia (*see also*
   Circulating anticoagulants) 286.5
Antitoxin complication or reaction —*see*
   Complications, vaccination
Anton (-Babinski) syndrome
   (hemiasomatognosia) 307.9
Antritis (chronic) 473.0
   acute 461.0

Antrum, antral —*see* condition
Anuria 788.5
   with
    abortion—*see* Abortion, by type, with renal
     failure
    ectopic pregnancy (*see also* categories
     633.0-633.9) 639.3
    molar pregnancy (*see also* categories
     630-632) 639.3
   calculus (impacted) (recurrent) 592.9
    kidney 592.0
    ureter 592.1
   congenital 753.3
   due to a procedure 997.5
   following
    abortion 639.3
    ectopic or molar pregnancy 639.3
   newborn 753.3
   postrenal 593.4
   puerperal, postpartum, childbirth 669.3
   specified as due to a procedure 997.5
   sulfonamide
    correct substance properly administered 788.5
    overdose or wrong substance given or taken
     961.0
   traumatic (following crushing) 958.5
Anus, anal —*see* condition
Anusitis 569.49
Anxiety (neurosis) (reaction) (state) 300.00
   alcohol-induced 291.89
   depression 300.4
   drug-induced 292.89
   due to or associated with physical condition
    293.84
   generalized 300.02
   hysteria 300.20
   in
    acute stress reaction 308.0
    transient adjustment reaction 309.24
   panic type 300.01
   separation, abnormal 309.21
   syndrome (organic) (transient) 293.84
Aorta, aortic —*see* condition
Aortectasia 441.9
Aortitis (nonsyphilitic) 447.6
   arteriosclerotic 440.0
   calcific 447.6
   Döhle-Heller 093.1
   luetic 093.1
   rheumatic (*see also* Endocarditis, acute,
    rheumatic) 391.1
   rheumatoid—*see* Arthritis, rheumatoid
   specific 093.1
   syphilitic 093.1
    congenital 090.5
Apathetic thyroid storm (*see also*
   Thyrotoxicosis) 242.9
Apepsia 536.8
   achlorhydric 536.0
   psychogenic 306.4
Aperistalsis, esophagus 530.0
Apert's syndrome (acrocephalosyndactyly)
   755.55
Apert-Gallais syndrome (adrenogenital) 255.2
Apertognathia 524.2
Aphagia 787.2
   psychogenic 307.1
Aphakia (acquired) (bilateral) (postoperative)
   (unilateral) 379.31
   congenital 743.35

Apoplexia, apoplexy, apoplectic—*continued*
hemiplegia (*see also* Disease, cerebrovascular, acute) 436
hemorrhagic (stroke) (*see also* Hemorrhage, brain) 432.9
ingravescent (*see also* Disease, cerebrovascular, acute) 436
late effect—*see* Late effect(s) (of) cerebrovascular disease
lung—*see* Embolism, pulmonary
meninges, hemorrhagic (*see also* Hemorrhage, subarachnoid) 430
neonatorum 767.0
newborn 767.0
pancreatitis 577.0
placenta 641.2
progressive (*see also* Disease, cerebrovascular, acute) 436
pulmonary (artery) (vein)—*see* Embolism, pulmonary
sanguineous (*see also* Disease, cerebrovascular, acute) 436
seizure (*see also* Disease, cerebrovascular, acute) 436
serous (*see also* Disease, cerebrovascular, acute) 436
spleen 289.59
stroke (*see also* Disease, cerebrovascular, acute) 436
thrombotic (*see also* Thrombosis, brain) 434.0
uremic—*see* Uremia
uteroplacental 641.2
Appendage
fallopian tube (cyst of Morgagni) 752.11
intestine (epiploic) 751.5
preauricular 744.1
testicular (organ of Morgagni) 752.8
Appendicitis 541
with
perforation, peritonitis (generalized), or rupture 540.0
with peritoneal abscess 540.1
peritoneal abscess 540.1
acute (catarrhal) (fulminating) (gangrenous) (inflammatory) (obstructive) (retrocecal) (suppurative) 540.9
with
perforation, peritonitis, or rupture 540.0
with peritoneal abscess 540.1
peritoneal abscess 540.1
amebic 006.8
chronic (recurrent) 542
exacerbation—*see* Appendicitis, acute
fulminating—*see* Appendicitis, acute
gangrenous—*see* Appendicitis, acute
healed (obliterative) 542
interval 542
neurogenic 542
obstructive 542
pneumococcal 541
recurrent 542
relapsing 542
retrocecal 541
subacute (adhesive) 542
subsiding 542
suppurative—*see* Appendicitis, acute
tuberculous (*see also* Tuberculosis) 014.8
Appendiclausis 543.9
Appendicolithiasis 543.9
Appendicopathia oxyurica 127.4

Appendix, appendicular —*see also* condition
Morgagni (male) 752.8
fallopian tube 752.11
Appetite
depraved 307.52
excessive 783.6
psychogenic 307.51
lack or loss (*see also* Anorexia) 783.0
nonorganic origin 307.59
perverted 307.52
hysterical 300.11
Apprehension, apprehensiveness (abnormal) (state) 300.00
specified type NEC 300.09
Approximal wear 521.1
Apraxia (classic) (ideational) (ideokinetic) (ideomotor) (motor) 784.69
oculomotor, congenital 379.51
verbal 784.69
Aptyalism 527.7
Aqueous misdirection 365.83
Arabicum elephantiasis (*see also* Infestation, filarial) 125.9
Arachnidism 989.5
Arachnitis —*see* Meningitis
Arachnodactyly 759.82
Arachnoidism 989.5
Arachnoiditis (acute) (adhesive) (basic) (brain) (cerebrospinal) (chiasmal) (chronic) (spinal) (*see also* Meningitis) 322.9
meningococcal (chronic) 036.0
syphilitic 094.2
tuberculous (*see also* Tuberculosis, meninges) 013.0
Araneism 989.5
Arboencephalitis, Australian 062.4
Arborization block (heart) 426.6
Arbor virus, arbovirus (infection) NEC 066.9
ARC 042
Arches —*see* condition
Arcuatus uterus 752.3
Arcus (cornea)
juvenilis 743.43
interfering with vision 743.42
senilis 371.41
Arc-welders' lung 503
Arc-welders' syndrome (photokeratitis) 370.24
Areflexia 796.1
Areola —*see* condition
Argentaffinoma (M8241/1)—*see also* Neoplasm, by site, uncertain behavior
benign (M8241/0)—*see* Neoplasm, by site, benign
malignant (M8241/3)—*see* Neoplasm, by site, malignant
syndrome 259.2
Argentinian hemorrhagic fever 078.7
Arginosuccinicaciduria 270.6
Argonz-Del Castillo syndrome (nonpuerperal galactorrhea and amenorrhea) 253.1
Argyll-Robertson phenomenon pupil, or syndrome (syphilitic) 094.89
atypical 379.45
nonluetic 379.45
nonsyphilitic 379.45
reversed 379.45
Argyria, argyriasis NEC 985.8
conjunctiva 372.55
cornea 371.16
from drug or medicinal agent

Argyria, argyriasis—*continued*
correct substance properly administered 709.09
overdose or wrong substance given or taken 961.2
Arhinencephaly 742.2
Arias-Stella phenomenon 621.3
Ariboflavinosis 266.0
Arizona enteritis 008.1
Arm —*see* condition
Armenian disease 277.3
Arnold-Chiari obstruction or syndrome (*see also* Spina bifida) 741.0
type I 348.4
type II (*see also* Spina bifida) 741.0
type III 742.0
type IV 742.2
Arrest, arrested
active phase of labor 661.1
affecting fetus or newborn 763.7
any plane in pelvis
complicating delivery 660.1
affecting fetus or newborn 763.1
bone marrow (*see also* Anemia, aplastic) 284.9
cardiac 427.5
with
abortion—*see* Abortion, by type, with specified complication NEC
ectopic pregnancy (*see also* categories 633.0-633.9) 639.8
molar pregnancy (*see also* categories 630-632) 639.8
complicating
anesthesia
correct substance properly administered 427.5
obstetric 668.1
overdose or wrong substance given 968.4
specified anesthetic—*see* Table of drugs and chemicals
delivery (cesarean) (instrumental) 669.4
ectopic or molar pregnancy 639.8
surgery (nontherapeutic) (therapeutic) 997.1
fetus or newborn 779.89
following
abortion 639.8
ectopic or molar pregnancy 639.8
postoperative (immediate) 997.1
long-term effect of cardiac surgery 429.4
cardiorespiratory (*see also* Arrest, cardiac) 427.5
deep transverse 660.3
affecting fetus or newborn 763.1
development or growth
bone 733.91
child 783.40
fetus 764.9
affecting management of pregnancy 656.5
tracheal rings 748.3
epiphyseal 733.91
granulopoiesis 288.0
heart—*see* Arrest, cardiac
respiratory 799.1
newborn 770.89
sinus 426.6
transverse (deep) 660.3
affecting fetus or newborn 763.1
Arrhenoblastoma (M8630.1)
benign (M8630/0)
specified site—*see* Neoplasm, by site, benign
unspecified site
female 220

Arrhenoblastoma—*continued*
male 222.0
malignant (M8630/3)
specified site— *see* Neoplasm, by site, malignant
unspecified site
female 183.0
male 186.9
specified site—*see* Neoplasm, by site, uncertain behavior
unspecified site
female 236.2
male 236.4
Arrhinencephaly 742.2
due to
trisomy 13 (13-15) 758.1
trisomy 18 (16-l8) 758.2
Arrhythmia (auricle) (cardiac) (cordis) (gallop rhythm) (juvenile) (nodal) (reflex) (sinus) (supraventricular) (transitory) (ventricle) 427.9
bigeminal rhythm 427.89
block 426.9
bradycardia 427.89
contractions, premature 427.60
coronary sinus 427.89
ectopic 427.89
extrasystolic 427.60
postoperative 997.1
psychogenic 306.2
vagal 780.2
Arrillaga-Ayerza syndrome (pulmonary artery sclerosis with pulmonary hypertension) 416.0
Arsenical
dermatitis 692.4
keratosis 692.4
pigmentation 985.1
from drug or medicinal agent
correct substance properly administered 709.09
overdose or wrong substance given or taken 961.1
Arsenism 985.1
from drug or medicinal agent
correct substance properly administered 692.4
overdose or wrong substance given or taken 961.1
Arterial —*see* condition
Arteriectasis 447.8
Arteriofibrosis —*see* Arteriosclerosis
Arteriolar sclerosis —*see* Arteriosclerosis
Arteriolith —*see* Arteriosclerosis
Arteriolitis 447.6
necrotizing, kidney 447.5
renal—*see* Hypertension, kidney
Arteriolosclerosis —*see* Arteriosclerosis
Arterionephrosclerosis (*see also* Hypertension, kidney) 403.90
Arteriopathy 447.9
Arteriosclerosis, arteriosclerotic (artery) (deformans) (diffuse) (disease) (endarteritis) (general) (obliterans) (obliterative) (occlusive) (senile) (with calcification) 440.9
with
gangrene 440.24
psychosis (*see also* Psychosis, arteriosclerotic) 290.40
ulceration 440.23
aorta 440.0
arteries of extremities NEC — *see* Arteriosclerosis, extremities

Arteriosclerosis, arteriosclerotic—*continued*
  basilar (artery) (*see also* Occlusion, artery,
      basilar) 433.0
  brain 437.0
  bypass graft
    coronary artery 414.05
      autologous artery (gastroepiploic) (internal
          mammary) 414.04
      autologous vein 414.02
      nonautologous biological 414.03
    extremity 440.30
      autologous vein 440.31
      nonautologous biological 440.32
  cardiac — *see* Arteriosclerosis, coronary
  cardiopathy — *see* Arteriosclerosis, coronary
  cardiorenal (*see also* Hypertension, cardiorenal)
      404.90
  cardiovascular (*see also* Disease,
      cardiovascular) 429.2
  carotid (artery) (common) (internal) (*see also*
      Occlusion, artery, carotid) 433.1
  central nervous system 437.0
  cerebral 437.0
    late effect—*see* Late effect(s) (of)
        cerebrovascular disease
  cerebrospinal 437.0
  cerebrovascular 437.0
  coronary (artery) 414.00
    graft—*see* Arteriosclerosis, bypass graft
    native artery 414.01
    of transplanted heart 414.06
  extremities (native artery) 440.20
    bypass graft 440.30
      autologous vein 440.31
      nonautologous biological 440.32
    claudication (intermittent) 440.21
      and
        gangrene 440.24
        rest pain 440.22
          and
            gangrene 440.24
            ulceration 440.23
              and gangrene 440.24
        ulceration 440.23
          and gangrene 440.24
    gangrene 440.24
    rest pain 440.22
      and
        gangrene 440.24
        ulceration 440.23
          and gangrene 440.24
    specified site NEC 440.29
    ulceration 440.23
      and gangrene 440.24
  heart (disease) — *see also* Arteriosclerosis,
      coronary
    valve 424.99
      aortic 424.1
      mitral 424.0
      pulmonary 424.3
      tricuspid 424.2
  kidney (*see also* Hypertension, kidney) 403.90
  labyrinth, labyrinthine 388.00
  medial NEC 440.20
  mesentery (artery) 557.1
  Mönckeberg's 440.20
  myocarditis 429.0

Arteriosclerosis, arteriosclerotic— *continued*
  nephrosclerosis (*see also* Hypertension, kidney)
      403.90
  peripheral (of extremities) *see* Arteriosclerosis,
      extremities
  precerebral 433.9
    specified artery NEC 433.8
  pulmonary (idiopathic) 416.0
  renal (*see also* Hypertension, kidney) 403.90
    arterioles (*see also* Hypertension, kidney)
        403.90
    artery 440.1
  retinal (vascular) 440.8 *[362.13]*
  specified artery NEC 440.8
    with gangrene 440.8 *[785.4]*
  spinal (cord) 437.0
  vertebral (artery) (*see also* Occlusion, artery,
      vertebral) 433.2
Arteriospasm 443.9
Arteriovenous —*see* condition
Arteritis 447.6
  allergic (*see also* Angiitis, hypersensitivity)
      446.20
  aorta (nonsyphilitic) 447.6
    syphilitic 093.1
  aortic arch 446.7
  brachiocephalica 446.7
  brain 437.4
    syphilitic 094.89
  branchial 446.7
  cerebral 437.4
    late effect—*see* Late effect(s) (of)
        cerebrovascular disease
    syphilitic 094.89
  coronary (artery) —*see also* Arteriosclerosis,
      coronary
    rheumatic 391.9
      chronic 398.99
    syphilitic 093.89
  cranial (left) (right) 446.5
  deformans—*see* Arteriosclerosis
  giant cell 446.5
  necrosing or necrotizing 446.0
  nodosa 446.0
  obliterans—*see also* Arteriosclerosis
    subclaviocarotica 446.7
  pulmonary 417.8
  retina 362.18
  rheumatic—*see* Fever, rheumatic
  senile—*see* Arteriosclerosis
  suppurative 447.2
  syphilitic (general) 093.89
    brain 094.89
    coronary 093.89
    spinal 094.89
  temporal 446.5
  young female, syndrome 446.7
Artery, arterial —*see* condition
Arthralgia (*see also* Pain, joint) 719.4
  allergic (*see also* Pain, joint) 719.4
  in caisson disease 993.3—
  psychogenic 307.89
  rubella 056.71
  Salmonella 003.23
  temporomandibular joint 524.62

Arthritis, arthritic (acute) (chronic) (subacute) 716.9

Note—Use the following fifth-digit subclassification with categories 711-712, 715-716:

0 *site unspecified*
1 *shoulder region*
2 *upper arm*
3 *forearm*
4 *hand*
5 *pelvic region and thigh*
6 *lower leg*
7 *ankle and foot*
8 *other specified sites*
9 *multiple sites*

allergic 716.2
ankylosing (crippling) (spine) 720.0
  sites other than spine 716.9
atrophic 714.0
  spine 720.9
back (*see also* Arthritis, spine) 721.90
Bechterew's (ankylosing spondylitis) 720.0
blennorrhagic 098.50
cervical, cervicodorsal (*see also* Spondylosis, cervical) 721.0
Charcot's 094.0 *[713.5]*
  diabetic 250.6 *[713.5]*
  syringomyelic 336.0 *[713.5]*
  tabetic 094.0 *[713.5]*
chylous (*see also* Filariasis) 125.9 *[711.7]*
climacteric NEC 716.3
coccyx 721.8
cricoarytenoid 478.79
crystal (-induced)—*see* Arthritis, due to crystals
deformans (*see also* Osteoarthrosis) 715.9
  spine 721.90
    with myelopathy 721.91
degenerative (*see also* Osteoarthrosis) 715.9
  idiopathic 715.09
  polyarticular 715.09
  spine 721.90
    with myelopathy 721.91
dermatoarthritis, lipoid 272.8 *[713.0]*
due to or associated with
  acromegaly 253.0 *[713.0]*
  actinomycosis 039.8 *[711.4]*
  amyloidosis 277.3 *[713.7]*
  bacterial disease NEC 040.89 *[711.4]*
  Behçet's syndrome 136.1 *[711.2]*
  blastomycosis 116.0 *[711.6]*
  brucellosis (*see also* Brucellosis) 023.9 *[711.4]*
  caisson disease 993.3
  coccidioidomycosis 114.3 *[711.6]*
  coliform (Escherichia coli) 711.0
  colitis, ulcerative (*see also* Colitis, ulcerative) 556.9 *[713.1]*
  cowpox 051.0 *[711.5]*
  crystals (*see also* Gout)
    dicalcium phosphate 275.49 *[712.1]*
    pyrophosphate 275.49 *[712.2]*
    specified NEC 275.49 *[712.8]*
  dermatoarthritis, lipoid 272.8 *[713.0]*
  dermatological disorder NEC 709.9 *[713.3]*
  diabetes 250.6 *[713.5]*
  diphtheria 032.89 *[711.4]*
  dracontiasis 125.7 *[711.7]*
  dysentery 009.0 *[711.3]*

Arthritis, arthritic—*continued*
  endocrine disorder NEC 259.9 *[713.0]*
  enteritis NEC 009.1 *[711.3]*
    infectious (*see also* Enteritis, infectious) 009.0 *[711.3]*
      specified organism NEC 008.8 *[711.3]*
    regional (*see also* Enteritis, regional) 555.9 *[713.1]*
    specified organism NEC 008.8 *[711.3]*
  epiphyseal slip, nontraumatic (old) 716.8
  erysipelas 035 *[711.4]*
  erythema
    epidemic 026.1
    multiforme 695.1 *[713.3]*
    nodosum 695.2 *[713.3]*
  Escherichia coli 711.0
  filariasis NEC 125.9 *[711.7]*
  gastrointestinal condition NEC 569.9 *[713.1]*
  glanders 024 *[711.4]*
  Gonococcus 098.50
  gout 274.0
  H. influenzae 711.0
  helminthiasis NEC 128.9 *[711.7]*
  hematological disorder NEC 289.9 *[713.2]*
  hemochromatosis 275.0 *[713.0]*
  hemoglobinopathy NEC (*see also* Disease, hemoglobin) 282.7 *[713.2]*
  hemophilia (*see also* Hemophilia) 286.0 *[713.2]*
  Hemophilus influenzae (H. influenzae) 711.0
  Henoch (-Schönlein) purpura 287.0 *[713.6]*
  histoplasmosis NEC (*see also* Histoplasmosis) 115.99 *[711.6]*
  hyperparathyroidism 252.0 *[713.0]*
  hypersensitivity reaction NEC 995.3 *[713.6]*
  hypogammaglobulinemia (*see also* Hypogammaglobulinemia) 279.00 *[713.0]*
  hypothyroidism NEC 244.9 *[713.0]*
  infection (*see also* Arthritis, infectious) 711.9
  infectious disease NEC 136.9 *[711.8]*
  leprosy (*see also* Leprosy) 030.9 *[711.4]*
  leukemia NEC (M9800/3) 208.9 *[713.2]*
  lipoid dermatoarthritis 272.8 *[713.0]*
  Lyme disease 088.81 *[711.8]*
  meaning Osteoarthritis—*see* Osteoarthrosis
  Mediterranean fever, familial 277.3 *[713.7]*
  meningococcal infection 036.82
  metabolic disorder NEC 277.9 *[713.0]*
  multiple myelomatosis (M9730/3) 203.0 *[713.2]*
  mumps 072.79 *[711.5]*
  mycobacteria 031.8 *[711.4]*
  mycosis NEC 117.9 *[711.6]*
  neurological disorder NEC 349.9 *[713.5]*
  ochronosis 270.2 *[713.0]*
  O'Nyong Nyong 066.3 *[711.5]*
  parasitic disease NEC 136.9 *[711.8]*
  paratyphoid fever (*see also* Fever, paratyphoid) 002.9 *[711.3]*
  Pneumococcus 711.0
  poliomyelitis (*see also* Poliomyelitis) 045.9 *[711.5]*
  Pseudomonas 711.0
  psoriasis 696.0
  pyogenic organism (E. coli) (H. influenzae) (Pseudomonas) (Streptococcus) 711.0
  rat-bite fever 026.1 *[711.4]*
  regional enteritis (*see also* Enteritis, regional) 555.9 *[713.1]*
  Reiter's disease 099.3 *[711.1]*
  respiratory disorder NEC 519.9 *[713.4]*

Arthritis, arthritic—*continued*
  reticulosis, malignant (M9720/3) 202.3
    [713.2]
  rubella 056.71
  salmonellosis 003.23
  sarcoidosis 135 *[713.7]*
  serum sickness 999.5 *[713.6]*
  Staphylococcus 711.0
  Streptococcus 711.0
  syphilis (*see also* Syphilis) 094.0 *[711.4]*
  syringomyelia 336.0 *[713.5]*
  thalassemia 282.4 *[713.2]*
  tuberculosis (*see also* Tuberculosis, arthritis)
    015.9 *[711.4]*
  typhoid fever 002.0 *[711.3]*
  ulcerative colitis (*see also* Colitis, ulcerative)
    556.9 *[713.1]*
  urethritis
    nongonococcal (*see also* Urethritis,
      nongonococcal) 099.40 *[711.1]*
    nonspecific (*see also* Urethritis,
      nongonococcal) 099.40 *[711.1]*
    Reiter's 099.3 *[711.1]*
  viral disease NEC 079.99 *[711.5]*
  erythema epidemic 026.1
  gonococcal 098.50
  gouty (acute) 274.0
  hypertrophic (*see also* Osteoarthrosis) 715.9
    spine 721.90
      with myelopathy 721.91
  idiopathic, blennorrheal 099.3
  in caisson disease 993.3 *[713.8]*
  infectious or infective (acute) (chronic)
    (subacute) NEC 711.9
    nonpyogenic 711.9
    spine 720.9
  inflammatory NEC 714.9
  juvenile rheumatoid (chronic) (polyarticular)
    714.30
    acute 714.31
    monoarticular 714.33
    pauciarticular 714.32
  lumbar (*see also* Spondylosis, lumbar) 721.3
  meningococcal 036.82
  menopausal NEC 716.3
  migratory—*see* Fever, rheumatic
  neuropathic (Charcot's) 094.0 *[713.5]*
    diabetic 250.6 *[713.5]*
    nonsyphilitic NEC 349.9 *[713.5]*
    syringomyelic 336.0 *[713.5]*
    tabetic 094.0 *[713.5]*
  nodosa (*see also* Osteoarthrosis) 715.9
    spine 721.90
      with myelopathy 721.91
  nonpyogenic NEC 716.9
    spine 721.90
      with myelopathy 721.91
  ochronotic 270.2 *[713.0]*
  palindromic (*see also* Rheumatism,
    palindromic) 719.3
  pneumococcal 711.0
  postdysenteric 009.0 *[711.3]*
  postrheumatic, chronic (Jaccoud's) 714.4
  primary progressive 714.0
    spine 720.9
  proliferative 714.0
    spine 720.0
  psoriatic 696.0
  purulent 711.0
  pyogenic or pyemic 711.0

Arthritis, arthritic—*continued*
  rheumatic 714.0
    acute or subacute—*see* Fever, rheumatic
    chronic 714.0
    spine 720.9
  rheumatoid (nodular) 714.0
    with
      splenoadenomegaly and leukopenia 714.1
      visceral or systemic involvement 714.2
    aortitis 714.89
    carditis 714.2
    heart disease 714.2
    juvenile (chronic) (polyarticular) 714.30
      acute 714.31
      monoarticular 714.33
      pauciarticular 714.32
    spine 720.0
  rubella 056.71
  sacral, sacroiliac, sacrococcygeal (*see also*
    Spondylosis, sacral) 721.3
  scorbutic 267
  senile or senescent (*see also* Osteoarthrosis)
    715.9
    spine 721.90
      with myelopathy 721.91
  septic 711.0
  serum (nontherapeutic) (therapeutic) 999.5
    [713.6]
  specified form NEC 716.8
  spine 721.90
    with myelopathy 721.91
    atrophic 720.9
    degenerative 721.90
      with myelopathy 721.91
    hypertrophic (with deformity) 721.90
      with myelopathy 721.91
    infectious or infective NEC 720.9
    Marie-Strümpell 720.0
    nonpyogenic 721.90
      with myelopathy 721.91
    pyogenic 720.9
    rheumatoid 720.0
    traumatic (old) 721.7
    tuberculous (*see also* Tuberculosis) 015.0
      [720.81]
  staphylococcal 711.0
  streptococcal 711.0
  suppurative 711.0
  syphilitic 094.0 *[713.5]*
    congenital 090.49 *[713.5]*
  syphilitica deformans (Charcot) 094.0 *[713.5]*
  temporomandibular joint 524.69
  thoracic (*see also* Spondylosis, thoracic) 721.2
  toxic of menopause 716.3
  transient 716.4
  traumatic (chronic) (old) (post) 716.1
    current injury—*see* nature of injury
  tuberculous (*see also* Tuberculosis, arthritis)
    015.9 *[711.4]*
  urethritica 099.3 *[711.1]*
  urica, uratic 274.0
  venereal 099.3 *[711.1]*
  vertebral (*see also* Arthritis, spine) 721.90
  villous 716.8
  von Bechterew's 720.0
Arthrocele (*see also* Effusion, joint) 719.0
Arthrochondritis —*see* Arthritis
Arthrodesis status V45.4
Arthrodynia (*see also* Pain, joint) 719.4
  psychogenic 307.89
Arthrodysplasia 755.9
Arthrofibrosis, joint (*see also* Ankylosis) 718.5

Arthrogryposis 728.3
  multiplex, congenita 754.89
Arthrokatadysis 715.35
Arthrolithiasis 274.0
Arthro-onychodysplasia 756.89
Arthro-osteo-onychodysplasia 756.89
Arthropathy (*see also* Arthritis) 716.9

---

*Note—Use the following fifth-digit
subclassification with categories 711-712, 716:*

0 site unspecified
1 shoulder region
2 upper arm
3 forearm
4 hand
5 pelvic region and thigh
6 lower leg
7 ankle and foot
8 other specified sites
9 multiple sites

  Behçet's 136.1 *[711.2]*
  Charcot's 094.0 *[713.5]*
    diabetic 250.6 *[713.5]*
    syringomyelic 336.0 *[713.5]*
    tabetic 094.0 *[713.5]*
  crystal (-induced)—*see* Arthritis, due to crystals
  gouty 274.0
  neurogenic, neuropathic (Charcot's) (tabetic)
      094.0 *[713.5]*
    diabetic 250.6 *[713.5]*
    nonsyphilitic NEC 349.9 *[713.5]*
    syringomyelic 336.0 *[713.5]*
  postdysenteric NEC 009.0 *[711.3]*
  postrheumatic, chronic (Jaccoud's) 714.4
  psoriatic 696.0
  pulmonary 731.2
  specified NEC 716.8
  syringomyelia 336.0 *[713.5]*
  tabes dorsalis 094.0 *[713.5]*
  tabetic 094.0 *[713.5]*
  transient 716.4
  traumatic 716.1
  uric acid 274.0
Arthrophyte (*see also* Loose, body, joint) 718.1
Arthrophytis 719.80
  ankle 719.87
  elbow 719.82
  foot 719.87
  hand 719.84
  hip 719.85
  knee 719.86
  multiple sites 719.89
  pelvic region 719.85
  shoulder (region) 719.81
  specified site NEC 719.88
  wrist 719.83
Arthropyosis (*see also* Arthritis, pyogenic) 711.0
Arthrosis (deformans) (degenerative) (*see also*
    Osteoarthrosis) 715.9
  Charcot's 094.0 *[713.5]*
  polyarticular 715.09
  spine (*see also* Spondylosis) 721.90
Arthus' phenomenon 995.2
  due to
    correct substance properly administered 995.2
    overdose or wrong substance given or taken
        977.9
      specified drug—*see* Table of drugs and
          chemicals
  serum 999.5

Articular —*see also* condition
  disc disorder (reducing or non-reducing) 524.63
  spondylolisthesis 756.12
Artificial
  device (prosthetic)—*see* Fitting, device
  insemination V26.1
  menopause (states) (symptoms) (syndrome)
      627.4
  opening status (functioning) (without
      complication) V44.9
    anus (colostomy) V44.3
    colostomy V44.3
    cystostomy V44.50
      appendico-vesicostomy V44.52
      cutaneous-vesicostomy V44.51
      specified type NEC V44.59
    enterostomy V44.4
    gastrostomy V44.1
    ileostomy V44.2
    intestinal tract NEC V44.4
    jejunostomy V44.4
    nephrostomy V44.6
    specified site NEC V44.8
    tracheostomy V44.0
    ureterostomy V44.6
    urethrostomy V44.6
    urinary tract NEC V44.6
    vagina V44.7
  vagina status V44.7
ARV (disease) (illness) (infection)—*see* Human
    immunodeficiency virus (disease) (illness)
    (infection)
Arytenoid —*see* condition
Asbestosis (occupational) 501
Asboe-Hansen's disease (incontinentia
    pigmenti) 757.33
Ascariasis (intestinal) (lung) 127.0
Ascaridiasis 127.0
Ascaridosis 127.0
Ascaris 127.0
  lumbricoides (infestation) 127.0
  pneumonia 127.0
Ascending —*see* condition
Aschoff's bodies (*see also* Myocarditis,
    rheumatic) 398.0
Ascites 789.5
  abdominal NEC 789.5
  cancerous (M8000/6) 197.6
  cardiac 428.0
  chylous (nonfilarial) 457.8
    filarial (*see also* Infestation, filarial) 125.9
  congenital 778.0
  due to S. japonicum 120.2
  fetal, causing fetopelvic disproportion 653.7
  heart 428.0
  joint (*see also* Effusion, joint) 719.0
  malignant (M8000/6) 197.6
  pseudochylous 789.5
  syphilitic 095.2
  tuberculous (*see also* Tuberculosis) 014.0
Ascorbic acid (vitamin C) deficiency (scurvy)
    267
ASCUS (atypical squamous cell changes of
    undetermined significance)
  favor benign 795.01
  favor dysplasia 795.02
ASCVD (arteriosclerotic cardiovascular disease)
    429.2
Aseptic —*see* condition
Asherman's syndrome 621.5
Asialia 527.7
Asiatic cholera (*see also* Cholera) 001.9

Asocial personality or trends 301.7
Asomatognosia 781.8
Aspergillosis 117.3
  with pneumonia 117.3 *[484.6]*
  allergic bronchopulmonary 518.6
  nonsyphilitic NEC 117.3
Aspergillus (flavus) (fumigatus) (infection)
  (terreus) 117.3
Aspermatogenesis 606.0
Aspermia (testis) 606.0
Asphyxia, asphyxiation (by) 799.0
  antenatal—*see* Distress, fetal
  bedclothes 994.7
  birth (*see also* Asphyxia, newborn) 768.9
  bunny bag 994.7
  carbon monoxide 986
  caul (*see also* Asphyxia, newborn) 768.9
  cave-in 994.7
    crushing—*see* Injury, internal, intrathoracic
      organs
  constriction 994.7
  crushing—*see* Injury, internal, intrathoracic
    organs
  drowning 994.1
  fetal, affecting newborn 768.9
  food or foreign body (in larynx) 933.1
    bronchioles 934.8
    bronchus (main) 934.1
    lung 934.8
    nasopharynx 933.0
    nose, nasal passages 932
    pharynx 933.0
    respiratory tract 934.9
      specified part NEC 934.8
    throat 933.0
    trachea 934.0
  gas, fumes, or vapor NEC 987.9
    specified—*see* Table of drugs and chemicals
  gravitational changes 994.7
  hanging 994.7
  inhalation—*see* Inhalation
  intrauterine
    fetal death (before onset of labor) 768.0
      during labor 768.1
    liveborn infant—*see* Distress, fetal, liveborn
      infant
  local 443.0
  mechanical 994.7
    during birth (*see also* Distress, fetal) 768.9
  mucus 933.1
    bronchus (main) 934.1
    larynx 933.1
    lung 934.8
    nasal passages 932
    newborn 770.1
    pharynx 933.0
    respiratory tract 934.9
      specified part NEC 934.8
    throat 933.0
    trachea 934.0
    vaginal (fetus or newborn) 770.1
  newborn 768.9
    blue 768.6
    livida 768.6
    mild or moderate 768.6
    pallida 768.5
    severe 768.5
    white 768.5
    with neurologic involvement 768.5
  pathological 799.0
  plastic bag 994.7

Asphyxia, Asphyxiation—*continued*
  postnatal (*see also* Asphyxia, newborn) 768.9
    mechanical 994.7
  pressure 994.7
  reticularis 782.61
  strangulation 994.7
  submersion 994.1
  traumatic NEC—*see* Injury, internal,
    intrathoracic organs
  vomiting, vomitus—*see* Asphyxia, food or
    foreign body
Aspiration
  acid pulmonary (syndrome) 997.3
    obstetric 668.0
  amniotic fluid 770.1
  bronchitis 507.0
  contents of birth canal 770.1
  fetal pneumonitis 770.1
  food, foreign body, or gasoline (with
    asphyxiation)—*see* Asphyxia, food or
    foreign body
  meconium 770.1
  mucus 933.1
    into
      bronchus (main) 934.1
      lung 934.8
      respiratory tract 934.9
        specified part NEC 934.8
      trachea 934.0
    newborn 770.1
    vaginal (fetus or newborn) 770.1
  newborn 770.1
  pneumonia 507.0
  pneumonitis 507.0
    fetus or newborn 770.1
    obstetric 668.0
  syndrome of newborn (massive) (meconium)
    770.1
  vernix caseosa 770.1
Asplenia 759.0
  with mesocardia 746.87
Assam fever 085.0
Assimilation, pelvis
  with disproportion 653.2
    affecting fetus or newborn 763.1
    causing obstructed labor 660.1
      affecting fetus or newborn 763.1
Assmann's focus (*see also* Tuberculosis) 011.0
Astasia (-abasia) 307.9
  hysterical 300.11
Asteatosis 706.8
  cutis 706.8
Astereognosis 780.99
Asterixis 781.3
  in liver disease 572.8
Asteroid hyalitis 379.22
Asthenia, asthenic 780.79
  cardiac (*see also* Failure, heart) 428.9
    psychogenic 306.2
  cardiovascular (*see also* Failure, heart) 428.9
    psychogenic 306.2
  heart (*see also* Failure, heart) 428.9
    psychogenic 306.2
  hysterical 300.11
  myocardial (*see also* Failure, heart) 428.9
    psychogenic 306.2
  nervous 300.5
  neurocirculatory 306.2
  neurotic 300.5
  psychogenic 300.5
  psychoneurotic 300.5

Asthenia, asthenic—*continued*
  psychophysiologic 300.5
  reaction, psychoneurotic 300.5
  senile 797
  Stiller's 780.79
  tropical anhidrotic 705.1
Asthenopia 368.13
  accommodative 367.4
  hysterical (muscular) 300.11
  psychogenic 306.7
Asthenospermia 792.2
Asthma, asthmatic (bronchial) (catarrh)
  (spasmodic) 493.9

---

*Note—Use the following fifth-digit
subclassification with category 493:*

*0 without mention of status asthmaticus or acute
exacerbation or unspecified*
1 with status asthmaticus
2 with acute exacerbation

---

  with
    chronic obstructive pulmonary disease
      (COPD) 493.2
    hay fever 493.0
    rhinitis, allergic 493.0
  allergic 493.9
    stated cause (external allergen) 493.0
  atopic 493.0
  cardiac (*see also* Failure, ventricular, left) 428.1
  cardiobronchial (*see also* Failure, ventricular,
    left) 428.1
  cardiorenal (*see also* Hypertension, cardiorenal)
    404.90
  childhood 493.0
  colliers' 500
  croup 493.9
  detergent 507.8
  due to
    detergent 507.8
    inhalation of fumes 506.3
    internal immunological process 493.0
  endogenous (intrinsic) 493.1
  eosinophilic 518.3
  exogenous (cosmetics) (dander or dust) (drugs)
    (dust) (feathers) (food) (hay) (platinum)
    (pollen) 493.0
  extrinsic 493.0
  grinders' 502
  hay 493.0
  heart (*see also* Failure, ventricular, left) 428.1
  IgE 493.0
  infective 493.1
  intrinsic 493.1
  Kopp's 254.8
  late-onset 493.1
  meat-wrappers' 506.9
  Millar's (laryngismus stridulus) 478.75
  millstone makers' 502
  miners' 500
  Monday morning 504
  New Orleans (epidemic) 493.0
  platinum 493.0
  pneumoconiotic (occupational) NEC 505
  potters' 502
  psychogenic 316 *[493.9]*
  pulmonary eosinophilic 518.3
  red cedar 495.8
  Rostan's (*see also* Failure, ventricular, left)
    428.1
  sandblasters' 502

Asthma, asthmatic—*continued*
  sequoiosis 495.8
  stonemasons' 502
  thymic 254.8
  tuberculous (*see also* Tuberculosis, pulmonary)
    011.9
  Wichmann's (laryngismus stridulus) 478.75
  wood 495.8
Astigmatism (compound) (congenital) 367.20
  irregular 367.22
  regular 367.21
Astroblastoma (M9430/3)
  nose 748.1
  specified site—*see* Neoplasm, by site,
    malignant
  unspecified site 191.9
Astrocytoma (cystic) (M9400/3)
  anaplastic type (M9401/3)
    specified site—*see* Neoplasm, by site,
      malignant
    unspecified site 191.9
  fibrillary (M9420/3)
    specified site—*see* Neoplasm, by site,
      malignant
    unspecified site 191.9
  fibrous (M9420/3)
    specified site—*see* Neoplasm, by site,
      malignant
    unspecified site 191.9
  gemistocytic (M9411/3)
    specified site—*see* Neoplasm, by site,
      malignant
    unspecified site 191.9
  juvenile (M9421/3)
    specified site—*see* Neoplasm, by site,
      malignant
    unspecified site 191.9
  nose 748.1
  pilocytic (M9421/3)
    specified site—*see* Neoplasm, by site,
      malignant
    unspecified site 191.9
  piloid (M9421/3)
    specified site—*see* Neoplasm, by site,
      malignant
    unspecified site 191.9
  protoplasmic (M9410/3)
    specified site—*see* Neoplasm, by site,
      malignant
    unspecified site 191.9
  specified site—*see* Neoplasm, by site, malignant
  subependymal (M9383/1) 237.5
    giant cell (M9384/1) 237.5
  unspecified site 191.9
Astroglioma (M9400/3)
  nose 748.1
  specified site—*see* Neoplasm, by site, malignant
  unspecified site 191.9
Asymbolia 784.60
Asymmetrical breathing 786.09
Asymmetry —*see also* Distortion
  chest 786.9
  face 754.0
  jaw NEC 524.12
    maxillary 524.11
  pelvis with disproportion 653.0
    affecting fetus or newborn 763.1
    causing obstructed labor 660.1
      affecting fetus or newborn 763.1
Asynergia 781.3
Asynergy 781.3
  ventricular 429.89

Asystole (heart) (*see also* Arrest, cardiac) 427.5
Ataxia, ataxy, ataxic 781.3
　acute 781.3
　brain 331.89
　cerebellar 334.3
　　hereditary (Marie's) 334.2
　　in
　　　alcoholism 303.9 *[334.4]*
　　　myxedema (*see also* Myxedema) 244.9
　　　　[334.4]
　　　neoplastic disease NEC 239.9 *[334.4]*
　cerebral 331.89
　family, familial 334.2
　　cerebral (Marie's) 334.2
　　spinal (Friedreich's) 334.0
　Friedreich's (heredofamilial) (spinal) 334.0
　frontal lobe 781.3
　gait 781.2
　　hysterical 300.11
　general 781.3
　hereditary NEC 334.2
　　cerebellar 334.2
　　spastic 334.1
　　spinal 334.0
　heredofamilial (Marie's) 334.2
　hysterical 300.11
　locomotor (progressive) 094.0
　　diabetic 250.6 *[337.1]*
　Marie's (cerebellar) (heredofamilial) 334.2
　nonorganic origin 307.9
　partial 094.0
　postchickenpox 052.7
　progressive locomotor 094.0
　psychogenic 307.9
　Sanger-Brown's 334.2
　spastic 094.0
　　hereditary 334.1
　　syphilitic 094.0
　spinal
　　hereditary 334.0
　　progressive locomotor 094.0
　telangiectasia 334.8
Ataxia-telangiectasia 334.8
Atelectasis (absorption collapse) (complete)
　　(compression) (massive) (partial)
　　(postinfective) (pressure collapse)
　　(pulmonary) (relaxation) 518.0
　newborn (congenital) (partial) 770.5
　　primary 770.4
　primary 770.4
　tuberculous (*see also* Tuberculosis, pulmonary)
　　011.9
Ateleiosis, ateliosis 253.3
Atelia —*see* Distortion
Ateliosis 253.3
Atelocardia 746.9
Atelomyelia 742.59
Athelia 757.6
Atheroembolism
　extremity
　　lower 445.02
　　upper 445.01
　kidney 445.81
　specified site NEC 445.89
Atheroma, atheromatous (*see also*
　　Arteriosclerosis) 440.9
　aorta, aortic 440.0
　　valve (*see also* Endocarditis, aortic) 424.1
　artery—*see* Arteriosclerosis
　basilar, (artery) (*see also* Occlusion, artery,
　　basilar) 433.0

Atheroma, atheromatous—*continued*
　carotid (artery) (common) (internal) (*see also*
　　Occlusion, artery, carotid) 433.1
　cerebral (arteries) 437.0
　coronary (artery)—*see* Arteriosclerosis,
　　coronary
　degeneration—*see* Arteriosclerosis
　heart, cardiac —*see* Arteriosclerosis, coronary
　mitral (valve) 424.0
　myocardium, myocardial —*see* Arteriosclerosis,
　　coronary
　pulmonary valve (heart) (*see also* Endocarditis,
　　pulmonary) 424.3
　skin 706.2
　tricuspid (heart) (valve) 424.2
　valve, valvular—*see* Endocarditis
　vertebral (artery) (*see also* Occlusion, artery,
　　vertebral) 433.2
Atheromatosis —*see also* Arteriosclerosis
　arterial, congenital 272.8
Atherosclerosis —*see* Arteriosclerosis
Athetosis (acquired) 781.0
　bilateral 333.7
　congenital (bilateral) 333.7
　double 333.7
　unilateral 781.0
Athlete's
　foot 110.4
　heart 429.3
Athletic team examination V70.3
Athrepsia 261
Athyrea (acquired) (*see also* Hypothyroidism)
　　244.9
　congenital 243
Athyreosis (congenital) 243
　acquired—*see* Hypothyroidism
Athyroidism (acquired) (*see also*
　　Hypothyroidism) 244.9
　congenital 243
Atmospheric pyrexia 992.0
Atonia, atony, atonic
　abdominal wall 728.2
　bladder (sphincter) 596.4
　　neurogenic NEC 596.54
　　　with cauda equina syndrome 344.61
　capillary 448.9
　cecum 564.89
　　psychogenic 306.4
　colon 564.89
　　psychogenic 306.4
　congenital 779.89
　dyspepsia 536.3
　　psychogenic 306.4
　intestine 564.89
　　psychogenic 306.4
　stomach 536.3
　　neurotic or psychogenic 306.4
　　psychogenic 306.4
　uterus 666.1
　　affecting fetus or newborn 763.7
　vesical 596.4
Atopy NEC V15.09
Atransferrinemia, congenital 273.8
Atresia, atretic (congenital) 759.89
　alimentary organ or tract NEC 751.8
　　lower 751.2
　　upper 750.8
　ani, anus, anal (canal) 751.2

Atresia, atretic—*continued*
aorta 747.22
  with hypoplasia of ascending aorta and
    defective development of left ventricle
    (with mitral valve atresia) 746.7
  arch 747.11
  ring 747.21
aortic (orifice) (valve) 746.89
  arch 747.11
aqueduct of Sylvius 742.3
  with spina bifida (*see also* Spina bifida) 741.0
artery NEC (*see also* Atresia, blood vessel)
  747.60
  cerebral 747.81
  coronary 746.85
  eye 743.58
  pulmonary 747.3
  umbilical 747.5
auditory canal (external) 744.02
bile, biliary duct (common) or passage 751.61
  acquired (*see also* Obstruction, biliary) 576.2
bladder (neck) 753.6
blood vessel (peripheral) NEC 747.60
  cerebral 747.81
  gastrointestinal 747.61
  lower limb 747.64
  pulmonary artery 747.3
  renal 747.62
  spinal 747.82
  upper limb 747.63
bronchus 748.3
canal, ear 744.02
cardiac
  valve 746.89
    aortic 746.89
    mitral 746.89
    pulmonary 746.01
    tricuspid 746.1
cecum 751.2
cervix (acquired) 622.4
  congenital 752.49
  in pregnancy or childbirth 654.6
    affecting fetus or newborn 763.89
    causing obstructed labor 660.2
      affecting fetus or newborn 763.1
choana 748.0
colon 751.2
cystic duct 751.61
  acquired 575.8
    with obstruction (*see also* Obstruction,
      gallbladder) 575.2
digestive organs NEC 751.8
duodenum 751.1
ear canal 744.02
ejaculatory duct 752.8
epiglottis 748.3
esophagus 750.3
Eustachian tube 744.24
fallopian tube (acquired) 628.2
  congenital 752.19
follicular cyst 620.0
foramen of
  Luschka 742.3
    with spina bifida (*see also* Spina bifida)
      741.0
  Magendie 742.3
    with spina bifida (*see also* Spina bifida)
      741.0
gallbladder 751.69
genital organ
  external

Atresia, atretic—*continued*
  female 752.49
    male NEC 752.8
      penis 752.69
  internal
    female 752.8
    male 752.8
glottis 748.3
gullet 750.3
heart
  valve NEC 746.89
    aortic 746.89
    mitral 746.89
    pulmonary 746.01
    tricuspid 746.1
hymen 752.42
  acquired 623.3
  postinfective 623.3
ileum 751.1
intestine (small) 751.1
  large 751.2
iris, filtration angle (*see also* Buphthalmia)
  743.20
jejunum 751.1
kidney 753.3
lacrimal, apparatus 743.65
  acquired—*see* Stenosis, lacrimal
larynx 748.3
ligament, broad 752.19
lung 748.5
meatus urinarius 753.6
mitral valve 746.89
  with atresia or hypoplasia of aortic orifice or
    valve, with hypoplasia of ascending aorta
    and defective development of left
    ventricle 746.7
nares (anterior) (posterior) 748.0
nasolacrimal duct 743.65
nasopharynx 748.8
nose, nostril 748.0
  acquired 738.0
organ or site NEC—*see* Anomaly, specified
  type NEC
osseous meatus (ear) 744.03
oviduct (acquired) 628.2
  congenital 752.19
parotid duct 750.23
  acquired 527.8
pulmonary (artery) 747.3
  valve 746.01
  vein 747.49
pulmonic 746.01
pupil 743.46
rectum 751.2
salivary duct or gland 750.23
  acquired 527.8
sublingual duct 750.23
  acquired 527.8
submaxillary duct or gland 750.23
  acquired 527.8
trachea 748.3
tricuspid valve 746.1
ureter 753.29
ureteropelvic junction 753.21
ureterovesical orifice 753.22
urethra (valvular) 753.6
urinary tract NEC 753.29
uterus 752.3
  acquired 621.8
vagina (acquired) 623.2
  congenital 752.49

Atresia, atretic—*continued*
   postgonococcal (old) 098.2
   postinfectional 623.2
   senile 623.2
   vascular NEC (*see also* Atresia, blood vessel)
      747.60
      cerebral 747.81
   vas deferens 752.8
   vein NEC (*see also* Atresia, blood vessel)
      747.60
      cardiac 746.89
      great 747.49
      portal 747.49
      pulmonary 747.49
   vena cava (inferior) (superior) 747.49
   vesicourethral orifice 753.6
   vulva 752.49
      acquired 624.8
Atrichia, atrichosis 704.00
   congenital (universal) 757.4
Atrioventricularis commune 745.69
Atrophia —*see also* Atrophy
   alba 709.09
   cutis 701.8
      idiopathica progressiva 701.8
      senilis 701.8
   dermatological, diffuse (idiopathic) 701.8
   flava hepatis (acuta) (subacuta) (*see also*
      Necrosis, liver) 570
   gyrata of choroid and retina (central) 363.54
      generalized 363.57
   senilis 797
      dermatological 701.8
   unguium 703.8
      congenita 757.5
Atrophoderma, atrophodermia 701.9
   diffusum (idiopathic) 701.8
   maculatum 701.3
      et striatum 701.3
         due to syphilis 095.8
      syphilitic 091.3
   neuriticum 701.8
   pigmentosum 757.33
   reticulatum symmetricum faciei 701.8
   senile 701.8
   symmetrical 701.8
   vermiculata 701.8
Atrophy, atrophic
   adrenal (autoimmune) (capsule) (cortex) (gland)
      255.4
      with hypofunction 255.4
   alveolar process or ridge (edentulous) 525.2
   appendix 543.9
   Aran-Duchenne muscular 335.21
   arm 728.2
   arteriosclerotic—*see* Arteriosclerosis
   arthritis 714.0
      spine 720.9
   bile duct (any) 576.8
   bladder 596.8
   blanche (of Milian) 701.3
   bone (senile) 733.99
      due to
         disuse 733.7
         infection 733.99
         tabes dorsalis (neurogenic) 094.0
      posttraumatic 733.99
   brain (cortex) (progressive) 331.9
      with dementia 290.10
      Alzheimer's 331.0
         with dementia—*see* Alzheimer's dementia

Atrophy, atrophic—*continued*
   circumscribed (Pick's) 331.1
      with dementia
         with behavioral disturbance 331.1 *[294.11]*
         without behavioral disturbance 331.1
            [294.10]
   congenital 742.4
   hereditary 331.9
   senile 331.2
   breast 611.4
      puerperal, postpartum 676.3
   buccal cavity 528.9
   cardiac (brown) (senile) (*see also* Degeneration,
      myocardial) 429.1
   cartilage (infectional) (joint) 733.99
   cast, plaster of Paris 728.2
   cerebellar—*see* Atrophy, brain
   cerebral—*see* Atrophy, brain
   cervix (endometrium) (mucosa) (myometrium)
      (senile) (uteri) 622.8
      menopausal 627.8
   Charcot-Marie-Tooth 356.1
   choroid 363.40
      diffuse secondary 363.42
      hereditary (*see also* Dystrophy, choroid)
         363.50
      gyrate
         central 363.54
         diffuse 363.57
         generalized 363.57
      senile 363.41
   ciliary body 364.57
   colloid, degenerative 701.3
   conjunctiva (senile) 372.89
   corpus cavernosum 607.89
   cortical (*see also* Atrophy, brain) 331.9
   Cruveilhier's 335.21
   cystic duct 576.8
   dacryosialadenopathy 710.2
   degenerative
      colloid 701.3
      senile 701.3
   Déjérine-Thomas 333.0
   diffuse idiopathic, dermatological 701.8
   disuse
      bone 733.7
      muscle 728.2
   Duchenne-Aran 335.21
   ear 388.9
   edentulous alveolar ridge 525.2
   emphysema, lung 492.8
   endometrium (senile) 621.8
      cervix 622.8
   enteric 569.89
   epididymis 608.3
   eyeball, cause unknown 360.41
   eyelid (senile) 374.50
   facial (skin) 701.9
   facioscapulohumeral (Landouzy-Déjérine) 359.1
   fallopian tube (senile), acquired 620.3
   fatty, thymus (gland) 254.8
   gallbladder 575.8
   gastric 537.89
   gastritis (chronic) 535.1
   gastrointestinal 569.89
   genital organ, male 608.89
   glandular 289.3
   globe (phthisis bulbi) 360.41
   gum 523.2
   hair 704.2

Atrophy, atrophic—*continued*
  heart (brown) (senile) (*see also* Degeneration,
      myocardial) 429.1
  hemifacial 754.0
    Romberg 349.89
  hydronephrosis 591
  infantile 261
    paralysis, acute (*see also* Poliomyelitis, with
        paralysis) 045.1
  intestine 569.89
  iris (generalized) (postinfectional) (sector
      shaped) 364.59
    essential 364.51
    progressive 364.51
    sphincter 364.54
  kidney (senile) (*see also* Sclerosis, renal) 587
    with hypertension (*see also* Hypertension,
        kidney) 403.90
    congenital 753.0
    hydronephrotic 591
    infantile 753.0
  lacrimal apparatus (primary) 375.13
    secondary 375.14
  Landouzy-Déjérine 359.1
  laryngitis, infection 476.0
  larynx 478.79
  Leber's optic 377.16
  lip 528.5
  liver (acute) (subacute) (*see also* Necrosis,
      liver) 570
    chronic (yellow) 571.8
    yellow (congenital) 570
      with
        abortion—*see* Abortion, by type, with
            specified complication NEC
        ectopic pregnancy (*see also* categories
            633.0-633.9) 639.8
        molar pregnancy (*see also* categories
            630-632) 639.8
      chronic 571.8
      complicating pregnancy 646.7
      following
        abortion 639.8
        ectopic or molar pregnancy 639.8
      from injection, inoculation or transfusion
          (onset within 8 months after
          administration)—*see* Hepatitis, viral
      healed 571.5
      obstetric 646.7
      postabortal 639.8
      postimmunization—*see* Hepatitis, viral
      posttransfusion—*see* Hepatitis, viral
      puerperal, postpartum 674.8
  lung (senile) 518.89
    congenital 748.69
  macular (dermatological) 701.3
    syphilitic, skin 091.3
      striated 095.8
  muscle, muscular 728.2
    disuse 728.2
    Duchenne-Aran 335.21
    extremity (lower) (upper) 728.2
    familial spinal 335.11
    general 728.2
    idiopathic 728.2
    infantile spinal 335.0
    myelopathic (progressive) 335.10
    myotonic 359.2
    neuritic 356.1
    neuropathic (peroneal) (progressive) 356.1
    peroneal 356.1

Atrophy, atrophic—*continued*
  primary (idiopathic) 728.2
  progressive (familial) (hereditary) (pure)
      335.21
    adult (spinal) 335.19
    infantile (spinal) 335.0
    juvenile (spinal) 335.11
    spinal 335.10
      adult 335.19
      hereditary or familial 335.11
      infantile 335.0
    pseudohypertrophic 359.1
    spinal (progressive) 335.10
      adult 335.19
      Aran-Duchenne 335.21
      familial 335.11
      hereditary 335.11
      infantile 335.0
      juvenile 335.11
    syphilitic 095.6
  myocardium (*see also* Degeneration,
      myocardial) 429.1
  myometrium (senile) 621.8
    cervix 622.8
  myotatic 728.2
  myotonia 359.2
  nail 703.8
    congenital 757.5
  nasopharynx 472.2
  nerve—*see also* Disorder, nerve
    abducens 378.54
    accessory 352.4
    acoustic or auditory 388.5
    cranial 352.9
      first (olfactory) 352.0
      second (optic) (*see also* Atrophy, optic
          nerve) 377.10
      third (oculomotor) (partial) 378.51
        total 378.52
      fourth (trochlear) 378.53
      fifth (trigeminal) 350.8
      sixth (abducens) 378.54
      seventh (facial) 351.8
      eighth (auditory) 388.5
      ninth (glossopharyngeal) 352.2
      tenth (pneumogastric) (vagus) 352.3
      eleventh (accessory) 352.4
      twelfth (hypoglossal) 352.5
    facial 351.8
    glossopharyngeal 352.2
    hypoglossal 352.5
    oculomotor (partial) 378.51
      total 378.52
    olfactory 352.0
    peripheral 355.9
    pneumogastric 352.3
    trigeminal 350.8
    trochlear 378.53
    vagus (pneumogastric) 352.3
  nervous system, congenital 742.8
  neuritic (*see also* Disorder, nerve) 355.9
  neurogenic NEC 355.9
    bone
      tabetic 094.0
  nutritional 261
  old age 797
  olivopontocerebellar 333.0
  optic nerve (ascending) (descending)
      (infectional) (nonfamilial) (papillomacular
      bundle) (postretinal) (secondary NEC)
      (simple) 377.10

Atrophy, atrophic—*continued*
  associated with retinal dystrophy 377.13
  dominant hereditary 377.16
  glaucomatous 377.14
  hereditary (dominant) (Leber's) 377.16
  Leber's (hereditary) 377.16
  partial 377.15
  postinflammatory 377.12
  primary 377.11
  syphilitic 094.84
    congenital 090.49
    tabes dorsalis 094.0
  orbit 376.45
  ovary (senile), acquired 620.3
  oviduct (senile), acquired 620.3
  palsy, diffuse 335.20
  pancreas (duct) (senile) 577.8
  papillary muscle 429.81
  paralysis 355.9
  parotid gland 527.0
  patches skin 701.3
    senile 701.8
  penis 607.89
  pharyngitis 472.1
  pharynx 478.29
  pluriglandular 258.8
  polyarthritis 714.0
  prostate 602.2
  pseudohypertrophic 359.1
  renal (*see also* Sclerosis, renal) 587
  reticulata 701.8
  retina (*see also* Degeneration, retina) 362.60
    hereditary (*see also* Dystrophy, retina) 362.70
  rhinitis 472.0
  salivary duct or gland 527.0
  scar NEC 709.2
  sclerosis, lobar (of brain) 331.0
    with dementia
      with behavioral disturbance 331.1 *[294.11]*
      without behavioral disturbance 331.1
        [294.10]
  scrotum 608.89
  seminal vesicle 608.89
  senile 797
    degenerative, of skin 701.3
  skin (patches) (senile) 701.8
  spermatic cord 608.89
  spinal (cord) 336.8
    acute 336.8
    muscular (chronic) 335.10
      adult 335.19
      familial 335.11
      juvenile 335.10
    paralysis 335.10
      acute (*see also* Poliomyelitis, with paralysis)
        045.1
  spine (column) 733.99
  spleen (senile) 289.59
  spots (skin) 701.3
    senile 701.8
  stomach 537.89
  striate and macular 701.3
    syphilitic 095.8
  subcutaneous 701.9
    due to injection 999.9
  sublingual gland 527.0
  submaxillary gland 527.0
  Sudeck's 733.7
  suprarenal (autoimmune) (capsule) (gland) 255.4
    with hypofunction 255.4
  tarso-orbital fascia, congenital 743.66

Atrophy, atrophic—*continued*
  testis 608.3
  thenar, partial 354.0
  throat 478.29
  thymus (fat) 254.8
  thyroid (gland) 246.8
    with
      cretinism 243
      myxedema 244.9
    congenital 243
  tongue (senile) 529.8
    papillae 529.4
    smooth 529.4
  trachea 519.1
  tunica vaginalis 608.89
  turbinate 733.99
  tympanic membrane (nonflaccid) 384.82
    flaccid 384.81
  ulcer (*see also* Ulcer, skin) 707.9
  upper respiratory tract 478.9
  uterus, uterine (acquired) (senile) 621.8
    cervix 622.8
    due to radiation (intended effect) 621.8
  vagina (senile) 627.3
  vascular 459.89
  vas deferens 608.89
  vertebra (senile) 733.99
  vulva (primary) (senile) 624.1
  Werdnig-Hoffmann 335.0
  yellow (acute) (congenital) (liver) (subacute)
    (*see also* Necrosis, liver) 570
    chronic 571.8
    resulting from administration of blood,
      plasma, serum, or other biological
      substance (within 8 months of
      administration)—*see* Hepatitis, viral

Attack
  akinetic (*see also* Epilepsy) 345.0
  angina—*see* Angina
  apoplectic (*see also* Disease, cerebrovascular,
    acute) 436
  benign shuddering 333.93
  bilious—*see* Vomiting
  cataleptic 300.11
  cerebral (*see also* Disease, cerebrovascular,
    acute) 436
  coronary (*see also* Infarct, myocardium) 410.9
  cyanotic, newborn 770.83
  epileptic (*see also* Epilepsy) 345.9
  epileptiform 780.39
  heart (*see also* Infarct, myocardium) 410.9
  hemiplegia (*see also* Disease, cerebrovascular,
    acute) 436
  hysterical 300.11
  jacksonian (*see also* Epilepsy) 345.5
  myocardium, myocardial (*see also* Infarct,
    myocardium) 410.9
  myoclonic (*see also* Epilepsy) 345.1
  panic 300.01
  paralysis (*see also* Disease, cerebrovascular,
    acute) 436
  paroxysmal 780.39
  psychomotor (*see also* Epilepsy) 345.4
  salaam (*see also* Epilepsy) 345.6
  schizophreniform (*see also* Schizophrenia) 295.4
  sensory and motor 780.39
  syncope 780.2
  toxic, cerebral 780.39
  transient ischemic (TIA) 435.9
  unconsciousness 780.2
    hysterical 300.11

Avulsion—*continued*
  nerve (root)—*see* Injury, nerve, by site
  scalp—*see* Wound, open, scalp
  skin and subcutaneous tissue—*see* Wound,
    open, by site
  symphyseal cartilage (inner), complicating
    delivery 665.6
  tendon—*see also* Sprain, by site
    with open wound—*see* Wound, open, by site
  toenail—*see* Wound, open, toe(s)
  tooth 873.63
    complicated 873.73
Awareness of heart beat 785.1
Axe grinders' disease 502
Axenfeld's anomaly or syndrome 743.44
Axilla, axillary —*see also* condition
  breast 757.6
Axonotmesis —*see* Injury, nerve, by site
Ayala's disease 756.89
Ayerza's disease or syndrome (pulmonary
  artery sclerosis with pulmonary hypertension)
  416.0
Azoospermia 606.0
Azorean disease (of the nervous system) 334.8
Azotemia 790.6
  meaning uremia (*see also* Uremia) 586
Aztec ear 744.29
Azygos lobe, lung (fissure) 748.69

B

Baader's syndrome (erythema multiforme exudativum) 695.1
Baastrup's syndrome 721.5
Babesiasis 088.82
Babesiosis 088.82
Babington's disease (familial hemorrhagic telangiectasia) 448.0
Babinski's syndrome (cardiovascular syphilis) 093.89
Babinski-Fröhlich syndrome (adiposogenital dystrophy) 253.8
Babinski-Nageotte syndrome 344.89
Bacillary —*see* condition
Bacilluria 791.9
  asymptomatic, in pregnancy or puerperium 646.5
  tuberculous (*see also* Tuberculosis) 016.9
Bacillus—*see also* **Infection, bacillus**
  abortus infection 023.1
  anthracis infection 022.9
  coli
    infection 041.4
      generalized 038.42
      intestinal 008.00
    pyemia 038.42
    septicemia 038.42
  Flexner's 004.1
  fusiformis infestation 101
  mallei infection 024
  Shiga's 004.0
  suipestifer infection (*see also* Infection, Salmonella) 003.9
Back —*see* condition
Backache (postural) 724.5
  psychogenic 307.89
  sacroiliac 724.6
Backflow (pyelovenous) (*see also* Disease, renal) 593.9
Backknee (*see also* Genu, recurvatum) 736.5
Bacteremia (*see also* Infection, bacillus) 790.7
  with
    sepsis—*see* Septicemia
  during
    labor 659.3
    pregnancy 647.8
  newborn 771.83
Bacteria
  in blood (*see also* Bacteremia) 790.7
  in urine (*see also* Bacteriuria) 599.0
Bacterial —*see* condition
Bactericholia (*see also* Cholecystitis, acute) 575.0
Bacterid, bacteride (Andrews' pustular) 686.8
Bacteriuria, bacteruria 791.9
  with
    urinary tract infection 599.0
  asymptomatic 791.9
    in pregnancy or puerperium 646.5
      affecting fetus or newborn 760.1
Bad
  breath 784.9
  heart—*see* Disease, heart
  trip (*see also* Abuse, drugs, nondependent) 305.3
Baehr-Schiffrin disease (thrombotic thrombocytopenic purpura) 446.6
Baelz's disease (cheilitis glandularis apostematosa) 528.5
Baerensprung's disease (eczema marginatum) 110.3

Bagassosis (occupational) 495.1
Baghdad boil 085.1
Bagratuni's syndrome (temporal arteritis) 446.5
Baker's
  cyst (knee) 727.51
    tuberculous (*see also* Tuberculosis) 015.2
  itch 692.89
Bakwin-Krida syndrome (craniometaphyseal dysplasia) 756.89
Balanitis (circinata) (gangraenosa) (infectious) (vulgaris) 607.1
  amebic 006.8
  candidal 112.2
  chlamydial 099.53
  due to Ducrey's bacillus 099.0
  erosiva circinata et gangraenosa 607.1
  gangrenous 607.1
  gonococcal (acute) 098.0
    chronic or duration of 2 months or over 098.2
  nongonococcal 607.1
  phagedenic 607.1
  venereal NEC 099.8
  xerotica obliterans 607.81
Balanoposthitis 607.1
  chlamydial 099.53
  gonococcal (acute) 098.0
    chronic or duration of 2 months or over 098.2
  ulcerative NEC 099.8
Balanorrhagia —*see* Balanitis
Balantidiasis 007.0
Balantidiosis 007.0
Balbuties, balbutio 307.0
Bald
  patches on scalp 704.00
  tongue 529.4
Baldness (*see also* Alopecia) 704.00
Balfour's disease (chloroma) 205.3
Balint's syndrome (psychic paralysis of visual fixation) 368.16
Balkan grippe 083.0
Ball
  food 938
  hair 938
Ballantyne (-Runge) **syndrome** (postmaturity) 766.2
Balloon disease (*see also* Effect, adverse, high altitude) 993.2
Ballooning posterior leaflet syndrome 424.0
Baló's disease or concentric sclerosis 341.1
Bamberger's disease (hypertrophic pulmonary osteoarthropathy) 731.2
Bamberger-Marie disease (hypertrophic pulmonary osteoarthropathy) 731.2
Bamboo spine 720.0
Bancroft's filariasis 125.0
Band(s)
  adhesive (*see also* Adhesions, peritoneum) 568.0
  amniotic 658.8
    affecting fetus or newborn 762.8
  anomalous or congenital—*see also* Anomaly, specified type NEC
    atrial 746.9
    heart 746.9
    intestine 751.4
    omentum 751.4
    ventricular 746.9
  cervix 622.3
  gallbladder (congenital) 751.69

Band(s)—*continued*
  intestinal (adhesive) (*see also* Adhesions,
    peritoneum) 568.0
    congenital 751.4
  obstructive (*see also* Obstruction, intestine)
    560.81
  periappendiceal (congenital) 751.4
  peritoneal (adhesive) (*see also* Adhesions,
    peritoneum) 568.0
    with intestinal obstruction 560.81
    congenital 751.4
  uterus 621.5
  vagina 623.2
Bandl's ring (contraction)
  complicating delivery 661.4
  affecting fetus or newborn 763.7
Bang's disease (Brucella abortus) 023.1
Bangkok hemorrhagic fever 065.4
Bannister's disease 995.1
Bantam-Albright-Martin disease
  (pseudohypoparathyroidism) 275.49
Banti's disease or syndrome (with cirrhosis)
  (with portal hypertension)—*see* Cirrhosis,
  liver
Bar
  calcaneocuboid 755.67
  calcaneonavicular 755.67
  cubonavicular 755.67
  prostate 600.9
  talocalcaneal 755.67
Baragnosis 780.99
Barasheh, barashek 266.2
Barcoo disease or rot (*see also* Ulcer, skin) 707.9
Bard-Pic syndrome (carcinoma, head of
  pancreas) 157.0
Bärensprung's disease (eczema marginatum)
  110.3
Baritosis 503
Barium lung disease 503
Barlow's syndrome (meaning mitral valve
  prolapse) 424.0
Barlow (-Möller) disease or syndrome (meaning
  infantile scurvy) 267
Barodontalgia 993.2
Baron Münchausen syndrome 301.51
Barosinusitis 993.1
Barotitis 993.0
Barotrauma 993.2
  odontalgia 993.2
  otitic 993.0
  sinus 993.1
Barraquer's disease or syndrome (progressive
  lipodystrophy) 272.6
Barré-Guillain syndrome 357.0
Barré-Liéou syndrome (posterior cervical
  sympathetic) 723.2
Barrel chest 738.3
Barrett's syndrome or ulcer (chronic peptic
  ulcer of esophagus) 530.2
Bársony-Polgár syndrome (corkscrew
  esophagus) 530.5
Bársony-Teschendorf syndrome (corkscrew
  esophagus) 530.5
Bartholin's
  adenitis (*see also* Bartholinitis) 616.8
  gland—*see* condition
Bartholinitis (suppurating) 616.8
  gonococcal (acute) 098.0
    chronic or duration of 2 months or over 098.2
Bartonellosis 088.0

Bartter's syndrome (secondary
  hyperaldosteronism with juxtaglomerular
  hyperplasia) 255.1
Basal—*see* **condition**
Basan's (hidrotic) ectodermal dysplasia 757.31
Baseball finger 842.13
Basedow's disease or syndrome (exophthalmic
  goiter) 242.0
Basic —*see* condition
Basilar —*see* condition
Bason's (hidrotic) ectodermal dysplasia 757.31
Basopenia 288.0
Basophilia 288.8
Basophilism (corticoadrenal) (Cushing's)
  (pituitary) (thymic) 255.0
Bassen-Kornzweig syndrome
  (abetalipoproteinemia) 272.5
Bat ear 744.29
Bateman's
  disease 078.0
  purpura (senile) 287.2
Bathing cramp 994.1
Bathophobia 300.23
Batten's disease, retina 330.1 *[362.71]*
Batten-Mayou disease 330.1 *[362.71]*
Batten-Steinert syndrome 359.2
Battered
  adult (syndrome) 995.81
  baby or child (syndrome) 995.54
  spouse (syndrome) 995.81
Battey mycobacterium infection 031.0
Battledore placenta —*see* Placenta, abnormal
Battle exhaustion (*see also* Reaction, stress,
  acute) 308.9
Baumgarten-Cruveilhier (cirrhosis) disease, or
  syndrome 571.5
Bauxite
  fibrosis (of lung) 503
  workers' disease 503
Bayle's disease (dementia paralytica) 094.1
Bazin's disease (primary) (*see also* Tuberculosis)
  017.1
Beach ear 380.12
Beaded hair (congenital) 757.4
Beard's disease (neurasthenia) 300.5
Bearn-Kunkel (-Slater) syndrome (lupoid
  hepatitis) 571.49
Beat
  elbow 727.2
  hand 727.2
  knee 727.2
Beats
  ectopic 427.60
  escaped, heart 427.60
    postoperative 997.1
  premature (nodal) 427.60
    atrial 427.61
    auricular 427.61
    postoperative 997.1
    specified type NEC 427.69
    supraventricular 427.61
    ventricular 427.69
Beau's
  disease or syndrome (*see also* Degeneration,
    myocardial) 429.1
  lines (transverse furrows on fingernails) 703.8
Bechterew's disease (ankylosing spondylitis)
  720.0
Bechterew-Strümpell-Marie syndrome
  (ankylosing spondylitis) 720.0

Beck's syndrome (anterior spinal artery occlusion) 433.8

Becker's
disease (idiopathic mural endomyocardial disease) 425.2
dystrophy 359.1

Beckwith (-Wiedemann) syndrome 759.89

Bedclothes, asphyxiation or suffocation by 994.7

Bednar's aphthae 528.2

Bedsore 707.0
with gangrene 707.0 *[785.4]*

Bedwetting (*see also* Enuresis) 788.36

Beer-drinkers' heart (disease) 425.5

Bee sting (with allergic or anaphylactic shock) 989.5

Begbie's disease (exophthalmic goiter) 242.0

Behavior disorder, disturbance —*see also* Disturbance, conduct
antisocial, without manifest psychiatric disorder
adolescent V71.02
adult V71.01
child V71.02
dyssocial, without manifest psychiatric disorder
adolescent V71.02
adult V71.01
child V71.02
high-risk—*see* Problem

Behçet's syndrome 136.1

Behr's disease 362.50

Beigel's disease or morbus (white piedra) 111.2

Bejel 104.0

Bekhterev's disease (ankylosing spondylitis) 720.0

Bekhterev-Strümpell-Marie syndrome (ankylosing spondylitis) 720.0

Belching (*see also* Eructation) 787.3

Bell's
disease (*see also* Psychosis, affective) 296.0
mania (*see also* Psychosis, affective) 296.0
palsy, paralysis 351.0
infant 767.5
newborn 767.5
syphilitic 094.89
spasm 351.0

Bence-Jones albuminuria, albuminosuria, or proteinuria 791.0

Bends 993.3

Benedikt's syndrome (paralysis) 344.89

Benign —*see also* condition
cellular changes, cervix 795.09
prostate
hyperplasia 600.0
neoplasm 222.2

Bennett's
disease (leukemia) 208.9
fracture (closed) 815.01
open 815.11

Benson's disease 379.22

Bent
back (hysterical) 300.11
nose 738.0
congenital 754.0

Bereavement V62.82
as adjustment reaction 309.0

Berger's paresthesia (lower limb) 782.0

Bergeron's disease (hysteroepilepsy) 300.11

Beriberi (acute) (atrophic) (chronic) (dry) (subacute) (wet) 265.0
with polyneuropathy 265.0 *[357.4]*
heart (disease) 265.0 *[425.7]*

Beriberi—*continued*
leprosy 030.1
neuritis 265.0 *[357.4]*

Berlin's disease or edema (traumatic) 921.3

Berloque dermatitis 692.72

Bernard-Horner syndrome (*see also* Neuropathy, peripheral, autonomic) 337.9

Bernard-Sergent syndrome (acute adrenocortical insufficiency) 255.4

Bernard-Soulier disease or thrombopathy 287.1

Bernhardt's disease or paresthesia 355.1

Bernhardt-Roth disease or syndrome (paresthesia) 355.1

Bernheim's syndrome (*see also* Failure, heart) 428.0

Bertielliasis 123.8

Bertolotti's syndrome (sacralization of fifth lumbar vertebra) 756.15

Berylliosis (acute) (chronic) (lung) (occupational) 503

Besnier's
lupus pernio 135
prurigo (atopic dermatitis) (infantile eczema) 691.8

Besnier-Boeck disease or sarcoid 135

Besnier-Boeck-Schaumann disease (sarcoidosis) 135

Best's disease 362.76

Bestiality 302.1

Beta-adrenergic hyperdynamic circulatory state 429.82

Beta-aminoisobutyric aciduria 277.2

Beta-mercaptolactate-cysteine disulfiduria 270.0

Beta thalassemia (major) (minor) (mixed) 282.4

Beurmann's disease (sporotrichosis) 117.1

Bezoar 938
intestine 936
stomach 935.2

Bezold's abscess (*see also* Mastoiditis) 383.01

Bianchi's syndrome (aphasia-apraxia-alexia) 784.69

Bicornuate or bicornis uterus 752.3
in pregnancy or childbirth 654.0
with obstructed labor 660.2
affecting fetus or newborn 763.1
affecting fetus or newborn 763.89

Bicuspid aortic valve 746.4

Biedl-Bardet syndrome 759.89

Bielschowsky's disease 330.1

Bielschowsky-Jansky
amaurotic familial idiocy 330.1
disease 330.1

Biemond's syndrome (obesity, polydactyly, and mental retardation) 759.89

Biermer's anemia or disease (pernicious anemia) 281.0

Biett's disease 695.4

Bifid (congenital)—*see also* Imperfect, closure
apex, heart 746.89
clitoris 752.49
epiglottis 748.3
kidney 753.3
nose 748.1
patella 755.64
scrotum 752.8
toe 755.66
tongue 750.13
ureter 753.4
uterus 752.3

Bifid — *continued*
uvula 749.02
 with cleft lip (*see also* Cleft, palate, with cleft
  lip) 749.20
Biforis uterus (suprasimplex) 752.3
Bifurcation (congenital)—*see also* Imperfect,
 closure
gallbladder 751.69
kidney pelvis 753.3
renal pelvis 753.3
rib 756.3
tongue 750.13
trachea 748.3
ureter 753.4
urethra 753.8
uvula 749.02
 with cleft lip (*see also* Cleft, palate, with cleft
  lip) 749.20
vertebra 756.19
Bigeminal pulse 427.89
Bigeminy 427.89
Big spleen syndrome 289.4
Bilateral —*see* condition
Bile duct —*see* condition
Bile pigments in urine 791.4
Bilharziasis (*see also* Schistosomiasis) 120.9
chyluria 120.0
cutaneous 120.3
galacturia 120.0
hematochyluria 120.0
intestinal 120.1
lipemia 120.9
lipuria 120.0
Oriental 120.2
piarhemia 120.9
pulmonary 120.2
tropical hematuria 120.0
vesical 120.0
Biliary —*see* condition
Bilious (attack)—*see also* Vomiting
fever, hemoglobinuric 084.8
Bilirubinuria 791.4
Biliuria 791.4
Billroth's disease
meningocele (*see also* Spina bifida) 741.9
Bilobate placenta —*see* Placenta, abnormal
Bilocular
heart 745.7
stomach 536.8
Bing-Horton syndrome (histamine cephalgia)
 346.2
Binswanger's disease or dementia 290.12
Biörck (-Thorson) syndrome (malignant
 carcinoid) 259.2
Biparta, bipartite —*see also* Imperfect, closure
carpal scaphoid 755.59
patella 755.64
placenta—*see* Placenta, abnormal
vagina 752.49
Bird
face 756.0
fanciers' lung or disease 495.2
Bird's disease (oxaluria) 271.8
Birth
abnormal fetus or newborn 763.9
accident, fetus or newborn—*see* Birth, injury
complications in mother—*see* Delivery,
 complicated
compression during NEC 767.9
defect—*see* Anomaly
delayed, fetus 763.9

Birth—*continued*
difficult NEC, affecting fetus or newborn 763.9
dry, affecting fetus or newborn 761.1
forced, NEC, affecting fetus or newborn 763.89
forceps, affecting fetus or newborn 763.2
hematoma of sternomastoid 767.8
immature 765.1
 extremely 765.0
inattention, after or at 995.52
induced, affecting fetus or newborn 763.89
infant—*see* Newborn
injury NEC 767.9
 adrenal gland 767.8
 basal ganglia 767.0
 brachial plexus (paralysis) 767.6
 brain (compression) (pressure) 767.0
 cerebellum 767.0
 cerebral hemorrhage 767.0
 conjunctiva 767.8
 eye 767.8
 fracture
  bone, any except clavicle or spine 767.3
  clavicle 767.2
  femur 767.3
  humerus 767.3
  long bone 767.3
  radius and ulna 767.3
  skeleton NEC 767.3
  skull 767.3
  spine 767.4
  tibia and fibula 767.3
 hematoma 767.8
  liver (subcapsular) 767.8
  mastoid 767.8
  skull 767.1
  sternomastoid 767.8
  testes 767.8
  vulva 767.8
 intracranial (edema) 767.0
 laceration
  brain 767.0
  by scalpel 767.8
  peripheral nerve 767.7
 liver 767.8
 meninges
  brain 767.0
  spinal cord 767.4
 nerves (cranial, peripheral) 767.7
  brachial plexus 767.6
  facial 767.5
 paralysis 767.7
  brachial plexus 767.6
  Erb (-Duchenne) 767.6
  facial nerve 767.5
  Klumpke (-Déjérine) 767.6
  radial nerve 767.6
  spinal (cord) (hemorrhage) (laceration)
   (rupture) 767.4
 rupture
  intracranial 767.0
  liver 767.8
  spinal cord 767.4
  spleen 767.8
  viscera 767.8
 scalp 767.1
 scalpel wound 767.8
 shock, newborn 779.89
 skeleton NEC 767.3
 specified NEC 767.8
 spinal cord 767.4
 spleen 767.8

Birth—*continued*
  subdural hemorrhage 767.0
  tentorial, tear 767.0
  testes 767.8
  vulva 767.8
  instrumental, NEC, affecting fetus or newborn
    763.2
  lack of care, after or at 995.52
  multiple
    affected by maternal complications of
      pregnancy 761.5
    healthy liveborn—*see* Newborn, multiple
  neglect, after or at 995.52
  newborn—*see* Newborn
  palsy or paralysis NEC 767.7
  precipitate, fetus or newborn 763.6
  premature (infant) 765.1
  prolonged, affecting fetus or newborn 763.9
  retarded, fetus or newborn 763.9
  shock, newborn 779.8
  strangulation or suffocation
    due to aspiration of amniotic fluid 770.1
    mechanical 767.8
  trauma NEC 767.9
  triplet
    affected by maternal complications of
      pregnancy 761.5
    healthy liveborn—*see* Newborn, multiple
  twin
    affected by maternal complications of
      pregnancy 761.5
    healthy liveborn—*see* Newborn, twin
  ventouse, affecting fetus or newborn 763.3
Birthmark 757.32
Bisalbuminemia 273.8
Biskra button 085.1
Bite (s)
  with intact skin surface—*see* Contusion
  animal—*see* Wound, open, by site
    intact skin surface—*see* Contusion
  centipede 989.5
  chigger 133.8
  fire ant 989.5
  flea—*see* Injury, superficial, by site
  human (open wound)—*see also* Wound, open,
    by site
    intact skin surface—*see* Contusion
  insect
    nonvenomous—*see* Injury, superficial, by site
    venomous 989.5
  mad dog (death from) 071
  poisonous 989.5
  red bug 133.8
  reptile 989.5
    nonvenomous—*see* Wound, open, by site
  snake 989.5
    nonvenomous—*see* Wound, open, by site
  spider (venomous) 989.5
    nonvenomous—*see* Injury, superficial, by site
  venomous 989.5
Biting
  cheek or lip 528.9
  nail 307.9
Black
  death 020.9
  eye NEC 921.0
  hairy tongue 529.3
  lung disease 500
Blackfan-Diamond anemia or syndrome
  (congenital hypoplastic anemia) 284.0
Blackhead 706.1
Blackout 780.2

Blackwater fever 084.8
Bladder —*see* Condition
Blast
  blindness 921.3
  concussion—*see* Blast, injury
  injury 869.0
    with open wound into cavity 869.1
    abdomen or thorax—*see* Injury, internal, by
      site
    brain (*see also* Concussion, brain) 850.9
      with skull fracture—*see* Fracture, skull
    ear (acoustic nerve trauma) 951.5
      with perforation, tympanic membrane—*see*
        Wound, open, ear, drum
    lung (*see also* Injury, internal, lung) 861.20
    otitic (explosive) 388.11
Blastomycosis, blastomycotic (chronic)
  (cutaneous) (disseminated) (lung)
  (pulmonary) (systemic) 116.0
  Brazilian 116.1
  European 117.5
  keloidal 116.2
  North American 116.0
  primary pulmonary 116.0
  South American 116.1
Bleb(s) 709.8
  emphysematous (bullous) (diffuse) (lung)
    (ruptured) (solitary) 492.0
  filtering, eye (postglaucoma) (status) V45.69
    with complication 997.99
    postcataract extraction (complication) 997.99
  lung (ruptured) 492.0
    congenital 770.5
  subpleural (emphysematous) 492.0
Bleeder (familial) (hereditary) (*see also* Defect,
  coagulation) 286.9
  nonfamilial 286.9
Bleeding (*see also* Hemorrhage) 459.0
  anal 569.3
  anovulatory 628.0
  atonic, following delivery 666.1
  capillary 448.9
  due to subinvolution 621.1
    puerperal 666.2
  ear 388.69
  excessive, associated with menopausal onset
    627.0
  familial (*see also* Defect, coagulation) 286.9
  following intercourse 626.7
  gastrointestinal 578.9
  gums 523.8
  hemorrhoids—*see* Hemorrhoids, bleeding
  intermenstrual
    irregular 626.6
    regular 626.5
  intraoperative 998.11
  irregular NEC 626.4
  menopausal 627.0
  mouth 528.9
  nipple 611.79
  nose 784.7
  ovulation 626.5
  postclimacteric 627.1
  postcoital 626.7
  postmenopausal 627.1
    following induced menopause 627.4
  postoperative 998.11
  preclimacteric 627.0
  puberty 626.3
    excessive, with onset of menstrual periods
      626.3

Bleeding—*continued*
  rectum, rectal 569.3
  tendencies (*see also* Defect, coagulation) 286.9
  throat 784.8
  umbilical stump 772.3
  umbilicus 789.9
  unrelated to menstrual cycle 626.6
  uterus, uterine 626.9
    climacteric 627.0
    dysfunctional 626.8
    functional 626.8
    unrelated to menstrual cycle 626.6
  vagina, vaginal 623.8
    functional 626.8
  vicarious 625.8
Blennorrhagia, blennorrhagic —*see*
  Blennorrhea
Blennorrhea (acute) 098.0
  adultorum 098.40
  alveolaris 523.4
  chronic or duration of 2 months or over 098.2
  gonococcal (neonatorum) 098.40
  inclusion (neonatal) (newborn) 771.6
  neonatorum 098.40
Blepharelosis (*see also* Entropion) 374.00
Blepharitis (eyelid) 373.00
  angularis 373.01
  ciliaris 373.00
    with ulcer 373.01
  marginal 373.00
    with ulcer 373.01
  scrofulous (*see also* Tuberculosis) 017.3
    [373.00]
  squamous 373.02
  ulcerative 373.01
Blepharochalasis 374.34
  congenital 743.62
Blepharoclonus 333.81
Blepharoconjunctivitis (*see also* Conjunctivitis)
  372.20
  angular 372.21
  contact 372.22
Blepharophimosis (eyelid) 374.46
  congenital 743.62
Blepharoplegia 374.89
Blepharoptosis 374.30
  congenital 743.61
Blepharopyorrhea 098.49
Blepharospasm 333.81
Blessig's cyst 362.62
Blighted ovum 631
Blind
  bronchus (congenital) 748.3
  eye—*see also* Blindness
    hypertensive 360.42
    hypotensive 360.41
  loop syndrome (postoperative) 579.2
  sac, fallopian tube (congenital) 752.19
  spot, enlarged 368.42
  tract or tube (congenital) NEC—*see* Atresia
Blindness (acquired) (congenital) (both eyes)
  369.00
  blast 921.3
  with nerve injury—*see* Injury, nerve, optic
  Bright's—*see* Uremia
  color (congenital) 368.59
    acquired 368.55
    blue 368.53
    green 368.52
    red 368.51
    total 368.54

Blindness—*continued*
  concussion 950.9
  cortical 377.75
  day 368.10
    acquired 368.10
    congenital 368.10
    hereditary 368.10
    specified type NEC 368.10
  due to
    injury NEC 950.9
    refractive error—*see* Error, refractive
  eclipse (total) 363.31
  emotional 300.11
  hysterical 300.11
  legal (both eyes) (USA definition) 369.4
    with impairment of better (less impaired) eye
      near-total 369.02
        with
          lesser eye impairment 369.02
            near-total 369.04
            total 369.03
        profound 369.05
          with
            lesser eye impairment 369.05
              near-total 369.07
              profound 369.08
              total 369.06
        severe 369.21
          with
            lesser eye impairment 369.21
              blind 369.11
              near-total 369.13
              profound 369.14
              severe 369.22
              total 369.12
      total
        with lesser eye impairment total 369.01
  mind 784.69
  moderate
    both eyes 369.25
      with impairment of lesser eye (specified as)
        blind, not further specified 369.15
        low vision, not further specified 369.23
        near-total 369.17
        profound 369.18
        severe 369.24
        total 369.16
    one eye 369.74
      with vision of other eye (specified as)
        near-normal 369.75
        normal 369.76
  near-total
    both eyes 369.04
      with impairment of lesser eye (specified as)
        blind, not further specified 369.02
        total 369.03
    one eye 369.64
      with vision of other eye (specified as)
        near-normal 369.65
        normal 369.66
  night 368.60
    acquired 368.62
    congenital (Japanese) 368.61
    hereditary 368.61
    specified type NEC 368.69
    vitamin A deficiency 264.5
  nocturnal—*see* Blindness, night
  one eye 369.60
    with low vision of other eye 369.10
  profound
    both eyes 369.08

Blindness—*continued*
  with impairment of lesser eye (specified as)
    blind, not further specified 369.05
    near-total 369.07
    total 369.06
  one eye 369.67
    with vision of other eye (specified as)
      near-normal 369.68
      normal 369.69
  psychic 784.69
  severe
    both eyes 369.22
      with impairment of lesser eye (specified as)
        blind, not further specified 369.11
        low vision, not further specified 369.21
        near-total 369.13
        profound 369.14
        total 369.12
    one eye 369.71
      with vision of other eye (specified as)
        near-normal 369.72
        normal 369.73
  snow 370.24
  sun 363.31
  temporary 368.12
  total
    both eyes 369.01
    one eye 369.61
      with vision of other eye (specified as)
        near-normal 369.62
        normal 369.63
  transient 368.12
  traumatic NEC 950.9
  word (developmental) 315.01
    acquired 784.61
    secondary to organic lesion 784.61
Blister —*see also* Injury, superficial, by site
  beetle dermatitis 692.89
  due to burn—*see* Burn, by site, second degree
  fever 054.9
  multiple, skin, nontraumatic 709.8
Bloating 787.3
Bloch-Siemens syndrome (incontinentia
    pigmenti) 757.33
Bloch-Stauffer dyshormonal dermatosis 757.33
Bloch-Sulzberger disease or syndrome
    (incontinentia pigmenti) (melanoblastosis)
    757.33
Block
  alveolar capillary 516.3
  arborization (heart) 426.6
  arrhythmic 426.9
  atrioventricular (AV) (incomplete) (partial)
    426.10
    with
      2:1 atrioventricular response block 426.13
      atrioventricular dissociation 426.0
    first degree (incomplete) 426.11
    second degree (Mobitz type I) 426.13
      Mobitz (type) II 426.12
    third degree 426.0
    complete 426.0
      congenital 746.86
    congenital 746.86
    Mobitz (incomplete)
      type I (Wenckebach's) 426.13
      type II 426.12
    partial 426.13
  auriculoventricular (*see also* Block,
    atrioventricular) 426.10
    complete 426.0

Block—*continued*
  congenital 746.86
  congenital 746.86
  bifascicular (cardiac) 426.53
  bundle branch (complete) (false) (incomplete)
    426.50
    bilateral 426.53
    left (complete) (main stem) 426.3
      with right bundle branch block 426.53
      anterior fascicular 426.2
        with
          posterior fascicular block 426.3
          right bundle branch block 426.52
      hemiblock 426.2
      incomplete 426.2
        with right bundle branch block 426.53
      posterior fascicular 426.2
        with
          anterior fascicular block 426.3
          right bundle branch block 426.51
    right 426.4
      with
        left bundle branch block (incomplete)
          (main stem) 426.53
        left fascicular block 426.53
          anterior 426.52
          posterior 426.51
    Wilson's type 426.4
  cardiac 426.9
  conduction 426.9
    complete 426.0
  Eustachian tube (*see also* Obstruction,
    Eustachian tube) 381.60
  fascicular (left anterior) (left posterior) 426.2
  foramen Magendie (acquired) 331.3
    congenital 742.3
      with spina bifida (*see also* Spina bifida)
        741.0
  heart 426.9
    first degree (atrioventricular) 426.11
    second degree (atrioventricular) 426.13
    third degree (atrioventricular) 426.0
    bundle branch (complete) (false) (incomplete)
      426.50
      bilateral 426.53
      left (*see also* Block, bundle branch, left)
        426.3
      right (*see also* Block, bundle branch, right)
        426.4
    complete (atrioventricular) 426.0
    congenital 746.86
    incomplete 426.13
    intra-atrial 426.6
    intraventricular NEC 426.6
    sinoatrial 426.6
    specified type NEC 426.6
  hepatic vein 453.0
  intraventricular (diffuse) (myofibrillar) 426.6
    bundle branch (complete) (false) (incomplete)
      426.50
      bilateral 426.53
      left (*see also* Block, bundle branch, left)
        426.3
      right (*see also* Block, bundle branch, right)
        426.4
  kidney (*see also* Disease, renal) 593.9
    postcystoscopic 997.5
  myocardial (*see also* Block, heart) 426.9
  nodal 426.10
  optic nerve 377.49
  organ or site (congenital) NEC—*see* Atresia

Block—*continued*
 parietal 426.6
 peri-infarction 426.6
 portal (vein) 452
 sinoatrial 426.6
 sinoauricular 426.6
 spinal cord 336.9
 trifascicular 426.54
 tubal 628.2
 vein NEC 453.9
Blocq's disease or syndrome (astasia-abasia)
  307.9
Blood
 constituents, abnormal NEC 790.6
 disease 289.9
  specified NEC 289.8
 donor V59.01
  other blood components V59.09
  stem cells V59.02
  whole blood V59.01
 dyscrasia 289.9
  with
   abortion—*see* Abortion, by type, with
    hemorrhage, delayed or excessive
   ectopic pregnancy (*see also* categories
    633.0-633.9) 639.1
   molar pregnancy (*see also* categories
    630-632) 639.1
  fetus or newborn NEC 776.9
  following
   abortion 639.1
   ectopic or molar pregnancy 639.1
  puerperal, postpartum 666.3
 flukes NEC (*see also* Infestation, Schistosoma)
  120.9
 in
  feces (*see also* Melena) 578.1
   occult 792.1
  urine (*see also* Hematuria) 599.7
 mole 631
 occult 792.1
 poisoning (*see also* Septicemia) 038.9
 pressure
  decreased, due to shock following injury 958.4
  fluctuating 796.4
  high (*see also* Hypertension) 401.9
   incidental reading (isolated) (nonspecific),
    without diagnosis of hypertension 796.2
  low (*see also* Hypotension) 458.9
   incidental reading (isolated) (nonspecific),
    without diagnosis of hypotension 796.3
 spitting (*see also* Hemoptysis) 786.3
 staining cornea 371.12
 transfusion
  without reported diagnosis V58.2
  donor V59.01
   stem cells V59.02
  reaction or complication—*see* Complications,
   transfusion
 tumor—*see* Hematoma
 vessel rupture—*see* Hemorrhage
 vomiting (*see also* Hematemesis) 578.0
Blood-forming organ disease 289.9
Bloodgood's disease 610.1
Bloodshot eye 379.93
Bloom (-Machacek) (-Torre) syndrome 757.39
Blotch, palpebral 372.55
Blount's disease (tibia vara) 732.4
Blount-Barber syndrome (tibia vara) 732.4

Blue
 baby 746.9
 bloater 491.20
  with acute bronchitis or exacerbation 491.21
 diaper syndrome 270.0
 disease 746.9
 dome cyst 610.0
 drum syndrome 381.02
 sclera 743.47
  with fragility of bone and deafness 756.51
 toe syndrome—*see* Atherosclerosis
Blueness (*see also* Cyanosis) 782.5
Blurring, visual 368.8
Blushing (abnormal) (excessive) 782.62
Boarder, hospital V65.0
 infant V65.0
Bockhart's impetigo (superficial folliculitis)
  704.8
Bodechtel-Guttmann disease (subacute
  sclerosing panencephalitis) 046.2
Boder-Sedgwick syndrome (ataxia-
  telangiectasia) 334.8
Body, bodies
 Aschoff (*see also* Myocarditis, rheumatic) 398.0
 asteroid, vitreous 379.22
 choroid, colloid (degenerative) 362.57
  hereditary 362.77
 cytoid (retina) 362.82
 drusen (retina) (*see also* Drusen) 362.57
  optic disc 377.21
 fibrin, pleura 511.0
 foreign—*see* Foreign body
 Hassall-Henle 371.41
 loose
  joint (*see also* Loose, body, joint) 718.1
   knee 717.6
  knee 717.6
  sheath, tendon 727.82
 Mallory's 034.1
 Mooser 081.0
 Negri 071
 rice (joint) (*see also* Loose, body, joint) 718.1
  knee 717.6
 rocking 307.3
Boeck's
 disease (sarcoidosis) 135
 lupoid (miliary) 135
 sarcoid 135
Boerhaave's syndrome (spontaneous esophageal
  rupture) 530.4
Boggy
 cervix 622.8
 uterus 621.8
Boil (*see also* Carbuncle) 680.9
 abdominal wall 680.2
 Aleppo 085.1
 ankle 680.6
 anus 680.5
 arm (any part, above wrist) 680.3
 auditory canal, external 680.0
 axilla 680.3
 back (any part) 680.2
 Baghdad 085.1
 breast 680.2
 buttock 680.5
 chest wall 680.2
 corpus cavernosum 607.2
 Delhi 085.1
 ear (any part) 680.0
 eyelid 373.13
 face (any part, except eye) 680.0

Boil —*continued*
finger (any) 680.4
flank 680.2
foot (any part) 680.7
forearm 680.3
Gafsa 085.1
genital organ, male 608.4
gluteal (region) 680.5
groin 680.2
hand (any part) 680.4
head (any part, except face) 680.8
heel 680.7
hip 680.6
knee 680.6
labia 616.4
lacrimal (*see also* Dacryocystitis) 375.30
gland (*see also* Dacryoadenitis) 375.00
passages (duct) (sac) (*see also* Dacryocystitis) 375.30
leg, any part except foot 680.6
multiple sites 680.9
Natal 085.1
neck 680.1
nose (external) (septum) 680.0
orbit, orbital 376.01
partes posteriores 680.5
pectoral region 680.2
penis 607.2
perineum 680.2
pinna 680.0
scalp (any part) 680.8
scrotum 608.4
seminal vesicle 608.0
shoulder 680.3
skin NEC 680.9
specified site NEC 680.8
spermatic cord 608.4
temple (region) 680.0
testis 608.4
thigh 680.6
thumb 680.4
toe (any) 680.7
tropical 085.1
trunk 680.2
tunica vaginalis 608.4
umbilicus 680.2
upper arm 680.3
vas deferens 608.4
vulva 616.4
wrist 680.4
Bold hives (*see also* Urticaria) 708.9
Bolivian hemorrhagic fever 078.7
Bombé, iris 364.74
Bomford-Rhoads anemia (refractory) 284.9
Bone —*see* condition
Bonnevie-Ullrich syndrome 758.6
Bonnier's syndrome 386.19
Bonvale Dam fever 780.79
Bony block of joint 718.80
ankle 718.87
elbow 718.82
foot 718.87
hand 718.84
hip 718.85
knee 718.86
multiple sites 718.89
pelvic region 718.85
shoulder (region) 718.81
specified site NEC 718.88
wrist 718.83

Borderline
intellectual functioning V62.89
pelvis 653.1
with obstruction during labor 660.1
affecting fetus or newborn 763.1
psychosis (*see also* Schizophrenia) 295.5
of childhood (*see also* Psychosis, childhood) 299.8
schizophrenia (*see also* Schizophrenia) 295.5
Borna disease 062.9
Bornholm disease (epidemic pleurodynia) 074.1
Borrelia vincentii (mouth) (pharynx) (tonsils) 101
Bostock's catarrh (*see also* Fever, hay) 477.9
Boston exanthem 048
Botalli, ductus (patent) (persistent) 747.0
Bothriocephalus latus infestation 123.4
Botulism 005.1
Bouba (*see also* Yaws) 102.9
Bouffée délirante 298.3
Bouillaud's disease or syndrome (rheumatic heart disease) 391.9
Bourneville's disease (tuberous sclerosis) 759.5
Boutonneuse fever 082.1
Boutonniere
deformity (finger) 736.21
hand (intrinsic) 736.21
Bouveret (-Hoffmann) disease or syndrome (paroxysmal tachycardia) 427.2
Bovine heart —*see* Hypertrophy, cardiac
Bowel —*see* condition
Bowen's
dermatosis (precancerous) (M8081/2)—*see* Neoplasm, skin, in situ
disease (M8081/2)—*see* Neoplasm, skin, in situ
epithelioma (M8081/2)—*see* Neoplasm, skin, in situ
type
epidermoid carcinoma in situ (M8081/2)—*see* Neoplasm, skin, in situ
intraepidermal squamous cell carcinoma (M8081/2)–*see* Neoplasm, skin, in situ
Bowing
femur 736.89
congenital 754.42
fibula 736.89
congenital 754.43
forearm 736.09
away from midline (cubitus valgus) 736.01
toward midline (cubitus varus) 736.02
leg(s), long bones, congenital 754.44
radius 736.09
away from midline (cubitus valgus) 736.01
toward midline (cubitus varus) 736.02
tibia 736.89
congenital 754.43
Bowleg (s) 736.42
congenital 754.44
rachitic 268.1
Boyd's dysentery 004.2
Brachial —*see* condition
Brachman-de Lange syndrome (Amsterdam dwarf, mental retardation, and brachycephaly) 759.89
Brachycardia 427.89
Brachycephaly 756.0
Brachymorphism and ectopia lentis 759.89
Bradley's disease (epidemic vomiting) 078.82
Bradycardia 427.89
chronic (sinus) 427.81
newborn 779.81

Bradycardia—*continued*
nodal 427.89
postoperative 997.1
reflex 337.0
sinoatrial 427.89
  with paroxysmal tachyarrhythmia or
    tachycardia 427.81
  chronic 427.81
sinus 427.89
  with paroxysmal tachyarrhythmia or
    tachycardia 427.81
  chronic 427.81
  persistent 427.81
  severe 427.81
tachycardia syndrome 427.81
vagal 427.89
Bradypnea 786.09
Brailsford's disease 732.3
radial head 732.3
tarsal scaphoid 732.5
Brailsford-Morquio disease or syndrome
  (mucopolysaccharidosis IV) 277.5
Brain —*see also* condition
death 348.8
syndrome (acute) (chronic) (nonpsychotic)
  (organic) (with neurotic reaction) (with
  behavioral reaction) (*see also* Syndrome,
  brain) 310.9
  with
    presenile brain disease 290.10
    psychosis, psychotic reaction (*see also*
      Psychosis, organic) 294.9
  congenital (*see also* Retardation, mental) 319
Branched-chain amino-acid disease 270.3
Branchial —*see* condition
Brandt's syndrome (acrodermatitis
  enteropathica) 686.8
Brash (water) 787.1
Brass-founders' ague 985.8
Bravais-Jacksonian epilepsy (*see also* Epilepsy)
  345.5
Braxton Hicks contractions 644.1
Braziers' disease 985.8
Brazilian
blastomycosis 116.1
leishmaniasis 085.5
Break
cardiorenal—*see* Hypertension, cardiorenal
retina (*see also* Defect, retina) 361.30
Breakbone fever 061
Breakdown
device, implant, or graft—*see* Complications,
  mechanical
nervous (*see also* Disorder, mental,
  nonpsychotic) 300.9
perineum 674.2
Breast —*see* condition
Breast feeding difficulties 676.8
Breath
foul 784.9
holder, child 312.81
holding spells 786.9
shortness 786.05
Breathing
asymmetrical 786.09
bronchial 786.09
exercises V57.0
labored 786.09
mouth 784.9
periodic 786.09
tic 307.20
Breathlessness 786.09

Breda's disease (*see also* Yaws) 102.9
Breech
delivery, affecting fetus or newborn 763.0
extraction, affecting fetus or newborn 763.0
presentation (buttocks) (complete) (frank) 652.2
  with successful version 652.1
  before labor, affecting fetus or newborn 761.7
  during labor, affecting fetus or newborn 763.0
Breisky's disease (kraurosis vulvae) 624.0
Brennemann's syndrome (acute mesenteric
  lymphadenitis) 289.2
Brenner's
tumor (benign) (M9000/0) 220
  borderline malignancy (M9000/1) 236.2
  malignant (M9000/3) 183.0
  proliferating (M9000/1) 236.2
Bretonneau's disease (diphtheritic malignant
  angina) 032.0
Breus' mole 631
Brevicollis 756.16
Bricklayers' itch 692.89
Brickmakers' anemia 126.9
Bridge
myocardial 746.85
Bright's
blindness—*see* Uremia
disease (*see also* Nephritis) 583.9
  arteriosclerotic (*see also* Hypertension,
    kidney) 403.90
Brill's disease (recrudescent typhus) 081.1
flea-borne 081.0
louse-borne 081.1
Brill-Symmers disease (follicular lymphoma)
  (M9690/3) 202.0
Brill-Zinsser disease (recrudescent typhus) 081.1
Brinton's disease (linitis plastica) (M8142/3)
  151.9
Brion-Kayser disease (*see also* Fever,
  paratyphoid) 002.9
Briquet's disorder or syndrome 300.81
Brissaud's
infantilism (infantile myxedema) 244.9
motor-verbal tic 307.23
Brissaud-Meige syndrome (infantile
  myxedema) 244.9
Brittle
bones (congenital) 756.51
nails 703.8
  congenital 757.5
Broad —*see also* condition
beta disease 272.2
ligament laceration syndrome 620.6
Brock's syndrome (atelectasis due to enlarged
  lymph nodes) 518.0
Brocq's disease 691.8
atopic (diffuse) neurodermatitis 691.8
lichen simplex chronicus 698.3
parakeratosis psoriasiformis 696.2
parapsoriasis 696.2
Brocq-Duhring disease (dermatitis
  herpetiformis) 694.0
Brodie's
abscess (localized) (chronic) (*see also*
  Osteomyelitis) 730.1
disease (joint) (*see also* Osteomyelitis) 730.1
Broken
arches 734
  congenital 755.67
back—*see* Fracture, vertebra, by site
bone—*see* Fracture, by site
compensation—*see* Disease, heart

Broken—*continued*
  implant or internal device—*see* listing under
    Complications, mechanical
  neck—*see* Fracture, vertebra, cervical
  nose 802.0
    open 802.1
  tooth, teeth 873.63
    complicated 873.73
Bromhidrosis 705.89
Bromidism, bromism
  acute 967.3
    correct substance properly administered
      349.82
    overdose or wrong substance given or taken
      967.3
  chronic (*see also* Dependence) 304.1
Bromidrosiphobia 300.23
Bromidrosis 705.89
Bronchi, bronchial —*see* condition
Bronchiectasis (cylindrical) (diffuse) (fusiform)
  (localized) (moniliform) (postinfectious)
  (recurrent) (saccular) 494.0
  with acute exacerbation 494.1
  congenital 748.61
  tuberculosis (*see also* Tuberculosis) 011.5
Bronchiolectasis —*see* Bronchiectasis
Bronchiolitis (acute) (infectious) (subacute)
  466.19
  with
    bronchospasm or obstruction 466.19
    influenza, flu, or grippe 487.1
  catarrhal (acute) (subacute) 466.19
  chemical 506.0
    chronic 506.4
  chronic (obliterative) 491.8
  due to external agent—*see* Bronchitis, acute,
    due to
  fibrosa obliterans 491.8
  influenzal 487.1
  obliterans 491.8
    status post lung transplant 996.84
    with organizing pneumonia (B.O.O.P.) 516.8
  obliterative (chronic) (diffuse) (subacute) 491.8
    due to fumes or vapors 506.4
  respiratory syncytial virus 466.11
  vesicular—*see* Pneumonia, broncho-
Bronchitis (diffuse) (hypostatic) (infectious)
  (inflammatory) (simple) 490
  with
    emphysema—*see* Emphysema
    influenza, flu, or grippe 487.1
    obstruction airway, chronic 491.20
      with acute exacerbation 491.21
    tracheitis 490
      acute or subacute 466.0
        with bronchospasm or obstruction 466.0
      chronic 491.8
  acute or subacute 466.0
    with
      bronchospasm 466.0
      chronic
        bronchitis (obstructive) 491.21
        obstructive pulmonary disease (COPD)
          491.21
      obstruction 466.0
      tracheitis 466.0
    chemical (due to fumes or vapors) 506.0
    due to
      fumes or vapors 506.0
      radiation 508.8
  allergic (acute) (*see also* Asthma) 493.9

Bronchitis—*continued*
  arachidic 934.1
  aspiration 507.0
    due to fumes or vapors 506.0
  asthmatic (acute) 493.90
    with
      acute exacerbation 493.92
      status asthmaticus 493.91
    chronic 493.2
  capillary 466.19
    with bronchospasm or obstruction 466.19
    chronic 491.8
  caseous (*see also* Tuberculosis) 011.3
  Castellani's 104.8
  catarrhal 490
    acute—*see* Bronchitis, acute
    chronic 491.0
  chemical (acute) (subacute) 506.0
    chronic 506.4
    due to fumes or vapors (acute) (subacute)
      506.0
      chronic 506.4
  chronic 491.9
    with
      tracheitis (chronic) 491.8
    asthmatic 493.2
    catarrhal 491.0
    chemical (due to fumes and vapors) 506.4
    due to
      fumes or vapors (chemical) (inhalation)
        506.4
      radiation 508.8
      tobacco smoking 491.0
    mucopurulent 491.1
    obstructive 491.20
      with acute bronchitis or acute exacerbation
        491.21
    purulent 491.1
    simple 491.0
    specified type NEC 491.8
  croupous 466.0
    with bronchospasm or obstruction 466.0
    due to fumes or vapors 506.0
  emphysematous 491.20
    with acute bronchitis or acute exacerbation
      491.21
  exudative 466.0
  fetid (chronic) (recurrent) 491.1
  fibrinous, acute or subacute 466.0
    with bronchospasm or obstruction 466.0
  grippal 487.1
  influenzal 487.1
  membranous, acute or subacute 466.0
    with bronchospasm or obstruction 466.0
  moulders' 502
  mucopurulent (chronic) (recurrent) 491.1
    acute or subacute 466.0
  non-obstructive 491.0
  obliterans 491.8
  obstructive (chronic) 491.20
    with acute bronchitis or acute exacerbation
      491.21
  pituitous 491.1
  plastic (inflammatory) 466.0
  pneumococcal, acute or subacute 466.0
    with bronchospasm or obstruction 466.0
  pseudomembranous 466.0

Bronchitis—*continued*
  purulent (chronic) (recurrent) 491.1
    acute or subacute 466.0
      with bronchospasm or obstruction 466.0
    putrid 491.1
    scrofulous (*see also* Tuberculosis) 011.3
    senile 491.9
    septic, acute or subacute 466.0
      with bronchospasm or obstruction 466.0
    smokers' 491.0
    spirochetal 104.8
    suffocative, acute or subacute 466.0
    summer (*see also* Asthma) 493.9
    suppurative (chronic) 491.1
      acute or subacute 466.0
    tuberculous (*see also* Tuberculosis) 011.3
    ulcerative 491.8
      Vincent's 101
    Vincent's 101
    viral, acute or subacute 466.0
      with bronchospasm or obstruction 466.0
Bronchoalveolitis 485
Bronchoaspergillosis 117.3
Bronchocele
  meaning
    dilatation of bronchus 519.1
    goiter 240.9
Bronchogenic carcinoma 162.9
Bronchohemisporosis 117.9
Broncholithiasis 518.89
  tuberculous (*see also* Tuberculosis) 011.3
Bronchomalacia 748.3
Bronchomoniliasis 112.89
Bronchomycosis 112.89
Bronchonocardiosis 039.1
Bronchopleuropneumonia —*see* Pneumonia, broncho-
Bronchopneumonia —*see* Pneumonia, broncho-
Bronchopneumonitis —*see* Pneumonia, broncho-
Bronchopulmonary —*see* condition
Bronchopulmonitis —*see* Pneumonia, broncho-
Bronchorrhagia 786.3
  newborn 770.3
  tuberculous (*see also* Tuberculosis) 011.3
Bronchorrhea (chronic) (purulent) 491.0
  acute 466.0
Bronchospasm 519.1
  with
    asthma—*see* Asthma
    bronchiolitis, acute 466.19
      due to respiratory syncytial virus 466.11
    bronchitis—*see* Bronchitis
    chronic obstructive pulmonary disease
      (COPD) 496
    emphysema—*see* Emphysema
      due to external agent—*see* Condition,
        respiratory, acture, due to
    due to external agent—*see* Condition,
      respiratory, acute, due to
Bronchospirochetosis 104.8
Bronchostenosis 519.1
Bronchus —*see* condition
Bronze, bronzed
  diabetes 275.0
  disease (Addison's) (skin) 255.4
    tuberculous (*see also* Tuberculosis) 017.6
Brooke's disease or tumor (M8100/0)—*see*
  Neoplasm, skin, benign
Brow presentation complicating delivery 652.4
Brown's tendon sheath syndrome 378.61
Brown enamel of teeth (hereditary) 520.5

Brown-Séquard's paralysis (syndrome) 344.89
Brucella, brucellosis (infection) 023.9
  abortus 023.1
  canis 023.3
  dermatitis, skin 023.9
  melitensis 023.0
  mixed 023.8
  suis 023.2
Bruck's disease 733.99
Bruck-de Lange disease or syndrome
  (Amsterdam dwarf, mental retardation, and
  brachycephaly) 759.89
Brugada syndrome 746.89
Brug's filariasis 125.1
Brugsch's syndrome (acropachyderma) 757.39
Bruhl's disease (splenic anemia with fever) 285.8
Bruise (skin surface intact)—*see also* Contusion
  with
    fracture—*see* Fracture, by site
    open wound—*see* Wound, open, by site
    internal organ (abdomen, chest, or pelvis)—*see*
      Injury, internal, by site
    umbilical cord 663.6
      affecting fetus or newborn 762.6
Bruit 785.9
  arterial (abdominal) (carotid) 785.9
  supraclavicular 785.9
Brushburn —*see* Injury, superficial, by site
Bruton's X-linked agammaglobulinemia 279.04
Bruxism 306.8
Bubbly lung syndrome 770.7
Bubo 289.3
  blennorrhagic 098.89
  chancroidal 099.0
  climatic 099.1
  due to Hemophilus ducreyi 099.0
  gonococcal 098.89
  indolent NEC 099.8
  inguinal NEC 099.8
    chancroidal 099.0
    climatic 099.1
    due to H. ducreyi 099.0
  scrofulous (*see also* Tuberculosis) 017.2
  soft chancre 099.0
  suppurating 683
  syphilitic 091.0
    congenital 090.0
  tropical 099.1
  venereal NEC 099.8
  virulent 099.0
Bubonic plague 020.0
Bubonocele —*see* Hernia, inguinal
Buccal —*see* condition
Buchanan's disease (juvenile osteochondrosis of
  iliac crest) 732.1
Buchem's syndrome (hyperostosis corticalis)
  733.3
Buchman's disease (osteochondrosis, juvenile)
  732.1
Bucket handle fracture (semilunar cartilage)
  (*see also* Tear, meniscus) 836.2
Budd-Chiari syndrome (hepatic vein
  thrombosis) 453.0
Budgerigar-fanciers' disease or lung 495.2
Büdinger-Ludloff-Läwen disease 717.89
Buerger's disease (thromboangiitis obliterans)
  443.1
Bulbar —*see* condition
Bulbus cordis 745.9
  persistent (in left ventricle) 745.8
Bulging fontanels (congenital) 756.0

Bulimia 783.6
  nonorganic origin 307.51
Bulky uterus 621.2
Bulla(e) 709.8
  lung (emphysematous) (solitary) 492.0
Bullet wound —*see also* Wound, open, by site
  fracture—*see* Fracture, by site, open
  internal organ (abdomen, chest, or pelvis)—*see*
    Injury, internal, by site, with open wound
  intracranial—*see* Laceration, brain, with open
    wound
Bullis fever 082.8
Bullying (*see also* Disturbance, conduct) 312.0
Bundle
  branch block (complete) (false) (incomplete)
    426.50
    bilateral 426.53
    left (*see also* Block, bundle branch, left) 426.3
      hemiblock 426.2
    right (*see also* Block, bundle branch, right)
      426.4
  of His—*see* condition
  of Kent syndrome (anomalous atrioventricular
    excitation) 426.7
Bungpagga 040.81
Bunion 727.1
Bunionette 727.1
Bunyamwera fever 066.3
Buphthalmia, buphthalmos (congenital) 743.20
  associated with
    keratoglobus, congenital 743.22
    megalocornea 743.22
    ocular anomalies NEC 743.22
  isolated 743.21
  simple 743.21
Bürger-Grütz disease or syndrome (essential
  familial hyperlipemia) 272.3
Buried roots 525.3
Burke's syndrome 577.8
Burkitt's
  tumor (M9750/3) 200.2
  type malignant, lymphoma, lymphoblastic, or
    undifferentiated (M9750/3) 200.2
Burn (acid) (cathode ray) (caustic) (chemical)
  (electric heating appliance) (electricity) (fire)
  (flame) (hot liquid or object) (irradiation)
  (lime) (radiation) (steam) (thermal) (x-ray)
  949.0

---

*Note—Use the following fifth-digit
subclassification with category 948 to indicate
the percent of body surface with third degree
burn:*

0 less than 10% or unspecified
1 10-19%
2 20-29%
3 30-39%
4 40-49%
5 50-59%
6 60-69%
7 70-79%
8 80-89%
9 90% or more of body surface

---

  with
    blisters—*see* Burn, by site, second degree
    erythema—*see* Burn, by site, first degree
    skin loss (epidermal)—*see also* Burn, by site,
      second degree
      full thickness—*see also* Burn, by site, third
        degree

Burn—*continued*
  with necrosis of underlying tissues—*see*
    Burn, by site, third degree, deep
  first degree—*see* Burn, by site, first degree
  second degree—*see* Burn, by site, second degree
  third degree—*see also* Burn, by site, third
    degree
    deep—*see* Burn, by site, third degree, deep
  abdomen, abdominal (muscle) (wall) 942.03
    with
      trunk—*see* Burn, trunk, multiple sites
    first degree 942.13
    second degree 942.23
    third degree 942.33
      deep 942.43
      with loss of body part 942.53
  ankle 945.03
    with
      lower limb(s)–*see* Burn, leg, multiple sites
    first degree 945.13
    second degree 945.23
    third degree 945.33
      deep 945.43
      with loss of body part 945.53
  anus—*see* Burn, trunk, specified site NEC
  arm(s) 943.00
    first degree 943.10
    second degree 943.20
    third degree 943.30
      deep 943.40
      with loss of body part 943.50
    lower—*see* Burn, forearm(s)
    multiple sites, except hand(s) or wrist(s)
      943.09
      first degree 943.19
      second degree 943.29
      third degree 943.39
        deep 943.49
        with loss of body part 943.59
    upper 943.03
      first degree 943.13
      second degree 943.23
      third degree 943.33
        deep 943.43
        with loss of body part 943.53
  auditory canal (external)—*see* Burn, ear
  auricle (ear)—*see* Burn, ear
  axilla 943.04
    with
      upper limb(s) except hand(s) or
        wrist(s)—*see* Burn, arm(s), multiple sites
    first degree 943.14
    second degree 943.24
    third degree 943.34
      deep 943.44
      with loss of body part 943.54
  back 942.04
    with
      trunk—*see* Burn, trunk, multiple sites
    first degree 942.14
    second degree 942.24
    third degree 942.34
      deep 942.44—
      with loss of body part 942.54
  biceps
    brachii—*see* Burn, arm(s), upper
    femoris—*see* Burn, thigh
  breast(s) 942.01
    with
      trunk—*see* Burn, trunk, multiple sites
    first degree 942.11

Burn—*continued*

second degree 942.21

third degree 942.31

deep 942.41

with loss of body part 942.51

brow—*see* Burn, forehead

buttock(s)—*see* Burn, back

canthus (eye) 940.1

chemical 940.0

cervix (uteri) 947.4

cheek (cutaneous) 941.07

with

face or head—*see* Burn, head, multiple sites

first degree 941.17

second degree 941.27

third degree 941.37

deep 941.47

with loss of body part 941.57

chest wall (anterior) 942.02

with

trunk—*see* Burn, trunk, multiple sites

first degree 942.12

second degree 942.22

third degree 942.32

deep 942.42

with loss of body part 942.52

chin 941.04

with

face or head—*see* Burn, head, multiple sites

first degree 941.14

second degree 941.24

third degree 941.34

deep 941.44

with loss of body part 941.54

clitoris—*see* Burn, genitourinary organs, external

colon 947.3

conjunctiva (and cornea) 940.4

chemical

acid 940.3

alkaline 940.2

cornea (and conjunctiva) 940.4

chemical

acid 940.3

alkaline 940.2

costal region—*see* Burn, chest wall

due to ingested chemical agent—*see* Burn, internal organs

ear (auricle) (canal) (drum) (external) 941.01

with

face or head—*see* Burn, head, multiple sites

first degree 941.11

second degree 941.21

third degree 941.31

deep 941.41

with loss of a body part 941.51

elbow 943.02

with

hand(s) and wrist(s)—*see* Burn, multiple specified sites

upper limb(s) except hand(s) or wrist(s)—*see also* Burn, arm(s), multiple sites

first degree 943.12

second degree 943.22

third degree 943.32

deep 943.42

with loss of body part 943.52

electricity, electric current—*see* Burn, by site

entire body—*see* Burn, multiple, specified sites

Burn—*continued*

epididymis—*see* Burn, genitourinary organs, external

epigastric region—*see* Burn, abdomen

epiglottis 947.1

esophagus 947.2

extent (percent of body surface)

less than 10 percent 948.0

10-19 percent 948.1

20-29 percent 948.2

30-39 percent 948.3

40-49 percent 948.4

50-59 percent 948.5

60-69 percent 948.6

70-79 percent 948.7

80-89 percent 948.8

90 percent or more 948.9

extremity

lower—*see* Burn, leg

upper—*see* Burn, arm(s)

eye(s) (and adnexa) (only) 940.9

with

face, head, or neck 941.02

first degree 941.12

second degree 941.22

third degree 941.32

deep 941.42

with loss of body part 941.52

other sites (classifiable to more than one category in 940-945)—*see* Burn, multiple, specified sites

resulting rupture and destruction of eyeball 940.5

specified part—*see* Burn, by site

eyeball—*see also* Burn, eye

with resulting rupture and destruction of eyeball 940.5

eyelid(s) 940.1

chemical 940.0

face—*see* Burn, head

finger (nail) (subungual) 944.01

with

hand(s)—*see* Burn, hand(s), multiple sites

other sites—*see* Burn, multiple, specified sites

thumb 944.04

first degree 944.14

second degree 944.24

third degree 944.34

deep 944.44

with loss of body part 944.54

first degree 944.11

second degree 944.21

third degree 944.31

deep 944.41

with loss of body part 944.51

multiple (digits) 944.03

with thumb—*see* Burn, finger, with thumb

first degree 944.13

second degree 944.23

third degree 944.33

deep 944.43

with loss of body part 944.53

flank—*see* Burn, abdomen

foot 945.02

with

lower limb(s)—*see* Burn, leg, multiple sites

first degree 945.12

second degree 945.22

third degree 945.32

deep 945.42

Burn—*continued*
  with loss of body part 945.52
 forearm(s) 943.01
  with
   upper limb(s) except hand(s) or
    wrist(s)—*see* Burn, arm(s), multiple sites
  first degree 943.11
  second degree 943.21
  third degree 943.31
   deep 943.41
    with loss of body part 943.51
 forehead 941.07
  with
   face or head—*see* Burn, head, multiple sites
  first degree 941.17
  second degree 941.27
  third degree 941.37
   deep 941.47
    with loss of body part 941.57
 fourth degree—*see* Burn, by site, third degree,
  deep
 friction—*see* Injury, superficial, by site
 from swallowing caustic or corrosive substance
  NEC—*see* Burn, internal organs
 full thickness—*see* Burn, by site, third degree
 gastrointestinal tract 947.3
 genitourinary organs
  external 942.05
   with
    trunk—*see* Burn, trunk, multiple sites
   first degree 942.15
   second degree 942.25
   third degree 942.35
    deep 942.45
     with loss of body part 942.55
  internal 947.8
 globe (eye)—*see* Burn, eyeball
 groin—*see* Burn, abdomen
 gum 947.0
 hand(s) (phalanges) (and wrist) 944.00
  first degree 944.10
  second degree 944.20
  third degree 944.30
   deep 944.40
    with loss of body part 944.50
  back (dorsal surface) 944.06
   first degree 944.16
   second degree 944.26
   third degree 944.36
    deep 944.46
     with loss of body part 944.56
  multiple sites 944.08
   first degree 944.18
   second degree 944.28
   third degree 944.38
    deep 944.48
     with loss of body part 944.58
 head (and face) 941.00
  eye(s) only 940.9
   specified part—*see* Burn, by site
  first degree 941.10
  second degree 941.20
  third degree 941.30
   deep 941.40
    with loss of body part 941.50
  multiple sites 941.09
   with eyes—*see* Burn, eyes, with face, head,
    or neck
   first degree 941.19
   second degree 941.29
   third degree 941.39

Burn—*continued*
  deep 941.49
   with loss of body part 941.59
 heel—*see* Burn, foot
 hip—*see* Burn, trunk, specified site NEC
 iliac region—*see* Burn, trunk, specified site NEC
 infected 958.3
 inhalation (*see also* Burn, internal organs) 947.9
 internal organs 947.9
  from caustic or corrosive substance
   (swallowing) NEC 947.9
  specified NEC (*see also* Burn, by site) 947.8
 interscapular region—*see* Burn, back
 intestine (large) (small) 947.3
 iris—*see* Burn, eyeball
 knee 945.05
  with
   lower limb(s)—*see* Burn, leg, multiple sites
  first degree 945.15
  second degree 945.25
  third degree 945.35
   deep 945.45
    with loss of body part 945.55
 labium (majus) (minus)—*see* Burn,
  genitourinary organs, external
 lacrimal apparatus, duct, gland, or sac 940.1
  chemical 940.0
 larynx 947.1
 late effect—*see* Late, effects (of), burn
 leg 945.00
  first degree 945.10
  second degree 945.20
  third degree 945.30
   deep 945.40
    with loss of body part 945.50
  lower 945.04
   with other part(s) of lower limb(s)—*see*
    Burn, leg, multiple sites
   first degree 945.14
   second degree 945.24
   third degree 945.34
    deep 945.44
     with loss of body part 945.54
  multiple sites 945.09
   first degree 945.19
   second degree 945.29
   third degree 945.39
    deep 945.49
     with loss of body part 945.59
  upper—*see* Burn, thigh
 lightning—*see* Burn, by site
 limb(s)
  lower (including foot or toe(s))—*see* Burn, leg
  upper (except wrist and hand)—*see* Burn,
   arm(s)
 lip(s) 941.03
  with
   face or head—*see* Burn, head, multiple sites
  first degree 941.13
  second degree 941.23
  third degree 941.33
   deep 941.43
    with loss of body part 941.53
 lumbar region—*see* Burn, back
 lung 947.1
 malar region—*see* Burn, cheek
 mastoid region—*see* Burn, scalp
 membrane, tympanic—*see* Burn, ear
 midthoracic region—*see* Burn, chest wall
 mouth 947.0

Burn—*continued*
  trachea 947.1
  trunk 942.00
    first degree 942.10
    second degree 942.20
    third degree 942.30
      deep 942.40
        with loss of body part 942.50
    multiple sites 942.09
      first degree 942.19
      second degree 942.29
      third degree 942.39
        deep 942.49
          with loss of body part 942.59
    specified site NEC 942.09
      first degree 942.19
      second degree 942.29
      third degree 942.39
        deep 942.49
          with loss of body part 942.59
  tunica vaginalis—*see* Burn, genitourinary
    organs, external
  tympanic membrane—*see* Burn, ear
  tympanum—*see* Burn, ear
  ultraviolet 692.82
  unspecified site (multiple) 949.0
    with extent of body surface involved specified
      less than 10 percent 948.0
      10-19 percent 948.1
      20-29 percent 948.2
      30-39 percent 948.3
      40-49 percent 948.4
      50-59 percent 948.5
      60-69 percent 948.6
      70-79 percent 948.7
      80-89 percent 948.8
      90 percent or more 948.9
    first degree 949.1
    second degree 949.2
    third degree 949.3
      deep 949.4
        with loss of body part 949.5
  uterus 947.4
  uvula 947.0
  vagina 947.4
  vulva—*see* Burn, genitourinary organs, external
  wrist(s) 944.07
    with
      hand(s)—*see* Burn, hand(s), multiple sites
    first degree 944.17
    second degree 944.27
    third degree 944.37
      deep 944.47
        with loss of body part 944.57
Burnett's syndrome (milk-alkali) 999.9
Burnier's syndrome (hypophyseal dwarfism)
  253.3
Burning
  feet syndrome 266.2
  sensation (*see also* Disturbance, sensation) 782.0
  tongue 529.6
Burns' disease (osteochondrosis, lower ulna)
  732.3
Bursa —*see also* condition
  pharynx 478.29
Bursitis NEC 727.3
  Achilles tendon 726.71
  adhesive 726.90
    shoulder 726.0
  ankle 726.79
  buttock 726.5

Bursitis—*continued*
  calcaneal 726.79
  collateral ligament
    fibular 726.63
    tibial 726.62
  Duplay's 726.2
  elbow 726.33
  finger 726.8
  foot 726.79
  gonococcal 098.52
  hand 726.4
  hip 726.5
  infrapatellar 726.69
  ischiogluteal 726.5
  knee 726.60
  occupational NEC 727.2
  olecranon 726.33
  pes anserinus 726.61
  pharyngeal 478.29
  popliteal 727.51
  prepatellar 726.65
  radiohumeral 727.3
  scapulohumeral 726.19
    adhesive 726.0
  shoulder 726.10
    adhesive 726.0
  subacromial 726.19
    adhesive 726.0
  subcoracoid 726.19
  subdeltoid 726.19
    adhesive 726.0
  subpatellar 726.69
  syphilitic 095.7
  Thornwaldt's, Tornwaldt's (pharyngeal) 478.29
  toe 726.79
  trochanteric area 726.5
  wrist 726.4
Burst stitches or sutures (complication of
  surgery) (external) 998.32
  internal 998.31
Buruli ulcer 031.1
Bury's disease (erythema elevatum diutinum)
  695.89
Buschke's disease or scleredema (adultorum)
  710.1
Busquet's disease (osteoperiostitis) (*see also*
  Osteomyelitis) 730.1
Busse-Buschke disease (cryptococcosis) 117.5
Buttock —*see* condition
Button
  Biskra 085.1
  Delhi 085.1
  oriental 085.1
Buttonhole hand (intrinsic) 736.21
Bwamba fever (encephalitis) 066.3
Byssinosis (occupational) 504
Bywaters' syndrome 958.5

C

Cacergasia 300.9
Cachexia 799.4
  cancerous (M8000/3) 199.1
  cardiac—*see* Disease, heart
  dehydration 276.5
    with
      hypernatremia 276.0
      hyponatremia 276.1
  due to malnutrition 261
  exophthalmic 242.0
  heart—*see* Disease, heart
  hypophyseal 253.2
  hypopituitary 253.2
  lead 984.9
    specified type of lead—*see* Table of drugs and
      chemicals
  malaria 084.9
  malignant (M8000/3) 199.1
  marsh 084.9
  nervous 300.5
  old age 797
  pachydermic—*see* Hypothyroidism
  paludal 084.9
  pituitary (postpartum) 253.2
  renal (*see also* Disease, renal) 593.9
  saturnine 984.9
    specified type of lead—*see* Table of drugs and
      chemicals
  senile 797
  Simmonds' (pituitary cachexia) 253.2
  splenica 289.59
  strumipriva (*see also* Hypothyroidism) 244.9
  tuberculous NEC (*see also* Tuberculosis) 011.9
café au lait spots 709.09
Caffey's disease or syndrome (infantile cortical
  hyperostosis) 756.59
Caisson disease 993.3
Caked breast (puerperal, postpartum) 676.2
Cake kidney 753.3
Calabar swelling 125.2
Calcaneal spur 726.73
Calcaneoapophysitis 732.5
Calcaneonavicular bar 755.67
Calcareous —*see* condition
Calcicosis (occupational) 502
Calciferol (vitamin D) deficiency 268.9
  with
    osteomalacia 268.2
    rickets (*see also* Rickets) 268.0
Calcification
  adrenal (capsule) (gland) 255.4
    tuberculous (*see also* Tuberculosis) 017.6
  aorta 440.0
  artery (annular)—*see* Arteriosclerosis
  auricle (ear) 380.89
  bladder 596.8
    due to S. hematobium 120.0
  brain (cortex)—*see* Calcification, cerebral
  bronchus 519.1
  bursa 727.82
  cardiac (*see also* Degeneration, myocardial)
    429.1
  cartilage (postinfectional) 733.99
  cerebral (cortex) 348.8
    artery 437.0
  cervix (uteri) 622.8
  choroid plexus 349.2
  conjunctiva 372.54

Calcification—*continued*
  corpora cavernosa (penis) 607.89
  cortex (brain)—*see* Calcification, cerebral
  dental pulp (nodular) 522.2
  dentinal papilla 520.4
  disc, intervertebral 722.90
    cervical, cervicothoracic 722.91
    lumbar, lumbosacral 722.93
    thoracic, thoracolumbar 722.92
  fallopian tube 620.8
  falx cerebri—*see* Calcification, cerebral
  fascia 728.89
  gallbladder 575.8
  general 275.40
  heart (*see also* Degeneration, myocardial) 429.1
    valve—*see* Endocarditis
  intervertebral cartilage or disc (postinfectional)
    722.90
    cervical, cervicothoracic 722.91
    lumbar, lumbosacral 722.93
    thoracic, thoracolumbar 722.92
  intracranial—*see* Calcification, cerebral
  intraspinal ligament 728.89
  joint 719.80
    ankle 719.87
    elbow 719.82
    foot 719.87
    hand 719.84
    hip 719.85
    knee 719.86
    multiple sites 719.89
    pelvic region 719.85
    shoulder (region) 719.81
    specified site NEC 719.88
    wrist 719.83
  kidney 593.89
    tuberculous (*see also* Tuberculosis) 016.0
  larynx (senile) 478.79
  lens 366.8
  ligament 728.89
    intraspinal 728.89
    knee (medial collateral) 717.89
  lung 518.89
    active 518.89
    postinfectional 518.89
    tuberculous (*see also* Tuberculosis,
      pulmonary) 011.9
  lymph gland or node (postinfectional) 289.3
    tuberculous (*see also* Tuberculosis, lymph
      gland) 017.2
  massive (paraplegic) 728.10
  medial NEC (*see also* Arteriosclerosis,
    extremities) 440.20
  meninges (cerebral) 349.2
  metastatic 275.40
  Mönckeberg's—*see* Arteriosclerosis
  muscle 728.10
    heterotopic, postoperative 728.13
  myocardium, myocardial (*see also*
    Degeneration, myocardial) 429.1
  ovary 620.8
  pancreas 577.8
  penis 607.99
  periarticular 728.89
  pericardium (*see also* Pericarditis) 423.8
  pineal gland 259.8
  pleura 511.0
    postinfectional 518.89

Note—The term "cancer" when modified by an
adjective or adjectival phrase indicating a
morphological type should be coded in the same
manner as "carcinoma" with that adjective or
phrase. Thus, "squamous-cell cancer" should
be coded in the same manner as
"squamous-cell carcinoma," which appears in
the list under "Carcinoma."

Candidiasis, candidal 112.9
  with pneumonia 112.4
  balanitis 112.2
  congenital 771.7
  disseminated 112.5
  endocarditis 112.81
  esophagus 112.84
  intertrigo 112.3
  intestine 112.85
  lung 112.4
  meningitis 112.83
  mouth 112.0
  nails 112.3
  neonatal 771.7
  onychia 112.3
  otitis externa 112.82
  otomycosis 112.82
  paronychia 112.3
  perionyxis 112.3
  pneumonia 112.4
  pneumonitis 112.4
  skin 112.3
  specified site NEC 112.89
  systemic 112.5
  urogenital site NEC 112.2
  vagina 112.1
  vulva 112.1
  vulvovaginitis 112.1
Candidiosis —*see* Candidiasis
Candiru infection or infestation 136.8
Canities (premature) 704.3
  congenital 757.4
Canker (mouth) (sore) 528.2
  rash 034.1
Cannabinosis 504
Canton fever 081.9
Cap
  cradle 690.11
Capillariasis 127.5
Capillary —*see* condition
Caplan's syndrome 714.81
Caplan-Colinet syndrome 714.81
Capsule —*see* condition
Capsulitis (joint) 726.90
  adhesive (shoulder) 726.0
  hip 726.5
  knee 726.60
  labyrinthine 387.8
  thyroid 245.9
  wrist 726.4
Caput
  crepitus 756.0
  medusae 456.8
  succedaneum 767.1
Carapata disease 087.1
Carate —*see* Pinta
Carboxyhemoglobinemia 986
Carbuncle 680.9
  abdominal wall 680.2
  ankle 680.6
  anus 680.5
  arm (any part, above wrist) 680.3
  auditory canal, external 680.0
  axilla 680.3
  back (any part) 680.2
  breast 680.2
  buttock 680.5
  chest wall 680.2
  corpus cavernosum 607.2
  ear (any part) (external) 680.0
  eyelid 373.13

Carbuncle—*continued*
  face (any part, except eye) 680.0
  finger (any) 680.4
  flank 680.2
  foot (any part) 680.7
  forearm 680.3
  genital organ (male) 608.4
  gluteal (region) 680.5
  groin 680.2
  hand (any part) 680.4
  head (any part, except face) 680.8
  heel 680.7
  hip 680.6
  kidney (*see also* Abscess, kidney) 590.2
  knee 680.6
  labia 616.4
  lacrimal
    gland (*see also* Dacryoadenitis) 375.00
    passages (duct) (sac) (*see also* Dacryocystitis) 375.30
  leg, any part except foot 680.6
  lower extremity, any part except foot 680.6
  malignant 022.0
  multiple sites 680.9
  neck 680.1
  nose (external) (septum) 680.0
  orbit, orbital 376.01
  partes posteriores 680.5
  pectoral region 680.2
  penis 607.2
  perineum 680.2
  pinna 680.0
  scalp (any part) 680.8
  scrotum 608.4
  seminal vesicle 608.0
  shoulder 680.3
  skin NEC 680.9
  specified site NEC 680.8
  spermatic cord 608.4
  temple (region) 680.0
  testis 608.4
  thigh 680.6
  thumb 680.4
  toe (any) 680.7
  trunk 680.2
  tunica vaginalis 608.4
  umbilicus 680.2
  upper arm 680.3
  urethra 597.0
  vas deferens 608.4
  vulva 616.4
  wrist 680.4
Carbunculus (*see also* Carbuncle) 680.9
Carcinoid (tumor) (M8240/1)—*see also*
  Neoplasm, by site, uncertain behavior
  and struma ovarii (M9091/1) 236.2
  argentaffin (M8241/1)—*see* Neoplasm, by site,
    uncertain behavior
    malignant (M8241/3)—*see* Neoplasm, by site,
      malignant
  benign (M9091/0) 220
  composite (M8244/3)—*see* Neoplasm, by site,
    malignant
  goblet cell (M8243/3)—*see* Neoplasm, by site,
    malignant
  malignant (M8240/3)—*see* Neoplasm, by site,
    malignant
  nonargentaffin (M8242/1)—*see also* Neoplasm,
    by site, uncertain behavior
    malignant (M8242/3)—*see* Neoplasm, by site,
      malignant

Carcinoid—*continued*
  strumal (M9091/1) 236.2
  syndrome (intestinal) (metastatic) 259.2
  type bronchial adenoma (M8240/3)—*see*
    Neoplasm, lung, malignant
Carcinoidosis 259.2
Carcinoma (M8010/3)—*see also* Neoplasm, by
  site, malignant

> *Note—Except where otherwise indicated, the*
> *morphological varieties of carcinoma in the list*
> *below should be coded by site as for*
> *"Neoplasm, malignant."*

  with
    apocrine metaplasia (M8573/3)
    cartilaginous (and osseous) metaplasia
      (M8571/3)
    osseous (and cartilaginous) metaplasia
      (M8571/3)
    productive fibrosis (M8141/3)
    spindle cell metaplasia (M8572/3)
    squamous metaplasia (M8570/3)
  acidophil (M8280/3)
    specified site—*see* Neoplasm, by site,
      malignant
    unspecified site 194.3
  acidophil-basophil, mixed (M8281/3)
    specified site—*see* Neoplasm, by site,
      malignant
    unspecified site 194.3
  acinar (cell) (M8550/3)
  acinic cell (M8550/3)
  adenocystic (M8200/3)
  adenoid
    cystic (M8200/3)
    squamous cell (M8075/3)
  adenosquamous (M8560/3)
  adnexal (skin) (M8390/3)—*see* Neoplasm, skin,
    malignant
  adrenal cortical (M8370/3) 194.0
  alveolar (M8251/3)
    cell (M8250/3)—*see* Neoplasm, lung,
      malignant
  anaplastic type (M8021/3)
  apocrine (M8401/3)
    breast—*see* Neoplasm, breast, malignant
    specified site NEC—*see* Neoplasm, skin,
      malignant
    unspecified site 173.9
  basal cell (pigmented) (M8090/3)—*see also*
    Neoplasm, skin, malignant
    fibro-epithelial type (M8093/3)—*see*
      Neoplasm, skin, malignant
    morphea type (M8092/3)—*see* Neoplasm,
      skin, malignant
    multicentric (M8091/3)—*see* Neoplasm, skin,
      malignant
  basaloid (M8123/3)
  basal-squamous cell, mixed (M8094/3)—*see*
    Neoplasm, skin, malignant
  basophil (M8300/3)
    specified site—*see* Neoplasm, by site,
      malignant
    unspecified site 194.3
  basophil-acidophil, mixed (M8281/3)
    specified site—*see* Neoplasm, by site,
      malignant
    unspecified site 194.3
  basosquamous (M8094/3)—*see* Neoplasm,
    skin, malignant

Carcinoma—*continued*
  bile duct type (M8160/3)
    and hepatocellular, mixed (M8180/3) 155.0
    liver 155.1
    specified site NEC—*see* Neoplasm, by site,
      malignant
    unspecified site 155.1
  branchial or branchiogenic 146.8
  bronchial or bronchogenic—*see* Neoplasm,
    lung, malignant
  bronchiolar (terminal) (M8250/3)—*see*
    Neoplasm, lung, malignant
  bronchiolo-alveolar (M8250/3)—*see* Neoplasm,
    lung, malignant
  bronchogenic (epidermoid) 162.9
  C cell (M8510/3)
    specified site—*see* Neoplasm, by site,
      malignant
    unspecified site 193
  ceruminous (M8420/3) 173.2
  chorionic (M9100/3)
    specified site—*see* Neoplasm, by site,
      malignant
    unspecified site
      female 181
      male 186.9
  chromophobe (M8270/3)
    specified site—*see* Neoplasm, by site,
      malignant
    unspecified site 194.3
  clear cell (mesonephroid type) (M8310/3)
  cloacogenic (M8124/3)
    specified site—*see* Neoplasm, by site,
      malignant
    unspecified site 154.8
  colloid (M8480/3)
  cribriform (M8201/3)
  cylindroid type (M8200/3)
  diffuse type (M8145/3)
    specified site—*see* Neoplasm, by site,
      malignant
    unspecified site 151.9
  duct (cell) (M8500/3)
    with Paget's disease (M8541/3)—*see*
      Neoplasm, breast, malignant
    infiltrating (M8500/3)
      specified site—*see* Neoplasm, by site,
        malignant
      unspecified site 174.9
  ductal (M8500/3)
  ductular, infiltrating (M8521/3)
  embryonal (M9070/3)
    and teratoma, mixed (M9081/3)
    combined with choriocarcinoma
      (M9101/3)—*see* Neoplasm, by site,
        malignant
    infantile type (M9071/3)
    liver 155.0
    polyembryonal type (M9072/3)
  endometrioid (M8380/3)
  eosinophil (M8280/3)
    specified site—*see* Neoplasm, by site,
      malignant
    unspecified site 194.3
  epidermoid (M8070/3)—*see also* Carcinoma,
    squamous cell
    and adenocarcinoma, mixed (M8560/3)
    in situ, Bowen's type (M8081/2)—*see*
      Neoplasm, skin, in situ
    intradermal—*see* Neoplasm, skin, in situ

Carcinoma—*continued*
  fibroepithelial type basal cell (M8093/3)—*see*
    Neoplasm, skin, malignant
  follicular (M8330/3)
    and papillary (mixed) (M8340/3) 193
    moderately differentiated type (M8332/3) 193
    pure follicle type (M8331/3) 193
    specified site—*see* Neoplasm, by site,
      malignant
    trabecular type (M8332/3) 193
    unspecified site 193
    well differentiated type (M8331/3) 193
  gelatinous (M8480/3)
  giant cell (M8031/3)
    and spindle cell (M8030/3)
  granular cell (M8320/3)
  granulosa cell (M8620/3) 183.0
  hepatic cell (M8170/3) 155.0
  hepatocellular (M8170/3) 155.0
    and bile duct, mixed (M8180/3)
      155.0
  hepatocholangiolitic (M8180/3) 155.0
  Hurthle cell (thyroid) 193
  hypernephroid (M8311/3)
  in
    adenomatous
      polyp (M8210/3)
      polyposis coli (M8220/3) 153.9
    pleomorphic adenoma (M8940/3)
    polypoid adenoma (M8210/3)
    situ (M8010/3)—*see* Carcinoma,
      in situ
    tubular adenoma (M8210/3)
    villous adenoma (M8261/3)
  infiltrating duct (M8500/3)
    with Paget's disease (M8541/3)—*see*
      Neoplasm, breast, malignant
    specified site—*see* Neoplasm, by site,
      malignant
    unspecified site 174.9
  inflammatory (M8530/3)
    specified site—*see* Neoplasm, by site,
      malignant
    unspecified site 174.9
  in situ (M8010/2)—*see also* Neoplasm, by site,
    in situ
    epidermoid (M8070/2)—*see also* Neoplasm,
      by site, in situ
      with questionable stromal invasion
        (M8076/2)
        specified site—*see* Neoplasm, by site, in
          situ
        unspecified site 233.1
      Bowen's type (M8081/2)—*see* Neoplasm,
        skin, in situ
    intraductal (M8500/2)
      specified site—*see* Neoplasm, by site, in situ
      unspecified site 233.0
    lobular (M8520/2)
      specified site—*see* Neoplasm, by site, in situ
      unspecified site 233.0
    papillary (M8050/2)—*see* Neoplasm, by site,
      in situ
    squamous cell (M8070/2)—*see also*
      Neoplasm, by site, in situ
    with questionable stromal invasion (M8076/2)
      specified site—*see* Neoplasm, by site, in
        situ
      unspecified site 233.1
    transitional cell (M8120/2)—*see* Neoplasm,
      by site, in situ

Carcinoma—*continued*
  intestinal type (M8144/3)
    specified site—*see* Neoplasm, by site,
      malignant
    unspecified site 151.9
  intraductal (noninfiltrating) (M8500/2)
    papillary (M8503/2)
      specified site—*see* Neoplasm, by site, in situ
      unspecified site 233.0
    specified site—*see* Neoplasm, by site, in situ
    unspecified site 233.0
  intraepidermal (M8070/2)—*see also* Neoplasm,
    skin, in situ
    squamous cell, Bowen's type (M8081/2)—*see*
      Neoplasm, skin, in situ
  intraepithelial (M8010/2)—*see also* Neoplasm,
    by site, in situ
    squamous cell (M8072/2)—*see* Neoplasm, by
      site, in situ
  intraosseous (M9270/3) 170.1
    upper jaw (bone) 170.0
  islet cell (M8150/3)
    and exocrine, mixed (M8154/3)
      specified site—*see* Neoplasm, by site,
        malignant
      unspecified site 157.9
    pancreas 157.4
    specified site NEC—*see* Neoplasm, by site,
      malignant
    unspecified site 157.4
  juvenile, breast (M8502/3)—*see* Neoplasm,
    breast, malignant
  Kulchitsky's cell (carcinoid tumor of intestine)
    259.2
  large cell (M8012/3)
    squamous cell, nonkeratinizing type
      (M8072/3)
  Leydig cell (testis) (M8650/3)
    specified site—*see* Neoplasm, by site,
      malignant
    unspecified site 186.9
      female 183.0
      male 186.9
  liver cell (M8170/3) 155.0
  lobular (infiltrating) (M8520/3)
    non-infiltrating (M8520/3)
      specified site—*see* Neoplasm, by site, in situ
      unspecified site 233.0
    specified site—*see* Neoplasm, by site,
      malignant
    unspecified site 174.9
  lymphoepithelial (M8082/3)
  medullary (M8510/3)
    with
      amyloid stroma (M8511/3)
        specified site—*see* Neoplasm, by site,
          malignant
        unspecified site 193
      lymphoid stroma (M8512/3)
        specified site—*see* Neoplasm, by site,
          malignant
        unspecified site 174.9
  mesometanephric (M9110/3)
  mesonephric (M9110/3)
  metastatic (M8010/6)—*see* Metastasis, cancer
  metatypical (M8095/3)—*see* Neoplasm, skin,
    malignant
  morphea type basal cell (M8092/3)—*see*
    Neoplasm, skin, malignant
  mucinous (M8480/3)
  mucin-producing (M8481/3)

Carcinoma—*continued*
mucin-secreting (M8481/3)
mucoepidermoid (M8430/3)
mucoid (M8480/3)
  cell (M8300/3)
    specified site—*see* Neoplasm, by site,
      malignant
    unspecified site 194.3
mucous (M8480/3)
nonencapsulated sclerosing (M8350/3) 193
noninfiltrating
  intracystic (M8504/2)—*see* Neoplasm, by
    site, in situ
  intraductal (M8500/2)
    papillary (M8503/2)
      specified site—*see* Neoplasm, by site, in
        situ
      unspecified site 233.0
    specified site—*see* Neoplasm, by site, in situ
    unspecified site 233.0
  lobular (M8520/2)
    specified site—*see* Neoplasm, by site, in situ
    unspecified site 233.0
oat cell (M8042/3)
  specified site—*see* Neoplasm, by site,
    malignant
  unspecified site 162.9
odontogenic (M9270/3) 170.1
  upper jaw (bone) 170.0
onocytic (M8290/3)
oxyphilic (M8290/3)
papillary (M8050/3)
  and follicular (mixed) (M8340/3) 193
  epidermoid (M8052/3)
  intraductal (noninfiltrating) (M8503/2)
    specified site—*see* Neoplasm, by site, in situ
    unspecified site 233.0
  serous (M8460/3)
    specified site—*see* Neoplasm, by site,
      malignant
    surface (M8461/3)
      specified site—*see* Neoplasm, by site,
        malignant
        unspecified site 183.0
    unspecified site 183.0
  squamous cell (M8052/3)
  transitional cell (M8130/3)
papillocystic (M8450/3)
  specified site—*see* Neoplasm, by site,
    malignant
  unspecified site 183.0
parafollicular cell (M8510/3)
  specified site—*see* Neoplasm, by site,
    malignant
  unspecified site 193
pleomorphic (M8022/3)
polygonal cell (M8034/3)
prickle cell (M8070/3)
pseudoglandular, squamous cell (M8075/3)
pseudomucinous (M8470/3)
  specified site—*see* Neoplasm, by site,
    malignant
  unspecified site 183.0
pseudosarcomatous (M8033/3)
regaud type (M8082/3)—*see* Neoplasm,
  nasopharynx, malignant
renal cell (M8312/3) 189.0
reserve cell (M8041/3)
round cell (M8041/3)
Schmincke (M8082/3)—*see* Neoplasm,
  nasopharynx, malignant

Carcinoma—*continued*
Schneiderian (M8121/3)
  specified site—*see* Neoplasm, by site,
    malignant
  unspecified site 160.0
scirrhous (M8141/3)
sebaceous (M8410/3)—*see* Neoplasm, skin,
  malignant
secondary (M8010/6)—*see* Neoplasm, by site,
  malignant, secondary
secretory, breast (M8502/3)—*see* Neoplasm,
  breast, malignant
serous (M8441/3)
  papillary (M8460/3)
    specified site—*see* Neoplasm, by site,
      malignant
    unspecified site 183.0
  surface, papillary (M8461/3)
    specified site—*see* Neoplasm, by site,
      malignant
    unspecified site 183.0
Sertoli cell (M8640/3)
  specified site—*see* Neoplasm, by site,
    malignant
  unspecified site 186.9
signet ring cell (M8490/3)
  metastatic (M8490/6)—*see* Neoplasm, by site,
    secondary
simplex (M8231/3)
skin appendage (M8390/3)—*see* Neoplasm,
  skin, malignant
small cell (M8041/3)
  fusiform cell type (M8043/3)
  squamous cell, non-keratinizing type
    (M8073/3)
solid (M8230/3)
  with amyloid stroma (M8511/3)
    specified site—*see* Neoplasm, by site,
      malignant
    unspecified site 193
spheroidal cell (M8035/3)
spindle cell (M8032/3)
  and giant cell (M8030/3)
spinous cell (M8070/3)
squamous (cell) (M8070/3)
  adenoid type (M8075/3)
  and adenocarcinoma, mixed (M8560/3)
  intraepidermal, Bowen's type—*see*
    Neoplasm, skin, in situ
  keratinizing type (large cell) (M8071/3)
  large cell, non-keratinizing type (M8072/3)
  microinvasive (M8076/3)
    specified site—*see* Neoplasm, by site,
      malignant
    unspecified site 180.9
  non-keratinizing type (M8072/3)
  papillary (M8052/3)
  pseudoglandular (M8075/3)
  small cell, non-keratinizing type (M8073/3)
  spindle cell type (M8074/3)
  verrucous (M8051/3)
superficial spreading (M8143/3)
sweat gland (M8400/3)—*see* Neoplasm, skin,
  malignant
theca cell (M8600/3) 183.0
thymic (M8580/3) 164.0
trabecular (M8190/3)
transitional (cell) (M8120/3)
  papillary (M8130/3)
  spindle cell type (M8122/3)

Carcinoma—*continued*
  tubular (M8211/3)
  undifferentiated type (M8020/3)
  urothelial (M8120/3)
  ventriculi 151.9
  verrucous (epidermoid) (squamous cell)
    (M8051/3)
  villous (M8262/3)
  water-clear cell (M8322/3) 194.1
  wolffian duct (M9110/3)
Carcinomaphobia 300.29
Carcinomatosis
  peritonei (M8010/6) 197.6
  specified site NEC (M8010/3)—*see* Neoplasm,
    by site, malignant
  unspecified site (M8010/6) 199.0
Carcinosarcoma (M8980/3)—*see also*
  Neoplasm, by site, malignant
  embryonal type (M8981/3)—*see* Neoplasm, by
    site, malignant
Cardia, cardial —*see* condition
Cardiac —*see also* condition
  death—*see* Disease, heart
  device
    defibrillator, automatic implantable V45.02
    in situ NEC V45.00
    pacemaker
      cardiac
        fitting or adjustment V53.3
        in situ V45.01
      carotid sinus
        fitting or adjustment V53.3
        in situ V45.09
  pacemaker—*see* Cardiac, device, pacemaker
  tamponade 423.9
Cardialgia (*see also* Pain, precordial) 786.51
Cardiectasis —*see* Hypertrophy, cardiac
Cardiochalasia 530.81
Cardiomalacia (*see also* Degeneration,
  myocardial) 429.1
Cardiomegalia glycogenica diffusa 271.0
Cardiomegaly (*see also* Hypertrophy, cardiac)
  429.3
  congenital 746.89
  glycogen 271.0
  hypertensive (*see also* Hypertension, heart)
    402.90
  idiopathic 429.3
Cardiomyoliposis (*see also* Degeneration,
  myocardial) 429.1
Cardiomyopathy (congestive) (constrictive)
  (familial) (infiltrative) (obstructive)
  (restrictive) (sporadic) 425.4
  alcoholic 425.5
  amyloid 277.3 *[425.7]*
  beriberi 265.0 *[425.7]*
  cobalt-beer 425.5
  congenital 425.3
  due to
    amyloidosis 277.3 *[425.7]*
    beriberi 265.0 *[425.7]*
    cardiac glycogenesis 271.0 *[425.7]*
    Chagas' disease 086.0
    Friedreich's ataxia 334.0 *[425.8]*
    mucopolysaccharidosis 277.5 *[425.7]*
    myotonia atrophica 359.2 *[425.8]*
    progressive muscular dystrophy 359.1 *[425.8]*
    sarcoidosis 135 *[425.8]*

Cardiomyopathy—*continued*
  glycogen storage 271.0 *[425.7]*
  hypertensive—*see* Hypertension, with, heart
    involvement
  hypertrophic
    nonobstructive 425.4
    obstructive 425.1
      congenital 746.84
  idiopathic (concentric) 425.4
  in
    Chagas' disease 086.0
    sarcoidosis 135 *[425.8]*
  ischemic 414.8
  metabolic NEC 277.9 *[425.7]*
    amyloid 277.3 *[425.7]*
    thyrotoxic (*see also* Thyrotoxicosis) 242.9
      [425.7]
    thyrotoxicosis (*see also* Thyrotoxicosis) 242.9
      [425.7]
  nutritional 269.9 *[425.7]*
    beriberi 265.0 *[425.7]*
  obscure of Africa 425.2
  postpartum 674.8
  primary 425.4
  secondary 425.9
  thyrotoxic (*see also* Thyrotoxicosis) 242.9
    [425.7]
  toxic NEC 425.9
  tuberculous (*see also* Tuberculosis) 017.9
    [425.8]
Cardionephritis —*see* Hypertension, cardiorenal
Cardionephropathy —*see* Hypertension,
  cardiorenal
Cardionephrosis —*see* Hypertension,
  cardiorenal
Cardioneurosis 306.2
Cardiopathia nigra 416.0
Cardiopathy (*see also* Disease, heart) 429.9
  hypertensive (*see also* Hypertension, heart)
    402.90
  idiopathic 425.4
  mucopolysaccharidosis 277.5 *[425.7]*
Cardiopericarditis (*see also* Pericarditis) 423.9
Cardiophobia 300.29
Cardioptosis 746.87
Cardiorenal —*see* condition
Cardiorrhexis (*see also* Infarct, myocardium)
  410.9
Cardiosclerosis —*see* Arteriosclerosis, coronary
Cardiosis —*see* Disease, heart
Cardiospasm (esophagus) (reflex) (stomach)
  530.0
  congenital 750.7
Cardiostenosis —*see* Disease, heart
Cardiosymphysis 423.1
Cardiothyrotoxicosis —*see* Hyperthyroidism
Cardiovascular —*see* condition
Carditis (acute) (bacterial) (chronic) (subacute)
  429.89
  Coxsackie 074.20
  hypertensive (*see also* Hypertension, heart)
    402.90
  meningococcal 036.40
  rheumatic—*see* Disease, heart, rheumatic
  rheumatoid 714.2
Care (of)
  child (routine) V20.1
  convalescent following V66.9
    chemotherapy V66.2
    medical NEC V66.5
    psychotherapy V66.3

Care—*continued*
  radiotherapy V66.1
  surgery V66.0
  surgical NEC V66.0
  treatment (for) V66.5
    combined V66.6
    fracture V66.4
    mental disorder NEC V66.3
    specified type NEC V66.5
  end-of-life care V66.7
  family member (handicapped) (sick)
    creating problem for family V61.49
    provided away from home for holiday relief
      V60.5
    unavailable, due to
      absence (person rendering care) (sufferer)
        V60.4
      inability (any reason) of person rendering
        care V60.4
  holiday relief V60.5
  hospice V66.7
  lack of (at or after birth) (infant) (child) 995.52
    adult 995.84
  lactation of mother V24.1
  palliative V66.7
  postpartum
    immediately after delivery V24.0
    routine follow-up V24.2
  prenatal V22.1
    first pregnancy V22.0
    high risk pregnancy V23.9
    specified problem NEC V23.8
  terminal V66.7
  unavailable, due to
    absence of person rendering care V60.4
    inability (any reason) of person rendering care
      V60.4
  well baby V20.1
Caries (bone) (*see also* Tuberculosis, bone)
    015.9 *[730.8]*
  arrested 521.04
  cementum 521.03
  cerebrospinal (tuberculous) 015.0 *[730.88]*
  dental (acute) (chronic) (incipient) (infected)
    521.09
    with pulp exposure 521.03
    extending to
      dentine 521.02
      pulp 521.03
    other specified NEC 521.09
  dentin (acute) (chronic) 521.02
  enamel (acute) (chronic) (incipient) 521.01
  external meatus 380.89
  hip (*see also* Tuberculosis) 015.1 *[730.85]*
  knee 015.2 *[730.86]*
  labyrinth 386.8
  limb NEC 015.7 *[730.88]*
  mastoid (chronic) (process) 383.1
  middle ear 385.89
  nose 015.7 *[730.88]*
  orbit 015.7 *[730.88]*
  ossicle 385.24
  petrous bone 383.20
  sacrum (tuberculous) 015.0 *[730.88]*
  spine, spinal (column) (tuberculous) 015.0
    [730.88]
  syphilitic 095.5
    congenital 090.0 *[730.8]*
  teeth (internal) 521.00
    initial 521.01
  vertebra (column) (tuberculous) 015.0 *[730.88]*
Carini's syndrome (ichthyosis congenita) 757.1

Carious teeth 521.00
Carneous mole 631
Carnosinemia 270.5
Carotid body or sinus syndrome 337.0
Carotidynia 337.0
Carotinemia (dietary) 278.3
Carotinosis (cutis) (skin) 278.3
Carpal tunnel syndrome 354.0
Carpenter's syndrome 759.89
Carpopedal spasm (*see also* Tetany) 781.7
Carpoptosis 736.05
Carrier (suspected) of
  amebiasis V02.2
  bacterial disease (meningococcal,
    staphylococcal, streptococcal) NEC V02.59
  cholera V02.0
  cystic fibrosis gene V83.81
  defective gene V83.89
  diphtheria V02.4
  dysentery (bacillary) V02.3
    amebic V02.2
  Endamoeba histolytica V02.2
  gastrointestinal pathogens NEC V02.3
  genetic defect V83.89
  gonorrhea V02.7
  group B streptococcus V02.51
  HAA (hepatitis Australian-antigen) V02.61
  hemophilia A (asymptomatic) V83.01
    symptomatic V83.02
  hepatitis V02.60
    Australian-antigen (HAA) V02.61
    B V02.61
    C V02.62
    serum V02.61
    specified type NEC V02.69
    viral V02.60
  infective organism NEC V02.9
  malaria V02.9
  paratyphoid V02.3
  Salmonella V02.3
    typhosa V02.1
  serum hepatitis V02.61
  Shigella V02.3
  Staphylococcus NEC V02.59
  Streptococcus NEC V02.52
    group B V02.51
  typhoid V02.1
  venereal disease NEC V02.8
Carrión's disease (Bartonellosis) 088.0
Car sickness 994.6
Carter's
  relapsing fever (Asiatic) 087.0
Cartilage —*see* condition
Caruncle (inflamed)
  abscess, lacrimal (*see also* Dacryocystitis)
    375.30
  conjunctiva 372.00
    acute 372.00
  eyelid 373.00
  labium (majus) (minus) 616.8
  lacrimal 375.30
  urethra (benign) 599.3
  vagina (wall) 616.8
Cascade stomach 537.6
Caseation lymphatic gland (*see also*
    Tuberculosis) 017.2
Caseous
  bronchitis—*see* Tuberculosis, pulmonary
  meningitis 013.0
  pneumonia—*see* Tuberculosis, pulmonary
Cassidy (-Scholte) syndrome (malignant
    carcinoid) 259.2

Castellani's bronchitis 104.8
Castleman's tumor or lymphoma (mediastinal
  lymph node hyperplasia) 785.6
Castration, traumatic 878.2
  complicated 878.3
Casts in urine 791.7
Cat's ear 744.29
Catalepsy 300.11
  catatonic (acute) (*see also* Schizophrenia) 295.2
  hysterical 300.11
  schizophrenic (*see also* Schizophrenia) 295.2
Cataphasia 307.0
Cataplexy (idiopathic) 347
Cataract (anterior cortical) (anterior polar)
    (black) (capsular) (central) (cortical)
    (hypermature) (immature) (incipient) (mature)
    366.9
  anterior
    and posterior axial embryonal 743.33
    pyramidal 743.31
    subcapsular polar
      infantile, juvenile, or presenile 366.01
      senile 366.13
  associated with
    calcinosis 275.40 *[366.42]*
    craniofacial dysostosis 756.0 *[366.44]*
    galactosemia 271.1 *[366.44]*
    hypoparathyroidism 252.1 *[366.42]*
    myotonic disorders 359.2 *[366.43]*
    neovascularization 366.33
  blue dot 743.39
  cerulean 743.39
  complicated NEC 366.30
  congenital 743.30
    capsular or subcapsular 743.31
    cortical 743.32
    nuclear 743.33
    specified type NEC 743.39
    total or subtotal 743.34
    zonular 743.32
  coronary (congenital) 743.39
    acquired 366.12
  cupuliform 366.14
  diabetic 250.5 *[366.41]*
  drug-induced 366.45
  due to
    chalcosis 360.24 *[366.34]*
    chronic choroiditis (*see also* Choroiditis)
      363.20 *[366.32]*
    degenerative myopia 360.21 *[366.34]*
    glaucoma (*see also* Glaucoma) 365.9 *[366.31]*
    infection, intraocular NEC 366.32
    inflammatory ocular disorder NEC 366.32
    iridocyclitis, chronic 364.10 *[366.33]*
    pigmentary retinal dystrophy 362.74 *[366.34]*
    radiation 366.46
  electric 366.46
  glassblowers' 366.46
  heat ray 366.46
  heterochromic 366.33
  in eye disease NEC 366.30
  infantile (*see also* Cataract, juvenile) 366.00
  intumescent 366.12
  irradiational 366.46
  juvenile 366.00
    anterior subcapsular polar 366.01
    combined forms 366.09
    cortical 366.03
    lamellar 366.03
    nuclear 366.04
    posterior subcapsular polar 366.02

Cataract—*continued*
  specified NEC 366.09
  zonular 366.03
  lamellar 743.32
    infantile, juvenile, or presenile 366.03
  morgagnian 366.18
  myotonic 359.2 *[366.43]*
  myxedema 244.9 *[366.44]*
  nuclear 366.16
  posterior, polar (capsular) 743.31
    infantile, juvenile, or presenile 366.02
    senile 366.14
  presenile (*see also* Cataract, juvenile) 366.00
  punctate
    acquired 366.12
    congenital 743.39
  secondary (membrane) 366.50
    obscuring vision 366.53
    specified type, not obscuring vision 366.52
  senile 366.10
    anterior subcapsular polar 366.13
    combined forms 366.19
    cortical 366.15
    hypermature 366.18
    immature 366.12
    incipient 366.12
    mature 366.17
    nuclear 366.16
    posterior subcapsular polar 366.14
    specified NEC 366.19
    total or subtotal 366.17
  snowflake 250.5 *[366.41]*
  specified NEC 366.8
  subtotal (senile) 366.17
    congenital 743.34
  sunflower 360.24 *[366.34]*
  tetanic NEC 252.1 *[366.42]*
  total (mature) (senile) 366.17
    congenital 743.34
    localized 366.21
    traumatic 366.22
  toxic 366.45
  traumatic 366.20
    partially resolved 366.23
    total 366.22
  zonular (perinuclear) 743.32
    infantile, juvenile, or presenile 366.03
Cataracta 366.10
  brunescens 366.16
  cerulea 743.39
  complicata 366.30
  congenita 743.30
  coralliformis 743.39
  coronaria (congenital) 743.39
    acquired 366.12
  diabetic 250.5 *[366.41]*
  floriformis 360.24 *[366.34]*
  membranacea
    accreta 366.50
    congenita 743.39
  nigra 366.16
Catarrh, catarrhal (inflammation) (*see also*
    condition) 460
  acute 460
  asthma, asthmatic (*see also* Asthma) 493.9
  Bostock's (*see also* Fever, hay) 477.9
  bowel—*see* Enteritis
  bronchial 490
    acute 466.0
    chronic 491.0
    subacute 466.0

Catarrh, catarrhal—*continued*
  cervix, cervical (canal) (uteri)—*see* Cervicitis
  chest (*see also* Bronchitis) 490
  chronic 472.0
  congestion 472.0
  conjunctivitis 372.03
  due to syphilis 095.9
    congenital 090.0
  enteric—*see* Enteritis
  epidemic 487.1
  Eustachian 381.50
  eye (acute) (vernal) 372.03
  fauces (*see also* Pharyngitis) 462
  febrile 460
  fibrinous acute 466.0
  gastroenteric—*see* Enteritis
  gastrointestinal—*see* Enteritis
  gingivitis 523.0
  hay (*see also* Fever, hay) 477.9
  infectious 460
  intestinal—*see* Enteritis
  larynx (*see also* Laryngitis, chronic) 476.0
  liver 070.1
    with hepatic coma 070.0
  lung (*see also* Bronchitis) 490
    acute 466.0
    chronic 491.0
  middle ear (chronic)—*see* Otitis media, chronic
  mouth 528.0
  nasal (chronic) (*see also* Rhinitis) 472.0
    acute 460
  nasobronchial 472.2
  nasopharyngeal (chronic) 472.2
    acute 460
  nose—*see* Catarrh, nasal
  ophthalmia 372.03
  pneumococcal, acute 466.0
  pulmonary (*see also* Bronchitis) 490
    acute 466.0
    chronic 491.0
  spring (eye) 372.13
  suffocating (*see also* Asthma) 493.9
  summer (hay) (*see also* Fever, hay) 477.9
  throat 472.1
  tracheitis 464.10
    with obstruction 464.11
  tubotympanal 381.4
    acute (*see also* Otitis media, acute,
      nonsuppurative) 381.00
    chronic 381.10
  vasomotor (*see also* Fever, hay) 477.9
  vesical (bladder)—*see* Cystitis
Catarrhus aestivus (*see also* Fever, hay) 477.9
Catastrophe, cerebral (*see also* Disease,
    cerebrovascular, acute) 436
Catatonia, catatonic (acute) 781.99
  agitation 295.2
  dementia (praecox) 295.2
  due to or associated with physical condition
    293.89
  excitation 295.2
  excited type 295.2
  schizophrenia 295.2
  stupor 295.2
  with
    affective psychosis —*see* Psychosis, affective)
Cat-scratch —*see also* Injury, superficial
  disease or fever 078.3
Cauda equina —*see also* condition syndrome
  344.60
Cauliflower ear 738.7
Caul over face 768.9

Causalgia 355.9
  lower limb 355.71
  upper limb 354.4
Cause
  external, general effects NEC 994.9
  not stated 799.9
  unknown 799.9
Caustic burn —*see also* Burn, by site
  from swallowing caustic or corrosive
    substance—*see* Burn, internal organs
Cavare's disease (familial periodic paralysis)
  359.3
Cave-in, injury
  crushing (severe) (*see also* Crush, by site) 869.1
  suffocation 994.7
Cavernitis (penis) 607.2
  lymph vessel—*see* Lymphangioma
Cavernositis 607.2
Cavernous —*see* condition
Cavitation of lung (*see also* Tuberculosis) 011.2
  nontuberculous 518.89
  primary, progressive 010.8
Cavity
  lung—*see* Cavitation of lung
  optic papilla 743.57
  pulmonary—*see* Cavitation of lung
  teeth 521.00
  vitreous (humor) 379.21
Cavovarus foot, congenital 754.59
Cavus foot (congenital) 754.71
  acquired 736.73
Cazenave's
  disease (pemphigus) NEC 694.4
  lupus (erythematosus) 695.4
Cecitis —*see* Appendicitis
Cecocele —*see* Hernia
Cecum —*see* condition
Celiac
  artery compression syndrome 447.4
  disease 579.0
  infantilism 579.0
Cell, cellular —*see also* condition
  anterior chamber (eye) (positive aqueous ray)
    364.04
Cellulitis (diffuse) (with lymphangitis) (*see also*
    Abscess) 682.9
  abdominal wall 682.2
  anaerobic (*see also* Gas gangrene) 040.0
  ankle 682.6
  anus 566
  areola 611.0
  arm (any part, above wrist) 682.3
  auditory canal (external) 380.10
  axilla 682.3
  back (any part) 682.2
  breast 611.0
    postpartum 675.1
  broad ligament (*see also* Disease, pelvis,
    inflammatory) 614.4
    acute 614.3
  buttock 682.5
  cervical (neck region) 682.1
  cervix (uteri) (*see also* Cervicitis) 616.0
  cheek, external 682.0
    internal 528.3
  chest wall 682.2
  chronic NEC 682.9
  colostomy 569.61
  corpus cavernosum 607.2
  digit 681.9

Cellulitis—*continued*
  Douglas' cul-de-sac or pouch (chronic) (*see also* Disease, pelvis, inflammatory) 614.4
    acute 614.3
  drainage site (following operation) 998.59
  ear, external 380.10
  enterostomy 569.61
  erysipelar (*see also* Erysipelas) 035
  eyelid 373.13
  face (any part, except eye) 682.0
  finger (intrathecal) (periosteal) (subcutaneous) (subcuticular) 681.00
  flank 682.2
  foot (except toe) 682.7
  forearm 682.3
  gangrenous (*see also* Gangrene) 785.4
  genital organ NEC
    female—*see* Abscess, genital organ, female
    male 608.4
  glottis 478.71
  gluteal (region) 682.5
  gonococcal NEC 098.0
  groin 682.2
  hand (except finger or thumb) 682.4
  head (except face) NEC 682.8
  heel 682.7
  hip 682.6
  jaw (region) 682.0
  knee 682.6
  labium (majus) (minus) (*see also* Vulvitis) 616.10
  larynx 478.71
  leg, except foot 682.6
  lip 528.5
  mammary gland 611.0
  mouth (floor) 528.3
  multiple sites NEC 682.9
  nasopharynx 478.21
  navel 682.2
    newborn NEC 771.4
  neck (region) 682.1
  nipple 611.0
  nose 478.1
    external 682.0
  orbit, orbital 376.01
  palate (soft) 528.3
  pectoral (region) 682.2
  pelvis, pelvic
    with
      abortion—*see* Abortion, by type, with sepsis
      ectopic pregnancy (*see also* categories 633.0-633.9) 639.0
      molar pregnancy (*see also* categories 630-632) 639.0
    female (*see also* Disease, pelvis, inflammatory) 614.4
      acute 614.3
    following
      abortion 639.0
      ectopic or molar pregnancy 639.0
    male (*see also* Abscess, peritoneum) 567.2
    puerperal, postpartum, childbirth 670
  penis 607.2
  perineal, perineum 682.2
  perirectal 566
  peritonsillar 475
  periurethral 597.0
  periuterine (*see also* Disease, pelvis, inflammatory) 614.4
    acute 614.3
  pharynx 478.21

Cellulitis—*continued*
  phlegmonous NEC 682.9
  rectum 566
  retromammary 611.0
  retroperitoneal (*see also* Peritonitis) 567.2
  round ligament (*see also* Disease, pelvis, inflammatory) 614.4
    acute 614.3
  scalp (any part) 682.8
    dissecting 704.8
  scrotum 608.4
  seminal vesicle 608.0
  septic NEC 682.9
  shoulder 682.3
  specified sites NEC 682.8
  spermatic cord 608.4
  submandibular (region) (space) (triangle) 682.0
    gland 527.3
  submaxillary 528.3
    gland 527.3
  submental (pyogenic) 682.0
    gland 527.3
  suppurative NEC 682.9
  testis 608.4
  thigh 682.6
  thumb (intrathecal) (periosteal) (subcutaneous) (subcuticular) 681.00
  toe (intrathecal) (periosteal) (subcutaneous) (subcuticular) 681.10
  tonsil 475
  trunk 682.2
  tuberculous (primary) (*see also* Tuberculosis) 017.0
  tunica vaginalis 608.4
  umbilical 682.2
    newborn NEC 771.4
  vaccinal 999.3
  vagina—*see* Vaginitis
  vas deferens 608.4
  vocal cords 478.5
  vulva (*see also* Vulvitis) 616.10
  wrist 682.4
Cementoblastoma, benign (M9273/0) 213.1
  upper jaw (bone) 213.0
Cementoma (M9273/0) 213.1
  gigantiform (M9276/0) 213.1
    upper jaw (bone) 213.0
  upper jaw (bone) 213.0
Cementoperiostitis 523.4
Cephalgia, cephalalgia (*see also* Headache) 784.0
  histamine 346.2
  nonorganic origin 307.81
  psychogenic 307.81
  tension 307.81
Cephalhematocele, cephalematocele
  due to birth injury 767.1
  fetus or newborn 767.1
  traumatic (*see also* Contusion, head) 920
Cephalhematoma, cephalematoma (calcified)
  due to birth injury 767.1
  fetus or newborn 767.1
  traumatic (*see also* Contusion, head) 920
Cephalic —*see* condition
Cephalitis —*see* Encephalitis
Cephalocele 742.0
Cephaloma —*see* Neoplasm, by site, malignant
Cephalomenia 625.8
Cephalopelvic —*see* condition
Cercomoniasis 007.3
Cerebellitis —*see* Encephalitis

Cerebellum (cerebellar)—*see* condition
Cerebral —*see* condition
Cerebritis —*see* Encephalitis
Cerebrohepatorenal syndrome 759.89
Cerebromacular degeneration 330.1
Cerebromalacia (*see also* Softening, brain) 434.9
Cerebrosidosis 272.7
Cerebrospasticity —*see* Palsy, cerebral
Cerebrospinal —*see* condition
Cerebrum —*see* condition
Ceroid storage disease 272.7
Cerumen (accumulation) (impacted) 380.4
Cervical —*see also* condition
  auricle 744.43
  rib 756.2
Cervicalgia 723.1
Cervicitis (acute) (chronic) (nonvenereal)
    (subacute) (with erosion or ectropion) 616.0
  with
    abortion—*see* Abortion, by type, with sepsis
    ectopic pregnancy (*see also* categories
      633.0-633.9) 639.0
    molar pregnancy (*see also* categories
      630-632) 639.0
    ulceration 616.0
  chlamydial 099.53
  complicating pregnancy or puerperium 646.6
    affecting fetus or newborn 760.8
  following
    abortion 639.0
    ectopic or molar pregnancy 639.0
  gonococcal (acute) 098.15
    chronic or duration of 2 months or more
      098.35
  senile (atrophic) 616.0
  syphilitic 095.8
  trichomonal 131.09
  tuberculous (*see also* Tuberculosis) 016.7
Cervicoaural fistula 744.49
Cervicocolpitis (emphysematosa) (*see also*
    Cervicitis) 616.0
Cervix —*see* condition
Cesarean delivery, operation or section NEC
    669.7
  affecting fetus or newborn 763.4
  post mortem, affecting fetus or newborn 761.6
  previous, affecting management of pregnancy
    654.2
Céstan's syndrome 344.89
Céstan-Chenais paralysis 344.89
Céstan-Raymond syndrome 433.8
Cestode infestation NEC 123.9
  specified type NEC 123.8
Cestodiasis 123.9
Chaberts' disease 022.9
Chacaleh 266.2
Chafing 709.8
Chagas' disease (*see also* Trypanosomiasis,
    American) 086.2
  with heart involvement 086.0
Chagres fever 084.0
Chalasia (cardiac sphincter) 530.81
Chalazion 373.2
Chalazoderma 757.39
Chalcosis 360.24
  cornea 371.15
  crystalline lens 360.24 *[366.34]*
  retina 360.24.
Chalicosis (occupational) (pulmonum) 502

Chancre (any genital site) (hard) (indurated)
    (infecting) (primary) (recurrent) 091.0
  congenital 090.0
  conjunctiva 091.2
  Ducrey's 099.0
  extragenital 091.2
  eyelid 091.2
  Hunterian 091.0
  lip (syphilis) 091.2
  mixed 099.8
  nipple 091.2
  Nisbet's 099.0
  of
    carate 103.0
    pinta 103.0
    yaws 102.0
  palate, soft 091.2
  phagedenic 099.0
  Ricord's 091.0
  Rollet's (syphilitic) 091.0
  seronegative 091.0
  seropositive 091.0
  simple 099.0
  soft 099.0
    bubo 099.0
  urethra 091.0
  yaws 102.0
Chancriform syndrome 114.1
Chancroid 099.0
  anus 099.0
  penis (Ducrey's bacillus) 099.0
  perineum 099.0
  rectum 099.0
  scrotum 099.0
  urethra 099.0
  vulva 099.0
Chandipura fever 066.8
Chandler's disease (osteochondritis dissecans,
    hip) 732.7
Change (s) (of)—*see also* Removal of
  arteriosclerotic—*see* Arteriosclerosis
  battery
    cardiac pacemaker V53.31
  bone 733.90
    diabetic 250.8 *[731.8]*
    in disease, unknown cause 733.90
  bowel habits 787.99
  cardiorenal (vascular) (*see also* Hypertension,
    cardiorenal) 404.90
  cardiovascular—*see* Disease, cardiovascular
  circulatory 459.9
  cognitive or personality change of other type,
    nonpsychotic 310.1
  color, teeth, tooth
    during formation 520.8
    posteruptive 521.7
  contraceptive device V25.42
  cornea, corneal
    degenerative NEC 371.40
    membrane NEC 371.30
    senile 371.41
  coronary (*see also* Ischemia, heart) 414.9
  degenerative
    chamber angle (anterior) (iris) 364.56
    ciliary body 364.57
    spine or vertebra (*see also* Spondylosis)
      721.90
  dental pulp, regressive 522.2
  dressing V58.3
  fixation device V54.89
    external V54.89

Change(s) (of)—*continued*
internal V54.0
heart—*see also* Disease, heart
hip joint 718.95
hyperplastic larynx 478.79
hypertrophic
nasal sinus (*see also* Sinusitis) 473.9
turbinate, nasal 478.0
upper respiratory tract 478.9
inflammatory—*see* Inflammation
joint (*see also* Derangement, joint) 718.90
sacroiliac 724.6
Kirschner wire V54.89
knee 717.9
macular, congenital 743.55
malignant (M——/3)—*see also* Neoplasm, by
site, malignant

---
*Note—for malignant change occurring in a
neoplasm, use the appropriate M code with
behavior digit /3 e.g., malignant change in
uterine fibroid—M8890/3. For malignant
change occurring in a nonneoplastic condition
(e.g., gastric ulcer) use the M code M8000/3.*

---

mental (status) NEC 780.99
due to or associated with physical
condition—*see* Syndrome, brain
myocardium, myocardial—*see* Degeneration,
myocardial
of life (*see also* Menopause) 627.2
pacemaker battery (cardiac) V53.31
peripheral nerve 355.9
personality (nonpsychotic) NEC 310.1
plaster cast V54.89
refractive, transient 367.81
regressive, dental pulp 522.2
retina 362.9
myopic (degenerative) (malignant) 360.21
vascular appearance 362.13
sacroiliac joint 724.6
scleral 379.19
degenerative 379.16
senile (*see also* Senility) 797
sensory (*see also* Disturbance, sensation) 782.0
skin texture 782.8
spinal cord 336.9
splint, external V54.89
subdermal implantable contraceptive V25.5
suture V58.3
traction device V54.89
trophic 355.9
arm NEC 354.9
leg NEC 355.8
lower extremity NEC 355.8
upper extremity NEC 354.9
vascular 459.9
vasomotor 443.9
voice 784.49
psychogenic 306.1
Changing sleep-work schedule, affecting sleep
307.45
Changuinola fever 066.0
Chapping skin 709.8
Character
depressive 301.12
Charcot's
arthropathy 094.0 *[713.5]*
cirrhosis—*see* Cirrhosis, biliary
disease 094.0
spinal cord 094.0

Charcot's—*continued*
fever (biliary) (hepatic) (intermittent)—*see*
Choledocholithiasis
joint (disease) 094.0 *[713.5]*
diabetic 250.6 *[713.5]*
syringomyelic 336.0 *[713.5]*
syndrome (intermittent claudication) 443.9
due to atherosclerosis 440.21
**Charcot-Marie-Tooth disease, paralysis, or syn-
drome** 356.1
Charleyhorse (quadriceps) 843.8
muscle, except quadriceps—*see* Sprain, by site
Charlouis' disease (*see also* Yaws) 102.9
Chauffeur's fracture —*see* Fracture, ulna,
lower end
Cheadle (-Möller) (-Barlow) disease or
syndrome (infantile scurvy) 267
Checking (of)
contraceptive device (intrauterine) V25.42
device
fixation V54.89
external V54.89
internal V54.0
traction V54.89
Kirschner wire V54.89
plaster cast V54.89
splint, external V54.89
Checkup
following treatment—*see* Examination
health V70.0
infant (not sick) V20.2
pregnancy (normal) V22.1
first V22.0
high risk pregnancy V23.9
specified problem NEC V23.8
Chédiak-Higashi (-Steinbrinck) anomaly,
disease, or syndrome (congenital gigantism of
peroxidase granules) 288.2
Cheek —*see also* condition
biting 528.9
Cheese itch 133.8
Cheese washers' lung 495.8
Cheilitis 528.5
actinic (due to sun) 692.72
chronic NEC 692.74
due to radiation, except from sun 692.82
due to radiation, except from sun 692.82
acute 528.5
angular 528.5
catarrhal 528.5
chronic 528.5
exfoliative 528.5
gangrenous 528.5
glandularis apostematosa 528.5
granulomatosa 351.8
infectional 528.5
membranous 528.5
Miescher's 351.8
suppurative 528.5
ulcerative 528.5
vesicular 528.5
Cheilodynia 528.5
Cheilopalatoschisis (*see also* Cleft, palate, with
cleft lip) 749.20
Cheilophagia 528.9
Cheiloschisis (*see also* Cleft, lip) 749.10
Cheilosis 528.5
with pellagra 265.2
angular 528.5
due to
dietary deficiency 266.0
vitamin deficiency 266.0

Cheiromegaly 729.89
Cheiropompholyx 705.81
Cheloid (*see also* Keloid) 701.4
Chemical burn —*see also* Burn, by site
  from swallowing chemical—*see* Burn, internal
    organs
Chemodectoma (M8693/1)—*see*
  Paraganglioma, nonchromaffin
Chemoprophylaxis NEC V07.39
Chemosis, conjunctiva 372.73
Chemotherapy
  convalescence V66.2
  encounter (for) V58.1
  maintenance V58.1
  prophylactic NEC V07.39
    fluoride V07.31
Cherubism 526.89
Chest —*see* condition
Cheyne-Stokes respiration (periodic) 786.04
Chiari's
  disease or syndrome (hepatic vein thrombosis)
    453.0
  malformation
    type I 348.4
    type II (*see also* Spina bifida) 741.0
    type III 742.0
    type IV 742.2
    network 746.89
Chiari-Frommel syndrome 676.6
Chicago disease (North American
  blastomycosis) 116.0
Chickenpox (*see also* Varicella) 052.9
  vaccination and inoculation (prophylactic) V05.4
Chiclero ulcer 085.4
Chiggers 133.8
Chignon 111.2
  fetus or newborn (from vacuum extraction)
    767.1
Chigoe disease 134.1
Chikungunya fever 066.3
Chilaiditi's syndrome (subphrenic displacement,
  colon) 751.4
Chilblains 991.5
  lupus 991.5
Child
  behavior causing concern V61.20
Childbed fever 670
Childbirth —*see also* Delivery
  puerperal complications—*see* Puerperal
Childhood, period of rapid growth V21.0
Chill (s) 780.99
  with fever 780.6
  congestive 780.99
    in malarial regions 084.6
  septic—*see* Septicemia
  urethral 599.84
Chilomastigiasis 007.8
Chin —*see* condition
Chinese dysentery 004.9
Chiropractic dislocation (*see also* Lesion,
  nonallopathic, by site) 739.9
Chitral fever 066.0
Chlamydia, chlamydial -*see* **condition**
Chloasma 709.09
  cachecticorum 709.09
  eyelid 374.52
    congenital 757.33
    hyperthyroid 242.0
  gravidarum 646.8
  idiopathic 709.09
  skin 709.09
  symptomatic 709.09

Chloroma (M9930/3) 205.3
Chlorosis 280.9
  Egyptian (*see also* Ancylostomiasis) 126.9
  miners' (*see also* Ancylostomiasis) 126.9
Chlorotic anemia 280.9
Chocolate cyst (ovary) 617.1
Choked
  disk or disc—*see* Papilledema
  on food, phlegm, or vomitus NEC (*see also*
    Asphyxia, food) 933.1
  phlegm 933.1
  while vomiting NEC (*see also* Asphyxia, food)
    933.1
Chokes (resulting from bends) 993.3
Choking sensation 784.9
Cholangiectasis (*see also* Disease, gallbladder)
  575.8
Cholangiocarcinoma (M8160/3)
  and hepatocellular carcinoma, combined
    (M8180/3) 155.0
  liver 155.1
  specified site NEC—*see* Neoplasm, by site,
    malignant
  unspecified site 155.1
Cholangiohepatitis 575.8
  due to fluke infestation 121.1
Cholangiohepatoma (M8180/3) 155.0
Cholangiolitis (acute) (chronic) (extrahepatic)
  (gangrenous) 576.1
  intrahepatic 575.8
  paratyphoidal (*see also* Fever, paratyphoid)
    002.9
  typhoidal 002.0
Cholangioma (M8160/0) 211.5
  malignant—*see* Cholangiocarcinoma
Cholangitis (acute) (ascending) (catarrhal)
  (chronic) (infective) (malignant) (primary)
  (recurrent) (sclerosing) (secondary)
  (stenosing) (suppurative) 576.1
  chronic nonsuppurative destructive 571.6
  nonsuppurative destructive (chronic) 571.6
Cholecystdocholithiasis —*see*
  Choledocholithiasis
Cholecystitis 575.10
  with
    calculus, stones in
      bile duct (common) (hepatic)—*see*
        Choledocholithiasis
      gallbladder—*see* Cholelithiasis
  acute and chronic 575.12
  chronic 575.11
  emphysematous (acute) (*see also* Cholecystitis,
    acute) 575.0
  gangrenous (*see also* Cholecystitis, acute) 575.0
  paratyphoidal, current (*see also* Fever,
    paratyphoid) 002.9
  suppurative (*see also* Cholecystitis, acute) 575.0
  typhoidal 002.0
Choledochitis (suppurative) 576.1
Choledocholith —*see* Choledocholithiasis
Choledocholithiasis 574.5

> *Note—Use the following fifth-digit
> subclassification with category 574:*
>
> *0 without mention of obstruction*
> *1 with obstruction*

  with
    cholecystitis 574.4
      acute 574.3
      chronic 574.4

Choledocholithiasis— *continued*
  cholelithiasis 574.9
    with
      cholecystitis 574.7
        acute 574.6
          and chronic 574.8
        chronic 574.7
Cholelithiasis (impacted) (multiple) 574.2

Note—Use the following fifth-digit subclassification with category 574:

0 without mention of obstruction
1 with obstruction

---

  with
    cholecystitis 574.1
      acute 574.0
      chronic 574.1
    choledocholithiasis 574.9
      with
        cholecystitis 574.7
          acute 574.6
            and chronic 574.8
        chronic cholecystitis 574.7
Cholemia (*see also* Jaundice) 782.4
  familial 277.4
  Gilbert's (familial nonhemolytic) 277.4
Cholemic gallstone —*see* Cholelithiasis
Choleperitoneum, choleperitonitis (*see also* Disease, gallbladder) 567.8
Cholera (algid) (Asiatic) (asphyctic) (epidemic) (gravis) (Indian) (malignant) (morbus) (pestilential) (spasmodic) 001.9
  antimonial 985.4
  carrier (suspected) of V02.0
  classical 001.0
  contact V01.0
  due to
    Vibrio
      cholerae (Inaba, Ogawa, Hikojima serotypes) 001.0
        El Tor 001.1
    El Tor 001.1
  exposure to V01.0
  vaccination, prophylactic (against) V03.0
Cholerine (*see also* Cholera) 001.9
Cholestasis 576.8
Cholesteatoma (ear) 385.30
  attic (primary) 385.31
  diffuse 385.35
  external ear (canal) 380.21
  marginal (middle ear) 385.32
    with involvement of mastoid cavity 385.33
    secondary (with middle ear involvement) 385.33
  mastoid cavity 385.30
  middle ear (secondary) 385.32
    with involvement of mastoid cavity 385.33
  postmastoidectomy cavity (recurrent) 383.32
  primary 385.31
  recurrent, postmastoidectomy cavity 383.32
  secondary (middle ear) 385.32
    with involvement of mastoid cavity 385.33
Cholesteatosis (middle ear) (*see also* Cholesteatoma) 385.30
  diffuse 385.35
Cholesteremia 272.0
Cholesterin
  granuloma, middle ear 385.82
  in vitreous 379.22

Cholesterol
  deposit
    retina 362.82
    vitreous 379.22
  imbibition of gallbladder (*see also* Disease, gallbladder) 575.6
Cholesterolemia 272.0
  essential 272.0
  familial 272.0
  hereditary 272.0
Cholesterosis, cholesterolosis (gallbladder) 575.6
  middle ear (*see also* Cholesteatoma) 385.30
  with
    cholecystitis—*see* Cholecystitis
    cholelithiasis—*see* Cholelithiasis
Cholocolic fistula (*see also* Fistula, gallbladder) 575.5
Choluria 791.4
Chondritis (purulent) 733.99
  costal 733.6
    Tietze's 733.6
  patella, posttraumatic 717.7
  posttraumatica patellae 717.7
  tuberculous (active) (*see also* Tuberculosis) 015.9
    intervertebral 015.0 *[730.88]*
Chondroangiopathia calcarea seu punctate 756.59
Chondroblastoma (M9230/0)—*see also* Neoplasm, bone, benign
  malignant (M9230/3)—*see* Neoplasm, bone, malignant
Chondrocalcinosis (articular) (crystal deposition) (dihydrate) (*see also* Arthritis, due to, crystals) 275.49 *[712.3]*
  due to
    calcium pyrophosphate 275.49 *[712.2]*
    dicalcium phosphate crystals 275.49 *[712.1]*
    pyrophosphate crystals 275.4 *[712.2]*
Chondrodermatitis nodularis helicis 380.00
Chondrodysplasia 756.4
  angiomatose 756.4
  calcificans congenita 756.59
  epiphysialis punctata 756.59
  hereditary deforming 756.4
Chondrodystrophia (fetalis) 756.4
  calcarea 756.4
  calcificans congenita 756.59
  fetalis hypoplastica 756.59
  hypoplastica calcinosa 756.59
  punctata 756.59
  tarda 277.5
Chondrodystrophy (familial) (hypoplastic) 756.4
Chondroectodermal dysplasia 756.55
Chondrolysis 733.99
Chondroma (M9220/0)—*see also* Neoplasm, cartilage, benign
  juxtacortical (M9221/0)—*see* Neoplasm, bone, benign
  periosteal (M9221/0)—*see* Neoplasm, bone, benign
Chondromalacia 733.92
  epiglottis (congenital) 748.3
  generalized 733.92
  knee 717.7
  larynx (congenital) 748.3
  localized, except patella 733.92
  patella, patellae 717.7
  systemic 733.92
  tibial plateau 733.92
  trachea (congenital) 748.3

Chromatopsia 368.59
Chromhidrosis, chromidrosis 705.89
Chromoblastomycosis 117.2
Chromomycosis 117.2
Chromophytosis 111.0
Chromotrichomycosis 111.8
Chronic —*see* condition
Churg-Strauss syndrome 446.4
Chyle cyst, mesentery 457.8
Chylocele (nonfilarial) 457.8
   filarial (*see also* Infestation, filarial) 125.9
   tunica vaginalis (nonfilarial) 608.84
      filarial (*see also* Infestation, filarial) 125.9
Chylomicronemia (fasting) (with
      hyperprebetalipoproteinemia) 272.3
Chylopericardium (acute) 420.90
Chylothorax (nonfilarial) 457.8
   filarial (*see also* Infestation, filarial) 125.9
Chylous
   ascites 457.8
   cyst of peritoneum 457.8
   hydrocele 603.9
   hydrothorax (nonfilarial) 457.8
      filarial (*see also* Infestation, filarial) 125.9
Chyluria 791.1
   bilharziasis 120.0
   due to
      Brugia (malayi) 125.1
      Wuchereria (bancrofti) 125.0
         malayi 125.1
   filarial (*see also* Infestation, filarial) 125.9
   filariasis (*see also* Infestation, filarial) 125.9
   nonfilarial 791.1
Cicatricial (deformity)—*see* Cicatrix
Cicatrix (adherent) (contracted) (painful)
      (vicious) 709.2
   adenoid 474.8
   alveolar process 525.8
   anus 569.49
   auricle 380.89
   bile duct (*see also* Disease, biliary) 576.8
   bladder 596.8
   bone 733.99
   brain 348.8
   cervix (postoperative) (postpartal) 622.3
      in pregnancy or childbirth 654.6
         causing obstructed labor 660.2
   chorioretinal 363.30
      disseminated 363.35
      macular 363.32
      peripheral 363.34
      posterior pole NEC 363.33
   choroid—*see* Cicatrix, chorioretinal
   common duct (*see also* Disease, biliary) 576.8
   congenital 757.39
   conjunctiva 372.64
   cornea 371.00
      tuberculous (*see also* Tuberculosis) 017.3
         [371.05]
   duodenum (bulb) 537.3
   esophagus 530.3
   eyelid 374.46
      with
         ectropion—*see* Ectropion
         entropion—*see* Entropion
      hypopharynx 478.29
   knee, semilunar cartilage 717.5
   lacrimal
      canaliculi 375.53
      duct
         acquired 375.56

Cicatrix—*continued*
      neonatal 375.55
      punctum 375.52
      sac 375.54
   larynx 478.79
   limbus (cystoid) 372.64
   lung 518.89
   macular 363.32
      disseminated 363.35
      peripheral 363.34
   middle ear 385.89
   mouth 528.9
   muscle 728.89
   nasolacrimal duct
      acquired 375.56
      neonatal 375.55
   nasopharynx 478.29
   palate (soft) 528.9
   penis 607.89
   prostate 602.8
   rectum 569.49
   retina 363.30
      disseminated 363.35
      macular 363.32
      peripheral 363.34
      posterior pole NEC 363.33
   semilunar cartilage—*see* Derangement,
      meniscus
   seminal vesicle 608.89
   skin 709.2
      infected 686.8
      postinfectional 709.2
      tuberculous (*see also* Tuberculosis) 017.0
   specified site NEC 709.2
   throat 478.29
   tongue 529.8
   tonsil (and adenoid) 474.8
   trachea 478.9
   tuberculous NEC (*see also* Tuberculosis) 011.9
   ureter 593.89
   urethra 599.84
   uterus 621.8
   vagina 623.4
      in pregnancy or childbirth 654.7
         causing obstructed labor 660.2
   vocal cord 478.5
   wrist, constricting (annular) 709.2
CIN I [cervical intraepithelial neoplasia I] 622.1
CIN II [cervical intraepithelial neoplasia II] 622.1
CIN III [cervical intraepithelial neoplasia III]
      233.1
Cinchonism
   correct substance properly administered 386.9
   overdose or wrong substance given or taken
      961.4
Circine herpes 110.5
Circle of Willis —*see* condition
Circular —*see also* condition
   hymen 752.49
Circulating anticoagulants 286.5
   following childbirth 666.3
   postpartum 666.3
Circulation
   collateral (venous), any site 459.89
   defective 459.9
      congenital 747.9
      lower extremity 459.89
   embryonic 747.9
   failure 799.8
      fetus or newborn 779.89
      peripheral 785.59

Circulation—*continued*
  fetal, persistent 747.83
  heart, incomplete 747.9
Circulatory system —*see* condition
Circulus senilis 371.41
Circumcision
  in absence of medical indication V50.2
  ritual V50.2
  routine V50.2
Circumscribed —*see* condition
Circumvallata placenta —*see* Placenta,
  abnormal
Cirrhosis, cirrhotic 571.5
  with alcoholism 571.2
  alcoholic (liver) 571.2
  atrophic (of liver)—*see* Cirrhosis, portal
  Baumgarten-Cruveilhier 571.5
  biliary (cholangiolitic) (cholangitic)
    (cholestatic) (extrahepatic) (hypertrophic)
    (intrahepatic) (nonobstructive) (obstructive)
    (pericholangiolitic) (posthepatic) (primary)
    (secondary) (xanthomatous) 571.6
   due to
    clonorchiasis 121.1
    flukes 121.3
  brain 331.9
  capsular—*see* Cirrhosis, portal
  cardiac 571.5
   alcoholic 571.2
  central (liver)—*see* Cirrhosis, liver
  Charcot's 571.6
  cholangiolitic—*see* Cirrhosis, biliary
  cholangitic—*see* Cirrhosis, biliary
  cholestatic—*see* Cirrhosis, biliary
  clitoris (hypertrophic) 624.2
  coarsely nodular 571.5
  congestive (liver)—*see* Cirrhosis, cardiac
  Cruveilhier-Baumgarten 571.5
  cryptogenic (of liver) 571.5
   alcoholic 571.2
  dietary (*see also* Cirrhosis, portal) 571.5
  due to
   bronzed diabetes 275.0
   congestive hepatomegaly—*see* Cirrhosis,
    cardiac
   cystic fibrosis 277.00
   hemochromatosis 275.0
   hepatolenticular degeneration 275.1
   passive congestion (chronic)—*see* Cirrhosis,
    cardiac
   Wilson's disease 275.1
   xanthomatosis 272.2
  extrahepatic (obstructive)—*see* Cirrhosis, biliary
  fatty 571.8
   alcoholic 571.0
  florid 571.2
  Glisson's—*see* Cirrhosis, portal
  Hanot's (hypertrophic)—*see* Cirrhosis, biliary
  hepatic—*see* Cirrhosis, liver
  hepatolienal—*see* Cirrhosis, liver
  hobnail—*see* Cirrhosis, portal
  hypertrophic—*see also* Cirrhosis, liver
   biliary—*see* Cirrhosis, biliary
   Hanot's—*see* Cirrhosis, biliary
  infectious NEC—*see* Cirrhosis, portal
  insular—*see* Cirrhosis, portal
  intrahepatic (obstructive) (primary)
   (secondary)—*see* Cirrhosis, biliary
  juvenile (*see also* Cirrhosis, portal) 571.5
  kidney (*see also* Sclerosis, renal) 587

Cirrhosis, cirrhotic—*continued*
  Laennec's (of liver) 571.2
   nonalcoholic 571.5
  liver (chronic) (hepatolienal) (hypertrophic)
   (nodular) (splenomegalic) (unilobar) 571.5
   with alcoholism 571.2
   alcoholic 571.2
   congenital (due to failure of obliteration of
    umbilical vein) 777.8
   cryptogenic 571.5
    alcoholic 571.2
   fatty 571.8
    alcoholic 571.0
   macronodular 571.5
    alcoholic 571.2
   micronodular 571.5
    alcoholic 571.2
   nodular, diffuse 571.5
    alcoholic 571.2
   pigmentary 275.0
   portal 571.5
    alcoholic 571.2
   postnecrotic 571.5
    alcoholic 571.2
   syphilitic 095.3
  lung (chronic) (*see also* Fibrosis, lung) 515
  macronodular (of liver) 571.5
   alcoholic 571.2
  malarial 084.9
  metabolic NEC 571.5
  micronodular (of liver) 571.5
   alcoholic 571.2
  monolobular—*see* Cirrhosis, portal
  multilobular—*see* Cirrhosis, portal
  nephritis (*see also* Sclerosis, renal) 587
  nodular—*see* Cirrhosis, liver
  nutritional (fatty) 571.5
  obstructive (biliary) (extrahepatic)
   (intrahepatic)—*see* Cirrhosis, biliary
  ovarian 620.8
  paludal 084.9
  pancreas (duct) 577.8
  pericholangiolitic—*see* Cirrhosis, biliary
  periportal—*see* Cirrhosis, portal
  pigment, pigmentary (of liver) 275.0
  portal (of liver) 571.5
   alcoholic 571.2
  posthepatitic (*see also* Cirrhosis, postnecrotic)
   571.5
  postnecrotic (of liver) 571.5
   alcoholic 571.2
  primary (intrahepatic)—*see* Cirrhosis, biliary
  pulmonary (*see also* Fibrosis, lung) 515
  renal (*see also* Sclerosis, renal) 587
  septal (*see also* Cirrhosis, postnecrotic) 571.5
  spleen 289.51
  splenomegalic (of liver)—*see* Cirrhosis, liver
  stasis (liver)—*see* Cirrhosis, liver
  stomach 535.4
  Todd's (*see also* Cirrhosis, biliary) 571.6
  toxic (nodular)—*see* Cirrhosis, postnecrotic
  trabecular—*see* Cirrhosis, postnecrotic
  unilobar—*see* Cirrhosis, liver
  vascular (of liver)—*see* Cirrhosis, liver
  xanthomatous (biliary) (*see also* Cirrhosis,
   biliary) 571.6
   due to xanthomatosis (familial) (metabolic)
    (primary) 272.2
Cistern, subarachnoid 793.0
Citrullinemia 270.6
Citrullinuria 270.6

Closure—*continued*
  congenital 743.65
    neonatal 375.55
  nose (congenital) 748.0
    acquired 738.0
  vagina 623.2
  valve—*see* Endocarditis
  vulva 624.8
Clot (blood)
  artery (obstruction) (occlusion) (*see also*
    Embolism) 444.9
  bladder 596.7
  brain (extradural or intradural) (*see also*
    Thrombosis, brain) 434.0
    late effect—*see* Late effect(s) (of)
      cerebrovascular disease
  circulation 444.9
  heart (*see also* Infarct, myocardium) 410.9
  vein (*see also* Thrombosis) 453.9
Clotting defect NEC (*see also* Defect,
    coagulation) 286.9
Clouded state 780.09
  epileptic (*see also* Epilepsy) 345.9
  paroxysmal (idiopathic) (*see also* Epilepsy)
    345.9
Clouding
  corneal graft 996.51
Cloudy
  antrum, antra 473.0
  dialysis effluent 792.5
Clouston's (hidrotic) ectodermal dysplasia 757.31
Clubbing of fingers 781.5
Clubfinger 736.29
  acquired 736.29
  congenital 754.89
Clubfoot (congenital) 754.70
  acquired 736.71
  equinovarus 754.51
  paralytic 736.71
Club hand (congenital) 754.89
  acquired 736.07
Clubnail (acquired) 703.8
  congenital 757.5
Clump kidney 753.3
Clumsiness 781.3
  syndrome 315.4
Cluttering 307.0
Clutton's joints 090.5
Coagulation, intravascular (diffuse)
    (disseminated) (*see also* Fibrinolysis) 286.6
  newborn 776.2
Coagulopathy (*see also* Defect, coagulation)
    286.9
  consumption 286.6
  intravascular (disseminated) NEC 286.6
    newborn 776.2
Coalition
  calcaneoscaphoid 755.67
  calcaneus 755.67
  tarsal 755.67
Coal miners'
  elbow 727.2
  lung 500
Coal workers' lung or pneumoconiosis 500
Coarctation
  aorta (postductal) (preductal) 747.10
  pulmonary artery 747.3
Coated tongue 529.3
Coats' disease 362.12
Cocainism (*see also* Dependence) 304.2
Coccidioidal granuloma 114.3

Coccidioidomycosis 114.9
  with pneumonia 114.0
  cutaneous (primary) 114.1
  disseminated 114.3
  extrapulmonary (primary) 114.1
  lung 114.5
    acute 114.0
    chronic 114.4
    primary 114.0
  meninges 114.2
  primary (pulmonary) 114.0
    acute 114.0
  prostate 114.3
  pulmonary 114.5
    acute 114.0
    chronic 114.4
    primary 114.0
  specified site NEC 114.3
Coccidioidosis 114.9
  lung 114.5
    acute 114.0
    chronic 114.4
    primary 114.0
  meninges 114.2
Coccidiosis (colitis) (diarrhea) (dysentery) 007.2
Cocciuria 791.9
Coccus in urine 791.9
Coccydynia 724.79
Coccygodynia 724.79
Coccyx —*see* condition
Cochin-China
  diarrhea 579.1
    anguilluliasis 127.2
  ulcer 085.1
Cock's peculiar tumor 706.2
Cockayne's disease or syndrome (microcephaly
    and dwarfism) 759.89
Cockayne-Weber syndrome (epidermolysis
    bullosa) 757.39
Cocked-up toe 735.2
Codman's tumor (benign chondroblastoma)
    (M9230/0)—*see* Neoplasm, bone, benign
Coenurosis 123.8
Coffee workers' lung 495.8
Cogan's syndrome 370.52
  congenital oculomotor apraxia 379.51
  nonsyphilitic interstitial keratitis 370.52
Coiling, umbilical cord —*see* Complications,
    umbilical cord
Coitus, painful (female) 625.0
  male 608.89
  psychogenic 302.76
Cold 460
  with influenza, flu, or grippe 487.1
  abscess—*see also* Tuberculosis, abscess
    articular—*see* Tuberculosis, joint
  agglutinin
    disease (chronic) or syndrome 283.0
    hemoglobinuria 283.0
      paroxysmal (cold) (nocturnal) 283.2
  allergic (*see also* Fever, hay) 477.9
  bronchus or chest—*see* Bronchitis
    with grippe or influenza 487.1
  common (head) 460
    vaccination, prophylactic (against) V04.7
  deep 464.10
  effects of 991.9
    specified effect NEC 991.8
  excessive 991.9
    specified effect NEC 991.8
  exhaustion from 991.8

Cold —*continued*
  exposure to 991.9
    specified effect NEC 991.8
  grippy 487.1
  head 460
  injury syndrome (newborn) 778.2
  intolerance 780.99
  on lung—*see* Bronchitis
  rose 477.0
  sensitivity, autoimmune 283.0
  virus 460
Coldsore (*see also* Herpes, simplex) 054.9
Colibacillosis 041.4
  generalized 038.42
Colibacilluria 791.9
Colic (recurrent) 789.0
  abdomen 789.0
    (recurrent)psychogenic 307.89
  appendicular 543.9
  appendix 543.9
  bile duct—*see* Choledocholithiasis
  biliary—*see* Cholelithiasis
  bilious—*see* Cholelithiasis
  common duct—*see* Choledocholithiasis
  Devonshire NEC 984.9
    specified type of lead—*see* Table of drugs and
      chemicals
  flatulent 787.3
  gallbladder or gallstone—*see* Cholelithiasis
  gastric 536.8
  hepatic (duct)—*see* Choledocholithiasis
  hysterical 300.11
  infantile 789.0
  intestinal 789.0
  kidney 788.0
  lead NEC 984.9
    specified type of lead—*see* Table of drugs and
      chemicals
  liver (duct)—*see* Choledocholithiasis
  mucous 564.9
    psychogenic 316 *[564.9]*
  nephritic 788.0
  painter's NEC 984.9
  pancreas 577.8
  psychogenic 306.4
  renal 788.0
  saturnine NEC 984.9
    specified type of lead—*see* Table of drugs and
      chemicals
  spasmodic 789.0
  ureter 788.0
  urethral 599.84
    due to calculus 594.2
  uterus 625.8
    menstrual 625.3
  vermicular 543.9
  virus 460
  worm NEC 128.9
Colicystitis (*see also* Cystitis) 595.9
Colitis (acute) (catarrhal) (croupous) (cystica
    superficialis) (exudative) (hemorrhagic)
    (noninfectious) (phlegmonous) (presumed
    noninfectious) 558.9
  adaptive 564.9
  allergic 558.3
  amebic (*see also* Amebiasis) 006.9
    nondysenteric 006.2
  anthrax 022.2
  bacillary (*see also* Infection, Shigella) 004.9
  balantidial 007.0
  chronic 558.9

Colitis—*continued*
  ulcerative (*see also* Colitis, ulcerative) 556.9
  coccidial 007.2
  dietetic 558.9
  due to radiation 558.1
  functional 558.9
  gangrenous 009.0
  giardial 007.1
  granulomatous 555.1
  gravis (*see also* Colitis, ulcerative) 556.9
  infectious (*see also* Enteritis, due to, specific
    organism) 009.0
    presumed 009.1
  ischemic 557.9
    acute 557.0
    chronic 557.1
    due to mesenteric artery insufficiency 557.1
  membranous 564.9
    psychogenic 316 *[564.9]*
  mucous 564.9
    psychogenic 316 *[564.9]*
  necrotic 009.0
  polyposa (*see also* Colitis, ulcerative) 556.9
  protozoal NEC 007.9
  pseudomembranous 008.45
  pseudomucinous 564.9
  regional 555.1
  segmental 555.1
  septic (*see also* Enteritis, due to, specific
    organism) 009.0
  spastic 564.9
    psychogenic 316 *[564.9]*
  staphylococcus 008.41
    food 005.0
  thromboulcerative 557.0
  toxic 558.2
  transmural 555.1
  trichomonal 007.3
  tuberculous (ulcerative) 014.8
  ulcerative (chronic) (idiopathic) (nonspecific)
    556.9
    entero- 556.0
    fulminant 557.0
    ileo- 556.1
    left-sided 556.5
    procto- 556.2
    proctosigmoid 556.3
    psychogenic 316 *[556]*
    specified NEC 556.8
    universal 556.6
Collagen disease NEC 710.9
  nonvascular 710.9
  vascular (allergic) (*see also* Angiitis,
    hypersensitivity) 446.20
Collagenosis (*see also* Collagen disease) 710.9
  cardiovascular 425.4
  mediastinal 519.3
Collapse 780.2
  adrenal 255.8
  cardiorenal (*see also* Hypertension, cardiorenal)
    404.90
  cardiorespiratory 785.51
    fetus or newborn 779.89
  cardiovascular (*see also* Disease, heart) 785.51
    fetus or newborn 779.89
  circulatory (peripheral) 785.59
    with
      abortion—*see* Abortion, by type, with shock
      ectopic pregnancy (*see also* categories
        633.0-633.9) 639.5

Collapse—*continued*
    molar pregnancy (*see also* categories
        630-632) 639.5
    during or after labor and delivery 669.1
    fetus or newborn 779.89
    following
        abortion 639.5
        ectopic or molar pregnancy 639.5
    during or after labor and delivery 669.1
    fetus or newborn 779.89
    external ear canal 380.50
      secondary to
        inflammation 380.53
        surgery 380.52
        trauma 380.51
    general 780.2
    heart—*see* Disease, heart
    heat 992.1
    hysterical 300.11
    labyrinth, membranous (congenital) 744.05
    lung (massive) (*see also* Atelectasis) 518.0
      pressure, during labor 668.0
    myocardial—*see* Disease, heart
    nervous (*see also* Disorder, mental,
        nonpsychotic) 300.9
    neurocirculatory 306.2
    nose 738.0
    postoperative (cardiovascular) 998.0
    pulmonary (*see also* Atelectasis) 518.0
      fetus or newborn 770.5
        partial 770.5
        primary 770.4
    thorax 512.8
      iatrogenic 512.1
      postoperative 512.1
    trachea 519.1
    valvular—*see* Endocarditis
    vascular (peripheral) 785.59
      with
        abortion—*see* Abortion, by type, with shock
        ectopic pregnancy (*see also* categories
          633.0-633.9) 639.5
        molar pregnancy (*see also* categories
          630-632) 639.5
      cerebral (*see also* Disease, cerebrovascular,
        acute) 436
      during or after labor and delivery 669.1
      fetus or newborn 779.89
      following
        abortion 639.5
        ectopic or molar pregnancy 639.5
    vasomotor 785.59
    vertebra 733.13
Collateral —*see also* condition
    circulation (venous) 459.89
    dilation, veins 459.89
Colles' fracture (closed) (reversed) (separation)
    813.41
    open 813.51
Collet's syndrome 352.6
Collet-Sicard syndrome 352.6
Colliculitis urethralis (*see also* Urethritis) 597.89
Colliers'
    asthma 500
    lung 500
    phthisis (*see also* Tuberculosis) 011.4
Collodion baby (ichthyosis congenita) 757.1
Colloid milium 709.3

Coloboma NEC 743.49
    choroid 743.59
    fundus 743.52
    iris 743.46
    lens 743.36
    lids 743.62
    optic disc (congenital) 743.57
      acquired 377.23
    retina 743.56
    sclera 743.47
Coloenteritis —*see* Enteritis
Colon —*see* condition
Coloptosis 569.89
Color
    amblyopia NEC 368.59
      acquired 368.55
    blindness NEC (congenital) 368.59
      acquired 368.55
Colostomy
    attention to V55.3
    fitting or adjustment V53.5
    malfunctioning 569.62
    status V44.3
Colpitis (*see also* Vaginitis) 616.10
Colpocele 618.6
Colpocystitis (*see also* Vaginitis) 616.10
Colporrhexis 665.4
Colpospasm 625.1
Column, spinal, vertebral —*see* condition
Coma 780.01
    apoplectic (*see also* Disease, cerebrovascular,
      acute) 436
    diabetic (with ketoacidosis) 250.3
      hyperosmolar 250.2
    eclamptic (*see also* Eclampsia) 780.39
    epileptic 345.3
    hepatic 572.2
    hyperglycemic 250.2
    hyperosmolar (diabetic) (nonketotic) 250.2
    hypoglycemic 251.0
      diabetic 250.3
    insulin 250.3
      hyperosmolar 250.2
      non-diabetic 251.0
      organic hyperinsulinism 251.0
    Kussmaul's (diabetic) 250.3
    liver 572.2
    newborn 779.2
    prediabetic 250.2
    uremic—*see* Uremia
Combat fatigue (*see also* Reaction, stress, acute)
    308.9
Combined —*see* condition
Comedo 706.1
Comedocarcinoma (M8501/3)—*see also*
    Neoplasm, breast, malignant
    noninfiltrating (M8501/2)
      specified site—*see* Neoplasm, by site, in situ
      unspecified site 233.0
Comedomastitis 610.4
Comedones 706.1
    lanugo 757.4
Comma bacillus, carrier (suspected) of V02.3
Comminuted fracture —*see* Fracture, by site
Common
    aortopulmonary trunk 745.0
    atrioventricular canal (defect) 745.69
    atrium 745.69
    cold (head) 460
      vaccination, prophylactic (against) V04.7
    truncus (arteriosus) 745.0
    ventricle 745.3

Commotio (current)
  cerebri (*see also* Concussion, brain) 850.9
    with skull fracture—*see* Fracture, skull, by site
  retinae 921.3
  spinalis—*see* Injury, spinal, by site
Commotion (current)
  brain (without skull fracture) (*see also*
    Concussion, brain) 850.9
    with skull fracture—*see* Fracture, skull, by site
  spinal cord—*see* Injury, spinal, by site
Communication
  abnormal—*see also* Fistula
    between
      base of aorta and pulmonary artery 745.0
      left ventricle and right atrium 745.4
      pericardial sac and pleural sac 748.8
      pulmonary artery and pulmonary vein 747.3
    congenital, between uterus and anterior
      abdominal wall 752.3
      bladder 752.3
      intestine 752.3
      rectum 752.3
  left ventricular-right atrial 745.4
  pulmonary artery-pulmonary vein 747.3
Compensation
  broken—*see* Failure, heart
  failure—*see* Failure, heart
  neurosis, psychoneurosis 300.11
Complaint —*see also* Disease
  bowel, functional 564.9
    psychogenic 306.4
  intestine, functional 564.9
    psychogenic 306.4
  kidney (*see also* Disease, renal) 593.9
  liver 573.9
  miners' 500
Complete —*see* condition
Complex
  cardiorenal (*see also* Hypertension, cardiorenal)
    404.90
  castration 300.9
  Costen's 524.60
  ego-dystonic homosexuality 302.0
  Eisenmenger's (ventricular septal defect) 745.4
  homosexual, ego-dystonic 302.0
  hypersexual 302.89
  inferiority 301.9
  jumped process
    spine—*see* Dislocation, vertebra
  primary, tuberculosis (*see also* Tuberculosis)
    010.0
  Taussig-Bing (transposition, aorta and
    overriding pulmonary artery) 745.11
Complications
  abortion NEC—*see* categories 634-639
  accidental puncture or laceration during a
    procedure 998.2
  amputation stump (late) (surgical) 997.60
    traumatic—*see* Amputation, traumatic
  anastomosis (and bypass)—*see also*
    Complications, due to (presence of) any
    device, implant, or graft classified to
    996.0-996.5 NEC
    hemorrhage NEC 998.11
    intestinal (internal) NEC 997.4
      involving urinary tract 997.5
    mechanical—*see* Complications, mechanical,
      graft
    urinary tract (involving intestinal tract) 997.5
  anesthesia, anesthetic NEC (*see also*
    Anesthesia, complication) 995.2

Complications—*continued*
  in labor and delivery 668.9
    affecting fetus or newborn 763.5
    cardiac 668.1
    central nervous system 668.2
    pulmonary 668.0
    specified type NEC 668.8
  aortocoronary (bypass) graft 996.03
    atherosclerosis —*see* Arteriosclerosis,
      coronary
    embolism 996.72
    occlusion NEC 996.72
    thrombus 996.72
  arthroplasty 996.4
  artificial opening
    cecostomy 569.60
    colostomy 569.6
    cystostomy 997.5
    enterostomy 569.60
    gastrostomy 536.40
    ileostomy 569.60
    jejunostomy 569.60
    nephrostomy 997.5
    tracheostomy 519.00
    ureterostomy 997.5
    urethrostomy 997.5
  bile duct implant (prosthetic) NEC 996.79
    infection or inflammation 996.69
    mechanical 996.59
  bleeding (intraoperative) (postoperative) 998.11
  blood vessel graft 996.1
    aortocoronary 996.03
      atherosclerosis —*see* Arteriosclerosis,
        coronary
      embolism 996.72
      occlusion NEC 996.72
      thrombus 996.72
    atherosclerosis —*see* Arteriosclerosis,
      extremities
    embolism 996.74
    occlusion NEC 996.74
    thrombus 996.74
  bone growth stimulator NEC 996.78
    infection or inflammation 996.67
  bone marrow transplant 996.85
  breast implant (prosthetic) NEC 996.79
    infection or inflammation 996.69
    mechanical 996.54
  bypass—*see also* Complications, anastomosis
    aortocoronary 996.03
      atherosclerosis —*see* Arteriosclerosis,
        coronary
      embolism 996.72
      occlusion NEC 996.72
      thrombus 996.72
    carotid artery 996.1
      atherosclerosis —*see* Arteriosclerosis,
        extremities
      embolism 996.74
      occlusion NEC 996.74
      thrombus 996.74
  cardiac (*see also* Disease, heart) 429.9
    device, implant, or graft NEC 996.72
      infection or inflammation 996.61
      long-term effect 429.4
      mechanical (*see also* Complications,
        mechanical, by type) 996.00
      valve prosthesis 996.71
        infection or inflammation 996.61
    postoperative NEC 997.1
      long-term effect 429.4

Complications—*continued*
  cardiorenal (*see also* Hypertension, cardiorenal)
      404.90
  carotid artery bypass graft 996.1
      atherosclerosis —*see* Arteriosclerosis,
          extremities
      embolism 996.74
      occlusion NEC 996.74
      thrombus 996.74
  cataract fragments in eye 998.82
  catheter device—*see also* Complications, due to
      (presence of) any device, implant, or graft
      classified to 996.0-996.5 NEC
      mechanical—*see* Complications, mechanical,
          catheter
  cecostomy 569.60
  cesarean section wound 674.3
  chin implant (prosthetic) NEC 996.79
      infection or inflammation 996.69
      mechanical 996.59
  colostomy (enterostomy) 569.60
      specified type NEC 569.69
  contraceptive device, intrauterine NEC 996.76
      infection 996.65
      inflammation 996.65
      mechanical 996.32
  cord (umbilical)—*see* Complications, umbilical
      cord
  cornea
      due to
          contact lens 371.82
  coronary (artery) bypass (graft) NEC 996.03
      atherosclerosis —*see* Arteriosclerosis,
          coronary
      embolism 996.72
      infection or inflammation 996.61
      mechanical 996.03
      occlusion NEC 996.72
      specified type NEC 996.72
      thrombus 996.72
  cystostomy 997.5
  delivery 669.9
      procedure (instrumental) (manual) (surgical)
          669.4
      specified type NEC 669.8
  dialysis (hemodialysis) (peritoneal) (renal) NEC
      999.9
      catheter NEC—*see also* Complications, due to
          (presence of) any device, implant or graft
          classified to 996.0-996.5 NEC
      infection or inflammation 996.62
          peritoneal 996.68
      mechanical 996.1
          peritoneal 996.56
  due to (presence of) any device, implant, or
      graft classified to 996.0-996.5
      with infection or inflammation—*see*
          Complications, infection or inflammation,
          due to (presence of) any device, implant,
          or graft classified to 996.0-996.5 NEC
      arterial NEC 996.74
          coronary NEC 996.03
              atherosclerosis —*see* Arteriosclerosis,
                  coronary
              embolism 996.72
              occlusion NEC 996.72
              specified type NEC 996.72
              thrombus 996.72
          renal dialysis 996.73
      arteriovenous fistula or shunt NEC 996.74
      bone growth stimulator 996.78

Complications—*continued*
  breast NEC 996.79
  cardiac NEC 996.72
      defibrillator 996.72
      pacemaker 996.72
      valve prosthesis 996.71
  catheter NEC 996.79
      spinal 996.75
      urinary, indwelling 996.76
      vascular NEC 996.74
          renal dialysis 996.73
      ventricular shunt 996.75
  coronary (artery) bypass (graft) NEC 996.03
      atherosclerosis —*see* Arteriosclerosis,
          coronary
      embolism 996.72
      occlusion NEC 996.72
      thrombus 996.72
  electrodes
      brain 996.75
      heart 996.72
  gastrointestinal NEC 996.79
  genitourinary NEC 996.76
  heart valve prosthesis NEC 996.71
  infusion pump 996.74
  internal
      joint prosthesis 996.77
      orthopedic NEC 996.78
      specified type NEC 996.79
  intrauterine contraceptive device NEC 996.76
  joint prosthesis, internal NEC 996.77
  mechanical—*see* Complications, mechanical
  nervous system NEC 996.75
  ocular lens NEC 996.79
  orbital NEC 996.79
  orthopedic NEC 996.78
      joint, internal 996.77
  renal dialysis 996.73
  specified type NEC 996.79
  urinary catheter, indwelling 996.76
  vascular NEC 996.74
  ventricular shunt 996.75
  during dialysis NEC 999.9
  ectopic or molar pregnancy NEC 639.9
  electroshock therapy NEC 999.9
  enterostomy 569.60
      specified type NEC 569.69
  external (fixation) device with internal
      component(s) NEC 996.78
      infection or inflammation 996.67
      mechanical 996.4
  extracorporeal circulation NEC 999.9
  eye implant (prosthetic) NEC 996.79
      infection or inflammation 996.69
      mechanical
          ocular lens 996.53
          orbital globe 996.59
  gastrointestinal, postoperative NEC (*see also*
      Complications, surgical procedures) 997.4
  gastrostomy 536.40
      specified type NEC 536.49
  genitourinary device, implant or graft NEC
      996.76
      infection or inflammation 996.65
          urinary catheter, indwelling 996.64
      mechanical (*see also* Complications,
          mechanical, by type) 996.30
          specified NEC 996.39
  graft (bypass) (patch)—*see also* Complications,
      due to (presence of) any device, implant, or
      graft classified to 996.0-996.5 NEC

Complications—*continued*
  bone marrow 996.85
  corneal NEC 996.79
    infection or inflammation 996.69
    rejection or reaction 996.51
    mechanical—*see* Complications, mechanical,
      graft
  organ (immune or nonimmune cause) (partial)
    (total) 996.80
    bone marrow 996.85
    heart 996.83
    intestines 996.87
    kidney 996.81
    liver 996.82
    lung 996.84
    pancreas 996.86
    specified NEC 996.89
  skin NEC 996.79
    infection or inflammation 996.69
    rejection 996.52
      artificial 996.55
      decellularized allodermis 996.55
  heart—*see also* Disease, heart
    transplant (immune or nonimmune cause)
      996.83
  hematoma (intraoperative) (postoperative)
    998.12
  hemorrhage (intraoperative) (postoperative)
    998.11
  hyperalimentation therapy NEC 999.9
  immunization (procedure)—*see* Complications,
    vaccination
  implant—*see also* Complications, due to
    (presence of) any device, implant, or graft
    classified to 996.0-996.5 NEC
    mechanical—*see* Complications, mechanical,
      implant
  infection and inflammation
    due to (presence of) any device, implant, or
      graft classified to 996.0-996.5 NEC 996.60
    arterial NEC 996.62
      coronary 996.61
      renal dialysis 996.62
    arteriovenous fistula or shunt 996.62
    bone growth stimulator 996.67
    breast 996.69
    cardiac 996.61
    catheter NEC 996.69
      peritoneal 996.68
      spinal 996.63
      urinary, indwelling 996.64
      vascular NEC 996.62
      ventricular shunt 996.63
    coronary artery bypass 996.61
    electrodes
      brain 996.63
      heart 996.61
    gastrointestinal NEC 996.69
    genitourinary NEC 996.65
      indwelling urinary catheter 996.64
    heart valve 996.61
    infusion pump 996.62
    intrauterine contraceptive device 996.65
    joint prosthesis, internal 996.66
    ocular lens 996.69
    orbital (implant) 996.69
    orthopedic NEC 996.67
      joint, internal 996.66
    specified type NEC 996.69
    urinary catheter, indwelling 996.64
    ventricular shunt 996.63

Complications—*continued*
  infusion (procedure) 999.9
    blood—*see* Complications, transfusion
    infection NEC 999.3
    sepsis NEC 999.3
  inhalation therapy NEC 999.9
  injection (procedure) 999.9
    drug reaction (*see also* Reaction, drug) 995.2
    infection NEC 999.3
    sepsis NEC 999.3
    serum (prophylactic) (therapeutic)—*see*
      Complications, vaccination
    vaccine (any)—*see* Complications, vaccination
  inoculation (any)—*see* Complications,
    vaccination
  internal device (catheter) (electronic) (fixation)
    (prosthetic) NEC—*see also* Complications,
    due to (presence of) any device, implant, or
    graft classified to 996.0-996.5 NEC
    mechanical—*see* Complications, mechanical
  intestinal transplant (immune or nonimmune
    cause) 996.87
  intraoperative bleeding or hemorrhage 998.11
  intrauterine contraceptive device (*see also*
    Complications, contraceptive device) 996.76
    infection or inflammation 996.65
    with fetal damage affecting management of
      pregnancy 655.8
  jejunostomy 569.60
  kidney transplant (immune or nonimmune
    cause) 996.81
  labor 669.9
    specified condition NEC 669.8
  liver transplant (immune or nonimmune cause)
    996.82
  lumbar puncture 349.0
  mechanical
    anastomosis—*see* Complications, mechanical,
      graft
    bypass—*see* Complications, mechanical, graft
    catheter NEC 996.59
      cardiac 996.09
      cystostomy 996.39
      dialysis (hemodialysis) 996.1
        peritoneal 996.56
      during a procedure 998.2
      urethral, indwelling 996.31
    colostomy 569.62
    device NEC 996.59
      balloon (counterpulsation), intra-aortic 996.1
      cardiac 996.00
        automatic implantable defibrillator 996.04
        long-term effect 429.4
        specified NEC 996.09
      contraceptive, intrauterine 996.32
      counterpulsation, intra-aortic 996.1
      fixation, external, with internal components
        996.4
      fixation, internal (nail, rod, plate) 996.4
      genitourinary 996.30
        specified NEC 996.39
      nervous system 996.2
      orthopedic, internal 996.4
      prosthetic NEC 996.59
      umbrella, vena cava 996.1
      vascular 996.1
    dorsal column stimulator 996.2
    electrode NEC 996.59
      brain 996.2
      cardiac 996.01
      spinal column 996.2

Complications—*continued*
  enterostomy 569.62
  fistula, arteriovenous, surgically created 996.1
  gastrostomy 536.42
  graft NEC 996.52
    aortic (bifurcation) 996.1
    aortocoronary bypass 996.03
    blood vessel NEC 996.1
    bone 996.4
    cardiac 996.00
    carotid artery bypass 996.1
    cartilage 996.4
    corneal 996.51
    coronary bypass 996.03
    decellularized allodermis 996.55
    genitourinary 996.30
      specified NEC 996.39
    muscle 996.4
    nervous system 996.2
    organ (immune or nonimmune cause) 996.80
      heart 996.83
      intestines 996.87
      kidney 996.81
      liver 996.82
      lung 996.84
      pancreas 996.86
      specified NEC 996.89
    orthopedic, internal 996.4
    peripheral nerve 996.2
    prosthetic NEC 996.59
    skin 996.52
      artificial 996.55
    specified NEC 996.59
    tendon 996.4
    tissue NEC 996.52
    tooth 996.59
    ureter, without mention of resection 996.39
    vascular 996.1
  heart valve prosthesis 996.02
    long-term effect 429.4
  implant NEC 996.59
    cardiac 996.00
      automatic implantable defibrillator 996.04
      long-term effect 429.4
      specified NEC 996.09
    electrode NEC 996.59
      brain 996.2
      cardiac 996.01
      spinal column 996.2
    genitourinary 996.30
    nervous system 996.2
    orthopedic, internal 996.4
    prosthetic NEC 996.59
      in
        bile duct 996.59
        breast 996.54
        chin 996.59
        eye
          ocular lens 996.53
          orbital globe 996.59
    vascular 996.1
  nonabsorbable surgical material 996.59
  pacemaker NEC 996.59
    brain 996.2
    cardiac 996.01
    nerve (phrenic) 996.2
  patch—*see* Complications, mechanical, graft
  prosthesis NEC 996.59
    bile duct 996.59
    breast 996.54
    chin 996.59

Complications—*continued*
    ocular lens 996.53
    reconstruction, vas deferens 996.39
    reimplant NEC 996.59
      extremity (*see also* Complications,
        reattached, extremity) 996.90
      organ (*see also* Complications, transplant,
        organ, by site) 996.80
      repair—*see* Complications, mechanical, graft
    shunt NEC 996.59
      arteriovenous, surgically created 996.1
      ventricular (communicating) 996.2
    stent NEC 996.59
    tracheostomy 519.02
    vas deferens reconstruction 996.39
  medical care NEC 999.9
    cardiac NEC 997.1
    gastrointestinal NEC 997.4
    nervous system NEC 997.00
    peripheral vascular NEC 997.2
    respiratory NEC 997.3
    urinary NEC 997.5
    vascular
      mesenteric artery 997.71
      other vessels 997.79
      peripheral vessels 997.2
      renal artery 997.72
  nephrostomy 997.5
  nervous system
    device, implant, or graft NEC 349.1
      mechanical 996.2
    postoperative NEC 997.00
  obstetric 669.9
    procedure (instrumental) (manual) (surgical)
      669.4
    specified NEC 669.8
    surgical wound 674.3
  ocular lens implant NEC 996.79
    infection or inflammation 996.69
    mechanical 996.53
  organ transplant—*see* Complications,
    transplant, organ, by site
  orthopedic device, implant, or graft
    internal (fixation) (nail) (plate) (rod) NEC
      996.78
      infection or inflammation 996.67
      joint prosthesis 996.77
        infection or inflammation 996.66
      mechanical 996.4
  pacemaker (cardiac) 996.72
    infection or inflammation 996.61
    mechanical 996.01
  pancreas transplant (immune or nonimmune
    cause) 996.86
  perfusion NEC 999.9
  perineal repair (obstetrical) 674.3
    disruption 674.2
  pessary (uterus) (vagina)—*see* Complications,
    contraceptive device
  phototherapy 990
  postcystoscopic 997.5
  postmastoidectomy NEC 383.30
  postoperative—*see* Complications, surgical
    procedures
  pregnancy NEC 646.9
    affecting fetus or newborn 761.9
  prosthetic device, internal—*see also*
    Complications, due to (presence of) any
    device, implant, or graft classified to
    996.0-996.5 NEC

Complications—*continued*
  mechanical NEC (*see also* Complications, mechanical) 996.59
  puerperium NEC (*see also* Puerperal) 674.9
  puncture, spinal 349.0
  pyelogram 997.5
  radiation 990
  radiotherapy 990
  reattached
    body part, except extremity 996.99
    extremity (infection) (rejection) 996.90
      arm(s) 996.94
      digit(s) (hand) 996.93
        foot 996.95
      finger(s) 996.93
      foot 996.95
      forearm 996.91
      hand 996.92
      leg 996.96
      lower NEC 996.96
      toe(s) 996.95
      upper NEC 996.94
  reimplant—*see also* Complications, due to (presence of) any device, implant, or graft classified to 996.0-996.5 NEC
    bone marrow 996.85
    extremity (*see also* Complications, reattached, extremity) 996.90
      due to infection 996.90
    mechanical—*see* Complications, mechanical, reimplant
    organ (immune or nonimmune cause) (partial) (total) (*see also* Complications, transplant, organ, by site) 996.80
  renal allograft 996.81
  renal dialysis—*see* Complications, dialysis
  respiratory 519.9
    device, implant or graft NEC 996.79
      infection or inflammation 996.69
      mechanical 996.59
    distress syndrome, adult, following trauma or surgery 518.5
    insufficiency, acute, postoperative 518.5
    postoperative NEC 997.3
    therapy NEC 999.9
  sedation during labor and delivery 668.9
    affecting fetus or newborn 763.5
    cardiac 668.1
    central nervous system 668.2
    pulmonary 668.0
    specified type NEC 668.8
  seroma (intraoperative) (postoperative) (noninfected) 998.13
    infected 998.51
  shunt—*see also* Complications, due to (presence of) any device, implant, or graft classified to 996.0-996.5 NEC
    mechanical—*see* Complications, mechanical, shunt
  specified body system NEC
    device, implant, or graft—*see* Complications, due to (presence of) any device, implant, or graft classified to 996.0-996.5 NEC
    postoperative NEC 997.99
  spinal puncture or tap 349.0
  stoma, external
    gastrointestinal tract
      colostomy 569.60
      enterostomy 569.60
      gastrostomy 536.40
    urinary tract 997.5

Complications— *continued*
  surgical procedures 998.9
    accidental puncture or laceration 998.2
    amputation stump (late) 997.60
    anastomosis—*see* Complications, anastomosis
    burst stitches or sutures (external) 998.32
      internal 998.31
    cardiac 997.1
      long-term effect following cardiac surgery 429.4
    cataract fragments in eye 998.82
    catheter device—*see* Complications, catheter device
    cecostomy malfunction 569.62
    colostomy malfunction 569.62
    cystostomy malfunction 997.5
    dehiscence (of incision) (external) 998.32
      internal 998.31
    dialysis NEC (*see also* Complications, dialysis) 999.9
    disruption
      anastomosis (internal)—*see* Complications, mechanical, graft
      internal suture (line) 998.31
      wound (external) 998.32
        internal 998.31
    dumping syndrome (postgastrectomy) 564.2
    elephantiasis or lymphedema 997.99
      postmastectomy 457.0
    emphysema (surgical) 998.81
    enterostomy malfunction 569.62
    evisceration 998.32
    fistula (persistent postoperative) 998.6
    foreign body inadvertently left in wound (sponge) (suture) (swab) 998.4
    from nonabsorbable surgical material (Dacron) (mesh) (permanent suture) (reinforcing) (Teflon)—*see* Complications, due to (presence of) any device, implant, or graft classified to 996.0-996.5 NEC
    gastrointestinal NEC 997.4
    gastrostomy malfunction 536.42
    hematoma 998.12
    hemorrhage 998.11
    ileostomy malfunction 569.62
    internal prosthetic device NEC (*see also* Complications, internal device) 996.70
      hemolytic anemia 283.19
      infection or inflammation 996.60
      malfunction—*see* Complications, mechanical
      mechanical complication—*see* Complications, mechanical
      thrombus 996.70
    jejunostomy malfunction 569.62
    nervous system NEC 997.00
    obstruction, internal anastomosis—*see* Complications, mechanical, graft
    other body system NEC 997.99
    peripheral vascular NEC 997.2
    postcardiotomy syndrome 429.4
    postcholecystectomy syndrome 576.0
    postcommissurotomy syndrome 429.4
    postgastrectomy dumping syndrome 564.2
    postmastectomy lymphedema syndrome 457.0
    postmastoidectomy 383.30
      cholesteatoma, recurrent 383.32
      cyst, mucosal 383.31
      granulation 383.33
      inflammation, chronic 383.33

Compression—*continued*
  with neurogenic bladder 344.61
  celiac (artery) (axis) 447.4
  cerebral—*see* Compression, brain
  cervical plexus 353.2
  cord (umbilical)—*see* Compression, umbilical
    cord
  cranial nerve 352.9
    second 377.49
    third (partial) 378.51
      total 378.52
    fourth 378.53
    fifth 350.8
    sixth 378.54
    seventh 351.8
  divers' squeeze 993.3
  duodenum (external) (*see also* Obstruction,
      duodenum) 537.3
  during birth 767.9
  esophagus 530.3
    congenital, external 750.3
  Eustachian tube 381.63
  facies (congenital) 754.0
  fracture—*see* Fracture, by site
  heart—*see* Disease, heart
  intestine (*see also* Obstruction, intestine) 560.9
    with hernia—*see* Hernia, by site, with
      obstruction
  laryngeal nerve, recurrent 478.79
  leg NEC 355.8
  lower extremity NEC 355.8
  lumbosacral plexus 353.1
  lung 518.89
  lymphatic vessel 457.1
  medulla—*see* Compression, brain
  nerve NEC—*see also* Disorder, nerve
    arm NEC 354.9
    autonomic nervous system (*see also*
      Neuropathy, peripheral, autonomic) 337.9
    axillary 353.0
    cranial NEC 352.9
    due to displacement of intervertebral disc
      722.2
      with myelopathy 722.70
      cervical 722.0
        with myelopathy 722.71
      lumbar, lumbosacral 722.10
        with myelopathy 722.73
      thoracic, thoracolumbar 722.11
        with myelopathy 722.72
    iliohypogastric 355.79
    ilioinguinal 355.79
    leg NEC 355.8
    lower extremity NEC 355.8
    median (in carpal tunnel) 354.0
    obturator 355.79
    optic 377.49
    plantar 355.6
    posterior tibial (in tarsal tunnel) 355.5
    root (by scar tissue) NEC 724.9
      cervical NEC 723.4
      lumbar NEC 724.4
      lumbosacral 724.4
      thoracic 724.4
    saphenous 355.79
    sciatic (acute) 355.0
    sympathetic 337.9
    traumatic—*see* Injury, nerve
    ulnar 354.2
    upper extremity NEC 354.9
  peripheral—*see* Compression, nerve

Compression—*continued*
  spinal (cord) (old or nontraumatic) 336.9
    by displacement of intervertebral disc—*see*
      Displacement, intervertebral disc
    nerve
      root NEC 724.9
        postoperative 722.80
          cervical region 722.81
          lumbar region 722.83
          thoracic region 722.82
        traumatic—*see* Injury, nerve, spinal
      traumatic—*see* Injury, nerve, spinal
    spondylogenic 721.91
      cervical 721.1
      lumbar, lumbosacral 721.42
      thoracic 721.41
    traumatic—*see also* Injury, spinal, by site
      with fracture, vertebra—*see* Fracture,
        vertebra, by site, with spinal cord injury
  spondylogenic—*see* Compression, spinal cord,
      spondylogenic
  subcostal nerve (syndrome) 354.8
  sympathetic nerve NEC 337.9
  syndrome 958.5
  thorax 512.8
    iatrogenic 512.1
    postoperative 512.1
  trachea 519.1
    congenital 748.3
  ulnar nerve (by scar tissue) 354.2
  umbilical cord
    affecting fetus or newborn 762.5
      cord prolapsed 762.4
    complicating delivery 663.2
      cord around neck 663.1
      cord prolapsed 663.0
  upper extremity NEC 354.9
  ureter 593.3
  urethra—*see* Stricture, urethra
  vein 459.2
  vena cava (inferior) (superior) 459.2
  vertebral NEC—*see* Compression, spinal (cord)
Compulsion, compulsive
  eating 307.51
  neurosis (obsessive) 300.3
  personality 301.4
  states (mixed) 300.3
  swearing 300.3
    in Gilles de la Tourette's syndrome 307.23
  tics and spasms 307.22
  water drinking NEC (syndrome) 307.9
Concato's disease (pericardial polyserositis)
    423.2
  peritoneal 568.82
  pleural—*see* Pleurisy
Concavity, chest wall 738.3
Concealed
  hemorrhage NEC 459.0
  penis 752.65
Concentric fading 368.12
Concern (normal) about sick person in family
    V61.49
Concrescence (teeth) 520.2
Concretio cordis 423.1
  rheumatic 393
Concretion —*see also* Calculus
  appendicular 543.9
  canaliculus 375.57
  clitoris 624.8
  conjunctiva 372.54
  eyelid 374.56

Concretion—*continued*
  intestine (impaction) (obstruction) 560.39
  lacrimal (passages) 375.57
  prepuce (male) 605
    female (clitoris) 624.8
  salivary gland (any) 527.5
  seminal vesicle 608.89
  stomach 537.89
  tonsil 474.8
Concussion (current) 850.9
  with
    loss of consciousness 850.5
      brief (less than one hour) 850.1
      moderate (1-24 hours) 850.2
      prolonged (more than 24 hours) (with
        complete recovery) (with return to
        pre-existing conscious level) 850.3
        without return to pre-existing conscious
        level 850.4
    mental confusion or disorientation (without
      loss of consciousness) 850.0
      with loss of consciousness—*see*
        Concussion, with, loss of consciousness
    without loss of consciousness 850.0
  blast (air) (hydraulic) (immersion) (underwater)
    869.0
    with open wound into cavity 869.1
    abdomen or thorax—*see* Injury, internal, by
      site
    brain—*see* Concussion, brain
    ear (acoustic nerve trauma) 951.5
      with perforation, tympanic membrane—*see*
        Wound, open, ear drum
    thorax—*see* Injury, internal, intrathoracic
      organs NEC
  brain or cerebral (without skull fracture) 850.9
    with
      loss of consciousness 850.5
        brief (less than one hour) 850.1
        moderate (1-24 hours) 850.2
        prolonged (more than 24 hours) (with
          complete recovery) (with return to
          pre-existing conscious level) 850.3
          without return to pre-existing conscious
          level 850.4
      mental confusion or disorientation (without
        loss of consciousness) 850.0
        with loss of consciousness—*see*
          Concussion, brain, with, loss of
          consciousness
    skull fracture—*see* Fracture, skull, by site
    without loss of consciousness 850.0
  cauda equina 952.4
  cerebral—*see* Concussion, brain
  conus medullaris (spine) 952.4
  hydraulic—*see* Concussion, blast
  internal organs—*see* Injury, internal, by site
  labyrinth—*see* Injury, intracranial
  ocular 921.3
  osseous labyrinth—*see* Injury, intracranial
  spinal (cord)—*see also* Injury, spinal, by site
    due to
      broken
        back—*see* Fracture, vertebra, by site, with
          spinal cord injury
        neck—*see* Fracture, vertebra, cervical,
          with spinal cord injury
      fracture, fracture dislocation, or
        compression fracture of spine or
        vertebra—*see* Fracture, vertebra, by site,
        with spinal cord injury

Concussion—*continued*
  syndrome 310.2
  underwater blast—*see* Concussion, blast
Condition —*see also* Disease
  psychiatric 298.9
  respiratory NEC 519.9
    acute or subacute NEC 519.9
      due to
        external agent 508.9
          specified type NEC 508.8
        fumes or vapors (chemical) (inhalation)
          506.3
        radiation 508.0
    chronic NEC 519.9
      due to
        external agent 508.9
          specified type NEC 508.8
        fumes or vapors (chemical) (inhalation)
          506.4
        radiation 508.1
    due to
      external agent 508.9
        specified type NEC 508.8
      fumes or vapors (chemical) (inhalation)
        506.9
Conduct disturbance (*see also* Disturbance,
  conduct) 312.9
  adjustment reaction 309.3
  hyperkinetic 314.2
Condyloma NEC 078.10
  acuminatum 078.11
  gonorrheal 098.0
  latum 091.3
  syphilitic 091.3
    congenital 090.0
  venereal, syphilitic 091.3
Confinement —*see* Delivery
Conflagration —*see also* Burn, by site
  asphyxia (by inhalation of smoke, gases, fumes,
    or vapors) 987.9
    specified agent—*see* Table of drugs and
      chemicals
Conflict
  family V61.9
    specified circumstance NEC V61.8
  interpersonal NEC V62.81
  marital V61.10
    involving divorce or estrangement V61.0
  parent-child V61.20
  partner V61.10
Confluent —*see* condition
Confusion, confused (mental) (state) (*see also*
  State, confusional) 298.9
  acute 293.0
  epileptic 293.0
  postoperative 293.9
  psychogenic 298.2
  reactive (from emotional stress, psychological
    trauma) 298.2
  subacute 293.1
Congelation 991.9
Congenital —*see also* condition
  aortic septum 747.29
  intrinsic factor deficiency 281.0
  malformation—*see* Anomaly
Congestion, congestive (chronic) (passive)
  asphyxia, newborn 768.9
  bladder 596.8
  bowel 569.89
  brain (*see also* Disease, cerebrovascular NEC)
    437.8

Congestion, congestive—*continued*
malarial 084.9
breast 611.79
bronchi 519.1
bronchial tube 519.1
catarrhal 472.0
cerebral—*see* Congestion, brain
cerebrospinal—*see* Congestion, brain
chest 514
chill 780.99
malarial (*see also* Malaria) 084.6
circulatory NEC 459.9
conjunctiva 372.71
due to disturbance of circulation 459.9
duodenum 537.3
enteritis—*see* Enteritis
eye 372.71
fibrosis syndrome (pelvic) 625.5
gastroenteritis—*see* Enteritis
general 799.8
glottis 476.0
heart (*see also* Failure, heart) 428.0
hepatic 573.0
hypostatic (lung) 514
intestine 569.89
intracranial—*see* Congestion, brain
kidney 593.89
labyrinth 386.50
larynx 476.0
liver 573.0
lung 514
active or acute (*see also* Pneumonia) 486
congenital 770.0
chronic 514
hypostatic 514
idiopathic, acute 518.5
passive 514
malaria, malarial (brain) (fever) (*see also* Malaria) 084.6
medulla—*see* Congestion, brain
nasal 478.1
orbit, orbital 376.33
inflammatory (chronic) 376.10
acute 376.00
ovary 620.8
pancreas 577.8
pelvic, female 625.5
pleural 511.0
prostate (active) 602.1
pulmonary—*see* Congestion, lung
renal 593.89
retina 362.89
seminal vesicle 608.89
spinal cord 336.1
spleen 289.51
chronic 289.51
stomach 537.89
trachea 464.11
urethra 599.84
uterus 625.5
with subinvolution 621.1
viscera 799.8
Congestive —*see* Congestion
Conical
cervix 622.6
cornea 371.60
teeth 520.2
Conjoined twins 759.4
causing disproportion (fetopelvic) 653.7
Conjugal maladjustment V61.10
involving divorce or estrangement V61.0
Conjunctiva —*see* condition

Conjunctivitis (exposure) (infectious)
(nondiphtheritic) (pneumococcal) (pustular)
(staphylococcal) (streptococcal) NEC 372.30
actinic 370.24
acute 372.00
atopic 372.05
contagious 372.03
follicular 372.02
hemorrhagic (viral) 077.4
adenoviral (acute) 077.3
allergic (chronic) 372.14
with hay fever 372.05
anaphylactic 372.05
angular 372.03
Apollo (viral) 077.4
atopic 372.05
blennorrhagic (neonatorum) 098.40
catarrhal 372.03
chemical 372.05
chlamydial 077.98
due to
Chlamydial trachomatis—*see* Trachoma
paratrachoma 077.0
chronic 372.10
allergic 372.14
follicular 372.12
simple 372.11
specified type NEC 372.14
vernal 372.13
diphtheritic 032.81
due to
dust 372.05
enterovirus type 70 077.4
erythema multiforme 695.1 *[372.33]*
filariasis (*see also* Filariasis) 125.9 *[372.15]*
mucocutaneous
disease NEC 372.33
leishmaniasis 085.5 *[372.15]*
Reiter's disease 099.3 *[372.33]*
syphilis 095.8 *[372.10]*
toxoplasmosis (acquired) 130.1
congenital (active) 771.2
trachoma—*see* Trachoma
dust 372.05
eczematous 370.31
epidemic 077.1
hemorrhagic 077.4
follicular (acute) 372.02
adenoviral (acute) 077.3
chronic 372.12
glare 370.24
gonococcal (neonatorum) 098.40
granular (trachomatous) 076.1
late effect 139.1
hemorrhagic (acute) (epidemic) 077.4
herpetic (simplex) 054.43
zoster 053.21
inclusion 077.0
infantile 771.6
influenzal 372.03
Koch-Weeks 372.03
light 372.05
medicamentosa 372.05
membranous 372.04
meningococcic 036.89
Morax-Axenfeld 372.02
mucopurulent NEC 372.03
neonatal 771.6
gonococcal 098.40
Newcastle's 077.8
nodosa 360.14

Conjunctivitis—*continued*
  of Beal 077.3
  parasitic 372.15
    filariasis (*see also* Filariasis) 125.9 *[372.15]*
    mucocutaneous leishmaniasis 085.5 *[372.15]*
  Parinaud's 372.02
  petrificans 372.39
  phlyctenular 370.31
  pseudomembranous 372.04
    diphtheritic 032.81
  purulent 372.03
  Reiter's 099.3 *[372.33]*
  rosacea 695.3 *[372.31]*
  serous 372.01
    viral 077.99
  simple chronic 372.11
  specified NEC 372.39
  sunlamp 372.04
  swimming pool 077.0
  trachomatous (follicular) 076.1
    acute 076.0
    late effect 139.1
  traumatic NEC 372.39
  tuberculous (*see also* Tuberculosis) 017.3
    [370.31]
  tularemic 021.3
  tularensis 021.3
  vernal 372.13
    limbar 372.13 *[370.32]*
  viral 077.99
    acute hemorrhagic 077.4
    specified NEC 077.8
Conjunctivochalasis 372.81
Conjunctoblepharitis —*see* Conjunctivitis
Conn (-Louis) syndrome (primary aldosteronism)
  255.1
Connective tissue —*see* condition
Conradi (-Hünermann) syndrome or disease
  (chondrodysplasia calcificans congenita)
  756.59
Consanguinity V19.7
Consecutive —*see* condition
Consolidated lung (base)—*see* Pneumonia, lobar
Constipation 564.00
  atonic 564.09
  drug induced
    correct substance properly administered
      564.09
    overdose or wrong substance given or taken
      977.9
      specified drug—*see* Table of drugs and
        chemicals
  neurogenic 564.09
  other specified NEC 564.09
  outlet dysfunction 564.02
  psychogenic 306.4
  simple 564.00
  slow transit 564.01
  spastic 564.09
Constitutional —*see also* condition
  arterial hypotension (*see also* Hypotension)
    458.9
  obesity 278.00
    morbid 278.01
  psychopathic state 301.9
  short stature in childhood 783.43
  state, developmental V21.9
    specified development NEC V21.8
  substandard 301.6
Constitutionally substandard 301.6

Constriction
  anomalous, meningeal bands or folds 742.8
  aortic arch (congenital) 747.10
  asphyxiation or suffocation by 994.7
  bronchus 519.1
  canal, ear (*see also* Stricture, ear canal,
    acquired) 380.50
  duodenum 537.3
  gallbladder (*see also* Obstruction, gallbladder)
    575.2
    congenital 751.69
  intestine (*see also* Obstruction, intestine) 560.9
  larynx 478.74
    congenital 748.3
  meningeal bands or folds, anomalous 742.8
  organ or site, congenital NEC—*see* Atresia
  prepuce (congenital) 605
  pylorus 537.0
    adult hypertrophic 537.0
    congenital or infantile 750.5
    newborn 750.5
  ring (uterus) 661.4
    affecting fetus or newborn 763.7
  spastic—*see also* Spasm
    ureter 593.3
    urethra—*see* Stricture, urethra
  stomach 537.89
  ureter 593.3
  urethra—*see* Stricture, urethra
  visual field (functional) (peripheral) 368.45
Constrictive —*see* condition
Consultation V65.9
  medical—*see also* Counseling, medical
    specified reason NEC V65.8
  without complaint or sickness V65.9
    feared complaint unfounded V65.5
    specified reason NEC V65.8
Consumption —*see* Tuberculosis
Contact
  with
    AIDS virus V01.7
    anthrax V01.81
    cholera V01.0
    communicable disease V01.9
      specified type NEC V01.89
      viral NEC V01.7
    German measles V01.4
    gonorrhea V01.6
    HIV V01.7
    human immunodeficiency virus V01.7
    parasitic disease NEC V01.89
    poliomyelitis V01.2
    rabies V01.5
    rubella V01.4
    smallpox V01.3
    syphilis V01.6
    tuberculosis V01.1
    venereal disease V01.6
    viral disease NEC V01.7
  dermatitis—*see* Dermatitis
Contamination, food (*see also* Poisoning, food)
  005.9
Contraception, contraceptive
  advice NEC V25.09
    family planning V25.09
    fitting of diaphragm V25.02
    prescribing or use of
      oral contraceptive agent V25.01
      specified agent NEC V25.02
  counseling NEC V25.09
    family planning V25.09

Contraception, contraceptive—*continued*
  fitting of diaphragm V25.02
  prescribing or use of
    oral contraceptive agent V25.01
    specified agent NEC V25.02
  device (in situ) V45.59
    causing menorrhagia 996.76
    checking V25.42
    complications 996.32
    insertion V25.1
    intrauterine V45.51
    reinsertion V25.42
    removal V25.42
    subdermal V45.52
  fitting of diaphragm V25.02
  insertion
    intrauterine contraceptive device V25.1
    subdermal implantable V25.5
  maintenance V25.40
    examination V25.40
      intrauterine device V25.42
      oral contraceptive V25.41
      specified method NEC V25.49
      subdermal implantable V25.43
    intrauterine device V25.42
    oral contraceptive V25.41
    specified method NEC V25.49
    subdermal implantable V25.43
  management NEC V25.49
  prescription
    oral contraceptive agent V25.01
      repeat V25.41
    specified agent NEC V25.02
      repeat V25.49
  sterilization V25.2
  surveillance V25.40
    intrauterine device V25.42
    oral contraceptive agent V25.41
    specified method NEC V25.49
    subdermal implantable V25.43
Contraction, contracture, contracted
  Achilles tendon (*see also* Short, tendon,
      Achilles) 727.81
  anus 564.89
  axilla 729.9
  bile duct (*see also* Disease, biliary) 576.8
  bladder 596.8
    neck or sphincter 596.0
  bowel (*see also* Obstruction, intestine) 560.9
  Braxton Hicks 644.1
  bronchus 519.1
  burn (old)—*see* Cicatrix
  cecum (*see also* Obstruction, intestine) 560.9
  cervix (*see also* Stricture, cervix) 622.4
    congenital 752.49
  cicatricial—*see* Cicatrix
  colon (*see also* Obstruction, intestine) 560.9
  conjunctiva trachomatous, active 076.1
    late effect 139.1
  Dupuytren's 728.6
  eyelid 374.41
  eye socket (after enucleation) 372.64
  face 729.9
  fascia (lata) (postural) 728.89
    Dupuytren's 728.6
    palmar 728.6
    plantar 728.71
  finger NEC 736.29
    congenital 755.59
    joint (*see also* Contraction, joint) 718.44
  flaccid, paralytic

Contraction—*continued*
  joint (*see also* Contraction, joint) 718.4
  muscle 728.85
    ocular 378.50
  gallbladder (*see also* Obstruction, gallbladder)
      575.2
  hamstring 728.89
    tendon 727.81
  heart valve—*see* Endocarditis
  Hicks' 644.1
  hip (*see also* Contraction, joint) 718.4
  hourglass
    bladder 596.8
      congenital 753.8
    gallbladder (*see also* Obstruction, gallbladder)
        575.2
      congenital 751.69
    stomach 536.8
      congenital 750.7
      psychogenic 306.4
    uterus 661.4
      affecting fetus or newborn 763.7
  hysterical 300.11
  infantile (*see also* Epilepsy) 345.6
  internal os (*see also* Stricture, cervix) 622.4
  intestine (*see also* Obstruction, intestine) 560.9
  joint (abduction) (acquired) (adduction)
      (flexion) (rotation) 718.40
    ankle 718.47
    congenital NEC 755.8
      generalized or multiple 754.89
        lower limb joints 754.89
      hip (*see also* Subluxation, congenital, hip)
          754.32
    lower limb (including pelvic girdle) not
        involving hip 754.89
    upper limb (including shoulder girdle) 755.59
    elbow 718.42
    foot 718.47
    hand 718.44
    hip 718.45
    hysterical 300.11
    knee 718.46
    multiple sites 718.49
    pelvic region 718.45
    shoulder (region) 718.41
    specified site NEC 718.48
    wrist 718.43
  kidney (granular) (secondary) (*see also*
      Sclerosis, renal) 587
    congenital 753.3
    hydronephritic 591
    pyelonephritic (*see also* Pyelitis, chronic)
        590.00
    tuberculous (*see also* Tuberculosis) 016.0
  ligament 728.89
    congenital 756.89
  liver—*see* Cirrhosis, liver
  muscle (postinfectional) (postural) NEC 728.85
    congenital 756.89
      sternocleidomastoid 754.1
    extraocular 378.60
    eye (extrinsic) (*see also* Strabismus) 378.9
      paralytic (*see also* Strabismus, paralytic)
          378.50
    flaccid 728.85
    hysterical 300.11
    ischemic (Volkmann's) 958.6
    paralytic 728.85
    posttraumatic 958.6
    psychogenic 306.0

Contraction—*continued*
    specified as conversion reaction 300.11
  myotonic 728.85
  neck (*see also* Torticollis) 723.5
    congenital 754.1
    psychogenic 306.0
  ocular muscle (*see also* Strabismus) 378.9
    paralytic (*see also* Strabismus, paralytic) 378.50
  organ or site, congenital NEC—*see* Atresia
  outlet (pelvis)—*see* Contraction, pelvis
  palmar fascia 728.6
  paralytic
    joint (*see also* Contraction, joint) 718.4
    muscle 728.85
      ocular (*see also* Strabismus, paralytic) 378.50
  pelvis (acquired) (general) 738.6
    affecting fetus or newborn 763.1
    complicating delivery 653.1
      causing obstructed labor 660.1
    generally contracted 653.1
      causing obstructed labor 660.1
    inlet 653.2
      causing obstructed labor 660.1
    midpelvic 653.8
      causing obstructed labor 660.1
    midplane 653.8
      causing obstructed labor 660.1
    outlet 653.3
      causing obstructed labor 660.1
  plantar fascia 728.71
  premature
    atrial 427.61
    auricular 427.61
    auriculoventricular 427.61
    heart (junctional) (nodal) 427.60
    supraventricular 427.61
    ventricular 427.69
  prostate 602.8
  pylorus (*see also* Pylorospasm) 537.81
  rectosigmoid (*see also* Obstruction, intestine) 560.9
  rectum, rectal (sphincter) 564.89
    psychogenic 306.4
  ring (Bandl's) 661.4
    affecting fetus or newborn 763.7
  scar—*see* Cicatrix
  sigmoid (*see also* Obstruction, intestine) 560.9
  socket, eye 372.64
  spine (*see also* Curvature, spine) 737.9
  stomach 536.8
    hourglass 536.8
      congenital 750.7
      psychogenic 306.4
    psychogenic 306.4
  tendon (sheath) (*see also* Short, tendon) 727.81
  toe 735.8
  ureterovesical orifice (postinfectional) 593.3
  urethra 599.84
  uterus 621.8
    abnormal 661.9
      affecting fetus or newborn 763.7
    clonic, hourglass or tetanic 661.4
      affecting fetus or newborn 763.7
    dyscoordinate 661.4
      affecting fetus or newborn 763.7
    hourglass 661.4
      affecting fetus or newborn 763.7
    hypotonic NEC 661.2
      affecting fetus or newborn 763.7

Contraction—*continued*
  incoordinate 661.4
    affecting fetus or newborn 763.7
  inefficient or poor 661.2
    affecting fetus or newborn 763.7
  irregular 661.2
    affecting fetus or newborn 763.7
  tetanic 661.4
    affecting fetus or newborn 763.7
  vagina (outlet) 623.2
  vesical 596.8
    neck or urethral orifice 596.0
  visual field, generalized 368.45
  Volkmann's (ischemic) 958.6
Contusion (skin surface intact) 924.9
  with
    crush injury—*see* Crush
    dislocation—*see* Dislocation, by site
    fracture—*see* Fracture, by site
    internal injury—*see also* Injury, internal, by site
    heart—*see* Contusion, cardiac
    kidney—*see* Contusion, kidney
    liver—*see* Contusion, liver
    lung—*see* Contusion, lung
    spleen—*see* Contusion, spleen
    intracranial injury—*see* Injury, intracranial
    nerve injury—*see* Injury, nerve
    open wound—*see* Wound, open, by site
  abdomen, abdominal (muscle) (wall) 922.2
    organ(s) NEC 868.00
  adnexa, eye NEC 921.9
  ankle 924.21
    with other parts of foot 924.20
  arm 923.9
    lower (with elbow) 923.10
    upper 923.03
      with shoulder or axillary region 923.09
  auditory canal (external) (meatus) (and other part(s) of neck, scalp, or face, except eye) 920
  auricle, ear (and other part(s) of neck, scalp, or face except eye) 920
  axilla 923.02
    with shoulder or upper arm 923.09
  back 922.31
  bone NEC 924.9
  brain (cerebral) (membrane) (with hemorrhage) 851.8

Note—Use the following fifth-digit subclassification with categories 851-854:

0 unspecified state of consciousness
1 with no loss of consciousness
2 with brief [less than one hour] loss of consciousness
3 with moderate [1-24 hours] loss of consciousness
4 with prolonged [more than 24 hours] loss of consciousness and return to pre-existing conscious level
5 with prolonged [more than 24 hours] loss of consciousness, without return to pre-existing conscious level
Use fifth-digit 5 to designate when a patient is unconscious and dies before regaining conciousness, regardless of the duration of the loss of conciousness
6 with loss of consciousness of unspecified duration
9 with concussion, unspecified

Contusion—*continued*
  with
    open intracranial wound 851.9
    skull fracture—*see* Fracture, skull, by site
  cerebellum 851.4
    with open intracranial wound 851.5
  cortex 851.0
    with open intracranial wound 851.1
  occipital lobe 851.4
    with open intracranial wound 851.5
  stem 851.4
    with open intracranial wound 851.5
  breast 922.0
  brow (and other part(s) of neck, scalp, or face, except eye) 920
  buttock 922.32
  canthus 921.1
  cardiac 861.01
    with open wound into thorax 861.11
  cauda equina (spine) 952.4
  cerebellum—*see* Contusion, brain, cerebellum
  cerebral—*see* Contusion, brain
  cheek(s) (and other part(s) of neck, scalp, or face, except eye) 920
  chest (wall) 922.1
  chin (and other part(s) of neck, scalp, or face, except eye) 920
  clitoris 922.4
  conjunctiva 921.1
  conus medullaris (spine) 952.4
  cornea 921.3
  corpus cavernosum 922.4
  cortex (brain) (cerebral)—*see* Contusion, brain, cortex
  costal region 922.1
  ear (and other part(s) of neck, scalp, or face except eye) 920
  elbow 923.11
    with forearm 923.10
  epididymis 922.4
  epigastric region 922.2
  eye NEC 921.9
  eyeball 921.3
  eyelid(s) (and periocular area) 921.1
  face (and neck, or scalp any part, except eye) 920
  femoral triangle 922.2
  fetus or newborn 772.6
  finger(s) (nail) (subungual) 923.3
  flank 922.2
  foot (with ankle) (excluding toe(s)) 924.20
  forearm (and elbow) 923.10
  forehead (and other part(s) of neck, scalp, or face, except eye) 920
  genital organs, external 922.4
  globe (eye) 921.3
  groin 922.2
  gum(s) (and other part(s) of neck, scalp, or face, except eye) 920
  hand(s) (except fingers alone) 923.20
  head (any part, except eye) (and face) (and neck) 920
  heart—*see* Contusion, cardiac
  heel 924.20
  hip 924.01
    with thigh 924.00
  iliac region 922.2
  inguinal region 922.2
  internal organs (abdomen, chest, or pelvis) NEC—*see* Injury, internal, by site
  interscapular region 922.33

Contusion—*continued*
  iris (eye) 921.3
  kidney 866.01
    with open wound into cavity 866.11
  knee 924.11
    with lower leg 924.10
  labium (majus) (minus) 922.4
  lacrimal apparatus, gland, or sac 921.1
  larynx (and other part(s) of neck, scalp, or face, except eye) 920
  late effect—*see* Late, effects (of), contusion
  leg 924.5
    lower (with knee) 924.10
  lens 921.3
  lingual (and other part(s) of neck, scalp, or face, except eye) 920
  lip(s) (and other part(s) of neck, scalp, or face, except eye) 920
  liver 864.01
    with
      laceration—*see* Laceration, liver
      open wound into cavity 864.11
  lower extremity 924.5
    multiple sites 924.4
  lumbar region 922.31
  lung 861.21
    with open wound into thorax 861.31
  malar region (and other part(s) of neck, scalp, or face, except eye) 920
  mandibular joint (and other part(s) of neck, scalp, or face, except eye) 920
  mastoid region (and other part(s) of neck, scalp, or face, except eye) 920
  membrane, brain—*see* Contusion, brain
  midthoracic region 922.1
  mouth (and other part(s) of neck, scalp, or face, except eye) 920
  multiple sites (not classifiable to same three-digit category) 924.8
    lower limb 924.4
    trunk 922.8
    upper limb 923.8
  muscle NEC 924.9
  myocardium—*see* Contusion, cardiac
  nasal (septum) (and other part(s) of neck, scalp, or face, except eye) 920
  neck (and scalp, or face any part, except eye) 920
  nerve—*see* Injury, nerve, by site
  continuednose (and other part(s) of neck, scalp, or face, except eye) 920
  occipital region (scalp) (and neck or face, except eye) 920
    lobe—*see* Contusion, brain, occipital lobe
  orbit (region) (tissues) 921.2
  palate (soft) (and other part(s) of neck, scalp, or face, except eye) 920
  parietal region (scalp) (and neck, or face, except eye) 920
    lobe—*see* Contusion, brain
  penis 922.4
  pericardium—*see* Contusion, cardiac
  perineum 922.4
  periocular area 921.1
  pharynx (and other part(s) of neck, scalp, or face, except eye) 920
  popliteal space (*see also* Contusion, knee) 924.11
  prepuce 922.4
  pubic region 922.4
  pudenda 922.4

Contusion—*continued*
pulmonary—*see* Contusion, lung
quadriceps femoralis 924.00
rib cage 922.1
sacral region 922.32
salivary ducts or glands (and other part(s) of neck, scalp, or face, except eye) 920
scalp (and neck, or face any part, except eye) 920
scapular region 923.01
with shoulder or upper arm 923.09
sclera (eye) 921.3
scrotum 922.4
shoulder 923.00
with upper arm or axillar regions 923.09
skin NEC 924.9
skull 920
spermatic cord 922.4
spinal cord—*see also* Injury, spinal, by site
cauda equina 952.4
conus medullaris 952.4
spleen 865.01
with open wound into cavity 865.11
sternal region 922.1
stomach—*see* Injury, internal, stomach
subconjunctival 921.1
subcutaneous NEC 924.9
submaxillary region (and other part(s) of neck, scalp, or face, except eye) 920
submental region (and other part(s) of neck, scalp, or face, except eye) 920
subperiosteal NEC 924.9
supraclavicular fossa (and other part(s) of neck, scalp, or face, except eye) 920
supraorbital (and other part(s) of neck, scalp, or face, except eye) 920
temple (region) (and other part(s) of neck, scalp, or face, except eye) 920
testis 922.4
thigh (and hip) 924.00
thorax 922.1
organ—*see* Injury, internal, intrathoracic
throat (and other part(s) of neck, scalp, or face, except eye) 920
thumb(s) (nail) (subungual) 923.3
toe(s) (nail) (subungual) 924.3
tongue (and other part(s) of neck, scalp, or face, except eye) 920
trunk 922.9
multiple sites 922.8
specified site—*see* Contusion, by site
tunica vaginalis 922.4
tympanum (membrane) (and other part(s) of neck, scalp, or face, except eye) 920
upper extremity 923.9
multiple sites 923.8
uvula (and other part(s) of neck, scalp, or face, except eye) 920
vagina 922.4
vocal cord(s) (and other part(s) of neck, scalp, or face, except eye) 920
vulva 922.4
wrist 923.21
with hand(s), except finger(s) alone 923.20
Conus (any type) (congenital) 743.57
acquired 371.60
medullaris syndrome 336.8
Convalescence (following) V66.9
chemotherapy V66.2
medical NEC V66.5
psychotherapy V66.3

Convalescence—*continued*
radiotherapy V66.1
surgery NEC V66.0
treatment (for) NEC V66.5
combined V66.6
fracture V66.4
mental disorder NEC V66.3
specified disorder NEC V66.5
Conversion
hysteria, hysterical, any type 300.11
laparoscopic surgical procedure to open procedure V64.4
neurosis, any 300.11
reaction, any 300.11
Converter, tuberculosis (test reaction) 795.5
Convulsions (idiopathic) 780.39
apoplectiform (*see also* Disease, cerebrovascular, acute) 436
brain 780.39
cerebral 780.39
cerebrospinal 780.39
due to trauma NEC—*see* Injury, intracranial
eclamptic (*see also* Eclampsia) 780.39
epileptic (*see also* Epilepsy) 345.9
epileptiform (*see also* Seizure, epileptiform) 780.39
epileptoid (*see also* Seizure, epileptiform) 780.39
ether
anesthetic
correct substance properly administered 780.39
overdose or wrong substance given 968.2
other specified type—*see* Table of drugs and chemicals
febrile 780.31
generalized 780.39
hysterical 300.11
infantile 780.39
epilepsy—*see* Epilepsy
internal 780.39
jacksonian (*see also* Epilepsy) 345.5
myoclonic 333.2
newborn 779.0
paretic 094.1
pregnancy (nephritic) (uremic)—*see* Eclampsia, pregnancy
psychomotor (*see also* Epilepsy) 345.4
puerperal, postpartum—*see* Eclampsia, pregnancy
recurrent 780.39
epileptic—*see* Epilepsy
reflex 781.0
repetitive 780.39
epileptic—*see* Epilepsy
salaam (*see also* Epilepsy) 345.6
scarlatinal 034.1
spasmodic 780.39
tetanus, tetanic (*see also* Tetanus) 037
thymic 254.8
uncinate 780.39
uremic 586
Convulsive —*see also* Convulsions
disorder or state 780.39
epileptic—*see* Epilepsy
equivalent, abdominal (*see also* Epilepsy) 345.5
Cooke-Apert-Gallais syndrome (adrenogenital) 255.2
Cooley's anemia (erythroblastic) 282.4
Coolie itch 126.9

Cooper's
  disease 610.1
  hernia—*see* Hernia, Cooper's
Coordination disturbance 781.3
Copper wire arteries, retina 362.13
Copra itch 133.8
Coprolith 560.39
Coprophilia 302.89
Coproporphyria, hereditary 277.1
Coprostasis 560.39
  with hernia—*see also* Hernia, by site, with
    obstruction
  gangrenous—*see* Hernia, by site, with
    gangrene
Cor
  biloculare 745.7
  bovinum—*see* Hypertrophy, cardiac
  bovis—*see also* Hypertrophy, cardiac
  pulmonale (chronic) 416.9
    acute 415.0
  triatriatum, triatrium 746.82
  triloculare 745.8
    biatriatum 745.3
    biventriculare 745.69
Corbus' disease 607.1
Cord —*see also* condition
  around neck (tightly) (with compression)
    affecting fetus or newborn 762.5
    complicating delivery 663.1
      without compression 663.3
        affecting fetus or newborn 762.6
  bladder NEC 344.61
    tabetic 094.0
  prolapse
    affecting fetus or newborn 762.4
    complicating delivery 663.0
Cord's angiopathy (*see also* Tuberculosis) 017.3
  [362.18]
Cordis ectopia 746.87
Corditis (spermatic) 608.4
Corectopia 743.46
Cori type glycogen storage disease —*see*
  Disease, glycogen storage
Cork-handlers' disease or lung 495.3
Corkscrew esophagus 530.5
Corlett's pyosis (impetigo) 684
Corn (infected) 700
Cornea—*see also* condition
  donor V59.5
  guttata (dystrophy) 371.57
  plana 743.41
Cornelia de Lange's syndrome (Amsterdam
  dwarf, mental retardation, and brachycephaly)
  759.89
Cornual gestation or pregnancy —*see*
  Pregnancy, cornual
Cornu cutaneum 702.8
Coronary (artery)—*see also* condition
  arising from aorta or pulmonary trunk 746.85
Corpora —*see also* condition
  amylacea (prostate) 602.8
  cavernosa—*see* condition
Corpulence (*see also* Obesity) 278.0
Corpus —*see* condition
Corrigan's disease —*see* Insufficiency, aortic
Corrosive burn —*see* Burn, by site
Corsican fever (*see also* Malaria) 084.6
Cortical —*see also* condition
  blindness 377.75
  necrosis, kidney (bilateral) 583.6
Corticoadrenal —*see* condition
Corticosexual syndrome 255.2

Coryza (acute) 460
  with grippe or influenza 487.1
  syphilitic 095.8
    congenital (chronic) 090.0
Costen's syndrome or complex 524.60
Costiveness (*see also* Constipation) 564.00
Costochondritis 733.6
Cotard's syndrome (paranoia) 297.1
Cot death 798.0
Cotungo's disease 724.3
Cough 786.2
  with hemorrhage (*see also* Hemoptysis) 786.3
  affected 786.2
  bronchial 786.2
    with grippe or influenza 487.1
  chronic 786.2
  epidemic 786.2
  functional 306.1
  hemorrhagic 786.3
  hysterical 300.11
  laryngeal, spasmodic 786.2
  nervous 786.2
  psychogenic 306.1
  smokers' 491.0
  tea tasters' 112.89
Counseling NEC V65.40
  without complaint or sickness V65.49
  abuse victim NEC V62.89
    child V61.21
    partner V61.11
    spouse V61.11
  child abuse, maltreatment, or neglect V61.21
  contraceptive NEC V25.09
    device (intrauterine) V25.02
    maintenance V25.40
      intrauterine contraceptive device V25.42
      oral contraceptive (pill) V25.41
      specified type NEC V25.49
      subdermal implantable V25.43
    management NEC V25.9
    oral contraceptive (pill) V25.01
    prescription NEC V25.02
      oral contraceptive (pill) V25.01
        repeat prescription V25.41
      repeat prescription V25.40
    subdermal implantable V25.43
    surveillance V25.40
  dietary V65.3
  exercise V65.41
  explanation of
    investigation finding NEC V65.49
    medication NEC V65.49
  family planning V25.09
  for nonattending third party V65.1
  genetic V26.3
  gonorrhea V65.45
  health (advice) (education) (instruction) NEC
    V65.49
  HIV V65.44
  human immunodeficiency virus V65.44
  injury prevention V65.43
  marital V61.10
  medical (for) V65.9
    boarding school resident V60.6
    condition not demonstrated V65.5
    feared complaint and no disease found V65.5
    institutional resident V60.6
    on behalf of another V65.1
    person living alone V60.3
  parent-child conflict V61.20
    specified problem NEC V61.29

Counseling—*continued*
  partner abuse
    perpetrator V61.12
    victim V61.11
  perpetrator of
    child abuse V62.83
      parental V61.22
    partner abuse V61.12
    spouse abuse V61.12
  procreative V65.49
  sex NEC V65.49
    transmitted disease NEC V65.45
      HIV V65.44
  specified reason NEC V65.49
  spousal abuse
    perpetrator V61.12
    victim V61.11
  substance use and abuse V65.42
  syphilis V65.45
  victim (of)
    abuse NEC V62.89
    child abuse V61.21
    partner abuse V61.11
    spousal abuse V61.11
Coupled rhythm 427.89
Couvelaire uterus (complicating delivery)—*see* Placenta, separation
Cowper's gland —*see* condition
Cowperitis (*see also* Urethritis) 597.89
  gonorrheal (acute) 098.0
    chronic or duration of 2 months or over 098.2
Cowpox (abortive) 051.0
  due to vaccination 999.0
  eyelid 051.0 *[373.5]*
    postvaccination 999.0 *[373.5]*
Coxa
  plana 732.1
  valga (acquired) 736.31
    congenital 755.61
    late effect of rickets 268.1
  vara (acquired) 736.32
    congenital 755.62
    late effect of rickets 268.1
Coxae malum senilis 715.25
Coxalgia (nontuberculous) 719.45
  tuberculous (*see also* Tuberculosis) 015.1 *[730.85]*
Coxalgic pelvis 736.30
Coxitis 716.65
Coxsackie (infection) (virus) 079.2
  central nervous system NEC 048
  endocarditis 074.22
  enteritis 008.67
  meningitis (aseptic) 047.0
  myocarditis 074.23
  pericarditis 074.21
  pharyngitis 074.0
  pleurodynia 074.1
  specific disease NEC 074.8
Crabs, meaning pubic lice 132.2
Crack baby 760.75
Cracked nipple 611.2
  puerperal, postpartum 676.1
Cradle cap 690.11
Craft neurosis 300.89
Craigiasis 007.8
Cramp (s) 729.82
  abdominal 789.0
  bathing 994.1
  colic 789.0
    psychogenic 306.4

Cramp(s)—*continued*
  due to immersion 994.1
  extremity (lower) (upper) NEC 729.82
  fireman 992.2
  heat 992.2
  hysterical 300.11
  immersion 994.1
  intestinal 789.0
    psychogenic 306.4
  linotypist's 300.89
    organic 333.84
  muscle (extremity) (general) 729.82
    due to immersion 994.1
    hysterical 300.11
  occupational (hand) 300.89
    organic 333.84
  psychogenic 307.89
  salt depletion 276.1
  stoker 992.2
  stomach 789.0
  telegraphers' 300.89
    organic 333.84
  typists' 300.89
    organic 333.84
  uterus 625.8
    menstrual 625.3
  writers' 333.84
    organic 333.84
    psychogenic 300.89
Cranial —*see* condition
Cranioclasis, fetal 763.89
Craniocleidodysostosis 755.59
Craniofenestria (skull) 756.0
Craniolacunia (skull) 756.0
Craniopagus 759.4
Craniopathy, metabolic 733.3
Craniopharyngeal —*see* condition
Craniopharyngioma (M9350/1) 237.0
Craniorachischisis (totalis) 740.1
Cranioschisis 756.0
Craniostenosis 756.0
Craniosynostosis 756.0
Craniotabes (cause unknown) 733.3
  rachitic 268.1
  syphilitic 090.5
Craniotomy, fetal 763.89
Cranium —*see* condition
Craw-craw 125.3
Creaking joint 719.60
  ankle 719.67
  elbow 719.62
  foot 719.67
  hand 719.64
  hip 719.65
  knee 719.66
  multiple sites 719.69
  pelvic region 719.65
  shoulder (region) 719.61
  specified site NEC 719.68
  wrist 719.63
Creeping
  eruption 126.9
  palsy 335.21
  paralysis 335.21
Crenated tongue 529.8
Creotoxism 005.9
Crepitus
  caput 756.0
  joint 719.60
    ankle 719.67
    elbow 719.62

Crepitus—*continued*
  foot 719.67
  hand 719.64
  hip 719.65
  knee 719.66
  multiple sites 719.69
  pelvic region 719.65
  shoulder (region) 719.61
  specified site NEC 719.68
  wrist 719.63
Crescent or conus choroid, congenital 743.57
Cretin, cretinism (athyrotic) (congenital)
    (endemic) (metabolic) (nongoitrous)
    (sporadic) 243
  goitrous (sporadic) 246.1
  pelvis (dwarf type) (male type) 243
    with disproportion (fetopelvic) 653.1
      affecting fetus or newborn 763.1
      causing obstructed labor 660.1
        affecting fetus or newborn 763.1
  pituitary 253.3
Cretinoid degeneration 243
Creutzfeldt-Jakob disease (syndrome) 046.1
  with dementia
    with behavioral disturbance 046.1 *[294.11]*
    without behavioral disturbance 046.1 *[294.10]*
Crib death 798.0
Cribriform hymen 752.49
Cri-du-chat syndrome 758.3
Crigler-Najjar disease or syndrome (congenital
    hyperbilirubinemia) 277.4
Crimean hemorrhagic fever 065.0
Criminalism 301.7
Crisis
  abdomen 789.0
  addisonian (acute adrenocortical insufficiency)
    255.4
  adrenal (cortical) 255.4
  asthmatic—*see* Asthma
  brain, cerebral (*see also* Disease,
    cerebrovascular, acute) 436
  celiac 579.0
  Dietl's 593.4
  emotional NEC 309.29
    acute reaction to stress 308.0
    adjustment reaction 309.9
    specific to childhood and adolescence 313.9
  gastric (tabetic) 094.0
  glaucomatocyclitic 364.22
  heart (*see also* Failure, heart) 428.9
  hypertensive—*see* Hypertension
  nitritoid
    correct substance properly administered 458.2
    overdose or wrong substance given or taken
      961.1
  oculogyric 378.87
    psychogenic 306.7
  Pel's 094.0
  psychosexual identity 302.6
  rectum 094.0
  renal 593.81
  sickle cell 282.62
  stomach (tabetic) 094.0
  tabetic 094.0
  thyroid (*see also* Thyrotoxicosis) 242.9
  thyrotoxic (*see also* Thyrotoxicosis) 242.9
  vascular—*see* Disease, cerebrovascular, acute
Crocq's disease (acrocyanosis) 443.89
Crohn's disease (*see also* Enteritis, regional)
    555.9
Cronkhite-Canada syndrome 211.3
Crooked septum, nasal 470

Cross
  birth (of fetus) complicating delivery 652.3
    with successful version 652.1
    causing obstructed labor 660.0
  bite, anterior or posterior 524.2
  eye (*see also* Esotropia) 378.00
Crossed ectopia of kidney 753.3
Crossfoot 754.50
Croup, croupous (acute) (angina) (catarrhal)
    (infective) (inflammatory) (laryngeal)
    (membranous) (nondiphtheritic)
    (pseudomembranous) 464.4
  asthmatic (*see also* Asthma) 493.9
  bronchial 466.0
  diphtheritic (membranous) 032.3
  false 478.75
  spasmodic 478.75
    diphtheritic 032.3
  stridulous 478.75
    diphtheritic 032.3
Crouzon's disease (craniofacial dysostosis) 756.0
Crowding, teeth 524.3
CRST syndrome (cutaneous systemic sclerosis)
    710.1
Cruchet's disease (encephalitis lethargica) 049.8
Cruelty in children (*see also* Disturbance,
    conduct) 312.9
Crural ulcer (*see also* Ulcer, lower extremity)
    707.10
Crush, crushed, crushing (injury) 929.9
  with
    fracture—*see* Fracture, by site
  abdomen 926.19
    internal—*see* Injury, internal, abdomen
  ankle 928.21
    with other parts of foot 928.20
  arm 927.9
    lower (and elbow) 927.10
    upper 927.03
      with shoulder or axillary region 927.09
  axilla 927.02
    with shoulder or upper arm 927.09
  back 926.11
  breast 926.19
  buttock 926.12
  cheek 925.1
  chest—*see* Injury, internal, chest
  ear 925.1
  elbow 927.11
    with forearm 927.10
  face 925.1
  finger(s) 927.3
    with hand(s) 927.20
    and wrist(s) 927.21
  flank 926.19
  foot, excluding toe(s) alone (with ankle) 928.20
  forearm (and elbow) 927.10
  genitalia, external (female) (male) 926.0
    internal—*see* Injury, internal, genital organ
      NEC
  hand, except finger(s) alone (and wrist) 927.20
  head—*see* Fracture, skull, by site
  heel 928.20
  hip 928.01
    with thigh 928.00
  internal organ (abdomen, chest, or pelvis)—*see*
    Injury, internal, by site
  knee 928.11
    with leg, lower 928.10
  labium (majus) (minus) 926.0
  larynx 925.2

Crush, crushed, crushing—*continued*
late effect—*see* Late, effects (of), crushing
leg 928.9
  lower 928.10
    and knee 928.11
  upper 928.00
limb
  lower 928.9
    multiple sites 928.8
  upper 927.9
    multiple sites 927.8
multiple sites NEC 929.0
neck 925.2
nerve—*see* Injury, nerve, by site
nose 802.0
  open 802.1
penis 926.0
pharynx 925.2
scalp 925.2
scapular region 927.01
  with shoulder or upper arm 927.09
scrotum 926.0
shoulder 927.00
  with upper arm or axillary region 927.09
skull or cranium—*see* Fracture, skull, by site
spinal cord—*see* Injury, spinal, by site
syndrome (complication of trauma) 958.5
testis 926.0
thigh (with hip) 928.00
throat 925.2
thumb(s) (and fingers) 927.3
toe(s) 928.3
  with foot 928.20
    and ankle 928.21
tonsil 925.2
trunk 926.9
  chest—*see* Injury, internal, intrathoracic
    organs NEC
  internal organ—*see* Injury, internal, by site
  multiple sites 926.8
  specified site NEC 926.19
vulva 926.0
wrist 927.21
  with hand(s), except fingers alone 927.20
Crusta lactea 690.11
Crusts 782.8
Crutch paralysis 953.4
Cruveilhier's disease 335.21
Cruveilhier-Baumgarten cirrhosis, disease, or syndrome 571.5
Cruz-Chagas disease (*see also* Trypanosomiasis) 086.2
Cryoglobulinemia (mixed) 273.2
Crypt (anal) (rectal) 569.49
Cryptitis (anal) (rectal) 569.49
Cryptococcosis (European) (pulmonary) (systemic) 117.5
Cryptococcus 117.5
  epidermicus 117.5
  neoformans, infection by 117.5
Cryptopapillitis (anus) 569.49
Cryptophthalmos (eyelid) 743.06
Cryptorchid, cryptorchism, cryptorchidism 752.51
Cryptosporidiosis 007.4
Cryptotia 744.29
Crystallopathy
  calcium pyrophosphate (*see also* Arthritis) 275.49 *[712.2]*
  dicalcium phosphate (*see also* Arthritis) 275.49 *[712.1]*

Crystallopathy—*continued*
gouty 274.0
pyrophosphate NEC (*see also* Arthritis) 275.49 *[712.2]*
uric acid 274.0
Crystalluria 791.9
Csillag's disease (lichen sclerosus et atrophicus) 701.0
Cuban itch 050.1
Cubitus
valgus (acquired) 736.01
  congenital 755.59
  late effect of rickets 268.1
varus (acquired) 736.02
  congenital 755.59
  late effect of rickets 268.1
Cultural deprivation V62.4
Cupping of optic disc 377.14
Curling's ulcer —*see* Ulcer, duodenum
Curling esophagus 530.5
Curschmann (-Batten) (-Steinert) disease or syndrome 359.2
Curvature
organ or site, congenital NEC—*see* Distortion
penis (lateral) 752.69
Pott's (spinal) (*see also* Tuberculosis) 015.0 *[737.43]*
radius, idiopathic, progressive (congenital) 755.54
spine (acquired) (angular) (idiopathic) (incorrect) (postural) 737.9
  congenital 754.2
  due to or associated with
    Charcot-Marie-Tooth disease 356.1 *[737.40]*
    mucopolysaccharidosis 277.5 *[737.40]*
    neurofibromatosis 237.71 *[737.40]*
    osteitis
      deformans 731.0 *[737.40]*
      fibrosa cystica 252.0 *[737.40]*
    osteoporosis (*see also* Osteoporosis) 733.00 *[737.40]*
    poliomyelitis (*see also* Poliomyelitis) 138 *[737.40]*
    tuberculosis (Pott's curvature) (*see also* Tuberculosis) 015.0 *[737.43]*
  kyphoscoliotic (*see also* Kyphoscoliosis) 737.30
  kyphotic (*see also* Kyphosis) 737.10
  late effect of rickets 268.1 *[737.40]*
  Pott's 015.0 *[737.40]*
  scoliotic (*see also* Scoliosis) 737.30
  specified NEC 737.8
  tuberculous 015.0 *[737.40]*
Cushing's
basophilism, disease, or syndrome (iatrogenic) (idiopathic) (pituitary basophilism) (pituitary dependent) 255.0
ulcer—*see* Ulcer, peptic
Cushingoid due to steroid therapy
correct substance properly administered 255.0
overdose or wrong substance given or taken 962.0
Cut (external)—*see* Wound, open, by site
Cutaneous —*see also* condition
hemorrhage 782.7
horn (cheek) (eyelid) (mouth) 702.8
larva migrans 126.9
Cutis —*see also* condition
hyperelastic 756.83
  acquired 701.8

Cutis—*continued*
  laxa 756.83
    senilis 701.8
  marmorata 782.61
  osteosis 709.3
  pendula 756.83
    acquired 701.8
  rhomboidalis nuchae 701.8
  verticis gyrata 757.39
    acquired 701.8
Cyanopathy, newborn 770.83
Cyanosis 782.5
  autotoxic 289.7
  common atrioventricular canal 745.69
  congenital 770.83
  conjunctiva 372.71
  due to
    endocardial cushion defect 745.60
    nonclosure, foramen botalli 745.5
    patent foramen botalli 745.5
    persistent foramen ovale 745.5
  enterogenous 289.7
  fetus or newborn 770.83
  ostium primum defect 745.61
  paroxysmal digital 443.0
  retina, retinal 362.10
Cycle
  anovulatory 628.0
  menstrual, irregular 626.4
Cyclencephaly 759.89
Cyclical vomiting 536.2
  psychogenic 306.4
Cyclitic membrane 364.74
Cyclitis (*see also* Iridocyclitis) 364.3
  acute 364.00
    primary 364.01
    recurrent 364.02
  chronic 364.10
    in
      sarcoidosis 135 *[364.11]*
      tuberculosis (*see also* Tuberculosis) 017.3
        [364.11]
  Fuchs' heterochromic 364.21
  granulomatous 364.10
  lens induced 364.23
  nongranulomatous 364.00
  posterior 363.21
  primary 364.01
  recurrent 364.02
  secondary (noninfectious) 364.04
    infectious 364.03
  subacute 364.00
    primary 364.01
    recurrent 364.02
Cyclokeratitis —*see* Keratitis
Cyclophoria 378.44
Cyclopia, cyclops 759.89
Cycloplegia 367.51
Cyclospasm 367.53
Cyclosporiasis 007.5
Cyclothymia 301.13
Cyclothymic personality 301.13
Cyclotropia 378.33
Cyesis —*see* Pregnancy
Cylindroma (M8200/3)—*see also* Neoplasm, by
  site, malignant
  eccrine dermal (M8200/0)—*see* Neoplasm,
    skin, benign
  skin (M8200/0)—*see* Neoplasm, skin, benign
Cylindruria 791.7
Cyllosoma 759.89

Cynanche
  diphtheritic 032.3
  tonsillaris 475
Cynorexia 783.6
Cyphosis —*see* Kyphosis
Cyprus fever (*see also* Brucellosis) 023.9
Cyriax's syndrome (slipping rib) 733.99
Cyst (mucus) (retention) (serous) (simple)

> *Note—In general, cysts are not neoplastic and are classified to the appropriate category for disease of the specified anatomical site. This generalization does not apply to certain types of cysts which are neoplastic in nature, for example, dermoid, nor does it apply to cysts of certain structures, for example, branchial cleft, which are classified as developmental anomalies. The following listing includes some of the most frequently reported sites of cysts as well as qualifiers which indicate the type of cyst. The latter qualifiers usually are not repeated under the anatomical sites. Since the code assignment for a given site may vary depending upon the type of cyst, the coder should refer to the listings under the specified type of cyst before consideration is given to the site.*

  accessory, fallopian tube 752.11
  adenoid (infected) 474.8
  adrenal gland 255.8
    congenital 759.1
  air, lung 518.89
  allantoic 753.7
  alveolar process (jaw bone) 526.2
  amnion, amniotic 658.8
  anterior chamber (eye) 364.60
    exudative 364.62
    implantation (surgical) (traumatic) 364.61
    parasitic 360.13
  anterior nasopalatine 526.1
  antrum 478.1
  anus 569.49
  apical (periodontal) (tooth) 522.8
  appendix 543.9
  arachnoid, brain 348.0
  arytenoid 478.79
  auricle 706.2
  Baker's (knee) 727.51
    tuberculous (*see also* Tuberculosis) 015.2
  Bartholin's gland or duct 616.2
  bile duct (*see also* Disease, biliary) 576.8
  bladder (multiple) (trigone) 596.8
  Blessig's 362.62
  blood, endocardial (*see also* Endocarditis)
    424.90
  blue dome 610.0
  bone (local) 733.20
    aneurysmal 733.22
    jaw 526.2
      developmental (odontogenic) 526.0
      fissural 526.1
      latent 526.89
    solitary 733.21
    unicameral 733.21
  brain 348.0
    congenital 742.4
    hydatid (*see also* Echinococcus) 122.9
    third ventricle (colloid) 742.4
  branchial (cleft) 744.42
  branchiogenic 744.42

Cyst —*continued*
  breast (benign) (blue dome) (pedunculated)
    (solitary) (traumatic) 610.0
    involution 610.4
    sebaceous 610.8
  broad ligament (benign) 620.8
    embryonic 752.11
  bronchogenic (mediastinal) (sequestration)
    518.89
    congenital 748.4
  buccal 528.4
  bulbourethral gland (Cowper's) 599.89
  bursa, bursal 727.49
    pharyngeal 478.26
  calcifying odontogenic (M9301/0) 213.1
    upper jaw (bone) 213.0
  canal of Nuck (acquired) (serous) 629.1
    congenital 752.41
  canthus 372.75
  carcinomatous (M8010/3)—*see* Neoplasm, by
    site, malignant
  cartilage (joint)—*see* Derangement, joint
  cauda equina 336.8
  cavum septi pellucidi NEC 348.0
  celomic (pericardium) 746.89
  cerebellopontine (angle)—*see* Cyst, brain
  cerebellum—*see* Cyst, brain
  cerebral—*see* Cyst, brain
  cervical lateral 744.42
  cervix 622.8
    embryonal 752.41
    nabothian (gland) 616.0
  chamber, anterior (eye) 364.60
    exudative 364.62
    implantation (surgical) (traumatic) 364.61
    parasitic 360.13
  chiasmal, optic NEC (*see also* Lesion,
    chiasmal) 377.54
  chocolate (ovary) 617.1
  choledochal (congenital) 751.69
    acquired 576.8
  choledochus 751.69
  chorion 658.8
  choroid plexus 348.0
  chyle, mesentery 457.8
  ciliary body 364.60
    exudative 364.64
    implantation 364.61
    primary 364.63
  clitoris 624.8
  coccyx (*see also* Cyst, bone) 733.20
  colloid
    third ventricle (brain) 742.4
    thyroid gland—*see* Goiter
  colon 569.89
  common (bile) duct (*see also* Disease, biliary)
    576.8
  congenital NEC 759.89
    adrenal glands 759.1
    epiglottis 748.3
    esophagus 750.4
    fallopian tube 752.11
    kidney 753.10
      multiple 753.19
      single 753.11
    larynx 748.3
    liver 751.62
    lung 748.4
    mediastinum 748.8
    ovary 752.0
    oviduct 752.11

Cyst —*continued*
  pancreas 751.7
  periurethral (tissue) 753.8
  prepuce NEC 752.69
    penis 752.69
  sublingual 750.26
  submaxillary gland 750.26
  thymus (gland) 759.2
  tongue 750.19
  ureterovesical orifice 753.4
  vulva 752.41
  conjunctiva 372.75
  cornea 371.23
  corpora quadrigemina 348.0
  corpus
    albicans (ovary) 620.2
    luteum (ruptured) 620.1
  Cowper's gland (benign) (infected) 599.89
  cranial meninges 348.0
  craniobuccal pouch 253.8
  craniopharyngeal pouch 253.8
  cystic duct (*see also* Disease, gallbladder) 575.8
  Cysticercus (any site) 123.1
  Dandy-Walker 742.3
    with spina bifida (*see also* Spina bifida) 741.0
  dental 522.8
    developmental 526.0
    eruption 526.0
    lateral periodontal 526.0
    primordial (keratocyst) 526.0
    root 522.8
  dentigerous 526.0
    mandible 526.0
    maxilla 526.0
  dermoid (M9084/0)—*see also* Neoplasm, by
    site, benign
    with malignant transformation (M9084/3)
      183.0
    implantation
      external area or site (skin) NEC 709.8
      iris 364.61
      skin 709.8
      vagina 623.8
      vulva 624.8
    mouth 528.4
    oral soft tissue 528.4
    sacrococcygeal 685.1
      with abscess 685.0
  developmental of ovary, ovarian 752.0
  dura (cerebral) 348.0
    spinal 349.2
  ear (external) 706.2
  echinococcal (*see also* Echinococcus) 122.9
  embryonal
    cervix uteri 752.41
    genitalia, female external 752.41
    uterus 752.3
    vagina 752.41
  endometrial 621.8
    ectopic 617.9
  endometrium (uterus) 621.8
    ectopic—*see* Endometriosis
  enteric 751.5
  enterogenous 751.5
  epidermal (inclusion) (*see also* Cyst, skin) 706.2
  epidermoid (inclusion) (*see also* Cyst, skin)
    706.2
    mouth 528.4
    not of skin—*see* Cyst, by site
    oral soft tissue 528.4
  epididymis 608.89

Cyst —*continued*
epiglottis 478.79
epiphysis cerebri 259.8
epithelial (inclusion) (*see also* Cyst, skin) 706.2
epoophoron 752.11
eruption 526.0
esophagus 530.89
ethmoid sinus 478.1
eye (retention) 379.8
  congenital 743.03
  posterior segment, congenital 743.54
eyebrow 706.2
eyelid (sebaceous) 374.84
  infected 373.13
  sweat glands or ducts 374.84
falciform ligament (inflammatory) 573.8
fallopian tube 620.8
female genital organs NEC 629.8
fimbrial (congenital) 752.11
fissural (oral region) 526.1
follicle (atretic) (graafian) (ovarian) 620.0
  nabothian (gland) 616.0
follicular (atretic) (ovarian) 620.0
  dentigerous 526.0
frontal sinus 478.1
gallbladder or duct 575.8
ganglion 727.43
Gartner's duct 752.11
gas, of mesentery 568.89
gingiva 523.8
gland of moll 374.84
globulomaxillary 526.1
graafian follicle 620.0
granulosal lutein 620.2
hemangiomatous (M9121/0) (*see also*
  Hemangioma) 228.00
hydatid (*see also* Echinococcus) 122.9
  fallopian tube (Morgagni) 752.11
  liver NEC 122.8
  lung NEC 122.9
  Morgagni 752.8
   fallopian tube 752.11
  specified site NEC 122.9
hymen 623.8
  embryonal 752.41
hypopharynx 478.26
hypophysis, hypophyseal (duct) (recurrent)
  253.8
  cerebri 253.8
implantation (dermoid)
  anterior chamber (eye) 364.61
  external area or site (skin) NEC 709.8
  iris 364.61
  vagina 623.8
  vulva 624.8
incisor, incisive canal 526.1
inclusion (epidermal) (epithelial) (epidermoid)
  (mucous) (squamous) (*see also* Cyst, skin)
  706.2
  not of skin—*see* Neoplasm, by site, benign
intestine (large) (small) 569.89
intracranial—*see* Cyst, brain
intraligamentous 728.89
  knee 717.89
intrasellar 253.8
iris (idiopathic) 364.60
  exudative 364.62
  implantation (surgical) (traumatic) 364.61
  miotic pupillary 364.55
  parasitic 360.13
Iwanoff's 362.62

Cyst —*continued*
jaw (bone) (aneurysmal) (extravasation)
  (hemorrhagic) (traumatic) 526.2
  developmental (odontogenic) 526.0
  fissural 526.1
keratin 706.2
kidney (congenital) 753.10
  acquired 593.2
  calyceal (*see also* Hydronephrosis) 591
  multiple 753.19
  pyelogenic (*see also* Hydronephrosis) 591
  simple 593.2
  single 753.11
  solitary (not congenital) 593.2
labium (majus) (minus) 624.8
  sebaceous 624.8
lacrimal
  apparatus 375.43
  gland or sac 375.12
larynx 478.79
lens 379.39
  congenital 743.39
lip (gland) 528.5
liver 573.8
  congenital 751.62
  hydatid (*see also* Echinococcus) 122.8
   granulosis 122.0
   multilocularis 122.5
lung 518.89
  congenital 748.4
  giant bullous 492.0
lutein 620.1
lymphangiomatous (M9173/0) 228.1
lymphoepithelial
  mouth 528.4
  oral soft tissue 528.4
macula 362.54
malignant (M8000/3)—*see* Neoplasm, by site,
  malignant
mammary gland (sweat gland) (*see also* Cyst,
  breast) 610.0
mandible 526.2
  dentigerous 526.0
  radicular 522.8
maxilla 526.2
  dentigerous 526.0
  radicular 522.8
median
  anterior maxillary 526.1
  palatal 526.1
mediastinum (congenital) 748.8
meibomian (gland) (retention) 373.2
  infected 373.12
membrane, brain 348.0
meninges (cerebral) 348.0
  spinal 349.2
meniscus knee 717.5
mesentery, mesenteric (gas) 568.89
  chyle 457.8
  gas 568.89
mesonephric duct 752.8
mesothelial
  peritoneum 568.89
  pleura (peritoneal) 568.89
milk 611.5
miotic pupillary (iris) 364.55
Morgagni (hydatid) 752.8
  fallopian tube 752.11
mouth 528.4
mullerian duct 752.8
multilocular (ovary) (M8000/1) 239.5

Cyst —*continued*
  myometrium 621.8
  nabothian (follicle) (ruptured) 616.0
  nasal sinus 478.1
  nasoalveolar 528.4
  nasolabial 528.4
  nasopalatine (duct) 526.1
    anterior 526.1
  nasopharynx 478.26
  neoplastic (M8000/1)—*see also* Neoplasm, by
    site, unspecified nature
    benign (M8000/0)—*see* Neoplasm, by site,
      benign
      uterus 621.8
  nervous system—*see* Cyst, brain
  neuroenteric 742.59
  neuroepithelial ventricle 348.0
  nipple 610.0
  nose 478.1
    skin of 706.2
  odontogenic, developmental 526.0
  omentum (lesser) 568.89
    congenital 751.8
  oral soft tissue (dermoid) (epidermoid)
    (lymphoepithelial) 528.4
  ora serrata 361.19
  orbit 376.81
  ovary, ovarian (twisted) 620.2
    adherent 620.2
    chocolate 617.1
    corpus
      albicans 620.2
      luteum 620.1
    dermoid (M9084/0) 220
    developmental 752.0
    due to failure of involution NEC 620.2
    endometrial 617.1
    follicular (atretic) (graafian) (hemorrhagic)
      620.0
    hemorrhagic 620.2
    in pregnancy or childbirth 654.4
      affecting fetus or newborn 763.89
      causing obstructed labor 660.2
        affecting fetus or newborn 763.1
    multilocular (M8000/1) 239.5
    pseudomucinous (M8470/0) 220
    retention 620.2
    serous 620.2
    theca lutein 620.2
    tuberculous (*see also* Tuberculosis) 016.6
    unspecified 620.2
  oviduct 620.8
  palatal papilla (jaw) 526.1
  palate 526.1
    fissural 526.1
    median (fissural) 526.1
  palatine, of papilla 526.1
  pancreas, pancreatic 577.2
    congenital 751.7
    false 577.2
    hemorrhagic 577.2
    true 577.2
  paranephric 593.2
  para ovarian 752.11
  paraphysis, cerebri 742.4
  parasitic NEC 136.9
  parathyroid (gland) 252.8
  paratubal (fallopian) 620.8
  paraurethral duct 599.89
  paroophoron 752.11

Cyst —*continued*
  parotid gland 527.6
    mucous extravasation or retention 527.6
  parovarian 752.11
  pars planus 364.60
    exudative 364.64
    primary 364.63
  pelvis, female
    in pregnancy or childbirth 654.4
      affecting fetus or newborn 763.89
      causing obstructed labor 660.2
        affecting fetus or newborn 763.1
  penis (sebaceous) 607.89
  periapical 522.8
  pericardial (congenital) 746.89
    acquired (secondary) 423.8
  pericoronal 526.0
  perineural (Tarlov's) 355.9
  periodontal 522.8
    lateral 526.0
  peripancreatic 577.2
  peripelvic (lymphatic) 593.2
  peritoneum 568.89
    chylous 457.8
  pharynx (wall) 478.26
  pilonidal (infected) (rectum) 685.1
    with abscess 685.0
    malignant (M9084/3) 173.5
  pituitary (duct) (gland) 253.8
  placenta (amniotic)—*see* Placenta, abnormal
  pleura 519.8
  popliteal 727.51
  porencephalic 742.4
    acquired 348.0
  postanal (infected) 685.1
    with abscess 685.0
  posterior segment of eye, congenital 743.54
  postmastoidectomy cavity 383.31
  preauricular 744.47
  prepuce 607.89
    congenital 752.69
  primordial (jaw) 526.0
  prostate 600.3
  pseudomucinous (ovary) (M8470/0) 220
  pudenda (sweat glands) 624.8
  pupillary, miotic 364.55
    sebaceous 624.8
  radicular (residual) 522.8
  radiculodental 522.8
  ranular 527.6
  Rathke's pouch 253.8
  rectum (epithelium) (mucous) 569.49
  renal—*see* Cyst, kidney
  residual (radicular) 522.8
  retention (ovary) 620.2
  retina 361.19
    macular 362.54
    parasitic 360.13
    primary 361.13
    secondary 361.14
  retroperitoneal 568.89
  sacrococcygeal (dermoid) 685.1
    with abscess 685.0
  salivary gland or duct 527.6
    mucous extravasation or retention 527.6
  Sampson's 617.1
  sclera 379.19
  scrotum (sebaceous) 706.2
    sweat glands 706.2
  sebaceous (duct) (gland) 706.2
    breast 610.8

Cyst —*continued*
   eyelid 374.84
   genital organ NEC
     female 629.8
     male 608.89
   scrotum 706.2
   semilunar cartilage (knee) (multiple) 717.5
   seminal vesicle 608.89
   serous (ovary) 620.2
   sinus (antral) (ethmoidal) (frontal) (maxillary)
     (nasal) (sphenoidal) 478.1
   Skene's gland 599.89
   skin (epidermal) (epidermoid, inclusion)
     (epithelial) (inclusion) (retention)
     (sebaceous) 706.2
     breast 610.8
     eyelid 374.84
     genital organ NEC
       female 629.8
       male 608.89
     neoplastic 216.3
     scrotum 706.2
     sweat gland or duct 705.89
   solitary
     bone 733.21
     kidney 593.2
   spermatic cord 608.89
   sphenoid sinus 478.1
   spinal meninges 349.2
   spine (*see also* Cyst, bone) 733.20
   spleen NEC 289.59
     congenital 759.0
     hydatid (*see also* Echinococcus) 122.9
   spring water (pericardium) 746.89
   subarachnoid 348.0
     intrasellar 793.0
   subdural (cerebral) 348.0
     spinal cord 349.2
   sublingual gland 527.6
     mucous extravasation or retention 527.6
   submaxillary gland 527.6
     mucous extravasation or retention 527.6
   suburethral 599.89
   suprarenal gland 255.8
   suprasellar—*see* Cyst, brain
   sweat gland or duct 705.89
   sympathetic nervous system 337.9
   synovial 727.40
     popliteal space 727.51
   Tarlov's 355.9
   tarsal 373.2
   tendon (sheath) 727.42
   testis 608.89
   theca-lutein (ovary) 620.2
   Thornwaldt's, Tornwaldt's 478.26
   thymus (gland) 254.8
   thyroglossal (duct) (infected) (persistent) 759.2
   thyroid (gland) 246.2
     adenomatous—*see* Goiter, nodular
     colloid (*see also* Goiter) 240.9
   thyrolingual duct (infected) (persistent) 759.2
   tongue (mucous) 529.8
   tonsil 474.8
   tooth (dental root) 522.8
   tubo-ovarian 620.8
     inflammatory 614.1
   tunica vaginalis 608.89
   turbinate (nose) (*see also* Cyst, bone) 733.20
   Tyson's gland (benign) (infected) 607.89
   umbilicus 759.89
   urachus 753.7

Cyst —*continued*
   ureter 593.89
   ureterovesical orifice 593.89
     congenital 753.4
   urethra 599.84
   urethral gland (Cowper's) 599.89
   uterine
     ligament 620.8
       embryonic 752.11
     tube 620.8
   uterus (body) (corpus) (recurrent) 621.8
     embryonal 752.3
   utricle (ear) 386.8
     prostatic 599.89
   utriculus masculinus 599.89
   vagina, vaginal (squamous cell) (wall) 623.8
     embryonal 752.41
     implantation 623.8
     inclusion 623.8
   vallecula, vallecular 478.79
   ventricle, neuroepithelial 348.0
   verumontanum 599.89
   vesical (orifice) 596.8
   vitreous humor 379.29
   vulva (sweat glands) 624.8
     congenital 752.41
     implantation 624.8
     inclusion 624.8
     sebaceous gland 624.8
   vulvovaginal gland 624.8
   wolffian 752.8

Cystadenocarcinoma (M8440/3)—*see also*
   Neoplasm, by site, malignant
   bile duct type (M8161/3) 155.1
   endometrioid (M8380/3)—*see* Neoplasm, by
     site, malignant
   mucinous (M8470/3)
     papillary (M8471/3)
       specified site—*see* Neoplasm, by site,
         malignant
       unspecified site 183.0
     specified site—*see* Neoplasm, by site,
       malignant
     unspecified site 183.0
   papillary (M8450/3)
     mucinous (M8471/3)
       specified site—*see* Neoplasm, by site,
         malignant
       unspecified site 183.0
     pseudomucinous (M8471/3)
       specified site—*see* Neoplasm, by site,
         malignant
       unspecified site 183.0
     serous (M8460/3)
       specified site—*see* Neoplasm, by site,
         malignant
       unspecified site 183.0
     specified site—*see* Neoplasm, by site,
       malignant
     unspecified 183.0
   pseudomucinous (M8470/3)
     papillary (M8471/3)
       specified site—*see* Neoplasm, by site,
         malignant
       unspecified site 183.0
     specified site—*see* Neoplasm, by site,
       malignant
     unspecified site 183.0
   serous (M8441/3)
     papillary (M8460/3)

Cystic—*continued*
  kidney, congenital 753.10
    medullary 753.16
    multiple 753.19
    polycystic—*see* Polycystic, kidney
    single 753.11
    specified NEC 753.19
  liver, congenital 751.62
  lung 518.89
    congenital 748.4
  mass—*see* Cyst
  mastitis, chronic 610.1
  ovary 620.2
  pancreas, congenital 751.7
Cysticerciasis 123.1
Cysticercosis (mammary) (subretinal) 123.1
Cysticercus 123.1
  cellulosae infestation 123.1
Cystinosis (malignant) 270.0
Cystinuria 270.0
Cystitis (bacillary) (colli) (diffuse) (exudative)
  (hemorrhagic) (purulent) (recurrent) (septic)
  (suppurative) (ulcerative) 595.9
  with
    abortion—*see* Abortion, by type, with urinary
      tract infection
    ectopic pregnancy (*see also* categories
      633.0-633.9) 639.8
    fibrosis 595.1
    leukoplakia 595.1
    malakoplakia 595.1
    metaplasia 595.1
    molar pregnancy (*see also* categories
      630-632) 639.8
  actinomycotic 039.8 *[595.4]*
  acute 595.0
    of trigone 595.3
  allergic 595.89
  amebic 006.8 *[595.4]*
  bilharzial 120.9 *[595.4]*
  blennorrhagic (acute) 098.11
    chronic or duration of 2 months or more
      098.31
  bullous 595.89
  calculus 594.1
  chlamydial 099.53
  chronic 595.2
    interstitial 595.1
    of trigone 595.3
  complicating pregnancy, childbirth, or
    puerperium 646.6
    affecting fetus or newborn 760.1
  cystic(a) 595.81
  diphtheritic 032.84
  echinococcal
    granulosus 122.3 *[595.4]*
    multilocularis 122.6 *[595.4]*
  emphysematous 595.89
  encysted 595.81
  follicular 595.3
  following
    abortion 639.8
    ectopic or molar pregnancy 639.8
  gangrenous 595.89
  glandularis 595.89
  gonococcal (acute) 098.11
    chronic or duration of 2 months or more
      098.31
  incrusted 595.89
  interstitial 595.1
  irradiation 595.82

Cystitis—*continued*
  irritation 595.89
  malignant 595.89
  monilial 112.2
  of trigone 595.3
  panmural 595.1
  polyposa 595.89
  prostatic 601.3
  radiation 595.82
  Reiter's (abacterial) 099.3
  specified NEC 595.89
  subacute 595.2
  submucous 595.1
  syphilitic 095.8
  trichomoniasis 131.09
  tuberculous (*see also* Tuberculosis) 016.1
  ulcerative 595.1
Cystocele (-rectocele)
  female (without uterine prolapse) 618.0
    with uterine prolapse 618.4
      complete 618.3
      incomplete 618.2
  in pregnancy or childbirth 654.4
    affecting fetus or newborn 763.89
    causing obstructed labor 660.2
      affecting fetus or newborn 763.1
  male 596.8
Cystoid
  cicatrix limbus 372.64
  degeneration macula 362.53
Cystolithiasis 594.1
Cystoma (M8440/0)—*see also* Neoplasm, by
  site, benign
  endometrial, ovary 617.1
  mucinous (M8470/0)
    specified site—*see* Neoplasm, by site, benign
    unspecified site 220
  serous (M8441/0)
    specified site—*see* Neoplasm, by site, benign
    unspecified site 220
  simple (ovary) 620.2
Cystoplegia 596.53
Cystoptosis 596.8
Cystopyelitis (*see also* Pyelitis) 590.80
Cystorrhagia 596.8
Cystosarcoma phyllodes (M9020/1) 238.3
  benign (M9020/0) 217
  malignant (M9020/3)—*see* Neoplasm, breast,
    malignant
Cystostomy status V44.50
  appendico-vesicostomy V44.52
  cutaneous-vesicostomy V44.51
  specified type NEC V44.59
  with complication 997.5
Cystourethritis (*see also* Urethritis) 597.89
Cystourethrocele (*see also* Cystocele)
  female (without uterine prolapse) 618.0
    with uterine prolapse 618.4
      complete 618.3
      incomplete 618.2
  male 596.8
Cytomegalic inclusion disease 078.5
  congenital 771.1
Cytomycosis, reticuloendothelial (*see also*
  Histoplasmosis, American) 115.00

D

Daae (-Finsen) disease (epidemic pleurodynia) 074.1
Dabney's grip 074.1
Da Costa's syndrome (neurocirculatory asthenia) 306.2
Dacryoadenitis, dacryadenitis 375.00
  acute 375.01
  chronic 375.02
Dacryocystitis 375.30
  acute 375.32
  chronic 375.42
  neonatal 771.6
  phlegmonous 375.33
  syphilitic 095.8
    congenital 090.0
  trachomatous, active 076.1
    late effect 139.1
  tuberculous (*see also* Tuberculosis) 017.3
Dacryocystoblennorrhea 375.42
Dacryocystocele 375.43
Dacryolith, dacryolithiasis 375.57
Dacryoma 375.43
Dacryopericystitis (acute) (subacute) 375.32
  chronic 375.42
Dacryops 375.11
Dacryosialadenopathy, atrophic 710.2
Dacryostenosis 375.56
  congenital 743.65
Dactylitis 686.9
  bone (*see also* Osteomyelitis) 730.2
  sickle-cell 282.61
  syphilitic 095.5
  tuberculous (*see also* Tuberculosis) 015.5
Dactylolysis spontanea 136.0
Dactylosymphysis (*see also* Syndactylism) 755.10
Damage
  arteriosclerotic—*see* Arteriosclerosis
  brain 348.9
    anoxic, hypoxic 348.1
      during or resulting from a procedure 997.01
    child NEC 343.9
    due to birth injury 767.0
    minimal (child) (*see also* Hyperkinesia) 314.9
    newborn 767.0
  cardiac—*see also* Disease, heart
  cardiorenal (vascular) (*see also* Hypertension, cardiorenal) 404.90
  central nervous system—*see* Damage, brain
  cerebral NEC—*see* Damage, brain
  coccyx, complicating delivery 665.6
  coronary (*see also* Ischemia, heart) 414.9
  eye, birth injury 767.8
  heart—*see also* Disease, heart
    valve—*see* Endocarditis
  hypothalamus NEC 348.9
  liver 571.9
    alcoholic 571.3
  myocardium (*see also* Degeneration, myocardial) 429.1
  pelvic
    joint or ligament, during delivery 665.6
    organ NEC
      with
        abortion—*see* Abortion, by type, with damage to pelvic organs
        ectopic pregnancy (*see also* categories 633.0-633.9) 639.2

Damage—*continued*
    molar pregnancy (*see also* categories 630-632) 639.2
  during delivery 665.5
  following
    abortion 639.2
    ectopic or molar pregnancy 639.2
  renal (*see also* Disease, renal) 593.9
  skin, solar 692.79
    acute 692.72
    chronic 692.74
  subendocardium, subendocardial (*see also* Degeneration, myocardial) 429.1
  vascular 459.9
Dameshek's syndrome (erythroblastic anemia) 282.4
Dana-Putnam syndrome (subacute combined sclerosis with pernicious anemia) 281.0 *[336.2]*
Danbolt (-Closs) syndrome (acrodermatitis enteropathica) 686.8
Dandruff 690.18
Dandy fever 061
Dandy-Walker deformity or syndrome (atresia, foramen of Magendie) 742.3
  with spina bifida (*see also* Spina bifida) 741.0
Dangle foot 736.79
Danielssen's disease (anesthetic leprosy) 030.1
Danlos' syndrome 756.83
Darier's disease (congenital) (keratosis follicularis) 757.39
  due to vitamin A deficiency 264.8
  meaning erythema annulare centrifugum 695.0
Darier-Roussy sarcoid 135
Darling's
  disease (*see also* Histoplasmosis, American) 115.00
  histoplasmosis (*see also* Histoplasmosis, American) 115.00
Dartre 054.9
Darwin's tubercle 744.29
Davidson's anemia (refractory) 284.9
Davies' disease 425.0
Davies-Colley syndrome (slipping rib) 733.99
Dawson's encephalitis 046.2
Day blindness (*see also* Blindness, day) 368.60
Dead
  fetus
    retained (in utero) 656.4
      early pregnancy (death before 22 completed weeks gestation) 632
      late (death after 22 completed weeks gestation) 656.4
    syndrome 641.3
  labyrinth 386.50
  ovum, retained 631
Deaf and dumb NEC 389.7
Deaf mutism (acquired) (congenital) NEC 389.7
  endemic 243
  hysterical 300.11
  syphilitic, congenital 090.0

Deafness (acquired) (bilateral) (both ears) (complete) (congenital) (hereditary) (middle ear) (partial) (unilateral) 389.9
  with blue sclera and fragility of bone 756.51
  auditory fatigue 389.9
  aviation 993.0
    nerve injury 951.5
  boilermakers' 951.5
  central 389.14
    with conductive hearing loss 389.2
  conductive (air) 389.00
    with sensorineural hearing loss 389.2
    combined types 389.08
    external ear 389.01
    inner ear 389.04
    middle ear 389.03
    multiple types 389.08
    tympanic membrane 389.02
  emotional (complete) 300.11
  functional (complete) 300.11
  high frequency 389.8
  hysterical (complete) 300.11
  injury 951.5
  low frequency 389.8
  mental 784.69
  mixed conductive and sensorineural 389.2
  nerve 389.12
    with conductive hearing loss 389.2
  neural 389.12
    with conductive hearing loss 389.2
  noise-induced 388.12
    nerve injury 951.5
  nonspeaking 389.7
  perceptive 389.10
    with conductive hearing loss 389.2
    central 389.14
    combined types 389.18
    multiple types 389.18
    neural 389.12
    sensory 389.11
  psychogenic (complete) 306.7
  sensorineural (*see also* Deafness, perceptive) 389.10
  sensory 389.11
    with conductive hearing loss 389.2
  specified type NEC 389.8
  sudden NEC 388.2
  syphilitic 094.89
  transient ischemic 388.02
  transmission—*see* Deafness, conductive
  traumatic 951.5
  word (secondary to organic lesion) 784.69
    developmental 315.31
Death
  after delivery (cause not stated) (sudden) 674.9
  anesthetic
    due to
      correct substance properly administered 995.4
      overdose or wrong substance given 968.4
        specified anesthetic—*see* Table of drugs and chemicals
    during delivery 668.9
  brain 348.8
  cardiac—*see* Disease, heart
  cause unknown 798.2
  cot (infant) 798.0
  crib (infant) 798.0

Death—*continued*
  fetus, fetal (cause not stated) (intrauterine) 779.9
    early, with retention (before 22 completed weeks gestation) 632
    from asphyxia or anoxia (before labor) 768.0
      during labor 768.1
    late, affecting management of pregnancy (after 22 completed weeks gestation) 656.4
  from pregnancy NEC 646.9
  instantaneous 798.1
  intrauterine (*see also* Death, fetus) 779.9
    complicating pregnancy 656.4
  maternal, affecting fetus or newborn 761.6
  neonatal NEC 779.9
  sudden (cause unknown) 798.1
    during delivery 669.9
      under anesthesia NEC 668.9
    infant, syndrome (SIDS) 798.0
    puerperal, during puerperium 674.9
  unattended (cause unknown) 798.9
  under anesthesia NEC
    due to
      correct substance properly administered 995.4
      overdose or wrong substance given 968.4
        specified anesthetic—*see* Table of drugs and chemicals
    during delivery 668.9
  violent 798.1
de Beurmann-Gougerot disease (sporotrichosis) 117.1
Debility (general) (infantile) (postinfectional) 799.3
  with nutritional difficulty 269.9
  congenital or neonatal NEC 779.9
  nervous 300.5
  old age 797
  senile 797
Débove's disease (splenomegaly) 789.2
Decalcification
  bone (*see also* Osteoporosis) 733.00
  teeth 521.8
Decapitation 874.9
  fetal (to facilitate delivery) 763.89
Decapsulation, kidney 593.89
Decay
  dental 521.00
  senile 797
  tooth, teeth 521.00
Decensus, uterus —*see* Prolapse, uterus
Deciduitis (acute)
  with
    abortion—*see* Abortion, by type, with sepsis
    ectopic pregnancy (*see also* categories 633.0-633.9) 639.0
    molar pregnancy (*see also* categories 630-632) 639.0
  affecting fetus or newborn 760.8
  following
    abortion 639.0
    ectopic or molar pregnancy 639.0
  in pregnancy 646.6
  puerperal, postpartum 670
Deciduoma malignum (M9100/3) 181
Deciduous tooth (retained) 520.6
Decline (general) (*see also* Debility) 799.3

Defect, defective—*continued*
  esophagus, congenital 750.9
  extensor retinaculum 728.9
  fibrin polymerization (*see also* Defect,
    coagulation) 286.3
  filling
    biliary tract 793.3
    bladder 793.5
    gallbladder 793.3
    kidney 793.5
    stomach 793.4
    ureter 793.5
  fossa ovalis 745.5
  gene, carrier (suspected) of V83.89
  Gerbode 745.4
  glaucomatous, without elevated tension 365.89
  Hageman (factor) (*see also* Defect, coagulation)
    286.3
  hearing (*see also* Deafness) 389.9
  high grade 317
  homogentisic acid 270.2
  interatrial septal 745.5
    acquired 429.71
  interauricular septal 745.5
    acquired 429.71
  interventricular septal 745.4
    with pulmonary stenosis or atresia,
      dextroposition of aorta, and hypertrophy
      of right ventricle 745.2
    acquired 429.71
    in tetralogy of Fallot 745.2
  iodide trapping 246.1
  iodotyrosine dehalogenase 246.1
  kynureninase 270.2
  learning, specific 315.2
  mental (*see also* Retardation, mental) 319
  osteochondral NEC 738.8
  ostium
    primum 745.61
    secundum 745.5
  pericardium 746.89
  peroxidase-binding 246.1
  placental blood supply—*see* Placenta,
    insufficiency
  platelet (qualitative) 287.1
    constitutional 286.4
  postural, spine 737.9
  protan 368.51
  pulmonic cusps, congenital 746.00
  renal pelvis 753.9
    obstructive 753.29
    specified type NEC 753.3
  respiratory system, congenital 748.9
    specified type NEC 748.8
  retina, retinal 361.30
    with detachment (*see also* Detachment, retina,
      with retinal defect) 361.00
    multiple 361.33
      with detachment 361.02
    nerve fiber bundle 362.85
    single 361.30
      with detachment 361.01
  septal (closure) (heart) NEC 745.9
    acquired 429.71
    atrial 745.5
    specified type NEC 745.8
  speech NEC 784.5
    developmental 315.39
    secondary to organic lesion 784.5
  Taussig-Bing (transposition, aorta and
    overriding pulmonary artery) 745.11

Defect, defective—*continued*
  teeth, wedge 521.2
  thyroid hormone synthesis 246.1
  tritan 368.53
  ureter 753.9
    obstructive 753.29
  vascular (acquired) (local) 459.9
    congenital (peripheral) NEC 747.60
      gastrointestinal 747.61
      lower limb 747.64
      renal 747.62
      specified NEC 747.69
      spinal 747.82
      upper limb 747.63
  ventricular septal 745.4
    with pulmonary stenosis or atresia,
      dextraposition of aorta, and hypertrophy
      of right ventricle 745.2
    acquired 429.71
    atrioventricular canal type 745.69
    between infundibulum and anterior portion
      745.4
    in tetralogy of Fallot 745.2
    isolated anterior 745.4
  vision NEC 369.9
  visual field 368.40
    arcuate 368.43
    heteronymous, bilateral 368.47
    homonymous, bilateral 368.46
    localized NEC 368.44
    nasal step 368.44
    peripheral 368.44
    sector 368.43
  voice 784.40
  wedge, teeth (abrasion) 521.2
Defeminization syndrome 255.2
Deferentitis 608.4
  gonorrheal (acute) 098.14
    chronic or duration of 2 months or over 098.34
Defibrination syndrome (*see also* Fibrinolysis)
  286.6
Deficiency, deficient
  3-beta-hydroxysteroid dehydrogenase 255.2
  6-phosphogluconic dehydrogenase (anemia)
    282.2
  11-beta-hydroxylase 255.2
  17-alpha-hydroxylase 255.2
  18-hydroxysteroid dehydrogenase 255.2
  20-alpha-hydroxylase 255.2
  21-hydroxylase 255.2
  abdominal muscle syndrome 756.79
  accelerator globulin (Ac G) (blood) (*see also*
    Defect, coagulation) 286.3
  AC globulin (congenital) (*see also* Defect,
    coagulation) 286.3
    acquired 286.7
  activating factor (blood) (*see also* Defect,
    coagulation) 286.3
  adenohypophyseal 253.2
  adenosine deaminase 277.2
  aldolase (hereditary) 271.2
  alpha-1-antitrypsin 277.6
  alpha-1-trypsin inhibitor 277.6
  alpha-fucosidase 271.8
  alpha-lipoprotein 272.5
  alpha-mannosidase 271.8
  amino acid 270.9
  anemia—*see* Anemia, deficiency
  aneurin 265.1
    with beriberi 265.0

Deficiency, deficient—*continued*
  antibody NEC 279.00
  antidiuretic hormone 253.5
  antihemophilic
    factor (A) 286.0
      B 286.1
      C 286.2
      globulin (AHG) NEC 286.0
  antitrypsin 277.6
  argininosuccinate synthetase or lyase 270.6
  ascorbic acid (with scurvy) 267
  autoprothrombin
    I (*see also* Defect, coagulation) 286.3
    II 286.1
    C (*see also* Defect, coagulation) 286.3
  bile salt 579.8
  biotin 266.2
  biotinidase 277.6
  bradykinase-1 277.6
  brancher enzyme (amylopectinosis) 271.0
  calciferol 268.9
    with
      osteomalacia 268.2
      rickets (*see also* Rickets) 268.0
  calcium 275.40
    dietary 269.3
  calorie, severe 261
  carbamyl phosphate synthetase 270.6
  cardiac (*see also* Insufficiency, myocardial)
    428.0
  carnitine palmityl transferase 791.3
  carotene 264.9
  Carr factor (*see also* Defect, coagulation) 286.9
  central nervous system 349.9
  ceruloplasmin 275.1
  cevitamic acid (with scurvy) 267
  choline 266.2
  Christmas factor 286.1
  chromium 269.3
  citrin 269.1
  clotting (blood) (*see also* Defect, coagulation)
    286.9
  coagulation factor NEC 286.9
    with
      abortion—*see* Abortion, by type, with
        hemorrhage
      ectopic pregnancy (*see also* categories
        634-638) 639.1
      molar pregnancy (*see also* categories
        630-632) 639.1
    acquired (any) 286.7
    antepartum or intrapartum 641.3
      affecting fetus or newborn 762.1
    due to
      liver disease 286.7
      vitamin K deficiency 286.7
    newborn, transient 776.3
    postpartum 666.3
    specified type NEC 286.3
  color vision (congenital) 368.59
    acquired 368.55
  combined, two or more coagulation factors (*see
    also* Defect, coagulation) 286.9
  complement factor NEC 279.8
  contact factor (*see also* Defect, coagulation)
    286.3
  copper NEC 275.1
  corticoadrenal 255.4
  craniofacial axis 756.0
  cyanocobalamin (vitamin B₁₂) 266.2

Deficiency, deficient—*continued*
  debrancher enzyme (limit dextrinosis) 271.0
  desmolase 255.2
  diet 269.9
  dihydrofolate reductase 281.2
  dihydropteridine reductase 270.1
  disaccharidase (intestinal) 271.3
  disease NEC 269.9
  ear(s) V48.8
  edema 262
  endocrine 259.9
  enzymes, circulating NEC (*see also* Deficiency,
    by specific enzyme) 277.6
  ergosterol 268.9
    with
      osteomalacia 268.2
      rickets (*see also* Rickets) 268.0
  erythrocytic glutathione (anemia) 282.2
  eyelid(s) V48.8
  factor (*see also* Defect, coagulation) 286.9
    I (congenital) (fibrinogen) 286.3
      antepartum or intrapartum 641.3
        affecting fetus or newborn 762.1
      newborn, transient 776.3
      postpartum 666.3
    II (congenital) (prothrombin) 286.3
    V (congenital) (labile) 286.3
    VII (congenital) (stable) 286.3
    VIII (congenital) (functional) 286.0
      with
        functional defect 286.0
        vascular defect 286.4
    IX (Christmas) (congenital) (functional) 286.1
    X (congenital) (Stuart-Prower) 286.3
    XI (congenital) (plasma thromboplastin
      antecedent) 286.2
    XII (congenital) (Hageman) 286.3
    XIII (congenital) (fibrin stabilizing) 286.3
    Hageman 286.3
    multiple (congenital) 286.9
      acquired 286.7
    fibrinase (*see also* Defect, coagulation) 286.3
    fibrinogen (congenital) (*see also* Defect,
      coagulation) 286.3
      acquired 286.6
    fibrin stabilizing factor (congenital) (*see also*
      Defect, coagulation) 286.3
      acquired 286.7
    finger—*see* Absence, finger
    Fletcher factor (*see also* Defect, coagulation)
      286.9
  fluorine 269.3
  folate, anemia 281.2
  folic acid (vitamin Bc) 266.2
    anemia 281.2
  follicle-stimulating hormone (FSH) 253.4
  fructokinase 271.2
  fructose-1, 6-diphosphate 271.2
  fructose-1-phosphate aldolase 271.2
  FSH (follicle-stimulating hormone) 253.4
  fucosidase 271.8
  galactokinase 271.1
  galactose-1-phosphate uridyl transferase 271.1
  gamma globulin in blood 279.00
  glass factor (*see also* Defect, coagulation) 286.3
  glucocorticoid 255.4
  glucose-6-phosphatase 271.0
  glucose-6-phosphate dehydrogenase anemia
    282.2
  glucuronyl transferase 277.4
  glutathione-reductase (anemia) 282.2

Deficiency, deficient—*continued*
  glycogen synthetase 271.0
  growth hormone 253.3
  Hageman factor (congenital) (*see also* Defect,
    coagulation) 286.3
  head V48.0
  hemoglobin (*see also* Anemia) 285.9
  hepatophosphorylase 271.0
  hexose monophosphate (HMP) shunt 282.2
  HGH (human growth hormone) 253.3
  HG-PRT 277.2
  homogentisic acid oxidase 270.2
  hormone—*see also* Deficiency, by specific
    hormone
    anterior pituitary (isolated) (partial) NEC
      253.4
    growth (human) 253.3
    follicle-stimulating 253.4
    growth (human) (isolated) 253.3
    human growth 253.3
    interstitial cell-stimulating 253.4
    luteinizing 253.4
    melanocyte-stimulating 253.4
    testicular 257.2
  human growth hormone 253.3
  humoral 279.00
    with
      hyper-IgM 279.05
        autosomal recessive 279.05
        X-linked 279.05
      increased IgM 279.05
    congenital hypogammaglobulinemia 279.04
      non-sex-linked 279.06
    selective immunoglobulin NEC 279.03
      IgA 279.01
      IgG 279.03
      IgM 279.02
        increased 279.05
    specified NEC 279.09
  hydroxylase 255.2
  hypoxanthine-guanine
    phosphoribosyltransferase (HG-PRT) 277.2
  ICSH (interstitial cell-stimulating hormone)
    253.4
  immunity NEC 279.3
    cell-mediated 279.10
      with
        hyperimmunoglobulinemia 279.2
        thrombocytopenia and eczema 279.12
      specified NEC 279.19
    combined (severe) 279.2
      syndrome 279.2
    common variable 279.06
    humoral NEC 279.00
    IgA (secretory) 279.01
    IgG 279.03
    IgM 279.02
  immunoglobulin, selective NEC 279.03
    IgA 279.01
    IgG 279.03
    IgM 279.02
  inositol (B complex) 266.2
  interferon 279.4
  internal organ V47.0
  interstitial cell-stimulating hormone (ICSH)
    253.4
  intrinsic (urethral) sphincter (ISD) 599.82
  intrinsic factor (Castle's) (congenital) 281.0
  invertase 271.3
  iodine 269.3
  iron, anemia 280.9

Deficiency, deficient—*continued*
  labile factor (congenital) (*see also* Defect,
    coagulation) 286.3
    acquired 286.7
  lacrimal fluid (acquired) 375.15
    congenital 743.64
  lactase 271.3
  Laki-Lorand factor (*see also* Defect,
    coagulation) 286.3
  lecithin-cholesterol acyltranferase 272.5
  LH (luteinizing hormone) 253.4
  limb V49.0
    lower V49.0
      congenital (*see also* Deficiency, lower limb,
        congenital) 755.30
    upper V49.0
      congenital (*see also* Deficiency, upper limb,
        congenital) 755.20
  lipocaic 577.8
  lipoid (high-density) 272.5
  lipoprotein (familial) (high density) 272.5
  liver phosphorylase 271.0
  lower limb V49.0
    congenital 755.30
      with complete absence of distal elements
        755.31
      longitudinal (complete) (partial) (with distal
        deficiencies, incomplete) 755.32
        with complete absence of distal elements
          755.31
        combined femoral, tibial, fibular
          (incomplete) 755.33
        femoral 755.34
        fibular 755.37
        metatarsal(s) 755.38
        phalange(s) 755.39
          meaning all digits 755.31
        tarsal(s) 755.38
        tibia 755.36
        tibiofibular 755.35
      transverse 755.31
  luteinizing hormone (LH) 253.4
  lysosomal alpha-1, 4 glucosidase 271.0
  magnesium 275.2
  mannosidase 271.8
  melanocyte-stimulating hormone (MSH) 253.4
  menadione (vitamin K) 269.0
    newborn 776.0
  mental (familial) (hereditary) (*see also*
    Retardation, mental) 319
  mineral NEC 269.3
  molybdenum 269.3
  moral 301.7
  multiple, syndrome 260
  myocardial (*see also* Insufficiency myocardial)
    428.0
  myophosphorylase 271.0
  NADH (DPNH) -methemoglobin-reductase
    (congenital) 289.7
  NADH diaphorase or reductase (congenital)
    289.7
  neck V48.1
  niacin (amide) (-tryptophan) 265.2
  nicotinamide 265.2
  nicotinic acid (amide) 265.2
  nose V48.8
  number of teeth (*see also* Anodontia) 520.0
  nutrition, nutritional 269.9
    specified NEC 269.8

Deformity—*continued*
  caruncle, lacrimal (congenital) 743.9
    acquired 375.69
  cascade, stomach 537.6
  cecum (congenital) 751.5
    acquired 569.89
  cerebral (congenital) 742.9
    acquired 348.8
  cervix (acquired) (uterus) 622.8
    congenital 752.40
  cheek (acquired) 738.19
    congenital 744.9
  chest (wall) (acquired) 738.3
    congenital 754.89
    late effect of rickets 268.1
  chin (acquired) 738.19
    congenital 744.9
  choroid (congenital) 743.9
    acquired 363.8
    plexus (congenital) 742.9
      acquired 349.2
  cicatricial—*see* Cicatrix
  cilia (congenital) 743.9
    acquired 374.89
  circulatory system (congenital) 747.9
  clavicle (acquired) 738.8
    congenital 755.51
  clitoris (congenital) 752.40
    acquired 624.8
  clubfoot—*see* Clubfoot
  coccyx (acquired) 738.6
    congenital 756.10
  colon (congenital) 751.5
    acquired 569.89
  concha (ear) (congenital) (*see also* Deformity,
      ear) 744.3
    acquired 380.32
  congenital, organ or site not listed (*see also*
      Anomaly) 759.9
  cornea (congenital) 743.9
    acquired 371.70
  coronary artery (congenital) 746.85
    acquired (*see also* Ischemia, heart) 414.9
  cranium (acquired) 738.19
    congenital (*see also* Deformity, skull,
      congenital) 756.0
  cricoid cartilage (congenital) 748.3
    acquired 478.79
  cystic duct (congenital) 751.60
    acquired 575.8
  Dandy-Walker 742.3
    with spina bifida (*see also* Spina bifida) 741.0
  diaphragm (congenital) 756.6
    acquired 738.8
  digestive organ(s) or system (congenital) NEC
      751.9
    specified type NEC 751.8
  ductus arteriosus 747.0
  duodenal bulb 537.89
  duodenum (congenital) 751.5
    acquired 537.89
  dura (congenital) 742.9
    brain 742.4
      acquired 349.2
    spinal 742.59
      acquired 349.2

Deformity—*continued*
  ear (congenital) 744.3
    acquired 380.32
    auricle 744.3
      causing impairment of hearing 744.02
    causing impairment of hearing 744.00
    external 744.3
      causing impairment of hearing 744.02
    internal 744.05
    lobule 744.3
    middle 744.03
      ossicles 744.04
    ossicles 744.04
  ectodermal (congenital) NEC 757.9
    specified type NEC 757.8
  ejaculatory duct (congenital) 752.9
    acquired 608.89
  elbow (joint) (acquired) 736.00
    congenital 755.50
    contraction 718.42
  endocrine gland NEC 759.2
  epididymis (congenital) 752.9
    acquired 608.89
    torsion 608.2
  epiglottis (congenital) 748.3
    acquired 478.79
  esophagus (congenital) 750.9
    acquired 530.89
  Eustachian tube (congenital) NEC 744.3
    specified type NEC 744.24
  extremity (acquired) 736.9
    congenital, except reduction deformity 755.9
      lower 755.60
      upper 755.50
    reduction—*see* Deformity, reduction
  eye (congenital) 743.9
    acquired 379.8
    muscle 743.9
  eyebrow (congenital) 744.89
  eyelid (congenital) 743.9
    acquired 374.89
    specified type NEC 743.62
  face (acquired) 738.19
    congenital (any part) 744.9
      due to intrauterine malposition and pressure
        754.0
  fallopian tube (congenital) 752.10
    acquired 620.8
  femur (acquired) 736.89
    congenital 755.60
  fetal
    with fetopelvic disproportion 653.7
      affecting fetus or newborn 763.1
    causing obstructed labor 660.1
      affecting fetus or newborn 763.1
    known or suspected, affecting management of
        pregnancy 655.9
  finger (acquired) 736.20
    boutonniere type 736.21
    congenital 755.50
    flexion contracture 718.44
    swan neck 736.22
  flexion (joint) (acquired) 736.9
    congenital NEC 755.9
    hip or thigh (acquired) 736.39
      congenital (*see also* Subluxation,
        congenital, hip) 754.32

Deformity—*continued*
  foot (acquired) 736.70
    cavovarus 736.75
      congenital 754.59
    congenital NEC 754.70
      specified type NEC 754.79
    valgus (acquired) 736.79
      congenital 754.60
        specified type NEC 754.69
    varus (acquired) 736.79
      congenital 754.50
        specified type NEC 754.59
  forearm (acquired) 736.00
    congenital 755.50
  forehead (acquired) 738.19
    congenital (*see also* Deformity, skull,
      congenital) 756.0
  frontal bone (acquired) 738.19
    congenital (*see also* Deformity, skull,
      congenital) 756.0
  gallbladder (congenital) 751.60
    acquired 575.8
  gastrointestinal tract (congenital) NEC 751.9
    acquired 569.89
    specified type NEC 751.8
  genitalia, genital organ(s) or system NEC
    congenital 752.9
    female (congenital) 752.9
      acquired 629.8
      external 752.40
      internal 752.9
    male (congenital) 752.9
      acquired 608.89
  globe (eye) (congenital) 743.9
    acquired 360.89
  gum (congenital) 750.9
    acquired 523.9
  gunstock 736.02
  hand (acquired) 736.00
    claw 736.06
    congenital 755.50
    minus (and plus) (intrinsic) 736.09
    pill roller (intrinsic) 736.09
    plus (and minus) (intrinsic) 736.09
    swan neck (intrinsic) 736.09
  head (acquired) 738.10
    congenital (*see also* Deformity, skull,
      congenital) 756.0
    specified NEC 738.19
  heart (congenital) 746.9
    auricle (congenital) 746.9
    septum 745.9
      auricular 745.5
      specified type NEC 745.8
      ventricular 745.4
    valve (congenital) NEC 746.9
      acquired—*see* Endocarditis
      pulmonary (congenital) 746.00
      specified type NEC 746.89
    ventricle (congenital) 746.9
  heel (acquired) 736.76
    congenital 755.67
  hepatic duct (congenital) 751.60
    acquired 576.8
    with calculus, choledocholithiasis, or
      stones—*see* Choledocholithiasis
  hip (joint) (acquired) 736.30
    congenital NEC 755.63
    flexion 718.45
      congenital (*see also* Subluxation,
      congenital, hip) 754.32

Deformity—*continued*
  hourglass—*see* Contraction, hourglass
  humerus (acquired) 736.89
    congenital 755.50
  hymen (congenital) 752.40
  hypophyseal (congenital) 759.2
  ileocecal (coil) (valve) (congenital) 751.5
    acquired 569.89
  ileum (intestine) (congenital) 751.5
    acquired 569.89
  ilium (acquired) 738.6
    congenital 755.60
  integument (congenital) 757.9
  intervertebral cartilage or disc (acquired)—*see*
    also Displacement, intervertebral disc
    congenital 756.10
  intestine (large) (small) (congenital) 751.5
    acquired 569.89
  iris (acquired) 364.75
    congenital 743.9
    prolapse 364.8
  ischium (acquired) 738.6
    congenital 755.60
  jaw (acquired) (congenital) NEC 524.9
    due to intrauterine malposition and pressure
      754.0
  joint (acquired) NEC 738.8
    congenital 755.9
    contraction (abduction) (adduction)
      (extension) (flexion)—*see* Contraction,
      joint
  kidney(s) (calyx) (pelvis) (congenital) 753.9
    acquired 593.89
    vessel 747.62
      acquired 459.9
  Klippel-Feil (brevicollis) 756.16
  knee (acquired) NEC 736.6
    congenital 755.64
  labium (majus) (minus) (congenital) 752.40
    acquired 624.8
  lacrimal apparatus or duct (congenital) 743.9
    acquired 375.69
  larynx (muscle) (congenital) 748.3
    acquired 478.79
    web (glottic) (subglottic) 748.2
  leg (lower) (upper) (acquired) NEC 736.89
    congenital 755.60
    reduction—*see* Deformity, reduction, lower
      limb
  lens (congenital) 743.9
    acquired 379.39
  lid (fold) (congenital) 743.9
    acquired 374.89
  ligament (acquired) 728.9
    congenital 756.9
  limb (acquired) 736.9
    congenital, except reduction deformity 755.9
      lower 755.60
        reduction (*see also* Deformity, reduction,
        lower limb) 755.30
      upper 755.50
        reduction (*see also* Deformity, reduction,
        lower limb) 755.20
    specified NEC 736.89
  lip (congenital) NEC 750.9
    acquired 528.5
    specified type NEC 750.26

Deformity—*continued*
  liver (congenital) 751.60
    acquired 573.8
    duct (congenital) 751.60
      acquired 576.8
      with calculus, choledocholithiasis, or
        stones—*see* Choledocholithiasis
  lower extremity—*see* Deformity, leg
  lumbosacral (joint) (region) (congenital) 756.10
    acquired 738.5
  lung (congenital) 748.60
    acquired 518.89
    specified type NEC 748.69
  lymphatic system, congenital 759.9
  Madelung's (radius) 755.54
  maxilla (acquired) (congenital) 524.9
  meninges or membrane (congenital) 742.9
    brain 742.4
      acquired 349.2
    spinal (cord) 742.59
      acquired 349.2
  mesentery (congenital) 751.9
    acquired 568.89
  metacarpus (acquired) 736.00
    congenital 755.50
  metatarsus (acquired) 736.70
    congenital 754.70
  middle ear, except ossicles (congenital) 744.03
    ossicles 744.04
  mitral (leaflets) (valve) (congenital) 746.9
    acquired—*see* Endocarditis, mitral
    Ebstein's 746.89
    parachute 746.5
    specified type NEC 746.89
    stenosis, congenital 746.5
  mouth (acquired) 528.9
    congenital NEC 750.9
      specified type NEC 750.26
  multiple, congenital NEC 759.7
    specified type NEC 759.89
  muscle (acquired) 728.9
    congenital 756.9
      specified type NEC 756.89
      sternocleidomastoid (due to intrauterine
        malposition and pressure) 754.1
  musculoskeletal system, congenital NEC 756.9
    specified type NEC 756.9
  nail (acquired) 703.9
    congenital 757.9
  nasal—*see* Deformity, nose
  neck (acquired) NEC 738.2
    congenital (any part) 744.9
      sternocleidomastoid 754.1
  nervous system (congenital) 742.9
  nipple (congenital) 757.9
    acquired 611.8
  nose, nasal (cartilage) (acquired) 738.0
    bone (turbinate) 738.0
    congenital 748.1
      bent 754.0
      squashed 754.0
    saddle 738.0
      syphilitic 090.5
    septum 470
      congenital 748.1
    sinus (wall) (congenital) 748.1
      acquired 738.0
    syphilitic (congenital) 090.5
      late 095.8
  ocular muscle (congenital) 743.9
    acquired 378.60

Deformity—*continued*
  opticociliary vessels (congenital) 743.9
  orbit (congenital) (eye) 743.9
    acquired NEC 376.40
      associated with craniofacial deformities
        376.44
      due to
        bone disease 376.43
        surgery 376.47
        trauma 376.47
  organ of Corti (congenital) 744.05
  ovary (congenital) 752.0
    acquired 620.8
  oviduct (congenital) 752.10
    acquired 620.8
  palate (congenital) 750.9
    acquired 526.89
    cleft (congenital) (*see also* Cleft, palate)
      749.00
    hard, acquired 526.89
    soft, acquired 528.9
  pancreas (congenital) 751.7
    acquired 577.8
  parachute, mitral valve 746.5
  parathyroid (gland) 759.2
  parotid (gland) (congenital) 750.9
    acquired 527.8
  patella (acquired) 736.6
    congenital 755.64
  pelvis, pelvic (acquired) (bony) 738.6
    with disproportion (fetopelvic) 653.0
      affecting fetus or newborn 763.1
      causing obstructed labor 660.1
        affecting fetus or newborn 763.1
    congenital 755.60
    rachitic (late effect) 268.1
  penis (glans) (congenital) 752.9
    acquired 607.89
  pericardium (congenital) 746.9
    acquired—*see* Pericarditis
  pharynx (congenital) 750.9
    acquired 478.29
  Pierre Robin (congenital) 756.0
  pinna (acquired) 380.32
    congenital 744.3
  pituitary (congenital) 759.2
  pleural folds (congenital) 748.8
  portal vein (congenital) 747.40
  posture—*see* Curvature, spine
  prepuce (congenital) 752.9
    acquired 607.89
  prostate (congenital) 752.9
    acquired 602.8
  pulmonary valve—*see* Endocarditis, pulmonary
  pupil (congenital) 743.9
    acquired 364.75
  pylorus (congenital) 750.9
    acquired 537.89
  rachitic (acquired), healed or old 268.1
  radius (acquired) 736.00
    congenital 755.50
      reduction—*see* Deformity, reduction, upper
        limb
  rectovaginal septum (congenital) 752.40
    acquired 623.8
  rectum (congenital) 751.5
    acquired 569.49

Deformity—*continued*

reduction (extremity) (limb) 755.4
  brain 742.2
  lower limb 755.30
    with complete absence of distal elements
      755.31
    longitudinal (complete) (partial) (with distal
      deficiencies, incomplete) 755.32
    with complete absence of distal elements
      755.31
    combined femoral, tibial, fibular
      (incomplete) 755.33
    femoral 755.34
    fibular 755.37
    metatarsal(s) 755.38
    phalange(s) 755.39
      meaning all digits 755.31
    tarsal(s) 755.38
    tibia 755.36
    tibiofibular 755.35
    transverse 755.31
  upper limb 755.20
    with complete absence of distal elements
      755.21
    longitudinal (complete) (partial) (with distal
      deficiencies, incomplete) 755.22
    with complete absence of distal elements
      755.21
    carpal(s) 755.28
    combined humeral, radial, ulnar
      (incomplete) 755.23
    humeral 755.24
    metacarpal(s) 755.28
    phalange(s) 755.29
      meaning all digits 755.21
    radial 755.26
    radioulnar 755.25
    ulnar 755.27
  transverse (complete) (partial) 755.21
renal—*see* Deformity, kidney
respiratory system (congenital) 748.9
  specified type NEC 748.8
rib (acquired) 738.3
  congenital 756.3
    cervical 756.2
rotation (joint) (acquired) 736.9
  congenital 755.9
  hip or thigh 736.39
    congenital (*see also* Subluxation,
      congenital, hip) 754.32
sacroiliac joint (congenital) 755.69
  acquired 738.5
sacrum (acquired) 738.5
  congenital 756.10
saddle
  back 737.8
  nose 738.0
    syphilitic 090.5
salivary gland or duct (congenital) 750.9
  acquired 527.8
scapula (acquired) 736.89
  congenital 755.50
scrotum (congenital) 752.9
  acquired 608.89
sebaceous gland, acquired 706.8
seminal tract or duct (congenital) 752.9
  acquired 608.89
septum (nasal) (acquired) 470
  congenital 748.1

Deformity—*continued*

shoulder (joint) (acquired) 736.89
  congenital 755.50
    specified type NEC 755.59
  contraction 718.41
sigmoid (flexure) (congenital) 751.5
  acquired 569.89
sinus of Valsalva 747.29
skin (congenital) 757.9
  acquired NEC 709.8
skull (acquired) 738.19
  congenital 756.0
    with
      anencephalus 740.0
      encephalocele 742.0
      hydrocephalus 742.3
        with spina bifida (*see also* Spina bifida)
          741.0
      microcephalus 742.1
    due to intrauterine malposition and pressure
      754.0
soft parts, organs or tissues (of pelvis)
  in pregnancy or childbirth NEC 654.9
    affecting fetus or newborn 763.89
    causing obstructed labor 660.2
      affecting fetus or newborn 763.1
spermatic cord (congenital) 752.9
  acquired 608.89
    torsion 608.2
spinal
  column—*see* Deformity, spine
  cord (congenital) 742.9
    acquired 336.8
    vessel (congenital) 747.82
  nerve root (congenital) 742.9
    acquired 724.9
  vessel 747.82
spine (acquired) NEC 738.5
  congenital 756.10
    due to intrauterine malposition and pressure
      754.2
  kyphoscoliotic (*see also* Kyphoscoliosis)
    737.30
  kyphotic (*see also* Kyphosis) 737.10
  lordotic (*see also* Lordosis) 737.20
  rachitic 268.1
  scoliotic (*see also* Scoliosis) 737.30
spleen
  acquired 289.59
  congenital 759.0
Sprengel's (congenital) 755.52
sternum (acquired) 738.3
  congenital 756.3
stomach (congenital) 750.9
  acquired 537.89
submaxillary gland (congenital) 750.9
  acquired 527.8
swan neck (acquired)
  finger 736.22
  hand 736.09
talipes—*see* Talipes
teeth, tooth NEC 520.9
testis (congenital) 752.9
  acquired 608.89
    torsion 608.2
thigh (acquired) 736.89
  congenital 755.60
thorax (acquired) (wall) 738.3
  congenital 754.89
  late effect of rickets 268.1

Deformity—*continued*
  thumb (acquired) 736.20
    congenital 755.50
  thymus (tissue) (congenital) 759.2
  thyroid (gland) (congenital) 759.2
    cartilage 748.3
      acquired 478.79
  tibia (acquired) 736.89
    congenital 755.60
    saber 090.5
  toe (acquired) 735.9
    congenital 755.66
    specified NEC 735.8
  tongue (congenital) 750.10
    acquired 529.8
  tooth, teeth NEC 520.9
  trachea (rings) (congenital) 748.3
    acquired 519.1
  transverse aortic arch (congenital) 747.21
  tricuspid (leaflets) (valve) (congenital) 746.9
    acquired—*see* Endocarditis, tricuspid
    atresia or stenosis 746.1
    specified type NEC 746.89
  trunk (acquired) 738.3
    congenital 759.9
  ulna (acquired) 736.00
    congenital 755.50
  upper extremity—*see* Deformity, arm
  urachus (congenital) 753.7
  ureter (opening) (congenital) 753.9
    acquired 593.89
  urethra (valve) (congenital) 753.9
    acquired 599.84
  urinary tract or system (congenital) 753.9
    urachus 753.7
  uterus (congenital) 752.3
    acquired 621.8
  uvula (congenital) 750.9
    acquired 528.9
  vagina (congenital) 752.40
    acquired 623.8
  valve, valvular (heart) (congenital) 746.9
    acquired—*see* Endocarditis
    pulmonary 746.00
    specified type NEC 746.89
  vascular (congenital) (peripheral) NEC 747.60
    acquired 459.9
    gastrointestinal 747.61
    lower limb 747.64
    renal 747.62
    specified site NEC 747.69
    spinal 747.82
    upper limb 747.63
  vas deferens (congenital) 752.9
    acquired 608.89
  vein (congenital) NEC (*see also* Deformity,
      vascular) 747.60
    brain 747.81
    coronary 746.9
    great 747.40
  vena cava (inferior) (superior) (congenital)
      747.40
  vertebra—*see* Deformity, spine
  vesicourethral orifice (acquired) 596.8
    congenital NEC 753.9
    specified type NEC 753.8
  vessels of optic papilla (congenital) 743.9
  visual field (contraction) 368.45
  vitreous humor (congenital) 743.9
    acquired 379.29

Deformity—*continued*
  vulva (congenital) 752.40
    acquired 624.8
  wrist (joint) (acquired) 736.00
    congenital 755.50
    contraction 718.43
    valgus 736.03
      congenital 755.59
    varus 736.04
      congenital 755.59

Degeneration, degenerative
  adrenal (capsule) (gland) 255.8
    with hypofunction 255.4
    fatty 255.8
    hyaline 255.8
    infectional 255.8
    lardaceous 277.3
  amyloid (any site) (general) 277.3
  anterior cornua, spinal cord 336.8
  aorta, aortic 440.0
    fatty 447.8
    valve (heart) (*see also* Endocarditis, aortic)
      424.1
  arteriovascular—*see* Arteriosclerosis
  artery, arterial (atheromatous) (calcareous)—*see*
      also Arteriosclerosis
    amyloid 277.3
    lardaceous 277.3
    medial NEC (*see also* Arteriosclerosis,
        extremities) 440.20
  articular cartilage NEC (*see also* Disorder,
      cartilage, articular) 718.0
    elbow 718.02
    knee 717.5
    patella 717.7
    shoulder 718.01
    spine (*see also* Spondylosis) 721.90
  atheromatous—*see* Arteriosclerosis
  bacony (any site) 277.3
  basal nuclei or ganglia NEC 333.0
  bone 733.90
  brachial plexus 353.0
  brain (cortical) (progressive) 331.9
    arteriosclerotic 437.0
    childhood 330.9
      specified type NEC 330.8
    congenital 742.4
    cystic 348.0
      congenital 742.4
    familial NEC 331.89
    grey matter 330.8
    heredofamilial NEC 331.89
    in
      alcoholism 303.9 [*331.7*]
      beriberi 265.0 [*331.7*]
      cerebrovascular disease 437.9 [*331.7*]
      congenital hydrocephalus 742.3 [*331.7*]
        with spina bifida (*see also* Spina bifida)
          741.0 [*331.7*]
      Fabry's disease 272.7 [*330.2*]
      Gaucher's disease 272.7 [*330.2*]
      Hunter's disease or syndrome 277.5 [*330.3*]
      lipidosis
        cerebral 330.1
        generalized 272.7 [*330.2*]
      mucopolysaccharidosis 277.5 [*330.3*]
      myxedema (*see also* Myxedema) 244.9
        [*331.7*]
      neoplastic disease NEC (M8000/1) 239.9
        [*331.7*]
      Niemann-Pick disease 272.7 [*330.2*]

Degeneration, degenerative—*continued*
- sphingolipidosis 272.7 *[330.2]*
- vitamin B$_{12}$ deficiency 266.2 *[331.7]*
- motor centers 331.89
- senile 331.2
- specified type NEC 331.89
- breast—*see* Disease, breast
- Bruch's membrane 363.40
- bundle of His 426.50
  - left 426.3
  - right 426.4
- calcareous NEC 275.49
- capillaries 448.9
  - amyloid 277.3
  - fatty 448.9
  - lardaceous 277.3
- cardiac (brown) (calcareous) (fatty) (fibrous)
  (hyaline) (mural) (muscular) (pigmentary)
  (senile) (with arteriosclerosis) (*see also*
  Degeneration, myocardial) 429.1
  - valve, valvular—*see* Endocarditis
- cardiorenal (*see also* Hypertension, cardiorenal)
  404.90
- cardiovascular (*see also* Disease,
  cardiovascular) 429.2
  - renal (*see also* Hypertension, cardiorenal)
    404.90
- cartilage (joint)—*see* Derangement, joint
- cerebellar NEC 334.9
  - primary (hereditary) (sporadic) 334.2
- cerebral—*see* Degeneration, brain
- cerebromacular 330.1
- cerebrovascular 437.1
  - due to hypertension 437.2
  - late effect—*see* Late effect(s) (of)
    cerebrovascular disease
- cervical plexus 353.2
- cervix 622.8
  - due to radiation (intended effect) 622.8
    - adverse effect or misadventure 622.8
- changes, spine or vertebra (*see also*
  Spondylosis) 721.90
- chitinous 277.3
- chorioretinal 363.40
  - congenital 743.53
  - hereditary 363.50
- choroid (colloid) (drusen) 363.40
  - hereditary 363.50
  - senile 363.41
    - diffuse secondary 363.42
- cochlear 386.8
- collateral ligament (knee) (medial) 717.82
  - lateral 717.81
- combined (spinal cord) (subacute) 266.2 *[336.2]*
  - with anemia (pernicious) 281.0 *[336.2]*
    - due to dietary deficiency 281.1 *[336.2]*
    - due to vitamin B$_{12}$ deficiency anemia (dietary)
      281.1 *[336.2]*
- conjunctiva 372.50
  - amyloid 277.3 *[372.50]*
- cornea 371.40
  - calcerous 371.44
  - familial (hereditary) (*see also* Dystrophy,
    cornea) 371.50
    - macular 371.55
    - reticular 371.54
  - hyaline (of old scars) 371.41
  - marginal (Terrien's) 371.48
  - mosaic (shagreen) 371.41
  - nodular 371.46
  - peripheral 371.48

Degeneration, degenerative—*continued*
- senile 371.41
- cortical (cerebellar) (parenchymatous) 334.2
  - alcoholic 303.9 *[334.4]*
  - diffuse, due to arteriopathy 437.0
- corticostriatal-spinal 334.8
- cretinoid 243
- cruciate ligament (knee) (posterior) 717.84
  - anterior 717.83
- cutis 709.3
  - amyloid 277.3
- dental pulp 522.2
- disc disease—*see* Degeneration, intervertebral
  disc
- dorsolateral (spinal cord)—*see* Degeneration,
  combined
- endocardial 424.90
- extrapyramidal NEC 333.90
- eye NEC 360.40
  - macular (*see also* Degeneration, macula)
    362.50
    - congenital 362.75
    - hereditary 362.76
- fatty (diffuse) (general) 272.8
  - liver 571.8
    - alcoholic 571.0
  - localized site—*see* Degeneration, by site, fatty
  - placenta—*see* Placenta, abnormal
- globe (eye) NEC 360.40
  - macular—*see* Degeneration, macula
- grey matter 330.8
- heart (brown) (calcareous) (fatty) (fibrous)
  (hyaline) (mural) (muscular) (pigmentary)
  (senile) (with arteriosclerosis) (*see also*
  Degeneration, myocardial) 429.1
  - amyloid 277.3 *[425.7]*
  - atheromatous —*see* Arteriosclerosis, coronary
  - gouty 274.82
  - hypertensive (*see also* Hypertension, heart)
    402.90
  - ischemic 414.9
  - valve, valvular—*see* Endocarditis
- hepatolenticular (Wilson's) 275.1
- hepatorenal 572.4
- heredofamilial
  - brain NEC 331.89
  - spinal cord NEC 336.8
- hyaline (diffuse) (generalized) 728.9
  - localized—*see also* Degeneration, by site
    - cornea 371.41
    - keratitis 371.41
- hypertensive vascular—*see* Hypertension
- infrapatellar fat pad 729.31
- internal semilunar cartilage 717.3
- intervertebral disc 722.6
  - with myelopathy 722.70
  - cervical, cervicothoracic 722.4
    - with myelopathy 722.71
  - lumbar, lumbosacral 722.52
    - with myelopathy 722.73
  - thoracic, thoracolumbar 722.51
    - with myelopathy 722.72
- intestine 569.89
  - amyloid 277.3
  - lardaceous 277.3
- iris (generalized) (*see also* Atrophy, iris) 364.59
  - pigmentary 364.53
  - pupillary margin 364.54
- ischemic—*see* Ischemia
- joint disease (*see also* Osteoarthrosis) 715.9
  - multiple sites 715.09

Degeneration, degenerative—*continued*
  spine (*see also* Spondylosis) 721.90
  kidney (*see also* Sclerosis, renal) 587
    amyloid 277.3 *[583.81]*
    cyst, cystic (multiple) (solitary) 593.2
      congenital (*see also* Cystic, disease, kidney)
        753.10
    fatty 593.89
    fibrocystic (congenital) 753.19
    lardaceous 277.3 *[583.81]*
    polycystic (congenital) 753.12
      adult type (APKD) 753.13
      autosomal dominant 753.13
      autosomal recessive 753.14
      childhood type (CPKD) 753.14
      infantile type 753.14
    waxy 277.3 *[583.81]*
  Kuhnt-Junius (retina) 362.52
  labyrinth, osseous 386.8
  lacrimal passages, cystic 375.12
  lardaceous (any site) 277.3
  lateral column (posterior), spinal cord (*see also*
    Degeneration, combined) 266.2 *[336.2]*
  lattice 362.63
  lens 366.9
    infantile, juvenile, or presenile 366.00
    senile 366.10
  lenticular (familial) (progressive) (Wilson's)
    (with cirrhosis of liver) 275.1
    striate artery 437.0
  lethal ball, prosthetic heart valve 996.02
  ligament
    collateral (knee) (medial) 717.82
      lateral 717.81
    cruciate (knee) (posterior) 717.84
      anterior 717.83
  liver (diffuse) 572.8
    amyloid 277.3
    congenital (cystic) 751.62
    cystic 572.8
      congenital 751.62
    fatty 571.8
      alcoholic 571.0
    hypertrophic 572.8
    lardaceous 277.3
    parenchymatous, acute or subacute (*see also*
      Necrosis, liver) 570
    pigmentary 572.8
    toxic (acute) 573.8
    waxy 277.3
  lung 518.8
  lymph gland 289.3
    hyaline 289.3
    lardaceous 277.3
  macula (acquired) (senile) 362.50
    atrophic 362.51
    Best's 362.76
    congenital 362.75
    cystic 362.54
    cystoid 362.53
    disciform 362.52
    dry 362.51
    exudative 362.52
    familial pseudoinflammatory 362.77
    hereditary 362.76
    hole 362.54
    juvenile (Stargardt's) 362.75
    nonexudative 362.51
    pseudohole 362.54
    wet 362.52

Degeneration, degenerative—*continued*
  medullary—*see* Degeneration, brain
  membranous labyrinth, congenital (causing
    impairment of hearing) 744.05
  meniscus—*see* Derangement, joint
  microcystoid 362.62
  mitral—*see* Insufficiency, mitral
  Mönckeberg's (*see also* Arteriosclerosis,
    extremities) 440.20
  moral 301.7
  motor centers, senile 331.2
  mural (*see also* Degeneration, myocardial) 429.1
    heart, cardiac (*see also* Degeneration,
      myocardial) 429.1
    myocardium, myocardial (*see also*
      Degeneration, myocardial) 429.1
  muscle 728.9
    fatty 728.9
    fibrous 728.9
    heart (*see also* Degeneration, myocardial)
      429.1
    hyaline 728.9
    muscular progressive 728.2
  myelin, central nervous system NEC 341.9
  myocardium, myocardial (brown) (calcareous)
    (fatty) (fibrous) (hyaline) (mural)
    (muscular) (pigmentary) (senile) (with
    arteriosclerosis) 429.1
    with rheumatic fever (conditions classifiable
      to 390) 398.0
      active, acute, or subacute 391.2
        with chorea 392.0
      inactive or quiescent (with chorea) 398.0
    amyloid 277.3 *[425.7]*
    congenital 746.89
    fetus or newborn 779.89
    gouty 274.82
    hypertensive (*see also* Hypertension, heart)
      402.90
    ischemic 414.8
    rheumatic (*see also* Degeneration,
      myocardium, with rheumatic fever) 398.0
    syphilitic 093.82
  nasal sinus (mucosa) (*see also* Sinusitis) 473.9
    frontal 473.1
    maxillary 473.0
  nerve—*see* Disorder, nerve
  nervous system 349.89
    amyloid 277.3 *[357.4]*
    autonomic (*see also* Neuropathy, peripheral,
      autonomic) 337.9
    fatty 349.89
    peripheral autonomic NEC (*see also*
      Neuropathy, peripheral, autonomic) 337.9
  nipple 611.9
  nose 478.1
  oculoacousticocerebral, congenital (progressive)
    743.8
  olivopontocerebellar (familial) (hereditary)
    333.0
  osseous labyrinth 386.8
  ovary 620.8
    cystic 620.2
    microcystic 620.2
  pallidal, pigmentary (progressive) 333.0
  pancreas 577.8
    tuberculous (*see also* Tuberculosis) 017.9
  papillary muscle 429.81
  paving stone 362.61
  penis 607.89
  peritoneum 568.89

Degeneration, degenerative—*continued*
  pigmentary (diffuse) (general)
    localized—*see* Degeneration, by site
    pallidal (progressive) 333.0
    secondary 362.65
  pineal gland 259.8
  pituitary (gland) 253.8
  placenta (fatty) (fibrinoid) (fibroid)—*see*
    Placenta, abnormal
  popliteal fat pad 729.31
  posterolateral (spinal cord) (*see also*
    Degeneration, combined) 266.2 *[336.2]*
  pulmonary valve (heart) (*see also* Endocarditis,
    pulmonary) 424.3
  pulp (tooth) 522.2
  pupillary margin 364.54
  renal (*see also* Sclerosis, renal) 587
    fibrocystic 753.19
    polycystic 753.12
      adult type (APKD) 753.13
      autosomal dominant 753.13
      autosomal recessive 753.14
      childhood type (CPKD) 753.14
      infantile type 753.14
  reticuloendothelial system 289.8
  retina (peripheral) 362.60
    with retinal defect (*see also* Detachment,
      retina, with retinal defect) 361.00
    cystic (senile) 362.50
    cystoid 362.53
    hereditary (*see also* Dystrophy, retina) 362.70
      cerebroretinal 362.71
      congenital 362.75
      juvenile (Stargardt's) 362.75
      macula 362.76
    Kuhnt-Junius 362.52
    lattice 362.63
    macular (*see also* Degeneration, macula)
      362.50
    microcystoid 362.62
    palisade 362.63
    paving stone 362.61
    pigmentary (primary) 362.74
      secondary 362.65
    posterior pole (*see also* Degeneration, macula)
      362.50
    secondary 362.66
    senile 362.60
      cystic 362.53
      reticular 362.64
  saccule, congenital (causing impairment of
    hearing) 744.05
  sacculocochlear 386.8
  senile 797
    brain 331.2
    cardiac, heart, or myocardium (*see also*
      Degeneration, myocardial) 429.1
    motor centers 331.2
    reticule 362.64
    retina, cystic 362.50
    vascular—*see* Arteriosclerosis
  silicone rubber poppet (prosthetic valve) 996.02
  sinus (cystic) (*see also* Sinusitis) 473.9
    polypoid 471.1
  skin 709.3
    amyloid 277.3
    colloid 709.3

Degeneration, degenerative—*continued*
  spinal (cord) 336.8
    amyloid 277.3
    column 733.90
    combined (subacute) (*see also* Degeneration,
      combined) 266.2 *[336.2]*
      with anemia (pernicious) 281.0 *[336.2]*
    dorsolateral (*see also* Degeneration,
      combined) 266.2 *[336.2]*
    familial NEC 336.8
    fatty 336.8
    funicular (*see also* Degeneration, combined)
      266.2 *[336.2]*
    heredofamilial NEC 336.8
    posterolateral (*see also* Degeneration,
      combined) 266.2 *[336.2]*
    subacute combined—*see* Degeneration,
      combined
    tuberculous (*see also* Tuberculosis) 013.8
  spine 733.90
  spleen 289.59
    amyloid 277.3
    lardaceous 277.3
  stomach 537.89
    lardaceous 277.3
  strionigral 333.0
  sudoriparous (cystic) 705.89
  suprarenal (capsule) (gland) 255.8
    with hypofunction 255.4
  sweat gland 705.89
  synovial membrane (pulpy) 727.9
  tapetoretinal 362.74
    adult or presenile form 362.50
  testis (postinfectional) 608.89
  thymus (gland) 254.8
    fatty 254.8
    lardaceous 277.3
  thyroid (gland) 246.8
  tricuspid (heart) (valve)—*see* Endocarditis,
    tricuspid
  tuberculous NEC (*see also* Tuberculosis) 011.9
  turbinate 733.90
  uterus 621.8
    cystic 621.8
  vascular (senile)—*see also* Arteriosclerosis
    hypertensive—*see* Hypertension
  vitreoretinal (primary) 362.73
    secondary 362.66
  vitreous humor (with infiltration) 379.21
  wallerian NEC—*see* Disorder, nerve
  waxy (any site) 277.3
  Wilson's hepatolenticular 275.1
Deglutition
  paralysis 784.9
    hysterical 300.11
  pneumonia 507.0
Degos' disease or syndrome 447.8
Degradation disorder, branched-chain
  amino-acid 270.3
Dehiscence
  anastomosis—*see* Complications, anastomosis
  cesarean wound 674.1
  episiotomy 674.2
  operation wound 998.32
    internal 998.31
  perineal wound (postpartum) 674.2
  postoperative 998.32
    abdomen 998.32
      internal 998.31
    internal 998.31
  uterine wound 674.1

Dehydration (cachexia) 276.5
　with
　　hypernatremia 276.0
　　hyponatremia 276.1
　newborn 775.5
Deiters' nucleus syndrome 386.19
Déjérine's disease 356.0
Déjérine-Klumpke paralysis 767.6
Déjérine-Roussy syndrome 348.8
Déjérine-Sottas disease or neuropathy
　　(hypertrophic) 356.0
Déjérine-Thomas atrophy or syndrome 333.0
de Lange's syndrome (Amsterdam dwarf,
　　mental retardation, and brachycephaly) 759.89
Delay, delayed
　adaptation, cones or rods 368.63
　any plane in pelvis
　　affecting fetus or newborn 763.1
　　complicating delivery 660.1
　birth or delivery NEC 662.1
　　affecting fetus or newborn 763.9
　　second twin, triplet, or multiple mate 662.3
　closure—*see also* Fistula
　　cranial suture 756.0
　　fontanel 756.0
　coagulation NEC 790.92
　conduction (cardiac) (ventricular) 426.9
　delivery NEC 662.1
　　second twin, triplet, etc. 662.3
　　　affecting fetus or newborn 763.89
　development
　　in childhood 783.40
　　　physiological 783.40
　　intellectual NEC 315.9
　　learning NEC 315.2
　　reading 315.00
　　sexual 259.0
　　speech 315.39
　　　associated with hyperkinesis 314.1
　　spelling 315.09
　gastric emptying 536.8
　menarche 256.39
　　due to pituitary hypofunction 253.4
　menstruation (cause unknown) 626.8
　milestone in childhood 783.42
　motility—*see* Hypomotility
　passage of meconium (newborn) 777.1
　primary respiration 768.9
　puberty 259.0
　sexual maturation, female 259.0
Del Castillo's syndrome (germinal aplasia) 606.0
Deleage's disease 359.89
Delhi (boil) (button) (sore) 085.1
Delinquency (juvenile) 312.9
　group (*see also* Disturbance, conduct) 312.2
　neurotic 312.4
Delirium, delirious 780.09
　acute (psychotic) 293.0
　alcoholic 291.0
　　acute 291.0
　　chronic 291.1
　alcoholicum 291.0
　chronic (*see also* Psychosis) 293.89
　　due to or associated with physical
　　　condition—*see* Psychosis, organic
　drug-induced 292.81
　eclamptic (*see also* Eclampsia) 780.39
　exhaustion (*see also* Reaction, stress, acute)
　　308.9
　hysterical 300.11

Delirium, delirious—*continued*
　in
　　presenile dementia 290.11
　　senile dementia 290.3
　induced by drug 292.81
　manic, maniacal (acute) (*see also* Psychosis,
　　affective) 296.0
　　recurrent episode 296.1
　　single episode 296.0
　puerperal 293.9
　senile 290.3
　subacute (psychotic) 293.1
　thyroid (*see also* Thyrotoxicosis) 242.9
　traumatic—*see also* Injury, intracranial
　　with
　　　lesion, spinal cord—*see* Injury, spinal, by
　　　　site
　　　shock, spinal—*see* Injury, spinal, by site
　tremens (impending) 291.0
　uremic—*see* Uremia
　withdrawal
　　alcoholic (acute) 291.0
　　　chronic 291.1
　　drug 292.0
Delivery

> Note—Use the following fifth-digit
> subclassification with categories 640-648,
> 651-676:
>
> *0　unspecified as to episode of care*
> *1　delivered, with or without mention of*
> *　　antepartum condition*
> *2　delivered, with mention of*
> *　　postpartum complication*
> *3　antepartum condition or complication*
> *4　postpartum condition or*
> *　　complication*

　breech (assisted) (spontaneous) 652.2
　　affecting fetus or newborn 763.0
　　extraction NEC 669.6
　cesarean (for) 669.7
　　abnormal
　　　cervix 654.6
　　　pelvic organs or tissues 654.9
　　　pelvis (bony) (major) NEC 653.0
　　　presentation or position 652.9
　　　　in multiple gestation 652.6
　　　size, fetus 653.5
　　　soft parts (of pelvis) 654.9
　　　uterus, congenital 654.0
　　　vagina 654.7
　　　vulva 654.8
　　abruptio placentae 641.2
　　acromion presentation 652.8
　　affecting fetus or newborn 763.4
　　anteversion, cervix or uterus 654.4
　　atony, uterus 666.1
　　bicornis or bicornuate uterus 654.0
　　breech presentation 652.2
　　brow presentation 652.4
　　cephalopelvic disproportion (normally formed
　　　fetus) 653.4
　　chin presentation 652.4
　　cicatrix of cervix 654.6
　　contracted pelvis (general) 653.1
　　　inlet 653.2
　　　outlet 653.3
　　cord presentation or prolapse 663.0
　　cystocele 654.4

Delivery—*continued*
 deformity (acquired) (congenital)
  pelvic organs or tissues NEC 654.9
  pelvis (bony) NEC 653.0
 displacement, uterus NEC 654.4
 disproportion NEC 653.9
 distress
  fetal 656.8
  maternal 669.0
 eclampsia 642.6
 face presentation 652.4
 failed
  forceps 660.7
  trial of labor NEC 660.6
  vacuum extraction 660.7
  ventouse 660.7
 fetal deformity 653.7
 fetal-maternal hemorrhage 656.0
 fetus, fetal
  distress 656.8
  prematurity 656.8
 fibroid (tumor) (uterus) 654.1
 footling 652.8
  with successful version 652.1
 hemorrhage (antepartum) (intrapartum) NEC
  641.9
 hydrocephalic fetus 653.6
 incarceration of uterus 654.3
 incoordinate uterine action 661.4
 inertia, uterus 661.2
  primary 661.0
  secondary 661.1
 lateroversion, uterus or cervix 654.4
 mal lie 652.9
 malposition
  fetus 652.9
   in multiple gestation 652.6
  pelvic organs or tissues NEC 654.9
  uterus NEC or cervix 654.4
 malpresentation NEC 652.9
  in multiple gestation 652.6
 maternal
  diabetes mellitus 648.0
  heart disease NEC 648.6
 meconium in liquor 656.8
  staining only 792.3
 oblique presentation 652.3
 oversize fetus 653.5
 pelvic tumor NEC 654.9
 placental insufficiency 656.5
 placenta previa 641.0
  with hemorrhage 641.1
 poor dilation, cervix 661.0
 pre-eclampsia 642.4
  severe 642.5
 previous
  cesarean delivery 654.2
  surgery (to)
   cervix 654.6
   gynecological NEC 654.9
   uterus NEC 654.9
    from previous cesarean delivery 654.2
   vagina 654.7
 prolapse
  arm or hand 652.7
  uterus 654.4
 prolonged labor 662.1
 rectocele 654.4
 retroversion, uterus or cervix 654.3

Delivery—*continued*
 rigid
  cervix 654.6
  pelvic floor 654.4
  perineum 654.8
  vagina 654.7
  vulva 654.8
 sacculation, pregnant uterus 654.4
 scar(s)
  cervix 654.6
  cesarean delivery 654.2
  uterus NEC 654.9
   due to previous cesarean delivery 654.2
 Shirodkar suture in situ 654.5
 shoulder presentation 652.8
 stenosis or stricture, cervix 654.6
 transverse presentation or lie 652.3
 tumor, pelvic organs or tissues NEC 654.4
 umbilical cord presentation or prolapse 663.0
 completely normal case—*see category* 650
 complicated (by) NEC 669.9
  abdominal tumor, fetal 653.7
   causing obstructed labor 660.1
  abnormal, abnormality of
   cervix 654.6
    causing obstructed labor 660.2
   forces of labor 661.9
   formation of uterus 654.0
   pelvic organs or tissues 654.9
    causing obstructed labor 660.2
   pelvis (bony) (major) NEC 653.0
    causing obstructed labor 660.1
   presentation or position NEC 652.9
    causing obstructed labor 660.0
   size, fetus 653.5
    causing obstructed labor 660.1
   soft parts (of pelvis) 654.9
    causing obstructed labor 660.2
   uterine contractions NEC 661.9
   uterus (formation) 654.0
    causing obstructed labor 660.2
   vagina 654.7
    causing obstructed labor 660.2
  abnormally formed uterus (any type)
   (congenital) 654.0
   causing obstructed labor 660.2
  acromion presentation 652.8
   causing obstructed labor 660.0
  adherent placenta 667.0
   with hemorrhage 666.0
  adhesions, uterus (to abdominal wall) 654.4
  advanced maternal age NEC 659.6
   multigravida 659.6
   primigravida 659.5
  air embolism 673.0
  amnionitis 658.4
  amniotic fluid embolism 673.1
  anesthetic death 668.9
  annular detachment, cervix 665.3
  antepartum hemorrhage—*see* Delivery,
   complicated, hemorrhage
  anteversion, cervix or uterus 654.4
   causing obstructed labor 660.2
  apoplexy 674.0
   placenta 641.2
  arrested active phase 661.1
  asymmetrical pelvis bone 653.0
   causing obstructed labor 660.1
  atony, uterus (hypotonic) (inertia) 666.1
   hypertonic 661.4
  Bandl's ring 661.4

Delivery—*continued*
    battledore placenta—*see* Placenta, abnormal
    bicornis or bicornuate uterus 654.0
        causing obstructed labor 660.2
    birth injury to mother NEC 665.9
    bleeding (*see also* Delivery, complicated,
            hemorrhage) 641.9
    breech presentation (assisted) (buttocks)
            (complete) (frank) (spontaneous) 652.2
        with successful version 652.1
    brow presentation 652.4
    cephalopelvic disproportion (normally formed
            fetus) 653.4
        causing obstructed labor 660.1
    cerebral hemorrhage 674.0
    cervical dystocia 661.0
    chin presentation 652.4
        causing obstructed labor 660.0
    cicatrix
        cervix 654.6
            causing obstructed labor 660.2
        vagina 654.7
            causing obstructed labor 660.2
    colporrhexis 665.4
        with perineal laceration 664.0
    compound presentation 652.8
        causing obstructed labor 660.0
    compression of cord (umbilical) 663.2
        around neck 663.1
        cord prolapsed 663.0
    contraction, contracted pelvis 653.1
        causing obstructed labor 660.1
        general 653.1
            causing obstructed labor 660.1
        inlet 653.2
            causing obstructed labor 660.1
        midpelvic 653.8
            causing obstructed labor 660.1
        midplane 653.8
            causing obstructed labor 660.1
        outlet 653.3
            causing obstructed labor 660.1
    contraction ring 661.4
    cord (umbilical) 663.9
        around neck, tightly or with compression
                663.1
            without compression 663.3
        bruising 663.6
        complication NEC 663.9
            specified type NEC 663.8
        compression NEC 663.2
        entanglement NEC 663.3
            with compression 663.2
        forelying 663.0
        hematoma 663.6
        marginal attachment 663.8
        presentation 663.0
        prolapse (complete) (occult) (partial) 663.0
        short 663.4
        specified complication NEC 663.8
        thrombosis (vessels) 663.6
        vascular lesion 663.6
        velamentous insertion 663.8
    Couvelaire uterus 641.2
    cretin pelvis (dwarf type) (male type) 653.1
        causing obstructed labor 660.1
    crossbirth 652.3
        with successful version 652.1
        causing obstructed labor 660.0
    cyst (Gartner's duct) 654.7

Delivery—*continued*
    cystocele 654.4
        causing obstructed labor 660.2
    death of fetus (near term) 656.4
        early (before 22 completed weeks'
                gestation) 632
    deformity (acquired) (congenital)
        fetus 653.7
            causing obstructed labor 660.1
        pelvic organs or tissues NEC 654.9
            causing obstructed labor 660.2
        pelvis (bony) NEC 653.0
            causing obstructed labor 660.1
    delay, delayed
        delivery in multiple pregnancy 662.3
        due to locked mates 660.5
        following rupture of membranes
                (spontaneous) 658.2
            artificial 658.3
    depressed fetal heart tones 659.7
    diastasis recti 665.8
    dilatation
        bladder 654.4
            causing obstructed labor 660.2
        cervix, incomplete, poor or slow 661.0
    diseased placenta 656.7
    displacement uterus NEC 654.4
        causing obstructed labor 660.2
    disproportion NEC 653.9
        causing obstructed labor 660.1
    disruptio uteri—*see* Delivery, complicated,
            rupture, uterus
    distress
        fetal 656.8
        maternal 669.0
    double uterus (congenital) 654.0
        causing obstructed labor 660.2
    dropsy amnion 657
    dysfunction, uterus 661.9
        hypertonic 661.4
        hypotonic 661.2
            primary 661.0
            secondary 661.1
        incoordinate 661.4
    dystocia
        cervical 661.0
        fetal—*see* Delivery, complicated, abnormal,
                presentation
        maternal—*see* Delivery, complicated,
                prolonged labor
        pelvic—*see* Delivery, complicated,
                contraction pelvis
        positional 652.8
        shoulder girdle 660.4
    eclampsia 642.6
    ectopic kidney 654.4
        causing obstructed labor 660.2
    edema, cervix 654.6
        causing obstructed labor 660.2
    effusion, amniotic fluid 658.1
    elderly multigravida 659.6
    elderly primigravida 659.5
    embolism (pulmonary) 673.2
        air 673.0
        amniotic fluid 673.1
        blood-clot 673.2
        cerebral 674.0
        fat 673.8
        pyemic 673.3
        septic 673.3

Delivery—*continued*

entanglement, umbilical cord 663.3
  with compression 663.2
  around neck (with compression) 663.1
eversion, cervix or uterus 665.2
excessive
  fetal growth 653.5
    causing obstructed labor 660.1
  size of fetus 653.5
    causing obstructed labor 660.1
face presentation 652.4
  causing obstructed labor 660.0
  to pubes 660.3
failure, fetal head to enter pelvic brim 652.5
  causing obstructed labor 660.0
fetal
  acid-base balance 656.8
  death (near term) NEC 656.4
    early (before 22 completed weeks'
      gestation) 632
  deformity 653.7
    causing obstructed labor 660.1
  distress 656.8
  heart rate or rhythm 659.7
fetopelvic disproportion 653.4
  causing obstructed labor 660.1
fever during labor 659.2
fibroid (tumor) (uterus) 654.1
  causing obstructed labor 660.2
fibromyomata 654.1
  causing obstructed labor 660.2
forelying umbilical cord 663.0
fracture of coccyx 665.6
hematoma 664.5
  broad ligament 665.7
  ischial spine 665.7
  pelvic 665.7
  perineum 664.5
  soft tissues 665.7
  subdural 674.0
  umbilical cord 663.6
  vagina 665.7
  vulva or perineum 664.5
hemorrhage (uterine) (antepartum)
    (intrapartum) (pregnancy) 641.9
  accidental 641.2
  associated with
    afibrinogenemia 641.3
    coagulation defect 641.3
      hyperfibrinolysis 641.3
      hypofibrinogenemia 641.3
  cerebral 674.0
  due to
    low-lying placenta 641.1
    placenta previa 641.1
    premature separation of placenta
      (normally implanted) 641.2
    retained placenta 666.0
    trauma 641.8
    uterine leiomyoma 641.8
  marginal sinus rupture 641.2
  placenta NEC 641.9
  postpartum (atonic) (immediate) (within 24
      hours) 666.1
    with retained or trapped placenta 666.0
  third stage 666.0
    delayed 666.2
    secondary 666.2
hourglass contraction, uterus 661.4
hydramnios 657

Delivery—*continued*

hydrocephalic fetus 653.6
  causing obstructed labor 660.1
hydrops fetalis 653.7
  causing obstructed labor 660.1
hypertension—*see* Hypertension,
    complicating pregnancy
hypertonic uterine dysfunction 661.4
hypotonic uterine dysfunction 661.2
impacted shoulders 660.4
incarceration, uterus 654.3
  causing obstructed labor 660.2
incomplete dilation (cervix) 661.0
incoordinate uterus 661.4
indication NEC 659.9
  specified type NEC 659.8
inertia, uterus 661.2
  hypertonic 661.4
  hypotonic 661.2
  primary 661.0
  secondary 661.1
infantile
  genitalia 654.4
    causing obstructed labor 660.2
  uterus (os) 654.4
    causing obstructed labor 660.2
injury (to mother) NEC 665.9
intrauterine fetal death (near term) NEC 656.4
  early (before 22 completed weeks'
      gestation) 632
inversion, uterus 665.2
kidney, ectopic 654.4
  causing obstructed labor 660.2
knot (true), umbilical cord 663.2
labor, premature (before 37 completed weeks
    gestation) 644.2
laceration 664.9
  anus (sphincter) 664.2
    with mucosa 664.3
  bladder (urinary) 665.5
  bowel 665.5
  central 664.4
  cervix (uteri) 665.3
  fourchette 664.0
  hymen 664.0
  labia (majora) (minora) 664.0
  pelvic
    floor 664.1
    organ NEC 665.5
  perineum, perineal 664.4
    first degree 664.0
    second degree 664.1
    third degree 664.2
    fourth degree 664.3
    central 664.4
    extensive NEC 664.4
    muscles 664.1
    skin 664.0
    slight 664.0
  peritoneum 665.5
  periurethral tissue 665.5
  rectovaginal (septum) (without perineal
      laceration) 665.4
    with perineum 664.2
      with anal or rectal mucosa 664.3
  skin (perineum) 664.0
  specified site or type NEC 664.8
  sphincter ani 664.2
    with mucosa 664.3
  urethra 665.5

Delivery—*continued*
  uterus 665.1
    before labor 665.0
    vagina, vaginal (deep) (high) (sulcus) (wall)
      (without perineal laceration) 665.4
    with perineum 664.0
      muscles, with perineum 664.1
    vulva 664.0
  lateroversion, uterus or cervix 654.4
    causing obstructed labor 660.2
  locked mates 660.5
  low implantation of placenta—*see* Delivery,
    complicated, placenta, previa
  mal lie 652.9
  malposition
    fetus NEC 652.9
      causing obstructed labor 660.0
    pelvic organs or tissues NEC 654.9
      causing obstructed labor 660.2
    placenta 641.1
      without hemorrhage 641.0
    uterus NEC or cervix 654.4
      causing obstructed labor 660.2
  malpresentation 652.9
    causing obstructed labor 660.0
  marginal sinus (bleeding) (rupture) 641.2
  maternal hypotension syndrome 669.2
  meconium in liquor 656.8
  membranes, retained—*see* Delivery,
    complicated, placenta, retained
  mentum presentation 652.4
    causing obstructed labor 660.0
  metrorrhagia (myopathia)—*see* Delivery,
    complicated, hemorrhage
  metrorrhexis—*see* Delivery, complicated,
    rupture, uterus
  multiparity (grand) 659.4
  myelomeningocele, fetus 653.7
    causing obstructed labor 660.1
  Nägele's pelvis 653.0
    causing obstructed labor 660.1
  nonengagement, fetal head 652.5
    causing obstructed labor 660.0
  oblique presentation 652.3
    causing obstructed labor 660.0
  obstetric
    shock 669.1
    trauma NEC 665.9
  obstructed labor 660.9
    due to
      abnormality pelvic organs or tissues
        (conditions classifiable to
        654.0-654.9) 660.2
      deep transverse arrest 660.3
      impacted shoulders 660.4
      locked twins 660.5
      malposition and malpresentation of fetus
        (conditions classifiable to
        652.0-652.9) 660.0
      persistent occipitoposterior 660.3
      shoulder dystocia 660.4
  occult prolapse of umbilical cord 663.0
  oversize fetus 653.5
    causing obstructed labor 660.1
  pathological retraction ring, uterus 661.4
  pelvic
    arrest (deep) (high) (of fetal head)
      (transverse) 660.3
    deformity (bone)—*see also* Deformity,
      pelvis, with disproportion

Delivery—*continued*
  soft tissue 654.9
    causing obstructed labor 660.2
  tumor NEC 654.9
    causing obstructed labor 660.2
  penetration, pregnant uterus by instrument
    665.1
  perforation—*see* Delivery, complicated,
    laceration
  persistent
    hymen 654.8
      causing obstructed labor 660.2
    occipitoposterior 660.3
  placenta, placental
    ablatio 641.2
    abnormality 656.7
      with hemorrhage 641.2
    abruptio 641.2
    accreta 667.0
      with hemorrhage 666.0
    adherent (without hemorrhage) 667.0
      with hemorrhage 666.0
    apoplexy 641.2
    battledore 663.8
    detachment (premature) 641.2
    disease 656.7
    hemorrhage NEC 641.9
    increta (without hemorrhage) 667.0
      with hemorrhage 666.0
    low (implantation) 641.1
      without hemorrhage 641.0
    malformation 656.7
      with hemorrhage 641.2
    malposition 641.1
      without hemorrhage 641.0
    marginal sinus rupture 641.2
    percreta 667.0
      with hemorrhage 666.0
    premature separation 641.2
    previa (central) (lateral) (marginal) (partial)
      641.1
      without hemorrhage 641.0
    retained (with hemorrhage) 666.0
      without hemorrhage 667.0
    rupture of marginal sinus 641.2
    separation (premature) 641.2
    trapped 666.0
      without hemorrhage 667.0
    vicious insertion 641.1
  polyhydramnios 657
  polyp, cervix 654.6
    causing obstructed labor 660.2
  precipitate labor 661.3
  premature
    labor (before 37 completed weeks gestation)
      644.2
    rupture, membranes 658.1
      delayed delivery following 658.2
  presenting umbilical cord 663.0
  previous
    cesarean delivery 654.2
    surgery
      cervix 654.6
        causing obstructed labor 660.2
      gynecological NEC 654.9
        causing obstructed labor 660.2
      perineum 654.8
      uterus NEC 654.9
        due to previous cesarean delivery 654.2
      vagina 654.7
        causing obstructed labor 660.2

Delivery—*continued*
    vulva 654.8
  primary uterine inertia 661.0
  primipara, elderly or old 659.5
  prolapse
    arm or hand 652.7
      causing obstructed labor 660.0
    cord (umbilical) 663.0
    fetal extremity 652.8
    foot or leg 652.8
      causing obstructed labor 660.0
    umbilical cord (complete) (occult) (partial)
      663.0
    uterus 654.4
      causing obstructed labor 660.2
  prolonged labor 662.1
    first stage 662.0
    second stage 662.2
    active phase 661.2
    due to
      cervical dystocia 661.0
      contraction ring 661.4
      tetanic uterus 661.4
      uterine inertia 661.2
        primary 661.0
        secondary 661.1
    latent phase 661.0
  pyrexia during labor 659.2
  rachitic pelvis 653.2
    causing obstructed labor 660.1
  rectocele 654.4
    causing obstructed labor 660.2
  retained membranes or portions of placenta
    666.2
    without hemorrhage 667.1
  retarded (prolonged) birth 662.1
  retention secundines (with hemorrhage) 666.2
    without hemorrhage 667.1
  retroversion, uterus or cervix 654.3
    causing obstructed labor 660.2
  rigid
    cervix 654.6
      causing obstructed labor 660.2
    pelvic floor 654.4
      causing obstructed labor 660.2
    perineum or vulva 654.8
      causing obstructed labor 660.2
    vagina 654.7
      causing obstructed labor 660.2
  Robert's pelvis 653.0
    causing obstructed labor 660.1
  rupture—*see also* Delivery, complicated,
    laceration
    bladder (urinary) 665.5
    cervix 665.3
    marginal sinus 641.2
    membranes, premature 658.1
    pelvic organ NEC 665.5
    perineum (without mention of other
      laceration)—*see* Delivery, complicated,
      laceration, perineum
    peritoneum 665.5
    urethra 665.5
    uterus (during labor) 665.1
      before labor 665.0
  sacculation, pregnant uterus 654.4
  sacral teratomas, fetal 653.7
    causing obstructed labor 660.1
  scar(s)
    cervix 654.6
      causing obstructed labor 660.2

Delivery—*continued*
  cesarean delivery 654.2
    causing obstructed labor 660.2
    perineum 654.8
      causing obstructed labor 660.2
    uterus NEC 654.9
      causing obstructed labor 660.2
      due to previous cesarean delivery 654.2
    vagina 654.7
      causing obstructed labor 660.2
    vulva 654.8
      causing obstructed labor 660.2
  scoliotic pelvis 653.0
    causing obstructed labor 660.1
  secondary uterine inertia 661.1
  secundines, retained—*see* Delivery,
    complicated, placenta, retained
  separation
    placenta (premature) 641.2
    pubic bone 665.6
    symphysis pubis 665.6
  septate vagina 654.7
    causing obstructed labor 660.2
  shock (birth) (obstetric) (puerperal) 669.1
  short cord syndrome 663.4
  shoulder
    girdle dystocia 660.4
    presentation 652.8
      causing obstructed labor 660.0
  Siamese twins 653.7
    causing obstructed labor 660.1
  slow slope active phase 661.2
  spasm
    cervix 661.4
    uterus 661.4
  spondylolisthesis, pelvis 653.3
    causing obstructed labor 660.1
  spondylolysis (lumbosacral) 653.3
    causing obstructed labor 660.1
  spondylosis 653.0
    causing obstructed labor 660.1
  stenosis or stricture
    cervix 654.6
      causing obstructed labor 660.2
    vagina 654.7
      causing obstructed labor 660.2
  sudden death, unknown cause 669.9
  tear (pelvic organ) (*see also* Delivery,
    complicated, laceration) 664.9
  teratomas, sacral, fetal 653.7
    causing obstructed labor 660.1
  tetanic uterus 661.4
  tipping pelvis 653.0
    causing obstructed labor 660.1
  transverse
    arrest (deep) 660.3
    presentation or lie 652.3
      with successful version 652.1
      causing obstructed labor 660.0
  trauma (obstetrical) NEC 665.9
  tumor
    abdominal, fetal 653.7
      causing obstructed labor 660.1
    pelvic organs or tissues NEC 654.9
      causing obstructed labor 660.2
  umbilical cord (*see also* Delivery,
    complicated, cord) 663.9
    around neck tightly, or with compression
      663.1
    entanglement NEC 663.3
      with compression 663.2

Delivery—*continued*
  prolapse (complete) (occult) (partial) 663.0
  unstable lie 652.0
    causing obstructed labor 660.0
  uterine
    inertia (*see also* Delivery, complicated,
      inertia, uterus) 661.2
    spasm 661.4
  vasa previa 663.5
  velamentous insertion of cord 663.8
  young maternal age 659.8
  delayed NEC 662.1
    following rupture of membranes
      (spontaneous) 658.2
      artificial 658.3
    second twin, triplet, etc. 662.3
  difficult NEC 669.9
    previous, affecting management of pregnancy
      or childbirth V23.49
    specified type NEC 669.8
  early onset (spontaneous) 644.2
  forceps NEC 669.5
    affecting fetus or newborn 763.2
  footling 652.8
    with successful version 652.1
  missed (at or near term) 656.4
  multiple gestation NEC 651.9
    with fetal loss and retention of one or more
      fetus(es) 651.6
    specified type NEC 651.8
      with fetal loss and retention of one or more
        fetus(es) 651.6
  nonviable infant 656.4
  normal—*see* category 650
  precipitate 661.3
    affecting fetus or newborn 763.6
  premature NEC (before 37 completed weeks
    gestation) 644.2
    previous, affecting management of pregnancy
      V23.41
  quadruplet NEC 651.2
    with fetal loss and retention of one or more
      fetus(es) 651.5
  quintuplet NEC 651.8
    with fetal loss and retention of one or more
      fetus(es) 651.6
  sextuplet NEC 651.8
    with fetal loss and retention of one or more
      fetus(es) 651.6
  specified complication NEC 669.8
  stillbirth (near term) NEC 656.4
    early (before 22 completed weeks' gestation)
      632
  term pregnancy (live birth) NEC—*see* category
    650
    stillbirth NEC 656.4
  threatened premature 644.2
  triplets NEC 651.1
    with fetal loss and retention of one or more
      fetus(es) 651.4
    delayed delivery (one or more mates) 662.3
    locked mates 660.5
  twins NEC 651.0
    with fetal loss and retention of one or more
      fetus(es) 651.3
    delayed delivery (one or more mates) 662.3
    locked mates 660.5
  uncomplicated—*see* category 650
  vacuum extractor NEC 669.5
    affecting fetus or newborn 763.3
  ventouse NEC 669.5
    affecting fetus or newborn 763.3

Dellen, cornea 371.41
Delusions (paranoid) 297.9
  grandiose 297.1
  parasitosis 300.29
  systematized 297.1
Dementia 294.8
  alcoholic (*see also* Psychosis, alcoholic) 291.2
  Alzheimer's—*see* Alzheimer's dementia
  arteriosclerotic (simple type) (uncomplicated)
    290.40
    with
      acute confusional state 290.41
      delirium 290.41
      delusional features 290.42
      depressive features 290.43
    depressed type 290.43
    paranoid type 290.42
  Binswanger's 290.12
  catatonic (acute) (*see also* Schizophrenia) 295.2
  congenital (*see also* Retardation, mental) 319
  degenerative 290.9
    presenile-onset—*see* Dementia, presenile
    senile-onset—*see* Dementia, senile
  developmental (*see also* Schizophrenia) 295.9
  dialysis 294.8
    transient 293.9
  due to or associated with condition(s) classified
    elsewhere
    Alzheimer's
      with behavioral disturbance 331.0 *[294.11]*
      without behavioral disturbance 331.0
        [294.10]
    cerebral lipidoses
      with behavioral disturbance 330.1 *[294.11]*
      without behavioral disturbance 330.1
        [294.10]
    epilepsy
      with behavioral disturbance 345.9 *[294.11]*
      without behavioral disturbance 345.9
        [294.10]
    hepatolenticular degeneration
      with behavioral disturbance 275.1 *[294.11]*
      without behavioral disturbance 275.1
        [294.10]
    HIV
      with behavioral disturbance 042 *[294.11]*
      without behavioral disturbance 042 *[294.10]*
    Huntington's chorea
      with behavioral disturbance 333.4 *[294.11]*
      without behavioral disturbance 333.4
        [294.10]
    Jakob-Creutzfeldt disease
      with behavioral disturbance 046.1 *[294.11]*
      without behavioral disturbance 046.1
        [294.10]
    multiple sclerosis
      with behavioral disturbance 340 *[294.11]*
      without behavioral disturbance 340 *[294.10]*
    neurosyphilis
      with behavioral disturbance 094.9 *[294.11]*
      without behavioral disturbance 094.9
        [294.10]
    Pelizaeus-Merzbacher disease
      with behavioral disturbance 333.0 *[294.11]*
      without behavioral disturbance 333.0
        [294.10]
    Pick's disease
      with behavioral disturbance 331.1 *[294.11]*
      without behavioral disturbance 331.1
        [294.10]

Dependence—*continued*
alphaprodine (hydrochloride) 304.0
Alurate 304.1
Alvodine 304.0
amethocaine 304.6
amidone 304.0
amidopyrine 304.6
aminopyrine 304.6
amobarbital 304.1
amphetamine(s) (type) (drugs classifiable to 969.7) 304.4
amylene hydrate 304.6
amylobarbitone 304.1
amylocaine 304.6
Amytal (sodium) 304.1
analgesic (drug) NEC 304.6
  synthetic with morphine-like effect 304.0
anesthetic (agent) (drug) (gas) (general) (local) NEC 304.6
Angel dust 304.6
anileridine 304.0
antipyrine 304.6
aprobarbital 304.1
aprobarbitone 304.1
atropine 304.6
Avertin (bromide) 304.6
barbenyl 304.1
barbital(s) 304.1
barbitone 304.1
barbiturate(s) (compounds) (drugs classifiable to 967.0) 304.1
barbituric acid (and compounds) 304.1
benzedrine 304.4
benzylmorphine 304.0
Beta-chlor 304.1
bhang 304.3
blue velvet 304.0
Brevital 304.1
bromal (hydrate) 304.1
bromide(s) NEC 304.1
bromine compounds NEC 304.1
bromisovalum 304.1
bromoform 304.1
Bromo-seltzer 304.1
bromural 304.1
butabarbital (sodium) 304.1
butabarpal 304.1
butallylonal 304.1
butethal 304.1
buthalitone (sodium) 304.1
Butisol 304.1
butobarbitone 304.1
butyl chloral (hydrate) 304.1
caffeine 304.4
cannabis (indica) (sativa) (resin) (derivatives) (type) 304.3
carbamazepine 304.6
Carbrital 304.1
carbromal 304.1
carisoprodol 304.6
Catha (edulis) 304.4
chloral (betaine) (hydrate) 304.1
chloralamide 304.1
chloralformamide 304.1
chloralose 304.1
chlordiazepoxide 304.1
Chloretone 304.1
chlorobutanol 304.1
chlorodyne 304.1
chloroform 304.6
Cliradon 304.0

Dependence—*continued*
coca (leaf) and derivatives 304.2
cocaine 304.2
  hydrochloride 304.2
  salt (any) 304.2
codeine 304.0
combination of drugs (excluding morphine or opioid type drug) NEC 304.8
  morphine or opioid type drug with any other drug 304.7
croton-chloral 304.1
cyclobarbital 304.1
cyclobarbitone 304.1
dagga 304.3
Delvinal 304.1
Demerol 304.0
desocodeine 304.0
desomorphine 304.0
desoxyephedrine 304.4
DET 304.5
dexamphetamine 304.4
dexedrine 304.4
dextromethorphan 304.0
dextromoramide 304.0
dextronorpseudophedrine 304.4
dextrorphan 304.0
diacetylmorphine 304.0
Dial 304.1
diallylbarbituric acid 304.1
diamorphine 304.0
diazepam 304.1
dibucaine 304.6
dichloroethane 304.6
diethyl barbituric acid 304.1
diethylsulfone-diethylmethane 304.1
difencloxazine 304.0
dihydrocodeine 304.0
dihydrocodeinone 304.0
dihydrohydroxycodeinone 304.0
dihydroisocodeine 304.0
dihydromorphine 304.0
dihydromorphinone 304.0
dihydroxcodeinone 304.0
Dilaudid 304.0
dimenhydrinate 304.6
dimethylmeperidine 304.0
dimethyltriptamine 304.5
Dionin 304.0
diphenoxylate 304.6
dipipanone 304.0
d-lysergic acid diethylamide 304.5
DMT 304.5
Dolophine 304.0
DOM 304.2
Doriden 304.1
dormiral 304.1
Dormison 304.1
Dromoran 304.0
drug NEC 304.9
  analgesic NEC 304.6
  combination (excluding morphine or opioid type drug) NEC 304.8
    morphine or opioid type drug with any other drug 304.7
  complicating pregnancy, childbirth, or puerperium 648.3
    affecting fetus or newborn 779.5
  hallucinogenic 304.5
  hypnotic NEC 304.1
  narcotic NEC 304.9
  psychostimulant NEC 304.4

Dependence—*continued*
Neravan 304.1
neurobarb 304.1
nicotine 305.1
Nisentil 304.0
nitrous oxide 304.6
Noctec 304.1
Noludar 304.1
nonbarbiturate sedatives and tranquilizers with
      similar effect 304.1
noptil 304.1
normorphine 304.0
noscapine 304.0
Novocaine 304.6
Numorphan 304.0
nunol 304.1
Nupercaine 304.6
Oblivon 304.1
on
    aspirator V46.0
    hyperbaric chamber V46.8
    iron lung V46.1
    machine (enabling) V46.9
        specified type NEC V46.8
    Possum (Patient-Operated-Selector-
        Mechanism) V46.8
    renal dialysis machine V45.1
    respirator V46.1
    supplemental oxygen V46.2
opiate 304.0
opioids 304.0
opioid type drug 304.0
    with any other drug 304.7
opium (alkaloids) (derivatives) (tincture) 304.0
ortal 304.1
Oxazepam 304.1
oxycodone 304.0
oxymorphone 304.0
Palfium 304.0
Panadol 304.6
pantopium 304.0
pantopon 304.0
papaverine 304.0
paracetamol 304.6
paracodin 304.0
paraldehyde 304.1
paregoric 304.0
Parzone 304.0
PCP (phencyclidine) 304.6
Pearly Gates 304.5
pentazocine 304.0
pentobarbital 304.1
pentobarbitone (sodium) 304.1
Pentothal 304.1
Percaine 304.6
Percodan 304.0
Perichlor 304.1
Pernocton 304.1
Pernoston 304.1
peronine 304.0
pethidine (hydrochloride) 304.0
petrichloral 304.1
peyote 304.5
Phanodorn 304.1
phenacetin 304.6
phenadoxone 304.0
phenaglycodol 304.1
phenazocine 304.0
phencyclidine 304.6
phenmetrazine 304.4
phenobal 304.1

Dependence—*continued*
phenobarbital 304.1
phenobarbitone 304.1
phenomorphan 304.0
phenonyl 304.1
phenoperidine 304.0
pholcodine 304.0
piminodine 304.0
Pipadone 304.0
Pitkin's solution 304.6
Placidyl 304.1
polysubstance 304.8
Pontocaine 304.6
pot 304.3
potassium bromide 304.1
Preludin 304.4
Prinadol 304.0
probarbital 304.1
procaine 304.6
propanal 304.1
propoxyphene 304.6
psilocibin 304.5
psilocin 304.5
psilocybin 304.5
psilocyline 304.5
psilocyn 304.5
psychedelic agents 304.5
psychostimulant NEC 304.4
psychotomimetic agents 304.5
pyrahexyl 304.3
Pyramidon 304.6
quinalbarbitone 304.1
racemoramide 304.0
racemorphan 304.0
Rela 304.6
scopolamine 304.6
secobarbital 304.1
Seconal 304.1
sedative NEC 304.1
    nonbarbiturate with barbiturate effect 304.1
Sedormid 304.1
sernyl 304.1
sodium bromide 304.1
Soma 304.6
Somnal 304.1
Somnos 304.1
Soneryl 304.1
soporific (drug) NEC 304.1
specified drug NEC 304.6
speed 304.4
spinocaine 304.6
Stovaine 304.6
STP 304.5
stramonium 304.6
Sulfonal 304.1
sulfonethylmethane 304.1
sulfonmethane 304.1
Surital 304.1
synthetic drug with morphine-like effect 304.0
talbutal 304.1
tetracaine 304.6
tetrahydrocannabinol 304.3
tetronal 304.1
THC 304.3
thebacon 304.0
thebaine 304.0
thiamil 304.1
thiamylal 304.1
thiopental 304.1
tobacco 305.1
toluene, toluol 304.6

Depressive reaction —*see also* Reaction, depressive
  acute (transient) 309.0
    with anxiety 309.28
  prolonged 309.1
  situational (acute) 309.0
    prolonged 309.1
Deprivation
  cultural V62.4
  emotional V62.89
    affecting
      adult 995.82
      infant or child 995.51
  food 994.2
    specific substance NEC 269.8
  protein (familial) (kwashiorkor) 260
  social V62.4
    affecting
      adult 995.82
      infant or child 995.51
  symptoms, syndrome
    alcohol 291.81
    drug 292.0
  vitamins (*see also* Deficiency, vitamin) 269.2
  water 994.3
de Quervain's
  disease (tendon sheath) 727.04
  thyroiditis (subacute granulomatous thyroiditis) 245.1
Derangement
  ankle (internal) 718.97
    current injury (*see also* Dislocation, ankle) 837.0
    recurrent 718.37
  cartilage (articular) NEC (*see also* Disorder, cartilage, articular) 718.0
    knee 717.9
      recurrent 718.36
    recurrent 718.3
  collateral ligament (knee) (medial) (tibial) 717.82
    current injury 844.1
      lateral (fibular) 844.0
    lateral (fibular) 717.81
      current injury 844.0
  cruciate ligament (knee) (posterior) 717.84
    anterior 717.83
      current injury 844.2
    current injury 844.2
  elbow (internal) 718.92
    current injury (*see also* Dislocation, elbow) 832.00
    recurrent 718.32
  gastrointestinal 536.9
  heart—*see* Disease, heart
  hip (joint) (internal) (old) 718.95
    current injury (*see also* Dislocation, hip) 835.00
    recurrent 718.35
  intervertebral disc—*see* Displacement, intervertebral disc
  joint (internal) 718.90
    ankle 718.97
    current injury—*see also* Dislocation, by site
      knee, meniscus or cartilage (*see also* Tear, meniscus) 836.2
    elbow 718.92
    foot 718.97
    hand 718.94
    hip 718.95
    knee 717.9

Derangement—*continued*
    multiple sites 718.99
    pelvic region 718.95
    recurrent 718.30
      ankle 718.37
      elbow 718.32
      foot 718.37
      hand 718.34
      hip 718.35
      knee 718.36
      multiple sites 718.39
      pelvic region 718.35
      shoulder (region) 718.31
      specified site NEC 718.38
      temporomandibular (old) 524.69
      wrist 718.33
    shoulder (region) 718.91
    specified site NEC 718.98
    spine NEC 724.9
    temporomandibular 524.69
    wrist 718.93
  knee (cartilage) (internal) 717.9
    current injury (*see also* Tear, meniscus) 836.2
    ligament 717.89
      capsular 717.85
      collateral—*see* Derangement, collateral ligament
      cruciate—*see* Derangement, cruciate ligament
      specified NEC 717.85
    recurrent 718.36
  low back NEC 724.9
  meniscus NEC (knee) 717.5
    current injury (*see also* Tear, meniscus) 836.2
    lateral 717.40
      anterior horn 717.42
      posterior horn 717.43
      specified NEC 717.49
    medial 717.3
      anterior horn 717.1
      posterior horn 717.2
    recurrent 718.3
    site other than knee—*see* Disorder, cartilage, articular
  mental (*see also* Psychosis) 298.9
  rotator cuff (recurrent) (tear) 726.10
    current 840.4
  sacroiliac (old) 724.6
    current—*see* Dislocation, sacroiliac
  semilunar cartilage (knee) 717.5
    current injury 836.2
      lateral 836.1
      medial 836.0
    recurrent 718.3
  shoulder (internal) 718.91
    current injury (*see also* Dislocation, shoulder) 831.00
    recurrent 718.31
  spine (recurrent) NEC 724.9
    current—*see* Dislocation, spine
  temporomandibular (internal) (joint) (old) 524.69
    current—*see* Dislocation, jaw
Dercum's disease or syndrome (adiposis dolorosa) 272.8
Derealization (neurotic) 300.6
Dermal —*see* condition
Dermaphytid —*see* Dermatophytosis
Dermatergosis —*see* Dermatitis

Dermatitis (allergic) (contact) (occupational)
  (venenata) 692.9
  ab igne 692.82
  acneiform 692.9
  actinic (due to sun) 692.70
    acute 692.72
    chronic NEC 692.74
    other than from sun NEC 692.82
  ambustionis
    due to
      burn or scald—*see* Burn, by site
      sunburn (*see also* Sunburn) 692.71
  amebic 006.6
  ammonia 691.0
  anaphylactoid NEC 692.9
  arsenical 692.4
  artefacta 698.4
    psychogenic 316 *[698.4]*
  asthmatic 691.8
  atopic (allergic) (intrinsic) 691.8
    psychogenic 316 *[691.8]*
  atrophicans 701.8
    diffusa 701.8
    maculosa 701.3
  berlock, berloque 692.72
  blastomycetic 116.0
  blister beetle 692.89
  Brucella NEC 023.9
  bullosa 694.9
    striata pratensis 692.6
  bullous 694.9
    mucosynechial, atrophic 694.60
      with ocular involvement 694.61
    seasonal 694.8
  calorica
    due to
      burn or scald—*see* Burn, by site
      cold 692.89
      sunburn (*see also* Sunburn) 692.71
  caterpillar 692.89
  cercarial 120.3
  combustionis
    due to
      burn or scald—*see* Burn, by site
      sunburn (*see also* Sunburn) 692.71
  congelationis 991.5
  contusiformis 695.2
  diabetic 250.8
  diaper 691.0
  diphtheritica 032.85
  due to
    acetone 692.2
    acids 692.4
    adhesive plaster 692.4
    alcohol (skin contact) (substances classifiable
      to 980.0-980.9) 692.4
      taken internally 693.8
    alkalis 692.4
    allergy NEC 692.9
    ammonia (household) (liquid) 692.4
    arnica 692.3
    arsenic 692.4
      taken internally 693.8
    blister beetle 692.89
    cantharides 692.3
    carbon disulphide 692.2
    caterpillar 692.89
    caustics 692.4
    cereal (ingested) 693.1
      contact with skin 692.5

Dermatitis—*continued*
  chemical(s) NEC 692.4
    internal 693.8
    irritant NEC 692.4
    taken internally 693.8
  chlorocompounds 692.2
  coffee (ingested) 693.1
    contact with skin 692.5
  cold weather 692.89
  cosmetics 692.81
  cyclohexanes 692.2
  deodorant 692.81
  detergents 692.0
  dichromate 692.4
  drugs and medicinals (correct substance
      properly administered) (internal use) 693.0
    external (in contact with skin) 692.3
      wrong substance given or taken 976.9
        specified substance—*see* Table of drugs
          and chemicals
    wrong substance given or taken 977.9
      specified substance—*see* Table of drugs
        and chemicals
  dyes 692.89
    hair 692.89
  epidermophytosis—*see* Dermatophytosis
  esters 692.2
  external irritant NEC 692.9
    specified agent NEC 692.89
  eye shadow 692.81
  fish (ingested) 693.1
    contact with skin 692.5
  flour (ingested) 693.1
    contact with skin 692.5
  food (ingested) 693.1
    in contact with skin 692.5
  fruit (ingested) 693.1
    contact with skin 692.5
  fungicides 692.3
  furs 692.89
  glycols 692.2
  greases NEC 692.1
  hair dyes 692.89
  hot
    objects and materials—*see* Burn, by site
    weather or places 692.89
  hydrocarbons 692.2
  infrared rays, except from sun 692.82
    solar NEC (*see* also Dermatitis, due to, sun)
      692.70
  ingested substance 693.9
    drugs and medicinals (*see also* Dermatitis,
      due to, drugs and medicinals) 693.0
    food 693.1
    specified substance NEC 693.8
  ingestion or injection of
    chemical 693.8
    drug (correct substance properly
      administered) 693.0
      wrong substance given or taken 977.9
        specified substance—*see* Table of drugs
          and chemicals
  insecticides 692.4
  internal agent 693.9
    drugs and medicinals (*see also* Dermatitis,
      due to, drugs and medicinals) 693.0
    food (ingested) 693.1
      in contact with skin 692.5
    specified agent NEC 693.8
  iodine 692.3
  iodoform 692.3

Dermatitis—*continued*
   juvenile 694.2
     senile 694.5
  hiemalis 692.89
  hypostatic, hypostatica 454.1
   with ulcer 454.2
  impetiginous 684
  infantile (acute) (chronic) (intertriginous)
    (intrinsic) (seborrheic) 690.12
  infectiosa eczematoides 690.8
  infectious (staphylococcal) (streptococcal) 686.9
   eczematoid 690.8
  infective eczematoid 690.8
  Jacquet's (diaper dermatitis) 691.0
  leptus 133.8
  lichenified NEC 692.9
  lichenoid, chronic 701.0
  lichenoides purpurica pigmentosa 709.1
  meadow 692.6
  medicamentosa (correct substance properly
    administered) (internal use) (*see also*
    Dermatitis, due to, drugs or medicinals)
    693.0
   due to contact with skin 692.3
  mite 133.8
  multiformis 694.0
   juvenile 694.2
    senile 694.5
  napkin 691.0
  neuro 698.3
  neurotica 694.0
  nummular NEC 692.9
  osteatosis, osteatotic 706.8
  papillaris capillitii 706.1
  pellagrous 265.2
  perioral 695.3
  perstans 696.1
  photosensitivity (sun) 692.72
   other light 692.82
  pigmented purpuric lichenoid 709.1
  polymorpha dolorosa 694.0
  primary irritant 692.9
  pruriginosa 694.0
  pruritic NEC 692.9
  psoriasiform nodularis 696.2
  psychogenic 316
  purulent 686.00
  pustular contagious 051.2
  pyococcal 686.00
  pyocyaneus 686.09
  pyogenica 686.00
  radiation 692.82
  repens 696.1
  Ritter's (exfoliativa) 695.81
  Schamberg's (progressive pigmentary
    dermatosis) 709.09
  schistosome 120.3
  seasonal bullous 694.8
  seborrheic 690.10
   infantile 690.12
  sensitization NEC 692.9
  septic (*see also* Septicemia) 686.00
   gonococcal 098.89
  solar, solare NEC (*see also* Dermatitis, due to,
    sun) 692.70
  stasis 459.81
   due to
    postphlebitic syndrome 459.12
     with ulcer 459.13
    varicose veins—*see* Varicose
   ulcerated or with ulcer (varicose) 454.2

Dermatitis—*continued*
  sunburn (*see also* Sunburn) 692.71
  suppurative 686.00
  traumatic NEC 709.8
  trophoneurotica 694.0
  ultraviolet, except from sun 692.82
   due to sun NEC (*see also* Dermatitis, due to,
    sun) 692.70
  varicose 454.1
   with ulcer 454.2
  vegetans 686.8
  verrucosa 117.2
  xerotic 706.8
Dermatoarthritis, lipoid 272.8 *[713.0]*
Dermatochalasia, dermatochalasis 374.87
Dermatofibroma (lenticulare) (M8832/0)—*see
   also* Neoplasm, skin, benign
  protuberans (M8832/1)—*see* Neoplasm, skin,
    uncertain behavior
Dermatofibrosarcoma (protuberans) (M8832/3)
  see Neoplasm, skin, malignant
Dermatographia 708.3
Dermatolysis (congenital) (exfoliativa) 757.39
  acquired 701.8
  eyelids 374.34
  palpebrarum 374.34
  senile 701.8
Dermatomegaly NEC 701.8
Dermatomucomyositis 710.3
Dermatomycosis 111.9
  furfuracea 111.0
  specified type NEC 111.8
Dermatomyositis (acute) (chronic) 710.3
Dermatoneuritis of children 985.0
Dermatophiliasis 134.1
Dermatophytide —*see* Dermatophytosis
Dermatophytosis (Epidermophyton) (infection)
   (microsporum) (tinea) (Trichophyton) 110.9
  beard 110.0
  body 110.5
  deep seated 110.6
  fingernails 110.1
  foot 110.4
  groin 110.3
  hand 110.2
  nail 110.1
  perianal (area) 110.3
  scalp 110.0
  scrotal 110.8
  specified site NEC 110.8
  toenails 110.1
  vulva 110.8
Dermatopolyneuritis 985.0
Dermatorrhexis 756.83
  acquired 701.8
Dermatosclerosis (*see also* Scleroderma) 710.1
  localized 701.0
Dermatosis 709.9
  Andrews' 686.8
  atopic 691.8
  Bowen's (M8081/2)—*see* Neoplasm, skin, in
   situ
  bullous 694.9
   specified type NEC 694.8
  erythematosquamous 690.8
  exfoliativa 695.89
  factitial 698.4
  gonococcal 098.89
  herpetiformis 694.0
   juvenile 694.2
    senile 694.5

Diarrhea, diarrheal—*continued*
dietetic 787.91
due to
  achylia gastrica 536.8
  Aerobacter aerogenes 008.2
  Bacillus coli—*see* Enteritis, E. coli
  bacteria NEC 008.5
  bile salts 579.8
  Capillaria
    hepatica 128.8
    philippinensis 127.5
  Clostridium perfringens (C) (F) 008.46
  Enterobacter aerogenes 008.2
  enterococci 008.49
  Escherichia coli—*see* Enteritis, E. coli
  Giardia lamblia 007.1
  Heterophyes heterophyes 121.6
  irritating foods 787.91
  Metagonimus yokogawai 121.5
  Necator americanus 126.1
  Paracolobactrum arizonae 008.1
  Paracolon bacillus NEC 008.47
    Arizona 008.1
  Proteus (bacillus) (mirabilis) (Morganii) 008.3
  Pseudomonas aeruginosa 008.42
  S. japonicum 120.2
  specified organism NEC 008.8
    bacterial 008.49
    viral NEC 008.69
  Staphylococcus 008.41
  Streptococcus 008.49
    anaerobic 008.46
  Strongyloides stercoralis 127.2
  Trichuris trichiuria 127.3
  virus NEC (*see also* Enteritis, viral) 008.69
dysenteric 009.2
  due to specified organism NEC 008.8
dyspeptic 787.91
endemic 009.3
epidemic 009.3
fermentative 787.91
flagellate 007.9
Flexner's (ulcerative) 004.1
functional 564.5
  following gastrointestinal surgery 564.4
  psychogenic 306.4
giardial 007.1
Giardia lamblia 007.1
hill 579.1
hyperperistalsis (nervous) 306.4
infectious 009.2
  presumed 009.3
inflammatory 787.91
  due to specified organism NEC 008.8
malarial (*see also* Malaria) 084.6
mite 133.8
mycotic 117.9
nervous 306.4
neurogenic 564.5
parenteral NEC 009.2
postgastrectomy 564.4
postvagotomy 564.4
prostaglandin induced 579.8
protozoal NEC 007.9
psychogenic 306.4
septic 009.2
  due to specified organism NEC 008.8
specified organism NEC 008.8
  bacterial 008.49
  viral NEC 008.69
Staphylococcus 008.41

Diarrhea, diarrheal—*continued*
Streptococcus 008.49
  anaerobic 088.46
toxic 558.2
travelers' 009.2
  due to specified organism NEC 008.8
trichomonal 007.3
tropical 579.1
tuberculous 014.8
ulcerative (chronic) (*see also* Colitis, ulcerative)
  556.9
viral (*see also* Enteritis, viral) 008.8
zymotic NEC 009.2
Diastasis
cranial bones 733.99
  congenital 756.0
joint (traumatic)—*see* Dislocation, by site
muscle 728.84
  congenital 756.89
recti (abdomen) 728.84
  complicating delivery 665.8
  congenital 756.79
Diastema, teeth, tooth 524.3
Diastematomyelia 742.51
Diataxia, cerebral, infantile 343.0
Diathesis
allergic V15.09
bleeding (familial) 287.9
cystine (familial) 270.0
gouty 274.9
hemorrhagic (familial) 287.9
  newborn NEC 776.0
oxalic 271.8
scrofulous (*see also* Tuberculosis) 017.2
spasmophilic (*see also* Tetany) 781.7
ulcer 536.9
uric acid 274.9
Diaz's disease or osteochondrosis 732.5
Dibothriocephaliasis 123.4
larval 123.5
Dibothriocephalus (infection) (infestation)
  (latus) 123.4
larval 123.5
Dicephalus 759.4
Dichotomy, teeth 520.2
Dichromat, dichromata (congenital) 368.59
Dichromatopsia (congenital) 368.59
Dichuchwa 104.0
Dicroceliasis 121.8
Didelphys, didelphic (*see also* Double uterus)
  752.2
Didymitis (*see also* Epididymitis) 604.90
Died —*see also* Death
without
  medical attention (cause unknown) 798.9
  sign of disease 798.2
Dientamoeba diarrhea 007.8
Dietary
inadequacy or deficiency 269.9
surveillance and counseling V65.3
Dietl's crisis 593.4
Dieulafoy lesion (hemorrhagic)
of
  duodenum 537.84
  intestine 569.86
  stomach 537.84
Dieulafoy's ulcer —*see* Ulcer, stomach
Difficult
birth, affecting fetus or newborn 763.9
delivery NEC 669.9

Difficulty
  feeding 783.3
    breast 676.8
    newborn 779.3
    nonorganic (infant) NEC 307.59
    mechanical, gastroduodenal stoma 537.89
  reading 315.00
  specific, spelling 315.09
  swallowing (*see also* Dysphagia) 787.2
  walking 719.7
Diffuse —*see* condition
Diffused ganglion 727.42
DiGeorge's syndrome (thymic hypoplasia)
    279.11
Digestive —*see* condition
Di Guglielmo's disease or syndrome (M9841/3)
    207.0
Diktyoma (M9051/3)—*see* Neoplasm, by site,
    malignant
Dilaceration, tooth 520.4
Dilatation
  anus 564.89
    venule—*see* Hemorrhoids
  aorta (focal) (general) (*see also* Aneurysm,
      aorta) 441.9
    congenital 747.29
    infectional 093.0
    ruptured 441.5
    syphilitic 093.0
  appendix (cystic) 543.9
  artery 447.8
  bile duct (common) (cystic) (congenital) 751.69
    acquired 576.8
  bladder (sphincter) 596.8
    congenital 753.8
    in pregnancy or childbirth 654.4
      causing obstructed labor 660.2
        affecting fetus or newborn 763.1
  blood vessel 459.89
  bronchus, bronchi 494.0
    with acute exacerbation 494.1
  calyx (due to obstruction) 593.89
  capillaries 448.9
  cardiac (acute) (chronic) (*see also* Hypertrophy,
      cardiac) 429.3
    congenital 746.89
      valve NEC 746.89
        pulmonary 746.09
    hypertensive (*see also* Hypertension, heart)
        402.90
  cavum septi pellucidi 742.4
  cecum 564.89
    psychogenic 306.4
  cervix (uteri)—*see also* Incompetency, cervix
    incomplete, poor, slow
      affecting fetus or newborn 763.7
      complicating delivery 661.0
        affecting fetus or newborn 763.7
  colon 564.7
    congenital 751.3
    due to mechanical obstruction 560.89
    psychogenic 306.4
  common bile duct (congenital) 751.69
    acquired 576.8
      with calculus, choledocholithiasis, or
        stones—*see* Choledocholithiasis
  cystic duct 751.69
    acquired (any bile duct) 575.8
  duct, mammary 610.4
  duodenum 564.89
  esophagus 530.89

Dilatation—*continued*
  congenital 750.4
  due to
    achalasia 530.0
    cardiospasm 530.0
  Eustachian tube, congenital 744.24
  fontanel 756.0
  gallbladder 575.8
    congenital 751.69
  gastric 536.8
    acute 536.1
    psychogenic 306.4
  heart (acute) (chronic) (*see also* Hypertrophy,
      cardiac) 429.3
    congenital 746.89
    hypertensive (*see also* Hypertension, heart)
        402.90
    valve—*see also* Endocarditis
      congenital 746.89
  ileum 564.89
    psychogenic 306.4
  inguinal rings—*see* Hernia, inguinal
  jejunum 564.89
    psychogenic 306.4
  kidney (calyx) (collecting structures) (cystic)
      (parenchyma) (pelvis) 593.89
  lacrimal passages 375.69
  lymphatic vessel 457.1
  mammary duct 610.4
  Meckel's diverticulum (congenital) 751.0
  meningeal vessels, congenital 742.8
  myocardium (acute) (chronic) (*see also*
      Hypertrophy, cardiac) 429.3
  organ or site, congenital NEC—*see* Distortion
  pancreatic duct 577.8
  pelvis, kidney 593.89
  pericardium—*see* Pericarditis
  pharynx 478.29
  prostate 602.8
  pulmonary
    artery (idiopathic) 417.8
      congenital 747.3
    valve, congenital 746.09
  pupil 379.43
  rectum 564.89
  renal 593.89
  saccule vestibularis, congenital 744.05
  salivary gland (duct) 527.8
  sphincter ani 564.89
  stomach 536.8
    acute 536.1
    psychogenic 306.4
  submaxillary duct 527.8
  trachea, congenital 748.3
  ureter (idiopathic) 593.89
    congenital 753.20
    due to obstruction 593.5
  urethra (acquired) 599.84
  vasomotor 443.9
  vein 459.89
  ventricular, ventricle (acute) (chronic) (*see also*
      Hypertrophy, cardiac) 429.3
    cerebral, congenital 742.4
    hypertensive (*see also* Hypertension, heart)
        402.90
  venule 459.89
    anus—*see* Hemorrhoids
  vesical orifice 596.8
Dilated, dilation —*see* Dilatation

Diminished
hearing (acuity) (*see also* Deafness) 389.9
pulse pressure 785.9
vision NEC 369.9
vital capacity 794.2
Diminuta taenia 123.6
Diminution, sense or sensation (cold) (heat)
(tactile) (vibratory) (*see also* Disturbance,
sensation) 782.0
Dimitri-Sturge-Weber disease
(encephalocutaneous angiomatosis) 759.6
Dimple
parasacral 685.1
with abscess 685.0
pilonidal 685.1
with abscess 685.0
postanal 685.1
with abscess 685.0
Dioctophyma renale (infection) (infestation)
128.8
Dipetalonemiasis 125.4
Diphallus 752.69
Diphtheria, diphtheritic (gangrenous)
(hemorrhagic) 032.9
carrier (suspected) of V02.4
cutaneous 032.85
cystitis 032.84
faucial 032.0
infection of wound 032.85
inoculation (anti) (not sick) V03.5
laryngeal 032.3
myocarditis 032.82
nasal anterior 032.2
nasopharyngeal 032.1
neurological complication 032.89
peritonitis 032.83
specified site NEC 032.89
Diphyllobothriasis (intestine) 123.4
larval 123.5
Diplacusis 388.41
Diplegia (upper limbs) 344.2
brain or cerebral 437.8
congenital 343.0
facial 351.0
congenital 352.6
infantile or congenital (cerebral) (spastic)
(spinal) 343.0
lower limbs 344.1
syphilitic, congenital 090.49
Diplococcus, diplococcal —*see* condition
Diplomyelia 742.59
Diplopia 368.2
refractive 368.15
Dipsomania (*see also* Alcoholism) 303.9
with psychosis (*see also* Psychosis, alcoholic)
291.9
Dipylidiasis 123.8
intestine 123.8
Direction, teeth, abnormal 524.3
Dirt-eating child 307.52
Disability
heart—*see* Disease, heart
learning NEC 315.2
special spelling 315.09
Disarticulation (*see also* Derangement, joint)
718.9
meaning
amputation
status—*see* Absence, by site
traumatic —*see* Amputation, traumatic
dislocation, traumatic or congenital—*see*
Dislocation

Disaster, cerebrovascular (*see also* Disease,
cerebrovascular, acute) 436
Discharge
anal NEC 787.99
breast (female) (male) 611.79
conjunctiva 372.89
continued locomotor idiopathic (*see also*
Epilepsy) 345.5
diencephalic autonomic idiopathic (*see also*
Epilepsy) 345.5
ear 388.60
blood 388.69
cerebrospinal fluid 388.61
excessive urine 788.42
eye 379.93
nasal 478.1
nipple 611.79
patterned motor idiopathic (*see also* Epilepsy)
345.5
penile 788.7
postnasal—*see* Sinusitis
sinus, from mediastinum 510.0
umbilicus 789.9
urethral 788.7
bloody 599.84
vaginal 623.5
Discitis 722.90
cervical, cervicothoracic 722.91
lumbar, lumbosacral 722.93
thoracic, thoracolumbar 722.92
Discogenic syndrome —*see* Displacement,
intervertebral disc
Discoid
kidney 753.3
meniscus, congenital 717.5
semilunar cartilage 717.5
Discoloration
mouth 528.9
nails 703.8
teeth 521.7
due to
drugs 521.7
metals (copper) (silver) 521.7
pulpal bleeding 521.7
during formation 520.8
posteruptive 521.7
Discomfort
chest 786.59
visual 368.13
Discomycosis —*see* Actinomycosis
Discontinuity, ossicles, ossicular chain 385.23
Discrepancy
leg length (acquired) 736.81
congenital 755.30
uterine size-date 646.8
Discrimination
political V62.4
racial V62.4
religious V62.4
sex V62.4
Disease, diseased —*see also* Syndrome
Abrami's (acquired hemolytic jaundice) 283.9
absorbent system 459.89
accumulation—*see* Thesaurismosis
acid-peptic 536.8
Acosta's 993.2
Adams-Stokes (-Morgagni) (syncope with heart
block) 426.9
Addison's (bronze) (primary adrenal
insufficiency) 255.4
anemia (pernicious) 281.0

Disease, diseased—*continued*
tuberculous (*see also* Tuberculosis) 017.6
Addison-Gull—*see* Xanthoma
adenoids (and tonsils) (chronic) 474.9
adrenal (gland) (capsule) (cortex) 255.9
hyperfunction 255.3
hypofunction 255.4
specified type NEC 255.8
ainhum (dactylolysis spontanea) 136.0
akamushi (scrub typhus) 081.2
Akureyri (epidemic neuromyasthenia) 049.8
Albarrán's (colibacilluria) 791.9
Albers-Schönberg's (marble bones) 756.52
Albert's 726.71
Albright (-Martin) (-Bantam) 275.49
Alibert's (mycosis fungoides) (M9700/3) 202.1
Alibert-Bazin (M9700/3) 202.1
alimentary canal 569.9
alligator skin (ichthyosis congenital) 757.1
acquired 701.1
Almeida's (Brazilian blastomycosis) 116.1
Alpers' 330.8
alpine 993.2
altitude 993.2
alveoli, teeth 525.9
Alzheimer's—*see* Alzheimer's
amyloid (any site) 277.3
anarthritic rheumatoid 446.5
Anders' (adiposis tuberosa simplex) 272.8
Andersen's (glycogenosis IV) 271.0
Anderson's (angiokeratoma corporis diffusum) 272.7
Andes 993.2
Andrews' (bacterid) 686.8
angiospastic, angiospasmodic 443.9
cerebral 435.9
with transient neurologic deficit 435.9
vein 459.89
anterior
chamber 364.9
horn cell 335.9
specified type NEC 335.8
antral (chronic) 473.0
acute 461.0
anus NEC 569.49
aorta (nonsyphilitic) 447.9
syphilitic NEC 093.89
aortic (heart) (valve) (*see also* Endocarditis, aortic) 424.1
apollo 077.4
aponeurosis 726.90
appendix 543.9
aqueous (chamber) 364.9
arc-welders' lung 503
Armenian 277.3
Arnold-Chiari (*see also* Spina bifida) 741.0
arterial 447.9
occlusive (*see also* Occlusion, by site) 444.22
with embolus or thrombus—*see* Occlusion, by site
due to stricture or stenosis 447.1
specified type NEC 447.8
arteriocardiorenal (*see also* Hypertension, cardiorenal) 404.90
arteriolar (generalized) (obliterative) 447.9
specified type NEC 447.8
arteriorenal—*see* Hypertension, kidney
arteriosclerotic—*see also* Arteriosclerosis
cardiovascular 429.2
coronary —*see* Arteriosclerosis, coronary
heart —*see* Arteriosclerosis, coronary

Disease, diseased—*continued*
vascular—*see* Arteriosclerosis
artery 447.9
cerebral 437.9
coronary —*see* Arteriosclerosis, coronary
specified type NEC 447.8
arthropod-borne NEC 088.9
specified type NEC 088.89
Asboe-Hansen's (incontinentia pigmenti) 757.33
atticoantral, chronic (with posterior or superior marginal perforation of ear drum) 382.2
auditory canal, ear 380.9
Aujeszky's 078.89
auricle, ear NEC 380.30
Australian X 062.4
autoimmune NEC 279.4
hemolytic (cold type) (warm type) 283.0
parathyroid 252.1
thyroid 245.2
aviators' (*see also* Effect, adverse, high altitude) 993.2
ax(e)-grinders' 502
Ayala's 756.89
Ayerza's (pulmonary artery sclerosis with pulmonary hypertension) 416.0
Azorean (of the nervous system) 334.8
Babington's (familial hemorrhagic telangiectasia) 448.0
back bone NEC 733.90
bacterial NEC 040.89
zoonotic NEC 027.9
specified type NEC 027.8
Baehr-Schiffrin (thrombotic thrombocytopenic purpura) 446.6
Baelz's (cheilitis glandularis apostematosa) 528.5
Baerensprung's (eczema marginatum) 110.3
Balfour's (chloroma) 205.3
balloon (*see also* Effect, adverse, high altitude) 993.2
Baló's 341.1
Bamberger (-Marie) (hypertrophic pulmonary osteoarthropathy) 731.2
Bang's (Brucella abortus) 023.1
Bannister's 995.1
Banti's (with cirrhosis) (with portal hypertension)—*see* Cirrhosis, liver
Barcoo (*see also* Ulcer, skin) 707.9
barium lung 503
Barlow (-Möller) (infantile scurvy) 267
barometer makers' 985.0
Barraquer (-Simons) (progressive lipodystrophy) 272.6
basal ganglia 333.90
degenerative NEC 333.0
specified NEC 333.89
Basedow's (exophthalmic goiter) 242.0
basement membrane NEC 583.89
with
pulmonary hemorrhage (Goodpasture's syndrome) 446.21 *[583.81]*
Bateman's 078.0
purpura (senile) 287.2
Batten's 330.1 *[362.71]*
Batten-Mayou (retina) 330.1 *[362.71]*
Batten-Steinert 359.2
Battey 031.0
Baumgarten-Cruveilhier (cirrhosis of liver) 571.5
bauxite-workers' 503
Bayle's (dementia paralytica) 094.1

Disease, diseased—*continued*
  Bazin's (primary) (*see also* Tuberculosis) 017.1
  Beard's (neurasthenia) 300.5
  Beau's (*see also* Degeneration, myocardial)
    429.1
  Bechterew's (ankylosing spondylitis) 720.0
  Becker's (idiopathic mural endomyocardial
    disease) 425.2
  Begbie's (exophthalmic goiter) 242.0
  Behr's 362.50
  Beigel's (white piedra) 111.2
  Bekhterev's (ankylosing spondylitis) 720.0
  Bell's (*see also* Psychosis, affective) 296.0
  Bennett's (leukemia) 208.9
  Benson's 379.22
  Bergeron's (hysteroepilepsy) 300.11
  Berlin's 921.3
  Bernard-Soulier (thrombopathy) 287.1
  Bernhardt (-Roth) 355.1
  beryllium 503
  Besnier-Boeck (-Schaumann) (sarcoidosis) 135
  Best's 362.76
  Beurmann's (sporotrichosis) 117.1
  Bielschowsky (-Jansky) 330.1
  Biermer's (pernicious anemia) 281.0
  Biett's (discoid lupus erythematosus) 695.4
  bile duct (*see also* Disease, biliary) 576.9
  biliary (duct) (tract) 576.9
    with calculus, choledocholithiasis, or
      stones—*see* Choledocholithiasis
  Billroth's (meningocele) (*see also* Spina bifida)
    741.9
  Binswanger's 290.12
  Bird's (oxaluria) 271.8
  bird fanciers' 495.2
  black lung 500
  bladder 596.9
    specified NEC 596.8
  bleeder's 286.0
  Bloch-Sulzberger (incontinentia pigmenti)
    757.33
  Blocq's (astasia-abasia) 307.9
  blood (-forming organs) 289.9
    specified NEC 289.8
    vessel 459.9
  Bloodgood's 610.1
  Blount's (tibia vara) 732.4
  blue 746.9
  Bodechtel-Guttmann (subacute sclerosing
    panencephalitis) 046.2
  Boeck's (sarcoidosis) 135
  bone 733.90
    fibrocystic NEC 733.29
      jaw 526.2
    marrow 289.9
    Paget's (osteitis deformans) 731.0
    specified type NEC 733.99
    von Recklinghausen's (osteitis fibrosa cystica)
      252.0
  Bonfils'—*see* Disease, Hodgkin's
  Borna 062.9
  Bornholm (epidemic pleurodynia) 074.1
  Bostock's (*see also* Fever, hay) 477.9
  Bouchard's (myopathic dilatation of the
    stomach) 536.1
  Bouillaud's (rheumatic heart disease) 391.9
  Bourneville (-Brissaud) (tuberous sclerosis)
    759.5
  Bouveret (-Hoffmann) (paroxysmal
    tachycardia) 427.2

Disease, diseased—*continued*
  bowel 569.9
    functional 564.9
      psychogenic 306.4
  Bowen's (M8081/2)—*see* Neoplasm, skin, in
    situ
  Bozzolo's (multiple myeloma) (M9730/3) 203.0
  Bradley's (epidemic vomiting) 078.82
  Brailsford's 732.3
    radius, head 732.3
    tarsal, scaphoid 732.5
  Brailsford-Morquio (mucopolysaccharidosis
    IV) 277.5
  brain 348.9
    Alzheimer's 331.0
      with dementia—*see* Alzheimer's, dementia
    arterial, artery 437.9
    arteriosclerotic 437.0
    congenital 742.9
    degenerative—*see* Degeneration, brain
    inflammatory—*see also* Encephalitis
      late effect—*see* category 326
    organic 348.9
      arteriosclerotic 437.0
    parasitic NEC 123.9
    Pick's 331.1
      with dementia
        with behavioral disturbance 331.1 *[294.11]*
        without behavioral disturbance 331.1
          [294.10]
    senile 331.2
  braziers' 985.8
  breast 611.9
    cystic (chronic) 610.1
    fibrocystic 610.1
    inflammatory 611.0
    Paget's (M8540/3) 174.0
    puerperal, postpartum NEC 676.3
    specified NEC 611.8
  Breda's (*see also* Yaws) 102.9
  Breisky's (kraurosis vulvae) 624.0
  Bretonneau's (diphtheritic malignant angina)
    032.0
  Bright's (*see also* Nephritis) 583.9
    arteriosclerotic (*see also* Hypertension,
      kidney) 403.90
  Brill's (recrudescent typhus) 081.1
    flea-borne 081.0
    louse-borne 081.1
  Brill-Symmers (follicular lymphoma)
    (M9690/3) 202.0
  Brill-Zinsser (recrudescent typhus) 081.1
  Brinton's (leather bottle stomach) (M8142/3)
    151.9
  Brion-Kayser (*see also* Fever, paratyphoid)
    002.9
  broad
    beta 272.2
    ligament, noninflammatory 620.9
      specified NEC 620.8
  Brocq's 691.8
    meaning
      atopic (diffuse) neurodermatitis 691.8
      dermatitis herpetiformis 694.0
      lichen simplex chronicus 698.3
      parapsoriasis 696.2
      prurigo 698.2
  Brocq-Duhring (dermatitis herpetiformis) 694.0
  Brodie's (joint) (*see also* Osteomyelitis) 730.1
  bronchi 519.1
  bronchopulmonary 519.1

Disease, diseased—*continued*
  bronze (Addison's) 255.4
    tuberculous (*see also* Tuberculosis) 017.6
  Brown-Séquard 344.89
  Bruck's 733.99
  Bruck-de Lange (Amsterdam dwarf, mental
      retardation, and brachycephaly) 759.89
  Bruhl's (splenic anemia with fever) 285.8
  Bruton's (X-linked agammaglobulinemia)
      279.04
  buccal cavity 528.9
  Buchanan's (juvenile osteochondrosis, iliac
      crest) 732.1
  Buchman's (osteochondrosis juvenile) 732.1
  Budgerigar-fanciers' 495.2
  Büdinger-Ludloff-Läwen 717.89
  Buerger's (thromboangiitis obliterans) 443.1
  Bürger-Grütz (essential familial hyperlipemia)
      272.3
  Burns' (lower ulna) 732.3
  bursa 727.9
  Bury's (erythema elevatum diutinum) 695.89
  Buschke's 710.1
  Busquet's (*see also* Osteomyelitis) 730.1
  Busse-Buschke (cryptococcosis) 117.5
  C₂ (*see also* Alcoholism) 303.9
  Caffey's (infantile cortical hyperostosis) 756.59
  caisson 993.3
  calculous 592.9
  California 114.0
  Calvé (-Perthes) (osteochondrosis, femoral
      capital) 732.1
  Camurati-Engelmann (diaphyseal sclerosis)
      756.59
  Canavan's 330.0
  capillaries 448.9
  Carapata 087.1
  cardiac-*see* Disease, heart
  cardiopulmonary, chronic 416.9
  cardiorenal (arteriosclerotic) (hepatic)
      (hypertensive) (vascular) (*see also*
      Hypertension, cardiorenal) 404.90
  cardiovascular (arteriosclerotic) 429.2
    congenital 746.9
    hypertensive (*see also* Hypertension, heart)
        402.90
      benign 402.10
      malignant 402.00
    renal (*see also* Hypertension, cardiorenal)
        404.90
    syphilitic (asymptomatic) 093.9
  carotid gland 259.8
  Carrión's (Bartonellosis) 088.0
  cartilage NEC 733.90
    specified NEC 733.99
  Castellani's 104.8
  cat-scratch 078.3
  Cavare's (familial periodic paralysis) 359.3
  Cazenave's (pemphigus) 694.4
  cecum 569.9
  celiac (adult) 579.0
    infantile 579.0
  cellular tissue NEC 709.9
  central core 359.0
  cerebellar, cerebellum—*see* Disease, brain
  cerebral (*see also* Disease, brain) 348.9
    arterial, artery 437.9
    degenerative—*see* Degeneration, brain
  cerebrospinal 349.9
  cerebrovascular NEC 437.9
    acute 436

Disease, diseased—*continued*
    embolic—*see* Embolism, brain
    late effect—*see* Late effect(s) (of)
        cerebrovascular disease
    puerperal, postpartum, childbirth 674.0
    thrombotic—*see* Thrombosis, brain
  arteriosclerotic 437.0
    embolic—*see* Embolism, brain
    ischemic, generalized NEC 437.1
    late effect—*see* Late effect(s) (of)
        cerebrovascular disease
    occlusive 437.1
    puerperal, postpartum, childbirth 674.0
    specified type NEC 437.8
    thrombotic—*see* Thrombosis, brain
  ceroid storage 272.7
  cervix (uteri)
    inflammatory 616.9
      specified NEC 616.8
    noninflammatory 622.9
      specified NEC 622.8
  Chabert's 022.9
  Chagas' (*see also* Trypanosomiasis, American)
      086.2
  Chandler's (osteochondritis dissecans, hip)
      732.7
  Charcot's (joint) 094.0 *[713.5]*
    spinal cord 094.0
  Charcot-Marie-Tooth 356.1
  Charlouis' (*see also* Yaws) 102.9
  Cheadle (-Möller) (-Barlow) (infantile scurvy)
      267
  Chédiak-Steinbrinck (-Higashi) (congenital
      gigantism of peroxidase granules) 288.2
  cheek, inner 528.9
  chest 519.9
  Chiari's (hepatic vein thrombosis) 453.0
  Chicago (North American blastomycosis) 116.0
  chignon (white piedra) 111.2
  chigoe, chigo (jigger) 134.1
  childhood granulomatous 288.1
  Chinese liver fluke 121.1
  chlamydial NEC 078.88
  cholecystic (*see also* Disease, gallbladder) 575.9
  choroid 363.9
    degenerative (*see also* Degeneration, choroid)
        363.40
    hereditary (*see also* Dystrophy, choroid)
        363.50
    specified type NEC 363.8
  Christian's (chronic histiocytosis X) 277.8
  Christian-Weber (nodular nonsuppurative
      panniculitis) 729.30
  Christmas 286.1
  ciliary body 364.9
  circulatory (system) NEC 459.9
    chronic, maternal, affecting fetus or newborn
        760.3
    specified NEC 459.89
    syphilitic 093.9
      congenital 090.5
  Civatte's (poikiloderma) 709.09
  climacteric 627.2
    male 608.89
  coagulation factor deficiency (congenital) (*see
      also* Defect, coagulation) 286.9
  Coats' 362.12
  coccidioidal pulmonary 114.5
    acute 114.0
    chronic 114.4
    primary 114.0

Disease, diseased—*continued*
  residual 114.4
  Cockayne's (microcephaly and dwarfism)
    759.89
  Cogan's 370.52
  cold
    agglutinin 283.0
      or hemoglobinuria 283.0
        paroxysmal (cold) (nocturnal) 283.2
    hemagglutinin (chronic) 283.0
  collagen NEC 710.9
    nonvascular 710.9
    specified NEC 710.8
    vascular (allergic) (*see also* Angiitis,
      hypersensitivity) 446.20
  colon 569.9
    functional 564.9
      congenital 751.3
    ischemic 557.0
  combined system (of spinal cord) 266.2 *[336.2]*
    with anemia (pernicious) 281.0 *[336.2]*
  compressed air 993.3
  Concato's (pericardial polyserositis) 423.2
    peritoneal 568.82
    pleural—*see* Pleurisy
  congenital NEC 799.8
  conjunctiva 372.9
    chlamydial 077.98
      specified NEC 077.8
    specified type NEC 372.89
    viral 077.99
      specified NEC 077.8
  connective tissue, diffuse (*see also* Disease,
    collagen) 710.9
  Conor and Bruch's (boutonneuse fever) 082.1
  Conradi (-Hünermann) 756.59
  Cooley's (erythroblastic anemia) 282.4
  Cooper's 610.1
  Corbus' 607.1
  cork-handlers' 495.3
  cornea (*see also* Keratopathy) 371.9
  coronary (*see also* Ischemia, heart) 414.9
    congenital 746.85
    ostial, syphilitic 093.20
      aortic 093.22
      mitral 093.21
      pulmonary 093.24
      tricuspid 093.23
  Corrigan's—*see* Insufficiency, aortic
  Cotugno's 724.3
  Coxsackie (virus) NEC 074.8
  cranial nerve NEC 352.9
  Creutzfeldt-Jakob 046.1
    with dementia
      with behavioral disturbance 046.1 *[294.11]*
      without behavioral disturbance 046.1
        [294.10]
  Crigler-Najjar (congenital hyperbilirubinemia)
    277.4
  Crocq's (acrocyanosis) 443.89
  Crohn's (intestine) (*see also* Enteritis, regional)
    555.9
  Crouzon's (craniofacial dysostosis) 756.0
  Cruchet's (encephalitis lethargica) 049.8
  Cruveilhier's 335.21
  Cruz-Chagas (*see also* Trypanosomiasis,
    American) 086.2
  crystal deposition (*see also* Arthritis, due to,
    crystals) 712.9
  Csillag's (lichen sclerosus et atrophicus) 701.0
  Curschmann's 359.2

Disease, diseased—*continued*
  Cushing's (pituitary basophilism) 255.0
  cystic
    breast (chronic) 610.1
    kidney, congenital (*see also* Cystic, disease,
      kidney) 753.10
    liver, congenital 751.62
    lung 518.89
      congenital 748.4
    pancreas 577.2
      congenital 751.7
    renal, congenital (*see also* Cystic, disease,
      kidney) 753.10
    semilunar cartilage 717.5
  cysticercus 123.1
  cystine storage (with renal sclerosis) 270.0
  cytomegalic inclusion (generalized) 078.5
    with
      pneumonia 078.5 *[484.1]*
    congenital 771.1
  Daae (-Finsen) (epidemic pleurodynia) 074.1
  dancing 297.8
  Danielssen's (anesthetic leprosy) 030.1
  Darier's (congenital) (keratosis follicularis)
    757.39
    erythema annulare centrifugum 695.0
    vitamin A deficiency 264.8
  Darling's (histoplasmosis) (*see also*
    Histoplasmosis, American) 115.00
  Davies' 425.0
  de Beurmann-Gougerot (sporotrichosis) 117.1
  Débove's (splenomegaly) 789.2
  deer fly (*see also* Tularemia) 021.9
  deficiency 269.9
  degenerative—*see also* Degeneration
    disc—*see* Degeneration, intervertebral disc
  Degos' 447.8
  Déjérine (-Sottas) 356.0
  Déleage's 359.89
  demyelinating, demyelinizating (brain stem)
    (central nervous system) 341.9
    multiple sclerosis 340
    specified NEC 341.8
  de Quervain's (tendon sheath) 727.04
    thyroid (subacute granulomatous thyroiditis)
      245.1
  Dercum's (adiposis dolorosa) 272.8
  Deutschländer's—*see* Fracture, foot
  Devergie's (pityriasis rubra pilaris) 696.4
  Devic's 341.0
  diaphorase deficiency 289.7
  diaphragm 519.4
  diarrheal, infectious 009.2
  diatomaceous earth 502
  Diaz's (osteochondrosis astragalus) 732.5
  digestive system 569.9
  Di Guglielmo's (erythemic myelosis)
    (M9841/3) 207.0
  Dimitri-Sturge-Weber (encephalocutaneous
    angiomatosis) 759.6
  disc, degenerative—*see* Degeneration,
    intervertebral disc
  discogenic (*see also* Disease, intervertebral
    disc) 722.90
  diverticular—*see* Diverticula
  Down's (mongolism) 758.0
  Dubini's (electric chorea) 049.8
  Dubois' (thymus gland) 090.5
  Duchenne's 094.0
    locomotor ataxia 094.0
    muscular dystrophy 359.1

Disease, diseased—*continued*
  kidney disease—*see* Hypertension,
    cardiorenal
  rheumatic fever (conditions classifiable to
    390)
    active 391.9
      with chorea 392.0
    inactive or quiescent (with chorea) 398.90
  amyloid 277.3 *[425.7]*
  aortic (valve) (*see also* Endocarditis, aortic)
    424.1
  arteriosclerotic or sclerotic (minimal)
    (senile)—*see* Arteriosclerosis, coronary
  artery, arterial —*see* Arteriosclerosis, coronary
  atherosclerotic —*see* Arteriosclerosis,
    coronary
  beer drinkers' 425.5
  beriberi 265.0 *[425.7]*
  black 416.0
  congenital NEC 746.9
    cyanotic 746.9
    maternal, affecting fetus or newborn 760.3
    specified type NEC 746.89
  congestive (*see also* Failure, heart) 428.0
  coronary 414.9
  cryptogenic 429.9
  due to
    amyloidosis 277.3 *[425.7]*
    beriberi 265.0 *[425.7]*
    cardiac glycogenosis 271.0 *[425.7]*
    Friedreich's ataxia 334.0 *[425.8]*
    gout 274.82
    mucopolysaccharidosis 277.5 *[425.7]*
    myotonia atrophica 359.2 *[425.8]*
    progressive muscular dystrophy 359.1
      [425.8]
    sarcoidosis 135 *[425.8]*
  fetal 746.9
    inflammatory 746.89
  fibroid (*see also* Myocarditis) 429.0
  functional 427.9
    postoperative 997.1
    psychogenic 306.2
  glycogen storage 271.0 *[425.7]*
  gonococcal NEC 098.85
  gouty 274.82
  hypertensive (*see also* Hypertension, heart)
    402.90
    benign 402.10
    malignant 402.00
  hyperthyroid (*see also* Hyperthyroidism)
    242.9 *[425.7]*
  incompletely diagnosed—*see* Disease, heart
  ischemic (chronic) (*see also* Ischemia, heart)
    414.9
    acute (*see also* Infarct, myocardium) 410.9
      without myocardial infarction 411.89
        with coronary (artery) occlusion 411.81
    asymptomatic 412
    diagnosed on ECG or other special
      investigation but currently presenting no
      symptoms 412
  kyphoscoliotic 416.1
  mitral (*see also* Endocarditis, mitral) 394.9
  muscular (*see also* Degeneration, myocardial)
    429.1
  postpartum 674.8
  psychogenic (functional) 306.2
  pulmonary (chronic) 416.9
    acute 415.0

Disease, diseased—*continued*
  specified NEC 416.8
  rheumatic (chronic) (inactive) (old)
    (quiescent) (with chorea) 398.90
    active or acute 391.9
      with chorea (active) (rheumatic)
        (Sydenham's) 392.0
      specified type NEC 391.8
    maternal, affecting fetus or newborn 760.3
  rheumatoid—*see* Arthritis, rheumatoid
  sclerotic —*see* Arteriosclerosis, coronary
  senile (*see also* Myocarditis) 429.0
  specified type NEC 429.89
  syphilitic 093.89
    aortic 093.1
      aneurysm 093.0
    asymptomatic 093.89
    congenital 090.5
  thyroid (gland) (*see also* Hyperthyroidism)
    242.9 *[425.7]*
  thyrotoxic (*see also* Thyrotoxicosis) 242.9
    [425.7]
  tuberculous (*see also* Tuberculosis) 017.9
    [425.8]
  valve, valvular (obstructive)
    (regurgitant)—*see also* Endocarditis
    congenital NEC (*see also* Anomaly, heart,
      valve) 746.9
    pulmonary 746.00
    specified type NEC 746.89
  vascular—*see* Disease, cardiovascular
  heavy-chain (gamma G) 273.2
  Heberden's 715.04
  Hebra's
    dermatitis exfoliativa 695.89
    erythema multiforme exudativum 695.1
    pityriasis
      maculata et circinata 696.3
      rubra 695.89
        pilaris 696.4
    prurigo 698.2
  Heerfordt's (uveoparotitis) 135
  Heidenhain's 290.10
    with dementia 290.10
  Heilmeyer-Schöner (M9842/3) 207.1
  Heine-Medin (*see also* Poliomyelitis) 045.9
  Heller's (*see also* Psychosis, childhood) 299.1
  Heller-Döhle (syphilitic aortitis) 093.1
  hematopoietic organs 289.9
  hemoglobin (Hb) 282.7
    with thalassemia 282.4
    abnormal (mixed) NEC 282.7
      with thalassemia 282.4
    AS genotype 282.5
    Bart's 282.7
    C (Hb-C) 282.7
      with other abnormal hemoglobin NEC 282.7
      elliptocytosis 282.7
      Hb-S 282.63
      sickle-cell 282.63
      thalassemia 282.4
    constant spring 282.7
    D (Hb-D) 282.7
      with other abnormal hemoglobin NEC 282.7
      Hb-S 282.69
      sickle-cell 282.69
      thalassemia 282.4
    E (Hb-E) 282.7
      with other abnormal hemoglobin NEC 282.7
      Hb-S 282.69
      sickle-cell 282.69

Disease, diseased—*continued*
  thalassemia 282.4
  elliptocytosis 282.7
  F (Hb-F) 282.7
  G (Hb-G) 282.7
  H (Hb-H) 282.4
  hereditary persistence, fetal (HPFH) ("Swiss
    variety") 282.7
  high fetal gene 282.7
  I thalassemia 282.4
  M 289.7
  S—*see* Disease, sickle-cell, Hb-S
  spherocytosis 282.7
  unstable, hemolytic 282.7
  Zurich (Hb-Zurich) 282.7
  hemolytic (fetus) (newborn) 773.2
  autoimmune (cold type) (warm type) 283.0
  due to or with
    incompatibility
      ABO (blood group) 773.1
      blood (group) (Duffy) (Kell) (Kidd)
        (Lewis) (M) (S) NEC 773.2
      Rh (blood group) (factor) 773.0
      Rh negative mother 773.0
    unstable hemoglobin 282.7
  hemorrhagic 287.9
  newborn 776.0
  Henoch (-Schönlein) (purpura nervosa) 287.0
  hepatic—*see* Disease, liver
  hepatolenticular 275.1
  heredodegenerative NEC
  brain 331.89
  spinal cord 336.8
  Hers' (glycogenosis VI) 271.0
  Herter (-Gee) (-Heubner) (nontropical sprue)
    579.0
  Herxheimer's (diffuse idiopathic cutaneous
    atrophy) 701.8
  Heubner's 094.89
  Heubner-Herter (nontropical sprue) 579.0
  high fetal gene or hemoglobin thalassemia 282.4
  Hildenbrand's (typhus) 081.9
  hip (joint) NEC 719.95
  congenital 755.63
  suppurative 711.05
  tuberculous (*see also* Tuberculosis) 015.1
    [730.85]
  Hippel's (retinocerebral angiomatosis) 759.6
  Hirschfeld's (acute diabetes mellitus) (*see also*
    Diabetes) 250.0
  Hirschsprung's (congenital megacolon) 751.3
  His (-Werner) (trench fever) 083.1
  HIV 042
  Hodgkin's (M9650/3) 201.9

---

*Note—Use the following fifth-digit
subclassification with categories 201:*

0 unspecified site
1 lymph nodes of head, face, and neck
2 intrathoracic lymph nodes
3 intra-abdominal lymph nodes
4 lymph nodes of axilla and upper limb
*5 lymph nodes of inguinal region and
    lower limb*
6 intrapelvic lymph nodes
7 spleen
8 lymph nodes of multiple sites

---

  lymphocytic
  depletion (M9653/3) 201.7
    diffuse fibrosis (M9654/3) 201.7

Disease, diseased—*continued*
  reticular type (M9655/3) 201.7
  predominance (M9651/3) 201.4
  lymphocytic-histiocytic predominance
    (M9651/3) 201.4
  mixed cellularity (M9652/3) 201.6
  nodular sclerosis (M9656/3) 201.5
  cellular phase (M9657/3) 201.5
  Hodgson's 441.9
  ruptured 441.5
  Hoffa (-Kastert) (liposynovitis prepatellaris)
    272.8
  Holla (*see also* Spherocytosis) 282.0
  homozygous-Hb-S 282.61
  hoof and mouth 078.4
  hookworm (*see also* Ancylostomiasis) 126.9
  Horton's (temporal arteritis) 446.5
  host-versus-graft (immune or nonimmune
    cause) 996.80
  bone marrow 996.85
  heart 996.83
  intestines 996.87
  kidney 996.81
  liver 996.82
  lung 996.84
  pancreas 996.86
  specified NEC 996.89
  HPFH (hereditary persistence of fetal
    hemoglobin) ("Swiss variety") 282.7
  Huchard's (continued arterial hypertension)
    401.9
  Huguier's (uterine fibroma) 218.9
  human immunodeficiency (virus) 042
  hunger 251.1
  Hunt's
  dyssynergia cerebellaris myoclonica 334.2
  herpetic geniculate ganglionitis 053.11
  Huntington's 333.4
  Huppert's (multiple myeloma) (M9730/3) 203.0
  Hurler's (mucopolysaccharidosis I) 277.5
  Hutchinson's, meaning
  angioma serpiginosum 709.1
  cheiropompholyx 705.81
  prurigo estivalis 692.72
  Hutchinson-Boeck (sarcoidosis) 135
  Hutchinson-Gilford (progeria) 259.8
  hyaline (diffuse) (generalized) 728.9
  membrane (lung) (newborn) 769
  hydatid (*see also* Echinococcus) 122.9
  Hyde's (prurigo nodularis) 698.3
  hyperkinetic (*see also* Hyperkinesia) 314.9
  heart 429.82
  hypertensive (*see also* Hypertension) 401.9
  hypophysis 253.9
  hyperfunction 253.1
  hypofunction 253.2
  Iceland (epidemic neuromyasthenia) 049.8
  I cell 272.7
  ill-defined 799.8
  immunologic NEC 279.9
  immunoproliferative 203.8
  inclusion 078.5
  salivary gland 078.5
  infancy, early NEC 779.9
  infective NEC 136.9
  inguinal gland 289.9
  internal semilunar cartilage, cystic 717.5
  intervertebral disc 722.90
  with myelopathy 722.70
  cervical, cervicothoracic 722.91
    with myelopathy 722.71

Disease, diseased—*continued*
  lumbar, lumbosacral 722.93
    with myelopathy 722.73
    thoracic, thoracolumbar 722.92
    with myelopathy 722.72
  intestine 569.9
    functional 564.9
      congenital 751.3
      psychogenic 306.4
    lardaceous 277.3
    organic 569.9
    protozoal NEC 007.9
  iris 364.9
  iron
    metabolism 275.0
    storage 275.0
  Isambert's (*see also* Tuberculosis, larynx) 012.3
  Iselin's (osteochondrosis, fifth metatarsal) 732.5
  Island (scrub typhus) 081.2
  itai-itai 985.5
  Jadassohn's (maculopapular erythroderma)
    696.2
  Jadassohn-Pellizari's (anetoderma) 701.3
  Jakob-Creutzfeldt 046.1
    with dementia
      with behavioral disturbance 046.1 *[294.11]*
      without behavioral disturbance 046.1
        [294.10]
  Jaksch (-Luzet) (pseudoleukemia infantum)
    285.8
  Janet's 300.89
  Jansky-Bielschowsky 330.1
  jaw NEC 526.9
    fibrocystic 526.2
  Jensen's 363.05
  Jeune's (asphyxiating thoracic dystrophy) 756.4
  jigger 134.1
  Johnson-Stevens (erythema multiforme
    exudativum) 695.1
  joint NEC 719.9
    ankle 719.97
    Charcot 094.0 *[713.5]*
    degenerative (*see also* Osteoarthrosis) 715.9
      multiple 715.09
      spine (*see also* Spondylosis) 721.90
    elbow 719.92
    foot 719.97
    hand 719.94
    hip 719.95
    hypertrophic (chronic) (degenerative) (*see
      also* Osteoarthrosis) 715.9
      spine (*see also* Spondylosis) 721.90
    knee 719.96
    Luschka 721.90
    multiple sites 719.99
    pelvic region 719.95
    sacroiliac 724.6
    shoulder (region) 719.91
    specified site NEC 719.98
    spine NEC 724.9
      pseudarthrosis following fusion 733.82
      sacroiliac 724.6
    wrist 719.93
  Jourdain's (acute gingivitis) 523.0
  Jüngling's (sarcoidosis) 135
  Kahler (-Bozzolo) (multiple myeloma)
    (M9730/3) 203.0
  Kalischer's 759.6
  Kaposi's 757.33
    lichen ruber 697.8
      acuminatus 696.4

Disease, diseased—*continued*
    moniliformis 697.8
    xeroderma pigmentosum 757.33
  Kaschin-Beck (endemic polyarthritis) 716.00
    ankle 716.07
    arm 716.02
      lower (and wrist) 716.03
      upper (and elbow) 716.02
    foot (and ankle) 716.07
    forearm (and wrist) 716.03
    hand 716.04
    leg 716.06
      lower 716.06
      upper 716.05
    multiple sites 716.09
    pelvic region (hip) (thigh) 716.05
    shoulder region 716.01
    specified site NEC 716.08
  Katayama 120.2
  Kawasaki 446.1
  Kedani (scrub typhus) 081.2
  kidney (functional) (pelvis) (*see also* Disease,
    renal) 593.9
    cystic (congenital) 753.10
      multiple 753.19
      single 753.11
      specified NEC 753.19
    fibrocystic (congenital) 753.19
    in gout 274.10
    polycystic (congenital) 753.12
      adult type (APKD) 753.13
      autosomal dominant 753.13
      autosomal recessive 753.14
      childhood type (CPKD) 753.14
      infantile type 753.14
  Kienböck's (carpal lunate) (wrist) 732.3
  Kimmelstiel (-Wilson) (intercapillary
    glomerulosclerosis) 250.4 *[581.81]*
  Kinnier Wilson's (hepatolenticular
    degeneration) 275.1
  kissing 075
  Kleb's (*see also* Nephritis) 583.9
  Klinger's 446.4
  Klippel's 723.8
  Klippel-Feil (brevicollis) 756.16
  knight's 911.1
  Köbner's (epidermolysis bullosa) 757.39
  Koenig-Wichmann (pemphigus) 694.4
  Köhler's
    first (osteoarthrosis juvenilis) 732.5
    second (Freiberg's infraction, metatarsal
      head) 732.5
    patellar 732.4
    tarsal navicular (bone) (osteoarthrosis
      juvenilis) 732.5
  Köhler-Freiberg (infraction, metatarsal head)
    732.5
  Köhler-Mouchet (osteoarthrosis juvenilis) 732.5
  Köhler-Pellegrini-Stieda (calcification, knee
    joint) 726.62
  König's (osteochondritis dissecans) 732.7
  Korsakoff's (nonalcoholic) 294.0
    alcoholic 291.1
  Kostmann's (infantile genetic agranulocytosis)
    288.0
  Krabbe's 330.0
  Kraepelin-Morel (*see also* Schizophrenia) 295.9
  Kraft-Weber-Dimitri 759.6
  Kufs' 330.1
  Kugelberg-Welander 335.11
  Kuhnt-Junius 362.52

Disease, diseased—*continued*
  Kümmell's (-Verneuil) (spondylitis) 721.7
  Kundrat's (lymphosarcoma) 200.1
  kuru 046.0
  Kussmaul (-Meier) (polyarteritis nodosa) 446.0
  Kyasanur Forest 065.2
  Kyrle's (hyperkeratosis follicularis in cutem
    penetrans) 701.1
  labia
    inflammatory 616.9
      specified NEC 616.8
    noninflammatory 624.9
      specified NEC 624.8
  labyrinth, ear 386.8
  lacrimal system (apparatus) (passages) 375.9
    gland 375.00
    specified NEC 375.89
  Lafora's 333.2
  Lagleyze-von Hippel (retinocerebral
    angiomatosis) 759.6
  Lancereaux-Mathieu (leptospiral jaundice) 100.0
  Landry's 357.0
  Lane's 569.89
  lardaceous (any site) 277.3
  Larrey-Weil (leptospiral jaundice) 100.0
  Larsen (-Johansson) (juvenile osteopathia
    patellae) 732.4
  larynx 478.70
  Lasègue's (persecution mania) 297.9
  Leber's 377.16
  Lederer's (acquired infectious hemolytic
    anemia) 283.19
  Legg's (capital femoral osteochondrosis) 732.1
  Legg-Calvé-Perthes (capital femoral
    osteochondrosis) 732.1
  Legg-Calvé-Waldenström (femoral capital
    osteochondrosis) 732.1
  Legg-Perthes (femoral capital osteochondrosis)
    732.1
  Legionnaires' 482.84
  Leigh's 330.8
  Leiner's (exfoliative dermatitis) 695.89
  Leloir's (lupus erythematosus) 695.4
  Lenegre's 426.0
  lens (eye) 379.39
  Leriche's (osteoporosis, posttraumatic) 733.7
  Letterer-Siwe (acute histiocytosis X) (M9722/3)
    202.5
  Lev's (acquired complete heart block) 426.0
  Lewandowski's (*see also* Tuberculosis) 017.0
  Lewandowski-Lutz (epidermodysplasia
    verruciformis) 078.19
  Leyden's (periodic vomiting) 536.2
  Libman-Sacks (verrucous endocarditis) 710.0
    [424.91]
  Lichtheim's (subacute combined sclerosis with
    pernicious anemia) 281.0 *[336.2]*
  ligament 728.9
  light chain 203.0
  Lightwood's (renal tubular acidosis) 588.8
  Lignac's (cystinosis) 270.0
  Lindau's (retinocerebral angiomatosis) 759.6
  Lindau-von Hippel (angiomatosis
    retinocerebellosa) 759.6
  lip NEC 528.5
  lipidosis 272.7
  lipoid storage NEC 272.7
  Lipschültz's 616.50
  Little's—*see* Palsy, cerebral

Disease, diseased—*continued*
  liver 573.9
    alcoholic 571.3
      acute 571.1
      chronic 571.3
    chronic 571.9
      alcoholic 571.3
    cystic, congenital 751.62
    drug-induced 573.3
    due to
      chemicals 573.3
      fluorinated agents 573.3
      hypersensitivity drugs 573.3
      isoniazids 573.3
    fibrocystic (congenital) 751.62
    glycogen storage 271.0
    organic 573.9
    polycystic (congenital) 751.62
  Lobo's (keloid blastomycosis) 116.2
  Lobstein's (brittle bones and blue sclera) 756.61
  locomotor system 334.9
  Lorain's (pituitary dwarfism) 253.3
  Lou Gehrig's 335.20
  Lucas-Championnière (fibrinous bronchitis)
    466.0
  Ludwig's (submaxillary cellulitis) 528.3
  luetic—*see* Syphilis
  lumbosacral region 724.6
  lung NEC 518.89
    black 500
    congenital 748.60
    cystic 518.89
      congenital 748.4
    fibroid (chronic) (*see also* Fibrosis, lung) 515
    fluke 121.2
      Oriental 121.2
    in
      amyloidosis 277.3 *[517.8]*
      polymyositis 710.4 *[517.8]*
      sarcoidosis 135 *[517.8]*
      Sjögren's syndrome 710.2 *[517.8]*
      syphilis 095.1
      systemic lupus erythematosus 710.0 *[517.8]*
      systemic sclerosis 710.1 *[517.2]*
    interstitial (chronic) 515
      acute 136.3
    nonspecific, chronic 496
    obstructive (chronic) (COPD) 496
      with
        acute exacerbation NEC 491.21
        alveolitis, allergic (*see also* Alveolitis,
          allergic) 495.9
        asthma (chronic) (obstructive) 493.2
        bronchiectasis 494.0
          with acute exacerbation 494.1
        bronchitis (chronic) 491.20
          with acute exacerbation 491.21
        emphysema NEC 492.8
      diffuse (with fibrosis) 496
    polycystic 518.89
      asthma (chronic) (obstructive) 493.2
      congenital 748.4
    purulent (cavitary) 513.0
    restrictive 518.89
    rheumatoid 714.81
      diffuse interstitial 714.81
    specified NEC 518.89
  Lutembacher's (atrial septal defect with mitral
    stenosis) 745.5
  Lutz-Miescher (elastosis perforans serpiginosa)
    701.1

Disease, diseased—*continued*
Lutz-Splendore-de Almeida (Brazilian
  blastomycosis) 116.1
Lyell's (toxic epidermal necrolysis) 695.1
  due to drug
    correct substance properly administered
      695.1
    overdose or wrong substance given or taken
      977.9
    specific drug—*see* Table of drugs and
      chemicals
Lyme 088.81
lymphatic (gland) (system) 289.9
  channel (noninfective) 457.9
  vessel (noninfective) 457.9
    specified NEC 457.8
lymphoproliferative (chronic) (M9970/1) 238.7
Machado-Joseph 334.8
Madelung's (lipomatosis) 272.8
Madura (actinomycotic) 039.9
  mycotic 117.4
Magitot's 526.4
Majocchi's (purpura annularis telangiectodes)
  709.1
malarial (*see also* Malaria) 084.6
Malassez's (cystic) 608.89
Malibu 919.8
  infected 919.9
malignant (M8000/3)—*see also* Neoplasm, by
  site, malignant
  previous, affecting management of pregnancy
    V23.8
Manson's 120.1
maple bark 495.6
maple syrup (urine) 270.3
Marburg (virus) 078.89
Marchiafava (-Bignami) 341.8
Marfan's 090.49
  congenital syphilis 090.49
  meaning Marfan's syndrome 759.82
Marie-Bamberger (hypertrophic pulmonary
  osteoarthropathy) (secondary) 731.2
  primary or idiopathic (acropachyderma)
    757.39
  pulmonary (hypertrophic osteoarthropathy)
    731.2
Marie-Strümpell (ankylosing spondylitis) 720.0
Marion's (bladder neck obstruction) 596.0
Marsh's (exophthalmic goiter) 242.0
Martin's 715.27
mast cell 757.33
  systemic (M9741/3) 202.6
mastoid (*see also* Mastoiditis) 383.9
  process 385.9
maternal, unrelated to pregnancy NEC,
  affecting fetus or newborn 760.9
Mathieu's (leptospiral jaundice) 100.0
Mauclaire's 732.3
Mauriac's (erythema nodosum syphiliticum)
  091.3
Maxcy's 081.0
McArdle (-Schmid-Pearson) (glycogenosis V)
  271.0
mediastinum NEC 519.3
Medin's (*see also* Poliomyelitis) 045.9
Mediterranean (with hemoglobinopathy) 282.4
medullary center (idiopathic) (respiratory) 348.8
Meige's (chronic hereditary edema) 757.0
Meleda 757.39
Ménétrier's (hypertrophic gastritis) 535.2

Disease, diseased—*continued*
Ménière's (active) 386.00
  cochlear 386.02
  cochleovestibular 386.01
  inactive 386.04
  in remission 386.04
  vestibular 386.03
meningeal—*see* Meningitis
mental (*see also* Psychosis) 298.9
Merzbacher-Pelizaeus 330.0
mesenchymal 710.9
mesenteric embolic 557.0
metabolic NEC 277.9
metal polishers' 502
metastatic—*see* Metastasis
Mibelli's 757.39
microdrepanocytic 282.4
Miescher's 709.3
Mikulicz's (dryness of mouth, absent or
  decreased lacrimation) 527.1
Milkman (-Looser) (osteomalacia with
  pseudofractures) 268.2
Miller's (osteomalacia) 268.2
Mills' 335.29
Milroy's (chronic hereditary edema) 757.0
Minamata 985.0
Minor's 336.1
Minot's (hemorrhagic disease, newborn) 776.0
Minot-von Willebrand-Jürgens
  (angiohemophilia) 286.4
Mitchell's (erythromelalgia) 443.89
mitral—*see* Endocarditis, mitral
Mljet (mal de Meleda) 757.39
Möbius', Moebius' 346.8
Moeller's 267
Möller (-Barlow) (infantile scurvy) 267
Mönckeberg's (*see also* arteriosclerosis,
  extremities) 440.20
Mondor's (thrombophlebitis of breast) 451.89
Monge's 993.2
Morel-Kraepelin (*see also* Schizophrenia) 295.9
Morgagni's (syndrome) (hyperostosis frontalis
  interna) 733.3
Morgagni-Adams-Stokes (syncope with heart
  block) 426.9
Morquio (-Brailsford) (-Ullrich)
  (mucopolysaccharidosis IV) 277.5
Morton's (with metatarsalgia) 355.6
Morvan's 336.0
motor neuron (bulbar) (mixed type) 335.20
Mouchet's (juvenile osteochondrosis, foot)
  732.5
mouth 528.9
Moyamoya 437.5
Mucha's (acute parapsoriasis varioliformis)
  696.2
mu-chain 273.2
mucolipidosis (I) (II) (III) 272.7
Münchmeyer's (exostosis luxurians) 728.11
Murri's (intermittent hemoglobinuria) 283.2
muscle 359.9
  inflammatory 728.9
  ocular 378.9
musculoskeletal system 729.9
mushroom workers' 495.5
Myà's (congenital dilation, colon) 751.3
  mycotic 117.9
myeloproliferative (chronic) (M9960/1) 238.7
myocardium, myocardial (*see also*
  Degeneration, myocardial) 429.1

Disease, diseased—*continued*
  hypertensive (*see also* Hypertension, heart)
      402.90
    primary (idiopathic) 425.4
  myoneural 358.9
  Naegeli's 287.1
  nail 703.9
    specified type NEC 703.8
  Nairobi sheep 066.1
  nasal 478.1
    cavity NEC 478.1
    sinus (chronic)—*see* Sinusitis
  navel (newborn) NEC 779.89
  nemaline body 359.0
  neoplastic, generalized (M8000/6) 199.0
  nerve—*see* Disorder, nerve
  nervous system (central) 349.9
    autonomic, peripheral (*see also* Neuropathy,
        peripheral, autonomic) 337.9
    congenital 742.9
    inflammatory—*see* Encephalitis
    parasympathetic (*see also* Neuropathy,
        peripheral, autonomic) 337.9
    peripheral NEC 355.9
    specified NEC 349.89
    sympathetic (*see also* Neuropathy, peripheral,
        autonomic) 337.9
    vegetative (*see also* Neuropathy, peripheral,
        autonomic) 337.9
  Nettleship's (urticaria pigmentosa) 757.33
  Neumann's (pemphigus vegetans) 694.4
  neurologic (central) NEC (*see also* Disease,
      nervous system) 349.9
    peripheral NEC 355.9
  neuromuscular system NEC 358.9
  Newcastle 077.8
  Nicolas (-Durand) -Favre (climatic bubo) 099.1
  Niemann-Pick (lipid histiocytosis) 272.7
  nipple 611.9
    Paget's (M8540/3) 174.0
  Nishimoto (-Takeuchi) 437.5
  nonarthropod-borne NEC 078.89
    central nervous system NEC 049.9
    enterovirus NEC 078.89
  non-autoimmune hemolytic NEC 283.10
  Nonne-Milroy-Meige (chronic hereditary
      edema) 757.0
  Norrie's (congenital progressive
      oculoacousticocerebral degeneration) 743.8
  nose 478.1
  nucleus pulposus—*see* Disease, intervertebral
      disc
  nutritional 269.9
    maternal, affecting fetus or newborn 760.4
  oasthouse, urine 270.2
  obliterative vascular 447.1
  Odelberg's (juvenile osteochondrosis) 732.1
  Oguchi's (retina) 368.61
  Ohara's (*see also* Tularemia) 021.9
  Ollier's (chondrodysplasia) 756.4
  Opitz's (congestive splenomegaly) 289.51
  Oppenheim's 358.8
  Oppenheim-Urbach (necrobiosis lipoidica
      diabeticorum) 250.8 *[709.3]*
  optic nerve NEC 377.49
  orbit 376.9
    specified NEC 376.89
  Oriental liver fluke 121.1
  Oriental lung fluke 121.2
  Ormond's 593.4
  Osgood's tibia (tubercle) 732.4

Disease, diseased—*continued*
  Osgood-Schlatter 732.4
  Osler (-Vaquez) (polycythemia vera) (M9950/1)
      238.4
  Osler-Rendu (familial hemorrhagic
      telangiectasia) 448.0
  osteofibrocystic 252.0
  Otto's 715.35
  outer ear 380.9
  ovary (noninflammatory) NEC 620.9
    cystic 620.2
    polycystic 256.4
    specified NEC 620.8
  Owren's (congenital) (*see also* Defect,
      coagulation) 286.3
  Paas' 756.59
  Paget's (osteitis deformans) 731.0
    with infiltrating duct carcinoma of the breast
        (M8541/3)—*see* Neoplasm, breast,
        malignant
    bone 731.0
      osteosarcoma in (M9184/3)—*see*
          Neoplasm, bone, malignant
    breast (M8540/3) 174.0
    extramammary (M8542/3)—*see also*
        Neoplasm, skin, malignant
      anus 154.3
      skin 173.5
    malignant (M8540/3)
      breast 174.0
      specified site NEC (M8542/3)—*see*
          Neoplasm, skin, malignant
      unspecified site 174.0
    mammary (M8540/3) 174.0
    nipple (M8540/3) 174.0
  palate (soft) 528.9
  Paltauf-Sternberg 201.9
  pancreas 577.9
    cystic 577.2
      congenital 751.7
    fibrocystic 277.00
  Panner's 732.3
    capitellum humeri 732.3
    head of humerus 732.3
    tarsal navicular (bone) (osteochondrosis) 732.5
  panvalvular—*see* Endocarditis, mitral
  parametrium 629.9
  parasitic NEC 136.9
    cerebral NEC 123.9
    intestinal NEC 129
    mouth 112.0
    skin NEC 134.9
    specified type—*see* Infestation
    tongue 112.0
  parathyroid (gland) 252.9
    specified NEC 252.8
  Parkinson's 332.0
  parodontal 523.9
  Parrot's (syphilitic osteochondritis) 090.0
  Parry's (exophthalmic goiter) 242.0
  Parson's (exophthalmic goiter) 242.0
  Pavy's 593.6
  Paxton's (white piedra) 111.2
  Payr's (splenic flexure syndrome) 569.89
  pearl-workers' (chronic osteomyelitis) (*see also*
      Osteomyelitis) 730.1
  Pel-Ebstein—*see* Disease, Hodgkin's

Disease, diseased—*continued*
  Pelizaeus-Merzbacher 330.0
    with dementia
      with behavioral disturbance 330.0 *[294.11]*
      without behavioral disturbance 330.0
        [294.10]
  Pellegrini-Stieda (calcification, knee joint)
    726.62
  pelvis, pelvic
    female NEC 629.9
      specified NEC 629.8
    gonococcal (acute) 098.19
      chronic or duration of 2 months or over
        098.39
    infection (*see also* Disease, pelvis,
      inflammatory) 614.9
    inflammatory (female) (PID) 614.9
      with
        abortion—*see* Abortion, by type, with
          sepsis
        ectopic pregnancy (*see also* categories
          633.0-633.9) 639.0
        molar pregnancy (*see also* categories
          630-632) 639.0
      acute 614.3
      chronic 614.4
      complicating pregnancy 646.6
        affecting fetus or newborn 760.8
      following
        abortion 639.0
        ectopic or molar pregnancy 639.0
      peritonitis (acute) 614.5
        chronic NEC 614.7
      puerperal, postpartum, childbirth 670
      specified NEC 614.8
    organ, female NEC 629.9
      specified NEC 629.8
    peritoneum, female NEC 629.9
      specified NEC 629.8
  penis 607.9
    inflammatory 607.2
  peptic NEC 536.9
    acid 536.8
  periapical tissues NEC 522.9
  pericardium 423.9
    specified type NEC 423.8
  perineum
    female
      inflammatory 616.9
        specified NEC 616.8
      noninflammatory 624.9
        specified NEC 624.8
    male (inflammatory) 682.2
  periodic (familial) (Reimann's) NEC 277.3
    paralysis 359.3
  periodontal NEC 523.9
    specified NEC 523.8
  periosteum 733.90
  peripheral
    arterial 443.9
    autonomic nervous system (*see also*
      Neuropathy, autonomic) 337.9
    nerve NEC (*see also* Neuropathy) 356.9
      multiple—*see* Polyneuropathy
    vascular 443.9
      specified type NEC 443.89
  peritoneum 568.9
    pelvic, female 629.9
      specified NEC 629.8
  Perrin-Ferraton (snapping hip) 719.65

Disease, diseased—*continued*
  persistent mucosal (middle ear) (with posterior
    or superior marginal perforation of ear
    drum) 382.2
  Perthes' (capital femoral osteochondrosis) 732.1
  Petit's (*see also* Hernia, lumbar) 553.8
  Peutz-Jeghers 759.6
  Peyronie's 607.89
  Pfeiffer's (infectious mononucleosis) 075
  pharynx 478.20
  Phocas' 610.1
  photochromogenic (acid-fast bacilli)
    (pulmonary) 031.0
    nonpulmonary 031.9
  Pick's
    brain 331.1
      with dementia
        with behavioral disturbance 331.1 *[294.11]*
        without behavioral disturbance 331.1
          [294.10]
    cerebral atrophy 331.1
      with dementia
        with behavioral disturbance 331.1 *[294.11]*
        without behavioral disturbance 331.1
          [294.10]
    lipid histiocytosis 272.7
    liver (pericardial pseudocirrhosis of liver)
      423.2
    pericardium (pericardial pseudocirrhosis of
      liver) 423.2
    polyserositis (pericardial pseudocirrhosis of
      liver) 423.2
  Pierson's (osteochondrosis) 732.1
  pigeon fancier's or breeders' 495.2
  pineal gland 259.8
  pink 985.0
  Pinkus' (lichen nitidus) 697.1
  pinworm 127.4
  pituitary (gland) 253.9
    hyperfunction 253.1
    hypofunction 253.2
  pituitary snuff-takers' 495.8
  placenta
    affecting fetus or newborn 762.2
    complicating pregnancy or childbirth 656.7
  pleura (cavity) (*see also* Pleurisy) 511.0
  Plummer's (toxic nodular goiter) 242.3
  pneumatic
    drill 994.9
    hammer 994.9
  policeman's 729.2
  Pollitzer's (hidradenitis suppurativa) 705.83
  polycystic (congenital) 759.89
    kidney or renal 753.12
      adult type (APKD) 753.13
      autosomal dominant 753.13
      autosomal recessive 753.14
      childhood type (CPKD) 753.14
      infantile type 753.14
    liver or hepatic 751.62
    lung or pulmonary 518.89
      congenital 748.4
    ovary, ovaries 256.4
    spleen 759.0
  Pompe's (glycogenosis II) 271.0
  Poncet's (tuberculous rheumatism) (*see also*
    Tuberculosis) 015.9
  Posada-Wernicke 114.9
  Potain's (pulmonary edema) 514

Disease, diseased—*continued*
    upper (acute) (infectious) NEC 465.9
        multiple sites NEC 465.8
        noninfectious NEC 478.9
        streptococcal 034.0
    retina, retinal NEC 362.9
        Batten's or Batten-Mayou 330.1 *[362.71]*
        degeneration 362.89
        vascular lesion 362.17
    rheumatic (*see also* Arthritis) 716.8
        heart—*see* Disease, heart, rheumatic
    rheumatoid (heart)—*see* Arthritis, rheumatoid
    rickettsial NEC 083.9
        specified type NEC 083.8
    Riedel's (ligneous thyroiditis) 245.3
    Riga (-Fede) (cachectic aphthae) 529.0
    Riggs' (compound periodontitis) 523.4
    Ritter's 695.81
    Rivalta's (cervicofacial actinomycosis) 039.3
    Robles' (onchocerciasis) 125.3 *[360.13]*
    Roger's (congenital interventricular septal
        defect) 745.4
    Rokitansky's (*see also* Necrosis, liver) 570
    Romberg's 349.89
    Rosenthal's (factor XI deficiency) 286.2
    Rossbach's (hyperchlorhydria) 536.8
        psychogenic 306.4
    Roth (-Bernhardt) 355.1
    Runeberg's (progressive pernicious anemia)
        281.0
    Rust's (tuberculous spondylitis) (*see also*
        Tuberculosis) 015.0 *[720.81]*
    Rustitskii's (multiple myeloma) (M9730/3)
        203.0
    Ruysch's (Hirschsprung's disease) 751.3
    Sachs (-Tay) 330.1
    sacroiliac NEC 724.6
    salivary gland or duct NEC 527.9
        inclusion 078.5
            streptococcal 034.0
        virus 078.5
    Sander's (paranoia) 297.1
    Sandhoff's 330.1
    sandworm 126.9
    Savill's (epidemic exfoliative dermatitis) 695.89
    Schamberg's (progressive pigmentary
        dermatosis) 709.09
    Schaumann's (sarcoidosis) 135
    Schenck's (sporotrichosis) 117.1
    Scheuermann's (osteochondrosis) 732.0
    Schilder (-Flatau) 341.1
    Schimmelbusch's 610.1
    Schlatter's tibia (tubercle) 732.4
    Schlatter-Osgood 732.4
    Schmorl's 722.30
        cervical 722.39
        lumbar, lumbosacral 722.32
        specified region NEC 722.39
        thoracic, thoracolumbar 722.31
    Scholz's 330.0
    Schönlein (-Henoch) (purpura rheumatica) 287.0
    Schottmüller's (*see also* Fever, paratyphoid)
        002.9
    Schüller-Christian (chronic histiocytosis X)
        277.8
    Schultz's (agranulocytosis) 288.0
    Schwalbe-Ziehen-Oppenheimer 333.6
    Schweninger-Buzzi (macular atrophy) 701.3
    sclera 379.19
    scrofulous (*see also* Tuberculosis) 017.2
    scrotum 608.9

Disease, diseased—*continued*
    sebaceous glands NEC 706.9
    Secretan's (posttraumatic edema) 782.3
    semilunar cartilage, cystic 717.5
    seminal vesicle 608.9
    Senear-Usher (pemphigus erythematosus) 694.4
    serum NEC 999.5
    Sever's (osteochondrosis calcaneum) 732.5
    Sézary's (reticulosis) (M9701/3) 202.2
    Shaver's (bauxite pneumoconiosis) 503
    Sheehan's (postpartum pituitary necrosis) 253.2
    shimamushi (scrub typhus) 081.2
    shipyard 077.1
    sickle-cell 282.60
        with
            crisis 282.62
            Hb-S disease 282.61
            other abnormal hemoglobin (Hb-D) (Hb-E)
                (Hb-G) (Hb-J) (Hb-K) (Hb-O) (Hb-P)
                (high fetal gene) 282.69
        elliptocytosis 282.60
        Hb-C 282.63
        Hb-S 282.61
            with
                crisis 282.62
                Hb-C 282.63
                other abnormal hemoglobin (Hb-D)
                    (Hb-E) (Hb-G) (Hb-J) (Hb-K) (Hb-O)
                    (Hb-P) (high fetal gene) 282.69
        spherocytosis 282.60
        thalassemia 282.4
    Siegal-Cattan-Mamou (periodic) 277.3
    silo fillers' 506.9
    Simian B 054.3
    Simmonds' (pituitary cachexia) 253.2
    Simons' (progressive lipodystrophy) 272.6
    Sinding-Larsen (juvenile osteopathia patellae)
        732.4
    sinus—*see also* Sinusitis
        brain 437.9
        specified NEC 478.1
    Sirkari's 085.0
    sixth 057.8
    Sjögren (-Gougerot) 710.2
        with lung involvement 710.2 *[517.8]*
    Skevas-Zerfus 989.5
    skin NEC 709.9
        due to metabolic disorder 277.9
        specified type NEC 709.8
    sleeping 347
        meaning sleeping sickness (*see also*
            Trypanosomiasis) 086.5
    small vessel 443.9
    Smith-Strang (oasthouse urine) 270.2
    Sneddon-Wilkinson (subcorneal pustular
        dermatosis) 694.1
    South African creeping 133.8
    Spencer's (epidemic vomiting) 078.82
    Spielmeyer-Stock 330.1
    Spielmeyer-Vogt 330.1
    spine, spinal 733.90
        combined system (*see also* Degeneration,
            combined) 266.2 *[336.2]*
            with pernicious anemia 281.0 *[336.2]*
        cord NEC 336.9
        congenital 742.9
        demyelinating NEC 341.8
        joint (*see also* Disease, joint, spine) 724.9
        tuberculous 015.0 *[730.8]*
    spinocerebellar 334.9
        specified NEC 334.8

Disease, diseased—*continued*
  spleen (organic) (postinfectional) 289.50
    amyloid 277.3
    lardaceous 277.3
    polycystic 759.0
    specified NEC 289.59
  sponge divers' 989.5
  Stanton's (melioidosis) 025
  Stargardt's 362.75
  Steinert's 359.2
  Sternberg's—*see* Disease, Hodgkin's
  Stevens-Johnson (erythema multiforme
    exudativum) 695.1
  Sticker's (erythema infectiosum) 057.0
  Stieda's (calcification, knee joint) 726.62
  Still's (juvenile rheumatoid arthritis) 714.30
  Stiller's (asthenia) 780.79
  Stokes' (exophthalmic goiter) 242.0
  Stokes-Adams (syncope with heart block) 426.9
  Stokvis (-Talma) (enterogenous cyanosis) 289.7
  stomach NEC (organic) 537.9
    functional 536.9
      psychogenic 306.4
    lardaceous 277.3
  stonemasons' 502
  storage
    glycogen (*see also* Disease, glycogen storage)
      271.0
    lipid 272.7
    mucopolysaccharide 277.5
  striatopallidal system 333.90
    specified NEC 333.89
  Strümpell-Marie (ankylosing spondylitis) 720.0
  Stuart's (congenital factor X deficiency) (*see*
    also Defect, coagulation) 286.3
  Stuart-Prower (congenital factor X deficiency)
    (*see also* Defect, coagulation) 286.3
  Sturge (-Weber) (-Dimitri) (encephalocutaneous
    angiomatosis) 759.6
  Stuttgart 100.89
  Sudeck's 733.7
  supporting structures of teeth NEC 525.9
  suprarenal (gland) (capsule) 255.9
    hyperfunction 255.3
    hypofunction 255.4
  Sutton's 709.09
  Sutton and Gull's—*see* Hypertension, kidney
  sweat glands NEC 705.9
    specified type NEC 705.89
  sweating 078.2
  Sweeley-Klionsky 272.4
  Swift (-Feer) 985.0
  swimming pool (bacillus) 031.1
  swineherd's 100.89
  Sylvest's (epidemic pleurodynia) 074.1
  Symmers (follicular lymphoma) (M9690/3)
    202.0
  sympathetic nervous system (*see also*
    Neuropathy, peripheral, autonomic) 337.9
  synovium 727.9
  syphilitic—*see* Syphilis
  systemic tissue mast cell (M9741/3) 202.6
  Taenzer's 757.4
  Takayasu's (pulseless) 446.7
  Talma's 728.85
  Tangier (familial high-density lipoprotein
    deficiency) 272.5
  Tarral-Besnier (pityriasis rubra pilaris) 696.4
  Tay-Sachs 330.1
  Taylor's 701.8
  tear duct 375.69

Disease, diseased—*continued*
  teeth, tooth 525.9
    hard tissues NEC 521.9
    pulp NEC 522.9
  tendon 727.9
    inflammatory NEC 727.9
  terminal vessel 443.9
  testis 608.9
  Thaysen-Gee (nontropical sprue) 579.0
  Thomsen's 359.2
  Thomson's (congenital poikiloderma) 757.33
  Thornwaldt's, Tornwaldt's (pharyngeal bursitis)
    478.29
  throat 478.20
    septic 034.0
  thromboembolic (*see also* Embolism) 444.9
  thymus (gland) 254.9
    specified NEC 254.8
  thyroid (gland) NEC 246.9
    heart (*see also* Hyperthyroidism) 242.9 *[425.7]*
    lardaceous 277.3
    specified NEC 246.8
  Tietze's 733.6
  Tommaselli's
    correct substance properly administered 599.7
    overdose or wrong substance given or taken
      961.4
  tongue 529.9
  tonsils, tonsillar (and adenoids) (chronic) 474.9
    specified NEC 474.8
  tooth, teeth 525.9
    hard tissues NEC 521.9
    pulp NEC 522.9
  Tornwaldt's (pharyngeal bursitis) 478.29
  Tourette's 307.23
  trachea 519.1
  tricuspid—*see* Endocarditis, tricuspid
  triglyceride-storage, type I, II, III 272.7
  triple vessel (coronary arteries) —*see*
    Arteriosclerosis, coronary
  trisymptomatic, Gougerot's 709.1
  trophoblastic (*see also* Hydatidiform mole) 630
    previous, affecting management of pregnancy
      V23.1
  tsutsugamushi (scrub typhus) 081.2
  tube (fallopian), noninflammatory 620.9
    specified NEC 620.8
  tuberculous NEC (*see also* Tuberculosis) 011.9
  tubo-ovarian
    inflammatory (*see also* Salpingo-oophoritis)
      614.2
    noninflammatory 620.9
      specified NEC 620.8
  tubotympanic, chronic (with anterior perforation
    of ear drum) 382.1
  tympanum 385.9
  Uhl's 746.84
  umbilicus (newborn) NEC 779.89
  Underwood's (sclerema neonatorum) 778.1
  undiagnosed 799.9
  Unna's (seborrheic dermatitis) 690.18
  unstable hemoglobin hemolytic 282.7
  Unverricht (-Lundborg) 333.2
  Urbach-Oppenheim (necrobiosis lipoidica
    diabeticorum) 250.8 *[709.3]*
  Urbach-Wiethe (lipoid proteinosis) 272.8
  ureter 593.9
  urethra 599.9
    specified type NEC 599.84
  urinary (tract) 599.9
    bladder 596.9

Disease, diseased—*continued*
  specified NEC 596.8
  maternal, affecting fetus or newborn 760.1
Usher-Senear (pemphigus erythematosus) 694.4
uterus (organic) 621.9
  infective (*see also* Endometritis) 615.9
  inflammatory (*see also* Endometritis) 615.9
  noninflammatory 621.9
    specified type NEC 621.8
uveal tract
  anterior 364.9
  posterior 363.9
vagabonds' 132.1
vagina, vaginal
  inflammatory 616.9
    specified NEC 616.8
  noninflammatory 623.9
    specified NEC 623.8
Valsuani's (progressive pernicious anemia, puerperal) 648.2
  complicating pregnancy or puerperium 648.2
valve, valvular—*see* Endocarditis
van Bogaert-Nijssen (-Peiffer) 330.0
van Creveld-von Gierke (glycogenosis I) 271.0
van den Bergh's (enterogenous cyanosis) 289.7
van Neck's (juvenile osteochondrosis) 732.1
Vaquez (-Osler) (polycythemia vera) (M9950/1) 238.4
vascular 459.9
  arteriosclerotic—*see* Arteriosclerosis
  hypertensive—*see* Hypertension
  obliterative 447.1
    peripheral 443.9
  occlusive 459.9
  peripheral (occlusive) 443.9
    in diabetes mellitus 250.7 *[443.81]*
    specified type NEC 443.89
vas deferens 608.9
vasomotor 443.9
vasospastic 443.9
vein 459.9
venereal 099.9
  fifth 099.1
  sixth 099.1
  chlamydial NEC 099.50
    anus 099.52
    bladder 099.53
    cervix 099.53
    epididymis 099.54
    genitourinary NEC 099.55
      lower 099.53
        specified NEC 099.54
    pelvic inflammatory disease 099.54
    perihepatic 099.56
    peritoneum 099.56
    pharynx 099.51
    rectum 099.52
    specified site NEC 099.59
    testis 099.54
    vagina 099.53
    vulva 099.53
  complicating pregnancy, childbirth, or puerperium 647.2
  specified nature or type NEC 099.8
    chlamydial—*see* Disease, venereal, chlamydial
Verneuil's (syphilitic bursitis) 095.7
Verse's (calcinosis intervertebralis) 275.49 *[722.90]*
vertebra, vertebral NEC 733.90
  disc—*see* Disease, Intervertebral disc

Disease, diseased—*continued*
vibration NEC 994.9
Vidal's (lichen simplex chronicus) 698.3
Vincent's (trench mouth) 101
Virchow's 733.99
virus (filterable) NEC 078.89
  arbovirus NEC 066.9
  arthropod-borne NEC 066.9
  central nervous system NEC 049.9
    specified type NEC 049.8
  complicating pregnancy, childbirth, or puerperium 647.6
  contact (with) V01.7
  exposure to V01.7
  Marburg 078.89
  maternal
    with fetal damage affecting management of pregnancy 655.3
  nonarthropod-borne NEC 078.89
    central nervous system NEC 049.9
      specified NEC 049.8
vitreous 379.29
vocal cords NEC 478.5
Vogt's (Cecile) 333.7
Vogt-Spielmeyer 330.1
Volhard-Fahr (malignant nephrosclerosis) 403.00
Volkmann's
  acquired 958.6
von Bechterew's (ankylosing spondylitis) 720.0
von Economo's (encephalitis lethargica) 049.8
von Eulenburg's (congenital paramyotonia) 359.2
von Gierke's (glycogenosis I) 271.0
von Graefe's 378.72
von Hippel's (retinocerebral angiomatosis) 759.6
von Hippel-Lindau (angiomatosis retinocerebellosa) 759.6
von Jaksch's (pseudoleukemia infantum) 285.8
von Recklinghausen's (M9540/1) 237.71
  bone (osteitis fibrosa cystica) 252.0
von Recklinghausen-Applebaum (hemochromatosis) 275.0
von Willebrand (-Jürgens) (angiohemophilia) 286.4
von Zambusch's (lichen sclerosus et atrophicus) 701.0
Voorhoeve's (dyschondroplasia) 756.4
Vrolik's (osteogenesis imperfecta) 756.51
vulva
  noninflammatory 624.9
    specified NEC 624.8
Wagner's (colloid milium) 709.3
Waldenström's (osteochondrosis capital femoral) 732.1
Wallgren's (obstruction of splenic vein with collateral circulation) 459.89
Wardrop's (with lymphangitis) 681.9
  finger 681.02
  toe 681.11
Wassilieff's (leptospiral jaundice) 100.0
wasting NEC 799.4
  due to malnutrition 261
  paralysis 335.21
Waterhouse-Friderichsen 036.3
waxy (any site) 277.3
Weber-Christian (nodular nonsuppurative panniculitis) 729.30
Wegner's (syphilitic osteochondritis) 090.0
Weil's (leptospiral jaundice) 100.0
  of lung 100.0

Disease, diseased—*continued*

Weir Mitchell's (erythromelalgia) 443.89
Werdnig-Hoffmann 335.0
Werlhof's (*see also* Purpura, thrombocytopenic)
    287.3
Wermer's 258.0
Werner's (progeria adultorum) 259.8
Werner-His (trench fever) 083.1
Werner-Schultz (agranulocytosis) 288.0
Wernicke's (superior hemorrhagic
    polioencephalitis) 265.1
Wernicke-Posadas 114.9
Whipple's (intestinal lipodystrophy) 040.2
whipworm 127.3
white
  blood cell 288.9
    specified NEC 288.8
  spot 701.0
White's (congenital) (keratosis follicularis)
    757.39
Whitmore's (melioidosis) 025
Widal-Abrami (acquired hemolytic jaundice)
    283.9
Wilkie's 557.1
Wilkinson-Sneddon (subcorneal pustular
    dermatosis) 694.1
Willis' (diabetes mellitus) (*see also* Diabetes)
    250.0
Wilson's (hepatolenticular degeneration) 275.1
Wilson-Brocq (dermatitis exfoliativa) 695.89
winter vomiting 078.82
Wise's 696.2
Wohlfart-Kugelberg-Welander 335.11
Woillez's (acute idiopathic pulmonary
    congestion) 518.5
Wolman's (primary familial xanthomatosis)
    272.7
wool-sorters' 022.1
Zagari's (xerostomia) 527.7
Zahorsky's (exanthem subitum) 057.8
Ziehen-Oppenheim 333.6
zoonotic, bacterial NEC 027.9
  specified type NEC 027.8
Disfigurement (due to scar) 709.2
  head V48.6
  limb V49.4
  neck V48.7
  trunk V48.7
Disgerminoma —*see* Dysgerminoma
Disinsertion, retina 361.04
Disintegration, complete, of the body 799.8
  traumatic 869.1
Disk kidney 753.3
Dislocatable hip, congenita l (*see also*
    Dislocation, hip, congenital) 754.30
Dislocation (articulation) (closed) (displacement)
    (simple) (subluxation) 839.8

---

*Note—"Closed" includes simple, complete,
partial, uncomplicated, and unspecified
dislocation. "Open" includes dislocation
specified as infected or compound and
dislocation with foreign body. "Chronic,"
"habitual," "old," or "recurrent" dislocations
should be coded as indicated under the entry
"Dislocation, recurrent"; and "pathological"
as indicated under the entry "Dislocation,
pathological." For late effect of dislocation see
Late, effect, dislocation.*

---

  with fracture—*see* Fracture, by site

Dislocation—*continued*

acromioclavicular (joint) (closed) 831.04
  open 831.14
anatomical site (closed)
  specified NEC 839.69
    open 839.79
  unspecified or ill-defined 839.8
    open 839.9
ankle (scaphoid bone) (closed) 837.0
  open 837.1
arm (closed) 839.8
  open 839.9
astragalus (closed) 837.0
  open 837.1
atlanto-axial (closed) 839.01
  open 839.11
atlas (closed) 839.01
  open 839.11
axis (closed) 839.02
  open 839.12
back (closed) 839.8
  open 839.9
Bell-Daly 723.8
breast bone (closed) 839.61
  open 839.71
capsule, joint—*see* Dislocation, by site
carpal (bone)—*see* Dislocation, wrist
carpometacarpal (joint) (closed) 833.04
  open 833.14
cartilage (joint)—*see also* Dislocation, by site
  knee—*see* Tear, meniscus
cervical, cervicodorsal, or cervicothoracic
    (spine) (vertebra)—*see* Dislocation,
    vertebra, cervical
chiropractic (*see also* Lesion, nonallopathic)
    739.9
chondrocostal—*see* Dislocation, costochondral
chronic—*see* Dislocation, recurrent
clavicle (closed) 831.04
  open 831.14
coccyx (closed) 839.41
  open 839.51
collar bone (closed) 831.04
  open 831.14
compound (open) NEC 839.9
congenital NEC 755.8
  hip (*see also* Dislocation, hip, congenital)
    754.30
  lens 743.37
  rib 756.3
  sacroiliac 755.69
  spine NEC 756.19
  vertebra 756.19
coracoid (closed) 831.09
  open 831.19
costal cartilage (closed) 839.69
  open 839.79
costochondral (closed) 839.69
  open 839.79
cricoarytenoid articulation (closed) 839.69
  open 839.79
cricothyroid (cartilage) articulation (closed)
    839.69
  open 839.79
dorsal vertebrae (closed) 839.21
  open 839.31
ear ossicle 385.23
elbow (closed) 832.00
  anterior (closed) 832.01
    open 832.11
  congenital 754.89

Dislocation—*continued*
    divergent (closed) 832.09
        open 832.19
    lateral (closed) 832.04
        open 832.14
    medial (closed) 832.03
        open 832.13
    open 832.10
    posterior (closed) 832.02
        open 832.12
    recurrent 718.32
    specified type NEC 832.09
        open 832.19
    eye 360.81
        lateral 376.36
    eyeball 360.81
        lateral 376.36
    femur
        distal end (closed) 836.50
            anterior 836.52
                open 836.62
            lateral 836.53
                open 836.63
            medial 836.54
                open 836.64
            open 836.60
            posterior 836.51
                open 836.61
        proximal end (closed) 835.00
            anterior (pubic) 835.03
                open 835.13
            obturator 835.02
                open 835.12
            open 835.10
            posterior 835.01
                open 835.11
    fibula
        distal end (closed) 837.0
            open 837.1
        proximal end (closed) 836.59
            open 836.69
    finger(s) (phalanx) (thumb) (closed) 834.00
        interphalangeal (joint) 834.02
            open 834.12
        metacarpal (bone), distal end 834.01
            open 834.11
        metacarpophalangeal (joint) 834.01
            open 834.11
        open 834.10
        recurrent 718.34
    foot (closed) 838.00
        open 838.10
        recurrent 718.37
    forearm (closed) 839.8
        open 839.9
    fracture—*see* Fracture, by site
    glenoid (closed) 831.09
        open 831.19
    habitual—*see* Dislocation, recurrent
    hand (closed) 839.8
        open 839.9
    hip (closed) 835.00
        anterior 835.03
            obturator 835.02
                open 835.12
            open 835.13
        congenital (unilateral) 754.30
            with subluxation of other hip 754.35
            bilateral 754.31
        developmental 718.75
        open 835.10

Dislocation—*continued*
    posterior 835.01
        open 835.11
        recurrent 718.35
    humerus (closed) 831.00
        distal end (*see also* Dislocation, elbow) 832.00
        open 831.10
        proximal end (closed) 831.00
            anterior (subclavicular) (subcoracoid)
                (subglenoid) (closed) 831.01
                open 831.11
            inferior (closed) 831.03
                open 831.13
            open 831.10
            posterior (closed) 831.02
                open 831.12
    implant—*see* Complications, mechanical
    incus 385.23
    infracoracoid (closed) 831.01
        open 831.11
    innominate (pubic junction) (sacral junction)
            (closed) 839.69
        acetabulum (*see also* Dislocation, hip) 835.00
        open 839.79
    interphalangeal (joint)
        finger or hand (closed) 834.02
            open 834.12
        foot or toe (closed) 838.06
            open 838.16
    jaw (cartilage) (meniscus) (closed) 830.0
        open 830.1
        recurrent 524.69
    joint NEC (closed) 839.8
        developmental 718.7
        open 839.9
        pathological—*see* Dislocation, pathological
        recurrent—*see* Dislocation, recurrent
    knee (closed) 836.50
        anterior 836.51
            open 836.61
        congenital (with genu recurvatum) 754.41
        habitual 718.36
        lateral 836.54
            open 836.64
        medial 836.53
            open 836.63
        old 718.36
        open 836.60
        posterior 836.52
            open 836.62
        recurrent 718.36
        rotatory 836.59
            open 836.69
    lacrimal gland 375.16
    leg (closed) 839.8
        open 839.9
    lens (crystalline) (complete) (partial) 379.32
        anterior 379.33
        congenital 743.37
        ocular implant 996.53
        posterior 379.34
        traumatic 921.3
    ligament—*see* Dislocation, by site
    lumbar (vertebrae) (closed) 839.20
        open 839.30
    lumbosacral (vertebrae) (closed) 839.20
        congenital 756.19
        open 839.30
    mandible (closed) 830.0
        open 830.1
    maxilla (inferior) (closed) 830.0

Dislocation—*continued*
 open 830.1
 meniscus (knee)—*see also* Tear, meniscus
  other sites—*see* Dislocation, by site
 metacarpal (bone)
  distal end (closed) 834.01
   open 834.11
  proximal end (closed) 833.05
   open 833.15
 metacarpophalangeal (joint) (closed) 834.01
  open 834.11
 metatarsal (bone) (closed) 838.04
  open 838.14
 metatarsophalangeal (joint) (closed) 838.05
  open 838.15
 midcarpal (joint) (closed) 833.03
  open 833.13
 midtarsal (joint) (closed) 838.02
  open 838.12
 Monteggia's—*see* Dislocation, hip
 multiple locations (except fingers only or toes
   only) (closed) 839.8
  open 839.9
 navicular (bone) foot (closed) 837.0
  open 837.1
 neck (*see also* Dislocation, vertebra, cervical)
   839.00
 Nélaton's—*see* Dislocation, ankle
 nontraumatic (joint)—*see* Dislocation,
   pathological
 nose (closed) 839.69
  open 839.79
 not recurrent, not current injury—*see*
   Dislocation, pathological
 occiput from atlas (closed) 839.01
  open 839.11
 old—*see* Dislocation, recurrent
 open (compound) NEC 839.9
 ossicle, ear 385.23
 paralytic (flaccid) (spastic)—*see* Dislocation,
   pathological
 patella (closed) 836.3
  congenital 755.64
  open 836.4
 pathological NEC 718.20
  ankle 718.27
  elbow 718.22
  foot 718.27
  hand 718.24
  hip 718.25
  knee 718.26
  lumbosacral joint 724.6
  multiple sites 718.29
  pelvic region 718.25
  sacroiliac 724.6
  shoulder (region) 718.21
  specified site NEC 718.28
  spine 724.8
   sacroiliac 724.6
  wrist 718.23
 pelvis (closed) 839.69
  acetabulum (*see also* Dislocation, hip) 835.00
  open 839.79
 phalanx
  foot or toe (closed) 838.09
   open 838.19
  hand or finger (*see also* Dislocation, finger)
   834.00
 postpoliomyelitic—*see* Dislocation, pathological
 prosthesis, internal—*see* Complications,
   mechanical

Dislocation—*continued*
 radiocarpal (joint) (closed) 833.02
  open 833.12
 radioulnar (joint)
  distal end (closed) 833.01
   open 833.11
  proximal end (*see also* Dislocation, elbow)
   832.00
 radius
  distal end (closed) 833.00
   open 833.10
  proximal end (closed) 832.01
   open 832.11
 recurrent (*see also* Derangement, joint,
   recurrent) 718.3
  elbow 718.32
  hip 718.35
  joint NEC 718.38
  knee 718.36
  lumbosacral (joint) 724.6
  patella 718.36
  sacroiliac 724.6
  shoulder 718.31
  temporomandibular 524.69
 rib (cartilage) (closed) 839.69
  congenital 756.3
  open 839.79
 sacrococcygeal (closed) 839.42
  open 839.52
 sacroiliac (joint) (ligament) (closed) 839.42
  congenital 755.69
  open 839.52
  recurrent 724.6
 sacrum (closed) 839.42
  open 839.52
 scaphoid (bone)
  ankle or foot (closed) 837.0
   open 837.1
  wrist (closed) (*see also* Dislocation, wrist)
   833.00
   open 833.10
 scapula (closed) 831.09
  open 831.19
 semilunar cartilage, knee—*see* Tear, meniscus
 septal cartilage (nose) (closed) 839.69
  open 839.79
 septum (nasal) (old) 470
 sesamoid bone—*see* Dislocation, by site
 shoulder (blade) (ligament) (closed) 831.00
  anterior (subclavicular) (subcoracoid)
    (subglenoid) (closed) 831.01
   open 831.11
  chronic 718.31
  inferior 831.03
   open 831.13
  open 831.10
  posterior (closed) 831.02
   open 831.12
  recurrent 718.31
 skull—*see* Injury, intracranial
 Smith's—*see* Dislocation, foot
 spine (articular process) (*see also* Dislocation,
   vertebra) (closed) 839.40
  atlanto-axial (closed) 839.01
   open 839.11
   recurrent 723.8
  cervical, cervicodorsal, cervicothoracic
    (closed) (*see also* Dislocation, vertebrae,
    cervical) 839.00
   open 839.10
   recurrent 723.8

Dislocation—*continued*
  coccyx 839.41
    open 839.51
  congenital 756.19
  due to birth trauma 767.4
    open 839.50
  recurrent 724.9
  sacroiliac 839.42
    recurrent 724.6
  sacrum (sacrococcygeal) (sacroiliac) 839.42
    open 839.52
  spontaneous—*see* Dislocation, pathological
  sternoclavicular (joint) (closed) 839.61
    open 839.71
  sternum (closed) 839.61
    open 839.71
  subastragalar—*see* Dislocation, foot
  subglenoid (closed) 831.01
    open 831.11
  symphysis
    jaw (closed) 830.0
      open 830.1
    mandibular (closed) 830.0
      open 830.1
    pubis (closed) 839.69
      open 839.79
  tarsal (bone) (joint) 838.01
    open 838.11
  tarsometatarsal (joint) 838.03
    open 838.13
  temporomandibular (joint) (closed) 830.0
    open 830.1
    recurrent 524.69
  thigh
    distal end (*see also* Dislocation, femur, distal
      end) 836.50
    proximal end (*see also* Dislocation, hip)
      835.00
  thoracic (vertebrae) (closed) 839.21
    open 839.31
  thumb(s) (*see also* Dislocation, finger) 834.00
  thyroid cartilage (closed) 839.69
    open 839.79
  tibia
    distal end (closed) 837.0
      open 837.1
    proximal end (closed) 836.50
      anterior 836.51
        open 836.61
      lateral 836.54
        open 836.64
      medial 836.53
        open 836.63
      open 836.60
      posterior 836.52
        open 836.62
      rotatory 836.59
        open 836.69
  tibiofibular
    distal (closed) 837.0
      open 837.1
    superior (closed) 836.59
      open 836.69
  toe(s) (closed) 838.09
    open 838.19
  trachea (closed) 839.69
    open 839.79
  ulna
    distal end (closed) 833.09
      open 833.19
    proximal end—*see* Dislocation, elbow

Dislocation—*continued*
  vertebra (articular process) (body) (closed)
    839.40
    cervical, cervicodorsal or cervicothoracic
      (closed) 839.00
      first (atlas) 839.01
        open 839.11
      second (axis) 839.02
        open 839.12
      third 839.03
        open 839.13
      fourth 839.04
        open 839.14
      fifth 839.05
        open 839.15
      sixth 839.06
        open 839.16
      seventh 839.07
        open 839.17
      congenital 756.19
      multiple sites 839.08
        open 839.18
      open 839.10
    congenital 756.19
    dorsal 839.21
      open 839.31
      recurrent 724.9
    lumbar, lumbosacral 839.20
      open 839.30
    open NEC 839.50
    recurrent 724.9
    specified region NEC 839.49
      open 839.59
    thoracic 839.21
      open 839.31
  wrist (carpal bone) (scaphoid) (semilunar)
    (closed) 833.00
    carpometacarpal (joint) 833.04
      open 833.14
    metacarpal bone, proximal end 833.05
      open 833.15
    midcarpal (joint) 833.03
      open 833.13
    open 833.10
    radiocarpal (joint) 833.02
      open 833.12
    radioulnar (joint) 833.01
      open 833.11
    recurrent 718.33
    specified site NEC 833.09
      open 833.19
  xiphoid cartilage (closed) 839.61
    open 839.71
Dislodgement
  artificial skin graft 996.55
  decellularized allodermis graft 996.55
Disobedience, hostile (covert) (overt) (*see also*
  Disturbance, conduct) 312.0
Disorder —*see also* Disease
  academic underachievement, childhood and
    adolescence 313.83
  accommodation 367.51
    drug-induced 367.89
    toxic 367.89
  adjustment (*see also* Reaction, adjustment) 309.9
  adrenal (capsule) (cortex) (gland) 255.9
    specified type NEC 255.8
  adrenogenital 255.2
  affective (*see also* Psychosis, affective) 296.90
    atypical 296.81

Disorder—*continued*

aggressive, unsocialized (*see also* Disturbance, conduct) 312.0
alcohol, alcoholic (*see also* Alcohol) 291.9
allergic—*see* Allergy
amino acid (metabolic) (*see also* Disturbance, metabolism, amino acid) 270.9
  albinism 270.2
  alkaptonuria 270.2
  argininosuccinicaciduria 270.6
  beta-amino-isobutyricaciduria 277.2
  cystathioninuria 270.4
  cystinosis 270.0
  cystinuria 270.0
  glycinuria 270.0
  homocystinuria 270.4
  imidazole 270.5
  maple syrup (urine) disease 270.3
  neonatal, transitory 775.8
  oasthouse urine disease 270.2
  ochronosis 270.2
  phenylketonuria 270.1
  phenylpyruvic oligophrenia 270.1
  purine NEC 277.2
  pyrimidine NEC 277.2
  renal transport NEC 270.0
  specified type NEC 270.8
  transport NEC 270.0
    renal 270.0
  xanthinuria 277.2
amnestic (*see also* Amnestic syndrome) 294.0
anaerobic glycolysis with anemia 282.3
anxiety (*see also* Anxiety) 300.00
  due to or associated with physical condition 293.84
arteriole 447.9
  specified type NEC 447.8
artery 447.9
  specified type NEC 447.8
articulation—*see* Disorder, joint
Asperger's 299.8
attachment of infancy 313.89
attention deficit 314.00
  with hyperactivity 314.01
  predominantly
    combined hyperactive/inattentive 314.01
    hyperactive/impulsive 314.01
    inattentive 314.00
  residual type 314.8
autistic 299.0
autoimmune NEC 279.4
  hemolytic (cold type) (warm type) 283.0
  parathyroid 252.1
  thyroid 245.2
avoidant, childhood or adolescence 313.21
balance
  acid-base 276.9
    mixed (with hypercapnia) 276.4
  electrolyte 276.9
  fluid 276.9
behavior NEC (*see also* Disturbance, conduct) 312.9
bilirubin excretion 277.4
bipolar (affective) (alternating) (Type I) (*see also* Psychosis, affective) 296.7
  atypical 296.7
  currently
    depressed 296.5
    hypomanic 296.4
    manic 296.4
    mixed 296.6

Disorder—*continued*

  Type II (recurrent major depressive episodes with hypomania) 296.89
bladder 596.9
  functional NEC 596.59
  specified NEC 596.8
bone NEC 733.90
  specified NEC 733.99
brachial plexus 353.0
branched-chain amino-acid degradation 270.3
breast 611.9
  puerperal, postpartum 676.3
  specified NEC 611.8
Briquet's 300.81
bursa 727.9
  shoulder region 726.10
carbohydrate metabolism, congenital 271.9
cardiac, functional 427.9
  postoperative 997.1
  psychogenic 306.2
cardiovascular, psychogenic 306.2
cartilage NEC 733.90
  articular 718.00
    ankle 718.07
    elbow 718.02
    foot 718.07
    hand 718.04
    hip 718.05
    knee 717.9
    multiple sites 718.09
    pelvic region 718.05
    shoulder region 718.01
    specified
      site NEC 718.08
      type NEC 733.99
    wrist 718.03
catatonic—*see* Catatonia
cervical region NEC 723.9
cervical root (nerve) NEC 353.2
character NEC (*see also* Disorder, personality) 301.9
coagulation (factor) (*see also* Defect, coagulation) 286.9
  factor VIII (congenital) (functional) 286.0
  factor IX (congenital) (functional) 286.1
  neonatal, transitory 776.3
coccyx 724.70
  specified NEC 724.79
cognitive 294.9
colon 569.9
  functional 564.9
    congenital 751.3
conduct (*see also* Disturbance, conduct) 312.9
  adjustment reaction 309.3
  adolescent onset type 312.82
  childhood onset type 312.81
  compulsive 312.30
    specified type NEC 312.39
  hyperkinetic 314.2
  socialized (type) 312.20
    aggressive 312.23
    unaggressive 312.21
  specified NEC 312.89
conduction, heart 426.9
  specified NEC 426.89
convulsive (secondary) (*see also* Convulsions) 780.39
  due to injury at birth 767.0
  idiopathic 780.39
coordination 781.3

Disorder—*continued*
cornea NEC 371.89
  due to contact lens 371.82
corticosteroid metabolism NEC 255.2
cranial nerve—*see* Disorder, nerve, cranial
cyclothymic 301.13
degradation, branched-chain amino acid 270.3
delusional 297.9
dentition 520.6
depressive NEC 311
  atypical 296.82
  major (*see also* Psychosis, affective) 296.2
    recurrent episode 296.3
    single episode 296.2
development, specific 315.9
  associated with hyperkinesia 314.1
  language 315.31
  learning 315.2
    arithmetical 315.1
    reading 315.00
  mixed 315.5
  motor coordination 315.4
  specified type NEC 315.8
  speech 315.39
diaphragm 519.4
digestive 536.9
  fetus or newborn 777.9
    specified NEC 777.8
  psychogenic 306.4
disintegrative (childhood) 299.1
dissociative 300.14
  identity 300.14
dysmorphic body 300.7
dysthymic 300.4
ear 388.9
  degenerative NEC 388.00
  external 380.9
    specified 380.89
  pinna 380.30
  specified type NEC 388.8
  vascular NEC 388.00
eating NEC 307.50
electrolyte NEC 276.9
  with
    abortion—*see* Abortion, by type, with
      metabolic disorder
    ectopic pregnancy (*see also* categories
      633.0-633.9) 639.4
    molar pregnancy (*see also* categories
      630-632) 639.4
  acidosis 276.2
    metabolic 276.2
    respiratory 276.2
  alkalosis 276.3
    metabolic 276.3
    respiratory 276.3
  following
    abortion 639.4
    ectopic or molar pregnancy 639.4
  neonatal, transitory NEC 775.5
emancipation as adjustment reaction 309.22
emotional (*see also* Disorder, mental,
  nonpsychotic) V40.9
endocrine 259.9
  specified type NEC 259.8
esophagus 530.9
  functional 530.5
  psychogenic 306.4
explosive
  intermittent 312.34
  isolated 312.35

Disorder—*continued*
expressive language 315.31
eye 379.90
  globe—*see* Disorder, globe
  ill-defined NEC 379.99
  limited duction NEC 378.63
  specified NEC 379.8
eyelid 374.9
  degenerative 374.50
  sensory 374.44
  specified type NEC 374.89
  vascular 374.85
factitious —*see* Illness, factitious
factor, coagulation (*see also* Defect,
  coagulation) 286.9
  VIII (congenital) (functional) 286.0
  IX (congenital) (functional) 286.1
fascia 728.9
feeding —*see* Feeding
female sexual arousal 302.72
fluid NEC 276.9
gastric (functional) 536.9
  motility 536.8
  psychogenic 306.4
  secretion 536.8
gastrointestinal (functional) NEC 536.9
  newborn (neonatal) 777.9
    specified NEC 777.8
  psychogenic 306.4
gender (child) 302.6
  adult 302.85
gender identity (childhood) 302.6
  adult-life 302.85
genitourinary system, psychogenic 306.50
globe 360.9
  degenerative 360.20
    specified NEC 360.29
  specified type NEC 360.89
hearing—*see also* Deafness
  conductive type (air) (*see also* Deafness,
    conductive) 389.00
  mixed conductive and sensorineural 389.2
  nerve 389.12
  perceptive (*see also* Deafness, perceptive)
    389.10
  sensorineural type NEC (*see also* Deafness,
    perceptive) 389.10
heart action 427.9
  postoperative 997.1
hematological, transient neonatal 776.9
  specified type NEC 776.8
hematopoietic organs 289.9
hemorrhagic NEC 287.9
  due to circulating anticoagulants 286.5
  specified type NEC 287.8
hemostasis (*see also* Defect, coagulation) 286.9
homosexual conflict 302.0
hypomanic (chronic) 301.11
identity
  childhood and adolescence 313.82
    gender 302.6
  gender 302.6
immune mechanism (immunity) 279.9
  single complement (C_1-C_9) 279.8
  specified type NEC 279.8
impulse control (*see also* Disturbance, conduct,
  compulsive) 312.30
infant sialic acid storage 271.8
integument, fetus or newborn 778.9
  specified type NEC 778.8

Disorder—*continued*
  interactional psychotic (childhood) (*see also* Psychosis, childhood) 299.1
  intermittent explosive 312.34
  intervertebral disc 722.90
    cervical, cervicothoracic 722.91
    lumbar, lumbosacral 722.93
    thoracic, thoracolumbar 722.92
  intestinal 569.9
    functional NEC 564.9
      congenital 751.3
      postoperative 564.4
    psychogenic 306.4
  introverted, of childhood and adolescence 313.22
  iron, metabolism 275.0
  isolated explosive 312.35
  joint NEC 719.90
    ankle 719.97
    elbow 719.92
    foot 719.97
    hand 719.94
    hip 719.95
    knee 719.96
    multiple sites 719.99
    pelvic region 719.95
    psychogenic 306.0
    shoulder (region) 719.91
    specified site NEC 719.98
    temporomandibular 524.60
      specified NEC 524.69
    wrist 719.93
  kidney 593.9
    functional 588.9
      specified NEC 588.8
  labyrinth, labyrinthine 386.9
    specified type NEC 386.8
  lactation 676.9
  language (developmental) (expressive) 315.31
    mixed (receptive) (receptive-expressive) 315.32
  ligament 728.9
  ligamentous attachments, peripheral—*see also* Enthesopathy
    spine 720.1
  limb NEC 729.9
    psychogenic 306.0
  lipid
    metabolism, congenital 272.9
    storage 272.7
  lipoprotein deficiency (familial) 272.5
  low back NEC 724.9
    psychogenic 306.0
  lumbosacral
    plexus 353.1
    root (nerve) NEC 353.4
  lymphoproliferative (chronic) NEC (M9970/1) 238.7
  major depressive (*see also* Psychosis, affective) 296.2
    recurrent episode 296.3
    single episode 296.2
  male erectile 302.72
    organic origin 607.84
  manic (*see also* Psychosis, affective) 296.0
    atypical 296.81
  meniscus NEC (*see also* Disorder, cartilage, articular) 718.0
  menopausal 627.9
    specified NEC 627.8

Disorder—*continued*
  menstrual 626.9
    psychogenic 306.52
    specified NEC 626.8
  mental (nonpsychotic) 300.9
    affecting management of pregnancy, childbirth, or puerperium 648.4
    drug-induced 292.9
      hallucinogen persistent perception 292.89
      specified type NEC 292.89
    due to or associated with
      alcoholism 291.9
      drug consumption NEC 292.9
        specified type NEC 292.89
      physical condition NEC 293.9
    induced by drug 292.9
      specified type NEC 292.89
    neurotic (*see also* Neurosis) 300.9
    presenile 310.1
      psychotic NEC 290.10
    previous, affecting management of pregnancy V23.8
    psychoneurotic (*see also* Neurosis) 300.9
    psychotic (*see also* Psychosis) 298.9
      senile 290.20
    specific, following organic brain damage 310.9
      cognitive or personality change of other type 310.1
      frontal lobe syndrome 310.0
      postconcussional syndrome 310.2
      specified type NEC 310.8
  metabolism NEC 277.9
    with
      abortion—*see* Abortion, by type, with metabolic disorder
      ectopic pregnancy (*see also* categories 633.0-633.9) 639.4
      molar pregnancy (*see also* categories 630-632) 639.4
    alkaptonuria 270.2
    amino acid (*see also* Disorder, amino acid) 270.9
      specified type NEC 270.8
    ammonia 270.6
    arginine 270.6
    argininosuccinic acid 270.6
    basal 794.7
    bilirubin 277.4
    calcium 275.40
    carbohydrate 271.9
      specified type NEC 271.8
    cholesterol 272.9
    citrulline 270.6
    copper 275.1
    corticosteroid 255.2
    cystine storage 270.0
    cystinuria 270.0
    fat 272.9
    following
      abortion 639.4
      ectopic or molar pregnancy 639.4
    fructosemia 271.2
    fructosuria 271.2
    fucosidosis 271.8
    galactose-1-phosphate uridyl transferase 271.1
    glutamine 270.7
    glycine 270.7
    glycogen storage NEC 271.0
      hepatorenal 271.0
    hemochromatosis 275.0
    in labor and delivery 669.0

Disorder—*continued*
  iron 275.0
  lactose 271.3
  lipid 272.9
    specified type NEC 272.8
    storage 272.7
  lipoprotein—*see also* Hyperlipemia
    deficiency (familial) 272.5
  lysine 270.7
  magnesium 275.2
  mannosidosis 271.8
  mineral 275.9
    specified type NEC 275.8
  mucopolysaccharide 277.5
  nitrogen 270.9
  ornithine 270.6
  oxalosis 271.8
  pentosuria 271.8
  phenylketonuria 270.1
  phosphate 275.3
  phosphorus 275.3
  plasma protein 273.9
    specified type NEC 273.8
  porphyrin 277.1
  purine 277.2
  pyrimidine 277.2
  serine 270.7
  sodium 276.9
  specified type NEC 277.8
  steroid 255.2
  threonine 270.7
  urea cycle 270.6
  xylose 271.8
  micturition NEC 788.69
    psychogenic 306.53
  misery and unhappiness, of childhood and
    adolescence 313.1
  mitral valve 424.0
  mood—*see* Psychosis, affective
  motor tic 307.20
    chronic 307.22
    transient, childhood 307.21
  movement NEC 333.90
    hysterical 300.11
    specified type NEC 333.99
    stereotypic 307.3
  mucopolysaccharide 277.5
  muscle 728.9
    psychogenic 306.0
    specified type NEC 728.3
  muscular attachments, peripheral—*see also*
    Enthesopathy
    spine 720.1
  musculoskeletal system NEC 729.9
    psychogenic 306.0
  myeloproliferative (chronic) NEC (M9960/1)
    238.7
  myoneural 358.9
    due to lead 358.2
    specified type NEC 358.8
    toxic 358.2
  myotonic 359.2
  neck region NEC 723.9
  nerve 349.9
    abducens NEC 378.54
    accessory 352.4
    acoustic 388.5
    auditory 388.5
    auriculotemporal 350.8
    axillary 353.0
    cerebral—*see* Disorder, nerve, cranial

Disorder—*continued*
  cranial 352.9
    first 352.0
    second 377.49
    third
      partial 378.51
      total 378.52
    fourth 378.53
    fifth 350.9
    sixth 378.54
    seventh NEC 351.9
    eighth 388.5
    ninth 352.2
    tenth 352.3
    eleventh 352.4
    twelfth 352.5
    multiple 352.6
  entrapment—*see* Neuropathy, entrapment
  facial 351.9
    specified NEC 351.8
  femoral 355.2
  glossopharyngeal NEC 352.2
  hypoglossal 352.5
  iliohypogastric 355.79
  ilioinguinal 355.79
  intercostal 353.8
  lateral
    cutaneous of thigh 355.1
    popliteal 355.3
  lower limb NEC 355.8
  medial, popliteal 355.4
  median NEC 354.1
  obturator 355.79
  oculomotor
    partial 378.51
    total 378.52
  olfactory 352.0
  optic 377.49
    ischemic 377.41
    nutritional 377.33
    toxic 377.34
  peroneal 355.3
  phrenic 354.8
  plantar 355.6
  pneumogastric 352.3
  posterior tibial 355.5
  radial 354.3
  recurrent laryngeal 352.3
  root 353.9
    specified NEC 353.8
  saphenous 355.79
  sciatic NEC 355.0
  specified NEC 355.9
    lower limb 355.79
    upper limb 354.8
  spinal 355.9
  sympathetic NEC 337.9
  trigeminal 350.9
    specified NEC 350.8
  trochlear 378.53
  ulnar 354.2
  upper limb NEC 354.9
  vagus 352.3
  nervous system NEC 349.9
    autonomic (peripheral) (*see also* Neuropathy,
      peripheral, autonomic) 337.9
    cranial 352.9
    parasympathetic (*see also* Neuropathy,
      peripheral, autonomic) 337.9
    specified type NEC 349.89

Disorder—*continued*

sympathetic (*see also* Neuropathy, peripheral, autonomic) 337.9

vegetative (*see also* Neuropathy, peripheral, autonomic) 337.9

neurohypophysis NEC 253.6

neurological NEC 781.99

  peripheral NEC 355.9

neuromuscular NEC 358.9

  hereditary NEC 359.1

  specified NEC 358.8

  toxic 358.2

neurotic 300.9

  specified type NEC 300.89

neutrophil, polymorphonuclear (functional) 288.1

obsessive-compulsive 300.3

oppositional, childhood and adolescence 313.81

optic

  chiasm 377.54

    associated with

      inflammatory disorders 377.54

      neoplasm NEC 377.52

        pituitary 377.51

      pituitary disorders 377.51

      vascular disorders 377.53

  nerve 377.49

  radiations 377.63

  tracts 377.63

orbit 376.9

  specified NEC 376.89

overanxious, of childhood and adolescence 313.0

pancreas, internal secretion (other than diabetes mellitus) 251.9

  specified type NEC 251.8

panic 300.01

  with agoraphobia 300.21

papillary muscle NEC 429.81

paranoid 297.9

  induced 297.3

  shared 297.3

parathyroid 252.9

  specified type NEC 252.8

paroxysmal, mixed 780.39

pentose phosphate pathway with anemia 282.2

personality 301.9

  affective 301.10

  aggressive 301.3

  amoral 301.7

  anancastic, anankastic 301.4

  antisocial 301.7

  asocial 301.7

  asthenic 301.6

  borderline 301.83

  compulsive 301.4

  cyclothymic 301.13

  dependent-passive 301.6

  dyssocial 301.7

  emotional instability 301.59

  epileptoid 301.3

  explosive 301.3

  following organic brain damage 310.1

  histrionic 301.50

  hyperthymic 301.11

  hypomanic (chronic) 301.11

  hypothymic 301.12

  hysterical 301.50

  immature 301.89

  inadequate 301.6

  introverted 301.21

Disorder—*continued*

  labile 301.59

  moral deficiency 301.7

  obsessional 301.4

  obsessive (-compulsive) 301.4

  overconscientious 301.4

  paranoid 301.0

  passive (-dependent) 301.6

  passive-aggressive 301.84

  pathological NEC 301.9

  pseudosocial 301.7

  psychopathic 301.9

  schizoid 301.20

    introverted 301.21

    schizotypal 301.22

  schizotypal 301.22

  seductive 301.59

  type A 301.4

  unstable 301.59

pervasive developmental, childhood-onset 299.8

pigmentation, choroid (congenital) 743.53

pinna 380.30

  specified type NEC 380.39

pituitary, thalamic 253.9

  anterior NEC 253.4

  iatrogenic 253.7

  postablative 253.7

  specified NEC 253.8

pityriasis-like NEC 696.8

platelets (blood) 287.1

polymorphonuclear neutrophils (functional) 288.1

porphyrin metabolism 277.1

postmenopausal 627.9

  specified type NEC 627.8

posttraumatic stress 309.81

  acute 308.3

  brief 308.3

  chronic 309.81

premenstrual dysphoric 625.4

psoriatic-like NEC 696.8

psychic, with diseases classified elsewhere 316

psychogenic NEC (*see also* condition) 300.9

  allergic NEC

    respiratory 306.1

  anxiety 300.00

    atypical 300.00

    generalized 300.02

  appetite 307.50

  articulation, joint 306.0

  asthenic 300.5

  blood 306.8

  cardiovascular (system) 306.2

  compulsive 300.3

  cutaneous 306.3

  depressive 300.4

  digestive (system) 306.4

  dysmenorrheic 306.52

  dyspneic 306.1

  eczematous 306.3

  endocrine (system) 306.6

  eye 306.7

  feeding 307.59

  functional NEC 306.9

  gastric 306.4

  gastrointestinal (system) 306.4

  genitourinary (system) 306.50

  heart (function) (rhythm) 306.2

  hemic 306.8

  hyperventilatory 306.1

  hypochondriacal 300.7

Disorder—*continued*
  hysterical 300.10
  intestinal 306.4
  joint 306.0
  learning 315.2
  limb 306.0
  lymphatic (system) 306.8
  menstrual 306.52
  micturition 306.53
  monoplegic NEC 306.0
  motor 307.9
  muscle 306.0
  musculoskeletal 306.0
  neurocirculatory 306.2
  obsessive 300.3
  occupational 300.89
  organ or part of body NEC 306.9
  organs of special sense 306.7
  paralytic NEC 306.0
  phobic 300.20
  physical NEC 306.9
  pruritic 306.3
  rectal 306.4
  respiratory (system) 306.1
  rheumatic 306.0
  sexual (function) 302.70
    specified type NEC 302.79
  skin (allergic) (eczematous) (pruritic) 306.3
  sleep 307.40
    initiation or maintenance 307.41
      persistent 307.42
      transient 307.41
    specified type NEC 307.49
  specified part of body NEC 306.8
  stomach 306.4
  psychomotor NEC 307.9
    hysterical 300.11
  psychoneurotic (*see also* Neurosis) 300.9
    mixed NEC 300.89
  psychophysiologic (*see also* Disorder,
    psychosomatic) 306.9
  psychosexual identity (childhood) 302.6
    adult-life 302.85
  psychosomatic NEC 306.9
    allergic NEC
      respiratory 306.1
    articulation, joint 306.0
    cardiovascular (system) 306.2
    cutaneous 306.3
    digestive (system) 306.4
    dysmenorrheic 306.52
    dyspneic 306.1
    endocrine (system) 306.6
    eye 306.7
    gastric 306.4
    gastrointestinal (system) 306.4
    genitourinary (system) 306.50
    heart (functional) (rhythm) 306.2
    hyperventilatory 306.1
    intestinal 306.4
    joint 306.0
    limb 306.0
    lymphatic (system) 306.8
    menstrual 306.52
    micturition 306.53
    monoplegic NEC 306.0
    muscle 306.0
    musculoskeletal 306.0
    neurocirculatory 306.2
    organs of special sense 306.7
    paralytic NEC 306.0

Disorder—*continued*
  pruritic 306.3
  rectal 306.4
  respiratory (system) 306.1
  rheumatic 306.0
  sexual (function) 302.70
    specified type NEC 302.79
  skin 306.3
  specified part of body NEC 306.8
  stomach 306.4
  psychotic—*see* Psychosis
  purine metabolism NEC 277.2
  pyrimidine metabolism NEC 277.2
  reactive attachment (of infancy or early
    childhood) 313.89
  reading, developmental 315.00
  reflex 796.1
  renal function, impaired 588.9
    specified type NEC 588.8
  renal transport NEC 588.8
  respiration, respiratory NEC 519.9
    due to
      aspiration of liquids or solids 508.9
      inhalation of fumes or vapors 506.9
    psychogenic 306.1
  retina 362.9
    specified type NEC 362.89
  sacroiliac joint NEC 724.6
  sacrum 724.6
  schizo-affective (*see also* Schizophrenia) 295.7
  schizoid, childhood or adolescence 313.22
  schizophreniform 295.4
  schizotypal personality 301.22
  secretion, thyrocalcitonin 246.0
  seizure 780.39
    recurrent 780.39
      epileptic—*see* Epilepsy
  sense of smell 781.1
    psychogenic 306.7
  separation anxiety 309.21
  sexual (*see also* Deviation, sexual) 302.9
    function, psychogenic 302.70
  shyness, of childhood and adolescence 313.21
  single complement (C_1-C_9) 279.8
  skin NEC 709.9
    fetus or newborn 778.9
      specified type 778.8
    psychogenic (allergic) (eczematous) (pruritic)
      306.3
    specified type NEC 709.8
    vascular 709.1
  sleep 780.50
    circadian rhythm 307.45
    initiation or maintenance (*see also* Insomnia)
      780.52
      nonorganic origin (transient) 307.41
        persistent 307.42
    nonorganic origin 307.40
      specified type NEC 307.49
    specified NEC 780.59
    with apnea—*see* Apnea, sleep
  social, of childhood and adolescence 313.22
    specified NEC 780.59
  soft tissue 729.9
  somatization 300.81
  somatoform (atypical) (undifferentiated) 300.82
    severe 300.81
  speech NEC 784.5
    nonorganic origin 307.9
  spine NEC 724.9

Displacement, displaced—*continued*

macula (congenital) 743.55

Meckel's diverticulum (congenital) 751.0

nail (congenital) 757.5

   acquired 703.8

opening of Wharton's duct in mouth 750.26

organ or site, congenital NEC—*see*

   Malposition, congenital

ovary (acquired) 620.4

   congenital 752.0

   free in peritoneal cavity (congenital) 752.0

   into hernial sac 620.4

oviduct (acquired) 620.4

   congenital 752.19

parathyroid (gland) 252.8

parotid gland (congenital) 750.26

punctum lacrimale (congenital) 743.65

sacroiliac (congenital) (joint) 755.69

   current injury—*see* Dislocation, sacroiliac

   old 724.6

spine (congenital) 756.19

spleen, congenital 759.0

stomach (congenital) 750.7

   acquired 537.89

subglenoid (closed) 831.01

sublingual duct (congenital) 750.26

teeth, tooth 524.3

tongue (congenital) (downward) 750.19

trachea (congenital) 748.3

ureter or ureteric opening or orifice (congenital) 753.4

uterine opening of oviducts or fallopian tubes 752.19

uterus, uterine (*see also* Malposition, uterus) 621.6

   congenital 752.3

ventricular septum 746.89

   with rudimentary ventricle 746.89

xyphoid bone (process) 738.3

Disproportion 653.9

affecting fetus or newborn 763.1

caused by

   conjoined twins 653.7

   contraction, pelvis (general) 653.1

     inlet 653.2

     midpelvic 653.8

     midplane 653.8

     outlet 653.3

   fetal

     ascites 653.7

     hydrocephalus 653.6

     hydrops 653.7

     meningomyelocele 653.7

     sacral teratoma 653.7

     tumor 653.7

   hydrocephalic fetus 653.6

   pelvis, pelvic, abnormality (bony) NEC 653.0

   unusually large fetus 653.5

causing obstructed labor 660.1

cephalopelvic, normally formed fetus 653.4

   causing obstructed labor 660.1

fetal NEC 653.5

   causing obstructed labor 660.1

fetopelvic, normally formed fetus 653.4

   causing obstructed labor 660.1

mixed maternal and fetal origin, normally formed fetus 653.4

pelvis, pelvic (bony) NEC 653.1

   causing obstructed labor 660.1

specified type NEC 653.8

Disruption

cesarean wound 674.1

family V61.0

gastrointestinal anastomosis 997.4

ligament(s)—*see also* Sprain

   knee

     current injury—*see* Dislocation, knee

     old 717.89

       capsular 717.85

       collateral (medial) 717.82

         lateral 717.81

       cruciate (posterior) 717.84

         anterior 717.83

       specified site NEC 717.85

marital V61.10

   involving divorce or estrangement V61.0

operation wound (external) 998.32

   internal 998.31

organ transplant, anastomosis site—*see*

   Complications, transplant, organ, by site

ossicles, ossicular chain 385.23

   traumatic—*see* Fracture, skull, base

parenchyma

   liver (hepatic)—*see* Laceration, liver, major

   spleen—*see* Laceration, spleen, parenchyma,

     massive

phase-shift, of 24-hour sleep-wake cycle 780.55

   nonorganic origin 307.45

sleep-wake cycle (24-hour) 780.55

   circadian rhythm 307.45

   nonorganic origin 307.45

suture line (external) 998.32

   internal 998.31

wound

   cesarean operation 674.1

   episiotomy 674.2

   operation 998.32

     cesarean 674.1

     internal 998.31

   perineal (obstetric) 674.2

   uterine 674.1

Disruptio uteri —*see also* Rupture, uterus

complicating delivery—*see* Delivery,

   complicated, rupture, uterus

Dissatisfaction with

employment V62.2

school environment V62.3

Dissecting —*see* condition

Dissection

aorta 441.00

   abdominal 441.02

   thoracic 441.01

   thoracoabdominal 441.03

artery, arterial

   carotid 443.21

   coronary 414.12

   iliac 443.22

   renal 443.23

   specified NEC 443.29

   vertebral 443.24

vascular 459.9

wound—*see* Wound, open, by site

Disseminated —*see* condition

Dissociated personality NEC 300.15

Dissociation

auriculoventricular or atrioventricular (any degree) (AV) 426.89

   with heart block 426.0

interference 426.89

isorhythmic 426.89

Dissociation—*continued*
  rhythm
    atrioventricular (AV) 426.89
    interference 426.89
Dissociative
  identity disorder 300.14
  reaction NEC 300.15
Dissolution, vertebra (*see also* Osteoporosis) 733.00
Distention
  abdomen (gaseous) 787.3
  bladder 596.8
  cecum 569.89
  colon 569.89
  gallbladder 575.8
  gaseous (abdomen) 787.3
  intestine 569.89
  kidney 593.89
  liver 573.9
  seminal vesicle 608.89
  stomach 536.8
    acute 536.1
    psychogenic 306.4
  ureter 593.5
  uterus 621.8
Distichia, distichiasis (eyelid) 743.63
Distoma hepaticum infestation 121.3
Distomiasis 121.9
  bile passages 121.3
    due to Clonorchis sinensis 121.1
  hemic 120.9
  hepatic (liver) 121.3
    due to Clonorchis sinensis (clonorchiasis) 121.1
  intestinal 121.4
  liver 121.3
    due to Clonorchis sinensis 121.1
  lung 121.2
  pulmonary 121.2
Distomolar (fourth molar) 520.1
  causing crowding 524.3
Disto-occlusion 524.2
Distortion (congenital)
  adrenal (gland) 759.1
  ankle (joint) 755.69
  anus 751.5
  aorta 747.29
  appendix 751.5
  arm 755.59
  artery (peripheral) NEC (*see also* Distortion, peripheral vascular system) 747.60
    cerebral 747.81
    coronary 746.85
    pulmonary 747.3
    retinal 743.58
    umbilical 747.5
  auditory canal 744.29
    causing impairment of hearing 744.02
  bile duct or passage 751.69
  bladder 753.8
  brain 742.4
  bronchus 748.3
  cecum 751.5
  cervix (uteri) 752.49
  chest (wall) 756.3
  clavicle 755.51
  clitoris 752.49
  coccyx 756.19
  colon 751.5
  common duct 751.69
  cornea 743.41

Distortion—*continued*
  cricoid cartilage 748.3
  cystic duct 751.69
  duodenum 751.5
  ear 744.29
    auricle 744.29
      causing impairment of hearing 744.02
      causing impairment of hearing 744.09
    external 744.29
      causing impairment of hearing 744.02
    inner 744.05
    middle, except ossicles 744.03
      ossicles 744.04
    ossicles 744.04
  endocrine (gland) NEC 759.2
  epiglottis 748.3
  Eustachian tube 744.24
  eye 743.8
    adnexa 743.69
  face bone(s) 756.0
  fallopian tube 752.19
  femur 755.69
  fibula 755.69
  finger(s) 755.59
  foot 755.67
  gallbladder 751.69
  genitalia, genital organ(s)
    female 752.8
      external 752.49
      internal NEC 752.8
    male 752.8
      penis 752.69
  glottis 748.3
  gyri 742.4
  hand bone(s) 755.59
  heart (auricle) (ventricle) 746.89
    valve (cusp) 746.89
  hepatic duct 751.69
  humerus 755.59
  hymen 752.49
  ileum 751.5
  intestine (large) (small) 751.5
    with anomalous adhesions, fixation or malrotation 751.4
  jaw NEC 524.8
  jejunum 751.5
  kidney 753.3
  knee (joint) 755.64
  labium (majus) (minus) 752.49
  larynx 748.3
  leg 755.69
  lens 743.36
  liver 751.69
  lumbar spine 756.19
    with disproportion (fetopelvic) 653.0
      affecting fetus or newborn 763.1
      causing obstructed labor 660.1
  lumbosacral (joint) (region) 756.19
  lung (fissures) (lobe) 748.69
  nerve 742.8
  nose 748.1
  organ
    of Corti 744.05
    or site not listed—*see* Anomaly, specified type NEC
  ossicles, ear 744.04
  ovary 752.0
  oviduct 752.19
  pancreas 751.7
  parathyroid (gland) 759.2
  patella 755.64

Distortion—*continued*
peripheral vascular system NEC 747.60
 gastrointestinal 747.61
 lower limb 747.64
 renal 747.62
 spinal 747.82
 upper limb 747.63
pituitary (gland) 759.2
radius 755.59
rectum 751.5
rib 756.3
sacroiliac joint 755.69
sacrum 756.19
scapula 755.59
shoulder girdle 755.59
site not listed—*see* Anomaly, specified type
 NEC
skull bone(s) 756.0
 with
  anencephalus 740.0
  encephalocele 742.0
  hydrocephalus 742.3
   with spina bifida (*see also* Spina bifida)
    741.0
  microcephalus 742.1
spinal cord 742.59
spine 756.19
spleen 759.0
sternum 756.3
thorax (wall) 756.3
thymus (gland) 759.2
thyroid (gland) 759.2
 cartilage 748.3
tibia 755.69
toe(s) 755.66
tongue 750.19
trachea (cartilage) 748.3
ulna 755.59
ureter 753.4
 causing obstruction 753.20
urethra 753.8
 causing obstruction 753.6
uterus 752.3
vagina 752.49
vein (peripheral) NEC (*see also* Distortion,
 peripheral vascular system) 747.60
 great 747.49
 portal 747.49
 pulmonary 747.49
 vena cava (inferior) (superior) 747.49
vertebra 756.19
visual NEC 368.15
 shape or size 368.14
vulva 752.49
wrist (bones) (joint) 755.59
Distress
abdomen 789.0
colon 789.0
emotional V40.9
epigastric 789.0
fetal (syndrome) 768.4
 affecting management of pregnancy or
  childbirth 656.8
 liveborn infant 768.4
  first noted
   before onset of labor 768.2
   during labor or delivery 768.3
 stillborn infant (death before onset of labor)
  768.0
  death during labor 768.1
gastrointestinal (functional) 536.9

Distress—*continued*
 psychogenic 306.4
intestinal (functional) NEC 564.9
 psychogenic 306.4
intrauterine (*see* Distress, fetal)
leg 729.5
maternal 669.0
mental V40.9
respiratory 786.09
 acute (adult) 518.82
 adult syndrome (following shock, surgery, or
  trauma) 518.5
  specified NEC 518.82
 fetus or newborn 770.89
 syndrome (idiopathic) (newborn) 769
stomach 536.9
 psychogenic 306.4
Distribution vessel, atypical NEC 747.60
 coronary artery 746.85
 spinal 747.82
Districhiasis 704.2
Disturbance —*see also* Disease
absorption NEC 579.9
 calcium 269.3
 carbohydrate 579.8
 fat 579.8
 protein 579.8
 specified type NEC 579.8
 vitamin (*see also* Deficiency, vitamin) 269.2
acid-base equilibrium 276.9
activity and attention, simple, with hyperkinesis
 314.01
amino acid (metabolic) (*see also* Disorder,
 amino acid) 270.9
 imidazole 270.5
 maple syrup (urine) disease 270.3
 transport 270.0
assimilation, food 579.9
attention, simple 314.00
 with hyperactivity 314.01
auditory, nerve, except deafness 388.5
behavior (*see also* Disturbance, conduct) 312.9
blood clotting (hypoproteinemia) (mechanism)
 (*see also* Defect, coagulation) 286.9
central nervous system NEC 349.9
cerebral nerve NEC 352.9
circulatory 459.9
conduct 312.9

---

*Note—Use the following fifth-digit
subclassification with categories 312.0-312.2:*

0 *unspecified*
1 *mild*
2 *moderate*
3 *severe*

---

   adjustment reaction 309.3
   adolescent onset type 312.82
   childhood onset type 312.81
   compulsive 312.30
    intermittent explosive disorder 312.34
    isolated explosive disorder 312.35
    kleptomania 312.32
    pathological gambling 312.31
    pyromania 312.33
   hyperkinetic 314.2
   intermittent explosive 312.34
   isolated explosive 312.35
   mixed with emotions 312.4
   socialized (type) 312.20
    aggressive 312.23

Disturbance—*continued*
   unaggressive 312.21
   specified type NEC 312.89
   undersocialized, unsocialized
      aggressive (type) 312.0
      unaggressive (type) 312.1
  coordination 781.3
  cranial nerve NEC 352.9
  deep sensibility—*see* Disturbance, sensation
  digestive 536.9
   psychogenic 306.4
  electrolyte—*see* Imbalance, electrolyte
  emotions specific to childhood and adolescence
    313.9
   with
     academic underachievement 313.83
     anxiety and fearfulness 313.0
     elective mutism 313.23
     identity disorder 313.82
     jealousy 313.3
     misery and unhappiness 313.1
     oppositional disorder 313.81
     overanxiousness 313.0
     sensitivity 313.21
     shyness 313.21
     social withdrawal 313.22
     withdrawal reaction 313.22
   involving relationship problems 313.3
   mixed 313.89
   specified type NEC 313.89
  endocrine (gland) 259.9
   neonatal, transitory 775.9
   specified NEC 775.8
  equilibrium 780.4
  feeding (elderly) (infant) 783.3
   newborn 779.3
   nonorganic origin NEC 307.59
   psychogenic NEC 307.59
  fructose metabolism 271.2
  gait 781.2
   hysterical 300.11
  gastric (functional) 536.9
   motility 536.8
   psychogenic 306.4
   secretion 536.8
  gastrointestinal (functional) 536.9
   psychogenic 306.4
  habit, child 307.9
  hearing, except deafness 388.40
  heart, functional (conditions classifiable to 426,
    427, 428)
   due to presence of (cardiac) prosthesis 429.4
   postoperative (immediate) 997.1
    long-term effect of cardiac surgery 429.4
   psychogenic 306.2
  hormone 259.9
  innervation uterus, sympathetic,
    parasympathetic 621.8
  keratinization NEC
   gingiva 523.1
   lip 528.5
   oral (mucosa) (soft tissue) 528.7
   tongue 528.7
  labyrinth, labyrinthine (vestibule) 386.9
  learning, specific NEC 315.2
  memory (*see also* Amnesia) 780.99
   mild, following organic brain damage 310.1
  mental (*see also* Disorder, mental) 300.9
   associated with diseases classified elsewhere
    316

Disturbance—*continued*
  metabolism (acquired) (congenital) (*see also*
    Disorder, metabolism) 277.9
   with
    abortion—*see* Abortion, by type, with
     metabolic disorder
    ectopic pregnancy (*see also* categories
     633.0-633.9) 639.4
    molar pregnancy (*see also* categories
     630-632) 639.4
   amino acid (*see also* Disorder, amino acid)
    270.9
    aromatic NEC 270.2
    branched-chain 270.3
    specified type NEC 270.8
    straight-chain NEC 270.7
    sulfur-bearing 270.4
    transport 270.0
   ammonia 270.6
   arginine 270.6
   argininosuccinic acid 270.6
   carbohydrate NEC 271.9
   cholesterol 272.9
   citrulline 270.6
   cystathionine 270.4
   fat 272.9
   following
    abortion 639.4
    ectopic or molar pregnancy 639.4
   general 277.7
    carbohydrate 271.9
    iron 275.0
    phosphate 275.3
    sodium 276.9
   glutamine 270.7
   glycine 270.7
   histidine 270.5
   homocystine 270.4
   in labor or delivery 669.0
   iron 275.0
   isoleucine 270.3
   leucine 270.3
   lipoid 272.9
    specified type NEC 272.8
   lysine 270.7
   methionine 270.4
   neonatal, transitory 775.9
    specified type NEC 775.8
   nitrogen 788.9
   ornithine 270.6
   phosphate 275.3
   phosphatides 272.7
   serine 270.7
   sodium NEC 276.9
   threonine 270.7
   tryptophan 270.2
   tyrosine 270.2
   urea cycle 270.6
   valine 270.3
  motor 796.1
  nervous functional 799.2
  neuromuscular mechanism (eye) due to syphilis
    094.84
  nutritional 269.9
   nail 703.8
  ocular motion 378.87
   psychogenic 306.7
  oculogyric 378.87
   psychogenic 306.7
  oculomotor NEC 378.87
   psychogenic 306.7

Disturbance—*continued*
  olfactory nerve 781.1
  optic nerve NEC 377.49
  oral epithelium, including tongue 528.7
  personality (pattern) (trait) (*see also* Disorder,
    personality) 301.9
    following organic brain damage 310.1
  polyglandular 258.9
  psychomotor 307.9
  pupillary 379.49
  reflex 796.1
  rhythm, heart 427.9
    postoperative (immediate) 997.1
      long-term effect of cardiac surgery 429.4
    psychogenic 306.2
  salivary secretion 527.7
  sensation (cold) (heat) (localization) (tactile
    discrimination localization) (texture)
    (vibratory) NEC 782.0
    hysterical 300.11
    skin 782.0
    smell 781.1
    taste 781.1
  sensory (*see also* Disturbance, sensation) 782.0
    innervation 782.0
  situational (transient) (*see also* Reaction,
    adjustment) 309.9
    acute 308.3
  sleep 780.50
    initiation or maintenance (*see also* Insomnia)
      780.52
      nonorganic origin 307.41
    nonorganic origin 307.40
      specified type NEC 307.49
    specified NEC 780.59
      nonorganic origin 307.49
    wakefulness (*see also* Hypersomnia) 780.54
      nonorganic origin 307.43
    with apnea—*see* Apnea, sleep
  sociopathic 301.7
  speech NEC 784.5
    developmental 315.39
      associated with hyperkinesis 314.1
    secondary to organic lesion 784.5
  stomach (functional) (*see also* Disturbance,
    gastric) 536.9
  sympathetic (nerve) (*see also* Neuropathy,
    peripheral, autonomic) 337.9
  temperature sense 782.0
    hysterical 300.11
  tooth
    eruption 520.6
    formation 520.4
    structure, hereditary NEC 520.5
  touch (*see also* Disturbance, sensation) 782.0
  vascular 459.9
    arteriosclerotic—*see* Arteriosclerosis
  vasomotor 443.9
  vasospastic 443.9
  vestibular labyrinth 386.9
  vision, visual NEC 368.9
    psychophysical 368.16
    specified NEC 368.8
    subjective 368.10
  voice 784.40
  wakefulness (initiation or maintenance) (*see
    also* Hypersomnia) 780.54
    nonorganic origin 307.43
Disulfiduria, beta-mercaptolactate-cysteine 270.0
Disuse atrophy, bone 733.7
Ditthomska syndrome 307.81
Diuresis 788.42

Divers'
  palsy or paralysis 993.3
  squeeze 993.3
Diverticula, diverticulosis, diverticulum (acute)
  (multiple) (perforated) (ruptured) 562.10
  with diverticulitis 562.11
  aorta (Kommerell's) 747.21
  appendix (noninflammatory) 543.9
  bladder (acquired) (sphincter) 596.3
    congenital 753.8
  broad ligament 620.8
  bronchus (congenital) 748.3
    acquired 494.0
      with acute exacerbation 494.1
  calyx, calyceal (kidney) 593.89
  cardia (stomach) 537.1
  cecum 562.10
    with
      diverticulitis 562.11
        with hemorrhage 562.13
      hemorrhage 562.12
    congenital 751.5
  colon (acquired) 562.10
    with
      diverticulitis 562.11
        with hemorrhage 562.13
      hemorrhage 562.12
    congenital 751.5
  duodenum 562.00
    with
      diverticulitis 562.01
        with hemorrhage 562.03
      hemorrhage 562.02
    congenital 751.5
  epiphrenic (esophagus) 530.6
  esophagus (congenital) 750.4
    acquired 530.6
    epiphrenic 530.6
    pulsion 530.6
    traction 530.6
    Zenker's 530.6
  Eustachian tube 381.89
  fallopian tube 620.8
  gallbladder (congenital) 751.69
  gastric 537.1
  heart (congenital) 746.89
  ileum 562.00
    with
      diverticulitis 562.01
        with hemorrhage 562.03
      hemorrhage 562.02
  intestine (large) 562.10
    with
      diverticulitis 562.11
        with hemorrhage 562.13
      hemorrhage 562.12
    congenital 751.5
    small 562.00
      with
        diverticulitis 562.01
          with hemorrhage 562.03
        hemorrhage 562.02
      congenital 751.5
  jejunum 562.00
    with
      diverticulitis 562.01
        with hemorrhage 562.03
      hemorrhage 562.02
  kidney (calyx) (pelvis) 593.89
    with calculus 592.0
  Kommerell's 747.21

Diverticula, diverticulosis—*continued*
  laryngeal ventricle (congenital) 748.3
  Meckel's (displaced) (hypertrophic) 751.0
  midthoracic 530.6
  organ or site, congenital NEC—*see* Distortion
  pericardium (congenital) (cyst) 746.89
    acquired (true) 423.8
  pharyngoesophageal (pulsion) 530.6
  pharynx (congenital) 750.27
  pulsion (esophagus) 530.6
  rectosigmoid 562.10
    with
      diverticulitis 562.11
        with hemorrhage 562.13
      hemorrhage 562.12
    congenital 751.5
  rectum 562.10
    with
      diverticulitis 562.11
        with hemorrhage 562.13
      hemorrhage 562.12
  renal (calyces) (pelvis) 593.89
    with calculus 592.0
  Rokitansky's 530.6
  seminal vesicle 608.0
  sigmoid 562.10
    with
      diverticulitis 562.11
        with hemorrhage 562.13
      hemorrhage 562.12
    congenital 751.5
  small intestine 562.00
    with
      diverticulitis 562.01
        with hemorrhage 562.03
      hemorrhage 562.02
  stomach (cardia) (juxtacardia) (juxtapyloric)
      (acquired) 537.1
    congenital 750.7
  subdiaphragmatic 530.6
  trachea (congenital) 748.3
    acquired 519.1
  traction (esophagus) 530.6
  ureter (acquired) 593.89
    congenital 753.4
  ureterovesical orifice 593.89
  urethra (acquired) 599.2
    congenital 753.8
  ventricle, left (congenital) 746.89
  vesical (urinary) 596.3
    congenital 753.8
  Zenker's (esophagus) 530.6
Diverticulitis (acute) (*see also* Diverticula)
    562.11
  with hemorrhage 562.13
  bladder (urinary) 596.3
  cecum (perforated) 562.11
    with hemorrhage 562.13
  colon (perforated) 562.11
    with hemorrhage 562.13
  duodenum 562.01
    with hemorrhage 562.03
  esophagus 530.6
  ileum (perforated) 562.01
    with hemorrhage 562.03
  intestine (large) (perforated) 562.11
    with hemorrhage 562.13
    small 562.01
      with hemorrhage 562.03
  jejunum (perforated) 562.01
    with hemorrhage 562.03

Diverticulitis—*continued*
  Meckel's (perforated) 751.0
  pharyngoesophageal 530.6
  rectosigmoid (perforated) 562.11
    with hemorrhage 562.13
  rectum 562.11
    with hemorrhage 562.13
  sigmoid (old) (perforated) 562.11
    with hemorrhage 562.13
  small intestine (perforated) 562.01
    with hemorrhage 562.03
  vesical (urinary) 596.3
Diverticulosis —*see* Diverticula
Division
  cervix uteri 622.8
    external os into two openings by frenum
      752.49
  external (cervical) into two openings by frenum
      752.49
  glans penis 752.69
  hymen 752.49
  labia minora (congenital) 752.49
  ligament (partial or complete) (current)—*see*
      also Sprain, by site
    with open wound—*see* Wound, open, by site
  muscle (partial or complete) (current)—*see also*
      Sprain, by site
    with open wound—*see* Wound, open, by site
  nerve—*see* Injury, nerve, by site
  penis glans 752.69
  spinal cord—*see* Injury, spinal, by site
  vein 459.9
  traumatic—*see* Injury, vascular, by site
Divorce V61.0
Dix-Hallpike neurolabyrinthitis 386.12
Dizziness 780.4
  hysterical 300.11
  psychogenic 306.9
Doan-Wiseman syndrome (primary splenic
    neutropenia) 288.0
Dog bite —*see* Wound, open, by site
Döhle-Heller aortitis 093.1
Döhle body-panmyelopathic syndrome 288.2
Dolichocephaly, dolichocephalus 754.0
Dolichocolon 751.5
Dolichostenomelia 759.82
Donohue's syndrome (leprechaunism) 259.8
Donor
  blood V59.01
    other blood components V59.09
    stem cells V59.02
    whole blood V59.01
  bone V59.2
    marrow V59.3
  cornea V59.5
  heart V59.8
  kidney V59.4
  liver V59.6
  lung V59.8
  lymphocyte V59.8
  organ V59.9
    specified NEC V59.8
  potential, examination of V70.8
  skin V59.1
  specified organ or tissue NEC V59.8
  stem cells V59.02
  tissue V59.9
    specified type NEC V59.8
Donovanosis (granuloma venereum) 099.2
DOPS (diffuse obstructive pulmonary syndrome)
    496

Dry, dryness—*continued*
  mouth 527.7
  nose 478.1
  skin syndrome 701.1
  socket (teeth) 526.5
  throat 478.29
DSAP (disseminated superficial actinic
    porokeratosis) 692.75
Duane's retraction syndrome 378.71
Duane-Stilling-Turk syndrome (ocular
    retraction syndrome) 378.71
Dubin-Johnson disease or syndrome 277.4
Dubini's disease (electric chorea) 049.8
Dubois' abscess or disease 090.5
Duchenne's
  disease 094.0
    locomotor ataxia 094.0
    muscular dystrophy 359.1
    pseudohypertrophy, muscles 359.1
  paralysis 335.22
  syndrome 335.22
Duchenne-Aran myelopathic muscular atrophy
    (nonprogressive) (progressive) 335.21
Duchenne-Griesinger disease 359.1
Ducrey's
  bacillus 099.0
  chancre 099.0
  disease (chancroid) 099.0
Duct, ductus —*see* condition
Duengero 061
Duhring's disease (dermatitis herpetiformis)
    694.0
Dukes (-Filatov) disease 057.8
Dullness
  cardiac (decreased) (increased) 785.3
Dumb ague (*see also* Malaria) 084.6
Dumbness (*see also* Aphasia) 784.3
Dumdum fever 085.0
Dumping syndrome (postgastrectomy) 564.2
  nonsurgical 536.8
Duodenitis (nonspecific) (peptic) 535.60
  due to
    Strongyloides stercoralis 127.2
  with hemorrhage 535.61
Duodenocholangitis 575.8
Duodenum, duodenal —*see* condition
Duplay's disease, periarthritis, or syndrome 726.2
Duplex —*see also* Accessory
  kidney 753.3
  placenta—*see* Placenta, abnormal
  uterus 752.2
Duplication —*see also* Accessory
  anus 751.5
  aortic arch 747.21
  appendix 751.5
  biliary duct (any) 751.69
  bladder 753.8
  cecum 751.5
    and appendix 751.5
  clitoris 752.49
  cystic duct 751.69
  digestive organs 751.8
  duodenum 751.5
  esophagus 750.4
  fallopian tube 752.19
  frontonasal process 756.0
  gallbladder 751.69
  ileum 751.5
  intestine (large) (small) 751.5
  jejunum 751.5
  kidney 753.3

Duplication—*continued*
  liver 751.69
  nose 748.1
  pancreas 751.7
  penis 752.69
  respiratory organs NEC 748.9
  salivary duct 750.22
  spinal cord (incomplete) 742.51
  stomach 750.7
  ureter 753.4
  vagina 752.49
  vas deferens 752.8
  vocal cords 748.3
Dupré's disease or syndrome (meningism) 781.6
Dupuytren's
  contraction 728.6
  disease (muscle contracture) 728.6
  fracture (closed) 824.4
    ankle (closed) 824.4
      open 824.5
    fibula (closed) 824.4
      open 824.5
    open 824.5
    radius (closed) 813.42
      open 813.52
  muscle contracture 728.6
Durand-Nicolas-Favre disease (climatic bubo)
    099.1
Duroziez's disease (congenital mitral stenosis)
    746.5
Dust
  conjunctivitis 372.05
  reticulation (occupational) 504
Dutton's
  disease (trypanosomiasis) 086.9
  relapsing fever (West African) 087.1
Dwarf, dwarfism 259.4
  with infantilism (hypophyseal) 253.3
  achondroplastic 756.4
  Amsterdam 759.89
  bird-headed 759.89
  congenital 259.4
  constitutional 259.4
  hypophyseal 253.3
  infantile 259.4
  Levi type 253.3
  Lorain-Levi (pituitary) 253.3
  Lorain type (pituitary) 253.3
  metatropic 756.4
  nephrotic-glycosuric, with hypophosphatemic
    rickets 270.0
  nutritional 263.2
  ovarian 758.6
  pancreatic 577.8
  pituitary 253.3
  polydystrophic 277.5
  primordial 253.3
  psychosocial 259.4
  renal 588.0
    with hypertension—*see* Hypertension, kidney
  Russell's (uterine dwarfism and craniofacial
    dysostosis) 759.89
Dyke-Young anemia or syndrome (acquired
    macrocytic hemolytic anemia) (secondary)
    (symptomatic) 283.9
Dynia abnormality (*see also* Defect,
    coagulation) 286.9
Dysacousis 388.40
Dysadrenocortism 255.9
  hyperfunction 255.3
  hypofunction 255.4
Dysarthria 784.5

Dysautonomia (*see also* Neuropathy, peripheral, autonomic) 337.9
    familial 742.8
Dysbarism 993.3
Dysbasia 719.7
    angiosclerotica intermittens 443.9
    due to atherosclerosis 440.21
    hysterical 300.11
    lordotica (progressiva) 333.6
    nonorganic origin 307.9
    psychogenic 307.9
Dysbetalipoproteinemia (familial) 272.2
Dyscalculia 315.1
Dyschezia (*see also* Constipation) 564.00
Dyschondroplasia (with hemangiomata) 756.4
    Voorhoeve's 756.4
Dyschondrosteosis 756.59
Dyschromia 709.00
Dyscollagenosis 710.9
Dyscoria 743.41
Dyscraniopyophalangy 759.89
Dyscrasia
    blood 289.9
        with antepartum hemorrhage 641.3
        fetus or newborn NEC 776.9
        hemorrhage, subungual 287.8
        puerperal, postpartum 666.3
    ovary 256.8
    plasma cell 273.9
    pluriglandular 258.9
    polyglandular 258.9
Dysdiadochokinesia 781.3
Dysectasia, vesical neck 596.8
Dysendocrinism 259.9
Dysentery, dysenteric (bilious) (catarrhal) (diarrhea) (epidemic) (gangrenous) (hemorrhagic) (infectious) (sporadic) (tropical) (ulcerative) 009.0
    abscess, liver (*see also* Abscess, amebic) 006.3
    amebic (*see also* Amebiasis) 006.9
        with abscess—*see* Abscess, amebic
        acute 006.0
        carrier (suspected) of V02.2
        chronic 006.1
    arthritis (*see also* Arthritis, due to, dysentery) 009.0 *[711.3]*
        bacillary 004.9 *[711.3]*
    asylum 004.9
    bacillary 004.9
        arthritis 004.9 *[711.3]*
        Boyd 004.2
        Flexner 004.1
        Schmitz (-Stutzer) 004.0
        Shiga 004.0
        Shigella 004.9
            group A 004.0
            group B 004.1
            group C 004.2
            group D 004.3
            specified type NEC 004.8
        Sonne 004.3
        specified type NEC 004.8
    bacterium 004.9
    balantidial 007.0
    Balantidium coli 007.0
    Boyd's 004.2
    Chilomastix 007.8
    Chinese 004.9
    choleriform 001.1
    coccidial 007.2
    Dientamoeba fragilis 007.8

Dysentery, dysenteric—*continued*
    due to specified organism NEC—*see* Enteritis, due to, by organism
    Embadomonas 007.8
    Endolimax nana—*see* Dysentery, amebic
    Entamoba, entamebic—*see* Dysentery, amebic
    Flexner's 004.1
    Flexner-Boyd 004.2
    giardial 007.1
    Giardia lamblia 007.1
    Hiss-Russell 004.1
    lamblia 007.1
    leishmanial 085.0
    malarial (*see also* Malaria) 084.6
    metazoal 127.9
    Monilia 112.89
    protozoal NEC 007.9
    Russell's 004.8
    salmonella 003.0
    schistosomal 120.1
    Schmitz (-Stutzer) 004.0
    Shiga 004.0
    Shigella NEC (*see also* Dysentery, bacillary) 004.9
        boydii 004.2
        dysenteriae 004.0
            Schmitz 004.0
            Shiga 004.0
        flexneri 004.1
        Group A 004.0
        Group B 004.1
        Group C 004.2
        Group D 004.3
        Schmitz 004.0
        Shiga 004.0
        Sonnei 004.3
    Sonne 004.3
    strongyloidiasis 127.2
    trichomonal 007.3
    tuberculous (*see also* Tuberculosis) 014.8
    viral (*see also* Enteritis, viral) 008.8
Dysequilibrium 780.4
Dysesthesia 782.0
    hysterical 300.11
Dysfibrinogenemia (congenital) (*see also* Defect, coagulation) 286.3
Dysfunction
    adrenal (cortical) 255.9
        hyperfunction 255.3
        hypofunction 255.4
    associated with sleep stages or arousal from sleep 780.56
        nonorganic origin 307.47
    bladder NEC 596.59
    bleeding, uterus 626.8
    brain, minimal (*see also* Hyperkinesia) 314.9
    cerebral 348.3
    colon 564.9
        psychogenic 306.4
    colostomy or enterostomy 569.62
    cystic duct 575.8
    diastolic 429.9
        with heart failure—*see* Failure, heart
        due to
            cardiomyopathy—*see* Cardiomyopathy
            hypertension—*see* Hypertension, heart
    endocrine NEC 259.9
    endometrium 621.8
    enteric stoma 569.62
    enterostomy 569.62
    Eustachian tube 381.81

Dysfunction—*continued*
  gallbladder 575.8
  gastrointestinal 536.9
  gland, glandular NEC 259.9
  heart 427.9
    postoperative (immediate) 997.1
      long-term effect of cardiac surgery 429.4
  hemoglobin 288.8
  hepatic 573.9
  hepatocellular NEC 573.9
  hypophysis 253.9
    hyperfunction 253.1
    hypofunction 253.2
    posterior lobe 253.6
      hypofunction 253.5
  kidney (*see also* Disease, renal) 593.9
  labyrinthine 386.50
    specified NEC 386.58
  liver 573.9
    constitutional 277.4
  minimal brain (child) (*see also* Hyperkinesia)
    314.9
  ovary, ovarian 256.9
    hyperfunction 256.1
      estrogen 256.0
    hypofunction 256.39
      postablative 256.2
    postablative 256.2
    specified NEC 256.8
  papillary muscle 429.81
    with myocardial infarction 410.8
  parathyroid 252.8
    hyperfunction 252.0
    hypofunction 252.1
  pineal gland 259.8
  pituitary (gland) 253.9
    hyperfunction 253.1
    hypofunction 253.2
    posterior 253.6
      hypofunction 253.5
  placental—*see* Placenta, insufficiency
  platelets (blood) 287.1
  polyglandular 258.9
    specified NEC 258.8
  psychosexual 302.70
    with
      dyspareunia (functional) (psychogenic)
        302.76
      frigidity 302.72
      impotence 302.72
      inhibition
        orgasm
          female 302.73
          male 302.74
        sexual
          desire 302.71
          excitement 302.72
      premature ejaculation 302.75
      sexual aversion 302.79
      specified disorder NEC 302.79
      vaginismus 306.51
  pylorus 537.9
  rectum 564.9
    psychogenic 306.4
  segmental (*see also* Dysfunction, somatic) 739.9
  senile 797
  sinoatrial node 427.81
  somatic 739.9
    abdomen 739.9
    acromioclavicular 739.7
    cervical 739.1

Dysfunction— *continued*
    cervicothoracic 739.1
    costochondral 739.8
    costovertebral 739.8
    extremities
      lower 739.6
      upper 739.7
    head 739.0
    hip 739.5
    umbar, lumbosacral 739.3
    occipitocervical 739.0
    pelvic 739.5
    pubic 739.5
    rib cage 739.8
    sacral 739.4
    sacrococcygeal 739.4
    sacroiliac 739.4
    specified site NEC 739.9
    sternochondral 739.8
    sternoclavicular 739.7
    temporomandibular 739.0
    thoracic, thoracolumbar 739.2
  stomach 536.9
    psychogenic 306.4
  suprarenal 255.9
    hyperfunction 255.3
    hypofunction 255.4
  symbolic NEC 784.60
    specified type NEC 784.69
  temporomandibular (joint)
      (joint-pain-syndrome) NEC 524.60
    specified NEC 524.69
  testicular 257.9
    hyperfunction 257.0
    hypofunction 257.2
    specified type NEC 257.8
  thymus 254.9
  thyroid 246.9
    complicating pregnancy, childbirth, or
      puerperium 648.1
    hyperfunction—*see* Hyperthyroidism
    hypofunction—*see* Hypothyroidism
  uterus, complicating delivery 661.9
    affecting fetus or newborn 763.7
    hypertonic 661.4
    hypotonic 661.2
      primary 661.0
      secondary 661.1
  velopharyngeal (acquired) 528.9
    congenital 750.29
  ventricular 429.9
    with congestive heart failure (*see also* Failure,
      heart) 428.0
    due to
      cardiomyopathy—*see* Cardiomyopathy
      hypertension—*see* Hypertension, heart
  vesicourethral NEC 596.59
  vestibular 386.50
    specified type NEC 386.58
Dysgammaglobulinemia 279.06
Dysgenesis
  gonadal (due to chromosomal anomaly) 758.6
    pure 752.7
  kidney(s) 753.0
  ovarian 758.6
  renal 753.0
  reticular 279.2
  seminiferous tubules 758.6
  tidal platelet 287.3

Dysgerminoma (M9060/3)
  specified site—*see* Neoplasm, by site, malignant
  unspecified site
    female 183.0
    male 186.9
Dysgeusia 781.1
Dysgraphia 781.3
Dyshidrosis 705.81
Dysidrosis 705.81
Dysinsulinism 251.8
Dyskaryotic cervical smear 795.09
Dyskeratosis (*see also* Keratosis) 701.1
  bullosa hereditaria 757.39
  cervix 622.1
  congenital 757.39
  follicularis 757.39
    vitamin A deficiency 264.8
  gingiva 523.8
  oral soft tissue NEC 528.7
  tongue 528.7
  uterus NEC 621.8
Dyskinesia 781.3
  biliary 575.8
  esophagus 530.5
  hysterical 300.11
  intestinal 564.89
  nonorganic origin 307.9
  orofacial 333.82
  psychogenic 307.9
  tardive (oral) 333.82
Dyslalia 784.5
  developmental 315.39
Dyslexia 784.61
  developmental 315.02
  secondary to organic lesion 784.61
Dysmaturity (*see also* Immaturity) 765.1
  lung 770.4
  pulmonary 770.4
Dysmenorrhea (essential) (exfoliative)
    (functional) (intrinsic) (membranous)
    (primary) (secondary) 625.3
  psychogenic 306.52
Dysmetabolic syndrome X 277.7
Dysmetria 781.3
Dysmorodystrophia mesodermalis congenita
    759.82
Dysnomia 784.3
Dysorexia 783.0
  hysterical 300.11
Dysostosis
  cleidocranial, cleidocranialis 755.59
  craniofacial 756.0
  Fairbank's (idiopathic familial generalized
    osteophytosis) 756.50
  mandibularis 756.0
  mandibulofacial, incomplete 756.0
  multiplex 277.5
  orodigitofacial 759.89
Dyspareunia (female) 625.0
  male 608.89
  psychogenic 302.76
Dyspepsia (allergic) (congenital) (fermentative)
    (flatulent) (functional) (gastric)
    (gastrointestinal) (neurogenic) (occupational)
    (reflex) 536.8
  acid 536.8
  atonic 536.3
    psychogenic 306.4
  diarrhea 787.91
    psychogenic 306.4
  intestinal 564.89

Dyspepsia—*continued*
  psychogenic 306.4
  nervous 306.4
  neurotic 306.4
  psychogenic 306.4
Dysphagia 787.2
  functional 300.11
  hysterical 300.11
  nervous 300.11
  psychogenic 306.4
  sideropenic 280.8
  spastica 530.5
Dysphagocytosis, congenital 288.1
Dysphasia 784.5
Dysphonia 784.49
  clericorum 784.49
  functional 300.11
  hysterical 300.11
  psychogenic 306.1
  spastica 478.79
Dyspigmentation —*see also* Pigmentation
  eyelid (acquired) 374.52
Dyspituitarism 253.9
  hyperfunction 253.1
  hypofunction 253.2
  posterior lobe 253.6
Dysplasia —*see also* Anomaly
  artery
    fibromuscular NEC 447.8
      carotid 447.8
      renal 447.3
  bladder 596.8
  bone (fibrous) NEC 733.29
    diaphyseal, progressive 756.59
    jaw 526.89
    monostotic 733.29
    polyostotic 756.54
    solitary 733.29
  brain 742.9
  bronchopulmonary, fetus or newborn 770.7
  cervix (uteri) 622.1
    cervical intraepithelial neoplasia I [CIN 1]
      622.1
    cervical intraepithelial neoplasia II [CIN II]
      622.1
    cervical intraepithelial neoplasia III [CIN III]
      233.1
    CIN I 622.1
    CIN II 622.1
    CIN III 233.1
  chondroectodermal 756.55
  chondromatose 756.4
  craniocarpotarsal 759.89
  craniometaphyseal 756.89
  dentinal 520.5
  diaphyseal, progressive 756.59
  ectodermal (anhidrotic) (Bason) (Clouston's)
    (congenital) (Feinmesser) (hereditary)
    (hidrotic) (Marshall) (Robinson's) 757.31
  epiphysealis 756.9
    multiplex 756.56
    punctata 756.59
  epiphysis 756.9
    multiple 756.56
  epithelial
    epiglottis 478.79
    uterine cervix 622.1
  erythroid NEC 289.8
  eye (*see also* Microphthalmos) 743.10
  familial metaphyseal 756.89

Dysplasia—*continued*
  fibromuscular, artery NEC 447.8
    carotid 447.8
    renal 447.3
  fibrous
    bone NEC 733.29
    diaphyseal, progressive 756.59
    jaw 526.89
    monostotic 733.29
    polyostotic 756.54
    solitary 733.29
  high grade squamous intraepithelial (HGSIL) 622.1
  hip (congenital) 755.63
    with dislocation (*see also* Dislocation, hip, congenital) 754.30
  hypohidrotic ectodermal 757.31
  joint 755.8
  kidney 753.15
  leg 755.69
  linguofacialis 759.89
  low grade squamous intraepithelial (LGSIL) 622.1
  lung 748.5
  macular 743.55
  mammary (benign) (gland) 610.9
    cystic 610.1
    specified type NEC 610.8
  metaphyseal 756.9
    familial 756.89
  monostotic fibrous 733.29
  muscle 756.89
  myeloid NEC 289.8
  nervous system (general) 742.9
  neuroectodermal 759.6
  oculoauriculovertebral 756.0
  oculodentodigital 759.89
  olfactogenital 253.4
  osteo-onycho-arthro (hereditary) 756.89
  periosteum 733.99
  polyostotic fibrous 756.54
  progressive diaphyseal 756.59
  prostate 602.3
    intraepithelial neoplasia I [PIN I] 602.3
    intraepithelial neoplasia II [PIN II] 602.3
    intraepithelial neoplasia III [PIN III] 233.4
  renal 753.15
  renofacialis 753.0
  retinal NEC 743.56
  retrolental 362.21
  spinal cord 742.9
  thymic, with immunodeficiency 279.2
  vagina 623.0
  vocal cord 478.5
  vulva 624.8
    intraepithelial neoplasia I [VIN I] 624.8
    intraepithelial neoplasia II [VIN II] 624.8
    intraepithelial neoplasia III [VIN III] 233.3
    VIN I 624.8
    VIN II 624.8
    VIN III 233.3
Dyspnea (nocturnal) (paroxysmal) 786.09
  asthmatic (bronchial) (*see also* Asthma) 493.9
    with bronchitis (*see also* Asthma) 493.9
      chronic 493.2
    cardiac (*see also* Failure, ventricular, left) 428.1
  cardiac (*see also* Failure, ventricular, left) 428.1
  functional 300.11
  hyperventilation 786.01
  hysterical 300.11

Dyspnea—*continued*
  Monday morning 504
  newborn 770.89
  psychogenic 306.1
  uremic—*see* Uremia
Dyspraxia 781.3
  syndrome 315.4
Dysproteinemia 273.8
  transient with copper deficiency 281.4
Dysprothrombinemia (constitutional) (*see also* Defect, coagulation) 286.3
Dysreflexia , autonomic 337.3
Dysrhythmia
  cardiac 427.9
    postoperative (immediate) 997.1
      long-term effect of cardiac surgery 429.4
    specified type NEC 427.89
  cerebral or cortical 348.3
Dyssecretosis, mucoserous 710.2
Dyssocial reaction without manifest psychiatric disorder
  adolescent V71.02
  adult V71.01
  child V71.02
Dyssomnia NEC 780.56
  nonorganic origin 307.47
Dyssplenism 289.4
Dyssynergia
  biliary (*see also* Disease, biliary) 576.8
  cerebellaris myoclonica 334.2
  detrusor sphincter (bladder) 596.55
  ventricular 429.89
Dystasia, hereditary areflexic 334.3
Dysthymia 300.4
Dysthymic disorder 300.4
Dysthyroidism 246.9
Dystocia 660.9
  affecting fetus or newborn 763.1
  cervical 661.0
    affecting fetus or newborn 763.7
  contraction ring 661.4
    affecting fetus or newborn 763.7
  fetal 660.9
    abnormal size 653.5
    affecting fetus or newborn 763.1
    deformity 653.7
  maternal 660.9
    affecting fetus or newborn 763.1
  positional 660.0
    affecting fetus or newborn 763.1
  shoulder (girdle) 660.4
    affecting fetus or newborn 763.1
  uterine NEC 661.4
    affecting fetus or newborn 763.7
Dystonia
  deformans progressiva 333.6
  due to drugs 333.7
  lenticularis 333.6
  musculorum deformans 333.6
  torsion (idiopathic) 333.6
    fragments (of) 333.89
    symptomatic 333.7
Dystonic
  movements 781.0
Dystopia kidney 753.3
Dystrophy, dystrophia 783.9
  adiposogenital 253.8
  asphyxiating thoracic 756.4
  Becker's type 359.1
  brevicollis 756.16
  Bruch's membrane 362.77

Dystrophy, dystrophia—*continued*
cervical (sympathetic) NEC 337.0
chondro-osseus with punctate epiphyseal
dysplasia 756.59
choroid (hereditary) 363.50
central (areolar) (partial) 363.53
total (gyrate) 363.54
circinate 363.53
circumpapillary (partial) 363.51
total 363.52
diffuse
partial 363.56
total 363.57
generalized
partial 363.56
total 363.57
gyrate
central 363.54
generalized 363.57
helicoid 363.52
peripapillary—*see* Dystrophy, choroid,
circumpapillary
serpiginous 363.54
cornea (hereditary) 371.50
anterior NEC 371.52
Cogan's 371.52
combined 371.57
crystalline 371.56
endothelial (Fuchs') 371.57
epithelial 371.50
juvenile 371.51
microscopic cystic 371.52
granular 371.53
lattice 371.54
macular 371.55
marginal (Terrien's) 371.48
Meesman's 371.51
microscopic cystic (epithelial) 371.52
nodular, Salzmann's 371.46
polymorphous 371.58
posterior NEC 371.58
ring-like 371.52
Salzmann's nodular 371.46
stromal NEC 371.56
dermatochondrocorneal 371.50
Duchenne's 359.1
due to malnutrition 263.9
Erb's 359.1
familial
hyperplastic periosteal 756.59
osseous 277.5
foveal 362.77
Fuchs', cornea 371.57
Gowers' muscular 359.1
hair 704.2
hereditary, progressive muscular 359.1
hypogenital, with diabetic tendency 759.81
Landouzy-Déjérine 359.1
Leyden-Möbius 359.1
mesodermalis congenita 759.82
muscular 359.1
congenital (hereditary) 359.0
myotonic 359.2
distal 359.1
Duchenne's 359.1
Erb's 359.1
fascioscapulohumeral 359.1
Gowers' 359.1
hereditary (progressive) 359.1
Landouzy-Déjérine 359.1
limb-girdle 359.1

Dystrophy, dystrophia—*continued*
myotonic 359.2
progressive (hereditary) 359.1
Charcot-Marie-Tooth 356.1
pseudohypertrophic (infantile) 359.1
myocardium, myocardial (*see also*
Degeneration, myocardial) 429.1
myotonic 359.2
myotonica 359.2
nail 703.8
congenital 757.5
neurovascular (traumatic) (*see also* Neuropathy,
peripheral, autonomic) 337.9
nutritional 263.9
ocular 359.1
oculocerebrorenal 270.8
oculopharyngeal 359.1
ovarian 620.8
papillary (and pigmentary) 701.1
pelvicrural atrophic 359.1
pigmentary (*see also* Acanthosis) 701.2
pituitary (gland) 253.8
polyglandular 258.8
posttraumatic sympathetic—*see* Dystrophy,
sympathetic
progressive ophthalmoplegic 359.1
retina, retinal (hereditary) 362.70
albipunctate 362.74
Bruch's membrane 362.77
cone, progressive 362.75
hyaline 362.77
in
Bassen-Kornzweig syndrome 272.5 *[362.72]*
cerebroretinal lipidosis 330.1 *[362.71]*
Refsum's disease 356.3 *[362.72]*
systemic lipidosis 272.7 *[362.71]*
juvenile (Stargardt's) 362.75
pigmentary 362.74
pigment epithelium 362.76
progressive cone (-rod) 362.75
pseudoinflammatory foveal 362.77
rod, progressive 362.75
sensory 362.75
vitelliform 362.76
Salzmann's nodular 371.46
scapuloperoneal 359.1
skin NEC 709.9
sympathetic (posttraumatic) (reflex) 337.20
lower limb 337.22
specified NEC 337.29
upper limb 337.21
tapetoretinal NEC 362.74
thoracic asphyxiating 756.4
unguium 703.8
congenital 757.5
vitreoretinal (primary) 362.73
secondary 362.66
vulva 624.0
Dysuria 788.1
psychogenic 306.53

E

Eagle-Barrett syndrome 756.71
Eales' disease (syndrome) 362.18
Ear —*see also* condition
  ache 388.70
    otogenic 388.71
    referred 388.72
  lop 744.29
  piercing V50.3
  swimmers' acute 380.12
  tank 380.12
  tropical 111.8 *[380.15]*
  wax 380.4
Earache 388.70
  otogenic 388.71
  referred 388.72
Eaton-Lambert syndrome (*see also* Neoplasm,
  by site, malignant) 199.1 *[358.1]*
Eberth's disease (typhoid fever) 002.0
Ebstein's
  anomaly or syndrome (downward displacement,
    tricuspid valve into right ventricle) 746.2
  disease (diabetes) 250.4 *[581.81]*
Eccentro-osteochondrodysplasia 277.5
Ecchondroma (M9210/0)—*see* Neoplasm, bone,
  benign
Ecchondrosis (M9210/1) 238.0
Ecchordosis physaliphora 756.0
Ecchymosis (multiple) 459.89
  conjunctiva 372.72
  eye (traumatic) 921.0
  eyelids (traumatic) 921.1
  newborn 772.6
  spontaneous 782.7
  traumatic—*see* Contusion
Echinococciasis —*see* Echinococcus
Echinococcosis —*see* Echinococcus
Echinococcus (infection) 122.9
  granulosus 122.4
    liver 122.0
    lung 122.1
    orbit 122.3 *[376.13]*
    specified site NEC 122.3
    thyroid 122.2
  liver NEC 122.8
    granulosus 122.0
    multilocularis 122.5
  lung NEC 122.9
    granulosus 122.1
    multilocularis 122.6
  multilocularis 122.7
    liver 122.5
    specified site NEC 122.6
  orbit 122.9 *[376.13]*
    granulosus 122.3 *[376.13]*
    multilocularis 122.6 *[376.13]*
  specified site NEC 122.9
    granulosus 122.3
    multilocularis 122.6 *[376.13]*
  thyroid NEC 122.9
    granulosus 122.2
    multilocularis 122.6
Echinorhynchiasis 127.7
Echinostomiasis 121.8
Echolalia 784.69
ECHO virus infection NEC 079.1

Eclampsia, eclamptic (coma) (convulsions)
  (delirium) 780.39
  female, child-bearing age NEC—*see* Eclampsia,
    pregnancy
  gravidarum—*see* Eclampsia, pregnancy
  male 780.39
  not associated with pregnancy or childbirth
    780.39
  pregnancy, childbirth or puerperium 642.6
    with pre-existing hypertension 642.7
    affecting fetus or newborn 760.0
  uremic 586
Eclipse blindness (total) 363.31
Economic circumstance affecting care V60.9
  specified type NEC V60.8
Economo's disease (encephalitis lethargica)
  049.8
Ectasia, ectasis
  aorta (*see also* Aneurysm, aorta) 441.9
    ruptured 441.5
  breast 610.4
  capillary 448.9
  cornea (marginal) (postinfectional) 371.71
  duct (mammary) 610.4
  kidney 593.89
  mammary duct (gland) 610.4
  papillary 448.9
  renal 593.89
  salivary gland (duct) 527.8
  scar, cornea 371.71
  sclera 379.11
Ecthyma 686.8
  contagiosum 051.2
  gangrenosum 686.09
  infectiosum 051.2
Ectocardia 746.87
Ectodermal dysplasia, congenital 757.31
Ectodermosis erosiva pluriorificialis 695.1
Ectopic, ectopia (congenital) 759.89
  abdominal viscera 751.8
    due to defect in anterior abdominal wall
      756.79
  ACTH syndrome 255.0
  adrenal gland 759.1
  anus 751.5
  auricular beats 427.61
  beats 427.60
  bladder 753.5
  bone and cartilage in lung 748.69
  brain 742.4
  breast tissue 757.6
  cardiac 746.87
  cerebral 742.4
  cordis 746.87
  endometrium 617.9
  gallbladder 751.69
  gastric mucosa 750.7
  gestation—*see* Pregnancy, ectopic
  heart 746.87
  hormone secretion NEC 259.3
  hyperparathyroidism 259.3
  kidney (crossed) (intrathoracic) (pelvis) 753.3
    in pregnancy or childbirth 654.4
      causing obstructed labor 660.2
  lens 743.37
  lentis 743.37
  mole—*see* Pregnancy, ectopic

Ectopic, ectopia—*continued*
   organ or site NEC—*see* Malposition, congenital
   ovary 752.0
   pancreas, pancreatic tissue 751.7
   pregnancy—*see* Pregnancy, ectopic
   pupil 364.75
   renal 753.3
   sebaceous glands of mouth 750.26
   secretion
      ACTH 255.0
      adrenal hormone 259.3
      adrenalin 259.3
      adrenocorticotropin 255.0
      antidiuretic hormone (ADH) 259.3
      epinephrine 259.3
      hormone NEC 259.3
      norepinephrine 259.3
      pituitary (posterior) 259.3
   spleen 759.0
   testis 752.51
   thyroid 759.2
   ureter 753.4
   ventricular beats 427.69
   vesicae 753.5
Ectrodactyly 755.4
   finger (*see also* Absence, finger, congenital)
      755.29
   toe (*see also* Absence, toe, congenital) 755.39
Ectromelia 755.4
   lower limb 755.30
   upper limb 755.20
Ectropion 374.10
   anus 569.49
   cervix 622.0
      with mention of cervicitis 616.0
   cicatricial 374.14
   congenital 743.62
   eyelid 374.10
      cicatricial 374.14
      congenital 743.62
      mechanical 374.12
      paralytic 374.12
      senile 374.11
      spastic 374.13
   iris (pigment epithelium) 364.54
   lip (congenital) 750.26
      acquired 528.5
   mechanical 374.12
   paralytic 374.12
   rectum 569.49
   senile 374.11
   spastic 374.13
   urethra 599.84
   uvea 364.54
Eczema (acute) (allergic) (chronic)
   (erythematous) (fissum) (occupational)
   (rubrum) (squamous) 692.9
   asteatotic 706.8
   atopic 691.8
   contact NEC 692.9
   dermatitis NEC 692.9
   due to specified cause—*see* Dermatitis, due to
   dyshidrotic 705.81
   external ear 380.22
   flexural 691.8
   gouty 274.89
   herpeticum 054.0
   hypertrophicum 701.8
   hypostatic—*see* Varicose, vein

Eczema—*continued*
   impetiginous 684
   infantile (acute) (chronic) (due to any
      substance) (intertriginous) (seborrheic)
      690.12
   intertriginous NEC 692.9
      infantile 690.12
   intrinsic 691.8
   lichenified NEC 692.9
   marginatum 110.3
   nummular 692.9
   pustular 686.8
   seborrheic 690.18
      infantile 690.12
   solare 692.72
   stasis (lower extremity) 454.1
      ulcerated 454.2
   vaccination, vaccinatum 999.0
   varicose (lower extremity)—*see* Varicose, vein
   verrucosum callosum 698.3
Eczematoid, exudative 691.8
Eddowes' syndrome (brittle bones and blue
   sclera) 756.51
Edema, edematous 782.3
   with nephritis (*see also* Nephrosis) 581.9
   allergic 995.1
   angioneurotic (allergic) (any site) (with
      urticaria) 995.1
      hereditary 277.6
   angiospastic 443.9
   Berlin's (traumatic) 921.3
   brain 348.5
      due to birth injury 767.8
      fetus or newborn 767.8
   cardiac (*see also* Failure, heart) 428.0
   cardiovascular (*see also* Failure, heart) 428.0
   cerebral—*see* Edema, brain
   cerebrospinal vessel—*see* Edema, brain
   cervix (acute) (uteri) 622.8
      puerperal, postpartum 674.8
   chronic hereditary 757.0
   circumscribed, acute 995.1
      hereditary 277.6
   complicating pregnancy (gestational) 646.1
      with hypertension—*see* Toxemia, of
         pregnancy
   conjunctiva 372.73
   connective tissue 782.3
   cornea 371.20
      due to contact lenses 371.24
      idiopathic 371.21
      secondary 371.22
   due to
      lymphatic obstruction—*see* Edema, lymphatic
      salt retention 276.0
   epiglottis—*see* Edema, glottis
   essential, acute 995.1
      hereditary 277.6
   extremities, lower—*see* Edema, legs
   eyelid NEC 374.82
   familial, hereditary (legs) 757.0
   famine 262
   fetus or newborn 778.5
   genital organs
      female 629.8
      male 608.86
   gestational 646.1
      with hypertension—*see* Toxemia, of
         pregnancy

Edema, edematous—*continued*
  glottis, glottic, glottides (obstructive) (passive) 478.6
    allergic 995.1
      hereditary 277.6
    due to external agent—*see* Condition, respiratory, acute, due to specified agent
  heart (*see also* Failure, heart) 428.0
    newborn 779.89
  heat 992.7
  hereditary (legs) 757.0
  inanition 262
  infectious 782.3
  intracranial 348.5
    due to injury at birth 767.8
  iris 364.8
  joint (*see also* Effusion, joint) 719.0
  larynx (*see also* Edema, glottis) 478.6
  legs 782.3
    due to venous obstruction 459.2
    hereditary 757.0
  localized 782.3
    due to venous obstruction 459.2
      lower extremity 459.2
  lower extremities—*see* Edema, legs
  lungs 514
    acute 518.4
      with heart disease or failure (*see also* Failure, ventricular, left) 428.1
        congestive 428.0
      chemical (due to fumes or vapors) 506.1
      due to
        external agent(s) NEC 508.9
          specified NEC 508.8
        fumes and vapors (chemical) (inhalation) 506.1
        radiation 508.0
    chemical (acute) 506.1
      chronic 506.4
    chronic 514
      chemical (due to fumes or vapors) 506.4
      due to
        external agent(s) NEC 508.9
          specified NEC 508.8
        fumes or vapors (chemical) (inhalation) 506.4
        radiation 508.1
    due to
      external agent 508.9
        specified NEC 508.8
      high altitude 993.2
      near drowning 994.1
    postoperative 518.4
    terminal 514
  lymphatic 457.1
    due to mastectomy operation 457.0
  macula 362.83
    cystoid 362.53
    diabetic 250.5 *[362.01]*
  malignant (*see also* Gangrene, gas) 040.0
  Milroy's 757.0
  nasopharynx 478.25
  neonatorum 778.5
  nutritional (newborn) 262
    with dyspigmentation, skin and hair 260
  optic disc or nerve—*see* Papilledema
  orbit 376.33
    circulatory 459.89
  palate (soft) (hard) 528.9
  pancreas 577.8
  penis 607.83

Edema, edematous—*continued*
  periodic 995.1
    hereditary 277.6
  pharynx 478.25
  pitting 782.3
  pulmonary—*see* Edema, lung
  Quincke's 995.1
    hereditary 277.6
  renal (*see also* Nephrosis) 581.9
  retina (localized) (macular) (peripheral) 362.83
    cystoid 362.53
    diabetic 250.5 *[362.01]*
  salt 276.0
  scrotum 608.86
  seminal vesicle 608.86
  spermatic cord 608.86
  spinal cord 336.1
  starvation 262
  stasis (*see also* Hypertension, venous) 459.30
  subconjunctival 372.73
  subglottic (*see also* Edema, glottis) 478.6
  supraglottic (*see also* Edema, glottis) 478.6
  testis 608.86
  toxic NEC 782.3
  traumatic NEC 782.3
  tunica vaginalis 608.86
  vas deferens 608.86
  vocal cord—*see* Edema, glottis
  vulva (acute) 624.8
Edentia (complete) (partial) (*see also* Absence, tooth) 520.0
  acquired 525.10
    due to
      caries 525.13
      extraction 525.10
      periodontal disease 525.12
      specified NEC 525.19
      trauma 525.11
  causing malocclusion 524.3
  congenital (deficiency of tooth buds) 520.0
Edentulism 525.10
Edsall's disease 992.2
Educational handicap V62.3
Edwards' syndrome 758.2
Effect, adverse NEC
  abnormal gravitational (G) forces or states 994.9
  air pressure—*see* Effect, adverse, atmospheric pressure
  altitude (high)—*see* Effect, adverse, high altitude
  anesthetic
    in labor and delivery NEC 668.9
      affecting fetus or newborn 763.5
  antitoxin—*see* Complications, vaccination
  atmospheric pressure 993.9
    due to explosion 993.4
    high 993.3
    low—*see* Effect, adverse, high altitude
    specified effect NEC 993.8
  biological, correct substance properly administered (*see also* Effect, adverse, drug) 995.2
  blood (derivatives) (serum) (transfusion)—*see* Complications, transfusion
  chemical substance NEC 989.9
    specified—*see* Table of drugs and chemicals
  cobalt, radioactive (*see also* Effect, adverse, radioactive substance) 990
  cold (temperature) (weather) 991.9
    chilblains 991.5
    frostbite—*see* Frostbite

Effect, adverse—*continued*
  specified effect NEC 991.8
  drugs and medicinals NEC 995.2
    correct substance properly administered 995.2
    overdose or wrong substance given or taken 977.9
      specified drug—*see* Table of drugs and chemicals
  electric current (shock) 994.8
    burn—*see* Burn, by site
  electricity (electrocution) (shock) 994.8
    burn—*see* Burn, by site
  exertion (excessive) 994.5
  exposure 994.9
    exhaustion 994.4
  external cause NEC 994.9
  fallout (radioactive) NEC 990
  fluoroscopy NEC 990
  foodstuffs
    allergic reaction (*see also* Allergy, food) 693.1
      anaphylactic shock due to food NEC 995.60
    noxious 988.9
      specified type NEC (*see also* Poisoning, by name of noxious foodstuff) 988.8
  gases, fumes, or vapors—*see* Table of drugs and chemicals
  glue (airplane) sniffing 304.6
  heat—*see* Heat
  high altitude NEC 993.2
    anoxia 993.2
    on
      fears 993.0
      sinuses 993.1
    polycythemia 289.0
  hot weather—*see* Heat
  hunger 994.2
  immersion, foot 991.4
  immunization—*see* Complications, vaccination
  immunological agents—*see* Complications, vaccination
  implantation (removable) of isotope or radium NEC 990
  infrared (radiation) (rays) NEC 990
    burn—*see* Burn, by site
    dermatitis or eczema 692.82
  infusion—*see* Complications, infusion
  ingestion or injection of isotope (therapeutic) NEC 990
  irradiation NEC (*see also* Effect, adverse, radiation) 990
  isotope (radioactive) NEC 990
  lack of care (child) (infant) (newborn) 995.52
    adult 995.84
  lightning 994.0
    burn—*see* Burn, by site
  Lirugin—*see* Complications, vaccination
  medicinal substance, correct, properly administered (*see also* Effect, adverse, drugs) 995.2
  mesothorium NEC 990
  motion 994.6
  noise, inner ear 388.10
  overheated places—*see* Heat
  polonium NEC 990
  psychosocial, of work environment V62.1
  radiation (diagnostic) (fallout) (infrared) (natural source) (therapeutic) (tracer) (ultraviolet) (x-ray) NEC 990

Effect, adverse—*continued*
  with pulmonary manifestations
    acute 508.0
    chronic 508.1
  dermatitis or eczema 692.82
    due to sun NEC (*see also* Dermatitis, due to, sun) 692.70
  fibrosis of lungs 508.1
  maternal with suspected damage to fetus
    affecting management of pregnancy 655.6
  pneumonitis 508.0
  radioactive substance NEC 990
    dermatitis or eczema 692.82
  radioactivity NEC 990
  radiotherapy NEC 990
    dermatitis or eczema 692.82
  radium NEC 990
  reduced temperature 991.9
    frostbite—*see* Frostbite
    immersion, foot (hand) 991.4
    specified effect NEC 991.8
  roentgenography NEC 990
  roentgenoscopy NEC 990
  roentgen rays NEC 990
  serum (prophylactic) (therapeutic) NEC 999.5
  specified NEC 995.89
    external cause NEC 994.9
  strangulation 994.7
  submersion 994.1
  teletherapy NEC 990
  thirst 994.3
  transfusion—*see* Complications, transfusion
  ultraviolet (radiation) (rays) NEC 990
    burn—*see also* Burn, by site
    from sun (*see also* Sunburn) 692.71
    dermatitis or eczema 692.82
    due to sun NEC (*see also* Dermatitis, due to, sun) 692.70
  uranium NEC 990
  vaccine (any)—*see* Complications, vaccination
  weightlessness 994.9
  whole blood—*see also* Complications, transfusion
    overdose or wrong substance given (*see also* Table of drugs and chemicals) 964.7
  working environment V62.1
  x-rays NEC 990
    dermatitis or eczema 692.82
Effect, remote
  of cancer, —*see* condition
Effects, late —*see* Late, effect (of)
Effluvium, telogen 704.02
Effort
  intolerance 306.2
  syndrome (aviators) (psychogenic) 306.2
Effusion
  Amniotic fluid (*see also* Rupture, membranes, premature) 658.1
  brain (serous) 348.5
  bronchial (*see also* Bronchitis) 490
  cerebral 348.5
  cerebrospinal (*see also* Meningitis) 322.9
    vessel 348.5
  chest—*see* Effusion, pleura
  intracranial 348.5
  joint 719.00
    ankle 719.07
    elbow 719.02
    foot 719.07
    hand 719.04

Effusion—*continued*
    hip 719.05
    knee 719.06
    multiple sites 719.09
    pelvic region 719.05
    shoulder (region) 719.01
    specified site NEC 719.08
    wrist 719.03
  meninges (*see also* Meningitis) 322.9
  pericardium, pericardial (*see also* Pericarditis)
        423.9
    acute 420.90
  peritoneal (chronic) 568.82
  pleura, pleurisy, pleuritic, pleuropericardial
        511.9
    bacterial, nontuberculous 511.1
    fetus or newborn 511.9
    malignant 197.2
    nontuberculous 511.9
      bacterial 511.1
    pneumococcal 511.1
    staphylococcal 511.1
    streptococcal 511.1
    tuberculous (*see also* Tuberculosis, pleura)
        012.0
      primary progressive 010.1
    traumatic 862.29
      with open wound 862.39
  pulmonary—*see* Effusion, pleura
  spinal (*see also* Meningitis) 322.9
  thorax, thoracic—*see* Effusion, pleura
Eggshell nails 703.8
  congenital 757.5
Ego-dystonic
  homosexuality 302.0
  lesbianism 302.0
Egyptian splenomegaly 120.1
Ehlers-Danlos syndrome 756.83
Ehrlichiosis 082.40
  chaffeensis 082.41
  specified type NEC 082.49
Eichstedt's disease (pityriasis versicolor) 111.0
Eisenmenger's complex or syndrome
    (ventricular septal defect) 745.4
Ejaculation, semen
  painful 608.89
    psychogenic 306.59
  premature 302.75
  retrograde 608.87
Ekbom syndrome (restless legs) 333.99
Ekman's syndrome (brittle bones and blue
    sclera) 756.51
Elastic skin 756.83
  acquired 701.8
Elastofibroma (M8820/0)—*see* Neoplasm,
    connective tissue, benign
Elastoidosis
  cutanea nodularis 701.8
  cutis cystica et comedonica 701.8
Elastoma 757.39
  juvenile 757.39
  Miescher's (elastosis perforans serpiginosa)
        701.1
Elastomyofibrosis 425.3
Elastosis 701.8
  atrophicans 701.8
  perforans serpiginosa 701.1
  reactive perforating 701.1
  senilis 701.8
  solar (actinic) 692.74
Elbow —*see* condition

Electric
  current, electricity, effects (concussion) (fatal)
      (nonfatal) (shock) 994.8
    burn—*see* Burn, by site
  feet (foot) syndrome 266.2
Electrocution 994.8
Electrolyte imbalance 276.9
  with
    abortion—*see* Abortion, by type, with
        metabolic disorder
    ectopic pregnancy (*see also* categories
        633.0-633.9) 639.4
    hyperemesis gravidarum (before 22 completed
        weeks gestation) 643.1
    molar pregnancy (*see also* categories
        630-632) 639.4
  following
    abortion 639.4
    ectopic or molar pregnancy 639.4
Elephant man syndrome 237.71
Elephantiasis (nonfilarial) 457.1
  arabicum (*see also* Infestation, filarial) 125.9
  congenita hereditaria 757.0
  congenital (any site) 757.0
  due to
    Brugia (malayi) 125.1
    mastectomy operation 457.0
    Wuchereria (bancrofti) 125.0
      malayi 125.1
  eyelid 374.83
  filarial (*see also* Infestation, filarial) 125.9
  filariensis (*see also* Infestation, filarial) 125.9
  gingival 523.8
  glandular 457.1
  graecorum 030.9
  lymphangiectatic 457.1
  lymphatic vessel 457.1
    due to mastectomy operation 457.0
  neuromatosa 237.71
  postmastectomy 457.0
  scrotum 457.1
  streptococcal 457.1
  surgical 997.99
    postmastectomy 457.0
  telangiectodes 457.1
  vulva (nonfilarial) 624.8
Elevated —*see* Elevation
Elevation
  17-ketosteroids 791.9
  acid phosphatase 790.5
  alkaline phosphatase 790.5
  amylase 790.5
  antibody titers 795.79
  basal metabolic rate (BMR) 794.7
  blood pressure (*see also* Hypertension) 401.9
    reading (incidental) (isolated) (nonspecific),
        no diagnosis of hypertension 796.2
  body temperature (of unknown origin) (*see also*
      Pyrexia) 780.6
  conjugate, eye 378.81
  diaphragm, congenital 756.6
  immunoglobulin level 795.79
  indolacetic acid 791.9
  lactic acid dehydrogenase (LDH) level 790.4
  lipase 790.5
  prostate specific antigen (PSA) 790.93
  renin 790.99
    in hypertension (*see also* Hypertension,
        renovascular) 405.91
  Rh titer 999.7
  scapula, congenital 755.52

Elevation—*continued*
  sedimentation rate 790.1
  SGOT 790.4
  SGPT 790.4
  transaminase 790.4
  vanillylmandelic acid 791.9
  venous pressure 459.89
  VMA 791.9
Elliptocytosis (congenital) (hereditary) 282.1
  Hb-C (disease) 282.7
  hemoglobin disease 282.7
  sickle-cell (disease) 282.60
    trait 282.5
Ellis-van Creveld disease or syndrome
  (chondroectodermal dysplasia) 756.55
Ellison-Zollinger syndrome (gastric
  hypersecretion with pancreatic islet cell
  tumor) 251.5
Elongation, elongated (congenital)—*see also*
  Distortion
  bone 756.9
  cervix (uteri) 752.49
    acquired 622.6
    hypertrophic 622.6
  colon 751.5
  common bile duct 751.69
  cystic duct 751.69
  frenulum, penis 752.69
  labia minora, acquired 624.8
  ligamentum patellae 756.89
  petiolus (epiglottidis) 748.3
  styloid bone (process) 733.99
  tooth, teeth 520.2
  uvula 750.26
    acquired 528.9
Elschnig bodies or pearls 366.51
El Tor cholera 001.1
Emaciation (due to malnutrition) 261
Emancipation disorder 309.22
Embadomoniasis 007.8
Embarrassment heart, cardiac —*see* Disease,
  heart
Embedded tooth, teeth 520.6
  with abnormal position (same or adjacent tooth)
    524.3
  root only 525.3
Embolic —*see* condition
Embolism 444.9
  with
    abortion—*see* Abortion, by type, with
      embolism
    ectopic pregnancy (*see also* categories
      633.0-633.9) 639.6
    molar pregnancy (*see also* categories
      630-632) 639.6
  air (any site) 958.0
    with
      abortion—*see* Abortion, by type, with
        embolism
      ectopic pregnancy (*see also* categories
        633.0-633.9) 639.6
      molar pregnancy (*see also* categories
        630-632) 639.6
    due to implanted device—*see* Complications,
      due to (presence of) any device, implant,
      or graft classified to 996.0-996.5 NEC
    following
      abortion 639.6
      ectopic or molar pregnancy 639.6
    infusion, perfusion, or transfusion 999.1

Embolism—*continued*
  in pregnancy, childbirth, or puerperium 673.0
    traumatic 958.0
  amniotic fluid (pulmonary) 673.1
    with
      abortion—*see* Abortion, by type, with
        embolism
      ectopic pregnancy (*see also* categories
        633.0-633.9) 639.6
      molar pregnancy (*see also* categories
        630-632) 639.6
    following
      abortion 639.6
      ectopic or molar pregnancy 639.6
  aorta, aortic 444.1
    abdominal 444.0
    bifurcation 444.0
    saddle 444.0
    thoracic 444.1
  artery 444.9
    auditory, internal 433.8
    basilar (*see also* Occlusion, artery, basilar)
      433.0
    bladder 444.89
    carotid (common) (internal) (*see also*
      Occlusion, artery, carotid) 433.1
    cerebellar (anterior inferior) (posterior
      inferior) (superior) 433.8
    cerebral (*see also* Embolism, brain) 434.1
    choroidal (anterior) 433.8
    communicating posterior 433.8
    coronary (*see also* Infarct, myocardium) 410.9
      without myocardial infarction 411.81
    extremity 444.22
      lower 444.22
      upper 444.21
    hypophyseal 433.8
    mesenteric (with gangrene) 557.0
    ophthalmic (*see also* Occlusion, retina) 362.30
    peripheral 444.22
    pontine 433.8
    precerebral NEC—*see* Occlusion, artery,
      precerebral
    pulmonary—*see* Embolism, pulmonary
    renal 593.81
    retinal (*see also* Occlusion, retina) 362.30
    specified site NEC 444.89
    vertebral (*see also* Occlusion, artery,
      vertebral) 433.2
  auditory, internal 433.8
  basilar (artery) (*see also* Occlusion, artery,
    basilar) 433.0
  birth, mother—*see* Embolism, obstetrical
  blood-clot
    with
      abortion—*see* Abortion, by type, with
        embolism
      ectopic pregnancy (*see also* categories
        633.0-633.9) 639.6
      molar pregnancy (*see also* categories
        630-632) 639.6
    following
      abortion 639.6
      ectopic or molar pregnancy 639.6
    in pregnancy, childbirth, or puerperium 673.2
  brain 434.1
    with
      abortion—*see* Abortion, by type, with
        embolism
      ectopic pregnancy (*see also* categories
        633.0-633.9) 639.6

Embolism—*continued*
  molar pregnancy (*see also* categories
    630-632) 639.6
  following
    abortion 639.6
    ectopic or molar pregnancy 639.6
  late effect—*see* Late effect(s) (of)
    cerebrovascular disease
  puerperal, postpartum, childbirth 674.0
capillary 448.9
cardiac (*see also* Infarct, myocardium) 410.9
carotid (artery) (common) (internal) (*see also*
  Occlusion, artery, carotid) 433.1
cavernous sinus (venous)—*see* Embolism,
  intracranial venous sinus
cerebral (*see also* Embolism, brain) 434.1
cholesterol —*see* Atheroembolism
choroidal (anterior) (artery) 433.8
coronary (artery or vein) (systemic) (*see also*
  Infarct, myocardium) 410.9
  without myocardial infarction 411.81
due to (presence of) any device, implant, or
  graft classifiable to 996.0-996.5 —*see*
  Complications, due to (presence of) any
  device, implant, or graft classified to
  996.0-996.5 NEC
encephalomalacia (*see also* Embolism, brain)
  434.1
extremities 444.22
  lower 444.22
  upper 444.21
eye 362.30
fat (cerebral) (pulmonary) (systemic) 958.1
  with
    abortion—*see* Abortion, by type, with
      embolism
    ectopic pregnancy (*see also* categories
      633.0-633.9) 639.6
    molar pregnancy (*see also* categories
      630-632) 639.6
  complicating delivery or puerperium 673.8
  following
    abortion 639.6
    ectopic or molar pregnancy 639.6
  in pregnancy, childbirth, or the puerperium
    673.8
femoral (artery) 444.22
  vein 453.8
following
  abortion 639.6
  ectopic or molar pregnancy 639.6
  infusion, perfusion, or transfusion
    air 999.1
    thrombus 999.2
heart (fatty) (*see also* Infarct, myocardium)
  410.9
hepatic (vein) 453.0
iliac (artery) 444.81
iliofemoral 444.81
in pregnancy, childbirth, or puerperium
  (pulmonary)—*see* Embolism, obstetrical
intestine (artery) (vein) (with gangrene) 557.0
intracranial (*see also* Embolism, brain) 434.1
  venous sinus (any) 325
    late effect—*see* category 326

Embolism—*continued*
  nonpyogenic 437.6
    in pregnancy or puerperium 671.5
kidney (artery) 593.81
lateral sinus (venous)—*see* Embolism,
  intracranial venous sinus
longitudinal sinus (venous)—*see* Embolism,
  intracranial venous sinus
lower extremity 444.22
lung (massive)—*see* Embolism, pulmonary
meninges (*see also* Embolism, brain) 434.1
mesenteric (artery) (with gangrene) 557.0
multiple NEC 444.9
obstetrical (pulmonary) 673.2
  air 673.0
  amniotic fluid (pulmonary) 673.1
  blood-clot 673.2
  cardiac 674.8
  fat 673.8
  heart 674.8
  pyemic 673.3
  septic 673.3
  specified NEC 674.8
ophthalmic (*see also* Occlusion, retina) 362.30
paradoxical NEC 444.9
penis 607.82
peripheral arteries NEC 444.22
  lower 444.22
  upper 444.21
pituitary 253.8
popliteal (artery) 444.22
portal (vein) 452
postoperative NEC 997.2
  cerebral 997.02
  mesenteric artery 997.71
  other vessels 997.79
  peripheral vascular 997.2
  pulmonary 415.11
  renal artery 997.72
precerebral artery (*see also* Occlusion, artery,
  precerebral) 433.9
puerperal—*see* Embolism, obstetrical
pulmonary (artery) (vein) 415.1
  with
    abortion—*see* Abortion, by type, with
      embolism
    ectopic pregnancy (*see also* categories
      633.0-633.9) 639.6
    molar pregnancy (*see also* categories
      630-632) 639.6
  following
    abortion 639.6
    ectopic or molar pregnancy 639.6
  iatrogenic 415.11
  in pregnancy, childbirth, or puerperium—*see*
    Embolism, obstetrical
  postoperative 415.11
pyemic (multiple) 038.9
  with
    abortion—*see* Abortion, by type, with
      embolism
    ectopic pregnancy (*see also* categories
      633.0-633.9) 639.6
    molar pregnancy (*see also* categories
      630-632) 639.6
  Aerobacter aerogenes 038.49
  enteric gram-negative bacilli 038.40
  Enterobacter aerogenes 038.49
  Escherichia coli 038.42

Embolism—*continued*
  following
    abortion 639.6
    ectopic or molar pregnancy 639.6
    Hemophilus influenzae 038.41
    pneumococcal 038.2
    Proteus vulgaris 038.49
    Pseudomonas (aeruginosa) 038.43
    puerperal, postpartum, childbirth (any
      organism) 673.3
    Serratia 038.44
    specified organism NEC 038.8
    staphylococcal 038.10
      aureus 038.11
      specified organism NEC 038.19
    streptococcal 038.0
  renal (artery) 593.81
    vein 453.3
  retina, retinal (*see also* Occlusion, retina) 362.30
  saddle (aorta) 444.0
  septicemic—*see* Embolism, pyemic
  sinus—*see* Embolism, intracranial venous sinus
  soap
    with
      abortion—*see* Abortion, by type, with
        embolism
      ectopic pregnancy (*see also* categories
        633.0-633.9) 639.6
      molar pregnancy (*see also* categories
        630-632) 639.6
    following
      abortion 639.6
      ectopic or molar pregnancy 639.6
  spinal cord (nonpyogenic) 336.1
    in pregnancy or puerperium 671.5
    pyogenic origin 324.1
      late effect—*see* category 326
  spleen, splenic (artery) 444.89
  thrombus (thromboembolism) following
    infusion, perfusion, or transfusion 999.2
  upper extremity 444.21
  vein 453.9
    with inflammation or phlebitis—*see*
      Thrombophlebitis
    cerebral (*see also* Embolism, brain) 434.1
    coronary (*see also* Infarct, myocardium) 410.9
      without myocardial infarction 411.81
    hepatic 453.0
    mesenteric (with gangrene) 557.0
    portal 452
    pulmonary—*see* Embolism, pulmonary
    renal 453.3
    specified NEC 453.8
      with inflammation or phlebitis—*see*
      Thrombophlebitis
  vena cava (inferior) (superior) 453.2
  vessels of brain (*see also* Embolism, brain)
    434.1
Embolization —*see* Embolism
Embolus —*see* Embolism
Embryoma (M9080/1)—*see also* Neoplasm, by
  site, uncertain behavior
  benign (M9080/0)—*see* Neoplasm, by site,
    benign
  kidney (M8960/3) 189.0
  liver (M8970/3) 155.0
  malignant (M9080/3)—*see also* Neoplasm, by
    site, malignant
  kidney (M8960/3) 189.0
  liver (M8970/3) 155.0
  testis (M9070/3) 186.9

Embryoma—*continued*
  undescended 186.0
  testis (M9070/3) 186.9
    undescended 186.0
Embryonic
  circulation 747.9
  heart 747.9
  vas deferens 752.8
Embryopathia NEC 759.9
Embryotomy, fetal 763.89
Embryotoxon 743.43
  interfering with vision 743.42
Emesis —*see also* Vomiting
  gravidarum—*see* Hyperemesis, gravidarum
Emissions, nocturnal (semen) 608.89
Emotional
  crisis—*see* Crisis, emotional
  disorder (*see also* Disorder, mental) 300.9
  instability (excessive) 301.3
  overlay—*see* Reaction, adjustment
  upset 300.9
Emotionality, pathological 301.3
Emotogenic disease (*see also* Disorder,
  psychogenic) 306.9
Emphysema (atrophic) (centriacinar)
  (centrilobular) (chronic) (diffuse) (essential)
  (hypertrophic) (interlobular) (lung)
  (obstructive) (panlobular) (paracicatricial)
  (paracinar) (postural) (pulmonary) (senile)
  (subpleural) (traction) (unilateral) (unilobular)
  (vesicular) 492.8
  with
    bronchitis
      acute and chronic 491.21
      chronic 491.20
        with acute bronchitis or acute
        exacerbation 491.21
  bullous (giant) 492.0
  cellular tissue 958.7
    surgical 998.81
  compensatory 518.2
  congenital 770.2
  conjunctiva 372.89
  connective tissue 958.7
    surgical 998.81
  due to fumes or vapors 506.4
  eye 376.89
  eyelid 374.85
    surgical 998.81
    traumatic 958.7
  fetus or newborn (interstitial) (mediastinal)
    (unilobular) 770.2
  heart 416.9
  interstitial 518.1
    congenital 770.2
    fetus or newborn 770.2
  laminated tissue 958.7
    surgical 998.81
  mediastinal 518.1
    fetus or newborn 770.2
  newborn (interstitial) (mediastinal) (unilobular)
    770.2
  obstructive diffuse with fibrosis 492.8
  orbit 376.89
  subcutaneous 958.7
    due to trauma 958.7
    nontraumatic 518.1
    surgical 998.81
  surgical 998.81
  thymus (gland) (congenital) 254.8
  traumatic 958.7

Emphysema—*continued*
  tuberculous (*see also* Tuberculosis, pulmonary)
    011.9
Employment examination (certification) V70.5
Empty sella (turcica) syndrome 253.8
Empyema (chest) (diaphragmatic) (double)
  (encapsulated) (general) (interlobar) (lung)
  (medial) (necessitatis) (perforating chest wall)
  (pleura) (pneumococcal) (residual)
  (sacculated) (streptococcal)
  (supradiaphragmatic) 510.9
  with fistula 510.0
  accessory sinus (chronic) (*see also* Sinusitis)
    473.9
  acute 510.9
    with fistula 510.0
  antrum (chronic) (*see also* Sinusitis, maxillary)
    473.0
  brain (any part) (*see also* Abscess, brain) 324.0
  ethmoidal (sinus) (chronic) (*see also* Sinusitis,
    ethmoidal) 473.2
  extradural (*see also* Abscess, extradural) 324.9
  frontal (sinus) (chronic) (*see also* Sinusitis,
    frontal) 473.1
  gallbladder (*see also* Cholecystitis, acute) 575.0
  mastoid (process) (acute) (*see also* Mastoiditis,
    acute) 383.00
  maxilla, maxillary 526.4
    sinus (chronic) (*see also* Sinusitis, maxillary)
      473.0
  nasal sinus (chronic) (*see also* Sinusitis) 473.9
  sinus (accessory) (nasal) (*see also* Sinusitis)
    473.9
  sphenoidal (chronic) (sinus) (*see also* Sinusitis,
    sphenoidal) 473.3
  subarachnoid (*see also* Abscess, extradural)
    324.9
  subdural (*see also* Abscess, extradural) 324.9
  tuberculous (*see also* Tuberculosis, pleura)
    012.0
  ureter (*see also* Ureteritis) 593.89
  ventricular (*see also* Abscess, brain) 324.0
Enameloma 520.2
Encephalitis (bacterial) (chronic) (hemorrhagic)
  (idiopathic) (nonepidemic) (spurious)
  (subacute) 323.9
  acute—*see also* Encephalitis, viral
    disseminated (postinfectious) NEC 136.9
      [323.6]
      postimmunization or postvaccination 323.5
    inclusional 049.8
    inclusion body 049.8
    necrotizing 049.8
  arboviral, arbovirus NEC 064
  arthropod-borne (*see also* Encephalitis, viral,
    arthropod-borne) 064
  Australian X 062.4
  Bwamba fever 066.3
  California (virus) 062.5
  Central European 063.2
  Czechoslovakian 063.2
  Dawson's (inclusion body) 046.2
  diffuse sclerosing 046.2
  due to
    actinomycosis 039.8 *[323.4]*
    cat-scratch disease 078.3 *[323.0]*
    infectious mononucleosis 075 *[323.0]*
    malaria (*see also* Malaria) 084.6 *[323.2]*
    Negishi virus 064
    ornithosis 073.7 *[323.0]*

Encephalitis—*continued*
  prophylactic inoculation against smallpox
    323.5
  rickettsiosis (*see also* Rickettsiosis) 083.9
    [323.1]
  rubella 056.01
  toxoplasmosis (acquired) 130.0
    congenital (active) 771.2 *[323.4]*
  typhus (fever) (*see also* Typhus) 081.9 *[323.1]*
  vaccination (smallpox) 323.5
  Eastern equine 062.2
  endemic 049.8
  epidemic 049.8
  equine (acute) (infectious) (viral) 062.9
    Eastern 062.2
    Venezuelan 066.2
    Western 062.1
  Far Eastern 063.0
  following vaccination or other immunization
    procedure 323.5
  herpes 054.3
  Ilheus (virus) 062.8
  inclusion body 046.2
  infectious (acute) (virus) NEC 049.8
  influenzal 487.8 *[323.4]*
    lethargic 049.8
  Japanese (B type) 062.0
  La Crosse 062.5
  Langat 063.8
  late effect—*see* Late, effect, encephalitis
  lead 984.9 *[323.7]*
  lethargic (acute) (infectious) (influenzal) 049.8
  lethargica 049.8
  louping ill 063.1
  lupus 710.0 *[323.8]*
  lymphatica 049.0
  Mengo 049.8
  meningococcal 036.1
  mumps 072.2
  Murray Valley 062.4
  myoclonic 049.8
  Negishi virus 064
  otitic NEC 382.4 *[323.4]*
  parasitic NEC 123.9 *[323.4]*
  periaxialis (concentrica) (diffusa) 341.1
  postchickenpox 052.0
  postexanthematous NEC 057.9 *[323.6]*
  postimmunization 323.5
  postinfectious NEC 136.9 *[323.6]*
  postmeasles 055.0
  posttraumatic 323.8
  postvaccinal (smallpox) 323.5
  postvaricella 052.0
  postviral NEC 079.99 *[323.6]*
    postexanthematous 057.9 *[323.6]*
    specified NEC 057.8 *[323.6]*
  Powassan 063.8
  progressive subcortical (Binswanger's) 290.12
  Rio Bravo 049.8
  rubella 056.01
  Russian
    autumnal 062.0
    spring-summer type (taiga) 063.0
  saturnine 984.9 *[323.7]*
  Semliki Forest 062.8
  serous 048
  slow-acting virus NEC 046.8
  specified cause NEC 323.8
  St. Louis type 062.3
  subacute sclerosing 046.2
  subcorticalis chronica 290.12

Encephalitis—*continued*
  summer 062.0
  suppurative 324.0
  syphilitic 094.81
    congenital 090.41
  tick-borne 063.9
  torula, torular 117.5 *[323.4]*
  toxic NEC 989.9 *[323.7]*
  toxoplasmic (acquired) 130.0
    congenital (active) 771.2 *[323.4]*
  trichinosis 124 *[323.4]*
  Trypanosomiasis (*see also* Trypanosomiasis)
    086.9 *[323.2]*
  tuberculous (*see also* Tuberculosis) 013.6
  type B (Japanese) 062.0
  type C 062.3
  van Bogaert's 046.2
  Venezuelan 066.2
  Vienna type 049.8
  viral, virus 049.9
    arthropod-borne NEC 064
      mosquito-borne 062.9
        Australian X disease 062.4
        California virus 062.5
        Eastern equine 062.2
        Ilheus virus 062.8
        Japanese (B type) 062.0
        Murray Valley 062.4
        specified type NEC 062.8
        St. Louis 062.3
        type B 062.0
        type C 062.3
        Western equine 062.1
      tick-borne 063.9
        biundulant 063.2
        Central European 063.2
        Czechoslovakian 063.2
        diphasic meningoencephalitis 063.2
        Far Eastern 063.0
        Langat 063.8
        louping ill 063.1
        Powassan 063.8
        Russian spring-summer (taiga) 063.0
        specified type NEC 063.8
      vector unknown 064
    slow acting NEC 046.8
    specified type NEC 049.8
    vaccination, prophylactic (against) V05.0
  von Economo's 049.8
  Western equine 062.1
  West Nile type 066.4
Encephalocele 742.0
  orbit 376.81
Encephalocystocele 742.0
Encephalomalacia (brain) (cerebellar) (cerebral)
    (cerebrospinal) (*see also* Softening, brain)
    434.9
  due to
    hemorrhage (*see also* Hemorrhage, brain) 431
    recurrent spasm of artery 435.9
  embolic (cerebral) (*see also* Embolism, brain)
    434.1
  subcorticalis chronica arteriosclerotica 290.12
  thrombotic (*see also* Thrombosis, brain) 434.0
Encephalomeningitis —*see* Meningoencephalitis
Encephalomeningocele 742.0
Encephalomeningomyelitis —*see*
    Meningoencephalitis
Encephalomeningopathy (*see also*
    Meningoencephalitis) 349.9

Encephalomyelitis (chronic) (granulomatous)
    (hemorrhagic necrotizing, acute) (myalgic,
    benign) (*see also* Encephalitis) 323.9
  abortive disseminated 049.8
  acute disseminated (postinfectious) 136.9
    [323.6]
    postimmunization 323.5
  due to or resulting from vaccination (any) 323.5
  equine (acute) (infectious) 062.9
    Eastern 062.2
    Venezuelan 066.2
    Western 062.1
  funicularis infectiosa 049.8
  late effect—*see* Late, effect, encephalitis
  Munch-Peterson's 049.8
  postchickenpox 052.0
  postimmunization 323.5
  postmeasles 055.0
  postvaccinal (smallpox) 323.5
  rubella 056.01
  specified cause NEC 323.8
  syphilitic 094.81
Encephalomyelocele 742.0
Encephalomyelomeningitis —*see*
    Meningoencephalitis
Encephalomyeloneuropathy 349.9
Encephalomyelopathy 349.9
  subacute necrotizing (infantile) 330.8
Encephalomyeloradiculitis (acute) 357.0
Encephalomyeloradiculoneuritis (acute) 357.0
Encephalomyeloradiculopathy 349.9
Encephalomyocarditis 074.23
Encephalopathia hyperbilirubinemica
    newborn 774.7
  due to isoimmunization (conditions classifiable
    to 773.0-773.2) 773.4
Encephalopathy (acute) 348.3
  alcoholic 291.2
  anoxic—*see* Damage, brain, anoxic
  arteriosclerotic 437.0
    late effect—*see* Late effect(s) (of)
      cerebrovascular disease
  bilirubin, newborn 774.7
    due to isoimmunization 773.4
  congenital 742.9
  demyelinating (callosal) 341.8
  due to
    birth injury (intracranial) 767.8
    dialysis 294.8
      transient 293.9
    hyperinsulinism—*see* Hyperinsulinism
    influenza (virus) 487.8
    lack of vitamin (*see also* Deficiency, vitamin)
      269.2
    nicotinic acid deficiency 291.2
    serum (nontherapeutic) (therapeutic) 999.5
    syphilis 094.81
    trauma (postconcussional) 310.2
      current (*see also* Concussion, brain) 850.9
        with skull fracture—*see* Fracture, skull, by
          site, with intracranial injury
    vaccination 323.5
  hepatic 572.2
  hyperbilirubinemic, newborn 774.7
    due to isoimmunization (conditions
      classifiable to 773.0-773.2) 773.4
  hypertensive 437.2
  hypoglycemic 251.2
  hypoxic—*see* Damage, brain, anoxic
  infantile cystic necrotizing (congenital) 341.8

Encephalopathy—*continued*
lead 984.9 *[323.7]*
leukopolio 330.0
metabolic (toxic)—*see* Delirium
necrotizing, subacute 330.8
pellagrous 265.2
portal-systemic 572.2
postcontusional 310.2
posttraumatic 310.2
saturnine 984.9 *[323.7]*
spongioform, subacute (viral) 046.1
subacute
necrotizing 330.8
spongioform 046.1
viral, spongioform 046.1
subcortical progressive (Schilder) 341.1
chronic (Binswanger's) 290.12
toxic 349.82
metabolic—*see* Delirium
traumatic (postconcussional) 310.2
current (*see also* Concussion, brain) 850.9
with skull fracture—*see* Fracture, skull, by
site, with intracranial injury
vitamin B deficiency NEC 266.9
Wernicke's (superior hemorrhagic
polioencephalitis) 265.1
Enchephalorrhagia (*see also* Hemorrhage,
brain) 432.9
healed or old V12.59
late effect—*see* Late effect(s) (of)
cerebrovascular disease
Encephalosis, posttraumatic 310.2
Enchondroma (M9220/0)—*see also* Neoplasm,
bone, benign
multiple, congenital 756.4
Enchondromatosis (cartilaginous) (congenital)
(multiple) 756.4
Enchondroses, multiple (cartilaginous)
(congenital) 756.4
Encopresis (*see also* Incontinence, feces) 787.6
nonorganic origin 307.7
Encounter for —*see also* Admission for
administrative purpose only V68.9
referral of patient without examination or
treatment V68.81
specified purpose NEC V68.89
chemotherapy V58.1
end-of-life care V66.7
hospice care V66.7
palliative care V66.7
radiotherapy V58.0
screening mammogram NEC V76.12
for high-risk patient V76.11
paternity testing V70.4
terminal care V66.7
Encystment —*see* Cyst
End-of-life care V66.7
Endamebiasis —*see* Amebiasis
Endamoeba —*see* Amebiasis
Endarteritis (bacterial, subacute) (infective)
(septic) 447.6
brain, cerebral or cerebrospinal 437.4
late effect—*see* Late effect(s) (of)
cerebrovascular disease
coronary (artery) —*see* Arteriosclerosis,
coronary
deformans—*see* Arteriosclerosis
embolic (*see also* Embolism) 444.9
obliterans—*see also* Arteriosclerosis
pulmonary 417.8
pulmonary 417.8

Endarteritis—*continued*
retina 362.18
senile—*see* Arteriosclerosis
syphilitic 093.89
brain or cerebral 094.89
congenital 090.5
spinal 094.89
tuberculous (*see also* Tuberculosis) 017.9
Endemic —*see* condition
Endocarditis (chronic) (indeterminate)
(interstitial) (marantis) (nonbacterial
thrombotic) (residual) (sclerotic) (sclerous)
(senile) (valvular) 424.90
with
rheumatic fever (conditions classifiable to 390)
active—*see* Endocarditis, acute, rheumatic
inactive or quiescent (with chorea) 397.9
acute or subacute 421.9
rheumatic (aortic) (mitral) (pulmonary)
(tricuspid) 391.1
with chorea (acute) (rheumatic)
(Sydenham's) 392.0
aortic (heart) (nonrheumatic) (valve) 424.1
with
mitral (valve) disease 396.9
active or acute 391.1
with chorea (acute) (rheumatic)
(Sydenham's) 392.0
rheumatic fever (conditions classifiable to
390)
active—*see* Endocarditis, acute, rheumatic
inactive or quiescent (with chorea) 395.9
with mitral disease 396.9
acute or subacute 421.9
arteriosclerotic 424.1
congenital 746.89
hypertensive 424.1
rheumatic (chronic) (inactive) 395.9
with mitral (valve) disease 396.9
active or acute 391.1
with chorea (acute) (rheumatic)
(Sydenham's) 392.0
active or acute 391.1
with chorea (acute) (rheumatic)
(Sydenham's) 392.0
specified cause, except rheumatic 424.1
syphilitic 093.22
arteriosclerotic or due to arteriosclerosis 424.99
atypical verrucous (Libman-Sacks) 710.0
[424.91]
bacterial (acute) (any valve) (chronic)
(subacute) 421.0
blastomycotic 116.0 *[421.1]*
candidal 112.81
congenital 425.3
constrictive 421.0
Coxsackie 074.22
due to
blastomycosis 116.0 *[421.1]*
candidiasis 112.81
Coxsackie (virus) 074.22
disseminated lupus erythematosus 710.0
[424.91]
histoplasmosis (*see also* Histoplasmosis)
115.94
hypertension (benign) 424.99
moniliasis 112.81
prosthetic cardiac valve 996.61
Q fever 083.0 *[421.1]*
serratia marcescens 421.0
typhoid (fever) 002.0 *[421.1]*

Endocarditis—*continued*
fetal 425.3
gonococcal 098.84
hypertensive 424.99
infectious or infective (acute) (any valve)
   (chronic) (subacute) 421.0
lenta (acute) (any valve) (chronic) (subacute)
   421.0
Libman-Sacks 710.0 *[424.91]*
Loeffler's (parietal fibroplastic) 421.0
malignant (acute) (any valve) (chronic)
   (subacute) 421.0
meningococcal 036.42
mitral (chronic) (double) (fibroid) (heart)
   (inactive) (valve) (with chorea) 394.9
  with
    aortic (valve) disease 396.9
     active or acute 391.1
      with chorea (acute) (rheumatic)
       (Sydenham's) 392.0
    rheumatic fever (conditions classifiable to
     390)
     active—*see* Endocarditis, acute, rheumatic
     inactive or quiescent (with chorea) 394.9
      with aortic valve disease 396.9
  active or acute 391.1
    bacterial 421.0
    with chorea (acute) (rheumatic)
     (Sydenham's) 392.0
  arteriosclerotic 424.0
  congenital 746.89
  hypertensive 424.0
  nonrheumatic 424.0
    acute or subacute 421.9
  syphilitic 093.21
monilial 112.81
mycotic (acute) (any valve) (chronic) (subacute)
   421.0
pneumococcic (acute) (any valve) (chronic)
   (subacute) 421.0
pulmonary (chronic) (heart) (valve) 424.3
  with
    rheumatic fever (conditions classifiable to
     390)
     active—*see* Endocarditis, acute, rheumatic
     inactive or quiescent (with chorea) 397.1
  acute or subacute 421.9
  rheumatic 391.1
    with chorea (acute) (rheumatic)
     (Sydenham's) 392.0
  arteriosclerotic or due to arteriosclerosis 424.3
  congenital 746.09
  hypertensive or due to hypertension (benign)
    424.3
  rheumatic (chronic) (inactive) (with chorea)
    397.1
    active or acute 391.1
    with chorea (acute) (rheumatic)
     (Sydenham's) 392.0
  syphilitic 093.24
purulent (acute) (any valve) (chronic)
   (subacute) 421.0
rheumatic (chronic) (inactive) (with chorea)
   397.9
  active or acute (aortic) (mitral) (pulmonary)
    (tricuspid) 391.1
    with chorea (acute) (rheumatic)
     (Sydenham's) 392.0
septic (acute) (any valve) (chronic) (subacute)
   421.0
specified cause, except rheumatic 424.99

Endocarditis—*continued*
streptococcal (acute) (any valve) (chronic)
   (subacute) 421.0
subacute—*see* Endocarditis, acute
suppurative (any valve) (acute) (chronic)
   (subacute) 421.0
syphilitic NEC 093.20
toxic (*see also* Endocarditis, acute) 421.9
tricuspid (chronic) (heart) (inactive) (rheumatic)
   (valve) (with chorea) 397.0
  with
    rheumatic fever (conditions classifiable to
     390)
     active—*see* Endocarditis, acute, rheumatic
     inactive or quiescent (with chorea) 397.0
  active or acute 391.1
    with chorea (acute) (rheumatic)
     (Sydenham's) 392.0
  arteriosclerotic 424.2
  congenital 746.89
  hypertensive 424.2
  nonrheumatic 424.2
    acute or subacute 421.9
  specified cause, except rheumatic 424.2
  syphilitic 093.23
tuberculous (*see also* Tuberculosis) 017.9
   [424.91]
typhoid 002.0 *[421.1]*
ulcerative (acute) (any valve) (chronic)
   (subacute) 421.0
vegetative (acute) (any valve) (chronic)
   (subacute) 421.0
verrucous (acute) (any valve) (chronic)
   (subacute) NEC 710.0 *[424.91]*
  nonbacterial 710.0 *[424.91]*
  nonrheumatic 710.0 *[424.91]*
Endocardium, endocardial —*see also* condition
cushion defect 745.60
  specified type NEC 745.69
Endocervicitis (*see also* Cervicitis) 616.0
due to
  intrauterine (contraceptive) device 996.65
gonorrheal (acute) 098.15
  chronic or duration of 2 months or over 098.35
hyperplastic 616.0
syphilitic 095.8
trichomonal 131.09
tuberculous (*see also* Tuberculosis) 016.7
Endocrine —*see* condition
Endocrinopathy, pluriglandular 258.9
Endodontitis 522.0
Endomastoiditis (*see also* Mastoiditis) 383.9
Endometrioma 617.9
Endometriosis 617.9
appendix 617.5
bladder 617.8
bowel 617.5
broad ligament 617.3
cervix 617.0
colon 617.5
cul-de-sac (Douglas') 617.3
exocervix 617.0
fallopian tube 617.2
female genital organ NEC 617.8
gallbladder 617.8
in scar of skin 617.6
internal 617.0
intestine 617.5
lung 617.8
myometrium 617.0
ovary 617.1

Endometriosis—*continued*
  parametrium 617.3
  pelvic peritoneum 617.3
  peritoneal (pelvic) 617.3
  rectovaginal septum 617.4
  rectum 617.5
  round ligament 617.3
  skin 617.6
  specified site NEC 617.8
  stromal (M8931/1) 236.0
  umbilicus 617.8
  uterus 617.0
    internal 617.0
  vagina 617.4
  vulva 617.8
Endometritis (nonspecific) (purulent) (septic)
    (suppurative) 615.9
  with
    abortion—*see* Abortion, by type, with sepsis
    ectopic pregnancy (*see also* categories
      633.0-633.9) 639.0
    molar pregnancy (*see also* categories
      630-632) 639.0
  acute 615.0
  blennorrhagic 098.16
    acute 098.16
    chronic or duration of 2 months or over 098.36
  cervix, cervical (*see also* Cervicitis) 616.0
    hyperplastic 616.0
  chronic 615.1
  complicating pregnancy 646.6
    affecting fetus or newborn 760.8
  decidual 615.9
  following
    abortion 639.0
    ectopic or molar pregnancy 639.0
  gonorrheal (acute) 098.16
    chronic or duration of 2 months or over 098.36
  hyperplastic 621.3
    cervix 616.0
  polypoid—*see* Endometritis, hyperplastic
  puerperal, postpartum, childbirth 670
  senile (atrophic) 615.9
  subacute 615.0
  tuberculous (*see also* Tuberculosis) 016.7
Endometrium —*see* condition
Endomyocardiopathy, South African 425.2
Endomyocarditis —*see* Endocarditis
Endomyofibrosis 425.0
Endomyometritis (*see also* Endometritis) 615.9
Endopericarditis —*see* Endocarditis
Endoperineuritis —*see* Disorder, nerve
Endophlebitis (*see also* Phlebitis) 451.9
  leg 451.2
    deep (vessels) 451.19
    superficial (vessels) 451.0
  portal (vein) 572.1
  retina 362.18
  specified site NEC 451.89
  syphilitic 093.89
Endophthalmia (*see also* Endophthalmitis)
    360.0
  gonorrheal 098.42
Endophthalmitis (globe) (infective) (metastatic)
    (purulent) (subacute) 360.00
  acute 360.01
  chronic 360.03
  parasitic 360.13
  phacoanaphylactic 360.19
  specified type NEC 360.19
  sympathetic 360.11

Endosalpingioma (M9111/1) 236.2
Endosteitis —*see* Osteomyelitis
Endothelioma, bone (M9260/3)—*see* Neoplasm,
    bone, malignant
Endotheliosis 287.8
  hemorrhagic infectional 287.8
Endotoxic shock 785.59
Endotrachelitis (*see also* Cervicitis) 616.0
Enema rash 692.89
Engel-von Recklinghausen disease or syndrome
    (osteitis fibrosa cystica) 252.0
Engelmann's disease (diaphyseal sclerosis)
    756.59
English disease (*see also* Rickets) 268.0
Engman's disease (infectious eczematoid
    dermatitis) 690.8
Engorgement
  breast 611.79
    newborn 778.7
    puerperal, postpartum 676.2
  liver 573.9
  lung 514
  pulmonary 514
  retina, venous 362.37
  stomach 536.8
  venous, retina 362.37
Enlargement, enlarged —*see also* Hypertrophy
  abdomen 789.3
  adenoids 474.12
    and tonsils 474.10
  alveolar process or ridge 525.8
  apertures of diaphragm (congenital) 756.6
  blind spot, visual field 368.42
  gingival 523.8
  heart, cardiac (*see also* Hypertrophy, cardiac)
    429.3
  lacrimal gland, chronic 375.03
  liver (*see also* Hypertrophy, liver) 789.1
  lymph gland or node 785.6
  orbit 376.46
  organ or site, congenital NEC—*see* Anomaly,
    specified type NEC
  parathyroid (gland) 252.0
  pituitary fossa 793.0
  prostate (simple) (soft) 600.0
  sella turcica 793.0
  spleen (*see also* Splenomegaly) 789.2
    congenital 759.0
  thymus (congenital) (gland) 254.0
  thyroid (gland) (*see also* Goiter) 240.9
  tongue 529.8
  tonsils 474.11
    and adenoids 474.10
  uterus 621.2
Enophthalmos 376.50
  due to
    atrophy of orbital tissue 376.51
    surgery 376.52
    trauma 376.52
Enostosis 526.89
Entamebiasis —*see* Amebiasis
Entamebic —*see* Amebiasis
Entanglement, umbilical cord (s) 663.3
  with compression 663.2
    affecting fetus or newborn 762.5
  around neck with compression 663.1
  twins in monoamniotic sac 663.2
Enteralgia 789.0
Enteric —*see* condition

Enteritis (acute) (catarrhal) (choleraic) (chronic)
(congestive) (diarrheal) (exudative)
(follicular) (hemorrhagic) (infantile)
(lienteric) (noninfectious) (perforative)
(phlegmonous) (presumed noninfectious)
(pseudomembranous) 558.9
adaptive 564.9
aertrycke infection 003.0
allergic 558.3
amebic (*see also* Amebiasis) 006.9
  with abscess—*see* Abscess, amebic
  acute 006.0
    with abscess—*see* Abscess, amebic
    nondysenteric 006.2
  chronic 006.1
    with abscess—*see* Abscess, amebic
    nondysenteric 006.2
  nondysenteric 006.2
anaerobic (cocci) (gram-negative)
  (gram-positive) (mixed) NEC 008.46
bacillary NEC 004.9
bacterial NEC 008.5
  specified NEC 008.49
Bacteroides (fragilis) (melaninogeniscus)
  (oralis) 008.46
Butyrivibrio (fibriosolvens) 008.46
Campylobacter 008.43
Candida 112.85
Chilomastix 007.8
choleriformis 001.1
chronic 558.9
  ulcerative (*see also* Colitis, ulcerative) 556.9
cicatrizing (chronic) 555.0
Clostridium
  botulinum 005.1
  difficile 008.45
  haemolyticum 008.46
  novyi 008.46
  perfringens (C) (F) 008.46
  specified type NEC 008.46
coccidial 007.2
dietetic 558.9
due to
  achylia gastrica 536.8
  adenovirus 008.62
  Aerobacter aerogenes 008.2
  anaerobes—*see* Enteritis, anaerobic 008.46
  Arizona (bacillus) 008.1
  astrovirus 008.66
  Bacillus coli—*see* Enteritis, E. coli 008.0
  bacteria NEC 008.5
    specified NEC 008.49
  Bacteroides 008.46
  Butyrivibrio (fibriosolvens) 008.46
  Calcivirus 008.65
  Campylobacter 008.43
  Clostridium—*see* Enteritis, Clostridium
  Cockle agent 008.64
  Coxsackie (virus) 008.67
  Ditchling agent 008.64
  ECHO virus 008.67
  Enterobacter aerogenes 008.2
  enterococci 008.49
  enterovirus NEC 008.67
  Escherichia coli—*see* Enteritis, E. coli
  Eubacterium 008.46
  Fusobacterium (nucleatum) 008.46
  gram-negative bacteria NEC 008.47
    anaerobic NEC 008.46

Enteritis—*continued*
  Hawaii agent 008.63
  irritating foods 558.9
  Klebsiella aerogenes 008.47
  Marin County agent 008.66
  Montgomery County agent 008.63
  Norwalk-like agent 008.63
  Norwalk virus 008.63
  Otofuke agent 008.63
  Paracolobactrum arizonae 008.1
  paracolon bacillus NEC 008.47
    Arizona 008.1
  Paramatta agent 008.64
  Peptococcus 008.46
  Peptostreptococcus 008.46
  Propionibacterium 008.46
  Proteus (bacillus) (mirabilis) (morganii) 008.3
  Pseudomonas aeruginosa 008.42
  radiation 558.1
  Rotavirus 008.61
  Sapporo agent 008.63
  small round virus (SRV) NEC 008.64
    featureless NEC 008.63
    structured NEC 008.63
  Snow Mountain (SM) agent 008.63
  specified
    bacteria NEC 008.49
    organism, nonbacterial NEC 008.8
    virus NEC 008.69
  Staphylococcus 008.41
  Streptococcus 008.49
    anaerobic 008.46
  Taunton agent 008.63
  Torovirus 008.69
  Treponema 008.46
  Veillonella 008.46
  virus 008.8
    specified type NEC 008.69
  Wollan (W) agent 008.64
  Yersinia enterocolitica 008.44
dysentery—*see* Dysentery
E. coli 008.00
  enterohemorrhagic 008.04
  enteroinvasive 008.03
  enteropathogenic 008.01
  enterotoxigenic 008.02
  specified type NEC 008.09
el tor 001.1
embadomonial 007.8
epidemic 009.0
Eubacterium 008.46
fermentative 558.9
fulminant 557.0
Fusobacterium (nucleatum) 008.46
gangrenous (*see also* Enteritis, due to, by
  organism) 009.0
giardial 007.1
gram-negative bacteria NEC 008.47
  anaerobic NEC 008.46
infectious NEC (*see also* Enteritis, due to, by
  organism) 009.0
  presumed 009.1
influenzal 487.8
ischemic 557.9
  acute 557.0
  chronic 557.1
  due to mesenteric artery insufficiency 557.1
membranous 564.9
mucous 564.9
myxomembranous 564.9

Enteritis—*continued*
  necrotic (*see also* Enteritis, due to, by organism) 009.0
  necroticans 005.2
  necrotizing of fetus or newborn 777.5
  neurogenic 564.9
  newborn 777.8
    necrotizing 777.5
  parasitic NEC 129
  paratyphoid (fever) (*see also* Fever, paratyphoid) 002.9
  Peptococcus 008.46
  Peptostreptococcus 008.46
  Propionibacterium 008.46
  protozoal NEC 007.9
  regional (of) 555.9
    intestine
      large (bowel, colon, or rectum) 555.1
        with small intestine 555.2
      small (duodenum, ileum, or jejunum) 555.0
        with large intestine 555.2
  Salmonella infection 003.0
  salmonellosis 003.0
  segmental (*see also* Enteritis, regional) 555.9
  septic (*see also* Enteritis, due to, by organism) 009.0
  Shigella 004.9
  simple 558.9
  spasmodic 564.9
  spastic 564.9
  staphylococcal 008.41
    due to food 005.0
  streptococcal 008.49
    anaerobic 008.46
  toxic 558.2
  Treponema (denticola) (macrodentium) 008.46
  trichomonal 007.3
  tuberculous (*see also* Tuberculosis) 014.8
  typhosa 002.0
  ulcerative (chronic) (*see also* Colitis, ulcerative) 556.9
  Veillonella 008.46
  viral 008.8
    adenovirus 008.62
    enterovirus 008.67
    specified virus NEC 008.69
  Yersinia enterocolitica 008.44
  zymotic 009.0
Enteroarticular syndrome 099.3
Enterobiasis 127.4
Enterobius vermicularis 127.4
Enterocele (*see also* Hernia) 553.9
  pelvis, pelvic (acquired) (congenital) 618.6
  vagina, vaginal (acquired) (congenital) 618.6
Enterocolitis —*see also* Enteritis
  fetus or newborn 777.8
    necrotizing 777.5
  fulminant 557.0
  granulomatous 555.2
  hemorrhagic (acute) 557.0
    chronic 557.1
  necrotizing (acute) (membranous) 557.0
  primary necrotizing 777.5
  pseudomembranous 008.45
  radiation 558.1
    newborn 777.5
  ulcerative 556.0
Enterocystoma 751.5
Enterogastritis —*see* Enteritis
Enterogenous cyanosis 289.7

Enterolith, enterolithiasis (impaction) 560.39
  with hernia—*see also* Hernia, by site, with obstruction
    gangrenous—*see* Hernia, by site, with gangrene
Enteropathy 569.9
  exudative (of Gordon) 579.8
  gluten 579.0
  hemorrhagic, terminal 557.0
  protein-losing 579.8
Enteroperitonitis (*see also* Peritonitis) 567.9
Enteroptosis 569.89
Enterorrhagia 578.9
Enterospasm 564.9
  psychogenic 306.4
Enterostenosis (*see also* Obstruction, intestine) 560.9
Enterostomy status V44.4
  with complication 569.60
Enthesopathy 726.39
  ankle and tarsus 726.70
  elbow region 726.30
    specified NEC 726.39
  hip 726.5
  knee 726.60
  peripheral NEC 726.8
  shoulder region 726.10
    adhesive 726.0
  spinal 720.1
  wrist and carpus 726.4
Entrance, air into vein —*see* Embolism, air
Entrapment, nerve —*see* Neuropathy, entrapment
Entropion (eyelid) 374.00
  cicatricial 374.04
  congenital 743.62
  late effect of trachoma (healed) 139.1
  mechanical 374.02
  paralytic 374.02
  senile 374.01
  spastic 374.03
Enucleation of eye (current) (traumatic) 871.3
Enuresis 788.30
  habit disturbance 307.6
  nocturnal 788.36
    psychogenic 307.6
  nonorganic origin 307.6
  psychogenic 307.6
Enzymopathy 277.9
Eosinopenia 288.0
Eosinophilia 288.3
  allergic 288.3
  hereditary 288.3
  idiopathic 288.3
  infiltrative 518.3
  Loeffler's 518.3
  myalgia syndrome 710.5
  pulmonary (tropical) 518.3
  secondary 288.3
  tropical 518.3
Eosinophilic —*see also* condition
  fasciitis 728.89
  granuloma (bone) 277.8
  infiltration lung 518.3
Ependymitis (acute) (cerebral) (chronic) (granular) (*see also* Meningitis) 322.9
Ependymoblastoma (M9392/3)
  specified site—*see* Neoplasm, by site, malignant
  unspecified site 191.9

Ependymoma (epithelial) (malignant) (M9391/3)
  anaplastic type (M9392/3)
    specified site—*see* Neoplasm, by site,
      malignant
    unspecified site 191.9
  benign (M9391/0)
    specified site—*see* Neoplasm, by site, benign
    unspecified site 225.0
  myxopapillary (M9394/1) 237.5
  papillary (M9393/1) 237.5
  specified site—*see* Neoplasm, by site, malignant
  unspecified site 191.9
Ependymopathy 349.2
  spinal cord 349.2
Ephelides, ephelis 709.09
Ephemeral fever (*see also* Pyrexia) 780.6
Epiblepharon (congenital) 743.62
Epicanthus, epicanthic fold (congenital)
  (eyelid) 743.63
Epicondylitis (elbow) (lateral) 726.32
  medial 726.31
Epicystitis (*see also* Cystitis) 595.9
Epidemic —*see* condition
Epidermidalization, cervix —*see* condition
Epidermidization, cervix *see* condition
Epidermis, epidermal —*see* condition
Epidermization, cervix —*see* condition
Epidermodysplasia verruciformis 078.19
Epidermoid
  cholesteatoma—*see* Cholesteatoma
  inclusion (*see also* Cyst, skin) 706.2
Epidermolysis
  acuta (combustiformis) (toxica) 695.1
  bullosa 757.39
  necroticans combustiformis 695.1
    due to drug
      correct substance properly administered
        695.1
      overdose or wrong substance given or taken
        977.9
      specified drug—*see* Table of drugs and
        chemicals
Epidermophytid —*see* Dermatophytosis
Epidermophytosis (infected)—*see*
  Dermatophytosis
Epidermosis, ear (middle) (*see also*
  Cholesteatoma) 385.30
Epididymis —*see* condition
Epididymitis (nonvenereal) 604.90
  with abscess 604.0
  acute 604.99
  blennorrhagic (acute) 098.0
    chronic or duration of 2 months or over 098.2
  caseous (*see also* Tuberculosis) 016.4
  chlamydial 099.54
  diphtheritic 032.89 *[604.91]*
  filarial 125.9 *[604.91]*
  gonococcal (acute) 098.0
    chronic or duration of 2 months or over 098.2
  recurrent 604.99
  residual 604.99
  syphilitic 095.8 *[604.91]*
  tuberculous (*see also* Tuberculosis) 016.4
Epididymo-orchitis (*see also* Epididymitis)
  604.90
  with abscess 604.0
  chlamydial 099.54
  gonococcal (acute) 098.13
    chronic or duration of 2 months or over 098.33
Epidural —*see* condition
Epigastritis (*see also* Gastritis) 535.5

Epigastrium, epigastric —*see* condition
Epigastrocele (*see also* Hernia, epigastric) 553.29
Epiglottiditis (acute) 464.30
  with obstruction 464.31
  chronic 476.1
  viral 464.30
    with obstruction 464.31
Epiglottis —*see* condition
Epiglottitis (acute) 464.30
  with obstruction 464.31
  chronic 476.1
  viral 464.30
    with obstruction 464.31
Epignathus 759.4
Epilepsia
  partialis continua (*see also* Epilepsy) 345.7
  procursiva (*see also* Epilepsy) 345.8
Epilepsy, epileptic (idiopathic) 345.9

---

*Note—use the following fifth-digit
subclassification with categories 345.0, 345.1,
345.4-345.9*

0 without mention of intractable epilepsy
1 with intractable epilepsy

---

  abdominal 345.5
  absence (attack) 345.0
  akinetic 345.0
    psychomotor 345.4
  automatism 345.4
  autonomic diencephalic 345.5
  brain 345.9
  Bravais-Jacksonian 345.5
  cerebral 345.9
  climacteric 345.9
  clonic 345.1
  clouded state 345.9
  coma 345.3
  communicating 345.4
  congenital 345.9
  convulsions 345.9
  cortical (focal) (motor) 345.5
  cursive (running) 345.8
  cysticercosis 123.1
  deterioration
    with behavioral disturbance 345.9 *[294.11]*
    without behavioral disturbance 345.9 *[294.10]*
  due to syphilis 094.89
  equivalent 345.5
  fit 345.9
  focal (motor) 345.5
  gelastic 345.8
  generalized 345.9
    convulsive 345.1
    flexion 345.1
    nonconvulsive 345.0
  grand mal (idiopathic) 345.1
  Jacksonian (motor) (sensory) 345.5
  Kojewnikoff's, Kojevnikov's, Kojevnikoff's
    345.7
  laryngeal 786.2
  limbic system 345.4
  major (motor) 345.1
  minor 345.0
  mixed (type) 345.9
  motor partial 345.5
  musicogenic 345.1
  myoclonus, myoclonic 345.1
    progressive (familial) 333.2
  nonconvulsive, generalized 345.0

Epilepsy, epileptic—*continued*
parasitic NEC 123.9
partial (focalized) 345.5
  with
    impairment of consciousness 345.4
    memory and ideational disturbances 345.4
  abdominal type 345.5
  motor type 345.5
  psychomotor type 345.4
  psychosensory type 345.4
  secondarily generalized 345.4
  sensory type 345.5
  somatomotor type 345.5
  somatosensory type 345.5
  temporal lobe type 345.4
  visceral type 345.5
  visual type 345.5
peripheral 345.9
petit mal 345.0
photokinetic 345.8
progressive myoclonic (familial) 333.2
psychic equivalent 345.5
psychomotor 345.4
psychosensory 345.4
reflex 345.1
seizure 345.9
senile 345.9
sensory-induced 345.5
sleep 347
somatomotor type 345.5
somatosensory 345.5
specified type NEC 345.8
status (grand mal) 345.3
  focal motor 345.7
  petit mal 345.2
  psychomotor 345.7
  temporal lobe 345.7
symptomatic 345.9
temporal lobe 345.4
tonic (-clonic) 345.1
traumatic (injury unspecified) 907.0
  injury specified—*see* Late, effect (of)
    specified injury
twilight 293.0
uncinate (gyrus) 345.4
Unverricht (-Lundborg) (familial myoclonic)
  333.2
visceral 345.5
visual 345.5
Epileptiform
convulsions 780.39
seizure 780.39
Epiloia 759.5
Epimenorrhea 626.2
Epipharyngitis (*see also* Nasopharyngitis) 460
Epiphora 375.20
due to
  excess lacrimation 375.21
  insufficient drainage 375.22
Epiphyseal arrest 733.91
femoral head 732.2
Epiphyseolysis, epiphysiolysis (*see also*
  Osteochondrosis) 732.9
Epiphysitis (*see also* Osteochondrosis) 732.9
juvenile 732.6
marginal (Scheuermann's) 732.0
os calcis 732.5
syphilitic (congenital) 090.0
vertebral (Scheuermann's) 732.0
Epiplocele (*see also* Hernia) 553.9
Epiploitis (*see also* Peritonitis) 567.9

Epiplosarcomphalocele (*see also* Hernia,
  umbilicus) 553.1
Episcleritis 379.00
gouty 274.89 *[379.09]*
nodular 379.02
periodica fugax 379.01
angioneurotic—*see* Edema, angioneurotic
specified NEC 379.09
staphylococcal 379.00
suppurative 379.00
syphilitic 095.0
tuberculous (*see also* Tuberculosis) 017.3
  [379.09]
Episode
brain (*see also* Disease, cerebrovascular, acute)
  436
cerebral (*see also* Disease, cerebrovascular,
  acute) 436
depersonalization (in neurotic state) 300.6
hyporesponsive 780.09
psychotic (*see also* Psychosis) 298.9
  organic, transient 293.9
schizophrenic (acute) NEC (*see also*
  Schizophrenia) 295.4
Epispadias
female 753.8
male 752.62
Episplenitis 289.59
Epistaxis (multiple) 784.7
hereditary 448.0
vicarious menstruation 625.8
Epithelioma (malignant) (M8011/3)—*see also*
  Neoplasm, by site, malignant
adenoides cysticum (M8100/0)—*see* Neoplasm,
  skin, benign
basal cell (M8090/3)—*see* Neoplasm, skin,
  malignant
benign (M8011/0)—*see* Neoplasm, by site,
  benign
Bowen's (M8081/2)—*see* Neoplasm, skin, in
  situ
calcifying (benign) (Malherbe's)
  (M8110/0)—*see* Neoplasm, skin, benign
external site—*see* Neoplasm, skin, malignant
intraepidermal, Jadassohn (M8096/0)—*see*
  Neoplasm, skin, benign
squamous cell (M8070/3)—*see* Neoplasm, by
  site, malignant
Epitheliopathy
pigment, retina 363.15
posterior multifocal placoid (acute) 363.15
Epithelium, epithelial —*see* condition
Epituberculosis (allergic) (with atelectasis) (*see
  also* Tuberculosis) 010.8
Eponychia 757.5
Epstein's
nephrosis or syndrome (*see also* Nephrosis)
  581.9
pearl (mouth) 528.4
Epstein-Barr infection (viral) 075
chronic 780.79 *[139.8]*
Epulis (giant cell) (gingiva) 523.8
Equinia 024
Equinovarus (congenital) 754.51
acquired 736.71
Equivalent
convulsive (abdominal) (*see also* Epilepsy)
  345.5
epileptic (psychic) (*see also* Epilepsy) 345.5

Erb's
  disease 359.1
  palsy, paralysis (birth) (brachial) (newborn)
    767.6
    spinal (spastic) syphilitic 094.89
  pseudohypertrophic muscular dystrophy 359.1
Erb (-Duchenne) paralysis (birth injury)
    (newborn) 767.6
Erb-Goldflam disease or syndrome 358.0
Erdheim's syndrome (acromegalic
    macrospondylitis) 253.0
Erection, painful (persistent) 607.3
Ergosterol deficiency (vitamin D) 268.9
  with
    osteomalacia 268.2
    rickets (see also Rickets) 268.0
Ergotism (ergotized grain) 988.2
  from ergot used as drug (migraine therapy)
    correct substance properly administered
      349.82
    overdose or wrong substance given or taken
      975.0
Erichsen's disease (railway spine) 300.16
Erlacher-Blount syndrome (tibia vara) 732.4
Erosio interdigitalis blastomycetica 112.3
Erosion
  arteriosclerotic plaque—see Arteriosclerosis, by
    site
  artery NEC 447.2
    without rupture 447.8
  bone 733.99
  bronchus 519.1
  cartilage (joint) 733.99
  cervix (uteri) (acquired) (chronic) (congenital)
    622.0
    with mention of cervicitis 616.0
  cornea (recurrent) (see also Keratitis) 371.42
    traumatic 918.1
  dental (idiopathic) (occupational) 521.3
  duodenum, postpyloric—see Ulcer, duodenum
  esophagus 530.89
  gastric 535.4
  intestine 569.89
  lymphatic vessel 457.8
  pylorus, pyloric (ulcer) 535,4
  sclera 379.16
  spine, aneurysmal 094.89
  spleen 289.59
  stomach 535.4
  teeth (idiopathic) (occupational) 521.3
    due to
      medicine 521.3
      persistent vomiting 521.3
  urethra 599.84
  uterus 621.8
  vertebra 733.99
Erotomania 302.89
  Clérambault's 297.8
Error
  in diet 269.9
  refractive 367.9
    astigmatism (see also Astigmatism) 367.20
    drug-induced 367.89
    hypermetropia 367.0
    hyperopia 367.0
    myopia 367.1
    presbyopia 367.4
    toxic 367.89
Eructation 787.3
  nervous 306.4
  psychogenic 306.4

Eruption
  creeping 126.9
  drug—see Dermatitis, due to, drug
  Hutchinson, summer 692.72
  Kaposi's varicelliform 054.0
  napkin (psoriasiform) 691.0
  polymorphous
    light (sun) 692.72
    other source 692.82
  psoriasiform, napkin 691.0
  recalcitrant pustular 694.8
  ringed 695.89
  skin (see also Dermatitis) 782.1
    creeping (meaning hookworm) 126.9
    due to
      chemical(s) NEC 692.4
        internal use 693.8
      drug—see Dermatitis, due to, drug
      prophylactic inoculation or vaccination
        against disease—see Dermatitis, due to,
        vaccine
      smallpox vaccination NEC—see Dermatitis,
        due to, vaccine
    erysipeloid 027.1
    feigned 698.4
    Hutchinson, summer 692.72
    Kaposi's, varicelliform 054.0
      vaccinia 999.0
    lichenoid, axilla 698.3
    polymorphous, due to light 692.72
    toxic NEC 695.0
    vesicular 709.8
  teeth, tooth
    accelerated 520.6
    delayed 520.6
    difficult 520.6
    disturbance of 520.6
    in abnormal sequence 520.6
    incomplete 520.6
    late 520.6
    natal 520.6
    neonatal 520.6
    obstructed 520.6
    partial 520.6
    persistent primary 520.6
    premature 520.6
  vesicular 709.8
Erysipelas (gangrenous) (infantile) (newborn)
    (phlegmonous) (suppurative) 035
  external ear 035 [380.13]
  puerperal, postpartum, childbirth 670
Erysipelatoid (Rosenbach's) 027.1
Erysipeloid (Rosenbach's) 027.1
Erythema, erythematous (generalized) 695.9
  ab igne—see Burn, by site, first degree
  annulare (centrifugum) (rheumaticum) 695.0
  arthriticum epidemicum 026.1
  brucellum (see also Brucellosis) 023.9
  bullosum 695.1
  caloricum—see Burn, by site, first degree
  chronicum migrans 088.81
    chronicum 088.81
  circinatum 695.1
  diaper 691.0
  due to
    chemical (contact) NEC 692.4
      internal 693.8
    drug (internal use) 693.0
      contact 692.3

Erythema, erythematous—*continued*
elevatum diutinum 695.89
endemic 265.2
epidemic, arthritic 026.1
figuratum perstans 695.0
gluteal 691.0
gyratum (perstans) (repens) 695.1
heat—*see* Burn, by site, first degree
ichthyosiforme congenitum 757.1
induratum (primary) (scrofulosorum) (*see also*
  Tuberculosis) 017.1
  nontuberculous 695.2
infantum febrile 057.8
infectional NEC 695.9
infectiosum 057.0
inflammation NEC 695.9
intertrigo 695.89
iris 695.1
lupus (discoid) (localized) (*see also* Lupus,
  erythematosus) 695.4
marginatum 695.0
  rheumaticum—*see* Fever, rheumatic
medicamentosum—*see* Dermatitis, due to, drug
migrans 529.1
multiforme 695.1
  bullosum 695.1
  conjunctiva 695.1
  exudativum (Hebra) 695.1
  pemphigoides 694.5
napkin 691.0
neonatorum 778.8
nodosum 695.2
  tuberculous (*see also* Tuberculosis) 017.1
nummular, nummulare 695.1
palmar 695.0
palmaris hereditarium 695.0
pernio 991.5
perstans solare 692.72
rash, newborn 778.8
scarlatiniform (exfoliative) (recurrent) 695.0
simplex marginatum 057.8
solare (*see also* Sunburn) 692.71
streptogenes 696.5
toxic, toxicum NEC 695.0
  newborn 778.8
tuberculous (primary) (*see also* Tuberculosis)
  017.0
venenatum 695.0
Erythematosus —*see* condition
Erythematous —*see* condition
Erythermalgia (primary) 443.89
Erythralgia 443.89
Erythrasma 039.0
Erythredema 985.0
polyneuritica 985.0
polyneuropathy 985.0
Erythremia (acute) (M9841/3) 207.0
chronic (M9842/3) 207.1
secondary 289.0
Erythroblastopenia (acquired) 284.8
congenital 284.0
Erythroblastophthisis 284.0
Erythroblastosis (fetalis) (newborn) 773.2
due to
  ABO
    antibodies 773.1
    incompatibility, maternal/fetal 773.1
    isoimmunization 773.1
  Rh
    antibodies 773.0
    incompatibility, maternal/fetal 773.0
    isoimmunization 773.0

Erythrocyanosis (crurum) 443.89
Erythrocythemia —*see* Erythremia
Erythrocytopenia 285.9
Erythrocytosis (megalosplenic)
familial 289.6
oval, hereditary (*see also* Elliptocytosis) 282.1
secondary 289.0
stress 289.0
Erythroderma (*see also* Erythema) 695.9
desquamativa (in infants) 695.89
exfoliative 695.89
ichthyosiform, congenital 757.1
infantum 695.89
maculopapular 696.2
neonatorum 778.8
psoriaticum 696.1
secondary 695.9
Erythrogenesis imperfecta 284.0
Erythroleukemia (M9840/3) 207.0
Erythromelalgia 443.89
Erythromelia 701.8
Erythropenia 285.9
Erythrophagocytosis 289.9
Erythrophobia 300.23
Erythroplakia
oral mucosa 528.7
tongue 528.7
Erythroplasia (Queyrat) (M8080/2)
specified site—*see* Neoplasm, skin, in situ
unspecified site 233.5
Erythropoiesis, idiopathic ineffective 285.0
Escaped beats, heart 427.60
postoperative 997.1
Esoenteritis —*see* Enteritis
Esophagalgia 530.89
Esophagectasis 530.89
due to cardiospasm 530.0
Esophagismus 530.5
Esophagitis (alkaline) (chemical) (chronic)
  (infectional) (necrotic) (postoperative) 530.10
acute 530.12
candidal 112.84
reflux 530.11
specified NEC 530.19
tuberculous (*see also* Tuberculosis) 017.8
ulcerative 530.19
Esophagocele 530.6
Esophagodynia 530.89
Esophagomalacia 530.89
Esophagoptosis 530.89
Esophagospasm 530.5
Esophagostenosis 530.3
Esophagostomiasis 127.7
Esophagotracheal —*see* condition
Esophagus —*see* condition
Esophoria 378.41
convergence, excess 378.84
divergence, insufficiency 378.85
Esotropia (nonaccommodative) 378.00
accommodative 378.35
alternating 378.05
  with
    A pattern 378.06
    specified noncomitancy NEC 378.08
    V pattern 378.07
    X pattern 378.08
    Y pattern 378.08
  intermittent 378.22
intermittent 378.20
  alternating 378.22

Esotropia—*continued*
  monocular 378.21
  monocular 378.01
  with
    A pattern 378.02
    specified noncomitancy NEC 378.04
    V pattern 378.03
    X pattern 378.04
    Y pattern 378.04
    intermittent 378.21
Espundia 085.5
Essential —*see* condition
Esterapenia 289.8
Esthesioneuroblastoma (M9522/3) 160.0
Esthesioneurocytoma (M9521/3) 160.0
Esthesioneuroepithelioma (M9523/3) 160.0
Esthiomene 099.1
Estivo-autumnal
  fever 084.0
  malaria 084.0
Estrangement V61.0
Estriasis 134.0
Ethanolaminuria 270.8
Ethanolism (*see also* Alcoholism) 303.9
Ether dependence, dependency (*see also*
  Dependence) 304.6
Etherism (*see also* Dependence) 304.6
Ethmoid, ethmoidal —*see* condition
Ethmoiditis (chronic) (nonpurulent) (purulent)
  (*see also* Sinusitis, ethmoidal) 473.2
  influenzal 487.1
  Woakes' 471.1
Ethylism (*see also* Alcoholism) 303.9
Eulenburg's disease (congenital paramyotonia)
  359.2
Eunuchism 257.2
Eunuchoidism 257.2
  hypogonadotropic 257.2
European blastomycosis 117.5
Eustachian —*see* condition
Euthyroid sick syndrome 790.94
Euthyroidism 244.9
Evaluation
  fetal lung maturity 659.8
  for suspected condition (*see also* Observation)
    V71.9
    abuse V71.81
    exposure
      anthrax V71.82
      biologic agent NEC V71.83
    neglect V71.81
    newborn—*see* Observation, suspected,
      condition, newborn
    specified condition NEC V71.89
  mental health V70.2
  requested by authority V70.1
  nursing care V63.8
  social service V63.8
Evan's syndrome (thrombocytopenic purpura)
  287.3
Eventration
  colon into chest—*see* Hernia, diaphragm
  diaphragm (congenital) 756.6
Eversion
  bladder 596.8
  cervix (uteri) 622.0
    with mention of cervicitis 616.0
  foot NEC 736.79
    congenital 755.67
  lacrimal punctum 375.51

Eversion—*continued*
  punctum lacrimale (postinfectional) (senile)
    375.51
  ureter (meatus) 593.89
  urethra (meatus) 599.84
  uterus 618.1
    complicating delivery 665.2
      affecting fetus or newborn 763.89
    puerperal, postpartum 674.8
Evisceration
  birth injury 767.8
  bowel (congenital)—*see* Hernia, ventral
  congenital (*see also* Hernia, ventral) 553.29
  operative wound 998.32
  traumatic NEC 869.1
    eye 871.3
Evulsion —*see* Avulsion
Ewing's
  angioendothelioma (M9260/3)—*see* Neoplasm,
    bone, malignant
  sarcoma (M9260/3)—*see* Neoplasm, bone,
    malignant
  tumor (M9260/3)—*see* Neoplasm, bone,
    malignant
Exaggerated lumbosacral angle (with
  impinging spine) 756.12
Examination (general) (routine) (of) (for) V70.9
  allergy V72.7
  annual V70.0
  cardiovascular preoperative V72.81
  cervical Papanicolaou smear V76.2
    as a part of routine gynecological examination
      V72.3
  child care (routine) V20.2
  clinical research investigation (normal control
    patient) (participant) V70.7
  dental V72.2
  developmental testing (child) (infant) V20.2
  donor (potential) V70.8
  ear V72.1
  eye V72.0
  following
    accident (motor vehicle) V71.4
    alleged rape or seduction (victim or culprit)
      V71.5
    inflicted injury (victim or culprit) NEC V71.6
    rape or seduction, alleged (victim or culprit)
      V71.5
    treatment (for) V67.9
      combined V67.6
      fracture V67.4
      involving high-risk medication NEC V67.51
      mental disorder V67.3
      specified condition NEC V67.59
  follow-up (routine) (following) V67.9
    cancer chemotherapy V67.2
    chemotherapy V67.2
    disease NEC V67.59
    high-risk medication NEC V67.51
    injury NEC V67.59
    population survey V70.6
    postpartum V24.2
    psychiatric V67.3
    psychotherapy V67.3
    radiotherapy V67.1
    specified surgery NEC V67.09
    surgery V67.00
      vaginal pap smear V67.01
  gynecological V72.3
    for contraceptive maintenance V25.40
      intrauterine device V25.42

Examination—*continued*
  pill V25.41
    specified method NEC V25.49
  health (of)
    armed forces personnel V70.5
    checkup V70.0
    child, routine V20.2
    defined subpopulation NEC V70.5
    inhabitants of institutions V70.5
    occupational V70.5
    pre-employment screening V70.5
    preschool children V70.5
      for admission to school V70.3
    prisoners V70.5
      for entrance into prison V70.3
    prostitutes V70.5
    refugees V70.5
    school children V70.5
    students V70.5
  hearing V72.1
  infant V20.2
  laboratory V72.6
  lactating mother V24.1
  medical (for) (of) V70.9
    administrative purpose NEC V70.3
    admission to
      old age home V70.3
      prison V70.3
      school V70.3
    adoption V70.3
    armed forces personnel V70.5
    at health care facility V70.0
    camp V70.3
    child, routine V20.2
    clinical research investigation (control)
      (normal comparison) (participant) V70.7
    defined subpopulation NEC V70.5
    donor (potential) V70.8
    driving license V70.3
    general V70.9
      routine V70.0
      specified reason NEC V70.8
    immigration V70.3
    inhabitants of institutions V70.5
    insurance certification V70.3
    marriage V70.3
    medicolegal reasons V70.4
    naturalization V70.3
    occupational V70.5
    population survey V70.6
    pre-employment V70.5
    preschool children V70.5
      for admission to school V70.3
    prison V70.3
    prisoners V70.5
      for entrance into prison V70.3
    prostitutes V70.5
    refugees V70.5
    school children V70.5
    specified reason NEC V70.8
    sport competition V70.3
    students V70.5
  medicolegal reason V70.4
  pelvic (annual) (periodic) V72.3
  periodic (annual) (routine) V70.0
  postpartum
    immediately after delivery V24.0
    routine follow-up V24.2
  pregnancy (unconfirmed) (possible) V72.4
  prenatal V22.1
    first pregnancy V22.0

Examination—*continued*
  high-risk pregnancy V23.9
    specified problem NEC V23.8
  preoperative V72.84
    cardiovascular V72.81
    respiratory V72.82
    specified NEC V72.83
  psychiatric V70.2
    follow-up not needing further care V67.3
    requested by authority V70.1
  radiological NEC V72.5
  respiratory preoperative V72.82
  screening—*see* Screening
  sensitization V72.7
  skin V72.7
    hypersensitivity V72.7
  special V72.9
  specified type or reason NEC V72.85
    preoperative V72.83
      specified NEC V72.83
  teeth V72.2
  vaginal Papanicolaou smear V76.47
    following hysterectomy for malignant
      condition V67.01
  victim or culprit following
    alleged rape or seduction V71.5
    inflicted injury NEC V71.6
  vision V72.0
  well baby V20.2
Exanthem, exanthema (*see also* Rash) 782.1
  Boston 048
  epidemic, with meningitis 048
  lichenoid psoriasiform 696.2
  subitum 057.8
  viral, virus NEC 057.9
    specified type NEC 057.8
Excess, excessive, excessively
  alcohol level in blood 790.3
  carbohydrate tissue, localized 278.1
  carotene (dietary) 278.3
  cold 991.9
    specified effect NEC 991.8
  convergence 378.84
  crying of infant (baby) 780.92
  development, breast 611.1
  diaphoresis 780.8
  divergence 378.85
  drinking (alcohol) NEC (*see also* Abuse, drugs,
    nondependent) 305.0
    continual (*see also* Alcoholism) 303.9
    habitual (*see also* Alcoholism) 303.9
  eating 783.6
  eyelid fold (congenital) 743.62
  fat 278.00
    in heart (*see also* Degeneration, myocardial)
      429.1
    tissue, localized 278.1
  foreskin 605
  gas 787.3
  gastrin 251.5
  glucagon 251.4
  heat (*see also* Heat) 992.9
  large
    colon 564.7
      congenital 751.3
    fetus or infant 766.0
      with obstructed labor 660.1
      affecting management of pregnancy 656.6
      causing disproportion 653.5
    newborn (weight of 4500 grams or more)
      766.0

Excess, excessive, excessively—*continued*
   organ or site, congenital NEC—*see* Anomaly,
      specified type NEC
   lid fold (congenital) 743.62
   long
     colon 751.5
     organ or site, congenital NEC—*see* Anomaly,
       specified type NEC
     umbilical cord (entangled)
      affecting fetus or newborn 762.5
      in pregnancy or childbirth 663.3
       with compression 663.2
   menstruation 626.2
   number of teeth 520.1
     causing crowding 524.3
   nutrients (dietary) NEC 783.6
   potassium (K) 276.7
   salivation (*see also* Ptyalism) 527.7
   secretion—*see also* Hypersecretion
     milk 676.6
     sputum 786.4
     sweat 780.8
   short
     organ or site, congenital NEC—*see* Anomaly,
       specified type NEC
     umbilical cord
      affecting fetus or newborn 762.6
      in pregnancy or childbirth 663.4
   skin NEC 701.9
     eyelid 743.62
      acquired 374.30
   sodium (Na) 276.0
   sputum 786.4
   sweating 780.8
   tearing (ducts) (eye) (*see also* Epiphora) 375.20
   thirst 783.5
     due to deprivation of water 994.3
   vitamin
     A (dietary) 278.2
      administered as drug (chronic) (prolonged
       excessive intake) 278.2
      reaction to sudden overdose 963.5
     D (dietary) 278.4
      administered as drug (chronic) (prolonged
       excessive intake) 278.4
      reaction to sudden overdose 963.5
   weight 278.00
     gain 783.1
      of pregnancy 646.1
     loss 783.21
Excitability, abnormal , under minor stress
   309.29
Excitation
   catatonic (*see also* Schizophrenia) 295.2
   psychogenic 298.1
   reactive (from emotional stress, psychological
     trauma) 298.1
Excitement
   manic (*see also* Psychosis, affective) 296.0
     recurrent episode 296.1
     single episode 296.0
   mental, reactive (from emotional stress,
     psychological trauma) 298.1
   state, reactive (from emotional stress,
     psychological trauma) 298.1
Excluded pupils 364.76
Excoriation (traumatic) (*see also* Injury,
   superficial, by site) 919.8
   neurotic 698.4
Excyclophoria 378.44
Excyclotropia 378.33
Exencephalus, exencephaly 742.0

Exercise
   breathing V57.0
   remedial NEC V57.1
   therapeutic NEC V57.1
Exfoliation, teeth due to systemic causes 525.0
Exfoliative —*see also* condition
   dermatitis 695.89
Exhaustion, exhaustive (physical NEC) 780.79
   battle (*see also* Reaction, stress, acute) 308.9
   cardiac (*see also* Failure, heart) 428.9
   delirium (*see also* Reaction, stress, acute) 308.9
   due to
     cold 991.8
     excessive exertion 994.5
     exposure 994.4
   fetus or newborn 779.89
   heart (*see also* Failure, heart) 428.9
   heat 992.5
     due to
      salt depletion 992.4
      water depletion 992.3
   manic (*see also* Psychosis, affective) 296.0
     recurrent episode 296.1
     single episode 296.0
   maternal, complicating delivery 669.8
     affecting fetus or newborn 763.89
   mental 300.5
   myocardium, myocardial (*see also* Failure,
     heart) 428.9
   nervous 300.5
   old age 797
   postinfectional NEC 780.79
   psychogenic 300.5
   psychosis (*see also* Reaction, stress, acute) 308.9
   senile 797
     dementia 290.0
Exhibitionism (sexual) 302.4
Exomphalos 756.79
Exophoria 378.42
   convergence, insufficiency 378.83
   divergence, excess 378.85
Exophthalmic
   cachexia 242.0
   goiter 242.0
   ophthalmoplegia 242.0 *[376.22]*
Exophthalmos 376.30
   congenital 743.66
   constant 376.31
   endocrine NEC 259.9 *[376.22]*
   hyperthyroidism 242.0 *[376.21]*
   intermittent NEC 376.34
   malignant 242.0 *[376.21]*
   pulsating 376.35
     endocrine NEC 259.9 *[376.22]*
   thyrotoxic 242.0 *[376.21]*
Exostosis 726.91
   cartilaginous (M9210/0)—*see* Neoplasm, bone,
     benign
   congenital 756.4
   ear canal, external 380.81
   gonococcal 098.89
   hip 726.5
   intracranial 733.3
   jaw (bone) 526.81
   luxurians 728.11
   multiple (cancellous) (congenital) (hereditary)
     756.4
   nasal bones 726.91
   orbit, orbital 376.42
   osteocartilaginous (M9210/0)—*see* Neoplasm,
     bone, benign

Exostosis—*continued*
  spine 721.8
    with spondylosis—*see* Spondylosis
  syphilitic 095.5
  wrist 726.4
Exotropia 378.10
  alternating 378.15
    with
      A pattern 378.16
      specified noncomitancy 378.18
      V pattern 378.17
      X pattern 378.18
      Y pattern 378.18
      intermittent 378.24
  intermittent 378.20
    alternating 378.24
    monocular 378.23
  monocular 378.11
    with
      A pattern 378.12
      specified noncomitancy NEC 378.14
      V pattern 378.13
      X pattern 378.14
      Y pattern 378.14
      intermittent 378.23
Explanation of
  investigation finding V65.4
  medication V65.4
Exposure 994.9
  cold 991.9
    specified effect NEC 991.8
  effects of 994.9
  exhaustion due to 994.4
  to
    AIDS virus V01.7
    anthrax V01.81
    asbestos V15.84
    body fluids (hazardous) V15.85
    cholera V01.0
    communicable disease V01.9
      specified type NEC V01.89
    German measles V01.4
    gonorrhea V01.6
    hazardous body fluids V15.85
    HIV V01.7
    human immunodeficiency virus V01.7
    lead V15.86
    parasitic disease V01.89
    poliomyelitis V01.2
    potentially hazardous body fluids V15.85
    rabies V01.5
    rubella V01.4
    smallpox V01.3
    syphilis V01.6
    tuberculosis V01.1
    venereal disease V01.6
    viral disease NEC V01.7
Exsanguination, fetal 772.0
Exstrophy
  abdominal content 751.8
  bladder (urinary) 753.5
Extensive —*see* condition
Extra —*see also* Accessory
  rib 756.3
    cervical 756.2
Extraction
  with hook 763.89
  breech NEC 669.6
    affecting fetus or newborn 763.0
  cataract postsurgical V45.61
  manual NEC 669.8
    affecting fetus or newborn 763.89

Extrasystole 427.60
  atrial 427.61
  postoperative 997.1
  ventricular 427.69
Extrauterine gestation or pregnancy —*see*
  Pregnancy, ectopic
Extravasation
  blood 459.0
    lower extremity 459.0
  chyle into mesentery 457.8
  pelvicalyceal 593.4
  pyelosinus 593.4
  urine 788.8
    from ureter 788.8
Extremity —*see* condition
Extrophy —*see* Exstrophy
Extroversion
  bladder 753.5
  uterus 618.1
    complicating delivery 665.2
      affecting fetus or newborn 763.89
    postpartal (old) 618.1
Extrusion
  breast implant (prosthetic) 996.54
  device, implant, or graft—*see* Complications,
    mechanical
  eye implant (ball) (globe) 996.59
  intervertebral disc—*see* Displacement,
    intervertebral disc
  lacrimal gland 375.43
  mesh (reinforcing) 996.59
  ocular lens implant 996.53
  prosthetic device NEC—*see* Complications,
    mechanical
  vitreous 379.26
Exudate, pleura —*see* Effusion, pleura
Exudates, retina 362.82
Exudative —*see* condition
Eye, eyeball, eyelid —*see* condition
Eyestrain 368.13
Eyeworm disease of Africa 125.2

F

Faber's anemia or syndrome (achlorhydric anemia) 280.9
Fabry's disease (angiokeratoma corporis diffusum) 272.7
Face, facial —*see* condition
Facet of cornea 371.44
Faciocephalalgia, autonomic (*see also* Neuropathy, peripheral, autonomic) 337.9
Facioscapulohumeral myopathy 359.1
Factitious disorder, illness —*see* Illness, factitious
Factor
  deficiency—*see* Deficiency, factor
  psychic, associated with diseases classified elsewhere 316
  risk—*see* Problem
Fahr-Volhard disease (malignant nephrosclerosis) 403.00
Failure, failed
  adenohypophyseal 253.2
  attempted abortion (legal) (*see also* Abortion, failed) 638.9
  bone marrow (anemia) 284.9
    acquired (secondary) 284.8
    congenital 284.0
    idiopathic 284.9
  cardiac (*see also* Failure, heart) 428.9
    newborn 779.89
  cardiorenal (chronic) 428.9
    hypertensive (*see also* Hypertension, cardiorenal) 404.93
  cardiorespiratory 799.1
    specified during or due to a procedure 997.1
    long-term effect of cardiac surgery 429.4
  cardiovascular (chronic) 428.9
  cerebrovascular 437.8
  cervical dilatation in labor 661.0
    affecting fetus or newborn 763.7
  circulation, circulatory 799.8
    fetus or newborn 779.89
    peripheral 785.50
  compensation—*see* Disease, heart
  congestive (*see also* Failure, heart) 428.0
  coronary (*see also* Insufficiency, coronary) 411.89
  descent of head (at term) 652.5
    affecting fetus or newborn 763.1
    in labor 660.0
      affecting fetus or newborn 763.1
  device, implant, or graft—*see* Complications, mechanical
  engagement of head NEC 652.5
    in labor 660.0
  extrarenal 788.9
  fetal head to enter pelvic brim 652.5
    affecting fetus or newborn 763.1
    in labor 660.0
      affecting fetus or newborn 763.1
  forceps NEC 660.7
    affecting fetus or newborn 763.1
  fusion (joint) (spinal) 996.4
  growth in childhood 783.43
  heart (acute) (sudden) 428.9
    with
      abortion—*see* Abortion, by type, with specified complication NEC

Failure, failed—*continued*
  acute pulmonary edema (*see also* Failure, ventricular, left) 428.1
    with congestion (*see also* Failure, heart) 428.0
  decompensation (*see also* Failure, heart) 428.0
  dilation—*see* Disease, heart
  ectopic pregnancy (*see also* categories 633.0-633.9) 639.8
  molar pregnancy (*see also* categories 630-632) 639.8
  arteriosclerotic 440.9
  combined left-right sided 428.0
  combined systolic and diastolic 428.40
    acute 428.41
    acute on chronic 428.43
    chronic 428.42
  compensated (*see also* Failure, heart) 428.0
  complicating
    abortion—*see* Abortion, by type, with specified complication NEC
    delivery (cesarean) (instrumental) 669.4
    ectopic pregnancy (*see also* categories 633.0-633.9) 639.8
    molar pregnancy (*see also* categories 630-632) 639.8
    obstetric anesthesia or sedation 668.1
    surgery 997.1
  congestive (compensated) (decompensated) (*see also* Failure, heart) 428.0
    with rheumatic fever (conditions classifiable to 390)
      active 391.8
      inactive or quiescent (with chorea) 398.91
    fetus or newborn 779.89
    hypertensive (*see also* Hypertension, heart) 402.91
      with renal disease (*see also* Hypertension, cardiorenal) 404.91
        with renal failure 404.93
      benign 402.11
      malignant 402.01
    rheumatic (chronic) (inactive) (with chorea) 398.91
      active or acute 391.8
        with chorea (Sydenham's) 392.0
  decompensated (*see also* Failure, heart) 428.0
  degenerative (*see also* Degeneration, myocardial) 429.1
  diastolic 428.30
    acute 428.31
    actue on chronic 428.33
    chronic 428.32
  due to presence of (cardiac) prosthesis 429.4
  fetus or newborn 779.89
  following
    abortion 639.8
    cardiac surgery 429.4
    ectopic or molar pregnancy 639.8
  high output NEC 428.9
  hypertensive (*see also* Hypertension, heart) 402.91
    with renal disease (*see also* Hypertension, cardiorenal) 404.91
      with renal failure 404.93
    benign 402.11

Failure, failed—*continued*
  malignant 402.01
  left (ventricular) (*see also* Failure, ventricular,
    left) 428.1
    with right-sided failure (*see also* Failure,
      heart) 428.0
  low output (syndrome) NEC 428.9
  organic—*see* Disease, heart
  postoperative (immediate) 997.1
    long term effect of cardiac surgery 429.4
  rheumatic (chronic) (congestive) (inactive)
    398.91
  right (secondary to left heart failure,
    conditions classifiable to 428.1)
    (ventricular) (*see also* Failure, heart) 428.0
  senile 797
  specified during or due to a procedure 997.1
    long-term effect of cardiac surgery 429.4
  systolic 428.20
    acute 428.21
    acute on chronic 428.23
    chronic 428.22
  thyrotoxic (*see also* Thyrotoxicosis) 242.9
    [425.7]
  valvular—*see* Endocarditis
  hepatic 572.8
    acute 570
    due to a procedure 997.4
  hepatorenal 572.4
  hypertensive heart (*see also* Hypertension,
    heart) 402.91
    benign 402.11
    malignant 402.01
  induction (of labor) 659.1
    abortion (legal) (*see also* Abortion, failed)
      638.9
    affecting fetus or newborn 763.89
    by oxytocic drugs 659.1
    instrumental 659.0
    mechanical 659.0
    medical 659.1
    surgical 659.0
  initial alveolar expansion, newborn 770.4
  involution, thymus (gland) 254.8
  kidney—*see* Failure, renal
  lactation 676.4
  Leydig's cell, adult 257.2
  liver 572.8
    acute 570
  medullary 799.8
  mitral—*see* Endocarditis, mitral
  myocardium, myocardial (*see also* Failure,
    heart) 428.9
    chronic (*see also* Failure, heart) 428.0
    congestive (*see also* Failure, heart) 428.0
  ovarian (primary) 256.39
    iatrogenic 256.2
    postablative 256.2
    postirradiation 256.2
    postsurgical 256.2
  ovulation 628.0
  prerenal 788.9
  renal 586
    with
      abortion—*see* Abortion, by type, with renal
        failure
      ectopic pregnancy (*see also* categories
        633.0-633.9) 639.3
      edema (*see also* Nephrosis) 581.9
      hypertension (*see also* Hypertension,
        kidney) 403.91

Failure, failed—*continued*
  hypertensive heart disease (conditions
    classifiable to 402) 404.92
    with heart failure 404.93
    benign 404.12
      with heart failure 404.13
    malignant 404.02
      with heart failure 404.03
    molar pregnancy (*see also* categories
      630-632) 639.3
    tubular necrosis (acute) 584.5
    acute 584.9
      with lesion of
        necrosis
          cortical (renal) 584.6
          medullary (renal) (papillary) 584.7
          tubular 584.5
        specified pathology NEC 584.8
    chronic 585
      hypertensive or with hypertension (*see also*
        Hypertension, kidney) 403.91
    due to a procedure 997.5
    following
      abortion 639.3
      crushing 958.5
      ectopic or molar pregnancy 639.3
      labor and delivery (acute) 669.3
    hypertensive (*see also* Hypertension, kidney)
      403.91
    puerperal, postpartum 669.3
  respiration, respiratory 518.81
    acute 518.81
    acute and chronic 518.84
    center 348.8
      newborn 770.84
    chronic 518.83
    due to trauma, surgery or shock 518.5
    newborn 770.84
  rotation
    cecum 751.4
    colon 751.4
    intestine 751.4
    kidney 753.3
  segmentation—*see also* Fusion
    fingers (*see also* Syndactylism, fingers) 755.11
    toes (*see also* Syndactylism, toes) 755.13
  seminiferous tubule, adult 257.2
  senile (general) 797
    with psychosis 290.20
  testis, primary (seminal) 257.2
  to progress 661.2
  to thrive
    adult 783.7
    child 783.41
  transplant 996.80
    bone marrow 996.85
    organ (immune or nonimmune cause) 996.80
      bone marrow 996.85
      heart 996.83
      intestines 996.87
      kidney 996.81
      liver 996.82
      lung 996.84
      pancreas 996.86
      specified NEC 996.89
    skin 996.52
      artificial 996.55
      decellularized allodermis 996.55
      temporary allograft or pigskin graft—*omit
        code*

Failure, failed—*continued*
trial of labor NEC 660.6
  affecting fetus or newborn 763.1
urinary 586
vacuum extraction
  abortion—*see* Abortion, failed
  delivery NEC 660.7
    affecting fetus or newborn 763.1
ventouse NEC 660.7
  affecting fetus or newborn 763.1
ventricular (*see also* Failure, heart) 428.9
  left 428.1
    with rheumatic fever (conditions classifiable
      to 390)
      active 391.8
        with chorea 392.0
      inactive or quiescent (with chorea) 398.91
    hypertensive (*see also* Hypertension, heart)
      402.91
      benign 402.11
      malignant 402.01
    rheumatic (chronic) (inactive) (with chorea)
      398.91
      active or acute 391.8
        with chorea 392.0
  right (*see also* Failure, heart) 428.0
vital centers, fetus or newborn 779.8
weight gain in childhood 783.41
Fainting (fit) (spell) 780.2
Falciform hymen 752.49
Fall, maternal, affecting fetus or newborn
  760.5
Fallen arches 734
Falling, any organ or part —*see* Prolapse
Fallopian
insufflation
  fertility testing V26.21
  following sterilization reversal V26.22
tube—*see* condition
Fallot's
pentalogy 745.2
tetrad or tetralogy 745.2
triad or trilogy 746.09
Fallout, radioactive (adverse effect) NEC 990
False —*see also* condition
bundle branch block 426.50
bursa 727.89
croup 478.75
joint 733.82
labor (pains) 644.1
opening, urinary, male 752.69
passage, urethra (prostatic) 599.4
positive
  serological test for syphilis 795.6
  Wassermann reaction 795.6
pregnancy 300.11
Family, familial —*see also* condition
disruption V61.0
planning advice V25.09
problem V61.9
specified circumstance NEC V61.8
Famine 994.2
edema 262
Fanconi's anemia (congenital pancytopenia)
  284.0
Fanconi (-de Toni) (-Debré) syndrome
  (cystinosis) 270.0
Farber (-Uzman) syndrome or disease
  (disseminated lipogranulomatosis) 272.8
Farcin 024
Farcy 024

Farmers '
lung 495.0
skin 692.74
Farsightedness 367.0
Fascia —*see* condition
Fasciculation 781.0
Fasciculitis optica 377.32
Fasciitis 729.4
eosinophilic 728.89
necrotizing 728.86
nodular 728.79
perirenal 593.4
plantar 728.71
pseudosarcomatous 728.79
traumatic (old) NEC 728.79
current—*see* Sprain, by site
Fasciola hepatica infestation 121.3
Fascioliasis 121.3
Fasciolopsiasis (small intestine) 121.4
Fasciolopsis (small intestine) 121.4
Fast pulse 785.0
Fat
embolism (cerebral) (pulmonary) (systemic)
  958.1
  with
    abortion—*see* Abortion, by type, with
      embolism
    ectopic pregnancy (*see also* categories
      633.0-633.9) 639.6
    molar pregnancy (*see also* categories
      630-632) 639.6
  complicating delivery or puerperium 673.8
  following
    abortion 639.6
    ectopic or molar pregnancy 639.6
  in pregnancy, childbirth, or the puerperium
    673.8
excessive 278.00
  in heart (*see also* Degeneration, myocardial)
    429.1
general 278.00
hernia, herniation 729.30
  eyelid 374.34
  knee 729.31
  orbit 374.34
  retro-orbital 374.34
  retropatellar 729.31
  specified site NEC 729.39
indigestion 579.8
in stool 792.1
localized (pad) 278.1
  heart (*see also* Degeneration, myocardial)
    429.1
  knee 729.31
  retropatellar 729.31
necrosis—*see also* Fatty, degeneration
  breast (aseptic) (segmental) 611.3
  mesentery 567.8
  omentum 567.8
pad 278.1
Fatal syncope 798.1
Fatigue 780.79
auditory deafness (*see also* Deafness) 389.9
chronic, syndrome 780.71
combat (*see also* Reaction, stress, acute) 308.9
during pregnancy 646.8
general 780.79
  psychogenic 300.5
heat (transient) 992.6
muscle 729.89
myocardium (*see also* Failure, heart) 428.9

Fetishism 302.81
  transvestic 302.3
Fetomaternal hemorrhage
  affecting management of pregnancy 656.0
  fetus or newborn 772.0
Fetus, fetal —*see also* condition
  papyraceous 779.89
  type lung tissue 770.4
Fever <u>780.6</u>
  with chills 780.6
    in malarial regions (*see also* Malaria) 084.6
  abortus NEC 023.9
  Aden 061
  African tick-borne 087.1
  American
    mountain tick 066.1
    spotted 082.0
  and ague (*see also* Malaria) 084.6
  aphthous 078.4
  arbovirus hemorrhagic 065.9
  Assam 085.0
  Australian A or Q 083.0
  Bangkok hemorrhagic 065.4
  biliary, Charcot's intermittent—*see*
      Choledocholithiasis
  bilious, hemoglobinuric 084.8
  blackwater 084.8
  blister 054.9
  Bonvale Dam 780.79
  boutonneuse 082.1
  brain 323.9
    late effect—*see* category 326
  breakbone 061
  Bullis 082.8
  Bunyamwera 066.3
  Burdwan 085.0
  Bwamba (encephalitis) 066.3
  Cameroon (*see also* Malaria) 084.6
  Canton 081.9
  catarrhal (acute) 460
    chronic 472.0
  cat-scratch 078.3
  cerebral 323.9
    late effect—*see* category 326
  cerebrospinal (meningococcal) (*see also*
      Meningitis, cerebrospinal) 036.0
  Chagres 084.0
  Chandipura 066.8
  changuinola 066.0
  Charcot's (biliary) (hepatic) (intermittent)—*see*
      Choledocholithiasis
  Chikungunya (viral) 066.3
    hemorrhagic 065.4
  childbed 670
  Chitral 066.0
  Colombo (*see also* Fever, paratyphoid) 002.9
  Colorado tick (virus) 066.1
  congestive
    malarial (*see also* Malaria) 084.6
    remittent (*see also* Malaria) 084.6
  Congo virus 065.0
  continued 780.6
    malarial 084.0
  Corsican (*see also* Malaria) 084.6
  Crimean hemorrhagic 065.0
  Cyprus (*see also* Brucellosis) 023.9
  dandy 061
  deer fly (*see also* Tularemia) 021.9
  dehydration, newborn 778.4
  dengue (virus) 061
    hemorrhagic 065.4

Fever—*continued*
  desert 114.0
  due to heat 992.0
  Dumdum 085.0
  enteric 002.0
  ephemeral (of unknown origin) (*see also*
      Pyrexia) 780.6
  epidemic, hemorrhagic of the Far East 065.0
  erysipelatous (*see also* Erysipelas) 035
  estivo-autumnal (malarial) 084.0
  etiocholanolone 277.3
  famine—*see also* Fever, relapsing
    meaning typhus—*see* Typhus
  Far Eastern hemorrhagic 065.0
  five day 083.1
  Fort Bragg 100.89
  gastroenteric 002.0
  gastromalarial (*see also* Malaria) 084.6
  Gibraltar (*see also* Brucellosis) 023.9
  glandular 075
  Guama (viral) 066.3
  Haverhill 026.1
  hay (allergic) (with rhinitis) 477.9
    with
      asthma (bronchial) (*see also* Asthma) 493.0
    due to
      dander 477.8
      dust 477.8
      fowl 477.8
      pollen, any plant or tree 477.0
      specified allergen other than pollen 477.8
  heat (effects) 992.0
  hematuric, bilious 084.8
  hemoglobinuric (malarial) 084.8
    bilious 084.8
  hemorrhagic (arthropod-borne) NEC 065.9
    with renal syndrome 078.6
    arenaviral 078.7
    Argentine 078.7
    Bangkok 065.4
    Bolivian 078.7
    Central Asian 065.0
    chikungunya 065.4
    Crimean 065.0
    dengue (virus) 065.4
    Ebola 065.8
    epidemic 078.6
      of Far East 065.0
    Far Eastern 065.0
    Junin virus 078.7
    Korean 078.6
    Kyasanur forest 065.2
    Machupo virus 078.7
    mite-borne NEC 065.8
    mosquito-borne 065.4
    Omsk 065.1
    Philippine 065.4
    Russian (Yaroslav) 078.6
    Singapore 065.4
    Southeast Asia 065.4
    Thailand 065.4
    tick-borne NEC 065.3
  hepatic (*see also* Cholecystitis) 575.8
    intermittent (Charcot's)—*see*
        Choledocholithiasis
  herpetic (*see also* Herpes) 054.9
  Hyalomma tick 065.0
  icterohemorrhagic 100.0
  inanition 780.6
    newborn 778.4
  infective NEC 136.9

Fever—*continued*
   intermittent (bilious) (*see also* Malaria) 084.6
      hepatic (Charcot)—*see* Choledocholithiasis
      of unknown origin (*see also* Pyrexia) 780.6
      pernicious 084.0
   iodide
      correct substance properly administered 780.6
      overdose or wrong substance given or taken
         975.5
   Japanese river 081.2
   jungle yellow 060.0
   Junin virus, hemorrhagic 078.7
   Katayama 120.2
   Kedani 081.2
   Kenya 082.1
   Korean hemorrhagic 078.6
   Lassa 078.89
   Lone Star 082.8
   lung—*see* Pneumonia
   Machupo virus, hemorrhagic 078.7
   malaria, malarial (*see also* Malaria) 084.6
   Malta (*see also* Brucellosis) 023.9
   Marseilles 082.1
   marsh (*see also* Malaria) 084.6
   Mayaro (viral) 066.3
   Mediterranean (*see also* Brucellosis) 023.9
      familial 277.3
      tick 082.1
   meningeal—*see* Meningitis
   metal fumes NEC 985.8
   Meuse 083.1
   Mexican—*see* Typhus, Mexican
   Mianeh 087.1
   miasmatic (*see also* Malaria) 084.6
   miliary 078.2
   milk, female 672
   mill 504
   mite-borne hemorrhagic 065.8
   Monday 504
   mosquito-borne NEC 066.3
      hemorrhagic NEC 065.4
   mountain 066.1
      meaning
         Rocky Mountain spotted 082.0
         undulant fever (*see also* Brucellosis) 023.9
      tick (American) 066.1
   Mucambo (viral) 066.3
   mud 100.89
   Neapolitan (*see also* Brucellosis) 023.9
   neutropenic 288.0
   nine-mile 083.0
   nonexanthematous tick 066.1
   North Asian tick-borne typhus 082.2
   Omsk hemorrhagic 065.1
   O'nyong-nyong (viral) 066.3
   Oropouche (viral) 066.3
   Oroya 088.0
   paludal (*see also* Malaria) 084.6
   Panama 084.0
   pappataci 066.0
   paratyphoid 002.9
      A 002.1
      B (Schottmüller's) 002.2
      C (Hirschfeld) 002.3
   parrot 073.9
   periodic 277.3
   pernicious, acute 084.0
   persistent (of unknown origin) (*see also*
      Pyrexia) 780.6
   petechial 036.0
   pharyngoconjunctival 077.2

Fever—*continued*
   adenoviral type 3 077.2
   Philippine hemorrhagic 065.4
   phlebotomus 066.0
   Piry 066.8
   Pixuna (viral) 066.3
   Plasmodium ovale 084.3
   pleural (*see also* Pleurisy) 511.0
   pneumonic—*see* Pneumonia
   polymer fume 987.8
   postoperative 998.89
      due to infection 998.59
   pretibial 100.89
   puerperal, postpartum 672
   putrid—*see* Septicemia
   pyemic—*see* Septicemia
   Q 083.0
      with pneumonia 083.0 [484.8]
   quadrilateral 083.0
   quartan (malaria) 084.2
   Queensland (coastal) 083.0
      seven-day 100.89
   Quintan (A) 083.1
   quotidian 084.0
   rabbit (*see also* Tularemia) 021.9
   rat-bite 026.9
      due to
         Spirillum minor or minus 026.0
         Spirochaeta morsus muris 026.0
         Streptobacillus moniliformis 026.1
   recurrent—*see* Fever, relapsing
   relapsing 087.9
      Carter's (Asiatic) 087.0
      Dutton's (West African) 087.1
      Koch's 087.9
      louse-borne (epidemic) 087.0
      Novy's (American) 087.1
      Obermeyer's (European) 087.0
      spirillum NEC 087.9
      tick-borne (endemic) 087.1
   remittent (bilious) (congestive) (gastric) (*see
      also* Malaria) 084.6
   rheumatic (active) (acute) (chronic) (subacute)
      390
      with heart involvement 391.9
         carditis 391.9
         endocarditis (aortic) (mitral) (pulmonary)
            (tricuspid) 391.1
         multiple sites 391.8
         myocarditis 391.2
         pancarditis, acute 391.8
         pericarditis 391.0
         specified type NEC 391.8
         valvulitis 391.1
      inactive or quiescent with cardiac hypertrophy
         398.99
         carditis 398.90
         endocarditis 397.9
            aortic (valve) 395.9
               with mitral (valve) disease 396.9
            mitral (valve) 394.9
               with aortic (valve) disease 396.9
            pulmonary (valve) 397.1
            tricuspid (valve) 397.0
         heart conditions (classifiable to 429.3,
            429.6, 429.9) 398.99
            failure (congestive) (conditions
               classifiable to 428.0, 428.9) 398.91
            left ventricular failure (conditions
               classifiable to 428.1) 398.91

Fever—*continued*
  myocardial degeneration (conditions
      classifiable to 429.1) 398.0
  myocarditis (conditions classifiable to
      429.0) 398.0
  pancarditis 398.99
  pericarditis 393
  Rift Valley (viral) 066.3
  Rocky Mountain spotted 082.0
  rose 477.0
  Ross river (viral) 066.3
  Russian hemorrhagic 078.6
  sandfly 066.0
  San Joaquin (valley) 114.0
  São Paulo 082.0
  scarlet 034.1
  septic—*see* Septicemia
  seven-day 061
    Japan 100.89
    Queensland 100.89
  shin bone 083.1
  Singapore hemorrhagic 065.4
  solar 061
  sore 054.9
  South African tick-bite 087.1
  Southeast Asia hemorrhagic 065.4
  spinal—*see* Meningitis
  spirillary 026.0
  splenic (*see also* Anthrax) 022.9
  spotted (Rocky Mountain) 082.0
    American 082.0
    Brazilian 082.0
    Colombian 082.0
    meaning
      cerebrospinal meningitis 036.0
      typhus 082.9
  spring 309.23
  steroid
    correct substance properly administered 780.6
    overdose or wrong substance given or taken
        962.0
  streptobacillary 026.1
  subtertian 084.0
  Sumatran mite 081.2
  sun 061
  swamp 100.89
  sweating 078.2
  swine 003.8
  sylvatic yellow 060.0
  Tahyna 062.5
  tertian—*see* Malaria, tertian
  Thailand hemorrhagic 065.4
  thermic 992.0
  three day 066.0
    with Coxsackie exanthem 074.8
  tick
    American mountain 066.1
    Colorado 066.1
    Kemerovo 066.1
    Mediterranean 082.1
    mountain 066.1
    nonexanthematous 066.1
    Quaranfil 066.1
  tick-bite NEC 066.1
  tick-borne NEC 066.1
    hemorrhagic NEC 065.3
  transitory of newborn 778.4
  trench 083.1
  tsutsugamushi 081.2
  typhogastric 002.0

Fever—*continued*
  typhoid (abortive) (ambulant) (any site)
      (hemorrhagic) (infection) (intermittent)
      (malignant) (rheumatic) 002.0
  typhomalarial (*see also* Malaria) 084.6
  typhus—*see* Typhus
  undulant (*see also* Brucellosis) 023.9
  unknown origin (*see also* Pyrexia) 780.6
  uremic—*see* Uremia
  uveoparotid 135
  valley (Coccidioidomycosis) 114.0
  Venezuelan equine 066.2
  Volhynian 083.1
  Wesselsbron (viral) 066.3
  West
    African 084.8
    Nile (viral) 066.4
  Whitmore's 025
  Wolhynian 083.1
  worm 128.9
  Yaroslav hemorrhagic 078.6
  yellow 060.9
    jungle 060.0
    sylvatic 060.0
    urban 060.1
    vaccination, prophylactic (against) V04.4
  Zika (viral) 066.3
Fibrillation
  atrial (established) (paroxysmal) 427.31
  auricular (atrial) (established) 427.31
  cardiac (ventricular) 427.41
  coronary (*see also* Infarct, myocardium) 410.9
  heart (ventricular) 427.41
  muscular 728.9
  postoperative 997.1
  ventricular 427.41
Fibrin
  ball or bodies, pleural (sac) 511.0
  chamber, anterior (eye) (gelatinous exudate)
      364.04
Fibrinogenolysis (hemorrhagic)—*see*
      Fibrinolysis
Fibrinogenopenia (congenital) (hereditary) (*see
      also* Defect, coagulation) 286.3
  acquired 286.6
Fibrinolysis (acquired) (hemorrhagic)
      (pathologic) 286.6
  with
    abortion—*see* Abortion, by type, with
        hemorrhage, delayed or excessive
    ectopic pregnancy (*see also* categories
        633.0-633.9) 639.1
    molar pregnancy (*see also* categories
        630-632) 639.1
  antepartum or intrapartum 641.3
    affecting fetus or newborn 762.1
  following
    abortion 639.1
    ectopic or molar pregnancy 639.1
  newborn, transient 776.2
  postpartum 666.3
Fibrinopenia (hereditary) (*see also* Defect,
      coagulation) 286.3
  acquired 286.6
Fibrinopurulent —*see* condition
Fibrinous —*see* condition
Fibroadenoma (M9010/0)
  cellular intracanalicular (M9020/0) 217
  giant (intracanalicular) (M9020/0) 217
  intracanalicular (M9011/0)
    cellular (M9020/0) 217

Fibroadenoma—*continued*
giant (M9020/0) 217
specified site—*see* Neoplasm, by site, benign
unspecified site 217
juvenile (M9030/0) 217
pericanalicular (M9012/0)
specified site—*see* Neoplasm, by site, benign
unspecified site 217
phyllodes (M9020/0) 217
prostate 600.2
specified site—*see* Neoplasm, by site, benign
unspecified site 217
Fibroadenosis, breast (chronic) (cystic) (diffuse)
(periodic) (segmental) 610.2
Fibroangioma (M9160/0)—*see also* Neoplasm,
by site, benign
juvenile (M9160/0)
specified site—*see* Neoplasm, by site, benign
unspecified site 210.7
Fibrocellulitis progressiva ossificans 728.11
Fibrochondrosarcoma (M9220/3)—*see*
Neoplasm, cartilage, malignant
Fibrocystic
disease 277.00
bone NEC 733.29
breast 610.1
jaw 526.2
kidney (congenital) 753.19
liver 751.62
lung 518.89
congenital 748.4
pancreas 277.00
kidney (congenital) 753.19
Fibrodysplasia ossificans multiplex
(progressiva) 728.11
Fibroelastosis (cordis) (endocardial)
(endomyocardial) 425.3
Fibroid (tumor) (M8890/0)—*see also* Neoplasm,
connective tissue, benign
disease, lung (chronic) (*see also* Fibrosis, lung)
515
heart (disease) (*see also* Myocarditis) 429.0
induration, lung (chronic) (*see also* Fibrosis,
lung) 515
in pregnancy or childbirth 654.1
affecting fetus or newborn 763.89
causing obstructed labor 660.2
affecting fetus or newborn 763.1
liver—*see* Cirrhosis, liver
lung (*see also* Fibrosis, lung) 515
pneumonia (chronic) (*see also* Fibrosis, lung)
515
uterus (M8890/0) (*see also* Leiomyoma, uterus)
218.9
Fibrolipoma (M8851/0) (*see also* Lipoma, by
site) 214.9
Fibroliposarcoma (M8850/3)—*see* Neoplasm,
connective tissue, malignant
Fibroma (M8810/0)—*see also* Neoplasm,
connective tissue, benign
ameloblastic (M9330/0) 213.1
upper jaw (bone) 213.0
bone (nonossifying) 733.99
ossifying (M9262/0)—*see* Neoplasm, bone,
benign
cementifying (M9274/0)—*see* Neoplasm, bone,
benign
chondromyxoid (M9241/0)—*see* Neoplasm,
bone, benign
desmoplastic (M8823/1)—*see* Neoplasm,
connective tissue, uncertain behavior

Fibroma—*continued*
facial (M8813/0)—*see* Neoplasm, connective
tissue, benign
invasive (M8821/1)—*see* Neoplasm, connective
tissue, uncertain behavior
molle (M8851/0) (*see also* Lipoma, by site)
214.9
myxoid (M8811/0)—*see* Neoplasm, connective
tissue, benign
nasopharynx, nasopharyngeal (juvenile)
(M9160/0) 210.7
nonosteogenic (nonossifying)—*see* Dysplasia,
fibrous
odontogenic (M9321/0) 213.1
upper jaw (bone) 213.0
ossifying (M9262/0)—*see* Neoplasm, bone,
benign
periosteal (M8812/0)—*see* Neoplasm, bone,
benign
prostate 600.2
soft (M8851/0) (*see also* Lipoma, by site) 214.9
Fibromatosis
abdominal (M8822/1)—*see* Neoplasm,
connective tissue, uncertain behavior
aggressive (M8821/1)—*see* Neoplasm,
connective tissue, uncertain behavior
Dupuytren's 728.6
gingival 523.8
plantar fascia 728.71
proliferative 728.79
pseudosarcomatous (proliferative)
(subcutaneous) 728.79
subcutaneous pseudosarcomatous (proliferative)
728.79
Fibromyalgia 729.1
Fibromyoma (M8890/0)—*see also* Neoplasm,
connective tissue, benign
uterus (corpus) (*see also* Leiomyoma, uterus)
218.9
in pregnancy or childbirth 654.1
affecting fetus or newborn 763.89
causing obstructed labor 660.2
affecting fetus or newborn 763.1
Fibromyositis (*see also* Myositis) 729.1
scapulohumeral 726.2
Fibromyxolipoma (M8852/0) (*see also* Lipoma,
by site) 214.9
Fibromyxoma (M8811/0)—*see* Neoplasm,
connective tissue, benign
Fibromyxosarcoma (M8811/3)—*see* Neoplasm,
connective tissue, malignant
Fibro-odontoma, ameloblastic (M9290/0) 213.1
upper jaw (bone) 213.0
Fibro-osteoma (M9262/0)—*see* Neoplasm,
bone, benign
Fibroplasia, retrolental 362.21
Fibropurulent —*see* condition
Fibrosarcoma (M8810/3)—*see also* Neoplasm,
connective tissue, malignant
ameloblastic (M9330/3) 170.1
upper jaw (bone) 170.0
congenital (M8814/3)—*see* Neoplasm,
connective tissue, malignant
fascial (M8813/3)—*see* Neoplasm, connective
tissue, malignant
infantile (M8814/3)—*see* Neoplasm, connective
tissue, malignant
odontogenic (M9330/3) 170.1
upper jaw (bone) 170.0
periosteal (M8812/3)—*see* Neoplasm, bone,
malignant

Fibrosclerosis
  breast 610.3
  corpora cavernosa (penis) 607.89
  familial multifocal NEC 710.8
  multifocal (idiopathic) NEC 710.8
  penis (corpora cavernosa) 607.89
Fibrosis, fibrotic
  adrenal (gland) 255.8
  alveolar (diffuse) 516.3
  amnion 658.8
  anal papillae 569.49
  anus 569.49
  appendix, appendiceal, noninflammatory 543.9
  arteriocapillary—*see* Arteriosclerosis
  bauxite (of lung) 503
  biliary 576.8
    due to Clonorchis sinensis 121.1
  bladder 596.8
    interstitial 595.1
    localized submucosal 595.1
    panmural 595.1
  bone, diffuse 756.59
  breast 610.3
  capillary—*see also* Arteriosclerosis
    lung (chronic) (*see also* Fibrosis, lung) 515
  cardiac (*see also* Myocarditis) 429.0
  cervix 622.8
  chorion 658.8
  corpus cavernosum 607.89
  cystic (of pancreas) 277.00
    with
      manifestations
        gastrointestinal 277.03
        pulmonary 277.02
        specified NEC 277.09
      meconium ileus 277.01
      pulmonary exacerbation 277.02
  due to (presence of) any device, implant, or
    graft—*see* Complications, due to (presence
    of) any device, implant, or graft classified to
    996.0-996.5 NEC
  ejaculatory duct 608.89
  endocardium (*see also* Endocarditis) 424.90
  endomyocardial (African) 425.0
  epididymis 608.89
  eye muscle 378.62
  graphite (of lung) 503
  heart (*see also* Myocarditis) 429.0
  hepatic—*see also* Cirrhosis, liver
    due to Clonorchis sinensis 121.1
  hepatolienal—*see* Cirrhosis, liver
  hepatosplenic—*see* Cirrhosis, liver
  infrapatellar fat pad 729.31
  interstitial pulmonary, newborn 770.7
  intrascrotal 608.89
  kidney (*see also* Sclerosis, renal) 587
  liver—*see* Cirrhosis, liver
  lung (atrophic) (capillary) (chronic) (confluent)
    (massive) (perialveolar) (peribronchial) 515
    with
      anthracosilicosis (occupational) 500
      anthracosis (occupational) 500
      asbestosis (occupational) 501
      bagassosis (occupational) 495.1
      bauxite 503
      berylliosis (occupational) 503
      byssinosis (occupational) 504
      calcicosis (occupational) 502
      chalicosis (occupational) 502
      dust reticulation (occupational) 504
      farmers' lung 495.0

Fibrosis, fibrotic—*continued*
    gannister disease (occupational) 502
    graphite 503
    pneumonoconiosis (occupational) 505
    pneumosiderosis (occupational) 503
    siderosis (occupational) 503
    silicosis (occupational) 502
    tuberculosis (*see also* Tuberculosis) 011.4
  diffuse (idiopathic) (interstitial) 516.3
  due to
    bauxite 503
    fumes or vapors (chemical) (inhalation)
      506.4
    graphite 503
    following radiation 508.1
    postinflammatory 515
    silicotic (massive) (occupational) 502
    tuberculous (*see also* Tuberculosis) 011.4
  lymphatic gland 289.3
  median bar 600.9
  mediastinum (idiopathic) 519.3
  meninges 349.2
  muscle NEC 728.2
    iatrogenic (from injection) 999.9
  myocardium, myocardial (*see also* Myocarditis)
    429.0
  oral submucous 528.8
  ovary 620.8
  oviduct 620.8
  pancreas 577.8
    cystic 277.00
      with
        manifestations
          gastrointestinal 277.03
          pulmonary 277.02
          specified NEC 277.09
        meconium ileus 277.01
        pulmonary exacerbation 277.02
  penis 607.89
  periappendiceal 543.9
  periarticular (*see also* Ankylosis) 718.5
  pericardium 423.1
  perineum, in pregnancy or childbirth 654.8
    affecting fetus or newborn 763.89
    causing obstructed labor 660.2
      affecting fetus or newborn 763.1
  perineural NEC 355.9
    foot 355.6
  periureteral 593.89
  placenta—*see* Placenta, abnormal
  pleura 511.0
  popliteal fat pad 729.31
  preretinal 362.56
  prostate (chronic) 600.9
  pulmonary (chronic) (*see also* Fibrosis, lung)
    515
    alveolar capillary block 516.3
    interstitial
      diffuse (idiopathic) 516.3
      newborn 770.7
  radiation—*see* Effect, adverse, radiation
  rectal sphincter 569.49
  retroperitoneal, idiopathic 593.4
  scrotum 608.89
  seminal vesicle 608.89
  senile 797
  skin NEC 709.2
  spermatic cord 608.89
  spleen 289.59
    bilharzial (*see also* Schistosomiasis) 120.9

Fibrosis, fibrotic—*continued*
  subepidermal nodular (M8832/0)—*see*
    Neoplasm, skin, benign
  submucous NEC 709.2
    oral 528.8
    tongue 528.8
  syncytium—*see* Placenta, abnormal
  testis 608.89
    chronic, due to syphilis 095.8
  thymus (gland) 254.8
  tunica vaginalis 608.89
  ureter 593.89
  urethra 599.84
  uterus (nonneoplastic) 621.8
    bilharzial (*see also* Schistosomiasis) 120.9
    neoplastic (*see also* Leiomyoma, uterus) 218.9
  vagina 623.8
  valve, heart (*see also* Endocarditis) 424.90
  vas deferens 608.89
  vein 459.89
    lower extremities 459.89
  vesical 595.1
Fibrositis (periarticular) (rheumatoid) 729.0
  humeroscapular region 726.2
  nodular, chronic
    Jaccoud's 714.4
    rheumatoid 714.4
  ossificans 728.11
  scapulohumeral 726.2
Fibrothorax 511.0
Fibrotic —*see* Fibrosis
Fibrous —*see* condition
Fibroxanthoma (M8831/0)—*see also* Neoplasm,
  connective tissue, benign
  atypical (M8831/1)—*see* Neoplasm, connective
    tissue, uncertain behavior
  malignant (M8831/3)—*see* Neoplasm,
    connective tissue, malignant
Fibroxanthosarcoma (M8831/3)—*see*
  Neoplasm, connective tissue, malignant
Fiedler's
  disease (leptospiral jaundice) 100.0
  myocarditis or syndrome (acute isolated
    myocarditis) 422.91
Fiessinger-Leroy (-Reiter) syndrome 099.3
Fiessinger-Rendu syndrome (erythema
  muliforme exudativum) 695.1
Fifth disease (eruptive) 057.0
  venereal 099.1
Filaria, filarial —*see* Infestation, filarial
Filariasis (*see also* Infestation, filarial) 125.9
  bancroftian 125.0
  Brug's 125.1
  due to
    bancrofti 125.0
    Brugia (Wuchereria) (malayi) 125.1
    Loa loa 125.2
    malayi 125.1
    organism NEC 125.6
    Wuchereria (bancrofti) 125.0
      malayi 125.1
  Malayan 125.1
  ozzardi 125.5
  specified type NEC 125.6
Filatoff's, Filatov's, Filatow's disease
  (infectious mononucleosis) 075
File-cutters' disease 984.9
  specified type of lead—*see* Table of drugs and
    chemicals

Filling defect
  biliary tract 793.3
  bladder 793.5
  duodenum 793.4
  gallbladder 793.3
  gastrointestinal tract 793.4
  intestine 793.4
  kidney 793.5
  stomach 793.4
  ureter 793.5
Filtering bleb, eye (postglaucoma) (status)
  V45.69
  with complication or rupture 997.99
  postcataract extraction (complication) 997.99
Fimbrial cyst (congenital) 752.11
Fimbriated hymen 752.49
Financial problem affecting care V60.2
Findings, abnormal, without diagnosis
  (examination) (laboratory test) 796.4
  17-ketosteroids, elevated 791.9
  acetonuria 791.6
  acid phosphatase 790.5
  albumin-globulin ratio 790.99
  albuminuria 791.0
  alcohol in blood 790.3
  alkaline phosphatase 790.5
  amniotic fluid 792.3
  amylase 790.5
  anisocytosis 790.09
  antenatal screening 796.5
  antibody titers, elevated 795.79
  anticardiolipin antibody 795.79
  antigen-antibody reaction 795.79
  antiphospholipid antibody 795.79
  anthrax, positive 795.31
  bacteriuria 791.9
  ballistocardiogram 794.39
  bicarbonate 276.9
  bile in urine 791.4
  bilirubin 277.4
  bleeding time (prolonged) 790.92
  blood culture, positive 790.7
  blood gas level 790.91
  blood sugar level 790.2
    high 790.2
    low 251.2
  calcium 275.40
  carbonate 276.9
  casts, urine 791.7
  catecholamines 791.9
  cells, urine 791.7
  cerebrospinal fluid (color) (content) (pressure)
    792.0
  chloride 276.9
  cholesterol 272.9
  chromosome analysis 795.2
  chyluria 791.1
  circulation time 794.39
  cloudy dialysis effluent 792.5
  cloudy urine 791.9
  coagulation study 790.92
  cobalt, blood 790.6
  color of urine (unusual) NEC 791.9
  copper, blood 790.6
  crystals, urine 791.9
  culture, positive NEC 795.39
    blood 790.7
    HIV V08
    human immunodeficiency virus V08
    nose 795.39
    skin lesion NEC 795.39

Findings, abnormal without diagnosis—*cont.*
  spinal fluid 792.0
  sputum 795.39
  stool 792.1
  throat 795.39
  urine 791.9
  viral
    human immunodeficiency V08
  wound 795.39
echocardiogram 793.2
echoencephalogram 794.01
echogram NEC—*see* Findings, abnormal,
  structure
electrocardiogram (ECG) (EKG) 794.31
electroencephalogram (EEG) 794.02
electrolyte level, urinary 791.9
electromyogram (EMG) 794.17
  ocular 794.14
electro-oculogram (EOG) 794.12
electroretinogram (ERG) 794.11
enzymes, serum NEC 790.5
fibrinogen titer coagulation study 790.92
filling defect—*see* Filling defect
function study NEC 794.9
  auditory 794.15
  bladder 794.9
  brain 794.00
  cardiac 794.30
  endocrine NEC 794.6
    thyroid 794.5
  kidney 794.4
  liver 794.8
  nervous system
    central 794.00
    peripheral 794.19
  oculomotor 794.14
  pancreas 794.9
  placenta 794.9
  pulmonary 794.2
  retina 794.11
  special senses 794.19
  spleen 794.9
  vestibular 794.16
gallbladder, nonvisualization 793.3
glucose 790.2
  tolerance test 790.2
glycosuria 791.5
heart
  shadow 793.2
  sounds 785.3
hematinuria 791.2
hematocrit
  drop (precipitous) 790.01
  elevated 282.7
  low 285.9
hematologic NEC 790.99
hematuria 599.7
hemoglobin
  elevated 282.7
  low 285.9
hemoglobinuria 791.2
histological NEC 795.4
hormones 259.9
immunoglobulins, elevated 795.79
indolacetic acid, elevated 791.9
iron 790.6
karyotype 795.2
ketonuria 791.6
lactic acid dehydrogenase (LDH) 790.4
lipase 790.5
lipids NEC 272.9

Findings, abnormal without diagnosis—*cont.*
lithium, blood 790.6
lung field (coin lesion) (shadow) 793.1
magnesium, blood 790.6
mammogram 793.80
  microcalcification 793.81
mediastinal shift 793.2
melanin, urine 791.9
microbiologic NEC 795.39
mineral, blood NEC 790.6
myoglobinuria 791.3
nasal swab, anthrax 795.31
nitrogen derivatives, blood 790.6
nonvisualization of gallbladder 793.3
nose culture, positive 795.39
odor of urine (unusual) NEC 791.9
oxygen saturation 790.91
Papanicolaou (smear) 795.1
  cervix 795.00
    atypical squamous cell changes of
      undetermined significance
      favor benign (ASCUS favor benign)
        795.01
      favor dysplasia (ASCUS favor dysplasia)
        795.02
    dyskaryotic 795.09
    nonspecific finding NEC 795.09
  other site 795.1
peritoneal fluid 792.9
phonocardiogram 794.39
phosphorus 275.3
pleural fluid 792.9
pneumoencephalogram 793.0
PO_2-oxygen ratio 790.91
poikilocytosis 790.09
potassium
  deficiency 276.8
  excess 276.7
PPD 795.5
prostate specific antigen (PSA) 790.93
protein, serum NEC 790.99
proteinuria 791.0
prothrombin time (partial) (prolonged) (PT)
  (PTT) 790.92
pyuria 791.9
radiologic (x-ray) 793.9
  abdomen 793.6
  biliary tract 793.3
  breast 793.89
    abnormal mammogram NOS 793.80
    mammographic microcalcification 793.81
  gastrointestinal tract 793.4
  genitourinary organs 793.5
  head 793.0
  intrathoracic organs NEC 793.2
  lung 793.1
  musculoskeletal 793.7
  placenta 793.9
  retroperitoneum 793.6
  skin 793.9
  skull 793.0
  subcutaneous tissue 793.9
red blood cell 790.09
  count 790.09
  morphology 790.09
  sickling 790.09
  volume 790.09
saliva 792.4
scan NEC 794.9
  bladder 794.9
  bone 794.9

Findings, abnormal without diagnosis—*cont.*
  brain 794.09
  kidney 794.4
  liver 794.8
  lung 794.2
  pancreas 794.9
  placental 794.9
  spleen 794.9
  thyroid 794.5
  sedimentation rate, elevated 790.1
  semen 792.2
  serological (for)
    human immunodeficiency virus (HIV)
      inconclusive 795.71
      positive V08
    syphilis—*see* Findings, serology for syphilis
  serology for syphilis
    false positive 795.6
    positive 097.1
      false 795.6
      follow-up of latent syphilis—*see* Syphilis,
        latent
      only finding—*see* Syphilis, latent
  serum 790.99
    blood NEC 790.99
    enzymes NEC 790.5
    proteins 790.99
  SGOT 790.4
  SGPT 790.4
  sickling of red blood cells 790.09
  skin test, positive 795.79
    tuberculin (without active tuberculosis) 795.5
  sodium 790.6
    deficiency 276.1
    excess 276.0
  spermatozoa 792.2
  spinal fluid 792.0
    culture, positive 792.0
  sputum culture, positive 795.39
    for acid-fast bacilli 795.39
  stool NEC 792.1
    bloody 578.1
      occult 792.1
    color 792.1
    culture, positive 792.1
    occult blood 792.1
  structure, body (echogram) (thermogram)
    (ultrasound) (x-ray) NEC 793.9
    abdomen 793.6
    breast 793.89
      abnormal mammogram 793.80
      mammographic microcalcification 793.81
    gastrointestinal tract 793.4
    genitourinary organs 793.5
    head 793.0
      echogram (ultrasound) 794.01
    intrathoracic organs NEC 793.2
    lung 793.1
    musculoskeletal 793.7
    placenta 793.9
    retroperitoneum 793.6
    skin 793.9
    subcutaneous tissue NEC 793.9
  synovial fluid 792.9
  thermogram—*see* Finding, abnormal, structure
  throat culture, positive 795.39
  thyroid (function) 794.5
    metabolism (rate) 794.5
    scan 794.5
    uptake 794.5
  total proteins 790.99

Findings, abnormal without diagnosis—*cont.*
  toxicology (drugs) (heavy metals) 796.0
  transaminase (level) 790.4
  triglycerides 272.9
  tuberculin skin test (without active tuberculosis)
    795.5
  ultrasound—*see also* Finding, abnormal,
    structure
    cardiogram 793.2
  uric acid, blood 790.6
  urine, urinary constituents 791.9
    acetone 791.6
    albumin 791.0
    bacteria 791.9
    bile 791.4
    blood 599.7
    casts or cells 791.7
    chyle 791.1
    culture, positive 791.9
    glucose 791.5
    hemoglobin 791.2
    ketone 791.6
    protein 791.0
    pus 791.9
    sugar 791.5
  vaginal fluid 792.9
  vanillylmandelic acid, elevated 791.9
  vectorcardiogram (VCG) 794.39
  ventriculogram (cerebral) 793.0
  VMA, elevated 791.9
  Wassermann reaction
    false positive 795.6
    positive 097.1
      follow-up of latent syphilis—*see* Syphilis,
        latent
      only finding—*see* Syphilis, latent
  white blood cell 288.9
    count 288.9
      elevated 288.8
      low 288.0
    differential 288.9
    morphology 288.9
  wound culture 795.39
  xerography 793.89
  zinc, blood 790.6
Finger —*see* condition
Fire, St. Anthony's (*see also* Erysipelas) 035
Fish
  hook stomach 537.89
  meal workers' lung 495.8
Fisher's syndrome 357.0
Fissure, fissured
  abdominal wall (congenital) 756.79
  anus, anal 565.0
    congenital 751.5
  buccal cavity 528.9
  clitoris (congenital) 752.49
  ear, lobule (congenital) 744.29
  epiglottis (congenital) 748.3
  larynx 478.79
    congenital 748.3
  lip 528.5
    congenital (*see also* Cleft, lip) 749.10
  nipple 611.2
    puerperal, postpartum 676.1
  palate (congenital) (*see also* Cleft, palate)
    749.00
  postanal 565.0
  rectum 565.0
  skin 709.8
    streptococcal 686.9

Fissure, fissured—*continued*
  spine (congenital) (*see also* Spina bifida) 741.9
  sternum (congenital) 756.3
  tongue (acquired) 529.5
    congenital 750.13
Fistula (sinus) 686.9
  abdomen (wall) 569.81
    bladder 596.2
    intestine 569.81
    ureter 593.82
    uterus 619.2
  abdominorectal 569.81
  abdominosigmoidal 569.81
  abdominothoracic 510.0
  abdominouterine 619.2
    congenital 752.3
  abdominovesical 596.2
  accessory sinuses (*see also* Sinusitis) 473.9
  actinomycotic—*see* Actinomycosis
  alveolar
    antrum (*see also* Sinusitis, maxillary) 473.0
    process 522.7
  anorectal 565.1
  antrobuccal (*see also* Sinusitis, maxillary) 473.0
  antrum (*see also* Sinusitis, maxillary) 473.0
  anus, anal (infectional) (recurrent) 565.1
    congenital 751.5
    tuberculous (*see also* Tuberculosis) 014.8
  aortic sinus 747.29
  aortoduodenal 447.2
  appendix, appendicular 543.9
  arteriovenous (acquired) 447.0
    brain 437.3
      congenital 747.81
        ruptured (*see also* Hemorrhage, subarachnoid) 430
      ruptured (*see also* Hemorrhage, subarachnoid) 430
    cerebral 437.3
      congenital 747.81
    congenital (peripheral) 747.60
      brain—*see* Fistula, arteriovenous, brain, congenital
      coronary 746.85
      gastrointestinal 747.61
      lower limb 747.64
      pulmonary 747.3
      renal 747.62
      specified NEC 747.69
      upper limb 747.63
    coronary 414.19
      congenital 746.85
    heart 414.19
    pulmonary (vessels) 417.0
      congenital 747.3
    surgically created (for dialysis) V45.1
      complication NEC 996.73
        atherosclerosis —*see* Arteriosclerosis, extremities
        embolism 996.74
        infection or inflammation 996.62
        mechanical 996.1
        occlusion NEC 996.74
        thrombus 996.74
    traumatic—*see* Injury, blood vessel, by site
  artery 447.2
  aural 383.81
    congenital 744.49
  auricle 383.81
    congenital 744.49
  Bartholin's gland 619.8

Fistula—*continued*
  bile duct (*see also* Fistula, biliary) 576.4
  biliary (duct) (tract) 576.4
    congenital 751.69
  bladder (neck) (sphincter) 596.2
    into seminal vesicle 596.2
  bone 733.99
  brain 348.8
    arteriovenous—*see* Fistula, arteriovenous, brain
  branchial (cleft) 744.41
  branchiogenous 744.41
  breast 611.0
    puerperal, postpartum 675.1
  bronchial 510.0
  bronchocutaneous, bronchomediastinal, bronchopleural, bronchopleuromediastinal (infective) 510.0
    tuberculous (*see also* Tuberculosis) 011.3
  bronchoesophageal 530.89
    congenital 750.3
  buccal cavity (infective) 528.3
  canal, ear 380.89
  carotid-cavernous
    congenital 747.81
      with hemorrhage 430
    traumatic 900.82
      with hemorrhage (see also Hemorrhage, brain, traumatic) 853.0
    late effect 908.3
  cecosigmoidal 569.81
  cecum 569.81
  cerebrospinal (fluid) 349.81
  cervical, lateral (congenital) 744.41
  cervicoaural (congenital) 744.49
  cervicosigmoidal 619.1
  cervicovesical 619.0
  cervix 619.8
  chest (wall) 510.0
  cholecystocolic (*see also* Fistula, gallbladder) 575.5
  cholecystocolonic (*see also* Fistula, gallbladder) 575.5
  cholecystoduodenal (*see also* Fistula, gallbladder) 575.5
  cholecystoenteric (*see also* Fistula, gallbladder) 575.5
  cholecystogastric (*see also* Fistula, gallbladder) 575.5
  cholecystointestinal (*see also* Fistula, gallbladder) 575.5
  choledochoduodenal 576.4
  cholocolic (*see also* Fistula, gallbladder) 575.5
  coccyx 685.1
    with abscess 685.0
  colon 569.81
  colostomy 569.69
  colovaginal (acquired) 619.1
  common duct (bile duct) 576.4
  congenital, NEC—*see* Anomaly, specified type NEC
  cornea, causing hypotony 360.32
  coronary, arteriovenous 414.19
    congenital 746.85
  costal region 510.0
  cul-de-sac, Douglas' 619.8
  cutaneous 686.9
  cystic duct (*see also* Fistula, gallbladder) 575.5
    congenital 751.69
  dental 522.7

Fistula—*continued*
  diaphragm 510.0
    bronchovisceral 510.0
    pleuroperitoneal 510.0
    pulmonoperitoneal 510.0
  duodenum 537.4
  ear (canal) (external) 380.89
  enterocolic 569.81
  enterocutaneous 569.81
  enteroenteric 569.81
  entero-uterine 619.1
    congenital 752.3
  enterovaginal 619.1
    congenital 752.49
  enterovesical 596.1
  epididymis 608.89
    tuberculous (*see also* Tuberculosis) 016.4
  esophagobronchial 530.89
    congenital 750.3
  esophagocutaneous 530.89
  esophagopleurocutaneous 530.89
  esophagotracheal 530.84
    congenital 750.3
  esophagus 530.89
    congenital 750.4
  ethmoid (*see also* Sinusitis, ethmoidal) 473.2
  eyeball (cornea) (sclera) 360.32
  eyelid 373.11
  fallopian tube (external) 619.2
  fecal 569.81
    congenital 751.5
  from periapical lesion 522.7
  frontal sinus (*see also* Sinusitis, frontal) 473.1
  gallbladder 575.5
    with calculus, cholelithiasis, stones (*see also*
      Cholelithiasis) 574.2
    congenital 751.69
  gastric 537.4
  gastrocolic 537.4
    congenital 750.7
    tuberculous (*see also* Tuberculosis) 014.8
  gastroenterocolic 537.4
  gastroesophageal 537.4
  gastrojejunal 537.4
  gastrojejunocolic 537.4
  genital
    organs
      female 619.9
        specified site NEC 619.8
      male 608.89
    tract-skin (female) 619.2
  hepatopleural 510.0
  hepatopulmonary 510.0
  horseshoe 565.1
  ileorectal 569.81
  ileosigmoidal 569.81
  ileostomy 569.69
  ileovesical 596.1
  ileum 569.81
  in ano 565.1
    tuberculous (*see also* Tuberculosis) 014.8
  inner ear (*see also* Fistula, labyrinth) 386.40
  intestine 569.81
  intestinocolonic (abdominal) 569.81
  intestinoureteral 593.82
  intestinouterine 619.1
  intestinovaginal 619.1
    congenital 752.49
  intestinovesical 596.1
  involving female genital tract 619.9
    digestive-genital 619.1

Fistula—*continued*
    genital tract-skin 619.2
    specified site NEC 619.8
    urinary-genital 619.0
  ischiorectal (fossa) 566
  jejunostomy 569.69
  jejunum 569.81
  joint 719.80
    ankle 719.87
    elbow 719.82
    foot 719.87
    hand 719.84
    hip 719.85
    knee 719.86
    multiple sites 719.89
    pelvic region 719.85
    shoulder (region) 719.81
    specified site NEC 719.88
    tuberculous—*see* Tuberculosis, joint
    wrist 719.83
  kidney 593.89
  labium (majus) (minus) 619.8
  labyrinth, labyrinthine NEC 386.40
    combined sites 386.48
    multiple sites 386.48
    oval window 386.42
    round window 386.41
    semicircular canal 386.43
  lacrimal, lachrymal (duct) (gland) (sac) 375.61
  lacrimonasal duct 375.61
  laryngotracheal 748.3
  larynx 478.79
  lip 528.5
    congenital 750.25
  lumbar, tuberculous (*see also* Tuberculosis)
    015.0 *[730.8]*
  lung 510.0
  lymphatic (node) (vessel) 457.8
  mamillary 611.0
  mammary (gland) 611.0
    puerperal, postpartum 675.1
  mastoid (process) (region) 383.1
  maxillary (*see also* Sinusitis, maxillary) 473.0
  mediastinal 510.0
  mediastinobronchial 510.0
  mediastinocutaneous 510.0
  middle ear 385.89
  mouth 528.3
  nasal 478.1
    sinus (*see also* Sinusitis) 473.9
  nasopharynx 478.29
  nipple—*see* Fistula, breast
  nose 478.1
  oral (cutaneous) 528.3
    maxillary (*see also* Sinusitis, maxillary) 473.0
    nasal (with cleft palate) (*see also* Cleft, palate)
      749.00
  orbit, orbital 376.10
  oro-antral (*see also* Sinusitis, maxillary) 473.0
  oval window (internal ear) 386.42
  oviduct (external) 619.2
  palate (hard) 526.89
    soft 528.9
  pancreatic 577.8
  pancreaticoduodenal 577.8
  parotid (gland) 527.4
    region 528.3
  pelvoabdominointestinal 569.81
  penis 607.89
  perianal 565.1

Fistula—*continued*

pericardium (pleura) (sac) (*see also* Pericarditis) 423.8
pericecal 569.81
perineal—*see* Fistula, perineum
perineorectal 569.81
perineosigmoidal 569.81
perineo-urethroscrotal 608.89
perineum, perineal (with urethral involvement) NEC 599.1
  tuberculous (*see also* Tuberculosis) 017.9
  ureter 593.82
perirectal 565.1
  tuberculous (*see also* Tuberculosis) 014.8
peritoneum (*see also* Peritonitis) 567.2
periurethral 599.1
pharyngo-esophageal 478.29
pharynx 478.29
  branchial cleft (congenital) 744.41
pilonidal (infected) (rectum) 685.1
  with abscess 685.0
pleura, pleural, pleurocutaneous, pleuroperitoneal 510.0
  stomach 510.0
  tuberculous (*see also* Tuberculosis) 012.0
pleuropericardial 423.8
postauricular 383.81
postoperative, persistent 998.6
preauricular (congenital) 744.46
prostate 602.8
pulmonary 510.0
  arteriovenous 417.0
    congenital 747.3
  tuberculous (*see also* Tuberculosis, pulmonary) 011.9
pulmonoperitoneal 510.0
rectolabial 619.1
rectosigmoid (intercommunicating) 569.81
rectoureteral 593.82
rectourethral 599.1
  congenital 753.8
rectouterine 619.1
  congenital 752.3
rectovaginal 619.1
  congenital 752.49
  old, postpartal 619.1
  tuberculous (*see also* Tuberculosis) 014.8
rectovesical 596.1
  congenital 753.8
rectovesicovaginal 619.1
rectovulvar 619.1
  congenital 752.49
rectum (to skin) 565.1
  tuberculous (*see also* Tuberculosis) 014.8
renal 593.89
retroauricular 383.81
round window (internal ear) 386.41
salivary duct or gland 527.4
  congenital 750.24
sclera 360.32
scrotum (urinary) 608.89
  tuberculous (*see also* Tuberculosis) 016.5
semicircular canals (internal ear) 386.43
sigmoid 569.81
  vesicoabdominal 596.1
sigmoidovaginal 619.1
  congenital 752.49
skin 686.9
  ureter 593.82
  vagina 619.2

Fistula—*continued*

sphenoidal sinus (*see also* Sinusitis, sphenoidal) 473.3
splenocolic 289.59
stercoral 569.81
stomach 537.4
sublingual gland 527.4
  congenital 750.24
submaxillary
  gland 527.4
    congenital 750.24
  region 528.3
thoracic 510.0
  duct 457.8
thoracicoabdominal 510.0
thoracicogastric 510.0
thoracicointestinal 510.0
thoracoabdominal 510.0
thoracogastric 510.0
thorax 510.0
thyroglossal duct 759.2
thyroid 246.8
trachea (congenital) (external) (internal) 748.3
tracheoesophageal 530.84
  congenital 750.3
  following tracheostomy 519.09
traumatic
  arteriovenous (*see also* Injury, blood vessel, by site) 904.9
  brain—*see* Injury, intracranial
tuberculous—*see* Tuberculosis, by site
typhoid 002.0
umbilical 759.89
umbilico-urinary 753.8
urachal, urachus 753.7
ureter (persistent) 593.82
ureteroabdominal 593.82
ureterocervical 593.82
ureterorectal 593.82
ureterosigmoido-abdominal 593.82
ureterovaginal 619.0
ureterovesical 596.2
urethra 599.1
  congenital 753.8
  tuberculous (*see also* Tuberculosis) 016.3
urethroperineal 599.1
urethroperineovesical 596.2
urethrorectal 599.1
  congenital 753.8
urethroscrotal 608.89
urethrovaginal 619.0
urethrovesical 596.2
urethrovesicovaginal 619.0
urinary (persistent) (recurrent) 599.1
uteroabdominal (anterior wall) 619.2
  congenital 752.3
uteroenteric 619.1
uterofecal 619.1
uterointestinal 619.1
  congenital 752.3
uterorectal 619.1
  congenital 752.3
uteroureteric 619.0
uterovaginal 619.8
uterovesical 619.0
  congenital 752.3
uterus 619.8
vagina (wall) 619.8
  postpartal, old 619.8
vaginocutaneous (postpartal) 619.2
vaginoileal (acquired) 619.1

Fistula—*continued*
vaginoperineal 619.2
vesical NEC 596.2
vesicoabdominal 596.2
vesicocervicovaginal 619.0
vesicocolic 596.1
vesicocutaneous 596.2
vesicoenteric 596.1
vesicointestinal 596.1
vesicometrorectal 619.1
vesicoperineal 596.2
vesicorectal 596.1
  congenital 753.8
vesicosigmoidal 596.1
vesicosigmoidovaginal 619.1
vesicoureteral 596.2
vesicoureterovaginal 619.0
vesicourethral 596.2
vesicourethrorectal 596.1
vesicouterine 619.0
  congenital 752.3
vesicovaginal 619.0
vulvorectal 619.1
  congenital 752.49
Fit   780.39
apoplectic (*see also* Disease, cerebrovascular,
    acute) 436
late effect—*see* Late effect(s) (of)
    cerebrovascular disease
epileptic (*see also* Epilepsy) 345.9
fainting 780.2
hysterical 300.11
newborn 779.0
Fitting (of)
artificial
  arm (complete) (partial) V52.0
  breast V52.4
  eye(s) V52.2
  leg(s) (complete) (partial) V52.1
brain neuropacemaker V53.02
cardiac pacemaker V53.31
carotid sinus pacemaker V53.39
cerebral ventricle (communicating) shunt
    V53.01
colostomy belt V53.5
contact lenses V53.1
cystostomy device V53.6
defibrillator, automatic implantable V53.32
dentures V52.3
device NEC V53.9
  abdominal V53.5
  cardiac
    defibrillator, automatic implantable V53.32
    pacemaker V53.31
    specified NEC V53.39
  cerebral ventricle (communicating) shunt
    V53.01
  intrauterine contraceptive V25.1
  nervous system V53.09
  orthodontic V53.4
  orthoptic V53.1
  prosthetic V52.9
    breast V52.4
    dental V52.3
    eye V52.2
    specified type NEC V52.8
  special senses V53.09
  substitution
    auditory V53.09
    nervous system V53.09
    visual V53.09

Fitting—*continued*
urinary V53.6
diaphragm (contraceptive) V25.02
glasses (reading) V53.1
hearing aid V53.2
ileostomy device V53.5
intestinal appliance or device NEC V53.5
intrauterine contraceptive device V25.1
neuropacemaker (brain) (peripheral nerve)
    (spinal cord) V53.02
orthodontic device V53.4
orthopedic (device) V53.7
  brace V53.7
  cast V53.7
  corset V53.7
  shoes V53.7
pacemaker (cardiac) V53.31
  brain V53.02
  carotid sinus V53.39
  peripheral nerve V53.02
  spinal cord V53.02
prosthesis V52.9
  arm (complete) (partial) V52.0
  breast V52.4
  dental V52.3
  eye V52.2
  leg (complete) (partial) V52.1
  specified type NEC V52.8
spectacles V53.1
wheelchair V53.8
Fitz's syndrome (acute hemorrhagic
    pancreatitis) 577.0
Fitz-Hugh and Curtis syndrome (gonococcal
    peritonitis) 098.86
Fixation
joint—*see* Ankylosis
larynx 478.79
pupil 364.76
stapes 385.22
  deafness (*see also* Deafness, conductive)
    389.04
uterus (acquired)—*see* Malposition, uterus
vocal cord 478.5
Flaccid —*see* condition
foot 736.79
forearm 736.09
palate, congenital 750.26
Flail
chest 807.4
  newborn 767.3
joint (paralytic) 718.80
  ankle 718.87
  elbow 718.82
  foot 718.87
  hand 718.84
  hip 718.85
  knee 718.86
  multiple sites 718.89
  pelvic region 718.85
  shoulder (region) 718.81
  specified site NEC 718.88
  wrist 718.83
Flajani (-Basedow) syndrome or disease
    (exophthalmic goiter) 242.0
Flap, liver 572.8
Flare, anterior chamber (aqueous) (eye) 364.04
Flashback phenomena (drug) (hallucinogenic)
    292.89

Flat
    chamber (anterior) (eye) 360.34
    chest, congenital 754.89
    electroencephalogram (EEG) 348.8
    foot (acquired) (fixed type) (painful) (postural)
        (spastic) 734
        congenital 754.61
            rocker bottom 754.61
            vertical talus 754.61
        rachitic 268.1
        rocker bottom (congenital) 754.61
        vertical talus, congenital 754.61
    organ or site, congenital NEC—*see* Anomaly,
        specified type NEC
    pelvis 738.6
        with disproportion (fetopelvic) 653.2
            affecting fetus or newborn 763.1
            causing obstructed labor 660.1
                affecting fetus or newborn 763.1
        congenital 755.69
Flatau-Schilder disease 341.1
Flattening
    head, femur 736.39
    hip 736.39
    lip (congenital) 744.89
    nose (congenital) 754.0
        acquired 738.0
Flatulence 787.3
Flatus 787.3
    vaginalis 629.8
Flax dressers' disease 504
Flea bite —*see* Injury, superficial, by site
Fleischer (-Kayser) ring (corneal pigmentation)
    275.1 [371.14]
Fleischner's disease 732.3
Fleshy mole 631
Flexibilitas cerea (*see also* Catalepsy) 300.11
Flexion
    cervix (*see also* Malposition, uterus) 621.6
    contracture, joint (*see also* Contraction, joint)
        718.4
    deformity, joint (*see also* Contraction, joint)
        718.4
        hip, congenital (*see also* Subluxation,
            congenital, hip) 754.32
    uterus (*see also* Malposition, uterus) 621.6
Flexner's
    bacillus 004.1
    diarrhea (ulcerative) 004.1
    dysentery 004.1
Flexner-Boyd dysentery 004.2
Flexure —*see* condition
Floater, vitreous 379.24
Floating
    cartilage (joint) (*see also* Disorder, cartilage,
        articular) 718.0
        knee 717.6
    gallbladder (congenital) 751.69
    kidney 593.0
        congenital 753.3
    liver (congenital) 751.69
    rib 756.3
    spleen 289.59
Flooding 626.2
Floor —*see* condition
Floppy
    infant NEC 781.99
    valve syndrome (mitral) 424.0
Flu —*see also* Influenza
    gastric NEC 008.8
Fluctuating blood pressure 796.4

Fluid
    abdomen 789.5
    chest (*see also* Pleurisy, with effusion) 511.9
    heart (*see also* Failure, heart) 428.0
    joint (*see also* Effusion, joint) 719.0
    loss (acute) 276.5
        with
            hypernatremia 276.0
            hyponatremia 276.1
    lung—*see also* Edema, lung
        encysted 511.8
    peritoneal cavity 789.5
    pleural cavity (*see also* Pleurisy, with effusion)
        511.9
    retention 276.6
Flukes NEC (*see also* Infestation, fluke) 121.9
    blood NEC (*see also* Infestation, Schistosoma)
        120.9
    liver 121.3
Fluor (albus) (vaginalis) 623.5
    trichomonal (Trichomonas vaginalis) 131.00
Fluorosis (dental) (chronic) 520.3
Flushing 782.62
    menopausal 627.2
Flush syndrome 259.2
Flutter
    atrial or auricular 427.32
    heart (ventricular) 427.42
        atrial 427.32
        impure 427.32
        postoperative 997.1
    ventricular 427.42
Flux (bloody) (serosanguineous) 009.0
Focal —*see* condition
Fochier's abscess —*see* Abscess, by site
Focus, Assmann's (*see also* Tuberculosis) 011.0
Fogo selvagem 694.4
Foix-Alajouanine syndrome 336.1
Folds, anomalous —*see also* Anomaly, specified
    type NEC
    Bowman's membrane 371.31
    Descemet's membrane 371.32
    epicanthic 743.63
    heart 746.89
    posterior segment of eye, congenital 743.54
Folie à deux 297.3
Follicle
    cervix (nabothian) (ruptured) 616.0
    graafian, ruptured, with hemorrhage 620.0
    nabothian 616.0
Folliclis (primary) (*see also* Tuberculosis) 017.0
Follicular —*see also* condition
    cyst (atretic) 620.0
Folliculitis 704.8
    abscedens et suffodiens 704.8
    decalvans 704.09
    gonorrheal (acute) 098.0
        chronic or duration of 2 months or more 098.2
    keloid, keloidalis 706.1
    pustular 704.8
    ulerythematosa reticulata 701.8
Folliculosis, conjunctival 372.02
Folling's disease (phenylketonuria) 270.1
Follow-up (examination) (routine) (following)
    V67.9
    cancer chemotherapy V67.2
    chemotherapy V67.2
    fracture V67.4
    high-risk medication V67.51
    injury NEC V67.59

Follow-up—*continued*
  postpartum
    immediately after delivery V24.0
    routine V24.2
  psychiatric V67.3
  psychotherapy V67.3
  radiotherapy V67.1
  specified condition NEC V67.59
  specified surgery NEC V67.09
  surgery V67.00
    vaginal pap smear V67.01
  treatment V67.9
    combined NEC V67.6
    fracture V67.4
    involving high-risk medication NEC V67.51
    mental disorder V67.3
    specified NEC V67.59
Fong's syndrome (hereditary
  osteoonychodysplasia) 756.89
Food
  allergy 693.1
  anaphylactic shock—*see* Anaphylactic shock,
    due to, food
  asphyxia (from aspiration or inhalation) (*see*
    also Asphyxia, food) 933.1
  choked on (*see also* Asphyxia, food) 933.1
  deprivation 994.2
    specified kind of food NEC 269.8
  intoxication (*see also* Poisoning, food) 005.9
  lack of 994.2
  poisoning (*see also* Poisoning, food) 005.9
  refusal or rejection NEC 307.59
  strangulation or suffocation (*see also* Asphyxia,
    food) 933.1
  toxemia (*see also* Poisoning, food) 005.9
Foot —*see also* condition
  and mouth disease 078.4
  process disease 581.3
Foramen ovale (nonclosure) (patent) (persistent)
  745.5
Forbes' (glycogen storage) disease 271.0
Forbes-Albright syndrome (nonpuerperal
  amenorrhea and lactation associated with
  pituitary tumor) 253.1
Forced birth or delivery NEC 669.8
  affecting fetus or newborn NEC 763.89
Forceps
  delivery NEC 669.5
  affecting fetus or newborn 763.2
Fordyce's disease (ectopic sebaceous glands)
  (mouth) 750.26
Fordyce-Fox disease (apocrine miliaria) 705.82
Forearm —*see* condition
Foreign body

> *Note*—*For foreign body with open wound or*
> *other injury, see Wound, open, or the type of*
> *injury specified.*

  accidentally left during a procedure 998.4
  anterior chamber (eye) 871.6
    magnetic 871.5
      retained or old 360.51
    retained or old 360.61
  ciliary body (eye) 871.6
    magnetic 871.5
      retained or old 360.52
    retained or old 360.62
  entering through orifice (current) (old)
    accessory sinus 932
    air passage (upper) 933.0
      lower 934.8

Foreign body—*continued*
  alimentary canal 938
  alveolar process 935.0
  antrum (Highmore) 932
  anus 937
  appendix 936
  asphyxia due to (*see also* Asphyxia, food)
    933.1
  auditory canal 931
  auricle 931
  bladder 939.0
  bronchioles 934.8
  bronchus (main) 934.1
  buccal cavity 935.0
  canthus (inner) 930.1
  cecum 936
  cervix (canal) uterine 939.1
  coil, ileocecal 936
  colon 936
  conjunctiva 930.1
  conjunctival sac 930.1
  cornea 930.0
  digestive organ or tract NEC 938
  duodenum 936
  ear (external) 931
  esophagus 935.1
  eye (external) 930.9
    combined sites 930.8
    intraocular—*see* Foreign body, by site
    specified site NEC 930.8
  eyeball 930.8
    intraocular—*see* Foreign body, intraocular
  eyelid 930.1
    retained or old 374.86
  frontal sinus 932
  gastrointestinal tract 938
  genitourinary tract 939.9
  globe 930.8
    penetrating 871.6
      magnetic 871.5
        retained or old 360.50
      retained or old 360.60
  gum 935.0
  Highmore's antrum 932
  hypopharynx 933.0
  ileocecal coil 936
  ileum 936
  inspiration (of) 933.1
  intestine (large) (small) 936
  lacrimal apparatus, duct, gland, or sac 930.2
  larynx 933.1
  lung 934.8
  maxillary sinus 932
  mouth 935.0
  nasal sinus 932
  nasopharynx 933.0
  nose (passage) 932
  nostril 932
  oral cavity 935.0
  palate 935.0
  penis 939.3
  pharynx 933.0
  pyriform sinus 933.0
  rectosigmoid 937
    junction 937
  rectum 937
  respiratory tract 934.9
    specified part NEC 934.8
  sclera 930.1
  sinus 932
    accessory 932

Formation—*continued*
  hyaline in cornea 371.49
  sequestrum in bone (due to infection) (*see also*
      Osteomyelitis) 730.1
  valve
    colon, congenital 751.5
    ureter (congenital) 753.29
Formication 782.0
Fort Bragg fever 100.89
Fossa —*see also* condition
  pyriform—*see* condition
Foster-Kennedy syndrome 377.04
Fothergill's
  disease, meaning scarlatina anginosa 034.1
  neuralgia (*see also* Neuralgia, trigeminal) 350.1
Foul breath 784.9
Found dead (cause unknown) 798.9
Foundling V20.0
Fournier's disease (idiopathic gangrene) 608.83
Fourth
  cranial nerve—*see* condition
  disease 057.8
  molar 520.1
Foville's syndrome 344.89
Fox's
  disease (apocrine miliaria) 705.82
  impetigo (contagiosa) 684
Fox-Fordyce disease (apocrine miliaria) 705.82
Fracture (abduction) (adduction) (avulsion)
  (compression) (crush) (dislocation) (oblique)
  (separation) (closed) 829.0

---

*Note—For fracture of any of the following sites
with fracture of other bones—see Fracture,
multiple.*

*"Closed" includes the following descriptions of
fractures, with or without delayed healing,
unless they are specified as open or compound:*

> *comminuted*
> *depressed*
> *elevated*
> *fissured*
> *greenstick*
> *impacted*
> *linear*
> *simple*
> *slipped epiphysis*
> *spiral*
> *unspecified*

*"Open" includes the following descriptions of
fractures, with or without delayed healing:*

> *compound*
> *infected*
> *missile*
> *puncture*
> *with foreign body*

*For late effect of fracture, see Late, effect,
fracture, by site.*

---

  with
    internal injuries in same region (conditions
      classifiable to 860-869)—*see also* Injury,
      internal, by site
    pelvic region—*see* Fracture, pelvis
  acetabulum (with visceral injury) (closed) 808.0
    open 808.1

Fracture—*continued*
  acromion (process) (closed) 811.01
    open 811.11
  alveolus (closed) 802.8
    open 802.9
  ankle (malleolus) (closed) 824.8
    bimalleolar (Dupuytren's) (Pott's) 824.4
      open 824.5
    bone 825.21
      open 825.31
    lateral malleolus only (fibular) 824.2
      open 824.3
    medial malleolus only (tibial) 824.0
      open 824.1
    open 824.9
    pathologic 733.16
    talus 825.21
      open 825.31
    trimalleolar 824.6
      open 824.7
  antrum—*see* Fracture, skull, base
  arm (closed) 818.0
    and leg(s) (any bones) 828.0
      open 828.1
    both (any bones) (with rib(s)) (with sternum)
      819.0
      open 819.1
    lower 813.80
      open 813.90
    open 818.1
    upper—*see* Fracture, humerus
  astragalus (closed) 825.21
    open 825.31
  atlas—*see* Fracture, vertebra, cervical, first
  axis—*see* Fracture, vertebra, cervical, second
  back—*see* Fracture, vertebra, by site
  Barton's—*see* Fracture, radius, lower end
  basal (skull)—*see* Fracture, skull, base
  Bennett's (closed) 815.01
    open 815.11
  bimalleolar (closed) 824.4
    open 824.5
  bone (closed) NEC 829.0
    birth injury NEC 767.3
    open 829.1
    pathologic NEC (*see also* Fracture,
      pathologic) 733.10
    stress NEC (*see also* Fracture, stress) 733.95
  boot top—*see* Fracture, fibula
  boxers'—*see* Fracture, metacarpal bone(s)
  breast bone—*see* Fracture, sternum
  bucket handle (semilunar cartilage)—*see* Tear,
    meniscus
  bursting—*see* Fracture, phalanx, hand, distal
  calcaneus (closed) 825.0
    open 825.1
  capitate (bone) (closed) 814.07
    open 814.17
  capitellum (humerus) (closed) 812.49
    open 812.59
  carpal bone(s) (wrist NEC) (closed) 814.00
    open 814.10
    specified site NEC 814.09
      open 814.19
  cartilage, knee (semilunar)—*see* Tear, meniscus
  cervical—*see* Fracture, vertebra, cervical
  chauffeur's—*see* Fracture, ulna, lower end
  chisel—*see* Fracture, radius, upper end
  clavicle (interligamentous part) (closed) 810.00
    acromial end 810.03
      open 810.13

Fracture—*continued*
  due to birth trauma 767.2
    open 810.10
    shaft (middle third) 810.02
      open 810.12
    sternal end 810.01
      open 810.11
  clayshovelers'—*see* Fracture, vertebra, cervical
  coccyx—*see also* Fracture, vertebra, coccyx
    complicating delivery 665.6
  collar bone—*see* Fracture, clavicle
  Colles' (reversed) (closed) 813.41
    open 813.51
  comminuted—*see* Fracture, by site
  compression—*see also* Fracture, by site
    nontraumatic—*see* Fracture, pathologic
  congenital 756.9
  coracoid process (closed) 811.02
    open 811.12
  coronoid process (ulna) (closed) 813.02
    mandible (closed) 802.23
      open 802.33
    open 813.12
  costochondral junction—*see* Fracture, rib
  costosternal junction—*see* Fracture, rib
  cranium—*see* Fracture, skull, by site
  cricoid cartilage (closed) 807.5
    open 807.6
  cuboid (ankle) (closed) 825.23
    open 825.33
  cuneiform
    foot (closed) 825.24
      open 825.34
    wrist (closed) 814.03
      open 814.13
  due to
    birth injury—*see* Birth injury, fracture
    gunshot—*see* Fracture, by site, open
    neoplasm—*see* Fracture, pathologic
    osteoporosis—*see* Fracture, pathologic
  Dupuytren's (ankle) (fibula) (closed) 824.4
    open 824.5
    radius 813.42
      open 813.52
  Duverney's—*see* Fracture, ilium
  elbow—*see also* Fracture, humerus, lower end
    olecranon (process) (closed) 813.01
      open 813.11
    supracondylar (closed) 812.41
      open 812.51
  ethmoid (bone) (sinus)—*see* Fracture, skull,
    base
  face bone(s) (closed) NEC 802.8
    with
      other bone(s)—*see also* Fracture, multiple,
        skull
      skull—*see also* Fracture, skull
        involving other bones—*see* Fracture,
          multiple, skull
    open 802.9
  fatigue—*see* Fracture, march
  femur, femoral (closed) 821.00
    cervicotrochanteric 820.03
      open 820.13
    condyles, epicondyles 821.21
      open 821.31
    distal end—*see* Fracture, femur, lower end
    epiphysis (separation)
      capital 820.01
        open 820.11
      head 820.01

Fracture—*continued*
    open 820.11
    lower 821.22
      open 821.32
    trochanteric 820.01
      open 820.11
    upper 820.01
      open 820.11
    head 820.09
      open 820.19
    lower end or extremity (distal end) (closed)
      821.20
      condyles, epicondyles 821.21
        open 821.31
      epiphysis (separation) 821.22
        open 821.32
      multiple sites 821.29
        open 821.39
      open 821.30
      specified site NEC 821.29
        open 821.39
      supracondylar 821.23
        open 821.33
      T-shaped 821.21
        open 821.31
    neck (closed) 820.8
      base (cervicotrochanteric) 820.03
        open 820.13
      extracapsular 820.20
        open 820.30
      intertrochanteric (section) 820.21
        open 820.31
      intracapsular 820.00
        open 820.10
      intratrochanteric 820.21
        open 821.31
      midcervical 820.02
        open 820.12
      open 820.9
      pathologic 733.14
        specified part NEC 733.15
      specified site NEC 820.09
        open 820.19
      transcervical 820.02
        open 820.12
      transtrochanteric 820.20
        open 820.30
    open 821.10
    pathologic 733.14
      specified part NEC 733.15
    peritrochanteric (section) 820.20
      open 820.30
    shaft (lower third) (middle third) (upper third)
      821.01
      open 821.11
    subcapital 820.09
      open 820.19
    subtrochanteric (region) (section) 820.22
      open 820.32
    supracondylar 821.23
      open 821.33
    transepiphyseal 820.01
      open 820.11
    trochanter (greater) (lesser) (*see also* Fracture,
      femur, neck, by site) 820.20
      open 820.30
    T-shaped, into knee joint 821.21
      open 821.31
    upper end 820.8
      open 820.9

Fracture—*continued*
  fibula (closed) 823.81
    with tibia 823.82
      open 823.92
    distal end 824.8
      open 824.9
    epiphysis
      lower 824.8
        open 824.9
      upper—*see* Fracture, fibula, upper end
    head—*see* Fracture, fibula, upper end
    involving ankle 824.2
      open 824.3
    lower end or extremity 824.8
      open 824.9
    malleolus (external) (lateral) 824.2
      open 824.3
    open NEC 823.91
    pathologic 733.16
    proximal end—*see* Fracture, fibula, upper end
    shaft 823.21
      with tibia 823.22
        open 823.32
      open 823.31
    stress 733.93
    torus 823.41
      with tibia 823.42
    upper end or extremity (epiphysis) (head)
      (proximal end) (styloid) 823.01
      with tibia 823.02
        open 823.12
      open 823.11
  finger(s), of one hand (closed) (*see also*
    Fracture, phalanx, hand) 816.00
    with
      metacarpal bone(s), of same hand 817.0
        open 817.1
      thumb of same hand 816.03
        open 816.13
    open 816.10
  foot, except toe(s) alone (closed) 825.20
    open 825.30
  forearm (closed) NEC 813.80
    lower end (distal end) (lower epiphysis)
      813.40
      open 813.50
    open 813.90
    shaft 813.20
      open 813.30
    upper end (proximal end) (upper epiphysis)
      813.00
      open 813.10
  fossa, anterior, middle, or posterior—*see*
    Fracture, skull, base
  frontal (bone)—*see also* Fracture, skull, vault
    sinus—*see* Fracture, skull base
  Galeazzi's—*see* Fracture, radius, lower end
  glenoid (cavity) (fossa) (scapula) (closed)
    811.03
    open 811.13
  Gosselin's—*see* Fracture, ankle
  greenstick—*see* Fracture, by site
  grenade-throwers'—*see* Fracture, humerus, shaft
  gutter—*see* Fracture, skull, vault
  hamate (closed) 814.08
    open 814.18
  hand, one (closed) 815.00
    carpals 814.00
      open 814.10
      specified site NEC 814.09
        open 814.19

Fracture—*continued*
  metacarpals 815.00
    open 815.10
  multiple, bones of one hand 817.0
    open 817.1
  open 815.10
  phalanges (*see also* Fracture, phalanx, hand)
    816.00
    open 816.10
  healing
    aftercare (*see also* Aftercare, fracture) V54.89
    change of cast V54.89
    complications—*see* condition
    convalescence V66.4
    removal of
      cast V54.89
      fixation device
        external V54.89
        internal V54.0
  heel bone (closed) 825.0
    open 825.1
  hip (closed) (*see also* Fracture, femur, neck)
    820.8
    open 820.9
    pathologic 733.14
  humerus (closed) 812.20
    anatomical neck 812.02
      open 812.12
    articular process (*see also* Fracture, humerus,
      condyle(s) 812.44
      open 812.54
    capitellum 812.49
      open 812.59
    condyle(s) 812.44
      lateral (external) 812.42
        open 812.52
      medial (internal epicondyle) 812.43
        open 812.53
      open 812.54
    distal end—*see* Fracture, humerus, lower end
    epiphysis
      lower (*see also* Fracture, humerus,
        condyle(s)) 812.44
        open 812.54
      upper 812.09
        open 812.19
    external condyle 812.42
      open 812.52
    great tuberosity 812.03
      open 812.13
    head 812.09
      open 812.19
    internal epicondyle 812.43
      open 812.53
    lesser tuberosity 812.09
      open 812.19
    lower end or extremity (distal end) (*see also*
      Fracture, humerus, by site) 812.40
      multiple sites NEC 812.49
        open 812.59
      open 812.50
      specified site NEC 812.49
        open 812.59
    neck 812.01
      open 812.11
    open 812.30
    pathologic 733.11
    proximal end—*see* Fracture, humerus, upper
      end
    shaft 812.21
      open 812.31

Fracture—*continued*
  supracondylar 812.41
    open 812.51
  surgical neck 812.01
    open 812.11
  trochlea 812.49
    open 812.59
  T-shaped 812.44
    open 812.54
  tuberosity—*see* Fracture, humerus, upper end
  upper end or extremity (proximal end) (*see
      also* Fracture, humerus, by site) 812.00
    open 812.10
    specified site NEC 812.09
      open 812.19
  hyoid bone (closed) 807.5
    open 807.6
  hyperextension—*see* Fracture, radius, lower end
  ilium (with visceral injury) (closed) 808.41
    open 808.51
  impaction, impacted—*see* Fracture, by site
  incus—*see* Fracture, skull, base
  innominate bone (with visceral injury) (closed)
      808.49
    open 808.59
  instep, of one foot (closed) 825.20
    with toe(s) of same foot 827.0
      open 827.1
    open 825.30
  internal
    ear—*see* Fracture, skull, base
    semilunar cartilage, knee—*see* Tear,
        meniscus, medial
  intertrochanteric—*see* Fracture, femur, neck,
      intertrochanteric .
  ischium (with visceral injury) (closed) 808.42
    open 808.52
  jaw (bone) (lower) (closed) (*see also* Fracture,
      mandible) 802.20
    angle 802.25
      open 802.35
    open 802.30
    upper—*see* Fracture, maxilla
  knee
    cap (closed) 822.0
      open 822.1
    cartilage (semilunar)—*see* Tear, meniscus
  labyrinth (osseous)—*see* Fracture, skull, base
  larynx (closed) 807.5
    open 807.6
  late effect—*see* Late, effects (of), fracture
  Le Fort's—*see* Fracture, maxilla
  leg (closed) 827.0
    with rib(s) or sternum 828.0
      open 828.1
    both (any bones) 828.0
      open 828.1
    lower—*see* Fracture, tibia
    open 827.1
    upper—*see* Fracture, femur
  limb
    lower (multiple) (closed) NEC 827.0
      open 827.1
    upper (multiple) (closed) NEC 818.0
      open 818.1
  long bones, due to birth trauma—*see* Birth
      injury, fracture
  lumbar—*see* Fracture, vertebra, lumbar
  lunate bone (closed) 814.02
    open 814.12

Fracture—*continued*
  malar bone (closed) 802.4
    open 802.5
  Malgaigne's (closed) 808.43
    open 808.53
  malleolus (closed)0 824.8
    bimalleolar 824.4
      open 824.5
    lateral 824.2
      and medial—*see also* Fracture, malleolus,
          bimalleolar
      with lip of tibia—*see* Fracture, malleolus,
          trimalleolar
      open 824.3
    medial (closed) 824.0
      and lateral—*see also* Fracture, malleolus,
          bimalleolar
      with lip of tibia—*see* Fracture, malleolus,
          trimalleolar
      open 824.1
    open 824.9
    trimalleolar (closed) 824.6
      open 824.7
  malleus—*see* Fracture, skull, base
  malunion 733.81
  mandible (closed) 802.20
    angle 802.25
      open 802.35
    body 802.28
      alveolar border 802.27
        open 802.37
      open 802.38
      symphysis 802.26
        open 802.36
    condylar process 802.21
      open 802.31
    coronoid process 802.23
      open 802.33
    multiple sites 802.29
      open 802.39
    open 802.30
    ramus NEC 802.24
      open 802.34
    subcondylar 802.22
      open 802.32
  manubrium—*see* Fracture, sternum
  march 733.95
    fibula 733.94
    metatarsals 733.94
    tibia 733.94
  maxilla, maxillary (superior) (upper jaw)
      (closed) 802.4
    inferior—*see* Fracture, mandible
    open 802.5
  meniscus, knee—*see* Tear, meniscus
  metacarpus, metacarpal (bone(s)), of one hand
      (closed) 815.00
    with phalanx, phalanges, hand (finger(s))
        (thumb) of same hand 817.0
      open 817.1
    base 815.02
      first metacarpal 815.01
        open 815.11
      open 815.12
      thumb 815.01
        open 815.11
    multiple sites 815.09
      open 815.19
    neck 815.04
      open 815.14
    open 815.10

Fracture—*continued*
  shaft 815.03
    open 815.13
  metatarsus, metatarsal (bone(s)), of one foot
    (closed) 825.25
    with tarsal bone(s) 825.29
      open 825.39
    open 825.35
  Montoggia's (closed) 813.03
    open 813.13
  Moore's—*see* Fracture, radius, lower end
  multangular bone (closed)
    larger 814.05
      open 814.15
    smaller 814.06
      open 814.16
  multiple (closed) 829.0

Note—Multiple fractures of sites classifiable to
the same three- or four-digit category are coded
to that category, except for sites classifiable to
810-818 or 820-827 in different limbs.

Multiple fractures of sites classifiable to
different fourth-digit subdivisions within the
same three- digit category should be dealt with
according to coding rules.

Multiple fractures of sites classifiable to
different three-digit categories (identifiable
from the listing under "Fracture"), and of sites
classifiable to 810-818 or 820-827 in different
limbs should be coded according to the
following list, which should be referred to in the
following priority order: skull or face bones,
pelvis or vertebral column, legs, arms.

  arm (multiple bones in same arm except in
    hand alone) (sites classifiable to 810-817
    with sites classifiable to a different
    three-digit category in 810-817 in same
    arm) (closed) 818.0
    open 818.1
  arms, both or arm(s) with rib(s) or sternum
    (sites classifiable to 810-818 with sites
    classifiable to same range of categories in
    other limb or to 807) (closed) 819.0
    open 819.1
  bones of trunk NEC (closed) 809.0
    open 809.1
  hand, metacarpal bone(s) with phalanx or
    phalanges of same hand (sites classifiable
    to 815 with sites classifiable to 816 in
    same hand) (closed) 817.0
    open 817.1
  leg (multiple bones in same leg) (sites
    classifiable to 820-826 with sites
    classifiable to a different three-digit
    category in that range in same leg)
    (closed) 827.0
    open 827.1
  legs, both or leg(s) with arm(s), rib(s), or
    sternum (sites classifiable to 820-
    827 with sites classifiable to same range
    of categories in other leg or to 807 or
    810-819) (closed) 828.0
    open 828.1
    open 829.1
  pelvis with other bones except skull or face
    bones (sites classifiable to 808 with sites
    classifiable to 805-807 or 810-829)
    (closed) 809.0

Fracture—*continued*
  open 809.1
  skull, specified or unspecified bones, or face
    bone(s) with any other bone(s) (sites
    classifiable to 800-803 with sites
    classifiable to 805-829) (closed) 804.0

Note—Use the following fifth-digit
subclassification with categories 800, 801, 803,
and 804:

0 unspecified state of consciousness
1 with no loss of consciousness
2 with brief [less than one hour] loss of
   consciousness
3 with moderate [1-24 hours] loss of
   consciousness
4 with prolonged [more than 24 hours] loss of
   consciousness and return to pre-existing
   conscious level
5 with prolonged [more than 24 hours] loss of
   consciousness, without return to pre-existing
   conscious level
Use fifth-digit 5 to designate when a patient is
unconcious and dies before regaining
conciousness, regardless of the duration of the
loss of conciousness
6 with loss of consciousness of unspecified
   duration
9 with concussion, unspecified

  with
    contusion, cerebral 804.1
    epidural hemorrhage 804.2
    extradural hemorrhage 804.2
    hemorrhage (intracranial) NEC 804.3
    intracranial injury NEC 804.4
    laceration, cerebral 804.1
    subarachnoid hemorrhage 804.2
    subdural hemorrhage 804.2
  open 804.5
    with
      contusion, cerebral 804.6
      epidural hemorrhage 804.7
      extradural hemorrhage 804.7
      hemorrhage (intracranial) NEC 804.8
      intracranial injury NEC 804.9
      laceration, cerebral 804.6
      subarachnoid hemorrhage 804.7
      subdural hemorrhage 804.7
  vertebral column with other bones, except
    skull or face bones (sites classifiable to
    805 or 806 with sites classifiable to
    807-808 or 810-829) (closed) 809.0
    open 809.1
  nasal (bone(s)) (closed) 802.0
    open 802.1
  sinus—Fracture, skull, base
  navicular
    carpal (wrist) (closed) 814.01
      open 814.11
    tarsal (ankle) (closed) 825.22
      open 825.32
  neck—*see* Fracture, vertebra, cervical
  neural arch—*see* Fracture, vertebra, by site
  nonunion 733.82
  nose, nasal, (bone) (septum) (closed) 802.0
    open 802.1
  occiput—*see* Fracture, skull, base
  odontoid process—*see* Fracture, vertebra,
    cervical

Fracture—*continued*

olecranon (process) (ulna) (closed) 813.01
  open 813.11
open 829.1
orbit, orbital (bone) (region) (closed) 802.8
  floor (blow-out) 802.6
    open 802.7
  open 802.9
  roof—*see* Fracture, skull, base
  specified part NEC 802.8
    open 802.9
os
  calcis (closed) 825.0
    open 825.1
  magnum (closed) 814.07
    open 814.17
  pubis (with visceral injury) (closed) 808.2
    open 808.3
  triquetrum (closed) 814.03
    open 814.13
osseous
  auditory meatus—*see* Fracture, skull, base
  labyrinth—*see* Fracture, skull, base
ossicles, auditory (incus) (malleus)
  (stapes)—*see* Fracture, skull, base
osteoporotic—*see* Fracture, pathologic
palate (closed) 802.8
  open 802.9
paratrooper—*see* Fracture, tibia, lower end
parietal bone—*see* Fracture, skull, vault
parry—*see* Fracture, Monteggia's
patella (closed) 822.0
  open 822.1
pathologic (cause unknown) 733.10
  ankle 733.16
  femur (neck) 733.14
    specified NEC 733.15
  fibula 733.16
  hip 733.14
  humerus 733.11
  radius 733.12
  specified site NEC 733.19
  tibia 733.16
  ulna 733.12
  vertebrae (collapse) 733.13
  wrist 733.12
pedicle (of vertebral arch)—*see* Fracture,
  vertebra, by site
pelvis, pelvic (bone(s)) (with visceral injury)
  (closed) 808.8
  multiple (with disruption of pelvic circle)
    808.43
    open 808.53
  open 808.9
  rim (closed) 808.49
    open 808.59
peritrochanteric (closed) 820.20
  open 820.30
phalanx, phalanges, of one
  foot (closed) 826.0
    with bone(s) of same lower limb 827.0
      open 827.1
    open 826.1

Fracture—*continued*

hand (closed) 816.00
  with metacarpal bone(s) of same hand 817.0
    open 817.1
  distal 816.02
    open 816.12
  middle 816.01
    open 816.11
  multiple sites NEC 816.03
    open 816.13
  open 816.10
  proximal 816.01
    open 816.11
pisiform (closed) 814.04
  open 814.14
pond—Fracture, skull, vault
Pott's (closed) 824.4
  open 824.5
prosthetic device, internal—*see* Complications,
  mechanical
pubis (with visceral injury) (closed) 808.2
  open 808.3
Quervain's (closed) 814.01
  open 814.11
radius (alone) (closed) 813.81
  with ulna NEC 813.83
    open 813.93
  distal end—*see* Fracture, radius, lower end
  epiphysis
    lower—*see* Fracture, radius, lower end
    upper—*see* Fracture, radius, upper end
  head—*see* Fracture, radius, upper end
  lower end or extremity (distal end) (lower
    epiphysis) 813.42
    with ulna (lower end) 813.44
      open 813.54
    open 813.52
    torus 813.45
  neck—*see* Fracture, radius, upper end
  open NEC 813.91
  pathologic 733.12
  proximal end—*see* Fracture, radius, upper end
  shaft (closed) 813.21
    with ulna (shaft) 813.23
      open 813.33
    open 813.31
  upper end 813.07
    with ulna (upper end) 813.08
      open 813.18
    epiphysis 813.05
      open 813.15
    head 813.05
      open 813.15
    multiple sites 813.07
      open 813.17
    neck 813.06
      open 813.16
    open 813.17
    specified site NEC 813.07
      open 813.17
ramus
  inferior or superior (with visceral injury)
    (closed) 808.2
    open 808.3
  ischium—*see* Fracture, ischium
  mandible 802.24
    open 802.34
rib(s) (closed) 807.0

Fracture—*continued*

> *Note—Use the following fifth-digit subclassification with categories 807.0-807.1:*
>
> 0 rib(s), unspecified
> 1 one rib
> 2 two ribs
> 3 three ribs
> 4 four ribs
> 5 five ribs
> 6 six ribs
> 7 seven ribs
> 8 eight or more ribs
> 9 multiple ribs, unspecified

  with flail chest (open) 807.4
  open 807.1
root, tooth 873.63
  complicated 873.73
sacrum—*see* Fracture, vertebra, sacrum
scaphoid
  ankle (closed) 825.22
    open 825.32
  wrist (closed) 814.01
    open 814.11
scapula (closed) 811.00
  acromial, acromion (process) 811.01
    open 811.11
  body 811.09
    open 811.19
  coracoid process 811.02
    open 811.12
  glenoid (cavity) (fossa) 811.03
    open 811.13
  neck 811.03
    open 811.13
  open 811.10
semilunar
  bone, wrist (closed) 814.02
    open 814.12
  cartilage (interior) (knee)—*see* Tear, meniscus
sesamoid bone—*see* Fracture, by site
Shepherd's (closed) 825.21
  open 825.31
shoulder—*see also* Fracture, humerus, upper end
  blade—*see* Fracture, scapula
silverfork—*see* Fracture, radius, lower end
sinus (ethmoid) (frontal) (maxillary) (nasal)
  (sphenoidal)—*see* Fracture, skull, base
  maxillary—*see* Fracture, maxilla
Skillern's—*see* Fracture, radius, shaft
skull (multiple NEC) (with face bones) (closed) 803.0

> *Note—Use the following fifth-digit subclassification with categories 800, 801, 803, and 804:*
>
> 0 unspecified state of consciousness
> 1 with no loss of consciousness
> 2 with brief [less than one hour] loss of consciousness
> 3 with moderate [1-24 hours] loss of consciousness
> 4 with prolonged [more than 24 hours] loss of consciousness and return to pre-existing conscious level
> 5 with prolonged [more than 24 hours] loss of consciousness, without return to pre-existing conscious level
> Use fifth-digit 5 to designate when a patient is unconscious and dies before regaining consciousness, regardless of the duration of the loss of consciousness
> 6 with loss of consciousness of unspecified duration
> 9 with concussion, unspecified

  with
    contusion, cerebral 803.1
    epidural hemorrhage 803.2
    extradural hemorrhage 803.2
    hemorrhage (intracranial) NEC 803.3
    intracranial injury NEC 803.4
    laceration, cerebral 803.1
    other bones—*see* Fracture, multiple, skull
    subarachnoid hemorrhage 803.2
    subdural hemorrhage 803.2
  base (antrum) (ethmoid bone) (fossa) (internal ear) (nasal sinus) (occiput) (sphenoid) (temporal bone) (closed) 801.0
    with
      contusion, cerebral 801.1
      epidural hemorrhage 801.2
      extradural hemorrhage 801.2
      hemorrhage (intracranial) NEC 801.3
      intracranial injury NEC 801.4
      laceration, cerebral 801.1
      subarachnoid hemorrhage 801.2
      subdural hemorrhage 801.2
    open 801.5
      with
        contusion, cerebral 801.6
        epidural hemorrhage 801.7
        extradural hemorrhage 801.7
        hemorrhage (intracranial) NEC 801.8
        intracranial injury NEC 801.9
        laceration, cerebral 801.6
        subarachnoid hemorrhage 801.7
        subdural hemorrhage 801.7
  birth injury 767.3
  face bones—*see* Fracture, face bones
  open 803.5
    with
      contusion, cerebral 803.6
      epidural hemorrhage 803.7
      extradural hemorrhage 803.7
      hemorrhage (intracranial) NEC 803.8
      intracranial injury NEC 803.9
      laceration, cerebral 803.6
      subarachnoid hemorrhage 803.7
      subdural hemorrhage 803.7
  vault (frontal bone) (parietal bone) (vertex) (closed) 800.0

Fracture—*continued*

ulna (alone) (closed) 813.82
  with radius NEC 813.83
    open 813.93
  coronoid process (closed) 813.02
    open 813.12
  distal end—*see* Fracture, ulna, lower end
  epiphysis
    lower—*see* Fracture, ulna, lower end
    upper—*see* Fracture, ulna, upper, end
  head—*see* Fracture, ulna, lower end
  lower end (distal end) (head) (lower
    epiphysis) (styloid process) 813.43
    with radius (lower end) 813.44
      open 813.54
    open 813.53
  olecranon process (closed) 813.01
    open 813.11
  open NEC 813.92
  pathologic 733.12
  proximal end—*see* Fracture, ulna, upper end
  shaft 813.22
    with radius (shaft) 813.23
      open 813.33
    open 813.32
  styloid process—*see* Fracture, ulna, lower end
  transverse—*see* Fracture, ulna, by site
  upper end (epiphysis) 813.04
    with radius (upper end) 813.08
      open 813.18
    multiple sites 813.04
      open 813.14
    open 813.14
    specified site NEC 813.04
      open 813.14
unciform (closed) 814.08
  open 814.18
vertebra, vertebral (back) (body) (column)
  (neural arch) (pedicle) (spine) (spinous
  process) (transverse process) (closed) 805.8
  with
    hematomyelia—*see* Fracture, vertebra, by
      site, with spinal cord injury
    injury to
      cauda equina—*see* Fracture, vertebra,
        sacrum, with spinal cord injury
      nerve—*see* Fracture, vertebra, by site,
        with spinal cord injury
      paralysis—*see* Fracture, vertebra, by site,
        with spinal cord injury
      paraplegia—*see* Fracture, vertebra, by site,
        with spinal cord injury
      quadriplegia—*see* Fracture, vertebra, by
        site, with spinal cord injury
      spinal concussion—*see* Fracture, vertebra,
        by site, with spinal cord injury
      spinal cord injury (closed) NEC 806.8

Fracture—*continued*

> *Note*—*Use the following fifth-digit
> subclassification with categories 806.0-806.3:*
>
> C_1-C_4 *or unspecified level and D_1-D_6 (T_1-T_6) or
> unspecified level with:*
>
> *0 unspecified spinal cord injury*
> *1 complete lesion of cord*
> *2 anterior cord syndrome*
> *3 central cord syndrome*
> *4 specified injury NEC*
>
> C_5-C_7 *level and D_7-D_{12} level with:*
>
> *5 unspecified spinal cord injury*
> *6 complete lesion of cord*
> *7 anterior cord syndrome*
> *8 central cord syndrome*
> *9 specified injury NEC*

    cervical 806.0
      open 806.1
    dorsal, dorsolumbar 806.2
      open 806.3
    open 806.9
    thoracic, thoracolumbar 806.2
      open 806.3
  atlanto-axial—*see* Fracture, vertebra, cervical
  cervical (hangman) (teardrop) (closed) 805.00
    with spinal cord injury—*see* Fracture,
      vertebra, with spinal cord injury, cervical
    first (atlas) 805.01
      open 805.11
    second (axis) 805.02
      open 805.12
    third 805.03
      open 805.13
    fourth 805.04
      open 805.14
    fifth 805.05
      open 805.15
    sixth 805.06
      open 805.16
    seventh 805.07
      open 805.17
    multiple sites 805.08
      open 805.18
    open 805.10
  coccyx (closed) 805.6
    with spinal cord injury (closed) 806.60
      cauda equina injury 806.62
        complete lesion 806.61
          open 806.71
        open 806.72
      open 806.70
      specified type NEC 806.69
        open 806.79
    open 805.7
  collapsed 733.13
  compression, not due to trauma 733.13
  dorsal (closed) 805.2
    with spinal cord injury—*see* Fracture,
      vertebra, with spinal cord injury, dorsal
    open 805.3
  dorsolumbar (closed) 805.2
    with spinal cord injury—*see* Fracture,
      vertebra, with spinal cord injury, dorsal
    open 805.3
  due to osteoporosis 733.13
  fetus or newborn 767.4

Fracture—*continued*
  lumbar (closed) 805.4
    with spinal cord injury (closed) 806.4
    open 806.5
    open 805.5
  nontraumatic 733.13
  open NEC 805.9
  pathologic 733.13
  sacrum (closed) 805.6
    with spinal cord injury 806.60
      cauda equina injury 806.62
      complete lesion 806.61
        open 806.71
        open 806.72
      open 806.70
      specified type NEC 806.69
        open 806.79
    open 805.7
  site unspecified (closed) 805.8
    with spinal cord injury (closed) 806.8
    open 806.9
    open 805.9
  stress (any site) 733.95
  thoracic (closed) 805.2
    with spinal cord injury—*see* Fracture,
      vertebra, with spinal cord injury, thoracic
    open 805.3
  vertex—*see* Fracture, skull, vault
  vomer (bone) 802.0
    open 802.1
  Wagstaffe's—*see* Fracture, ankle
  wrist (closed) 814.00
    open 814.10
    pathologic 733.12
  xiphoid (process)—*see* Fracture, sternum
  zygoma (zygomatic arch) (closed) 802.4
    open 802.5
Fragile X syndrome 759.83
Fragilitas
  crinium 704.2
  hair 704.2
  ossium 756.51
    with blue sclera 756.51
  unguium 703.8
    congenital 757.5
Fragility
  bone 756.51
    with deafness and blue sclera 756.51
  capillary (hereditary) 287.8
  hair 704.2
  nails 703.8
Fragmentation —*see* Fracture, by site
Frambesia, frambesial (tropica) (*see also* Yaws)
  102.9
  initial lesion or ulcer 102.0
  primary 102.0
Frambeside
  gummatous 102.4
  of early yaws 102.2
Frambesioma 102.1
Franceschetti's syndrome (mandibulofacial
  dysostosis) 756.0
Francis' disease (*see also* Tularemia) 021.9
Frank's essential thrombocytopenia (*see also*
  Purpura, thrombocytopenic) 287.3
Franklin's disease (heavy chain) 273.2
Fraser's syndrome 759.89
Freckle 709.09
  malignant melanoma in (M8742/3)—*see*
    Melanoma
  melanotic (of Hutchinson) (M8742/2)—*see*
    Neoplasm, skin, in situ

Freeman-Sheldon syndrome 759.89
Freezing 991.9
  specified effect NEC 991.8
Frei's disease (climatic bubo) 099.1
Freiberg's
  disease (osteochondrosis, second metatarsal)
    732.5
  infraction of metatarsal head 732.5
  osteochondrosis 732.5
Fremitus, friction, cardiac 785.3
Frenulum lingua 750.0
Frenum
  external os 752.49
  tongue 750.0
Frequency (urinary) NEC 788.41
  micturition 788.41
  nocturnal 788.43
  psychogenic 306.53
Frey's syndrome (auriculotemporal syndrome)
  350.8
Friction
  burn (*see also* Injury, superficial, by site) 919.0
  fremitus, cardiac 785.3
  precordial 785.3
  sounds, chest 786.7
Friderichsen-Waterhouse syndrome or disease
  036.3
Friedländer's
  B (bacillus) NEC (*see also* condition) 041.3
    sepsis or septicemia 038.49
  disease (endarteritis obliterans)—*see*
    Arteriosclerosis
Friedreich's
  ataxia 334.0
  combined systemic disease 334.0
  disease 333.2
    combined systemic 334.0
  myoclonia 333.2
  sclerosis (spinal cord) 334.0
Friedrich-Erb-Arnold syndrome
  (acropachyderma) 757.39
Frigidity 302.72
  psychic or psychogenic 302.72
Fröhlich's disease or syndrome (adiposogenital
  dystrophy) 253.8
Froin's syndrome 336.8
Frommel's disease 676.6
Frommel-Chiari syndrome 676.6
Frontal —*see also* condition
  lobe syndrome 310.0
Frostbite 991.3
  face 991.0
  foot 991.2
  hand 991.1
  specified site NEC 991.3
Frotteurism 302.89
Frozen 991.9
  pelvis 620.8
  shoulder 726.0
Fructosemia 271.2
Fructosuria (benign) (essential) 271.2
Fuchs'
  black spot (myopic) 360.21
  corneal dystrophy (endothelial) 371.57
  heterochromic cyclitis 364.21
Fucosidosis 271.8
Fugue 780.99
  hysterical (dissociative) 300.13
  reaction to exceptional stress (transient) 308.1
Fuller Albright's syndrome (osteitis fibrosa
  disseminata) 756.59
Fuller's earth disease 502

Fulminant, fulminating —*see* condition
Functional —*see* condition
Fundus —*see also* condition
  flavimaculatus 362.76
Fungemia 117.9
Fungus, fungous
  cerebral 348.8
  disease NEC 117.9
  infection—*see* Infection, fungus
  testis (*see also* Tuberculosis) 016.5 *[608.81]*
Funiculitis (acute) 608.4
  chronic 608.4
  endemic 608.4
  gonococcal (acute) 098.14
    chronic or duration of 2 months or over 098.34
  tuberculous (*see also* Tuberculosis) 016.5
F.U.O. (*see also* Pyrexia) 780.6
Funnel
  breast (acquired) 738.3
    congenital 754.81
    late effect of rickets 268.1
  chest (acquired) 738.3
    congenital 754.81
    late effect of rickets 268.1
  pelvis (acquired) 738.6
    with disproportion (fetopelvic) 653.3
      affecting fetus or newborn 763.1
      causing obstructed labor 660.1
        affecting fetus or newborn 763.1
    congenital 755.69
    tuberculous (*see also* Tuberculosis) 016.9
Furfur 690.18
  microsporon 111.0
Furor, paroxysmal (idiopathic) (*see also* Epilepsy) 345.8
Furriers' lung 495.8
Furrowed tongue 529.5
  congenital 750.13
Furrowing nail (s) (transverse) 703.8
  congenital 757.5
Furuncle 680.9
  abdominal wall 680.2
  ankle 680.6
  anus 680.5
  arm (any part, above wrist) 680.3
  auditory canal, external 680.0
  axilla 680.3
  back (any part) 680.2
  breast 680.2
  buttock 680.5
  chest wall 680.2
  corpus cavernosum 607.2
  ear (any part) 680.0
  eyelid 373.13
  face (any part, except eye) 680.0
  finger (any) 680.4
  flank 680.2
  foot (any part) 680.7
  forearm 680.3
  gluteal (region) 680.5
  groin 680.2
  hand (any part) 680.4
  head (any part, except face) 680.8
  heel 680.7
  hip 680.6
  kidney (*see also* Abscess, kidney) 590.2
  knee 680.6
  labium (majus) (minus) 616.4
  lacrimal
    gland (*see also* Dacryoadenitis) 375.00

Furuncle—*continued*
  passages (duct) (sac) (see *also* Dacryocystitis) 375.30
  leg, any part except foot 680.6
  malignant 022.0
  multiple sites 680.9
  neck 680.1
  nose (external) (septum) 680.0
  orbit 376.01
  partes posteriores 680.5
  pectoral region 680.2
  penis 607.2
  perineum 680.2
  pinna 680.0
  scalp (any part) 680.8
  scrotum 608.4
  seminal vesicle 608.0
  shoulder 680.3
  skin NEC 680.9
  specified site NEC 680.8
  spermatic cord 608.4
  temple (region) 680.0
  testis 604.90
  thigh 680.6
  thumb 680.4
  toe (any) 680.7
  trunk 680.2
  tunica vaginalis 608.4
  umbilicus 680.2
  upper arm 680.3
  vas deferens 608.4
  vulva 616.4
  wrist 680.4
Furunculosis (*see also* Furuncle) 680.9
  external auditory meatus 680.0 *[380.13]*
Fusarium (infection) 118
Fusion, fused (congenital)
  anal (with urogenital canal) 751.5
  aorta and pulmonary artery 745.0
  astragaloscaphoid 755.67
  atria 745.5
  atrium and ventricle 745.69
  auditory canal 744.02
  auricles, heart 745.5
  binocular, with defective stereopsis 368.33
  bone 756.9
  cervical spine—*see* Fusion, spine
  choanal 748.0
  commissure, mitral valve 746.5
  cranial sutures, premature 756.0
  cusps, heart valve NEC 746.89
    mitral 746.5
    tricuspid 746.89
  ear ossicles 744.04
  fingers (*see also* Syndactylism, fingers) 755.11
  hymen 752.42
  hymeno-urethral 599.89
    causing obstructed labor 660.1
      affecting fetus or newborn 763.1
  joint (acquired)—*see also* Ankylosis
    congenital 755.8
  kidneys (incomplete) 753.3
  labium (majus) (minus) 752.49
  larynx and trachea 748.3
  limb 755.8
    lower 755.69
    upper 755.59
  lobe, lung 748.5
  lumbosacral (acquired) 724.6
    congenital 756.15
    surgical V45.4

Fusion, fused—*continued*
  nares (anterior) (posterior) 748.0
  nose, nasal 748.0
  nostril(s) 748.0
  organ or site NEC—*see* Anomaly, specified
    type NEC
  ossicles 756.9
    auditory 744.04
  pulmonary valve segment 746.02
  pulmonic cusps 746.02
  ribs 756.3
  sacroiliac (acquired) (joint) 724.6
    congenital 755.69
    surgical V45.4
  skull, imperfect 756.0
  spine (acquired) 724.9
    arthrodesis status V45.4
    congenital (vertebra) 756.15
    postoperative status V45.4
  sublingual duct with submaxillary duct at
    opening in mouth 750.26
  talonavicular (bar) 755.67
  teeth, tooth 520.2
  testes 752.8
  toes (*see also* Syndactylism, toes) 755.13
  trachea and esophagus 750.3
  twins 759.4
  urethral-hymenal 599.89
  vagina 752.49
  valve cusps—*see* Fusion, cusps, heart valve
  ventricles, heart 745.4
  vertebra (arch)—*see* Fusion, spine
  vulva 752.49
Fusospirillosis (mouth) (tongue) (tonsil) 101
Fussy infant (baby) 780.91

G

Gafsa boil 085.1
Gain, weight (abnormal) (excessive) (*see also* Weight, gain) 783.1
Gaisböck's disease or syndrome (polycythemia hypertonica) 289.0
Gait
  abnormality 781.2
    hysterical 300.11
  ataxic 781.2
    hysterical 300.11
  disturbance 781.2
    hysterical 300.11
  paralytic 781.2
  scissor 781.2
  spastic 781.2
  staggering 781.2
    hysterical 300.11
Galactocele (breast) (infected) 611.5
  puerperal, postpartum 676.8
Galactophoritis 611.0
  puerperal, postpartum 675.2
Galactorrhea 676.6
  not associated with childbirth 611.6
Galactosemia (classic) (congenital) 271.1
Galactosuria 271.1
Galacturia 791.1
  bilharziasis 120.0
Galen's vein —*see* condition
Gallbladder —*see also* condition
  acute (*see also* Disease, gallbladder) 575.0
Gall duct —*see* condition
Gallop rhythm 427.89
Gallstone (cholemic) (colic) (impacted)—*see also* Cholelithiasis
  causing intestinal obstruction 560.31
Gambling, pathological 312.31
Gammaloidosis 277.3
Gammopathy 273.9
  macroglobulinemia 273.3
  monoclonal (benign) (essential) (idiopathic) (with lymphoplasmacytic dyscrasia) 273.1
Gamna's disease (siderotic splenomegaly) 289.51
Gampsodactylia (congenital) 754.71
Gamstorp's disease (adynamia episodica hereditaria) 359.3
Gandy-Nanta disease (siderotic splenomegaly) 289.51
Gang activity without manifest psychiatric disorder V71.09
  adolescent V71.02
  adult V71.01
  child V71.02
Gangliocytoma (M9490/0)—*see* Neoplasm, connective tissue, benign
Ganglioglioma (M9505/1)—*see* Neoplasm, by site, uncertain behavior
Ganglion 727.43
  joint 727.41
  of yaws (early) (late) 102.6
  periosteal (*see also* Periostitis) 730.3
  tendon sheath (compound) (diffuse) 727.42
  tuberculous (*see also* Tuberculosis) 015.9
Ganglioneuroblastoma (M9490/3)—*see* Neoplasm, connective tissue, malignant

Ganglioneuroma (M9490/0)—*see also* Neoplasm, connective tissue, benign
  malignant (M9490/3)—*see* Neoplasm, connective tissue, malignant
Ganglioneuromatosis (M9491/0)—*see* Neoplasm, connective tissue, benign
Ganglionitis
  fifth nerve (*see also* Neuralgia, trigeminal) 350.1
  gasserian 350.1
  geniculate 351.1
    herpetic 053.11
    newborn 767.5
  herpes zoster 053.11
  herpetic geniculate (Hunt's syndrome) 053.11
Gangliosidosis 330.1
Gangosa 102.5
Gangrene, gangrenous (anemia) (artery) (cellulitis) (dermatitis) (dry) (infective) (moist) (pemphigus) (septic) (skin) (stasis) (ulcer) 785.4
  with
    arteriosclerosis (native artery) 440.24
      bypass graft 440.30
        autologous vein 440.31
        nonautologous biological 440.32
    diabetes (mellitus) 250.7 *[785.4]*
  abdomen (wall) 785.4
    arteriosclerotic 440.29 *[785.4]*
  adenitis 683
  alveolar 526.5
  angina 462
    diphtheritic 032.0
  anus 569.49
  appendices epiploicae—*see* Gangrene, mesentery
  appendix—*see* Appendicitis, acute
  arteriosclerotic —*see* Arteriosclerosis, with, gangrene
  auricle 785.4
  Bacillus welchii (*see also* Gangrene, gas) 040.0
  bile duct (*see also* Cholangitis) 576.8
  bladder 595.89
  bowel—*see* Gangrene, intestine
  cecum—*see* Gangrene, intestine
  Clostridium perfringens or welchii (*see also* Gangrene, gas) 040.0
  colon—*see* Gangrene, intestine
  connective tissue 785.4
  cornea 371.40
  corpora cavernosa (infective) 607.2
    noninfective 607.89
  cutaneous, spreading 785.4
  decubital 707.0 *[785.4]*
  diabetic (any site) 250.7 *[785.4]*
  dropsical 785.4
  emphysematous (*see also* Gangrene, gas) 040.0
  epidemic (ergotized grain) 988.2
  epididymis (infectional) (*see also* Epididymitis) 604.99
  erysipelas (*see also* Erysipelas) 035
  extremity (lower) (upper) 785.4
  gallbladder or duct (*see also* Cholecystitis, acute) 575.0
  gas (bacillus) 040.0

Gangrene, gangrenous—*continued*
  with
    abortion—*see* Abortion, by type, with sepsis
    ectopic pregnancy (*see also* categories
      633.0-633.9) 639.0
    molar pregnancy (*see also* categories
      630-632) 639.0
  following
    abortion 639.0
    ectopic or molar pregnancy 639.0
  puerperal, postpartum, childbirth 670
  glossitis 529.0
  gum 523.8
  hernia—*see* Hernia, by site, with gangrene
  hospital noma 528.1
  intestine, intestinal (acute) (hemorrhagic)
    (massive) 557.0
  with
    hernia—*see* Hernia, by site, with gangrene
    mesenteric embolism or infarction 557.0
    obstruction (*see also* Obstruction, intestine)
      560.9
  laryngitis 464.00
    with obstruction 464.01
  liver 573.8
  lung 513.0
    spirochetal 104.8
  lymphangitis 457.2
  Meleney's (cutaneous) 686.09
  mesentery 557.0
  with
    embolism or infarction 557.0
    intestinal obstruction (*see also* Obstruction,
      intestine) 560.9
  mouth 528.1
  noma 528.1
  orchitis 604.90
  ovary (*see also* Salpingo-oophoritis) 614.2
  pancreas 577.0
  penis (infectional) 607.2
    noninfective 607.89
  perineum 785.4
  pharynx 462
    septic 034.0
  pneumonia 513.0
  Pott's 440.24
  presenile 443.1
  pulmonary 513.0
  pulp, tooth 522.1
  quinsy 475
  Raynaud's (symmetric gangrene) 443.0 *[785.4]*
  rectum 569.49
  retropharyngeal 478.24
  rupture—*see* Hernia, by site, with gangrene
  scrotum 608.4
    noninfective 608.83
  senile 440.24
  sore throat 462
  spermatic cord 608.4
    noninfective 608.89
  spine 785.4
  spirochetal NEC 104.8
  spreading cutaneous 785.4
  stomach 537.89
  stomatitis 528.1
  symmetrical 443.0 *[785.4]*
  testis (infectional) (*see also* Orchitis) 604.99
    noninfective 608.89
  throat 462
    diphtheritic 032.0
  thyroid (gland) 246.8

Gangrene, gangrenous—*continued*
  tonsillitis (acute) 463
  tooth (pulp) 522.1
  tuberculous NEC (*see also* Tuberculosis) 011.9
  tunica vaginalis 608.4
    noninfective 608.89
  umbilicus 785.4
  uterus (*see also* Endometritis) 615.9
  uvulitis 528.3
  vas deferens 608.4
    noninfective 608.89
  vulva (*see also* Vulvitis) 616.10
Gannister disease (occupational) 502
  with tuberculosis—*see* Tuberculosis, pulmonary
Ganser's syndrome, hysterical 300.16
Gardner-Diamond syndrome (autoerythrocyte
  sensitization) 287.2
Gargoylism 277.5
Garré's
  disease (*see also* Osteomyelitis) 730.1
  osteitis (sclerosing) (*see also* Osteomyelitis)
    730.1
  osteomyelitis (*see also* Osteomyelitis) 730.1
Garrod's pads, knuckle 728.79
Gartner's duct
  cyst 752.11
  persistent 752.11
Gas
  asphyxia, asphyxiation, inhalation, poisoning,
    suffocation NEC 987.9
    specified gas—*see* Table of drugs and
      chemicals
  bacillus gangrene or infection—*see* Gas,
    gangrene
  cyst, mesentery 568.89
  excessive 787.3
  gangrene 040.0
  with
    abortion—*see* Abortion, by type, with sepsis
    ectopic pregnancy (*see also* categories
      633.0-633.9) 639.0
    molar pregnancy (*see also* categories
      630-632) 639.0
  following
    abortion 639.0
    ectopic or molar pregnancy 639.0
  puerperal, postpartum, childbirth 670
  on stomach 787.3
  pains 787.3
Gastradenitis 535.0
Gastralgia 536.8
  psychogenic 307.89
Gastrectasis, gastrectasia 536.1
  psychogenic 306.4
Gastric —*see* condition
Gastrinoma (M8153/1)
  malignant (M8153/3)
    pancreas 157.4
    specified site NEC—*see* Neoplasm, by site,
      malignant
    unspecified site 157.4
  specified site—*see* Neoplasm, by site,
    uncertain behavior
  unspecified site 235.5

Gastritis 535.5

Note—Use the following fifth-digit
subclassification for category 535:

0 without mention of hemorrhage
1 with hemorrhage
---

acute 535.0
alcoholic 535.3
allergic 535.4
antral 535.4
atrophic 535.1
atrophic-hyperplastic 535.1
bile-induced 535.4
catarrhal 535.0
chronic (atrophic) 535.1
cirrhotic 535.4
corrosive (acute) 535.4
dietetic 535.4
due to diet deficiency 269.9 [535.4]
eosinophilic 535.4
erosive 535.4
follicular 535.4
    chronic 535.1
giant hypertrophic 535.2
glandular 535.4
    chronic 535.1
hypertrophic (mucosa) 535.2
    chronic giant 211.1
irritant 535.4
nervous 306.4
phlegmonous 535.0
psychogenic 306.4
sclerotic 535.4
spastic 536.8
subacute 535.0
superficial 535.4
suppurative 535.0
toxic 535.4
tuberculous (see also Tuberculosis) 017.9
Gastrocarcinoma (M8010/3) 151.9
Gastrocolic —see condition
Gastrocolitis —see Enteritis
Gastrodisciasis 121.8
Gastroduodenitis (see also Gastritis) 535.5
catarrhal 535.0
infectional 535.0
virus, viral 008.8
    specified type NEC 008.69
Gastrodynia 536.8
Gastroenteritis (acute) (catarrhal) (congestive)
(hemorrhagic) (noninfectious) (see also
Enteritis) 558.9
aertrycke infection 003.0
allergic 558.3
chronic 558.9
    ulcerative (see also Colitis, ulcerative) 556.9
dietetic 558.9
due to
    food poisoning (see also Poisoning, food)
        005.9
    radiation 558.1
epidemic 009.0
functional 558.9
infectious (see also Enteritis, due to, by
    organism) 009.0
    presumed 009.1
salmonella 003.0
septic (see also Enteritis, due to, by organism)
    009.0
toxic 558.2

Gastroenteritis—continued
tuberculous (see also Tuberculosis) 014.8
ulcerative (see also Colitis, ulcerative) 556.9
viral NEC 008.8
    specified type NEC 008.69
zymotic 009.0
Gastroenterocolitis —see Enteritis
Gastroenteropathy, protein-losing 579.8
Gastroenteroptosis 569.89
**Gastroesophageal laceration-hemorrhage
    syndrome** 530.7
Gastroesophagitis 530.19
Gastrohepatitis (see also Gastritis) 535.5
Gastrointestinal —see condition
Gastrojejunal —see condition
Gastrojejunitis (see also Gastritis) 535.5
Gastrojejunocolic —see condition
Gastroliths 537.89
Gastromalacia 537.89
Gastroparalysis 536.8
diabetic 250.6 [337.1]
Gastroparesis 536.3
diabetic 250.6 [536.3]
Gastropathy, exudative 579.8
Gastroptosis 537.5
Gastrorrhagia 578.0
Gastrorrhea 536.8
psychogenic 306.4
Gastroschisis (congenital) 756.79
acquired 569.89
Gastrospasm (neurogenic) (reflex) 536.8
neurotic 306.4
psychogenic 306.4
Gastrostaxis 578.0
Gastrostenosis 537.89
Gastrostomy
attention to V55.1
complication 536.40
    specified type 536.49
infection 536.41
malfunctioning 536.42
status V44.1
Gastrosuccorrhea (continuous) (intermittent)
536.8
neurotic 306.4
psychogenic 306.4
Gaucher's
disease (adult) (cerebroside lipidosis) (infantile)
    272.7
hepatomegaly 272.7
splenomegaly (cerebroside lipidosis) 272.7
Gayet's disease (superior hemorrhagic
polioencephalitis) 265.1
Gayet-Wernicke's syndrome (superior
hemorrhagic polioencephalitis) 265.1
Gee (-Herter) (-Heubner) (-Thaysen) disease or
syndrome (nontropical sprue) 579.0
Gélineau's syndrome 347
Gemination, teeth 520.2
Gemistocytoma (M9411/3)
specified site—see Neoplasm, by site, malignant
unspecified site 191.9
General, generalized —see condition
Genital —see condition
Genito-anorectal syndrome 099.1
Genitourinary system —see condition
Genu
congenital 755.64
extrorsum (acquired) 736.42
    congenital 755.64
    late effects of rickets 268.1

Genu—*continued*
  introrsum (acquired) 736.41
    congenital 755.64
    late effects of rickets 268.1
  rachitic (old) 268.1
  recurvatum (acquired) 736.5
    congenital 754.40
      with dislocation of knee 754.41
    late effects of rickets 268.1
  valgum (acquired) (knock-knee) 736.41
    congenital 755.64
    late effects of rickets 268.1
  varum (acquired) (bowleg) 736.42
    congenital 755.64
    late effects of rickets 268.1
Geographic tongue 529.1
Geophagia 307.52
Geotrichosis 117.9
  intestine 117.9
  lung 117.9
  mouth 117.9
Gephyrophobia 300.29
Gerbode defect 745.4
Gerhardt's
  disease (erythromelalgia) 443.89
  syndrome (vocal cord paralysis) 478.30
Gerlier's disease (epidemic vertigo) 078.81
German measles 056.9
  exposure to V01.4
Germinoblastoma (diffuse) (M9614/3) 202.8
  follicular (M9692/3) 202.0
Germinoma (M9064/3)—*see* Neoplasm, by site,
    malignant
Gerontoxon 371.41
Gerstmann's syndrome (finger agnosia) 784.69
Gestation (period)—*see also* Pregnancy
  ectopic NEC (*see also* Pregnancy, ectopic)
    633.90
    with intrauterine pregnancy 633.91
Gestational proteinuria 646.2
  with hypertension—*see* Toxemia, of pregnancy
Ghon tubercle primary infection (*see also*
    Tuberculosis) 010.0
Ghost
  teeth 520.4
  vessels, cornea 370.64
Ghoul hand 102.3
Giant
  cell
    epulis 523.8
    peripheral (gingiva) 523.8
    tumor, tendon sheath 727.02
  colon (congenital) 751.3
  esophagus (congenital) 750.4
  kidney 753.3
  urticaria 995.1
    hereditary 277.6
Giardia lamblia infestation 007.1
Giardiasis 007.1
Gibert's disease (pityriasis rosea) 696.3
Gibraltar fever —*see* Brucellosis
Giddiness 780.4
  hysterical 300.11
  psychogenic 306.9
Gierke's disease (glycogenosis I) 271.0
Gigantism (cerebral) (hypophyseal) (pituitary)
    253.0
Gilbert's disease or cholemia (familial
    nonhemolytic jaundice) 277.4
Gilchrist's disease (North American
    blastomycosis) 116.0

Gilford (-Hutchinson) disease or syndrome
    (progeria) 259.8
Gilles de la Tourette's disease (motor-verbal tic)
    307.23
Gillespie's syndrome (dysplasia
    oculodentodigitalis) 759.89
Gingivitis 523.1
  acute 523.0
    necrotizing 101
  catarrhal 523.0
  chronic 523.1
  desquamative 523.1
  expulsiva 523.4
  hyperplastic 523.1
  marginal, simple 523.1
  necrotizing, acute 101
  pellagrous 265.2
  ulcerative 523.1
    acute necrotizing 101
  Vincent's 101
Gingivoglossitis 529.0
Gingivopericementitis 523.4
Gingivosis 523.1
Gingivostomatitis 523.1
  herpetic 054.2
Giovannini's disease 117.9
Gland, glandular —*see* condition
Glanders 024
Glanzmann (-Naegeli) disease or thrombasthenia
    287.1
Glassblowers' disease 527.1
Glaucoma (capsular) (inflammatory)
    (noninflammatory) (primary) 365.9
  with increased episcleral venous pressure 365.82
  absolute 360.42
  acute 365.22
    narrow angle 365.22
    secondary 365.60
  angle closure 365.20
    acute 365.22
    chronic 365.23
    intermittent 365.21
    interval 365.21
    residual stage 365.24
    subacute 365.21
  border line 365.00
  chronic 365.11
    noncongestive 365.11
    open angle 365.11
    simple 365.11
  closed angle—*see* Glaucoma, angle closure
  congenital 743.20
    associated with other eye anomalies 743.22
    simple 743.21
  congestive—*see* Glaucoma, narrow angle
  corticosteroid-induced (glaucomatous stage)
    365.31
    residual stage 365.32
  hemorrhagic 365.60
  hypersecretion 365.81
  in or with
    aniridia 743.45 *[365.42]*
    Axenfeld's anomaly 743.44 *[365.41]*
    concussion of globe 921.3 *[365.65]*
    congenital syndromes NEC 759.89 *[365.44]*
    dislocation of lens
      anterior 379.33 *[365.59]*
      posterior 379.34 *[365.59]*
    disorder of lens NEC 365.59
    epithelial down-growth 364.61 *[365.64]*
    glaucomatocyclitic crisis 364.22 *[365.62]*

Glaucoma—*continued*
  hypermature cataract 366.18 *[365.51]*
  hyphema 364.41 *[365.63]*
  inflammation, ocular 365.62
  iridocyclitis 364.3 *[365.62]*
  iris
    anomalies NEC 743.46 *[365.42]*
    atrophy, essential 364.51 *[365.42]*
    bombé 364.74 *[365.61]*
    rubeosis 364.42 *[365.63]*
  microcornea 743.41 *[365.43]*
  neurofibromatosis 237.71 *[365.44]*
  ocular
    cysts NEC 365.64
    disorders NEC 365.60
    trauma 365.65
    tumors NEC 365.64
  postdislocation of lens
    anterior 379.33 *[365.59]*
    posterior 379.34 *[365.59]*
  pseudoexfoliation of capsule 366.11 *[365.52]*
  pupillary block or seclusion 364.74 *[365.61]*
  recession of chamber angle 364.77 *[365.65]*
  retinal vein occlusion 362.35 *[365.63]*
  Rieger's anomaly or syndrome 743.44
    [365.41]
  rubeosis of iris 364.42 *[365.63]*
  seclusion of pupil 364.74 *[365.61]*
  spherophakia 743.36 *[365.59]*
  Sturge-Weber (-Dimitri) syndrome 759.6
    [365.44]
  systemic syndrome NEC 365.44
  tumor of globe 365.64
  vascular disorders NEC 365.63
  infantile 365.14
    congenital 743.20
      associated with other eye anomalies 743.22
      simple 743.21
  juvenile 365.14
  low tension 365.12
  malignant 365.83
  narrow angle (primary) 365.20
    acute 365.22
    chronic 365.23
    intermittent 365.21
    interval 365.21
    residual stage 365.24
    subacute 365.21
  newborn 743.20
    associated with other eye anomalies 743.22
    simple 743.21
  noncongestive (chronic) 365.11
  nonobstructive (chronic) 365.11
  obstructive 365.60
    due to lens changes 365.59
  open angle 365.10
    with
      borderline intraocular pressure 365.01
      cupping of optic discs 365.01
    primary 365.11
    residual stage 365.15
  phacolytic 365.51
    with hypermature cataract 366.18 *[365.51]*
  pigmentary 365.13
  postinfectious 365.60
  pseudoexfoliation 365.52
    with pseudoexfoliation of capsule 366.11
      [365.52]
  secondary NEC 365.60
  simple (chronic) 365.11
  simplex 365.11

Glaucoma—*continued*
  steroid responders 365.03
  suspect 365.00
  syphilitic 095.8
  traumatic NEC 365.65
    newborn 767.8
  tuberculous (*see also* Tuberculosis) 017.3
    [365.62]
  wide angle (*see also* Glaucoma, open angle)
    365.10
Glaucomatous flecks (subcapsular) 366.31
Glazed tongue 529.4
Gleet 098.2
Glénard's disease or syndrome (enteroptosis)
  569.89
Glinski-Simmonds syndrome (pituitary
  cachexia) 253.2
Glioblastoma (multiforme) (M9440/3)
  with sarcomatous component (M9442/3)
    specified site—*see* Neoplasm, by site,
      malignant
    unspecified site 191.9
  giant cell (M9441/3)
    specified site—*see* Neoplasm, by site,
      malignant
    unspecified site 191.9
  specified site—*see* Neoplasm, by site, malignant
  unspecified site 191.9
Glioma (malignant) (M9380/3)
  astrocytic (M9400/3)
    specified site—*see* Neoplasm, by site,
      malignant
    unspecified site 191.9
  mixed (M9382/3)
    specified site—*see* Neoplasm, by site,
      malignant
    unspecified site 191.9
  nose 748.1
  specified site NEC—*see* Neoplasm, by site,
    malignant
  subependymal (M9383/1) 237.5
  unspecified site 191.9
Gliomatosis cerebri (M9381/3) 191.0
Glioneuroma (M9505/1)—*see* Neoplasm, by
  site, uncertain behavior
Gliosarcoma (M9380/3)
  specified site—*see* Neoplasm, by site, malignant
  unspecified site 191.9
Gliosis (cerebral) 349.89
  spinal 336.0
Glisson's
  cirrhosis—*see* Cirrhosis, portal
  disease (*see also* Rickets) 268.0
Glissonitis 573.3
Globinuria 791.2
Globus 306.4
  hystericus 300.11
Glomangioma (M8712/0) (*see also*
  Hemangioma) 228.00
Glomangiosarcoma (M8710/3)—*see* Neoplasm,
  connective tissue, malignant
Glomerular nephritis (*see also* Nephritis) 583.9
Glomerulitis (*see also* Nephritis) 583.9
Glomerulonephritis (*see also* Nephritis) 583.9
  with
    edema (*see also* Nephrosis) 581.9
    lesion of
      exudative nephritis 583.89
      interstitial nephritis (diffuse) (focal) 583.89
      necrotizing glomerulitis 583.4
        acute 580.4

Glomerulonephritis—*continued*
    chronic 582.4
      renal necrosis 583.9
        cortical 583.6
        medullary 583.7
      specified pathology NEC 583.89
        acute 580.89
        chronic 582.89
    necrosis, renal 583.9
      cortical 583.6
      medullary (papillary) 583.7
    specified pathology or lesion NEC 583.89
    acute 580.9
      with
        exudative nephritis 580.89
        interstitial nephritis (diffuse) (focal) 580.89
        necrotizing glomerulitis 580.4
      extracapillary with epithelial crescents 580.4
      poststreptococcal 580.0
      proliferative (diffuse) 580.0
      rapidly progressive 580.4
      specified pathology NEC 580.89
    arteriolar (*see also* Hypertension, kidney) 403.90
    arteriosclerotic (*see also* Hypertension, kidney) 403.90
    ascending (*see also* Pyelitis) 590.80
    basement membrane NEC 583.89
      with
        pulmonary hemorrhage (Goodpasture's syndrome) 446.21 *[583.81]*
    chronic 582.9
      with
        exudative nephritis 582.89
        interstitial nephritis (diffuse) (focal) 582.89
        necrotizing glomerulitis 582.4
        specified pathology or lesion NEC 582.89
      endothelial 582.2
      extracapillary with epithelial crescents 582.4
      hypocomplementemic persistent 582.2
      lobular 582.2
      membranoproliferative 582.2
      membranous 582.1
        and proliferative (mixed) 582.2
        sclerosing 582.1
      mesangiocapillary 582.2
      mixed membranous and proliferative 582.2
      proliferative (diffuse) 582.0
      rapidly progressive 582.4
      sclerosing 582.1
    cirrhotic—*see* Sclerosis, renal
    desquamative—*see* Nephrosis
    due to or associated with
      amyloidosis 277.3 *[583.81]*
        with nephrotic syndrome 277.3 *[581.81]*
        chronic 277.3 *[582.81]*
      diabetes mellitus 250.4 *[583.81]*
        with nephrotic syndrome 250.4 *[581.81]*
      diphtheria 032.89 *[580.81]*
      gonococcal infection (acute) 098.19 *[583.81]*
        chronic or duration or 2 months or over 098.39 *[583.81]*
      infectious hepatitis 070.9 *[580.81]*
      malaria (with nephrotic syndrome) 084.9 *[581.81]*
      mumps 072.79 *[580.81]*
      polyarteritis (nodosa) (with nephrotic syndrome) 446.0 *[581.81]*
      specified pathology NEC 583.89
        acute 580.89
        chronic 582.89
      streptotrichosis 039.8 *[583.81]*

Glomerulonephritis—*continued*
      subacute bacterial endocarditis 421.0 *[580.81]*
      syphilis (late) 095.4
        congenital 090.5 *[583.81]*
        early 091.69 *[583.81]*
      systemic lupus erythematosus 710.0 *[583.81]*
        with nephrotic syndrome 710.0 *[581.81]*
        chronic 710.0 *[582.81]*
      tuberculosis (*see also* Tuberculosis) 016.0 *[583.81]*
      typhoid fever 002.0 *[580.81]*
    extracapillary with epithelial crescents 583.4
      acute 580.4
      chronic 582.4
    exudative 583.89
      acute 580.89
      chronic 582.89
    focal (*see also* Nephritis) 583.9
      embolic 580.4
    granular 582.89
    granulomatous 582.89
    hydremic (*see also* Nephrosis) 581.9
    hypocomplementemic persistent 583.2
      with nephrotic syndrome 581.2
      chronic 582.2
    immune complex NEC 583.89
    infective (*see also* Pyelitis) 590.80
    interstitial (diffuse) (focal) 583.89
      with nephrotic syndrome 581.89
      acute 580.89
      chronic 582.89
    latent or quiescent 582.9
    lobular 583.2
      with nephrotic syndrome 581.2
      chronic 582.2
    membranoproliferative 583.2
      with nephrotic syndrome 581.2
      chronic 582.2
    membranous 583.1
      with nephrotic syndrome 581.1
      and proliferative (mixed) 583.2
        with nephrotic syndrome 581.2
        chronic 582.2
      chronic 582.1
      sclerosing 582.1
        with nephrotic syndrome 581.1
    mesangiocapillary 583.2
      with nephrotic syndrome 581.2
      chronic 582.2
    minimal change 581.3
    mixed membranous and proliferative 583.2
      with nephrotic syndrome 581.2
      chronic 582.2
    necrotizing 583.4
      acute 580.4
      chronic 582.4
    nephrotic (*see also* Nephrosis) 581.9
    old—*see* Glomerulonephritis, chronic
    parenchymatous 581.89
    poststreptococcal 580.0
    proliferative (diffuse) 583.0
      with nephrotic syndrome 581.0
      acute 580.0
      chronic 582.0
    purulent (*see also* Pyelitis) 590.80
    quiescent—*see* Nephritis, chronic
    rapidly progressive 583.4
      acute 580.4
      chronic 582.4
    sclerosing membranous (chronic) 582.1
      with nephrotic syndrome 581.1

Glomerulonephritis—*continued*
  septic (*see also* Pyelitis) 590.80
  specified pathology or lesion NEC 583.89
    with nephrotic syndrome 581.89
    acute 580.89
    chronic 582.89
  suppurative (acute) (disseminated) (*see also*
    Pyelitis) 590.80
  toxic—*see* Nephritis, acute
  tubal, tubular—*see* Nephrosis, tubular
  type II (Ellis)—*see* Nephrosis
  vascular—*see* Hypertension, kidney
Glomerulosclerosis (*see also* Sclerosis, renal)
  587
  focal 582.1
    with nephrotic syndrome 581.1
  intercapillary (nodular) (with diabetes) 250.4
    [581.81]
Glossagra 529.6
Glossalgia 529.6
Glossitis 529.0
  areata exfoliativa 529.1
  atrophic 529.4
  benign migratory 529.1
  gangrenous 529.0
  Hunter's 529.4
  median rhomboid 529.2
  Moeller's 529.4
  pellagrous 265.2
Glossocele 529.8
Glossodynia 529.6
  exfoliativa 529.4
Glossoncus 529.8
Glossophytia 529.3
Glossoplegia 529.8
Glossoptosis 529.8
Glossopyrosis 529.6
Glossotrichia 529.3
Glossy skin 701.9
Glottis —*see* condition
Glottitis —*see* Glossitis
Glucagonoma (M8152/0)
  malignant (M8152/3)
    pancreas 157.4
    specified site NEC—*see* Neoplasm, by site,
      malignant
    unspecified site 157.4
  pancreas 211.7
  specified site NEC—*see* Neoplasm, by site,
    benign
  unspecified site 211.7
Glucoglycinuria 270.7
Glue ear syndrome 381.20
Glue sniffing (airplane glue) (*see also*
  Dependence) 304.6
Glycinemia (with methylmalonic acidemia) 270.7
Glycinuria (renal) (with ketosis) 270.0
Glycogen
  infiltration (*see also* Disease, glycogen storage)
    271.0
  storage disease (*see also* Disease, glycogen
    storage) 271.0
Glycogenosis (*see also* Disease, glycogen
  storage) 271.0
  cardiac 271.0 *[425.7]*
  Cori, types I-VII 271.0
  diabetic, secondary 250.8 *[259.8]*
  diffuse (with hepatic cirrhosis) 271.0
  generalized 271.0
  glucose-6-phosphatase deficiency 271.0
  hepatophosphorylase deficiency 271.0

Glycogenosis—*continued*
  hepatorenal 271.0
  myophosphorylase deficiency 271.0
Glycopenia 251.2
Glycoprolinuria 270.8
Glycosuria 791.5
  renal 271.4
Gnathostoma (spinigerum) (infection)
  (infestation) 128.1
  wandering swellings from 128.1
Gnathostomiasis 128.1
Goiter (adolescent) (colloid) (diffuse) (dipping)
  (due to iodine deficiency) (endemic)
  (euthyroid) (heart) (hyperplastic) (internal)
  (intrathoracic) (juvenile) (mixed type)
  (nonendemic) (parenchymatous) (plunging)
  (sporadic) (subclavicular) (substernal) 240.9
  with
    hyperthyroidism (recurrent) (*see also* Goiter,
      toxic) 242.0
    thyrotoxicosis (*see also* Goiter, toxic) 242.0
  adenomatous (*see also* Goiter, nodular) 241.9
  cancerous (M8000/3) 193
  complicating pregnancy, childbirth, or
    puerperium 648.1
  congenital 246.1
  cystic (*see also* Goiter, nodular) 241.9
  due to enzyme defect in synthesis of thyroid
    hormone (butane-insoluble iodine)
    (coupling) (deiodinase) (iodide trapping or
    organification) (iodotyrosine dehalogenase)
    (peroxidase) 246.1
  dyshormonogenic 246.1
  exophthalmic (*see also* Goiter, toxic) 242.0
  familial (with deaf-mutism) 243
  fibrous 245.3
  lingual 759.2
  lymphadenoid 245.2
  malignant (M8000/3) 193
  multinodular (nontoxic) 241.1
    toxic or with hyperthyroidism (*see also*
      Goiter, toxic) 242.2
  nodular (nontoxic) 241.9
    with
      hyperthyroidism (*see also* Goiter, toxic)
        242.3
      thyrotoxicosis (*see also* Goiter, toxic) 242.3
    endemic 241.9
    exophthalmic (diffuse) (*see also* Goiter, toxic)
      242.0
    multinodular (nontoxic) 241.1
    sporadic 241.9
    toxic (*see also* Goiter, toxic) 242.3
    uninodular (nontoxic) 241.0
  nontoxic (nodular) 241.9
    multinodular 241.1
    uninodular 241.0
  pulsating (*see also* Goiter, toxic) 242.0
  simple 240.0
  toxic 242.0

Note—Use the following fifth-digit
subclassification with category 242:

0 without mention of thyrotoxic crisis
*   or storm*
1 with mention of thyrotoxic crisis or storm

---

    adenomatous 242.3
      multinodular 242.2
      uninodular 242.1
    multinodular 242.2

Goiter—*continued*
  nodular 242.3
    multinodular 242.2
    uninodular 242.1
  uninodular 242.1
  uninodular (nontoxic) 241.0
    toxic or with hyperthyroidism (*see also*
      Goiter, toxic) 242.1
Goldberg (-Maxwell) (-Morris) syndrome
  (testicular feminization) 257.8
Goldblatt's
  hypertension 440.1
  kidney 440.1
Goldenhar's syndrome (oculoauriculovertebral
  dysplasia) 756.0
Goldflam-Erb disease or syndrome 358.0
Goldscheider's disease (epidermolysis bullosa)
  757.39
Goldstein's disease (familial hemorrhagic
  telangiectasia) 448.0
Golfer's elbow 726.32
Goltz-Gorlin syndrome (dermal hypoplasia)
  757.39
Gonadoblastoma (M9073/1)
  specified site—*see* Neoplasm, by site uncertain
    behavior
  unspecified site
    female 236.2
    male 236.4
Gonecystitis (*see also* Vesiculitis) 608.0
Gongylonemiasis 125.6
  mouth 125.6
Goniosynechiae 364.73
Gonococcemia 098.89
Gonococcus, gonococcal (disease) (infection)
  (*see also* condition) 098.0
  anus 098.7
  bursa 098.52
  chronic NEC 098.2
  complicating pregnancy, childbirth, or
    puerperium 647.1
    affecting fetus or newborn 760.2
  conjunctiva, conjunctivitis (neonatorum) 098.40
  dermatosis 098.89
  endocardium 098.84
  epididymo-orchitis 098.13
    chronic or duration of 2 months or over 098.33
  eye (newborn) 098.40
  fallopian tube (chronic) 098.37
    acute 098.17
  genitourinary (acute) (organ) (system) (tract)
    (*see also* Gonorrhea) 098.0
    lower 098.0
      chronic 098.2
    upper 098.10
      chronic 098.30
  heart NEC 098.85
  joint 098.50
  keratoderma 098.81
  keratosis (blennorrhagica) 098.81
  lymphatic (gland) (node) 098.89
  meninges 098.82
  orchitis (acute) 098.13
    chronic or duration of 2 months or over 098.33
  pelvis (acute) 098.19
    chronic or duration of 2 months or over 098.39
  pericarditis 098.83
  peritonitis 098.86
  pharyngitis 098.6
  pharynx 098.6

Gonococcus, gonococcal—*continued*
  proctitis 098.7
  pyosalpinx (chronic) 098.37
    acute 098.17
  rectum 098.7
  septicemia 098.89
  skin 098.89
  specified site NEC 098.89
  synovitis 098.51
  tendon sheath 098.51
  throat 098.6
  urethra (acute) 098.0
    chronic or duration of 2 months or over 098.2
  vulva (acute) 098.0
    chronic or duration of 2 months or over 098.2
Gonocytoma (M9073/1)
  specified site—*see* Neoplasm, by site, uncertain
    behavior
  unspecified site
    female 236.2
    male 236.4
Gonorrhea 098.0
  acute 098.0
  Bartholin's gland (acute) 098.0
    chronic or duration of 2 months or over 098.2
  bladder (acute) 098.11
    chronic or duration of 2 months or over 098.31
  carrier (suspected of) V02.7
  cervix (acute) 098.15
    chronic or duration of 2 months or over 098.35
  chronic 098.2
  complicating pregnancy, childbirth, or
    puerperium 647.1
    affecting fetus or newborn 760.2
  conjunctiva, conjunctivitis (neonatorum) 098.40
  contact V01.6
  Cowper's gland (acute) 098.0
    chronic or duration of 2 months or over 098.2
  duration of two months or over 098.2
  exposure to V01.6
  fallopian tube (chronic) 098.37
    acute 098.17
  genitourinary (acute) (organ) (system) (tract)
    098.0
    chronic 098.2
    duration of two months or over 098.2
  kidney (acute) 098.19
    chronic or duration of 2 months or over 098.39
  ovary (acute) 098.19
    chronic or duration of 2 months or over 098.39
  pelvis (acute) 098.19
    chronic or duration of 2 months or over 098.39
  penis (acute) 098.0
    chronic or duration of 2 months or over 098.2
  prostate (acute) 098.12
    chronic or duration of 2 months or over 098.32
  seminal vesicle (acute) 098.14
    chronic or duration of 2 months or over 098.34
  specified site NEC—*see* Gonococcus
  spermatic cord (acute) 098.14
    chronic or duration of 2 months or over 098.34
  urethra (acute) 098.0
    chronic or duration of 2 months or over 098.2
  vagina (acute) 098.0
    chronic or duration of 2 months or over 098.2
  vas deferens (acute) 098.14
    chronic or duration of 2 months or over 098.34
  vulva (acute) 098.0
    chronic or duration of 2 months or over 098.2
Goodpasture's syndrome (pneumorenal) 446.21

Gopalan's syndrome (burning feet) 266.2
Gordon's disease (exudative enteropathy) 579.8
Gorlin-Chaudhry-Moss syndrome 759.89
Gougerot's syndrome (trisymptomatic) 709.1
Gougerot-Blum syndrome (pigmented purpuric
 lichenoid dermatitis) 709.1
Gougerot-Carteaud disease or syndrome
 (confluent reticulate papillomatosis) 701.8
Gougerot-Hailey-Hailey disease (benign
 familial chronic pemphigus) 757.39
Gougerot (-Houwer) -Sjögren syndrome
 (keratoconjunctivitis sicca) 710.2
Gouley's syndrome (constrictive pericarditis)
 423.2
Goundou 102.6
Gout, gouty 274.9
 with specified manifestations NEC 274.89
 arthritis (acute) 274.0
 arthropathy 274.0
 degeneration, heart 274.82
 diathesis 274.9
 eczema 274.89
 episcleritis 274.89 [379.09]
 external ear (tophus) 274.81
 glomerulonephritis 274.10
 iritis 274.89 [364.11]
 joint 274.0
 kidney 274.10
 lead 984.9
  specified type of lead—see Table of drugs and
   chemicals
 nephritis 274.10
 neuritis 274.89 [357.4]
 phlebitis 274.89 [451.9]
 rheumatic 714.0
 saturnine 984.9
  specified type of lead—see Table of drugs and
   chemicals
 spondylitis 274.0
 synovitis 274.0
 syphilitic 095.8
 tophi 274.0
  ear 274.81
  heart 274.82
  specified site NEC 274.82
Gowers'
 muscular dystrophy 359.1
 syndrome (vasovagal attack) 780.2
Gowers-Paton-Kennedy syndrome 377.04
Gradenigo's syndrome 383.02
Graft-versus-host disease (bone marrow) 996.85
 due to organ transplant NEC—see
  Complications, transplant, organ
Graham Steell's murmur (pulmonic
 regurgitation) (see also Endocarditis,
 pulmonary) 424.3
Grain-handlers' disease or lung 495.8
Grain mite (itch) 133.8
Grand
 mal (idiopathic) (see also Epilepsy) 345.1
  hysteria of Charcot 300.11
  nonrecurrent or isolated 780.39
 multipara
  affecting management of labor and delivery
   659.4
  status only (not pregnant) V61.5
Granite workers' lung 502

Granular —see also condition
 inflammation, pharynx 472.1
 kidney (contracting) (see also Sclerosis, renal)
  587
 liver—see Cirrhosis, liver
 nephritis—see Nephritis
Granulation tissue, abnormal —see also
 Granuloma
 abnormal or excessive 701.5
 postmastoidectomy cavity 383.33
 postoperative 701.5
 skin 701.5
Granulocytopenia, granulocytopenic (primary)
 288.0
 malignant 288.0
Granuloma NEC 686.1
 abdomen (wall) 568.89
  skin (pyogenicum) 686.1
   from residual foreign body 709.4
 annulare 695.89
 anus 569.49
 apical 522.6
 appendix 543.9
 aural 380.23
 beryllium (skin) 709.4
  lung 503
 bone (see also Osteomyelitis) 730.1
  eosinophilic 277.8
  from residual foreign body 733.99
 canaliculus lacrimalis 375.81
 cerebral 348.8
 cholesterin, middle ear 385.82
 coccidioidal (progressive) 114.3
  lung 114.4
  meninges 114.2
  primary (lung) 114.0
 colon 569.89
 conjunctiva 372.61
 dental 522.6
 ear, middle (cholesterin) 385.82
  with otitis media—see Otitis media
 eosinophilic 277.8
  bone 277.8
  lung 277.8
  oral mucosa 528.9
 exuberant 701.5
 eyelid 374.89
 facial
  lethal midline 446.3
  malignant 446.3
 faciale 701.8
 fissuratum (gum) 523.8
 foot NEC 686.1
 foreign body (in soft tissue) NEC 728.82
  bone 733.99
  in operative wound 998.4
  muscle 728.82
  skin 709.4
  subcutaneous tissue 709.4
 fungoides 202.1
 gangraenescens 446.3
 giant cell (central) (jaw) (reparative) 526.3
  gingiva 523.8
  peripheral (gingiva) 523.8
 gland (lymph) 289.3
 Hodgkin's (M9661/3) 201.1
 ileum 569.89
 infectious NEC 136.9
 inguinale (Donovan) 099.2
  venereal 099.2
 intestine 569.89

Granuloma—*continued*
  iridocyclitis 364.10
  jaw (bone) 526.3
    reparative giant cell 526.3
  kidney (*see also* Infection, kidney) 590.9
  lacrimal sac 375.81
  larynx 478.79
  lethal midline 446.3
  lipid 277.8
  lipoid 277.8
  liver 572.8
  lung (infectious) (*see also* Fibrosis, lung) 515
    coccidioidal 114.4
    eosinophilic 277.8
  lymph gland 289.3
  Majocchi's 110.6
  malignant, face 446.3
  mandible 526.3
  mediastinum 519.3
  midline 446.3
  monilial 112.3
  muscle 728.82
    from residual foreign body 728.82
  nasal sinus (*see also* Sinusitis) 473.9
  operation wound 998.59
    foreign body 998.4
    stitch (external) 998.89
      internal organ 998.89
    talc 998.7
  oral mucosa, eosinophilic or pyogenic 528.9
  orbit, orbital 376.11
  paracoccidioidal 116.1
  penis, venereal 099.2
  periapical 522.6
  peritoneum 568.89
    due to ova of helminths NEC (*see also*
      Helminthiasis) 128.9
  postmastoidectomy cavity 383.33
  postoperative–*see* Granuloma, operation wound
  prostate 601.8
  pudendi (ulcerating) 099.2
  pudendorum (ulcerative) 099.2
  pulp, internal (tooth) 521.4
  pyogenic, pyogenicum (skin) 686.1
    maxillary alveolar ridge 522.6
    oral mucosa 528.9
  rectum 569.49
  reticulohistiocytic 277.8
  rubrum nasi 705.89
  sarcoid 135
  Schistosoma 120.9
  septic (skin) 686.1
  silica (skin) 709.4
  sinus (accessory) (infectional) (nasal) (*see also*
    Sinusitis) 473.9
  skin (pyogenicum) 686.1
    from foreign body or material 709.4
  sperm 608.89
  spine
    syphilitic (epidural) 094.89
    tuberculous (*see also* Tuberculosis) 015.0
      [730.88]
  stitch (postoperative) 998.89
    internal wound 998.89
  suppurative (skin) 686.1
  suture (postoperative) 998.89
    internal wound 998.89
  swimming pool 031.1
  talc 728.82
    in operation wound 998.7

Granuloma—*continued*
  telangiectaticum (skin) 686.1
  trichophyticum 110.6
  tropicum 102.4
  umbilicus 686.1
    newborn 771.4
  urethra 599.84
  uveitis 364.10
  vagina 099.2
  venereum 099.2
  vocal cords 478.5
  Wegener's (necrotizing respiratory
    granulomatosis) 446.4
Granulomatosis NEC 686.1
  disciformis chronica et progressiva 709.3
  infantiseptica 771.2
  lipoid 277.8
  lipophagic, intestinal 040.2
  miliary 027.0
  necrotizing, respiratory 446.4
  progressive, septic 288.1
  Wegener's (necrotizing respiratory) 446.4
Granulomatous tissue —*see* Granuloma
Granulosis rubra nasi 705.89
Graphite fibrosis (of lung) 503
Graphospasm 300.89
  organic 333.84
Grating scapula 733.99
Gravel (urinary) (*see also* Calculus) 592.9
Graves' disease (exophthalmic goiter) (*see also*
  Goiter, toxic) 242.0
Gravis —*see* condition
Grawitz's tumor (hypernephroma) (M8312/3)
  189.0
Grayness, hair (premature) 704.3
  congenital 757.4
Gray or grey syndrome (chloramphenicol)
  (newborn) 779.4
Greenfield's disease 330.0
Green sickness 280.9
Greenstick fracture —*see* Fracture, by site
Greig's syndrome (hypertelorism) 756.0
Griesinger's disease (*see also* Ancylostomiasis)
  126.9
Grinder's
  asthma 502
  lung 502
  phthisis (*see also* Tuberculosis) 011.4
Grinding, teeth 306.8
Grip
  Dabney's 074.1
  devil's 074.1
Grippe, grippal —*see also* Influenza
  Balkan 083.0
  intestinal 487.8
  summer 074.8
Grippy cold 487.1
Grisel's disease 723.5
Groin —*see* condition
Grooved
  nails (transverse) 703.8
  tongue 529.5
    congenital 750.13
Ground itch 126.9
Growing pains, children 781.99

Growth (fungoid) (neoplastic) (new)
    (M8000/1)—*see also* Neoplasm, by site,
    unspecified nature
  adenoid (vegetative) 474.12
  benign (M8000/0)—*see* Neoplasm, by site,
    benign
  fetal, poor 764.9
    affecting management of pregnancy 656.5
  malignant (M8000/3)—*see* Neoplasm, by site
    malignant
  rapid, childhood V21.0
  secondary (M8000/6)—*see* Neoplasm, by site,
    malignant, secondary
Gruber's hernia —*see* Hernia, Gruber's
Gruby's disease (tinea tonsurans) 110.0
G-trisomy 758.0
Guama fever 066.3
Gubler (-Millard) paralysis or syndrome 344.89
Guérin-Stern syndrome (arthrogryposis
  multiplex congenita) 754.89
Guertin's disease (electric chorea) 049.8
Guillain-Barré disease or syndrome 357.0
Guinea worms (infection) (infestation) 125.7
Guinon's disease (motor-verbal tic) 307.23
Gull's disease (thyroid atrophy with myxedema)
  244.8
Gull and Sutton's disease —*see* Hypertension,
  kidney
Gum —*see* condition
Gumboil 522.7
Gumma (syphilitic) 095.9
  artery 093.89
    cerebral or spinal 094.89
  bone 095.5
    of yaws (late) 102.6
  brain 094.89
  cauda equina 094.89
  central nervous system NEC 094.9
  ciliary body 095.8 *[364.11]*
  congenital 090.5
    testis 090.5
  eyelid 095.8 *[373.5]*
  heart 093.89
  intracranial 094.89
  iris 095.8 *[364.11]*
  kidney 095.4
  larynx 095.8
  leptomeninges 094.2
  liver 095.3
  meninges 094.2
  myocardium 093.82
  nasopharynx 095.8
  neurosyphilitic 094.9
  nose 095.8
  orbit 095.8
  palate (soft) 095.8
  penis 095.8
  pericardium 093.81
  pharynx 095.8
  pituitary 095.8
  scrofulous (*see also* Tuberculosis) 017.0
  skin 095.8
  specified site NEC 095.8
  spinal cord 094.89
  tongue 095.8
  tonsil 095.8
  trachea 095.8
  tuberculous (*see also* Tuberculosis) 017.0

Gumma—*continued*
  ulcerative due to yaws 102.4
  ureter 095.8
  yaws 102.4
    bone 102.6
Gunn's syndrome (jaw-winking syndrome)
  742.8
Gunshot wound —*see also* Wound, open, by site
  fracture—*see* Fracture, by site, open
  internal organs (abdomen, chest, or pelvis)—*see*
    Injury, internal, by site, with open wound
  intracranial—*see* Laceration, brain, with open
    intracranial wound
Günther's disease or syndrome (congenital
  erythropoietic porphyria) 277.1
Gustatory hallucination 780.1
Gynandrism 752.7
Gynandroblastoma (M8632/1)
  specified site—*see* Neoplasm, by site, uncertain
    behavior
  unspecified site
    female 236.2
    male 236.4
Gynandromorphism 752.7
Gynatresia (congenital) 752.49
Gynecoid pelvis, male 738.6
Gynecological examination V72.3
  for contraceptive maintenance V25.40
Gynecomastia 611.1
Gynephobia 300.29
Gyrate scalp 757.39

H

Haas' disease (osteochondrosis head of humerus) 732.3
Habermann's disease (acute parapsoriasis varioliformis) 696.2
Habit, habituation
  chorea 307.22
  disturbance, child 307.9
  drug (*see also* Dependence) 304.9
  laxative (*see also* Abuse, drugs, nondependent) 305.9
  spasm 307.20
    chronic 307.22
    transient of childhood 307.21
  tic 307.20
    chronic 307.22
    transient of childhood 307.21
  use of
    nonprescribed drugs (*see also* Abuse, drugs, nondependent) 305.9
    patent medicines (*see also* Abuse, drugs, nondependent) 305.9
  vomiting 536.2
Hadfield-Clarke syndrome (pancreatic infantilism) 577.8
Haff disease 985.1
Hageman factor defect, deficiency, or disease (*see also* Defect, coagulation) 286.3
Haglund's disease (osteochondrosis os tibiale externum) 732.5
Haglund-Läwen-Fründ syndrome 717.89
Hagner's disease (hypertrophic pulmonary osteoarthropathy) 731.2
Hag teeth, tooth 524.3
Hailey-Hailey disease (benign familial chronic pemphigus) 757.39
Hair —*see also* condition
  plucking 307.9
Hairball in stomach 935.2
Hairy black tongue 529.3
Half vertebra 756.14
Halitosis 784.9
Hallermann-Streiff syndrome 756.0
Hallervorden-Spatz disease or syndrome 333.0
Hallopeau's
  acrodermatitis (continua) 696.1
  disease (lichen sclerosis et atrophicus) 701.0
Hallucination (auditory) (gustatory) (olfactory) (tactile) 780.1
  alcoholic 291.3
  drug-induced 292.12
  visual 368.16
Hallucinosis 298.9
  alcoholic (acute) 291.3
  drug-induced 292.12
Hallus —*see* Hallux
Hallux 735.9
  malleus (acquired) 735.3
  rigidus (acquired) 735.2
    congenital 755.66
    late effects of rickets 268.1
  valgus (acquired) 735.0
    congenital 755.66
  varus (acquired) 735.1
    congenital 755.66
Halo, visual 368.15
Hamartoblastoma 759.6

Hamartoma 759.6
  epithelial (gingival), odontogenic, central, or peripheral (M9321/0) 213.1
  upper jaw (bone) 213.0
  vascular 757.32
Hamartosis, hamartoses NEC 759.6
Hamman's disease or syndrome (spontaneous mediastinal emphysema) 518.1
Hamman-Rich syndrome (diffuse interstitial pulmonary fibrosis) 516.3
Hammer toe (acquired) 735.4
  congenital 755.66
  late effects of rickets 268.1
Hand —*see* condition
Hand-Schüller-Christian disease or syndrome (chronic histiocytosis x) 277.8
Hand-foot syndrome 282.61
Hanging (asphyxia) (strangulation) (suffocation) 994.7
Hangnail (finger) (with lymphangitis) 681.02
Hangover (alcohol) (*see also* Abuse, drugs, nondependent) 305.0
Hanot's cirrhosis or disease —*see* Cirrhosis, biliary
Hanot-Chauffard (-Troisier) syndrome (bronze diabetes) 275.0
Hansen's disease (leprosy) 030.9
  benign form 030.1
  malignant form 030.0
Harada's disease or syndrome 363.22
Hard chancre 091.0
Hard firm prostate 600.1
Hardening
  artery—*see* Arteriosclerosis
  brain 348.8
  liver 571.8
Hare's syndrome (M8010/3) (carcinoma, pulmonary apex) 162.3
Harelip (*see also* Cleft, lip) 749.10
Harkavy's syndrome 446.0
Harlequin (fetus) 757.1
  color change syndrome 779.89
Harley's disease (intermittent hemoglobinuria) 283.2
Harris'
  lines 733.91
  syndrome (organic hyperinsulinism) 251.1
Hart's disease or syndrome (pellagra-cerebellar ataxia-renal aminoaciduria) 270.0
Hartmann's pouch (abnormal sacculation of gallbladder neck) 575.8
  of intestine V44.3
    attention to V55.3
Hartnup disease (pellagra-cerebellar ataxia-renal aminoaciduria) 270.0
Harvester lung 495.0
Hashimoto's disease or struma (struma lymphomatosa) 245.2
Hassall-Henle bodies (corneal warts) 371.41
Haut mal (*see also* Epilepsy) 345.1
Haverhill fever 026.1
Hawaiian wood rose dependence 304.5
Hawkins' keloid 701.4
Hay
  asthma (*see also* Asthma) 493.0
  fever (allergic) (with rhinitis) 477.9
    with asthma (bronchial) (*see also* Asthma) 493.0

Hay —*continued*
  allergic, due to grass, pollen, ragweed, or tree
    477.0
  conjunctivitis 372.05
  due to
    dander 477.8
    dust 477.8
    fowl 477.8
    pollen 477.0
    specified allergen other than pollen 477.8
Hayem-Faber syndrome (achlorhydric anemia)
  280.9
Hayem-Widal syndrome (acquired hemolytic
  jaundice) 283.9
Haygarth's nodosities 715.04
Hazard-Crile tumor (M8350/3) 193
Hb (abnormal)
  disease—*see* Disease, hemoglobin
  trait—*see* Trait
H disease 270.0
Head —*see also* condition
  banging 307.3
Headache 784.0
  allergic 346.2
  cluster 346.2
  due to
    loss, spinal fluid 349.0
    lumbar puncture 349.0
    saddle block 349.0
  emotional 307.81
  histamine 346.2
  lumbar puncture 349.0
  menopausal 627.2
  migraine 346.9
  nonorganic origin 307.81
  postspinal 349.0
  psychogenic 307.81
  psychophysiologic 307.81
  sick 346.1
  spinal 349.0
    complicating labor and delivery 668.8
    postpartum 668.8
  spinal fluid loss 349.0
  tension 307.81
  vascular 784.0
    migraine type 346.9
  vasomotor 346.9
Health
  advice V65.4
  audit V70.0
  checkup V70.0
  education V65.4
  hazard (*see also* History of) V15.9
    specified cause NEC V15.89
  instruction V65.4
  services provided because (of)
    boarding school residence V60.6
    holiday relief for person providing home care
      V60.5
    inadequate
      housing V60.1
      resources V60.2
    lack of housing V60.0
    no care available in home V60.4
    person living alone V60.3
    poverty V60.3
    residence in institution V60.6
    specified cause NEC V60.8
    vacation relief for person providing home care
      V60.5

Healthy
  donor (*see also* Donor) V59.9
  infant or child
    accompanying sick mother V65.0
    receiving care V20.1
  person
    accompanying sick relative V65.0
    admitted for sterilization V25.2
    receiving prophylactic inoculation or
      vaccination (*see also* Vaccination,
      prophylactic) V05.9
Hearing examination V72.1
Heart —*see* condition
Heartburn 787.1
  psychogenic 306.4
Heat (effects) 992.9
  apoplexy 992.0
  burn—*see also* Burn, by site
    from sun (*see also* Sunburn) 692.71
  collapse 992.1
  cramps 992.2
  dermatitis or eczema 692.89
  edema 992.7
  erythema—*see* Burn, by site
  excessive 992.9
    specified effect NEC 992.8
  exhaustion 992.5
    anhydrotic 992.3
    due to
      salt (and water) depletion 992.4
      water depletion 992.3
  fatigue (transient) 992.6
  fever 992.0
  hyperpyrexia 992.0
  prickly 705.1
  prostration—*see* Heat, exhaustion
  pyrexia 992.0
  rash 705.1
  specified effect NEC 992.8
  stroke 992.0
  sunburn (*see also* Sunburn) 692.71
  syncope 992.1
Heavy-chain disease 273.2
Heavy-for-dates (fetus or infant) 766.1
  4500 grams or more 766.0
  exceptionally 766.0
Hebephrenia, hebephrenic (acute) (*see also*
  Schizophrenia) 295.1
  dementia (praecox) (*see also* Schizophrenia)
    295.1
  schizophrenia (*see also* Schizophrenia) 295.1
Heberden's
  disease or nodes 715.04
  syndrome (angina pectoris) 413.9
Hebra's disease
  dermatitis exfoliativa 695.89
  erythema multiforme exudativum 695.1
  pityriasis 695.89
    maculata et circinata 696.3
    rubra 695.89
      pilaris 696.4
  prurigo 698.2
Hebra, nose 040.1
Hedinger's syndrome (malignant carcinoid)
  259.2
Heel —*see* condition
Heerfordt's disease or syndrome
  (uveoparotitis) 135
Hegglin's anomaly or syndrome 288.2
Heidenhain's disease 290.10
  with dementia 290.10

Heilmeyer-Schöner disease (M9842/3) 207.1
Heine-Medin disease (*see also* Poliomyelitis) 045.9
Heinz-body anemia, congenital 282.7
Heller's disease or syndrome (infantile psychosis) (*see also* Psychosis, childhood) 299.1
H.E.L.L.P. 642.5
Helminthiasis (*see also* Infestation, by specific parasite) 128.9
  Ancylostoma (*see also* Ancylostoma) 126.9
  intestinal 127.9
    mixed types (types classifiable to more than one of the titles 120.0-127.7) 127.8
    specified type 127.7
  mixed types (intestinal) (types classifiable to more than one of the titles 120.0-127.7) 127.8
  Necator americanus 126.1
  specified type NEC 128.8
  Trichinella 124
Heloma 700
Hemangioblastoma (M9161/1)—*see also* Neoplasm, connective tissue, uncertain behavior
  malignant (M9161//3)—*see* Neoplasm, connective tissue, malignant
Hemangioblastomatosis, cerebelloretinal 759.6
Hemangioendothelioma (M9130/1)—*see also* Neoplasm, by site, uncertain behavior
  benign (M9130/0) 228.00
  bone (diffuse) (M9130/3)—*see* Neoplasm, bone, malignant
  malignant (M9130/3)—*see* Neoplasm, connective tissue, malignant
  nervous system (M9130/0) 228.09
Hemangioendotheliosarcoma (M9130/3)—*see* Neoplasm, connective tissue, malignant
Hemangiofibroma (M9160/0)—*see* Neoplasm, by site, benign
Hemangiolipoma (M8861/0)—*see* Lipoma
Hemangioma (M9120/0) 228.00
  arteriovenous (M9123/0)—*see* Hemangioma, by site
  brain 228.02
  capillary (M9131/0)—*see* Hemangioma, by site
  cavernous (M9121/0)—*see* Hemangioma, by site
  central nervous system NEC 228.09
  choroid 228.09
  heart 228.09
  infantile (M9131/0)—*see* Hemangioma, by site
  intra-abdominal structures 228.04
  intracranial structures 228.02
  intramuscular (M9132/0)—*see* Hemangioma, by site
  iris 228.09
  juvenile (M9131/0)—*see* Hemangioma, by site
  malignant (M9120/3)—*see* Neoplasm, connective tissue, malignant
  meninges 228.09
    brain 228.02
    spinal cord 228.09
  peritoneum 228.04
  placenta—*see* Placenta, abnormal
  plexiform (M9131/0)—*see* Hemangioma, by site
  racemose (M9123/0)—*see* Hemangioma, by site
  retina 228.03
  retroperitoneal tissue 228.04
  sclerosing (M8832/0)—*see* Neoplasm, skin, benign

Hemangioma—*continued*
  simplex (M9131/0)—*see* Hemangioma, by site
  skin and subcutaneous tissue 228.01
  specified site NEC 228.09
  spinal cord 228.09
  venous (M9122/0)—*see* Hemangioma, by site
  verrucous keratotic (M9142/0)—*see* Hemangioma, by site
Hemangiomatosis (systemic) 757.32
  involving single site—*see* Hemangioma
Hemangiopericytoma (M9150/1)—*see also* Neoplasm, connective tissue, uncertain behavior
  benign (M9150/0)—*see* Neoplasm, connective tissue, benign
  malignant (M9150/3)—*see* Neoplasm, connective tissue, malignant
Hemangiosarcoma (M9120/3)—*see* Neoplasm, connective tissue, malignant
Hemarthrosis (nontraumatic) 719.0
  ankle 719.17
  elbow 719.12
  foot 719.17
  hand 719.14
  hip 719.15
  knee 719.16
  multiple sites 719.19
  pelvic region 719.15
  shoulder (region) 719.11
  specified site NEC 719.18
  traumatic—*see* Sprain, by site
  wrist 719.13
Hematemesis 578.0
  with ulcer—*see* Ulcer, by site, with hemorrhage
  due to S. japonicum 120.2
  Goldstein's (familial hemorrhagic telangiectasia) 448.0
  newborn 772.4
    due to swallowed maternal blood 777.3
Hematidrosis 705.89
Hematinuria (*see also* Hemoglobinuria) 791.2
  malarial 084.8
  paroxysmal 283.2
Hematite miners' lung 503
Hematobilia 576.8
Hematocele (congenital) (diffuse) (idiopathic) 608.83
  broad ligament 620.7
  canal of Nuck 629.0
  cord, male 608.83
  fallopian tube 620.8
  female NEC 629.0
  ischiorectal 569.89
  male NEC 608.83
  ovary 629.0
  pelvis, pelvic
    female 629.0
      with ectopic pregnancy (*see also* Pregnancy, ectopic) 633.90
      with intrauterine pregnancy 633.91
    male 608.83
  periuterine 629.0
  retrouterine 629.0
  scrotum 608.83
  spermatic cord (diffuse) 608.83
  testis 608.84
  traumatic—*see* Injury, internal, pelvis
  tunica vaginalis 608.83
  uterine ligament 629.0
  uterus 621.4
  vagina 623.6
  vulva 624.5

Hematoma—*continued*
intracranial—*see* Hematoma, brain
kidney, cystic 593.81
 traumatic 866.01
  with open wound into cavity 866.11
labia (nontraumatic) 624.5
lingual (and other parts of neck, scalp, or face, except eye) 920
liver (subcapsular) 573.8
 birth injury 767.8
 fetus or newborn 767.8
 traumatic NEC 864.01
  with
   laceration—*see* Laceration, liver
   open wound into cavity 864.11
mediastinum—*see* Injury, internal, mediastinum
meninges, meningeal (brain)—*see also* Hematoma, brain, subarachnoid
 spinal—*see* Injury, spinal, by site
mesosalpinx (nontraumatic) 620.8
 traumatic—*see* Injury, internal, pelvis
muscle (traumatic)—*see* Contusion, by site
nasal (septum) (and other part(s) of neck, scalp, or face, except eye) 920
obstetrical surgical wound 674.3
orbit, orbital (nontraumatic) 376.32
 traumatic 921.2
ovary (corpus luteum) (nontraumatic) 620.1
 traumatic—*see* Injury, internal, ovary
pelvis (female) (nontraumatic) 629.8
 complicating delivery 665.7
 male 608.83
 traumatic—*see also* Injury, internal, pelvis
  specified organ NEC (*see also* Injury, internal, pelvis) 867.6
penis (nontraumatic) 607.82
pericranial (and neck, or face any part, except eye) 920
 due to injury at birth 767.1
perineal wound (obstetrical) 674.3
 complicating delivery 664.5
perirenal, cystic 593.81
pinna 380.31
placenta—*see* Placenta, abnormal
postoperative 998.12
retroperitoneal (nontraumatic) 568.81
 traumatic—*see* Injury, internal, retroperitoneum
retropubic, male 568.81
scalp (and neck, or face any part, except eye) 920
 fetus or newborn 767.1
scrotum (nontraumatic) 608.83
 traumatic 922.4
seminal vesicle (nontraumatic) 608.83
 traumatic—*see* Injury, internal, seminal vesicle
spermatic cord—*see also* Injury, internal, spermatic cord
 nontraumatic 608.83
spinal (cord) (meninges)—*see also* Injury, spinal, by site
 fetus or newborn 767.4
 nontraumatic 336.1
spleen 865.01
 with
  laceration—*see* Laceration, spleen
  open wound into cavity 865.11
sternocleidomastoid, birth injury 767.8

Hematoma—*continued*
sternomastoid, birth injury 767.8
subarachnoid—*see also* Hematoma, brain, subarachnoid
 fetus or newborn 772.2
 nontraumatic (*see also* Hemorrhage, subarachnoid) 430
 newborn 772.2
subdural—*see also* Hematoma, brain, subdural
 fetus or newborn (localized) 767.0
 nontraumatic (*see also* Hemorrhage, subdural) 432.1
subperiosteal (syndrome) 267
 traumatic—*see* Hematoma, by site
superficial, fetus or newborn 772.6
syncytium—*see* Placenta, abnormal
testis (nontraumatic) 608.83
 birth injury 767.8
 traumatic 922.4
tunica vaginalis (nontraumatic) 608.83
umbilical cord 663.6
 affecting fetus or newborn 762.6
uterine ligament (nontraumatic) 620.7
 traumatic—*see* Injury, internal, pelvis
uterus 621.4
 traumatic—*see* Injury, internal, pelvis
vagina (nontraumatic) (ruptured) 623.6
 complicating delivery 665.7
 traumatic 922.4
vas deferens (nontraumatic) 608.83
 traumatic—*see* Injury, internal, vas deferens
vitreous 379.23
vocal cord 920
vulva (nontraumatic) 624.5
 complicating delivery 664.5
 fetus or newborn 767.8
 traumatic 922.4
Hematometra 621.4
Hematomyelia 336.1
 with fracture of vertebra (*see also* Fracture, vertebra, by site, with spinal cord injury) 806.8
 fetus or newborn 767.4
Hematomyelitis 323.9
 late effect—*see* category 326
Hematoperitoneum (*see also* Hemoperitoneum) 568.81
Hematopneumothorax (*see also* Hemothorax) 511.8
Hematoporphyria (acquired) (congenital) 277.1
Hematoporphyrinuria (acquired) (congenital) 277.1
Hematorachis, hematorrhachis 336.1
 fetus or newborn 767.4
Hematosalpinx 620.8
 with
  ectopic pregnancy (*see also* categories 633.0-633.9) 639.2
  molar pregnancy (*see also* categories 630-632) 639.2
 infectional (*see also* Salpingo-oophoritis) 614.2
Hematospermia 608.82
Hematothorax (*see also* Hemothorax) 511.8
Hematotympanum 381.03
Hematuria (benign) (essential) (idiopathic) 599.7
 due to S. hematobium 120.0
 endemic 120.0
 intermittent 599.7
 malarial 084.8
 paroxysmal 599.7

Hematuria—*continued*
  sulfonamide
    correct substance properly administered 599.7
    overdose or wrong substance given or taken
      961.0
  tropical (bilharziasis) 120.0
  tuberculous (*see also* Tuberculosis) 016.9
Hematuric bilious fever 084.8
Hemeralopia 368.10
Hemiabiotrophy 799.8
Hemi-akinesia 781.8
Hemianalgesia (*see also* Disturbance, sensation)
  782.0
Hemianencephaly 740.0
Hemianesthesia (*see also* Disturbance,
  sensation) 782.0
Hemianopia, hemianopsia (altitudinal)
  (homonymous) 368.46
  binasal 368.47
  bitemporal 368.47
  heteronymous 368.47
  syphilitic 095.8
Hemiasomatognosia 307.9
Hemiathetosis 781.0
Hemiatrophy 799.8
  cerebellar 334.8
  face 349.89
    progressive 349.89
  fascia 728.9
  leg 728.2
  tongue 529.8
Hemiballism (us) 333.5
Hemiblock (cardiac) (heart) (left) 426.2
Hemicardia 746.89
Hemicephalus, hemicephaly 740.0
Hemichorea 333.5
Hemicrania 346.9
  congenital malformation 740.0
Hemidystrophy —*see* Hemiatrophy
Hemiectromelia 755.4
Hemihypalgesia (*see also* Disturbance,
  sensation) 782.0
Hemihypertrophy (congenital) 759.89
  cranial 756.0
Hemihypesthesia (*see also* Disturbance,
  sensation) 782.0
Hemi-inattention 781.8
Hemimelia 755.4
  lower limb 755.30
    paraxial (complete) (incomplete) (intercalary)
      (terminal) 755.32
      fibula 755.37
      tibia 755.36
    transverse (complete) (partial) 755.31
  upper limb 755.20
    paraxial (complete) (incomplete) (intercalary)
      (terminal) 755.22
      radial 755.26
      ulnar 755.27
    transverse (complete) (partial) 755.21
Hemiparalysis (*see also* Hemiplegia) 342.9
Hemiparesis (*see also* Hemiplegia) 342.9
Hemiparesthesia (*see also* Disturbance,
  sensation) 782.0

Hemiplegia 342.9
  acute (*see also* Disease, cerebrovascular, acute)
    436
  alternans facialis 344.89
  apoplectic (*see also* Disease, cerebrovascular,
    acute) 436
    late effect or residual
      affecting
        dominant side 438.21
        nondominant side 438.22
        unspecfied side 438.20
  arteriosclerotic 437.0
    late effect or residual
      affecting
        dominant side 438.21
        nondominant side 438.22
        unspecified side 438.20
  ascending (spinal) NEC 344.89
  attack (*see also* Disease, cerebrovascular, acute)
    436
  brain, cerebral (current episode) 437.8
    congenital 343.1
  cerebral—*see* Hemiplegia, brain
  congenital (cerebral) (spastic) (spinal) 343.1
  conversion neurosis (hysterical) 300.11
  cortical—*see* Hemiplegia, brain
  due to
    arteriosclerosis 437.0
      late effect or residual
        affecting
          dominant side 438.21
          nondominant side 438.22
          unspecified side 438.20
    cerebrovascular lesion (*see also* Disease,
      cerebrovascular, acute) 436
      late effect
        affecting
          dominant side 438.21
          nondominant side 438.22
          unspecified side 438.20
  embolic (current) (*see also* Embolism, brain)
    434.1
    late effect
      affecting
        dominant side 438.21
        nondominant side 438.22
        unspecified side 438.20
  flaccid 342.0
  hypertensive (current episode) 437.8
  infantile (postnatal) 343.4
  late effect
    birth injury, intracranial or spinal 343.4
    cerebrovascular lesion—*see* Late effect(s) (of)
      cerebrovascular disease
    viral encephalitis 139.0
  middle alternating NEC 344.89
  newborn NEC 767.0
  seizure (current episode) (*see also* Disease,
    cerebrovascular, acute) 436
  spastic 342.1
    congenital or infantile 343.1
  specified NEC 342.8
  thrombotic (current) (*see also* Thrombosis,
    brain) 434.0
    late effect—*see* late effect(s) (of)
      cerebrovascular disease
Hemisection, spinal cord —*see* Fracture,
  vertebra, by site, with spinal cord injury
Hemispasm 781.0
  facial 781.0
Hemispatial neglect 781.8

Hemisporosis 117.9
Hemitremor 781.0
Hemivertebra 756.14
Hemobilia 576.8
Hemocholecyst 575.8
Hemochromatosis (acquired) (diabetic)
  (hereditary) (liver) (myocardium) (primary
  idiopathic) (secondary) 275.0
  with refractory anemia 285.0
Hemodialysis V56.0
Hemoglobin —*see also* condition
  abnormal (disease)—*see* Disease, hemoglobin
  AS genotype 282.5
  fetal, hereditary persistence 282.7
  high-oxygen-affinity 289.0
  low NEC 285.9
  S (Hb-S), heterozygous 282.5
Hemoglobinemia 283.2
  due to blood transfusion NEC 999.8
    bone marrow 996.85
  paroxysmal 283.2
Hemoglobinopathy (mixed) (*see also* Disease,
  hemoglobin) 282.7
  with thalassemia 282.4
  sickle-cell 282.60
    with thalassemia 282.4
Hemoglobinuria, hemoglobinuric 791.2
  with anemia, hemolytic, acquired (chronic)
    NEC 283.2
  cold (agglutinin) (paroxysmal) (with Raynaud's
    syndrome) 283.2
  due to
    exertion 283.2
    hemolysis (from external causes) NEC 283.2
  exercise 283.2
  fever (malaria) 084.8
  infantile 791.2
  intermittent 283.2
  malarial 084.8
  march 283.2
  nocturnal (paroxysmal) 283.2
  paroxysmal (cold) (nocturnal) 283.2
Hemolymphangioma (M9175/0) 228.1
Hemolysis
  fetal—*see* Jaundice, fetus or newborn
  intravascular (disseminated) NEC 286.6
  with
    abortion—*see* Abortion, by type, with
      hemorrhage, delayed or excessive
    ectopic pregnancy (*see also* categories
      633.0-633.9) 639.1
    hemorrhage of pregnancy 641.3
      affecting fetus or newborn 762.1
    molar pregnancy (*see also* categories
      630-632) 639.1
  acute 283.2
  following
    abortion 639.1
    ectopic or molar pregnancy 639.1
  neonatal—*see* Jaundice, fetus or newborn
  transfusion NEC 999.8
    bone marrow 996.85
Hemolytic —*see also* condition
  anemia—*see* Anemia, hemolytic
  uremic syndrome 283.11
Hemometra 621.4
Hemopericardium (with effusion) 423.0
  newborn 772.8
  traumatic (*see also* Hemothorax, traumatic)
    860.2
    with open wound into thorax 860.3

Hemoperitoneum 568.81
  infectional (*see also* Peritonitis) 567.2
  traumatic—*see* Injury, internal, peritoneum
Hemophilia (familial) (hereditary) 286.0
  A 286.0
    carrier (asymptomatic) V83.01
      symptomatic V83.02
  acquired 286.5
  B (Leyden) 286.1
  C 286.2
  calcipriva (*see also* Fibrinolysis) 286.7
  classical 286.0
  nonfamilial 286.7
  vascular 286.4
Hemophilus influenzae NEC 041.5
  arachnoiditis (basic) (brain) (spinal) 320.0
    late effect—*see* category 326
  bronchopneumonia 482.2
  cerebral ventriculitis 320.0
    late effect—*see* category 326
  cerebrospinal inflammation 320.0
    late effect—*see* category 326
  infection NEC 041.5
  leptomeningitis 320.0
    late effect—*see* category 326
  meningitis (cerebral) (cerebrospinal) (spinal)
    320.0
    late effect—*see* category 326
  meningomyelitis 320.0
    late effect—*see* category 326
  pachymeningitis (adhesive) (fibrous)
    (hemorrhagic) (hypertrophic) (spinal) 320.0
    late effect—*see* category 326
  pneumonia (broncho-) 482.2
Hemophthalmos 360.43
Hemopneumothorax (*see also* Hemothorax)
  511.8
  traumatic 860.4
    with open wound into thorax 860.5
Hemoptysis 786.3
  due to Paragonimus (westermani) 121.2
  newborn 770.3
  tuberculous (*see also* Tuberculosis, pulmonary)
    011.9
Hemorrhage, hemorrhagic (nontraumatic) 459.0
  abdomen 459.0
  accidental (antepartum) 641.2
    affecting fetus or newborn 762.1
  adenoid 474.8
  adrenal (capsule) (gland) (medulla) 255.4
    newborn 772.5
  after labor—*see* Hemorrhage, postpartum
  alveolar
    lung, newborn 770.3
    process 525.8
  alveolus 525.8
  amputation stump (surgical) 998.11
    secondary, delayed 997.69
  anemia (chronic) 280.0
    acute 285.1
  antepartum—*see* Hemorrhage, pregnancy
  anus (sphincter) 569.3
  apoplexy (stroke) 432.9
  arachnoid—*see* Hemorrhage, subarachnoid
  artery NEC 459.0
    brain (*see also* Hemorrhage, brain) 431
    middle meningeal—*see* Hemorrhage,
      subarachnoid
  basilar (ganglion) (*see also* Hemorrhage, brain)
    431
  bladder 596.8

Hemorrhage, hemorrhagic—*continued*
  blood dyscrasia 289.9
  bowel 578.9
    newborn 772.4
  brain (miliary) (nontraumatic) 431
    with
      birth injury 767.0
      arachnoid—*see* Hemorrhage, subarachnoid
    due to
      birth injury 767.0
      rupture of aneurysm (congenital) (*see also*
        Hemorrhage, subarachnoid) 430
        mycotic 431
      syphilis 094.89
    epidural or extradural—*see* Hemorrhage,
        extradural
    fetus or newborn (anoxic) (hypoxic) (due to
        birth trauma) (nontraumatic) 767.0
    intraventricular 772.10
      grade I 772.11
      grade II 772.12
      grade III 772.13
      grade IV 772.14
    iatrogenic 997.02
    postoperative 997.02
    puerperal, postpartum, childbirth 674.0
    stem 431
    subarachnoid, arachnoid or meningeal—*see*
        Hemorrhage, subarachnoid
    subdural—*see* Hemorrhage, subdural
    traumatic NEC 853.0

---

*Note—Use the following fifth-digit
subclassification with categories 851-854:*

0 unspecified state of consciousness
1 with no loss of consciousness
*2 with brief [less than one hour] loss of
consciousness*
*3 with moderate [1-24 hours] loss of
consciousness*
*4 with prolonged [more than 24 hours] loss of
consciousness and return to pre-existing
conscious level*
*5 with prolonged [more than 24 hours] loss of
consciousness, without return to pre-existing
conscious level*
*Use fifth-digit 5 to designate when a patient is
unconscious and dies before regaining
consciousness, regardless of the duration of the
loss of consciousness*
*6 with loss of consciousness of unspecified
duration*
9 with concussion, unspecified

---

      with
        cerebral
          contusion—*see* Contusion, brain
          laceration—*see* Laceration, brain
          open intracranial wound 853.1
          skull fracture—*see* Fracture, skull, by site
        extradural or epidural 852.4
          with open intracranial wound 852.5
        subarachnoid 852.0
          with open intracranial wound 852.1
        subdural 852.2
          with open intracranial wound 852.3
  breast 611.79
  bronchial tube—*see* Hemorrhage, lung
  bronchopulmonary—*see* Hemorrhage, lung
  bronchus (cause unknown) (*see also*
      Hemorrhage, lung) 786.3

Hemorrhage, hemorrhagic—*continued*
  bulbar (*see also* Hemorrhage, brain) 431
  bursa 727.89
  capillary 448.9
    primary 287.8
  capsular—*see* Hemorrhage, brain
  cardiovascular 429.89
  cecum 578.9
  cephalic (*see also* Hemorrhage, brain) 431
  cerebellar (*see also* Hemorrhage, brain) 431
  cerebellum (*see also* Hemorrhage, brain) 431
  cerebral (*see also* Hemorrhage, brain) 431
    fetus or newborn (anoxic) (traumatic) 767.0
  cerebromeningeal (*see also* Hemorrhage, brain)
      431
  cerebrospinal (*see also* Hemorrhage, brain) 431
  cerebrum (*see also* Hemorrhage, brain) 431
  cervix (stump) (uteri) 622.8
  cesarean section wound 674.3
  chamber, anterior (eye) 364.41
  childbirth—*see* Hemorrhage, complicating,
      delivery
  choroid 363.61
    expulsive 363.62
  ciliary body 364.41
  cochlea 386.8
  colon—*see* Hemorrhage, intestine
  complicating
    delivery 641.9
      affecting fetus or newborn 762.1
      associated with
        afibrinogenemia 641.3
          affecting fetus or newborn 763.89
        coagulation defect 641.3
          affecting fetus or newborn 763.89
        hyperfibrinolysis 641.3
          affecting fetus or newborn 763.89
        hypofibrinogenemia 641.3
          affecting fetus or newborn 763.89
      due to
        low-lying placenta 641.1
          affecting fetus or newborn 762.0
        placenta previa 641.1
          affecting fetus or newborn 762.0
        premature separation of placenta 641.2
          affecting fetus or newborn 762.1
        retained
          placenta 666.0
          secundines 666.2
        trauma 641.8
          affecting fetus or newborn 763.89
        uterine leiomyoma 641.8
          affecting fetus or newborn 763.89
    surgical procedure 998.11
  concealed NEC 459.0
  congenital 772.9
  conjunctiva 372.72
    newborn 772.8
  cord, newborn 772.0
    slipped ligature 772.3
    stump 772.3
  corpus luteum (ruptured) 620.1
  cortical (*see also* Hemorrhage, brain) 431
  cranial 432.9
  cutaneous 782.7
    newborn 772.6
  cyst, pancreas 577.2
  cystitis—*see* Cystitis
  delayed
    with

Hemorrhage, hemorrhagic—*continued*
   abortion—*see* Abortion, by type, with
      hemorrhage, delayed or excessive
      ectopic pregnancy (*see also* categories
         633.0-633.9) 639.1
      molar pregnancy (*see also* categories
         630-632) 639.1
   following
      abortion 639.1
      ectopic or molar pregnancy 639.1
      postpartum 666.2
   diathesis (familial) 287.9
      newborn 776.0
   disease 287.9
      newborn 776.0
      specified type NEC 287.8
   disorder 287.9
      due to circulating anticoagulants 286.5
      specified type NEC 287.8
   due to
      any device, implant, or graft (presence of)
         classifiable to 996.0-996.5—*see*
         Complications, due to (presence of) any
         device, implant, or graft classified to
         996.0—996.5 NEC
      circulating anticoagulant 286.5
   duodenum, duodenal 537.89
      ulcer—*see* Ulcer, duodenum, with hemorrhage
   dura mater—*see* Hemorrhage, subdural
   endotracheal—*see* Hemorrhage, lung
   epidural—*see* Hemorrhage, extradural
   episiotomy 674.3
   esophagus 530.82
      varix (*see also* Varix, esophagus, bleeding)
         456.0
   excessive
      with
         abortion—*see* Abortion, by type, with
            hemorrhage, delayed or excessive
         ectopic pregnancy (*see also* categories
            633.0-633.9) 639.1
         molar pregnancy (*see also* categories
            630-632) 639.1
      following
         abortion 639.1
         ectopic or molar pregnancy 639.1
   external 459.0
   extradural (traumatic)—*see also* Hemorrhage,
      brain, traumatic, extradural
      birth injury 767.0
      fetus or newborn (anoxic) (traumatic) 767.0
      nontraumatic 432.0
   eye 360.43
      chamber (anterior) (aqueous) 364.41
      fundus 362.81
   eyelid 374.81
   fallopian tube 620.8
   fetomaternal 772.0
      affecting management of pregnancy or
         puerperium 656.0
   fetus, fetal 772.0
      from
         cut end of co-twin's cord 772.0
         placenta 772.0
         ruptured cord 772.0
         vasa previa 772.0
      into
         co-twin 772.0
         mother's circulation 772.0
            affecting management of pregnancy or
               puerperium 656.0

Hemorrhage, hemorrhagic—*continued*
   fever (*see also* Fever, hemorrhagic) 065.9
      with renal syndrome 078.6
      arthropod-borne NEC 065.9
      Bangkok 065.4
      Crimean 065.0
      dengue virus 065.4
      epidemic 078.6
      Junin virus 078.7
      Korean 078.6
      Machupo virus 078.7
      mite-borne 065.8
      mosquito-borne 065.4
      Philippine 065.4
      Russian (Yaroslav) 078.6
      Singapore 065.4
      southeast Asia 065.4
      Thailand 065.4
      tick-borne NEC 065.3
   fibrinogenolysis (*see also* Fibrinolysis) 286.6
   fibrinolytic (acquired) (*see also* Fibrinolysis)
      286.6
   fontanel 767.1
   from tracheostomy stoma 519.09
   fundus, eye 362.81
   funis
      affecting fetus or newborn 772.0
      complicating delivery 663.8
   gastric (*see also* Hemorrhage, stomach) 578.9
   gastroenteric 578.9
      newborn 772.4
   gastrointestinal (tract) 578.9
      newborn 772.4
   genitourinary (tract) NEC 599.89
   gingiva 523.8
   globe 360.43
   gravidarum—*see* Hemorrhage, pregnancy
   gum 523.8
   heart 429.89
   hypopharyngeal (throat) 784.8
   intermenstrual 626.6
      irregular 626.6
      regular 626.5
   internal (organs) 459.0
      capsule (*see also* Hemorrhage brain) 431
      ear 386.8
      newborn 772.8
   intestine 578.9
      congenital 772.4
      newborn 772.4
   into
      bladder wall 596.7
      bursa 727.89
      corpus luysii (*see also* Hemorrhage, brain) 431
   intra-abdominal 459.0
      during or following surgery 998.11
   intra-alveolar, newborn (lung) 770.3
   intracerebral (*see also* Hemorrhage, brain) 431
   intracranial NEC 432.9
      puerperal, postpartum, childbirth 674.0
      traumatic—*see* Hemorrhage, brain, traumatic
   intramedullary NEC 336.1
   intraocular 360.43
   intraoperative 998.11
   intrapartum—*see* Hemorrhage, complicating,
      delivery
   intrapelvic
      female 629.8
      male 459.0
   intraperitoneal 459.0
   intrapontine (*see also* Hemorrhage, brain) 431

Hemorrhage, hemorrhagic—*continued*
  intrauterine 621.4
    complicating delivery—*see* Hemorrhage,
      complicating, delivery
    in pregnancy or childbirth—*see* Hemorrhage,
      pregnancy
    postpartum (*see also* Hemorrhage,
      postpartum) 666.1
  intraventricular (*see also* Hemorrhage, brain)
    431
    fetus or newborn (anoxic) (traumatic) 772.10
      grade I 772.11
      grade II 772.12
      grade III 772.13
      grade IV 772.14
  intravesical 596.7
  iris (postinfectional) (postinflammatory) (toxic)
    364.41
  joint (nontraumatic) 719.10
    ankle 719.17
    elbow 719.12
    foot 719.17
    forearm 719.13
    hand 719.14
    hip 719.15
    knee 719.16
    lower leg 719.16
    multiple sites 719.19
    pelvic region 719.15
    shoulder (region) 719.11
    specified site NEC 719.18
    thigh 719.15
    upper arm 719.12
    wrist 719.13
  kidney 593.81
  knee (joint) 719.16
  labyrinth 386.8
  leg NEC 459.0
  lenticular striate artery (*see also* Hemorrhage,
    brain) 431
  ligature, vessel 998.11
  liver 573.8
  lower extremity NEC 459.0
  lung 786.3
    newborn 770.3
    tuberculous (*see also* Tuberculosis,
      pulmonary) 011.9
  malaria 084.8
  marginal sinus 641.2
  massive subaponeurotic, birth injury 767.1
  maternal, affecting fetus or newborn 762.1
  mediastinum 786.3
  medulla (*see also* Hemorrhage, brain) 431
  membrane (brain) (*see also* Hemorrhage,
    subarachnoid) 430
    spinal cord—*see* Hemorrhage, spinal cord
  meninges, meningeal (brain) (middle) (*see also*
    Hemorrhage, subarachnoid) 430
    spinal cord—*see* Hemorrhage, spinal cord
  mesentery 568.81
  metritis 626.8
  midbrain (*see also* Hemorrhage, brain) 431
  mole 631
  mouth 528.9
  mucous membrane NEC 459.0
    newborn 772.8
  muscle 728.89
  nail (subungual) 703.8
  nasal turbinate 784.7
    newborn 772.8
  nasopharynx 478.29

Hemorrhage, hemorrhagic—*continued*
  navel, newborn 772.3
  newborn 772.9
    adrenal 772.5
    alveolar (lung) 770.3
    brain (anoxic) (hypoxic) (due to birth trauma)
      767.0
    cerebral (anoxic) (hypoxic) (due to birth
      trauma) 767.0
    conjunctiva 772.8
    cutaneous 772.6
    diathesis 776.0
    due to vitamin K deficiency 776.0
    gastrointestinal 772.4
    internal (organs) 772.8
    intestines 772.4
    intra-alveolar (lung) 770.3
    intracranial (from any perinatal cause) 767.0
    intraventricular (from any perinatal cause)
      772.10
      grade I 772.11
      grade II 772.12
      grade III 772.13
      grade IV 772.14
    lung 770.3
    pulmonary (massive) 770.3
    spinal cord, traumatic 767.4
    stomach 772.4
    subaponeurotic (massive) 767.1
    subarachnoid (from any perinatal cause) 772.2
    subconjunctival 772.8
    umbilicus 772.0
      slipped ligature 772.3
      vasa previa 772.0
  nipple 611.79
  nose 784.7
    newborn 772.8
  obstetrical surgical wound 674.3
  omentum 568.89
    newborn 772.4
  optic nerve (sheath) 377.42
  orbit 376.32
  ovary 620.1
  oviduct 620.8
  pancreas 577.8
  parathyroid (gland) (spontaneous) 252.8
  parturition—*see* Hemorrhage, complicating,
    delivery
  penis 607.82
  pericardium, pericarditis 423.0
  perineal wound (obstetrical) 674.3
  peritoneum, peritoneal 459.0
  peritonsillar tissue 474.8
    after operation on tonsils 998.11
    due to infection 475
  petechial 782.7
  pituitary (gland) 253.8
  placenta NEC 641.9
    affecting fetus or newborn 762.1
    from surgical or instrumental damage 641.8
      affecting fetus or newborn 762.1
    previa 641.1
      affecting fetus or newborn 762.0
  pleura—*see* Hemorrhage, lung
  polioencephalitis, superior 265.1
  polymyositis—*see* Polymyositis
  pons (*see also* Hemorrhage, brain) 431
  pontine (*see also* Hemorrhage, brain) 431
  popliteal 459.0
  postcoital 626.7
  postextraction (dental) 998.11

Hemorrhage, hemorrhagic—*continued*
  postmenopausal 627.1
  postnasal 784.7
  postoperative 998.11
  postpartum (atonic) (following delivery of placenta) 666.1
    delayed or secondary (after 24 hours) 666.2
    retained placenta 666.0
    third stage 666.0
  pregnancy (concealed) 641.9
    accidental 641.2
      affecting fetus or newborn 762.1
    affecting fetus or newborn 762.1
    before 22 completed weeks gestation 640.9
      affecting fetus or newborn 762.1
    due to
      abruptio placenta 641.2
        affecting fetus or newborn 762.1
      afibrinogenemia or other coagulation defect (conditions classifiable to 286.0-286.9) 641.3
        affecting fetus or newborn 762.1
      coagulation defect 641.3
        affecting fetus or newborn 762.1
      hyperfibrinolysis 641.3
        affecting fetus or newborn 762.1
      hypofibrinogenemia 641.3
        affecting fetus or newborn 762.1
      leiomyoma, uterus 641.8
        affecting fetus or newborn 762.1
      low-lying placenta 641.1
        affecting fetus or newborn 762.1
      marginal sinus (rupture) 641.2
        affecting fetus or newborn 762.1
      placenta previa 641.1
        affecting fetus or newborn 762.0
      premature separation of placenta (normally implanted) 641.2
        affecting fetus or newborn 762.1
      threatened abortion 640.0
        affecting fetus or newborn 762.1
      trauma 641.8
        affecting fetus or newborn 762.1
    early (before 22 completed weeks gestation) 640.9
      affecting fetus or newborn 762.1
    previous, affecting management of pregnancy or childbirth V23.49
    unavoidable—*see* Hemorrhage, pregnancy, due to placenta previa
  prepartum (mother)—*see* Hemorrhage, pregnancy
  preretinal, cause unspecified 362.81
  prostate 602.1
  puerperal (*see also* Hemorrhage, postpartum) 666.1
  pulmonary—*see also* Hemorrhage, lung
    newborn (massive) 770.3
    renal syndrome 446.21
  purpura (primary) (*see also* Purpura, thrombocytopenic) 287.3
  rectum (sphincter) 569.3
  recurring, following initial hemorrhage at time of injury 958.2
  renal 593.81
    pulmonary syndrome 446.21
  respiratory tract (*see also* Hemorrhage, lung) 786.3
  retina, retinal (deep) (superficial) (vessels) 362.81
    diabetic 250.5 *[362.01]*

Hemorrhage, hemorrhagic—*continued*
  due to birth injury 772.8
  retrobulbar 376.89
  retroperitoneal 459.0
  retroplacental (*see also* Placenta, separation) 641.2
  scalp 459.0
    due to injury at birth 767.1
  scrotum 608.83
  secondary (nontraumatic) 459.0
    following initial hemorrhage at time of injury 958.2
  seminal vesicle 608.83
  skin 782.7
    newborn 772.6
  spermatic cord 608.83
  spinal (cord) 336.1
    aneurysm (ruptured) 336.1
      syphilitic 094.89
    due to birth injury 767.4
    fetus or newborn 767.4
  spleen 289.59
  spontaneous NEC 459.0
    petechial 782.7
  stomach 578.9
    newborn 772.4
    ulcer—*see* Ulcer, stomach, with hemorrhage
  subaponeurotic, newborn 767.1
    massive (birth injury) 767.1
  subarachnoid (nontraumatic) 430
    fetus or newborn (anoxic) (traumatic) 772.2
    puerperal, postpartum, childbirth 674.0
    traumatic—*see* Hemorrhage, brain, traumatic, subarachnoid
  subconjunctival 372.72
    due to birth injury 772.8
    newborn 772.8
  subcortical (*see also* Hemorrhage, brain) 431
  subcutaneous 782.7
  subdiaphragmatic 459.0
  subdural (nontraumatic) 432.1
    due to birth injury 767.0
    fetus or newborn (anoxic) (hypoxic) (due to birth trauma) 767.0
    puerperal, postpartum, childbirth 674.0
    spinal 336.1
    traumatic—*see* Hemorrhage, brain, traumatic, subdural
  subhyaloid 362.81
  subperiosteal 733.99
  subretinal 362.81
  subtentorial (*see also* Hemorrhage, subdural) 432.1
  subungual 703.8
    due to blood dyscrasia 287.8
  suprarenal (capsule) (gland) 255.4
    fetus or newborn 772.5
  tentorium (traumatic)—*see also* Hemorrhage, brain, traumatic
    fetus or newborn 767.0
    nontraumatic—*see* Hemorrhage, subdural
  testis 608.83
  thigh 459.0
  third stage 666.0
  thorax—*see* Hemorrhage, lung
  throat 784.8
  thrombocythemia 238.7
  thymus (gland) 254.8
  thyroid (gland) 246.3
    cyst 246.3
  tongue 529.8

Hemorrhage, hemorrhagic—*continued*
tonsil 474.8
postoperative 998.11
tooth socket (postextraction) 998.11
trachea—*see* Hemorrhage, lung
traumatic—*see also* nature of injury
brain—*see* Hemorrhage, brain, traumatic
recurring or secondary (following initial
hemorrhage at time of injury) 958.2
tuberculous NEC (*see also* Tuberculosis,
pulmonary) 011.9
tunica vaginalis 608.83
ulcer—*see* Ulcer, by site, with hemorrhage
umbilicus, umbilical cord 772.0
after birth, newborn 772.3
complicating delivery 663.8
affecting fetus or newborn 772.0
slipped ligature 772.3
stump 772.3
unavoidable (due to placenta previa) 641.1
affecting fetus or newborn 762.0
upper extremity 459.0
urethra (idiopathic) 599.84
uterus, uterine (abnormal) 626.9
climacteric 627.0
complicating delivery—*see* Hemorrhage,
complicating, delivery
due to
intrauterine contraceptive device 996.76
perforating uterus 996.32
functional or dysfunctional 626.8
in pregnancy—*see* Hemorrhage, pregnancy
intermenstrual 626.6
irregular 626.6
regular 626.5
postmenopausal 627.1
postpartum (*see also* Hemorrhage,
postpartum) 666.1
prepubertal 626.8
pubertal 626.3
puerperal (immediate) 666.1
vagina 623.8
vasa previa 663.5
affecting fetus or newborn 772.0
vas deferens 608.83
ventricular (*see also* Hemorrhage, brain) 431
vesical 596.8
viscera 459.0
newborn 772.8
vitreous (humor) (intraocular) 379.23
vocal cord 478.5
vulva 624.8
Hemorrhoids (anus) (rectum) (without
complication) 455.6
bleeding, prolapsed, strangulated, or ulcerated
NEC 455.8
external 455.5
internal 455.2
complicated NEC 455.8
complicating pregnancy and puerperium 671.8
external 455.3
with complication NEC 455.5
bleeding, prolapsed, strangulated, or ulcerated
455.5
thrombosed 455.4
internal 455.0
with complication NEC 455.2
bleeding, prolapsed, strangulated, or ulcerated
455.2
thrombosed 455.1
residual skin tag 455.9

Hemorrhoids—*continued*
sentinel pile 455.9
thrombosed NEC 455.7
external 455.4
internal 455.1
Hemosalpinx 620.8
Hemosiderosis 275.0
dietary 275.0
pulmonary (idiopathic) 275.0 *[516.1]*
transfusion NEC 999.8
bone marrow 996.85
Hemospermia 608.82
Hemothorax 511.8
bacterial, nontuberculous 511.1
newborn 772.8
nontuberculous 511.8
bacterial 511.1
pneumococcal 511.1
postoperative 998.11
staphylococcal 511.1
streptococcal 511.1
traumatic 860.2
with
open wound into thorax 860.3
pneumothorax 860.4
with open wound into thorax 860.5
tuberculous (*see also* Tuberculosis, pleura)
012.0
Hemotympanum 385.89
Hench-Rosenberg syndrome (palindromic
arthritis) (*see also* Rheumatism, palindromic)
719.3
Henle's warts 371.41
Henoch (-Schönlein)
disease or syndrome (allergic purpura) 287.0
purpura (allergic) 287.0
Henpue, henpuye 102.6
Heparitinuria 277.5
Hepar lobatum 095.3
Hepatalgia 573.8
Hepatic —*see also* condition
flexure syndrome 569.89
Hepatitis 573.3
acute (*see also* Necrosis, liver) 570
alcoholic 571.1
infective 070.1
with hepatic coma 070.0
alcoholic 571.1
amebic—*see* Abscess, liver, amebic
anicteric (acute)—*see* Hepatitis, viral
antigen-associated (HAA) *see* Hepatitis, viral,
type B
Australian antigen (positive) *see* Hepatitis, viral,
type B
catarrhal (acute) 070.1
with hepatic coma 070.0
chronic 571.40
newborn 070.1
with hepatic coma 070.0
chemical 573.3
cholangiolitic 573.8
cholestatic 573.8
chronic 571.40
active 571.49
viral—*see* Hepatitis, viral
aggressive 571.49
persistent 571.41
viral—*see* Hepatitis, viral
cytomegalic inclusion virus 078.5 *[573.1]*
diffuse 573.3
"dirty needle"—*see* Hepatitis, viral

Hepatitis—*continued*
  with hepatic coma 070.2
  drug-induced 573.3
  due to
    Coxsackie 074.8 *[573.1]*
    cytomegalic inclusion virus 078.5 *[573.1]*
    infectious mononucleosis 075 *[573.1]*
    malaria 084.9 *[573.2]*
    mumps 072.71
    secondary syphilis 091.62
    toxoplasmosis (acquired) 130.5
      congenital (active) 771.2
  epidemic—*see* Hepatitis, viral, type A
  fetus or newborn 774.4
  fibrous (chronic) 571.49
    acute 570
  from injection, inoculation, or transfusion
      (blood) (other substance) (plasma) (serum)
      (onset within 8 months after administration)
      see Hepatitis, viral
  fulminant (viral) (*see also* Hepatitis, viral) 070.9
    with hepatic coma 070.6
    type A 070.1
      with hepatic coma 070.0
    type B—*see* Hepatitis, viral, Type B
  giant cell (neonatal) 774.4
  hemorrhagic 573.8
  homologous serum—*see* Hepatitis, viral
  hypertrophic (chronic) 571.49
    acute 570
  infectious, infective (acute) (chronic) (subacute)
      070.1
    with hepatic coma 070.0
  inoculation—*see* Hepatitis, viral
  interstitial (chronic) 571.49
    acute 570
  lupoid 571.49
  malarial 084.9 *[573.2]*
  malignant (*see also* Necrosis, liver) 570
  neonatal (toxic) 774.4
  newborn 774.4
  parenchymatous (acute) (*see also* Necrosis,
      liver) 570
  peliosis 573.3
  persistent, chronic 571.41
  plasma cell 571.49
  postimmunization—*see* Hepatitis, viral
  postnecrotic 571.49
  posttransfusion—*see* Hepatitis, viral
  recurrent 571.49
  septic 573.3
  serum—*see* Hepatitis, viral
    carrier (suspected) of V02.61
  subacute (*see also* Necrosis, liver) 570
  suppurative (diffuse) 572.0
  syphilitic (late) 095.3
    congenital (early) 090.0 *[573.2]*
      late 090.5 *[573.2]*
    secondary 091.62
  toxic (noninfectious) 573.3
    fetus or newborn 774.4
  tuberculous (*see also* Tuberculosis) 017.9
  viral (acute) (anicteric) (cholangiolitic)
      (cholestatic) (chronic) (subacute) 070.9
    with hepatic coma 070.6
    AU-SH type virus—*see* Hepatitis, viral, type B
    Australian antigen—*see* Hepatitis, viral, type
      B
    B-antigen—*see* Hepatitis, viral, type B
    Coxsackie 074.8 *[573.1]*
    cytomegalic inclusion 078.5 *[573.1]*

Hepatitis—*continued*
  IH (virus)—*see* Hepatitis, viral, type A
  infectious hepatitis virus—*see* Hepatitis, viral,
      type A
  serum hepatitis virus—*see* Hepatitis, viral,
      type B
  SH—*see* Hepatitis, viral, type B
  specified type NEC 070.59
    with hepatic coma 070.49
  type A 070.1
    with hepatic coma 070.0
  type B (acute) 070.30
    with
      hepatic coma 070.20
        with hepatitis delta 070.21
      hepatitis delta 070.31
        with hepatic coma 070.21
    carrier status V02.61
    chronic 070.32
      with
        hepatic coma 070.22
          with hepatitis delta 070.23
        hepatitis delta 070.33
          with hepatic coma 070.23
  type C (acute) 070.51
    with hepatic coma 070.41
    carrier status V02.62
    chronic 070.54
      with hepatic coma 070.44
  type delta (with hepatitis B carrier state)
      070.52
    with
      active hepatitis B disease—*see* Hepatitis,
        viral, type B
      hepatic coma 070.42
  type E 070.53
    with hepatic coma 070.43
  vaccination and inoculation (prophylactic)
      V05.3
  Waldenström's (lupoid hepatitis) 571.49
Hepatization, lung (acute)—*see also*
    Pneumonia, lobar
  chronic (*see also* Fibrosis, lung) 515
Hepatoblastoma (M8970/3) 155.0
Hepatocarcinoma (M8170/3) 155.0
Hepatocholangiocarcinoma (M8180/3) 155.0
Hepatocholangioma, benign (M8180/0) 211.5
Hepatocholangitis 573.8
Hepatocystitis (*see also* Cholecystitis) 575.10
Hepatodystrophy 570
Hepatolenticular degeneration 275.1
Hepatolithiasis —*see* Choledocholithiasis
Hepatoma (malignant) (M8170/3) 155.0
  benign (M8170/0) 211.5
  congenital (M8970/3) 155.0
  embryonal (M8970/3) 155.0
Hepatomegalia glycogenica diffusa 271.0
Hepatomegaly (*see also* Hypertrophy, liver)
    789.1
  congenital 751.69
    syphilitic 090.0
  due to Clonorchis sinensis 121.1
  Gaucher's 272.7
  syphilitic (congenital) 090.0
Hepatoptosis 573.8
Hepatorrhexis 573.8
Hepatosis, toxic 573.8
Hepatosplenomegaly 571.8
  due to S. japonicum 120.2
  hyperlipemic (Burger-Grutz type) 272.3
Herald patch 696.3
Hereditary —*see* condition

Heredodegeneration 330.9
  macular 362.70
Heredopathia atactica polyneuritiformis 356.3
Heredosyphilis (*see also* Syphilis, congenital)
  090.9
Hermaphroditism (true) 752.7
  with specified chromosomal anomaly—*see*
    Anomaly, chromosomes, sex
Hernia, hernial (acquired) (recurrent) 553.9
  with
    gangrene (obstructed) NEC 551.9
    obstruction NEC 552.9
      and gangrene 551.9
  abdomen (wall)—*see* Hernia, ventral
  abdominal, specified site NEC 553.8
    with
      gangrene (obstructed) 551.8
      obstruction 552.8
        and gangrene 551.8
  appendix 553.8
    with
      gangrene (obstructed) 551.8
      obstruction 552.8
        and gangrene 551.8
  bilateral (inguinal)—*see* Hernia, inguinal
  bladder (sphincter)
    congenital (female) (male) 756.71
    female 618.0
    male 596.8
  brain 348.4
    congenital 742.0
  broad ligament 553.8
  cartilage, vertebral—*see* Displacement,
    intervertebral disc
  cerebral 348.4
    congenital 742.0
    endaural 742.0
  ciliary body 364.8
    traumatic 871.1
  colic 553.9
    with
      gangrene (obstructed) 551.9
      obstruction 552.9
        and gangrene 551.9
  colon 553.9
    with
      gangrene (obstructed) 551.9
      obstruction 552.9
        and gangrene 551.9
  colostomy (stoma) 569.69
  Cooper's (retroperitoneal) 553.8
    with
      gangrene (obstructed) 551.8
      obstruction 552.8
        and gangrene 551.8
  crural—*see* Hernia, femoral
  diaphragm, diaphragmatic 553.3
    with
      gangrene (obstructed) 551.3
      obstruction 552.3
        and gangrene 551.3
    congenital 756.6
    due to gross defect of diaphragm 756.6
    traumatic 862.0
      with open wound into cavity 862.1
  direct (inguinal)—*see* Hernia, inguinal
  disc, intervertebral—*see* Displacement,
    intervertebral disc
  diverticulum, intestine 553.9
    with
      gangrene (obstructed) 551.9

Hernia, hernial—*continued*
  obstruction 552.9
    and gangrene 551.9
  double (inguinal)—*see* Hernia, inguinal
  duodenojejunal 553.8
    with
      gangrene (obstructed) 551.8
      obstruction 552.8
        and gangrene 551.8
  en glissade—*see* Hernia, inguinal
  enterostomy (stoma) 569.69
  epigastric 553.29
    with
      gangrene (obstruction) 551.29
      obstruction 552.29
        and gangrene 551.29
    recurrent 553.21
      with
        gangrene (obstructed) 551.21
        obstruction 552.21
          and gangrene 551.21
  esophageal hiatus (sliding) 553.3
    with
      gangrene (obstructed) 551.3
      obstruction 552.3
        and gangrene 551.3
    congenital 750.6
  external (inguinal)—*see* Hernia, inguinal
  fallopian tube 620.4
  fascia 728.89
  fat 729.30
    eyelid 374.34
    orbital 374.34
    pad 729.30
      eye, eyelid 374.34
      knee 729.31
      orbit 374.34
      popliteal (space) 729.31
      specified site NEC 729.39
  femoral (unilateral) 553.00
    with
      gangrene (obstructed) 551.00
      obstruction 552.00
        with gangrene 551.00
    bilateral 553.02
      gangrenous (obstructed) 551.02
      obstructed 552.02
        with gangrene 551.02
      recurrent 553.03
        gangrenous (obstructed) 551.03
        obstructed 552.03
          with gangrene 551.03
    recurrent (unilateral) 553.01
      bilateral 553.03
        gangrenous (obstructed) 551.03
        obstructed 552.03
          with gangrene 551.03
      gangrenous (obstructed) 551.01
      obstructed 552.01
        with gangrene 551.01
  foramen
    Bochdalek 553.3
      with
        gangrene (obstructed) 551.3
        obstruction 552.3
          and gangrene 551.3
      congenital 756.6
    magnum 348.4
    Morgagni, morgagnian 553.3
      with
        gangrene 551.3

Hernia, hernial—*continued*
    obstruction 552.3
      and gangrene 551.3
    congenital 756.6
  funicular (umbilical) 553.1
    with
      gangrene (obstructed) 551.1
      obstruction 552.1
        and gangrene 551.1
    spermatic cord—*see* Hernia, inguinal
  gangrenous—*see* Hernia, by site, with gangrene
  gastrointestinal tract 553.9
    with
      gangrene (obstructed) 551.9
      obstruction 552.9
        and gangrene 551.9
  gluteal—*see* Hernia, femoral
  Gruber's (internal mesogastric) 553.8
    with
      gangrene (obstructed) 551.8
      obstruction 552.8
        and gangrene 551.8
  Hesselbach's 553.8
    with
      gangrene (obstructed) 551.8
      obstruction 552.8
        and gangrene 551.8
  hiatal (esophageal) (sliding) 553.3
    with
      gangrene (obstructed) 551.3
      obstruction 552.3
        and gangrene 551.3
    congenital 750.6
  incarcerated (*see also* Hernia, by site, with
    obstruction) 552.9
    gangrenous (*see also* Hernia, by site, with
      gangrene) 551.9
  incisional 553.21
    with
      gangrene (obstructed) 551.21
      obstruction 552.21
        and gangrene 551.21
    lumbar—*see* Hernia, lumbar
    recurrent 553.21
      with
        gangrene (obstructed) 551.21
        obstruction 552.21
          and gangrene 551.21
  indirect (inguinal)—*see* Hernia, inguinal
  infantile—*see* Hernia, inguinal
  infrapatellar fat pad 729.31
  inguinal (direct) (double) (encysted) (external)
    (funicular) (indirect) (infantile) (internal)
    (interstitial) (oblique) (scrotal) (sliding)
    550.9

Note—*Use the following fifth-digit
subclassification with category 550:*

*0 unilateral or unspecified (not specified as
    recurrent)*
1 unilateral or unspecified, recurrent
2 bilateral (not specified as recurrent)
3 bilateral, recurrent

---

    with
      gangrene (obstructed) 550.0
      obstruction 550.1
        and gangrene 550.0
  internal 553.8
    with
      gangrene (obstructed) 551.8

Hernia, hernial—*continued*
    obstruction 552.8
      and gangrene 551.8
    inguinal—*see* Hernia, inguinal
  interstitial 553.9
    with
      gangrene (obstructed) 551.9
      obstruction 552.9
        and gangrene 551.9
    inguinal—*see* Hernia, inguinal
  intervertebral cartilage or disc—*see*
    Displacement, intervertebral disc
  intestine, intestinal 553.9
    with
      gangrene (obstructed) 551.9
      obstruction 552.9
        and gangrene 551.9
  intra-abdominal 553.9
    with
      gangrene (obstructed) 551.9
      obstruction 552.9
        and gangrene 551.9
  intraparietal 553.9
    with
      gangrene (obstructed) 551.9
      obstruction 552.9
        and gangrene 551.9
  iris 364.8
    traumatic 871.1
  irreducible (*see also* Hernia, by site, with
    obstruction) 552.9
    gangrenous (with obstruction) (*see also*
      Hernia, by site, with gangrene) 551.9
  ischiatic 553.8
    with
      gangrene (obstructed) 551.8
      obstruction 552.8
        and gangrene 551.8
  ischiorectal 553.8
    with
      gangrene (obstructed) 551.8
      obstruction 552.8
        and gangrene 551.8
  lens 379.32
    traumatic 871.1
  linea
    alba—*see* Hernia, epigastric
    semilunaris—*see* Hernia, spigelian
  Littre's (diverticular) 553.9
    with
      gangrene (obstructed) 551.9
      obstruction 552.9
        and gangrene 551.9
  lumbar 553.8
    with
      gangrene (obstructed) 551.8
      obstruction 552.8
        and gangrene 551.8
    intervertebral disc 722.10
  lung (subcutaneous) 518.89
    congenital 748.69
  mediastinum 519.3
  mesenteric (internal) 553.8
    with
      gangrene (obstructed) 551.8
      obstruction 552.8
        and gangrene 551.8
  mesocolon 553.8
    with
      gangrene (obstructed) 551.8
      obstruction 552.8

Hernia, hernial—*continued*
 ventral 553.20
   with
     gangrene (obstructed) 551.20
     obstruction 552.20
       and gangrene 551.20
   recurrent 553.21
     with
       gangrene (obstructed) 551.21
       obstruction 552.21
         and gangrene 551.21
   vesical
     congenital (female) (male) 756.71
     female 618.0
     male 596.8
   vitreous (into anterior chamber) 379.21
     traumatic 871.1
Herniation —*see also* Hernia
 brain (stem) 348.4
 cerebral 348.4
 gastric mucosa (into duodenal bulb) 537.89
 mediastinum 519.3
 nucleus pulposus—*see* Displacement,
   intervertebral disc
Herpangina 074.0
Herpes, herpetic 054.9
 auricularis (zoster) 053.71
   simplex 054.73
 blepharitis (zoster) 053.20
   simplex 054.41
 circinate 110.5
 circinatus 110.5
   bullous 694.5
 conjunctiva (simplex) 054.43
   zoster 053.21
 cornea (simplex) 054.43
   disciform (simplex) 054.43
   zoster 053.21
 encephalitis 054.3
 eye (zoster) 053.29
   simplex 054.40
 eyelid (zoster) 053.20
   simplex 054.41
 febrilis 054.9
 fever 054.9
 geniculate ganglionitis 053.11
 genital, genitalis 054.10
   specified site NEC 054.19
 gestationis 646.8
 gingivostomatitis 054.2
 iridocyclitis (simplex) 054.44
   zoster 053.22
 iris (any site) 695.1
 iritis (simplex) 054.44
 keratitis (simplex) 054.43
   dendritic 054.42
   disciform 054.43
   interstitial 054.43
     zoster 053.21
 keratoconjunctivitis (simplex) 054.43
   zoster 053.21
 labialis 054.9
   meningococcal 036.89
 lip 054.9
 meningitis (simplex) 054.72
   zoster 053.0
 ophthalmicus (zoster) 053.20
   simplex 054.40
 otitis externa (zoster) 053.71
   simplex 054.73
 penis 054.13

Herpes, herpetic—*continued*
 perianal 054.10
 pharyngitis 054.79
 progenitalis 054.10
 scrotum 054.19
 septicemia 054.5
 simplex 054.9
   complicated 054.8
     ophthalmic 054.40
       specified NEC 054.49
     specified NEC 054.79
   congenital 771.2
   external ear 054.73
   keratitis 054.43
     dendritic 054.42
   meningitis 054.72
   neuritis 054.79
   specified complication NEC 054.79
     ophthalmic 054.49
   visceral 054.71
 stomatitis 054.2
 tonsurans 110.0
   maculosus (of Hebra) 696.3
 visceral 054.71
 vulva 054.12
 vulvovaginitis 054.11
 whitlow 054.6
 zoster 053.9
   auricularis 053.71
   complicated 053.8
     specified NEC 053.79
   conjunctiva 053.21
   cornea 053.21
   ear 053.71
   eye 053.29
   geniculate 053.11
   keratitis 053.21
     interstitial 053.21
   neuritis 053.10
   ophthalmicus(a) 053.20
   oticus 053.71
   otitis externa 053.71
   specified complication NEC 053.79
   specified site NEC 053.9
 zosteriform, intermediate type 053.9
Herrick's
 anemia (hemoglobin S disease) 282.61
 syndrome (hemoglobin S disease) 282.61
Hers' disease (glycogenosis VI) 271.0
Herter's infantilism (nontropical sprue) 579.0
Herter (-Gee) disease or syndrome (nontropical
   sprue) 579.0
Herxheimer's disease (diffuse idiopathic
   cutaneous atrophy) 701.8
Herxheimer's reaction 995.0
Hesselbach's hernia —*see* Hernia, Hesselbach's
Heterochromia (congenital) 743.46
 acquired 364.53
 cataract 366.33
 cyclitis 364.21
 hair 704.3
 iritis 364.21
 retained metallic foreign body 360.62
   magnetic 360.52
 uveitis 364.21
Heterophoria 378.40
 alternating 378.45
 vertical 378.43
Heterophyes, small intestine 121.6
Heterophyiasis 121.6
Heteropsia 368.8

Heterotopia, heterotopic —*see also*
Malposition, congenital
cerebralis 742.4
pancreas, pancreatic 751.7
spinalis 742.59
Heterotropia 378.30
intermittent 378.20
vertical 378.31
vertical (constant) (intermittent) 378.31
Heubner's disease 094.89
Heubner-Herter disease or syndrome
(nontropical sprue) 579.0
Hexadactylism 755.00
Heyd's syndrome (hepatorenal) 572.4
HGSIL (high grade squamous intraepithelial
dysplasia) 622.1
Hibernoma (M8880/0)—*see* Lipoma
Hiccough 786.8
epidemic 078.89
psychogenic 306.1
Hiccup (*see also* Hiccough) 786.8
Hicks (-Braxton) contractures 644.1
Hidden penis 752.65
Hidradenitis (axillaris) (suppurative) 705.83
Hidradenoma (nodular) (M8400/0)—*see also*
Neoplasm, skin, benign
clear cell (M8402/0)—*see* Neoplasm, skin,
benign
papillary (M8405/0)—*see* Neoplasm, skin,
benign
Hidrocystoma (M8404/0)—*see* Neoplasm, skin,
benign
High
A$_2$ anemia 282.4
altitude effects 993.2
anoxia 993.2
on
ears 993.0
sinuses 993.1
polycythemia 289.0
arch
foot 755.67
palate 750.26
artery (arterial) tension (*see also* Hypertension)
401.9
without diagnosis of hypertension 796.2
basal metabolic rate (BMR) 794.7
blood pressure (*see also* Hypertension) 401.9
incidental reading (isolated) (nonspecific), no
diagnosis of hypertension 796.2
compliance bladder 596.4
diaphragm (congenital) 756.6
frequency deafness (congenital) (regional) 389.8
head at term 652.5
output failure (cardiac) (*see also* Failure, heart)
428.9
oxygen-affinity hemoglobin 289.0
palate 750.26
risk
behavior —*see* Problem
family situation V61.9
specified circumstance NEC V61.8
individual NEC V62.89
infant NEC V20.1
patient taking drugs (prescribed) V67.51
nonprescribed (*see also* Abuse, drugs,
nondependent) 305.9
pregnancy V23.9
inadequate prenatal care V23.7
specified problem NEC V23.8

High—*continued*
temperature (of unknown origin) (*see also*
Pyrexia) 780.6
thoracic rib 756.3
Hildenbrand's disease (typhus) 081.9
Hilger's syndrome 337.0
Hill diarrhea 579.1
Hilliard's lupus (*see also* Tuberculosis) 017.0
Hilum —*see* condition
Hip —*see* condition
Hippel's disease (retinocerebral angiomatosis)
759.6
Hippus 379.49
Hirschfeld's disease (acute diabetes mellitus)
(*see also* Diabetes) 250.0
Hirschsprung's disease or megacolon
(congenital) 751.3
Hirsuties (*see also* Hypertrichosis) 704.1
Hirsutism (*see also* Hypertrichosis) 704.1
Hirudiniasis (external) (internal) 134.2
His-Werner disease (trench fever) 083.1
Hiss-Russell dysentery 004.1
Histamine cephalgia 346.2
Histidinemia 270.5
Histidinuria 270.5
Histiocytoma (M8832/0)—*see also* Neoplasm,
skin, benign
fibrous (M8830/0)—*see also* Neoplasm, skin,
benign
atypical (M8830/1)—*see* Neoplasm,
connective tissue, uncertain behavior
malignant (M8830/0)—*see* Neoplasm,
connective tissue, malignant
Histiocytosis (acute) (chronic) (subacute) 277.8
acute differentiated progressive (M9722/3) 202.5
cholesterol 277.8
essential 277.8
lipid, lipoid (essential) 272.7
lipochrome (familial) 288.1
malignant (M9720/3) 202.3
X (chronic) 277.8
acute (progressive) (M9722/3) 202.5
Histoplasmosis 115.90
with
endocarditis 115.94
meningitis 115.91
pericarditis 115.93
pneumonia 115.95
retinitis 115.92
specified manifestation NEC 115.99
African (due to Histoplasma duboisii) 115.10
with
endocarditis 115.14
meningitis 115.11
pericarditis 115.13
pneumonia 115.15
retinitis 115.12
specified manifestation NEC 115.19
American (due to Histoplasma capsulatum)
115.00
with
endocarditis 115.04
meningitis 115.01
pericarditis 115.03
pneumonia 115.05
retinitis 115.02
specified manifestation NEC 115.09
Darling's—*see* Histoplasmosis, American
large form (*see also* Histoplasmosis, African)
115.10

Histoplasmosis—*continued*
lung 115.05
small form (*see also* Histoplasmosis, American)
115.00
History (personal) of
abuse
emotional V15.42
neglect V15.42
physical V15.41
sexual V15.41
affective psychosis V11.1
alcoholism V11.3
specified as drinking problem (*see also*
Abuse, drugs, nondependent) 305.0
allergy to
analgesic agent NEC V14.6
anesthetic NEC V14.4
antibiotic agent NEC V14.1
penicillin V14.0
anti-infective agent NEC V14.3
diathesis V15.09
drug V14.9
specified type NEC V14.8
eggs V15.03
food additives V15.05
insect bite V15.06
latex V15.07
medicinal agents V14.9
specified type NEC V14.8
milk products V15.02
narcotic agent NEC V14.5
nuts V15.05
peanuts V15.01
penicillin V14.0
radiographic dye V15.08
seafood V15.04
serum V14.7
specified food NEC V15.05
specified nonmedicinal agents NEC V15.09
spider bite V15.06
sulfa V14.2
sulfonamides V14.2
therapeutic agent NEC V15.09
vaccine V14.7
anemia V12.3
arthritis V13.4
benign neoplasm of brain V12.41
blood disease V12.3
calculi, urinary V13.01
cardiovascular disease V12.50
myocardial infarction 412
child abuse V15.41
cigarette smoking V15.82
circulatory system disease V12.50
myocardial infarction 412
congenital malformation V13.69
contraception V15.7
diathesis, allergic V15.09
digestive system disease V12.70
peptic ulcer V12.71
polyps, colonic V12.72
specified NEC V12.79
disease (of) V13.9
blood V12.3
blood-forming organs V12.3
cardiovascular system V12.50
circulatory system V12.50
digestive system V12.70
peptic ulcer V12.71
polyps, colonic V12.72
specified NEC V12.79

History—*continued*
infectious V12.00
malaria V12.03
poliomyelitis V12.02
specified NEC V12.09
tuberculosis V12.01
parasitic V12.00
specified NEC V12.09
respiratory system V12.6
skin V13.3
specified site NEC V13.8
subcutaneous tissue V13.3
trophoblastic V13.1
affecting management of pregnancy V23.1
disorder (of) V13.9
endocrine V12.2
genital system V13.29
hematological V12.3
immunity V12.2
mental V11.9
affective type V11.1
manic-depressive V11.1
neurosis V11.2
schizophrenia V11.0
specified type NEC V11.8
metabolic V12.2
musculoskeletal NEC V13.5
nervous system V12.40
specified type NEC V12.49
obstetric V13.29
affecting management of current pregnancy
V23.49
pre-term labor V23.41
pre-term labor V13.21
sense organs V12.40
specified type NEC V12.49
specified site NEC V13.8
urinary system V13.00
calculi V13.01
specified NEC V13.09
drug use
nonprescribed (*see also* Abuse, drugs,
nondependent) 305.9
patent (*see also* Abuse, drugs, nondependent)
305.9
effect NEC of external cause V15.89
embolism (pulmonary) V12.51
emotional abuse V15.42
endocrine disorder V12.2
family
allergy V19.6
anemia V18.2
arteriosclerosis V17.4
arthritis V17.7
asthma V17.5
blindness V19.0
blood disorder NEC V18.3
cardiovascular disease V17.4
cerebrovascular disease V17.1
chronic respiratory condition NEC V17.6
congenital anomalies V19.5
consanguinity V19.7
coronary artery disease V17.3
cystic fibrosis V18.1
deafness V19.2
diabetes mellitus V18.0
digestive disorders V18.5
disease or disorder (of)
allergic V19.6
blood NEC V18.3
cardiovascular NEC V17.4

History—*continued*
  colon V10.05
  connective tissue NEC V10.89
  corpus uteri V10.42
  digestive system V10.00
    specified part NEC V10.09
  duodenum V10.09
  endocrine gland NEC V10.88
  epididymis V10.48
  esophagus V10.03
  eye V10.84
  fallopian tube V10.44
  female genital organ V10.40
    specified site NEC V10.44
  gallbladder V10.09
  gastrointestinal tract V10.00
  gum V10.02
  hematopoietic NEC V10.79
  hypopharynx V10.02
  ileum V10.09
  intrathoracic organs NEC V10.20
  jejunum V10.09
  kidney V10.52
  large intestine V10.05
  larynx V10.21
  lip V10.02
  liver V10.07
  lung V10.11
  lymphatic NEC V10.79
  lymph glands or nodes NEC V10.79
  male genital organ V10.45
    specified site NEC V10.49
  mediastinum V10.29
  melanoma (of skin) V10.82
  middle ear V10.22
  mouth V10.02
    specified part NEC V10.02
  nasal cavities V10.22
  nasopharynx V10.02
  nervous system NEC V10.86
  nose V10.22
  oropharynx V10.02
  ovary V10.43
  pancreas V10.09
  parathyroid V10.88
  penis V10.49
  pharynx V10.02
  pineal V10.88
  pituitary V10.88
  placenta V10.44
  pleura V10.29
  prostate V10.46
  rectosigmoid junction V10.06
  rectum V10.06
  renal pelvis V10.53
  respiratory organs NEC V10.20
  salivary gland V10.02
  skin V10.83
    melanoma V10.82
  small intestine NEC V10.09
  soft tissue NEC V10.89
  specified site NEC V10.89
  stomach V10.04
  testis V10.47
  thymus V10.29
  thyroid V10.87
  tongue V10.01
  trachea V10.12
  ureter V10.59
  urethra V10.59
  urinary organ V10.50

History—*continued*
  uterine adnexa V10.44
  uterus V10.42
  vagina V10.44
  vulva V10.44
  manic-depressive psychosis V11.1
  mental disorder V11.9
    affective type V11.1
    manic-depressive V11.1
    neurosis V11.2
    schizophrenia V11.0
    specified type NEC V11.8
  metabolic disorder V12.2
  musculoskeletal disorder NEC V13.5
  myocardial infarction 412
  neglect (emotional) V15.42
  nervous system disorder V12.40
    specified type NEC V12.49
  neurosis V11.2
  noncompliance with medical treatment V15.81
  nutritional deficiency V12.1
  obstetric disorder V13.29
    affecting management of current pregnancy V23.49
      pre-term labor V23.41
    pre-term labor V13.41
  parasitic disease V12.00
    specified NEC V12.09
  perinatal problems V13.7
    low birth weight (*see also* Status, low birth weight) V21.30
  physical abuse V15.41
  poisoning V15.6
  poliomyelitis V12.02
  polyps, colonic V12.72
  poor obstetric V23.49
    affecting management of current pregnancy V23.49
      pre-term labor V23.41
    pre-term labor V13.41
  psychiatric disorder V11.9
    affective type V11.1
    manic-depressive V11.1
    neurosis V11.2
    schizophrenia V11.0
    specified type NEC V11.8
  psychological trauma V15.49
    emotional abuse V15.42
    neglect V15.42
    physical abuse V15.41
    rape V15.41
  psychoneurosis V11.2
  radiation therapy V15.3
  rape V15.41
  respiratory system disease V12.6
  reticulosarcoma V10.71
  schizophrenia V11.0
  skin disease V13.3
  smoking (tobacco) V15.82
  subcutaneous tissue disease V13.3
  surgery (major) to
    great vessels V15.1
    heart V15.1
    major organs NEC V15.2
  thrombophlebitis V12.52
  thrombosis V12.51
  tobacco use V15.82
  trophoblastic disease V13.1
    affecting management of pregnancy V23.1
  tuberculosis V12.01
  ulcer, peptic V12.71

History—*continued*
  urinary system disorder V13.00
    calculi V13.01
    specified NEC V13.09
HIV infection (disease) (illness)—*see* Human immunodeficiency virus (disease) (illness) (infection)
Hives (bold) (*see also* Urticaria) 708.9
Hoarseness 784.49
Hobnail liver —*see* Cirrhosis, portal
Hobo, hoboism V60.0
Hodgkin's
  disease (M9650/3) 201.9
    lymphocytic
      depletion (M9653/3) 201.7
        diffuse fibrosis (M9654/3) 201.7
        reticular type (M9655/3) 201.7
      predominance (M9651/3) 201.4
    lymphocytic-histiocytic predominance (M9651/3) 201.4
    mixed cellularity (M9652/3) 201.6
    nodular sclerosis (M9656/3) 201.5
      cellular phase (M9657/3) 201.5
  granuloma (M9661/3) 201.1
  lymphogranulomatosis (M9650/3) 201.9
  lymphoma (M9650/3) 201.9
  lymphosarcoma (M9650/3) 201.9
  paragranuloma (M9660/3) 201.0
  sarcoma (M9662/3) 201.2
Hodgson's disease (aneurysmal dilatation of aorta) 441.9
  ruptured 441.5
Hodi-potsy 111.0
Hoffa -(Kastert) disease or syndrome (liposynovitis prepatellaris) 272.8
Hoffmann's syndrome 244.9 *[359.5]*
Hoffmann-Bouveret syndrome (paroxysmal tachycardia) 427.2
Hole
  macula 362.54
  optic disc, crater-like 377.22
  retina (macula) 362.54
    round 361.31
      with detachment 361.01
Holla disease (*see also* Spherocytosis) 282.0
Holländer-Simons syndrome (progressive lipodystrophy) 272.6
Hollow foot (congenital) 754.71
  acquired 736.73
Holmes' syndrome (visual disorientation) 368.16
Holoprosencephaly 742.2
  due to
    trisomy 13 758.1
    trisomy 18 758.2
Holthouse's hernia —*see* Hernia, inguinal
Homesickness 309.89
Homocystinemia 270.4
Homocystinuria 270.4
Homologous serum jaundice (prophylactic) (therapeutic)—*see* Hepatitis, viral
Homosexuality —*omit code*
  ego-dystonic 302.0
  pedophilic 302.2
  problems with 302.0
Homozygous Hb-S disease 282.61
Honeycomb lung 518.89
  congenital 748.4
Hong Kong ear 117.3
HOOD (hereditary osteo-onychodysplasia) 756.89

Hooded
  clitoris 752.49
  penis 752.69
Hookworm (anemia) (disease) (infestation)—*see* Ancylostomiasis
Hoppe-Goldflam syndrome 358.0
Hordeolum (external) (eyelid) 373.11
  internal 373.12
Horn
  cutaneous 702.8
    cheek 702.8
    eyelid 702.8
    penis 702.8
  iliac 756.89
  nail 703.8
    congenital 757.5
  papillary 700
Horner's
  syndrome (*see also* Neuropathy, peripheral, autonomic) 337.9
    traumatic 954.0
  teeth 520.4
Horseshoe kidney (congenital) 753.3
Horton's
  disease (temporal arteritis) 446.5
  headache or neuralgia 346.2
Hospice care V66.7
Hospitalism (in children) NEC 309.83
Hourglass contraction, contracture
  bladder 596.8
  gallbladder 575.2
    congenital 751.69
  stomach 536.8
    congenital 750.7
    psychogenic 306.4
  uterus 661.4
    affecting fetus or newborn 763.7
Household circumstance affecting care V60.9
  specified type NEC V60.8
Housemaid's knee 727.2
Housing circumstance affecting care V60.9
  specified type NEC V60.8
Huchard's disease (continued arterial hypertension) 401.9
Hudson-Ståhli lines 371.11
Huguier's disease (uterine fibroma) 218.9
Hum, venous —*omit code*
Human bite (open wound)—*see also* Wound, open, by site
  intact skin surface—*see* Contusion
Human immunodeficiency virus (disease) (illness) 042
  infection V08
    with symptoms, symptomatic 042
Human immunodeficiency virus-2 infection 079.53
Human immunovirus (disease) (illness) (infection)—*see* Human immunodeficiency virus (disease) (illness) (infection)
Human papillomavirus 079.4
Human T-cell lymphotrophic virus I infection 079.51
Human T-cell lymphotrophic virus II infection 079.52
Human T-cell lymphotropic virus-III (disease) (illness) (infection)—*see* Human immunodeficiency virus (disease) (illness) (infection)
HTLV-I infection 079.51
HTLV-II infection 079.52

HTLV-III (disease) (illness) (infection)—*see* Human immunodeficiency virus (disease) (illness) (infection)
HTLV-III/LAV (disease) (illness) (infection)—*see* Human immunodeficiency virus (disease) (illness) (infection)
Humpback (acquired) 737.9
  congenital 756.19
Hunchback (acquired) 737.9
  congenital 756.19
Hunger 994.2
  air, psychogenic 306.1
  disease 251.1
Hunner's ulcer (*see also* Cystitis) 595.1
Hunt's
  neuralgia 053.11
  syndrome (herpetic geniculate ganglionitis) 053.11
  dyssynergia cerebellaris myoclonica 334.2
Hunter's glossitis 529.4
Hunter (-Hurler) syndrome (mucopolysaccharidosis II) 277.5
Hunterian chancre 091.0
Huntington's
  chorea 333.4
  disease 333.4
Huppert's disease (multiple myeloma) (M9730/3) 203.0
Hurler (-Hunter) disease or syndrome (mucopolysaccharidosis II) 277.5
Hürthle cell
  adenocarcinoma (M8290/3) 193
  adenoma (M8290/0) 226
  carcinoma (M8290/3) 193
  tumor (M8290/0) 226
Hutchinson's
  disease meaning
    angioma serpiginosum 709.1
    cheiropompholyx 705.81
    prurigo estivalis 692.72
    summer eruption, or summer prurigo 692.72
  incisors 090.5
  melanotic freckle (M8742/2)—*see also* Neoplasm, skin, in situ
    malignant melanoma in (M8742/3)—*see* Melanoma
  teeth or incisors (congenital syphilis) 090.5
Hutchinson-Boeck disease or syndrome (sarcoidosis) 135
Hutchinson-Gilford disease or syndrome (progeria) 259.8
Hyaline
  degeneration (diffuse) (generalized) 728.9
    localized—*see* Degeneration, by site
  membrane (disease) (lung) (newborn) 769
Hyalinosis cutis et mucosae 272.8
Hyalin plaque, sclera, senile 379.16
Hyalitis (asteroid) 379.22
  syphilitic 095.8
Hydatid
  cyst or tumor—*see also* Echinococcus
    fallopian tube 752.11
Hydatid—*continued*
  mole—*see* Hydatidiform mole
  Morgagni (congenital) 752.8
    fallopian tube 752.11
Hydatidiform mole (benign) (complicating pregnancy) (delivered) (undelivered) 630
  invasive (M9100/1) 236.1
  malignant (M9100/1) 236.1

Hydatidiform mole—*continued*
  previous, affecting management of pregnancy V23.1
Hydatidosis —*see* Echinococcus
Hyde's disease (prurigo nodularis) 698.3
Hydradenitis 705.83
Hydradenoma (M8400/0)—*see* Hidradenoma
Hydralazine lupus or syndrome
  correct substance properly administered 695.4
  overdose or wrong substance given or taken 972.6
Hydramnios 657
  affecting fetus or newborn 761.3
Hydrancephaly 742.3
  with spina bifida (*see also* Spina bifida) 741.0
Hydranencephaly 742.3
  with spina bifida (*see also* Spina bifida) 741.0
Hydrargyrism NEC 985.0
Hydrarthrosis (*see also* Effusion, joint) 719.0
  gonococcal 098.50
  intermittent (*see also* Rheumatism, palindromic) 719.3
  of yaws (early) (late) 102.6
  syphilitic 095.8
    congenital 090.5
Hydremia 285.9
Hydrencephalocele (congenital) 742.0
Hydrencephalomeningocele (congenital) 742.0
Hydroa 694.0
  aestivale 692.72
  gestationis 646.8
  herpetiformis 694.0
  pruriginosa 694.0
  vacciniforme 692.72
Hydroadenitis 705.83
Hydrocalycosis (*see also* Hydronephrosis) 591
  congenital 753.29
Hydrocalyx (*see also* Hydronephrosis) 591
Hydrocele (calcified) (chylous) (idiopathic) (infantile) (inguinal canal) (recurrent) (senile) (spermatic cord) (testis) (tunica vaginalis) 603.9
  canal of Nuck (female) 629.1
    male 603.9
  congenital 778.6
  encysted 603.0
    congenital 778.6
  female NEC 629.8
  infected 603.1
  round ligament 629.8
  specified type NEC 603.8
    congenital 778.6
  spinalis (*see also* Spina bifida) 741.9
  vulva 624.8
Hydrocephalic fetus
  affecting management of pregnancy 655.0
  causing disproportion 653.6
    with obstructed labor 660.1
      affecting fetus or newborn 763.1
Hydrocephalus (acquired) (external) (internal) (malignant) (noncommunicating) (obstructive) (recurrent) 331.4
  aqueduct of Sylvius stricture 742.3
    with spina bifida (*see also* Spina bifida) 741.0
  chronic 742.3
    with spina bifida (*see also* Spina bifida) 741.0
  communicating 331.3
  congenital (external) (internal) 742.3
    with spina bifida (*see also* Spina bifida) 741.0
  due to
    stricture of aqueduct of Sylvius 742.3

Hydrocephalus—*continued*
  with spina bifida (*see also* Spina bifida)
    741.0
  toxoplasmosis (congenital) 771.2
  fetal affecting management of pregnancy 655.0
  foramen Magendie block (acquired) 331.3
    congenital 742.3
      with spina bifida (*see also* Spina bifida)
        741.0
  newborn 742.3
    with spina bifida (*see also* Spina bifida) 741.0
  otitic 331.4
  syphilitic, congenital 090.49
  tuberculous (*see also* Tuberculosis) 013.8
Hydrocolpos (congenital) 623.8
Hydrocystoma (M8404/0)—*see* Neoplasm, skin,
  benign
Hydroencephalocele (congenital) 742.0
Hydroencephalomeningocele (congenital) 742.0
Hydrohematopneumothorax (*see also*
  Hemothorax) 511.8
Hydromeningitis —*see* Meningitis
Hydromeningocele (spinal) (*see also* Spina
  bifida) 741.9
  cranial 742.0
Hydrometra 621.8
Hydrometrocolpos 623.8
Hydromicrocephaly 742.1
Hydromphalus (congenital) (since birth) 757.39
Hydromyelia 742.53
Hydromyelocele (*see also* Spina bifida) 741.9
Hydronephrosis 591
  atrophic 591
  congenital 753.29
  due to S. hematobium 120.0
  early 591
  functionless (infected) 591
  infected 591
  intermittent 591
  primary 591
  secondary 591
  tuberculous (*see also* Tuberculosis) 016.0
Hydropericarditis (*see also* Pericarditis) 423.9
Hydropericardium (*see also* Pericarditis) 423.9
Hydroperitoneum 789.5
Hydrophobia 071
Hydrophthalmos (*see also* Buphthalmia) 743.20
Hydropneumohemothorax (*see also*
  Hemothorax) 511.8
Hydropneumopericarditis (*see also*
  Pericarditis) 423.9
Hydropneumopericardium (*see also*
  Pericarditis) 423.9
Hydropneumothorax 511.8
  nontuberculous 511.8
    bacterial 511.1
    pneumococcal 511.1
    staphylococcal 511.1
    streptococcal 511.1
  traumatic 860.0
    with open wound into thorax 860.1
  tuberculous (*see also* Tuberculosis, pleural)
    012.0
Hydrops 782.3
  abdominis 789.5
  amnii (complicating pregnancy) (*see also*
    Hydramnios) 657
  articulorum intermittens (*see also* Rheumatism,
    palindromic) 719.3
  cardiac (*see also* Failure, heart) 428.0
  congenital—*see* Hydrops, fetalis

Hydrops—*continued*
  endolymphatic (*see also* Disease, Ménière's)
    386.00
  fetal(is) or newborn 778.0
    due to isoimmunization 773.3
    not due to isoimmunization 778.0
  gallbladder 575.3
  idiopathic (fetus or newborn) 778.0
  joint (*see also* Effusion, joint) 719.0
  labyrinth (*see also* Disease, Ménière's) 386.00
  meningeal NEC 331.4
  nutritional 262
  pericardium—*see* Pericarditis
  pleura (*see also* Hydrothorax) 511.8
  renal (*see also* Nephrosis) 581.9
  spermatic cord (*see also* Hydrocele) 603.9
Hydropyonephrosis (*see also* Pyelitis) 590.80
  chronic 590.00
Hydrorachis 742.53
Hydrorrhea (nasal) 478.1
  gravidarum 658.1
  pregnancy 658.1
Hydrosadenitis 705.83
Hydrosalpinx (fallopian tube) (follicularis) 614.1
Hydrothorax (double) (pleural) 511.8
  chylous (nonfilarial) 457.8
    filaria (*see also* Infestation, filarial) 125.9
  nontuberculous 511.8
    bacterial 511.1
    pneumococcal 511.1
    staphylococcal 511.1
    streptococcal 511.1
  traumatic 862.29
    with open wound into thorax 862.39
  tuberculous (*see also* Tuberculosis, pleura)
    012.0
Hydroureter 593.5
  congenital 753.22
Hydroureteronephrosis (*see also*
  Hydronephrosis) 591
Hydrourethra 599.84
Hydroxykynureninuria 270.2
Hydroxyprolinemia 270.8
Hydroxyprolinuria 270.8
Hygroma (congenital) (cystic) (M9173/0) 228.1
  prepatellar 727.3
  subdural—*see* Hematoma, subdural
Hymen —*see* condition
Hymenolepiasis (diminuta) (infection)
  (infestation) (nana) 123.6
Hymenolepis (diminuta) (infection) (infestation)
  (nana) 123.6
Hypalgesia (*see also* Disturbance, sensation)
  782.0
Hyperabduction syndrome 447.8
Hyperacidity, gastric 536.8
  psychogenic 306.4
Hyperactive, hyperactivity
  basal cell, uterine cervix 622.1
  bladder 596.51
  bowel (syndrome) 564.9
    sounds 787.5
  cervix epithelial (basal) 622.1
  child 314.01
  colon 564.9
  gastrointestinal 536.8
    psychogenic 306.4
  intestine 564.9
  labyrinth (unilateral) 386.51
    with loss of labyrinthine reactivity 386.58
    bilateral 386.52

Hyperactive, hyperactivity—*continued*
nasal mucous membrane 478.1
stomach 536.8
thyroid (gland) (*see also* Thyrotoxicosis) 242.9
Hyperacusis 388.42
Hyperadrenalism (cortical) 255.3
medullary 255.6
Hyperadrenocorticism 255.3
congenital 255.2
iatrogenic
correct substance properly administered 255.3
overdose or wrong substance given or taken
962.0
Hyperaffectivity 301.11
Hyperaldosteronism (atypical) (hyperplastic)
(normoaldosteronal) (normotensive) (primary)
(secondary) 255.1
Hyperalgesia (*see also* Disturbance, sensation)
782.0
Hyperalimentation 783.6
carotene 278.3
specified NEC 278.8
vitamin A 278.2
vitamin D 278.4
Hyperaminoaciduria 270.9
arginine 270.6
citrulline 270.6
cystine 270.0
glycine 270.0
lysine 270.7
ornithine 270.6
renal (types I, II, III) 270.0
Hyperammonemia (congenital) 270.6
Hyperamnesia 780.99
Hyperamylasemia 790.5
Hyperaphia 782.0
Hyperazotemia 791.9
Hyperbetalipoproteinemia (acquired)
(essential) (familial) (hereditary) (primary)
(secondary) 272.0
with prebetalipoproteinemia 272.2
Hyperbilirubinemia 782.4
congenital 277.4
constitutional 277.4
neonatal (transient) (*see also* Jaundice, fetus or
newborn) 774.6
of prematurity 774.2
**Hyperbilirubinemica encephalopathia, new-
born** 774.7
due to isoimmunization 773.4
Hypercalcemia, hypercalcemic (idiopathic)
275.42
nephropathy 588.8
Hypercalcinuria 275.40
Hypercapnia 786.09
with mixed acid-base disorder 276.4
fetal, affecting newborn 770.89
Hypercarotinemia 278.3
Hypercementosis 521.5
Hyperchloremia 276.9
Hyperchlorhydria 536.8
neurotic 306.4
psychogenic 306.4
Hypercholesterinemia —*see*
Hypercholesterolemia
Hypercholesterolemia 272.0
with hyperglyceridemia, endogenous 272.2
essential 272.0
familial 272.0
hereditary 272.0
primary 272.0
pure 272.0

Hypercholesterolosis 272.0
Hyperchylia gastricsa 536.8
psychogenic 306.4
Hyperchylomicronemia (familial) (with
hyperbetalipoproteinemia) 272.3
Hypercoagulation syndrome 289.8
Hypercorticosteronism
correct substance properly administered 255.3
overdose or wrong substance given or taken
962.0
Hypercortisonism
correct substance properly administered 255.3
overdose or wrong substance given or taken
962.0
**Hyperdynamic beta-adrenergic state or syn-
drome** (circulatory) 429.82
Hyperelectrolytemia 276.9
Hyperemesis 536.2
arising during pregnancy—*see* Hyperemesis,
gravidarum
gravidarum (mild) (before 22 completed weeks
gestation) 643.0
with
carbohydrate depletion 643.1
dehydration 643.1
electrolyte imbalance 643.1
metabolic disturbance 643.1
affecting fetus or newborn 761.8
severe (with metabolic disturbance) 643.1
psychogenic 306.4
Hyperemia (acute) 780.99
anal mucosa 569.49
bladder 596.7
cerebral 437.8
conjunctiva 372.71
ear, internal, acute 386.30
enteric 564.89
eye 372.71
eyelid (active) (passive) 374.82
intestine 564.89
iris 364.41
kidney 593.81
labyrinth 386.30
liver (active) (passive) 573.8
lung 514
ovary 620.8
passive 780.99
pulmonary 514
renal 593.81
retina 362.89
spleen 289.59
stomach 537.89
Hyperesthesia (body surface) (*see also*
Disturbance, sensation) 782.0
larynx (reflex) 478.79
hysterical 300.11
pharynx (reflex) 478.29
Hyperestrinism 256.0
Hyperestrogenism 256.0
Hyperestrogenosis 256.0
Hyperextension, joint 718.80
ankle 718.87
elbow 718.82
foot 718.87
hand 718.84
hip 718.85
knee 718.86
multiple sites 718.89
pelvic region 718.85
shoulder (region) 718.81
specified site NEC 718.88
wrist 718.83

Hyperfibrinolysis —*see* Fibrinolysis
Hyperfolliculinism 256.0
Hyperfructosemia 271.2
Hyperfunction
　adrenal (cortex) 255.3
　　androgenic, acquired benign 255.3
　　medulla 255.6
　　virilism 255.2
　corticoadrenal NEC 255.3
　labyrinth—*see* Hyperactive, labyrinth
　medulloadrenal 255.6
　ovary 256.1
　　estrogen 256.0
　pancreas 577.8
　parathyroid (gland) 252.0
　pituitary (anterior) (gland) (lobe) 253.1
　testicular 257.0
Hypergammaglobulinemia 289.8
　monoclonal, benign (BMH) 273.1
　polyclonal 273.0
　Waldenström's 273.0
Hyperglobulinemia 273.8
Hyperglycemia 790.6
　maternal
　　affecting fetus or newborn 775.0
　　manifest diabetes in infant 775.1
　postpancreatectomy (complete) (partial) 251.3
Hyperglyceridemia 272.1
　endogenous 272.1
　essential 272.1
　familial 272.1
　hereditary 272.1
　mixed 272.3
　pure 272.1
Hyperglycinemia 270.7
Hypergonadism
　ovarian 256.1
　testicular (infantile) (primary) 257.0
Hyperheparinemia (*see also* Circulating
　anticoagulants) 286.5
Hyperhidrosis, hyperidrosis 780.8
　psychogenic 306.3
Hyperhistidinemia 270.5
Hyperinsulinism (ectopic) (functional) (organic)
　NEC 251.1
　iatrogenic 251.0
　reactive 251.2
　spontaneous 251.2
　therapeutic misadventure (from administration
　　of insulin) 962.3
Hyperiodemia 276.9
Hyperirritability (cerebral), in newborn 779.1
Hyperkalemia 276.7
Hyperkeratosis (*see also* Keratosis) 701.1
　cervix 622.1
　congenital 757.39
　cornea 371.89
　due to yaws (early) (late) (palmar or plantar)
　　102.3
　eccentrica 757.39
　figurata centrifuga atrophica 757.39
　follicularis 757.39
　　in cutem penetrans 701.1
　limbic (cornea) 371.89
　palmoplantaris climacterica 701.1
　pinta (carate) 103.1
　senile (with pruritus) 702.0
　tongue 528.7
　universalis congenita 757.1
　vagina 623.1
　vocal cord 478.5
　vulva 624.0

Hyperkinesia, hyperkinetic (disease) (reaction)
　(syndrome) 314.9
　with
　　attention deficit —*see* Disorder, attention
　　　deficit
　　conduct disorder 314.2
　　developmental delay 314.1
　　simple disturbance of activity and attention
　　　314.01
　　specified manifestation NEC 314.8
　heart (disease) 429.82
　of childhood or adolescence NEC 314.9
Hyperlacrimation (*see also* Epiphora) 375.20
Hyperlipemia (*see also* Hyperlipidemia) 272.4
Hyperlipidemia 272.4
　carbohydrate-induced 272.1
　combined 272.4
　endogenous 272.1
　exogenous 272.3
　fat-induced 272.3
　group
　　A 272.0
　　B 272.1
　　C 272.2
　　D 272.3
　mixed 272.2
　specified type NEC 272.4
Hyperlipidosis 272.7
　hereditary 272.7
Hyperlipoproteinemia (acquired) (essential)
　(familial) (hereditary) (primary) (secondary)
　272.4
　Fredrickson type
　　I 272.3
　　IIa 272.0
　　IIb 272.2
　　III 272.2
　　IV 272.1
　　V 272.3
　low-density-lipoid-type (LDL) 272.0
　very-low-density-lipoid-type [VLDL] 272.1
Hyperlucent lung, unilateral 492.8
Hyperluteinization 256.1
Hyperlysinemia 270.7
Hypermagnesemia 275.2
　neonatal 775.5
Hypermaturity (fetus or newborn) 766.2
Hypermenorrhea 626.2
Hypermetabolism 794.7
Hypermethioninemia 270.4
Hypermetropia (congenital) 367.0
Hypermobility
　cecum 564.9
　coccyx 724.71
　colon 564.9
　　psychogenic 306.4
　ileum 564.9
　joint (acquired) 718.80
　　ankle 718.87
　　elbow 718.82
　　foot 718.87
　　hand 718.84
　　hip 718.85
　　knee 718.86
　　multiple sites 718.89
　　pelvic region 718.85
　　shoulder (region) 718.81
　　specified site NEC 718.88
　　wrist 718.83
　kidney, congenital 753.3
　meniscus (knee) 717.5

Hypermobility—*continued*
  scapula 718.81
  stomach 536.8
    psychogenic 306.4
  syndrome 728.5
  testis, congenital 752.52
  urethral 599.81
Hypermotility
  gastrointestinal 536.8
  intestine 564.9
    psychogenic 306.4
  stomach 536.8
Hypernasality 784.49
Hypernatremia 276.0
  with water depletion 276.0
Hypernephroma (M8312/3) 189.0
Hyperopia 367.0
Hyperorexia 783.6
Hyperornithinemia 270.6
Hyperosmia (*see also* Disturbance, sensation)
  781.1
Hyperosmolality 276.0
Hyperosteogenesis 733.99
Hyperostosis 733.99
  calvarial 733.3
  cortical 733.3
    infantile 756.59
  frontal, internal of skull 733.3
  interna frontalis 733.3
  monomelic 733.99
  skull 733.3
    congenital 756.0
  vertebral 721.8
    with spondylosis—*see* Spondylosis
    ankylosing 721.6
Hyperovarianism 256.1
Hyperovarism, hyperovaria 256.1
Hyperoxaluria (primary) 271.8
Hyperoxia 987.8
Hyperparathyroidism 252.0
  ectopic 259.3
  secondary, of renal origin 588.8
Hyperpathia (*see also* Disturbance, sensation)
  782.0
  psychogenic 307.80
Hyperperistalsis 787.4
  psychogenic 306.4
Hyperpermeability, capillary 448.9
Hyperphagia 783.6
Hyperphenylalaninemia 270.1
Hyperphoria 378.40
  alternating 378.45
Hyperphosphatemia 275.3
Hyperpiesia (*see also* Hypertension) 401.9
Hyperpiesis (*see also* Hypertension) 401.9
Hyperpigmentation —*see* Pigmentation
Hyperpinealism 259.8
Hyperpipecolatemia 270.7
Hyperpituitarism 253.1
Hyperplasia, hyperplastic
  adenoids (lymphoid tissue) 474.12
    and tonsils 474.10
  adrenal (capsule) (cortex) (gland) 255.8
    with
      sexual precocity (male) 255.2
      virilism, adrenal 255.2
      virilization (female) 255.2
    congenital 255.2
    due to excess ACTH (ectopic) (pituitary) 255.0
    medulla 255.8
  alpha cells (pancreatic)

Hyperplasia, hyperplastic—*continued*
  with
    gastrin excess 251.5
    glucagon excess 251.4
  appendix (lymphoid) 543.0
  artery, fibromuscular NEC 447.8
    carotid 447.8
    renal 447.3
  bone 733.99
    marrow 289.9
  breast (*see also* Hypertrophy, breast) 611.1
  carotid artery 447.8
  cementation, cementum (teeth) (tooth) 521.5
  cervical gland 785.6
  cervix (uteri) 622.1
    basal cell 622.1
    congenital 752.49
    endometrium 622.1
    polypoid 622.1
  chin 524.05
  clitoris, congenital 752.49
  dentin 521.5
  endocervicitis 616.0
  endometrium, endometrial (adenomatous)
    (atypical) (cystic) (glandular) (polypoid)
    (uterus) 621.3
    cervix 622.1
  epithelial 709.8
    focal, oral, including tongue 528.7
    mouth (focal) 528.7
    nipple 611.8
    skin 709.8
    tongue (focal) 528.7
    vaginal wall 623.0
  erythroid 289.9
  fascialis ossificans (progressiva) 728.11
  fibromuscular, artery NEC 447.8
    carotid 447.8
    renal 447.3
  genital
    female 629.8
    male 608.89
  gingiva 523.8
  glandularis
    cystica uteri 621.3
    endometrium (uterus) 621.3
    interstitialis uteri 621.3
  granulocytic 288.8
  gum 523.8
  hymen, congenital 752.49
  islands of Langerhans 251.1
  islet cell (pancreatic) 251.9
    alpha cells
      with excess
        gastrin 251.5
        glucagon 251.4
    beta cells 251.1
  juxtaglomerular (complex) (kidney) 593.89
  kidney (congenital) 753.3
  liver (congenital) 751.69
  lymph node (gland) 785.6
  lymphoid (diffuse) (nodular) 785.6
    appendix 543.0
    intestine 569.89
  mandibular 524.02
    alveolar 524.72
    unilateral condylar 526.89
  Marchand multiple nodular (liver)—*see*
    Cirrhosis, postnecrotic
  maxillary 524.01
    alveolar 524.71

Hyperplasia, hyperplastic—*continued*
medulla, adrenal 255.8
myometrium, myometrial 621.2
nose (lymphoid) (polypoid) 478.1
oral soft tissue (inflammatory) (irritative)
   (mucosa) NEC 528.9
  gingiva 523.8
  tongue 529.8
organ or site, congenital NEC—*see* Anomaly,
   specified type NEC
ovary 620.8
palate, papillary 528.9
pancreatic islet cells 251.9
  alpha
    with excess
      gastrin 251.5
      glucagon 251.4
  beta 251.1
parathyroid (gland) 252.0
persistent, vitreous (primary) 743.51
pharynx (lymphoid) 478.29
prostate 600.9
  adenofibromatous 600.2
  nodular 600.1
renal artery (fibromuscular) 447.3
reticuloendothelial (cell) 289.9
salivary gland (any) 527.1
Schimmelbusch's 610.1
suprarenal (capsule) (gland) 255.8
thymus (gland) (persistent) 254.0
thyroid (*see also* Goiter) 240.9
  primary 242.0
  secondary 242.2
tonsil (lymphoid tissue) 474.11
  and adenoids 474.10
urethrovaginal 599.89
uterus, uterine (myometrium) 621.2
  endometrium 621.3
vitreous (humor), primary persistent 743.51
vulva 624.3
zygoma 738.11
Hyperpnea (*see also* Hyperventilation) 786.01
Hyperpotassemia 276.7
Hyperprebetalipoproteinemia 272.1
  with chylomicronemia 272.3
  familial 272.1
Hyperprolactinemia 253.1
Hyperprolinemia 270.8
Hyperproteinemia 273.8
Hyperprothrombinemia 289.8
Hyperpselaphesia 782.0
Hyperpyrexia 780.6
  heat (effects of) 992.0
  malarial (*see also* Malaria) 084.6
  malignant, due to anesthetic 995.86
  rheumatic—*see* Fever, rheumatic
  unknown origin (*see also* Pyrexia) 780.6
Hyperreactor, vascular 780.2
Hyperreflexia 796.1
  bladder, autonomic 596.54
    with cauda equina 344.61
  detrusor 344.61
Hypersalivation (*see also* Ptyalism) 527.7
Hypersarcosinemia 270.8
Hypersecretion
  ACTH 255.3
  androgens (ovarian) 256.1
  calcitonin 246.0
  corticoadrenal 255.3
  cortisol 255.0
  estrogen 256.0

Hypersecretion—*continued*
  gastric 536.8
    psychogenic 306.4
  gastrin 251.5
  glucagon 251.4
  hormone
    ACTH 255.3
    anterior pituitary 253.1
    growth NEC 253.0
    ovarian androgen 256.1
    testicular 257.0
    thyroid stimulating 242.8
  insulin—*see* Hyperinsulinism
  lacrimal glands (*see also* Epiphora) 375.20
  medulloadrenal 255.6
  milk 676.6
  ovarian androgens 256.1
  pituitary (anterior) 253.1
  salivary gland (any) 527.7
  testicular hormones 257.0
  thyrocalcitonin 246.0
  upper respiratory 478.9
Hypersegmentation, hereditary 288.2
  eosinophils 288.2
  neutrophil nuclei 288.2
Hypersensitive, hypersensitiveness
  hypersensitivity —*see also* Allergy
  angiitis 446.20
    specified NEC 446.29
  carotid sinus 337.0
  colon 564.9
    psychogenic 306.4
  DNA (deoxyribonucleic acid) NEC 287.2
  drug (*see also* Allergy, drug) 995.2
  esophagus 530.89
  insect bites—*see* Injury, superficial, by site
  labyrinth 386.58
  pain (*see also* Disturbance, sensation) 782.0
  pneumonitis NEC 495.9
  reaction (*see also* Allergy) 995.3
    upper respiratory tract NEC 478.8
  stomach (allergic) (nonallergic) 536.8
    psychogenic 306.4
Hypersomatotropism (classic) 253.0
Hypersomnia 780.54
  with sleep apnea 780.53
  nonorganic origin 307.43
    persistent (primary) 307.44
    transient 307.43
Hypersplenia 289.4
Hypersplenism 289.4
Hypersteatosis 706.3
Hyperstimulation, ovarian 256.1
Hypersuprarenalism 255.3
Hypersusceptibility —*see* Allergy
Hyper-TBG-nemia 246.8
Hypertelorism 756.0
  orbit, orbital 376.41

— "H" listing resumes after
Hypertension table...

Hypertension, hypertensive

	Malignant	Benign	Unspecified
(arterial) (arteriolar) (crisis) (degeneration) (disease) (essential) (fluctuating) (idiopathic) (intermittent) (labile) (low renin) (orthostatic) (paroxysmal) (primary) (systemic) (uncontrolled) (vascular)	401.0	401.1	401.9
with			
heart involvement (conditions classifiable to 425.8, 428, 429.0-429.3, 429.8, 429.9 due to hypertension) (*see also* Hypertension, heart)	402.00	402.10	402.90
with kidney involvement—*see* Hypertension, cardiorenal			
renal involvement (only conditions classifiable to 585, 586, 587) (excludes conditions classifiable to 584) (*see also* Hypertension, kidney)	403.00	403.10	403.90
with heart involvement—*see* Hypertension, cardiorenal			
failure (and sclerosis) (*see also* Hypertension, kidney) .	403.01	403.11	403.91
sclerosis without failure (*see also* Hypertension, kidney) .	403.00	403.10	403.90
accelerated (*see also* Hypertension, by type, malignant) . .	401.0	—	—
antepartum—*see* Hypertension complicating pregnancy, childbirth, or the puerperium			
cardiorenal (disease)	404.00	404.10	404.90
with			
heart failure	404.01	404.11	404.91
and renal failure	404.03	404.13	404.93
renal failure	404.02	404.12	404.92
and heart failure	404.03	404.13	404.93
cardiovascular disease (arteriosclerotic) (sclerotic)	402.00	402.10	402.90
with			
heart failure	402.01	402.11	402.91
renal involvement (conditions classifiable to 403) (*see also* Hypertension, cardiorenal)	404.00	404.10	404.90
cardiovascular renal (disease) (sclerosis) (*see also* Hypertension cardiorenal)	404.00	404.10	404.90
cerebrovascular disease NEC	437.2	437.2	437.2
complicating pregnancy, childbirth, or the puerperium . . .	642.2	642.0	642.9
with			
albuminuria (and edema) (mild)	—	—	642.4
severe	—	—	642.5
edema (mild)	—	—	642.4
severe	—	—	642.5
heart disease	642.2	642.2	642.2
and renal disease	642.2	642.2	642.2
renal disease	642.2	642.2	642.2
and heart disease	642.2	642.2	642.2
chronic	642.2	642.0	642.0
with pre-eclampsia or eclampsia	642.7	642.7	642.7
fetus or newborn	760.0	760.0	760.0
essential	—	642.0	642.0
with pre-eclampsia or eclampsia	—	642.7	642.7
fetus or newborn	760.0	760.0	760.0
fetus or newborn	760.0	760.0	760.0
gestational	—	—	642.3
pre-existing	642.2	642.0	642.0
with pre-eclampsia or eclampsia	642.7	642.7	642.7
fetus or newborn	760.0	760.0	760.0
secondary to renal disease	642.1	642.1	642.1
with pre-eclampsia or eclampsia	642.7	642.7	642.7
fetus or newborn	760.0	760.0	760.0
transient	—	—	642.3
due to			
aldosteronism, primary	405.09	405.19	405.99
brain tumor	405.09	405.19	405.99
bulbar poliomyelitis	405.09	405.19	405.99
calculus			
kidney	405.09	405.19	405.99
ureter	405.09	405.19	405.99
coarctation, aorta	405.09	405.19	405.99
Cushing's disease	405.09	405.19	405.99
glomerulosclerosis (*see also* Hypertension, kidney) . . .	403.00	403.10	403.90
periarteritis nodosa	405.09	405.19	405.99
pheochromocytoma	405.09	405.19	405.99
polycystic kidney(s)	405.09	405.19	405.99
polycythemia	405.09	405.19	405.99
porphyria	405.09	405.19	405.99
pyelonephritis	405.09	405.19	405.99

	Malignant	Benign	Unspecified
renal (artery)			
aneurysm	405.01	405.11	405.91
anomaly	405.01	405.11	405.91
embolism	405.01	405.11	405.91
fibromuscular hyperplasia	405.01	405.11	405.91
occlusion	405.01	405.11	405.91
stenosis	405.01	405.11	405.91
thrombosis	405.01	405.11	405.91
encephalopathy	437.2	437.2	437.2
gestational (transient) NEC	—	—	642.3
Goldblatt's	440.1	440.1	440.1
heart (disease) (conditions classifiable to 425.8, 428, 429.0-429.3, 429.8, 429.9 due to hypertension)	402.00	402.10	402.90
with			
heart failure	402.01	402.11	402.91
of newborn	—	—	747.83
hypertensive kidney disease (conditions classifiable to 403)			
(*see also* Hypertension, cardiorenal)	404.00	404.10	404.90
renal sclerosis (*see also* Hypertension, cardiorenal)	404.00	404.10	404.90
intracranial, benign	—	348.2	—
intraocular	—	—	365.04
kidney	403.00	403.10	403.90
with			
heart involvement (conditions classifiable to 425.8, 428, 429.0-429.3, 429.8, 429.9 due to hypertension) (*see also* Hypertension cardiorenal)	404.00	404.10	404.90
hypertensive heart (disease) (conditions classifiable to 402)			
(*see also* Hypertension, cardiorenal)	404.00	404.10	404.90
lesser circulation	—	—	416.0
necrotizing	401.0	—	—
ocular	—	—	365.04
portal (due to chronic liver disease)	—	—	572.3
postoperative 997.91			
psychogenic	—	—	306.2
puerperal, postpartum—*see* Hypertension, complicating pregnancy, childbirth, or the puerperium			
pulmonary (artery)	—	—	416.8
idiopathic	—	—	416.0
primary	—	—	416.0
with cor pulmonale (chronic)	—	—	416.8
acute	—	—	415.0
secondary	—	—	416.8
renal (disease) (*see also* Hypertension, kidney)	403.00	403.10	403.90
renovascular NEC	405.01	405.11	405.91
secondary NEC	405.09	405.19	405.99
due to			
aldosteronism, primary	405.09	405.19	405.99
brain tumor	405.09	405.19	405.99
bulbar poliomyelitis	405.09	405.19	405.99
calculus			
kidney	405.09	405.19	405.99
ureter	405.09	405.19	405.99
coarctation, aorta	405.09	405.19	405.99
Cushing's disease	405.09	405.19	405.99
glomerulosclerosis (*see also* Hypertension, kidney)	403.00	403.10	403.90
periarteritis nodosa	405.09	405.19	405.99
pheochromocytoma	405.09	405.19	405.99
polycystic kidney(s)	405.09	405.19	405.99
polycythemia	405.09	405.19	405.99
porphyria	405.09	405.19	405.99
pyelonephritis	405.09	405.19	405.99
renal (artery)			
aneurysm	405.01	405.11	405.91
anomaly	405.01	405.11	405.91
embolism	405.01	405.11	405.91
fibromuscular hyperplasia	405.01	405.11	405.91
occlusion	405.01	405.11	405.91
stenosis	405.01	405.11	405.91
thrombosis	405.01	405.11	405.91
transient	—	—	796.2
of pregnancy	—	—	642.3
venous, chronic (asymptomatic) (idiopathic)	—	—	459.30
due to			
deep vein thrombosis (*see also* Syndrome, postphlebetic)	—	—	459.10
with			
complication NEC	—	—	459.39
inflammation	—	—	459.32

	Malignant	Benign	Unspecified
with ulcer	—	—	459.33
ulcer	—	—	459.31
with inflammation	—	—	459.33

This page intentionally left blank

Hyperthecosis, ovary 256.8
Hyperthermia (of unknown origin) (*see also*
  Pyrexia) 780.6
  malignant (due to anesthesia) 995.86
  newborn 778.4
Hyperthymergasia (*see also* Psychosis,
  affective) 296.0
  reactive (from emotional stress, psychological
    trauma) 298.1
  recurrent episode 296.1
  single episode 296.0
Hyperthymism 254.8
Hyperthyroid (recurrent)—*see* Hyperthyroidism
Hyperthyroidism (latent) (preadult) (recurrent)
  (without goiter) 242.9

Note—Use the following fifth-digit
subclassification with category 242:

0 *without mention of thyrotoxic crisis or storm*
1 *with mention of thyrotoxic crisis or storm*

---

  with
    goiter (diffuse) 242.0
      adenomatous 242.3
        multinodular 242.2
        uninodular 242.1
      nodular 242.3
        multinodular 242.2
        uninodular 242.1
      thyroid nodule 242.1
    complicating pregnancy, childbirth, or
      puerperium 648.1
    neonatal (transient) 775.3
Hypertonia —Hypertonicity
Hypertonicity
  bladder 596.51
  fetus or newborn 779.89
  gastrointestinal (tract) 536.8
  infancy 779.89
    due to electrolyte imbalance 779.89
  muscle 728.85
  stomach 536.8
    psychogenic 306.4
  uterus, uterine (contractions) 661.4
    affecting fetus or newborn 763.7
Hypertony —*see* Hypertonicity
Hypertransaminemia 790.4
Hypertrichosis 704.1
  congenital 757.4
  eyelid 374.54
  lanuginosa 757.4
    acquired 704.1
Hypertriglyceridemia, essential 272.1
Hypertrophy, hypertrophic
  adenoids (infectional) 474.12
    and tonsils (faucial) (infective) (lingual)
      (lymphoid) 474.10
  adrenal 255.8
  alveolar process or ridge 525.8
  anal papillae 569.49
  apocrine gland 705.82
  artery NEC 447.8
    carotid 447.8
    congenital (peripheral) NEC 747.60
    gastrointestinal 747.61
    lower limb 747.64
    renal 747.62
    specified NEC 747.69
    spinal 747.82
    upper limb 747.63

Hypertrophy, hypertrophic—*continued*
  arthritis (chronic) (*see also* Osteoarthrosis) 715.9
    spine (*see also* Spondylosis) 721.90
  arytenoid 478.79
  asymmetrical (heart) 429.9
  auricular—*see* Hypertrophy, cardiac
  Bartholin's gland 624.8
  bile duct 576.8
  bladder (sphincter) (trigone) 596.8
  blind spot, visual field 368.42
  bone 733.99
  brain 348.8
  breast 611.1
    cystic 610.1
    fetus or newborn 778.7
    fibrocystic 610.1
    massive pubertal 611.1
    puerperal, postpartum 676.3
    senile (parenchymatous) 611.1
  cardiac (chronic) (idiopathic) 429.3
    with
      rheumatic fever (conditions classifiable to
        390)
        active 391.8
          with chorea 392.0
        inactive or quiescent (with chorea) 398.99
    congenital NEC 746.89
    fatty (*see also* Degeneration, myocardial)
      429.1
    hypertensive (*see also* Hypertension, heart)
      402.90
    rheumatic (with chorea) 398.99
      active or acute 391.8
        with chorea 392.0
    valve (*see also* Endocarditis) 424.90
      congenital NEC 746.89
  cartilage 733.99
  cecum 569.89
  cervix (uteri) 622.6
    congenital 752.49
    elongation 622.6
  clitoris (cirrhotic) 624.2
    congenital 752.49
  colon 569.89
    congenital 751.3
  conjunctiva, lymphoid 372.73
  cornea 371.89
  corpora cavernosa 607.89
  duodenum 537.89
  endometrium (uterus) 621.3
    cervix 622.6
  epididymis 608.89
  esophageal hiatus (congenital) 756.6
    with hernia—*see* Hernia, diaphragm
  eyelid 374.30
  falx, skull 733.99
  fat pad 729.30
    infrapatellar 729.31
    knee 729.31
    orbital 374.34
    popliteal 729.31
    prepatellar 729.31
    retropatellar 729.31
    specified site NEC 729.39
  foot (congenital) 755.67
  frenum, frenulum (tongue) 529.8
    linguae 529.8
    lip 528.5
  gallbladder or cystic duct 575.8
  gastric mucosa 535.2
  gingiva 523.8

Hypertrophy, hypertrophic—*continued*
  gland, glandular (general) NEC 785.6
  gum (mucous membrane) 523.8
  heart (idiopathic)—*see also* Hypertrophy,
      cardiac
    valve—*see also* Endocarditis
      congenital NEC 746.89
  hemifacial 754.0
  hepatic—*see* Hypertrophy, liver
  hiatus (esophageal) 756.6
  hilus gland 785.6
  hymen, congenital 752.49
  ileum 569.89
  infrapatellar fat pad 729.31
  intestine 569.89
  jejunum 569.89
  kidney (compensatory) 593.1
    congenital 753.3
  labial frenulum 528.5
  labium (majus) (minus) 624.3
  lacrimal gland, chronic 375.03
  ligament 728.9
    spinal 724.8
  linguae frenulum 529.8
  lingual tonsil (infectional) 474.11
  lip (frenum) 528.5
    congenital 744.81
  liver 789.1
    acute 573.8
    cirrhotic—*see* Cirrhosis, liver
    congenital 751.69
    fatty—*see* Fatty, liver
  lymph gland 785.6
    tuberculous—*see* Tuberculosis, lymph gland
  mammary gland—*see* Hypertrophy, breast
  maxillary frenulum 528.5
  Meckel's diverticulum (congenital) 751.0
  medial meniscus, acquired 717.3
  median bar 600.9
  mediastinum 519.3
  meibomian gland 373.2
  meniscus, knee, congenital 755.64
  metatarsal head 733.99
  metatarsus 733.99
  mouth 528.9
  mucous membrane
    alveolar process 523.8
    nose 478.1
    turbinate (nasal) 478.0
  muscle 728.9
  muscular coat, artery NEC 447.8
    carotid 447.8
    renal 447.3
  myocardium (*see also* Hypertrophy, cardiac)
      429.3
    idiopathic 425.4
  myometrium 621.2
  nail 703.8
    congenital 757.5
  nasal 478.1
    alae 478.1
    bone 738.0
    cartilage 478.1
    mucous membrane (septum) 478.1
    sinus (*see also* Sinusitis) 473.9
    turbinate 478.0
  nasopharynx, lymphoid (infectional) (tissue)
      (wall) 478.29
  neck, uterus 622.6
  nipple 611.1
  normal aperture diaphragm (congenital) 756.6

Hypertrophy, hypertrophic—*continued*
  nose (*see also* Hypertrophy, nasal) 478.1
  orbit 376.46
  organ or site, congenital NEC—*see* Anomaly,
      specified type NEC
  osteoarthropathy (pulmonary) 731.2
  ovary 620.8
  palate (hard) 526.89
    soft 528.9
  pancreas (congenital) 751.7
  papillae
    anal 569.49
    tongue 529.3
  parathyroid (gland) 252.0
  parotid gland 527.1
  penis 607.89
  phallus 607.89
    female (clitoris) 624.2
  pharyngeal tonsil 474.12
  pharyngitis 472.1
  pharynx 478.29
    lymphoid (infectional) (tissue) (wall) 478.29
  pituitary (fossa) (gland) 253.8
  popliteal fat pad 729.31
  preauricular (lymph) gland (Hampstead) 785.6
  prepuce (congenital) 605
    female 624.2
  prostate (asymptomatic) (early) (recurrent)
      600.9
    adenofibromatous 600.2
    benign 600.0
    congenital 752.8
  psuedoedematous hypodermal 757.0
  pseudomuscular 359.1
  pylorus (muscle) (sphincter) 537.0
    congenital 750.5
    infantile 750.5
  rectal sphincter 569.49
  rectum 569.49
  renal 593.1
  rhinitis (turbinate) 472.0
  salivary duct or gland 527.1
    congenital 750.26
  scaphoid (tarsal) 733.99
  scar 701.4
  scrotum 608.89
  sella turcica 253.8
  seminal vesicle 608.89
  sigmoid 569.89
  skin condition NEC 701.9
  spermatic cord 608.89
  spinal ligament 728.9
  spleen—*see* Splenomegaly
  spondylitis (spine) (*see also* Spondylosis) 721.90
  stomach 537.89
  subaortic stenosis (idiopathic) 425.1
  sublingual gland 527.1
    congenital 750.26
  submaxillary gland 527.1
  suprarenal (gland) 255.8
  tendon 727.9
  testis 608.89
    congenital 752.8
  thymic, thymus (congenital) (gland) 254.0
  thyroid (gland) (*see also* Goiter) 240.9
    primary 242.0
    secondary 242.2
  toe (congenital) 755.65
    acquired 735.8
  tongue 529.8
    congenital 750.15

Hypertrophy, hypertrophic—*continued*
frenum 529.8
papillae (foliate) 529.3
tonsil (faucial) (infective) (lingual) (lymphoid) 474.11
and adenoids 474.10
with
adenoiditis 474.01
tonsillitis 474.00
and adenoiditis 474.02
tunica vaginalis 608.89
turbinate (mucous membrane) 478.0
ureter 593.89
urethra 599.84
uterus 621.2
puerperal, postpartum 674.8
uvula 528.9
vagina 623.8
vas deferens 608.89
vein 459.89
ventricle, ventricular (heart) (left) (right)—*see also* Hypertrophy, cardiac
congenital 746.89
due to hypertension (left) (right) (*see also* Hypertension, heart) 402.90
benign 402.10
malignant 402.00
right with ventricular septal defect, pulmonary stenosis or atresia, and dextraposition of aorta 745.2
verumontanum 599.89
vesical 596.8
vocal cord 478.5
vulva 624.3
stasis (nonfilarial) 624.3
Hypertropia (intermittent) (periodic) 378.31
Hypertyrosinemia 270.2
Hyperuricemia 790.6
Hypervalinemia 270.3
Hyperventilation (tetany) 786.01
hysterical 300.11
psychogenic 306.1
syndrome 306.1
Hyperviscidosis 277.00
Hyperviscosity (of serum) (syndrome) NEC 273.3
polycythemic 289.0
sclerocythemic 282.8
Hypervitaminosis (dietary) NEC 278.8
A (dietary) 278.2
D (dietary) 278.4
from excessive administration or use of vitamin preparations (chronic) 278.8
reaction to sudden overdose 963.5
vitamin A 278.2
reaction to sudden overdose 963.5
vitamin D 278.4
reaction to sudden overdose 963.5
vitamin K
correct substance properly administered 278.8
overdose or wrong substance given or taken 964.3
Hypervolemia 276.6
Hypesthesia (*see also* Disturbance, sensation) 782.0
cornea 371.81
Hyphema (anterior chamber) (ciliary body) (iris) 364.41
traumatic 921.3
Hyphemia —*see* Hyphema

Hypoacidity, gastric 536.8
psychogenic 306.4
Hypoactive labyrinth (function)—*see* Hypofunction, labyrinth
Hypoadrenalism 255.4
tuberculous (*see also* Tuberculosis) 017.6
Hypoadrenocorticism 255.4
pituitary 253.4
Hypoalbuminemia 273.8
Hypoalphalipoproteinemia 272.5
Hypobarism 993.2
Hypobaropathy 993.2
Hypobetalipoproteinemia (familial) 272.5
Hypocalcemia 275.41
cow's milk 775.4
dietary 269.3
neonatal 775.4
phosphate-loading 775.4
Hypocalcification, teeth 520.4
Hypochloremia 276.9
Hypochlorhydria 536.8
neurotic 306.4
psychogenic 306.4
Hypocholesteremia 272.5
Hypochondria (reaction) 300.7
Hypochondriac 300.7
Hypochondriasis 300.7
Hypochromasia blood cells 280.9
Hypochromic anemia 280.9
due to blood loss (chronic) 280.0
acute 285.1
microcytic 280.9
Hypocoagulability (*see also* Defect, coagulation) 286.9
Hypocomplementemia 279.8
Hypocythemia (progressive) 284.9
Hypodontia (*see also* Anodontia) 520.0
Hypoeosinophilia 288.8
Hypoesthesia (*see also* Disturbance, sensation) 782.0
cornea 371.81
tactile 782.0
Hypoestrinism 256.39
Hypoestrogenism 256.39
Hypoferremia 280.9
due to blood loss (chronic) 280.0
Hypofertility
female 628.9
male 606.1
Hypofibrinogenemia) 286.3
acquired 286.6
congenital 286.3
Hypofunction
adrenal (gland) 255.4
cortex 255.4
medulla 255.5
specified NEC 255.5
cerebral 331.9
corticoadrenal NEC 255.4
intestinal 564.89
labyrinth (unilateral) 386.53
with loss of labyrinthine reactivity 386.55
bilateral 386.54
with loss of labyrinthine reactivity 386.56
Leydig cell 257.2
ovary 256.39
postablative 256.2
pituitary (anterior) (gland) (lobe) 253.2
posterior 253.5
testicular 257.2
iatrogenic 257.1

Hypofunction—*continued*
  postablative 257.1
  postirradiation 257.1
  postsurgical 257.1
Hypogammaglobulinemia 279.00
  acquired primary 279.06
  non-sex-linked, congenital 279.06
  sporadic 279.06
  transient of infancy 279.09
Hypogenitalism (congenital) (female) (male) 752.8
  penis 752.69
Hypoglycemia (spontaneous) 251.2
  coma 251.0
    diabetic 250.3
  diabetic 250.8
  due to insulin 251.0
    therapeutic misadventure 962.3
  familial (idiopathic) 251.2
  following gastrointestinal surgery 579.3
  infantile (idiopathic) 251.2
  in infant of diabetic mother 775.0
  leucine-induced 270.3
  neonatal 775.6
  reactive 251.2
  specified NEC 251.1
Hypoglycemic shock 251.0
  diabetic 250.8
  due to insulin 251.0
  functional (syndrome) 251.1
Hypogonadism
  female 256.39
  gonadotrophic (isolated) 253.4
  hypogonadotropic (isolated) (with anosmia) 253.4
  isolated 253.4
  male 257.2
  ovarian (primary) 256.39
  pituitary (secondary) 253.4
  testicular (primary) (secondary) 257.2
Hypohidrosis 705.0
Hypohidrotic ectodermal dysplasia 757.31
Hypoidrosis 705.0
Hypoinsulinemia, postsurgical 251.3
  postpancreatectomy (complete) (partial) 251.3
Hypokalemia 276.8
Hypokinesia 780.99
Hypoleukia splenica 289.4
Hypoleukocytosis 288.8
Hypolipidemia 272.5
Hypolipoproteinemia 272.5
Hypomagnesemia 275.2
  neonatal 775.4
Hypomania, hypomanic reaction (*see also* Psychosis, affective) 296.0
  recurrent episode 296.1
  single episode 296.0
Hypomastia (congenital) 757.6
Hypomenorrhea 626.1
Hypometabolism 783.9
Hypomotility
  gastrointestinal tract 536.8
    psychogenic 306.4
  intestine 564.89
    psychogenic 306.4
  stomach 536.8
    psychogenic 306.4
Hyponasality 784.49
Hyponatremia 276.1
Hypo-ovarianism 256.39
Hypo-ovarism 256.39

Hypoparathyroidism (idiopathic) (surgically induced) 252.1
  neonatal 775.4
Hypopharyngitis 462
Hypophoria 378.40
Hypophosphatasia 275.3
Hypophosphatemia (acquired) (congenital) (familial) 275.3
  renal 275.3
Hypophyseal, hypophysis —*see also* condition
  dwarfism 253.3
  gigantism 253.0
  syndrome 253.8
Hypophyseothalamic syndrome 253.8
Hypopiesis —*see* Hypotension
Hypopigmentation 709.00
  eyelid 374.53
Hypopinealism 259.8
Hypopituitarism (juvenile) (syndrome) 253.2
  due to
    hormone therapy 253.7
    hypophysectomy 253.7
    radiotherapy 253.7
  postablative 253.7
  postpartum hemorrhage 253.2
Hypoplasia, hypoplasis 759.89
  adrenal (gland) 759.1
  alimentary tract 751.8
    lower 751.2
    upper 750.8
  anus, anal (canal) 751.2
  aorta 747.22
  aortic
    arch (tubular) 747.10
    orifice or valve with hypoplasia of ascending aorta and defective development of left ventricle (with mitral valve atresia) 746.7
  appendix 751.2
  areola 757.6
  arm (*see also* Absence, arm, congenital) 755.20
  artery (congenital) (peripheral) NEC 747.60
    brain 747.81
    cerebral 747.81
    coronary 746.85
    gastrointestinal 747.61
    lower limb 747.64
    pulmonary 747.3
    renal 747.62
    retinal 743.58
    specified NEC 747.69
    spinal 747.82
    umbilical 747.5
    upper limb 747.63
  auditory canal 744.29
    causing impairment of hearing 744.02
  biliary duct (common) or passage 751.61
  bladder 753.8
  bone NEC 756.9
    face 756.0
    malar 756.0
    mandible 524.04
      alveolar 524.74
    marrow 284.9
      acquired (secondary) 284.8
      congenital 284.0
      idiopathic 284.9
    maxilla 524.03
      alveolar 524.73
    skull (*see also* Hypoplasia, skull) 756.0
  brain 742.1
    gyri 742.2

Hypoplasia, hypoplasis—*continued*
  specified part 742.2
  breast (areola) 757.6
  bronchus (tree) 748.3
  cardiac 746.89
    valve—*see* Hypoplasia, heart, valve
    vein 746.89
  carpus (*see also* Absence, carpal, congenital)
    755.28
  cartilaginous 756.9
  cecum 751.2
  cementum 520.4
    hereditary 520.5
  cephalic 742.1
  cerebellum 742.2
  cervix (uteri) 752.49
  chin 524.06
  clavicle 755.51
  coccyx 756.19
  colon 751.2
  corpus callosum 742.2
  cricoid cartilage 748.3
  dermal, focal (Goltz) 757.39
  digestive organ(s) or tract NEC 751.8
    lower 751.2
    upper 750.8
  ear 744.29
    auricle 744.23
    lobe 744.29
    middle, except ossicles 744.03
      ossicles 744.04
    ossicles 744.04
  enamel of teeth (neonatal) (postnatal) (prenatal)
    520.4
    hereditary 520.5
  endocrine (gland) NEC 759.2
  endometrium 621.8
  epididymis 752.8
  epiglottis 748.3
  erythroid, congenital 284.0
  erythropoietic, chronic acquired 284.8
  esophagus 750.3
  Eustachian tube 744.24
  eye (*see also* Microphthalmos) 743.10
    lid 743.62
  face 744.89
    bone(s) 756.0
  fallopian tube 752.19
  femur (*see also* Absence, femur, congenital)
    755.34
  fibula (*see also* Absence, fibula, congenital)
    755.37
  finger (*see also* Absence, finger, congenital)
    755.29
  focal dermal 757.39
  foot 755.31
  gallbladder 751.69
  genitalia, genital organ(s)
    female 752.8
      external 752.49
      internal NEC 752.8
    in adiposogenital dystrophy 253.8
    male 752.8
      penis 752.69
  glottis 748.3
  hair 757.4
  hand 755.21
  heart 746.89
    left (complex) (syndrome) 746.7
    valve NEC 746.89
      pulmonary 746.01

Hypoplasia, hypoplasis—*continued*
  humerus (*see also* Absence, humerus,
    congenital) 755.24
  hymen 752.49
  intestine (small) 751.1
    large 751.2
  iris 743.46
  jaw 524.09
  kidney(s) 753.0
  labium (majus) (minus) 752.49
  labyrinth, membranous 744.05
  lacrimal duct (apparatus) 743.65
  larynx 748.3
  leg (*see also* Absence, limb, congenital, lower)
    755.30
  limb 755.4
    lower (*see also* Absence, limb, congenital,
      lower) 755.30
    upper (*see also* Absence, limb, congenital,
      upper) 755.20
  liver 751.69
  lung (lobe) 748.5
  mammary (areolar) 757.6
  mandibular 524.04
    alveolar 524.74
    unilateral condylar 526.89
  maxillary 524.03
    alveolar 524.73
  medullary 284.9
  megakaryocytic 287.3
  metacarpus (*see also* Absence, metacarpal,
    congenital) 755.28
  metatarsus (*see also* Absence, metatarsal,
    congenital) 755.38
  muscle 756.89
    eye 743.69
  myocardium (congenital) (Uhl's anomaly)
    746.84
  nail(s) 757.5
  nasolacrimal duct 743.65
  nervous system NEC 742.8
  neural 742.8
  nose, nasal 748.1
  ophthalmic (*see also* Microphthalmos) 743.10
  organ
    of Corti 744.05
    or site NEC—*see* Anomaly, by site
  osseous meatus (ear) 744.03
  ovary 752.0
  oviduct 752.19
  pancreas 751.7
  parathyroid (gland) 759.2
  parotid gland 750.26
  patella 755.64
  pelvis, pelvic girdle 755.69
  penis 752.69
  peripheral vascular system (congenital) NEC
    747.60
    gastrointestinal 747.61
    lower limb 747.64
    renal 747.62
    specified NEC 747.69
    spinal 747.82
    upper limb 747.63
  pituitary (gland) 759.2
  pulmonary 748.5
    arteriovenous 747.3
    artery 747.3
    valve 746.01
  punctum lacrimale 743.65

Hypoplasia, hypoplasis—*continued*
radioulnar (*see also* Absence, radius,
    congenital, with ulna) 755.25
radius (*see also* Absence, radius, congenital)
    755.26
rectum 751.2
respiratory system NEC 748.9
rib 756.3
sacrum 756.19
scapula 755.59
shoulder girdle 755.59
skin 757.39
skull (bone) 756.0
    with
        anencephalus 740.0
        encephalocele 742.0
        hydrocephalus 742.3
            with spina bifida (*see also* Spina bifida)
                741.0
        microcephalus 742.1
spinal (cord) (ventral horn cell) 742.59
    vessel 747.82
spine 756.19
spleen 759.0
sternum 756.3
tarsus (*see also* Absence, tarsal, congenital)
    755.38
testis, testicle 752.8
thymus (gland) 279.11
thyroid (gland) 243
    cartilage 748.3
tibiofibular (*see also* Absence, tibia, congenital,
    with fibula) 755.35
toe (*see also* Absence, toe, congenital) 755.39
tongue 750.16
trachea (cartilage) (rings) 748.3
Turner's (tooth) 520.4
ulna (*see also* Absence, ulna, congenital) 755.27
umbilical artery 747.5
ureter 753.29
uterus 752.3
vagina 752.49
vascular (peripheral) NEC (*see also* Hypoplasia,
    peripheral vascular system) 747.60
    brain 747.81
vein(s) (peripheral) NEC (*see also* Hypoplasia,
    peripheral vascular system 747.60
    brain 747.81
    cardiac 746.89
    great 747.49
    portal 747.49
    pulmonary 747.49
vena cava (inferior) (superior) 747.49
vertebra 756.19
vulva 752.49
zonule (ciliary) 743.39
zygoma 738.12
Hypopotassemia 276.8
Hypoproaccelerinemia (*see also* Defect,
    coagulation) 286.3
Hypoproconvertinemia (congenital) (*see also*
    Defect, coagulation) 286.3
Hypoproteinemia (essential) (hypermetabolic)
    (idiopathic) 273.8
Hypoproteinosis 260
Hypoprothrombinemia (congenital) (hereditary)
    (idiopathic) (*see also* Defect, coagulation)
    286.3
    acquired 286.7
    newborn 776.3
Hypopselaphesia 782.0

Hypopyon (anterior chamber) (eye) 364.05
    iritis 364.05
    ulcer (cornea) 370.04
Hypopyrexia 780.99
Hyporeflex 796.1
Hyporeninemia, extreme 790.99
    in primary aldosteronism 255.1
Hyporesponsive episode 780.09
Hyposecretion
    ACTH 253.4
        ovary 256.39
        postablative 256.2
    salivary gland (any) 527.7
Hyposegmentation of neutrophils, hereditary
    288.2
Hyposiderinemia 280.9
Hyposmolality 276.1
    syndrome 276.1
Hyposomatotropism 253.3
Hyposomnia (*see also* Insomnia) 780.52
Hypospadias (male) 752.61
    female 753.8
Hypospermatogenesis 606.1
Hyposphagma 372.72
Hyposplenism 289.59
Hypostasis, pulmonary 514
Hypostatic —*see* condition
Hyposthenuria 593.89
Hyposuprarenalism 255.4
Hypo-TBG-nemia 246.8
Hypotension (arterial) (constitutional) 458.9
    chronic 458.1
    iatrogenic 458.2
    maternal, syndrome (following labor and
        delivery) 669.2
    orthostatic (chronic) 458.0
        dysautonomic-dyskinetic syndrome 333.0
    permanent idiopathic 458.1
    postoperative 458.2
    postural 458.0
    specified type NEC 458.8
    transient 796.3
Hypothermia (accidental) 991.6
    anesthetic 995.89
    newborn NEC 778.3
    not associated with low environmental
        temperature 780.99
Hypothymergasia (*see also* Psychosis, affective)
    296.2
    recurrent episode 296.3
    single episode 296.2
Hypothyroidism (acquired) 244.9
    complicating pregnancy, childbirth, or
        puerperium 648.1
    congenital 243
    due to
        ablation 244.1
            radioactive iodine 244.1
            surgical 244.0
        iodine (administration) (ingestion) 244.2
            radioactive 244.1
        irradiation therapy 244.1
        p-aminosalicylic acid (PAS) 244.3
        phenylbutazone 244.3
        resorcinol 244.3
        specified cause NEC 244.8
        surgery 244.0
    goitrous (sporadic) 246.1
    iatrogenic NEC 244.3
    iodine 244.2
    pituitary 244.8

Hypothyroidism—*continued*
   postablative NEC 244.1
   postsurgical 244.0
   primary 244.9
   secondary NEC 244.8
   specified cause NEC 244.8
   sporadic goitrous 246.1
Hypotonia, hypotonicity, hypotony 781.3
   benign congenital 358.8
   bladder 596.4
   congenital 779.89
      benign 358.8
   eye 360.30
      due to
         fistula 360.32
         ocular disorder NEC 360.33
      following loss of aqueous or vitreous 360.33
      primary 360.31
   infantile muscular (benign) 359.0
   muscle 728.9
   uterus, uterine (contractions)—*see* Inertia, uterus
Hypotrichosis 704.09
   congenital 757.4
   lid (congenital) 757.4
      acquired 374.55
   postinfectional NEC 704.09
Hypotropia 378.32
Hypoventilation 786.09
Hypovitaminosis (*see also* Deficiency, vitamin)
      269.2
Hypovolemia 276.5
   surgical shock 998.0
   traumatic (shock) 958.4
Hypoxemia (*see also* Anoxia) 799.0
Hypoxia (*see also* Anoxia) 799.0
   cerebral 348.1
      during or resulting from a procedure 997.01
      newborn 768.9
         mild or moderate 768.6
         severe 768.5
   fetal, affecting newborn 768.9
   intrauterine—*see* Distress, fetal
   myocardial (*see also* Insufficiency, coronary)
      411.89
      arteriosclerotic —*see* Arteriosclerosis,
         coronary
   newborn 768.9
Hypsarrhythmia (*see also* Epilepsy) 345.6
Hysteralgia, pregnant uterus 646.8
Hysteria, hysterical 300.10
   anxiety 300.20
   Charcot's gland 300.11
   conversion (any manifestation) 300.11
   dissociative type NEC 300.15
   psychosis, acute 298.1
Hysteroepilepsy 300.11
Hysterotomy , affecting fetus or newborn
      763.89

I

Iatrogenic syndrome of excess cortisol 255.0
Iceland disease (epidemic neuromyasthenia)
   049.8
Ichthyosis (congenita) 757.1
  acquired 701.1
  fetalis gravior 757.1
  follicularis 757.1
  hystrix 757.39
  lamellar 757.1
  lingual 528.6
  palmaris and plantaris 757.39
  simplex 757.1
  vera 757.1
  vulgaris 757.1
Ichthyotoxism 988.0
  bacterial (*see also* Poisoning, food) 005.9
Icteroanemia, hemolytic (acquired) 283.9
  congenital (*see also* Spherocytosis) 282.0
Icterus (*see also* Jaundice) 782.4
  catarrhal—*see* Icterus, infectious
  conjunctiva 782.4
    newborn 774.6
  epidemic—*see* Icterus, infectious
  febrilis—*see* Icterus, infectious
  fetus or newborn—*see* Jaundice, fetus or
    newborn
  gravis (*see also* Necrosis, liver) 570
    complicating pregnancy 646.7
      affecting fetus or newborn 760.8
    fetus or newborn NEC 773.0
    obstetrical 646.7
      affecting fetus or newborn 760.8
  hematogenous (acquired) 283.9
  hemolytic (acquired) 283.9
    congenital (*see also* Spherocytosis) 282.0
  hemorrhagic (acute) 100.0
    leptospiral 100.0
    newborn 776.0
    spirochetal 100.0
  infectious 070.1
    with hepatic coma 070.0
    leptospiral 100.0
    spirochetal 100.0
  intermittens juvenilis 277.4
  malignant (*see also* Necrosis, liver) 570
  neonatorum (*see also* Jaundice, fetus or
    newborn) 774.6
  pernicious (*see also* Necrosis, liver) 570
  spirochetal 100.0
Ictus solaris, solis 992.0
Identity disorder 313.82
  dissociative 300.14
  gender role (child) 302.6
    adult 302.85
  psychosexual (child) 302.6
    adult 302.85
Idioglossia 307.9
Idiopathic —*see* condition
Idiosyncrasy (*see also* Allergy) 995.3
  drug, medicinal substance, and biological—*see*
    Allergy, drug
Idiot, idiocy (congenital) 318.2
  amaurotic (Bielschowsky) (-Jansky) (family)
    (infantile (late)) (juvenile (late))
    (Vogt-Spielmeyer) 330.1
  microcephalic 742.1
  Mongolian 758.0
  oxycephalic 756.0
Id reaction (due to bacteria) 692.89

IgE asthma 493.0
Ileitis (chronic) (*see also* Enteritis) 558.9
  infectious 009.0
  noninfectious 558.9
  regional (ulcerative) 555.0
    with large intestine 555.2
  segmental 555.0
    with large intestine 555.2
  terminal (ulcerative) 555.0
    with large intestine 555.2
Ileocolitis (*see also* Enteritis) 558.9
  infectious 009.0
  regional 555.2
  ulcerative 556.1
Ileostomy status V44.2
  with complication 569.60
Ileotyphus 002.0
Ileum —*see* condition
Ileus (adynamic) (bowel) (colon) (inhibitory)
    (intestine) (neurogenic) (paralytic) 560.1
  arteriomesenteric duodenal 537.2
  due to gallstone (in intestine) 560.31
  duodenal, chronic 537.2
  following gastrointestinal surgery 997.4
  gallstone 560.31
  mechanical (*see also* Obstruction, intestine)
    560.9
  meconium 777.1
    due to cystic fibrosis 277.01
  myxedema 564.89
  postoperative 997.4
  transitory, newborn 777.4
Iliac —*see* condition
Iliotibial band friction syndrome 728.89
Ill, louping 063.1
Illegitimacy V61.6
Illness —*see also* Disease
  factitious 300.19
    with
      combined physical and psychological
        symptoms 300.19
      physical symptoms 300.19
      psychological symptoms 300.16
    chronic (with physical symptoms) 301.51
  heart—*see* Disease, heart
  manic-depressive (*see also* Psychosis, affective)
    296.80
  mental (*see also* Disorder, mental) 300.9
Imbalance 781.2
  autonomic (*see also* Neuropathy, peripheral,
    autonomic) 337.9
  electrolyte 276.9
    with
      abortion—*see* Abortion, by type, with
        metabolic disorder
      ectopic pregnancy (*see also* categories
        633.0-633.9) 639.4
      hyperemesis gravidarum (before 22
        completed weeks gestation) 643.1
      molar pregnancy (*see also* categories
        630-632) 639.4
    following
      abortion 639.4
      ectopic or molar pregnancy 639.4
    neonatal, transitory NEC 775.5
  endocrine 259.9
  eye muscle NEC 378.9
    heterophoria—*see* Heterophoria

Imbalance—*continued*
glomerulotubular NEC 593.89
hormone 259.9
hysterical (*see also* Hysteria) 300.10
labyrinth NEC 386.50
posture 729.9
sympathetic (*see also* Neuropathy, peripheral,
  autonomic) 337.9
Imbecile, imbecility 318.0
moral 301.7
old age 290.9
senile 290.9
specified IQ—*see* IQ
unspecified IQ 318.0
Imbedding, intrauterine device 996.32
Imbibition, cholesterol (gallbladder) 575.6
Imerslund (-Gräsbeck) syndrome (anemia due to
  familial selective vitamin B_{12} malabsorption)
  281.1
Iminoacidopathy 270.8
Iminoglycinuria, familial 270.8
Immature —*see also* Immaturity
personality 301.89
Immaturity 765.1
extreme 765.0
fetus or infant light-for-dates—*see*
  Light-for-dates
lung, fetus or newborn 770.4
organ or site NEC—*see* Hypoplasia
pulmonary, fetus or newborn 770.4
reaction 301.89
sexual (female) (male) 259.0
Immersion 994.1
foot 991.4
hand 991.4
Immobile, immobility
intestine 564.89
joint—*see* Ankylosis
syndrome (paraplegic) 728.3
Immunization
ABO
  affecting management of pregnancy 656.2
  fetus or newborn 773.1
complication—*see* Complications, vaccination
Rh factor
  affecting management of pregnancy 656.1
  fetus or newborn 773.0
  from transfusion 999.7
Immunodeficiency 279.3
with
  adenosine-deaminase deficiency 279.2
  defect, predominant
    B-cell 279.00
    T-cell 279.10
  hyperimmunoglobulinemia 279.2
  lymphopenia, hereditary 279.2
  thrombocytopenia and eczema 279.12
  thymic
    aplasia 279.2
    dysplasia 279.2
autosomal recessive, Swiss-type 279.2
common variable 279.06
severe combined (SCID) 279.2
to Rh factor
  affecting management of pregnancy 656.1
  fetus or newborn 773.0
X-linked, with increased IgM 279.05
Immunotherapy, prophylactic V07.2

Impaction, impacted
bowel, colon, rectum 560.30
  with hernia—*see also* Hernia, by site, with
    obstruction
    gangrenous—*see* Hernia, by site, with
      gangrene
  by
    calculus 560.39
    gallstone 560.31
  fecal 560.39
  specified type NEC 560.39
calculus—*see* Calculus
cerumen (ear) (external) 380.4
cuspid 520.6
  with abnormal position (same or adjacent
    tooth) 524.3
dental 520.6
  with abnormal position (same or adjacent
    tooth) 524.3
fecal, feces 560.39
  with hernia—*see also* Hernia, by site, with
    obstruction
    gangrenous—*see* Hernia, by site, with
      gangrene
fracture—*see* Fracture, by site
gallbladder—*see* Cholelithiasis
gallstone(s)—*see* Cholelithiasis
  in intestine (any part) 560.31
intestine(s) 560.30
  with hernia—*see also* Hernia, by site, with
    obstruction
    gangrenous—*see* Hernia, by site, with
      gangrene
  by
    calculus 560.39
    gallstone 560.31
  fecal 560.39
  specified type NEC 560.39
intrauterine device (IUD) 996.32
molar 520.6
  with abnormal position (same or adjacent
    tooth) 524.3
shoulder 660.4
  affecting fetus or newborn 763.1
tooth, teeth 520.6
  with abnormal position (same or adjacent
    tooth) 524.3
turbinate 733.99
Impaired, impairment (function)
arm V49.1
  movement, involving
    musculoskeletal system V49.1
    nervous system V49.2
auditory discrimination 388.43
back V48.3
body (entire) V49.89
hearing (*see also* Deafness) 389.9
heart—*see* Disease, heart
kidney (*see also* Disease, renal) 593.9
  disorder resulting from 588.9
  specified NEC 588.8
leg V49.1
  movement, involving
    musculoskeletal system V49.1
    nervous system V49.2
limb V49.1
  movement, involving
    musculoskeletal system V49.1
    nervous system V49.2
liver 573.8
mastication 524.9

Impaired, impairment—*continued*
mobility
  ear ossicles NEC 385.22
  incostapedial joint 385.22
  malleus 385.21
myocardium, myocardial (*see also*
  Insufficiency, myocardial) 428.0
neuromusculoskeletal NEC V49.89
  back V48.3
  head V48.2
  limb V49.2
  neck V48.3
  spine V48.3
  trunk V48.3
rectal sphincter 787.99
renal (*see also* Disease, renal) 593.9
  disorder resulting from 588.9
    specified NEC 588.8
spine V48.3
vision NEC 369.9
  both eyes NEC 369.3
  moderate 369.74
    both eyes 369.25
      with impairment of lesser eye (specified
        as)
        blind, not further specified 369.15
        low vision, not further specified 369.23
        near-total 369.17
        profound 369.18
        severe 369.24
        total 369.16
    one eye 369.74
      with vision of other eye (specified as)
        near-normal 369.75
        normal 369.76
  near-total 369.64
    both eyes 369.04
      with impairment of lesser eye (specified
        as)
        blind, not further specified 369.02
        total 369.03
    one eye 369.64
      with vision of other eye (specified as)
        near-normal 369.65
        normal 369.66
  one eye 369.60
    with low vision of other eye 369.10
  profound 369.67
    both eyes 369.08
      with impairment of lesser eye (specified
        as)
        blind, not further specified 369.05
        near-total 369.07
        total 369.06
    one eye 369.67
      with vision of other eye (specified as)
        near-normal 369.68
        normal 369.69
  severe 369.71
    both eyes 369.22
      with impairment of lesser eye (specified
        as)
        blind, not further specified 369.11
        low vision, not further specified 369.21
        near-total 369.13
        profound 369.14
        total 369.12
    one eye 369.71
      with vision of other eye (specified as)
        near-normal 369.72
        normal 369.73

Impaired, impairment—*continued*
total
  both eyes 369.01
  one eye 369.61
    with vision of other eye (specified as)
      near-normal 369.62
      normal 369.63
Impaludism —*see* Malaria
Impediment, speech NEC 784.5
psychogenic 307.9
secondary to organic lesion 784.5
Impending
cerebrovascular accident or attack 435.9
coronary syndrome 411.1
delirium tremens 291.0
myocardial infarction 411.1
Imperception, auditory (acquired) (congenital)
389.9
Imperfect
aeration, lung (newborn) 770.5
closure (congenital)
  alimentary tract NEC 751.8
    lower 751.5
    upper 750.8
  atrioventricular ostium 745.69
  atrium (secundum) 745.5
    primum 745.61
  branchial cleft or sinus 744.41
  choroid 743.59
  cricoid cartilage 748.3
  cusps, heart valve NEC 746.89
    pulmonary 746.09
  ductus
    arteriosus 747.0
    Botalli 747.0
  ear drum 744.29
    causing impairment of hearing 744.03
  endocardial cushion 745.60
  epiglottis 748.3
  esophagus with communication to bronchus
    or trachea 750.3
  Eustachian valve 746.89
  eyelid 743.62
  face, facial (*see also* Cleft, lip) 749.10
  foramen
    Botalli 745.5
    ovale 745.5
  genitalia, genital organ(s) or system
    female 752.8
      external 752.49
      internal NEC 752.8
      uterus 752.3
    male 752.8
      penis 752.69
  glottis 748.3
  heart valve (cusps) NEC 746.89
  interatrial ostium or septum 745.5
  interauricular ostium or septum 745.5
  interventricular ostium or septum 745.4
  iris 743.46
  kidney 753.3
  larynx 748.3
  lens 743.36
  lip (*see also* Cleft, lip) 749.10
  nasal septum or sinus 748.1
  nose 748.1
  omphalomesenteric duct 751.0
  optic nerve entry 743.57
  organ or site NEC—*see* Anomaly, specified
    type, by site

Inebriety (*see also* Abuse, drugs, nondependent) 305.0
Inefficiency
  kidney (*see also* Disease, renal) 593.9
  thyroid (acquired) (gland) 244.9
Inelasticity, skin 782.8
Inequality, leg (acquired) (length) 736.81
  congenital 755.30
Inertia
  bladder 596.4
    neurogenic 596.54
      with cauda equina syndrome 344.61
  stomach 536.8
    psychogenic 306.4
  uterus, uterine 661.2
    affecting fetus or newborn 763.7
    primary 661.0
    secondary 661.1
  vesical 596.4
    neurogenic 596.54
      with cauda equina 344.61
Infant —*see also* condition
  excessive crying of 780.92
  fussy (baby) 780.91
  held for adoption V68.89
  newborn—*see* Newborn
  syndrome of diabetic mother 775.0
"Infant Hercules" syndrome 255.2
Infantile —*see also* condition
  genitalia, genitals 259.0
    in pregnancy or childbirth NEC 654.4
      affecting fetus or newborn 763.89
      causing obstructed labor 660.2
        affecting fetus or newborn 763.1
  heart 746.9
  kidney 753.3
  lack of care 995.52
  macula degeneration 362.75
  melanodontia 521.05
  os, uterus (*see also* Infantile, genitalia) 259.0
  pelvis 738.6
    with disproportion (fetopelvic) 653.1
      affecting fetus or newborn 763.1
      causing obstructed labor 660.1
        affecting fetus or newborn 763.1
  penis 259.0
  testis 257.2
  uterus (*see also* Infantile, genitalia) 259.0
  vulva 752.49
Infantilism 259.9
  with dwarfism (hypophyseal) 253.3
  Brissaud's (infantile myxedema) 244.9
  celiac 579.0
  Herter's (nontropical sprue) 579.0
  hypophyseal 253.3
  hypothalamic (with obesity) 253.8
  idiopathic 259.9
  intestinal 579.0
  pancreatic 577.8
  pituitary 253.3
  renal 588.0
  sexual (with obesity) 259.0
Infants, healthy liveborn —*see* Newborn
Infarct, infarction
  adrenal (capsule) (gland) 255.4
  amnion 658.8
  anterior (with contiguous portion of intraventricular septum) NEC (*see also* Infarct, myocardium) 410.1
  appendices epiploicae 557.0
  bowel 557.0

Infarct, infarction—*continued*
  brain (stem) 434.91
    embolic (*see also* Embolism, brain) 434.11
    healed or old, without residuals V12.59
    iatrogenic 997.02
    postoperative 997.02
    puerperal, postpartum, childbirth 674.0
    thrombotic (*see also* Thrombosis, brain) 434.01
  breast 611.8
  Brewer's (kidney) 593.81
  cardiac (*see also* Infarct, myocardium) 410.9
  cerebellar (*see also* Infarct, brain) 434.91
    embolic (*see also* Embolism, brain) 434.11
  cerebral (*see also* Infarct, brain) 434.91
    embolic (*see also* Embolism, brain) 434.11
  chorion 658.8
  colon (acute) (agnogenic) (embolic) (hemorrhagic) (nonocclusive) (nonthrombotic) (occlusive) (segmental) (thrombotic) (with gangrene) 557.0
  coronary artery (*see also* Infarct, myocardium) 410.9
  embolic (*see also* Embolism) 444.9
  fallopian tube 620.8
  gallbladder 575.8
  heart (*see also* Infarct, myocardium) 410.9
  hepatic 573.4
  hypophysis (anterior lobe) 253.8
  impending (myocardium) 411.1
  intestine (acute) (agnogenic) (embolic) (hemorrhagic) (nonocclusive) (nonthrombotic) (occlusive) (thrombotic) (with gangrene) 557.0
  kidney 593.81
  liver 573.4
  lung (embolic) (thrombotic) 415.19
    with
      abortion—*see* Abortion, by type, with, embolism
      ectopic pregnancy (*see also* categories 633.0-633.9) 639.6
      molar pregnancy (*see also* categories 630-632) 639.6
    following
      abortion 639.6
      ectopic or molar pregnancy 639.6
    iatrogenic 415.11
    in pregnancy, childbirth, or puerperium—*see* Embolism, obstetrical
    postoperative 415.11
  lymph node or vessel 457.8
  medullary (brain)—*see* Infarct, brain
  meibomian gland (eyelid) 374.85
  mesentery, mesenteric (embolic) (thrombotic) (with gangrene) 557.0
  midbrain—*see* Infarct, brain
  myocardium, myocardial (acute or with a stated duration of 8 weeks or less) (with hypertension) 410.9

Note—use the following fifth-digit subclassification with category 410

0 *episode unspecified*
1 *initial episode*
2 *subsequent episode without recurrence*

Infarct, infarction—*continued*
with symptoms after 8 weeks from date of
infarction 414.8
anterior (wall) (with contiguous portion of
intraventricular septum) NEC 410.1
anteroapical (with contiguous portion of
intraventricular septum) 410.1
anterolateral (wall) 410.0
anteroseptal (with contiguous portion of
intraventricular septum) 410.1
apical-lateral 410.5
atrial 410.8
basal-lateral 410.5
chronic (with symptoms after 8 weeks from
date of infarction) 414.8
diagnosed on ECG, but presenting no
symptoms 412
diaphragmatic wall (with contiguous portion
of intraventricular septum) 410.4
healed or old, currently presenting no
symptoms 412
high lateral 410.5
impending 411.1
inferior (wall) (with contiguous portion of
intraventricular septum) 410.4
inferolateral (wall) 410.2
inferoposterior wall 410.3
lateral wall 410.5
nontransmural 410.7
papillary muscle 410.8
past (diagnosed on ECG or other special
investigation, but correctly presenting no
symptoms) 412
with symptoms NEC 414.8
posterior (strictly) (true) (wall) 410.6
posterobasal 410.6
posteroinferior 410.3
posterolateral 410.5
previous, currently presenting no symptoms
412
septal 410.8
specified site NEC 410.8
subendocardial 410.7
syphilitic 093.82
nontransmural 410.7
omentum 557.0
ovary 620.8
pancreas 577.8
papillary muscle (*see also* Infarct, myocardium)
410.8
parathyroid gland 252.8
pituitary (gland) 253.8
placenta (complicating pregnancy) 656.7
affecting fetus or newborn 762.2
pontine—*see* Infarct, brain
posterior NEC (*see also* Infarct, myocardium)
410.6
prostate 602.8
pulmonary (artery) (hemorrhagic) (vein) 415.19
with
abortion—*see* Abortion, by type, with
embolism
ectopic pregnancy (*see also* categories
633.0-633.9) 639.6
molar pregnancy (*see also* categories
630-632) 639.6
following
abortion 639.6
ectopic or molar pregnancy 639.6
iatrogenic 415.11

Infarct, infarction—*continued*
in pregnancy, childbirth, or puerperium—*see*
Embolism, obstetrical
postoperative 415.11
renal 593.81
embolic or thrombotic 593.81
retina, retinal 362.84
with occlusion—*see* Occlusion, retina
spinal (acute) (cord) (embolic) (nonembolic)
336.1
spleen 289.59
embolic or thrombotic 444.89
subchorionic—*see* Infarct, placenta
subendocardial (*see also* Infarct, myocardium)
410.7
suprarenal (capsule) (gland) 255.4
syncytium—*see* Infarct, placenta
testis 608.83
thrombotic (*see also* Thrombosis) 453.9
artery, arterial—*see* Embolism
thyroid (gland) 246.3
ventricle (heart) (*see also* Infarct, myocardium)
410.9
Infecting —*see* condition
Infection, infected, infective (opportunistic)
136.9
with lymphangitis—*see* Lymphangitis
abortion—*see* Abortion, by type, with sepsis
abscess (skin)—*see* Abscess, by site
Absidia 117.7
Acanthocheilonema (perstans) 125.4
streptocerca 125.6
accessory sinus (chronic) (*see also* Sinusitis)
473.9
Achorion—*see* Dermatophytosis
Acremonium falciforme 117.4
acromioclavicular (joint) 711.91
actinobacillus
lignieresii 027.8
mallei 024
muris 026.1
actinomadura—*see* Actinomycosis
Actinomyces (israelii)—*see also* Actinomycosis
muris-ratti 026.1
Actinomycetales (actinomadura) (Actinomyces)
(Nocardia) (Streptomyces)—*see*
Actinomycosis
actinomycotic NEC (*see also* Actinomycosis)
039.9
adenoid (chronic) 474.01
acute 463
and tonsil (chronic) 474.02
acute or subacute 463
adenovirus NEC 079.0
in diseases classified elsewhere—*see* category
079
unspecified nature or site 079.0
Aerobacter aerogenes NEC 041.85
enteritis 008.2
aerogenes capsulatus (*see also* Gangrene, gas)
040.0
aertrycke (*see also* Infection, Salmonella) 003.9
ajellomyces dermatitidis 116.0
alimentary canal NEC (*see also* Enteritis, due
to, by organism) 009.0
Allescheria boydii 117.6
Alternaria 118
alveolus, alveolar (process) (pulpal origin) 522.4
ameba, amebic (histolytica) (*see also*
Amebiasis) 006.9
acute 006.0

Infection, infected, infective—*continued*
  chronic 006.1
  free-living 136.2
  hartmanni 007.8
  specified
    site NEC 006.8
    type NEC 007.8
  amniotic fluid or cavity 658.4
    affecting fetus or newborn 762.7
  anaerobes (cocci) (gram-negative) (gram
    positive) (mixed) NEC 041.84
  anal canal 569.49
  Ancylostoma braziliense 126.2
  Angiostrongylus cantonensis 128.8
  anisakiasis 127.1
  Anisakis larva 127.1
  anthrax (*see also* Anthrax) 022.9
  antrum (chronic) (*see also* Sinusitis, maxillary)
    473.0
  anus (papillae) (sphincter) 569.49
  arbor virus NEC 066.9
  arbovirus NEC 066.9
  argentophil-rod 027.0
  Ascaris lumbricoides 127.0
  ascomycetes 117.4
  Aspergillus (flavus) (fumigatus) (terreus) 117.3
  atypical
    acid-fast (bacilli) (*see also* Mycobacterium,
      atypical) 031.9
    mycobacteria (*see also* Mycobacterium,
      atypical) 031.9
  auditory meatus (circumscribed) (diffuse)
    (external) (*see also* Otitis, externa) 380.10
  auricle (ear) (*see also* Otitis, externa) 380.10
  axillary gland 683
  Babesiasis 088.82
  Babesiosis 088.82
  Bacillus NEC 041.89
    abortus 023.1
    anthracis (*see also* Anthrax) 022.9
    cereus (food poisoning) 005.89
    coli—*see* Infection, Escherichia coli
    coliform NEC 041.85
    Ducrey's (any location) 099.0
    Flexner's 004.1
    fragilis NEC 041.82
    Friedländer's NEC 041.3
    fusiformis 101
    gas (gangrene) (*see also* Gangrene, gas) 040.0
    mallei 024
    melitensis 023.0
    paratyphoid, paratyphosus 002.9
      A 002.1
      B 002.2
      C 002.3
    Schmorl's 040.3
    Shiga 004.0
    suipestifer (*see also* Infection, Salmonella)
      003.9
    swimming pool 031.1
    typhosa 002.0
    welchii (*see also* Gangrene, gas) 040.0
    Whitmore's 025
  bacterial NEC 041.9
    specified NEC 041.89
      anaerobic NEC 041.84
      gram-negative NEC 041.85
      anaerobic NEC 041.84
  Bacterium
    paratyphosum 002.9
      A 002.1

Infection, infected, infective—*continued*
      B 002.2
      C 002.3
    typhosum 002.0
  Bacteroides (fragilis) (melaninogenicus) (oralis)
    NEC 041.84
  balantidium coli 007.0
  Bartholin's gland 616.8
  Basidiobolus 117.7
  Bedsonia 079.98
    specified NEC 079.88
  bile duct 576.1
  bladder (*see also* Cystitis) 595.9
  Blastomyces, blastomycotic 116.0
    brasiliensis 116.1
    dermatitidis 116.0
    European 117.5
    Loboi 116.2
    North American 116.0
    South American 116.1
  blood stream—*see* Septicemia
  bone 730.9
    specified—*see* Osteomyelitis
  Bordetella 033.9
    bronchiseptica 033.8
    parapertussis 033.1
    pertussis 033.0
  Borrelia
    bergdorfi 088.81
    vincentii (mouth) (pharynx) (tonsil) 101
  brain (*see also* Encephalitis) 323.9
    late effect—*see* category 326
    membranes—(*see also* Meningitis) 322.9
    septic 324.0
      late effect—*see* category 326
      meninges (*see also* Meningitis) 320.9
  branchial cyst 744.42
  breast 611.0
    puerperal, postpartum 675.2
      with nipple 675.9
        specified type NEC 675.8
      nonpurulent 675.2
      purulent 675.1
  bronchus (*see also* Bronchitis) 490
    fungus NEC 117.9
  Brucella 023.9
    abortus 023.1
    canis 023.3
    melitensis 023.0
    mixed 023.8
    suis 023.2
  Brugia (Wuchereria) malayi 125.1
  bursa—*see* Bursitis
  buttocks (skin) 686.9
  Candida (albicans) (tropicalis) (*see also*
    Candidiasis) 112.9
    congenital 771.7
  Candiru 136.8
  Capillaria
    hepatica 128.8
    philippinensis 127.5
  cartilage 733.99
  cat liver fluke 121.0
  cellulitis—*see* Cellulitis, by site
  Cephalosporum falciforme 117.4
  Cercomonas hominis (intestinal) 007.3
  cerebrospinal (*see also* Meningitis) 322.9
    late effect—*see* category 326
  cervical gland 683
  cervix (*see also* Cervicitis) 616.0
  cesarean section wound 674.3

Infection, infected, infective—*continued*
  Chilomastix (intestinal) 007.8
  Chlamydia 079.98
    specified NEC 079.88
  Cholera (*see also* Cholera) 001.9
  chorionic plate 658.8
  Cladosporium
    bantianum 117.8
    carrionii 117.2
    mansoni 111.1
    trichoides 117.8
    wernecki 111.1
  Clonorchis (sinensis) (liver) 121.1
  Clostridium (haemolyticum) (novyi) NEC
      041.84
    botulinum 005.1
    congenital 771.89
    histolyticum (*see also* Gangrene, gas) 040.0
    oedematiens (*see also* Gangrene, gas) 040.0
    perfringens 041.83
      due to food 005.2
    septicum (*see also* Gangrene, gas) 040.0
    sordelii (*see also* Gangrene, gas) 040.0
    welchii (*see also* Gangrene, gas) 040.0
      due to food 005.2
  Coccidioides (immitis) (*see also*
      Coccidioidomycosis) 114.9
  coccus NEC 041.89
  colon (*see also* Enteritis, due to, by organism)
      009.0
    bacillus—*see* Infection, Escherichia coli
  colostomy or enterostomy 569.61
  common duct 576.1
  complicating pregnancy, childbirth, or
      puerperium NEC 647.9
    affecting fetus or newborn 760.2
  Condiobolus 117.7
  congenital NEC 771.89
    Candida albicans 771.7
    chronic 771.2
    clostridial 771.89
    Cytomegalovirus 771.1
    Escherichia coli 771.89
    hepatitis, viral 771.2
    Herpes simplex 771.2
    listeriosis 771.2
    malaria 771.2
    poliomyelitis 771.2
    rubella 771.0
    Salmonella 771.89
    streptococcal 771.89
    toxoplasmosis 771.2
    tuberculosis 771.2
    urinary (tract) 771.82
    vaccinia 771.2
  corpus luteum (*see also* Salpingo-oophoritis)
      614.2
  Corynebacterium diphtheriae—*see* Diphtheria
  Coxsackie (*see also* Coxsackie) 079.2
    endocardium 074.22
    heart NEC 074.20
    in diseases classified elsewhere—*see* category
        079
    meninges 047.0
    myocardium 074.23
    pericardium 074.21
    pharynx 074.0
    specified disease NEC 074.8
    unspecified nature or site 079.2
  Cryptococcus neoformans 117.5
  Cryptosporidia 007.4

Infection, infected, infective—*continued*
  Cunninghamella 117.7
  cyst—*see* Cyst
  Cysticercus cellulosae 123.1
  cytomegalovirus 078.5
    congenital 771.1
  dental (pulpal origin) 522.4
  deuteromycetes 117.4
  Dicrocoelium dendriticum 121.8
  Dipetalonema (perstans) 125.4
    streptocerca 125.6
  diphtherial—*see* Diphtheria
  Diphyllobothrium (adult) (latum) (pacificum)
      123.4
    larval 123.5
  Diplogonoporus (grandis) 123.8
  Dipylidium (caninum) 123.8
  Dirofilaria 125.6
  dog tapeworm 123.8
  Dracunculus medinensis 125.7
  Dreschlera 118
    hawaiiensis 117.8
  Ducrey's bacillus (any site) 099.0
  due to or resulting from
    device, implant, or graft (any) (presence
        of)—*see* Complications, infection and
        inflammation, due to (presence of) any
        device, implant, or graft classified to
        996.0-996.5 NEC
    injection, inoculation, infusion, transfusion, or
        vaccination (prophylactic) (therapeutic)
        999.3
    injury NEC—*see* Wound, open, by site,
        complicated
    surgery 998.59
  duodenum 535.6
  ear—*see also* Otitis
    external (*see also* Otitis, externa) 380.10
    inner (*see also* Labyrinthitis) 386.30
    middle —*see* Otitis, media
  Eaton's agent NEC 041.81
  Eberthella typhosa 002.0
  Ebola 065.8
  echinococcosis 122.9
  Echinococcus (*see also* Echinococcus) 122.9
  Echinostoma 121.8
  ECHO virus 079.1
    in diseases classified elsewhere—*see* category
        079
    unspecified nature or site 079.1
  Ehrlichiosis 082.40
    chaffeensis 082.41
    specified type NEC 082.49
  Endamoeba—*see* Infection, ameba
  endocardium (*see also* Endocarditis) 421.0
  endocervix (*see also* Cervicitis) 616.0
  Entamoeba—*see* Infection, ameba
  enteric (*see also* Enteritis, due to, by organism)
      009.0
  Enterobacter aerogenes NEC 041.85
  Enterobius vermicularis 127.4
  enterococcus NEC 041.04
  enterovirus NEC 079.89
    central nervous system NEC 048
    enteritis 008.67
    meningitis 047.9
  Entomophthora 117.7
  Epidermophyton—*see* Dermatophytosis
  epidermophytosis—*see* Dermatophytosis
  episiotomy 674.3

Infection, infected, infective—*continued*
  Epstein-Barr virus 075
    chronic 780.79 *[139.8]*
  erysipeloid 027.1
  Erysipelothrix (insidiosa) (rhusiopathiae) 027.1
  erythema infectiosum 057.0
  Escherichia coli NEC 041.4
    congenital 771.89
    enteritis—*see* Enteritis, E. coli
    generalized 038.42
    intestinal—*see* Enteritis, E. coli
  ethmoidal (chronic) (sinus) (*see also* Sinusitis,
      ethmoidal) 473.2
  Eubacterium 041.84
  Eustachian tube (ear) 381.50
    acute 381.51
    chronic 381.52
  exanthema subitum 057.8
  external auditory canal (meatus) (*see also* Otitis,
      externa) 380.10
  eye NEC 360.00
  eyelid 373.9
    specified NEC 373.8
  fallopian tube (*see also* Salpingo-oophoritis)
      614.2
  fascia 728.89
  Fasciola
    gigantica 121.3
    hepatica 121.3
  Fasciolopsis (buski) 121.4
  fetus (intra-amniotic)—*see* Infection, congenital
  filarial—*see* Infestation, filarial
  finger (skin) 686.9
    abscess (with lymphangitis) 681.00
      pulp 681.01
    cellulitis (with lymphangitis) 681.00
    distal closed space (with lymphangitis) 681.00
    nail 681.02
      fungus 110.1
  fish tapeworm 123.4
    larval 123.5
  flagellate, intestinal 007.9
  fluke—*see* Infestation, fluke
  focal
    teeth (pulpal origin) 522.4
    tonsils 474.00
      and adenoids 474.02
  Fonsecaea
    compactum 117.2
    pedrosoi 117.2
  food (*see also* Poisoning, food) 005.9
  foot (skin) 686.9
    fungus 110.4
  Francisella tularensis (*see also* Tularemia) 021.9
  frontal sinus (chronic) (*see also* Sinusitis,
      frontal) 473.1
  fungus NEC 117.9
    beard 110.0
    body 110.5
    dermatiacious NEC 117.8
    foot 110.4
    groin 110.3
    hand 110.2
    nail 110.1
    pathogenic to compromised host only 118
    perianal (area) 110.3
    scalp 110.0
    scrotum 110.8
    skin 111.9
      foot 110.4
      hand 110.2

Infection, infected, infective—*continued*
  toenails 110.1
  trachea 117.9
  Fusarium 118
  Fusobacterium 041.84
  gallbladder (*see also* Cholecystitis, acute) 575.0
  Gardnerella vaginalis 041.89
  gas bacillus (*see also* Gas, gangrene) 040.0
  gastric (*see also* Gastritis) 535.5
  Gastrodiscoides hominis 121.8
  gastroenteric (*see also* Enteritis, due to, by
      organism) 009.0
  gastrointestinal (*see also* Enteritis, due to, by
      organism) 009.0
  gastrostomy 536.41
  generalized NEC (*see also* Septicemia) 038.9
  genital organ or tract NEC
    female 614.9
      with
        abortion—*see* Abortion, by type, with
          sepsis
        ectopic pregnancy (*see also* categories
          633.0-633.9) 639.0
        molar pregnancy (*see also* categories
          630-632) 639.0
      complicating pregnancy 646.6
        affecting fetus or newborn 760.8
      following
        abortion 639.0
        ectopic or molar pregnancy 639.0
      puerperal, postpartum, childbirth 670
        minor or localized 646.6
          affecting fetus or newborn 760.8
    male 608.4
  genitourinary tract NEC 599.0
  Ghon tubercle, primary (*see also* Tuberculosis)
      010.0
  Giardia lamblia 007.1
  gingival (chronic) 523.1
    acute 523.0
    Vincent's 101
  glanders 024
  Glenosporopsis amazonica 116.2
  Gnathostoma spinigerum 128.1
  Gongylonema 125.6
  gonococcal NEC (*see also* Gonococcus) 098.0
  gram-negative bacilli NEC 041.85
    anaerobic 041.84
  guinea worm 125.7
  gum (*see also* Infection, gingival) 523.1
  Hantavirus 079.81
  heart 429.89
  Helicobacter pylori (H. pylori) 041.86
  helminths NEC 128.9
    intestinal 127.9
      mixed (types classifiable to more than one
        category in 120.0-127.7) 127.8
      specified type NEC 127.7
    specified type NEC 128.8
  Hemophilus influenzae NEC 041.5
    generalized 038.41
  Herpes (simplex) (*see also* Herpes, simplex)
      054.9
    congenital 771.2
    zoster (*see also* Herpes, zoster) 053.9
      eye NEC 053.29
  Heterophyes heterophyes 121.6
  Histoplasma (*see also* Histoplasmosis) 115.90
    capsulatum (*see also* Histoplasmosis,
      American) 115.00

Infection, infected, infective—*continued*
  duboisii (*see also* Histoplasmosis, African)
    115.10
  HIV V08
    with symptoms, symptomatic 042
  hookworm (*see also* Ancylostomiasis) 126.9
  human immunodeficiency virus V08
    with symptoms, symptomatic 042
  human papillomavirus 079.4
  hydrocele 603.1
  hydronephrosis 591
  Hymenolepis 123.6
  hypopharynx 478.29
  inguinal glands 683
    due to soft chancre 099.0
  intestine, intestinal (*see also* Enteritis, due to, by organism) 009.0
  intrauterine (*see also* Endometritis) 615.9
    complicating delivery 646.6
  isospora belli or hominis 007.2
  Japanese B encephalitis 062.0
  jaw (bone) (acute) (chronic) (lower) (subacute) (upper) 526.4
  joint—*see* Arthritis, infectious or infective
  kidney (cortex) (hematogenous) 590.9
    with
      abortion—*see* Abortion, by type, with urinary tract infection
      calculus 592.0
      ectopic pregnancy (*see also* categories 633.0-633.9) 639.8
      molar pregnancy (*see also* categories 630-632) 639.8
    complicating pregnancy or puerperium 646.6
      affecting fetus or newborn 760.1
    following
      abortion 639.8
      ectopic or molar pregnancy 639.8
    pelvis and ureter 590.3
  Klebsiella pneumoniae NEC 041.3
  knee (skin) NEC 686.9
    joint—*see* Arthritis, infectious
  Koch's (*see also* Tuberculosis, pulmonary) 011.9
  labia (majora) (minora) (*see also* Vulvitis) 616.10
  lacrimal
    gland (*see also* Dacryoadenitis) 375.00
    passages (duct) (sac) (*see also* Dacryocystitis) 375.30
  larynx NEC 478.79
  leg (skin) NEC 686.9
  Leishmania (*see also* Leishmaniasis) 085.9
    braziliensis 085.5
    donovani 085.0
    Ethiopica 085.3
    furunculosa 085.1
    infantum 085.0
    mexicana 085.4
    tropica (minor) 085.1
      major 085.2
  Leptosphaeria senegalensis 117.4
  leptospira (*see also* Leptospirosis) 100.9
    Australis 100.89
    Bataviae 100.89
    pyrogenes 100.89
    specified type NEC 100.89
  leptospirochetal NEC (*see also* Leptospirosis) 100.9
  Leptothrix—*see* Actinomycosis

Infection, infected, infective—*continued*
  Listeria monocytogenes (listeriosis) 027.0
    congenital 771.2
  liver fluke—*see* Infestation, fluke, liver
  Loa loa 125.2
    eyelid 125.2 *[373.6]*
  Loboa loboi 116.2
  local, skin (staphylococcal) (streptococcal) NEC 686.9
    abscess—*see* Abscess, by site
    cellulitis—*see* Cellulitis, by site
    ulcer (*see also* Ulcer, skin) 707.9
  Loefflerella
    mallei 024
    whitmori 025
  lung 518.89
    atypical Mycobacterium 031.0
      tuberculous (*see also* Tuberculosis, pulmonary) 011.9
    basilar 518.89
    chronic 518.89
    fungus NEC 117.9
    spirochetal 104.8
    virus—*see* Pneumonia, virus
  lymph gland (axillary) (cervical) (inguinal) 683
    mesenteric 289.2
  lymphoid tissue, base of tongue or posterior pharynx, NEC 474.00
  madurella
    grisea 117.4
    mycetomii 117.4
  major
    with
      abortion—*see* Abortion, by type, with sepsis
      ectopic pregnancy (*see also* categories 633.0-633.9) 639.0
      molar pregnancy (*see also* categories 630-632) 639.0
    following
      abortion 639.0
      ectopic or molar pregnancy 639.0
    puerperal, postpartum, childbirth 670
  malarial—*see* Malaria
  Malassezia furfur 111.0
  Malleomyces
    mallei 024
    pseudomallei 025
  mammary gland 611.0
    puerperal, postpartum 675.2
  Mansonella (ozzardi) 125.5
  mastoid (suppurative)—*see* Mastoiditis
  maxilla, maxillary 526.4
    sinus (chronic) (*see also* Sinusitis, maxillary) 473.0
  mediastinum 519.2
  medina 125.7
  meibomian
    cyst 373.12
    gland 373.12
  melioidosis 025
  meninges (*see also* Meningitis) 320.9
  meningococcal (*see also* condition) 036.9
    brain 036.1
    cerebrospinal 036.0
    endocardium 036.42
    generalized 036.2
    meninges 036.0
    meningococcemia 036.2
    specified site NEC 036.89
  mesenteric lymph nodes or glands NEC 289.2
  Metagonimus 121.5

Infection, infected, infective—*continued*
metatarsophalangeal 711.97
microorganism resistant to drugs—*see*
Resistance (to), drugs by microorganisms
Microsporidia 136.8
microsporum, microsporic—*see*
Dermatophytosis
Mima polymorpha NEC 041.85
mixed flora NEC 041.89
Monilia (*see also* Candidiasis) 112.9
neonatal 771.7
Monosporium apiospermum 117.6
mouth (focus) NEC 528.9
parasitic 112.0
Mucor 117.7
muscle NEC 728.89
mycelium NEC 117.9
mycetoma
actinomycotic NEC (*see also* Actinomycosis)
039.9
mycotic NEC 117.4
Mycobacterium, mycobacterial (*see also*
Mycobacterium) 031.9
mycoplasma NEC 041.81
mycotic NEC 117.9
pathogenic to compromised host only 118
skin NEC 111.9
systemic 117.9
myocardium NEC 422.90
nail (chronic) (with lymphangitis) 681.9
finger 681.02
fungus 110.1
ingrowing 703.0
toe 681.11
fungus 110.1
nasal sinus (chronic) (*see also* Sinusitis) 473.9
nasopharynx (chronic) 478.29
acute 460
navel 686.9
newborn 771.4
Neisserian—*see* Gonococcus
Neotestudina rosatii 117.4
newborn, generalized 771.89
nipple 611.0
puerperal, postpartum 675.0
with breast 675.9
specified type NEC 675.8
Nocardia—*see* Actinomycosis
nose 478.1
nostril 478.1
obstetrical surgical wound 674.3
Oesophagostomum (apiostomum) 127.7
Oestrus ovis 134.0
Oidium albicans (*see also* Candidiasis) 112.9
Onchocerca (volvulus) 125.3
eye 125.3 *[360.13]*
eyelid 125.3 *[373.6]*
operation wound 998.59
Opisthorchis (felineus) (tenuicollis) (viverrini)
121.0
orbit 376.00
chronic 376.10
ovary (*see also* Salpingo-oophoritis) 614.2
Oxyuris vermicularis 127.4
pancreas 577.0
Paracoccidioides brasiliensis 116.1
Paragonimus (westermani) 121.2
parainfluenza virus 079.89
parameningococcus NEC 036.9
with meningitis 036.0
parasitic NEC 136.9

Infection, infected, infective—*continued*
paratyphoid 002.9
Type A 002.1
Type B 002.2
Type C 002.3
paraurethral ducts 597.89
parotid gland 527.2
Pasteurella NEC 027.2
multocida (cat-bite) (dog-bite) 027.2
pestis (*see also* Plague) 020.9
pseudotuberculosis 027.2
septica (cat-bite) (dog-bite) 027.2
tularensis (*see also* Tularemia) 021.9
pelvic, female (*see also* Disease, pelvis,
inflammatory) 614.9
penis (glans) (retention) NEC 607.2
herpetic 054.13
Peptococcus 041.84
Peptostreptococcus 041.84
periapical (pulpal origin) 522.4
peridental 523.3
perineal wound (obstetrical) 674.3
periodontal 523.3
periorbital 376.00
chronic 376.10
perirectal 569.49
perirenal (*see also* Infection, kidney) 590.9
peritoneal (*see also* Peritonitis) 567.9
periureteral 593.89
periurethral 597.89
Petriellidium boydii 117.6
pharynx 478.29
Coxsackie virus 074.0
phlegmonous 462
posterior, lymphoid 474.00
Phialophora
gougerotii 117.8
jeanselmei 117.8
verrucosa 117.2
Piedraia hortai 111.3
pinna, acute 380.11
pinta 103.9
intermediate 103.1
late 103.2
mixed 103.3
primary 103.0
pinworm 127.4
pityrosporum furfur 111.0
pleuropneumonia-like organisms NEC (PPLO)
041.81
pneumococcal NEC 041.2
generalized (purulent) 038.2
Pneumococcus NEC 041.2
postoperative wound 998.59
posttraumatic NEC 958.3
postvaccinal 999.3
prepuce NEC 607.1
Propionibacterium 041.84
prostate (capsule) (*see also* Prostatitis) 601.9
Proteus (mirabilis) (morganii) (vulgaris) NEC
041.6
enteritis 008.3
protozoal NEC 136.8
intestinal NEC 007.9
Pseudomonas NEC 041.7
mallei 024
pneumonia 482.1
pseudomallei 025
psittacosis 073.9
puerperal, postpartum (major) 670
minor 646.6

Infection, infected, infective—*continued*
pulmonary—*see* Infection, lung
purulent—*see* Abscess
putrid, generalized—*see* Septicemia
pyemic—*see* Septicemia
Pyrenochaeta romeroi 117.4
Q fever 083.0
rabies 071
rectum (sphincter) 569.49
renal (*see also* Infection, kidney) 590.9
  pelvis and ureter 590.3
resistant to drugs—*see* Resistance (to), drugs by
    microorganisms
respiratory 519.8
  chronic 519.8
  influenzal (acute) (upper) 487.1
  lung 518.89
  rhinovirus 460
  syncytial virus 079.6
  upper (acute) (infectious) NEC 465.9
    with flu, grippe, or influenza 487.1
    influenzal 487.1
    multiple sites NEC 465.8
    streptococcal 034.0
    viral NEC 465.9
respiratory syncytial virus (RSV) 079.6
resulting from presence of shunt or other
    internal prosthetic device—*see*
    Complications, infection and inflammation,
    due to (presence of) any device, implant, or
    graft classified to 996.0-996.5 NEC
retrovirus 079.50
  human immunodeficiency virus type 2
    [HIV-2] 079.53
  human T-cell lymphotrophic virus type I
    [HTLV-I] 079.51
  human T-cell lymphotrophic virus type II
    [HTLV-II] 079.52
  specified NEC 079.59
Rhinocladium 117.1
Rhinosporidium (seeberi) 117.0
rhinovirus
  in diseases classified elsewhere—*see* category
    079
  unspecified nature or site 079.3
Rhizopus 117.7
rickettsial 083.9
rickettsialpox 083.2
rubella (*see also* Rubella) 056.9
  congenital 771.0
Saccharomyces (*see also* Candidiasis) 112.9
Saksenaea 117.7
salivary duct or gland (any) 527.2
Salmonella (aertrycke) (callinarum)
    (choleraesuis) (enteritidis) (suipestifer)
    (typhimurium) 003.9
  with
    arthritis 003.23
    gastroenteritis 003.0
    localized infection 003.20
      specified type NEC 003.29
    meningitis 003.21
    osteomyelitis 003.24
    pneumonia 003.22
    septicemia 003.1
    specified manifestation NEC 003.8
  congenital 771.89
  due to food (poisoning) (any serotype) (*see*
    also Poisoning, food, due to, Salmonella)
  hirschfeldii 002.3
  localized 003.20

Infection, infected, infective—*continued*
  specified type NEC 003.29
  paratyphi 002.9
    A 002.1
    B 002.2
    C 002.3
  schottmuelleri 002.2
  specified type NEC 003.8
  typhi 002.0
  typhosa 002.0
saprophytic 136.8
Sarcocystis, lindemanni 136.5
scabies 133.0
Schistosoma—*see* Infestation, Schistosoma
Schmorl's bacillus 040.3
scratch or other superficial injury—*see* Injury,
    superficial, by site
scrotum (acute) NEC 608.4
secondary, burn or open wound (dislocation)
    (fracture) 958.3
seminal vesicle (*see also* Vesiculitis) 608.0
septic
  generalized—*see* Septicemia
  localized, skin (*see also* Abscess) 682.9
septicemic—*see* Septicemia
seroma 998.51
Serratia (marcescens) 041.85
  generalized 038.44
sheep liver fluke 121.3
Shigella 004.9
  boydii 004.2
  dysenteriae 004.0
  Flexneri 004.1
  group
    A 004.0
    B 004.1
    C 004.2
    D 004.3
  Schmitz (-Stutzer) 004.0
  Schmitzii 004.0
  Shiga 004.0
  Sonnei 004.3
  specified type NEC 004.8
Sin Nombre virus 079.81
sinus (*see also* Sinusitis) 473.9
  pilonidal 685.1
    with abscess 685.0
  skin NEC 686.9
Skene's duct or gland (*see also* Urethritis)
    597.89
skin (local) (staphylococcal) (streptococcal)
    NEC 686.9
  abscess—*see* Abscess, by site
  cellulitis—*see* Cellulitis, by site
  due to fungus 111.9
    specified type NEC 111.8
  mycotic 111.9
    specified type NEC 111.8
  ulcer (*see also* Ulcer, skin) 707.9
slow virus 046.9
  specified condition NEC 046.8
Sparganum (mansoni) (proliferum) 123.5
spermatic cord NEC 608.4
sphenoidal (chronic) (sinus) (*see also* Sinusitis,
    sphenoidal) 473.3
Spherophorus necrophorus 040.3
spinal cord NEC (*see also* Encephalitis) 323.9
  abscess 324.1
    late effect—*see* category 326
  late effect—*see* category 326
  meninges—*see* Meningitis

Infection, infected, infective—*continued*
  streptococcal 320.2
  Spirillum
    minus or minor 026.0
    morsus muris 026.0
    obermeieri 087.0
  spirochetal NEC 104.9
    lung 104.8
    specified nature or site NEC 104.8
  spleen 289.59
  Sporothrix schenckii 117.1
  Sporotrichum (schenckii) 117.1
  Sporozoa 136.8
  staphylococcal NEC 041.10
    aureus 041.11
    food poisoning 005.0
    generalized (purulent) 038.10
      aureus 038.11
      specified organism NEC 038.19
    pneumonia 482.40
      aureus 482.41
      specified type NEC 482.49
    septicemia 038.10
      aureus 038.11
      specified organism NEC 038.19
    specified NEC 041.19
  steatoma 706.2
  Stellantchasmus falcatus 121.6
  Streptobacillus moniliformis 026.1
  streptococcal NEC 041.00
    congenital 771.89
    generalized (purulent) 038.0
    group
      A 041.01
      B 041.02
      C 041.03
      D [enterococcus] 041.04
      G 041.05
    pneumonia—*see* Pneumonia, streptococcal
      482.3
    septicemia 038.0
    sore throat 034.0
    specified NEC 041.09
  Streptomyces—*see* Actinomycosis
  streptotrichosis—*see* Actinomycosis
  Strongyloides (stercoralis) 127.2
  stump (amputation) (posttraumatic) (surgical)
    997.62
    traumatic—*see* Amputation, traumatic, by
      site, complicated
  subcutaneous tissue, local NEC 686.9
  submaxillary region 528.9
  suipestifer (*see also* Infection, Salmonella) 003.9
  swimming pool bacillus 031.1
  syphilitic—*see* Syphilis
  systemic—*see* Septicemia
  Taenia—*see* Infestation, Taenia
  Taeniarhynchus saginatus 123.2
  tapeworm—*see* Infestation, tapeworm
  tendon (sheath) 727.89
  Ternidens diminutus 127.7
  testis (*see also* Orchitis) 604.90
  thigh (skin) 686.9
  threadworm 127.4
  throat 478.29
    pneumococcal 462
    staphylococcal 462
    streptococcal 034.0
    viral NEC (*see also* Pharyngitis) 462
  thumb (skin) 686.9
    abscess (with lymphangitis) 681.00

Infection, infected, infective—*continued*
    pulp 681.01
    cellulitis (with lymphangitis) 681.00
    nail 681.02
  thyroglossal duct 529.8
  toe (skin) 686.9
    abscess (with lymphangitis) 681.10
    cellulitis (with lymphangitis) 681.10
    nail 681.11
      fungus 110.1
  tongue NEC 529.0
    parasitic 112.0
  tonsil (faucial) (lingual) (pharyngeal) 474.00
    acute or subacute 463
    and adenoid 474.02
    tag 474.00
  tooth, teeth 522.4
    periapical (pulpal origin) 522.4
    peridental 523.3
    periodontal 523.3
    pulp 522.0
    socket 526.5
  Torula histolytica 117.5
  Toxocara (cani) (cati) (felis) 128.0
  Toxoplasma gondii (*see also* Toxoplasmosis)
    130.9
  trachea, chronic 491.8
    fungus 117.9
  traumatic NEC 958.3
  trematode NEC 121.9
  trench fever 083.1
  Treponema
    denticola 041.84
    macrodenticum 041.84
    pallidum (*see also* Syphilis) 097.9
  Trichinella (spiralis) 124
  Trichomonas 131.9
    bladder 131.09
    cervix 131.09
    hominis 007.3
    intestine 007.3
    prostate 131.03
    specified site NEC 131.8
    urethra 131.02
    urogenitalis 131.00
    vagina 131.01
    vulva 131.01
  Trichophyton, trichophytid—*see*
    Dermatophytosis
  Trichosporon (beigelii) cutaneum 111.2
  Trichostrongylus 127.6
  Trichuris (trichiuria) 127.3
  Trombicula (irritans) 133.8
  Trypanosoma (*see also* Trypanosomiasis) 086.9
    cruzi 086.2
  tubal (*see also* Salpingo-oophoritis) 614.2
  tuberculous NEC (*see also* Tuberculosis) 011.9
  tubo-ovarian (*see also* Salpingo-oophoritis)
    614.2
  tunica vaginalis 608.4
  tympanic membrane—*see* Myringitis
  typhoid (abortive) (ambulant) (bacillus) 002.0
  typhus 081.9
    flea-borne (endemic) 081.0
    louse-borne (epidemic) 080
    mite-borne 081.2
    recrudescent 081.1
    tick-borne 082.9
      African 082.1
      North Asian 082.2
  umbilicus (septic) 686.9

Infection, infected, infective—*continued*
 newborn NEC 771.4
 ureter 593.89
 urethra (*see also* Urethritis) 597.80
 urinary (tract) NEC 599.0
  with
   abortion—*see* Abortion, by type, with
    urinary tract infection
   ectopic pregnancy (*see also* categories
    633.0-633.9) 639.8
   molar pregnancy (*see also* categories
    630-632) 639.8
  candidal 112.2
  complicating pregnancy, childbirth, or
   puerperium 646.6
   affecting fetus or newborn 760.1
   asymptomatic 646.5
    affecting fetus or newborn 760.1
  diplococcal (acute) 098.0
   chronic 098.2
  due to Trichomonas (vaginalis) 131.00
  following
   abortion 639.8
   ectopic or molar pregnancy 639.8
  gonococcal (acute) 098.0
   chronic or duration of 2 months or over
    098.2
  newborn 771.82
  trichomonal 131.00
  tuberculous (*see also* Tuberculosis) 016.3
 uterus, uterine (*see also* Endometritis) 615.9
 utriculus masculinus NEC 597.89
 vaccination 999.3
 vagina (granulation tissue) (wall) (*see also*
  Vaginitis) 616.10
 varicella 052.9
 varicose veins—*see* Varicose, veins
 variola 050.9
  major 050.0
  minor 050.1
 vas deferens NEC 608.4
 Veillonella 041.84
 verumontanum 597.89
 vesical (*see also* Cystitis) 595.9
 Vibrio
  cholerae 001.0
   El Tor 001.1
  parahaemolyticus (food poisoning) 005.4
  vulnificus 041.85
 Vincent's (gums) (mouth) (tonsil) 101
 virus, viral 079.99
  adenovirus
   in diseases classified elsewhere—*see*
    category 079
   unspecified nature or site 079.0
  central nervous system NEC 049.9
   enterovirus 048
    meningitis 047.9
     specified type NEC 047.8
   slow virus 046.9
    specified condition NEC 046.8
  chest 519.8
  conjunctivitis 077.99
   specified type NEC 077.8
  Coxsackie (*see also* Infection, Coxsackie)
   079.2
  Ebola 065.8
  ECHO
   in diseases classified elsewhere—*see*
    category 079
   unspecified nature or site 079.1

Infection, infected, infective—*continued*
 encephalitis 049.9
  arthropod-borne NEC 064
  tick-borne 063.9
   specified type NEC 063.8
 enteritis NEC (*see also* Enteritis, viral) 008.8
 exanthem NEC 057.9
 Hantavirus 079.81
 human papilloma 079.4
 in diseases classified elsewhere—*see* category
  079
 intestine (*see also* Enteritis, viral) 008.8
 lung—*see* Pneumonia, viral
 respiratory syncytial virus (RSV) 079.6
 rhinovirus
  in diseases classified elsewhere—*see*
   category 079
  unspecified nature or site 079.3
 salivary gland disease 078.5
 slow 046.9
  specified condition NEC 046.8
 specified type NEC 079.89
  in diseases classified elsewhere—*see*
   category 079
  unspecified nature or site 079.99
 warts 078.10
 vulva (*see also* Vulvitis) 616.10
 whipworm 127.3
 Whitmore's bacillus 025
 wound (local) (posttraumatic) NEC 958.3
  with
   dislocation—*see* Dislocation, by site, open
   fracture—*see* Fracture, by site, open
   open wound—*see* Wound, open, by site,
    complicated
  postoperative 998.59
  surgical 998.59
 Wuchereria 125.0
  bancrofti 125.0
  malayi 125.1
 yaws—*see* Yaws
 yeast (*see also* Candidiasis) 112.9
 yellow fever (*see also* Fever, yellow) 060.9
 Yersinia pestis (*see also* Plague) 020.9
 Zeis' gland 373.12
 zoonotic bacterial NEC 027.9
 Zopfia senegalensis 117.4
Infective, infectious —*see* condition
Inferiority complex 301.9
 constitutional psychopathic 301.9
Infertility
 female 628.9
  associated with
   adhesions, peritubal 614.6 *[628.2]*
   anomaly
    cervical mucus 628.4
    congenital
     cervix 628.4
     fallopian tube 628.2
     uterus 628.3
     vagina 628.4
   anovulation 628.0
   dysmucorrhea 628.4
   endometritis, tuberculous (*see also*
    Tuberculosis) 016.7 *[628.3]*
   Stein-Leventhal syndrome 256.4 *[628.0]*
  due to
   adiposogenital dystrophy 253.8 *[628.1]*
   anterior pituitary disorder NEC 253.4
    [628.1]
    hyperfunction 253.1 *[628.1]*

Infestation—*continued*
  Gasterophilus (intestinalis) 134.0
  Gastrodiscoides hominis 121.8
  Giardia lamblia 007.1
  Gnathostoma (spinigerum) 128.1
  Gongylonema 125.6
  guinea worm 125.7
  helminth NEC 128.9
    intestinal 127.9
      mixed (types classifiable to more than one
        category in 120.0-127.7) 127.8
      specified type NEC 127.7
    specified type NEC 128.8
  Heterophyes heterophyes (small intestine) 121.6
  hookworm (*see also* Infestation, ancylostoma)
    126.9
  Hymenolepis (diminuta) (nana) 123.6
  intestinal NEC 129
  leeches (aquatic) (land) 134.2
  Leishmania—*see* Leishmaniasis
  lice (*see also* infestation, pediculus) 132.9
  Linguatulidae, linguatula (pentastoma) (serrata)
    134.1
  Loa loa 125.2
    eyelid 125.2 *[373.6]*
  louse (*see also* Infestation, pediculus) 132.9
    body 132.1
    head 132.0
    pubic 132.2
  maggots 134.0
  Mansonella (ozzardi) 125.5
  medina 125.7
  Metagonimus yokogawai (small intestine) 121.5
  Microfilaria streptocerca 125.3
    eye 125.3 *[360.13]*
    eyelid 125.3 *[373.6]*
  Microsporon furfur 111.0
  microsporum—*see* Dermatophytosis
  mites 133.9
    scabic 133.0
    specified type NEC 133.8
  Monilia (albicans) (*see also* Candidiasis) 112.9
    vagina 112.1
    vulva 112.1
  mouth 112.0
  Necator americanus 126.1
  nematode (intestinal) 127.9
    Ancylostoma (*see also* Ancylostoma) 126.9
    Ascaris lumbricoides 127.0
    conjunctiva NEC 128.9
    Dioctophyma 128.8
    Enterobius vermicularis 127.4
    Gnathostoma spinigerum 128.1
    Oesophagostomum (apiostomum) 127.7
    Physaloptera 127.4
    specified type NEC 127.7
    Strongyloides stercoralis 127.2
    Ternidens diminutus 127.7
    Trichinella spiralis 124
    Trichostrongylus 127.6
    Trichuris (trichiuria) 127.3
  Oesophagostomum (apiostomum) 127.7
  Oestrus ovis 134.0
  Onchocerca (volvulus) 125.3
    eye 125.3 *[360.13]*
    eyelid 125.3 *[373.6]*
  Opisthorchis (felineus) (tenuicollis) (viverrini)
    121.0
  Oxyuris vermicularis 127.4
  Paragonimus (westermani) 121.2
  parasite, parasitic NEC 136.9

Infestation—*continued*
  eyelid 134.9 *[373.6]*
  intestinal 129
  mouth 112.0
  orbit 376.13
  skin 134.9
  tongue 112.0
  pediculus 132.9
    capitis (humanus) (any site) 132.0
    corporis (humanus) (any site) 132.1
    eyelid 132.0 *[373.6]*
    mixed (classifiable to more than one category
      in 132.0-132.2) 132.3
    pubis (any site) 132.2
  phthirus (pubis) (any site) 132.2
    with any infestation classifiable to 132.0 and
      132.1 132.3
  pinworm 127.4
  pork tapeworm (adult) 123.0
  protozoal NEC 136.8
  pubic louse 132.2
  rat tapeworm 123.6
  red bug 133.8
  roundworm (large) NEC 127.0
  sand flea 134.1
  saprophytic NEC 136.8
  Sarcoptes scabiei 133.0
  scabies 133.0
  Schistosoma 120.9
    bovis 120.8
    cercariae 120.3
    hematobium 120.0
    intercalatum 120.8
    japonicum 120.2
    mansoni 120.1
    mattheii 120.8
    specified
      site—*see* Schistosomiasis
      type NEC 120.8
    spindale 120.8
  screw worms 134.0
  skin NEC 134.9
  Sparganum (mansoni) (proliferum) 123.5
    larval 123.5
  specified type NEC 134.8
  Spirometra larvae 123.5
  Sporozoa NEC 136.8
  Stellantchasmus falcatus 121.6
  Strongyloides 127.2
  Strongylus (gibsoni) 127.7
  Taenia 123.3
    diminuta 123.6
    Echinococcus (*see also* Echinococcus) 122.9
    mediocanellata 123.2
    nana 123.6
    saginata (mediocanellata) 123.2
    solium (intestinal form) 123.0
      larval form 123.1
  Taeniarhynchus saginatus 123.2
  tapeworm 123.9
    beef 123.2
    broad 123.4
      larval 123.5
    dog 123.8
    dwarf 123.6
    fish 123.4
      larval 123.5
    pork 123.0
    rat 123.6
  Ternidens diminutus 127.7
  Tetranychus molestissimus 133.8

Infestation—*continued*
threadworm 127.4
tongue 112.0
Toxocara (cani) (cati) (felis) 128.0
trematode(s) NEC 121.9
Trichina spiralis 124
Trichinella spiralis 124
Trichocephalus 127.3
Trichomonas 131.9
  bladder 131.09
  cervix 131.09
  intestine 007.3
  prostate 131.03
  specified site NEC 131.8
  urethra (female) (male) 131.02
  urogenital 131.00
  vagina 131.01
  vulva 131.01
Trichophyton—*see* Dermatophytosis
Trichostrongylus instabilis 127.6
Trichuris (trichiuria) 127.3
Trombicula (irritans) 133.8
Trypanosoma—*see* Trypanosomiasis
Tunga penetrans 134.1
Uncinaria americana 126.1
whipworm 127.3
worms NEC 128.9
  intestinal 127.9
Wuchereria 125.0
  bancrofti 125.0
  malayi 125.1
Infiltrate, infiltration
with an iron compound 275.0
amyloid (any site) (generalized) 277.3
calcareous (muscle) NEC 275.49
  localized—*see* Degeneration, by site
calcium salt (muscle) 275.49
corneal (*see also* Edema, cornea) 371.20
eyelid 373.9
fatty (diffuse) (generalized) 272.8
  localized—*see* Degeneration, by site, fatty
glycogen, glycogenic (*see also* Disease,
    glycogen storage) 271.10
heart, cardiac
  fatty (*see also* Degeneration, myocardial)
    429.1
  glycogenic 271.0 *[425.7]*
inflammatory in vitreous 379.29
kidney (*see also* Disease, renal) 593.9
leukemic (M9800/3)—*see* Leukemia
liver 573.8
  fatty—*see* Fatty, liver
  glycogen (*see also* Disease, glycogen storage)
    271.0
lung (*see also* Infiltrate, pulmonary) 518.3
  eosinophilic 518.3
  x-ray finding only 793.1
lymphatic (*see also* Leukemia, lymphatic) 204.9
  gland, pigmentary 289.3
muscle, fatty 728.9
myelogenous (*see also* Leukemia, myeloid)
    205.9
myocardium, myocardial
  fatty (*see also* Degeneration, myocardial)
    429.1
  glycogenic 271.0 *[425.7]*
pulmonary 518.3
  with
    eosinophilia 518.3
    pneumonia—*see* Pneumonia, by type
  x-ray finding only 793.1

Infiltrate, infiltration—*continued*
Ranke's primary (*see also* Tuberculosis) 010.0
skin, lymphocyctic (benign) 709.8
thymus (gland) (fatty) 254.8
urine 788.8
vitreous humor 379.29
Infirmity 799.8
senile 797
Inflammation, inflamed, inflammatory (with
    exudation)
abducens (nerve) 378.54
accessory sinus (chronic) (*see also* Sinusitis)
    473.9
adrenal (gland) 255.8
alimentary canal—*see* Enteritis
alveoli (teeth) 526.5
  scorbutic 267
amnion—*see* Amnionitis
anal canal 569.49
antrum (chronic) (*see also* Sinusitis, maxillary)
    473.0
anus 569.49
appendix (*see also* Appendicitis) 541
arachnoid—*see* Meningitis
areola 611.0
  puerperal, postpartum 675.0
areolar tissue NEC 686.9
artery—*see* Arteritis
auditory meatus (external) (*see also* Otitis,
    externa) 380.10
Bartholin's gland 616.8
bile duct or passage 576.1
bladder (*see also* Cystitis) 595.9
bone—*see* Osteomyelitis
bowel (*see also* Enteritis) 558.9
brain (*see also* Encephalitis) 323.9
  late effect—*see* category 326
  membrane—*see* Meningitis
breast 611.0
  puerperal, postpartum 675.2
broad ligament (*see also* Disease, pelvis,
    inflammatory) 614.4
  acute 614.3
bronchus—*see* Bronchitis
bursa—*see* Bursitis
capsule
  liver 573.3
  spleen 289.59
catarrhal (*see also* Catarrh) 460
  vagina 616.10
cecum (*see also* Appendicitis) 541
cerebral (*see also* Encephalitis) 323.9
  late effect—*see* category 326
  membrane—*see* Meningitis
cerebrospinal (*see also* Meningitis) 322.9
  late effect—*see* category 326
  meningococcal 036.0
  tuberculous (*see also* Tuberculosis) 013.6
cervix (uteri) (*see also* Cervicitis) 616.0
chest 519.9
choroid NEC (*see also* Choroiditis) 363.20
cicatrix (tissue)—*see* Cicatrix
colon (*see also* Enteritis) 558.9
  granulomatous 555.1
  newborn 558.9
connective tissue (diffuse) NEC 728.9
cornea (*see also* Keratitis) 370.9
  with ulcer (*see also* Ulcer, cornea) 370.00
corpora cavernosa (penis) 607.2
cranial nerve—*see* Disorder, nerve, cranial
diarrhea—*see* Diarrhea

Inflammation, inflamed, inflammatory—*cont.*
  disc (intervertebral) (space) 722.90
    cervical, cervicothoracic 722.91
    lumbar, lumbosacral 722.93
    thoracic, thoracolumbar 722.93
  Douglas' cul-de-sac or pouch (chronic) (*see also* Disease, pelvis, inflammatory) 614.4
    acute 614.3
  due to (presence of) any device, implant, or graft classifiable to 996.0-996.5—*see* Complications, infection and inflammation, due to (presence of) any device, implant, or graft classified to 996.0-996.5 NEC
  duodenum 535.6
  dura mater—*see* Meningitis
  ear—*see also* Otitis
    external (*see also* Otitis, externa) 380.10
    inner (*see also* Labyrinthitis) 386.30
    middle—*see* Otitis media
  esophagus 530.10
  ethmoidal (chronic) (sinus) (*see also* Sinusitis, ethmoidal) 473.2
  Eustachian tube (catarrhal) 381.50
    acute 381.51
    chronic 381.52
  extrarectal 569.49
  eye 379.99
  eyelid 373.9
    specified NEC 373.8
  fallopian tube (*see also* Salpingo-oophoritis) 614.2
  fascia 728.9
  fetal membranes (acute) 658.4
    affecting fetus or newborn 762.7
  follicular, pharynx 472.1
  frontal (chronic) (sinus) (*see also* Sinusitis, frontal) 473.1
  gallbladder (*see also* Cholecystitis, acute) 575.0
  gall duct (*see also* Cholecystitis) 575.10
  gastrointestinal (*see also* Enteritis) 558.9
  genital organ (diffuse) (internal)
    female 614.9
      with
        abortion—*see* Abortion, by type, with sepsis
        ectopic pregnancy (*see also* categories 633.0-633.9) 639.0
        molar pregnancy (*see also* categories 630-632) 639.0
        complicating pregnancy, childbirth, or puerperium 646.6
          affecting fetus or newborn 760.8
        following
          abortion 639.0
          ectopic or molar pregnancy 639.0
    male 608.4
  gland (lymph) (*see also* Lymphadenitis) 289.3
  glottis (*see also* Laryngitis) 464.00
    with obstruction 464.01
  granular, pharynx 472.1
  gum 523.1
  heart (*see also* Carditis) 429.89
  hepatic duct 576.8
  hernial sac—*see* Hernia, by site
  ileum (*see also* Enteritis) 558.9
    terminal or regional 555.0
      with large intestine 555.2
  intervertebral disc 722.90
    cervical, cervicothoracic 722.91
    lumbar, lumbosacral 722.93
    thoracic, thoracolumbar 722.92

Inflammation, inflamed, inflammatory—*cont.*
  intestine (*see also* Enteritis) 558.9
  jaw (acute) (bone) (chronic) (lower) (suppurative) (upper) 526.4
  jejunum—*see* Enteritis
  joint NEC (*see also* Arthritis) 716.9
    sacroiliac 720.2
  kidney (*see also* Nephritis) 583.9
  knee (joint) 716.66
    tuberculous (active) (*see also* Tuberculosis) 015.2
  labium (majus) (minus) (*see also* Vulvitis) 616.10
  lacrimal
    gland (*see also* Dacryoadenitis) 375.00
    passages (duct) (sac) (*see also* Dacryocystitis) 375.30
  larynx (*see also* Laryngitis) 464.00
    with obstruction 464.01
    diphtheritic 032.3
  leg NEC 686.9
  lip 528.5
  liver (capsule) (*see also* Hepatitis) 573.3
    acute 570
    chronic 571.40
    suppurative 572.0
  lung (acute) (*see also* Pneumonia) 486
    chronic (interstitial) 518.89
  lymphatic vessel (*see also* Lymphangitis) 457.2
  lymph node or gland (*see also* Lymphadenitis) 289.3
  mammary gland 611.0
    puerperal, postpartum 675.2
  maxilla, maxillary 526.4
    sinus (chronic) (*see also* Sinusitis, maxillary) 473.0
  membranes of brain or spinal cord—*see* Meningitis
  meninges—*see* Meningitis
  mouth 528.0
  muscle 728.9
  myocardium (*see also* Myocarditis) 429.0
  nasal sinus (chronic) (*see also* Sinusitis) 473.9
  nasopharynx—*see* Nasopharyngitis
  navel 686.9
    newborn NEC 771.4
  nerve NEC 729.2
  nipple 611.0
    puerperal, postpartum 675.0
  nose 478.1
    suppurative 472.0
  oculomotor nerve 378.51
  optic nerve 377.30
  orbit (chronic) 376.10
    acute 376.00
    chronic 376.10
  ovary (*see also* Salpingo-oophoritis) 614.2
  oviduct (*see also* Salpingo-oophoritis) 614.2
  pancreas—*see* Pancreatitis
  parametrium (chronic) (*see also* Disease, pelvis, inflammatory) 614.4
    acute 614.3
  parotid region 686.9
    gland 527.2
  pelvis, female (*see also* Disease, pelvis, inflammatory) 614.9
  penis (corpora cavernosa) 607.2
  perianal 569.49
  pericardium (*see also* Pericarditis) 423.9
  perineum (female) (male) 686.9
  perirectal 569.49

Inflammation, inflamed, inflammatory—*cont.*
peritoneum (*see also* Peritonitis) 567.9
periuterine (*see also* Disease, pelvis, inflammatory) 614.9
perivesical (*see also* Cystitis) 595.9
petrous bone (*see also* Petrositis) 383.20
pharynx (*see also* Pharyngitis) 462
follicular 472.1
granular 472.1
pia mater—*see* Meningitis
pleura—*see* Pleurisy
postmastoidectomy cavity 383.30
chronic 383.33
prostate (*see also* Prostatitis) 601.9
rectosigmoid—*see* Rectosigmoiditis
rectum (*see also* Proctitis) 569.49
respiratory, upper (*see also* Infection, respiratory, upper) 465.9
chronic, due to external agent—*see* Condition, respiratory, chronic, due to, external agent
due to
fumes or vapors (chemical) (inhalation) 506.2
radiation 508.1
retina (*see also* Retinitis) 363.20
retrocecal (*see also* Appendicitis) 541
retroperitoneal (*see also* Peritonitis) 567.9
salivary duct or gland (any) (suppurative) 527.2
scorbutic, alveoli, teeth 267
scrotum 608.4
sigmoid—*see* Enteritis
sinus (*see also* Sinusitis) 473.9
Skene's duct or gland (*see also* Urethritis) 597.89
skin 686.9
spermatic cord 608.4
sphenoidal (sinus) (*see also* Sinusitis, sphenoidal) 473.3
spinal
cord (*see also* Encephalitis) 323.9
late effect—*see* category 326
membrane—*see* Meningitis
nerve—*see* Disorder, nerve
spine (*see also* Spondylitis) 720.9
spleen (capsule) 289.59
stomach—*see* Gastritis
stricture, rectum 569.49
subcutaneous tissue NEC 686.9
suprarenal (gland) 255.8
synovial (fringe) (membrane)—*see* Bursitis
tendon (sheath) NEC 726.90
testis (*see also* Orchitis) 604.90
thigh 686.9
throat (*see also* Sore throat) 462
thymus (gland) 254.8
thyroid (gland) (*see also* Thyroiditis) 245.9
tongue 529.0
tonsil—*see* Tonsillitis
trachea—*see* Tracheitis
trochlear nerve 378.53
tubal (*see also* Salpingo-oophoritis) 614.2
tuberculous NEC (*see also* Tuberculosis) 011.9
tubo-ovarian (*see also* Salpingo-oophoritis) 614.2
tunica vaginalis 608.4
tympanic membrane—*see* Myringitis
umbilicus, umbilical 686.9
newborn NEC 771.4
uterine ligament (*see also* Disease, pelvis, inflammatory) 614.4
acute 614.3

Inflammation, inflamed, inflammatory—*cont.*
uterus (catarrhal) (*see also* Endometritis) 615.9
uveal tract (anterior) (*see also* Iridocyclitis) 364.3
posterior—*see* Chorioretinitis
sympathetic 360.11
vagina (*see also* Vaginitis) 616.10
vas deferens 608.4
vein (*see also* Phlebitis) 451.9
thrombotic 451.9
cerebral (*see also* Thrombosis, brain) 434.0
leg 451.2
deep (vessels) NEC 451.19
superficial (vessels) 451.0
lower extremity 451.2
deep (vessels) NEC 451.19
superficial (vessels) 451.0
vocal cord 478.5
vulva (*see also* Vulvitis) 616.10
Inflation, lung imperfect (newborn) 770.5
Influenza, influenzal 487.1
with
bronchitis 487.1
bronchopneumonia 487.0
cold (any type) 487.1
digestive manifestations 487.8
hemoptysis 487.1
involvement of
gastrointestinal tract 487.8
nervous system 487.8
laryngitis 487.1
manifestations NEC 487.8
respiratory 487.1
pneumonia 487.0
pharyngitis 487.1
pneumonia (any form classifiable to 480-483, 485-486) 487.0
respiratory manifestations NEC 487.1
sinusitis 487.1
sore throat 487.1
tonsillitis 487.1
tracheitis 487.1
upper respiratory infection (acute) 487.1
abdominal 487.8
Asian 487.1
bronchial 487.1
bronchopneumonia 487.0
catarrhal 487.1
epidemic 487.1
gastric 487.8
intestinal 487.8
laryngitis 487.1
maternal affecting fetus or newborn 760.2
manifest influenza in infant 771.2
pharyngitis 487.1
pneumonia (any form) 487.0
respiratory (upper) 487.1
stomach 487.8
vaccination, prophylactic (against) V04.8
Influenza-like disease 487.1
Infraction, Freiberg's (metatarsal head) 732.5
Infusion complication, misadventure or reaction —*see* Complication, infusion
Ingestion
chemical—*see* Table of drugs and chemicals
drug or medicinal substance
overdose or wrong substance given or taken 977.9
specified drug—*see* Table of drugs and chemicals
foreign body NEC (*see also* Foreign body) 938

Ingrowing
hair 704.8
nail (finger) (toe) (infected) 703.0
Inguinal —*see also* condition
testis 752.51
Inhalation
carbon monoxide 986
flame
mouth 947.0
lung 947.1
food or foreign body (*see also* Asphyxia, food
or foreign body) 933.1
gas, fumes, or vapor (noxious) 987.9
specified agent—*see* Table of drugs and
chemicals
liquid or vomitus (*see also* Asphyxia, food or
foreign body) 933.1
lower respiratory tract NEC 934.9
meconium (fetus or newborn) 770.1
mucus (*see also* Asphyxia, mucus) 933.1
oil (causing suffocation) (*see also* Asphyxia,
food or foreign body) 933.1
pneumonia—*see* Pneumonia, aspiration
smoke 987.9
steam 987.9
stomach contents or secretions (*see also*
Asphyxia, food or foreign body) 933.1
in labor and deliver 668.0
Inhibition, inhibited
academic as adjustment reaction 309.23
orgasm
female 302.73
male 302.74
sexual
desire 302.71
excitement 302.72
work as adjustment reaction 309.23
Inhibitor, systemic lupus erythematosus
(presence of) 286.5
Iniencephalus, iniencephaly 740.2
Injected eye 372.74
Injury 959.9

*Note—For abrasion, insect bite (nonvenomous),
blister, or scratch, see Injury, superficial. For
laceration, traumatic rupture, tear, or
penetrating wound of internal organs, such as
heart, lung, liver, kidney, pelvic organs,
whether or not accompanied by open wound in
the same region, see Injury, internal. For nerve
injury, see Injury, nerve. For late effect of
injuries classifiable to 850-854, 860-869,
900-919, 950-959, see Late, effect, injury, by
type.*

abdomen, abdominal (viscera)—*see also* Injury,
internal, abdomen
muscle or wall 959.1
acoustic, resulting in deafness 951.5
adenoid 959.09
adrenal (gland)—*see* Injury, internal, adrenal
alveolar (process) 959.09
ankle (and foot) (and knee) (and leg, except
thigh) 959.7
anterior chamber, eye 921.3
anus 959.1
aorta (thoracic) 901.0
abdominal 902.0
appendix—*see* Injury, internal, appendix
arm, upper (and shoulder) 959.2
artery (complicating trauma) (*see also* Injury,
blood vessel, by site) 904.9

Injury—*continued*
cerebral or meningeal (*see also* Hemorrhage,
brain, traumatic, subarachnoid) 852.0
auditory canal (external) (meatus) 959.09
auricle, auris, ear 959.09
axilla 959.2
back 959.1
bile duct—*see* Injury, internal, bile duct
birth—*see also* Birth, injury
canal NEC, complicating delivery 665.9
bladder (sphincter)—*see* Injury, internal, bladder
blast (air) (hydraulic) (immersion) (underwater)
NEC 869.0
with open wound into cavity NEC 869.1
abdomen or thorax—*see* Injury, internal, by
site
brain—*see* Concussion, brain
ear (acoustic nerve trauma) 951.5
with perforation of tympanic
membrane—*see* Wound, open, ear, drum
blood vessel NEC 904.9
abdomen 902.9
multiple 902.87
specified NEC 902.89
aorta (thoracic) 901.0
abdominal 902.0
arm NEC 903.9
axillary 903.00
artery 903.01
vein 903.02
azygos vein 901.89
basilic vein 903.1
brachial (artery) (vein) 903.1
bronchial 901.89
carotid artery 900.00
common 900.01
external 900.02
internal 900.03
celiac artery 902.20
specified branch NEC 902.24
cephalic vein (arm) 903.1
colica dextra 902.26
cystic
artery 902.24
vein 902.39
deep plantar 904.6
digital (artery) (vein) 903.5
due to accidental puncture or laceration during
procedure 998.2
extremity
lower 904.8
multiple 904.7
specified NEC 904.7
upper 903.9
multiple 903.8
specified NEC 903.8
femoral
artery (superficial) 904.1
above profunda origin 904.0
common 904.0
vein 904.2
gastric
artery 902.21
vein 902.39
head 900.9
intracranial—*see* Injury, intracranial
multiple 900.82
specified NEC 900.89
hemiazygos vein 901.89
hepatic
artery 902.22

Injury—*continued*
 diaphragm—*see* Injury, internal, diaphragm
 duodenum—*see* Injury, internal, duodenum
 ear (auricle) (canal) (drum) (external) 959.09
 elbow (and forearm) (and wrist) 959.3
 epididymis 959.1
 epigastric region 959.1
 epiglottis 959.09
 epiphyseal, current—*see* Fracture, by site
 esophagus—*see* Injury, internal, esophagus
 Eustachian tube 959.09
 extremity (lower) (upper) NEC 959.8
 eye 921.9
  penetrating eyeball—*see* Injury, eyeball,
    penetrating
  superficial 918.9
 eyeball 921.3
  penetrating 871.7
   with
    partial loss (of intraocular tissue) 871.12
    prolapse or exposure (of intraocular
     tissue) 871.1
   without prolapse 871.0
   foreign body (nonmagnetic) 871.6
    magnetic 871.5
  superficial 918.9
 eyebrow 959.09
 eyelid(s) 921.1
  laceration—*see* Laceration, eyelid
  superficial 918.0
 face (and neck) 959.09
 fallopian tube—*see* Injury, internal, fallopian
   tube
 finger(s) (nail) 959.5
 flank 959.1
 foot (and ankle) (and knee) (and leg except
   thigh) 959.7
 forceps NEC 767.9
  scalp 767.1
 forearm (and elbow) (and wrist) 959.3
 forehead 959.09
 gallbladder—*see* Injury, internal, gallbladder
 gasserian ganglion 951.2
 gastrointestinal tract—*see* Injury, internal,
   gastrointestinal tract
 genital organ(s)
  with
   abortion—*see* Abortion, by type, with,
     damage to pelvic organs
   ectopic pregnancy (*see also* categories
     633.0-633.9) 639.2
   molar pregnancy (*see also* categories
     630-632) 639.2
  external 959.1
  following
   abortion 639.2
   ectopic or molar pregnancy 639.2
  internal—*see* Injury, internal, genital organs
  obstetrical trauma NEC 665.9
   affecting fetus or newborn 763.89
 gland
  lacrimal 921.1
   laceration 870.8
  parathyroid 959.09
  salivary 959.09
  thyroid 959.09
 globe (eye) (*see also* Injury, eyeball) 921.3
 grease gun—*see* Wound, open, by site,
   complicated
 groin 959.1

Injury—*continued*
 gum 959.09
 hand(s) (except fingers) 959.4
 head NEC 959.01
  with
   loss of consciousness 850.5
   skull fracture—*see* Fracture, skull, by site
 heart—*see* Injury, internal, heart
 heel 959.7
 hip (and thigh) 959.6
 hymen 959.1
 hyperextension (cervical) (vertebra) 847.0
 ileum—*see* Injury, internal, ileum
 iliac region 959.1
 infrared rays NEC 990
 instrumental (during surgery) 998.2
  birth injury—*see* Birth, injury
  nonsurgical (*see also* Injury, by site) 959.9
  obstetrical 665.9
   affecting fetus or newborn 763.89
   bladder 665.5
   cervix 665.3
   high vaginal 665.4
   perineal NEC 664.9
   urethra 665.5
   uterus 665.5
 internal 869.0

---

*Note—For injury of internal organ(s) by foreign
body entering through a natural orifice (e.g.,
inhaled, ingested, or swallowed)—see Foreign
body, entering through orifice.*

*For internal injury of any of the following sites
with internal injury of any other of the sites—
see Injury, internal, multiple.*

---

  with
   fracture
    pelvis—*see* Fracture, pelvis
    specified site, except pelvis—*see* Injury,
      internal, by site
   open wound into cavity 869.1
  abdomen, abdominal (viscera) NEC 868.00
   with
    fracture, pelvis—*see* Fracture, pelvis
    open wound into cavity 868.10
   specified site NEC 868.09
    with open wound into cavity 868.19
  adrenal (gland) 868.01
   with open wound into cavity 868.11
  aorta (thoracic) 901.0
   abdominal 902.0
  appendix 863.85
   with open wound into cavity 863.95
  bile duct 868.02
   with open wound into cavity 868.12
  bladder (sphincter) 867.0
   with
    abortion—*see* Abortion, by type, with,
      damage to pelvic organs
    ectopic pregnancy (*see also* categories
      633.0-633.9) 639.2
    molar pregnancy (*see also* categories
      630-632) 639.2
    open wound into cavity 867.1
   following
    abortion 639.2
    ectopic or molar pregnancy 639.2
   obstetrical trauma 665.5
    affecting fetus or newborn 763.89
  blood vessel—*see* Injury, blood vessel, by site

Injury—*continued*

broad ligament 867.6
  with open wound into cavity 867.7
bronchus, bronchi 862.21
  with open wound into cavity 862.31
cecum 863.89
  with open wound into cavity 863.99
cervix (uteri) 867.4
  with
    abortion—*see* Abortion, by type, with
      damage to pelvic organs
    ectopic pregnancy (*see also* categories
      633.0-633.9) 639.2
    molar pregnancy (*see also* categories
      630-632) 639.2
    open wound into cavity 867.5
  following
    abortion 639.2
    ectopic or molar pregnancy 639.2
    obstetrical trauma 665.3
      affecting fetus or newborn 763.89
chest (*see also* Injury, internal, intrathoracic
  organs) 862.8
  with open wound into cavity 862.9
colon 863.40
  with
    open wound into cavity 863.50
    rectum 863.46
      with open wound into cavity 863.56
  ascending (right) 863.41
    with open wound into cavity 863.51
  descending (left) 863.43
    with open wound into cavity 863.53
  multiple sites 863.46
    with open wound into cavity 863.56
  sigmoid 863.44
    with open wound into cavity 863.54
  specified site NEC 863.49
    with open wound into cavity 863.59
  transverse 863.42
    with open wound into cavity 863.52
common duct 868.02
  with open wound into cavity 868.12
complicating delivery 665.9
  affecting fetus or newborn 763.89
diaphragm 862.0
  with open wound into cavity 862.1
duodenum 863.21
  with open wound into cavity 863.31
esophagus (intrathoracic) 862.22
  with open wound into cavity 862.32
  cervical region 874.4
    complicated 874.5
fallopian tube 867.6
  with open wound into cavity 867.7
gallbladder 868.02
  with open wound into cavity 868.12
gastrointestinal tract NEC 863.80
  with open wound into cavity 863.90
genital organ NEC 867.6
  with open wound into cavity 867.7
heart 861.00
  with open wound into thorax 861.10
ileum 863.29
  with open wound into cavity 863.39
intestine NEC 863.89
  with open wound into cavity 863.99
  large NEC 863.40
    with open wound into cavity 863.50
  small NEC 863.20
    with open wound into cavity 863.30

Injury—*continued*

intra-abdominal (organ) 868.00
  with open wound into cavity 868.10
  multiple sites 868.09
    with open wound into cavity 868.19
  specified site NEC 868.09
    with open wound into cavity 868.19
intrathoracic organs (multiple) 862.8
  with open wound into cavity 862.9
  diaphragm (only)—*see* Injury, internal,
    diaphragm
  heart (only)—*see* Injury, internal, heart
  lung (only)—*see* Injury, internal, lung
  specified site NEC 862.29
    with open wound into cavity 862.39
intrauterine (*see also* Injury, internal, uterus)
  867.4
  with open wound into cavity 867.5
jejunum 863.29
  with open wound into cavity 863.39
kidney (subcapsular) 866.00
  with
    disruption of parenchyma (complete)
      866.03
      with open wound into cavity 866.13
    hematoma (without rupture of capsule)
      866.01
      with open wound into cavity 866.11
    laceration 866.02
      with open wound into cavity 866.12
    open wound into cavity 866.10
liver 864.00
  with
    contusion 864.01
      with open wound into cavity 864.11
    hematoma 864.01
      with open wound into cavity 864.11
    laceration 864.05
      with open wound into cavity 864.15
    major (disruption of hepatic
      parenchyma) 864.04
      with open wound into cavity 864.14
    minor (capsule only) 864.02
      with open wound into cavity 864.12
    moderate (involving parenchyma) 864.03
      with open wound into cavity 864.13
    multiple 864.04
    stellate 864.04
      with open wound in cavity 864.14
  open wound into cavity 864.10
lung 861.20
  with open wound into thorax 861.30
  hemopneumothorax—*see*
    Hemopneumothorax, traumatic
  hemothorax—*see* Hemothorax, traumatic
  pneumohemothorax—*see*
    Pneumohemothorax, traumatic
  pneumothorax—*see* Pneumothorax,
    traumatic
mediastinum 862.29
  with open wound into cavity 862.39
mesentery 863.89
  with open wound into cavity 863.99
mesosalpinx 867.6
  with open wound into cavity 867.7

Injury—*continued*
multiple 869.0

> *Note—Multiple internal injuries of sites*
> *classifiable to the same three- or four- digit*
> *category should be classified to that category.*
> *Multiple injuries classifiable to different*
> *fourth-digit subdivisions of 861 (heart and lung*
> *injuries) should be dealt with according to*
> *coding rules.*

    with open wound into cavity 869.1
    intra-abdominal organ (sites classifiable to
        863-868)
      with
        intrathoracic organ(s) (sites classifiable
            to 861-862) 869.0
          with open wound into cavity 869.1
        other intra-abdominal organ(s) (sites
            classifiable to 863-868, except
            where classifiable to the same
            three-digit category) 868.09
          with open wound into cavity 868.19
    intrathoracic organ (sites classifiable to
        861-862)
      with
        intra-abdominal organ(s) (sites
            classifiable to 863-868) 869.0
          with open wound into cavity 869.1
        other intrathoracic organ(s) (sites
            classifiable to 861-862, except
            where classifiable to the same
            three-digit category) 862.8
          with open wound into cavity 862.9
    myocardium—*see* Injury, internal, heart
    ovary 867.6
      with open wound into cavity 867.7
    pancreas (multiple sites) 863.84
      with open wound into cavity 863.94
      body 863.82
        with open wound into cavity 863.92
      head 863.81
        with open wound into cavity 863.91
      tail 863.83
        with open wound into cavity 863.93
    pelvis, pelvic (organs) (viscera) 867.8
      with
        fracture, pelvis—*see* Fracture, pelvis
        open wound into cavity 867.9
      specified site NEC 867.6
        with open wound into cavity 867.7
    peritoneum 868.03
      with open wound into cavity 868.13
    pleura 862.29
      with open wound into cavity 862.39
    prostate 867.6
      with open wound into cavity 867.7
    rectum 863.45
      with
        colon 863.46
          with open wound into cavity 863.56
        open wound into cavity 863.55
    retroperitoneum 868.04
      with open wound into cavity 868.14
    round ligament 867.6
      with open wound into cavity 867.7
    seminal vesicle 867.6
      with open wound into cavity 867.7
    spermatic cord 867.6
      with open wound into cavity 867.7
      scrotal—*see* Wound, open, spermatic cord

Injury—*continued*
  spleen 865.00
    with
      disruption of parenchyma (massive)
          865.04
        with open wound into cavity 865.14
      hematoma (without rupture of capsule)
          865.01
        with open wound into cavity 865.11
      open wound into cavity 865.10
      tear, capsular 865.02
        with open wound into cavity 865.12
        extending into parenchyma 865.03
          with open wound into cavity 865.13
  stomach 863.0
    with open wound into cavity 863.1
  suprarenal gland (multiple) 868.01
    with open wound into cavity 868.11
  thorax, thoracic (cavity) (organs) (multiple)
      (*see also* Injury, internal, intrathoracic
      organs) 862.8
    with open wound into cavity 862.9
  thymus (gland) 862.29
    with open wound into cavity 862.39
  trachea (intrathoracic) 862.29
    with open wound into cavity 862.39
    cervical region (*see also* Wound, open,
        trachea) 874.02
  ureter 867.2
    with open wound into cavity 867.3
  urethra (sphincter) 867.0
    with
      abortion—*see* Abortion, by type, with,
          damage to pelvic organs
      ectopic pregnancy (*see also* categories
          633.0-633.9) 639.2
      molar pregnancy (*see also* categories
          630-632) 639.2
      open wound into cavity 867.1
    following
      abortion 639.2
      ectopic or molar pregnancy 639.2
    obstetrical trauma 665.5
      affecting fetus or newborn 763.89
  uterus 867.4
    with
      abortion—*see* Abortion, by type, with,
          damage to pelvic organs
      ectopic pregnancy (*see also* categories
          633.0-633.9) 639.2
      molar pregnancy (*see also* categories
          630-632) 639.2
      open wound into cavity 867.5
    following
      abortion 639.2
      ectopic or molar pregnancy 639.2
    obstetrical trauma NEC 665.5
      affecting fetus or newborn 763.89
  vas deferens 867.6
    with open wound into cavity 867.7
  vesical (sphincter) 867.0
    with open wound into cavity 867.1
  viscera (abdominal) (*see also* Injury, internal,
      multiple) 868.00
    with
      fracture, pelvis—*see* Fracture, pelvis
      open wound into cavity 868.10
      thoracic NEC (*see also* Injury, internal,
          intrathoracic organs) 862.8
        with open wound into cavity 862.9

Injury—*continued*
  interscapular region 959.1
  intervertebral disc 959.1
  intestine—*see* Injury, internal, intestine
  intra-abdominal (organs) NEC—*see* Injury,
    internal, intra-abdominal
  intracranial 854.0

---

*Note—Use the following fifth-digit
subclassification with categories 851-854:*

0 unspecified state of consciousness
1 with no loss of consciousness
*2 with brief [less than one hour] loss of
    consciousness*
*3 with moderate [1-24 hours] loss of
    consciousness*
*4 with prolonged [more than 24 hours] loss of
    consciousness and return to pre-existing
    conscious level*
*5 with prolonged [more than 24 hours] loss of
    consciousness, without return to pre-existing
    conscious level*
*Use fifth-digit 5 to designate when a patient is
unconscious and dies before regaining
consciousness, regardless of the duration of the
loss of consciousness*
*6 with loss of consciousness of unspecified
    duration*
9 with concussion, unspecified

---

  with
    open intracranial wound 854.1
    skull fracture—*see* Fracture, skull, by site
  contusion 851.8
    with open intracranial wound 851.9
    brain stem 851.4
      with open intracranial wound 851.5
    cerebellum 851.4
      with open intracranial wound 851.5
    cortex (cerebral) 851.0
      with open intracranial wound 851.2
  hematoma—*see* Injury, intracranial,
      hemorrhage
  hemorrhage 853.0
    with
      laceration—*see* Injury, intracranial,
        laceration
      open intracranial wound 853.1
    extradural 852.4
      with open intracranial wound 852.5
    subarachnoid 852.0
      with open intracranial wound 852.1
    subdural 852.2
      with open intracranial wound 852.3
  laceration 851.8
    with open intracranial wound 851.9
    brain stem 851.6
      with open intracranial wound 851.7
    cerebellum 851.6
      with open intracranial wound 851.7
    cortex (cerebral) 851.2
      with open intracranial wound 851.3
  intraocular—*see* Injury, eyeball, penetrating
  intrathoracic organs (multiple)—*see* Injury,
      internal, intrathoracic organs
  intrauterine—*see* Injury, internal, intrauterine
  iris 921.3
    penetrating—*see* Injury, eyeball, penetrating
  jaw 959.09
  jejunum—*see* Injury, internal, jejunum

Injury—*continued*
  joint NEC 959.9
    old or residual 718.80
      ankle 718.87
      elbow 718.82
      foot 718.87
      hand 718.84
      hip 718.85
      knee 718.86
      multiple sites 718.89
      pelvic region 718.85
      shoulder (region) 718.81
      specified site NEC 718.88
      wrist 718.83
  kidney—*see* Injury, internal, kidney
  knee (and ankle) (and foot) (and leg, except
      thigh) 959.7
  labium (majus) (minus) 959.1
  labyrinth, ear 959.09
  lacrimal apparatus, gland, or sac 921.1
    laceration 870.8
  larynx 959.09
  late effect—*see* Late, effects (of), injury
  leg except thigh (and ankle) (and foot) (and
      knee) 959.7
    upper or thigh 959.6
  lens, eye 921.3
    penetrating—*see* Injury, eyeball, penetrating
  lid, eye—*see* Injury, eyelid
  lip 959.09
  liver—*see* Injury, internal, liver
  lobe, parietal—*see* Injury, intracranial
  lumbar (region) 959.1
    plexus 953.5
  lumbosacral (region) 959.1
    plexus 953.5
  lung—*see* Injury, internal, lung
  malar region 959.09
  mastoid region 959.09
  maternal, during pregnancy, affecting fetus or
      newborn 760.5
  maxilla 959.09
  mediastinum—*see* Injury, internal, mediastinum
  membrane
    brain (*see also* Injury, intracranial) 854.0
    tympanic 959.09
  meningeal artery—*see* Hemorrhage, brain,
      traumatic, subarachnoid
  meninges (cerebral)—*see* Injury, intracranial
  mesenteric
    artery—*see* Injury, blood vessel, mesenteric,
      artery
    plexus, inferior 954.1
    vein—*see* Injury, blood vessel, mesenteric,
      vein
  mesentery—*see* Injury, internal, mesentery
  mesosalpinx—*see* Injury, internal, mesosalpinx
  middle ear 959.09
  midthoracic region 959.1
  mouth 959.09
  multiple (sites not classifiable to the same
      four-digit category in 959.0-959.7) 959.8
    internal 869.0
      with open wound into cavity 869.1
  musculocutaneous nerve 955.4
  nail
    finger 959.5
    toe 959.7
  nasal (septum) (sinus) 959.09
  nasopharynx 959.09

Injury—*continued*
spleen—*see* Injury, internal, spleen
stellate ganglion 954.1
sternal region 959.1
stomach—*see* Injury, internal, stomach
subconjunctival 921.1
subcutaneous 959.9
subdural—*see* Injury, intracranial
submaxillary region 959.09
submental region 959.09
subungual
    fingers 959.5
    toes 959.7
superficial 919

---

*Note—Use the following fourth-digit
subdivisions with categories 910-919:*

*.0 Abrasion or friction burn without mention of
    infection*
.1 Abrasion or friction burn, infected
.2 Blister without mention of infection
.3 Blister, infected
*.4 Insect bite, nonvenomous, without mention
    of infection*
.5 Insect bite, nonvenomous, infected
*.6 Superficial foreign body (splinter) without
    major open wound and without mention of
    infection*
*.7 Superficial foreign body (splinter) without
    major open wound, infected*
*.8 Other and unspecified superficial injury
    without mention of infection*
*.9 Other and unspecified superficial injury,
    infected*

For late effects of superficial injury, *see*
category 906.2.

---

abdomen, abdominal (muscle) (wall) (and
    other part(s) of trunk) 911
ankle (and hip, knee, leg, or thigh) 916
anus (and other part(s) of trunk) 911
arm 913
    upper (and shoulder) 912
auditory canal (external) (meatus) (and other
    part(s) of face, neck, or scalp, except eye)
    910
axilla (and upper arm) 912
back (and other part(s) of trunk) 911
breast (and other part(s) of trunk) 911
brow (and other part(s) of face, neck or scalp,
    except eye) 910
buttock (and other part(s) of trunk) 911
canthus, eye 918.0
cheek(s) (and other part(s) of face, neck, or
    scalp, except eye) 910
chest wall (and other part(s) of trunk) 911
chin (and other part(s) of face, neck, or scalp,
    except eye) 910
clitoris (and other part(s) of trunk) 911
conjunctiva 918.2
cornea 918.1
    due to contact lens 371.82
costal region (and other part(s) of trunk) 911
ear(s) (auricle) (canal) (drum) (external) (and
    other part(s) of face, neck, or scalp, except
    eye) 910
elbow (and forearm) (and wrist) 913
epididymis (and other part(s) of trunk) 911

Injury—*continued*
epigastric region (and other part(s) of trunk)
    911
epiglottis (and other part(s) of face, neck, or
    scalp, except eye) 910
eye(s) (and adnexa) NEC 918.9
eyelid(s) (and periocular area) 918.0
face (any part(s), except eye) (and neck or
    scalp) 910
finger(s) (nail) (any) 915
flank (and other part(s) of trunk) 911
foot (phalanges) (and toe(s)) 917
forearm (and elbow) (and wrist) 913
forehead (and other part(s) of face, neck, or
    scalp, except eye) 910
globe (eye) 918.9
groin (and other part(s) of trunk) 911
gum(s) (and other part(s) of face, neck, or
    scalp, except eye) 910
hand(s) (except fingers alone) 914
head (and other part(s) of face, neck, or scalp,
    except eye) 910
heel (and foot or toe) 917
hip (and ankle, knee, leg, or thigh) 916
iliac region (and other part(s) of trunk) 911
interscapular region (and other part(s) of
    trunk) 911
iris 918.9
knee (and ankle, hip, leg, or thigh) 916
labium (majus) (minus) (and other part(s) of
    trunk) 911
lacrimal (apparatus) (gland) (sac) 918.0
leg (lower) (upper) (and ankle, hip, knee, or
    thigh) 916
lip(s) (and other part(s) of face, neck, or scalp,
    except eye) 910
lower extremity (except foot) 916
lumbar region (and other part(s) of trunk) 911
malar region (and other part(s) of face, neck,
    or scalp, except eye) 910
mastoid region (and other part(s) of face,
    neck, or scalp, except eye) 910
midthoracic region (and other part(s) of trunk)
    911
mouth (and other part(s) of face, neck, or
    scalp, except eye) 910
multiple sites (not classifiable to the same
    three-digit category) 919
nasal (septum) (and other part(s) of face,
    neck, or scalp, except eye) 910
neck (and face or scalp, any part(s), except
    eye) 910
nose (septum) (and other part(s) of face, neck,
    or scalp, except eye) 910
occipital region (and other part(s) of face,
    neck, or scalp, except eye) 910
orbital region 918.0
palate (soft) (and other part(s) of face, neck,
    or scalp, except eye) 910
parietal region (and other part(s) of face, neck,
    or scalp, except eye) 910
penis (and other part(s) of trunk) 911
perineum (and other part(s) of trunk) 911
periocular area 918.0
pharynx (and other part(s) of face, neck, or
    scalp, except eye) 910
popliteal space (and ankle, hip, leg, or thigh)
    916
prepuce (and other part(s) of trunk) 911
pubic region (and other part(s) of trunk) 911

Injury—*continued*
  pudenda (and other part(s) of trunk) 911
  sacral region (and other part(s) of trunk) 911
  salivary (ducts) (glands) (and other part(s) of
    face, neck, or scalp, except eye) 910
  scalp (and other part(s) of face or neck, except
    eye) 910
  scapular region (and upper arm) 912
  sclera 918.2
  scrotum (and other part(s) of trunk) 911
  shoulder (and upper arm) 912
  skin NEC 919
  specified site(s) NEC 919
  sternal region (and other part(s) of trunk) 911
  subconjunctival 918.2
  subcutaneous NEC 919
  submaxillary region (and other part(s) of face,
    neck, or scalp, except eye) 910
  submental region (and other part(s) of face,
    neck, or scalp, except eye) 910
  supraclavicular fossa (and other part(s) of
    face, neck or scalp, except eye) 910
  supraorbital 918.0
  temple (and other part(s) of face, neck, or
    scalp, except eye) 910
  temporal region (and other part(s) of face,
    neck, or scalp, except eye) 910
  testis (and other part(s) of trunk) 911
  thigh (and ankle, hip, knee, or leg) 916
  thorax, thoracic (external) (and other part(s) of
    trunk) 911
  throat (and other part(s) of face, neck, or
    scalp, except eye) 910
  thumb(s) (nail) 915
  toe(s) (nail) (subungual) (and foot) 917
  tongue (and other part(s) of face, neck, or
    scalp, except eye) 910
  tooth, teeth 521.2
  trunk (any part(s)) 911
  tunica vaginalis (and other part(s) of trunk)
    911
  tympanum, tympanic membrane (and other
    part(s) of face, neck, or scalp, except eye)
    910
  upper extremity NEC 913
  uvula (and other part(s) of face, neck, or
    scalp, except eye) 910
  vagina (and other part(s) of trunk) 911
  vulva (and other part(s) of trunk) 911
  wrist (and elbow) (and forearm) 913
  supraclavicular fossa 959.1
  supraorbital 959.09
  surgical complication (external or internal site)
    998.2
  symphysis pubis 959.1
    complicating delivery 665.6
    affecting fetus or newborn 763.89
  temple 959.09
  temporal region 959.09
  testis 959.1
  thigh (and hip) 959.6
  thorax, thoracic (external) 959.1
    cavity—*see* Injury, internal, thorax
    internal—*see* Injury, internal, intrathoracic
      organs
  throat 959.09
  thumb(s) (nail) 959.5
  thymus—*see* Injury, internal, thymus
  thyroid (gland) 959.09
  toe (nail) (any) 959.7

Injury—*continued*
  tongue 959.09
  tonsil 959.09
  tooth NEC 873.63
    complicated 873.73
  trachea—*see* Injury, internal, trachea
  trunk 959.1
  tunica vaginalis 959.1
  tympanum, tympanic membrane 959.09
  ultraviolet rays NEC 990
  ureter—*see* Injury, internal, ureter
  urethra (sphincter)—*see* Injury, internal, urethra
  uterus—*see* Injury, internal, uterus
  uvula 959.09
  vagina 959.1
  vascular—*see* Injury, blood vessel
  vas deferens—*see* Injury, internal, vas deferens
  vein (*see also* Injury, blood vessel, by site) 904.9
  vena cava
    inferior 902.10
    superior 901.2
  vesical (sphincter)—*see* Injury, internal, vesical
  viscera (abdominal)—*see* Injury, internal,
    viscera
    with fracture, pelvis—*see* Fracture, pelvis
  visual 950.9
    cortex 950.3
  vitreous (humor) 871.2
  vulva 959.1
  whiplash (cervical spine) 847.0
  wringer—*see* Crush, by site
  wrist (and elbow) (and forearm) 959.3
  x-ray NEC 990
Inoculation —*see also* Vaccination
  complication or reaction—*see* Complication,
    vaccination
Insanity, insane (*see also* Psychosis) 298.9
  adolescent (*see also* Schizophrenia) 295.9
  alternating (*see also* Psychosis, affective,
    circular) 296.7
  confusional 298.9
    acute 293.0
    subacute 293.1
  delusional 298.9
  paralysis, general 094.1
    progressive 094.1
  paresis, general 094.1
  senile 290.20
Insect
  bite—*see* Injury, superficial, by site
  venomous, poisoning by 989.5
Insemination, artificial V26.1
Insertion
  cord (umbilical) lateral or velamentous 663.8
    affecting fetus or newborn 762.6
  intrauterine contraceptive device V25.1
  placenta, vicious—*see* Placenta, previa
  subdermal implantable contraceptive V25.5
  velamentous, umbilical cord 663.8
    affecting fetus or newborn 762.6
Insolation 992.0
  meaning sunstroke 992.0
Insomnia 780.52
  with sleep apnea 780.51
  nonorganic origin 307.41
    persistent (primary) 307.42
    transient 307.41
  subjective complaint 307.49

Inspiration
  food or foreign body (*see also* Asphyxia, food
      or foreign body) 933.1
  mucus (*see also* Asphyxia, mucus) 933.1
Inspissated bile syndrome, newborn 774.4
Instability
  detrusor 596.59
  emotional (excessive) 301.3
  joint (posttraumatic) 718.80
      ankle 718.87
      elbow 718.82
      foot 718.87
      hand 718.84
      hip 718.85
      knee 718.86
      lumbosacral 724.6
      multiple sites 718.89
      pelvic region 718.85
      sacroiliac 724.6
      shoulder (region) 718.81
      specified site NEC 718.88
      wrist 718.83
  lumbosacral 724.6
  nervous 301.89
  personality (emotional) 301.59
  thyroid, paroxysmal 242.9
  urethral 599.83
  vasomotor 780.2
Insufficiency, insufficient
  accommodation 367.4
  adrenal (gland) (acute) (chronic) 255.4
      medulla 255.5
      primary 255.4
      specified NEC 255.5
  adrenocortical 255.4
  anus 569.49
  aortic (valve) 424.1
      with
          mitral (valve) disease 396.1
              insufficiency, incompetence, or
                  regurgitation 396.3
              stenosis or obstruction 396.1
          stenosis or obstruction 424.1
              with mitral (valve) disease 396.8
      congenital 746.4
      rheumatic 395.1
          with
              mitral (valve) disease 396.1
                  insufficiency, incompetence, or
                      regurgitation 396.3
                  stenosis or obstruction 396.1
              stenosis or obstruction 395.2
                  with mitral (valve) disease 396.8
      specified cause NEC 424.1
      syphilitic 093.22
  arterial 447.1
      basilar artery 435.0
      carotid artery 435.8
      cerebral 437.1
      coronary (acute or subacute) 411.89
      mesenteric 557.1
      peripheral 443.9
      precerebral 435.9
      vertebral artery 435.1
      vertibrobasilar 435.3
  arteriovenous 459.9
  basilar artery 435.0
  biliary 575.8

Insufficiency, insufficient—*continued*
  cardiac (*see also* Insufficiency, myocardial)
      428.0
      complicating surgery 997.1
      due to presence of (cardiac) prosthesis 429.4
      postoperative 997.1
          long-term effect of cardiac surgery 429.4
      specified during or due to a procedure 997.1
          long-term effect of cardiac surgery 429.4
  cardiorenal (*see also* Hypertension, cardiorenal)
      404.90
  cardiovascular (*see also* Disease,
      cardiovascular) 429.2
      renal (*see also* Hypertension, cardiorenal)
          404.90
  carotid artery 435.8
  cerebral (vascular) 437.9
  cerebrovascular 437.9
      with transient focal neurological signs and
          symptoms 435.9
      acute 437.1
          with transient focal neurological signs and
              symptoms 435.9
  circulatory NEC 459.9
      fetus or newborn 779.89
  convergence 378.83
  coronary (acute or subacute) 411.89
      chronic or with a stated duration of over 8
          weeks 414.8
  corticoadrenal 255.4
  dietary 269.9
  divergence 378.85
  food 994.2
  gastroesophageal 530.89
  gonadal
      ovary 256.39
      testis 257.2
  gonadotropic hormone secretion 253.4
  heart—*see also* Insufficiency, myocardial
      fetus or newborn 779.89
      valve (*see also* Endocarditis) 424.90
          congenital NEC 746.89
  hepatic 573.8
  idiopathic autonomic 333.0
  kidney (acute) (chronic) 593.9
  labyrinth, labyrinthine (function) 386.53
      bilateral 386.54
      unilateral 386.53
  lacrimal 375.15
  liver 573.8
  lung (acute) (*see also* Insufficiency, pulmonary)
      518.82
      following trauma, surgery, or shock 518.5
      newborn 770.89
  mental (congenital) (*see also* Retardation,
      mental) 319
  mesenteric 557.1
  mitral (valve) 424.0
      with
          aortic (valve) disease 396.3
              insufficiency, incompetence, or
                  regurgitation 396.3
              stenosis or obstruction 396.2
          obstruction or stenosis 394.2
              with aortic valve disease 396.8
      congenital 746.6

Insufficiency, insufficient—*continued*
  rheumatic 394.1
    with
      aortic (valve) disease 396.3
        insufficiency, incompetence, or
          regurgitation 396.3
        stenosis or obstruction 396.2
      obstruction or stenosis 394.2
        with aortic valve disease 396.8
      active or acute 391.1
        with chorea, rheumatic (Sydenham's)
          392.0
    specified cause, except rheumatic 424.0
  muscle
    heart—*see* Insufficiency, myocardial
    ocular (*see also* Strabismus) 378.9
  myocardial, myocardium (with arteriosclerosis)
    428.0
    with rheumatic fever (conditions classifiable
      to 390)
      active, acute, or subacute 391.2
        with chorea 392.0
      inactive or quiescent (with chorea) 398.0
    congenital 746.89
    due to presence of (cardiac) prosthesis 429.4
    fetus or newborn 779.89
    following cardiac surgery 429.4
    hypertensive (*see also* Hypertension, heart)
      402.91
      benign 402.11
      malignant 402.01
    postoperative 997.1
      long-term effect of cardiac surgery 429.4
    rheumatic 398.0
      active, acute, or subacute 391.2
        with chorea (Sydenham's) 392.0
    syphilitic 093.82
  nourishment 994.2
  organic 799.8
  ovary 256.39
    postablative 256.2
  pancreatic 577.8
  parathyroid (gland) 252.1
  peripheral vascular (arterial) 443.9
  pituitary (anterior) 253.2
    posterior 253.5
  placental—*see* Placenta, insufficiency
  platelets 287.5
  prenatal care in current pregnancy V23.7
  progressive pluriglandular 258.9
  pseudocholinesterase 289.8
  pulmonary (acute) 518.82
    following
      shock 518.5
      surgery 518.5
      trauma 518.5
    newborn 770.89
    valve (*see also* Endocarditis, pulmonary) 424.3
    congenital 746.09
  pyloric 537.0
  renal (acute) (chronic) 593.9
    due to a procedure 997.5
  respiratory 786.09
    acute 518.82
      following shock, surgery, or trauma 518.5
    newborn 770.89
  rotation—*see* Malrotation
  suprarenal 255.4
    medulla 255.5
  tarso-orbital fascia, congenital 743.66

Insufficiency, insufficient—*continued*
  tear film 375.15
  testis 257.2
  thyroid (gland) (acquired)—*see also*
    Hypothyroidism
    congenital 243
  tricuspid (*see also* Endocarditis, tricuspid) 397.0
    congenital 746.89
    syphilitic 093.23
  urethral sphincter 599.84
  valve, valvular (heart) (*see also* Endocarditis)
    424.90
  vascular 459.9
    intestine NEC 557.9
    mesenteric 557.1
    peripheral 443.9
    renal (*see also* Hypertension, kidney) 403.90
  velopharyngeal
    acquired 528.9
    congenital 750.29
  venous (peripheral) 459.81
  ventricular—*see* Insufficiency, myocardial
  vertebral artery 435.1
  vertibrobasilar artery 435.3
  weight gain during pregnancy 646.8
  zinc 269.3
Insufflation
  fallopian
    fertility testing V26.21
    following sterilization reversal V26.22
  meconium 770.1
Insular —*see* condition
Insulinoma (M8151/0)
  malignant (M8151/3)
    pancreas 157.4
    specified site—*see* Neoplasm, by site,
      malignant
    unspecified site 157.4
  pancreas 211.7
  specified site—*see* Neoplasm, by site, benign
  unspecified site 211.7
Insuloma —*see* Insulinoma
Insult
  brain 437.9
    acute 436
  cerebral 437.9
    acute 436
  cerebrovascular 437.9
    acute 436
  vascular NEC 437.9
    acute 436
Insurance examination (certification) V70.3
Intemperance (*see also* Alcoholism) 303.9
Interception of pregnancy (menstrual
  extraction) V25.3
Intermenstrual
  bleeding 626.6
    irregular 626.6
    regular 626.5
  hemorrhage 626.6
    irregular 626.6
    regular 626.5
  pain(s) 625.2
Intermittent— *see* condition
Internal —*see* condition
Interproximal wear 521.1
Interruption
  aortic arch 747.11
  bundle of His 426.50
  fallopian tube (for sterilization) V25.2

Interruption—*continued*
  phase-shift, sleep cycle 307.45
  repeated REM-sleep 307.48
  sleep
    due to perceived environmental disturbances 307.48
    phase-shift, of 24-hour sleep-wake cycle 307.45
    repeated REM-sleep type 307.48
  vas deferens (for sterilization) V25.2
Intersexuality 752.7
Interstitial —*see* condition
Intertrigo 695.89
  labialis 528.5
Intervertebral disc —*see* condition
Intestine, intestinal —*see also* condition
  flu 487.8
Intolerance
  carbohydrate NEC 579.8
  cardiovascular exercise, with pain (at rest) (with less than ordinary activity) (with ordinary activity) V47.2
  cold 780.99
  disaccharide (hereditary) 271.3
  drug
    correct substance properly administered 995.2
    wrong substance given or taken in error 977.9
    specified drug—*see* Table of drugs and chemicals
  effort 306.2
  fat NEC 579.8
  foods NEC 579.8
  fructose (hereditary) 271.2
  glucose (-galactose) (congenital) 271.3
  gluten 579.0
  lactose (hereditary) (infantile) 271.3
  lysine (congenital) 270.7
  milk NEC 579.8
  protein (familial) 270.7
  starch NEC 579.8
  sucrose (-isomaltose) (congenital) 271.3
Intoxicated NEC (*see also* Alcoholism) 305.0
Intoxication
  acid 276.2
  acute
    alcoholic 305.0
      with alcoholism 303.0
      hangover effects 305.0
    caffeine 305.9
    hallucinogenic (*see also* Abuse, drugs, nondependent) 305.3
  alcohol (acute) 305.0
    with alcoholism 303.0
    hangover effects 305.0
    idiosyncratic 291.4
    pathological 291.4
  alimentary canal 558.2
  ammonia (hepatic) 572.2
  chemical—*see also* Table of drugs and chemicals
  via placenta or breast milk 760.70
    alcohol 760.71
    anti-infective agents 760.74
    cocaine 760.75
    "crack" 760.75
    hallucinogenic agents NEC 760.73
    medicinal agents NEC 760.79
    narcotics 760.72
    obstetric anesthetic or analgesic drug 763.5
    specified agent NEC 760.79

Intoxication—*continued*
    suspected, affecting management of pregnancy 655.5
  cocaine, through placenta or breast milk 760.75
  delirium
    alcohol 291.0
    drug 292.81
  drug
    with delirium 292.81
    correct substance properly administered (*see also* Allergy, drug) 995.2
    newborn 779.4
    obstetric anesthetic or sedation 668.9
      affecting fetus or newborn 763.5
    overdose or wrong substance given or taken—*see* Table of drugs and chemicals
    pathologic 292.2
    specific to newborn 779.4
    via placenta or breast milk 760.70
      alcohol 760.71
      anti-infective agents 760.74
      cocaine 760.75
      "crack" 760.75
      hallucinogenic agents 760.73
      medicinal agents NEC 760.79
      narcotics 760.72
      obstetric anesthetic or analgesic drug 763.5
      specified agent NEC 760.79
      suspected, affecting management of pregnancy 655.5
  enteric—*see* Intoxication, intestinal
  fetus or newborn, via placenta or breast milk 760.70
    alcohol 760.71
    anti-infective agents 760.74
    cocaine 760.75
    "crack" 760.75
    hallucinogenic agents 760.73
    medicinal agents NEC 760.79
    narcotics 760.72
    obstetric anesthetic or analgesic drug 763.5
    specified agent NEC 760.79
    suspected, affecting management of pregnancy 655.5
  food—*see* Poisoning, food
  gastrointestinal 558.2
  hallucinogenic (acute) 305.3
  hepatocerebral 572.2
  idiosyncratic alcohol 291.4
  intestinal 569.89
    due to putrefaction of food 005.9
  methyl alcohol (*see also* Alcoholism) 305.0
    with alcoholism 303.0
  pathologic 291.4
    drug 292.2
  potassium (K) 276.7
  septic
    with
      abortion—*see* Abortion, by type, with sepsis
      ectopic pregnancy (*see also* categories 633.0-633.9) 639.0
      molar pregnancy (*see also* categories 630-632) 639.0
    during labor 659.3
    following
      abortion 639.0
      ectopic or molar pregnancy 639.0
    generalized—*see* Septicemia
    puerperal, postpartum, childbirth 670
  serum (prophylactic) (therapeutic) 999.5
  uremic—*see* Uremia
  water 276.6

Iritis—*continued*
  gouty 274.89 *[364.11]*
  granulomatous 364.10
  hypopyon 364.05
  lens induced 364.23
  nongranulomatous 364.00
  papulosa 095.8 *[364.11]*
  primary 364.01
  recurrent 364.02
  rheumatic 364.10
  secondary 364.04
    infectious 364.03
    noninfectious 364.04
  subacute 364.00
    primary 364.01
    recurrent 364.02
  sympathetic 360.11
  syphilitic (secondary) 091.52
    congenital 090.0 *[364.11]*
    late 095.8 *[364.11]*
  tuberculous (*see also* Tuberculosis) 017.3
    [364.11]
  uratic 274.89 *[364.11]*
Iron
  deficiency anemia 280.9
  metabolism disease 275.0
  storage disease 275.0
Iron-miners' lung 503
Irradiated enamel (tooth, teeth) 521.8
Irradiation
  burn—*see* Burn, by site
  effects, adverse 990
Irreducible, irreducibility —*see* condition
Irregular, irregularity
  action, heart 427.9
  alveolar process 525.8
  bleeding NEC 626.4
  breathing 786.09
  colon 569.89
  contour of cornea 743.41
    acquired 371.70
  dentin in pulp 522.3
  eye movements NEC 379.59
  menstruation (cause unknown) 626.4
  periods 626.4
  prostate 602.9
  pupil 364.75
  respiratory 786.09
  septum (nasal) 470
  shape, organ or site, congenital NEC—*see*
    Distortion
  sleep-wake rhythm (non-24-hour) 780.55
    nonorganic origin 307.45
  vertebra 733.99
Irritability (nervous) 799.2
  bladder 596.8
    neurogenic 596.54
      with cauda equina syndrome 344.61
  bowel (syndrome) 564.1
  bronchial (*see also* Bronchitis) 490
  cerebral, newborn 779.1
  colon 564.1
    psychogenic 306.4
  duodenum 564.89
  heart (psychogenic) 306.2
  ileum 564.89
  jejunum 564.89
  myocardium 306.2
  rectum 564.89
  stomach 536.9
    psychogenic 306.4

Irritability—*continued*
  sympathetic (nervous system) (*see also*
    Neuropathy, peripheral, autonomic) 337.9
  urethra 599.84
  ventricular (heart) (psychogenic) 306.2
Irritable —*see* Irritability
Irritation
  anus 569.49
  axillary nerve 353.0
  bladder 596.8
  brachial plexus 353.0
  brain (traumatic) (*see also* Injury, intracranial)
    854.0
    nontraumatic—*see* Encephalitis
  bronchial (*see also* Bronchitis) 490
  cerebral (traumatic) (*see also* Injury,
    intracranial) 854.0
    nontraumatic—*see* Encephalitis
  cervical plexus 353.2
  cervix (*see also* Cervicitis) 616.0
  choroid, sympathetic 360.11
  cranial nerve—*see* Disorder, nerve, cranial
  digestive tract 536.9
    psychogenic 306.4
  gastric 536.9
    psychogenic 306.4
  gastrointestinal (tract) 536.9
    functional 536.9
    psychogenic 306.4
  globe, sympathetic 360.11
  intestinal (bowel) 564.9
  labyrinth 386.50
  lumbosacral plexus 353.1
  meninges (traumatic) (*see also* Injury,
    intracranial) 854.0
    nontraumatic—*see* Meningitis
  myocardium 306.2
  nerve—*see* Disorder, nerve
  nervous 799.2
  nose 478.1
  penis 607.89
  perineum 709.9
  peripheral
    autonomic nervous system (*see also*
      Neuropathy, peripheral, autonomic) 337.9
    nerve—*see* Disorder, nerve
  peritoneum (*see also* Peritonitis) 567.9
  pharynx 478.29
  plantar nerve 355.6
  spinal (cord) (traumatic)—*see also* Injury,
    spinal, by site
    nerve—*see also* Disorder, nerve
      root NEC 724.9
      traumatic—*see* Injury, nerve, spinal
    nontraumatic—*see* Myelitis
  stomach 536.9
    psychogenic 306.4
  sympathetic nerve NEC (*see also* Neuropathy,
    peripheral, autonomic) 337.9
  ulnar nerve 354.2
  vagina 623.9
Isambert's disease 012.3
Ischemia, ischemic 459.9
  basilar artery (with transient neurologic deficit)
    435.0
  bone NEC 733.40
  bowel (transient) 557.9
    acute 557.0
    chronic 557.1
    due to mesenteric artery insufficiency 557.1

Ischemia, ischemic—*continued*
  brain—*see also* Ischemia, cerebral
    recurrent focal 435.9
  cardiac (*see also* Ischemia, heart) 414.9
  cardiomyopathy 414.8
  carotid artery (with transient neurologic deficit)
    435.8
  cerebral (chronic) (generalized) 437.1
    arteriosclerotic 437.0
    intermittent (with transient neurologic deficit)
      435.9
    puerperal, postpartum, childbirth 674.0
    recurrent focal (with transient neurologic
      deficit) 435.9
    transient (with transient neurologic deficit)
      435.9
  colon 557.9
    acute 557.0
    chronic 557.1
    due to mesenteric artery insufficiency 557.1
  coronary (chronic) (*see also* Ischemia, heart)
    414.9
  heart (chronic or with a stated duration of over 8
    weeks) 414.9
    acute or with a stated duration of 8 weeks or
      less (*see also* Infarct, myocardium) 410.9
      without myocardial infarction 411.89
        with coronary (artery) occlusion 411.81
    subacute 411.89
  intestine (transient) 557.9
    acute 557.0
    chronic 557.1
    due to mesenteric artery insufficiency 557.1
  kidney 593.81
  labyrinth 386.50
  muscles, leg 728.89
  myocardium, myocardial (chronic or with a
    stated duration of over 8 weeks) 414.8
    acute (*see also* Infarct, myocardium) 410.9
      without myocardial infarction 411.89
        with coronary (artery) occlusion 411.81
  renal 593.81
  retina, retinal 362.84
  small bowel 557.9
    acute 557.0
    chronic 557.1
    due to mesenteric artery insufficiency 557.1
  spinal cord 336.1
  subendocardial (*see also* Insufficiency,
    coronary) 411.89
  vertebral artery (with transient neurologic
    deficit) 435.1
Ischialgia (*see also* Sciatica) 724.3
Ischiopagus 759.4
Ischium, ischial —*see* condition
Ischomenia 626.8
Ischuria 788.5
Iselin's disease or osteochondrosis 732.5
Islands of
  parotid tissue in
    lymph nodes 750.26
    neck structures 750.26
  submaxillary glands in
    fascia 750.26
    lymph nodes 750.26
    neck muscles 750.26
Islet cell tumor, pancreas (M8150/0) 211.7
Isoimmunization NEC (*see also* Incompatibility)
  656.2
  fetus or newborn 773.2
    ABO blood groups 773.1
    Rhesus (Rh) factor 773.0

Isolation V07.0
  social V62.4
Isosporosis 007.2
Issue
  medical certificate NEC V68.0
    cause of death V68.0
    fitness V68.0
    incapacity V68.0
  repeat prescription NEC V68.1
    appliance V68.1
    contraceptive V25.40
      device NEC V25.49
        intrauterine V25.42
        specified type NEC V25.49
      pill V25.41
    glasses V68.1
    medicinal substance V68.1
Itch (*see also* Pruritus) 698.9
  bakers' 692.89
  barbers' 110.0
  bricklayers' 692.89
  cheese 133.8
  clam diggers' 120.3
  coolie 126.9
  copra 133.8
  Cuban 050.1
  dew 126.9
  dhobie 110.3
  eye 379.99
  filarial (*see also* Infestation, filarial) 125.9
  grain 133.8
  grocers' 133.8
  ground 126.9
  harvest 133.8
  jock 110.3
  Malabar 110.9
    beard 110.0
    foot 110.4
    scalp 110.0
  meaning scabies 133.0
  Norwegian 133.0
  perianal 698.0
  poultrymen's 133.8
  sarcoptic 133.0
  scrub 134.1
  seven year V61.10
    meaning scabies 133.0
  straw 133.8
  swimmers' 120.3
  washerwoman's 692.4
  water 120.3
  winter 698.8
Itsenko-Cushing syndrome (pituitary
  basophilism) 255.0
Ivemark's syndrome (asplenia with congenital
  heart disease) 759.0
Ivory bones 756.52
Ixodes 134.8
Ixodiasis 134.8

Jaccoud's nodular fibrositis, chronic
(Jaccoud's syndrome) 714.4
Jackson's
membrane 751.4
paralysis or syndrome 344.89
veil 751.4
Jacksonian
epilepsy (*see also* Epilepsy) 345.5
seizures (focal) (*see also* Epilepsy) 345.5
Jacob's ulcer (M8090/3)—*see* Neoplasm, skin,
malignant, by site
Jacquet's dermatitis (diaper dermatitis) 691.0
Jadassohn's
blue nevus (M8780/0)—*see* Neoplasm, skin,
benign
disease (maculopapular erythroderma) 696.2
intraepidermal epithelioma (M8096/0)—*see*
Neoplasm, skin, benign
Jadassohn-Lewandowski syndrome
(pachyonychia congenita) 757.5
Jadassohn-Pellizari's disease (anetoderma)
701.3
Jadassohn-Tièche nevus (M8780/0)—*see*
Neoplasm, skin, benign
Jaffe-Lichtenstein (-Uehlinger) syndrome 252.0
Jahnke's syndrome (encephalocutaneous
angiomatosis) 759.6
Jakob-Creutzfeldt disease or syndrome 046.1
with dementia
with behavioral disturbance 046.1 *[294.11]*
without behavioral disturbance 046.1 *[294.10]*
Jaksch (-Luzet) disease or syndrome
(pseudoleukemia infantum) 285.8
Jamaican
neuropathy 349.82
paraplegic tropical ataxic-spastic syndrome
349.82
Janet's disease (psychasthenia) 300.89
Janiceps 759.4
Jansky-Bielschowsky amaurotic familial idiocy
330.1
Japanese
B type encephalitis 062.0
river fever 081.2
seven-day fever 100.89
Jaundice (yellow) 782.4
acholuric (familial) (splenomegalic) (*see also*
Spherocytosis) 282.0
acquired 283.9
breast milk 774.39
catarrhal (acute) 070.1
with hepatic coma 070.0
chronic 571.9
epidemic—*see* Jaundice, epidemic
cholestatic (benign) 782.4
chronic idiopathic 277.4
epidemic (catarrhal) 070.1
with hepatic coma 070.0
leptospiral 100.0
spirochetal 100.0
febrile (acute) 070.1
with hepatic coma 070.0
leptospiral 100.0
spirochetal 100.0

Jaundice—*continued*
fetus or newborn 774.6
due to or associated with
ABO
antibodies 773.1
incompatibility, maternal/fetal 773.1
isoimmunization 773.1
absence or deficiency of enzyme system for
bilirubin conjugation (congenital) 774.39
blood group incompatibility NEC 773.2
breast milk inhibitors to conjugation 774.39
associated with preterm delivery 774.2
bruising 774.1
Crigler-Najjar syndrome 277.4 *[774.31]*
delayed conjugation 774.30
associated with preterm delivery 774.2
development 774.39
drugs or toxins transmitted from mother
774.1
G-6-PD deficiency 282.2 *[774.0]*
galactosemia 271.1 *[774.5]*
Gilbert's syndrome 277.4 *[774.31]*
hepatocellular damage 774.4
hereditary hemolytic anemia (*see also*
Anemia, hemolytic) 282.9 *[774.0]*
hypothyroidism, congenital 243 *[774.31]*
incompatibility, maternal/fetal NEC 773.2
infection 774.1
inspissated bile syndrome 774.4
isoimmunization NEC 773.2
mucoviscidosis 277.01 *[774.5]*
obliteration of bile duct, congenital 751.61
[774.5]
polycythemia 774.1
preterm delivery 774.2
red cell defect 282.9 *[774.0]*
Rh
antibodies 773.0
incompatibility, maternal/fetal 773.0
isoimmunization 773.0
spherocytosis (congenital) 282.0 *[774.0]*
swallowed maternal blood 774.1
physiological NEC 774.6
from injection, inoculation, infusion, or
transfusion (blood) (plasma) (serum) (other
substance) (onset within 8 months after
administration)—*see* Hepatitis, viral
Gilbert's (familial nonhemolytic) 277.4
hematogenous 283.9
hemolytic (acquired) 283.9
congenital (*see also* Spherocytosis) 282.0
hemorrhagic (acute) 100.0
leptospiral 100.0
newborn 776.0
spirochetal 100.0
hepatocellular 573.8
homologous (serum)—*see* Hepatitis, viral
idiopathic, chronic 277.4
infectious (acute) (subacute) 070.1
with hepatic coma 070.0
leptospiral 100.0
spirochetal 100.0
leptospiral 100.0
malignant (*see also* Necrosis, liver) 570
newborn (physiological) (*see also* Jaundice,
fetus or newborn) 774.6

Jaundice—*continued*
  nonhemolytic, congenital familial (Gilbert's)
    277.4
  nuclear, newborn (*see also* Kernicterus of
    newborn) 774.7
  obstructive NEC (*see also* Obstruction, biliary)
    576.8
  postimmunization—*see* Hepatitis, viral
  posttransfusion—*see* Hepatitis, viral
  regurgitation (*see also* Obstruction, biliary)
    576.8
  serum (homologous) (prophylactic)
    (therapeutic)—*see* Hepatitis, viral
  spirochetal (hemorrhagic) 100.0
  symptomatic 782.4
    newborn 774.6
Jaw —*see* condition
Jaw-blinking 374.43
  congenital 742.8
Jaw-winking phenomenon or syndrome 742.8
Jealousy
  alcoholic 291.5
  childhood 313.3
  sibling 313.3
Jejunitis (*see also* Enteritis) 558.9
Jejunostomy status V44.4
Jejunum, jejunal —*see* condition
Jensen's disease 363.05
Jericho boil 085.1
Jerks, myoclonic 333.2
Jeune's disease or syndrome (asphyxiating
    thoracic dystrophy) 756.4
Jigger disease 134.1
Job's syndrome (chronic granulomatous disease)
    288.1
Jod-Basedow phenomenon 242.8
Johnson-Stevens disease (erythema multiforme
    exudativum) 695.1
Joint —*see also* condition
  Charcot's 094.0 *[713.5]*
  false 733.82
  flail—*see* Flail, joint
  mice—*see* Loose, body, joint, by site
  sinus to bone 730.9
  von Gies' 095.8
Jordan's anomaly or syndrome 288.2
Josephs-Diamond-Blackfan anemia (congenital
    hypoplastic) 284.0
Joubert syndrome 759.89
Jumpers' knee 727.2
Jungle yellow fever 060.0
Jüngling's disease (sarcoidosis) 135
Junin virus hemorrhagic fever 078.7
Juvenile —*see also* condition
  delinquent 312.9
    group (*see also* Disturbance, conduct) 312.2
    neurotic 312.4

K

Kahler (-Bozzolo) disease (multiple myeloma)
(M9730/3) 203.0
Kakergasia 300.9
Kakke 265.0
Kala-azar (Indian) (infantile) (Mediterranean)
(Sudanese) 085.0
Kalischer's syndrome (encephalocutaneous
angiomatosis) 759.6
Kallmann's syndrome (hypogonadotropic
hypogonadism with anosmia) 253.4
Kanner's syndrome (autism) (*see also*
Psychosis, childhood) 299.0
Kaolinosis 502
Kaposi's
disease 757.33
lichen ruber 696.4
acuminatus 696.4
moniliformis 697.8
xeroderma pigmentosum 757.33
sarcoma (M9140/3) 176.9
adipose tissue 176.1
aponeurosis 176.1
artery 176.1
blood vessel 176.1
bursa 176.1
connective tissue 176.1
external genitalia 176.8
fascia 176.1
fatty tissue 176.1
fibrous tissue 176.1
gastrointestinal tract NEC 176.3
ligament 176.1
lung 176.4
lymph
gland(s) 176.5
node(s) 176.5
lymphatic(s) NEC 176.1
muscle (skeletal) 176.1
oral cavity NEC 176.8
palate 176.2
scrotum 176.8
skin 176.0
soft tissue 176.1
specified site NEC 176.8
subcutaneous tissue 176.1
synovia 176.1
tendon (sheath) 176.1
vein 176.1
vessel 176.1
viscera NEC 176.9
vulva 176.8
varicelliform eruption 054.0
vaccinia 999.0
Kartagener's syndrome or triad (sinusitis,
bronchiectasis, situs inversus) 759.3
Kasabach-Merritt syndrome (capillary
hemangioma associated with
thrombocytopenic purpura) 287.3
Kaschin-Beck disease (endemic
polyarthritis)—*see* Disease, Kaschin-Beck
Kast's syndrome (dyschondroplasia with
hemangiomas) 756.4
Katatonia (*see also* Schizophrenia) 295.2
Katayama disease or fever 120.2
Kathisophobia 781.0
Kawasaki disease 446.1
Kayser-Fleischer ring (cornea)
(pseudosclerosis) 275.1 *[371.14]*

Kaznelson's syndrome (congenital hypoplastic
anemia) 284.0
Kedani fever 081.2
Kelis 701.4
Kelly (-Patterson) syndrome (sideropenic
dysphagia) 280.8
Keloid, cheloid 701.4
Addison's (morphea) 701.0
cornea 371.00
Hawkins' 701.4
scar 701.4
Keloma 701.4
Kenya fever 082.1
Keratectasia 371.71
congenital 743.41
Keratitis (nodular) (nonulcerative) (simple)
(zonular) NEC 370.9
with ulceration (*see also* Ulcer, cornea) 370.00
actinic 370.24
arborescens 054.42
areolar 370.22
bullosa 370.8
deep—*see* Keratitis, interstitial
dendritic(a) 054.42
desiccation 370.34
diffuse interstitial 370.52
disciform(is) 054.43
varicella 052.7 *[370.44]*
epithelialis vernalis 372.13 *[370.32]*
exposure 370.34
filamentary 370.23
gonococcal (congenital) (prenatal) 098.43
herpes, herpetic (simplex) NEC 054.43
zoster 053.21
hypopyon 370.04
in
chickenpox 052.7 *[370.44]*
exanthema (*see also* Exanthem) 057.9
[370.44]
paravaccinia (*see also* Paravaccinia) 051.9
[370.44]
smallpox (*see also* Smallpox) 050.9 *[370.44]*
vernal conjunctivitis 372.13 *[370.32]*
interstitial (nonsyphilitic) 370.50
with ulcer (*see also* Ulcer, cornea) 370.00
diffuse 370.52
herpes, herpetic (simplex) 054.43
zoster 053.21
syphilitic (congenital) (hereditary) 090.3
tuberculous (*see also* Tuberculosis) 017.3
[370.59]
lagophthalmic 370.34
macular 370.22
neuroparalytic 370.35
neurotrophic 370.35
nummular 370.22
oyster-shuckers' 370.8
parenchymatous—*see* Keratitis, interstitial
petrificans 370.8
phlyctenular 370.31
postmeasles 055.71
punctata, punctate 370.21
leprosa 030.0 *[370.21]*
profunda 090.3
superficial (Thygeson's) 370.21
purulent 370.8
pustuliformis profunda 090.3

Keratitis—*continued*
  rosacea 695.3 *[370.49]*
  sclerosing 370.54
  specified type NEC 370.8
  stellate 370.22
  striate 370.22
  superficial 370.20
    with conjunctivitis (*see also*
        Keratoconjunctivitis) 370.40
      punctate (Thygeson's) 370.21
  suppurative 370.8
  syphilitic (congenital) (prenatal) 090.3
  trachomatous 076.1
    late effect 139.1
  tuberculous (phlyctenular) (*see also*
        Tuberculosis) 017.3 *[370.31]*
  ulcerated (*see also* Ulcer, cornea) 370.00
  vesicular 370.8
  welders' 370.24
  xerotic (*see also* Keratomalacia) 371.45
    vitamin A deficiency 264.4
Keratoacanthoma 238.2
Keratocele 371.72
Keratoconjunctivitis (*see also* Keratitis) 370.40
  adenovirus type 8 077.1
  epidemic 077.1
  exposure 370.34
  gonococcal 098.43
  herpetic (simplex) 054.43
    zoster 053.21
  in
    chickenpox 052.7 *[370.44]*
    exanthema (*see also* Exanthem) 057.9
        [370.44]
    paravaccinia (*see also* Paravaccinia) 051.9
        [370.44]
    smallpox (*see also* Smallpox) 050.9 *[370.44]*
  infectious 077.1
  neurotrophic 370.35
  phlyctenular 370.31
  postmeasles 055.71
  shipyard 077.1
  sicca (Sjögren's syndrome) 710.2
    not in Sjögren's syndrome 370.33
  specified type NEC 370.49
  tuberculous (phlyctenular) (*see also*
        Tuberculosis) 017.3 *[370.31]*
Keratoconus 371.60
  acute hydrops 371.62
  congenital 743.41
  stable 371.61
Keratocyst (dental) 526.0
Keratoderma, keratodermia (congenital)
      (palmaris et plantaris) (symmetrical) 757.39
  acquired 701.1
  blennorrhagica 701.1
    gonococcal 098.81
  climacterium 701.1
  eccentrica 757.39
  gonorrheal 098.81
  punctata 701.1
  tylodes, progressive 701.1
Keratodermatocele 371.72
Keratoglobus 371.70
  congenital 743.41
    associated with buphthalmos 743.22
Keratohemia 371.12
Keratoiritis (*see also* Iridocyclitis) 364.3
  syphilitic 090.3
  tuberculous (*see also* Tuberculosis) 017.3
      [364.11]

Keratolysis exfoliativa (congenital) 757.39
  acquired 695.89
  neonatorum 757.39
Keratoma 701.1
  congenital 757.39
  malignum congenitale 757.1
  palmaris et plantaris hereditarium 757.39
  senile 702.0
Keratomalacia 371.45
  vitamin A deficiency 264.4
Keratomegaly 743.41
Keratomycosis 111.1
  nigricans (palmaris) 111.1
Keratopathy 371.40
  band (*see also* Keratitis) 371.43
  bullous (*see also* Keratitis) 371.23
  degenerative (*see also* Degeneration, cornea)
        371.40
    hereditary (*see also* Dystrophy, cornea) 371.50
  discrete colliquative 371.49
Keratoscleritis, tuberculous (*see also*
      Tuberculosis) 017.3 *[370.31]*
Keratosis 701.1
  actinic 702.0
  arsenical 692.4
  blennorrhagica 701.1
    gonococcal 098.81
  congenital (any type) 757.39
  ear (middle) (*see also* Cholesteatoma) 385.30
  female genital (external) 629.8
  follicular, vitamin A deficiency 264.8
  follicularis 757.39
    acquired 701.1
    congenital (acneiformis) (Siemens') 757.39
    spinulosa (decalvans) 757.39
    vitamin A deficiency 264.8
  gonococcal 098.81
  larynx, laryngeal 478.79
  male genital (external) 608.89
  middle ear (*see also* Cholesteatoma) 385.30
  nigricans 701.2
    congenital 757.39
  obturans 380.21
  palmaris et plantaris (symmetrical) 757.39
  penile 607.89
  pharyngeus 478.29
  pilaris 757.39
    acquired 701.1
  punctata (palmaris et plantaris) 701.1
  scrotal 608.89
  seborrheic 702.19
    inflamed 702.11
  senilis 702.0
  solar 702.0
  suprafollicularis 757.39
  tonsillaris 478.29
  vagina 623.1
  vegetans 757.39
  vitamin A deficiency 264.8
Kerato-uveitis (*see also* Iridocyclitis) 364.3
Keraunoparalysis 994.0
Kerion (celsi) 110.0
Kernicterus of newborn (not due to
      isoimmunization) 774.7
  due to isoimmunization (conditions classifiable
      to 773.0-773.2) 773.4
Ketoacidosis 276.2
  diabetic 250.1
Ketonuria 791.6
  branched-chain, intermittent 270.3
Ketosis 276.2
  diabetic 250.1

Kidney —*see* condition
Kienböck's
    disease 732.3
        adult 732.8
    osteochondrosis 732.3
Kimmelstiel (-Wilson) disease or syndrome
    (intercapillary glomerulosclerosis) 250.4
    [581.81]
Kink, kinking
    appendix 543.9
    artery 447.1
    cystic duct, congenital 751.61
    hair (acquired) 704.2
    ileum or intestine (*see also* Obstruction,
        intestine) 560.9
    Lane's (*see also* Obstruction, intestine) 560.9
    organ or site, congenital NEC—*see* Anomaly,
        specified type NEC, by site
    ureter (pelvic junction) 593.3
        congenital 753.20
    vein(s) 459.2
        caval 459.2
        peripheral 459.2
Kinnier Wilson's disease (hepatolenticular
    degeneration) 275.1
Kissing
    osteophytes 721.5
    spine 721.5
    vertebra 721.5
Klauder's syndrome (erythema multiforme
    exudativum) 695.1
Kleb's disease (*see also* Nephritis) 583.9
Klein-Waardenburg syndrome
    (ptosisepicanthus) 270.2
Kleine-Levin syndrome 349.89
Kleptomania 312.32
Klinefelter's syndrome 758.7
Klinger's disease 446.4
Klippel's disease 723.8
Klippel-Feil disease or syndrome (brevicollis)
    756.16
Klippel-Trenaunay syndrome 759.89
Klumpke (-Déjérine) palsy, paralysis (birth)
    (newborn) 767.6
Klüver-Bucy (-Terzian) syndrome 310.0
Knee —*see* condition
Knifegrinders' rot (*see also* Tuberculosis) 011.4
Knock-knee (acquired) 736.41
    congenital 755.64
Knot
    intestinal, syndrome (volvulus) 560.2
    umbilical cord (true) 663.2
        affecting fetus or newborn 762.5
Knots, surfer 919.8
    infected 919.9
Knotting (of)
    hair 704.2
    intestine 560.2
Knuckle pads (Garrod's) 728.79
Köbner's disease (epidermolysis bullosa) 757.39
Koch's
    infection (*see also* Tuberculosis, pulmonary)
        011.9
    relapsing fever 087.9
Koch-Weeks conjunctivitis 372.03
Koenig-Wichman disease (pemphigus) 694.4

Köhler's disease (osteochondrosis) 732.5
    first (osteochondrosis juvenilis) 732.5
    second (Freiburg's infarction, metatarsal head)
        732.5
    patellar 732.4
    tarsal navicular (bone) (osteoarthosis juvenilis)
        732.5
Köhler-Mouchet disease (osteoarthrosis
    juvenilis) 732.5
Köhler-Pellegrini-Stieda disease or syndrome
    (calcification, knee joint) 726.62
Koilonychia 703.8
    congenital 757.5
Kojevnikov's, Kojewnikoff's epilepsy (*see also*
    Epilepsy) 345.7
König's
    disease (osteochondritis dissecans) 732.7
    syndrome 564.89
Koniophthisis (*see also* Tuberculosis) 011.4
Koplik's spots 055.9
Kopp's asthma 254.8
Korean hemorrhagic fever 078.6
Korsakoff (-Wernicke) disease, psychosis, or
    syndrome (nonalcoholic) 294.0
    alcoholic 291.1
Korsakov's disease —*see* Korsakoff's disease
Korsakow's disease —*see* Korsakoff's disease
Kostmann's disease or syndrome (infantile
    genetic agranulocytosis) 288.0
Krabbe's
    disease (leukodystrophy) 330.0
    syndrome
        congenital muscle hypoplasia 756.89
        cutaneocerebral angioma 759.6
Kraepelin-Morel disease (*see also*
    Schizophrenia) 295.9
Kraft-Weber-Dimitri disease 759.6
Kraurosis
    ani 569.49
    penis 607.0
    vagina 623.8
    vulva 624.0
Kreotoxism 005.9
Krukenberg's
    spindle 371.13
    tumor (M8490/6) 198.6
Kufs' disease 330.1
Kugelberg-Welander disease 335.11
Kuhnt-Junius degeneration or disease 362.52
Kulchitsky's cell carcinoma (carcinoid tumor of
    intestine) 259.2
Kümmell's disease or spondylitis 721.7
Kundrat's disease (lymphosarcoma) 200.1
Kunekune —*see* Dermatophytosis
Kunkel syndrome (lupoid hepatitis) 571.49
Kupffer cell sarcoma (M9124/3) 155.0
Kuru 046.0
Kussmaul's
    coma (diabetic) 250.3
    disease (polyarteritis nodosa) 446.0
    respiration (air hunger) 786.09
Kwashiorkor (marasmus type) 260
Kyasanur Forest disease 065.2
Kyphoscoliosis, kyphoscoliotic (acquired) (*see
    also* Scoliosis) 737.30
    congenital 756.19
    due to radiation 737.33
    heart (disease) 416.1

Kyphoscoliosis, kyphoscoliotic—*continued*
 idiopathic 737.30
  infantile
   progressive 737.32
   resolving 737.31
 late effect of rickets 268.1 *[737.43]*
 specified NEC 737.39
 thoracogenic 737.34
 tuberculous (*see also* Tuberculosis) 015.0
   [737.43]
Kyphosis, kyphotic (acquired) (postural) 737.10
 adolescent postural 737.0
 congenital 756.19
 dorsalis juvenilis 732.0
 due to or associated with
  Charcot-Marie-Tooth disease 356.1 *[737.41]*
  mucopolysaccharidosis 277.5 *[737.41]*
  neurofibromatosis 237.71 *[737.41]*
  osteitis
   deformans 731.0 *[737.41]*
   fibrosa cystica 252.0 *[737.41]*
  osteoporosis (*see also* Osteoporosis) 733.0
    [737.41]
  poliomyelitis (*see also* Poliomyelitis) 138
    [737.41]
  radiation 737.11
  tuberculosis (*see also* Tuberculosis) 015.0
    [737.41]
 Kümmell's 721.7
 late effect of rickets 268.1 *[737.41]*
 Morquio-Brailsford type (spinal) 277.5 *[737.41]*
 pelvis 738.6
 postlaminectomy 737.12
 specified cause NEC 737.19
 syphilitic, congenital 090.5 *[737.41]*
 tuberculous (*see also* Tuberculosis) 015.0
   [737.41]
Kyrle's disease (hyperkeratosis follicularis in
  cutem penetrans) 701.1

L

Labia, labium —*see* condition
Labiated hymen 752.49
Labile
  blood pressure 796.2
  emotions, emotionality 301.3
  vasomotor system 443.9
Labioglossal paralysis 335.22
Labium leporinum (*see also* Cleft, lip) 749.10
Labor (*see also* Delivery)
  with complications—*see* Delivery, complicated
  abnormal NEC 661.9
    affecting fetus or newborn 763.7
  arrested active phase 661.1
    affecting fetus or newborn 763.7
  desultory 661.2
    affecting fetus or newborn 763.7
  dyscoordinate 661.4
    affecting fetus or newborn 763.7
  early onset (22-36 weeks gestation) 644.2
  failed
    induction 659.1
      mechanical 659.0
      medical 659.1
      surgical 659.0
    trial (vaginal delivery) 660.6
  false 644.1
  forced or induced, affecting fetus or newborn
    763.89
  hypertonic 661.4
    affecting fetus or newborn 763.7
  hypotonic 661.2
    affecting fetus or newborn 763.7
    primary 661.0
      affecting fetus or newborn 763.7
    secondary 661.1
      affecting fetus or newborn 763.7
  incoordinate 661.4
    affecting fetus or newborn 763.7
  irregular 661.2
    affecting fetus or newborn 763.7
  long—*see* Labor, prolonged
  missed (at or near term) 656.4
  obstructed NEC 660.9
    affecting fetus or newborn 763.1
    specified cause NEC 660.8
      affecting fetus or newborn 763.1
  pains, spurious 644.1
  precipitate 661.3
    affecting fetus or newborn 763.6
  premature 644.2
    threatened 644.0
  prolonged or protracted 662.1
    affecting fetus or newborn 763.89
    first stage 662.0
      affecting fetus or newborn 763.89
    second stage 662.2
      affecting fetus or newborn 763.89
  threatened NEC 644.1
  undelivered 644.1

Labored breathing (*see also* Hyperventilation)
  786.09
Labyrinthitis (inner ear) (destructive) (latent)
  386.30
  circumscribed 386.32
  diffuse 386.31
  focal 386.32
  purulent 386.33
  serous 386.31
  suppurative 386.33
  syphilitic 095.8
  toxic 386.34
  viral 386.35
Laceration —*see also* Wound, open, by site
  accidental, complicating surgery 998.2
  Achilles tendon 845.09
    with open wound 892.2
  anus (sphincter) 863.89
    with
      abortion—*see* Abortion, by type, with
        damage to pelvic organs
      ectopic pregnancy (*see also* categories
        633.0-633.9) 639.2
      molar pregnancy (*see also* categories
        630-632) 639.2
    complicating delivery 664.2
      with laceration of anal or rectal mucosa
        664.3
    following
      abortion 639.2
      ectopic or molar pregnancy 639.2
    nontraumatic, nonpuerperal 565.0
  bladder (urinary)
    with
      abortion—*see* Abortion, by type, with
        damage to pelvic organs
      ectopic pregnancy (*see also* categories
        633.0-633.9) 639.2
      molar pregnancy (*see also* categories
        630-632) 639.2
    following
      abortion 639.2
      ectopic or molar pregnancy 639.2
    obstetrical trauma 665.5
  blood vessel—*see* Injury, blood vessel, by site
  bowel
    with
      abortion—*see* Abortion, by type, with
        damage to pelvic organs
      ectopic pregnancy (*see also* categories
        633.0-633.9) 639.2
      molar pregnancy (*see also* categories
        630-632) 639.2
    following
      abortion 639.2
      ectopic or molar pregnancy 639.2
    obstetrical trauma 665.5

Laceration—*continued*
  brain (with hemorrhage) (cerebral) (membrane) 851.8

Note—Use the following fifth-digit subclassification with categories 851-854:

0 unspecified state of consciousness
1 with no loss of consciousness
2 with brief [less than one hour] loss of consciousness
3 with moderate [1-24 hours] loss of consciousness
4 with prolonged [more than 24 hours] loss of consciousness and return to pre-existing conscious level
5 with prolonged [more than 24 hours] loss of consciousness, without return to pre-existing conscious level
Use fifth-digit 5 to designate when a patient is unconscious and dies before regaining consciousness, regardless of the duration of the loss of consciousness
6 with loss of consciousness of unspecified duration
9 with concussion, unspecified

---

  with
    open intracranial wound 851.9
    skull fracture—see Fracture, skull, by site
  cerebellum 851.6
    with open intracranial wound 851.7
  cortex 851.2
    with open intracranial wound 851.3
    during birth 767.0
  stem 851.6
    with open intracranial wound 851.7
broad ligament
  with
    abortion—*see* Abortion, by type, with damage to pelvic organs
    ectopic pregnancy (*see also* categories 633.0-633.9) 639.2
    molar pregnancy (*see also* categories 630-632) 639.2
  following
    abortion 639.2
    ectopic or molar pregnancy 639.2
  nontraumatic 620.6
  obstetrical trauma 665.6
  syndrome (nontraumatic) 620.6
capsule, joint—*see* Sprain, by site
cardiac—*see* Laceration, heart
causing eversion of cervix uteri (old) 622.0
central, complicating delivery 664.4
cerebellum—*see* Laceration, brain, cerebellum
cerebral—*see also* Laceration, brain
  during birth 767.0
cervix (uteri)
  with
    abortion—*see* Abortion, by type, with damage to pelvic organs
    ectopic pregnancy (*see also* categories 633.0-633.9) 639.2
    molar pregnancy (*see also* categories 630-632) 639.2
  following
    abortion 639.2
    ectopic or molar pregnancy 639.2
  nonpuerperal, nontraumatic 622.3
  obstetrical trauma (current) 665.3
  old (postpartal) 622.3

Laceration—*continued*
  traumatic—*see* Injury, internal, cervix
chordae heart 429.5
complicated 879.9
cornea—*see* Laceration, eyeball
  superficial 918.1
cortex (cerebral)—*see* Laceration, brain, cortex
esophagus 530.89
eye(s)—*see* Laceration, ocular
eyeball NEC 871.4
  with prolapse or exposure of intraocular tissue 871.1
  penetrating—*see* Penetrating wound, eyeball
  specified as without prolapse of intraocular tissue 871.0
eyelid NEC 870.8
  full thickness 870.1
    involving lacrimal passages 870.2
  skin (and periocular area) 870.0
  penetrating—*see* Penetrating wound, orbit
fourchette
  with
    abortion—*see* Abortion, by type, with damage to pelvic organs
    ectopic pregnancy (*see also* categories 633.0-633.9) 639.2
    molar pregnancy (*see also* categories 630-632) 639.2
  complicating delivery 664.0
  following
    abortion 639.2
    ectopic or molar pregnancy 639.2
heart (without penetration of heart chambers) 861.02
  with
    open wound into thorax 861.12
    penetration of heart chambers 861.03
      with open wound into thorax 861.13
hernial sac—*see* Hernia, by site
internal organ (abdomen) (chest) (pelvis) NEC—*see* Injury, internal, by site
kidney (parenchyma) 866.02
  with
    complete disruption of parenchyma (rupture) 866.03
      with open wound into cavity 866.13
    open wound into cavity 866.12
labia
  complicating delivery 664.0
ligament—*see also* Sprain, by site
  with open wound—*see* Wound, open, by site
liver 864.05
  with open wound into cavity 864.15
  major (disruption of hepatic parenchyma) 864.04
    with open wound into cavity 864.14
  minor (capsule only) 864.02
    with open wound into cavity 864.12
  moderate (involving parenchyma without major disruption) 864.03
    with open wound into cavity 864.13
  multiple 864.04
    with open wound into cavity 864.14
  stellate 864.04
    with open wound into cavity 864.14
lung 861.22
  with open wound into thorax 861.32
meninges—*see* Laceration, brain
meniscus (knee) (*see also* Tear, meniscus) 836.2
  old 717.5
  site other than knee—*see also* Sprain, by site

Laceration—*continued*
    old NEC (*see also* Disorder, cartilage,
        articular) 718.0
    muscle—*see also* Sprain, by site
    with open wound—*see* Wound, open, by site
    myocardium—*see* Laceration, heart
    nerve—*see* Injury, nerve, by site
    ocular NEC (*see also* Laceration, eyeball) 871.4
    adnexa NEC 870.8
      penetrating 870.3
        with foreign body 870.4
    orbit (eye) 870.8
      penetrating 870.3
        with foreign body 870.4
    pelvic
      floor (muscles)
        with
          abortion—*see* Abortion, by type, with
            damage to pelvic organs
          ectopic pregnancy (*see also* categories
            633.0-633.9) 639.2
          molar pregnancy (*see also* categories
            630-632) 639.2
        complicating delivery 664.1
        following
          abortion 639.2
          ectopic or molar pregnancy 639.2
        nonpuerperal 618.7
        old (postpartal) 618.7
      organ NEC
        with
          abortion—*see* Abortion, by type, with
            damage to pelvic organs
          ectopic pregnancy (*see also* categories
            633.0-633.9) 639.2
          molar pregnancy (*see also* categories
            630-632) 639.2
        complicating delivery 665.5
          affecting fetus or newborn 763.89
        following
          abortion 639.2
          ectopic or molar pregnancy 639.2
        obstetrical trauma 665.5
    perineum, perineal (old) (postpartal) 618.7
      with
        abortion—*see* Abortion, by type, with
          damage to pelvic floor
        ectopic pregnancy (*see also* categories
          633.0-633.9) 639.2
        molar pregnancy (*see also* categories
          630-632) 639.2
      complicating delivery 664.4
        first degree 664.0
        second degree 664.1
        third degree 664.2
        fourth degree 664.3
        central 664.4
        involving
          anal sphincter 664.2
          fourchette 664.0
          hymen 664.0
          labia 664.0
          pelvic floor 664.1
          perineal muscles 664.1
          rectovaginal septum 664.2
            with anal mucosa 664.3
          skin 664.0
          sphincter (anal) 664.2
            with anal mucosa 664.3
          vagina 664.0
          vaginal muscles 664.1

Laceration—*continued*
      vulva 664.0
      secondary 674.2
      following
        abortion 639.2
        ectopic or molar pregnancy 639.2
      male 879.6
        complicated 879.7
      muscles, complicating delivery 664.1
      nonpuerperal, current injury 879.6
        complicated 879.7
      secondary (postpartal) 674.2
    peritoneum
      with
        abortion—*see* Abortion, by type, with
          damage to pelvic organs
        ectopic pregnancy (*see also* categories
          633.0-633.9) 639.2
        molar pregnancy (*see also* categories
          630-632) 639.2
      following
        abortion 639.2
        ectopic or molar pregnancy 639.2
      obstetrical trauma 665.5
    periurethral tissue
      with
        abortion—*see* Abortion, by type, with
          damage to pelvic organs
        ectopic pregnancy (*see also* categories
          633.0-633.9) 639.2
        molar pregnancy (*see also* categories
          630-632) 639.2
      following
        abortion 639.2
        ectopic or molar pregnancy 639.2
      obstetrical trauma 665.5
    rectovaginal (septum)
      with
        abortion—*see* Abortion, by type, with
          damage to pelvic organs
        ectopic pregnancy (*see also* categories
          633.0-633.9) 639.2
        molar pregnancy (*see also* categories
          630-632) 639.2
      complicating delivery 665.4
        with perineum 664.2
          involving anal or rectal mucosa 664.3
      following
        abortion 639.2
        ectopic or molar pregnancy 639.2
      nonpuerperal 623.4
      old (postpartal) 623.4
    spinal cord (meninges)—*see also* Injury, spinal,
      by site
      due to injury at birth 767.4
      fetus or newborn 767.4
    spleen 865.09
      with
        disruption of parenchyma (massive) 865.04
          with open wound into cavity 865.14
        open wound into cavity 865.19
      capsule (without disruption of parenchyma)
        865.02
        with open wound into cavity 865.12
      parenchyma 865.03
        with open wound into cavity 865.13
        massive disruption (rupture) 865.04
          with open wound into cavity 865.14

Laceration—*continued*
  tendon 848.9
    with open wound–*see* Wound, open, by site
    Achilles 845.09
      with open wound 892.2
    lower limb NEC 844.9
      with open wound NEC 894.2
    upper limb NEC 840.9
      with open wound NEC 884.2
  tentorium cerebelli—*see* Laceration, brain,
    cerebellum
  tongue 873.64
    complicated 873.74
  urethra
    with
      abortion—*see* Abortion, by type, with
        damage to pelvic organs
      ectopic pregnancy (*see also* categories
        633.0- 633.9) 639.2
      molar pregnancy (*see also* categories
        630-632) 639.2
    following
      abortion 639.2
      ectopic or molar pregnancy 639.2
    nonpuerperal, nontraumatic 599.84
    obstetrical trauma 665.5
  uterus
    with
      abortion—*see* Abortion, by type, with
        damage to pelvic organs
      ectopic pregnancy (*see also* categories
        633.0-633.9) 639.2
      molar pregnancy (*see also* categories
        630-632) 639.2
    following
      abortion 639.2
      ectopic or molar pregnancy 639.2
    nonpuerperal, nontraumatic 621.8
    obstetrical trauma NEC 665.8
    old (postpartal) 621.8
  vagina
    with
      abortion—*see* Abortion, by type, with
        damage to pelvic organs
      ectopic pregnancy (*see also* categories
        633.0-633.9) 639.2
      molar pregnancy (*see also* categories
        630-632) 639.2
      perineal involvement, complicating delivery
        664.0
    complicating delivery 665.4
      first degree 664.0
      second degree 664.1
      third degree 664.2
      fourth degree 664.3
      high 665.4
      muscles 664.1
      sulcus 665.4
      wall 665.4
    following
      abortion 639.2
      ectopic or molar pregnancy 639.2
    nonpuerperal, nontraumatic 623.4
    old (postpartal) 623.4
  valve, heart—*see* Endocarditis
  vulva
    with
      abortion—*see* Abortion, by type, with
        damage to pelvic organs
      ectopic pregnancy (*see also* categories
        633.0-633.9) 639.2

Laceration— *continued*
      molar pregnancy (*see also* categories
        630-632) 639.2
    complicating delivery 664.0
    following
      abortion 639.2
      ectopic or molar pregnancy 639.2
    nonpuerperal, nontraumatic 624.4
    old (postpartal) 624.4
Lachrymal —*see* condition
Lachrymonasal duct —*see* condition
Lack of
  appetite (*see also* Anorexia) 783.0
  care
    in home V60.4
    of adult 995.84
    of infant (at or after birth) 995.52
  coordination 781.3
  development—*see also* Hypoplasia
    physiological in childhood 783.40
  education V62.3
  energy 780.79
  financial resources V60.2
  food 994.2
    in environment V60.8
  growth in childhood 783.43
  heating V60.1
  housing (permanent) (temporary) V60.0
    adequate V60.1
  material resources V60.2
  medical attention 799.8
  memory (*see also* Amnesia) 780.99
    mild, following organic brain damage 310.1
  ovulation 628.0
  person able to render necessary care V60.4
  physical exercise V69.0
  physiologic development in childhood 783.40
  prenatal care in current pregnancy V23.7
  shelter V60.0
  water 994.3
Lacrimal —*see* condition
Lacrimation, abnormal (*see also* Epiphora)
  375.20
Lacrimonasal duct —*see* condition
Lactation, lactating (breast) (puerperal)
  (postpartum)
  defective 676.4
  disorder 676.9
    specified type NEC 676.8
  excessive 676.6
  failed 676.4
  mastitis NEC 675.2
  mother (care and/or examination) V24.1
  nonpuerperal 611.6
  suppressed 676.5
Lacticemia 271.3
  excessive 276.2
Lactosuria 271.3
Lacunar skull 756.0
Laennec's cirrhosis (alcoholic) 571.2
  nonalcoholic 571.5
Lafora's disease 333.2
Lag, lid (nervous) 374.41
Lagleyze-von Hippel disease (retinocerebral
  angiomatosis) 759.6
Lagophthalmos (eyelid) (nervous) 374.20
  cicatricial 374.23
  keratitis (*see also* Keratitis) 370.34
  mechanical 374.22
  paralytic 374.21

La grippe —*see* Influenza
Lahore sore 085.1
Lakes, venous (cerebral) 437.8
Laki-Lorand factor deficiency (*see also* Defect, coagulation) 286.3
Lalling 307.9
Lambliasis 007.1
Lame back 724.5
Lancereaux's diabetes (diabetes mellitus with marked emaciation) 250.8 *[261]*
Landouzy-Déjérine dystrophy (fascioscapulohumeral atrophy) 359.1
Landry's disease or paralysis 357.0
Landry-Guillain-Barré syndrome 357.0
Lane's
  band 751.4
  disease 569.89
  kink (*see also* Obstruction, intestine) 560.9
Langdon Down's syndrome (mongolism) 758.0
Language abolition 784.69
Lanugo (persistent) 757.4
Laparoscopic surgical procedure converted to open procedure V64.4
Lardaceous
  degeneration (any site) 277.3
  disease 277.3
  kidney 277.3 *[583.81]*
  liver 277.3
Large
  baby (regardless of gestational age) 766.1
    exceptionally (weight of 4500 grams or more) 766.0
    of diabetic mother 775.0
  ear 744.22
  fetus—*see also* Oversize, fetus
    causing disproportion 653.5
      with obstructed labor 660.1
  for dates
    fetus or newborn (regardless of gestational age) 766.1
      affecting management of pregnancy 656.6
      exceptionally (weight of 4500 grams or more) 766.0
  physiological cup 743.57
  waxy liver 277.3
  white kidney—*see* Nephrosis
Larsen's syndrome (flattened facies and multiple congenital dislocations) 755.8
Larsen-Johansson disease (juvenile osteopathia patellae) 732.4
Larva migrans
  cutaneous NEC 126.9
    ancylostoma 126.9
  of Diptera in vitreous 128.0
  visceral NEC 128.0
Laryngeal —*see also* condition
  syncope 786.2
Laryngismus (acute) (infectious) (stridulous) 478.75
  congenital 748.3
  diphtheritic 032.3
Laryngitis (acute) (edematous) (fibrinous) (gangrenous) (infective) (infiltrative) (malignant) (membranous) (phlegmonous) (pneumococcal) (pseudomembranous) (septic) (subglottic) (suppurative) (ulcerative) (viral) 464.00
  with
    influenza, flu, or grippe 487.1
    obstruction 464.01
    tracheitis (*see also* Laryngotracheitis) 464.20

Laryngitis— *continued*
    with obstruction 464.21
  acute 464.20
    with obstruction 464.21
    chronic 476.1
  atrophic 476.0
  Borrelia vincentii 101
  catarrhal 476.0
  chronic 476.0
    with tracheitis (chronic) 476.1
    due to external agent—*see* Condition, respiratory, chronic, due to
  diphtheritic (membranous) 032.3
  due to external agent—*see* Inflammation, respiratory, upper, due to
  H. influenzae 464.00
    with obstruction 464.01
  Hemophilus influenzae 464.00
    with obstruction 464.01
  hypertrophic 476.0
  influenzal 487.1
  pachydermic 478.79
  sicca 476.0
  spasmodic 478.75
    acute 464.00
      with obstruction 464.01
  streptococcal 034.0
  stridulous 478.75
  syphilitic 095.8
    congenital 090.5
  tuberculous (*see also* Tuberculosis, larynx) 012.3
  Vincent's 101
Laryngocele (congenital) (ventricular) 748.3
Laryngofissure 478.79
  congenital 748.3
Laryngomalacia (congenital) 748.3
Laryngopharyngitis (acute) 465.0
  chronic 478.9
  due to external agent—*see* Condition, respiratory, chronic, due to
  due to external agent—*see* Inflammation, respiratory, upper, due to
  septic 034.0
Laryngoplegia (*see also* Paralysis, vocal cord) 478.30
Laryngoptosis 478.79
Laryngospasm 478.75
  due to external agent—*see* Condition, respiratory, acute, due to
Laryngostenosis 478.74
  congenital 748.3
Laryngotracheitis (acute) (infectional) (viral) (*see also* Laryngitis) 464.20
  with obstruction 464.21
  atrophic 476.1
  Borrelia vincentii 101
  catarrhal 476.1
  chronic 476.1
  due to external agent—*see* Condition, respiratory, chronic, due to
  diphtheritic (membranous) 032.3
  due to external agent—*see* Inflammation, respiratory, upper, due to
  H. influenzae 464.20
    with obstruction 464.21
  hypertrophic 476.1
  influenzal 487.1
  pachydermic 478.75
  sicca 476.1
  spasmodic 478.75

Laryngotracheitis— *continued*
   acute 464.20
     with obstruction 464.21
   streptococcal 034.0
   stridulous 478.75
   syphilitic 095.8
    congenital 090.5
   tuberculous (*see also* Tuberculosis, larynx)
     012.3
   Vincent's 101
Laryngotracheobronchitis (*see also* Bronchitis)
   490
   acute 466.0
   chronic 491.8
   viral 466.0
Laryngotracheobronchopneumonitis —*see*
   Pneumonia, broncho-
Larynx, laryngeal —*see* condition
Lasègue's disease (persecution mania) 297.9
Lassa fever 078.89
Lassitude (*see also* Weakness) 780.79
Late —*see also* condition
   effect(s) (of)—*see also* condition
    abscess
     intracranial or intraspinal (conditions
      classifiable to 324)–*see* category 326
    adverse effect of drug, medicinal or biological
     substance 909.5
    allergic reaction 909.9
    amputation
     postoperative (late) 997.60
     traumatic (injury classifiable to 885-887 and
      895-897) 905.9
    burn (injury classifiable to 948-949) 906.9
     extremities NEC (injury classifiable to 943
      or 945) 906.7
     hand or wrist (injury classifiable to 944)
      906.6
     eye (injury classifiable to 940) 906.5
     face, head, and neck (injury classifiable to
      941) 906.5
     specified site NEC (injury classifiable to
      942 and 946-947) 906.8
    cerebrovascular disease (conditions
     classifiable to 430-437) 438.9
    with
     alterations of sensations 438.6
     aphasia 438.11
     apraxia 438.81
     ataxia 438.84
     cognitive deficits 438.0
     disturbances of vision 438.7
     dysphagia 438.82
     dysphasia 438.12
     facial droop 438.83
     facial weakness 438.83
     hemiplegia/hemiparesis
      affecting
       dominant side 438.21
       nondominant side 438.22
       unspecified side 438.20
     monoplegia of lower limb
      affecting
       dominant side 438.41
       nondominant side 438.42
       unspecified side 438.40
     monoplegia of upper limb
      affecting
       dominant side 438.31
       nondominant side 438.32
       unspecified side 438.30

Late —*continued*
    paralytic syndrome NEC
     affecting
      bilateral 438.53
      dominant side 438.51
      nondominant side 438.52
      unspecified side 438.50
     speech and language deficit 438.10
      specified type NEC 438.19
     vertigo 438.85
    specified type NEC 438.89
   childbirth complication(s) 677
   complication(s) of
    childbirth 677
    delivery 677
    pregnancy 677
    puerperium 677
    surgical and medical care (conditions
     classifiable to 996-999) 909.3
    trauma (conditions classifiable to 958) 908.6
   contusion (injury classifiable to 920-924)
    906.3
   crushing (injury classifiable to 925-929) 906.4
   delivery complication(s) 677
   dislocation (injury classifiable to 830-839)
    905.6
   encephalitis or encephalomyelitis (conditions
    classifiable to 323)—*see* category 326
    in infectious diseases 139.8
     viral (conditions classifiable to 049.8,
      049.9, 062-064) 139.0
   external cause NEC (conditions classifiable to
    995) 909.9
    certain conditions classifiable to categories
     991-994 909.4
   foreign body in orifice (injury classifiable to
    930-939) 908.5
   fracture (multiple) (injury classifiable to
    828-829) 905.5
    extremity
     lower (injury classifiable to 821-827)
      905.4
      neck of femur (injury classifiable to
       820) 905.3
      upper (injury classifiable to 810-819)
       905.2
    face and skull (injury classifiable to
     800-804) 905.0
    skull and face (injury classifiable to
     800-804) 905.0
    spine and trunk (injury classifiable to 805
     and 807-809) 905.1
     with spinal cord lesion (injury classifiable
      to 806) 907.2
   infection
    pyogenic, intracranial—*see* category 326
   infectious diseases (conditions classifiable to
    001-136) NEC 139.8
   injury (injury classifiable to 959) 908.9
    blood vessel 908.3
     abdomen and pelvis (injury classifiable to
      902) 908.4
     extremity (injury classifiable to 903-904)
      908.3
     head and neck (injury classifiable to 900)
      908.3
      intracranial (injury classifiable to
       850-854) 907.0
       with skull fracture 905.0
     thorax (injury classifiable to 901) 908.4

Late —*continued*
- internal organ NEC (injury classifiable to 867 and 869) 908.2
  - abdomen (injury classifiable to 863-866 and 868) 908.1
  - thorax (injury classifiable to 860-862) 908.0
- intracranial (injury classifiable to 850-854) 907.0
  - with skull fracture (injury classifiable to 800-801 and 803-804) 905.0
- nerve NEC (injury classifiable to 957) 907.9
  - cranial (injury classifiable to 950-951) 907.1
  - peripheral NEC (injury classifiable to 957) 907.9
    - lower limb and pelvic girdle (injury classifiable to 956) 907.5
    - upper limb and shoulder girdle (injury classifiable to 955) 907.4
  - roots and plexus(es), spinal (injury classifiable to 953) 907.3
  - trunk (injury classifiable to 954) 907.3
- pregnancy complication(s) 677
- puerperal complication(s) 677
- spinal
  - cord (injury classifiable to 806 and 952) 907.2
  - nerve root(s) and plexus(es) (injury classifiable to 953) 907.3
- superficial (injury classifiable to 910-919) 906.2
- tendon (tendon injury classifiable to 840-848, 880-884 with .2, and 890-894 with .2) 905.8
- meningitis
  - bacterial (conditions classifiable to 320)—*see* category 326
  - unspecified cause (conditions classifiable to 322)—*see* category 326
- myelitis (*see also* Late, effect(s) (of), encephalitis)—*see* category 326
- parasitic diseases (conditions classifiable to 001-136 NEC) 139.8
- phlebitis or thrombophlebitis of intracranial venous sinuses (conditions classifiable to 325)—*see* category 326
- poisoning due to drug, medicinal or biological substance (conditions classifiable to 960-979) 909.0
- poliomyelitis, acute (conditions classifiable to 045) 138
- radiation (conditions classifiable to 990) 909.2
- rickets 268.1
- sprain and strain without mention of tendon injury (injury classifiable to 840-848, except tendon injury) 905.7
  - tendon involvement 905.8
- toxic effect of
  - drug, medicinal or biological substance (conditions classifiable to 960-979) 909.0
  - nonmedical substance (conditions classifiable to 980-989) 909.1
- trachoma (conditions classifiable to 076) 139.1
- tuberculosis 137.0
  - bones and joints (conditions classifiable to 015) 137.3
  - central nervous system (conditions classifiable to 013) 137.1

Late —*continued*
- genitourinary (conditions classifiable to 016) 137.2
- pulmonary (conditions classifiable to 010-012) 137.0
- specified organs NEC (conditions classifiable to 014, 017-018) 137.4
- viral encephalitis (conditions classifiable to 049.8, 049.9, 062-064) 139.0
- wound, open
  - extremity (injury classifiable to 880-884 and 890-894, except .2) 906.1
  - tendon (injury classifiable to 880-884 with .2 and 890-894 with .2) 905.8
  - head, neck, and trunk (injury classifiable to 870-879) 906.0

Latent —*see* condition
Lateral —*see* condition
Laterocession —*see* Lateroversion
Lateroflexion —*see* Lateroversion
Lateroversion
- cervix—*see* Lateroversion, uterus
- uterus, uterine (cervix) (postinfectional) (postpartal, old) 621.6
  - congenital 752.3
  - in pregnancy or childbirth 654.4
    - affecting fetus or newborn 763.89
Lathyrism 988.2
Launois' syndrome (pituitary gigantism) 253.0
Launois-Bensaude's lipomatosis 272.8
Launois-Cléret syndrome (adiposogenital dystrophy) 253.8
Laurence-Moon-Biedl syndrome (obesity, polydactyly, and mental retardation) 759.89
LAV (disease) (illness) (infection)—*see* Human immunodeficiency virus (disease) (illness) (infection)
LAV/HTLV-III (disease) (illness) (infection)—*see* Human immunodeficiency virus (disease) (illness) (infection)
Lawford's syndrome (encephalocutaneous angiomatosis) 759.6
Lax, laxity —*see also* Relaxation
- ligament 728.4
- skin (acquired) 701.8
  - congenital 756.83
Laxative habit (*see also* Abuse, drugs, nondependent) 305.9
Lazy leukocyte syndrome 288.0
Lead —*see also* condition
- exposure to V15.86
- incrustation of cornea 371.15
- poisoning 984.9
  - specified type of lead—*see* Table of drugs and chemicals
Lead miner's lung 503
Leakage
- amniotic fluid 658.1
  - with delayed delivery 658.2
  - affecting fetus or newborn 761.1
- bile from drainage tube (T tube) 997.4
- blood (microscopic), fetal, into maternal circulation 656.0
  - affecting management of pregnancy or puerperium 656.0
- device, implant, or graft—*see* Complications, mechanical
- spinal fluid at lumbar puncture site 997.09
- urine, continuous 788.37
Leaky heart —*see* Endocarditis
Learning defect, specific NEC (strephosymbolia) 315.2

Leather bottle stomach (M8142/3) 151.9
Leber's
  congenital amaurosis 362.76
  optic atrophy (hereditary) 377.16
Lederer's anemia or disease (acquired
  infectious hemolytic anemia) 283.19
Lederer-Brill syndrome (acquired infectious
  hemolytic anemia) 283.19
Leeches (aquatic) (land) 134.2
Left-sided neglect 781.8
Leg —*see* condition
Legal investigation V62.5
Legg (-Calvé) -Perthes disease or syndrome
  (osteochondrosis, femoral capital) 732.1
Legionnaires' disease 482.84
Leigh's disease 330.8
Leiner's disease (exfoliative dermatitis) 695.89
Leiofibromyoma (M8890/0)—*see also*
  Leiomyoma
  uterus (cervix) (corpus) (*see also* Leiomyoma,
    uterus) 218.9
Leiomyoblastoma (M8891/1)—*see* Neoplasm,
  connective tissue, uncertain behavior
Leiomyofibroma (M8890/0)—*see also*
  Neoplasm, connective tissue, benign
  uterus (cervix) (corpus) (*see also* Leiomyoma,
    uterus) 218.9
Leiomyoma (M8890/0)—*see also* Neoplasm,
  connective tissue, benign
  bizarre (M8893/0)—*see* Neoplasm, connective
    tissue, benign
  cellular (M8892/1)—*see* Neoplasm, connective
    tissue, uncertain behavior
  epithelioid (M8891/1)—*see* Neoplasm,
    connective tissue, uncertain behavior
  prostate (polypoid) 600.2
  uterus (cervix) (corpus) 218.9
    interstitial 218.1
    intramural 218.1
    submucous 218.0
    subperitoneal 218.2
    subserous 218.2
    vascular (M8894/0)—*see* Neoplasm,
      connective tissue, benign
Leiomyomatosis (intravascular) (M8890/1)—*see*
  Neoplasm, connective tissue, uncertain
  behavior
Leiomyosarcoma (M8890/3)—*see also*
  Neoplasm, connective tissue, malignant
  epithelioid (M8891/3)—*see* Neoplasm,
    connective tissue, malignant
Leishmaniasis 085.9
  American 085.5
    cutaneous 085.4
    mucocutaneous 085.5
  Asian desert 085.2
  Brazilian 085.5
  cutaneous 085.9
    acute necrotizing 085.2
    American 085.4
    Asian desert 085.2
    diffuse 085.3
    dry form 085.1
    Ethiopian 085.3
    eyelid 085.5 *[373.6]*
    late 085.1
    lepromatous 085.3
    recurrent 085.1
    rural 085.2
    ulcerating 085.1
    urban 085.1

Leishmaniasis—*continued*
  wet form 085.2
  zoonotic form 085.2
  dermal—*see also* Leishmaniasis, cutaneous
    post kala-azar 085.0
  eyelid 085.5 *[373.6]*
  infantile 085.0
  Mediterranean 085.0
  mucocutaneous (American) 085.5
  naso-oral 085.5
  nasopharyngeal 085.5
  Old World 085.1
  tegumentaria diffusa 085.4
  vaccination, prophylactic (against) V05.2
  visceral (Indian) 085.0
Leishmanoid, dermal —*see also* Leishmaniasis,
  cutaneous
  post kala-azar 085.0
Leloir's disease 695.4
Lenegre's disease 426.0
Lengthening, leg 736.81
Lennox's syndrome (*see also* Epilepsy) 345.0
Lens —*see* condition
Lenticonus (anterior) (posterior) (congenital)
  743.36
Lenticular degeneration, progressive 275.1
Lentiglobus (posterior) (congenital) 743.36
Lentigo (congenital) 709.09
  juvenile 709.09
  Maligna (M8742/2)—*see also* Neoplasm, skin,
    in situ
    melanoma (M8742/3)—*see* Melanoma
  senile 709.09
Leonine leprosy 030.0
Leontiasis
  ossium 733.3
  syphilitic 095.8
    congenital 090.5
Léopold-Lévi's syndrome (paroxysmal thyroid
  instability) 242.9
Lepore hemoglobin syndrome 282.4
Lepothrix 039.0
Lepra 030.9
  Willan's 696.1
Leprechaunism 259.8
Lepromatous leprosy 030.0
Leprosy 030.9
  anesthetic 030.1
  beriberi 030.1
  borderline (group B) (infiltrated) (neuritic) 030.3
  cornea (*see also* Leprosy, by type) 030.9
    [371.89]
  dimorphous (group B) (infiltrated)
    (lepromatous) (neuritic) (tuberculoid) 030.3
  eyelid 030.0 *[373.4]*
  indeterminate (group I) (macular) (neuritic)
    (uncharacteristic) 030.2
  leonine 030.0
  lepromatous (diffuse) (infiltrated) (macular)
    (neuritic) (nodular) (type L) 030.0
  macular (early) (neuritic) (simple) 030.2
  maculoanesthetic 030.1
  mixed 030.0
  neuro 030.1
  nodular 030.0
  primary neuritic 030.3
  specified type or group NEC 030.8
  tubercular 030.1
  tuberculoid (macular) (maculoanesthetic)
    (major) (minor) (neuritic) (type T) 030.1
Leptocytosis, hereditary 282.4

Leptomeningitis (chronic) (circumscribed)
   (hemorrhagic) (nonsuppurative) (*see also*
   Meningitis) 322.9
   aseptic 047.9
      adenovirus 049.1
      Coxsackie virus 047.0
      ECHO virus 047.1
      enterovirus 047.9
      lymphocytic choriomeningitis 049.0
   epidemic 036.0
   late effect—*see* category 326
   meningococcal 036.0
   pneumococcal 320.1
   syphilitic 094.2
   tuberculous (*see also* Tuberculosis, meninges)
      013.0
Leptomeningopathy (*see also* Meningitis) 322.9
Leptospiral —*see* condition
Leptospirochetal —*see* condition
Leptospirosis 100.9
   autumnalis 100.89
   canicula 100.89
   grippotyphosa 100.89
   hebdomidis 100.89
   icterohemorrhagica 100.0
   nanukayami 100.89
   pomona 100.89
   Weil's disease 100.0
Leptothricosis —*see* Actinomycosis
Leptothrix infestation —*see* Actinomycosis
Leptotricosis —*see* Actinomycosis
Leptus dermatitis 133.8
Léri's pleonosteosis 756.89
Léri-Weill syndrome 756.59
Leriche syndrome (aortic bifurcation occlusion)
   444.0
Lermoyez's syndrome (*see also* Disease,
   Ménière's) 386.00
Lesbianism —*omit code*
   egodystonic 302.0
   problems with 302.0
Lesch-Nyhan syndrome (hypoxanthine-guanine-
   phosphoribosyltransferase deficiency) 277.2
Lesion
   abducens nerve 378.54
   alveolar process 525.8
   anorectal 569.49
   aortic (valve)—*see* Endocarditis, aortic
   auditory nerve 388.5
   basal ganglion 333.90
   bile duct (*see also* Disease, biliary) 576.8
   bladder 596.9
   bone 733.90
   brachial plexus 353.0
   brain 348.8
      congenital 742.9
      vascular (*see also* Lesion, cerebrovascular)
         437.9
         degenerative 437.1
         healed or old without residuals V12.59
         hypertensive 437.2
         late effect—*see* Late effect(s) (of)
            cerebrovascular disease
   buccal 528.9
   calcified—*see* Calcification
   canthus 373.9
   carate—*see* Pinta, lesions
   cardia 537.89
   cardiac—*see also* Disease, heart congenital
      746.9
      valvular—*see* Endocarditis

Lesion—*continued*
   cauda equina 344.60
      with neurogenic bladder 344.61
   cecum 569.89
   cerebral—*see* Lesion, brain
   cerebrovascular (*see also* Disease,
      cerebrovascular NEC) 437.9
      degenerative 437.1
      healed or old without residuals V12.59
      hypertensive 437.2
      specified type NEC 437.8
   cervical root (nerve) NEC 353.2
   chiasmal 377.54
      associated with
         inflammatory disorders 377.54
         neoplasm NEC 377.52
         pituitary 377.51
         pituitary disorders 377.51
         vascular disorders 377.53
   chorda tympani 351.8
   coin, lung 793.1
   colon 569.89
   congenital—*see* Anomaly
   conjunctiva 372.9
   coronary artery (*see also* Ischemia, heart) 414.9
   cranial nerve 352.9
      first 352.0
      second 377.49
      third
         partial 378.51
         total 378.52
      fourth 378.53
      fifth 350.9
      sixth 378.54
      seventh 351.9
      eighth 388.5
      ninth 352.2
      tenth 352.3
      eleventh 352.4
      twelfth 352.5
   cystic—*see* Cyst
   degenerative—*see* Degeneration
   dermal (skin) 709.9
   Dieulafoy (hemorrhagic)
      of
         duodenum 537.84
         intestine 569.86
         stomach 537.84
   duodenum 537.89
      with obstruction 537.3
   eyelid 373.9
   gasserian ganglion 350.8
   gastric 537.89
   gastroduodenal 537.89
   gastrointestinal 569.89
   glossopharyngeal nerve 352.2
   heart (organic)—*see also* Disease, heart
      vascular—*see* Disease, cardiovascular
   helix (ear) 709.9
   hyperchromic, due to pinta (carate) 103.1
   hyperkeratotic (*see also* Hyperkeratosis) 701.1
   hypoglossal nerve 352.5
   hypopharynx 478.29
   hypothalamic 253.9
   ileocecal coil 569.89
   ileum 569.89
   iliohypogastric nerve 355.79
   ilioinguinal nerve 355.79
   in continuity—*see* Injury, nerve, by site
   inflammatory—*see* Inflammation
   intestine 569.89

Lesion—*continued*
  intracerebral—*see* Lesion, brain
  intrachiasmal (optic) (*see also* Lesion,
    chiasmal) 377.54
  intracranial, space-occupying NEC 784.2
  joint 719.90
    ankle 719.97
    elbow 719.92
    foot 719.97
    hand 719.94
    hip 719.95
    knee 719.96
    multiple sites 719.99
    pelvic region 719.95
    sacroiliac (old) 724.6
    shoulder (region) 719.91
    specified site NEC 719.98
    wrist 719.93
  keratotic (*see also* Keratosis) 701.1
  kidney (*see also* Disease, renal) 593.9
  laryngeal nerve (recurrent) 352.3
  leonine 030.0
  lip 528.5
  liver 573.8
  lumbosacral
    plexus 353.1
    root (nerve) NEC 353.4
  lung 518.89
    coin 793.1
  maxillary sinus 473.0
  mitral—*see* Endocarditis, mitral
  motor cortex 348.8
  nerve (*see also* Disorder, nerve) 355.9
  nervous system 349.9
    congenital 742.9
  nonallopathic NEC 739.9
    in region (of)
      abdomen 739.9
      acromioclavicular 739.7
      cervical, cervicothoracic 739.1
      costochondral 739.8
      costovertebral 739.8
      extremity
        lower 739.6
        upper 739.7
      head 739.0
      hip 739.5
      lower extremity 739.6
      lumbar, lumbosacral 739.3
      occipitocervical 739.0
      pelvic 739.5
      pubic 739.5
      rib cage 739.8
      sacral, sacrococcygeal, sacroiliac 739.4
      sternochondral 739.8
      sternoclavicular 739.7
      thoracic, thoracolumbar 739.2
      upper extremity 739.7
  nose (internal) 478.1
  obstructive—*see* Obstruction
  obturator nerve 355.79
  occlusive
    artery—*see* Embolism, artery
  organ or site NEC—*see* Disease, by site
  osteolytic 733.90
  paramacular, of retina 363.32
  peptic 537.89
  periodontal, due to traumatic occlusion 523.8
  perirectal 569.49
  peritoneum (granulomatous) 568.89
  pigmented (skin) 709.00

Lesion—*continued*
  pinta—*see* Pinta, lesions
  polypoid—*see* Polyp
  prechiasmal (optic) (*see also* Lesion, chiasmal)
    377.54
  primary—*see also* Syphilis, primary
    carate 103.0
    pinta 103.0
    yaws 102.0
  pulmonary 518.89
    valve (*see also* Endocarditis, pulmonary) 424.3
  pylorus 537.89
  radiation NEC 990
  radium NEC 990
  rectosigmoid 569.89
  retina, retinal—*see also* Retinopathy
    vascular 362.17
  retroperitoneal 568.89
  romanus 720.1
  sacroiliac (joint) 724.6
  salivary gland 527.8
    benign lymphoepithelial 527.8
  saphenous nerve 355.79
  secondary—*see* Syphilis, secondary
  sigmoid 569.89
  sinus (accessory) (nasal) (*see also* Sinusitis)
    473.9
  skin 709.9
    suppurative 686.00
  SLAP (superior glenoid labrum) 840.7
  space-occupying, intracranial NEC 784.2
  spinal cord 336.9
    congenital 742.9
    traumatic (complete) (incomplete)
      (transverse)—*see also* Injury, spinal, by
      site
      with
        broken
          back—*see* Fracture, vertebra, by site,
            with spinal cord injury
          neck—*see* Fracture, vertebra, cervical,
            with spinal cord injury
        fracture, vertebra—*see* Fracture, vertebra,
          by site, with spinal cord injury
  spleen 289.50
  stomach 537.89
  superior glenoid labrum (SLAP) 840.7
  syphilitic—*see* Syphilis
  tertiary—*see* Syphilis, tertiary
  thoracic root (nerve) 353.3
  tonsillar fossa 474.9
  tooth, teeth 525.8
    white spot 521.01
  traumatic NEC (*see also* nature and site of
    injury) 959.9
  tricuspid (valve)—*see* Endocarditis, tricuspid
  trigeminal nerve 350.9
  ulcerated or ulcerative—*see* Ulcer
  uterus NEC 621.9
  vagina 623.8
  vagus nerve 352.3
  valvular—*see* Endocarditis
  vascular 459.9
    affecting central nervous system (*see also*
      Lesion, cerebrovascular) 437.9
    following trauma (*see also* Injury, blood
      vessel, by site) 904.9
    retina 362.17
    traumatic—*see* Injury, blood vessel, by site
  umbilical cord 663.6
    affecting fetus or newborn 762.6

Lesion—*continued*
  visual
    cortex NEC (*see also* Disorder, visual, cortex)
      377.73
    pathway NEC (*see also* Disorder, visual,
      pathway) 377.63
    warty—*see* Verruca
    white spot, on teeth 521.01
    x-ray NEC 990
Lethargic —*see* condition
Lethargy 780.79
Letterer-Siwe disease (acute histiocytosis X)
  (M9722/3) 202.5
Leucinosis 270.3
Leucocoria 360.44
Leucosarcoma (M9850/3) 207.8
Leukasmus 270.2
Leukemia, leukemic (congenital) (M9800/3)
  208.9

> *Note—Use the following fifth-digit*
> *subclassification for categories 203-208:*
>
> *0 without mention of remission*
> *1 with remission*

  acute NEC (M9801/3) 208.0
  aleukemic NEC (M9804/3) 208.8
    granulocytic (M9864/3) 205.8
  basophilic (M9870/3) 205.1
  blast (cell) (M9801/3) 208.0
  blastic (M9801/3) 208.0
    granulocytic (M9861/3) 205.0
  chronic NEC (M9803/3) 208.1
  compound (M9810/3) 207.8
  eosinophilic (M9880/3) 205.1
  giant cell (M9910/3) 207.2
  granulocytic (M9860/3) 205.9
    acute (M9861/3) 205.0
    aleukemic (M9864/3) 205.8
    blastic (M9861/3) 205.0
    chronic (M9863/3) 205.1
    subacute (M9862/3) 205.2
    subleukemic (M9864/3) 205.8
  hairy cell (M9940/3) 202.4
  hemoblastic (M9801/3) 208.0
  histiocytic (M9890/3) 206.9
  lymphatic (M9820/3) 204.9
    acute (M9821/3) 204.0
    aleukemic (M9824/3) 204.8
    chronic (M9823/3) 204.1
    subacute (M9822/3) 204.2
    subleukemic (M9824/3) 204.8
  lymphoblastic (M9821/3) 204.0
  lymphocytic (M9820/3) 204.9
    acute (M9821/3) 204.0
    aleukemic (M9824/3) 204.8
    chronic (M9823/3) 204.1
    subacute (M9822/3) 204.2
    subleukemic (M9824/3) 204.8
  lymphogenous (M9820/3)—*see* Leukemia,
    lymphoid
  lymphoid (M9820/3) 204.9
    acute (M9821/3) 204.0
    aleukemic (M9824/3) 204.8
    blastic (M9821/3) 204.0
    chronic (M9823/3) 204.1
    subacute (M9822/3) 204.2
    subleukemic (M9824/3) 204.8
  lymphosarcoma cell (M9850/3) 207.8
  mast cell (M9900/3) 207.8
  megakaryocytic (M9910/3) 207.2

Leukemia, leukemic—*continued*
  megakaryocytoid (M9910/3) 207.2
  mixed (cell) (M9810/3) 207.8
  monoblastic (M9891/3) 206.0
  monocytic (Schilling-type) (M9890/3) 206.9
    acute (M9891/3) 206.0
    aleukemic (M9894/3) 206.8
    chronic (M9893/3) 206.1
    Naegeli-type (M9863/3) 205.1
    subacute (M9892/3) 206.2
    subleukemic (M9894/3) 206.8
  monocytoid (M9890/3) 206.9
    acute (M9891/3) 206.0
    aleukemic (M9894/3) 206.8
    chronic (M9893/3) 206.1
    myelogenous (M9863/3) 205.1
    subacute (M9892/3) 206.2
    subleukemic (M9894/3) 206.8
  monomyelocytic (M9860/3)—*see* Leukemia,
    myelomonocytic
  myeloblastic (M9861/3) 205.0
  myelocytic (M9863/3) 205.1
    acute (M9861/3) 205.0
  myelogenous (M9860/3) 205.9
    acute (M9861/3) 205.0
    aleukemic (M9864/3) 205.8
    chronic (M9863/3) 205.1
    monocytoid (M9863/3) 205.1
    subacute (M9862/3) 205.2
    subleukemic (M9864) 205.8
  myeloid (M9860/3) 205.9
    acute (M9861/3) 205.0
    aleukemic (M9864/3) 205.8
    chronic (M9863/3) 205.1
    subacute (M9862/3) 205.2
    subleukemic (M9864/3) 205.8
  myelomonocytic (M9860/3) 205.9
    acute (M9861/3) 205.0
    chronic (M9863/3) 205.1
  Naegeli-type monocytic (M9863/3) 205.1
  neutrophilic (M9865/3) 205.1
  plasma cell (M9830/3) 203.1
  plasmacytic (M9830/3) 203.1
  prolymphocytic (M9825/3)—*see* Leukemia,
    lymphoid
  promyelocytic, acute (M9866/3) 205.0
  Schilling-type monocytic (M9890/3)—*see*
    Leukemia, monocytic
  stem cell (M9801/3) 208.0
  subacute NEC (M9802/3) 208.2
  subleukemic NEC (M9804/3) 208.8
  thrombocytic (M9910/3) 207.2
  undifferentiated (M9801/3) 208.0
Leukemoid reaction (lymphocytic) (monocytic)
  (myelocytic) 288.8
Leukoclastic vasculitis 446.29
Leukocoria 360.44
Leukocythemia —*see* Leukemia
Leukocytosis 288.8
  basophilic 288.8
  eosinophilic 288.3
  lymphocytic 288.8
  monocytic 288.8
  neutrophilic 288.8
Leukoderma 709.09
  syphilitic 091.3
    late 095.8
Leukodermia (*see also* Leukoderma) 709.09
Leukodystrophy (cerebral) (globoid cell)
  (metachromatic) (progressive) (sudanophilic)
  330.0
Leukoedema, mouth or tongue 528.7

Leukoencephalitis
  acute hemorrhagic (postinfectious) NEC 136.9
    [323.6]
    postimmunization or postvaccinal 323.5
  subacute sclerosing 046.2
    van Bogaert's 046.2
  van Bogaert's (sclerosing) 046.2
Leukoencephalopathy (*see also* Encephalitis)
  323.9
  acute necrotizing hemorrhagic (postinfectious)
    136.9 *[323.6]*
    postimmunization or postvaccinal 323.5
  metachromatic 330.0
  multifocal (progressive) 046.3
  progressive multifocal 046.3
Leukoerythroblastosis 289.0
Leukoerythrosis 289.0
Leukokeratosis (*see also* Leukoplakia) 702.8
  mouth 528.6
  nicotina palati 528.7
  tongue 528.6
Leukokoria 360.44
Leukokoraurosis vulva, vulvae 624.0
Leukolymphosarcoma (M9850/3) 207.8
Leukoma (cornea) (interfering with central
  vision) 371.03
  adherent 371.04
Leukomalacia, periventricular 779.7
Leukomelanopathy, hereditary 288.2
Leukonychia (punctata) (striata) 703.8
  congenital 757.5
Leukopathia
  unguium 703.8
    congenital 757.5
Leukopenia 288.0
  cyclic 288.0
  familial 288.0
  malignant 288.0
  periodic 288.0
  transitory neonatal 776.7
Leukopenic —*see* condition
Leukoplakia 702.8
  anus 569.49
  bladder (postinfectional) 596.8
  buccal 528.6
  cervix (uteri) 622.2
  esophagus 530.83
  gingiva 528.6
  kidney (pelvis) 593.89
  larynx 478.79
  lip 528.6
  mouth 528.6
  oral soft tissue (including tongue) (mucosa)
    528.6
  palate 528.6
  pelvis (kidney) 593.89
  penis (infectional) 607.0
  rectum 569.49
  syphilitic 095.8
  tongue 528.6
  tonsil 478.29
  ureter (postinfectional) 593.89
  urethra (postinfectional) 599.84
  uterus 621.8
  vagina 623.1
  vesical 596.8
  vocal cords 478.5
  vulva 624.0
Leukopolioencephalopathy 330.0
Leukorrhea (vagina) 623.5
  due to trichomonas (vaginalis) 131.00
  trichomonal (Trichomonas vaginalis) 131.00

Leukosarcoma (M9850/3) 207.8
Leukosis (M9800/3)—*see* Leukemia
Lev's disease or syndrome (acquired complete
  heart block) 426.0
Levi's syndrome (pituitary dwarfism) 253.3
Levocardia (isolated) 746.87
  with situs inversus 759.3
Levulosuria 271.2
Lewandowski's disease (primary) (*see also*
  Tuberculosis) 017.0
Lewandowski-Lutz disease (epidermodysplasia
  verruciformis) 078.19
Leyden's disease (periodic vomiting) 536.2
Leyden's-Möbius dystrophy 359.1
Leydig cell
  carcinoma (M8650/3)
    specified site—*see* Neoplasm, by site,
      malignant
    unspecified site
      female 183.0
      male 186.9
  tumor (M8650/1)
    benign (M8650/0)
      specified site—*see* Neoplasm, by site,
        benign
      unspecified site
        female 220
        male 222.0
    malignant (M8650/3)
      specified site—*see* Neoplasm, by site,
        malignant
      unspecified site
        female 183.0
        male 186.9
    specified site—*see* Neoplasm, by site,
      uncertain behavior
    unspecified site
      female 236.2
      male 236.4
Leydig-Sertoli cell tumor (M8631/0)
  specified site—*see* Neoplasm, by site, benign
  unspecified site
    female 220
    male 222.0
LGSIL (low grade squamous intraepithelial
  dysplasia) 622.1
Liar, pathologic 301.7
Libman-Sacks disease or syndrome 710.0
  [424.91]
Lice (infestation) 132.9
  body (pediculus corporis) 132.1
  crab 132.2
  head (pediculus capitis) 132.0
  mixed (classifiable to more than one of the
    categories 132.0-132.2) 132.3
  pubic (pediculus pubis) 132.2
Lichen 697.9
  albus 701.0
  annularis 695.89
  atrophicus 701.0
  corneus obtusus 698.3
  myxedematous 701.8
  nitidus 697.1
  pilaris 757.39
    acquired 701.1
  planopilaris 697.0
  planus (acute) (chronicus) (hypertrophic)
    (verrucous) 697.0
    morphoeicus 701.0
    sclerosus (et atrophicus) 701.0
  ruber 696.4

Lichen—*continued*
acuminatus 696.4
moniliformis 697.8
obtusus corneus 698.3
of Wilson 697.0
planus 697.0
sclerosus (et atrophicus) 701.0
scrofulosus (primary) (*see also* Tuberculosis)
017.0
simplex (Vidal's) 698.3
chronicus 698.3
circumscriptus 698.3
spinulosus 757.39
mycotic 117.9
striata 697.8
urticatus 698.2
Lichenification 698.3
nodular 698.3
Lichenoides tuberculosis (primary) (*see also*
Tuberculosis) 017.0
Lichtheim's disease or syndrome (subacute
combined sclerosis with pernicious anemia)
281.0 *[336.2]*
Lien migrans 289.59
Lientery (*see also* Diarrhea) 787.91
infectious 009.2
Life circumstance problem NEC V62.89
Ligament —*see* condition
Light-for-dates (infant) 764.0
with signs of fetal malnutrition 764.1
affecting management of pregnancy 656.5
Light-headedness 780.4
Lightning (effects) (shock) (stroke) (struck by)
994.0
burn—*see* Burn, by site
foot 266.2
Lightwood's disease or syndrome (renal tubular
acidosis) 588.8
Lignac's disease (cystinosis) 270.0
Lignac (-de Toni) (-Fanconi) (-Debré) syndrome
(cystinosis) 270.0
Lignac (-Fanconi) syndrome (cystinosis) 270.0
Ligneous thyroiditis 245.3
Likoff's syndrome (angina in menopausal
women) 413.9
Limb —*see* condition
Limitation of joint motion (*see also* Stiffness,
joint) 719.5
sacroiliac 724.6
Limit dextrinosis 271.0
Limited
cardiac reserve—*see* Disease, heart
duction, eye NEC 378.63
Lindau's disease (retinocerebral angiomatosis)
759.6
Lindau (-von Hippel) disease (angiomatosis
retinocerebellosa) 759.6
Linea corneae senilis 371.41
Lines
Beau's (transverse furrows on fingernails) 703.8
Harris' 733.91
Hudson-Stähli 371.11
Stähli's 371.11
Lingua
geographical 529.1
nigra (villosa) 529.3
plicata 529.5
congenital 750.13
tylosis 528.6
Lingual (tongue)—*see also* condition
thyroid 759.2

Linitis (gastric) 535.4
plastica (M8142/3) 151.9
Lioderma essentialis (cum melanosis et
telangiectasia) 757.33
Lip —*see also* condition
biting 528.9
Lipalgia 272.8
Lipedema —*see* Edema
Lipemia (*see also* Hyperlipidemia) 272.4
retina, retinalis 272.3
Lipidosis 272.7
cephalin 272.7
cerebral (infantile) (juvenile) (late) 330.1
cerebroretinal 330.1 *[362.71]*
cerebroside 272.7
cerebrospinal 272.7
chemically-induced 272.7
cholesterol 272.7
diabetic 250.8 *[272.7]*
dystopic (hereditary) 272.7
glycolipid 272.7
hepatosplenomegalic 272.3
hereditary, dystopic 272.7
sulfatide 330.0
Lipoadenoma (M8324/0)—*see* Neoplasm, by
site, benign
Lipoblastoma (M8881/0)—*see* Lipoma, by site
Lipoblastomatosis (M8881/0)—*see* Lipoma, by
site
Lipochondrodystrophy 277.5
Lipochrome histiocytosis (familial) 288.1
Lipodystrophia progressiva 272.6
Lipodystrophy (progressive) 272.6
insulin 272.6
intestinal 040.2
Lipofibroma (M8851/0)—*see* Lipoma, by site
Lipoglycoproteinosis 272.8
Lipogranuloma, sclerosing 709.8
Lipogranulomatosis (disseminated) 272.8
kidney 272.8
Lipoid —*see* condition
histiocytosis 272.7
essential 272.7
nephrosis (*see also* Nephrosis) 581.3
proteinosis of Urbach 272.8
Lipoidemia (*see also* Hyperlipidemia) 272.4
Lipoidosis (*see also* Lipidosis) 272.7
Lipoma (M8850/0) 214.9
breast (skin) 214.1
face 214.0
fetal (M8881/0)—*see also* Lipoma, by site
fat cell (M8880/0)—*see* Lipoma, by site
infiltrating (M8856/0)—*see* Lipoma, by site
intra-abdominal 214.3
intramuscular (M8856/0)—*see* Lipoma, by site
intrathoracic 214.2
kidney 214.3
mediastinum 214.2
muscle 214.8
peritoneum 214.3
retroperitoneum 214.3
skin 214.1
face 214.0
spermatic cord 214.4
spindle cell (M8857/0)—*see* Lipoma, by site
stomach 214.3
subcutaneous tissue 214.1
face 214.0
thymus 214.2
thyroid gland 214.2

Lipomatosis (dolorosa) 272.8
  epidural 214.8
  fetal (M8881/0)—*see* Lipoma, by site
  Launois-Bensaude's 272.8
Lipomyohemangioma (M8860/0)
  specified site—*see* Neoplasm, connective
    tissue, benign
  unspecified site 223.0
Lipomyoma (M8860/0)
  specified site—*see* Neoplasm, connective
    tissue, benign
  unspecified site 223.0
Lipomyxoma (M8852/0)—*see* Lipoma, by site
Lipomyxosarcoma (M8852/3)—*see* Neoplasm,
  connective tissue, malignant
Lipophagocytosis 289.8
Lipoproteinemia (alpha) 272.4
  broad-beta 272.2
  floating-beta 272.2
  hyper-pre-beta 272.1
Lipoproteinosis (Rössle-Urbach-Wiethe) 272.8
Liposarcoma (M8850/3)—*see also* Neoplasm,
  connective tissue, malignant
  differentiated type (M8851/3)—*see* Neoplasm,
    connective tissue, malignant
  embryonal (M8852/3)—*see* Neoplasm,
    connective tissue, malignant
  mixed type (M8855/3)—*see* Neoplasm,
    connective tissue, malignant
  myxoid (M8852/3)—*see* Neoplasm, connective
    tissue, malignant
  pleomorphic (M8854/3)—*see* Neoplasm,
    connective tissue, malignant
  round cell (M8853/3)—*see* Neoplasm,
    connective tissue, malignant
  well differentiated type (M8851/3)—*see*
    Neoplasm, connective tissue, malignant
Liposynovitis prepatellaris 272.8
Lipping
  cervix 622.0
  spine (*see also* Spondylosis) 721.90
  vertebra (*see also* Spondylosis) 721.90
Lip pits (mucus), congenital 750.25
Lipschütz disease or ulcer 616.50
Lipuria 791.1
  bilharziasis 120.0
Liquefaction, vitreous humor 379.21
Lisping 307.9
Lissauer's paralysis 094.1
Lissencephalia, lissencephaly 742.2
Listerellose 027.0
Listeriose 027.0
Listeriosis 027.0
  congenital 771.2
  fetal 771.2
  suspected fetal damage affecting management
    of pregnancy 655.4
Listlessness 780.79
Lithemia 790.6
Lithiasis —*see also* Calculus
  hepatic (duct)—*see* Choledocholithiasis
  urinary 592.9
Lithopedion 779.9
  affecting management of pregnancy 656.8
Lithosis (occupational) 502
  with tuberculosis—*see* Tuberculosis, pulmonary
Lithuria 791.9
Litigation V62.5
Little
  league elbow 718.82
  stroke syndrome 435.9
Little's disease —*see* Palsy, cerebral

Littre's
  gland—*see* condition
  hernia—*see* Hernia, Littre's
Littritis (*see also* Urethritis) 597.89
Livedo 782.61
  annularis 782.61
  racemose 782.61
  reticularis 782.61
Live flesh 781.0
Liver —*see also* condition
  donor V59.6
Livida, asphyxia
  newborn 768.6
Living
  alone V60.3
    with handicapped person V60.4
Lloyd's syndrome 258.1
Loa loa 125.2
Loasis 125.2
Lobe, lobar —*see* condition
Lobo's disease or blastomycosis 116.2
Lobomycosis 116.2
Lobotomy syndrome 310.0
Lobstein's disease (brittle bones and blue sclera)
  756.51
Lobster-claw hand 755.58
Lobulation (congenital)—*see also* Anomaly,
  specified type NEC, by site
  kidney, fetal 753.3
  liver, abnormal 751.69
  spleen 759.0
Lobule, lobular —*see* condition
Local, localized —*see* condition
Locked bowel or intestine (*see also* Obstruction,
  intestine) 560.9
Locked twins 660.5
  affecting fetus or newborn 763.1
Locked-in state 344.81
Locking
  joint (*see also* Derangement, joint) 718.90
  knee 717.9
Lockjaw (*see also* Tetanus) 037
Locomotor ataxia (progressive) 094.0
Löffler's
  endocarditis 421.0
  eosinophilia or syndrome 518.3
  pneumonia 518.3
  syndrome (eosinophilic pneumonitis) 518.3
Löfgren's syndrome (sarcoidosis) 135
Loiasis 125.2
  eyelid 125.2 *[373.6]*
Loneliness V62.89
Lone star fever 082.8
Long labor 662.1
  affecting fetus or newborn 763.89
  first stage 662.0
  second stage 662.2
Long-term (current) drug use V58.69
  antibiotics V58.62
  anticoagulants V58.61
Longitudinal stripes or grooves, nails 703.8
  congenital 757.5
Loop
  intestine (*see also* Volvulus) 560.2
  intrascleral nerve 379.29
  vascular on papilla (optic) 743.57
Loose —*see also* condition
  body
    in tendon sheath 727.82
    joint 718.10
      ankle 718.17

Loose—*continued*
  elbow 718.12
  foot 718.17
  hand 718.14
  hip 718.15
  knee 717.6
  multiple sites 718.19
  pelvic region 718.15
  prosthetic implant—*see* Complications,
    mechanical
  shoulder (region) 718.11
  specified site NEC 718.18
  wrist 718.13
  cartilage (joint) (*see also* Loose, body, joint)
    718.1
    knee 717.6
  facet (vertebral) 724.9
  prosthetic implant—*see* Complications,
    mechanical
  sesamoid, joint (*see also* Loose, body, joint)
    718.1
  tooth, teeth 525.8
Loosening epiphysis 732.9
Looser (-Debray) -Milkman syndrome
  (osteomalacia with pseudofractures) 268.2
Lop ear (deformity) 744.29
Lorain's disease or syndrome (pituitary
  dwarfism) 253.3
Lorain-Levi syndrome (pituitary dwarfism)
  253.3
Lordosis (acquired) (postural) 737.20
  congenital 754.2
  due to or associated with
    Charcot-Marie-Tooth disease 356.1 *[737.42]*
    mucopolysaccharidosis 277.5 *[737.42]*
    neurofibromatosis 237.71 *[737.42]*
    osteitis
      deformans 731.0 *[737.42]*
      fibrosa cystica 252.0 *[737.42]*
    osteoporosis (*see also* Osteoporosis) 733.00
      [737.42]
    poliomyelitis (*see also* Poliomyelitis) 138
      [737.42]
    tuberculosis (*see also* Tuberculosis) 015.0
      [737.42]
  late effect of rickets 268.1 *[737.42]*
  postlaminectomy 737.21
  postsurgical NEC 737.22
  rachitic 268.1 *[737.42]*
  specified NEC 737.29
  tuberculous (*see also* Tuberculosis) 015.0
    [737.42]
Loss
  appetite 783.0
    hysterical 300.11
    nonorganic origin 307.59
    psychogenic 307.59
  blood—*see* Hemorrhage
  central vision 368.41
  consciousness 780.09
    transient 780.2
  control, sphincter, rectum 787.6
    nonorganic origin 307.7
  ear ossicle, partial 385.24
  elasticity, skin 782.8
  extremity or member, traumatic, current—*see*
    Amputation, traumatic
  fluid (acute) 276.5
    with
      hypernatremia 276.0
      hyponatremia 276.1

Loss —*continued*
  fetus or newborn 775.5
  hair 704.00
  hearing—*see also* Deafness
    central 389.14
    conductive (air) 389.00
      with sensorineural hearing loss 389.2
      combined types 389.08
      external ear 389.01
      inner ear 389.04
      middle ear 389.03
      multiple types 389.08
      tympanic membrane 389.02
    mixed type 389.2
    nerve 389.12
    neural 389.12
    noise-induced 388.12
    perceptive NEC (*see also* Loss, hearing,
      sensorineural) 389.10
    sensorineural 389.10
      with conductive hearing loss 389.2
      central 389.14
      combined types 389.18
      multiple types 389.18
      neural 389.12
      sensory 389.11
    sensory 389.11
    specified type NEC 389.8
    sudden NEC 388.2
  height 781.91
  labyrinthine reactivity (unilateral) 386.55
    bilateral 386.56
  memory (*see also* Amnesia) 780.99
    mild, following organic brain damage 310.1
  mind (*see also* Psychosis) 298.9
  organ or part—*see* Absence, by site, acquired
  sensation 782.0
  sense of
    smell (*see also* Disturbance, sensation) 781.1
    taste (*see also* Disturbance, sensation) 781.1
    touch (*see also* Disturbance, sensation) 781.1
  sight (acquired) (complete) (congenital)—*see*
    Blindness
  spinal fluid
    headache 349.0
  substance of
    bone (*see also* Osteoporosis) 733.00
    cartilage 733.99
    ear 380.32
    vitreous (humor) 379.26
  tooth, teeth
    acquired 525.10
      due to
        caries 525.13
        extraction 525.10
        periodontal disease 525.12
        specified NEC 525.19
        trauma 525.11
  vision, visual (*see also* Blindness) 369.9
    both eyes (*see also* Blindness, both eyes) 369.3
    complete (*see also* Blindness, both eyes)
      369.00
    one eye 369.8
    sudden 368.11
    transient 368.12
  vitreous 379.26
  voice (*see also* Aphonia) 784.41
  weight (cause unknown) 783.21
Lou Gehrig's disease 335.20
Louis-Bar syndrome (ataxia-telangiectasia)
  334.8
Louping ill 063.1

Lousiness —*see* Lice
Low
back syndrome 724.2
basal metabolic rate (BMR) 794.7
birthweight 765.1
extreme (less than 1000 grams) 765.0
for gestational age 764.0
status (*see also* Status, low birth weight)
V21.30
bladder compliance 596.52
blood pressure (*see also* Hypotension) 458.9
reading (incidental) (isolated) (nonspecific)
796.3
cardiac reserve—*see* Disease, heart
compliance bladder 596.52
frequency deafness—*see* Disorder, hearing
function—*see also* Hypofunction
kidney (*see also* Disease, renal) 593.9
liver 573.9
hemoglobin 285.9
implantation, placenta—*see* Placenta, previa
insertion, placenta—*see* Placenta, previa
lying
kidney 593.0
organ or site, congenital—*see* Malposition,
congenital
placenta—*see* Placenta, previa
output syndrome (cardiac) (*see also* Failure,
heart) 428.9
platelets (blood) (*see also* Thrombocytopenia)
287.5
reserve, kidney (*see also* Disease, renal) 593.9
salt syndrome 593.9
tension glaucoma 365.12
vision 369.9
both eyes 369.20
one eye 369.70
Lowe (-Terrey-MacLachlan) syndrome
(oculocerebrorenal dystrophy) 270.8
Lower extremity —*see* condition
Lown (-Ganong)-Levine syndrome (short P-R
interval, normal QRS complex, and
paroxysmal supraventricular tachycardia)
426.81
LSD reaction (*see also* Abuse, drugs,
nondependent) 305.3
L-shaped kidney 753.3
Lucas-Championnière disease (fibrinous
bronchitis) 466.0
Lucey-Driscoll syndrome (jaundice due to
delayed conjugation) 774.30
Ludwig's
angina 528.3
disease (submaxillary cellulitis) 528.3
Lues (venerea), luetic—*see* Syphilis
Luetscher's syndrome (dehydration) 276.5
Lumbago 724.2
due to displacement, intervertebral disc 722.10
Lumbalgia 724.2
due to displacement, intervertebral disc 722.10
Lumbar —*see* condition
Lumbarization, vertebra 756.15
Lumbermen's itch 133.8
Lump —*see also* Mass
abdominal 789.3
breast 611.72
chest 786.6
epigastric 789.3
head 784.2
kidney 753.3
liver 789.1

Lump—*continued*
lung 786.6
mediastinal 786.6
neck 784.2
nose or sinus 784.2
pelvic 789.3
skin 782.2
substernal 786.6
throat 784.2
umbilicus 789.3
Lunacy (*see also* Psychosis) 298.9
Lunatomalacia 732.3
Lung —*see also* condition
donor V59.8
drug addict's 417.8
mainliners' 417.8
vanishing 492.0
Lupoid (miliary) of Boeck 135
Lupus 710.0
Cazenave's (erythematosus) 695.4
discoid (local) 695.4
disseminated 710.0
erythematodes (discoid) (local) 695.4
erythematosus (discoid) (local) <u>695.4</u>
disseminated 710.0
eyelid 373.34
systemic 710.0
with
encephalitis 710.0 *[323.8]*
lung involvement <u>710.0 *[517.8]*</u>
inhibitor (presence of) 286.5
exedens 017.0
eyelid (*see also* Tuberculosis) 017.0 *[373.4]*
Hilliard's 017.0
hydralazine
correct substance properly administered 695.4
overdose or wrong substance given or taken
972.6
miliaris disseminatus faciei 017.0
nephritis 710.0 *[583.81]*
acute 710.0 *[580.81]*
chronic 710.0 *[582.81]*
nontuberculous, not disseminated 695.4
pernio (Besnier) 135
tuberculous (*see also* Tuberculosis) 017.0
eyelid (*see also* Tuberculosis) 017.0 *[373.4]*
vulgaris 017.0
Luschka's joint disease 721.90
Luteinoma (M8610/0) 220
Lutembacher's disease or syndrome (atrial
septal defect with mitral stenosis) 745.5
Luteoma (M8610/0) 220
Lutz-Miescher disease (elastosis perforans
serpiginosa) 701.1
Lutz-Splendore-de Almeida disease (Brazilian
blastomycosis) 116.1
Luxatio
bulbi due to birth injury 767.8
coxae congenita (*see also* Dislocation, hip,
congenital) 754.30
erecta—*see* Dislocation, shoulder
imperfecta—*see* Sprain, by site
perinealis—*see* Dislocation, hip
Luxation —*see also* Dislocation, by site
eyeball 360.81
due to birth injury 767.8
lateral 376.36
genital organs (external) NEC—*see* Wound,
open, genital organs
globe (eye) 360.81
lateral 376.36

Luxation—*continued*
  lacrimal gland (postinfectional) 375.16
  lens (old) (partial) 379.32
    congenital 743.37
      syphilitic 090.49 *[379.32]*
    Marfan's disease 090.49
    spontaneous 379.32
  penis—*see* Wound, open, penis
  scrotum—*see* Wound, open, scrotum
  testis—*see* Wound, open, testis
L-xyloketosuria 271.8
Lycanthropy (*see also* Psychosis) 298.9
Lyell's disease or syndrome (toxic epidermal
  necrolysis) 695.1
  due to drug
    correct substance properly administered 695.1
    overdose or wrong substance given or taken
      977.9
      specified drug—*see* Table of drugs and
        chemicals
Lyme disease 088.81
Lymph
  gland or node—*see* condition
  scrotum (*see also* Infestation, filarial) 125.9
Lymphadenitis 289.3
  with
    abortion—*see* Abortion, by type, with sepsis
    ectopic pregnancy (*see also* categories
      633.0-633.9) 639.0
    molar pregnancy (*see also* categories
      630-632) 639.0
  acute 683
    mesenteric 289.2
  any site, except mesenteric 289.3
    acute 683
    chronic 289.1
    mesenteric (acute) (chronic) (nonspecific)
      (subacute) 289.2
    subacute 289.1
      mesenteric 289.2
  breast, puerperal, postpartum 675.2
  chancroidal (congenital) 099.0
  chronic 289.1
    mesenteric 289.2
  dermatopathic 695.89
  due to
    anthracosis (occupational) 500
    Brugia (Wuchereria) malayi 125.1
    diphtheria (toxin) 032.89
    lymphogranuloma venereum 099.1
    Wuchereria bancrofti 125.0
  following
    abortion 639.0
    ectopic or molar pregnancy 639.0
  generalized 289.3
  gonorrheal 098.89
  granulomatous 289.1
  infectional 683
  mesenteric (acute) (chronic) (nonspecific)
    (subacute) 289.2
    due to Bacillus typhi 002.0
    tuberculous (*see also* Tuberculosis) 014.8
  mycobacterial 031.8
  purulent 683
  pyogenic 683
  regional 078.3
  septic 683
  streptococcal 683
  subacute, unspecified site 289.1
  suppurative 683
  syphilitic (early) (secondary) 091.4

Lymphadenitis—*continued*
  late 095.8
  tuberculous—*see* Tuberculosis, lymph gland
  venereal 099.1
Lymphadenoid goiter 245.2
Lymphadenopathy (general) 785.6
  due to toxoplasmosis (acquired) 130.7
  congenital (active) 771.2
Lymphadenopathy-associated virus (disease)
  (illness) (infection)—*see* Human
  Immunodeficiency virus (disease) (illness)
  (infection)
Lymphadenosis 785.6
  acute 075
Lymphangiectasis 457.1
  conjunctiva 372.89
  postinfectional 457.1
  scrotum 457.1
Lymphangiectatic elephantiasis, nonfilarial
  457.1
Lymphangioendothelioma (M9170/0) 228.1
  malignant (M9170/3)—*see* Neoplasm,
    connective tissue, malignant
Lymphangioma (M9170/0) 228.1
  capillary (M9171/0) 228.1
  cavernous (M9172/0) 228.1
  cystic (M9173/0) 228.1
  malignant (M9170/3)—*see* Neoplasm,
    connective tissue, malignant
Lymphangiomyoma (M9174/0) 228.1
Lymphangiomyomatosis (M9174/1)—*see*
  Neoplasm, connective tissue, uncertain
  behavior
Lymphangiosarcoma (M9170/3)—*see*
  Neoplasm, connective tissue, malignant
Lymphangitis 457.2
  with
    abortion—*see* Abortion, by type, with sepsis
    abscess—*see* Abscess, by site
    cellulitis—*see* Abscess, by site
    ectopic pregnancy (*see also* categories
      633.0-633.9) 639.0
    molar pregnancy (*see also* categories
      630-632) 639.0
  acute (with abscess or cellulitis) 682.9
    specified site—*see* Abscess, by site
  breast, puerperal, postpartum 675.2
  chancroidal 099.0
  chronic (any site) 457.2
  due to
    Brugia (Wuchereria) malayi 125.1
    Wuchereria bancrofti 125.0
  following
    abortion 639.0
    ectopic or molar pregnancy 639.0
  gangrenous 457.2
  penis
    acute 607.2
    gonococcal (acute) 098.0
      chronic or duration of 2 months or more
        098.2
  puerperal, postpartum, childbirth 670
  strumous, tuberculous (*see also* Tuberculosis)
    017.2
  subacute (any site) 457.2
  tuberculous—*see* Tuberculosis, lymph gland
Lymphatic (vessel)—*see* condition
Lymphatism 254.8
  scrofulous (*see also* Tuberculosis) 017.2
Lymphectasia 457.1

Lymphedema (*see also* Elephantiasis) 457.1
  acquired (chronic) 457.1
  chronic hereditary 757.0
  congenital 757.0
  idiopathic hereditary 757.0
  praecox 457.1
  secondary 457.1
  surgical NEC 997.99
    postmastectomy (syndrome) 457.0
Lymph-hemangioma (M9120/0)—*see*
  Hemangioma, by site
Lymphoblastic —*see* condition
Lymphoblastoma (diffuse) (M9630/3) 200.1
  giant follicular (M9690/3) 202.0
  macrofollicular (M9690/3) 202.0
Lymphoblastosis, acute benign 075
Lymphocele 457.8
Lymphocythemia 288.8
Lymphocytic —*see also* condition
  chorioencephalitis (acute) (serous) 049.0
  choriomeningitis (acute) (serous) 049.0
Lymphocytoma (diffuse) (malignant) (M9620/3)
  200.1
Lymphocytomatosis (M9620/3) 200.1
Lymphocytopenia 288.8
Lymphocytosis (symptomatic) 288.8
  infectious (acute) 078.89
Lymphoepithelioma (M8082/3)—*see*
  Neoplasm, by site, malignant
Lymphogranuloma (malignant) (M9650/3) 201.9
  inguinale 099.1
  venereal (any site) 099.1
    with stricture of rectum 099.1
  venereum 099.1
Lymphogranulomatosis (malignant) (M9650/3)
  201.9
  benign (Boeck's sarcoid) (Schaumann's) 135
  Hodgkin's (M9650/3) 201.9
Lymphoid —*see* condition
Lympholeukoblastoma (M9850/3) 207.8
Lympholeukosarcoma (M9850/3) 207.8
Lymphoma (malignant) (M9590/3) 202.8

*Note—Use the following fifth-digit
subclassification with categories 200-202:*

0 unspecified site
1 lymph nodes of head, face and neck
2 intrathoracic lymph nodes
3 intra-abdominal lymph nodes
4 lymph nodes of axilla and upper limb
*5 lymph nodes of inguinal region and
   lower limb*
6 intrapelvic lymph nodes
7 spleen
8 lymph nodes of multiple sites

  benign (M9590/0)—*see* Neoplasm, by site,
    benign
  Burkitt's type (lymphoblastic) (undifferentiated)
    (M9750/3) 200.2
  Castleman's (mediastinal lymph node
    hyperplasia) 785.6
  centroblastic-centrocytic
    diffuse (M9614/3) 202.8
    follicular (M9692/3) 202.0
  centroblastic type (diffuse) (M9632/3) 202.8
    follicular (M9697/3) 202.0
  centrocytic (M9622/3) 202.8
  compound (M9613/3) 200.8
  convoluted cell type (lymphoblastic) (M9602/3)
    202.8

Lymphoma—*continued*
  diffuse NEC (M9590/3) 202.8
  follicular (giant) (M9690/3) 202.0
    center cell (diffuse) (M9615/3) 202.8
      cleaved (diffuse) (M9623/3) 202.8
        follicular (M9695/3) 202.0
      non-cleaved (diffuse) (M9633/3) 202.8
        follicular (M9698/3) 202.0
    centroblastic-centrocytic (M9692/3) 202.0
    centroblastic type (M9697/3) 202.0
    lymphocytic
      intermediate differentiation (M9694/3) 202.0
      poorly differentiated (M9696/3) 202.0
    mixed (cell type) (lymphocytic-histiocytic)
      (small cell and large cell) (M9691/3) 202.0
  germinocytic (M9622/3) 202.8
  giant, follicular or follicle (M9690/3) 202.0
  histiocytic (diffuse) (M9640/3) 200.0
    nodular (M9642/3) 200.0
    pleomorphic cell type (M9641/3) 200.0
  Hodgkin's (M9650/3) (*see also* Disease,
    Hodgkin's) 201.9
  immunoblastic (type) (M9612/3) 200.8
  large cell (M9640/3) 200.0
    nodular (M9642/3) 200.0
    pleomorphic cell type (M9641/3) 200.0
  lymphoblastic (diffuse) (M9630/3) 200.1
    Burkitt's type (M9750/3) 200.2
    convoluted cell type (M9602/3) 202.8
  lymphocytic (cell type) (diffuse) (M9620/3)
    200.1
    with plasmacytoid differentiation, diffuse
      (M9611/3) 200.8
    intermediate differentiation (diffuse)
      (M9621/3) 200.1
      follicular (M9694/3) 202.0
      nodular (M9694/3) 202.0
    nodular (M9690/3) 202.0
    poorly differentiated (diffuse) (M9630/3)
      200.1
      follicular (M9696/3) 202.0
      nodular (M9696/3) 202.0
    well differentiated (diffuse) (M9620/3) 200.1
      follicular (M9693/3) 202.0
      nodular (M9693/3) 202.0
  lymphocytic-histiocytic, mixed (diffuse)
    (M9613/3) 200.8
    follicular (M9691/3) 202.0
    nodular (M9691/3) 202.0
  lymphoplasmacytoid type (M9611/3) 200.8
  lymphosarcoma type (M9610/3) 200.1
  macrofollicular (M9690/3) 202.0
  mixed cell type (diffuse) (M9613/3) 200.8
    follicular (M9691/3) 202.0
    nodular (M9691/3) 202.0
  nodular (M9690/3) 202.0
    histiocytic (M9642/3) 200.0
    lymphocytic (M9690.3) 202.0
      intermediate differentiation (M9694/3) 202.0
      poorly differentiated (M9696/3) 202.0
    mixed (cell type) (lymphocytic-histiocytic)
      (small cell and large cell) (M9691/3) 202.0
  non-Hodgkin's type NEC (M9591/3) 202.8
  reticulum cell (type) (M9640/3) 200.0
  small cell and large cell, mixed (diffuse)
    (M9613/3) 200.8
    follicular (M9691/3) 202.0
    nodular (9691/3) 202.0
  stem cell (type) (M9601/3) 202.8
  T-cell 202.1

Lymphoma—*continued*
  undifferentiated (cell type) (non-Burkitt's)
      (M9600/3) 202.8
    Burkitt's type (M9750/3) 200.2
Lymphomatosis (M9590/3)—*see also*
    Lymphoma
  granulomatous 099.1
Lymphopathia
  venereum 099.1
  veneris 099.1
Lymphopenia 288.8
  familial 279.2
Lymphoreticulosis, benign (of inoculation)
    078.3
Lymphorrhea 457.8
Lymphosarcoma (M9610/3) 200.1
  diffuse (M9610/3) 200.1
    with plasmacytoid differentiation (M9611/3)
        200.8
    lymphoplasmacytic (M9611/3) 200.8
  follicular (giant) (M9690/3) 202.0
    lymphoblastic (M9696/3) 202.0
    lymphocytic, intermediate differentiation
        (M9694/3) 202.0
    mixed cell type (M9691/3) 202.0
  giant follicular (M9690/3) 202.0
  Hodgkin's (M9650/3) 201.9
  immunoblastic (M9612/3) 200.8
  lymphoblastic (diffuse) (M9630/3) 200.1
    follicular (M9696/3) 202.0
    nodular (M9696/3) 202.0
  lymphocytic (diffuse) (M9620/3) 200.1
    intermediate differentiation (diffuse)
        (M9621/3) 200.1
      follicular (M9694/3) 202.0
      nodular (M9694/3) 202.0
  mixed cell type (diffuse) (M9613/3) 200.8
    follicular (M9691/3) 202.0
    nodular (M9691/3) 202.0
  nodular (M9690/3) 202.0
    lymphoblastic (M9696/3) 202.0
    lymphocytic, intermediate differentiation
        (M9694/3) 202.0
    mixed cell type (M9691/3) 202.0
  prolymphocytic (M9631/3) 200.1
  reticulum cell (M9640/3) 200.0
Lymphostasis 457.8
Lypemania (*see also* Melancholia) 296.2
Lyssa 071

M

Macacus ear 744.29
Maceration
  fetus (cause not stated) 779.9
  wet feet, tropical (syndrome) 991.4
Machado-Joseph disease 334.8
Machupo virus hemorrhagic fever 078.7
Macleod's syndrome (abnormal transradiancy, one lung) 492.8
Macrocephalia, macrocephaly 756.0
Macrocheilia (congenital) 744.81
Macrochilia (congenital) 744.81
Macrocolon (congenital) 751.3
Macrocornea 743.41
  associated with buphthalmos 743.22
Macrocytic —*see* condition
Macrocytosis 289.8
Macrodactylia, macrodactylism (fingers) (thumbs) 755.57
  toes 755.65
Macrodontia 520.2
Macroencephaly 742.4
Macrogenia 524.05
Macrogenitosomia (female) (male) (praecox) 255.2
Macrogingivae 523.8
Macroglobulinemia (essential) (idiopathic) (monoclonal) (primary) (syndrome) (Waldenström's) 273.3
Macroglossia (congenital) 750.15
  acquired 529.8
Macrognathia, macrognathism (congenital) 524.00
  mandibular 524.02
    alveolar 524.72
  maxillary 524.01
    alveolar 524.71
Macrogyria (congenital) 742.4
Macrohydrocephalus (*see also* Hydrocephalus) 331.4
Macromastia (*see also* Hypertrophy, breast) 611.1
Macropsia 368.14
Macrosigmoid 564.7
  congenital 751.3
Macrospondylitis, acromegalic 253.0
Macrostomia (congenital) 744.83
Macrotia (external ear) (congenital) 744.22
Macula
  cornea, corneal
    congenital 743.43
      interfering with vision 743.42
    interfering with central vision 371.03
    not interfering with central vision 371.02
  degeneration (*see also* Degeneration, macula) 362.50
  hereditary (*see also* Dystrophy, retina) 362.70
  edema, cystoid 362.53
Maculae ceruleae 132.1
Macules and papules 709.8
Maculopathy, toxic 362.55
Madarosis 374.55
Madelung's
  deformity (radius) 755.54
  disease (lipomatosis) 272.8
  lipomatosis 272.8
Madness (*see also* Psychosis) 298.9
  myxedema (acute) 293.0
  subacute 293.1

Madura
  disease (actinomycotic) 039.9
    mycotic 117.4
  foot (actinomycotic) 039.4
    mycotic 117.4
Maduromycosis (actinomycotic) 039.9
  mycotic 117.4
Maffucci's syndrome (dyschondroplasia with hemangiomas) 756.4
Magenblase syndrome 306.4
Main en griffe (acquired) 736.06
  congenital 755.59
Maintenance
  chemotherapy regimen or treatment V58.1
  dialysis regimen or treatment
    extracorporeal (renal) V56.0
    peritoneal V56.8
    renal V56.0
  drug therapy or regimen V58.1
  external fixation NEC V54.89
  radiotherapy V58.0
  traction NEC V54.89
Majocchi's
  disease (purpura annularis telangiectodes) 709.1
  granuloma 110.6
Major —*see* condition
Mal
  cerebral (idiopathic) (*see also* Epilepsy) 345.9
  comital (*see also* Epilepsy) 345.9
  de los pintos (*see also* Pinta) 103.9
  de Meleda 757.39
  de mer 994.6
  lie—*see* Presentation, fetal
  perforant (*see also* Ulcer, lower extremity) 707.15
Malabar itch 110.9
  beard 110.0
  foot 110.4
  scalp 110.0
Malabsorption 579.9
  calcium 579.8
  carbohydrate 579.8
  disaccharide 271.3
  drug-induced 579.8
  due to bacterial overgrowth 579.8
  fat 579.8
  folate, congenital 281.2
  galactose 271.1
  glucose-galactose (congenital) 271.3
  intestinal 579.9
  isomaltose 271.3
  lactose (hereditary) 271.3
  methionine 270.4
  monosaccharide 271.8
  postgastrectomy 579.3
  postsurgical 579.3
  protein 579.8
  sucrose (-isomaltose) (congenital) 271.3
  syndrome 579.9
    postgastrectomy 579.3
    postsurgical 579.3
Malacia, bone 268.2
  juvenile (*see also* Rickets) 268.0
  Kienböck's (juvenile) (lunate) (wrist) 732.3
    adult 732.8

Malacoplakia
bladder 596.8
colon 569.89
pelvis (kidney) 593.89
ureter 593.89
urethra 599.84
Malacosteon 268.2
juvenile (*see also* Rickets) 268.0
Maladaptation —*see* Maladjustment
Maladie de Roger 745.4
Maladjustment
conjugal V61.10
involving divorce or estrangement V61.0
educational V62.3
family V61.9
specified circumstance NEC V61.8
marital V61.10
involving divorce or estrangement V61.0
occupational V62.2
simple, adult (*see also* Reaction, adjustment)
309.9
situational acute (*see also* Reaction, adjustment)
309.9
social V62.4
Malaise 780.79
Malakoplakia —*see* Malacoplakia
Malaria, malarial (fever) 084.6
algid 084.9
any type, with
algid malaria 084.9
blackwater fever 084.8
fever
blackwater 084.8
hemoglobinuric (bilious) 084.8
hemoglobinuria, malarial 084.8
hepatitis 084.9 *[573.2]*
nephrosis 084.9 *[581.81]*
pernicious complication NEC 084.9
cardiac 084.9
cerebral 084.9
cardiac 084.9
carrier (suspected) of V02.9
cerebral 084.9
complicating pregnancy, childbirth, or
puerperium 647.4
congenital 771.2
congestion, congestive 084.6
brain 084.9
continued 084.0
estivo-autumnal 084.0
falciparum (malignant tertian) 084.0
hematinuria 084.8
hematuria 084.8
hemoglobinuria 084.8
hemorrhagic 084.6
induced (therapeutically) 084.7
accidental—*see* Malaria, by type
liver 084.9 *[573.2]*
malariae (quartan) 084.2
malignant (tertian) 084.0
mixed infections 084.5
monkey 084.4
ovale 084.3
pernicious, acute 084.0
Plasmodium, P.
falciparum 084.0
malariae 084.2
ovale 084.3
vivax 084.1

Malaria, malarial—*continued*
quartan 084.2
quotidian 084.0
recurrent 084.6
induced (therapeutically) 084.7
accidental—*see* Malaria, by type
remittent 084.6
specified types NEC 084.4
spleen 084.6
subtertian 084.0
tertian (benign) 084.1
malignant 084.0
tropical 084.0
typhoid 084.6
vivax (benign tertian) 084.1
Malassez's disease (testicular cyst) 608.89
Malassimilation 579.9
Maldescent, testis 752.51
Maldevelopment —*see also* Anomaly, by site
brain 742.9
colon 751.5
hip (joint) 755.63
congenital dislocation (*see also* Dislocation,
hip, congenital) 754.30
mastoid process 756.0
middle ear, except ossicles 744.03
ossicles 744.04
newborn (not malformation) 764.9
ossicles, ear 744.04
spine 756.10
toe 755.66
Male type pelvis 755.69
with disproportion (fetopelvic) 653.2
affecting fetus or newborn 763.1
causing obstructed labor 660.1
affecting fetus or newborn 763.1
Malformation (congenital)—*see also* Anomaly
bone 756.9
bursa 756.9
Chiari
type I 348.4
type II (*see also* Spina bifida) 741.0
type III 742.0
type IV 742.2
circulatory system NEC 747.9
specified type NEC 747.89
cochlea 744.05
digestive system NEC 751.9
lower 751.5
specified type NEC 751.8
upper 750.9
eye 743.9
gum 750.9
heart NEC 746.9
specified type NEC 746.89
valve 746.9
internal ear 744.05
joint NEC 755.9
specified type NEC 755.8
Mondini's (congenital) (malformation, cochlea)
744.05
muscle 756.9
nervous system (central) 742.9
pelvic organs or tissues
in pregnancy or childbirth 654.9
affecting fetus or newborn 763.89
causing obstructed labor 660.2
affecting fetus or newborn 763.1
placenta (*see also* Placenta, abnormal) 656.7

Malformation—*continued*
respiratory organs 748.9
  specified type NEC 748.8
Rieger's 743.44
sense organs NEC 742.9
  specified type NEC 742.8
skin 757.9
  specified type NEC 757.8
spinal cord 742.9
teeth, tooth NEC 520.9
tendon 756.9
throat 750.9
umbilical cord (complicating delivery) 663.9
  affecting fetus or newborn 762.6
umbilicus 759.9
urinary system NEC 753.9
  specified type NEC 753.8
Malfunction —*see also* Dysfunction
arterial graft 996.1
cardiac pacemaker 996.01
catheter device—*see* Complications,
    mechanical, catheter
colostomy 569.62
cystostomy 997.5
device, implant, or graft NEC—*see*
    Complications, mechanical
enteric stoma 569.62
enterostomy 569.62
gastroenteric 536.8
gastrostomy 536.42
nephrostomy 997.5
pacemaker—*see* Complications, mechanical,
    pacemaker
prosthetic device, internal—*see* Complications,
    mechanical
tracheostomy 519.02
vascular graft or shunt 996.1
Malgaigne's fracture (closed) 808.43
open 808.53
Malherbe's
calcifying epithelioma (M8110/0)—*see*
    Neoplasm, skin, benign
tumor (M8110/0)—*see* Neoplasm, skin, benign
Malibu disease 919.8
infected 919.9
Malignancy (M8000/3)—*see* Neoplasm, by site,
    malignant
Malignant —*see* condition
Malingerer, malingering V65.2
Mallet, finger (acquired) 736.1
congenital 755.59
late effect of rickets 268.1
Malleus 024
Mallory's bodies 034.1
Mallory-Weiss syndrome 530.7
Malnutrition (calorie) 263.9
complicating pregnancy 648.9
degree
  first 263.1
  second 263.0
  third 262
  mild 263.1
  moderate 263.0
  severe 261
    protein-calorie 262
fetus 764.2
  "light-for-dates" 764.1
following gastrointestinal surgery 579.3
intrauterine or fetal 764.2
  fetus or infant "light-for-dates" 764.1

Malnutrition—*continued*
lack of care, or neglect (child) (infant) 995.52
  adult 995.84
malignant 260
mild 263.1
moderate 263.0
protein 260
protein-calorie 263.9
  severe 262
  specified type NEC 263.8
severe 261
  protein-calorie NEC 262
Malocclusion (teeth) 524.4
due to
  abnormal swallowing 524.5
  accessory teeth (causing crowding) 524.3
  dentofacial abnormality NEC 524.8
  impacted teeth (causing crowding) 524.3
  missing teeth 524.3
  mouth breathing 524.5
  supernumerary teeth (causing crowding) 524.3
  thumb sucking 524.5
  tongue, lip, or finger habits 524.5
temporomandibular (joint) 524.69
Malposition
cardiac apex (congenital) 746.87
cervix—*see* Malposition, uterus
congenital
  adrenal (gland) 759.1
  alimentary tract 751.8
    lower 751.5
    upper 750.8
  aorta 747.21
  appendix 751.5
  arterial trunk 747.29
  artery (peripheral) NEC (*see also* Malposition,
      congenital, peripheral vascular system)
      747.60
    coronary 746.85
    pulmonary 747.3
  auditory canal 744.29
    causing impairment of hearing 744.02
  auricle (ear) 744.29
    causing impairment of hearing 744.02
    cervical 744.43
  biliary duct or passage 751.69
  bladder (mucosa) 753.8
    exteriorized or extroverted 753.5
  brachial plexus 742.8
  brain tissue 742.4
  breast 757.6
  bronchus 748.3
  cardiac apex 746.87
  cecum 751.5
  clavicle 755.51
  colon 751.5
  digestive organ or tract NEC 751.8
    lower 751.5
    upper 750.8
  ear (auricle) (external) 744.29
    ossicles 744.04
  endocrine (gland) NEC 759.2
  epiglottis 748.3
  Eustachian tube 744.24
  eye 743.8
  facial features 744.89
  fallopian tube 752.19
  finger(s) 755.59
    supernumerary 755.01

Malposition—*continued*
  foot 755.67
  gallbladder 751.69
  gastrointestinal tract 751.8
  genitalia, genital organ(s) or tract
    female 752.8
      external 752.49
      internal NEC 752.8
    male 752.8
      penis 752.69
  glottis 748.3
  hand 755.59
  heart 746.87
    dextrocardia 746.87
      with complete transposition of viscera
        759.3
  hepatic duct 751.69
  hip (joint) (*see also* Dislocation, hip,
    congenital) 754.30
  intestine (large) (small) 751.5
    with anomalous adhesions, fixation, or
      malrotation 751.4
  joint NEC 755.8
  kidney 753.3
  larynx 748.3
  limb 755.8
    lower 755.69
    upper 755.59
  liver 751.69
  lung (lobe) 748.69
  nail(s) 757.5
  nerve 742.8
  nervous system NEC 742.8
  nose, nasal (septum) 748.1
  organ or site NEC—*see* Anomaly, specified
    type NEC, by site
  ovary 752.0
  pancreas 751.7
  parathyroid (gland) 759.2
  patella 755.64
  peripheral vascular system 747.60
    gastrointestinal 747.61
    lower limb 747.64
    renal 747.62
    specified NEC 747.69
    spinal 747.82
    upper limb 747.63
  pituitary (gland) 759.2
  respiratory organ or system NEC 748.9
  rib (cage) 756.3
    supernumerary in cervical region 756.2
  scapula 755.59
  shoulder 755.59
  spinal cord 742.59
  spine 756.19
  spleen 759.0
  sternum 756.3
  stomach 750.7
  symphysis pubis 755.69
  testis (undescended) 752.51
  thymus (gland) 759.2
  thyroid (gland) (tissue) 759.2
    cartilage 748.3
  toe(s) 755.66
    supernumerary 755.02
  tongue 750.19
  trachea 748.3
  uterus 752.3

Malposition—*continued*
  vein(s) (peripheral) NEC (*see also*
    Malposition, congenital, peripheral
    vascular system) 747.60
    great 747.49
    portal 747.49
    pulmonary 747.49
  vena cava (inferior) (superior) 747.49
  device, implant, or graft—*see* Complications,
    mechanical
  fetus NEC (*see also* Presentation, fetal) 652.9
    with successful version 652.1
    affecting fetus or newborn 763.1
    before labor, affecting fetus or newborn 761.7
    causing obstructed labor 660.0
    in multiple gestation (one fetus or more) 652.6
      with locking 660.5
      causing obstructed labor 660.0
  gallbladder (*see also* Disease, gallbladder) 575.8
  gastrointestinal tract 569.89
    congenital 751.8
  heart (*see also* Malposition, congenital, heart)
    746.87
  intestine 569.89
    congenital 751.5
  pelvic organs or tissues
    in pregnancy or childbirth 654.4
      affecting fetus or newborn 763.89
      causing obstructed labor 660.2
        affecting fetus or newborn 763.1
  placenta—*see* Placenta, previa
  stomach 537.89
    congenital 750.7
  tooth, teeth (with impaction) 524.3
  uterus or cervix (acquired) (acute) (adherent)
    (any degree) (asymptomatic)
    (postinfectional) (postpartal, old) 621.6
    anteflexion or anteversion (*see also*
      Anteversion, uterus) 621.6
    congenital 752.3
    flexion 621.6
      lateral (*see also* Lateroversion, uterus) 621.6
    in pregnancy or childbirth 654.4
      affecting fetus or newborn 763.89
      causing obstructed labor 660.2
        affecting fetus or newborn 763.1
    inversion 621.6
    lateral (flexion) (version) (*see also*
      Lateroversion, uterus) 621.6
    lateroflexion (*see also* Lateroversion, uterus)
      621.6
    lateroversion (*see also* Lateroversion, uterus)
      621.6
    retroflexion or retroversion (*see also*
      Retroversion, uterus) 621.6
Malposture 729.9
Malpresentation, fetus (*see also* Presentation,
  fetal) 652.9
Malrotation
  cecum 751.4
  colon 751.4
  intestine 751.4
  kidney 753.3
Malta fever (*see also* Brucellosis) 023.9
Maltosuria 271.3
Maltreatment (of)
  adult 995.80
    emotional 995.82
    multiple forms 995.85
    neglect (nutritional) 995.84
    physical 995.81

Maltreatment—*continued*
  psychological 995.82
  sexual 995.83
 child 995.50
  emotional 995.51
  multiple forms 995.59
  neglect (nutritional) 995.52
  psychological 995.51
  physical 995.54
   shaken infant syndrome 995.55
  sexual 995.53
 spouse 995.80—*(see also* Maltreatment, adult)
Malt workers' lung 495.4
Malum coxae senilis 715.25
Malunion, fracture 733.81
Mammillitis (*see also* Mastitis) 611.0
 puerperal, postpartum 675.2
Mammitis (*see also* Mastitis) 611.0
 puerperal, postpartum 675.2
Mammographic microcalcification 793.81
Mammoplasia 611.1
Management
 contraceptive V25.9
  specified type NEC V25.8
 procreative V26.9
  specified type NEC V26.8
Mangled NEC (*see also* nature and site of injury)
 959.9
Mania (monopolar) (*see also* Psychosis,
 affective) 296.0
 alcoholic (acute) (chronic) 291.9
 Bell's—*see* Mania, chronic
 chronic 296.0
  recurrent episode 296.1
  single episode 296.0
 compulsive 300.3
 delirious (acute) 296.0
  recurrent episode 296.1
  single episode 296.0
 epileptic (*see also* Epilepsy) 345.4
 hysterical 300.10
 inhibited 296.89
 puerperal (after delivery) 296.0
  recurrent episode 296.1
  single episode 296.0
 recurrent episode 296.1
 senile 290.8
 single episode 296.0
 stupor 296.89
 stuporous 296.89
 unproductive 296.89
**Manic-depressive insanity, psychosis reaction,
 or syndrome** (*see also* Psychosis, affective)
 296.80
 circular (alternating) 296.7
  currently
   depressed 296.5
   episode unspecified 296.7
   hypomanic, previously depressed 296.4
   manic 296.4
  mixed 296.6
 depressed (type), depressive 296.2
  atypical 296.82
  recurrent episode 296.3
  single episode 296.2
 hypomanic 296.0
  recurrent episode 296.1
  single episode 296.0
 manic 296.0
  atypical 296.81
  recurrent episode 296.1

Manic-depressive...—*continued*
 single episode 296.0
 mixed NEC 296.89
 perplexed 296.89
 stuporous 296.89
Manifestations, rheumatoid
 lungs 714.81
 pannus—*see* Arthritis, rheumatoid
 subcutaneous nodules—*see* Arthritis,
  rheumatoid
Mankowsky's syndrome (familial dysplastic
 osteopathy) 731.2
Mannoheptulosuria 271.8
Mannosidosis 271.8
Manson's
 disease (schistosomiasis) 120.1
 pyosis (pemphigus contagiosus) 684
 schistosomiasis 120.1
Mansonellosis 125.5
Manual —*see* condition
Maple bark disease 495.6
Maple bark-strippers' lung 495.6
Maple syrup (urine) disease or syndrome 270.3
Marable's syndrome (celiac artery compression)
 447.4
Marasmus 261
 brain 331.9
 due to malnutrition 261
 intestinal 569.89
 nutritional 261
 senile 797
 tuberculous NEC (*see also* Tuberculosis) 011.9
Marble
 bones 756.52
 skin 782.61
Marburg disease (virus) 078.89
March
 foot 733.94
 hemoglobinuria 283.2
Marchand multiple nodular hyperplasia (liver)
 571.5
Marchesani (-Weill) syndrome
 (brachymorphism and ectopia lentis) 759.89
Marchiafava (-Bignami) disease or syndrome
 341.8
Marchiafava-Micheli syndrome (paroxysmal
 nocturnal hemoglobinuria) 283.2
Marcus Gunn's syndrome (jaw-winking
 syndrome) 742.8
Marfan's
 congenital syphilis 090.49
 disease 090.49
 syndrome (arachnodactyly) 759.82
  meaning congenital syphilis 090.49
  with luxation of lens 090.49 *[379.32]*
Marginal
 implantation, placenta—*see* Placenta, previa
 placenta—*see* Placenta, previa
 sinus (hemorrhage) (rupture) 641.2
  affecting fetus or newborn 762.1
Marie's
 cerebellar ataxia 334.2
 syndrome (acromegaly) 253.0
Marie-Bamberger disease or syndrome
 (hypertrophic) (pulmonary) (secondary) 731.2
 idiopathic (acropachyderma) 757.39
 primary (acropachyderma) 757.39
**Marie-Charcot-Tooth neuropathic atrophy,
 muscle** 356.1
Marie-Strümpell arthritis or disease
 (ankylosing spondylitis) 720.0

Marihuana, marijuana
  abuse (*see also* Abuse, drugs, nondependent)
      305.2
  dependence (*see also* Dependence) 304.3
Marion's disease (bladder neck obstruction)
      596.0
Marital conflict V61.10
Mark
  port wine 757.32
  raspberry 757.32
  strawberry 757.32
  stretch 701.3
  tattoo 709.09
Maroteaux-Lamy syndrome
      (mucopolysaccharidosis VI) 277.5
Marriage license examination V70.3
Marrow (bone)
  arrest 284.9
  megakaryocytic 287.3
  poor function 289.9
Marseilles fever 082.1
Marsh's disease (exophthalmic goiter) 242.0
Marshall's (hidrotic) ectodermal dysplasia 757.31
Marsh fever (*see also* Malaria) 084.6
Martin's disease 715.27
Martin-Albright syndrome
      (pseudohypoparathyroidism) 275.49
Martorell-Fabre syndrome (pulseless disease)
      446.7
**Masculinization, female with adrenal
      hyperplasia** 255.2
Masculinovoblastoma (M8670/0) 220
Masochism 302.83
Masons' lung 502
Mass
  abdominal 789.3
  anus 787.99
  bone 733.90
  breast 611.72
  cheek 784.2
  chest 786.6
  cystic—*see* Cyst
  ear 388.8
  epigastric 789.3
  eye 379.92
  female genital organ 625.8
  gum 784.2
  head 784.2
  intracranial 784.2
  joint 719.60
    ankle 719.67
    elbow 719.62
    foot 719.67
    hand 719.64
    hip 719.65
    knee 719.66
    multiple sites 719.69
    pelvic region 719.65
    shoulder (region) 719.61
    specified site NEC 719.68
    wrist 719.63
  kidney (*see also* Disease, kidney) 593.9
  lung 786.6
  lymph node 785.6
  malignant (M8000/3)—*see* Neoplasm, by site,
      malignant
  mediastinal 786.6
  mouth 784.2
  muscle (limb) 729.89
  neck 784.2
  nose or sinus 784.2

Mass—*continued*
  palate 784.2
  pelvis, pelvic 789.3
  penis 607.89
  perineum 625.8
  rectum 787.99
  scrotum 608.89
  skin 782.2
  specified organ NEC—*see* Disease of specified
      organ or site
  splenic 789.2
  substernal 786.6
    thyroid (*see also* Goiter) 240.9
  superficial (localized) 782.2
  testes 608.89
  throat 784.2
  tongue 784.2
  umbilicus 789.3
  uterus 625.8
  vagina 625.8
  vulva 625.8
Massive —*see* condition
Mastalgia 611.71
  psychogenic 307.89
Mast cell
  disease 757.33
    systemic (M9741/3) 202.6
  leukemia (M9900/3) 207.8
  sarcoma (M9742/3) 202.6
  tumor (M9740/1) 238.5
    malignant (M9740/3) 202.6
Masters-Allen syndrome 620.6
Mastitis (acute) (adolescent) (diffuse)
      (interstitial) (lobular) (nonpuerperal)
      (nonsuppurative) (parenchymatous)
      (phlegmonous) (simple) (subacute)
      (suppurative) 611.0
  chronic (cystic) (fibrocystic) 610.1
  cystic 610.1
    Schimmelbusch's type 610.1
  fibrocystic 610.1
  infective 611.0
  lactational 675.2
  lymphangitis 611.0
  neonatal (noninfective) 778.7
    infective 771.5
  periductal 610.4
  plasma cell 610.4
  puerperal, postpartum, (interstitial)
      (nonpurulent) (parenchymatous) 675.2
    purulent 675.1
    stagnation 676.2
  puerperalis 675.2
  retromammary 611.0
    puerperal, postpartum 675.1
  submammary 611.0
    puerperal, postpartum 675.1
Mastocytoma (M9740/1) 238.5
  malignant (M9740/3) 202.6
Mastocytosis 757.33
  malignant (M9741/3) 202.6
  systemic (M9741/3) 202.6
Mastodynia 611.71
  psychogenic 307.89
Mastoid —*see* condition
Mastoidalgia (*see also* Otalgia) 388.70
Mastoiditis (coalescent) (hemorrhagic)
      (pneumococcal) (streptococcal) (suppurative)
      383.9
  acute or subacute 383.00

Measles—*continued*
　liberty 056.9
　otitis media 055.2
　pneumonia 055.1
　specified complications NEC 055.79
　vaccination, prophylactic (against) V04.2
Meatitis, urethral (*see also* Urethritis) 597.89
Meat poisoning —*see* Poisoning, food
Meatus, meatal —*see* condition
Meat-wrappers' asthma 506.9
Meckel's
　diverticulitis 751.0
　diverticulum (displaced) (hypertrophic) 751.0
Meconium
　aspiration 770.1
　delayed passage in newborn 777.1
　ileus 777.1
　　due to cystic fibrosis 277.01
　in liquor 792.3
　　noted during delivery 656.8
　insufflation 770.1
　obstruction
　　fetus or newborn 777.1
　　in mucoviscidosis 277.01
　passage of 792.3
　　noted during delivery—*omit code*
　peritonitis 777.6
　plug syndrome (newborn) NEC 777.1
Median —*see also* condition
　arcuate ligament syndrome 447.4
　bar (prostate) 600.9
　　vesical orifice 600.9
　rhomboid glossitis 529.2
Mediastinal shift 793.2
Mediastinitis (acute) (chronic) 519.2
　actinomycotic 039.8
　syphilitic 095.8
　tuberculous (*see also* Tuberculosis) 012.8
Mediastinopericarditis (*see also* Pericarditis)
　423.9
　acute 420.90
　chronic 423.8
　　rheumatic 393
　rheumatic, chronic 393
Mediastinum, mediastinal —*see* condition
Medical services provided for —*see* Health,
　services provided because (of)
Medicine poisoning (by overdose) (wrong
　substance given or taken in error) 977.9
　specified drug or substance—*see* Table of drugs
　　and chemicals
Medin's disease (poliomyelitis) 045.9
Mediterranean
　anemia (with other hemoglobinopathy) 282.4
　disease or syndrome (hemipathic) 282.4
　fever (*see also* Brucellosis) 023.9
　　familial 277.3
　kala-azar 085.0
　leishmaniasis 085.0
　tick fever 082.1
Medulla —*see* condition
Medullary
　cystic kidney 753.16
　sponge kidney 753.17
Medullated fibers
　optic (nerve) 743.57
　retina 362.85
Medulloblastoma (M9470/3)
　desmoplastic (M9471/3) 191.6
　specified site—*see* Neoplasm, by site, malignant
　unspecified site 191.6

Medulloepithelioma (M9501/3)—*see also*
　Neoplasm, by site, malignant
　teratoid (M9502/3)—*see* Neoplasm, by site,
　　malignant
Medullomyoblastoma (M9472/3)
　specified site—*see* Neoplasm, by site, malignant
　unspecified site 191.6
Meekeren-Ehlers-Danlos syndrome 756.83
Megacaryocytic —*see* condition
Megacolon (acquired) (functional) (not
　Hirschsprung's disease) 564.7
　aganglionic 751.3
　congenital, congenitum 751.3
　Hirschsprung's (disease) 751.3
　psychogenic 306.4
　toxic (*see also* Colitis, ulcerative) 556.9
Megaduodenum 537.3
Megaesophagus (functional) 530.0
　congenital 750.4
Megakaryocytic —*see* condition
Megalencephaly 742.4
Megalerythema (epidermicum) (infectiosum)
　057.0
Megalia, cutis et ossium 757.39
Megaloappendix 751.5
Megalocephalus, megalocephaly NEC 756.0
Megalocornea 743.41
　associated with buphthalmos 743.22
Megalocytic anemia 281.9
Megalodactylia (fingers) (thumbs) 755.57
　toes 755.65
Megaloduodenum 751.5
Megaloesophagus (functional) 530.0
　congenital 750.4
Megalogastria (congenital) 750.7
Megalomania 307.9
Megalophthalmos 743.8
Megalopsia 368.14
Megalosplenia (*see also* Splenomegaly) 789.2
Megaloureter 593.89
　congenital 753.22
Megarectum 569.49
Megasigmoid 564.7
　congenital 751.3
Megaureter 593.89
　congenital 753.22
Megrim 346.9
Meibomian
　cyst 373.2
　　infected 373.12
　gland—*see* condition
　infarct (eyelid) 374.85
　stye 373.11
Meibomitis 373.12
Meige
　-Milroy disease (chronic hereditary edema)
　　757.0
　syndrome (blepharospasm-oromandibular
　　dystonia) 333.82
Melalgia, nutritional 266.2
Melancholia (*see also* Psychosis, affective)
　296.90
　climacteric 296.2
　　recurrent episode 296.3
　　single episode 296.2
　hypochondriac 300.7
　intermittent 296.2
　　recurrent episode 296.3
　　single episode 296.2
　involutional 296.2
　　recurrent episode 296.3

Melancholia—*continued*
  single episode 296.2
  menopausal 296.2
    recurrent episode 296.3
    single episode 296.2
  puerperal 296.2
  reactive (from emotional stress, psychological
      trauma) 298.0
  recurrent 296.3
  senile 290.21
  stuporous 296.2
    recurrent episode 296.3
    single episode 296.2
Melanemia 275.0
Melanoameloblastoma (M9363/0)—*see*
    Neoplasm, bone, benign
Melanoblastoma (M8720/3)—*see* Melanoma
Melanoblastosis
  Block-Sulzberger 757.33
  cutis linearis sive systematisata 757.33
Melanocarcinoma (M8720/3)—*see* Melanoma
Melanocytoma, eyeball (M8726/0) 224.0
Melanoderma, melanodermia 709.09
  Addison's (primary adrenal insufficiency) 255.4
Melanodontia, infantile 521.05
Melanodontoclasia 521.05
Melanoepithelioma (M8720/3)—*see* Melanoma
Melanoma (malignant) (M8720/3) 172.9

> *Note—Except where otherwise indicated, the
> morphological varieties of melanoma in the list
> below should be coded by site as for
> "Melanoma (malignant)." Internal sites should
> be coded to malignant neoplasm of those sites.*

  abdominal wall 172.5
  ala nasi 172.3
  amelanotic (M8730/3)—*see* Melanoma, by site
  ankle 172.7
  anus, anal 154.3
    canal 154.2
  arm 172.6
  auditory canal (external) 172.2
  auricle (ear) 172.2
  auricular canal (external) 172.2
  axilla 172.5
  axillary fold 172.5
  back 172.5
  balloon cell (M8722/3)—*see* Melanoma, by site
  benign (M8720/0)—*see* Neoplasm, skin, benign
  breast (female) (male) 172.5
  brow 172.3
  buttock 172.5
  canthus (eye) 172.1
  cheek (external) 172.3
  chest wall 172.5
  chin 172.3
  choroid 190.6
  conjunctiva 190.3
  ear (external) 172.2
  epithelioid cell (M8771/3)—*see also*
      Melanoma, by site
    and spindle cell, mixed (M8775/3)—*see*
      Melanoma, by site
  external meatus (ear) 172.2
  eye 190.9
  eyebrow 172.3
  eyelid (lower) (upper) 172.1
  face NEC 172.3
  female genital organ (external) NEC 184.4
  finger 172.6
  flank 172.5

Melanoma—*continued*
  foot 172.7
  forearm 172.6
  forehead 172.3
  foreskin 187.1
  gluteal region 172.5
  groin 172.5
  hand 172.6
  heel 172.7
  helix 172.2
  hip 172.7
  in
    giant pigmented nevus (M8761/3)—*see*
        Melanoma, by site
    Hutchinson's melanotic freckle
        (M8742/3)—*see* Melanoma, by site
    junctional nevus (M8740/3)—*see* Melanoma,
        by site
    precancerous melanosis (M8741/3)—*see*
        Melanoma, by site
  interscapular region 172.5
  iris 190.0
  jaw 172.3
  juvenile (M8770/0)—*see* Neoplasm, skin,
      benign
  knee 172.7
  labium
    majus 184.1
    minus 184.2
  lacrimal gland 190.2
  leg 172.7
  lip (lower) (upper) 172.0
  liver 197.7
  lower limb NEC 172.7
  male genital organ (external) NEC 187.9
  meatus, acoustic (external) 172.2
  meibomian gland 172.1
  metastatic
    of or from specified site—*see* Melanoma, by
        site
    site not of skin—*see* Neoplasm, by site,
        malignant, secondary
    to specified site—*see* Neoplasm, by site,
        malignant, secondary
    unspecified site 172.9
  nail 172.9
    finger 172.6
    toe 172.7
  neck 172.4
  nodular (M8721/3)—*see* Melanoma, by site
  nose, external 172.3
  orbit 190.1
  penis 187.4
  perianal skin 172.5
  perineum 172.5
  pinna 172.2
  popliteal (fossa) (space) 172.7
  prepuce 187.1
  pubes 172.5
  pudendum 184.4
  retina 190.5
  scalp 172.4
  scrotum 187.7
  septum nasal (skin) 172.3
  shoulder 172.6
  skin NEC 172.8
  spindle cell (M8772/3)—*see also* Melanoma, by
      site
    type A (M8773/3) 190.0
    type B (M8774/3) 190.0
  submammary fold 172.5

Melanoma—*continued*
  superficial spreading (M8743/3)—*see*
    Melanoma, by site
  temple 172.3
  thigh 172.7
  toe 172.7
  trunk NEC 172.5
  umbilicus 172.5
  upper limb NEC 172.6
  vagina vault 184.0
  vulva 184.4
Melanoplakia 528.9
Melanosarcoma (M8720/3)—*see also* Melanoma
  epithelioid cell (M8771/3)—*see* Melanoma
Melanosis 709.09
  addisonian (primary adrenal insufficiency) 255.4
    tuberculous (*see also* Tuberculosis) 017.6
  adrenal 255.4
  colon 569.89
  conjunctiva 372.55
    congenital 743.49
  corii degenerativa 757.33
  cornea (presenile) (senile) 371.12
    congenital 743.43
      interfering with vision 743.42
    prenatal 743.43
      interfering with vision 743.42
  eye 372.55
    congenital 743.49
  jute spinners' 709.09
  lenticularis progressiva 757.33
  liver 573.8
  precancerous (M8741/2)—*see also* Neoplasm,
    skin, in situ
    malignant melanoma in (M8741/3)—*see*
      Melanoma
  Riehl's 709.09
  sclera 379.19
    congenital 743.47
  suprarenal 255.4
  tar 709.09
  toxic 709.09
Melanuria 791.9
MELAS 758.89
Melasma 709.09
  adrenal (gland) 255.4
  suprarenal (gland) 255.4
Melena 578.1
  due to
    swallowed maternal blood 777.3
    ulcer—*see* Ulcer, by site, with hemorrhage
  newborn 772.4
    due to swallowed maternal blood 777.3
Meleney's
  gangrene (cutaneous) 686.09
  ulcer (chronic undermining) 686.09
Melioidosis 025
Melitensis, febris 023.0
Melitococcosis 023.0
Melkersson (-Rosenthal) syndrome 351.8
Mellitus, diabetes —*see* Diabetes
Melorheostosis (bone) (leri) 733.99
Meloschisis 744.83
Melotia 744.29
Membrana
  capsularis lentis posterior 743.39
  epipapillaris 743.57
Membranacea placenta —*see* Placenta,
  abnormal
Membranaceous uterus 621.8

Membrane, membranous —*see also* condition
  folds, congenital—*see* Web
  Jackson's 751.4
  over face (causing asphyxia), fetus or newborn
    768.9
  premature rupture—*see* Rupture, membranes,
    premature
  pupillary 364.74
    persistent 743.46
  retained (complicating delivery) (with
    hemorrhage) 666.2
    without hemorrhage 667.1
  secondary (eye) 366.50
  unruptured (causing asphyxia) 768.9
  vitreous humor 379.25
Membranitis, fetal 658.4
  affecting fetus or newborn 762.7
Memory disturbance, loss or lack (*see also*
  Amnesia) 780.99
  mild, following organic brain damage 310.1
Menadione (vitamin K) deficiency 269.0
Menarche, precocious 259.1
Mendacity, pathologic 301.7
Mende's syndrome (ptosis-epicanthus) 270.2
Mendelson's syndrome (resulting from a
  procedure) 997.3
  obstetric 668.0
Ménétrier's disease or syndrome (hypertrophic
  gastritis) 535.2
Ménière's disease, syndrome, or vertigo 386.00
  cochlear 386.02
  cochleovestibular 386.01
  inactive 386.04
  in remission 386.04
  vestibular 386.03
Meninges, meningeal —*see* condition
Meningioma (M9530/0)—*see also* Neoplasm,
  meninges, benign
  angioblastic (M9535/0)—*see* Neoplasm,
    meninges, benign
  angiomatous (M9534/0)—*see* Neoplasm,
    meninges, benign
  endotheliomatous (M9531/0)—*see* Neoplasm,
    meninges, benign
  fibroblastic (M9532/0)—*see* Neoplasm,
    meninges, benign
  fibrous (M9532/0)—*see* Neoplasm, meninges,
    benign
  hemangioblastic (M9535/0)—*see* Neoplasm,
    meninges, benign
  hemangiopericytic (M9536/0)—*see* Neoplasm,
    meninges, benign
  malignant (M9530/3)—*see* Neoplasm,
    meninges, malignant
  meningiothelial (M9531/0)—*see* Neoplasm,
    meninges, benign
  meningotheliomatous (M9531/0)—*see*
    Neoplasm, meninges, benign
  mixed (M9537/0)—*see* Neoplasm, meninges,
    benign
  multiple (M9530/1) 237.6
  papillary (M9538/1) 237.6
  psammomatous (M9533/0)—*see* Neoplasm,
    meninges, benign
  syncytial (M9531/0)—*see* Neoplasm, meninges,
    benign
  transitional (M9537/0)—*see* Neoplasm,
    meninges, benign
Meningiomatosis (diffuse) (M9530/1) 237.6
Meningism (*see also* Meningismus) 781.6

Meningismus (infectional) (pneumococcal) 781.6
  due to serum or vaccine 997.09 *[321.8]*
  influenzal NEC 487.8
Meningitis (basal) (basic) (basilar) (brain)
    (cerebral) (cervical) (congestive) (diffuse)
    (hemorrhagic) (infantile) (membranous)
    (metastatic) (nonspecific) (pontine)
    (progressive) (simple) (spinal) (subacute)
    (sympathetica) (toxic) 322.9
  abacterial NEC (*see also* Meningitis, aseptic)
    047.9
  actinomycotic 039.8 *[320.7]*
  adenoviral 049.1
  Aerobacter aerogenes 320.82
  anaerobes (cocci) (gram-negative)
    (gram-positive) (mixed) (NEC) 320.81
  arbovirus NEC 066.9 *[321.2]*
    specified type NEC 066.8 *[321.2]*
  aseptic (acute) NEC 047.9
    adenovirus 049.1
    Coxsackie virus 047.0
    due to
      adenovirus 049.1
      Coxsackie virus 047.0
      ECHO virus 047.1
      enterovirus 047.9
      mumps 072.1
      poliovirus (*see also* Poliomyelitis) 045.2
        [321.2]
    ECHO virus 047.1
    herpes (simplex) virus 054.72
      zoster 053.0
    leptospiral 100.81
    lymphocytic choriomeningitis 049.0
    noninfective 322.0
  Bacillus pyocyaneus 320.89
  bacterial NEC 320.9
    anaerobic 320.81
    gram-negative 320.82
      anaerobic 320.81
  Bacteroides (fragilis) (oralis) (melaninogenicus)
    320.81
  cancerous (M8000/6) 198.4
  candidal 112.83
  carcinomatous (M8010/6) 198.4
  caseous (*see also* Tuberculosis, meninges) 013.0
  cerebrospinal (acute) (chronic) (diplococcal)
    (endemic) (epidemic) (fulminant)
    (infectious) (malignant) (meningococcal)
    (sporadic) 036.0
    carrier (suspected) of V02.59
  chronic NEC 322.2
  clear cerebrospinal fluid NEC 322.0
  Clostridium (haemolyticum) (novyi) NEC
    320.81
  coccidioidomycosis 114.2
  Coxsackie virus 047.0
  cryptococcal 117.5 *[321.0]*
  diplococcal 036.0
    gram-negative 036.0
    gram-positive 320.1
  Diplococcus pneumoniae 320.1
  due to
    actinomycosis 039.8 *[320.7]*
    adenovirus 049.1
    coccidiomycosis 114.2
    enterovirus 047.9
      specified NEC 047.8
    histoplasmosis (*see also* Histoplasmosis)
      115.91
    Listerosis 027.0 *[320.7]*

Meningitis—*continued*
  Lyme disease 088.81 *[320.7]*
  moniliasis 112.83
  mumps 072.1
  neurosyphilis 094.2
  nonbacterial organisms NEC 321.8
  oidiomycosis 112.83
  poliovirus (*see also* Poliomyelitis) 045.2
    [321.2]
  preventive immunization, inoculation, or
    vaccination 997.09 *[321.8]*
  sarcoidosis 135 *[321.4]*
  sporotrichosis 117.1 *[321.1]*
  syphilis 094.2
    acute 091.81
    congenital 090.42
    secondary 091.81
  trypanosomiasis (*see also* Trypanosomiasis)
    086.9 *[321.3]*
  whooping cough 033.9 *[320.7]*
  E. coli 320.82
  ECHO virus 047.1
  endothelial-leukocytic, benign, recurrent 047.9
  Enterobacter aerogenes 320.82
  enteroviral 047.9
    specified type NEC 047.8
  enterovirus 047.9
    specified NEC 047.8
  eosinophilic 322.1
  epidemic NEC 036.0
  Escherichia coli (E. coli) 320.82
  Eubacterium 320.81
  fibrinopurulent NEC 320.9
    specified type NEC 320.89
  Friedländer (bacillus) 320.82
  fungal NEC 117.9 *[321.1]*
  Fusobacterium 320.81
  gonococcal 098.82
  gram-negative bacteria NEC 320.82
    anaerobic 320.81
    cocci 036.0
      specified NEC 320.82
  gram-negative cocci NEC 036.0
    specified NEC 320.82
  gram-positive cocci NEC 320.9
  H. influenzae 320.0
  herpes (simplex) virus 054.72
    zoster 053.0
  infectious NEC 320.9
  influenzal 320.0
  Klebsiella pneumoniae 320.82
  late effect—*see* Late, effect, meningitis
  leptospiral (aseptic) 100.81
  Listerella (monocytogenes) 027.0 *[320.7]*
  Listeria monocytogenes 027.0 *[320.7]*
  lymphocytic (acute) (benign) (serous) 049.0
    choriomeningitis virus 049.0
  meningococcal (chronic) 036.0
  Mima polymorpha 320.82
  Mollaret's 047.9
  monilial 112.83
  mumps (virus) 072.1
  mycotic NEC 117.9 *[321.1]*
  Neisseria 036.0
  neurosyphilis 094.2
  nonbacterial NEC (*see also* Meningitis, aseptic)
    047.9
  nonpyogenic NEC 322.0
  oidiomycosis 112.83
  ossificans 349.2
  Peptococcus 320.81

Meningitis—*continued*
  Peptostreptococcus 320.81
  pneumococcal 320.1
  poliovirus (*see also* Poliomyelitis) 045.2 *[321.2]*
  Proprionibacterium 320.81
  Proteus morganii 320.82
  Pseudomonas (aeruginosa) (pyocyaneus) 320.82
  purulent NEC 320.9
    specified organism NEC 320.89
  pyogenic NEC 320.9
    specified organism NEC 320.89
  Salmonella 003.21
  septic NEC 320.9
    specified organism NEC 320.89
  serosa circumscripta NEC 322.0
  serous NEC (*see also* Meningitis, aseptic) 047.9
    lymphocytic 049.0—
    syndrome 348.2
  Serratia (marcescens) 320.82
  specified organism NEC 320.89
  sporadic cerebrospinal 036.0
  sporotrichosis 117.1 *[321.1]*
  staphylococcal 320.3
  sterile 997.09
  streptococcal (acute) 320.2
  suppurative 320.9
    specified organism NEC 320.89
  syphilitic 094.2
    acute 091.81
    congenital 090.42
    secondary 091.81
  torula 117.5 *[321.0]*
  traumatic (complication of injury) 958.8
  Treponema (denticola) (macrodenticum) 320.81
  trypanosomiasis 086.1 *[321.3]*
  tuberculous (*see also* Tuberculosis, meninges)
    013.0
  typhoid 002.0 *[320.7]*
  Veillonella 320.81
  Vibrio vulnificus 320.82
  viral, virus NEC (*see also* Meningitis, aseptic)
    047.9
  Wallgren's (*see also* Meningitis, aseptic) 047.9
Meningocele (congenital) (spinal) (*see also*
    Spina bifida) 741.9
  acquired (traumatic) 349.2
  cerebral 742.0
  cranial 742.0
Meningocerebritis —*see* Meningoencephalitis
Meningococcemia (acute) (chronic) 036.2
Meningococcus, meningococcal (*see also*
    condition) 036.9
  adrenalitis, hemorrhagic 036.3
  carditis 036.40
  carrier (suspected) of V02.59
  cerebrospinal fever 036.0
  encephalitis 036.1
  endocarditis 036.42
  infection NEC 036.9
  meningitis (cerebrospinal) 036.0
  myocarditis 036.43
  optic neuritis 036.81
  pericarditis 036.41
  septicemia (chronic) 036.2
Meningoencephalitis (*see also* Encephalitis)
    323.9
  acute NEC 048
  bacterial, purulent, pyogenic, or septic—*see*
    Meningitis
  chronic NEC 094.1
  diffuse NEC 094.1

Meningoencephalitis—*continued*
  diphasic 063.2
  due to
    actinomycosis 039.8 *[320.7]*
    blastomycosis NEC (*see also* Blastomycosis)
      116.0 *[323.4]*
    free-living amebae 136.2
    Listeria monocytogenes 027.0 *[320.7]*
    Lyme disease 088.81 *[320.7]*
    mumps 072.2
    Naegleria (amebae) (gruberi) (organisms)
      136.2
    rubella 056.01
    sporotrichosis 117.1 *[321.1]*
    toxoplasmosis (acquired) 130.0
      congenital (active) 771.2 *[323.4]*
    Trypanosoma 086.1 *[323.2]*
  epidemic 036.0
  herpes 054.3
  herpetic 054.3
  H. influenzae 320.0
  infectious (acute) 048
  influenzal 320.0
  late effect—*see* category 326
  Listeria monocytogenes 027.0 *[320.7]*
  lymphocytic (serous) 049.0
  mumps 072.2
  parasitic NEC 123.9 *[323.4]*
  pneumococcal 320.1
  primary amebic 136.2
  rubella 056.01
  serous 048
    lymphocytic 049.0
  specific 094.2
  staphylococcal 320.3
  streptococcal 320.2
  syphilitic 094.2
  toxic NEC 989.9 *[323.7]*
    due to
      carbon tetrachloride 987.8 *[323.7]*
      hydroxyquinoline derivatives poisoning
        961.3 *[323.7]*
      lead 984.9 *[323.7]*
      mercury 985.0 *[323.7]*
      thallium 985.8 *[323.7]*
  toxoplasmosis (acquired) 130.0
  trypanosomic 086.1 *[323.2]*
  tuberculous (*see also* Tuberculosis, meninges)
    013.0
  virus NEC 048
Meningoencephalocele 742.0
  syphilitic 094.89
    congenital 090.49
Meningoencephalomyelitis (*see also*
    Meningoencephalitis) 323.9
  acute NEC 048
    disseminated (postinfectious) 136.9 *[323.6]*
      postimmunization or postvaccination 323.5
  due to
    actinomycosis 039.8 *[320.7]*
    torula 117.5 *[323.4]*
    toxoplasma or toxoplasmosis (acquired) 130.0
      congenital (active) 771.2 *[323.4]*
  late effect—*see* category 326
Meningoencephalomyelopathy (*see also*
    Meningoencephalomyelitis) 349.9
Meningoencephalopathy (*see also*
    Meningoencephalitis) 348.3
Meningoencephalopoliomyelitis (*see also*
    Poliomyelitis, bulbar) 045.0
  late effect 138

Meningomyelitis (*see also* Meningoencephalitis) 323.9
  blastomycotic NEC (*see also* Blastomycosis) 116.0 *[323.4]*
  due to
    actinomycosis 039.8 *[320.7]*
    blastomycosis (*see also* Blastomycosis) 116.0 *[323.4]*
    Meningococcus 036.0
    sporotrichosis 117.1 *[323.4]*
    torula 117.5 *[323.4]*
  late effect—*see* category 326
  lethargic 049.8
  meningococcal 036.0
  syphilitic 094.2
  tuberculous (*see also* Tuberculosis, meninges) 013.0
Meningomyelocele (*see also* Spina bifida) 741.9
  syphilitic 094.89
Meningomyeloneuritis —*see* Meningoencephalitis
Meningoradiculitis —*see* Meningitis
Meningovascular —*see* condition
Meniscocytosis 282.60
Menkes' syndrome —*see* Syndrome, Menkes'
Menolipsis 626.0
Menometrorrhagia 626.2
Menopause, menopausal (symptoms) (syndrome) 627.2
  arthritis (any site) NEC 716.3
  artificial 627.4
  bleeding 627.0
  crisis 627.2
  depression (*see also* Psychosis, affective) 296.2
    agitated 296.2
      recurrent episode 296.3
      single episode 296.2
    psychotic 296.2
      recurrent episode 296.3
      single episode 296.2
    recurrent episode 296.3
    single episode 296.2
    melancholia (*see also* Psychosis, affective) 296.2
      recurrent episode 296.3
      single episode 296.2
  paranoid state 297.2
  paraphrenia 297.2
  postsurgical 627.4
  premature 256.31
    postirradiation 256.2
    postsurgical 256.2
  psychoneurosis 627.2
  psychosis NEC 298.8
  surgical 627.4
  toxic polyarthritis NEC 716.39
Menorrhagia (primary) 626.2
  climacteric 627.0
  menopausal 627.0
  postclimacteric 627.1
  postmenopausal 627.1
  preclimacteric 627.0
  premenopausal 627.0
  puberty (menses retained) 626.3
Menorrhalgia 625.3
Menoschesis 626.8
Menostaxis 626.2
Menses, retention 626.8
Menstrual —*see* Menstruation
  cycle, irregular 626.4
  disorders NEC 626.9

Menstrual—*continued*
  extraction V25.3
  fluid, retained 626.8
  molimen 625.4
  period, normal V65.5
  regulation V25.3
Menstruation
  absent 626.0
  anovulatory 628.0
  delayed 626.8
  difficult 625.3
  disorder 626.9
    psychogenic 306.52
    specified NEC 626.8
  during pregnancy 640.8
  excessive 626.2
  frequent 626.2
  infrequent 626.1
  irregular 626.4
  latent 626.8
  membranous 626.8
  painful (primary) (secondary) 625.3
    psychogenic 306.52
  passage of clots 626.2
  precocious 626.8
  protracted 626.8
  retained 626.8
  retrograde 626.8
  scanty 626.1
  suppression 626.8
  vicarious (nasal) 625.8
Mentagra (*see also* Sycosis) 704.8
Mental —*see also* condition
  deficiency (*see also* Retardation, mental) 319
  deterioration (*see also* Psychosis) 298.9
  disorder (*see also* Disorder, mental) 300.9
  exhaustion 300.5
  insufficiency (congenital) (*see also* Retardation, mental) 319
  observation without need for further medical care NEC V71.09
  retardation (*see also* Retardation, mental) 319
  subnormality (*see also* Retardation, mental) 319
    mild 317
    moderate 318.0
    profound 318.2
    severe 318.1
  upset (*see also* Disorder, mental) 300.9
Meralgia paresthetica 355.1
Mercurial —*see* condition
Mercurialism NEC 985.0
Merergasia 300.9
MERFF 758.89
Merkel cell tumor —*see* Neoplasm, by site, malignant
Merocele (*see also* Hernia, femoral) 553.00
Meromelia 755.4
  lower limb 755.30
    intercalary 755.32
      femur 755.34
        tibiofibular (complete) (incomplete) 755.33
      fibula 755.37
      metatarsal(s) 755.38
      tarsal(s) 755.38
      tibia 755.36
      tibiofibular 755.35
    terminal (complete) (partial) (transverse) 755.31
      longitudinal 755.32
        metatarsal(s) 755.38
        phalange(s) 755.39

Meromelia—*continued*
  tarsal(s) 755.38
  transverse 755.31
  upper limb 755.20
    intercalary 755.22
      carpal(s) 755.28
      humeral 755.24
        radioulnar (complete) (incomplete) 755.23
      metacarpal(s) 755.28
      phalange(s) 755.29
      radial 755.26
      radioulnar 755.25
      ulnar 755.27
    terminal (complete) (partial) (transverse)
      755.21
      longitudinal 755.22
        carpal(s) 755.28
        metacarpal(s) 755.28
        phalange(s) 755.29
    transverse 755.21
Merosmia 781.1
Merycism (*see also* Rumination)—*see also*
  Vomiting
  psychogenic 307.53
Merzbacher-Pelizaeus disease 330.0
Mesaortitis —*see* Aortitis
Mesarteritis —*see* Arteritis
Mesencephalitis (*see also* Encephalitis) 323.9
  late effect—*see* category 326
Mesenchymoma (M8990/1)—*see also*
  Neoplasm, connective tissue, uncertain
  behavior
  benign (M8990/0)—*see* Neoplasm, connective
    tissue, benign
  malignant (M8990/3)—*see* Neoplasm,
    connective tissue, malignant
Mesentery, mesenteric —*see* condition
Mesiodens, mesiodentes 520.1
  causing crowding 524.3
Mesio-occlusion 524.2
Mesocardia (with asplenia) 746.87
Mesocolon —*see* condition
Mesonephroma (malignant) (M9110/3)—*see*
  also Neoplasm, by site, malignant
  benign (M9110/0)—*see* Neoplasm, by site,
    benign
Mesophlebitis —*see* Phlebitis
Mesostromal dysgenesis 743.51
Mesothelioma (malignant) (M9050/3)—*see also*
  Neoplasm, by site, malignant
  benign (M9050/0)—*see* Neoplasm, by site,
    benign
  biphasic type (M9053/3)—*see also* Neoplasm,
    by site, malignant
  benign (M9053/0)—*see* Neoplasm, by site,
    benign
  epithelioid (M9052/3)—*see also* Neoplasm, by
    site, malignant
  benign (M9052/0)—*see* Neoplasm, by site,
    benign
  fibrous (M9051/3)—*see also* Neoplasm, by site,
    malignant
  benign (M9051/0)—*see* Neoplasm, by site,
    benign
Metabolism disorder 277.9
  specified type NEC 277.8
Metagonimiasis 121.5
Metagonimus infestation (small intestine) 121.5
Metal
  pigmentation (skin) 709.00
  polishers' disease 502
Metalliferous miners' lung 503

Metamorphopsia 368.14
Metaplasia
  bone, in skin 709.3
  breast 611.8
  cervix—*omit code*
  endometrium (squamous) 621.8
  intestinal, of gastric mucosa 537.89
  kidney (pelvis) (squamous) (*see also* Disease,
    renal) 593.89
  myelogenous 289.8
  myeloid (agnogenic) (megakaryocytic) 289.8
  spleen 289.59
  squamous cell
    amnion 658.8
    bladder 596.8
    cervix—*see* condition
    trachea 519.1
    tracheobronchial tree 519.1
    uterus 621.8
    cervix—*see* condition
Metastasis, metastatic
  abscess—*see* Abscess
  calcification 275.40
  cancer, neoplasm, or disease
    from specified site (M8000/3)—*see*
      Neoplasm, by site, malignant
    to specified site (M8000/6)—*see* Neoplasm,
      by site, secondary
  deposits (in) (M8000/6)—*see* Neoplasm, by
    site, secondary
  pneumonia 038.8 *[484.8]*
  spread (to) (M8000/6)—*see* Neoplasm, by site,
    secondary
Metatarsalgia 726.70
  anterior 355.6
  due to Freiberg's disease 732.5
  Morton's 355.6
Metatarsus, metatarsal —*see also* condition
  abductus valgus (congenital) 764.60
  abductus varus (congenital) 754.53
  adductus valgus (congenital) 754.60
  adductus varus (congenital) 754.53
  primus varus 754.52
  valgus (adductus) (congenital) 754.60
  varus (abductus) (congenital) 754.53
    primus 754.52
Methemoglobinemia 289.7
  acquired (with sulfhemoglobinemia) 289.7
  congenital 289.7
  enzymatic 289.7
  Hb-M disease 289.7
  hereditary 289.7
  toxic 289.7
Methemoglobinuria (*see also* Hemoglobinuria)
  791.2
Methioninemia 270.4
Metritis (catarrhal) (septic) (suppurative) (*see*
  also Endometritis) 615.9
  blennorrhagic 098.16
    chronic or duration of 2 months or over 098.36
  cervical (*see also* Cervicitis) 616.0
  gonococcal 098.16
    chronic or duration of 2 months or over 098.36
  hemorrhagic 626.8
  puerperal, postpartum, childbirth 670
  tuberculous (*see also* Tuberculosis) 016.7
Metropathia hemorrhagica 626.8
Metroperitonitis (*see also* Peritonitis, pelvic,
  female) 614.5

Metrorrhagia 626.6
　arising during pregnancy—*see* Hemorrhage,
　　pregnancy
　postpartum NEC 666.2
　primary 626.6
　psychogenic 306.59
　puerperal 666.2
Metrorrhexis —*see* Rupture, uterus
Metrosalpingitis (*see also* Salpingo-oophoritis)
　614.2
Metrostaxis 626.6
Metrovaginitis (*see also* Endometritis) 615.9
　gonococcal (acute) 098.16
　　chronic or duration of 2 months or over 098.36
Mexican fever —*see* Typhus, Mexican
Meyenburg-Altherr-Uehlinger syndrome
　733.99
Meyer-Schwickerath and Weyers syndrome
　(dysplasia oculodentodigitalis) 759.89
Meynert's amentia (nonalcoholic) 294.0
　alcoholic 291.1
Mibelli's disease 757.39
Mice, joint (*see also* Loose, body, joint) 718.1
　knee 717.6
Micheli-Rietti syndrome (thalassemia minor)
　282.4
Michotte's syndrome 721.5
Micrencephalon, micrencephaly 742.1
Microaneurysm, retina 362.14
　diabetic 250.5 *[362.01]*
Microangiopathy 443.9
　diabetic (peripheral) 250.7 *[443.81]*
　　retinal 250.5 *[362.01]*
　peripheral 443.9
　　diabetic 250.7 *[443.81]*
　retinal 362.18
　　diabetic 250.5 *[362.01]*
　thrombotic 446.6
　　Moschcowitz's (thrombotic thrombocytopenic
　　　purpura) 446.6
Microcalcification, mammographic 793.81
Microcephalus, microcephalic, microcephaly
　742.1
　due to toxoplasmosis (congenital) 771.2
Microcheilia 744.82
Microcolon (congenital) 751.5
Microcornea (congenital) 743.41
Microcytic —*see* condition
Microdontia 520.2
Microdrepanocytosis (thalassemia-Hb-S
　disease) 282.4
Microembolism
　atherothrombotic —*see* Atheroembolism
　retina 362.33
Microencephalon 742.1
Microfilaria streptocerca infestation 125.3
Microgastria (congenital) 750.7
Microgenia 524.06
Microgenitalia (congenital) 752.8
　penis 752.64
Microglioma (M9710/3)
　specified site—*see* Neoplasm, by site, malignant
　unspecified site 191.9
Microglossia (congenital) 750.16
Micrognathia, micrognathism (congenital)
　524.00
　mandibular 524.04
　　alveolar 524.74
　maxillary 524.03
　　alveolar 524.73
Microgyria (congenital) 742.2

Microinfarct, heart (*see also* Insufficiency,
　coronary) 411.89
Microlithiasis, alveolar, pulmonary 516.2
Micromyelia (congenital) 742.59
Micropenis 752.64
Microphakia (congenital) 743.36
Microphthalmia (congenital) (*see also*
　Microphthalmos) 743.10
Microphthalmos (congenital) 743.10
　associated with eye and adnexal anomalies NEC
　　743.12
　due to toxoplasmosis (congenital) 771.2
　isolated 743.11
　simple 743.11
　syndrome 759.89
Micropsia 368.14
Microsporidiosis 136.8
Microsporon furfur infestation 111.0
Microsporosis (*see also* Dermatophytosis) 110.9
　nigra 111.1
Microstomia (congenital) 744.84
Microthelia 757.6
Microthromboembolism —*see* Embolism
Microtia (congenital) (external ear) 744.23
Microtropia 378.34
Micturition
　disorder NEC 788.69
　　psychogenic 306.53
　frequency 788.41
　　psychogenic 306.53
　nocturnal 788.43
　painful 788.1
　　psychogenic 306.53
Middle
　ear—*see* condition
　lobe (right) syndrome 518.0
Midplane —*see* condition
Miescher's disease 709.3
　cheilitis 351.8
　granulomatosis disciformis 709.3
Miescher-Leder syndrome or granulomatosis
　709.3
Mieten's syndrome 759.89
Migraine (idiopathic) 346.9
　with aura 346.0
　abdominal (syndrome) 346.2
　allergic (histamine) 346.2
　atypical 346.1
　basilar 346.2
　classical 346.0
　common 346.1
　hemiplegic 346.8
　lower-half 346.2
　menstrual 625.4
　ophthalmic 346.8
　ophthalmoplegic 346.8
　retinal 346.2
　variant 346.2
Migrant, social V60.0
Migratory, migrating —*see also* condition
　person V60.0
　testis, congenital 752.52
Mikulicz's disease or syndrome (dryness of
　mouth, absent or decreased lacrimation) 527.1
Milian atrophia blanche 701.3
Miliaria (crystallina) (rubra) (tropicalis) 705.1
　apocrine 705.82
Miliary —*see* condition
Milium (*see also* Cyst, sebaceous) 706.2
　colloid 709.3
　eyelid 374.84

Milk
  crust 690.11
  excess secretion 676.6
  fever, female 672
  poisoning 988.8
  retention 676.2
  sickness 988.8
  spots 423.1
Milkers' nodes 051.1
Milk-leg (deep vessels) 671.4
  complicating pregnancy 671.3
  nonpuerperal 451.19
  puerperal, postpartum, childbirth 671.4
Milkman (-Looser) disease or syndrome
    (osteomalacia with pseudofractures) 268.2
Milky urine (see also Chyluria) 791.1
Millar's asthma (laryngismus stridulus) 478.75
Millard-Gubler paralysis or syndrome 344.89
Millard-Gubler-Foville paralysis 344.89
Miller's disease (osteomalacia) 268.2
Miller Fisher's syndrome 357.0
Milles' syndrome (encephalocutaneous
    angiomatosis) 759.6
Mills' disease 335.29
Millstone makers' asthma or lung 502
Milroy's disease (chronic hereditary edema)
    757.0
Miners' —see also condition
  asthma 500
  elbow 727.2
  knee 727.2
  lung 500
  nystagmus 300.89
  phthisis (see also Tuberculosis) 011.4
  tuberculosis (see also Tuberculosis) 011.4
Minkowski-Chauffard syndrome (see also
    Spherocytosis) 282.0
Minor —see condition
Minor's disease 336.1
Minot's disease (hemorrhagic disease, newborn)
    776.0
Minot-von Willebrand (-Jürgens) disease or
    syndrome (angiohemophilia) 286.4
Minus (and plus) hand (intrinsic) 736.09
Miosis (persistent) (pupil) 379.42
Mirizzi's syndrome (hepatic duct stenosis) (see
    also Obstruction, biliary) 576.2
  with calculus, cholelithiasis, or stones—see
      Choledocholithiasis
Mirror writing 315.09
  secondary to organic lesion 784.69
Misadventure (prophylactic) (therapeutic) (see
    also Complications) 999.9
  administration of insulin 962.3
  infusion—see Complications, infusion
  local applications (of fomentations, plasters,
      etc.) 999.9
  burn or scald—see Burn, by site
  medical care (early) (late) NEC 999.9
    adverse effect of drugs or chemicals—see
        Table of drugs and chemicals
    burn or scald—see Burn, by site
  radiation NEC 990
  radiotherapy NEC 990
  surgical procedure (early) (late)—see
      Complications, surgical procedure
  transfusion—see Complications, transfusion
  vaccination or other immunological
      procedure—see Complications, vaccination
Misanthropy 301.7
Miscarriage —see Abortion, spontaneous

Mischief, malicious, child (see also Disturbance,
    conduct) 312.0
Misdirection , aqueous 365.83
Mismanagement, feeding 783.3
Misplaced, misplacement
  kidney (see also Disease, renal) 593.0
    congenital 753.3
  organ or site, congenital NEC—see
      Malposition, congenital
Missed
  abortion 632
  delivery (at or near term) 656.4
  labor (at or near term) 656.4
Missing —see also Absence
  teeth (acquired) 525.10
    congenital (see also Anodontia) 520.0
    due to
      caries 525.13
      extraction 525.10
      periodontal disease 525.12
      specified NEC 525.19
      trauma 525.11
  vertebrae (congenital) 756.13
Misuse of drugs NEC (see also Abuse, drug,
    nondependent) 305.9
Mitchell's disease (erythromelalgia) 443.89
Mite (s)
  diarrhea 133.8
  grain (itch) 133.8
  hair follicle (itch) 133.8
  in sputum 133.8
Mitral —see condition
Mittelschmerz 625.2
Mixed —see condition
Mljet disease (mal de Meleda) 757.39
Mobile, mobility
  cecum 751.4
  coccyx 733.99
  excessive—see Hypermobility
  gallbladder 751.69
  kidney 593.0
    congenital 753.3
  organ or site, congenital NEC—see
      Malposition, congenital
  spleen 289.59
Mobitz heart block (atrioventricular) 426.10
  type I (Wenckebach's) 426.13
  type II 426.12
Möbius'
  disease 346.8
  syndrome
    congenital oculofacial paralysis 352.6
    ophthalmoplegic migraine 346.8
Moeller (-Barlow) disease (infantile scurvy) 267
  glossitis 529.4
Mohr's syndrome (Types I and II) 759.89
Mola destruens (M9100/1) 236.1
Molarization, premolars 520.2
Molar pregnancy 631
  hydatidiform (delivered) (undelivered) 630
Mold (s) in vitreous 117.9
Molding, head (during birth) 767.3
Mole (pigmented) (M8720/0)—see also
    Neoplasm, skin, benign
  blood 631
  Breus' 631
  cancerous (M8720/3)—see Melanoma
  carneous 631
  destructive (M9100/1) 236.1
  ectopic—see Pregnancy, ectopic
  fleshy 631

Mole—*continued*
hemorrhagic 631
hydatid, hydatidiform (benign) (complicating pregnancy) (delivered) (undelivered) (*see also* Hydatidiform mole) 630
  invasive (M9100/1) 236.1
  malignant (M9100/1) 236.1
  previous, affecting management of pregnancy V23.1
invasive (hydatidiform) (M9100/1) 236.1
malignant
  meaning
    malignant hydatidiform mole (M9100/1) 236.1
    melanoma (M8720/3)—*see* Melanoma
nonpigmented (M8730/0)—*see* Neoplasm, skin, benign
pregnancy NEC 631
skin (M8720/0)—*see* Neoplasm, skin, benign
tubal—*see* Pregnancy, tubal
vesicular (*see also* Hydatidiform mole) 630
Molimen, molimina (menstrual) 625.4
Mollaret's meningitis 047.9
Mollities (cerebellar) (cerebral) 437.8
ossium 268.2
Molluscum
contagiosum 078.0
epitheliale 078.0
fibrosum (M8851/0)—*see* Lipoma, by site
pendulum (M8851/0)—*see* Lipoma, by site
Mönckeberg's arteriosclerosis, degeneration disease, or sclerosis (*see also* Arteriosclerosis, extremities) 440.20
Monday fever 504
Monday morning dyspnea or asthma 504
Mondini's malformation (cochlea) 744.05
Mondor's disease (thrombophlebitis of breast) 451.89
Mongolian, mongolianism, mongolism mongoloid 758.0
spot 757.33
Monilethrix (congenital) 757.4
Monilia infestation —*see* Candidiasis
Moniliasis —*see also* Candidiasis
neonatal 771.7
vulvovaginitis 112.1
Monoarthritis 716.60
ankle 716.67
arm 716.62
  lower (and wrist) 716.63
  upper (and elbow) 716.62
foot (and ankle) 716.67
forearm (and wrist) 716.63
hand 716.64
leg 716.66
  lower 716.66
  upper 716.65
pelvic region (hip) (thigh) 716.65
shoulder (region) 716.61
specified site NEC 716.68
Monoblastic —*see* condition
Monochromatism (cone) (rod) 368.54
Monocytic —*see* condition
Monocytosis (symptomatic) 288.8
Monofixation syndrome 378.34
Monomania (*see also* Psychosis) 298.9
Mononeuritis 355.9
cranial nerve—*see* Disorder, nerve, cranial
femoral nerve 355.2
lateral
  cutaneous nerve of thigh 355.1

Mononeuritis—*continued*
popliteal nerve 355.3
lower limb 355.8
  specified nerve NEC 355.79
medial popliteal nerve 355.4
median nerve 354.1
multiplex 354.5
plantar nerve 355.6
posterior tibial nerve 355.5
radial nerve 354.3
sciatic nerve 355.0
ulnar nerve 354.2
upper limb 354.9
  specified nerve NEC 354.8
vestibular 388.5
Mononeuropathy (*see also* Mononeuritis) 355.9
diabetic NEC 250.6 *[355.9]*
  lower limb 250.6 *[355.8]*
  upper limb 250.6 *[354.9]*
iliohypogastric nerve 355.79
ilioinguinal nerve 355.79
obturator nerve 355.79
saphenous nerve 355.79
Mononucleosis, infectious 075
with hepatitis 075 *[573.1]*
Monoplegia 344.5
brain (current episode) (*see also* Paralysis, brain) 437.8
  fetus or newborn 767.8
cerebral (current episode) (*see also* Paralysis, brain) 437.8
congenital or infantile (cerebral) (spastic) (spinal) 343.3
embolic (current) (*see also* Embolism, brain) 434.1
  late effect—*see* Late effect(s) (of) cerebrovascular disease
infantile (cerebral) (spastic) (spinal) 343.3
lower limb 344.30
  affecting
    dominant side 344.31
    nondominant side 344.32
  due to late effect of cerebrovascular accident —*see* Late effect(s) (of) cerebrovascular accident
newborn 767.8
psychogenic 306.0
  specified as conversion reaction 300.11
thrombotic (current) (*see also* Thrombosis, brain) 434.0
  late effect—*see* Late effect(s) (of) cerebrovascular disease
transient 781.4
upper limb 344.40
  affecting
    dominant side 344.41
    nondominant side 344.42
  due to late effect of cerebrovascular accident —*see* Late effect(s) (of) cerebrovascular accident
Monorchism, monorchidism 752.8
Monteggia's fracture (closed) 813.03
open 813.13
Mood swings
brief compensatory 296.99
rebound 296.99
Moore's syndrome (*see also* Epilepsy) 345.5
Mooren's ulcer (cornea) 370.07
Mooser-Neill reaction 081.0
Mooser bodies 081.0

Moral
  deficiency 301.7
  imbecility 301.7
Morax-Axenfeld conjunctivitis 372.03
Morbilli (*see also* Measles) 055.9
Morbus
  anglicus, anglorum 268.0
  Beigel 111.2
  caducus (*see also* Epilepsy) 345.9
  caeruleus 746.89
  celiacus 579.0
  comitialis (*see also* Epilepsy) 345.9
  cordis—*see also* Disease, heart
    valvulorum—*see* Endocarditis
  coxae 719.95
  tuberculous (*see also* Tuberculosis) 015.1
  hemorrhagicus neonatorum 776.0
  maculosus neonatorum 772.6
  renum 593.0
  senilis (*see also* Osteoarthrosis) 715.9
Morel-Kraepelin disease (*see also* Schizophrenia) 295.9
Morel-Moore syndrome (hyperostosis frontalis interna) 733.3
Morel-Morgagni syndrome (hyperostosis frontalis interna) 733.3
Morgagni
  cyst, organ, hydatid, or appendage 752.8
  fallopian tube 752.11
  disease or syndrome (hyperostosis frontalis interna) 733.3
Morgagni-Adams-Stokes syndrome (syncope with heart block) 426.9
Morgagni-Stewart-Morel syndrome (hyperostosis frontalis interna) 733.3
Moria (*see also* Psychosis) 298.9
Morning sickness 643.0
Moron 317
Morphea (guttate) (linear) 701.0
Morphine dependence (*see also* Dependence) 304.0
Morphinism (*see also* Dependence) 304.0
Morphinomania (*see also* Dependence) 304.0
Morphoea 701.0
Morquio (-Brailsford) (-Ullrich) disease or syndrome (mucopolysaccharidosis IV) 277.5
  kyphosis 277.5
Morris syndrome (testicular feminization) 257.8
Morsus humanus (open wound)—*see also* Wound, open, by site
  skin surface intact—*see* Contusion
Mortification (dry) (moist) (*see also* Gangrene) 785.4
Morton's
  disease 355.6
  foot 355.6
  metatarsalgia (syndrome) 355.6
  neuralgia 355.6
  neuroma 355.6
  syndrome (metatarsalgia) (neuralgia) 355.6
  toe 355.6
Morvan's disease 336.0
Mosaicism, mosaic (chromosomal) 758.9
  autosomal 758.5
  sex 758.81
Moschcowitz's syndrome (thrombotic thrombocytopenic purpura) 446.6
Mother yaw 102.0
Motion sickness (from travel, any vehicle) (from roundabouts or swings) 994.6
Mottled teeth (enamel) (endemic) (nonendemic) 520.3

Mottling enamel (endemic) (nonendemic) (teeth) 520.3
Mouchet's disease 732.5
Mould (s) (in vitreous) 117.9
Moulders'
  bronchitis 502
  tuberculosis (*see also* Tuberculosis) 011.4
Mounier-Kuhn syndrome 494.0
  with acute exacerbation 494.1
Mountain
  fever—*see* Fever, mountain
  sickness 993.2
    with polycythemia, acquired 289.0
    acute 289.0
  tick fever 066.1
Mouse, joint (*see also* Loose, body, joint) 718.1
  knee 717.6
Mouth —*see* condition
Movable
  coccyx 724.71
  kidney (*see also* Disease, renal) 593.0
    congenital 753.3
  organ or site, congenital NEC—*see* Malposition, congenital
  spleen 289.59
Movement
  abnormal (dystonic) (involuntary) 781.0
  decreased fetal 655.7
  paradoxical facial 374.43
Moya Moya disease 437.5
Mozart's ear 744.29
Mucha's disease (acute parapsoriasis varioliformis) 696.2
Mucha-Haberman syndrome (acute parapsoriasis varioliformis) 696.2
Mu-chain disease 273.2
Mucinosis (cutaneous) (papular) 701.8
Mucocele
  appendix 543.9
  buccal cavity 528.9
  gallbladder (*see also* Disease, gallbladder) 575.3
  lacrimal sac 375.43
  orbit (eye) 376.81
  salivary gland (any) 527.6
  sinus (accessory) (nasal) 478.1
  turbinate (bone) (middle) (nasal) 478.1
  uterus 621.8
Mucocutaneous lymph node syndrome (acute) (febrile) (infantile) 446.1
Mucoenteritis 564.9
Mucolipidosis I, II, III 272.7
Mucopolysaccharidosis (types 1-6) 277.5
  cardiopathy 277.5 *[425.7]*
Mucormycosis (lung) 117.7
Mucositis —*see also* Inflammation by site
  necroticans agranulocytica 288.0
Mucous —*see also* condition
  patches (syphilitic) 091.3
    congenital 090.0
Mucoviscidosis 277.00
  with meconium obstruction 277.01
Mucus
  asphyxia or suffocation (*see also* Asphyxia, mucus) 933.1
    newborn 770.1
  in stool 792.1
  plug (*see also* Asphyxia, mucus) 933.1
    aspiration, of newborn 770.1
    tracheobronchial 519.1
      newborn 770.1
Muguet 112.0
Mulberry molars 090.5

Mullerian mixed tumor (M8950/3)—*see* Neoplasm, by site, malignant
Multicystic kidney 753.19
Multilobed placenta —*see* Placenta, abnormal
Multinodular prostate 600.1
Multiparity V61.5
  affecting
    fetus or newborn 763.89
    management of
      labor and delivery 659.4
      pregnancy V23.3
  requiring contraceptive management (*see also* Contraception) V25.9
Multipartita placenta —*see* Placenta, abnormal
Multiple, multiplex —*see also* condition
  birth
    affecting fetus or newborn 761.5
    healthy liveborn—*see* Newborn, multiple
  digits (congenital) 755.00
    fingers 755.01
    toes 755.02
  organ or site NEC—*see* Accessory
  personality 300.14
  renal arteries 747.62
Mumps 072.9
  with complication 072.8
    specified type NEC 072.79
  encephalitis 072.2
  hepatitis 072.71
  meningitis (aseptic) 072.1
  meningoencephalitis 072.2
  oophoritis 072.79
  orchitis 072.0
  pancreatitis 072.3
  polyneuropathy 072.72
  vaccination, prophylactic (against) V04.6
Mumu (*see also* Infestation, filarial) 125.9
Münchausen syndrome 301.51
Münchmeyer's disease or syndrome (exostosis luxurians) 728.11
Mural —*see* condition
Murmur (cardiac) (heart) (nonorganic) (organic) 785.2
  abdominal 787.5
  aortic (valve) (*see also* Endocarditis, aortic) 424.1
  benign—*omit code*
  cardiorespiratory 785.2
  diastolic—*see* condition
  Flint (*see also* Endocarditis, aortic) 424.1
  functional—*omit code*
  Graham Steell (pulmonic regurgitation) (*see also* Endocarditis, pulmonary) 424.3
  innocent—*omit code*
  insignificant—*omit code*
  midsystolic 785.2
  mitral (valve)—*see* stenosis, mitral
  physiologic—*see* condition
  presystolic, mitral—*see* Insufficiency, mitral
  pulmonic (valve) (*see also* Endocarditis, pulmonary) 424.3
  Still's (vibratory)—*omit code*
  systolic (valvular)—*see* condition
  tricuspid (valve)—*see* Endocarditis, tricuspid
  valvular—*see* condition
  vibratory—*omit code*
  undiagnosed 785.2
Murri's disease (intermittent hemoglobinuria) 283.2
Muscae volitantes 379.24
Muscle, muscular —*see* condition
Musculoneuralgia 729.1

Mushrooming hip 718.95
Mushroom workers' (pickers') lung 495.5
Mutism (*see also* Aphasia) 784.3
  akinetic 784.3
  deaf (acquired) (congenital) 389.7
  elective (selective) 313.23
    adjustment reaction 309.83
  hysterical 300.11
Myà's disease (congenital dilation, colon) 751.3
Myalgia (intercostal) 729.1
  eosinophilia syndrome 710.5
  epidemic 074.1
    cervical 078.89
  psychogenic 307.89
  traumatic NEC 959.9
Myasthenia, myasthenic 358.0
  cordis—*see* Failure, heart
  gravis 358.0
    neonatal 775.2
    pseudoparalytica 358.0
  stomach 536.8
    psychogenic 306.4
  syndrome in
    botulism 005.1 *[358.1]*
    diabetes mellitus 250.6 *[358.1]*
    hypothyroidism (*see also* Hypothyroidism) 244.9 *[358.1]*
    malignant neoplasm NEC 199.1 *[358.1]*
    pernicious anemia 281.0 *[358.1]*
    thyrotoxicosis (*see also* Thyrotoxicosis) 242.9 *[358.1]*
Mycelium infection NEC 117.9
Mycetismus 988.1
Mycetoma (actinomycotic) 039.9
  bone 039.8
    mycotic 117.4
  foot 039.4
    mycotic 117.4
  madurae 039.9
    mycotic 117.4
  maduromycotic 039.9
    mycotic 117.4
  mycotic 117.4
  nocardial 039.9
Mycobacteriosis —*see* Mycobacterium
Mycobacterium, mycobacterial (infection) 031.9
  acid-fast (bacilli) 031.9
  anonymous (*see also* Mycobacterium, atypical) 031.9
  atypical (acid-fast bacilli) 031.9
    cutaneous 031.1
    pulmonary 031.0
      tuberculous (*see also* Tuberculosis, pulmonary) 011.9
    specified site NEC 031.8
  avium 031.0
    intracellulare complex bacteremia (MAC) 031.2
  balnei 031.1
  Battey 031.0
  cutaneous 031.1
  disseminated 031.2
    avium-intracellulare complex (DMAC) 031.2
  fortuitum 031.0
  intracellulare (battey bacillus) 031.0
  kakerifu 031.8
  kansasii 031.0
  kasongo 031.8
  leprae—*see* Leprosy
  luciflavum 031.0

Mycobacterium, mycobacterial—*continued*
  marinum 031.1
  pulmonary 031.0
    tuberculous (*see also* Tuberculosis,
      pulmonary) 011.9
  scrofulaceum 031.1
  tuberculosis (human, bovine)—*see also*
    Tuberculosis
  avian type 031.0
  ulcerans 031.1
  xenopi 031.0
Mycosis, mycotic 117.9
  cutaneous NEC 111.9
  ear 111.8 *[380.15]*
  fungoides (M9700/3) 202.1
  mouth 112.0
  pharynx 117.9
  skin NEC 111.9
  stomatitis 112.0
  systemic NEC 117.9
  tonsil 117.9
  vagina, vaginitis 112.1
Mydriasis (persistent) (pupil) 379.43
Myelatelia 742.59
Myelinoclasis, perivascular, acute
    (postinfectious) NEC 136.9 *[323.6]*
  postimmunization or postvaccinal 323.5
Myelinosis, central pontine 341.8
Myelitis (acute) (ascending) (cerebellar)
    (childhood) (chronic) (descending) (diffuse)
    (disseminated) (pressure) (progressive) (spinal
    cord) (subacute) (transverse) (*see also*
    Encephalitis) 323.9
  late effect—*see* category 326
  optic neuritis in 341.0
  postchickenpox 052.7
  postvaccinal 323.5
  syphilitic (transverse) 094.89
  tuberculous (*see also* Tuberculosis) 013.6
  virus 049.9
Myeloblastic —*see* condition
Myelocele (*see also* Spina bifida) 741.9
  with hydrocephalus 741.0
Myelocystocele (*see also* Spina bifida) 741.9
Myelocytic —*see* condition
Myelocytoma 205.1
Myelodysplasia (spinal cord) 742.59
  meaning myelodysplastic syndrome—*see*
    Syndrome, myelodysplastic
Myeloencephalitis —*see* Encephalitis
Myelofibrosis (osteosclerosis) 289.8
Myelogenous —*see* condition
Myeloid —*see* condition
Myelokathexis 288.0
Myeloleukodystrophy 330.0
Myelolipoma (M8870/0)—*see* Neoplasm, by
    site, benign
Myeloma (multiple) (plasma cell) (plasmacytic)
    (M9730/3) 203.0
  monostotic (M9731/1) 238.6
  solitary (M9731/1) 238.6
Myelomalacia 336.8
Myelomata, multiple (M9730/3) 203.0
Myelomatosis (M9730/3) 203.0
Myelomeningitis —*see* Meningoencephalitis
Myelomeningocele (spinal cord) (*see also* Spina
    bifida) 741.9
  fetal, causing fetopelvic disproportion 653.7
Myelo-osteo-musculodysplasia hereditaria
    756.89
Myelopathic —*see* condition

Myelopathy (spinal cord) 336.9
  cervical 721.1
  diabetic 250.6 *[336.3]*
  drug-induced 336.8
  due to or with
    carbon tetrachloride 987.8 *[323.7]*
    degeneration or displacement, intervertebral
      disc 722.70
    cervical, cervicothoracic 722.71
    lumbar, lumbosacral 722.73
    thoracic, thoracolumbar 722.72
    hydroxyquinoline derivatives 961.3 *[323.7]*
    infection—*see* Encephalitis
    intervertebral disc disorder 722.70
    cervical, cervicothoracic 722.71
    lumbar, lumbosacral 722.73
    thoracic, thoracolumbar 722.72
    lead 984.9 *[323.7]*
    mercury 985.0 *[323.7]*
    neoplastic disease (*see also* Neoplasm, by
      site) 239.9 *[336.3]*
    pernicious anemia 281.0 *[336.3]*
    spondylosis 721.91
    cervical 721.1
    lumbar, lumbosacral 721.42
    thoracic 721.41
    thallium 985.8 *[323.7]*
  lumbar, lumbosacral 721.42
  necrotic (subacute) 336.1
  radiation-induced 336.8
  spondylogenic NEC 721.91
    cervical 721.1
    lumbar, lumbosacral 721.42
    thoracic 721.41
  thoracic 721.41
  toxic NEC 989.9 *[323.7]*
  transverse (*see also* Encephalitis) 323.9
  vascular 336.1
Myeloproliferative disease (M9960/1) 238.7
Myeloradiculitis (*see also* Polyneuropathy) 357.0
Myeloradiculodysplasia (spinal) 742.59
Myelosarcoma (M9930/3) 205.3
Myelosclerosis 289.8
  with myeloid metaplasia (M9961/1) 238.7
  disseminated, of nervous system 340
  megakaryocytic (M9961/1) 238.7
Myelosis (M9860/3) (*see also* Leukemia,
    myeloid) 205.9
  acute (M9861/3) 205.0
  aleukemic (M9864/3) 205.8
  chronic (M9863/3) 205.1
  erythremic (M9840/3) 207.0
    acute (M9841/3) 207.0
  megakaryocytic (M9920/3) 207.2
  nonleukemic (chronic) 288.8
  subacute (M9862/3) 205.2
Myesthenia —*see* Myasthenia
Myiasis (cavernous) 134.0
  orbit 134.0 *[376.13]*
Myoadenoma, prostate 600.2
Myoblastoma
  granular cell (M9580/0)—*see also* Neoplasm,
    connective tissue, benign
    malignant (M9580/3)—*see* Neoplasm,
      connective tissue, malignant
  tongue (M9580/0) 210.1
Myocardial —*see* condition

Myocardiopathy (congestive) (constrictive) (familial) (hypertrophic nonobstructive) (idiopathic) (infiltrative) (obstructive) (primary) (restrictive) (sporadic) 425.4
alcoholic 425.5
amyloid 277.3 *[425.7]*
beriberi 265.0 *[425.7]*
cobalt-beer 425.5
due to
  amyloidosis 277.3 *[425.7]*
  beriberi 265.0 *[425.7]*
  cardiac glycogenosis 271.0 *[425.7]*
  Chagas' disease 086.0
  Friedreich's ataxia 334.0 *[425.8]*
  influenza 487.8 *[425.8]*
  mucopolysaccharidosis 277.5 *[425.7]*
  myotonia atrophica 359.2 *[425.8]*
  progressive muscular dystrophy 359.1 *[425.8]*
  sarcoidosis 135 *[425.8]*
glycogen storage 271.0 *[425.7]*
hypertrophic obstructive 425.1
metabolic NEC 277.9 *[425.7]*
nutritional 269.9 *[425.7]*
obscure (African) 425.2
postpartum 674.8
secondary 425.9
thyrotoxic (*see also* Thyrotoxicosis) 242.9 *[425.7]*
toxic NEC 425.9
Myocarditis (fibroid) (interstitial) (old) (progressive) (senile) (with arteriosclerosis) 429.0
with
  rheumatic fever (conditions classifiable to 390) 398.0
    active (*see also* Myocarditis, acute, rheumatic) 391.2
    inactive or quiescent (with chorea) 398.0
active (nonrheumatic) 422.90
  rheumatic 391.2
    with chorea (acute) (rheumatic) (Sydenham's) 392.0
acute or subacute (interstitial) 422.90
  due to Streptococcus (beta-hemolytic) 391.2
  idiopathic 422.91
  rheumatic 391.2
    with chorea (acute) (rheumatic) (Sydenham's) 392.0
  specified type NEC 422.99
aseptic of newborn 074.23
bacterial (acute) 422.92
chagasic 086.0
chronic (interstitial) 429.0
congenital 746.89
constrictive 425.4
Coxsackie (virus) 074.23
diphtheritic 032.82
due to or in
  Coxsackie (virus) 074.23
  diphtheria 032.82
  epidemic louse-borne typhus 080 *[422.0]*
  influenza 487.8 *[422.0]*
  Lyme disease 088.81 *[422.0]*
  scarlet fever 034.1 *[422.0]*
  toxoplasmosis (acquired) 130.3
  tuberculosis (*see also* Tuberculosis) 017.9 *[422.0]*
  typhoid 002.0 *[422.0]*
  typhus NEC 081.9 *[422.0]*
eosinophilic 422.91
epidemic of newborn 074.23

Myocarditis—*continued*
Fiedler's (acute) (isolated) (subacute) 422.91
giant cell (acute) (subacute) 422.91
gonococcal 098.85
granulomatous (idiopathic) (isolated) (nonspecific) 422.91
hypertensive (*see also* Hypertension, heart) 402.90
idiopathic 422.91
  granulomatous 422.91
infective 422.92
influenzal 487.8 *[422.0]*
isolated (diffuse) (granulomatous) 422.91
malignant 422.99
meningococcal 036.43
nonrheumatic, active 422.90
parenchymatous 422.90
pneumococcal (acute) (subacute) 422.92
rheumatic (chronic) (inactive) (with chorea) 398.0
  active or acute 391.2
    with chorea (acute) (rheumatic) (Sydenham's) 392.0
septic 422.92
specific (giant cell) (productive) 422.91
staphylococcal (acute) (subacute) 422.92
suppurative 422.92
syphilitic (chronic) 093.82
toxic 422.93
  rheumatic (*see also* Myocarditis, acute rheumatic) 391.2
tuberculous (*see also* Tuberculosis) 017.9 *[422.0]*
typhoid 002.0 *[422.0]*
valvular—*see* Endocarditis
viral, except Coxsackie 422.91
  Coxsackie 074.23
  of newborn (Coxsackie) 074.23
Myocardium, myocardial —*see* condition
Myocardosis (*see also* Cardiomyopathy) 425.4
Myoclonia (essential) 333.2
epileptica 333.2
Friedrich's 333.2
massive 333.2
Myoclonic
epilepsy, familial (progressive) 333.2
jerks 333.2
Myoclonus (familial essential) (multifocal) (simplex) 333.2
facial 351.8
massive (infantile) 333.2
pharyngeal 478.29
Myodiastasis 728.84
Myoendocarditis —*see also* Endocarditis
acute or subacute 421.9
Myoepithelioma (M8982/0)—*see* Neoplasm, by site, benign
Myofascitis (acute) 729.1
low back 724.2
Myofibroma (M8890/0)—*see also* Neoplasm, connective tissue, benign
uterus (cervix) (corpus) (*see also* Leiomyoma) 218.9
Myofibrosis 728.2
heart (*see also* Myocarditis) 429.0
humeroscapular region 726.2
scapulohumeral 726.2
Myofibrositis (*see also* Myositis) 729.1
scapulohumeral 726.2
Myogelosis (occupational) 728.89
Myoglobinuria 791.3
Myoglobulinuria, primary 791.3

Myokymia —*see also* Myoclonus
  facial 351.8
Myolipoma (M8860/0)
  specified site—*see* Neoplasm, connective
    tissue, benign
  unspecified site 223.0
Myoma (M8895/0)—*see also* Neoplasm,
    connective tissue, benign
  cervix (stump) (uterus) (*see also* Leiomyoma)
    218.9
  malignant (M8895/3)—*see* Neoplasm,
    connective tissue, malignant
  prostate 600.2
  uterus (cervix) (corpus) (*see also* Leiomyoma)
    218.9
    in pregnancy or childbirth 654.1
      affecting fetus or newborn 763.89
      causing obstructed labor 660.2
        affecting fetus or newborn 763.1
Myomalacia 728.9
  cordis, heart (*see also* Degeneration,
    myocardial) 429.1
Myometritis (*see also* Endometritis) 615.9
Myometrium —*see* condition
Myonecrosis, clostridial 040.0
Myopathy 359.9
  alcoholic 359.4
  amyloid 277.3 *[359.6]*
  benign congenital 359.0
  central core 359.0
  centronuclear 359.0
  congenital (benign) 359.0
  critical illness 359.81
  distal 359.1
  due to drugs 359.4
  endocrine 259.9 *[359.5]*
    specified type NEC 259.8 *[359.5]*
  extraocular muscles 376.82
  facioscapulohumeral 359.1
  in
    Addison's disease 255.4 *[359.5]*
    amyloidosis 277.3 *[359.6]*
    cretinism 243 *[359.5]*
    Cushing's syndrome 255.0 *[359.5]*
    disseminated lupus erythematosus 710.0
      [359.6]
    giant cell arteritis 446.5 *[359.6]*
    hyperadrenocorticism NEC 255.3 *[359.5]*
    hyperparathyroidism 252.0 *[359.5]*
    hypopituitarism 253.2 *[359.5]*
    hypothyroidism (*see also* Hypothyroidism)
      244.9 *[359.5]*
    malignant neoplasm NEC (M8000/3) 199.1
      [359.6]
    myxedema (*see also* Myxedema) 244.9
      [359.5]
    polyarteritis nodosa 446.0 *[359.6]*
    rheumatoid arthritis 714.0 *[359.6]*
    sarcoidosis 135 *[359.6]*
    scleroderma 710.1 *[359.6]*
    Sjögren's disease 710.2 *[359.6]*
    thyrotoxicosis (*see also* Thyrotoxicosis) 242.9
      [359.5]
  inflammatory 359.89
  intensive care (ICU) 359.81
  limb-girdle 359.1
  myotubular 359.0
  necrotizing, acute 359.81
  nemaline 359.0
  ocular 359.1
  oculopharyngeal 359.1
  of critical illness 359.81

Myopathy—*continued*
  primary 359.89
  progressive NEC 359.89
  rod body 359.0
  quadriplegic, acute 359.81
  scapulohumeral 359.1
  specified type NEC 359.89
  toxic 359.4
Myopericarditis (*see also* Pericarditis) 423.9
Myopia (axial) (congenital) (increased curvature
    or refraction, nucleus of lens) 367.1
  degenerative, malignant 360.21
  malignant 360.21
  progressive high (degenerative) 360.21
Myosarcoma (M8895/3)—*see* Neoplasm,
    connective tissue, malignant
Myosis (persistent) 379.42
  stromal (endolymphatic) (M8931/1) 236.0
Myositis 729.1
  clostridial 040.0
  due to posture 729.1
  epidemic 074.1
  fibrosa or fibrous (chronic) 728.2
    Volkmann's (complicating trauma) 958.6
  infective 728.0
  interstitial 728.81
  multiple—*see* Polymyositis
  occupational 729.1
  orbital, chronic 376.12
  ossificans 728.12
    circumscribed 728.12
    progressive 728.11
    traumatic 728.12
  progressive fibrosing 728.11
  purulent 728.0
  rheumatic 729.1
  rheumatoid 729.1
  suppurative 728.0
  syphilitic 095.6
  traumatic (old) 729.1
Myospasia impulsiva 307.23
Myotonia (acquisita) (intermittens) 728.85
  atrophica 359.2
  congenita 359.2
  dystrophica 359.2
Myotonic pupil 379.46
Myriapodiasis 134.1
Myringitis
  with otitis media—*see* Otitis media
  acute 384.00
    specified type NEC 384.09
  bullosa hemorrhagica 384.01
  bullous 384.01
  chronic 384.1
Mysophobia 300.29
Mytilotoxism 988.0
Myxadenitis labialis 528.5
Myxedema (adult) (idiocy) (infantile) (juvenile)
    (thyroid gland) (*see also* Hypothyroidism)
    244.9
  circumscribed 242.9
  congenital 243
  cutis 701.8
  localized (pretibial) 242.9
  madness (acute) 293.0
    subacute 293.1
  papular 701.8
  pituitary 244.8
  postpartum 674.8
  pretibial 242.9
  primary 244.9

Myxochondrosarcoma (M9220/3)—*see*
　Neoplasm, cartilage, malignant
Myxofibroma (M8811/0)—*see also* Neoplasm,
　connective tissue, benign
　odontogenic (M9320/0) 213.1
　upper jaw (bone) 213.0
Myxofibrosarcoma (M8811/3)—*see* Neoplasm,
　connective tissue, malignant
Myxolipoma (M8852/0) (*see also* Lipoma, by
　site) 214.9
Myxoliposarcoma (M8852/3)—*see* Neoplasm,
　connective tissue, malignant
Myxoma (M8840/0)—*see also* Neoplasm,
　connective tissue, benign
　odontogenic (M9320/0) 213.1
　upper jaw (bone) 213.0
Myxosarcoma (M8840/3)—*see* Neoplasm,
　connective tissue, malignant

N

Naegeli's
disease (hereditary hemorrhagic thrombasthenia) 287.1
leukemia, monocytic (M9863/3) 205.1
syndrome (incontinentia pigmenti) 757.33
Naffziger's syndrome 353.0
Naga sore (*see also* Ulcer, skin) 707.9
Nägele's pelvis 738.6
with disproportion (fetopelvic) 653.0
affecting fetus or newborn 763.1
causing obstructed labor 660.1
affecting fetus or newborn 763.1
Nager-de Reynier syndrome (dysostosis mandibularis) 756.0
Nail —*see also* condition
biting 307.9
patella syndrome (hereditary osteo-onychodysplasia) 756.89
Nanism, nanosomia (*see also* Dwarfism) 259.4
hypophyseal 253.3
pituitary 253.3
renis, renalis 588.0
Nanukayami 100.89
Napkin rash 691.0
Narcissism 301.81
Narcolepsy 347
Narcosis
carbon dioxide (respiratory) 786.09
due to drug
correct substance properly administered 780.09
overdose or wrong substance given or taken 977.9
specified drug—*see* Table of drugs and chemicals
Narcotism (chronic) (*see also* listing under Dependence) 304.9
acute
correct substance properly administered 349.82
overdose or wrong substance given or taken 967.8
specified drug—*see* Table of drugs and chemicals
Narrow
anterior chamber angle 365.02
pelvis (inlet) (outlet)—*see* Contraction, pelvis
Narrowing
artery NEC 447.1
auditory, internal 433.8
basilar 433.0
with other precerebral artery 433.3
bilateral 433.3
carotid 433.1
with other precerebral artery 433.3
bilateral 433.3
cerebellar 433.8
choroidal 433.8
communicating posterior 433.8
coronary —*see also* Arteriosclerosis, coronary
congenital 746.85
due to syphilis 090.5
hypophyseal 433.8
pontine 433.8
precerebral NEC 433.9
multiple or bilateral 433.3
specified NEC 433.8

Narrowing—*continued*
vertebral 433.2
with other precerebral artery 433.3
bilateral 433.3
auditory canal (external) (*see also* Stricture, ear canal, acquired) 380.50
cerebral arteries 437.0
cicatricial—*see* Cicatrix
congenital—*see* Anomaly, congenital
coronary artery—*see* Narrowing, artery, coronary
ear, middle 385.22
Eustachian tube (*see also* Obstruction, Eustachian tube) 381.60
eyelid 374.46
congenital 743.62
intervertebral disc or space NEC—*see* Degeneration, intervertebral disc
joint space, hip 719.85
larynx 478.74
lids 374.46
congenital 743.62
mesenteric artery (with gangrene) 557.0
palate 524.8
palpebral fissure 374.46
retinal artery 362.13
ureter 593.3
urethra (*see also* Stricture, urethra) 598.9
Narrowness, abnormal, eyelid 743.62
Nasal —*see* condition
Nasolacrimal —*see* condition
Nasopharyngeal —*see also* condition
bursa 478.29
pituitary gland 759.2
torticollis 723.5
Nasopharyngitis (acute) (infective) (subacute) 460
chronic 472.2
due to external agent—*see* Condition, respiratory, chronic, due to
due to external agent—*see* Condition, respiratory, due to
septic 034.0
streptococcal 034.0
suppurative (chronic) 472.2
ulcerative (chronic) 472.2
Nasopharynx, nasopharyngeal —*see* condition
Natal tooth, teeth 520.6
Nausea (*see also* Vomiting) 787.02
epidemic 078.82
gravidarum—*see* Hyperemesis, gravidarum
marina 994.6
with vomiting 787.01
Naval —*see* condition
Neapolitan fever (*see also* Brucellosis) 023.9
Nearsightedness 367.1
Near-syncope 780.2
Nebécourt's syndrome 253.3
Nebula, cornea (eye) 371.01
congenital 743.43
interfering with vision 743.42
Necator americanus infestation 126.1
Necatoriasis 126.1
Neck —*see* condition
Necrencephalus (*see also* Softening, brain) 437.8
Necrobacillosis 040.3

Necrobiosis 799.8
  brain or cerebral (*see also* Softening, brain)
    437.8
  lipoidica 709.3
    diabeticorum 250.8 *[709.3]*
Necrodermolysis 695.1
Necrolysis, toxic epidermal 695.1
  due to drug
    correct substance properly administered 695.1
    overdose or wrong substance given or taken
      977.9
      specified drug—*see* Table of drugs and
        chemicals
Necrophilia 302.89
Necrosis, necrotic
  adrenal (capsule) (gland) 255.8
  antrum, nasal sinus 478.1
  aorta (hyaline) (*see also* Aneurysm, aorta) 441.9
    cystic medial 441.00
      abdominal 441.02
      thoracic 441.01
      thoracoabdominal 441.03
    ruptured 441.5
  arteritis 446.0
  artery 447.5
  aseptic, bone 733.40
    femur (head) (neck) 733.42
      medial condyle 733.43
    humoral head 733.41
    medial femoral condyle 733.43
    specified site NEC 733.49
    talus 733.44
  avascular, bone NEC (*see also* Necrosis,
    aseptic, bone) 733.40
  bladder (aseptic) (sphincter) 596.8
  bone (*see also* Osteomyelitis) 730.1
    acute 730.0
    aseptic or avascular 733.40
      femur (head) (neck) 733.42
        medial condyle 733.43
      humoral head 733.41
      medial femoral condyle 733.43
      specified site NEC 733.49
      talus 733.44
    ethmoid 478.1
    ischemic 733.40
    jaw 526.4
    marrow 289.8
    Paget's (osteitis deformans) 731.0
    tuberculous—*see* Tuberculosis, bone
  brain (softening) (*see also* Softening, brain)
    437.8
  breast (aseptic) (fat) (segmental) 611.3
  bronchus, bronchi 519.1
  central nervous system NEC (*see also*
    Softening, brain) 437.8
  cerebellar (*see also* Softening, brain) 437.8
  cerebral (softening) (*see also* Softening, brain)
    437.8
  cerebrospinal (softening) (*see also* Softening,
    brain) 437.8
  cornea (*see also* Keratitis) 371.40
  cortical, kidney 583.6
  cystic medial (aorta) 441.00
    abdominal 441.02
    thoracic 441.01
    thoracoabdominal 441.03
  dental 521.09
    pulp 522.1

Necrosis, necrotic—*continued*
  due to swallowing corrosive substance—*see*
    Burn, by site
  ear (ossicle) 385.24
  esophagus 530.89
  ethmoid (bone) 478.1
  eyelid 374.50
  fat, fatty (generalized) (*see also* Degeneration,
    fatty) 272.8
    breast (aseptic) (segmental) 611.3
    intestine 569.89
    localized—*see* Degeneration, by site, fatty
    mesentery 567.8
    omentum 567.8
    pancreas 577.8
    peritoneum 567.8
    skin (subcutaneous) 709.3
      newborn 778.1
  femur (aseptic) (avascular) 733.42
    head 733.42
    medial condyle 733.43
    neck 733.42
  gallbladder (*see also* Cholecystitis, acute) 575.0
  gangrenous 785.4
  gastric 537.89
  glottis 478.79
  heart (myocardium)—*see* Infarct, myocardium
  hepatic (*see also* Necrosis, liver) 570
  hip (aseptic) (avascular) 733.42
  intestine (acute) (hemorrhagic) (massive) 557.0
  ischemic 785.4
  jaw 526.4
  kidney (bilateral) 583.9
    acute 584.9
    cortical 583.6
      acute 584.6
        with
          abortion—*see* Abortion, by type, with
            renal failure
          ectopic pregnancy (*see also* categories
            633.0-633.9) 639.3
          molar pregnancy (*see also* categories
            630-632) 639.3
        complicating pregnancy 646.2
          affecting fetus or newborn 760.1
        following labor and delivery 669.3
    medullary (papillary) (*see also* Pyelitis) 590.80
      in
        acute renal failure 584.7
        nephritis, nephropathy 583.7
    papillary (*see also* Pyelitis) 590.80
      in
        acute renal failure 584.7
        nephritis, nephropathy 583.7
    tubular 584.5
      with
        abortion—*see* Abortion, by type, with
          renal failure
        ectopic pregnancy (*see also* categories
          633.0-633.9) 639.3
        molar pregnancy (*see also* categories
          630-632) 639.3
      complicating
        abortion 639.3
        ectopic or molar pregnancy 639.3
        pregnancy 646.2
          affecting fetus or newborn 760.1
      following labor and delivery 669.3
      traumatic 958.5
  larynx 478.79

Necrosis, necrotic—*continued*
  liver (acute) (congenital) (diffuse) (massive)
      (subacute) 570
    with
      abortion—*see* Abortion, by type, with
          specified complication NEC
      ectopic pregnancy (*see also* categories
          633.0-633.9) 639.8
      molar pregnancy (*see also* categories
          630-632) 639.8
      complicating pregnancy 646.7
        affecting fetus or newborn 760.8
      following
        abortion 639.8
        ectopic or molar pregnancy 639.8
      obstetrical 646.7
      postabortal 639.8
      puerperal, postpartum 674.8
      toxic 573.3
  lung 513.0
  lymphatic gland 683
  mammary gland 611.3
  mastoid (chronic) 383.1
  mesentery 557.0
    fat 567.8
  mitral valve—*see* Insufficiency, mitral
  myocardium, myocardial—*see* Infarct,
      myocardium
  nose (septum) 478.1
  omentum 557.0
    with mesenteric infarction 557.0
    fat 567.8
  orbit, orbital 376.10
  ossicles, ear (aseptic) 385.24
  ovary (*see also* Salpingo-oophoritis) 614.2
  pancreas (aseptic) (duct) (fat) 577.8
    acute 577.0
    infective 577.0
  papillary, kidney (*see also* Pyelitis) 590.80
  peritoneum 557.0
    with mesenteric infarction 557.0
    fat 567.8
  pharynx 462
    in granulocytopenia 288.0
  phosphorus 983.9
  pituitary (gland) (postpartum) (Sheehan) 253.2
  placenta (*see also* Placenta, abnormal) 656.7
  pneumonia 513.0
  pulmonary 513.0
  pulp (dental) 522.1
  pylorus 537.89
  radiation—*see* Necrosis, by site
  radium—*see* Necrosis, by site
  renal—*see* Necrosis, kidney
  sclera 379.19
  scrotum 608.89
  skin or subcutaneous tissue 709.8
    due to burn—*see* Burn, by site
    gangrenous 785.4
  spine, spinal (column) 730.18
    acute 730.18
    cord 336.1
  spleen 289.59
  stomach 537.89
  stomatitis 528.1
  subcutaneous fat 709.3
    fetus or newborn 778.1
  subendocardial—*see* Infarct, myocardium
  suprarenal (capsule) (gland) 255.8

Necrosis, necrotic—*continued*
  teeth, tooth 521.09
  testis 608.89
  thymus (gland) 254.8
  tonsil 474.8
  trachea 519.1
  tuberculous NEC—*see* Tuberculosis
  tubular (acute) (anoxic) (toxic) 584.5
    due to a procedure 997.5
  umbilical cord, affecting fetus or newborn 762.6
  vagina 623.8
  vertebra (lumbar) 730.18
    acute 730.18
    tuberculous (*see also* Tuberculosis) 015.0
        [730.8]
  vesical (aseptic) (bladder) 596.8
  x-ray—*see* Necrosis, by site
Necrospermia 606.0
Necrotizing angiitis 446.0
Negativism 301.7
Neglect (child) (newborn) NEC 995.52
  adult 995.84
  after or at birth 995.52
  hemispatial 781.8
  left-sided 781.8
  sensory 781.8
  visuospatial 781.8
Negri bodies 071
Neill-Dingwall syndrome (microcephaly and
    dwarfism) 759.89
Neisserian infection NEC—*see* Gonococcus
Nematodiasis NEC (*see also* Infestation,
    Nematode) 127.9
  ancylostoma (*see also* Ancylostomiasis) 126.9
Neoformans cryptococcus infection 117.5
Neonatal —*see also* condition
  teeth, tooth 520.6
Neonatorum —*see* condition

> *"N" listing resumes after*
> *"Neoplasm, neoplastic" table…*

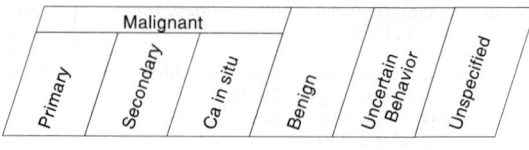

| | Malignant | | | | |
	Primary	Secondary	Ca in situ	Benign	Uncertain Behavior	Unspecified
Neoplasm, neoplastic	**199.1**	**199.1**	**234.9**	**229.9**	**238.9**	**239.9**

> *Note—1. The list below gives the code numbers for neoplasms by anatomical site. For each site there are six possible code numbers according to whether the neoplasm in question is malignant, benign, in situ, of uncertain behavior, or of unspecified nature. The description of the neoplasm will often indicate which of the six columns is appropriate; e.g., malignant melanoma of skin, benign fibroadenoma of breast, carcinoma in situ of cervix uteri.*
>
> *Where such descriptors are not present, the remainder of the Index should be consulted where guidance is given to the appropriate column for each morphological (histological) variety listed; e.g., Mesonephroma—see Neoplasm, malignant; Embryoma—see also Neoplasm, uncertain behavior; Disease, Bowen's—see Neoplasm, skin, in situ. However, the guidance in the Index can be overridden if one of the descriptors mentioned above is present; e.g., malignant adenoma of colon is coded to 153.9 and not to 211.3 as the adjective "malignant" overrides the Index entry "Adenoma—see also Neoplasm, benign."*
>
> *Note—2. Sites marked with the sign * (e.g., face NEC*) should be classified to malignant neoplasm of skin of these sites if the variety of neoplasm is a squamous cell carcinoma or an epidermoid carcinoma and to benign neoplasm of skin of these sites if the variety of neoplasm is a papilloma (any type).*

	Primary	Secondary	Ca in situ	Benign	Uncertain Behavior	Unspecified
abdomen, abdominal	195.2	198.89	234.8	229.8	238.8	239.8
cavity	195.2	198.89	234.8	229.8	238.8	239.8
organ	195.2	198.89	234.8	229.8	238.8	239.8
viscera	195.2	198.89	234.8	229.8	238.8	239.8
wall	173.5	198.2	232.5	216.5	238.2	239.2
connective tissue	171.5	198.89	—	215.5	238.1	239.2
abdominopelvic	195.8	198.89	234.8	229.8	238.8	239.8
accessory sinus—*see* Neoplasm, sinus						
acoustic nerve	192.0	198.4	—	225.1	237.9	239.7
acromion (process)	170.4	198.5	—	213.4	238.0	239.2
adenoid (pharynx) (tissue)	147.1	198.89	230.0	210.7	235.1	239.0
adipose tissue *(see also* Neoplasm,						
connective tissue)	171.9	198.89	—	215.9	238.1	239.2
adnexa (uterine)	183.9	198.82	233.3	221.8	236.3	239.5
adrenal (cortex) (gland) (medulla)	194.0	198.7	234.8	227.0	237.2	239.7
ala nasi (external)	173.3	198.2	232.3	216.3	238.2	239.2
alimentary canal or tract NEC	159.9	197.8	230.9	211.9	235.5	239.0
alveolar	143.9	198.89	230.0	210.4	235.1	239.0
mucosa	143.9	198.89	230.0	210.4	235.1	239.0
lower	143.1	198.89	230.0	210.4	235.1	239.0
upper	143.0	198.89	230.0	210.4	235.1	239.0
ridge or process	170.1	198.5	—	213.1	238.0	239.2
carcinoma	143.9	—	—	—	—	—
lower	143.1	—	—	—	—	—
upper	143.0	—	—	—	—	—
lower	170.1	198.5	—	213.1	238.0	239.2
mucosa	143.9	198.89	230.0	210.4	235.1	239.0
lower	143.1	198.89	230.0	210.4	235.1	239.0
upper	143.0	198.89	230.0	210.4	235.1	239.0
upper	170.0	198.5	—	213.0	238.0	239.2
sulcus	145.1	198.89	230.0	210.4	235.1	239.0
alveolus	143.9	198.89	230.0	210.4	235.1	239.0
lower	143.1	198.89	230.0	210.4	235.1	239.0
upper	143.0	198.89	230.0	210.4	235.1	239.0
ampulla of Vater	156.2	197.8	230.8	211.5	235.3	239.0
ankle NEC*	195.5	198.89	232.7	229.8	238.8	239.8
anorectum, anorectal (junction)	154.8	197.5	230.7	211.4	235.2	239.0
antecubital fossa or space*	195.4	198.89	232.6	229.8	238.8	239.8
antrum (Highmore) (maxillary)	160.2	197.3	231.8	212.0	235.9	239.1
pyloric	151.2	197.8	230.2	211.1	235.2	239.0
tympanicum	160.1	197.3	231.8	212.0	235.9	239.1
anus, anal	154.3	197.5	230.6	211.4	235.5	239.0
canal	154.2	197.5	230.5	211.4	235.5	239.0

	Malignant					
	Primary	Secondary	Ca in situ	Benign	Uncertain Behavior	Unspecified
anus, anal—*continued*						
contiguous sites with rectosigmoid						
junction or rectum	154.8	—	—	—	—	—
margin	173.5	198.2	232.5	216.5	238.2	239.2
skin	173.5	198.2	232.5	216.5	238.2	239.2
sphincter	154.2	197.5	230.5	211.4	235.5	239.0
aorta (thoracic)	171.4	198.89	—	215.4	238.1	239.2
abdominal	171.5	198.89	—	215.5	238.1	239.2
aortic body	194.6	198.89	—	227.6	237.3	239.7
aponeurosis	171.9	198.89	—	215.9	238.1	239.2
palmar	171.2	198.89	—	215.2	238.1	239.2
plantar	171.3	198.89	—	215.3	238.1	239.2
appendix	153.5	197.5	230.3	211.3	235.2	239.0
arachnoid (cerebral)	192.1	198.4	—	225.2	237.6	239.7
spinal	192.3	198.4	—	225.4	237.6	239.7
areola (female)	174.0	198.81	233.0	217	238.3	239.3
male	175.0	198.81	233.0	217	238.3	239.3
arm NEC*	195.4	198.89	232.6	229.8	238.8	239.8
artery—*see* Neoplasm, connective tissue						
aryepiglottic fold	148.2	198.89	230.0	210.8	235.1	239.0
hypopharyngeal aspect	148.2	198.89	230.0	210.8	235.1	239.0
laryngeal aspect	161.1	197.3	231.0	212.1	235.6	239.1
marginal zone	148.2	198.89	230.0	210.8	235.1	239.0
arytenoid (cartilage)	161.3	197.3	231.0	212.1	235.6	239.1
fold—*see* Neoplasm, aryepiglottic						
atlas	170.2	198.5	—	213.2	238.0	239.2
atrium, cardiac	164.1	198.89	—	212.7	238.8	239.8
auditory						
canal (external) (skin)	173.2	198.2	232.2	216.2	238.2	239.2
internal	160.1	197.3	231.8	212.0	235.9	239.1
nerve	192.0	198.4	—	225.1	237.9	239.7
tube	160.1	197.3	231.8	212.0	235.9	239.1
opening	147.2	198.89	230.0	210.7	235.1	239.0
auricle, ear	173.2	198.2	232.2	216.2	238.2	239.2
cartilage	171.0	198.89	—	215.0	238.1	239.2
auricular canal (external)	173.2	198.2	232.2	216.2	238.2	239.2
internal	160.1	197.3	231.8	212.0	235.9	239.1
autonomic nerve or nervous system NEC	171.9	198.89	—	215.9	238.1	239.2
axilla, axillary	195.1	198.89	234.8	229.8	238.8	239.8
fold	173.5	198.2	232.5	216.5	238.2	239.2
back NEC*	195.8	198.89	232.5	229.8	238.8	239.8
Bartholin's gland	184.1	198.82	233.3	221.2	236.3	239.5
basal ganglia	191.0	198.3	—	225.0	237.5	239.6
basis pedunculi	191.7	198.3	—	225.0	237.5	239.6
bile or biliary (tract)	156.9	197.8	230.8	211.5	235.3	239.0
canaliculi (biliferi) (intrahepatic)	155.1	197.8	230.8	211.5	235.3	239.0
canals, interlobular	155.1	197.8	230.8	211.5	235.3	239.0
contiguous sites	156.8	—	—	—	—	—
duct or passage (common) (cyst)						
(extrahepatic)	156.1	197.8	230.8	211.5	235.3	239.0
contiguous sites with gallbladder	156.8	—	—	—	—	—
interlobular	155.1	197.8	230.8	211.5	235.3	239.0
intrahepatic	155.1	197.8	230.8	211.5	235.3	239.0
and extrahepatic	156.9	197.8	230.8	211.5	235.3	239.0
bladder (urinary)	188.9	198.1	233.7	223.3	236.7	239.4
contiguous sites	188.8	—	—	—	—	—
dome	188.1	198.1	233.7	223.3	236.7	239.4
neck	188.5	198.1	233.7	223.3	236.7	239.4
orifice	188.9	198.1	233.7	223.3	236.7	239.4
ureteric	188.6	198.1	233.7	223.3	236.7	239.4
urethral	188.5	198.1	233.7	223.3	236.7	239.4
sphincter	188.8	198.1	233.7	223.3	236.7	239.4
trigone	188.0	198.1	233.7	223.3	236.7	239.4

| | Malignant | | | | | |
	Primary	Secondary	Ca in situ	Benign	Uncertain Behavior	Unspecified
urachus	188.7	—	233.7	223.3	236.7	239.4
wall	188.9	198.1	233.7	223.3	236.7	239.4
anterior	188.3	198.1	233.7	223.3	236.7	239.4
lateral	188.2	198.1	233.7	223.3	236.7	239.4
posterior	188.4	198.1	233.7	223.3	236.7	239.4
blood vessel—*see* Neoplasm, connective tissue						

Note—Carcinomas and adenocarcinomas, of any type other than intraosseous or odontogenic, of the sites listed under "Neoplasm, bone" should be considered as constituting metastatic spread from an unspecified primary site and coded to 198.5 for morbidity coding and to 199.1 for underlying cause of death coding.

bone (periosteum)	170.9	198.5	—	213.9	238.0	239.2
acetabulum	170.6	198.5	—	213.6	238.0	239.2
acromion (process)	170.4	198.5	—	213.4	238.0	239.2
ankle	170.8	198.5	—	213.8	238.0	239.2
arm NEC	170.4	198.5	—	213.4	238.0	239.2
astragalus	170.8	198.5	—	213.8	238.0	239.2
atlas	170.2	198.5	—	213.2	238.0	239.2
axis	170.2	198.5	—	213.2	238.0	239.2
back NEC	170.2	198.5	—	213.2	238.0	239.2
calcaneus	170.8	198.5	—	213.8	238.0	239.2
calvarium	170.0	198.5	—	213.0	238.0	239.2
carpus (any)	170.5	198.5	—	213.5	238.0	239.2
cartilage NEC	170.9	198.5	—	213.9	238.0	239.2
clavicle	170.3	198.5	—	213.3	238.0	239.2
clivus	170.0	198.5	—	213.0	238.0	239.2
coccygeal vertebra	170.6	198.5	—	213.6	238.0	239.2
coccyx	170.6	198.5	—	213.6	238.0	239.2
costal cartilage	170.3	198.5	—	213.3	238.0	239.2
costovertebral joint	170.3	198.5	—	213.3	238.0	239.2
cranial	170.0	198.5	—	213.0	238.0	239.2
cuboid	170.8	198.5	—	213.8	238.0	239.2
cuneiform	170.9	198.5	—	213.9	238.0	239.2
ankle	170.8	198.5	—	213.8	238.0	239.2
wrist	170.5	198.5	—	213.5	238.0	239.2
digital	170.9	198.5	—	213.9	238.0	239.2
finger	170.5	198.5	—	213.5	238.0	239.2
toe	170.8	198.5	—	213.8	238.0	239.2
elbow	170.4	198.5	—	213.4	238.0	239.2
ethmoid (labyrinth)	170.0	198.5	—	213.0	238.0	239.2
face	170.0	198.5	—	213.0	238.0	239.2
lower jaw	170.1	198.5	—	213.1	238.0	239.2
femur (any part)	170.7	198.5	—	213.7	238.0	239.2
fibula (any part)	170.7	198.5	—	213.7	238.0	239.2
finger (any)	170.5	198.5	—	213.5	238.0	239.2
foot	170.8	198.5	—	213.8	238.0	239.2
forearm	170.4	198.5	—	213.4	238.0	239.2
frontal	170.0	198.5	—	213.0	238.0	239.2
hand	170.5	198.5	—	213.5	238.0	239.2
heel	170.8	198.5	—	213.8	238.0	239.2
hip	170.6	198.5	—	213.6	238.0	239.2
humerus (any part)	170.4	198.5	—	213.4	238.0	239.2
hyoid	170.0	198.5	—	213.0	238.0	239.2
ilium	170.6	198.5	—	213.6	238.0	239.2
innominate	170.6	198.5	—	213.6	238.0	239.2
intervertebral cartilage or disc	170.2	198.5	—	213.2	238.0	239.2
ischium	170.6	198.5	—	213.6	238.0	239.2
jaw (lower)	170.1	198.5	—	213.1	238.0	239.2
upper	170.0	198.5	—	213.0	238.0	239.2
knee	170.7	198.5	—	213.7	238.0	239.2
leg NEC	170.7	198.5	—	213.7	238.0	239.2
limb NEC	170.9	198.5	—	213.9	238.0	239.2
lower (long bones)	170.7	198.5	—	213.7	238.0	239.2

	Malignant					
	Primary	Secondary	Ca in situ	Benign	Uncertain Behavior	Unspecified
bone—*continued*						
short bones	170.8	198.5	—	213.8	238.0	239.2
upper (long bones)	170.4	198.5	—	213.4	238.0	239.2
short bones	170.5	198.5	—	213.5	238.0	239.2
long	170.9	198.5	—	213.9	238.0	239.2
lower limbs NEC.	170.7	198.5	—	213.7	238.0	239.2
upper limbs NEC.	170.4	198.5	—	213.4	238.0	239.2
malar	170.0	198.5	—	213.0	238.0	239.2
mandible	170.1	198.5	—	213.1	238.0	239.2
marrow NEC	202.9	198.5	—	—	—	238.7
mastoid	170.0	198.5	—	213.0	238.0	239.2
maxilla, maxillary (superior)	170.0	198.5	—	213.0	238.0	239.2
inferior	170.1	198.5	—	213.1	238.0	239.2
metacarpus (any)	170.5	198.5	—	213.5	238.0	239.2
metatarsus (any)	170.8	198.5	—	213.8	238.0	239.2
navicular (ankle)	170.8	198.5	—	213.8	238.0	239.2
hand	170.5	198.5	—	213.5	238.0	239.2
nose, nasal	170.0	198.5	—	213.0	238.0	239.2
occipital	170.0	198.5	—	213.0	238.0	239.2
orbit	170.0	198.5	—	213.0	238.0	239.2
parietal	170.0	198.5	—	213.0	238.0	239.2
patella	170.8	198.5	—	213.8	238.0	239.2
pelvic	170.6	198.5	—	213.6	238.0	239.2
phalanges	170.9	198.5	—	213.9	238.0	239.2
foot	170.8	198.5	—	213.8	238.0	239.2
hand	170.5	198.5	—	213.5	238.0	239.2
pubic	170.6	198.5	—	213.6	238.0	239.2
radius (any part)	170.4	198.5	—	213.4	238.0	239.2
rib	170.3	198.5	—	213.3	238.0	239.2
sacral vertebra	170.6	198.5	—	213.6	238.0	239.2
sacrum	170.6	198.5	—	213.6	238.0	239.2
scaphoid (of hand)	170.5	198.5	—	213.5	238.0	239.2
of ankle	170.8	198.5	—	213.8	238.0	239.2
scapula (any part)	170.4	198.5	—	213.4	238.0	239.2
sella turcica	170.0	198.5	—	213.0	238.0	239.2
short	170.9	198.5	—	213.9	238.0	239.2
lower limb	170.8	198.5	—	213.8	238.0	239.2
upper limb	170.5	198.5	—	213.5	238.0	239.2
shoulder	170.4	198.5	—	213.4	238.0	239.2
skeleton, skeletal NEC	170.9	198.5	—	213.9	238.0	239.2
skull	170.0	198.5	—	213.0	238.0	239.2
sphenoid	170.0	198.5	—	213.0	238.0	239.2
spine, spinal (column)	170.2	198.5	—	213.2	238.0	239.2
coccyx	170.6	198.5	—	213.6	238.0	239.2
sacrum	170.6	198.5	—	213.6	238.0	239.2
sternum	170.3	198.5	—	213.3	238.0	239.2
tarsus (any)	170.8	198.5	—	213.8	238.0	239.2
temporal	170.0	198.5	—	213.0	238.0	239.2
thumb	170.5	198.5	—	213.5	238.0	239.2
tibia (any part)	170.7	198.5	—	213.7	238.0	239.2
toe (any)	170.8	198.5	—	213.8	238.0	239.2
trapezium	170.5	198.5	—	213.5	238.0	239.2
trapezoid	170.5	198.5	—	213.5	238.0	239.2
turbinate	170.0	198.5	—	213.0	238.0	239.2
ulna (any part)	170.4	198.5	—	213.4	238.0	239.2
unciform	170.5	198.5	—	213.5	238.0	239.2
vertebra (column)	170.2	198.5	—	213.2	238.0	239.2
coccyx	170.6	198.5	—	213.6	238.0	239.2
sacrum	170.6	198.5	—	213.6	238.0	239.2
vomer	170.0	198.5	—	213.0	238.0	239.2
wrist	170.5	198.5	—	213.5	238.0	239.2
xiphoid process	170.3	198.5	—	213.3	238.0	239.2
zygomatic	170.0	198.5	—	213.0	238.0	239.2

	Malignant					
	Primary	Secondary	Ca in situ	Benign	Uncertain Behavior	Unspecified
book-leaf (mouth)	145.8	198.89	230.0	210.4	235.1	239.0
bowel—*see* Neoplasm, intestine						
brachial plexus	171.2	198.89	—	215.2	238.1	239.2
brain NEC	191.9	198.3	—	225.0	237.5	239.6
basal ganglia	191.0	198.3	—	225.0	237.5	239.6
cerebellopontine angle	191.6	198.3	—	225.0	237.5	239.6
cerebellum NOS	191.6	198.3	—	225.0	237.5	239.6
cerebrum	191.0	198.3	—	225.0	237.5	239.6
choroid plexus	191.5	198.3	—	225.0	237.5	239.6
contiguous sites	191.8	—	—	—	—	—
corpus callosum	191.8	198.3	—	225.0	237.5	239.6
corpus striatum	191.0	198.3	—	225.0	237.5	239.6
cortex (cerebral)	191.0	198.3	—	225.0	237.5	239.6
frontal lobe	191.1	198.3	—	225.0	237.5	239.6
globus pallidus	191.0	198.3	—	225.0	237.5	239.6
hippocampus	191.2	198.3	—	225.0	237.5	239.6
hypothalamus	191.0	198.3	—	225.0	237.5	239.6
internal capsule	191.0	198.3	—	225.0	237.5	239.6
medulla oblongata	191.7	198.3	—	225.0	237.5	239.6
meninges	192.1	198.4	—	225.2	237.6	239.7
midbrain	191.7	198.3	—	225.0	237.5	239.6
occipital lobe	191.4	198.3	—	225.0	237.5	239.6
parietal lobe	191.3	198.3	—	225.0	237.5	239.6
peduncle	191.7	198.3	—	225.0	237.5	239.6
pons	191.7	198.3	—	225.0	237.5	239.6
stem	191.7	198.3	—	225.0	237.5	239.6
tapetum	191.8	198.3	—	225.0	237.5	239.6
temporal lobe	191.2	198.3	—	225.0	237.5	239.6
thalamus	191.0	198.3	—	225.0	237.5	239.6
uncus	191.2	198.3	—	225.0	237.5	239.6
ventricle (floor)	191.5	198.3	—	225.0	237.5	239.6
branchial (cleft) (vestiges)	146.8	198.89	230.0	210.6	235.1	239.0
breast (connective tissue) (female)						
(glandular tissue) (soft parts)	174.9	198.81	233.0	217	238.3	239.3
areola	174.0	198.81	233.0	217	238.3	239.3
male	175.0	198.81	233.0	217	238.3	239.3
axillary tail	174.6	198.81	233.0	217	238.3	239.3
central portion	174.1	198.81	233.0	217	238.3	239.3
contiguous sites	174.8	—	—	—	—	—
ectopic sites	174.8	198.81	233.0	217	238.3	239.3
inner	174.8	198.81	233.0	217	238.3	239.3
lower	174.8	198.81	233.0	217	238.3	239.3
lower-inner quadrant	174.3	198.81	233.0	217	238.3	239.3
lower-outer quadrant	174.5	198.81	233.0	217	238.3	239.3
male	175.9	198.81	233.0	217	238.3	239.3
areola	175.0	198.81	233.0	217	238.3	239.3
ectopic tissue	175.9	198.81	233.0	217	238.3	239.3
nipple	175.0	198.81	233.0	217	238.3	239.3
mastectomy site (skin)	173.5	198.2	—	—	—	—
specified as breast tissue	174.8	198.81	—	—	—	—
midline	174.8	198.81	233.0	217	238.3	239.3
nipple	174.0	198.81	233.0	217	238.3	239.3
male	175.0	198.81	233.0	217	238.3	239.3
outer	174.8	198.81	233.0	217	238.3	239.3
skin	173.5	198.2	232.5	216.5	238.2	239.2
tail (axillary)	174.6	198.81	233.0	217	238.3	239.3
upper	174.8	198.81	233.0	217	238.3	239.3
upper-inner quadrant	174.2	198.81	233.0	217	238.3	239.3
upper-outer quadrant	174.4	198.81	233.0	217	238.3	239.3
broad ligament	183.3	198.82	233.3	221.0	236.3	239.5
bronchiogenic, bronchogenic (lung)	162.9	197.0	231.2	212.3	235.7	239.1
bronchiole	162.9	197.0	231.2	212.3	235.7	239.1

	Malignant					
	Primary	Secondary	Ca in situ	Benign	Uncertain Behavior	Unspecified
bronchus	162.9	197.0	231.2	212.3	235.7	239.1
carina	162.2	197.0	231.2	212.3	235.7	239.1
contiguous sites with lung or trachea	162.8	—	—	—	—	—
lower lobe of lung	162.5	197.0	231.2	212.3	235.7	239.1
main	162.2	197.0	231.2	212.3	235.7	239.1
middle lobe of lung	162.4	197.0	231.2	212.3	235.7	239.1
upper lobe of lung	162.3	197.0	231.2	212.3	235.7	239.1
brow	173.3	198.2	232.3	216.3	238.2	239.2
buccal (cavity)	145.9	198.89	230.0	210.4	235.1	239.0
commissure	145.0	198.89	230.0	210.4	235.1	239.0
groove (lower) (upper)	145.1	198.89	230.0	210.4	235.1	239.0
mucosa	145.0	198.89	230.0	210.4	235.1	239.0
sulcus (lower) (upper)	145.1	198.89	230.0	210.4	235.1	239.0
bulbourethral gland	189.3	198.1	233.9	223.81	236.99	239.5
bursa—see Neoplasm, connective tissue						
buttock NEC*	195.3	198.89	232.5	229.8	238.8	239.8
calf*	195.5	198.89	232.7	229.8	238.8	239.8
calvarium	170.0	198.5	—	213.0	238.0	239.2
calyx, renal	189.1	198.0	233.9	223.1	236.91	239.5
canal						
anal	154.2	197.5	230.5	211.4	235.5	239.0
auditory (external)	173.2	198.2	232.2	216.2	238.2	239.2
auricular (external)	173.2	198.2	232.2	216.2	238.2	239.2
canaliculi, biliary (biliferi) (intrahepatic)	155.1	197.8	230.8	211.5	235.3	239.0
canthus (eye) (inner) (outer)	173.1	198.2	232.1	216.1	238.2	239.2
capillary—see Neoplasm, connective tissue						
caput coli	153.4	197.5	230.3	211.3	235.2	239.0
cardia (gastric)	151.0	197.8	230.2	211.1	235.2	239.0
cardiac orifice (stomach)	151.0	197.8	230.2	211.1	235.2	239.0
cardio-esophageal junction	151.0	197.8	230.2	211.1	235.2	239.0
cardio-esophagus	151.0	197.8	230.2	211.1	235.2	239.0
carina (bronchus)	162.2	197.0	231.2	212.3	235.7	239.1
carotid (artery)	171.0	198.89	—	215.0	238.1	239.2
body	194.5	198.89	—	227.5	237.3	239.7
carpus (any bone)	170.5	198.5	—	213.5	238.0	239.2
cartilage (articular) (joint) NEC—see also						
Neoplasm, bone	170.9	198.5	—	213.9	238.0	239.2
arytenoid	161.3	197.3	231.0	212.1	235.6	239.1
auricular	171.0	198.89	—	215.0	238.1	239.2
bronchi	162.2	197.3	—	212.3	235.7	239.1
connective tissue—see Neoplasm, connective tissue						
costal	170.3	198.5	—	213.3	238.0	239.2
cricoid	161.3	197.3	231.0	212.1	235.6	239.1
cuneiform	161.3	197.3	231.0	212.1	235.6	239.1
ear (external)	171.0	198.89	—	215.0	238.1	239.2
ensiform	170.3	198.5	—	213.3	238.0	239.2
epiglottis	161.1	197.3	231.0	212.1	235.6	239.1
anterior surface	146.4	198.89	230.0	210.6	235.1	239.0
eyelid	171.0	198.89	—	215.0	238.1	239.2
intervertebral	170.2	198.5	—	213.2	238.0	239.2
larynx, laryngeal	161.3	197.3	231.0	212.1	235.6	239.1
nose, nasal	160.0	197.3	231.8	212.0	235.9	239.1
pinna	171.0	198.89	—	215.0	238.1	239.2
rib	170.3	198.5	—	213.3	238.0	239.2
semilunar (knee)	170.7	198.5	—	213.7	238.0	239.2
thyroid	161.3	197.3	231.0	212.1	235.6	239.1
trachea	162.0	197.3	231.1	212.2	235.7	239.1
cauda equina	192.2	198.3	—	225.3	237.5	239.7
cavity						
buccal	145.9	198.89	230.0	210.4	235.1	239.0
nasal	160.0	197.3	231.8	212.0	235.9	239.1
oral	145.9	198.89	230.0	210.4	235.1	239.0

| | Malignant | | | | | |
	Primary	Secondary	Ca in situ	Benign	Uncertain Behavior	Unspecified
cavity—*continued*						
peritoneal	158.9	197.6	—	211.8	235.4	239.0
tympanic	160.1	197.3	231.8	212.0	235.9	239.1
cecum	153.4	197.5	230.3	211.3	235.2	239.0
central						
nervous system—*see* Neoplasm,						
nervous system						
white matter	191.0	198.3	—	225.0	237.5	239.6
cerebellopontine (angle)	191.6	198.3	—	225.0	237.5	239.6
cerebellum, cerebellar	191.6	198.3	—	225.0	237.5	239.6
cerebrum, cerebral (cortex) (hemisphere)						
(white matter)	191.0	198.3	—	225.0	237.5	239.6
meninges	192.1	198.4	—	225.2	237.6	239.7
peduncle	191.7	198.3	—	225.0	237.5	239.6
ventricle (any)	191.5	198.3	—	225.0	237.5	239.6
cervical region	195.0	198.89	234.8	229.8	238.8	239.8
cervix (cervical) (uteri) (uterus)	180.9	198.82	233.1	219.0	236.0	239.5
canal	180.0	198.82	233.1	219.0	236.0	239.5
contiguous sites	180.8	—	—	—	—	—
endocervix (canal) (gland)	180.0	198.82	233.1	219.0	236.0	239.5
exocervix	180.1	198.82	233.1	219.0	236.0	239.5
external os	180.1	198.82	233.1	219.0	236.0	239.5
internal os	180.0	198.82	233.1	219.0	236.0	239.5
nabothian gland	180.0	198.82	233.1	219.0	236.0	239.5
squamocolumnar junction	180.8	198.82	233.1	219.0	236.0	239.5
stump	180.8	198.82	233.1	219.0	236.0	239.5
cheek	195.0	198.89	234.8	229.8	238.8	239.8
external	173.3	198.2	232.3	216.3	238.2	239.2
inner aspect	145.0	198.89	230.0	210.4	235.1	239.0
internal	145.0	198.89	230.0	210.4	235.1	239.0
mucosa	145.0	198.89	230.0	210.4	235.1	239.0
chest (wall) NEC	195.1	198.89	234.8	229.8	238.8	239.8
chiasma opticum	192.0	198.4	—	225.1	237.9	239.7
chin	173.3	198.2	232.3	216.3	238.2	239.2
choana	147.3	198.89	230.0	210.7	235.1	239.0
cholangiole	155.1	197.8	230.8	211.5	235.3	239.0
choledochal duct	156.1	197.8	230.8	211.5	235.3	239.0
choroid	190.6	198.4	234.0	224.6	238.8	239.8
plexus	191.5	198.3	—	225.0	237.5	239.6
ciliary body	190.0	198.4	234.0	224.0	238.8	239.8
clavicle	170.3	198.5	—	213.3	238.0	239.2
clitoris	184.3	198.82	233.3	221.2	236.3	239.5
clivus	170.0	198.5	—	213.0	238.0	239.2
cloacogenic zone	154.8	197.5	230.7	211.4	235.5	239.0
coccygeal						
body or glomus	194.6	198.89	—	227.6	237.3	239.7
vertebra	170.6	198.5	—	213.6	238.0	239.2
coccyx	170.6	198.5	—	213.6	238.0	239.2
colon—*see also* Neoplasm, intestine, large						
and rectum	154.0	197.5	230.4	211.4	235.2	239.0
column, spinal—*see* Neoplasm, spine						
columnella	173.3	198.2	232.3	216.3	238.2	239.2
commissure						
labial, lip	140.6	198.89	230.0	210.4	235.1	239.0
laryngeal	161.0	197.3	231.0	212.1	235.6	239.1
common (bile) duct	156.1	197.8	230.8	211.5	235.3	239.0
concha	173.2	198.2	232.2	216.2	238.2	239.2
nose	160.0	197.3	231.8	212.0	235.9	239.1
conjunctiva	190.3	198.4	234.0	224.3	238.8	239.8

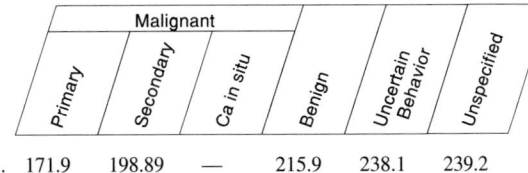

| | Malignant | | | | |
	Primary	Secondary	Ca in situ	Benign	Uncertain Behavior	Unspecified
connective tissue NEC	171.9	198.89	—	215.9	238.1	239.2

> *Note—For neoplasms of connective tissue (blood vessel, bursa, fasica, ligament, muscle, peripheral nerves, sympathetic and parasympathetic nerves, and ganglia, synovia, tendon, etc.) or of morphological types that indicate connective tissue, code according to the list under "Neoplasm, connective tissue;" for sites that do not appear in this list, code to neoplasm of that site; e.g.: liposarcoma, shoulder 171.2; leiomyosarcoma, stomach 151.9; neurofibroma, chest wall 215.4.*
>
> *Morphological types that indicate connective tissue appear in their proper place in the alphabetic index with the instruction "see Neoplasm, connective tissue..."*

	Primary	Secondary	Ca in situ	Benign	Uncertain Behavior	Unspecified
abdomen	171.5	198.89	—	215.5	238.1	239.2
abdominal wall	171.5	198.89	—	215.5	238.1	239.2
ankle	171.3	198.89	—	215.3	238.1	239.2
antecubital fossa or space	171.2	198.89	—	215.2	238.1	239.2
arm	171.2	198.89	—	215.2	238.1	239.2
auricle (ear)	171.0	198.89	—	215.0	238.1	239.2
axilla	171.4	198.89	—	215.4	238.1	239.2
back	171.7	198.89	—	215.7	238.1	239.2
breast (female) *(see also* Neoplasm, breast)	174.9	198.81	233.0	217	238.3	239.3
male	175.9	198.81	233.0	217	238.3	239.3
buttock	171.6	198.89	—	215.6	238.1	239.2
calf	171.3	198.89	—	215.3	238.1	239.2
cervical region	171.0	198.89	—	215.0	238.1	239.2
cheek	171.0	198.89	—	215.0	238.1	239.2
chest (wall)	171.4	198.89	—	215.4	238.1	239.2
chin	171.0	198.89	—	215.0	238.1	239.2
contiguous sites	171.8	—	—	—	—	—
diaphragm	171.4	198.89	—	215.4	238.1	239.2
ear (external)	171.0	198.89	—	215.0	238.1	239.2
elbow	171.2	198.89	—	215.2	238.1	239.2
extrarectal	171.6	198.89	—	215.6	238.1	239.2
extremity	171.8	198.89	—	215.8	238.1	239.2
lower	171.3	198.89	—	215.3	238.1	239.2
upper	171.2	198.89	—	215.2	238.1	239.2
eyelid	171.0	198.89	—	215.0	238.1	239.2
face	171.0	198.89	—	215.0	238.1	239.2
finger	171.2	198.89	—	215.2	238.1	239.2
flank	171.7	198.89	—	215.7	238.1	239.2
foot	171.3	198.89	—	215.3	238.1	239.2
forearm	171.2	198.89	—	215.2	238.1	239.2
forehead	171.0	198.89	—	215.0	238.1	239.2
gluteal region	171.6	198.89	—	215.6	238.1	239.2
great vessels NEC	171.4	198.89	—	215.4	238.1	239.2
groin	171.6	198.89	—	215.6	238.1	239.2
hand	171.2	198.89	—	215.2	238.1	239.2
head	171.0	198.89	—	215.0	238.1	239.2
heel	171.3	198.89	—	215.3	238.1	239.2
hip	171.3	198.89	—	215.3	238.1	239.2
hypochondrium	171.5	198.89	—	215.5	238.1	239.2
iliopsoas muscle	171.6	198.89	—	215.5	238.1	239.2
infraclavicular region	171.4	198.89	—	215.4	238.1	239.2
inguinal (canal) (region)	171.6	198.89	—	215.6	238.1	239.2
intrathoracic	171.4	198.89	—	215.4	238.1	239.2
ischorectal fossa	171.6	198.89	—	215.6	238.1	239.2
jaw	143.9	198.89	230.0	210.4	235.1	239.0
knee	171.3	198.89	—	215.3	238.1	239.2
leg	171.3	198.89	—	215.3	238.1	239.2

	Malignant					
	Primary	Secondary	Ca in situ	Benign	Uncertain Behavior	Unspecified
connective tissue—*continued*						
limb NEC	171.9	198.89	—	215.8	238.1	239.2
lower	171.3	198.89	—	215.3	238.1	239.2
upper	171.2	198.89	—	215.2	238.1	239.2
nates	171.6	198.89	—	215.6	238.1	239.2
neck	171.0	198.89	—	215.0	238.1	239.2
orbit	190.1	198.4	234.0	224.1	238.8	239.8
pararectal	171.6	198.89	—	215.6	238.1	239.2
para-urethral	171.6	198.89	—	215.6	238.1	239.2
paravaginal	171.6	198.89	—	215.6	238.1	239.2
pelvis (floor)	171.6	198.89	—	215.6	238.1	239.2
pelvo-abdominal	171.8	198.89	—	215.8	238.1	239.2
perineum	171.6	198.89	—	215.6	238.1	239.2
perirectal (tissue)	171.6	198.89	—	215.6	238.1	239.2
periurethral (tissue)	171.6	198.89	—	215.6	238.1	239.2
popliteal fossa or space	171.3	198.89	—	215.3	238.1	239.2
presacral	171.6	198.89	—	215.6	238.1	239.2
psoas muscle	171.5	198.89	—	215.5	238.1	239.2
pterygoid fossa	171.0	198.89	—	215.0	238.1	239.2
rectovaginal septum or wall	171.6	198.89	—	215.6	238.1	239.2
rectovesical	171.6	198.89	—	215.6	238.1	239.2
retroperitoneum	158.0	197.6	—	211.8	235.4	239.0
sacrococcygeal region	171.6	198.89	—	215.6	238.1	239.2
scalp	171.0	198.89	—	215.0	238.1	239.2
scapular region	171.4	198.89	—	215.4	238.1	239.2
shoulder	171.2	198.89	—	215.2	238.1	239.2
skin (dermis) NEC	173.9	198.2	232.9	216.9	238.2	239.2
submental	171.0	198.89	—	215.0	238.1	239.2
supraclavicular region	171.0	198.89	—	215.0	238.1	239.2
temple	171.0	198.89	—	215.0	238.1	239.2
temporal region	171.0	198.89	—	215.0	238.1	239.2
thigh	171.3	198.89	—	215.3	238.1	239.2
thoracic (duct) (wall)	171.4	198.89	—	215.4	238.1	239.2
thorax	171.4	198.89	—	215.4	238.1	239.2
thumb	171.2	198.89	—	215.2	238.1	239.2
toe	171.3	198.89	—	215.3	238.1	239.2
trunk	171.7	198.89	—	215.7	238.1	239.2
umbilicus	171.5	198.89	—	215.5	238.1	239.2
vesicorectal	171.6	198.89	—	215.6	238.1	239.2
wrist	171.2	198.89	—	215.2	238.1	239.2
conus medullaris	192.2	198.3	—	225.3	237.5	239.7
cord (true) (vocal)	161.0	197.3	231.0	212.1	235.6	239.1
false	161.1	197.3	231.0	212.1	235.6	239.1
spermatic	187.6	198.82	233.6	222.8	236.6	239.5
spinal (cervical) (lumbar) (thoracic)	192.2	198.3	—	225.3	237.5	239.7
cornea (limbus)	190.4	198.4	234.0	224.4	238.8	239.8
corpus						
albicans	183.0	198.6	233.3	220	236.2	239.5
callosum, brain	191.8	198.3	—	225.0	237.5	239.6
cavernosum	187.3	198.82	233.5	222.1	236.6	239.5
gastric	151.4	197.8	230.2	211.1	235.2	239.0
penis	187.3	198.82	233.5	222.1	236.6	239.5
striatum, cerebrum	191.0	198.3	—	225.0	237.5	239.6
uteri	182.0	198.82	233.2	219.1	236.0	239.5
isthmus	182.1	198.82	233.2	219.1	236.0	239.5
cortex						
adrenal	194.0	198.7	234.8	227.0	237.2	239.7
cerebral	191.0	198.3	—	225.0	237.5	239.6
costal cartilage	170.3	198.5	—	213.3	238.0	239.2
costovertebral joint	170.3	198.5	—	213.3	238.0	239.2

	Malignant					
	Primary	Secondary	Ca in situ	Benign	Uncertain Behavior	Unspecified
Cowper's gland	189.3	198.1	233.9	223.81	236.99	239.5
cranial (fossa, any)	191.9	198.3	—	225.0	237.5	239.6
meninges	192.1	198.4	—	225.2	237.6	239.7
nerve (any)	192.0	198.4	—	225.1	237.9	239.7
craniobuccal pouch	194.3	198.89	234.8	227.3	237.0	239.7
craniopharyngeal (duct) (pouch)	194.3	198.89	234.8	227.3	237.0	239.7
cricoid	148.0	198.89	230.0	210.8	235.1	239.0
cartilage	161.3	197.3	231.0	212.1	235.6	239.1
cricopharynx	148.0	198.89	230.0	210.8	235.1	239.0
crypt of Morgagni	154.8	197.5	230.7	211.4	235.2	239.0
crystalline lens	190.0	198.4	234.0	224.0	238.8	239.8
cul-de-sac (Douglas')	158.8	197.6	—	211.8	235.4	239.0
cuneiform cartilage	161.3	197.3	231.0	212.1	235.6	239.1
cutaneous—*see* Neoplasm, skin						
cutis—*see* Neoplasm, skin						
cystic (bile) duct (common)	156.1	197.8	230.8	211.5	235.3	239.0
dermis—*see* Neoplasm, skin						
diaphragm	171.4	198.89	—	215.4	238.1	239.2
digestive organs, system, tube, tract NEC	159.9	197.8	230.9	211.9	235.5	239.0
contiguous sites with peritoneum	159.8	—	—	—	—	—
disc, intervertebral	170.2	198.5	—	213.2	238.0	239.2
disease, generalized	199.0	199.0	234.9	229.9	238.9	199.0
disseminated	199.0	199.0	234.9	229.9	238.9	199.0
Douglas' cul-de-sac or pouch	158.8	197.6	—	211.8	235.4	239.0
duodenojejunal junction	152.8	197.4	230.7	211.2	235.2	239.0
duodenum	152.0	197.4	230.7	211.2	235.2	239.0
dura (cranial) (mater)	192.1	198.4	—	225.2	237.6	239.7
cerebral	192.1	198.4	—	225.2	237.6	239.7
spinal	192.3	198.4	—	225.4	237.6	239.7
ear (external)	173.2	198.2	232.2	216.2	238.2	239.2
auricle or auris	173.2	198.2	232.2	216.2	238.2	239.2
canal, external	173.2	198.2	232.2	216.2	238.2	239.2
cartilage	171.0	198.89	—	215.0	238.1	239.2
external meatus	173.2	198.2	232.2	216.2	238.2	239.2
inner	160.1	197.3	231.8	212.0	235.9	239.8
lobule	173.2	198.2	232.2	216.2	238.2	239.2
middle	160.1	197.3	231.8	212.0	235.9	239.8
contiguous sites with accessory sinuses or nasal cavities	160.8	—	—	—	—	—
skin	173.2	198.2	232.2	216.2	238.2	239.2
earlobe	173.2	198.2	232.2	216.2	238.2	239.2
ejaculatory duct	187.8	198.82	233.6	222.8	236.6	239.5
elbow NEC*	195.4	198.89	232.6	229.8	238.8	239.8
endocardium	164.1	198.89	—	212.7	238.8	239.8
endocervix (canal) (gland)	180.0	198.82	233.1	219.0	236.0	239.5
endocrine gland NEC	194.9	198.89	—	227.9	237.4	239.7
pluriglandular NEC	194.8	198.89	234.8	227.8	237.4	239.7
endometrium (gland) (stroma)	182.0	198.82	233.2	219.1	236.0	239.5
ensiform cartilage	170.3	198.5	—	213.3	238.0	239.2
enteric—*see* Neoplasm, intestine						
ependyma (brain)	191.5	198.3	—	225.0	237.5	239.6
epicardium	164.1	198.89	—	212.7	238.8	239.8
epididymis	187.5	198.82	233.6	222.3	236.6	239.5
epidural	192.9	198.4	—	225.9	237.9	239.7
epiglottis	161.1	197.3	231.0	212.1	235.6	239.1
anterior aspect or surface	146.4	198.89	230.0	210.6	235.1	239.0
cartilage	161.3	197.3	231.0	212.1	235.6	239.1
free border (margin)	146.4	198.89	230.0	210.6	235.1	239.0
junctional region	146.5	198.89	230.0	210.6	235.1	239.0
posterior (laryngeal) surface	161.1	197.3	231.0	212.1	235.6	239.1
suprahyoid portion	161.1	197.3	231.0	212.1	235.6	239.1

| | Malignant | | | | | |
	Primary	Secondary	Ca in situ	Benign	Uncertain Behavior	Unspecified
esophagogastric junction	151.0	197.8	230.2	211.1	235.2	239.0
esophagus	150.9	197.8	230.1	211.0	235.5	239.0
abdominal	150.2	197.8	230.1	211.0	235.5	239.0
cervical	150.0	197.8	230.1	211.0	235.5	239.0
contiguous sites	150.8	—	—	—	—	—
distal (third)	150.5	197.8	230.1	211.0	235.5	239.0
lower (third)	150.5	197.8	230.1	211.0	235.5	239.0
middle (third)	150.4	197.8	230.1	211.0	235.5	239.0
proximal (third)	150.3	197.8	230.1	211.0	235.5	239.0
specified part NEC	150.8	197.8	230.1	211.0	235.5	239.0
thoracic	150.1	197.8	230.1	211.0	235.5	239.0
upper (third)	150.3	197.8	230.1	211.0	235.5	239.0
ethmoid (sinus)	160.3	197.3	231.8	212.0	235.9	239.1
bone or labyrinth	170.0	198.5	—	213.0	238.0	239.2
Eustachian tube	160.1	197.3	231.8	212.0	235.9	239.1
exocervix	180.1	198.82	233.1	219.0	236.0	239.5
external						
meatus (ear)	173.2	198.2	232.2	216.2	238.2	239.2
os, cervix uteri	180.1	198.82	233.1	219.0	236.0	239.5
extradural	192.9	198.4	—	225.9	237.9	239.7
extrahepatic (bile) duct	156.1	197.8	230.8	211.5	235.3	239.0
contiguous sites with gallbladder	156.8	—	—	—	—	—
extraocular muscle	190.1	198.4	234.0	224.1	238.8	239.8
extrarectal	195.3	198.89	234.8	229.8	238.8	239.8
extremity*	195.8	198.89	232.8	229.8	238.8	239.8
lower*	195.5	198.89	232.7	229.8	238.8	239.8
upper*	195.4	198.89	232.6	229.8	238.8	239.8
eye NEC	190.9	198.4	234.0	224.9	238.8	239.8
contiguous sites	190.8	—	—	—	—	—
specified sites NEC	190.8	198.4	234.0	224.8	238.8	239.8
eyeball	190.0	198.4	234.0	224.0	238.8	239.8
eyebrow	173.3	198.2	232.3	216.3	238.2	239.2
eyelid (lower) (skin) (upper)	173.1	198.2	232.1	216.1	238.2	239.2
cartilage	171.0	198.89	—	215.0	238.1	239.2
face NEC*	195.0	198.89	232.3	229.8	238.8	239.8
fallopian tube (accessory)	183.2	198.82	233.3	221.0	236.3	239.5
falx (cerebelli) (cerebri)	192.1	198.4	—	225.2	237.6	239.7
fascia—*see also* Neoplasm, connective tissue						
palmar	171.2	198.89	—	215.2	238.1	239.2
plantar	171.3	198.89	—	215.3	238.1	239.2
fatty tissue—*see* Neoplasm, connective tissue						
fauces, faucial NEC	146.9	198.89	230.0	210.6	235.1	239.0
pillars	146.2	198.89	230.0	210.6	235.1	239.0
tonsil	146.0	198.89	230.0	210.5	235.1	239.0
femur (any part)	170.7	198.5	—	213.7	238.0	239.2
fetal membrane	181	198.82	233.2	219.8	236.1	239.5
fibrous tissue—*see* Neoplasm, connective tissue						
fibula (any part)	170.7	198.5	—	213.7	238.0	239.2
filum terminale	192.2	198.3	—	225.3	237.5	239.7
finger NEC*	195.4	198.89	232.6	229.8	238.8	239.8
flank NEC*	195.8	198.89	232.5	229.8	238.8	239.8
follicle, nabothian	180.0	198.82	233.1	219.0	236.0	239.5
foot NEC*	195.5	198.89	232.7	229.8	238.8	239.8
forearm NEC*	195.4	198.89	232.6	229.8	238.8	239.8
forehead (skin)	173.3	198.2	232.3	216.3	238.2	239.2
foreskin	187.1	198.82	233.5	222.1	236.6	239.5

	Malignant					
	Primary	Secondary	Ca in situ	Benign	Uncertain Behavior	Unspecified
fornix						
pharyngeal	147.3	198.89	230.0	210.7	235.1	239.0
vagina	184.0	198.82	233.3	221.1	236.3	239.5
fossa (of)						
anterior (cranial)	191.9	198.3	—	225.0	237.5	239.6
cranial	191.9	198.3	—	225.0	237.5	239.6
ischiorectal	195.3	198.89	234.8	229.8	238.8	239.8
middle (cranial)	191.9	198.3	—	225.0	237.5	239.6
pituitary	194.3	198.89	234.8	227.3	237.0	239.7
posterior (cranial)	191.9	198.3	—	225.0	237.5	239.6
pterygoid	171.0	198.89	—	215.0	238.1	239.2
pyriform	148.1	198.89	230.0	210.8	235.1	239.0
Rosenmüller	147.2	198.89	230.0	210.7	235.1	239.0
tonsillar	146.1	198.89	230.0	210.6	235.1	239.0
fourchette	184.4	198.82	233.3	221.2	236.3	239.5
frenulum						
labii—*see* Neoplasm, lip, internal						
linguae	141.3	198.89	230.0	210.1	235.1	239.0
frontal						
bone	170.0	198.5	—	213.0	238.0	239.2
lobe, brain	191.1	198.3	—	225.0	237.5	239.6
meninges	192.1	198.4	—	225.2	237.6	239.7
pole	191.1	198.3	—	225.0	237.5	239.6
sinus	160.4	197.3	231.8	212.0	235.9	239.1
fundus						
stomach	151.3	197.8	230.2	211.1	235.2	239.0
uterus	182.0	198.82	233.2	219.1	236.0	239.5
gall duct (extrahepatic)	156.1	197.8	230.8	211.5	235.3	239.0
intrahepatic	155.1	197.8	230.8	211.5	235.3	239.0
gallbladder	156.0	197.8	230.8	211.5	235.3	239.0
contiguous sites with extrahepatic						
bile ducts	156.8	—	—	—	—	—
ganglia (*see also* Neoplasm, connective						
tissue)	171.9	198.89	—	215.9	238.1	239.2
basal	191.0	198.3	—	225.0	237.5	239.6
ganglion (*see also* Neoplasm, connective						
tissue)	171.9	198.89	—	215.9	238.1	239.2
cranial nerve	192.0	198.4	—	225.1	237.9	239.7
Gartner's duct	184.0	198.82	233.3	221.1	236.3	239.5
gastric—*see* Neoplasm, stomach						
gastrocolic	159.8	197.8	230.9	211.9	235.5	239.0
gastroesophageal junction	151.0	197.8	230.2	211.1	235.2	239.0
gastrointestinal (tract) NEC	159.9	197.8	230.9	211.9	235.5	239.0
generalized	199.0	199.0	234.9	229.9	238.9	199.0
genital organ or tract						
female NEC	184.9	198.82	233.3	221.9	236.3	239.5
contiguous sites	184.8	—	—	—	—	—
specified site NEC	184.8	198.82	233.3	221.8	236.3	239.5
male NEC	187.9	198.82	233.6	222.9	236.6	239.5
contiguous sites	187.8	—	—	—	—	—
specified site NEC	187.8	198.82	233.6	222.8	236.6	239.5
genitourinary tract						
female	184.9	198.82	233.3	221.9	236.3	239.5
male	187.9	198.82	233.6	222.9	236.6	239.5
gingiva (alveolar) (marginal)	143.9	198.89	230.0	210.4	235.1	239.0
lower	143.1	198.89	230.0	210.4	235.1	239.0
mandibular	143.1	198.89	230.0	210.4	235.1	239.0
maxillary	143.0	198.89	230.0	210.4	235.1	239.0
upper	143.0	198.89	230.0	210.4	235.1	239.0

	Malignant					
	Primary	Secondary	Ca in situ	Benign	Uncertain Behavior	Unspecified
gland, glandular (lymphatic) (system)—						
see also Neoplasm, lymph gland						
endocrine NEC	194.9	198.89	—	227.9	237.4	239.7
salivary—see Neoplasm, salivary,						
gland						
glans penis	187.2	198.82	233.5	222.1	236.6	239.5
globus pallidus	191.0	198.3	—	225.0	237.5	239.6
glomus						
coccygeal	194.6	198.89	—	227.6	237.3	239.7
jugularis.	194.6	198.89	—	227.6	237.3	239.7
glosso-epiglottic fold(s)	146.4	198.89	230.0	210.6	235.1	239.0
glossopalatine fold	146.2	198.89	230.0	210.6	235.1	239.0
glossopharyngeal sulcus	146.1	198.89	230.0	210.6	235.1	239.0
glottis	161.0	197.3	231.0	212.1	235.6	239.1
gluteal region*	195.3	198.89	232.5	229.8	238.8	239.8
great vessels NEC	171.4	198.89	—	215.4	238.1	239.2
groin NEC*	195.3	198.89	232.5	229.8	238.8	239.8
gum	143.9	198.89	230.0	210.4	235.1	239.0
contiguous sites	143.8	—	—	—	—	—
lower	143.1	198.89	230.0	210.4	235.1	239.0
upper	143.0	198.89	230.0	210.4	235.1	239.0
hand NEC*	195.4	198.89	232.6	229.8	238.8	239.8
head NEC*	195.0	198.89	232.4	229.8	238.8	239.8
heart.	164.1	198.89	—	212.7	238.8	239.8
contiguous sites with mediastinum or						
thymus	164.8	—	—	—	—	—
heel NEC*	195.5	198.89	232.7	229.8	238.8	239.8
helix.	173.2	198.2	232.2	216.2	238.2	239.2
hematopoietic, hemopoietic tissue NEC .	202.8	198.89	—	—	—	238.7
hemisphere, cerebral	191.0	198.3	—	225.0	237.5	239.6
hemorrhoidal zone	154.2	197.5	230.5	211.4	235.5	239.0
hepatic	155.2	197.7	230.8	211.5	235.3	239.0
duct (bile).	156.1	197.8	230.8	211.5	235.3	239.0
flexure (colon)	153.0	197.5	230.3	211.3	235.2	239.0
primary	155.0	—	—	—	—	—
hilus of lung	162.2	197.0	231.2	212.3	235.7	239.1
hip NEC*	195.5	198.89	232.7	229.8	238.8	239.8
hippocampus, brain	191.2	198.3	—	225.0	237.5	239.6
humerus (any part)	170.4	198.5	—	213.4	238.0	239.2
hymen.	184.0	198.82	233.3	221.1	236.3	239.5
hypopharynx, hypopharyngeal NEC . . .	148.9	198.89	230.0	210.8	235.1	239.0
contiguous sites	148.8	—	—	—	—	—
postcricoid region	148.0	198.89	230.0	210.8	235.1	239.0
posterior wall	148.3	198.89	230.0	210.8	235.1	239.0
pyriform fossa (sinus)	148.1	198.89	230.0	210.8	235.1	239.0
specified site NEC	148.8	198.89	230.0	210.8	235.1	239.0
wall	148.9	198.89	230.0	210.8	235.1	239.0
posterior.	148.3	198.89	230.0	210.8	235.1	239.0
hypophysis	194.3	198.89	234.8	227.3	237.0	239.7
hypothalamus	191.0	198.3	—	225.0	237.5	239.6
ileocecum, ileocecal (coil, junction, valve)	153.4	197.5	230.3	211.3	235.2	239.0
ileum	152.2	197.4	230.7	211.2	235.2	239.0
ilium	170.6	198.5	—	213.6	238.0	239.2
immunoproliferative NEC	203.8	—	—	—	—	—
infraclavicular (region)*	195.1	198.89	232.5	229.8	238.8	239.8
inguinal (region)*	195.3	198.89	232.5	229.8	238.8	239.8
insula	191.0	198.3	—	225.0	237.5	239.6
insular tissue (pancreas)	157.4	197.8	230.9	211.7	235.5	239.0
brain.	191.0	198.3	—	225.0	237.5	239.6

	Malignant					
	Primary	Secondary	Ca in situ	Benign	Uncertain Behavior	Unspecified
interarytenoid fold	148.2	198.89	230.0	210.8	235.1	239.0
hypopharyngeal aspect	148.2	198.89	230.0	210.8	235.1	239.0
laryngeal aspect	161.1	197.3	231.0	212.1	235.6	239.1
marginal zone	148.2	198.89	230.0	210.8	235.1	239.0
interdental papillae	143.9	198.89	230.0	210.4	235.1	239.0
lower	143.1	198.89	230.0	210.4	235.1	239.0
upper	143.0	198.89	230.0	210.4	235.1	239.0
internal						
capsule	191.0	198.3	—	225.0	237.5	239.6
os (cervix)	180.0	198.82	233.1	219.0	236.0	239.5
intervertebral cartilage or disc	170.2	198.5	—	213.2	238.0	239.2
intestine, intestinal	159.0	197.8	230.7	211.9	235.2	239.0
large	153.9	197.5	230.3	211.3	235.2	239.0
appendix	153.5	197.5	230.3	211.3	235.2	239.0
caput coli	153.4	197.5	230.3	211.3	235.2	239.0
cecum	153.4	197.5	230.3	211.3	235.2	239.0
colon	153.9	197.5	230.3	211.3	235.2	239.0
and rectum	154.0	197.5	230.4	211.4	235.2	239.0
ascending	153.6	197.5	230.3	211.3	235.2	239.0
caput	153.4	197.5	230.3	211.3	235.2	239.0
contiguous sites	153.8	—	—	—	—	—
descending	153.2	197.5	230.3	211.3	235.2	239.0
distal	153.2	197.5	230.3	211.3	235.2	239.0
left	153.2	197.5	230.3	211.3	235.2	239.0
pelvic	153.3	197.5	230.3	211.3	235.2	239.0
right	153.6	197.5	230.3	211.3	235.2	239.0
sigmoid (flexure)	153.3	197.5	230.3	211.3	235.2	239.0
transverse	153.1	197.5	230.3	211.3	235.2	239.0
contiguous sites	153.8	—	—	—	—	—
hepatic flexure	153.0	197.5	230.3	211.3	235.2	239.0
ileocecum,ileocecal (coil, valve)	153.4	197.5	230.3	211.3	235.2	239.0
sigmoid flexure (lower) (upper)	153.3	197.5	230.3	211.3	235.2	239.0
splenic flexure	153.7	197.5	230.3	211.3	235.2	239.0
small	152.9	197.4	230.7	211.2	235.2	239.0
contiguous sites	152.8	—	—	—	—	—
duodenum	152.0	197.4	230.7	211.2	235.2	239.0
ileum	152.2	197.4	230.7	211.2	235.2	239.0
jejunum	152.1	197.4	230.7	211.2	235.2	239.0
tract NEC	159.0	197.8	230.7	211.9	235.2	239.0
intra-abdominal	195.2	198.89	234.8	229.8	238.8	239.8
intracranial NEC	191.9	198.3	—	225.0	237.5	239.6
intrahepatic (bile) duct	155.1	197.8	230.8	211.5	235.3	239.0
intraocular	190.0	198.4	234.0	224.0	238.8	239.8
intraorbital	190.1	198.4	234.0	224.1	238.8	239.8
intrasellar	194.3	198.89	234.8	227.3	237.0	239.7
intrathoracic (cavity) (organs NEC)	195.1	198.89	234.8	229.8	238.8	239.8
contiguous sites with respiratory						
organs	165.8	—	—	—	—	—
iris	190.0	198.4	234.0	224.0	238.8	239.8
ischiorectal (fossa)	195.3	198.89	234.8	229.8	238.8	239.8
ischium	170.6	198.5	—	213.6	238.0	239.2
island of Reil	191.0	198.3	—	225.0	237.5	239.6
islands or islets of Langerhans	157.4	197.8	230.9	211.7	235.5	239.0
isthmus uteri	182.1	198.82	233.2	219.1	236.0	239.5
jaw	195.0	198.89	234.8	229.8	238.8	239.8
bone	170.1	198.5	—	213.1	238.0	239.2
carcinoma	143.9	—	—	—	—	—
lower	143.1	—	—	—	—	—
upper	143.0	—	—	—	—	—
lower	170.1	198.5	—	213.1	238.0	239.2
upper	170.0	198.5	—	213.0	238.0	239.2

| | Malignant | | | | | |
	Primary	Secondary	Ca in situ	Benign	Uncertain Behavior	Unspecified
jaw—*continued*						
carcinoma (any type) (lower) (upper)	195.0	—	—	—	—	—
skin	173.3	198.2	232.3	216.3	238.2	239.2
soft tissues	143.9	198.89	230.0	210.4	235.1	239.0
lower	143.1	198.89	230.0	210.4	235.1	239.0
upper	143.0	198.89	230.0	210.4	235.1	239.0
jejunum	152.1	197.4	230.7	211.2	235.2	239.0
joint NEC *(see also* Neoplasm, bone)	170.9	198.5	—	213.9	238.0	239.2
acromioclavicular	170.4	198.5	—	213.4	238.0	239.2
bursa or synovial membrane—*see* Neoplasm, connective tissue						
costovertebral	170.3	198.5	—	213.3	238.0	239.2
sternocostal	170.3	198.5	—	213.3	238.0	239.2
temporomandibular	170.1	198.5	—	213.1	238.0	239.2
junction						
anorectal	154.8	197.5	230.7	211.4	235.5	239.0
cardioesophageal	151.0	197.8	230.2	211.1	235.2	239.0
esophagogastric	151.0	197.8	230.2	211.1	235.2	239.0
gastroesophageal	151.0	197.8	230.2	211.1	235.2	239.0
hard and soft palate	145.5	198.89	230.0	210.4	235.1	239.0
ileocecal	153.4	197.5	230.3	211.3	235.2	239.0
pelvirectal	154.0	197.5	230.4	211.4	235.2	239.0
pelviureteric	189.1	198.0	233.9	223.1	236.91	239.5
rectosigmoid	154.0	197.5	230.4	211.4	235.2	239.0
squamocolumnar, of cervix	180.8	198.82	233.1	219.0	236.0	239.5
kidney (parenchyma)	189.0	198.0	233.9	223.0	236.91	239.5
calyx	189.1	198.0	233.9	223.1	236.91	239.5
hilus	189.1	198.0	233.9	223.1	236.91	239.5
pelvis	189.1	198.0	233.9	223.1	236.91	239.5
knee NEC*	195.5	198.89	232.7	229.8	238.8	239.8
labia (skin)	184.4	198.82	233.3	221.2	236.3	239.5
majora	184.1	198.82	233.3	221.2	236.3	239.5
minora	184.2	198.82	233.3	221.2	236.3	239.5
labial—*see also* Neoplasm, lip						
sulcus (lower) (upper)	145.1	198.89	230.0	210.4	235.1	239.0
labium (skin)	184.4	198.82	233.3	221.2	236.3	239.5
majus	184.1	198.82	233.3	221.2	236.3	239.5
minus	184.2	198.82	233.3	221.2	236.3	239.5
lacrimal						
canaliculi	190.7	198.4	234.0	224.7	238.8	239.8
duct (nasal)	190.7	198.4	234.0	224.7	238.8	239.8
gland	190.2	198.4	234.0	224.2	238.8	239.8
punctum	190.7	198.4	234.0	224.7	238.8	239.8
sac	190.7	198.4	234.0	224.7	238.8	239.8
Langerhans, islands or islets	157.4	197.8	230.9	211.7	235.5	239.0
laryngopharynx	148.9	198.89	230.0	210.8	235.1	239.0
larynx, laryngeal NEC	161.9	197.3	231.0	212.1	235.6	239.1
aryepiglottic fold	161.1	197.3	231.0	212.1	235.6	239.1
cartilage (arytenoid) (cricoid) (cuneiform) (thyroid)	161.3	197.3	231.0	212.1	235.6	239.1
commissure (anterior) (posterior)	161.0	197.3	231.0	212.1	235.6	239.1
contiguous sites	161.8	—	—	—	—	—
extrinsic NEC	161.1	197.3	231.0	212.1	235.6	239.1
meaning hypopharynx	148.9	198.89	230.0	210.8	235.1	239.0
interarytenoid fold	161.1	197.3	231.0	212.1	235.6	239.1
intrinsic	161.0	197.3	231.0	212.1	235.6	239.1
ventricular band	161.1	197.3	231.0	212.1	235.6	239.1
leg NEC*	195.5	198.89	232.7	229.8	238.8	239.8
lens, crystalline	190.0	198.4	234.0	224.0	238.8	239.8

| | Malignant | | | | |
	Primary	Secondary	Ca in situ	Benign	Uncertain Behavior	Unspecified
lid (lower) (upper)	173.1	198.2	232.1	216.1	238.2	239.2
ligament—*see also* Neoplasm, connective tissue						
broad	183.3	198.82	233.3	221.0	236.3	239.5
Mackenrodt's	183.8	198.82	233.3	221.8	236.3	239.5
non-uterine—*see* Neoplasm, connective tissue						
round	183.5	198.82	—	221.0	236.3	239.5
sacro-uterine	183.4	198.82	—	221.0	236.3	239.5
uterine	183.4	198.82	—	221.0	236.3	239.5
utero-ovarian	183.8	198.82	233.3	221.8	236.3	239.5
uterosacral	183.4	198.82	—	221.0	236.3	239.5
limb*	195.8	198.89	232.8	229.8	238.8	239.8
lower*	195.5	198.89	232.7	229.8	238.8	239.8
upper*	195.4	198.89	232.6	229.8	238.8	239.8
limbus of cornea	190.4	198.4	234.0	224.4	238.8	239.8
lingual NEC *(see also* Neoplasm, tongue)	141.9	198.89	230.0	210.1	235.1	239.0
lingula, lung	162.3	197.0	231.2	212.3	235.7	239.1
lip (external) (lipstick area) (vermillion border)	140.9	198.89	230.0	210.0	235.1	239.0
buccal aspect—*see* Neoplasm, lip, internal						
commissure	140.6	198.89	230.0	210.4	235.1	239.0
contiguous sites	140.8	—	—	—	—	—
with oral cavity or pharynx	149.8	—	—	—	—	—
frenulum—*see* Neoplasm, lip, internal						
inner aspect—*see* Neoplasm, lip, internal						
internal (buccal) (frenulum) (mucosa) (oral)	140.5	198.89	230.0	210.0	235.1	239.0
lower	140.4	198.89	230.0	210.0	235.1	239.0
upper	140.3	198.89	230.0	210.0	235.1	239.0
lower	140.1	198.89	230.0	210.0	235.1	239.0
internal (buccal) (frenulum) (mucosa) (oral)	140.4	198.89	230.0	210.0	235.1	239.0
mucosa—*see* Neoplasm, lip, internal						
oral aspect—*see* Neoplasm, lip, internal						
skin (commissure) (lower) (upper) . .	173.0	198.2	232.0	216.0	238.2	239.2
upper	140.0	198.89	230.0	210.0	235.1	239.0
internal (buccal) (frenulum) (mucosa) (oral)	140.3	198.89	230.0	210.0	235.1	239.0
liver	155.2	197.7	230.8	211.5	235.3	239.0
primary	155.0	—	—	—	—	—
lobe						
azygos	162.3	197.0	231.2	212.3	235.7	239.1
frontal	191.1	198.3	—	225.0	237.5	239.6
lower	162.5	197.0	231.2	212.3	235.7	239.1
middle	162.4	197.0	231.2	212.3	235.7	239.1
occipital	191.4	198.3	—	225.0	237.5	239.6
parietal	191.3	198.3	—	225.0	237.5	239.6
temporal	191.2	198.3	—	225.0	237.5	239.6
upper	162.3	197.0	231.2	212.3	235.7	239.1
lumbosacral plexus	171.6	198.4	—	215.6	238.1	239.2
lung	162.9	197.0	231.2	212.3	235.7	239.1
azygos lobe	162.3	197.0	231.2	212.3	235.7	239.1
carina	162.2	197.0	231.2	212.3	235.7	239.1
contiguous sites with bronchus or trachea	162.8	—	—	—	—	—
hilus	162.2	197.0	231.2	212.3	235.7	239.1

| | Malignant | | | | | |
	Primary	Secondary	Ca in situ	Benign	Uncertain Behavior	Unspecified
lung—*continued*						
lingula	162.3	197.0	231.2	212.3	235.7	239.1
lobe NEC	162.9	197.0	231.2	212.3	235.7	239.1
lower lobe	162.5	197.0	231.2	212.3	235.7	239.1
main bronchus	162.2	197.0	231.2	212.3	235.7	239.1
middle lobe	162.4	197.0	231.2	212.3	235.7	239.1
upper lobe	162.3	197.0	231.2	212.3	235.7	239.1
lymph, lymphatic						
channel NEC *(see also* Neoplasm,						
connective tissue)	171.9	198.89	—	215.9	238.1	239.2
gland (secondary)	—	196.9	—	229.0	238.8	239.8
abdominal	—	196.2	—	229.0	238.8	239.8
aortic	—	196.2	—	229.0	238.8	239.8
arm	—	196.3	—	229.0	238.8	239.8
auricular (anterior) (posterior)	—	196.0	—	229.0	238.8	239.8
axilla, axillary	—	196.3	—	229.0	238.8	239.8
brachial	—	196.3	—	229.0	238.8	239.8
bronchial	—	196.1	—	229.0	238.8	239.8
bronchopulmonary	—	196.1	—	229.0	238.8	239.8
celiac	—	196.2	—	229.0	238.8	239.8
cervical	—	196.0	—	229.0	238.8	239.8
cervicofacial	—	196.0	—	229.0	238.8	239.8
Cloquet	—	196.5	—	229.0	238.8	239.8
colic	—	196.2	—	229.0	238.8	239.8
common duct	—	196.2	—	229.0	238.8	239.8
cubital	—	196.3	—	229.0	238.8	239.8
diaphragmatic	—	196.1	—	229.0	238.8	239.8
epigastric, inferior	—	196.6	—	229.0	238.8	239.8
epitrochlear	—	196.3	—	229.0	238.8	239.8
esophageal	—	196.1	—	229.0	238.8	239.8
face	—	196.0	—	229.0	238.8	239.8
femoral	—	196.5	—	229.0	238.8	239.8
gastric	—	196.2	—	229.0	238.8	239.8
groin	—	196.5	—	229.0	238.8	239.8
head	—	196.0	—	229.0	238.8	239.8
hepatic	—	196.2	—	229.0	238.8	239.8
hilar (pulmonary)	—	196.1	—	229.0	238.8	239.8
splenic	—	196.2	—	229.0	238.8	239.8
hypogastric	—	196.6	—	229.0	238.8	239.8
ileocolic	—	196.2	—	229.0	238.8	239.8
iliac	—	196.6	—	229.0	238.8	239.8
infraclavicular	—	196.3	—	229.0	238.8	239.8
inguina, inguinal	—	196.5	—	229.0	238.8	239.8
innominate	—	196.1	—	229.0	238.8	239.8
intercostal	—	196.1	—	229.0	238.8	239.8
intestinal	—	196.2	—	229.0	238.8	239.8
intrabdominal	—	196.2	—	229.0	238.8	239.8
intrapelvic	—	196.6	—	229.0	238.8	239.8
intrathoracic	—	196.1	—	229.0	238.8	239.9
jugular	—	196.0	—	229.0	238.8	239.8
leg	—	196.5	—	229.0	238.8	239.8
limb						
lower	—	196.5	—	229.0	238.8	239.8
upper	—	196.3	—	229.0	238.8	239.8
lower limb	—	196.5	—	229.0	238.8	238.9
lumbar	—	196.2	—	229.0	238.8	239.8
mandibular	—	196.0	—	229.0	238.8	239.8
mediastinal	—	196.1	—	229.0	238.8	239.8
mesenteric (inferior) (superior)	—	196.2	—	229.0	238.8	239.8
midcolic	—	196.2	—	229.0	238.8	239.8

| | Malignant | | | | | |
	Primary	Secondary	Ca in situ	Benign	Uncertain Behavior	Unspecified
lymph, lymphatic—*continued*						
multiple sites in categories						
196.0-196.6	—	196.8	—	229.0	238.8	239.8
neck	—	196.0	—	229.0	238.8	239.8
obturator	—	196.6	—	229.0	238.8	239.8
occipital	—	196.0	—	229.0	238.8	239.8
pancreatic	—	196.2	—	229.0	238.8	239.8
para-aortic	—	196.2	—	229.0	238.8	239.8
paracervical	—	196.6	—	229.0	238.8	239.8
parametrial	—	196.6	—	229.0	238.8	239.8
parasternal	—	196.1	—	229.0	238.8	239.8
parotid	—	196.0	—	229.0	238.8	239.8
pectoral	—	196.3	—	229.0	238.8	239.8
pelvic	—	196.6	—	229.0	238.8	239.8
peri-aortic	—	196.2	—	229.0	238.8	239.8
peripancreatic	—	196.2	—	229.0	238.8	239.8
popliteal	—	196.5	—	229.0	238.8	239.8
porta hepatis	—	196.2	—	229.0	238.8	239.8
portal	—	196.2	—	229.0	238.8	239.8
preauricular	—	196.0	—	229.0	238.8	239.8
prelaryngeal	—	196.0	—	229.0	238.8	239.8
presymphysial	—	196.6	—	229.0	238.8	239.8
pretracheal	—	196.0	—	229.0	238.8	239.8
primary (any site) NEC	202.9	—	—	—	—	—
pulmonary (hiler)	—	196.1	—	229.0	238.8	239.8
pyloric	—	196.2	—	229.0	238.8	239.8
retroperitoneal	—	196.2	—	229.0	238.8	239.8
retropharyngeal	—	196.0	—	229.0	238.8	239.8
Rosenmüller's	—	196.5	—	229.0	238.8	239.8
sacral	—	196.6	—	229.0	238.8	239.8
scalene	—	196.0	—	229.0	238.8	239.8
site NEC	—	196.9	—	229.0	238.8	239.8
splenic (hilar)	—	196.2	—	229.0	238.8	239.8
subclavicular	—	196.3	—	229.0	238.8	239.8
subinguinal	—	196.5	—	229.0	238.8	239.8
sublingual	—	196.0	—	229.0	238.8	239.8
submandibular	—	196.0	—	229.0	238.8	239.8
submaxillary	—	196.0	—	229.0	238.8	239.8
submental	—	196.0	—	229.0	238.8	239.8
subscapular	—	196.3	—	229.0	238.8	239.8
supraclavicular	—	196.0	—	229.0	238.8	239.8
thoracic	—	196.1	—	229.0	238.8	239.8
tibial	—	196.5	—	229.0	238.8	239.8
tracheal	—	196.1	—	229.0	238.8	239.8
tracheobronchial	—	196.1	—	229.0	238.8	239.8
upper limb	—	196.3	—	229.0	238.8	239.8
Virchow's	—	196.0	—	229.0	238.8	239.8
node—*see also* Neoplasm, lymph gland						
primary NEC	202.9	—	—	—	—	—
vessel (*see also* Neoplasm, connective						
tissue)	171.9	198.89	—	215.9	238.1	239.2
Mackenrodt's ligament	183.8	198.82	233.3	221.8	236.3	239.5
malar	170.0	198.5	—	213.0	238.0	239.2
region—*see* Neoplasm, cheek						
mammary gland—*see* Neoplasm, breast						
mandible	170.1	198.5	—	213.1	238.0	239.2
alveolar						
mucose	143.1	198.89	230.0	210.4	235.1	239.0
ridge or process	170.1	198.5	—	213.1	238.0	239.2
carcinoma	143.1	—	—	—	—	—
carcinoma	143.1	—	—	—	—	—

		Malignant				
	Primary	Secondary	Ca in situ	Benign	Uncertain Behavior	Unspecified
marrow (bone) NEC	202.9	198.5	—	—	—	238.7
mastectomy site (skin)	173.5	198.2	—	—	—	—
specified as breast tissue	174.8	198.81	—	—	—	—
mastoid (air cells) (antrum) (cavity)	160.1	197.3	231.8	212.0	235.9	239.1
bone or process	170.0	198.5	—	213.0	238.0	239.2
maxilla, maxillary (superior)	170.0	198.5	—	213.0	238.0	239.2
alveolar						
mucosa	143.0	198.89	230.0	210.4	235.1	239.0
ridge or process	170.0	198.5	—	213.0	238.0	239.2
carcinoma	143.0	—	—	—	—	—
antrum	160.2	197.3	231.8	212.0	235.9	239.1
carcinoma	143.0	—	—	—	—	—
inferior—*see* Neoplasm, mandible						
sinus	160.2	197.3	231.8	212.0	235.9	239.1
meatus						
external (ear)	173.2	198.2	232.2	216.2	238.2	239.2
Meckel's diverticulum	152.3	197.4	230.7	211.2	235.2	239.0
mediastinum, mediastinal	164.9	197.1	—	212.5	235.8	239.8
anterior	164.2	197.1	—	212.5	235.8	239.8
contiguous sites with heart and						
thymus	164.8	—	—	—	—	—
posterior	164.3	197.1	—	212.5	235.8	239.8
medulla						
adrenal	194.0	198.7	234.8	227.0	237.2	239.7
oblongata	191.7	198.3	—	225.0	237.5	239.6
meibomian gland	173.1	198.2	232.1	216.1	238.2	239.2
melanoma —*see* Melanoma						
meninges (brain) (cerebral) (cranial)						
(intracranial)	192.1	198.4	—	225.2	237.6	239.7
spinal (cord)	192.3	198.4	—	225.4	237.6	239.7
meniscus, knee joint (lateral) (medial)	170.7	198.5	—	213.7	238.0	239.2
mesentery, mesenteric	158.8	197.6	—	211.8	235.4	239.0
mesoappendix	158.8	197.6	—	211.8	235.4	239.0
mesocolon	158.8	197.6	—	211.8	235.4	239.0
mesopharynx—*see* Neoplasm, oropharynx						
mesosalpinx	183.3	198.82	233.3	221.0	236.3	239.5
mesovarium	183.3	198.82	233.3	221.0	236.3	239.5
metacarpus (any bone)	170.5	198.5	—	213.5	238.0	239.2
metastatic NEC—*see also* Neoplasm,						
by site, secondary	—	199.1	—	—	—	—
metatarsus (any bone)	170.8	198.5	—	213.8	238.0	239.2
midbrain	191.7	198.3	—	225.0	237.5	239.6
milk duct—*see* Neoplasm, breast						
mons						
pubis	184.4	198.82	233.3	221.2	236.3	239.5
veneris	184.4	198.82	233.3	221.2	236.3	239.5
motor tract	192.9	198.4	—	225.9	237.9	239.7
brain	191.9	198.3	—	225.0	237.5	239.6
spinal	192.2	198.3	—	225.3	237.5	239.7
mouth	145.9	198.89	230.0	210.4	235.1	239.0
contiguous sites	145.8	—	—	—	—	—
floor	144.9	198.89	230.0	210.3	235.1	239.0
anterior portion	144.0	198.89	230.0	210.3	235.1	239.0
contiguous sites	144.8	—	—	—	—	—
lateral portion	144.1	198.89	230.0	210.3	235.1	239.0
roof	145.5	198.89	230.0	210.4	235.1	239.0
specified part NEC	145.8	198.89	230.0	210.4	235.1	239.0
vestibule	145.1	198.89	230.0	210.4	235.1	239.0
mucosa						
alveolar (ridge or process)	143.9	198.89	230.0	210.4	235.1	239.0
lower	143.1	198.89	230.0	210.4	235.1	239.0
upper	143.0	198.89	230.0	210.4	235.1	239.0

| | Malignant | | | | | |
	Primary	Secondary	Ca in situ	Benign	Uncertain Behavior	Unspecified
mucosa—*continued*						
buccal	145.0	198.89	230.0	210.4	235.1	239.0
cheek	145.0	198.89	230.0	210.4	235.1	239.0
lip—*see* Neoplasm, lip, internal						
nasal	160.0	197.3	231.8	212.0	235.9	239.1
oral	145.0	198.89	230.0	210.4	235.1	239.0
Müllerian duct						
female	184.8	198.82	233.3	221.8	236.3	239.5
male	187.8	198.82	233.6	222.8	236.6	239.5
multiple sites NEC	199.0	199.0	234.9	229.9	238.9	199.0
muscle—*see also* Neoplasm, connective tissue						
extraocular	190.1	198.4	234.0	224.1	238.8	239.8
myocardium	164.1	198.89	—	212.7	238.8	239.8
myometrium	182.0	198.82	233.2	219.1	236.0	239.5
myopericardium	164.1	198.89	—	212.7	238.8	239.8
nabothian gland (follicle)	180.0	198.82	233.1	219.0	236.0	239.5
nail	173.9	198.2	232.9	216.9	238.2	239.2
finger	173.6	198.2	232.6	216.6	238.2	239.2
toe	173.7	198.2	232.7	216.7	238.2	239.2
nares, naris (anterior) (posterior)	160.0	197.3	231.8	212.0	235.9	239.1
nasal—*see* Neoplasm, nose						
nasolabial groove	173.3	198.2	232.3	216.3	238.2	239.2
nasolacrimal duct	190.7	198.4	234.0	224.7	238.8	239.8
nasopharynx, nasopharyngeal	147.9	198.89	230.0	210.7	235.1	239.0
contiguous sites	147.8	—	—	—	—	—
floor	147.3	198.89	230.0	210.7	235.1	239.0
roof	147.0	198.89	230.0	210.7	235.1	239.0
specified site NEC	147.8	198.89	230.0	210.7	235.1	239.0
wall	147.9	198.89	230.0	210.7	235.1	239.0
anterior	147.3	198.89	230.0	210.7	235.1	239.0
lateral	147.2	198.89	230.0	210.7	235.1	239.0
posterior	147.1	198.89	230.0	210.7	235.1	239.0
superior	147.0	198.89	230.0	210.7	235.1	239.0
nates	173.5	198.2	232.5	216.5	238.2	239.2
neck NEC*	195.0	198.89	234.8	229.8	238.8	239.8
nerve (autonomic) (ganglion) (parasympathetic) (peripheral) (sympathetic)—*see also* Neoplasm, connective tissue						
abducens	192.0	198.4	—	225.1	237.9	239.7
accessory (spinal)	192.0	198.4	—	225.1	237.9	239.7
acoustic	192.0	198.4	—	225.1	237.9	239.7
auditory	192.0	198.4	—	225.1	237.9	239.7
brachial	171.2	198.89	—	215.2	238.1	239.2
cranial (any)	192.0	198.4	—	225.1	237.9	239.7
facial	192.0	198.4	—	225.1	237.9	239.7
femoral	171.3	198.89	—	215.3	238.1	239.2
glossopharyngeal	192.0	198.4	—	225.1	237.9	239.7
hypoglossal	192.0	198.4	—	225.1	237.9	239.7
intercostal	171.4	198.89	—	215.4	238.1	239.2
lumbar	171.7	198.89	—	215.7	238.1	239.2
median	171.2	198.89	—	215.2	238.1	239.2
obturator	171.3	198.89	—	215.3	238.1	239.2
oculomotor	192.0	198.4	—	225.1	237.9	239.7
olfactory	192.0	198.4	—	225.1	237.9	239.7
optic	192.0	198.4	—	225.1	237.9	239.7
peripheral NEC	171.9	198.89	—	215.9	238.1	239.2
radial	171.2	198.89	—	215.2	238.1	239.2
sacral	171.6	198.89	—	215.6	238.1	239.2
sciatic	171.3	198.89	—	215.3	238.1	239.2
spinal NEC	171.9	198.89	—	215.9	238.1	239.2

	Malignant					
	Primary	Secondary	Ca in situ	Benign	Uncertain Behavior	Unspecified
nerve—*continued*						
trigeminal	192.0	198.4	—	225.1	237.9	239.7
trochlear	192.0	198.4	—	225.1	237.9	239.7
ulnar	171.2	198.89	—	215.2	238.1	239.2
vagus	192.0	198.4	—	225.1	237.9	239.7
nervous system (central) NEC	192.9	198.4	—	225.9	237.9	239.7
autonomic NEC	171.9	198.89	—	215.9	238.1	239.2
brain—*see also* Neoplasm, brain						
membrane or meninges	192.1	198.4	—	225.2	237.6	239.7
contiguous sites	192.8	—	—	—	—	—
parasympathetic NEC	171.9	198.89	—	215.9	238.1	239.2
sympathetic NEC	171.9	198.89	—	215.9	238.1	239.2
nipple (female)	174.0	198.81	233.0	217	238.3	239.3
male	175.0	198.81	233.0	217	238.3	239.3
nose, nasal	195.0	198.89	234.8	229.8	238.8	239.8
ala (external)	173.3	198.2	232.3	216.3	238.2	239.2
bone	170.0	198.5	—	213.0	238.0	239.2
cartilage	160.0	197.3	231.8	212.0	235.9	239.1
cavity	160.0	197.3	231.8	212.0	235.9	239.1
contiguous sites with accessory sinuses or middle ear	160.8	—	—	—	—	—
choana	147.3	198.89	230.0	210.7	235.1	239.0
external (skin)	173.3	198.2	232.3	216.3	238.2	239.2
fossa	160.0	197.3	231.8	212.0	235.9	239.1
internal	160.0	197.3	231.8	212.0	235.9	239.1
mucosa	160.0	197.3	231.8	212.0	235.9	239.1
septum	160.0	197.3	231.8	212.0	235.9	239.1
posterior margin	147.3	198.89	230.0	210.7	235.1	239.0
sinus—*see* Neoplasm, sinus						
skin	173.3	198.2	232.3	216.3	238.2	239.2
turbinate (mucosa)	160.0	197.3	231.8	212.0	235.9	239.1
bone	170.0	198.5	—	213.0	238.0	239.2
vestibule	160.0	197.3	231.8	212.0	235.9	239.1
nostril	160.0	197.3	231.8	212.0	235.9	239.1
nucleus pulposus	170.2	198.5	—	213.2	238.0	239.2
occipital						
bone	170.0	198.5	—	213.0	238.0	239.2
lobe or pole, brain	191.4	198.3	—	225.0	237.5	239.6
odontogenic—*see* Neoplasm, jaw bone						
oesophagus—*see* Neoplasm, esophagus						
olfactory nerve or bulb	192.0	198.4	—	225.1	237.9	239.7
olive (brain)	191.7	198.3	—	225.0	237.5	239.6
omentum	158.8	197.6	—	211.8	235.4	239.0
operculum (brain)	191.0	198.3	—	225.0	237.5	239.6
optic nerve, chiasm, or tract	192.0	198.4	—	225.1	237.9	239.7
oral (cavity)	145.9	198.89	230.0	210.4	235.1	239.0
contiguous sites with lip or pharynx	149.8	—	—	—	—	—
ill-defined	149.9	198.89	230.0	210.4	235.1	239.0
mucosa	145.9	198.89	230.0	210.4	235.1	239.0
orbit	190.1	198.4	234.0	224.1	238.8	239.8
bone	170.0	198.5	—	213.0	238.0	239.2
eye	190.1	198.4	234.0	224.1	238.8	239.8
soft parts	190.1	198.4	234.0	224.1	238.8	239.8
organ of Zuckerkandl	194.6	198.89	—	227.6	237.3	239.7
oropharynx	146.9	198.89	230.0	210.6	235.1	239.0
branchial cleft (vestige)	146.8	198.89	230.0	210.6	235.1	239.0
contiguous sites	146.8	—	—	—	—	—
junctional region	146.5	198.89	230.0	210.6	235.1	239.0
lateral wall	146.6	198.89	230.0	210.6	235.1	239.0
pillars of fauces	146.2	198.89	230.0	210.6	235.1	239.0

	Malignant					
	Primary	Secondary	Ca in situ	Benign	Uncertain Behavior	Unspecified
oropharynx—*continued*						
posterior wall	146.7	198.89	230.0	210.6	235.1	239.0
specified part NEC	146.8	198.89	230.0	210.6	235.1	239.0
vallecula	146.3	198.89	230.0	210.6	235.1	239.0
os						
external	180.1	198.82	233.1	219.0	236.0	239.5
internal	180.0	198.82	233.1	219.0	236.0	239.5
ovary	183.0	198.6	233.3	220	236.2	239.5
oviduct	183.2	198.82	233.3	221.0	236.3	239.5
palate	145.5	198.89	230.0	210.4	235.1	239.0
hard	145.2	198.89	230.0	210.4	235.1	239.0
junction of hard and soft palate	145.5	198.89	230.0	210.4	235.1	239.0
soft	145.3	198.89	230.0	210.4	235.1	239.0
nasopharyngeal surface	147.3	198.89	230.0	210.7	235.1	239.0
posterior surface	147.3	198.89	230.0	210.7	235.1	239.0
superior surface	147.3	198.89	230.0	210.7	235.1	239.0
palatoglossal arch	146.2	198.89	230.0	210.6	235.1	239.0
palatopharyngeal arch	146.2	198.89	230.0	210.6	235.1	239.0
pallium	191.0	198.3	—	225.0	237.5	239.6
palpebra	173.1	198.2	232.1	216.1	238.2	239.2
pancreas	157.9	197.8	230.9	211.6	235.5	239.0
body	157.1	197.8	230.9	211.6	235.5	239.0
contiguous sites	157.8	—	—	—	—	—
duct (of Santorini) (of Wirsung)	157.3	197.8	230.9	211.6	235.5	239.0
ectopic tissue	157.8	197.8	230.9	211.6	235.5	239.0
head	157.0	197.8	230.9	211.6	235.5	239.0
islet cells	157.4	197.8	230.9	211.7	235.5	239.0
neck	157.8	197.8	230.9	211.6	235.5	239.0
tail	157.2	197.8	230.9	211.6	235.5	239.0
para-aortic body	194.6	198.89	—	227.6	237.3	239.7
paraganglion NEC	194.6	198.89	—	227.6	237.3	239.7
parametrium	183.4	198.82	—	221.0	236.3	239.5
paranephric	158.0	197.6	—	211.8	235.4	239.0
pararectal	195.3	198.89	—	229.8	238.8	239.8
parasagittal (region)	195.0	198.89	234.8	229.8	238.8	239.8
parasellar	192.9	198.4	—	225.9	237.9	239.7
parathyroid (gland)	194.1	198.89	234.8	227.1	237.4	239.7
paraurethral	195.3	198.89	—	229.8	238.8	239.8
gland	189.4	198.1	233.9	223.89	236.99	239.5
paravaginal	195.3	198.89	—	229.8	238.8	239.8
parenchyma, kidney	189.0	198.0	233.9	223.0	236.91	239.5
parietal						
bone	170.0	198.5	—	213.0	238.0	239.2
lobe, brain	191.3	198.3	—	225.0	237.5	239.6
paroophoron	183.3	198.82	233.3	221.0	236.3	239.5
parotid (duct) (gland)	142.0	198.89	230.0	210.2	235.0	239.0
parovarium	183.3	198.82	233.3	221.0	236.3	239.5
patella	170.8	198.5	—	213.8	238.0	239.2
peduncle, cerebral	191.7	198.3	—	225.0	237.5	239.6
pelvirectal junction	154.0	197.5	230.4	211.4	235.2	239.0
pelvis, pelvic	195.3	198.89	234.8	229.8	238.8	239.8
bone	170.6	198.5	—	213.6	238.0	239.2
floor	195.3	198.89	234.8	229.8	238.8	239.8
renal	189.1	198.0	233.9	223.1	236.91	239.5
viscera	195.3	198.89	234.8	229.8	238.8	239.8
wall	195.3	198.89	234.8	229.8	238.8	239.8
pelvo-abdominal	195.8	198.89	234.8	229.8	238.8	239.8
penis	187.4	198.82	233.5	222.1	236.6	239.5
body	187.3	198.82	233.5	222.1	236.6	239.5
corpus (cavernosum)	187.3	198.82	233.5	222.1	236.6	239.5
glans	187.2	198.82	233.5	222.1	236.6	239.5
skin NEC	187.4	198.82	233.5	222.1	236.6	239.5

	Malignant					
	Primary	Secondary	Ca in situ	Benign	Uncertain Behavior	Unspecified
periadrenal (tissue)	158.0	197.6	—	211.8	235.4	239.0
perianal (skin)	173.5	198.2	232.5	216.5	238.2	239.2
pericardium	164.1	198.89	—	212.7	238.8	239.8
perinephric	158.0	197.6	—	211.8	235.4	239.0
perineum	195.3	198.89	234.8	229.8	238.8	239.8
periodontal tissue NEC	143.9	198.89	230.0	210.4	235.1	239.0
periosteum—see Neoplasm, bone						
peripancreatic	158.0	197.6	—	211.8	235.4	239.0
peripheral nerve NEC	171.9	198.89	—	215.9	238.1	239.2
perirectal (tissue)	195.3	198.89	—	229.8	238.8	239.8
perirenal (tissue)	158.0	197.6	—	211.8	235.4	239.0
peritoneum, peritoneal (cavity)	158.9	197.6	—	211.8	235.4	239.0
contiguous sites	158.8	—	—	—	—	—
with digestive organs	159.8	—	—	—	—	—
parietal	158.8	197.6	—	211.8	235.4	239.0
pelvic	158.8	197.6	—	211.8	235.4	239.0
specified part NEC	158.8	197.6	—	211.8	235.4	239.0
peritonsillar (tissue)	195.0	198.89	234.8	229.8	238.8	239.8
periurethral tissue	195.3	198.89	—	229.8	238.8	239.8
phalanges	170.9	198.5	—	213.9	238.0	239.2
foot	170.8	198.5	—	213.8	238.0	239.2
hand	170.5	198.5	—	213.5	238.0	239.2
pharynx, pharyngeal	149.0	198.89	230.0	210.9	235.1	239.0
bursa	147.1	198.89	230.0	210.7	235.1	239.0
fornix	147.3	198.89	230.0	210.7	235.1	239.0
recess	147.2	198.89	230.0	210.7	235.1	239.0
region	149.0	198.89	230.0	210.9	235.1	239.0
tonsil	147.1	198.89	230.0	210.7	235.1	239.0
wall (lateral) (posterior)	149.0	198.89	230.0	210.9	235.1	239.0
pia mater (cerebral) (cranial)	192.1	198.4	—	225.2	237.6	239.7
spinal	192.3	198.4	—	225.4	237.6	239.7
pillars of fauces	146.2	198.89	230.0	210.6	235.1	239.0
pineal (body) (gland)	194.4	198.89	234.8	227.4	237.1	239.7
pinna (ear) NEC	173.2	198.2	232.2	216.2	238.2	239.2
cartilage	171.0	198.89	—	215.0	238.1	239.2
piriform fossa or sinus	148.1	198.89	230.0	210.8	235.1	239.0
pituitary (body) (fossa) (gland) (lobe) . .	194.3	198.89	234.8	227.3	237.0	239.7
placenta	181	198.82	233.2	219.8	236.1	239.5
pleura, pleural (cavity)	163.9	197.2	—	212.4	235.8	239.1
contiguous sites	163.8	—	—	—	—	—
parietal	163.0	197.2	—	212.4	235.8	239.1
visceral	163.1	197.2	—	212.4	235.8	239.1
plexus						
brachial	171.2	198.89	—	215.2	238.1	239.2
cervical	171.0	198.89	—	215.0	238.1	239.2
choroid	191.5	198.3	—	225.0	237.5	239.6
lumbosacral	171.6	198.89	—	215.6	238.1	239.2
sacral	171.6	198.89	—	215.6	238.1	239.2
pluri-endocrine	194.8	198.89	234.8	227.8	237.4	239.7
pole						
frontal	191.1	198.3	—	225.0	237.5	239.6
occipital	191.4	198.3	—	225.0	237.5	239.6
pons (varolii)	191.7	198.3	—	225.0	237.5	239.6
popliteal fossa or space*	195.5	198.89	234.8	229.8	238.8	239.8
postcricoid (region)	148.0	198.89	230.0	210.8	235.1	239.0
posterior fossa (cranial)	191.6	198.3	—	225.0	237.5	239.6
postnasal space	147.9	198.89	230.0	210.7	235.1	239.0
prepuce	187.1	198.82	233.5	222.1	236.6	239.5
prepylorus	151.1	197.8	230.2	211.1	235.2	239.0
presacral (region)	195.3	198.89	—	229.8	238.8	239.8

	Malignant					
	Primary	Secondary	Ca in situ	Benign	Uncertain Behavior	Unspecified
prostate (gland)	185	198.82	233.4	222.2	236.5	239.5
utricle	189.3	198.1	233.9	223.81	236.99	239.5
pterygoid fossa	171.0	198.89	—	215.0	238.1	239.2
pubic bone	170.6	198.5	—	213.6	238.0	239.2
pudenda, pudendum (female)	184.4	198.82	233.3	221.2	236.3	239.5
pulmonary	162.9	197.0	231.2	212.3	235.7	239.1
putamen	191.0	198.3	—	225.0	237.5	239.6
pyloric						
antrum	151.2	197.8	230.2	211.1	235.2	239.0
canal	151.1	197.8	230.2	211.1	235.2	239.0
pylorus	151.1	197.8	230.2	211.1	235.2	239.0
pyramid (brain)	191.7	198.3	—	225.0	237.5	239.6
pyriform fossa or sinus	148.1	198.89	230.0	210.8	235.1	239.0
radius (any part)	170.4	198.5	—	213.4	238.0	239.2
Rathke's pouch	194.3	198.89	234.8	227.3	237.0	239.7
rectosigmoid (colon) (junction)	154.0	197.5	230.4	211.4	235.2	239.0
contiguous sites with anus or rectum .	154.8	—	—	—	—	—
rectouterine pouch	158.8	197.6	—	211.8	235.4	239.0
rectovaginal septum or wall	195.3	198.89	234.8	229.8	238.8	239.8
rectovesical septum	195.3	198.89	234.8	229.8	238.8	239.8
rectum (ampulla)	154.1	197.5	230.4	211.4	235.2	239.0
and colon	154.0	197.5	230.4	211.4	235.2	239.0
contiguous sites with anus or						
rectosigmoid junction	154.8	—	—	—	—	—
renal	189.0	198.0	233.9	223.0	236.91	239.5
calyx	189.1	198.0	233.9	223.1	236.91	239.5
hilus	189.1	198.0	233.9	223.1	236.91	239.5
parenchyma	189.0	198.0	233.9	223.0	236.91	239.5
pelvis	189.1	198.0	233.9	223.1	236.91	239.5
respiratory						
organs or system NEC	165.9	197.3	231.9	212.9	235.9	239.1
contiguous sites with intrathoracic						
organs	165.8	—	—	—	—	—
specified sites NEC	165.8	197.3	231.8	212.8	235.9	239.1
tract NEC	165.9	197.3	231.9	212.9	235.9	239.1
upper	165.0	197.3	231.9	212.9	235.9	239.1
retina	190.5	198.4	234.0	224.5	238.8	239.8
retrobulbar	190.1	198.4	—	224.1	238.8	239.8
retrocecal	158.0	197.6	—	211.8	235.4	239.0
retromolar (area) (triangle) (trigone) . .	145.6	198.89	230.0	210.4	235.1	239.0
retro-orbital	195.0	198.89	234.8	229.8	238.8	239.8
retroperitoneal (space) (tissue)	158.0	197.6	—	211.8	235.4	239.0
contiguous sites	158.8	—	—	—	—	—
retroperitoneum	158.0	197.6	—	211.8	235.4	239.0
contiguous sites	158.8	—	—	—	—	—
retropharyngeal	149.0	198.89	230.0	210.9	235.1	239.0
retrovesical (septum)	195.3	198.89	234.8	229.8	238.8	239.8
rhinencephalon	191.0	198.3	—	225.0	237.5	239.6
rib	170.3	198.5	—	213.3	238.0	239.2
Rosenmüller's fossa	147.2	198.89	230.0	210.7	235.1	239.0
round ligament	183.5	198.82	—	221.0	236.3	239.5
sacrococcyx, sacrococcygeal	170.6	198.5	—	213.6	238.0	239.2
region	195.3	198.89	234.8	229.8	238.8	239.8
sacrouterine ligament	183.4	198.82	—	221.0	236.3	239.5
sacrum, sacral (vertebra)	170.6	198.5	—	213.6	238.0	239.2
salivary gland or duct (major)	142.9	198.89	230.0	210.2	235.0	239.0
contiguous sites	142.8	—	—	—	—	—
minor NEC	145.9	198.89	230.0	210.4	235.1	239.0
parotid	142.0	198.89	230.0	210.2	235.0	239.0
pluriglandular	142.8	198.89	230.0	210.2	235.0	239.0

	Malignant					
	Primary	Secondary	Ca in situ	Benign	Uncertain Behavior	Unspecified
salivary gland or duct (major)—*continued*						
sublingual	142.2	198.89	230.0	210.2	235.0	239.0
submandibular	142.1	198.89	230.0	210.2	235.0	239.0
submaxillary	142.1	198.89	230.0	210.2	235.0	239.0
salpinx (uterine)	183.2	198.82	233.3	221.0	236.3	239.5
Santorini's duct	157.3	197.8	230.9	211.6	235.5	239.0
scalp	173.4	198.2	232.4	216.4	238.2	239.2
scapula (any part)	170.4	198.5	—	213.4	238.0	239.2
scapular region	195.1	198.89	234.8	229.8	238.8	239.8
scar NEC *(see also* Neoplasm, skin) . .	173.9	198.2	232.9	216.9	238.2	239.2
sciatic nerve	171.3	198.89	—	215.3	238.1	239.2
sclera	190.0	198.4	234.0	224.0	238.8	239.8
scrotum (skin)	187.7	198.82	233.6	222.4	236.6	239.5
sebaceous gland—*see* Neoplasm, skin						
sella turcica	194.3	198.89	234.8	227.3	237.0	239.7
bone	170.0	198.5	—	213.0	238.0	239.2
semilunar cartilage (knee)	170.7	198.5	—	213.7	238.0	239.2
seminal vesicle	187.8	198.82	233.6	222.8	236.6	239.5
septum						
nasal	160.0	197.3	231.8	212.0	235.9	239.1
posterior margin	147.3	198.89	230.0	210.7	235.1	239.0
rectovaginal	195.3	198.89	234.8	229.8	238.8	239.8
rectovesical	195.3	198.89	234.8	229.8	238.8	239.8
urethrovaginal	184.9	198.82	233.3	221.9	236.3	239.5
vesicovaginal	184.9	198.82	233.3	221.9	236.3	239.5
shoulder NEC*	195.4	198.89	232.6	229.8	238.8	239.8
sigmoid flexure (lower) (upper)	153.3	197.5	230.3	211.3	235.2	239.0
sinus (accessory)	160.9	197.3	231.8	212.0	235.9	239.1
bone (any)	170.0	198.5	—	213.0	238.0	239.2
contiguous sites with middle ear or nasal cavities	160.8	—	—	—	—	—
ethmoidal	160.3	197.3	231.8	212.0	235.9	239.1
frontal	160.4	197.3	231.8	212.0	235.9	239.1
maxillary	160.2	197.3	231.8	212.0	235.9	239.1
nasal, paranasal NEC	160.9	197.3	231.8	212.0	235.9	239.1
pyriform	148.1	198.89	230.0	210.8	235.1	239.0
sphenoidal	160.5	197.3	231.8	212.0	235.9	239.1
skeleton, skeletal NEC	170.9	198.5	—	213.9	238.0	239.2
Skene's gland	189.4	198.1	233.9	223.89	236.99	239.5
skin NEC	173.9	198.2	232.9	216.9	238.2	239.2
abdominal wall	173.5	198.2	232.5	216.5	238.2	239.2
ala nasi	173.3	198.2	232.3	216.3	238.2	239.2
ankle	173.7	198.2	232.7	216.7	238.2	239.2
antecubital space	173.6	198.2	232.6	216.6	238.2	239.2
anus	173.5	198.2	232.5	216.5	238.2	239.2
arm	173.6	198.2	232.6	216.6	238.2	239.2
auditory canal (external)	173.2	198.2	232.2	216.2	238.2	239.2
auricle (ear)	173.2	198.2	232.2	216.2	238.2	239.2
auricular canal (external)	173.2	198.2	232.2	216.2	238.2	239.2
axilla, axillary fold	173.5	198.2	232.5	216.5	238.2	239.2
back	173.5	198.2	232.5	216.5	238.2	239.2
breast	173.5	198.2	232.5	216.5	238.2	239.2
brow	173.3	198.2	232.3	216.3	238.2	239.2
buttock	173.5	198.2	232.5	216.5	238.2	239.2
calf	173.7	198.2	232.7	216.7	238.2	239.2
canthus (eye) (inner) (outer)	173.1	198.2	232.1	216.1	238.2	239.2
cervical region	173.4	198.2	232.4	216.4	238.2	239.2
cheek (external)	173.3	198.2	232.3	216.3	238.2	239.2
chest (wall)	173.5	198.2	232.5	216.5	238.2	239.2
chin	173.3	198.2	232.3	216.3	238.2	239.2

| | Malignant | | | | |
	Primary	Secondary	Ca in situ	Benign	Uncertain Behavior	Unspecified
skin NEC—*continued*						
clavicular area	173.5	198.2	232.5	216.5	238.2	239.2
clitoris	184.3	198.82	233.3	221.2	236.3	239.5
columnella	173.3	198.2	232.3	216.3	238.2	239.2
concha	173.2	198.2	232.2	216.2	238.2	239.2
contiguous sites	173.8	—	—	—	—	—
ear (external)	173.2	198.2	232.2	216.2	238.2	239.2
elbow	173.6	198.2	232.6	216.6	238.2	239.2
eyebrow	173.3	198.2	232.3	216.3	238.2	239.2
eyelid	173.1	198.2	232.1	216.1	238.2	239.2
face NEC	173.3	198.2	232.3	216.3	238.2	239.2
female genital organs (external)	184.4	198.82	233.3	221.2	236.3	239.5
clitoris	184.3	198.82	233.3	221.2	236.3	239.5
labium NEC	184.4	198.82	233.3	221.2	236.3	239.5
majus	184.1	198.82	233.3	221.2	236.3	239.5
minus	184.2	198.82	233.3	221.2	236.3	239.5
pudendum	184.4	198.82	233.3	221.2	236.3	239.5
vulva	184.4	198.82	233.3	221.2	236.3	239.5
finger	173.6	198.2	232.6	216.6	238.2	239.2
flank	173.5	198.2	232.5	216.5	238.2	239.2
foot	173.7	198.2	232.7	216.7	238.2	239.2
forearm	173.6	198.2	232.6	216.6	238.2	239.2
forehead	173.3	198.2	232.3	216.3	238.2	239.2
glabella	173.3	198.2	232.3	216.3	238.2	239.2
gluteal region	173.5	198.2	232.5	216.5	238.2	239.2
groin	173.5	198.2	232.5	216.5	238.2	239.2
hand	173.6	198.2	232.6	216.6	238.2	239.2
head NEC	173.4	198.2	232.4	216.4	238.2	239.2
heel	173.7	198.2	232.7	216.7	238.2	239.2
helix	173.2	198.2	232.2	216.2	238.2	239.2
hip	173.7	198.2	232.7	216.7	238.2	239.2
infraclavicular region	173.5	198.2	232.5	216.5	238.2	239.2
inguinal region	173.5	198.2	232.5	216.5	238.2	239.2
jaw	173.3	198.2	232.3	216.3	238.2	239.2
knee	173.7	198.2	232.7	216.7	238.2	239.2
labia						
majora	184.1	198.82	233.3	221.2	236.3	239.5
minora	184.2	198.82	233.3	221.2	236.3	239.5
leg	173.7	198.2	232.7	216.7	238.2	239.2
lid (lower) (upper)	173.1	198.2	232.1	216.1	238.2	239.2
limb NEC	173.9	198.2	232.9	216.9	238.2	239.5
lower	173.7	198.2	232.7	216.7	238.2	239.2
upper	173.6	198.2	232.6	216.6	238.2	239.2
lip (lower) (upper)	173.0	198.2	232.0	216.0	238.2	239.2
male genital organs	187.9	198.82	233.6	222.9	236.6	239.5
penis	187.4	198.82	233.5	222.1	236.6	239.5
prepuce	187.1	198.82	233.5	222.1	236.6	239.5
scrotum	187.7	198.82	233.6	222.4	236.6	239.5
mastectomy site	173.5	198.2	—	—	—	—
specified as breast tissue	174.8	198.81	—	—	—	—
meatus, acoustic (external)	173.2	198.2	232.2	216.2	238.2	239.2
melanoma —*see* Melanoma						
nates	173.5	198.2	232.5	216.5	238.2	239.2
neck	173.4	198.2	232.4	216.4	238.2	239.2
nose (external)	173.3	198.2	232.3	216.3	238.2	239.2
palm	173.6	198.2	232.6	216.6	238.2	239.2
palpebra	173.1	198.2	232.1	216.1	238.2	239.2
penis NEC	187.4	198.82	233.5	222.1	236.6	239.5
perianal	173.5	198.2	232.5	216.5	238.2	239.2
perineum	173.5	198.2	232.5	216.5	238.2	239.2

| | Malignant | | | | | |
	Primary	Secondary	Ca in situ	Benign	Uncertain Behavior	Unspecified
skin NEC—*continued*						
pinna	173.2	198.2	232.2	216.2	238.2	239.2
plantar	173.7	198.2	232.7	216.7	238.2	239.2
popliteal fossa or space	173.7	198.2	232.7	216.7	238.2	239.2
prepuce	187.1	198.82	233.5	222.1	236.6	239.5
pubes	173.5	198.2	232.5	216.5	238.2	239.2
sacrococcygeal region	173.5	198.2	232.5	216.5	238.2	239.2
scalp	173.4	198.2	232.4	216.4	238.2	239.2
scapular region	173.5	198.2	232.5	216.5	238.2	239.2
scrotum	187.7	198.82	233.6	222.4	236.6	239.5
shoulder	173.6	198.2	232.6	216.6	238.2	239.2
sole (foot)	173.7	198.2	232.7	216.7	238.2	239.2
specified sites NEC	173.8	198.2	232.8	216.8	232.8	239.2
submammary fold	173.5	198.2	232.5	216.5	238.2	239.2
supraclavicular region	173.4	198.2	232.4	216.4	238.2	239.2
temple	173.3	198.2	232.3	216.3	238.2	239.2
thigh	173.7	198.2	232.7	216.7	238.2	239.2
thoracic wall	173.5	198.2	232.5	216.5	238.2	239.2
thumb	173.6	198.2	232.6	216.6	238.2	239.2
toe	173.7	198.2	232.7	216.7	238.2	239.2
tragus	173.2	198.2	232.2	216.2	238.2	239.2
trunk	173.5	198.2	232.5	216.5	238.2	239.2
umbilicus	173.5	198.2	232.5	216.5	238.2	239.2
vulva	184.4	198.82	233.3	221.2	236.3	239.5
wrist	173.6	198.2	232.6	216.6	238.2	239.2
skull	170.0	198.5	—	213.0	238.0	239.2
soft parts or tissues—*see* Neoplasm, connective tissue						
specified site NEC	195.8	198.89	234.8	229.8	238.8	239.8
spermatic cord	187.6	198.82	233.6	222.8	236.6	239.5
sphenoid	160.5	197.3	231.8	212.0	235.9	239.1
bone	170.0	198.5	—	213.0	238.0	239.2
sinus	160.5	197.3	231.8	212.0	235.9	239.1
sphincter						
anal	154.2	197.5	230.5	211.4	235.5	239.0
of Oddi	156.1	197.8	230.8	211.5	235.3	239.0
spine, spinal (column)	170.2	198.5	—	213.2	238.0	239.2
bulb	191.7	198.3	—	225.0	237.5	239.6
coccyx	170.6	198.5	—	213.6	238.0	239.2
cord (cervical) (lumbar) (sacral) (thoracic)	192.2	198.3	—	225.3	237.5	239.7
dura mater	192.3	198.4	—	225.4	237.6	239.7
lumbosacral	170.2	198.5	—	213.2	238.0	239.2
membrane	192.3	198.4	—	225.4	237.6	239.7
meninges	192.3	198.4	—	225.4	237.6	239.7
nerve (root)	171.9	198.89	—	215.9	238.1	239.2
pia mater	192.3	198.4	—	225.4	237.6	239.7
root	171.9	198.89	—	215.9	238.1	239.2
sacrum	170.6	198.5	—	213.6	238.0	239.2
spleen, splenic NEC	159.1	197.8	230.9	211.9	235.5	239.0
flexure (colon)	153.7	197.5	230.3	211.3	235.2	239.0
stem, brain	191.7	198.3	—	225.0	237.5	239.6
Stensen's duct	142.0	198.89	230.0	210.2	235.0	239.0
sternum	170.3	198.5	—	213.3	238.0	239.2
stomach	151.9	197.8	230.2	211.1	235.2	239.0
antrum (pyloric)	151.2	197.8	230.2	211.1	235.2	239.0
body	151.4	197.8	230.2	211.1	235.2	239.0
cardia	151.0	197.8	230.2	211.1	235.2	239.0
cardiac orifice	151.0	197.8	230.2	211.1	235.2	239.0
contiguous sites	151.8	—	—	—	—	—
corpus	151.4	197.8	230.2	211.1	235.2	239.0

	Malignant			Benign	Uncertain Behavior	Unspecified
	Primary	Secondary	Ca in situ	Benign	Uncertain Behavior	Unspecified
stomach—*continued*						
fundus	151.3	197.8	230.2	211.1	235.2	239.0
greater curvature NEC	151.6	197.8	230.2	211.1	235.2	239.0
lesser curvature NEC	151.5	197.8	230.2	211.1	235.2	239.0
prepylorus	151.1	197.8	230.2	211.1	235.2	239.0
pylorus	151.1	197.8	230.2	211.1	235.2	239.0
wall NEC	151.9	197.8	230.2	211.1	235.2	239.0
anterior NEC	151.8	197.8	230.2	211.1	235.2	239.0
posterior NEC	151.8	197.8	230.2	211.1	235.2	239.0
stroma, endometrial	182.0	198.82	233.2	219.1	236.0	239.5
stump, cervical	180.8	198.82	233.1	219.0	236.0	239.5
subcutaneous (nodule) (tissue) NEC—*see* Neoplasm, connective tissue						
subdural	192.1	198.4	—	225.2	237.6	239.7
subglottis, subglottic	161.2	197.3	231.0	212.1	235.6	239.1
sublingual	144.9	198.89	230.0	210.3	235.1	239.0
gland or duct	142.2	198.89	230.0	210.2	235.0	239.0
submandibular gland	142.1	198.89	230.0	210.2	235.0	239.0
submaxillary gland or duct	142.1	198.89	230.0	210.2	235.0	239.0
submental	195.0	198.89	234.8	229.8	238.8	239.8
subpleural	162.9	197.0	—	212.3	235.7	239.1
substernal	164.2	197.1	—	212.5	235.8	239.8
sudoriferous, sudoriparous gland, site unspecified	173.9	198.2	232.9	216.9	238.2	239.2
specified site—*see* Neoplasm, skin						
supraclavicular region	195.0	198.89	234.8	229.8	238.8	239.8
supraglottis	161.1	197.3	231.0	212.1	235.6	239.1
suprarenal (capsule) (cortex) (gland) (medulla)	194.0	198.7	234.8	227.0	237.2	239.7
suprasellar (region)	191.9	198.3	—	225.0	237.5	239.6
sweat gland (apocrine) (eccrine), site unspecified	173.9	198.2	232.9	216.9	238.2	239.2
specified site—*see* Neoplasm, skin						
sympathetic nerve or nervous system NEC	171.9	198.89	—	215.9	238.1	239.2
symphysis pubis	170.6	198.5	—	213.6	238.0	239.2
synovial membrane—*see* Neoplasm, connective tissue						
tapetum, brain	191.8	198.3	—	225.0	237.5	239.6
tarsus (any bone)	170.8	198.5	—	213.8	238.0	239.2
temple (skin)	173.3	198.2	232.3	216.3	238.2	239.2
temporal						
bone	170.0	198.5	—	213.0	238.0	239.2
lobe or pole	191.2	198.3	—	225.0	237.5	239.6
region	195.0	198.89	234.8	229.8	238.8	239.8
skin	173.3	198.2	232.3	216.3	238.2	239.2
tendon (sheath)—*see* Neoplasm, connective tissue						
tentorium (cerebelli)	192.1	198.4	—	225.2	237.6	239.7
testis, testes (descended) (scrotal)	186.9	198.82	233.6	222.0	236.4	239.5
ectopic	186.0	198.82	233.6	222.0	236.4	239.5
retained	186.0	198.82	233.6	222.0	236.4	239.5
undescended	186.0	198.82	233.6	222.0	236.4	239.5
thalamus	191.0	198.3	—	225.0	237.5	239.6
thigh NEC*	195.5	198.89	234.8	229.8	238.8	239.8
thorax, thoracic (cavity) (organs NEC)	195.1	198.89	234.8	229.8	238.8	239.8
duct	171.4	198.89	—	215.4	238.1	239.2
wall NEC	195.1	198.89	234.8	229.8	238.8	239.8
throat	149.0	198.89	230.0	210.9	235.1	239.0
thumb NEC*	195.4	198.89	232.6	229.8	238.8	239.8

	Malignant					
	Primary	Secondary	Ca in situ	Benign	Uncertain Behavior	Unspecified
thymus (gland)	164.0	198.89	—	212.6	235.8	239.8
contiguous sites with heart and						
mediastinum	164.8	—	—	—	—	—
thyroglossal duct	193	198.89	234.8	226	237.4	239.7
thyroid (gland)	193	198.89	234.8	226	237.4	239.7
cartilage	161.3	197.3	231.0	212.1	235.6	239.1
tibia (any part)	170.7	198.5	—	213.7	238.0	239.2
toe NEC*	195.5	198.89	232.7	229.8	238.8	239.8
tongue	141.9	198.89	230.0	210.1	235.1	239.0
anterior (two-thirds) NEC	141.4	198.89	230.0	210.1	235.1	239.0
dorsal surface	141.1	198.89	230.0	210.1	235.1	239.0
ventral surface	141.3	198.89	230.0	210.1	235.1	239.0
base (dorsal surface)	141.0	198.89	230.0	210.1	235.1	239.0
border (lateral)	141.2	198.89	230.0	210.1	235.1	239.0
contiguous sites	141.8	—	—	—	—	—
dorsal surface NEC	141.1	198.89	230.0	210.1	235.1	239.0
fixed part NEC	141.0	198.89	230.0	210.1	235.1	239.0
foramen cecum	141.1	198.89	230.0	210.1	235.1	239.0
frenulum linguae	141.3	198.89	230.0	210.1	235.1	239.0
junctional zone	141.5	198.89	230.0	210.1	235.1	239.0
margin (lateral)	141.2	198.89	230.0	210.1	235.1	239.0
midline NEC	141.1	198.89	230.0	210.1	235.1	239.0
mobile part NEC	141.4	198.89	230.0	210.1	235.1	239.0
posterior (third)	141.0	198.89	230.0	210.1	235.1	239.0
root	141.0	198.89	230.0	210.1	235.1	239.0
surface (dorsal)	141.1	198.89	230.0	210.1	235.1	239.0
base	141.0	198.89	230.0	210.1	235.1	239.0
ventral	141.3	198.89	230.0	210.1	235.1	239.0
tip	141.2	198.89	230.0	210.1	235.1	239.0
tonsil	141.6	198.89	230.0	210.1	235.1	239.0
tonsil	146.0	198.89	230.0	210.5	235.1	239.0
fauces, faucial	146.0	198.89	230.0	210.5	235.1	239.0
lingual	141.6	198.89	230.0	210.1	235.1	239.0
palatine	146.0	198.89	230.0	210.5	235.1	239.0
pharyngeal	147.1	198.89	230.0	210.7	235.1	239.0
pillar (anterior) (posterior)	146.2	198.89	230.0	210.6	235.1	239.0
tonsillar fossa	146.1	198.89	230.0	210.6	235.1	239.0
tooth socket NEC	143.9	198.89	230.0	210.4	235.1	239.0
trachea (cartilage) (mucosa)	162.0	197.3	231.1	212.2	235.7	239.1
contiguous sites with bronchus or lung	162.8	—	—	—	—	—
tracheobronchial	162.8	197.3	231.1	212.2	235.7	239.1
contiguous sites with lung	162.8	—	—	—	—	—
tragus	173.2	198.2	232.2	216.2	238.2	239.2
trunk NEC*	195.8	198.89	232.5	229.8	238.8	239.8
tubo-ovarian	183.8	198.82	233.3	221.8	236.3	239.5
tunica vaginalis	187.8	198.82	233.6	222.8	236.6	239.5
turbinate (bone)	170.0	198.5	—	213.0	238.0	239.2
nasal	160.0	197.3	231.8	212.0	235.9	239.1
tympanic cavity	160.1	197.3	231.8	212.0	235.9	239.1
ulna (any part)	170.4	198.5	—	213.4	238.0	239.2
umbilicus, umbilical	173.5	198.2	232.5	216.5	238.2	239.2
uncus, brain	191.2	198.3	—	225.0	237.5	239.6
unknown site or unspecified	199.1	199.1	234.9	229.9	238.9	239.9
urachus	188.7	198.1	233.7	223.3	236.7	239.4
ureter, ureteral	189.2	198.1	233.9	223.2	236.91	239.5
orifice (bladder)	188.6	198.1	233.7	223.3	236.7	239.4
ureter-bladder (junction)	188.6	198.1	233.7	223.3	236.7	239.4
urethra, urethral (gland)	189.3	198.1	233.9	223.81	236.99	239.5
orifice, internal	188.5	198.1	233.7	223.3	236.7	239.4
urethrovaginal (septum)	184.9	198.82	233.3	221.9	236.3	239.5

	Malignant					
	Primary	Secondary	Ca in situ	Benign	Uncertain Behavior	Unspecified
urinary organ or system NEC	189.9	198.1	233.9	223.9	236.99	239.5
bladder—*see* Neoplasm, bladder						
contiguous sites	189.8	—	—	—	—	—
specified sites NEC	189.8	198.1	233.9	223.89	236.99	239.5
utero-ovarian	183.8	198.82	233.3	221.8	236.3	239.5
ligament	183.3	198.82	—	221.0	236.3	239.5
uterosacral ligament	183.4	198.82	—	221.0	236.3	239.5
uterus, uteri, uterine	179	198.82	233.2	219.9	236.0	239.5
adnexa NEC	183.9	198.82	233.3	221.8	236.3	239.5
contiguous sites	183.8	—	—	—	—	—
body	182.0	198.82	233.2	219.1	236.0	239.5
contiguous sites	182.8	—	—	—	—	—
cervix	180.9	198.82	233.1	219.0	236.0	239.5
cornu	182.0	198.82	233.2	219.1	236.0	239.5
corpus	182.0	198.82	233.2	219.1	236.0	239.5
endocervix (canal) (gland)	180.0	198.82	233.1	219.0	236.0	239.5
endometrium	182.0	198.82	233.2	219.1	236.0	239.5
exocervix	180.1	198.82	233.1	219.0	236.0	239.5
external os	180.1	198.82	233.1	219.0	236.0	239.5
fundus	182.0	198.82	233.2	219.1	236.0	239.5
internal os	180.0	198.82	233.1	219.0	236.0	239.5
isthmus	182.1	198.82	233.2	219.1	236.0	239.5
ligament	183.4	198.82	—	221.0	236.3	239.5
broad	183.3	198.82	233.3	221.0	236.3	239.5
round	183.5	198.82	—	221.0	236.3	239.5
lower segment	182.1	198.82	233.2	219.1	236.0	239.5
myometrium	182.0	198.82	233.2	219.1	236.0	239.5
squamocolumnar junction	180.8	198.82	233.1	219.0	236.0	239.5
tube	183.2	198.82	233.3	221.0	236.3	239.5
utricle, prostatic	189.3	198.1	233.9	223.81	236.99	239.5
uveal tract	190.0	198.4	234.0	224.0	238.8	239.8
uvula	145.4	198.89	230.0	210.4	235.1	239.0
vagina, vaginal (fornix) (vault) (wall)	184.0	198.82	233.3	221.1	236.3	239.5
vaginovesical	184.9	198.82	233.3	221.9	236.3	239.5
septum	194.9	198.82	233.3	221.9	236.3	239.5
vallecula (epiglottis)	146.3	198.89	230.0	210.6	235.1	239.0
vascular—*see* Neoplasm, connective tissue						
vas deferens	187.6	198.82	233.6	222.8	236.6	239.5
Vater's ampulla	156.2	197.8	230.8	211.5	235.3	239.0
vein, venous—*see* Neoplasm, connective tissue						
vena cava (abdominal) (inferior)	171.5	198.89	—	215.5	238.1	239.2
superior	171.4	198.89	—	215.4	238.1	239.2
ventricle (cerebral) (floor) (fourth) (lateral) (third)	191.5	198.3	—	225.0	237.5	239.6
cardiac (left) (right)	164.1	198.89	—	212.7	238.8	239.8
ventricular band of larynx	161.1	197.3	231.0	212.1	235.6	239.1
ventriculus—*see* Neoplasm, stomach						
vermillion border—*see* Neoplasm, lip						
vermis, cerebellum	191.6	198.3	—	225.0	237.5	239.6
vertebra (column)	170.2	198.5	—	213.2	238.0	239.2
coccyx	170.6	198.5	—	213.6	238.0	239.2
sacrum	170.6	198.5	—	213.6	238.0	239.2
vesical—*see* Neoplasm, bladder						
vesicle, seminal	187.8	198.82	233.6	222.8	236.6	239.5
vesicocervical tissue	184.9	198.82	233.3	221.9	236.3	239.5
vesicorectal	195.3	198.89	234.8	229.8	238.8	239.8
vesicovaginal	184.9	198.82	233.3	221.9	236.3	239.5
septum	184.9	198.82	233.3	221.9	236.3	239.5
vessel (blood)—*see* Neoplasm, connective tissue						

	Malignant					
	Primary	Secondary	Ca in situ	Benign	Uncertain Behavior	Unspecified
vestibular gland, greater	184.1	198.82	233.3	221.2	236.3	239.5
vestibule						
mouth	145.1	198.89	230.0	210.4	235.1	239.0
nose	160.0	197.3	231.8	212.0	235.9	239.1
Virchow's gland	—	196.0	—	229.0	238.8	239.8
viscera NEC	195.8	198.89	234.8	229.8	238.8	239.8
vocal cords (true)	161.0	197.3	231.0	212.1	235.6	239.1
false	161.1	197.3	231.0	212.1	235.6	239.1
vomer	170.0	198.5	—	213.0	238.0	239.2
vulva	184.4	198.82	233.3	221.2	236.3	239.5
vulvovaginal gland	184.4	198.82	233.3	221.2	236.3	239.5
Waldeyer's ring	149.1	198.89	230.0	210.9	235.1	239.0
Wharton's duct	142.1	198.89	230.0	210.2	235.0	239.0
white matter (central) (cerebral)	191.0	198.3	—	225.0	237.5	239.6
windpipe	162.0	197.3	231.1	212.2	235.7	239.1
Wirsung's duct	157.3	197.8	230.9	211.6	235.5	239.0
wolffian (body) (duct)						
female	184.8	198.82	233.3	221.8	236.3	239.5
male	187.8	198.82	233.6	222.8	236.6	239.5
womb—*see* Neoplasm, uterus						
wrist NEC*	195.4	198.89	232.6	229.8	238.8	239.8
xiphoid process	170.3	198.5	—	213.3	238.0	239.2
Zuckerkandl's organ	194.6	198.89	—	227.6	237.3	239.7

Neovascularization
choroid 362.16
ciliary body 364.42
cornea 370.60
  deep 370.63
  localized 370.61
iris 364.42
retina 362.16
subretinal 362.16
Nephralgia 788.0
Nephritis, nephritic (albuminuric) (azotemic)
  (congenital) (degenerative) (diffuse)
  (disseminated) (epithelial) (familial) (focal)
  (granulomatous) (hemorrhagic) (infantile)
  (nonsuppurative, excretory) (uremic) 583.9
with
  edema—*see* Nephrosis
  lesion of
    glomerulonephritis
      hypocomplementemic persistent 583.2
        with nephrotic syndrome 581.2
        chronic 582.2
      lobular 583.2
        with nephrotic syndrome 581.2
        chronic 582.2
      membranoproliferative 583.2
        with nephrotic syndrome 581.2
        chronic 582.2
      membranous 583.1
        with nephrotic syndrome 581.1
        chronic 582.1
      mesangiocapillary 583.2
        with nephrotic syndrome 581.2
        chronic 582.2
      mixed membranous and proliferative 583.2
        with nephrotic syndrome 581.2
        chronic 582.2
      proliferative (diffuse) 583.0
        with nephrotic syndrome 581.0
        acute 580.0
        chronic 582.0
      rapidly progressive 583.4
        acute 580.4
        chronic 582.4
    interstitial nephritis (diffuse) (focal) 583.89
      with nephrotic syndrome 581.89
      acute 580.89
      chronic 582.89
    necrotizing glomerulitis 583.4
      acute 580.4
      chronic 582.4
    renal necrosis 583.9
      cortical 583.6
      medullary 583.7
    specified pathology NEC 583.89
      with nephrotic syndrome 581.89
      acute 580.89
      chronic 582.89
  necrosis, renal 583.9
    cortical 583.6
    medullary (papillary) 583.7
  nephrotic syndrome (*see also* Nephrosis) 581.9
  papillary necrosis 583.7
  specified pathology NEC 583.89
acute 580.9
  extracapillary with epithelial crescents 580.4
  hypertensive (*see also* Hypertension, kidney)
    403.90
  necrotizing 580.4
  poststreptococcal 580.0
  proliferative (diffuse) 580.0

Nephritis, nephritic—*continued*
  rapidly progressive 580.4
  specified pathology NEC 580.89
amyloid 277.3 *[583.81]*
  chronic 277.3 *[582.81]*
arteriolar (*see also* Hypertension, kidney) 403.90
arteriosclerotic (*see also* Hypertension, kidney)
  403.90
ascending (*see also* Pyelitis) 590.80
atrophic 582.9
basement membrane NEC 583.89
  with
    pulmonary hemorrhage (Goodpasture's
      syndrome) 446.21 *[583.81]*
calculous, calculus 592.0
cardiac (*see also* Hypertension, kidney) 403.90
cardiovascular (*see also* Hypertension, kidney)
  403.90
chronic 582.9
  arteriosclerotic (*see also* Hypertension,
    kidney) 403.90
  hypertensive (*see also* Hypertension, kidney)
    403.90
cirrhotic (*see also* Sclerosis, renal) 587
complicating pregnancy, childbirth, or
  puerperium 646.2
  with hypertension 642.1
    affecting fetus or newborn 760.0
  affecting fetus or newborn 760.1
croupous 580.9
desquamative—*see* Nephrosis
due to
  amyloidosis 277.3 *[583.81]*
    chronic 277.3 *[582.81]*
  arteriosclerosis (*see also* Hypertension,
    kidney) 403.90
  diabetes mellitus 250.4 *[583.81]*
    with nephrotic syndrome 250.4 *[581.81]*
  diphtheria 032.89 *[580.81]*
  gonococcal infection (acute) 098.19 *[583.81]*
    chronic or duration of 2 months or over
      098.39 *[583.81]*
  gout 274.10
  infectious hepatitis 070.9 *[580.81]*
  mumps 072.79 *[580.81]*
  specified kidney pathology NEC 583.89
    acute 580.89
    chronic 582.89
  streptotrichosis 039.8 *[583.81]*
  subacute bacterial endocarditis 421.0 *[580.81]*
  systemic lupus erythematosus 710.0 *[583.81]*
    chronic 710.0 *[582.81]*
  typhoid fever 002.0 *[580.81]*
endothelial 582.2
end stage (chronic) (terminal) NEC 585
epimembranous 581.1
exudative 583.89
  with nephrotic syndrome 581.89
  acute 580.89
  chronic 582.89
gonococcal (acute) 098.19 *[583.81]*
  chronic or duration of 2 months or over
    098.39 *[583.81]*
gouty 274.10
hereditary (Alport's syndrome) 759.89
hydremic—*see* Nephrosis
hypertensive (*see also* Hypertension, kidney)
  403.90
hypocomplementemic persistent 583.2
  with nephrotic syndrome 581.2
  chronic 582.2

Nephritis, nephritic—*continued*
  immune complex NEC 583.89
  infective (*see also* Pyelitis) 590.80
  interstitial (diffuse) (focal) 583.89
    with nephrotic syndrome 581.89
    acute 580.89
    chronic 582.89
  latent or quiescent—*see* Nephritis, chronic
  lead 984.9
    specified type of lead—*see* Table of drugs and
      chemicals
  lobular 583.2
    with nephrotic syndrome 581.2
    chronic 582.2
  lupus 710.0 *[583.81]*
    acute 710.0 *[580.81]*
    chronic 710.0 *[582.81]*
  membranoproliferative 583.2
    with nephrotic syndrome 581.2
    chronic 582.2
  membranous 583.1
    with nephrotic syndrome 581.1
    chronic 582.1
  mesangiocapillary 583.2
    with nephrotic syndrome 581.2
    chronic 582.2
  minimal change 581.3
  mixed membranous and proliferative 583.2
    with nephrotic syndrome 581.2
    chronic 582.2
  necrotic, necrotizing 583.4
    acute 580.4
    chronic 582.4
  nephrotic—*see* Nephrosis
  old—*see* Nephritis, chronic
  parenchymatous 581.89
  polycystic 753.12
    adult type (APKD) 753.13
    autosomal dominant 753.13
    autosomal recessive 753.14
    childhood type (CPKD) 753.14
    infantile type 753.14
  poststreptococcal 580.0
  pregnancy—*see* Nephritis, complicating
    pregnancy
  proliferative 583.0
    with nephrotic syndrome 581.0
    acute 580.0
    chronic 582.0
  purulent (*see also* Pyelitis) 590.80
  rapidly progressive 583.4
    acute 580.4
    chronic 582.4
  salt-losing or salt-wasting (*see also* Disease,
    renal) 593.9
  saturnine 984.9
    specified type of lead—*see* Table of drugs and
      chemicals
  septic (*see also* Pyelitis) 590.80
  specified pathology NEC 583.89
    acute 580.89
    chronic 582.89
  staphylococcal (*see also* Pyelitis) 590.80
  streptotrichosis 039.8 *[583.81]*
  subacute (*see also* Nephrosis) 581.9
  suppurative (*see also* Pyelitis) 590.80
  syphilitic (late) 095.4
    congenital 090.5 *[583.81]*
    early 091.69 *[583.81]*
  terminal (chronic) (end-stage) NEC 585
  toxic—*see* Nephritis, acute

Nephritis, nephritic—*continued*
  tubal, tubular—*see* Nephrosis, tubular
  tuberculous (*see also* Tuberculosis) 016.0
    [583.81]
  type II (Ellis)—*see* Nephrosis
  vascular—*see* Hypertension, kidney
  war 580.9
Nephroblastoma (M8960/3) 189.0
  epithelial (M8961/3) 189.0
  mesenchymal (M8962/3) 189.0
Nephrocalcinosis 275.49
Nephrocystitis, pustular (*see also* Pyelitis)
  590.80
Nephrolithiasis (congenital) (pelvis) (recurrent)
  592.0
  uric acid 274.11
Nephroma (M8960/3) 189.0
  mesoblastic (M8960/1) 236.9
Nephronephritis (*see also* Nephrosis) 581.9
Nephronopthisis 753.16
Nephropathy (*see also* Nephritis) 583.9
  with
    exudative nephritis 583.89
    interstitial nephritis (diffuse) (focal) 583.89
    medullary necrosis 583.7
    necrosis 583.9
      cortical 583.6
      medullary or papillary 583.7
    papillary necrosis 583.7
    specified lesion or cause NEC 583.89
  analgesic 583.89
    with medullary necrosis, acute 584.7
  arteriolar (*see also* Hypertension, kidney) 403.90
  arteriosclerotic (*see also* Hypertension, kidney)
    403.90
  complicating pregnancy 646.2
  diabetic 250.4 *[583.81]*
  gouty 274.10
    specified type NEC 274.19
  hypercalcemic 588.8
  hypertensive (*see also* Hypertension, kidney)
    403.90
  hypokalemic (vacuolar) 588.8
  obstructive 593.89
    congenital 753.20
  phenacetin 584.7
  phosphate-losing 588.0
  potassium depletion 588.8
  proliferative (*see also* Nephritis, proliferative)
    583.0
  protein-losing 588.8
  salt-losing or salt-wasting (*see also* Disease,
    renal) 593.9
  sickle-cell (*see also* Disease, sickle-cell) 282.60
    [583.81]
  toxic 584.5
  vasomotor 584.5
  water-losing 588.8
Nephroptosis (*see also* Disease, renal) 593.0
  congenital (displaced) 753.3
Nephropyosis (*see also* Abscess, kidney) 590.2
Nephrorrhagia 593.81
Nephrosclerosis (arteriolar) (arteriosclerotic)
  (chronic) (hyaline) (*see also* Hypertension,
  kidney) 403.90
  gouty 274.10
  hyperplastic (arteriolar) (*see also* Hypertension,
    kidney) 403.90
  senile (*see also* Sclerosis, renal) 587

Neuralgia, neuralgic—*continued*
  trigeminal 053.12
  pubic region 355.8
  radial (nerve) 723.4
  rectum 787.99
  sacroiliac joint 724.3
  sciatic (nerve) 724.3
  scrotum 608.9
  seminal vesicle 608.9
  shoulder 354.9
  Sluder's 337.0
  specified nerve NEC—*see* Disorder, nerve
  spermatic cord 608.9
  sphenopalatine (ganglion) 337.0
  subscapular (nerve) 723.4
  suprascapular (nerve) 723.4
  testis 608.89
  thenar (median) 354.1
  thigh 355.8
  tongue 352.5
  trifacial (nerve) (*see also* Neuralgia, trigeminal)
    350.1
  trigeminal (nerve) 350.1
    postherpetic 053.12
  tympanic plexus 388.71
  ulnar (nerve) 723.4
  vagus (nerve) 352.3
  wrist 354.9
  writers' 300.89
    organic 333.84
Neurapraxia —*see* Injury, nerve
Neurasthenia 300.5
  cardiac 306.2
  gastric 306.4
  heart 306.2
  postfebrile 780.79
  postviral 780.79
Neurilemmoma (M9560/0)—*see also* Neoplasm,
    connective tissue, benign
  acoustic (nerve) 225.1
  malignant (M9560/3)—*see also* Neoplasm,
    connective tissue, malignant
    acoustic (nerve) 192.0
Neurilemmosarcoma (M9560/3)—*see*
    Neoplasm, connective tissue, malignant
Neurilemoma —*see* Neurilemmoma
Neurinoma (M9560/0)—*see* Neurilemmoma
Neurinomatosis (M9560/1)—*see also*
    Neoplasm, connective tissue, uncertain
    behavior
  centralis 759.5
Neuritis (*see also* Neuralgia) 729.2
  abducens (nerve) 378.54
  accessory (nerve) 352.4
  acoustic (nerve) 388.5
    syphilitic 094.86
  alcoholic 357.5
    with psychosis 291.1
  amyloid, any site 277.3 *[357.4]*
  anterior crural 355.8
  arising during pregnancy 646.4
  arm 723.4
  ascending 355.2
  auditory (nerve) 388.5
  brachial (nerve) NEC 723.4
    due to displacement, intervertebral disc 722.0
  cervical 723.4
  chest (wall) 353.8
  costal region 353.8

Neuritis—*continued*
  cranial nerve—*see also* Disorder, nerve, cranial
    first or olfactory 352.0
    second or optic 377.30
    third or oculomotor 378.52
    fourth or trochlear 378.53
    fifth or trigeminal (*see also* Neuralgia,
      trigeminal) 350.1
    sixth or abducens 378.54
    seventh or facial 351.8
      newborn 767.5
    eighth or acoustic 388.5
    ninth or glossopharyngeal 352.1
    tenth or vagus 352.3
    eleventh or accessory 352.4
    twelfth or hypoglossal 352.5
  Déjérine-Sottas 356.0
  diabetic 250.6 *[357.2]*
  diphtheritic 032.89 *[357.4]*
  due to
    beriberi 265.0 *[357.4]*
    displacement, prolapse, protrusion, or rupture
      of intervertebral disc 722.2
      cervical 722.0
      lumbar, lumbosacral 722.10
      thoracic, thoracolumbar 722.11
    herniation, nucleus pulposus 722.2
      cervical 722.0
      lumbar, lumbosacral 722.10
      thoracic, thoracolumbar 722.11
  endemic 265.0 *[357.4]*
  facial 351.8
    newborn 767.5
  general—*see* Polyneuropathy
  geniculate ganglion 351.1
    due to herpes 053.11
  glossopharyngeal (nerve) 352.1
  gouty 274.89 *[357.4]*
  hypoglossal (nerve) 352.5
  ilioinguinal (nerve) 355.8
  in diseases classified elsewhere—*see*
    Polyneuropathy, in
  infectious (multiple) 357.0
  intercostal (nerve) 353.8
  interstitial hypertrophic progressive NEC 356.9
  leg 355.8
  lumbosacral NEC 724.4
  median (nerve) 354.1
    thenar 354.1
  multiple (acute) (infective) 356.9
    endemic 265.0 *[357.4]*
  multiplex endemica 265.0 *[357.4]*
  nerve root (*see also* Radiculitis) 729.2
  oculomotor (nerve) 378.52
  olfactory (nerve) 352.0
  optic (nerve) 377.30
    in myelitis 341.0
    meningococcal 036.81
  pelvic 355.8
  peripheral (nerve)—*see also* Neuropathy,
    peripheral
    complicating pregnancy or puerperium 646.4
    specified nerve NEC—*see* Mononeuritis
  pneumogastric (nerve) 352.3
  postchickenpox 052.7
  postherpetic 053.19
  progressive hypertrophic interstitial NEC 356.9
  puerperal, postpartum 646.4
  radial (nerve) 723.4
  retrobulbar 377.32
    syphilitic 094.85

Neuritis—*continued*
  rheumatic (chronic) 729.2
  sacral region 355.8
  sciatic (nerve) 724.3
    due to displacement of intervertebral disc
      722.10
  serum 999.5
  specified nerve NEC—*see* Disorder, nerve
  spinal (nerve) 355.9
    root (*see also* Radiculitis) 729.2
  subscapular (nerve) 723.4
  suprascapular (nerve) 723.4
  syphilitic 095.8
  thenar (median) 354.1
  thoracic NEC 724.4
  toxic NEC 357.7
  trochlear (nerve) 378.53
  ulnar (nerve) 723.4
  vagus (nerve) 352.3
Neuroangiomatosis, encephalofacial 759.6
Neuroastrocytoma (M9505/1)—*see* Neoplasm,
  by site, uncertain behavior
Neuro-avitaminosis 269.2
Neuroblastoma (M9500/3)
  olfactory (M9522/3) 160.0
  specified site—*see* Neoplasm, by site, malignant
  unspecified site 194.0
Neurochorioretinitis (*see also* Chorioretinitis)
  363.20
Neurocirculatory asthenia 306.2
Neurocytoma (M9506/0)—*see* Neoplasm, by
  site, benign
Neurodermatitis (circumscribed) (circumscripta)
  (local) 698.3
  atopic 691.8
  diffuse (Brocq) 691.8
  disseminated 691.8
  nodulosa 698.3
Neuroencephalomyelopathy, optic 341.0
Neuroepithelioma (M9503/3)—*see also*
  Neoplasm, by site, malignant
  olfactory (M9521/3) 160.0
Neurofibroma (M9540/0)—*see also* Neoplasm,
  connective tissue, benign
  melanotic (M9541/0)—*see* Neoplasm,
    connective tissue, benign
  multiple (M9540/1) 237.70
    Type 1 237.71
    Type 2 237.72
  plexiform (M9550/0)—*see* Neoplasm,
    connective tissue, benign
Neurofibromatosis (multiple) (M9540/1) 237.70
  acoustic 237.72
  malignant (M9540/3)—*see* Neoplasm,
    connective tissue, malignant
  Type 1 237.71
  Type 2 237.72
  von Recklinghausen's 237.71
Neurofibrosarcoma (M9540/3)—*see* Neoplasm,
  connective tissue, malignant
Neurogenic —*see also* condition
  bladder (atonic) (automatic) (autonomic)
    (flaccid) (hypertonic) (hypotonic) (inertia)
    (infranuclear) (irritable) (motor) (nonreflex)
    (nuclear) (paralysis) (reflex) (sensory)
    (spastic) (supranuclear) (uninhibited) 596.54
    with cauda equina syndrome 344.61
  bowel 564.81
  heart 306.2
Neuroglioma (M9505/1)—*see* Neoplasm, by
  site, uncertain behavior
Neurolabyrinthitis (of Dix and Hallpike) 386.12

Neurolathyrism 988.2
Neuroleprosy 030.1
Neuroleptic malignant syndrome 333.92
Neurolipomatosis 272.8
Neuroma (M9570/0)—*see also* Neoplasm,
  connective tissue, benign
  acoustic (nerve) (M9560/0) 225.1
  amputation (traumatic)—*see also* Injury, nerve,
    by site
    surgical complication (late) 997.61
  appendix 211.3
  auditory nerve 225.1
  digital 355.6
    toe 355.6
  interdigital (toe) 355.6
  intermetatarsal 355.6
  Morton's 355.6
  multiple 237.70
    Type 1 237.71
    Type 2 237.72
  nonneoplastic 355.9
    arm NEC 354.9
    leg NEC 355.8
    lower extremity NEC 355.8
    specified site NEC—*see* Mononeuritis, by site
    upper extremity NEC 354.9
  optic (nerve) 225.1
  plantar 355.6
  plexiform (M9550/0)—*see* Neoplasm,
    connective tissue, benign
  surgical (nonneoplastic) 355.9
    arm NEC 354.9
    leg NEC 355.8
    lower extremity NEC 355.8
    upper extremity NEC 354.9
  traumatic—*see also* Injury, nerve, by site
    old—*see* Neuroma, nonneoplastic
Neuromyalgia 729.1
Neuromyasthenia (epidemic) 049.8
Neuromyelitis 341.8
  ascending 357.0
  optica 341.0
Neuromyopathy NEC 358.9
Neuromyositis 729.1
Neuronevus (M8725/0)—*see* Neoplasm, skin,
  benign
Neuronitis 357.0
  ascending (acute) 355.2
  vestibular 386.12
Neuroparalytic —*see* condition
Neuropathy, neuropathic (*see also* Disorder,
  nerve) 355.9
  acute motor 357.82
  alcoholic 357.5
    with psychosis 291.1
  arm NEC 354.9
  autonomic (peripheral)—*see* Neuropathy,
    peripheral, autonomic
  axillary nerve 353.0
  brachial plexus 353.0
  cervical plexus 353.2
  chronic
    progressive segmentally demyelinating 357.89
    relapsing demyelinating 357.89
  congenital sensory 356.2
  Déjérine-Sottas 356.0
  diabetic 250.6 *[357.2]*
  entrapment 355.9
    iliohypogastric nerve 355.79
    ilioinguinal nerve 355.79
    lateral cutaneous nerve of thigh 355.1

Neurosis, neurotic—*continued*
  chronic 309.81
  psychasthenic (type) 300.89
  railroad 300.16
  rectum 306.4
  respiratory 306.1
  rumination 306.4
  senile 300.89
  sexual 302.70
  situational 300.89
  specified type NEC 300.89
  state 300.9
    with depersonalization episode 300.6
  stomach 306.4
  vasomotor 306.2
  visceral 306.4
  war 300.16
Neurospongioblastosis diffusa 759.5
Neurosyphilis (arrested) (early) (inactive) (late)
    (latent) (recurrent) 094.9
  with ataxia (cerebellar) (locomotor) (spastic)
    (spinal) 094.0
  acute meningitis 094.2
  aneurysm 094.89
  arachnoid (adhesive) 094.2
  arteritis (any artery) 094.89
  asymptomatic 094.3
  congenital 090.40
  dura (mater) 094.89
  general paresis 094.1
  gumma 094.9
  hemorrhagic 094.9
  juvenile (asymptomatic) (meningeal) 090.40
  leptomeninges (aseptic) 094.2
  meningeal 094.2
  meninges (adhesive) 094.2
  meningovascular (diffuse) 094.2
  optic atrophy 094.84
  parenchymatous (degenerative) 094.1
  paresis (*see also* Paresis, general) 094.1
  paretic (*see also* Paresis, general) 094.1
  relapse 094.9
  remission in (sustained) 094.9
  serological 094.3
  specified nature or site NEC 094.89
  tabes (dorsalis) 094.0
    juvenile 090.40
  tabetic 094.0
    juvenile 090.40
  taboparesis 094.1
    juvenile 090.40
  thrombosis 094.89
  vascular 094.89
Neurotic (*see also* Neurosis) 300.9
  excoriation 698.4
  psychogenic 306.3
Neurotmesis —*see* Injury, nerve, by site
Neurotoxemia —*see* Toxemia
Neutroclusion 524.2
Neutropenia, neutropenic (chronic) (cyclic)
    (drug-induced) (genetic) (idiopathic)
    (immune) (infantile) (malignant) (periodic)
    (pernicious) (primary) (splenic)
    (splenomegaly) (toxic) 288.0
  chronic hypoplastic 288.0
  congenital (nontransient) 288.0
  fever 288.0
  neonatal, transitory (isoimmune) (maternal
    transfer) 776.7
Neutrophilia, hereditary giant 288.2
Nevocarcinoma (M8720/3)—*see* Melanoma

Nevus (M8720/0)—*see also* Neoplasm, skin,
  benign

*Note—Except where otherwise indicated, the
varieties of nevus in the list below that are
followed by a morphology code number (M——
-/0) should be coded by site as for "Neoplasm,
skin, benign."*

  acanthotic 702.8
  achromic (M8730/0)
  amelanotic (M8730/0)
  anemic, anemicus 709.09
  angiomatous (M9120/0) (*see also*
    Hemangioma) 228.00
  araneus 448.1
  avasculosus 709.09
  balloon cell (M8722/0)
  bathing trunk (M8761/1) 238.2
  blue (M8780/0)
    cellular (M8790/0)
    giant (M8790/0)
    Jadassohn's (M8780/0)
    malignant (M8780/3)—*see* Melanoma
  capillary (M9131/0) (*see also* Hemangioma)
    228.00
  cavernous (M9121/0) (*see also* Hemangioma)
    228.00
  cellular (M8720/0)
    blue (M8790/0)
  comedonicus 757.33
  compound (M8760/0)
  conjunctiva (M8720/0) 224.3
  dermal (M8750/0)
    and epidermal (M8760/0)
  epithelioid cell (and spindle cell) (M8770/0)
  flammeus 757.32
    osteohypertrophic 759.89
  hairy (M8720/0)
  halo (M8723/0)
  hemangiomatous (M9120/0) (*see also*
    Hemangioma) 228.00
  intradermal (M8750/0)
  intraepidermal (M8740/0)
  involuting (M8724/0)
  Jadassohn's (blue) (M8780/0)
  junction, junctional (M8740/0)
    malignant melanoma in (M8740/3)—*see*
      Melanoma
  juvenile (M8770/0)
  lymphatic (M9170/0) 228.1
  magnocellular (M8726/0)
    specified site—*see* Neoplasm, by site, benign
    unspecified site 224.0
  malignant (M8720/3)—*see* Melanoma
  meaning hemangioma (M9120/0) (*see also*
    Hemangioma) 228.00
  melanotic (pigmented) (M8720/0)
  multiplex 759.5
  nonneoplastic 448.1
  nonpigmented (M8730/0)
  nonvascular (M8720/0)
  oral mucosa, white sponge 750.26
  osteohypertrophic, flammeus 759.89
  papillaris (M8720/0)
  papillomatosus (M8720/0)
  pigmented (M8720/0)
    giant (M8761/1)—*see also* Neoplasm, skin,
      uncertain behavior
      malignant melanoma in (M8761/3)—*see*
        Melanoma
    systematicus 757.33

Nevus—*continued*
pilosus (M8720/0)
port wine 757.32
sanguineous 757.32
sebaceous (senile) 702.8
senile 448.1
spider 448.1
spindle cell (and epithelioid cell) (M8770/0)
stellar 448.1
strawberry 757.32
syringocystadenomatous papilliferous
    (M8406/0)
unius lateris 757.33
Unna's 757.32
vascular 757.32
verrucous 757.33
white sponge (oral mucosa) 750.26
Newborn (infant) (liveborn)
gestation
    24 completed weeks 765.22
    25-26 completed weeks 765.23
    27-28 completed weeks 765.24
    29-30 completed weeks 765.25
    31-32 completed weeks 765.26
    33-34 completed weeks 765.27
    35-36 completed weeks 765.28
    37 or more completed weeks 765.29
    less than 24 completed weeks 765.21
    unspecified completed weeks 765.20
multiple NEC
    born in hospital (without mention of cesarean
      delivery or section) V37.00
    with cesarean delivery or section V37.01
    born outside hospital
      hospitalized V37.1
      not hospitalized V37.2
    mates all liveborn
      born in hospital (without mention of
        cesarean delivery or section) V34.00
      with cesarean delivery or section V34.01
      born outside hospital
        hospitalized V34.1
        not hospitalized V34.2
    mates all stillborn
      born in hospital (without mention of
        cesarean delivery or section) V35.00
      with cesarean delivery or section V35.01
      born outside hospital
        hospitalized V35.1
        not hospitalized V35.2
    mates liveborn and stillborn
      born in hospital (without mention of
        cesarean delivery or section) V36.00
      with cesarean delivery or section V36.01
      born outside hospital
        hospitalized V36.1
        not hospitalized V36.2
single
    born in hospital (without mention of cesarean
      delivery or section) V30.00
    with cesarean delivery or section V30.01
    born outside hospital
      hospitalized V30.1
      not hospitalized V30.2
twin NEC
    born in hospital (without mention of cesarean
      delivery or section) V33.00
    with cesarean delivery or section V33.01
    born outside hospital
      hospitalized V33.1
      not hospitalized V33.2

Newborn—*continued*
mate liveborn
    born in hospital V31.0
    born outside hospital
      hospitalized V31.1
      not hospitalized V31.2
mate stillborn
    born in hospital V32.0
    born outside hospital
      hospitalized V32.1
      not hospitalized V32.2
unspecified as to single or multiple birth
    born in hospital (without mention of cesarean
      delivery or section) V39.00
    with cesarean delivery or section V39.01
    born outside hospital
      hospitalized V39.1
      not hospitalized V39.2
Newcastle's conjunctivitis or disease 077.8
Nezelof's syndrome (pure alymphocytosis)
    279.13
Niacin (amide) deficiency 265.2
Nicolas-Durand-Favre disease (climatic bubo)
    099.1
Nicolas-Favre disease (climatic bubo) 099.1
Nicotinic acid (amide) deficiency 265.2
Niemann-Pick disease (lipid histiocytosis)
    (splenomegaly) 272.7
Night
blindness (*see also* Blindness, night) 368.60
    congenital 368.61
    vitamin A deficiency 264.5
cramps 729.82
sweats 780.8
terrors, child 307.46
Nightmare 307.47
REM-sleep type 307.47
Nipple —*see* condition
Nisbet's chancre 099.0
Nishimoto (-Takeuchi) disease 437.5
Nitritoid crisis or reaction —*see* Crisis, nitritoid
Nitrogen retention, extrarenal 788.9
Nitrosohemoglobinemia 289.8
Njovera 104.0
No
diagnosis 799.9
disease (found) V71.9
room at the inn V65.0
Nocardiasis —*see* Nocardiosis
Nocardiosis 039.9
with pneumonia 039.1
lung 039.1
specified type NEC 039.8
Nocturia 788.43
psychogenic 306.53
Nocturnal —*see also* condition
dyspnea (paroxysmal) 786.09
emissions 608.89
enuresis 788.36
    psychogenic 307.6
frequency (micturition) 788.43
    psychogenic 306.53
Nodal rhythm disorder 427.89
Nodding of head 781.0
Node (s)—*see also* Nodule
Heberden's 715.04
larynx 478.79
lymph—*see* condition
milkers' 051.1
Osler's 421.0
rheumatic 729.89

Node(s)—*continued*
Schmorl's 722.30
  lumbar, lumbosacral 722.32
  specified region NEC 722.39
  thoracic, thoracolumbar 722.31
singers' 478.5
skin NEC 782.2
tuberculous—*see* Tuberculosis, lymph gland
vocal cords 478.5
Nodosities, Haygarth's 715.04
Nodule(s), nodular
actinomycotic (*see also* Actinomycosis) 039.9
arthritic—*see* Arthritis, nodosa
cutaneous 782.2
Haygarth's 715.04
inflammatory—*see* Inflammation
juxta-articular 102.7
  syphilitic 095.7
  yaws 102.7
larynx 478.79
lung, solitary 518.89
  emphysematous 492.8
milkers' 051.1
prostate 600.1
rheumatic 729.89
rheumatoid—*see* Arthritis rheumatoid
scrotum (inflammatory) 608.4
singers' 478.5
skin NEC 782.2
solitary, lung 518.89
  emphysematous 492.8
subcutaneous 782.2
thyroid (gland) (nontoxic) (uninodular) 241.0
  with
    hyperthyroidism 242.1
    thyrotoxicosis 242.1
  toxic or with hyperthyroidism 242.1
vocal cords 478.5
Noma (gangrenous) (hospital) (infective) 528.1
auricle (*see also* Gangrene) 785.4
mouth 528.1
pudendi (*see also* Vulvitis) 616.10
vulvae (*see also* Vulvitis) 616.10
Nomadism V60.0
Non-adherence
artificial skin graft 996.55
decellularized allodermis graft 996.55
Non-autoimmune hemolytic anemia NEC
283.10
Nonclosure —*see also* Imperfect, closure
ductus
  arteriosus 747.0
  Botalli 747.0
Eustachian valve 746.89
foramen
  Botalli 745.5
  ovale 745.5
Noncompliance with medical treatment V15.81
Nondescent (congenital)—*see also* Malposition,
  congenital
cecum 751.4
colon 751.4
testis 752.51
Nondevelopment
brain 742.1
  specified part 742.2
heart 746.89
organ or site, congenital NEC—*see* Hypoplasia
Nonengagement
head NEC 652.5
  in labor 660.1
    affecting fetus or newborn 763.1

Nonexanthematous tick fever 066.1
Nonexpansion, lung (newborn) NEC 770.4
Nonfunctioning
cystic duct (*see also* Disease, gallbladder) 575.8
gallbladder (*see also* Disease, gallbladder) 575.8
kidney (*see also* Disease, renal) 593.9
labyrinth 386.58
Nonhealing
stump (surgical) 997.60
wound, surgical 998.83
Nonimplantation of ovum, causing infertility
628.3
Noninsufflation, fallopian tube 628.2
Nonne-Milroy-Meige syndrome (chronic
  hereditary edema) 757.0
Nonovulation 628.0
Nonpatent fallopian tube 628.2
Nonpneumatization, lung NEC 770.4
Nonreflex bladder 596.54
  with cauda equina 344.61
Nonretention of food —*see also* Vomiting
Nonrotation —*see* Malrotation
Nonsecretion, urine (*see also* Anuria) 788.5
newborn 753.3
Nonunion
fracture 733.82
organ or site, congenital NEC—*see* Imperfect,
  closure
symphysis pubis, congenital 755.69
top sacrum, congenital 756.19
Nonviability 765.0
Nonvisualization, gallbladder 793.3
Nonvitalized tooth 522.9
Normal
delivery—*see* category 650
menses V65.5
state (feared complaint unfounded) V65.5
Normoblastosis 289.8
Normocytic anemia (infectional) 285.9
due to blood loss (chronic) 280.0
  acute 285.1
Norrie's disease (congenital) (progressive
  oculoacousticocerebral degeneration) 743.8
North American blastomycosis 116.0
Norwegian itch 133.0
Nose, nasal —*see* condition
Nosebleed 784.7
Nosomania 298.9
Nosophobia 300.29
Nostalgia 309.89
Notch of iris 743.46
Notched lip, congenital (*see also* Cleft, lip)
749.10
Notching nose, congenital (tip) 748.1
Nothnagel's
syndrome 378.52
vasomotor acroparesthesia 443.89
Novy's relapsing fever (American) 087.1
Noxious
foodstuffs, poisoning by
  fish 988.0
  fungi 988.1
  mushrooms 988.1
  plants (food) 988.2
  shellfish 988.0
  specified type NEC 988.8
  toadstool 988.1
substances transmitted through placenta or
  breast milk 760.70
  alcohol 760.71
  anti-infective agents 760.74

Noxious—*continued*
    cocaine 760.75
    "crack" 760.75
    diethylstilbestrol (DES) 760.76
    hallucinogenic agents NEC 760.73
    medicinal agents NEC 760.79
    narcotics 760.72
    obstetric anesthetic or analgesic 763.5
    specified agent NEC 760.79
    suspected, affecting management of
        pregnancy 655.5
Nuchal hitch (arm) 652.8
Nucleus pulposus —*see* condition
Numbness 782.0
Nuns' knee 727.2
Nursemaid's
  elbow 832.0
  shoulder 831.0
Nutmeg liver 573.8
Nutrition, deficient or insufficient (particular
    kind of food) 269.9
  due to
    insufficient food 994.2
    lack of
      care (child) (infant) 995.52
        adult 995.84
      food 994.2
Nyctalopia (*see also* Blindness, night) 368.60
  vitamin A deficiency 264.5
Nycturia 788.43
  psychogenic 306.53
Nymphomania 302.89
Nystagmus 379.50
  associated with vestibular system disorders
    379.54
  benign paroxysmal positional 386.11
  central positional 386.2
  congenital 379.51
  deprivation 379.53
  dissociated 379.55
  latent 379.52
  miners' 300.89
  positional
    benign paroxysmal 386.11
    central 386.2
  specified NEC 379.56
  vestibular 379.54
  visual deprivation 379.53

O

Oasthouse urine disease 270.2
Obermeyer's relapsing fever (European) 087.0
Obesity (constitutional) (exogenous) (familial)
(nutritional) (simple) 278.00
adrenal 255.8
due to hyperalimentation 278.00
endocrine NEC 259.9
endogenous 259.9
Fröhlich's (adiposogenital dystrophy) 253.8
glandular NEC 259.9
hypothyroid (*see also* Hypothyroidism) 244.9
morbid 278.01
of pregnancy 646.1
pituitary 253.8
thyroid (*see also* Hypothyroidism) 244.9
Oblique —*see also* condition
lie before labor, affecting fetus or newborn 761.7
Obliquity, pelvis 738.6
Obliteration
abdominal aorta 446.7
appendix (lumen) 543.9
artery 447.1
ascending aorta 446.7
bile ducts 576.8
with calculus, choledocholithiasis, or
stones—*see* Choledocholithiasis
congenital 751.61
jaundice from 751.61 *[774.5]*
common duct 576.8
with calculus, choledocholithiasis, or
stones—*see* Choledocholithiasis
congenital 751.61
cystic duct 575.8
with calculus, choledocholithiasis, or
stones—*see* Choledocholithiasis
disease, arteriolar 447.1
endometrium 621.8
eye, anterior chamber 360.34
fallopian tube 628.2
lymphatic vessel 457.1
postmastectomy 457.0
organ or site, congenital NEC—*see* Atresia
placental blood vessels—*see* Placenta, abnormal
supra-aortic branches 446.7
ureter 593.89
urethra 599.84
vein 459.9
vestibule (oral) 525.8
Observation (for) V71.9
without need for further medical care V71.9
accident NEC V71.4
at work V71.3
criminal assault V71.6
deleterious agent ingestion V71.89
disease V71.9
cardiovascular V71.7
heart V71.7
mental V71.09
specified condition NEC V71.89
foreign body ingestion V71.89
growth and development variations V21.8
injuries (accidental) V71.4
inflicted NEC V71.6
during alleged rape or seduction V71.5
malignant neoplasm, suspected V71.1
postpartum
immediately after delivery V24.0
routine follow-up V24.2

Observation—*continued*
pregnancy
high-risk V23.9
specified problem NEC V23.8
normal (without complication) V22.1
with nonobstetric complication V22.2
first V22.0
rape or seduction, alleged V71.5
injury during V71.5
suicide attempt, alleged V71.89
suspected (undiagnosed) (unproven)
abuse V71.81
cardiovascular disease V71.7
child or wife battering victim V71.6
concussion (cerebral) V71.6
condition NEC V71.89
infant—*see* Observation, suspected,
condition, newborn
newborn V29.9
cardiovascular disease V29.8
congenital anomaly V29.8
genetic V29.3
infectious V29.0
ingestion foreign object V29.8
injury V29.8
metabolic V29.3
neoplasm V29.8
neurological V29.1
poison, poisoning V29.8
respiratory V29.2
specified NEC V29.8
exposure
anthrax V71.82
biologic agent NEC V71.83
infectious disease not requiring isolation
V71.89
malignant neoplasm V71.1
mental disorder V71.09
neglect V71.81
neoplasm
benign V71.89
malignant V71.1
specified condition NEC V71.89
tuberculosis V71.2
tuberculosis, suspected V71.2
Obsession, obsessional 300.3
ideas and mental images 300.3
impulses 300.3
neurosis 300.3
phobia 300.3
psychasthenia 300.3
ruminations 300.3
state 300.3
syndrome 300.3
Obsessive-compulsive 300.3
neurosis 300.3
reaction 300.3
Obstetrical trauma NEC (complicating
delivery) 665.9
with
abortion—*see* Abortion, by type, with damage
to pelvic organs
ectopic pregnancy (*see also* categories
633.0-633.9) 639.2
molar pregnancy (*see also* categories
630-632) 639.2
affecting fetus or newborn 763.89

Obstetrical trauma—*continued*
  following
    abortion 639.2
    ectopic or molar pregnancy 639.2
Obstipation (*see also* Constipation) 564.00
  psychogenic 306.4
Obstruction, obstructed, obstructive
  airway NEC 519.8
    with
      allergic alveolitis NEC 495.9
      asthma NEC (*see also* Asthma) 493.9
      bronchiectasis 494.0
        with acute exacerbation 494.1
      bronchitis (*see also* Bronchitis, with,
          obstruction) 491.20
      emphysema NEC 492.8
    chronic 496
      with
        allergic alveolitis NEC 495.5
        asthma NEC (*see also* Asthma) 493.2
        bronchiectasis 494.0
          with acute exacerbation 494.1
        bronchitis (*see also* Bronchitis, chronic,
            obstructive) 491.20
        emphysema NEC 492.8
    due to
      bronchospasm 519.1
      foreign body 934.9
      inhalation of fumes or vapors 506.9
      laryngospasm 478.75
  alimentary canal (*see also* Obstruction,
      intestine) 560.9
  ampulla of Vater 576.2
    with calculus, cholelithiasis, or stones—*see*
        Choledocholithiasis
  aortic (heart) (valve) (*see also* Stenosis, aortic)
      424.1
    rheumatic (*see also* Stenosis, aortic,
        rheumatic) 395.0
  aortoiliac 444.0
  aqueduct of Sylvius 331.4
    congenital 742.3
      with spina bifida (*see also* Spina bifida)
          741.0
  Arnold-Chiari (*see also* Spina bifida) 741.0
  artery (*see also* Embolism, artery) 444.9
    basilar (complete) (partial) (*see also*
        Occlusion, artery, basilar) 433.0
    carotid (complete) (partial) (*see also*
        Occlusion, artery, carotid) 433.1
    precerebral—*see* Occlusion, artery,
        precerebral NEC
    retinal (central) (*see also* Occlusion, retina)
        362.30
    vertebral (complete) (partial) (*see also*
        Occlusion, artery, vertebral) 433.2
  asthma (chronic) (with obstructive pulmonary
      disease) 493.2
  band (intestinal) 560.81
  bile duct or passage (*see also* Obstruction,
      biliary) 576.2
    congenital 751.61
      jaundice from 751.61 [774.5]
  biliary (duct) (tract) 576.2
    with calculus 574.51
      with cholecystitis (chronic) 574.41
        acute 574.31
    congenital 751.61
      jaundice from 751.61 [774.5]
  gallbladder 575.2
    with calculus 574.21

Obstruction, obstructed, . . .—*continued*
    with cholecystitis (chronic) 574.11
      acute 574.01
  bladder neck (acquired) 596.0
    congenital 753.6
  bowel (*see also* Obstruction, intestine) 560.9
  bronchus 519.1
  canal, ear (*see also* Stricture, ear canal,
      acquired) 380.50
  cardia 537.89
  caval veins (inferior) (superior) 459.2
  cecum (*see also* Obstruction, intestine) 560.9
  circulatory 459.9
  colon (*see also* Obstruction, intestine) 560.9
    sympathicotonic 560.89
  common duct (*see also* Obstruction, biliary)
      576.2
    congenital 751.61
  coronary (*see also* Arteriosclerosis, coronary)
    acute (*see also* Infarct, myocardium) 410.9
      without myocardial infarction 411.81
  cystic duct (*see also* Obstruction, gallbladder)
      575.2
    congenital 751.61
  device, implant, or graft—*see* Complications,
      due to (presence of) any device, implant, or
      graft classified to 996.0-996.5 NEC
  due to foreign body accidentally left in
      operation wound 998.4
  duodenum 537.3
    congenital 751.1
    due to
      compression NEC 537.3
      cyst 537.3
      intrinsic lesion or disease NEC 537.3
      scarring 537.3
      torsion 537.3
      ulcer 532.91
      volvulus 537.3
  ejaculatory duct 608.89
  endocardium 424.90
    arteriosclerotic 424.99
    specified cause, except rheumatic 424.99
  esophagus 530.3
  Eustachian tube (complete) (partial) 381.60
    cartilaginous
      extrinsic 381.63
      intrinsic 381.62
    due to
      cholesteatoma 381.61
      osseous lesion NEC 381.61
      polyp 381.61
    osseous 381.61
  fallopian tube (bilateral) 628.2
  fecal 560.39
    with hernia—*see also* Hernia, by site, with
        obstruction
    gangrenous—*see* Hernia, by site, with
        gangrene
  foramen of Monro (congenital) 742.3
    with spina bifida (*see also* Spina bifida) 741.0
  foreign body—*see* Foreign body
  gallbladder 575.2
    with calculus, cholelithiasis, or stones 574.21
      with cholecystitis (chronic) 574.11
        acute 574.01
    congenital 751.69
      jaundice from 751.69 [774.5]
  gastric outlet 537.0
  gastrointestinal (*see also* Obstruction, intestine)
      560.9

Obstruction, obstructed, . . .—*continued*
glottis 478.79
hepatic 573.8
  duct (*see also* Obstruction, biliary) 576.2
    congenital 751.61
icterus (*see also* Obstruction, biliary) 576.8
  congenital 751.61
ileocecal coil (*see also* Obstruction, intestine)
  560.9
ileum (*see also* Obstruction, intestine) 560.9
iliofemoral (artery) 444.81
internal anastomosis—*see* Complications,
  mechanical, graft
intestine (mechanical) (neurogenic)
  (paroxysmal) (postinfectional) (reflex) 560.9
  with
    adhesions (intestinal) (peritoneal) 560.81
    hernia—*see also* Hernia, by site, with
      obstruction
      gangrenous—*see* Hernia, by site, with
        gangrene
  adynamic (*see also* Ileus) 560.1
  by gallstone 560.31
  congenital or infantile (small) 751.1
    large 751.2
  due to
    Ascaris lumbricoides 127.0
    mural thickening 560.89
    procedure 997.4
      involving urinary tract 997.5
  impaction 560.39
  infantile—*see* Obstruction, intestine,
    congenital
  newborn
    due to
      fecaliths 777.1
      inspissated milk 777.2
      meconium (plug) 777.1
        in mucoviscidosis 277.01
      transitory 777.4
  specified cause NEC 560.89
  transitory, newborn 777.4
  volvulus 560.2
intracardiac ball valve prosthesis 996.02
jaundice (*see also* Obstruction, biliary) 576.8
  congenital 751.61
jejunum (*see also* Obstruction, intestine) 560.9
kidney 593.89
labor 660.9
  affecting fetus or newborn 763.1
  by
    bony pelvis (conditions classifiable to
      653.0-653.9) 660.1
    deep transverse arrest 660.3
    impacted shoulder 660.4
    locked twins 660.5
    malposition (fetus) (conditions classifiable
      to 652.0-652.9) 660.0
      head during labor 660.3
    persistent occipitoposterior position 660.3
    soft tissue, pelvic (conditions classifiable to
      654.0-654.9) 660.2
lacrimal
  canaliculi 375.53
  congenital 743.65
  punctum 375.52
  sac 375.54
lacrimonasal duct 375.56
  congenital 743.65
  neonatal 375.55
lacteal, with steatorrhea 579.2

Obstruction, obstructed, . . .—*continued*
laryngitis (*see also* Laryngitis) 464.01
larynx 478.79
  congenital 748.3
liver 573.8
  cirrhotic (*see also* Cirrhosis, liver) 571.5
lung 518.89
  with
    asthma—*see* Asthma
    bronchitis (chronic) 491.2
    emphysema NEC 492.8
  airway, chronic 496
  chronic NEC 496
    with
      asthma (chronic) (obstructive) 493.2
  disease, chronic 496
    with
      asthma (chronic) (obstructive) 493.2
  emphysematous 492.8
lymphatic 457.1
meconium
  fetus or newborn 777.1
    in mucoviscidosis 277.01
  newborn due to fecaliths 777.1
mediastinum 519.3
mitral (rheumatic)—*see* Stenosis, mitral
nasal 478.1
  duct 375.56
    neonatal 375.55
  sinus—*see* Sinusitis
nasolacrimal duct 375.56
  congenital 743.65
  neonatal 375.55
nasopharynx 478.29
nose 478.1
organ or site, congenital NEC—*see* Atresia
pancreatic duct 577.8
parotid gland 527.8
pelviureteral junction (*see also* Obstruction,
  ureter) 593.4
pharynx 478.29
portal (circulation) (vein) 452
prostate 600.9
  valve (urinary) 596.0
pulmonary
  valve (heart) (*see also* Endocarditis,
    pulmonary) 424.3
  vein, isolated 747.49
pyemic—*see* Septicemia
pylorus (acquired) 537.0
  congenital 750.5
  infantile 750.5
rectosigmoid (*see also* Obstruction, intestine)
  560.9
rectum 569.49
renal 593.89
respiratory 519.8
  chronic 496
retinal (artery) (vein) (central) (*see also*
  Occlusion, retina) 362.30
salivary duct (any) 527.8
  with calculus 527.5
sigmoid (*see also* Obstruction, intestine) 560.9
sinus (accessory) (nasal) (*see also* Sinusitis)
  473.9
Stensen's duct 527.8
stomach 537.89
  acute 536.1
  congenital 750.7
submaxillary gland 527.8
  with calculus 527.5

Obstruction, obstructed, . . .—*continued*
thoracic duct 457.1
thrombotic—*see* Thrombosis
tooth eruption 520.6
trachea 519.1
tracheostomy airway 519.09
tricuspid—*see* Endocarditis, tricuspid
upper respiratory, congenital 748.8
ureter (functional) 593.4
   congenital 753.20
   due to calculus 592.1
ureteropelvic junction, congenital 753.21
ureterovesical junction, congenital 753.22
urethra 599.6
   congenital 753.6
urinary (moderate) 599.6
   organ or tract (lower) 599.6
   prostatic valve 596.0
uropathy 599.6
uterus 621.8
vagina 623.2
valvular—*see* Endocarditis
vascular graft or shunt 996.1
   atherosclerosis —*see* Arteriosclerosis,
      coronary
   embolism 996.74
   occlusion NEC 996.74
   thrombus 996.74
vein, venous 459.2
   caval (inferior) (superior) 459.2
   thrombotic—*see* Thrombosis
vena cava (inferior) (superior) 459.2
ventricular shunt 996.2
vesical 596.0
vesicourethral orifice 596.0
vessel NEC 459.9
Obturator —*see* condition
Occlusal wear, teeth 521.1
Occlusion
anus 569.49
   congenital 751.2
   infantile 751.2
aortoiliac (chronic) 444.0
aqueduct of Sylvius 331.4
   congenital 742.3
      with spina bifida (*see also* Spina bifida)
         741.0
arteries of extremities, lower 444.22
   without thrombus or embolus (*see also*
      Arteriosclerosis, extremities) 440.20
   due to stricture or stenosis 447.1
   upper 444.21
      without thrombus or embolus (*see also*
        Arteriosclerosis, extremities) 440.20
      due to stricture or stenosis 447.1
artery NEC (*see also* Embolism, artery) 444.9
   auditory, internal 433.8
   basilar 433.0
      with other precerebral artery 433.3
      bilateral 433.3
   brain or cerebral (*see also* Infarct, brain) 434.9
   carotid 433.1
      with other precerebral artery 433.3
      bilateral 433.3
   cerebellar (anterior inferior) (posterior
      inferior) (superior) 433.8
   cerebral (*see also* Infarct, brain) 434.9
   choroidal (anterior) 433.8
   communicating posterior 433.8
   coronary (thrombotic) (*see also* Infarct,
      myocardium) 410.9

Occlusion—*continued*
   acute 410.9
      without myocardial infarction 411.81
      healed or old 412
   hypophyseal 433.8
   iliac 444.81
   mesenteric (embolic) (thrombotic) (with
      gangrene) 557.0
   pontine 433.8
   precerebral NEC 433.9
      late effect—*see* Late effect(s) (of)
         cerebrovascular disease
      multiple or bilateral 433.3
      puerperal, postpartum, childbirth 674.0
      specified NEC 433.8
   renal 593.81
   retinal—*see* Occlusion, retina, artery
   spinal 433.8
   vertebral 433.2
      with other precerebral artery 433.3
      bilateral 433.3
basilar (artery)—*see* Occlusion, artery, basilar
bile duct (any) (*see also* Obstruction, biliary)
   576.2
bowel (*see also* Obstruction, intestine) 560.9
brain (artery) (vascular) (*see also* Infarct, brain)
   434.9
breast (duct) 611.8
carotid (artery) (common) (internal)—*see*
   Occlusion, artery, carotid
cerebellar (anterior inferior) (artery) (posterior
   inferior) (superior) 433.8
cerebral (artery) (*see also* Infarct, brain) 434.9
cerebrovascular (*see also* Infarct, brain) 434.9
   diffuse 437.0
cervical canal (*see also* Stricture, cervix) 622.4
   by falciparum malaria 084.0
cervix (uteri) (*see also* Stricture, cervix) 622.4
choanal 748.0
choroidal (artery) 433.8
colon (*see also* Obstruction, intestine) 560.9
communicating posterior artery 433.8
coronary (artery) (thrombotic) (*see also* Infarct,
   myocardium) 410.9
   acute 410.9
      without myocardial infarction 411.81
      healed or old 412
   without myocardial infarction 411.81
cystic duct (*see also* Obstruction, gallbladder)
   575.2
   congenital 751.69
embolic—*see* Embolism
fallopian tube 628.2
   congenital 752.19
gallbladder (*see also* Obstruction, gallbladder)
   575.2
   congenital 751.69
      jaundice from 751.69 *[774.5]*
gingiva, traumatic 523.8
hymen 623.3
   congenital 752.42
hypophyseal (artery) 433.8
iliac artery 444.81
intestine (*see also* Obstruction, intestine) 560.9
kidney 593.89
lacrimal apparatus—*see* Stenosis, lacrimal
lung 518.89
lymph or lymphatic channel 457.1
mammary duct 611.8
mesenteric artery (embolic) (thrombotic) (with
   gangrene) 557.0

Occlusion—*continued*
  nose 478.1
    congenital 748.0
  organ or site, congenital NEC—*see* Atresia
  oviduct 628.2
    congenital 752.19
  periodontal, traumatic 523.8
  peripheral arteries (lower extremity) 444.22
    without thrombus or embolus (*see also*
      Arteriosclerosis, extremities) 440.20
    due to stricture or stenosis 447.1
    upper extremity 444.21
      without thrombus or embolus (*see also*
        Arteriosclerosis, extremities) 440.20
      due to stricture or stenosis 447.1
  pontine (artery) 433.8
  posterior lingual, of mandibular teeth 524.2
  precerebral artery—*see* Occlusion, artery,
    precerebral NEC
  puncta lacrimalia 375.52
  pupil 364.74
  pylorus (*see also* Stricture, pylorus) 537.0
  renal artery 593.81
  retina, retinal (vascular) 362.30
    artery, arterial 362.30
      branch 362.32
      central (total) 362.31
      partial 362.33
      transient 362.34
      tributary 362.32
    vein 362.30
      branch 362.36
      central (total) 362.35
      incipient 362.37
      partial 362.37
      tributary 362.36
  spinal artery 433.8
  stent
    coronary 996.72
  teeth (mandibular) (posterior lingual) 524.2
  thoracic duct 457.1
  tubal 628.2
  ureter (complete) (partial) 593.4
    congenital 753.29
  urethra (*see also* Stricture, urethra) 598.9
    congenital 753.6
  uterus 621.8
  vagina 623.2
  vascular NEC 459.9
  vein—*see* Thrombosis
  vena cava (inferior) (superior) 453.2
  ventricle (brain) NEC 331.4
  vertebral (artery)—*see* Occlusion, artery,
    vertebral
  vessel (blood) NEC 459.9
  vulva 624.8
Occlusio pupillae 364.74
Occupational
  problems NEC V62.2
  therapy V57.21
Ochlophobia 300.29
Ochronosis (alkaptonuric) (congenital)
    (endogenous) 270.2
  with chloasma of eyelid 270.2
Ocular muscle —*see also* condition
  myopathy 359.1
  torticollis 781.93
Oculoauriculovertebral dysplasia 756.0
Oculogyric
  crisis or disturbance 378.87
    psychogenic 306.7
Oculomotor syndrome 378.81

Oddi's sphincter spasm 576.5
Odelberg's disease (juvenile osteochondrosis)
    732.1
Odontalgia 525.9
Odontoameloblastoma (M9311/0) 213.1
  upper jaw (bone) 213.0
Odontoclasia 521.05
Odontoclasis 873.63
  complicated 873.73
Odontodysplasia, regional 520.4
Odontogenesis imperfecta 520.5
Odontoma (M9280/0) 213.1
  ameloblastic (M9311/0) 213.1
    upper jaw (bone) 213.0
  calcified (M9280/0) 213.1
    upper jaw (bone) 213.0
  complex (M9282/0) 213.1
    upper jaw (bone) 213.0
  compound (M9281/0) 213.1
    upper jaw (bone) 213.0
  fibroameloblastic (M9290/0) 213.1
    upper jaw (bone) 213.0
  follicular 526.0
  upper jaw (bone) 213.0
Odontomyelitis (closed) (open) 522.0
Odontonecrosis 521.09
Odontorrhagia 525.8
Odontosarcoma, ameloblastic (M9290/3) 170.1
  upper jaw (bone) 170.0
Odynophagia 787.2
Oesophagostomiasis 127.7
Oesophagostomum infestation 127.7
Oestriasis 134.0
Ogilvie's syndrome (sympathicotonic colon
    obstruction) 560.89
Oguchi's disease (retina) 368.61
Ohara's disease (*see also* Tularemia) 021.9
Oidiomycosis (*see also* Candidiasis) 112.9
Oidiomycotic meningitis 112.83
Oidium albicans infection (*see also* Candidiasis)
    112.9
Old age 797
  dementia (of) 290.0
Olfactory —*see* condition
Oligemia 285.9
Oligergasia (*see also* Retardation, mental) 319
Oligoamnios 658.0
  affecting fetus or newborn 761.2
Oligoastrocytoma, mixed (M9382/3)
  specified site—*see* Neoplasm, by site, malignant
  unspecified site 191.9
Oligocythemia 285.9
Oligodendroblastoma (M9460/3)
  specified site—*see* Neoplasm, by site, malignant
  unspecified site 191.9
Oligodendroglioma (M9450/3)
  anaplastic type (M9451/3)
    specified site—*see* Neoplasm, by site,
      malignant
    unspecified site 191.9
  specified site—*see* Neoplasm, by site, malignant
  unspecified site 191.9
Oligodendroma —*see* Oligodendroglioma
Oligodontia (*see also* Anodontia) 520.0
Oligoencephalon 742.1
Oligohydramnios 658.0
  affecting fetus or newborn 761.2
  due to premature rupture of membranes 658.1
    affecting fetus or newborn 761.2
Oligohydrosis 705.0
Oligomenorrhea 626.1

Oligophrenia (*see also* Retardation, mental) 319
  phenylpyruvic 270.1
Oligospermia 606.1
Oligotrichia 704.09
  congenita 757.4
Oliguria 788.5
  with
    abortion—*see* Abortion, by type, with renal
      failure
    ectopic pregnancy (*see also* categories
      633.0-633.9) 639.3
    molar pregnancy (*see also* categories
      630-632) 639.3
    complicating
      abortion 639.3
      ectopic or molar pregnancy 639.3
      pregnancy 646.2
        with hypertension—*see* Toxemia, of
          pregnancy
    due to a procedure 997.5
    following labor and delivery 669.3
    heart or cardiac—*see* Failure, heart
    puerperal, postpartum 669.3
    specified due to a procedure 997.5
Ollier's disease (chondrodysplasia) 756.4
Omentitis (*see also* Peritonitis) 567.9
Omentocele (*see also* Hernia, omental) 553.8
Omentum, omental —*see* condition
Omphalitis (congenital) (newborn) 771.4
  not of newborn 686.9
  tetanus 771.3
Omphalocele 756.79
Omphalomesenteric duct, persistent 751.0
Omphalorrhagia, newborn 772.3
Omsk hemorrhagic fever 065.1
Onanism 307.9
Onchocerciasis 125.3
  eye 125.3 *[360.13]*
Onchocercosis 125.3
Oncocytoma (M8290/0)—*see* Neoplasm, by site,
  benign
Ondine's curse 348.8
Oneirophrenia (*see also* Schizophrenia) 295.4
Onychauxis 703.8
  congenital 757.5
Onychia (with lymphangitis) 681.9
  dermatophytic 110.1
  finger 681.02
  toe 681.11
Onychitis (with lymphangitis) 681.9
  finger 681.02
  toe 681.11
Onychocryptosis 703.0
Onychodystrophy 703.8
  congenital 757.5
Onychogryphosis 703.8
Onychogryposis 703.8
Onycholysis 703.8
Onychomadesis 703.8
Onychomalacia 703.8
Onychomycosis 110.1
  finger 110.1
  toe 110.1
Onycho-osteodysplasia 756.89
Onychophagy 307.9
Onychoptosis 703.8
Onychorrhexis 703.8
  congenital 757.5
Onychoschizia 703.8
Onychotrophia (*see also* Atrophy, nail) 703.8
O'nyong-nyong fever 066.3
Onyxis (finger) (toe) 703.0

Onyxitis (with lymphangitis) 681.9
  finger 681.02
  toe 681.11
Oophoritis (cystic) (infectional) (interstitial) (*see*
    also Salpingo-oophoritis) 614.2
  complicating pregnancy 646.6
  fetal (acute) 752.0
  gonococcal (acute) 098.19
    chronic or duration of 2 months or over 098.39
  tuberculous (*see also* Tuberculosis) 016.6
Opacity, opacities
  cornea 371.00
    central 371.03
    congenital 743.43
      interfering with vision 743.42
    degenerative (*see also* Degeneration, cornea)
      371.40
    hereditary (*see also* Dystrophy, cornea) 371.50
    inflammatory (*see also* Keratitis) 370.9
    late effect of trachoma (healed) 139.1
    minor 371.01
    peripheral 371.02
  enamel (fluoride) (nonfluoride) (teeth) 520.3
  lens (*see also* Cataract) 366.9
  snowball 379.22
  vitreous (humor) 379.24
    congenital 743.51
Opalescent dentin (hereditary) 520.5
Open, opening
  abnormal, organ or site, congenital—*see*
    Imperfect, closure
  angle with
    borderline intraocular pressure 365.01
    cupping of discs 365.01
  bite (anterior) (posterior) 524.2
  false—*see* Imperfect, closure
  wound—*see* Wound, open, by site
Operation
  causing mutilation of fetus 763.89
  destructive, on live fetus, to facilitate birth
    763.89
  for delivery, fetus or newborn 763.89
  maternal, unrelated to current delivery, affecting
    fetus or newborn 760.6
Operational fatigue 300.89
Operative —*see* condition
Operculitis (chronic) 523.4
  acute 523.3
Operculum, retina 361.32
  with detachment 361.01
Ophiasis 704.01
Ophthalmia (*see also* Conjunctivitis) 372.30
  actinic rays 370.24
  allergic (acute) 372.05
    chronic 372.14
  blennorrhagic (neonatorum) 098.40
  catarrhal 372.03
  diphtheritic 032.81
  Egyptian 076.1
  electric, electrica 370.24
  gonococcal (neonatorum) 098.40
  metastatic 360.11
  migraine 346.8
  neonatorum, newborn 771.6
    gonococcal 098.40
  nodosa 360.14
  phlyctenular 370.31
    with ulcer (*see also* Ulcer, cornea) 370.00
  sympathetic 360.11
Ophthalmitis —*see* Ophthalmia
Ophthalmocele (congenital) 743.66
Ophthalmoneuromyelitis 341.0

Ophthalmopathy , infiltrative with
   thyrotoxicosis 242.0
Ophthalmoplegia (*see also* Strabismus) 378.9
   anterior internuclear 378.86
   ataxia-areflexia syndrome 357.0
   bilateral 378.9
   diabetic 250.5 *[378.86]*
   exophthalmic 242.0 *[376.22]*
   external 378.55
      progressive 378.72
      total 378.56
   interna(l) (complete) (total) 367.52
   internuclear 378.86
   migraine 346.8
   painful 378.55
   Parinaud's 378.81
   progressive external 378.72
   supranuclear, progressive 333.0
   total (external) 378.56
      internal 367.52
   unilateral 378.9
Opisthognathism 524.00
Opisthorchiasis (felineus) (tenuicollis)
   (viverrini) 121.0
Opisthotonos, opisthotonus 781.0
Opitz's disease (congestive splenomegaly)
   289.51
Opiumism (*see also* Dependence) 304.0
Oppenheim's disease 358.8
Oppenheim-Urbach disease or syndrome
   (necrobiosis lipoidica diabeticorum) 250.8
   [709.3]
Opsoclonia 379.59
Optic nerve —*see* condition
Orbit —*see* condition
Orchioblastoma (M9071/3) 186.9
Orchitis (nonspecific) (septic) 604.90
   with abscess 604.0
   blennorrhagic (acute) 098.13
      chronic or duration of 2 months or over 098.33
   diphtheritic 032.89 *[604.91]*
   filarial 125.9 *[604.91]*
   gangrenous 604.99
   gonococcal (acute) 098.13
      chronic or duration of 2 months or over 098.33
   mumps 072.0
   parotidea 072.0
   suppurative 604.99
   syphilitic 095.8 *[604.91]*
   tuberculous (*see also* Tuberculosis) 016.5
      [608.81]
Orf 051.2
Organic —*see also* condition
   heart—*see* Disease, heart
   insufficiency 799.8
Oriental
   bilharziasis 120.2
   schistosomiasis 120.2
   sore 085.1
Orifice —*see* condition
Origin, both great vessels from right ventricle
   745.11
Ormond's disease or syndrome 593.4
Ornithosis 073.9
   with
      complication 073.8
         specified NEC 073.7
      pneumonia 073.0
      pneumonitis (lobular) 073.0
Orodigitofacial dysostosis 759.89
Oropouche fever 066.3

Orotaciduria, oroticaciduria (congenital)
   (hereditary) (pyrimidine deficiency) 281.4
Oroya fever 088.0
Orthodontics V58.5
   adjustment V53.4
   aftercare V58.5
   fitting V53.4
Orthopnea 786.02
Orthoptic training V57.4
Os, uterus —*see* condition
Osgood-Schlatter
   disease 732.4
   osteochondrosis 732.4
Osler's
   disease (M9950/1) (polycythemia vera) 238.4
   nodes 421.0
Osler-Rendu disease (familial hemorrhagic
   telangiectasia) 448.0
Osler-Vaquez disease (M9950/1) (polycythemia
   vera) 238.4
Osler-Weber-Rendu syndrome (familial
   hemorrhagic telangiectasia) 448.0
Osmidrosis 705.89
Osseous —*see* condition
Ossification
   artery—*see* Arteriosclerosis
   auricle (ear) 380.39
   bronchus 519.1
   cardiac (*see also* Degeneration, myocardial)
      429.1
   cartilage (senile) 733.99
   coronary —*see* Arteriosclerosis, coronary
   diaphragm 728.10
   ear 380.39
      middle (*see also* Otosclerosis) 387.9
   falx cerebri 349.2
   fascia 728.10
   fontanel
      defective or delayed 756.0
      premature 756.0
   heart (*see also* Degeneration, myocardial) 429.1
      valve—*see* Endocarditis
   larynx 478.79
   ligament
      posterior longitudinal 724.8
         cervical 723.7
   meninges (cerebral) 349.2
      spinal 336.8
   multiple, eccentric centers 733.99
   muscle 728.10
      heterotopic, postoperative 728.13
   myocardium, myocardial (*see also*
      Degeneration, myocardial) 429.1
   penis 607.81
   periarticular 728.89
   sclera 379.16
   tendon 727.82
   trachea 519.1
   tympanic membrane (*see also*
      Tympanosclerosis) 385.00
   vitreous (humor) 360.44
Osteitis (*see also* Osteomyelitis) 730.2
   acute 730.0
   alveolar 526.5
   chronic 730.1
   condensans (ilii) 733.5
   deformans (Paget's) 731.0
      due to or associated with malignant neoplasm
         (*see also* Neoplasm, bone, malignant)
         170.9 *[731.1]*
   due to yaws 102.6

Osteitis—*continued*
  fibrosa NEC 733.29
    cystica (generalisata) 252.0
    disseminata 756.59
    osteoplastica 252.0
  fragilitans 756.51
  Garré's (sclerosing) 730.1
  infectious (acute) (subacute) 730.0
    chronic or old 730.1
  jaw (acute) (chronic) (lower) (neonatal)
      (suppurative) (upper) 526.4
  parathyroid 252.0
  petrous bone (*see also* Petrositis) 383.20
  pubis 733.5
  sclerotic, nonsuppurative 730.1
  syphilitic 095.5
  tuberculosa
    cystica (of Jüngling) 135
    multiplex cystoides 135
Osteoarthritica spondylitis (spine) (*see also*
    Spondylosis) 721.90
Osteoarthritis (*see also* Osteoarthrosis) 715.9
  distal interphalangeal 715.9
  hyperplastic 731.2
  interspinalis (*see also* Spondylosis) 721.90
  spine, spinal NEC (*see also* Spondylosis) 721.90
Osteoarthropathy (*see also* Osteoarthrosis)
    715.9
  chronic idiopathic hypertrophic 757.39
  familial idiopathic 757.39
  hypertrophic pulmonary 731.2
    secondary 731.2
  idiopathic hypertrophic 757.39
  primary hypertrophic 731.2
  pulmonary hypertrophic 731.2
  secondary hypertrophic 731.2
Osteoarthrosis (degenerative) (hypertrophic)
    (rheumatoid) 715.9

---

*Note—Use the following fifth-digit
subclassification with category 715:*

0 site unspecified
1 shoulder region
2 upper arm
3 forearm
4 hand
5 pelvic region and thigh
6 lower leg
7 ankle and foot
8 other specified sites except spine
9 multiple sites

---

  deformans alkaptonurica 270.2
  generalized 715.09
  juvenilis (Köhler's) 732.5
  localized 715.3
    idiopathic 715.1
    primary 715.1
    secondary 715.2
  multiple sites, not specified as generalized
      715.89
  polyarticular 715.09
  spine (*see also* Spondylosis) 721.90
  temperomandibular joint 524.69
Osteoblastoma (M9200/0)—*see* Neoplasm,
    bone, benign
Osteochondritis (*see also* Osteochondrosis)
    732.9
  dissecans 732.7
  hip 732.7
  ischiopubica 732.1

Osteochondritis—*continued*
  multiple 756.59
  syphilitic (congenital) 090.0
Osteochondrodermodysplasia 756.59
Osteochondrodystrophy 277.5
  deformans 277.5
  familial 277.5
  fetalis 756.4
Osteochondrolysis 732.7
Osteochondroma (M9210/0)—*see also*
    Neoplasm, bone, benign
  multiple, congenital 756.4
Osteochondromatosis (M9210/1) 238.0
  synovial 727.82
Osteochondromyxosarcoma (M9180/3)—*see*
    Neoplasm, bone, malignant
Osteochondropathy NEC 732.9
Osteochondrosarcoma (M9180/3)—*see*
    Neoplasm, bone, malignant
Osteochondrosis 732.9
  acetabulum 732.1
  adult spine 732.8
  astragalus 732.5
  Blount's 732.4
  Buchanan's (juvenile osteochondrosis of iliac
      crest) 732.1
  Buchman's (juvenile osteochondrosis) 732.1
  Burns' 732.3
  calcaneus 732.5
  capitular epiphysis (femur) 732.1
  carpal
    lunate (wrist) 732.3
    scaphoid 732.3
  coxae juvenilis 732.1
  deformans juvenilis (coxae) (hip) 732.1
    Scheuermann's 732.0
    spine 732.0
    tibia 732.4
    vertebra 732.0
  Diaz's (astragalus) 732.5
  dissecans (knee) (shoulder) 732.7
  femoral capital epiphysis 732.1
  femur (head) (juvenile) 732.1
  foot (juvenile) 732.5
  Freiberg's (disease) (second metatarsal) 732.5
  Haas' 732.3
  Haglund's (os tibiale externum) 732.5
  hand (juvenile) 732.3
  head of
    femur 732.1
    humerus (juvenile) 732.3
  hip (juvenile) 732.1
  humerus (juvenile) 732.3
  iliac crest (juvenile) 732.1
  ilium (juvenile) 732.1
  ischiopubic synchondrosis 732.1
  Iselin's (osteochondrosis fifth metatarsal) 732.5
  juvenile, juvenilis 732.6
    arm 732.3
    capital femoral epiphysis 732.1
    capitellum humeri 732.3
    capitular epiphysis 732.1
    carpal scaphoid 732.3
    clavicle, sternal epiphysis 732.6
    coxae 732.1
    deformans 732.1
    foot 732.5
    hand 732.3
    hip and pelvis 732.1
    lower extremity, except foot 732.4
    lunate, wrist 732.3

Osteochondrosis—*continued*
  medial cuneiform bone 732.5
  metatarsal (head) 732.5
  metatarsophalangeal 732.5
  navicular, ankle 732.5
  patella 732.4
  primary patellar center (of Köhler) 732.4
  specified site NEC 732.6
  spine 732.0
  tarsal scaphoid 732.5
  tibia (epiphysis) (tuberosity) 732.4
  upper extremity 732.3
  vertebra (body) (Calvé) 732.0
    epiphyseal plates (of Scheuermann) 732.0
  Kienböck's (disease) 732.3
  Köhler's (disease) (navicular, ankle) 732.5
    patellar 732.4
    tarsal navicular 732.5
  Legg-Calvé-Perthes (disease) 732.1
  lower extremity (juvenile) 732.4
  lunate bone 732.3
  Mauclaire's 732.3
  metacarpal heads (of Mauclaire) 732.3
  metatarsal (fifth) (head) (second) 732.5
  navicular, ankle 732.5
  os calcis 732.5
  Osgood-Schlatter 732.4
  os tibiale externum 732.5
  Panner's 732.3
  patella (juvenile) 732.4
  patellar center
    primary (of Köhler) 732.4
    secondary (of Sinding-Larsen) 732.4
  pelvis (juvenile) 732.1
  Pierson's 732.1
  radial head (juvenile) 732.3
  Scheuermann's 732.0
  Sever's (calcaneum) 732.5
  Sinding-Larsen (secondary patellar center) 732.4
  spine (juvenile) 732.0
    adult 732.8
  symphysis pubis (of Pierson) (juvenile) 732.1
  syphilitic (congenital) 090.0
  tarsal (navicular) (scaphoid) 732.5
  tibia (proximal) (tubercle) 732.4
  tuberculous—*see* Tuberculosis, bone
  ulna 732.3
  upper extremity (juvenile) 732.3
  van Neck's (juvenile osteochondrosis) 732.1
  vertebral (juvenile) 732.0
    adult 732.8
Osteoclastoma (M9250/1) 238.0
  malignant (M9250/3)—*see* Neoplasm, bone,
    malignant
Osteocopic pain 733.90
Osteodynia 733.90
Osteodystrophy
  azotemic 588.0
  chronica deformans hypertrophica 731.0
  congenital 756.50
    specified type NEC 756.59
  deformans 731.0
  fibrosa localisata 731.0
  parathyroid 252.0
  renal 588.0
Osteofibroma (M9262/0)—*see* Neoplasm, bone,
    benign
Osteofibrosarcoma (M9182/3)—*see* Neoplasm,
    bone, malignant
Osteogenesis imperfecta 756.51
Osteogenic —*see* condition

Osteoma (M9180/0)—*see also* Neoplasm, bone,
    benign
  osteoid (M9191/0)—*see also* Neoplasm, bone,
    benign
  giant (M9200/0)—*see* Neoplasm, bone, benign
Osteomalacia 268.2
  chronica deformans hypertrophica 731.0
  due to vitamin D deficiency 268.2
  infantile (*see also* Rickets) 268.0
  juvenile (*see also* Rickets) 268.0
  pelvis 268.2
  vitamin D-resistant 275.3
Osteomalacic bone 268.2
Osteomalacosis 268.2
Osteomyelitis (general) (infective) (localized)
    (neonatal) (purulent) (pyogenic) (septic)
    (staphylococcal) (streptococcal) (suppurative)
    (with periostitis) 730.2

*Note—Use the following fifth-digit
subclassification with category 730:*

0   site unspecified
1   shoulder region
2   upper arm
3   forearm
4   hand
5   pelvic region and thigh
6   lower leg
7   ankle and foot
8   other specified sites
9   multiple sites

  acute or subacute 730.0
  chronic or old 730.1
  due to or associated with
    diabetes mellitus 250.8 *[731.8]*
    tuberculosis (*see also* Tuberculosis, bone)
      015.9 *[730.8]*
      limb bones 015.5 *[730.8]*
      specified bones NEC 015.7 *[730.8]*
      spine 015.0 *[730.8]*
    typhoid 002.0 *[730.8]*
  Garré's 730.1
  jaw (acute) (chronic) (lower) (neonatal)
    (suppurative) (upper) 526.4
  nonsuppurating 730.1
  orbital 376.03
  petrous bone (*see also* Petrositis) 383.20
  Salmonella 003.24
  sclerosing, nonsuppurative 730.1
  sicca 730.1
  syphilitic 095.5
    congenital 090.0 *[730.8]*
  tuberculous—*see* Tuberculosis, bone
  typhoid 002.0 *[730.8]*
Osteomyelofibrosis 289.8
Osteomyelosclerosis 289.8
Osteonecrosis 733.40
  meaning osteomyelitis 730.1
Osteo-onycho-arthro dysplasia 756.89
Osteo-onychodysplasia, hereditary 756.89
Osteopathia
  condensans disseminata 756.53
  hyperostotica multiplex infantilis 756.59
  hypertrophica toxica 731.2
  striata 756.4
Osteopathy resulting from poliomyelitis (*see
    also* Poliomyelitis) 045.9 *[730.7]*
  familial dysplastic 731.2
Osteopecilia 756.53
Osteopenia 733.90

Osteoperiostitis (*see also* Osteomyelitis) 730.2
  ossificans toxica 731.2
  toxica ossificans 731.2
Osteopetrosis (familial) 756.52
Osteophyte —*see* Exostosis
Osteophytosis —*see* Exostosis
Osteopoikilosis 756.53
Osteoporosis (generalized) 733.00
  circumscripta 731.0
  disuse 733.03
  drug-induced 733.09
  idiopathic 733.02
  postmenopausal 733.01
  posttraumatic 733.7
  screening V82.81
  senile 733.01
  specified type NEC 733.09
Osteoporosis-osteomalacia syndrome 268.2
Osteopsathyrosis 756.51
Osteoradionecrosis, jaw 526.89
Osteosarcoma (M9180/3)—*see also* Neoplasm,
    bone, malignant
  chondroblastic (M9181/3)—*see* Neoplasm,
    bone, malignant
  fibroblastic (M9182/3)—*see* Neoplasm, bone,
    malignant
  in Paget's disease of bone (M9184/3)—*see*
    Neoplasm, bone, malignant
  juxtacortical (M9190/3)—*see* Neoplasm, bone,
    malignant
  parosteal (M9190/3)—*see* Neoplasm, bone,
    malignant
  telangiectatic (M9183/3)—*see* Neoplasm, bone,
    malignant
Osteosclerosis 756.52
  fragilis (generalisata) 756.52
  myelofibrosis 289.8
Osteosclerotic anemia 289.8
Osteosis
  acromegaloid 757.39
  cutis 709.3
  parathyroid 252.0
  renal fibrocystic 588.0
Österreicher-Turner syndrome 756.89
Ostium
  atrioventriculare commune 745.69
  primum (arteriosum) (defect) (persistent) 745.61
  secundum (arteriosum) (defect) (patent)
    (persistent) 745.5
Ostrum-Furst syndrome 756.59
Otalgia 388.70
  otogenic 388.71
  referred 388.72
Othematoma 380.31
Otitic hydrocephalus 348.2
Otitis 382.9
  with effusion 381.4
    purulent 382.4
    secretory 381.4
    serous 381.4
    suppurative 382.4
  acute 382.9
  adhesive (*see also* Adhesions, middle ear)
    385.10
  chronic 382.9
    with effusion 381.3
    mucoid, mucous (simple) 381.20
    purulent 382.3
    secretory 381.3
    serous 381.10
    suppurative 382.3

Otitis—*continued*
  diffuse parasitic 136.8
  externa (acute) (diffuse) (hemorrhagica) 380.10
    actinic 380.22
    candidal 112.82
    chemical 380.22
    chronic 380.23
      mycotic—*see* Otitis, externa, mycotic
      specified type NEC 380.23
    circumscribed 380.10
    contact 380.22
    due to
      erysipelas 035 *[380.13]*
      impetigo 684 *[380.13]*
      seborrheic dermatitis 690.10 *[380.13]*
    eczematoid 380.22
    furuncular 680.0 *[380.13]*
    infective 380.10
      chronic 380.16
    malignant 380.14
    mycotic (chronic) 380.15
      due to
        aspergillosis 117.3 *[380.15]*
        moniliasis 112.82
        otomycosis 111.8 *[380.15]*
    reactive 380.22
    specified type NEC 380.22
    tropical 111.8 *[380.15]*
  insidiosa (*see also* Otosclerosis) 387.9
  interna (*see also* Labyrinthitis) 386.30
  media (hemorrhagic) (staphylococcal)
      (streptococcal) 382.9
    acute 382.9
      with effusion 381.00
        allergic 381.04
          mucoid 381.05
          sanguineous 381.06
          serous 381.04
      catarrhal 381.00
      exudative 381.00
      mucoid 381.02
        allergic 381.05
      necrotizing 382.00
        with spontaneous rupture of ear drum
            382.01
      in
        influenza 487.8 *[382.02]*
        measles 055.2
        scarlet fever 034.1 *[382.02]*
      nonsuppurative 381.00
      purulent 382.00
        with spontaneous rupture of ear drum
            382.01
      sanguineous 381.03
        allergic 381.06
      secretory 381.01
      seromucinous 381.02
      serous 381.01
        allergic 381.04
      suppurative 382.00
        with spontaneous rupture of ear drum
            382.01
        due to
          influenza 487.8 *[382.02]*
          scarlet fever 034.1 *[382.02]*
      transudative 381.00
    adhesive (*see also* Adhesions, middle ear)
      385.10
    allergic 381.4
      acute 381.04
        mucoid 381.05

Otitis—*continued*
> sanguineous 381.06
> serous 381.04
> > chronic 381.3
> catarrhal 381.4
> > acute 381.00
> > chronic (simple) 381.10
> chronic 382.9
> > with effusion 381.3
> > adhesive (*see also* Adhesions, middle ear) 385.10
> > allergic 381.3
> > atticoantral, suppurative (with posterior or superior marginal perforation of ear drum) 382.2
> > benign suppurative (with anterior perforation of ear drum) 382.1
> > catarrhal 381.10
> > exudative 381.3
> > mucinous 381.20
> > mucoid, mucous (simple) 381.20
> > mucosanguineous 381.29
> > nonsuppurative 381.3
> > purulent 382.3
> > secretory 381.3
> > seromucinous 381.3
> > serosanguineous 381.19
> > serous (simple) 381.10
> > suppurative 382.3
> > > atticoantral (with posterior or superior marginal perforation of ear drum) 382.2
> > > benign (with anterior perforation of ear drum) 382.1
> > > tuberculous (*see also* Tuberculosis) 017.4
> > > tubotympanic 382.1
> > transudative 381.3
> exudative 381.4
> > acute 381.00
> > chronic 381.3
> fibrotic (*see also* Adhesions, middle ear) 385.10
> mucoid, mucous 381.4
> > acute 381.02
> > chronic (simple) 381.20
> mucosanguineous, chronic 381.29
> nonsuppurative 381.4
> > acute 381.00
> > chronic 381.3
> postmeasles 055.2
> purulent 382.4
> > acute 382.00
> > > with spontaneous rupture of ear drum 382.01
> > chronic 382.3
> sanguineous, acute 381.03
> > allergic 381.06
> secretory 381.4
> > acute or subacute 381.01
> > chronic 381.3
> seromucinous 381.4
> > acute or subacute 381.02
> > chronic 381.3
> serosanguineous, chronic 381.19
> serous 381.4
> > acute or subacute 381.01
> > chronic (simple) 381.10
> subacute—*see* Otitis, media, acute
> suppurative 382.4
> > acute 382.00

Otitis—*continued*
> with spontaneous rupture of ear drum 382.01
> > chronic 382.3
> > atticoantral 382.2
> > benign 382.1
> > tuberculous (*see also* Tuberculosis) 017.4
> > tubotympanic 382.1
> transudative 381.4
> > acute 381.00
> > chronic 381.3
> tuberculous (*see also* Tuberculosis) 017.4
> postmeasles 055.2
Otoconia 386.8
Otolith syndrome 386.19
Otomycosis 111.8 *[380.15]*
> in
> > aspergillosis 117.3 *[380.15]*
> > moniliasis 112.82
Otopathy 388.9
Otoporosis (*see also* Otosclerosis) 387.9
Otorrhagia 388.69
> traumatic—*see* nature of injury
Otorrhea 388.60
> blood 388.69
> cerebrospinal (fluid) 388.61
Otosclerosis (general) 387.9
> cochlear (endosteal) 387.2
> involving
> > otic capsule 387.2
> > oval window
> > > nonobliterative 387.0
> > > obliterative 387.1
> > round window 387.2
> nonobliterative 387.0
> obliterative 387.1
> specified type NEC 387.8
Otospongiosis (*see also* Otosclerosis) 387.9
Otto's disease or pelvis 715.35
Outburst, aggressive (*see also* Disturbance, conduct) 312.0
> in children and adolescents 313.9
Outcome of delivery
> multiple birth NEC V27.9
> > all liveborn V27.5
> > all stillborn V27.7
> > some liveborn V27.6
> > unspecified V27.9
> single V27.9
> > liveborn V27.0
> > stillborn V27.1
> twins V27.9
> > both liveborn V27.2
> > both stillborn V27.4
> > one liveborn, one stillborn V27.3
Outlet —*see also* condition
> syndrome (thoracic) 353.0
Outstanding ears (bilateral) 744.29
Ovalocytosis (congenital) (hereditary) (*see also* Elliptocytosis) 282.1
Ovarian —*see also* condition
> pregnancy—*see* Pregnancy, ovarian
> remnant syndrome 620.8
> vein syndrome 593.4
Ovaritis (cystic) (*see also* Salpingo-oophoritis) 614.2
Ovary, ovarian —*see* condition
Overactive —*see also* Hyperfunction
> bladder 596.51
> eye muscle (*see also* Strabismus) 378.9
> hypothalamus 253.8
> thyroid (*see also* Thyrotoxicosis) 242.9

Overactivity, child 314.01
Overbite (deep) (excessive) (horizontal)
  (vertical) 524.2
Overbreathing (*see also* Hyperventilation)
  786.01
Overconscientious personality 301.4
Overdevelopment —*see also* Hypertrophy
  breast (female) (male) 611.1
  nasal bones 738.0
  prostate, congenital 752.8
Overdistention —*see* Distention
Overdose overdosage (drug) 977.9
  specified drug or substance—*see* Table of drugs
    and chemicals
Overeating 783.6
  with obesity 278.0
  nonorganic origin 307.51
Overexertion (effects) (exhaustion) 994.5
Overexposure (effects) 994.9
  exhaustion 994.4
Overfeeding (*see also* Overeating) 783.6
Overgrowth, bone NEC 733.99
Overheated (effects) (places)—*see* Heat
Overinhibited child 313.0
Overjet 524.2
Overlaid, overlying (suffocation) 994.7
Overlapping toe (acquired) 735.8
  congenital (fifth toe) 755.66
Overload
  fluid 276.6
  potassium (K) 276.7
  sodium (Na) 276.0
Overnutrition (*see also* Hyperalimentation)
  783.6
Overproduction —*see also* Hypersecretion
  ACTH 255.3
  cortisol 255.0
  growth hormone 253.0
  thyroid-stimulating hormone (TSH) 242.8
Overriding
  aorta 747.21
  finger (acquired) 736.29
    congenital 755.59
  toe (acquired) 735.8
    congenital 755.66
Oversize
  fetus (weight of 4500 grams or more) 766.0
    affecting management of pregnancy 656.6
    causing disproportion 653.5
      with obstructed labor 660.1
      affecting fetus or newborn 763.1
Overstimulation, ovarian 256.1
Overstrained 780.79
  heart—*see* Hypertrophy, cardiac
Overweight (*see also* Obesity) 278.00
Overwork 780.79
Oviduct —*see* condition
Ovotestis 752.7
Ovulation (cycle)
  failure or lack of 628.0
  pain 625.2
Ovum
  blighted 631
  dropsical 631
  pathologic 631
Owren's disease or syndrome (parahemophilia)
  (*see also* Defect, coagulation) 286.3
Oxalosis 271.8
Oxaluria 271.8
Ox heart —*see* Hypertrophy, cardiac

OX syndrome 758.6
Oxycephaly, oxycephalic 756.0
  syphilitic, congenital 090.0
Oxyuriasis 127.4
Oxyuris vermicularis (infestation) 127.4
Ozena 472.0

P

Pacemaker syndrome 429.4
Pachyderma, pachydermia 701.8
  laryngis 478.5
  laryngitis 478.79
  larynx (verrucosa) 478.79
Pachydermatitis 701.8
Pachydermatocele (congenital) 757.39
  acquired 701.8
Pachydermatosis 701.8
Pachydermoperiostitis
  secondary 731.2
Pachydermoperiostosis
  primary idiopathic 757.39
  secondary 731.2
Pachymeningitis (adhesive) (basal) (brain)
  (cerebral) (cervical) (chronic) (circumscribed)
  (external) (fibrous) (hemorrhagic)
  (hypertrophic) (internal) (purulent) (spinal)
  (suppurative) (*see also* Meningitis) 322.9
  gonococcal 098.82
Pachyonychia (congenital) 757.5
  acquired 703.8
Pachyperiosteodermia
  primary or idiopathic 757.39
  secondary 731.2
Pachyperiostosis
  primary or idiopathic 757.39
  secondary 731.2
Pacinian tumor (M9507/0)—*see* Neoplasm,
  skin, benign
Pads, knuckle or Garrod's 728.79
Paget's disease (osteitis deformans) 731.0
  with infiltrating duct carcinoma of the breast
    (M8541/3)—*see* Neoplasm, breast,
    malignant
  bone 731.0
    osteosarcoma in (M9184/3)—*see* Neoplasm,
      bone, malignant
  breast (M8540/3) 174.0
  extramammary (M8542/3)—*see also* Neoplasm,
    skin, malignant
    anus 154.3
    skin 173.5
  malignant (M8540/3)
    breast 174.0
    specified site NEC (M8542/3)—*see*
      Neoplasm, skin, malignant
    unspecified site 174.0
  mammary (M8540/3) 174.0
  necrosis of bone 731.0
  nipple (M8540/3) 174.0
  osteitis deformans 731.0
Paget-Schroetter syndrome (intermittent venous
  claudication) 453.8
Pain(s)
  abdominal 789.0
  adnexa (uteri) 625.9
  alimentary, due to vascular insufficiency 557.9
  anginoid (*see also* Pain, precordial) 786.51
  anus 569.42
  arch 729.5
  arm 729.5
  back (postural) 724.5
    low 724.2
    psychogenic 307.89
  bile duct 576.9
  bladder 788.9

Pain(s)—*continued*
  bone 733.90
  breast 611.71
    psychogenic 307.89
  broad ligament 625.9
  cartilage NEC 733.90
  cecum 789.0
  cervicobrachial 723.3
  chest (central) 786.50
    atypical 786.59
    midsternal 786.51
    musculoskeletal 786.59
    noncardiac 786.59
    substernal 786.51
    wall (anterior) 786.52
  coccyx 724.79
  colon 789.0
  common duct 576.9
  coronary—*see* Angina
  costochondral 786.52
  diaphragm 786.52
  due to (presence of) any device, implant, or
    graft classifiable to 996.0-996.5—*see*
    Complications, due to (presence of) any
    device, implant, or graft classified to
    996.0-996.5 NEC
  ear (*see also* Otalgia) 388.70
  epigastric, epigastrium 789.0
  extremity (lower) (upper) 729.5
  eye 379.91
  face, facial 784.0
    atypical 350.2
    nerve 351.8
  false (labor) 644.1
  female genital organ NEC 625.9
    psychogenic 307.89
  finger 729.5
  flank 789.0
  foot 729.5
  gallbladder 575.9
  gas (intestinal) 787.3
  gastric 536.8
  generalized 780.99
  genital organ
    female 625.9
    male 608.9
    psychogenic 307.89
  groin 789.0
  growing 781.99
  hand 729.5
  head (*see also* Headache) 784.0
  heart (*see also* Pain, precordial) 786.51
  infraorbital (*see also* Neuralgia, trigeminal)
    350.1
  intermenstrual 625.2
  jaw 526.9
  joint 719.40
    ankle 719.47
    elbow 719.42
    foot 719.47
    hand 719.44
    hip 719.45
    knee 719.46
    multiple sites 719.49
    pelvic region 719.45
    psychogenic 307.89
    shoulder (region) 719.41
    specified site NEC 719.48

Pain(s)—*continued*
  wrist 719.43
  kidney 788.0
  labor, false or spurious 644.1
  laryngeal 784.1
  leg 729.5
  limb 729.5
  low back 724.2
  lumbar region 724.2
  mastoid (*see also* Otalgia) 388.70
  maxilla 526.9
  metacarpophalangeal (joint) 719.44
  metatarsophalangeal (joint) 719.47
  mouth 528.9
  muscle 729.1
    intercostal 786.59
  nasal 478.1
  nasopharynx 478.29
  neck NEC 723.1
    psychogenic 307.89
  nerve NEC 729.2
  neuromuscular 729.1
  nose 478.1
  ocular 379.91
  ophthalmic 379.91
  orbital region 379.91
  osteocopic 733.90
  ovary 625.9
    psychogenic 307.89
  over heart (*see also* Pain, precordial) 786.51
  ovulation 625.2
  pelvic (female) 625.9
    male NEC 789.0
      psychogenic 307.89
    psychogenic 307.89
  penis 607.9
    psychogenic 307.89
  pericardial (*see also* Pain, precordial) 786.51
  perineum
    female 625.9
    male 608.9
  pharynx 478.29
  pleura, pleural, pleuritic 786.52
  post-operative —*see* Pain, by site
  preauricular 388.70
  precordial (region) 786.51
    psychogenic 307.89
  psychogenic 307.80
    cardiovascular system 307.89
    gastrointestinal system 307.89
    genitourinary system 307.89
    heart 307.89
    musculoskeletal system 307.89
    respiratory system 307.89
    skin 306.3
  radicular (spinal) (*see also* Radiculitis) 729.2
  rectum 569.42
  respiration 786.52
  retrosternal 786.51
  rheumatic NEC 729.0
    muscular 729.1
  rib 786.50
  root (spinal) (*see also* Radiculitis) 729.2
  round ligament (stretch) 625.9
  sacroiliac 724.6
  sciatic 724.3
  scrotum 608.9
    psychogenic 307.89
  seminal vesicle 608.9
  sinus 478.1
  skin 782.0

Pain(s)—*continued*
  spermatic cord 608.9
  spinal root (*see also* Radiculitis) 729.2
  stomach 536.8
    psychogenic 307.89
  substernal 786.51
  temporomandibular (joint) 524.62
  temporomaxillary joint 524.62
  testis 608.9
    psychogenic 307.89
  thoracic spine 724.1
    with radicular and visceral pain 724.4
  throat 784.1
  tibia 733.90
  toe 729.5
  tongue 529.6
  tooth 525.9
  trigeminal (*see also* Neuralgia, trigeminal) 350.1
  umbilicus 789.0
  ureter 788.0
  urinary (organ) (system) 788.0
  uterus 625.9
    psychogenic 307.89
  vagina 625.9
  vertebrogenic (syndrome) 724.5
  vesical 788.9
  vulva 625.9
  xiphoid 733.90
Painful —*see also* Pain
  arc syndrome 726.19
  coitus
    female 625.0
    male 608.89
    psychogenic 302.76
  ejaculation (semen) 608.89
    psychogenic 302.79
  erection 607.3
  feet syndrome 266.2
  menstruation 625.3
    psychogenic 306.52
  micturition 788.1
  ophthalmoplegia 378.55
  respiration 786.52
  scar NEC 709.2
  urination 788.1
  wire sutures 998.89
Painters' colic 984.9
  specified type of lead—*see* Table of drugs and chemicals
Palate —*see* condition
Palatoplegia 528.9
Palatoschisis (*see also* Cleft, palate) 749.00
Palilalia 784.69
Palindromic arthritis (*see also* Rheumatism, palindromic) 719.3
Palliative care V66.7
Pallor 782.61
  temporal, optic disc 377.15
Palmar —*see also* condition
  fascia—*see* condition
Palpable
  cecum 569.89
  kidney 593.89
  liver 573.9
  lymph nodes 785.6
  ovary 620.8
  prostate 602.9
  spleen (*see also* Splenomegaly) 789.2
  uterus 625.8
Palpitation (heart) 785.1
  psychogenic 306.2

Palsy (*see also* Paralysis) 344.9
   atrophic diffuse 335.20
   Bell's 351.0
      newborn 767.5
   birth 767.7
   brachial plexus 353.0
      fetus or newborn 767.6
   brain—*see also* Palsy, cerebral
      noncongenital or noninfantile 344.89
         due to vascular lesion—*see* category 438
         late effect—*see* Late effect(s) (of)
            cerebrovascular disease
      syphilitic 094.89
         congenital 090.49
   bulbar (chronic) (progressive) 335.22
      pseudo NEC 335.23
      supranuclear NEC 344.89
   cerebral (congenital) (infantile) (spastic) 343.9
      athetoid 333.7
      diplegic 343.0
         due to previous vascular lesion—*see*
            category 438
         late effect—*see* Late effect(s) (of)
            cerebrovascular disease
      hemiplegic 343.1
      monoplegic 343.3
      noncongenital or noninfantile 437.8
         due to previous vascular lesion—*see*
            category 438
         late effect—*see* Late effect(s) (of)
            cerebrovascular disease
      paraplegic 343.0
      quadriplegic 343.2
      spastic, not congenital or infantile 344.89
      syphilitic 094.89
         congenital 090.49
      tetraplegic 343.2
   cranial nerve—*see also* Disorder, nerve, cranial
      multiple 352.6
   creeping 335.21
   divers' 993.3
   Erb's (birth injury) 767.6
   facial 351.0
      newborn 767.5
   glossopharyngeal 352.2
   Klumpke (-Déjérine) 767.6
   lead 984.9
      specified type of lead—*see* Table of drugs and
         chemicals
   median nerve (tardy) 354.0
   peroneal nerve (acute) (tardy) 355.3
   progressive supranuclear 333.0
   pseudobulbar NEC 335.23
   radial nerve (acute) 354.3
   seventh nerve 351.0
      newborn 767.5
   shaking (*see also* Parkinsonism) 332.0
   spastic (cerebral) (spinal) 343.9
      hemiplegic 343.1
   specified nerve NEC—*see* Disorder, nerve
   supranuclear NEC 356.8
      progressive 333.0
   ulnar nerve (tardy) 354.2
   wasting 335.21
Paltauf-Sternberg disease 201.9
Paludism —*see* Malaria
Panama fever 084.0
Panaris (with lymphangitis) 681.9
   finger 681.02
   toe 681.11

Panaritium (with lymphangitis) 681.9
   finger 681.02
   toe 681.11
Panarteritis (nodosa) 446.0
   brain or cerebral 437.4
Pancake heart 793.2
   with cor pulmonale (chronic) 416.9
Pancarditis (acute) (chronic) 429.89
   with
      rheumatic
         fever (active) (acute) (chronic) (subacute)
            391.8
         inactive or quiescent 398.99
   rheumatic, acute 391.8
      chronic or inactive 398.99
Pancoast's syndrome or tumor (carcinoma,
   pulmonary apex) (M8010/3) 162.3
Pancoast-Tobias syndrome (M8010/3)
   (carcinoma, pulmonary apex) 162.3
Pancolitis 556.6
Pancreas, pancreatic —*see* condition
Pancreatitis 577.0
   acute (edematous) (hemorrhagic) (recurrent)
      577.0
   annular 577.0
   apoplectic 577.0
   calcereous 577.0
   chronic (infectious) 577.1
      recurrent 577.1
   cystic 577.2
   fibrous 577.8
   gangrenous 577.0
   hemorrhagic (acute) 577.0
   interstitial (chronic) 577.1
      acute 577.0
   malignant 577.0
   mumps 072.3
   painless 577.1
   recurrent 577.1
   relapsing 577.1
   subacute 577.0
   suppurative 577.0
   syphilitic 095.8
Pancreatolithiasis 577.8
Pancytolysis 289.9
Pancytopenia (acquired) 284.8
   with malformations 284.0
   congenital 284.0
Panencephalitis —*see also* Encephalitis
   subacute, sclerosing 046.2
Panhematopenia 284.8
   congenital 284.0
   constitutional 284.0
   splenic, primary 289.4
Panhemocytopenia 284.8
   congenital 284.0
   constitutional 284.0
Panhypogonadism 257.2
Panhypopituitarism 253.2
   prepubertal 253.3
Panic (attack) (state) 300.01
   reaction to exceptional stress (transient) 308.0
Panmyelopathy, familial constitutional 284.0
Panmyelophthisis 284.9
   acquired (secondary) 284.8
   congenital 284.0
   idiopathic 284.9
Panmyelosis (acute) (M9951/1) 238.7
Panner's disease 732.3
   capitellum humeri 732.3
   head of humerus 732.3
   tarsal navicular (bone) (osteochondrosis) 732.5

Panneuritis endemica 265.0 *[357.4]*
Panniculitis 729.30
  back 724.8
  knee 729.31
  neck 723.6
  nodular, nonsuppurative 729.30
  sacral 724.8
  specified site NEC 729.39
Panniculus adiposus (abdominal) 278.1
Pannus 370.62
  allergic eczematous 370.62
  degenerativus 370.62
  keratic 370.62
  rheumatoid—*see* Arthritis, rheumatoid
  trachomatosus, trachomatous (active) 076.1
    [370.62]
    late effect 139.1
Panophthalmitis 360.02
Panotitis —*see* Otitis media
Pansinusitis (chronic) (hyperplastic)
    (nonpurulent) (purulent) 473.8
  acute 461.8
  due to fungus NEC 117.9
  tuberculous (*see also* Tuberculosis) 012.8
Panuveitis 360.12
  sympathetic 360.11
Panvalvular disease —*see* Endocarditis, mitral
Papageienkrankheit 073.9
Papanicolaou smear
  cervix (screening test) V76.2
    as part of gynecological examination V72.3
    for suspected malignant neoplasm V76.2
      no disease found V71.1
    nonspecific abnormal finding 795.00
      atypical squamous cell changes of
        undetermined significance
        favor benign (ASCUS favor benign)
          795.01
        favor dysplasia (ASCUS favor dysplasia)
          795.02
      nonspecific finding NEC 795.09
      unsatisfactory 795.09
  other specified site—*see also* Screening,
      malignant neoplasm
    for suspected malignant neoplasm—*see also*
      Screening, malignant neoplasm
    no disease found V71.1
    nonspecific abnormal finding 795.1
  vagina V76.47
    following hysterectomy for malignant
      condition V67.01
Papilledema 377.00
  associated with
    decreased ocular pressure 377.02
    increased intracranial pressure 377.01
    retinal disorder 377.03
  choked disc 377.00
  infectional 377.00
Papillitis 377.31
  anus 569.49
  chronic lingual 529.4
  necrotizing, kidney 584.7
  optic 377.31
  rectum 569.49
  renal, necrotizing 584.7
  tongue 529.0

Papilloma (M8050/0)—*see also* Neoplasm, by
    site, benign

> *Note—Except where otherwise indicated, the
> morphological varieties of papilloma in the list
> below should be coded by site as for
> "Neoplasm, benign."*

  acuminatum (female) (male) 078.11
  bladder (urinary) (transitional cell) (M8120/1)
    236.7
    benign (M8120/0) 223.3
  choroid plexus (M9390/0) 225.0
    anaplastic type (M9390/3) 191.5
    malignant (M9390/3) 191.5
  ductal (M8503/0)
  dyskeratotic (M8052/0)
  epidermoid (M8052/0)
  hyperkeratotic (M8052/0)
  intracystic (M8504/0)
  intraductal (M8503/0)
  inverted (M8053/0)
  keratotic (M8052/0)
  parakeratotic (M8052/0)
  pinta (primary) 103.0
  renal pelvis (transitional cell) (M8120/1) 236.99
    benign (M8120/0) 223.1
  Schneiderian (M8121/0)
    specified site—*see* Neoplasm, by site, benign
    unspecified site 212.0
  serous surface (M8461/0)
    borderline malignancy (M8461/1)
      specified site—*see* Neoplasm, by site,
        uncertain behavior
      unspecified site 236.2
    specified site—*see* Neoplasm, by site, benign
    unspecified site 220
  squamous (cell) (M8052/0)
  transitional (cell) (M8120/0)
    bladder (urinary) (M8120/1) 236.7
    inverted type (M8121/1)—*see* Neoplasm, by
      site, uncertain behavior
    renal pelvis (M8120/1) 236.91
    ureter (M8120/1) 236.91
  ureter (transitional cell) (M8120/1) 236.91
    benign (M8120/0) 223.2
  urothelial (M8120/1)—*see* Neoplasm, by site,
    uncertain behavior
  verrucous (M8051/0)
  villous (M8261/1)—*see* Neoplasm, by site,
    uncertain behavior
  yaws, plantar or palmar 102.1
Papillomata, multiple, of yaws 102.1
Papillomatosis (M8060/0)—*see also* Neoplasm,
    by site, benign
  confluent and reticulate 701.8
  cutaneous 701.8
  ductal, breast 610.1
  Gougerot-Carteaud (confluent reticulate) 701.8
  intraductal (diffuse) (M8505/0)—*see* Neoplasm,
    by site, benign
  subareolar duct (M8506/0) 217
Papillon-Léage and Psaume syndrome
    (orodigitofacial dysostosis) 759.89
Papule 709.8
  carate (primary) 103.0
  fibrous, of nose (M8724/0) 216.3
  pinta (primary) 103.0
Papulosis, malignant 447.8
Papyraceous fetus 779.89
  complicating pregnancy 646.0
Paracephalus 759.7
Parachute mitral valve 746.5

Paracoccidioidomycosis 116.1
  mucocutaneous-lymphangitic 116.1
  pulmonary 116.1
  visceral 116.1
Paracoccidiomycosis *—see*
  Paracoccidioidomycosis
Paracusis 388.40
Paradentosis 523.5
Paradoxical facial movements 374.43
Paraffinoma 999.9
Paraganglioma (M8680/1)
  adrenal (M8700/0) 227.0
    malignant (M8700/3) 194.0
  aortic body (M8691/1) 237.3
    malignant (M8691/3) 194.6
  carotid body (M8692/1) 237.3
    malignant (M8692/3) 194.5
  chromaffin (M8700/0)—*see also* Neoplasm, by
    site, benign
    malignant (M8700/3)—*see* Neoplasm, by site,
      malignant
  extra-adrenal (M8693/1)
    malignant (M8693/3)
      specified site—*see* Neoplasm, by site,
        malignant
      unspecified site 194.6
    specified site—*see* Neoplasm, by site,
      uncertain behavior
    unspecified site 237.3
  glomus jugulare (M8690/1) 237.3
    malignant (M8690/3) 194.6
  jugular (M8690/1) 237.3
    malignant (M8680/3)
      specified site—*see* Neoplasm, by site,
        malignant
      unspecified site 194.6
  nonchromaffin (M8693/1)
    malignant (M8693/3)
      specified site—*see* Neoplasm, by site,
        malignant
      unspecified site 194.6
    specified site—*see* Neoplasm, by site,
      uncertain behavior
    unspecified site 237.3
  parasympathetic (M8682/1)
    specified site—*see* Neoplasm, by site,
      uncertain behavior
    unspecified site 237.3
  specified site—*see* Neoplasm, by site, uncertain
    behavior
  sympathetic (M8681/1)
    specified site—*see* Neoplasm, by site,
      uncertain behavior
    unspecified site 237.3
  unspecified site 237.3
Parageusia 781.1
  psychogenic 306.7
Paragonimiasis 121.2
Paragranuloma, Hodgkin's (M9660/3) 201.0
Parahemophilia (*see also* Defect, coagulation)
  286.3
Parakeratosis 690.8
  psoriasiformis 696.2
  variegata 696.2
Paralysis, paralytic (complete) (incomplete)
  344.9
  with
    broken
      back—*see* Fracture, vertebra, by site, with
        spinal cord injury

Paralysis, paralytic—*continued*
  neck—*see* Fracture, vertebra, cervical, with
    spinal cord injury
  fracture, vertebra—*see* Fracture, vertebra, by
    site, with spinal cord injury
  syphilis 094.89
  abdomen and back muscles 355.9
  abdominal muscles 355.9
  abducens (nerve) 378.54
  abductor 355.9
    lower extremity 355.8
    upper extremity 354.9
  accessory nerve 352.4
  accommodation 367.51
    hysterical 300.11
  acoustic nerve 388.5
  agitans 332.0
    arteriosclerotic 332.0
  alternating 344.89
    oculomotor 344.89
  amyotrophic 335.20
  ankle 355.8
  anterior serratus 355.9
  anus (sphincter) 569.49
  apoplectic (current episode) (*see also* Disease,
    cerebrovascular, acute) 436
    late effect—*see* Late effect(s) (of)
      cerebrovascular disease
    category 438
  arm 344.40
    affecting
      dominant side 344.41
      nondominant side 344.42
    both 344.2
    due to old CVA—*see* category 438
    hysterical 300.11
    late effect—*see* Late effect(s) (of)
      cerebrovascular disease
    psychogenic 306.0
    transient 781.4
      traumatic NEC (*see also* Injury, nerve,
        upper limb) 955.9
  arteriosclerotic (current episode) 437.0
    late effect—*see* Late effect(s) (of)
      cerebrovascular disease
  ascending (spinal), acute 357.0
  associated, nuclear 344.89
  asthenic bulbar 358.0
  ataxic NEC 334.9
    general 094.1
  athetoid 333.7
  atrophic 356.9
    infantile, acute (*see also* Poliomyelitis, with
      paralysis) 045.1
    muscle NEC 355.9
    progressive 335.21
    spinal (acute) (*see also* Poliomyelitis, with
      paralysis) 045.1
  attack (*see also* Disease, cerebrovascular, acute)
    436
  axillary 353.0
  Babinski-Nageotte's 344.89
  Bell's 351.0
    newborn 767.5
  Benedikt's 344.89
  birth (injury) 767.7
    brain 767.0
    intracranial 767.0
    spinal cord 767.4
  bladder (sphincter) 596.53
    neurogenic 596.54

Paralysis, paralytic—*continued*
   with cauda equina syndrome 344.61
   puerperal, postpartum, childbirth 665.5
   sensory 596.54
      with cauda equina 344.61
   spastic 596.54
      with cauda equina 344.61
  bowel, colon, or intestine (*see also* Ileus) 560.1
  brachial plexus 353.0
   due to birth injury 767.6
   newborn 767.6
  brain
   congenital—*see* Palsy, cerebral
   current episode 437.8
   diplegia 344.2
   due to previous vascular lesion—*see* category
      438
   hemiplegia 342.9
     due to previous vascular lesion—*see*
       category 438
     late effect—*see* Late effect(s) (of)
       cerebrovascular disease
   infantile—*see* Palsy, cerebral
   late effect—*see* Late effect(s) (of)
     cerebrovascular disease
   monoplegia—*see also* Monoplegia
     due to previous vascular lesion—*see*
       category 438
     late effect—*see* Late effect(s) (of)
       cerebrovascular disease
   paraplegia 344.1
   quadriplegia —*see* Quadriplegia
   syphilitic, congenital 090.49
   triplegia 344.89
  bronchi 519.1
  Brown-Séquard's 344.89
  bulbar (chronic) (progressive) 335.22
   infantile (*see also* Poliomyelitis, bulbar) 045.0
   poliomyelitic (*see also* Poliomyelitis, bulbar)
     045.0
   pseudo 335.23
   supranuclear 344.89
  bulbospinal 358.0
  cardiac (*see also* Failure, heart) 428.9
  cerebral
   current episode 437.8
   spastic, infantile—*see* Palsy, cerebral
  cerebrocerebellar 437.8
   diplegic infantile 343.0
  cervical
   plexus 353.2
   sympathetic NEC 337.0
  Céstan-Chenais 344.89
  Charcot-Marie-Tooth type 356.1
  childhood—*see* Palsy, cerebral
  Clark's 343.9
  colon (*see also* Ileus) 560.1
  compressed air 993.3
  compression
   arm NEC 354.9
   cerebral—*see* Paralysis, brain
   leg NEC 355.8
   lower extremity NEC 355.8
   upper extremity NEC 354.9
  congenital (cerebral) (spastic) (spinal)—*see*
    Palsy, cerebral
  conjugate movement (of eye) 378.81
   cortical (nuclear) (supranuclear) 378.81
  convergence 378.83
  cordis (*see also* Failure, heart) 428.9
  cortical (*see also* Paralysis, brain) 437.8

Paralysis, paralytic—*continued*
  cranial or cerebral nerve (*see also* Disorder,
    nerve, cranial) 352.9
  creeping 335.21
  crossed leg 344.89
  crutch 953.4
  deglutition 784.9
   hysterical 300.11
  dementia 094.1
  descending (spinal) NEC 335.9
  diaphragm (flaccid) 519.4
   due to accidental section of phrenic nerve
     during procedure 998.2
  digestive organs NEC 564.89
  diplegic—*see* Diplegia
  divergence (nuclear) 378.85
  divers' 993.3
  Duchenne's 335.22
  due to intracranial or spinal birth injury—*see*
    Palsy, cerebral
  embolic (current episode) (*see also* Embolism,
    brain) 434.1
   late effect —*see* Late effect(s) (of)
     cerebrovascular disease
  enteric (*see also* Ileus) 560.1
   with hernia—*see* Hernia, by site, with
     obstruction
  Erb's syphilitic spastic spinal 094.89
  Erb (-Duchenne) (birth) (newborn) 767.6
  esophagus 530.89
  essential, infancy (*see also* Poliomyelitis) 045.9
  extremity
   lower —*see* Paralysis, leg
   spastic (hereditary) 343.3
    noncongenital or noninfantile 344.1
   transient (cause unknown) 781.4
   upper —*see* Paralysis, arm
  eye muscle (extrinsic) 378.55
   intrinsic 367.51
  facial (nerve) 351.0
   birth injury 767.5
   congenital 767.5
   following operation NEC 998.2
   newborn 767.5
  familial 359.3
   periodic 359.3
   spastic 334.1
  fauces 478.29
  finger NEC 354.9
  foot NEC 355.8
  gait 781.2
  gastric nerve 352.3
  gaze 378.81
  general 094.1
   ataxic 094.1
   insane 094.1
   juvenile 090.40
   progressive 094.1
   tabetic 094.1
  glossopharyngeal (nerve) 352.2
  glottis (*see also* Paralysis, vocal cord) 478.30
  gluteal 353.4
  Gubler (-Millard) 344.89
  hand 354.9
   hysterical 300.11
   psychogenic 306.0
  heart (*see also* Failure, heart) 428.9
  hemifacial, progressive 349.89
  hemiplegic—*see* Hemiplegia
  hyperkalemic periodic (familial) 359.3
  hypertensive (current episode) 437.8

Paralysis, paralytic—*continued*
  hypoglossal (nerve) 352.5
  hypokalemic periodic 359.3
  Hyrtl's sphincter (rectum) 569.49
  hysterical 300.11
  ileus (*see also* Ileus) 560.1
  infantile (*see also* Poliomyelitis) 045.9
    atrophic acute 045.1
    bulbar 045.0
    cerebral—*see* Palsy, cerebral
    paralytic 045.1
    progressive acute 045.9
    spastic—*see* Palsy, cerebral
    spinal 045.9
  infective (*see also* Poliomyelitis) 045.9
  inferior nuclear 344.9
  insane, general or progressive 094.1
  internuclear 378.86
  interosseous 355.9
  intestine (*see also* Ileus) 560.1
  intracranial (current episode) (*see also*
      Paralysis, brain) 437.8
    due to birth injury 767.0
  iris 379.49
    due to diphtheria (toxin) 032.81 *[379.49]*
  ischemic, Volkmann's (complicating trauma)
      958.6
  Jackson's 344.89
  jake 357.7
  Jamaica ginger (jake) 357.7
  juvenile general 090.40
  Klumpke (-Déjérine) (birth) (newborn) 767.6
  labioglossal (laryngeal) (pharyngeal) 335.22
  Landry's 357.0
  laryngeal nerve (recurrent) (superior) (*see also*
      Paralysis, vocal cord) 478.30
  larynx (*see also* Paralysis, vocal cord) 478.30
    due to diphtheria (toxin) 032.3
  late effect
    due to
      birth injury, brain or spinal (cord)—*see*
          Palsy, cerebral
      edema, brain or cerebral—*see* Paralysis,
          brain
      lesion
        cerebrovascular—*see* category 438
        late effect—*see* Late effect(s) (of)
            cerebrovascular disease
      spinal (cord)—*see* Paralysis, spinal
  lateral 335.24
  lead 984.9
    specified type of lead—*see* Table of drugs and
        chemicals
  left side—*see* Hemiplegia
  leg 344.30
    affecting
      dominant side 344.31
      nondominant side 344.32
    both (*see also* Paraplegia) 344.1
    crossed 344.89
    hysterical 300.11
    psychogenic 306.0
    transient or transitory 781.4
      traumatic NEC (*see also* Injury, nerve,
          lower limb) 956.9
  levator palpebrae superioris 374.31
  limb NEC 344.5
    all four—*see* Quadriplegia
    quadriplegia—*see* Quadriplegia
  lip 528.5
  Lissauer's 094.1

Paralysis, paralytic—*continued*
  local 355.9
  lower limb—*see also* Paralysis, leg
    both (*see also* Paraplegia) 344.1
  lung 518.89
    newborn 770.89
  median nerve 354.1
  medullary (tegmental) 344.89
  mesencephalic NEC 344.89
    tegmental 344.89
  middle alternating 344.89
  Millard-Gubler-Foville 344.89
  monoplegic—*see* Monoplegia
  motor NEC 344.9
    cerebral—*see* Paralysis, brain
    spinal—*see* Paralysis, spinal
  multiple
    cerebral—*see* Paralysis, brain
    spinal—*see* Paralysis, spinal
  muscle (flaccid) 359.9
    due to nerve lesion NEC 355.9
    eye (extrinsic) 378.55
      intrinsic 367.51
      oblique 378.51
    iris sphincter 364.8
    ischemic (complicating trauma) (Volkmann's)
        958.6
    pseudohypertrophic 359.1
  muscular (atrophic) 359.9
    progressive 335.21
  musculocutaneous nerve 354.9
  musculospiral 354.9
  nerve—*see also* Disorder, nerve
    third or oculomotor (partial) 378.51
      total 378.52
    fourth or trochlear 378.53
    sixth or abducens 378.54
    seventh or facial 351.0
      birth injury 767.5
      due to
        injection NEC 999.9
        operation NEC 997.09
      newborn 767.5
    accessory 352.4
    auditory 388.5
    birth injury 767.7
    cranial or cerebral (*see also* Disorder, nerve,
        cranial) 352.9
    facial 351.0
      birth injury 767.5
      newborn 767.5
    laryngeal (*see also* Paralysis, vocal cord)
        478.30
    newborn 767.7
    phrenic 354.8
      newborn 767.7
    radial 354.3
      birth injury 767.6
      newborn 767.6
    syphilitic 094.89
    traumatic NEC (*see also* Injury, nerve, by
        site) 957.9
    trigeminal 350.9
    ulnar 354.2
  newborn NEC 767.0
  normokalemic periodic 359.3
  obstetrical, newborn 767.7
  ocular 378.9
  oculofacial, congenital 352.6
  oculomotor (nerve) (partial) 378.51
    alternating 344.89

Paralysis, paralytic—*continued*
  external bilateral 378.55
    total 378.52
  olfactory nerve 352.0
  palate 528.9
  palatopharyngolaryngeal 352.6
  paratrigeminal 350.9
  periodic (familial) (hyperkalemic)
    (hypokalemic) (normokalemic) (secondary)
    359.3
  peripheral
    autonomic nervous system—*see* Neuropathy,
      peripheral, autonomic
    nerve NEC 355.9
  peroneal (nerve) 355.3
  pharynx 478.29
  phrenic nerve 354.8
  plantar nerves 355.6
  pneumogastric nerve 352.3
  poliomyelitis (current) (*see also* Poliomyelitis,
    with paralysis) 045.1
    bulbar 045.0
  popliteal nerve 355.3
  pressure (*see also* Neuropathy, entrapment)
    355.9
  progressive 335.21
    atrophic 335.21
    bulbar 335.22
    general 094.1
    hemifacial 349.89
    infantile, acute (*see also* Poliomyelitis) 045.9
    multiple 335.20
  pseudobulbar 335.23
  pseudohypertrophic 359.1
    muscle 359.1
  psychogenic 306.0
  pupil, pupillary 379.49
  quadriceps 355.8
  quadriplegic (*see also* Quadriplegia) 344.0
  radial nerve 354.3
    birth injury 767.6
  rectum (sphincter) 569.49
  rectus muscle (eye) 378.55
  recurrent laryngeal nerve (*see also* Paralysis,
    vocal cord) 478.30
  respiratory (muscle) (system) (tract) 786.09
    center NEC 344.89
      fetus or newborn 770.89
    congenital 768.9
    newborn 768.9
  right side—*see* Hemiplegia
  Saturday night 354.3
  saturnine 984.9
    specified type of lead—*see* Table of drugs and
      chemicals
  sciatic nerve 355.0
  secondary—*see* Paralysis, late effect
  seizure (cerebral) (current episode) (*see also*
    Disease, cerebrovascular, acute) 436
    late effect—*see* Late effect(s) (of)
      cerebrovascular disease
  senile NEC 344.9
  serratus magnus 355.9
  shaking (*see also* Parkinsonism) 332.0
  shock (*see also* Disease, cerebrovascular, acute)
    436
    late effect—*see* Late effect(s) (of)
      cerebrovascular disease
  shoulder 354.9
  soft palate 528.9
  spasmodic—*see* Paralysis, spastic

Paralysis, paralytic— *continued*
  spastic 344.9
    cerebral infantile—*see* Palsy, cerebral
    congenital (cerebral)—*see* Palsy, cerebral
    familial 334.1
    hereditary 334.1
    infantile 343.9
    noncongenital or noninfantile, cerebral 344.9
    syphilitic 094.0
      spinal 094.89
  sphincter, bladder (*see also* Paralysis, bladder)
    596.53
  spinal (cord) NEC 344.1
    accessory nerve 352.4
    acute (*see also* Poliomyelitis) 045.9
    ascending acute 357.0
    atrophic (acute) (*see also* Poliomyelitis, with
      paralysis) 045.1
      spastic, syphilitic 094.89
    congenital NEC 343.9
    hemiplegic —*see* Hemiplegia
    hereditary 336.8
    infantile (*see also* Poliomyelitis) 045.9
    late effect NEC 344.89
    monoplegic—*see* Monoplegia
    nerve 355.9
    progressive 335.10
    quadriplegic —*see* Quadriplegia
    spastic NEC 343.9
    traumatic—*see* Injury, spinal, by site
  sternomastoid 352.4
  stomach 536.3
    nerve 352.3
  stroke (current episode) (*see also* Disease,
    cerebrovascular, acute) 436
    late effect—*see* Late effect(s) (of)
      cerebrovascular disease
  subscapularis 354.8
  superior nuclear NEC 334.9
  supranuclear 356.8
  sympathetic
    cervical NEC 337.0
    nerve NEC (*see also* Neuropathy, peripheral,
      autonomic) 337.9
    nervous system—*see* Neuropathy, peripheral,
      autonomic
  syndrome 344.9
    specified NEC 344.89
  syphilitic spastic spinal (Erb's) 094.89
  tabetic general 094.1
  thigh 355.8
  throat 478.29
    diphtheritic 032.0
    muscle 478.29
  thrombotic (current episode) (*see also*
    Thrombosis, brain) 434.0
    late effect—*see* Late effect(s) (of)
      cerebrovascular disease
  thumb NEC 354.9
  tick (-bite) 989.5
  Todd's (postepileptic transitory paralysis)
    344.89
  toe 355.6
  tongue 529.8
  transient
    arm or leg NEC 781.4
    traumatic NEC (*see also* Injury, nerve, by
      site) 957.9
  trapezius 352.4
  traumatic, transient NEC (*see also* Injury, nerve,
    by site) 957.9

Paralysis, paralytic—*continued*
  trembling (*see also* Parkinsonism) 332.0
  triceps brachii 354.9
  trigeminal nerve 350.9
  trochlear nerve 378.53
  ulnar nerve 354.2
  upper limb —*see also* Paralysis, arm
    both (*see also* Diplegia) 344.2
  uremic—*see* Uremia
  uveoparotitic 135
  uvula 528.9
    hysterical 300.11
    postdiphtheritic 032.0
  vagus nerve 352.3
  vasomotor NEC 337.9
  velum palati 528.9
  vesical (*see also* Paralysis, bladder) 596.53
  vestibular nerve 388.5
  visual field, psychic 368.16
  vocal cord 478.30
    bilateral (partial) 478.33
      complete 478.34
    complete (bilateral) 478.34
    unilateral (partial) 478.31
      complete 478.32
  Volkmann's (complicating trauma) 958.6
  wasting 335.21
  Weber's 344.89
  wrist NEC 354.9
Paramedial orifice, urethrovesical 753.8
Paramenia 626.9
Parametritis (chronic) (*see also* Disease, pelvis,
    inflammatory) 614.4
  acute 614.3
  puerperal, postpartum, childbirth 670
Parametrium, parametric —*see* condition
Paramnesia (*see also* Amnesia) 780.99
Paramolar 520.1
  causing crowding 524.3
Paramyloidosis 277.3
Paramyoclonus multiplex 333.2
Paramyotonia 359.2
  congenita 359.2
Paraneoplastic syndrome —*see* condition
Parangi (*see also* Yaws) 102.9
Paranoia 297.1
  alcoholic 291.5
  querulans 297.8
  senile 290.20
Paranoid
  dementia (*see also* Schizophrenia) 295.3
    praecox (acute) 295.3
    senile 290.20
  personality 301.0
  psychosis 297.9
    alcoholic 291.5
    climacteric 297.2
    drug-induced 292.11
    involutional 297.2
    menopausal 297.2
    protracted reactive 298.4
    psychogenic 298.4
      acute 298.3
    senile 290.20
  reaction (chronic) 297.9
    acute 298.3
  schizophrenia (acute) (*see also* Schizophrenia)
    295.3
  state 297.9
    alcohol-induced 291.5
    climacteric 297.2

Paranoid—*continued*
  drug-induced 292.11
  due to or associated with
    arteriosclerosis (cerebrovascular) 290.42
    presenile brain disease 290.12
    senile brain disease 290.20
  involutional 297.2
  menopausal 297.2
  senile 290.20
  simple 297.0
  specified type NEC 297.8
  tendencies 301.0
  traits 301.0
  trends 301.0
  type, psychopathic personality 301.0
Paraparesis (*see also* Paralysis) 344.9
Paraphasia 784.3
Paraphilia (*see also* Deviation, sexual) 302.9
Paraphimosis (congenital) 605
  chancroidal 099.0
Paraphrenia, paraphrenic (late) 297.2
  climacteric 297.2
  dementia (*see also* Schizophrenia) 295.3
  involutional 297.2
  menopausal 297.2
  schizophrenia (acute) (*see also* Schizophrenia)
    295.3
Paraplegia 344.1
  with
    broken back—*see* Fracture, vertebra, by site,
      with spinal cord injury
    fracture, vertebra—*see* Fracture, vertebra, by
      site, with spinal cord injury
  ataxic—*see* Degeneration, combined, spinal cord
  brain (current episode) (*see also* Paralysis,
    brain) 437.8
  cerebral (current episode) (*see also* Paralysis,
    brain) 437.8
  congenital or infantile (cerebral) (spastic)
    (spinal) 343.0
  cortical—*see* Paralysis, brain
  familial spastic 334.1
  functional (hysterical) 300.11
  hysterical 300.11
  infantile 343.0
  late effect 344.1
  Pott's (*see also* Tuberculosis) 015.0 *[730.88]*
  psychogenic 306.0
  spastic
    Erb's spinal 094.89
    hereditary 334.1
    not infantile or congenital 344.1
  spinal (cord)
    traumatic NEC—*see* Injury, spinal, by site
  syphilitic (spastic) 094.89
  traumatic NEC—*see* Injury, spinal, by site
Paraproteinemia 273.2
  benign (familial) 273.1
  monoclonal 273.1
  secondary to malignant or inflammatory disease
    273.1
Parapsoriasis 696.2
  en plaques 696.2
  guttata 696.2
  lichenoides chronica 696.2
  retiformis 696.2
  varioliformis (acuta) 696.2
Parascarlatina 057.8

Parasitic —*see also* condition
  disease NEC (*see also* Infestation, parasitic)
      136.9
    contact V01.89
    exposure to V01.89
    intestinal NEC 129
    skin NEC 134.9
  stomatitis 112.0
  sycosis 110.0
    beard 110.0
    scalp 110.0
  twin 759.4
Parasitism NEC 136.9
  intestinal NEC 129
  skin NEC 134.9
  specified—*see* Infestation
Parasitophobia 300.29
Parasomnia 780.59
  nonorganic origin 307.47
Paraspadias 752.69
Paraspasm facialis 351.8
Parathyroid gland —*see* condition
Parathyroiditis (autoimmune) 252.1
Parathyroprival tetany 252.1
Paratrachoma 077.0
Paratyphilitis (*see also* Appendicitis) 541
Paratyphoid (fever)—*see* Fever, paratyphoid
Paratyphus —*see* Fever, paratyphoid
Paraurethral duct 753.8
Para-urethritis 597.89
  gonococcal (acute) 098.0
    chronic or duration of 2 months or over 098.2
Paravaccinia NEC 051.9
  milkers' node 051.1
Paravaginitis (*see also* Vaginitis) 616.10
Parencephalitis (*see also* Encephalitis) 323.9
  late effect—*see* category 326
Parergasia 298.9
Paresis (*see also* Paralysis) 344.9
  accommodation 367.51
  bladder (spastic) (sphincter) (*see also* Paralysis,
      bladder) 596.53
    tabetic 094.0
  bowel, colon, or intestine (*see also* Ileus) 560.1
  brain or cerebral—*see* Paralysis, brain
  extrinsic muscle, eye 378.55
  general 094.1
    arrested 094.1
    brain 094.1
    cerebral 094.1
    insane 094.1
    juvenile 090.40
      remission 090.49
    progressive 094.1
    remission (sustained) 094.1
    tabetic 094.1
  heart (*see also* Failure, heart) 428.9
  infantile (*see also* Poliomyelitis) 045.9
  insane 094.1
  juvenile 090.40
  late effect—*see* Paralysis, late effect
  luetic (general) 094.1
  peripheral progressive 356.9
  pseudohypertrophic 359.1
  senile NEC 344.9
  stomach 536.3
  syphilitic (general) 094.1
    congenital 090.40
  transient, limb 781.4
  vesical (sphincter) NEC 596.53

Paresthesia (*see also* Disturbance, sensation)
      782.0
  Berger's (paresthesia of lower limb) 782.0
  Bernhardt 355.1
  Magnan's 782.0
Paretic —*see* condition
Parinaud's
  conjunctivitis 372.02
  oculoglandular syndrome 372.02
  ophthalmoplegia 378.81
  syndrome (paralysis of conjugate upward gaze)
      378.81
Parkes Weber and Dimitri syndrome
      (encephalocutaneous angiomatosis) 759.6
Parkinson's disease, syndrome, or tremor
      —*see* Parkinsonism
Parkinsonism (arteriosclerotic) (idiopathic)
      (primary) 332.0
  associated with orthostatic hypotension
      (idiopathic) (symptomatic) 333.0
  due to drugs 332.1
  secondary 332.1
  syphilitic 094.82
Parodontitis 523.4
Parodontosis 523.5
Paronychia (with lymphangitis) 681.9
  candidal (chronic) 112.3
  chronic 681.9
    candidal 112.3
    finger 681.02
    toe 681.11
  finger 681.02
  toe 681.11
  tuberculous (primary) (*see also* Tuberculosis)
      017.0
Parorexia NEC 307.52
  hysterical 300.11
Parosmia 781.1
  psychogenic 306.7
Parotid gland —*see* condition
Parotiditis (*see also* Parotitis) 527.2
  epidemic 072.9
  infectious 072.9
Parotitis 527.2
  allergic 527.2
  chronic 527.2
  epidemic (*see also* Mumps) 072.9
  infectious (*see also* Mumps) 072.9
  noninfectious 527.2
  nonspecific toxic 527.2
  not mumps 527.2
  postoperative 527.2
  purulent 527.2
  septic 527.2
  suppurative (acute) 527.2
  surgical 527.2
  toxic 527.2
Paroxysmal —*see also* condition
  dyspnea (nocturnal) 786.09
Parrot's disease (syphilitic osteochondritis) 090.0
Parrot fever 073.9
Parry's disease or syndrome (exophthalmic
      goiter) 242.0
Parry-Romberg syndrome 349.89
Parson's disease (exophthalmic goiter) 242.0
Parsonage-Aldren-Turner syndrome 353.5
Parsonage-Turner syndrome 353.5
Pars planitis 363.21
Particolored infant 757.39
Parturition —*see* Delivery

Passage
    false, urethra 599.4
    of sounds or bougies (*see also* Attention to
        artificial opening) V55.9
Passive —*see* condition
Pasteurella septica 027.2
Pasteurellosis (*see also* Infection, Pasteurella)
    027.2
PAT (paroxysmal atrial tachycardia) 427.0
Patau's syndrome (trisomy D₁) 758.1
Patch
    herald 696.3
Patches
    mucous (syphilitic) 091.3
        congenital 090.0
    smokers' (mouth) 528.6
Patellar —*see* condition
Patellofemoral syndrome 719.46
Patent —*see also* Imperfect closure
    atrioventricular ostium 745.69
    canal of Nuck 752.41
    cervix 622.5
        complicating pregnancy 654.5
            affecting fetus or newborn 761.0
    ductus arteriosus or Botalli 747.0
    Eustachian
        tube 381.7
        valve 746.89
    foramen
        Botalli 745.5
        ovale 745.5
    interauricular septum 745.5
    interventricular septum 745.4
    omphalomesenteric duct 751.0
    os (uteri)—*see* Patent, cervix
    ostium secundum 745.5
    urachus 753.7
    vitelline duct 751.0
Paternity testing V70.4
Paterson's syndrome (sideropenic dysphagia)
    280.8
Paterson (-Brown) (-Kelly) syndrome
    (sideropenic dysphagia) 280.8
Paterson-Kelly syndrome or web (sideropenic
    dysphagia) 280.8
Pathologic, pathological —*see also* condition
    asphyxia 799.0
    drunkenness 291.4
    emotionality 301.3
    liar 301.7
    personality 301.9
    resorption, tooth 521.4
    sexuality (*see also* Deviation, sexual) 302.9
Pathology (of)—*see* Disease
Patterned motor discharges, idiopathic (*see
    also* Epilepsy) 345.5
Patulous —*see also* Patent
    anus 569.49
    Eustachian tube 381.7
Pause, sinoatrial 427.81
Pavor nocturnus 307.46
Pavy's disease 593.6
Paxton's disease (white piedra) 111.2
Payr's disease or syndrome (splenic flexure
    syndrome) 569.89
Pearls
    Elschnig 366.51
    enamel 520.2
Pearl-workers' disease (chronic osteomyelitis)
    (*see also* Osteomyelitis) 730.1
Pectenitis 569.49
Pectenosis 569.49

Pectoral —*see* condition
Pectus
    carinatum (congenital) 754.82
        acquired 738.3
        rachitic (*see also* Rickets) 268.0
    excavatum (congenital) 754.81
        acquired 738.3
        rachitic (*see also* Rickets) 268.0
    recurvatum (congenital) 754.81
        acquired 738.3
Pedatrophia 261
Pederosis 302.2
Pediculosis (infestation) 132.9
    capitis (head louse) (any site) 132.0
    corporis (body louse) (any site) 132.1
    eyelid 132.0 *[373.6]*
    mixed (classifiable to more than one category in
        132.0-132.2) 132.3
    pubis (pubic louse) (any site) 132.2
    vestimenti 132.1
    vulvae 132.2
Pediculus (infestation)—*see* Pediculosis
Pedophilia 302.2
Peg-shaped teeth 520.2
Pel's crisis 094.0
Pel-Ebstein disease —*see* Disease, Hodgkin's
Pelade 704.01
Pelger-Huët anomaly or syndrome (hereditary
    hyposegmentation) 288.2
Peliosis (rheumatica) 287.0
Pelizaeus-Merzbacher
    disease 330.0
    sclerosis, diffuse cerebral 330.0
Pellagra (alcoholic or with alcoholism) 265.2
    with polyneuropathy 265.2 *[357.4]*
Pellagra-cerebellar-ataxia-renal aminoaciduria
    syndrome 270.0
Pellegrini's disease (calcification, knee joint)
    726.62
Pellegrini (-Stieda) disease or syndrome
    (calcification, knee joint) 726.62
Pellizzi's syndrome (pineal) 259.8
Pelvic —*see also* condition
    congestion-fibrosis syndrome 625.5
    kidney 753.3
Pelvioectasis 591
Pelviolithiasis 592.0
Pelviperitonitis
    female (*see also* Peritonitis, pelvic, female)
        614.5
    male (*see also* Peritonitis) 567.2
Pelvis, pelvic —*see also* condition or type
    infantile 738.6
    Nägele's 738.6
    obliquity 738.6
    Robert's 755.69
Pemphigoid 694.5
    benign, mucous membrane 694.60
        with ocular involvement 694.61
    bullous 694.5
    cicatricial 694.60
        with ocular involvement 694.61
    juvenile 694.2
Pemphigus 694.4
    benign 694.5
        chronic familial 757.39
    Brazilian 694.4
    circinatus 694.0
    congenital, traumatic 757.39
    conjunctiva 694.61
    contagiosus 684

Pemphigus—*continued*
  erythematodes 694.4
  erythematosus 694.4
  foliaceus 694.4
  frambesiodes 694.4
  gangrenous (*see also* Gangrene) 785.4
  malignant 694.4
  neonatorum, newborn 684
  ocular 694.61
  papillaris 694.4
  seborrheic 694.4
  South American 694.4
  syphilitic (congenital) 090.0
  vegetans 694.4
  vulgaris 694.4
  wildfire 694.4
Pendred's syndrome (familial goiter with
    deaf-mutism) 243
Pendulous
  abdomen 701.9
    in pregnancy or childbirth 654.4
      affecting fetus or newborn 763.89
  breast 611.8
Penetrating wound —*see also* Wound, open, by
    site
  with internal injury—*see* Injury, internal, by
    site, with open wound
  eyeball 871.7
    with foreign body (nonmagnetic) 871.6
      magnetic 871.5
  ocular (*see also* Penetrating wound, eyeball)
    871.7
    adnexa 870.3
      with foreign body 870.4
    orbit 870.3
      with foreign body 870.4
Penetration, pregnant uterus by instrument
  with
    abortion—*see* Abortion, by type, with damage
      to pelvic organs
    ectopic pregnancy (*see also* categories
      633.0-633.9) 639.2
    molar pregnancy (*see also* categories
      630-632) 639.2
  complication of delivery 665.1
    affecting fetus or newborn 763.89
  following
    abortion 639.2
    ectopic or molar pregnancy 639.2
Penfield's syndrome (*see also* Epilepsy) 345.5
Penicilliosis of lung 117.3
Penis —*see* condition
Penitis 607.2
Penta X syndrome 758.81
Pentalogy (of Fallot) 745.2
Pentosuria (benign) (essential) 271.8
Peptic acid disease 536.8
Peregrinating patient V65.2
Perforated —*see* Perforation
Perforation, perforative (nontraumatic)
  antrum (*see also* Sinusitis, maxillary) 473.0
  appendix 540.0
    with peritoneal abscess 540.1
  atrial septum, multiple 745.5
  attic, ear 384.22
    healed 384.81
  bile duct, except cystic (*see also* Disease,
    biliary) 576.3
    cystic 575.4
  bladder (urinary) 596.6
    with

Perforation, perforative—*continued*
    abortion—*see* Abortion, by type, with
      damage to pelvic organs
    ectopic pregnancy (*see also* categories
      633.0-633.9) 639.2
    molar pregnancy (*see also* categories
      630-632) 639.2
  following
    abortion 639.2
    ectopic or molar pregnancy 639.2
  obstetrical trauma 665.5
  bowel 569.83
    with
      abortion—*see* Abortion, by type, with
        damage to pelvic organs
      ectopic pregnancy (*see also* categories
        633.0-633.9) 639.2
      molar pregnancy (*see also* categories
        630-632) 639.2
    fetus or newborn 777.6
    following
      abortion 639.2
      ectopic or molar pregnancy 639.2
    obstetrical trauma 665.5
  broad ligament
    with
      abortion—*see* Abortion, by type, with
        damage to pelvic organs
      ectopic pregnancy (*see also* categories
        633.0-633.9) 639.2
      molar pregnancy (*see also* categories
        630-632) 639.2
    following
      abortion 639.2
      ectopic or molar pregnancy 639.2
    obstetrical trauma 665.6
  by
    device, implant, or graft—*see* Complications,
      mechanical
    foreign body left accidentally in operation
      wound 998.4
    instrument (any) during a procedure,
      accidental 998.2
  cecum 540.0
    with peritoneal abscess 540.1
  cervix (uteri)—*see also* Injury, internal, cervix
    with
      abortion—*see* Abortion, by type, with
        damage to pelvic organs
      ectopic pregnancy (*see also* categories
        633.0-633.9) 639.2
      molar pregnancy (*see also* categories
        630-632) 639.2
    following
      abortion 639.2
      ectopic or molar pregnancy 639.2
    obstetrical trauma 665.3
  colon 569.83
  common duct (bile) 576.3
  cornea (*see also* Ulcer, cornea) 370.00
    due to ulceration 370.06
  cystic duct 575.4
  diverticulum (*see also* Diverticula) 562.10
    small intestine 562.00
  duodenum, duodenal (ulcer)—*see* Ulcer,
    duodenum, with perforation
  ear drum—*see* Perforation, tympanum
  enteritis—*see* Enteritis
  esophagus 530.4
  ethmoidal sinus (*see also* Sinusitis, ethmoidal)
    473.2

Perforation, perforative—*continued*
  foreign body (external site)—*see also* Wound,
    open, by site, complicated
    internal site, by ingested object—*see* Foreign
      body
  frontal sinus (*see also* Sinusitis, frontal) 473.1
  gallbladder or duct (*see also* Disease,
    gallbladder) 575.4
  gastric (ulcer)—*see* Ulcer, stomach, with
    perforation
  heart valve—*see* Endocarditis
  ileum (*see also* Perforation, intestine) 569.83
  instrumental
    external—*see* Wound, open, by site
    pregnant uterus, complicating delivery 665.9
    surgical (accidental) (blood vessel) (nerve)
      (organ) 998.2
  intestine 569.83
    with
      abortion—*see* Abortion, by type, with
        damage to pelvic organs
      ectopic pregnancy (*see also* categories
        633.0-633.9) 639.2
      molar pregnancy (*see also* categories
        630-632) 639.2
      fetus or newborn 777.6
      obstetrical trauma 665.5
      ulcerative NEC 569.83
  jejunum, jejunal 569.83
    ulcer—*see* Ulcer, gastrojejunal, with
      perforation
  mastoid (antrum) (cell) 383.89
  maxillary sinus (*see also* Sinusitis, maxillary)
    473.0
  membrana tympani—*see* Perforation, tympanum
  nasal
    septum 478.1
      congenital 748.1
      syphilitic 095.8
    sinus (*see also* Sinusitis) 473.9
      congenital 748.1
  palate (hard) 526.89
    soft 528.9
      syphilitic 095.8
    syphilitic 095.8
  palatine vault 526.89
    syphilitic 095.8
      congenital 090.5
  pelvic
    floor
      with
        abortion—*see* Abortion, by type, with
          damage to pelvic organs
        ectopic pregnancy (*see also* categories
          633.0-633.9) 639.2
        molar pregnancy (*see also* categories
          630-632) 639.2
        obstetrical trauma 664.1
    organ
      with
        abortion—*see* Abortion, by type, with
          damage to pelvic organs
        ectopic pregnancy (*see also* categories
          633.0-633.9) 639.2
        molar pregnancy (*see also* categories
          630-632) 639.2
      following
        abortion 639.2
        ectopic or molar pregnancy 639.2
      obstetrical trauma 665.5
  perineum—*see* Laceration, perineum

Perforation, perforative— *continued*
  periurethral tissue
    with
      abortion—*see* Abortion, by type, with
        damage to pelvic organs
      ectopic pregnancy (*see also* categories
        630-632) 639.2
      molar pregnancy (*see also* categories
        630-632) 639.2
  pharynx 478.29
  pylorus, pyloric (ulcer)—*see* Ulcer, stomach,
    with perforation
  rectum 569.49
  sigmoid 569.83
  sinus (accessory) (chronic) (nasal) (*see also*
    Sinusitis) 473.9
  sphenoidal sinus (*see also* Sinusitis, sphenoidal)
    473.3
  stomach (due to ulcer)—*see* Ulcer, stomach,
    with perforation
  surgical (accidental) (by instrument) (blood
    vessel) (nerve) (organ) 998.2
  traumatic
    external—*see* Wound, open, by site
    eye (*see also* Penetrating wound, ocular) 871.7
    internal organ—*see* Injury, internal, by site
  tympanum (membrane) (persistent
    posttraumatic) (postinflammatory) 384.20
    with
      otitis media—*see* Otitis media
    attic 384.22
    central 384.21
    healed 384.81
    marginal NEC 384.23
    multiple 384.24
    pars flaccida 384.22
    total 384.25
    traumatic—*see* Wound, open, ear, drum
  typhoid, gastrointestinal 002.0
  ulcer—*see* Ulcer, by site, with perforation
  ureter 593.89
  urethra
    with
      abortion—*see* Abortion, by type, with
        damage to pelvic organs
      ectopic pregnancy (*see also* categories
        633.0-633.9) 639.2
      molar pregnancy (*see also* categories
        630-632) 639.2
    following
      abortion 639.2
      ectopic or molar pregnancy 639.2
    obstetrical trauma 665.5
  uterus—*see also* Injury, internal, uterus
    with
      abortion—*see* Abortion, by type, with
        damage to pelvic organs
      ectopic pregnancy (*see also* categories
        633.0-633.9) 639.2
      molar pregnancy (*see also* categories
        630-632) 639.2
    by intrauterine contraceptive device 996.32
    following
      abortion 639.2
      ectopic or molar pregnancy 639.2
    obstetrical trauma—*see* Injury, internal,
      uterus, obstetrical trauma
  uvula 528.9
    syphilitic 095.8
  vagina—*see* Laceration, vagina
  viscus NEC 799.8

Perforation, perforative—*continued*
  traumatic 868.00
    with open wound into cavity 868.10
Periadenitis mucosa necrotica recurrens 528.2
Periangiitis 446.0
Periantritis 535.4
Periappendicitis (acute) (*see also* Appendicitis)
    541
Periarteritis (disseminated) (infectious)
    (necrotizing) (nodosa) 446.0
Periarthritis (joint) 726.90
  Duplay's 726.2
  gonococcal 098.50
  humeroscapularis 726.2
  scapulohumeral 726.2
  shoulder 726.2
  wrist 726.4
Periarthrosis (angioneural)—*see* Periarthritis
Peribronchitis 491.9
  tuberculous (*see also* Tuberculosis) 011.3
Pericapsulitis, adhesive (shoulder) 726.0
Pericarditis (granular) (with decompensation)
    (with effusion) 423.9
  with
    rheumatic fever (conditions classifiable to 390)
      active (*see also* Pericarditis, rheumatic)
        391.0
      inactive or quiescent 393
  actinomycotic 039.8 *[420.0]*
  acute (nonrheumatic) 420.90
    with chorea (acute) (rheumatic) (Sydenham's)
        392.0
    bacterial 420.99
    benign 420.91
    hemorrhagic 420.90
    idiopathic 420.91
    infective 420.90
    nonspecific 420.91
    rheumatic 391.0
      with chorea (acute) (rheumatic)
        (Sydenham's) 392.0
    sicca 420.90
    viral 420.91
  adhesive or adherent (external) (internal) 423.1
    acute—*see* Pericarditis, acute
    rheumatic (external) (internal) 393
  amebic 006.8 *[420.0]*
  bacterial (acute) (subacute) (with serous or
      seropurulent effusion) 420.99
  calcareous 423.2
  cholesterol (chronic) 423.8
    acute 420.90
  chronic (nonrheumatic) 423.8
    rheumatic 393
  constrictive 423.2
  Coxsackie 074.21
  due to
    actinomycosis 039.8 *[420.0]*
    amebiasis 006.8 *[420.0]*
    Coxsackie (virus) 074.21
    histoplasmosis (*see also* Histoplasmosis)
        115.93
    nocardiosis 039.8 *[420.0]*
    tuberculosis (*see also* Tuberculosis) 017.9
        [420.0]
  fibrinocaseous (*see also* Tuberculosis) 017.9
      [420.0]
  fibrinopurulent 420.99
  fibrinous—*see* Pericarditis, rheumatic
  fibropurulent 420.99
  fibrous 423.1

Pericarditis—*continued*
  gonococcal 098.83
  hemorrhagic 423.0
  idiopathic (acute) 420.91
  infective (acute) 420.90
  meningococcal 036.41
  neoplastic (chronic) 423.8
    acute 420.90
  nonspecific 420.91
  obliterans, obliterating 423.1
  plastic 423.1
  pneumococcal (acute) 420.99
  postinfarction 411.0
  purulent (acute) 420.99
  rheumatic (active) (acute) (with effusion) (with
      pneumonia) 391.0
    with chorea (acute) (rheumatic) (Sydenham's)
        392.0
    chronic or inactive (with chorea) 393
  septic (acute) 420.99
  serofibrinous—*see* Pericarditis, rheumatic
  staphylococcal (acute) 420.99
  streptococcal (acute) 420.99
  suppurative (acute) 420.99
  syphilitic 093.81
  tuberculous (acute) (chronic) (*see also*
      Tuberculosis) 017.9 *[420.0]*
  uremic 585 *[420.0]*
  viral (acute) 420.91
Pericardium, pericardial —*see* condition
Pericellulitis (*see also* Cellulitis) 682.9
Pericementitis 523.4
  acute 523.3
  chronic (suppurative) 523.4
Pericholecystitis (*see also* Cholecystitis) 575.10
Perichondritis
  auricle 380.00
    acute 380.01
    chronic 380.02
  bronchus 491.9
  ear (external) 380.00
    acute 380.01
    chronic 380.02
  larynx 478.71
    syphilitic 095.8
    typhoid 002.0 *[478.71]*
  nose 478.1
  pinna 380.00
    acute 380.01
    chronic 380.02
  trachea 478.9
Periclasia 523.5
Pericolitis 569.89
Pericoronitis (chronic) 523.4
  acute 523.3
Pericystitis (*see also* Cystitis) 595.9
Pericytoma (M9150/1)—*see also* Neoplasm,
    connective tissue, uncertain behavior
  benign (M9150/0)—*see* Neoplasm, connective
    tissue, benign
  malignant (M9150/3)—*see* Neoplasm,
    connective tissue, malignant
Peridacryocystitis, acute 375.32
Peridiverticulitis (*see also* Diverticulitis) 562.11
Periduodenitis 535.6
Periendocarditis (*see also* Endocarditis) 424.90
  acute or subacute 421.9
Periepididymitis (*see also* Epididymitis) 604.90
Perifolliculitis (abscedens) 704.8
  capitis, abscedens et suffodiens 704.8
  dissecting, scalp 704.8

Perifolliculitis—*continued*
scalp 704.8
superficial pustular 704.8
Perigastritis (acute) 535.0
Perigastrojejunitis (acute) 535.0
Perihepatitis (acute) 573.3
chlamydial 099.56
gonococcal 098.86
Peri-ileitis (subacute) 569.89
Perilabyrinthitis (acute)—*see* Labyrinthitis
Perimeningitis —*see* Meningitis
Perimetritis (*see also* Endometritis) 615.9
Perimetrosalpingitis (*see also*
Salpingo-oophoritis) 614.2
Perinephric —*see* condition
Perinephritic —*see* condition
Perinephritis (*see also* Infection, kidney) 590.9
purulent (*see also* Abscess, kidney) 590.2
Perineum, perineal —*see* condition
Perineuritis NEC 729.2
Periodic —*see also* condition
disease (familial) 277.3
edema 995.1
hereditary 277.6
fever 277.3
paralysis (familial) 359.3
peritonitis 277.3
polyserositis 277.3
somnolence 347
Periodontal
cyst 522.8
pocket 523.8
Periodontitis (chronic) (complex) (compound)
(local) (simplex) 523.4
acute 523.3
apical 522.6
acute (pulpal origin) 522.4
Periodontoclasia 523.5
Periodontosis 523.5
Periods —*see also* Menstruation
heavy 626.2
irregular 626.4
Perionychia (with lymphangitis) 681.9
finger 681.02
toe 681.11
Perioophoritis (*see also* Salpingo-oophoritis)
614.2
Periorchitis (*see also* Orchitis) 604.90
Periosteum, periosteal —*see* condition
Periostitis (circumscribed) (diffuse) (infective)
730.3

---

*Note—Use the following fifth-digit
subclassification with category 730:*

0 site unspecified
1 shoulder region
2 upper arm
3 forearm
4 hand
5 pelvic region and thigh
6 lower leg
7 ankle and foot
8 other specified sites
9 multiple sites

---

with osteomyelitis (*see also* Osteomyelitis)
730.2
acute or subacute 730.0
chronic or old 730.1
albuminosa, albuminosus 730.3
alveolar 526.5

Periostitis—*continued*
alveolodental 526.5
dental 526.5
gonorrheal 098.89
hyperplastica, generalized 731.2
jaw (lower) (upper) 526.4
monomelic 733.99
orbital 376.02
syphilitic 095.5
congenital 090.0 *[730.8]*
secondary 091.61
tuberculous (*see also* Tuberculosis, bone) 015.9
[730.8]
yaws (early) (hypertrophic) (late) 102.6
Periostosis (*see also* Periostitis) 730.3
with osteomyelitis (*see also* Osteomyelitis)
730.2
acute or subacute 730.0
chronic or old 730.1
hyperplastic 756.59
Periphlebitis (*see also* Phlebitis) 451.9
lower extremity 451.2
deep (vessels) 451.19
superficial (vessels) 451.0
portal 572.1
retina 362.18
superficial (vessels) 451.0
tuberculous (*see also* Tuberculosis) 017.9
retina 017.3 *[362.18]*
Peripneumonia —*see* Pneumonia
Periproctitis 569.49
Periprostatitis (*see also* Prostatitis) 601.9
Perirectal —*see* condition
Perirenal —*see* condition
Perisalpingitis (*see also* Salpingo-oophoritis)
614.2
Perisigmoiditis 569.89
Perisplenitis (infectional) 289.59
Perispondylitis —*see* Spondylitis
Peristalsis reversed or visible 787.4
Peritendinitis (*see also* Tenosynovitis) 726.90
adhesive (shoulder) 726.0
Perithelioma (M9150/1)—*see* Pericytoma
Peritoneum, peritoneal —*see also* condition
equilibration test V56.32
Peritonitis (acute) (adhesive) (fibrinous)
(hemorrhagic) (idiopathic) (localized)
(perforative) (primary) (with adhesions) (with
effusion) 567.9
with or following
abortion—*see* Abortion, by type, with sepsis
abscess 567.2
appendicitis 540.0
with peritoneal abscess 540.1
ectopic pregnancy (*see also* categories
633.0-633.9) 639.0
molar pregnancy (*see also* categories
630-632) 639.0
aseptic 998.7
bacterial 567.2
bile, biliary 567.8
chemical 998.7
chlamydial 099.56
chronic proliferative 567.8
congenital NEC 777.6
diaphragmatic 567.2
diffuse NEC 567.2
diphtheritic 032.83
disseminated NEC 567.2
due to
bile 567.8

Peritonitis—*continued*
  foreign
    body or object accidentally left during a
      procedure (instrument) (sponge) (swab)
      998.4
    substance accidentally left during a
      procedure (chemical) (powder) (talc)
      998.7
    talc 998.7
    urine 567.8
  fibrinopurulent 567.2
  fibrinous 567.2
  fibrocaseous (*see also* Tuberculosis) 014.0
  fibropurulent 567.2
  general, generalized (acute) 567.2
  gonococcal 098.86
  in infective disease NEC 136.9 *[567.0]*
  meconium (newborn) 777.6
  pancreatic 577.8
  paroxysmal, benign 277.3
  pelvic
    female (acute) 614.5
      chronic NEC 614.7
        with adhesions 614.6
      puerperal, postpartum, childbirth 670
    male (acute) 567.2
  periodic (familial) 277.3
  phlegmonous 567.2
  pneumococcal 567.1
  postabortal 639.0
  proliferative, chronic 567.8
  puerperal, postpartum, childbirth 670
  purulent 567.2
  septic 567.2
  staphylococcal 567.2
  streptococcal 567.2
  subdiaphragmatic 567.2
  subphrenic 567.2
  suppurative 567.2
  syphilitic 095.2
    congenital 090.0 *[567.0]*
  talc 998.7
  tuberculous (*see also* Tuberculosis) 014.0
  urine 567.8
Peritonsillar —*see* condition
Peritonsillitis 475
Perityphlitis (*see also* Appendicitis) 541
Periureteritis 593.89
Periurethral —*see* condition
Periurethritis (gangrenous) 597.89
Periuterine —*see* condition
Perivaginitis (*see also* Vaginitis) 616.10
Perivasculitis, retinal 362.18
Perivasitis (chronic) 608.4
Periventricular leukomalacia 779.7
Perivesiculitis (seminal) (*see also* Vesiculitis)
  608.0
Perlèche 686.8
  due to
    moniliasis 112.0
    riboflavin deficiency 266.0
Pernicious —*see* condition
Pernio, perniosis 991.5
Persecution
  delusion 297.9
  social V62.4
Perseveration (tonic) 784.69
Persistence, persistent (congenital) 759.89
  anal membrane 751.2
  arteria stapedia 744.04
  atrioventricular canal 745.69

Persistence, persistent—*continued*
  bloody ejaculate 792.2
  branchial cleft 744.41
  bulbus cordis in left ventricle 745.8
  canal of Cloquet 743.51
  capsule (opaque) 743.51
  cilioretinal artery or vein 743.51
  cloaca 751.5
  communication—*see* Fistula, congenital
  convolutions
    aortic arch 747.21
    fallopian tube 752.19
    oviduct 752.19
    uterine tube 752.19
  double aortic arch 747.21
  ductus
    arteriosus 747.0
    Botalli 747.0
  fetal
    circulation 747.83
    form of cervix (uteri) 752.49
    hemoglobin (hereditary) ("Swiss variety")
      282.7
    pulmonary hypertension 747.83
  foramen
    Botalli 745.5
    ovale 745.5
  Gartner's duct 752.11
  hemoglobin, fetal (hereditary) (HPFH) 282.7
  hyaloid
    artery (generally incomplete) 743.51
    system 743.51
  hymen (tag)
    in pregnancy or childbirth 654.8
      causing obstructed labor 660.2
  lanugo 757.4
  left
    posterior cardinal vein 747.49
    root with right arch of aorta 747.21
    superior vena cava 747.49
  Meckel's diverticulum 751.0
  mesonephric duct 752.8
    fallopian tube 752.11
  mucosal disease (middle ear) (with posterior or
    superior marginal perforation of ear drum)
    382.2
  nail(s), anomalous 757.5
  occiput, anterior or posterior 660.3
    fetus or newborn 763.1
  omphalomesenteric duct 751.0
  organ or site NEC—*see* Anomaly, specified
    type NEC
  ostium
    atrioventriculare commune 745.69
    primum 745.61
    secundum 745.5
  ovarian rests in fallopian tube 752.19
  pancreatic tissue in intestinal tract 751.5
  primary (deciduous)
    teeth 520.6
    vitreous hyperplasia 743.51
  pulmonary hypertension 747.83
  pupillary membrane 743.46
    iris 743.46
  Rhesus (Rh) titer 999.7
  right aortic arch 747.21
  sinus
    urogenitalis 752.8
    venosus with imperfect incorporation in right
      auricle 747.49
  thymus (gland) 254.8

Persistence, persistent—*continued*
  hyperplasia 254.0
  thyroglossal duct 759.2
  thyrolingual duct 759.2
  truncus arteriosus or communis 745.0
  tunica vasculosa lentis 743.39
  umbilical sinus 753.7
  urachus 753.7
  vegetative state 780.03
  vitelline duct 751.0
  wolffian duct 752.8
Person (with)
  admitted for clinical research, as participant or
    control subject V70.7
  awaiting admission to adequate facility
    elsewhere V63.2
    undergoing social agency investigation V63.8
  concern (normal) about sick person in family
    V61.49
  consulting on behalf of another V65.1
  feared
    complaint in whom no diagnosis was made
      V65.5
    condition not demonstrated V65.5
  feigning illness V65.2
  healthy, accompanying sick person V65.0
  living (in)
    alone V60.3
    boarding school V60.6
    residence remote from hospital or medical
      care facility V63.0
    residential institution V60.6
    without
      adequate
        financial resources V60.2
        housing (heating) (space) V60.1
      housing (permanent) (temporary) V60.0
      material resources V60.2
      person able to render necessary care V60.4
      shelter V60.0
  medical services in home not available V63.1
  on waiting list V63.2
    undergoing social agency investigation V63.8
  sick or handicapped in family V61.49
  "worried well" V65.5
Personality
  affective 301.10
  aggressive 301.3
  amoral 301.7
  anancastic, anankastic 301.4
  antisocial 301.7
  asocial 301.7
  asthenic 301.6
  avoidant 301.82
  borderline 301.83
  change 310.1
  compulsive 301.4
  cycloid 301.13
  cyclothymic 301.13
  dependent 301.6
  depressive (chronic) 301.12
  disorder, disturbance NEC 301.9
    with
      antisocial disturbance 301.7
      pattern disturbance NEC 301.9
      sociopathic disturbance 301.7
      trait disturbance 301.9
  dual 300.14
  dyssocial 301.7
  eccentric 301.89
    "haltlose" type 301.89

Personality—*continued*
  emotionally unstable 301.59
  epileptoid 301.3
  explosive 301.3
  fanatic 301.0
  histrionic 301.50
  hyperthymic 301.11
  hypomanic 301.11
  hypothymic 301.12
  hysterical 301.50
  immature 301.89
  inadequate 301.6
  labile 301.59
  masochistic 301.89
  morally defective 301.7
  multiple 300.14
  narcissistic 301.81
  obsessional 301.4
  obsessive (-compulsive) 301.4
  overconscientious 301.4
  paranoid 301.0
  passive (-dependent) 301.6
  passive-aggressive 301.84
  pathologic NEC 301.9
  pattern defect or disturbance 301.9
  pseudosocial 301.7
  psychoinfantile 301.59
  psychoneurotic NEC 301.89
  psychopathic 301.9
    with
      amoral trend 301.7
      antisocial trend 301.7
      asocial trend 301.7
      pathologic sexuality (*see also* Deviation,
        sexual) 302.9
      mixed types 301.9
    schizoid 301.20
      introverted 301.21
      schizotypal 301.22
      with sexual deviation (*see also* Deviation,
        sexual) 302.9
    antisocial 301.7
    dyssocial 301.7
  type A 301.4
  unstable (emotional) 301.59
Perthes' disease (capital femoral
  osteochondrosis) 732.1
Pertussis (*see also* Whooping cough) 033.9
  vaccination, prophylactic (against) V03.6
Peruvian wart 088.0
Perversion, perverted
  appetite 307.52
    hysterical 300.11
  function
    pineal gland 259.8
    pituitary gland 253.9
      anterior lobe
        deficient 253.2
        excessive 253.1
      posterior lobe 253.6
    placenta—*see* Placenta, abnormal
  sense of smell or taste 781.1
    psychogenic 306.7
  sexual (*see also* Deviation, sexual) 302.9
Pervious, congenital —*see also* Imperfect,
  closure
  ductus arteriosus 747.0
Pes (congenital) (*see also* Talipes) 754.70
  abductus (congenital) 754.60
    acquired 736.79
  acquired NEC 736.79

Pes *—continued*
planus 734
adductus (congenital) 754.79
acquired 736.79
cavus 754.71
acquired 736.73
planovalgus (congenital) 754.69
acquired 736.79
planus (acquired) (any degree) 734
congenital 754.61
rachitic 268.1
valgus (congenital) 754.61
acquired 736.79
varus (congenital) 754.50
acquired 736.79
Pest *(see also* Plague) 020.9
Pestis *(see also* Plague) 020.9
bubonica 020.0
fulminans 020.0
minor 020.8
pneumonica—*see* Plague, pneumonic
Petechia, petechiae 782.7
fetus or newborn 772.6
Petechial
fever 036.0
typhus 081.9
Petges-Cléjat or Petges-Clégat syndrome
(poikilodermatomyositis) 710.3
Petit's
disease *(see also* Hernia, lumbar) 553.8
Petit mal (idiopathic) *(see also* Epilepsy) 345.0
status 345.2
Petrellidosis 117.6
Petrositis 383.20
acute 383.21
chronic 383.22
Peutz-Jeghers disease or syndrome 759.6
Peyronie's disease 607.89
Pfeiffer's disease 075
Phacentocele 379.32
traumatic 921.3
Phacoanaphylaxis 360.19
Phacocele (old) 379.32
traumatic 921.3
Phaehyphomycosis 117.8
Phagedena (dry) (moist) *(see also* Gangrene)
785.4
arteriosclerotic 440.24
geometric 686.09
penis 607.89
senile 440.24
sloughing 785.4
tropical *(see also* Ulcer, skin) 707.9
vulva 616.50
Phagedenic *—see also* condition
abscess—*see also* Abscess
chancroid 099.0
bubo NEC 099.8
chancre 099.0
ulcer (tropical) *(see also* Ulcer, skin) 707.9
Phagomania 307.52
Phakoma 362.89
Phantom limb (syndrome) 353.6
Pharyngeal *—see also* condition
arch remnant 744.41
pouch syndrome 279.11

Pharyngitis (acute) (catarrhal) (gangrenous)
(infective) (malignant) (membranous)
(phlegmonous) (pneumococcal)
(pseudomembranous) (simple)
(staphylococcal) (subacute) (suppurative)
(ulcerative) (viral) 462
with influenza, flu, or grippe 487.1
aphthous 074.0
atrophic 472.1
chlamydial 099.51
chronic 472.1
Coxsackie virus 074.0
diphtheritic (membranous) 032.0
follicular 472.1
fusospirochetal 101
gonococcal 098.6
granular (chronic) 472.1
herpetic 054.79
hypertrophic 472.1
infectional, chronic 472.1
influenzal 487.1
lymphonodular, acute 074.8
septic 034.0
streptococcal 034.0
tuberculous *(see also* Tuberculosis) 012.8
vesicular 074.0
Pharyngoconjunctival fever 077.2
Pharyngoconjunctivitis, viral 077.2
Pharyngolaryngitis (acute) 465.0
chronic 478.9
septic 034.0
Pharyngoplegia 478.29
Pharyngotonsillitis 465.8
tuberculous 012.8
Pharyngotracheitis (acute) 465.8
chronic 478.9
Pharynx, pharyngeal *—see* condition
Phase of life problem NEC V62.89
Phenomenon
Arthus'—*see* Arthus' phenomenon
flashback (drug) 292.89
jaw-winking 742.8
Jod-Basedow 242.8
L. E. cell 710.0
lupus erythematosus cell 710.0
Pelger-Huët (hereditary hyposegmentation)
288.2
Raynaud's (paroxysmal digital cyanosis)
(secondary) 443.0
Reilly's *(see also* Neuropathy, peripheral,
autonomic) 337.9
vasomotor 780.2
vasospastic 443.9
vasovagal 780.2
Wenckebach's, heart block (second degree)
426.13
Phenylketonuria (PKU) 270.1
Phenylpyruvicaciduria 270.1
Pheochromoblastoma (M8700/3)
specified site—*see* Neoplasm, by site, malignant
unspecified site 194.0
Pheochromocytoma (M8700/0)
malignant (M8700/3)
specified site—*see* Neoplasm, by site,
malignant
unspecified site 194.0
specified site—*see* Neoplasm, by site, benign
unspecified site 227.0
Phimosis (congenital) 605
chancroidal 099.0
due to infection 605

Phlebectasia (*see also* Varicose, vein) 454.9
  congenital NEC 747.60
  esophagus (*see also* Varix, esophagus) 456.1
    with hemorrhage (*see also* Varix, esophagus,
      bleeding) 456.0
Phlebitis (infective) (pyemic) (septic)
  (suppurative) 451.9
  antecubital vein 451.82
  arm NEC 451.84
    axillary vein 451.89
    basilic vein 451.82
    deep 451.83
    superficial 451.82
  basilic vein 451.82
  blue 451.19
  brachial vein 451.83
  breast, superficial 451.89
  cavernous (venous) sinus—*see* Phlebitis,
    intracranial sinus
  cephalic vein 451.82
  cerebral (venous) sinus—*see* Phlebitis,
    intracranial sinus
  chest wall, superficial 451.89
  complicating pregnancy or puerperium 671.9
    affecting fetus or newborn 760.3
  cranial (venous) sinus—*see* Phlebitis,
    intracranial sinus
  deep (vessels) 451.19
    femoral vein 451.11
    specified vessel NEC 451.19
  due to implanted device—*see* Complications,
    due to (presence of) any device, implant, or
    graft classified to 996.0-996.5 NEC
  during or resulting from a procedure 997.2
  femoral vein (deep) (superficial) 451.11
  femoropopliteal 451.19
  following infusion, perfusion, or transfusion
    999.2
  gouty 274.89 *[451.9]*
  hepatic veins 451.89
  iliac vein 451.81
  iliofemoral 451.11
  intracranial sinus (any) (venous) 325
    late effect—*see* category 326
    nonpyogenic 437.6
      in pregnancy or puerperium 671.5
  jugular vein 451.89
  lateral (venous) sinus—*see* Phlebitis,
    intracranial sinus
  leg 451.2
    deep (vessels) 451.19
      femoral vein 451.11
      specified vessel NEC 451.19
    superficial (vessels) 451.0
      femoral vein 451.11
  longitudinal sinus—*see* Phlebitis, intracranial
    sinus
  lower extremity 451.2
    deep (vessels) 451.19
      femoral vein 451.11
      specified vessel NEC 451.19
    superficial (vessels) 451.0
      femoral vein 451.11
  migrans, migrating (superficial) 453.1
  pelvic
    with
      abortion—*see* Abortion, by type, with sepsis
      ectopic pregnancy (*see also* categories
        633.0-633.9) 639.0
      molar pregnancy (*see also* categories
        630-632) 639.0

Phlebitis—*continued*
  following
    abortion 639.0
    ectopic or molar pregnancy 639.0
    puerperal, postpartum 671.4
  popliteal vein 451.19
  portal (vein) 572.1
  postoperative 997.2
  pregnancy 671.9
    deep 671.3
    specified type NEC 671.5
    superficial 671.2
  puerperal, postpartum, childbirth 671.9
    deep 671.4
    lower extremities 671.2
    pelvis 671.4
    specified site NEC 671.5
    superficial 671.2
  radial vein 451.83
  retina 362.18
  saphenous (great) (long) 451.0
    accessory or small 451.0
  sinus (meninges)—*see* Phlebitis, intracranial
    sinus
  specified site NEC 451.89
  subclavian vein 451.89
  syphilitic 093.89
  tibial vein 451.19
  ulcer, ulcerative 451.9
    leg 451.2
      deep (vessels) 451.19
        femoral vein 451.11
        specified vessel NEC 451.19
      superficial (vessels) 451.0
        femoral vein 451.11
    lower extremity 451.2
      deep (vessels) 451.19
        femoral vein 451.11
        specified vessel NEC 451.19
      superficial (vessels) 451.0
  ulnar vein 451.83
  umbilicus 451.89
  upper extremity—*see* Phlebitis, arm
  uterus (septic) (*see also* Endometritis) 615.9
  varicose (leg) (lower extremity) (*see also*
    Varicose, vein) 454.1
Phlebofibrosis 459.89
Phleboliths 459.89
Phlebosclerosis 459.89
Phlebothrombosis —*see* Thrombosis
Phlebotomus fever 066.0
Phlegm, choked on 933.1
Phlegmasia
  alba dolens (deep vessels) 451.19
    complicating pregnancy 671.3
    nonpuerperal 451.19
    puerperal, postpartum, childbirth 671.4
  cerulea dolens 451.19
Phlegmon (*see also* Abscess) 682.9
  erysipelatous (*see also* Erysipelas) 035
  iliac 682.2
    fossa 540.1
  throat 478.29
Phlegmonous —*see* condition
Phlyctenulosis (allergic) (keratoconjunctivitis)
  (nontuberculous) 370.31
  cornea 370.31
    with ulcer (*see also* Ulcer, cornea) 370.00
  tuberculous (*see also* Tuberculosis) 017.3
    [370.31]

Placenta, placental—*continued*
  hormone disturbance or malfunction—*see* Placenta, abnormal
  hyperplasia—*see* Placenta, abnormal
  increta (without hemorrhage) 667.0
    with hemorrhage 666.0
  infarction 656.7
    affecting fetus or newborn 762.2
  insertion, vicious—*see* Placenta, previa
  insufficiency
    affecting
      fetus or newborn 762.2
      management of pregnancy 656.5
  lateral—*see* Placenta, previa
  low implantation or insertion—*see* Placenta, previa
  low-lying—*see* Placenta, previa
  malformation—*see* Placenta, abnormal
  malposition—*see* Placenta, previa
  marginalis, marginata—*see* Placenta, previa
  marginal sinus (hemorrhage) (rupture) 641.2
    affecting fetus or newborn 762.1
  membranacea—*see* Placenta, abnormal
  multilobed—*see* Placenta, abnormal
  multipartita—*see* Placenta, abnormal
  necrosis—*see* Placenta, abnormal
  percreta (without hemorrhage) 667.0
    with hemorrhage 666.0
  polyp 674.4
  previa (central) (centralis) (complete) (lateral) (marginal) (marginalis) (partial) (partialis) (total) (with hemorrhage) 641.1
    affecting fetus or newborn 762.0
    noted
      before labor, without hemorrhage (with cesarean delivery) 641.0
      during pregnancy (without hemorrhage) 641.0
    without hemorrhage (before labor and delivery) (during pregnancy) 641.0
  retention (with hemorrhage) 666.0
    fragments, complicating puerperium (delayed hemorrhage) 666.2
      without hemorrhage 667.1
    postpartum, puerperal 666.2
      without hemorrhage 667.0
  separation (normally implanted) (partial) (premature) (with hemorrhage) 641.2
    affecting fetus or newborn 762.1
  septuplex—*see* Placenta, abnormal
  small—*see* Placenta, insufficiency
  softening (premature)—*see* Placenta, abnormal
  spuria—*see* Placenta, abnormal
  succenturiata—*see* Placenta, abnormal
  syphilitic 095.8
  transfusion syndromes 762.3
  transmission of chemical substance—*see* Absorption, chemical, through placenta
  trapped (with hemorrhage) 666.0
    without hemorrhage 667.0
  trilobate—*see* Placenta, abnormal
  tripartita—*see* Placenta, abnormal
  triplex—*see* Placenta, abnormal
  varicose vessel—*see* Placenta, abnormal
  vicious insertion—*see* Placenta, previa
Placentitis
  affecting fetus or newborn 762.7
  complicating pregnancy 658.4
Plagiocephaly (skull) 754.0

Plague 020.9
  abortive 020.8
  ambulatory 020.8
  bubonic 020.0
  cellulocutaneous 020.1
  lymphatic gland 020.0
  pneumonic 020.5
    primary 020.3
    secondary 020.4
  pulmonary—*see* Plague, pneumonic
  pulmonic—*see* Plague, pneumonic
  septicemic 020.2
  tonsillar 020.9
    septicemic 020.2
  vaccination, prophylactic (against) V03.3
Planning, family V25.09
  contraception V25.9
  procreation V26.4
Plaque
  artery, arterial—*see* Arteriosclerosis
  calcareous—*see* Calcification
  Hollenhorst's (retinal) 362.33
  tongue 528.6
Plasma cell myeloma 203.0
Plasmacytoma, plasmocytoma (solitary) (M9731/1) 238.6
  benign (M9731/0)—*see* Neoplasm, by site, benign
  malignant (M9731/3) 203.8
Plasmacytosis 288.8
Plaster ulcer (*see also* Decubitus) 707.0
Platybasia 756.0
Platyonychia (congenital) 757.5
  acquired 703.8
Platypelloid pelvis 738.6
  with disproportion (fetopelvic) 653.2
    affecting fetus or newborn 763.1
    causing obstructed labor 660.1
      affecting fetus or newborn 763.1
  congenital 755.69
Platyspondylia 756.19
Plethora 782.62
  newborn 776.4
Pleura, pleural —*see* condition
Pleuralgia 786.52
Pleurisy (acute) (adhesive) (chronic) (costal) (diaphragmatic) (double) (dry) (fetid) (fibrinous) (fibrous) (interlobar) (latent) (lung) (old) (plastic) (primary) (residual) (sicca) (sterile) (subacute) (unresolved) (with adherent pleura) 511.0
  with
    effusion (without mention of cause) 511.9
      bacterial, nontuberculous 511.1
        nontuberculous NEC 511.9
          bacterial 511.1
        pneumococcal 511.1
        specified type NEC 511.8
        staphylococcal 511.1
        streptococcal 511.1
      tuberculous (*see also* Tuberculosis, pleura) 012.0
        primary, progressive 010.1
    influenza, flu, or grippe 487.1
    tuberculosis—*see* Pleurisy, tuberculous
  encysted 511.8
  exudative (*see also* Pleurisy, with effusion) 511.9
    bacterial, nontuberculous 511.1
  fibrinopurulent 510.9
    with fistula 510.0

Pleurisy—*continued*
  fibropurulent 510.9
    with fistula 510.0
  hemorrhagic 511.8
  influenzal 487.1
  pneumococcal 511.0
    with effusion 511.1
  purulent 510.9
    with fistula 510.0
  septic 510.9
    with fistula 510.0
  serofibrinous (*see also* Pleurisy, with effusion)
    511.9
    bacterial, nontuberculous 511.1
  seropurulent 510.9
    with fistula 510.0
  serous (*see also* Pleurisy, with effusion) 511.9
    bacterial, nontuberculous 511.1
  staphylococcal 511.0
    with effusion 511.1
  streptococcal 511.0
    with effusion 511.1
  suppurative 510.9
    with fistula 510.0
  traumatic (post) (current) 862.29
    with open wound into cavity 862.39
  tuberculous (with effusion) (*see also*
    Tuberculosis, pleura) 012.0
    primary, progressive 010.1
Pleuritis sicca —*see* Pleurisy
Pleurobronchopneumonia (*see also* Pneumonia,
  broncho-) 485
Pleurodynia 786.52
  epidemic 074.1
  viral 074.1
Pleurohepatitis 573.8
Pleuropericarditis (*see also* Pericarditis) 423.9
  acute 420.90
Pleuropneumonia (acute) (bilateral) (double)
  (septic) (*see also* Pneumonia) 486
  chronic (*see also* Fibrosis, lung) 515
Pleurorrhea (*see also* Hydrothorax) 511.8
Plexitis, brachial 353.0
Plica
  knee 727.83
  polonica 132.0
  tonsil 474.8
Plicae dysphonia ventricularis 784.49
Plicated tongue 529.5
  congenital 750.13
Plug
  bronchus NEC 519.1
  meconium (newborn) NEC 777.1
  mucus—*see* Mucus, plug
Plumbism 984.9
  specified type of lead—*see* Table of drugs and
    chemicals
Plummer's disease (toxic nodular goiter) 242.3
Plummer-Vinson syndrome (sideropenic
  dysphagia) 280.8
Pluricarential syndrome of infancy 260
Plurideficiency syndrome of infancy 260
Plus (and minus) hand (intrinsic) 736.09
PMS 625.4
Pneumathemia —*see* Air, embolism, by type
Pneumatic drill or hammer disease 994.9
Pneumatocele (lung) 518.89
  intracranial 348.8
  tension 492.0

Pneumatosis
  cystoides intestinalis 569.89
  peritonei 568.89
  pulmonum 492.8
Pneumaturia 599.84
Pneumoblastoma (M8981/3)—*see* Neoplasm,
  lung, malignant
Pneumocephalus 348.8
Pneumococcemia 038.2
Pneumococcus, pneumococcal —*see* condition
Pneumoconiosis (due to) (inhalation of) 505
  aluminum 503
  asbestos 501
  bagasse 495.1
  bauxite 503
  beryllium 503
  carbon electrode makers' 503
  coal
    miners' (simple) 500
    workers' (simple) 500
  cotton dust 504
  diatomite fibrosis 502
  dust NEC 504
    inorganic 503
    lime 502
    marble 502
    organic NEC 504
  fumes or vapors (from silo) 506.9
  graphite 503
  hard metal 503
  mica 502
  moldy hay 495.0
  rheumatoid 714.81
  silica NEC 502
    and carbon 500
  silicate NEC 502
  talc 502
Pneumocystis carinii pneumonia 136.3
Pneumocystosis 136.3
  with pneumonia 136.3
Pneumoenteritis 025
Pneumohemopericardium (*see also*
  Pericarditis) 423.9
Pneumohemothorax (*see also* Hemothorax)
  511.8
  traumatic 860.4
    with open wound into thorax 860.5
Pneumohydropericardium (*see also*
  Pericarditis) 423.9
Pneumohydrothorax (*see also* Hydrothorax)
  511.8
Pneumomediastinum 518.1
  congenital 770.2
  fetus or newborn 770.2
Pneumomycosis 117.9
Pneumonia (acute) (Alpenstich) (benign)
  (bilateral) (brain) (cerebral) (circumscribed)
  (congestive) (creeping) (delayed resolution)
  (double) (epidemic) (fever) (flash) (fulminant)
  (fungoid) (granulomatous) (hemorrhagic)
  (incipient) (infantile) (infectious) (infiltration)
  (insular) (intermittent) (latent) (lobe)
  (migratory) (newborn) (organized)
  (overwhelming) (primary) (progressive)
  (pseudolobar) (purulent) (resolved)
  (secondary) (senile) (septic) (suppurative)
  (terminal) (true) (unresolved) (vesicular) 486
  with influenza, flu, or grippe 487.0
  adenoviral 480.0
  adynamic 514
  alba 090.0

Pneumonia—*continued*
  allergic 518.3
  alveolar—*see* Pneumonia, lobar
  anaerobes 482.81
  anthrax 022.1 *[484.5]*
  apex, apical—*see* Pneumonia, lobar
  ascaris 127.0 *[484.8]*
  aspiration 507.0
    due to
      aspiration of microorganisms
        bacterial 482.9
          specified type NEC 482.89
        specified organism NEC 483.8
          bacterial NEC 482.89
        viral 480.9
          specified type NEC 480.8
      food (regurgitated) 507.0
      gastric secretions 507.0
      milk 507.0
      oils, essences 507.1
      solids, liquids NEC 507.8
      vomitus 507.0
    newborn 770.1
  asthenic 514
  atypical (disseminated, focal) (primary) 486
    with influenza 487.0
  bacillus 482.9
    specified type NEC 482.89
  bacterial 482.9
    specified type NEC 482.89
  Bacteroides (fragilis) (oralis) (melaninogenicus)
      482.81
  basal, basic, basilar—*see* Pneumonia, lobar
  broncho-, bronchial (confluent) (croupous)
      (diffuse) (disseminated) (hemorrhagic)
      (involving lobes) (lobar) (terminal) 485
    with influenza 487.0
    allergic 518.3
    aspiration (*see also* Pneumonia, aspiration)
        507.0
    bacterial 482.9
      specified type NEC 482.89
    capillary 466.19
      with bronchospasm or obstruction 466.19
    chronic (*see also* Fibrosis, lung) 515
    congenital (infective) 770.0
    diplococcal 481
    Eaton's agent 483.0
    Escherichia coli (E. coli) 482.82
    Friedländer's bacillus 482.0
    Hemophilus influenzae 482.2
    hiberno-vernal 083.0 *[484.8]*
    hypostatic 514
    influenzal 487.0
    inhalation (*see also* Pneumonia, aspiration)
        507.0
      due to fumes or vapors (chemical) 506.0
    Klebsiella 482.0
    lipid 507.1
      endogenous 516.8
    Mycoplasma (pneumoniae) 483.0
    ornithosis 073.0
    pleuropneumonia-like organisms (PPLO)
        483.0
    pneumococcal 481
    Proteus 482.83
    pseudomonas 482.1
    specified organism NEC 483.8
      bacterial NEC 482.89
    staphylococcal 482.40
      aureus 482.41

Pneumonia—*continued*
    specified type NEC 482.49
    streptococcal—*see* Pneumonia, streptococcal
    typhoid 002.0 *[484.8]*
    viral, virus (*see also* Pneumonia, viral) 480.9
  Butyrivibrio (fibriosolvens) 482.81
  Candida 112.4
  capillary 466.19
    with bronchospasm or obstruction 466.19
  caseous (*see also* Tuberculosis) 011.6
  catarrhal—*see* Pneumonia, broncho-
  central—*see* Pneumonia, lobar
  Chlamydia, chlamydial 483.1
    pneumoniae 483.1
    psittaci 073.0
    specified type NEC 483.1
    trachomatis 483.1
  cholesterol 516.8
  chronic (*see also* Fibrosis, lung) 515
  cirrhotic (chronic) (*see also* Fibrosis, lung) 515
  Clostridium (haemolyticum) (novyi) NEC
      482.81
  confluent—*see* Pneumonia, broncho-
  congenital (infective) 770.0
    aspiration 770.1
  croupous—*see* Pneumonia, lobar
  cytomegalic inclusion 078.5 *[484.1]*
  deglutition (*see also* Pneumonia, aspiration)
      507.0
  desquamative interstitial 516.8
  diffuse—*see* Pneumonia, broncho-
  diplococcal, diplococcus (broncho-) (lobar) 481
  disseminated (focal)—*see* Pneumonia, broncho-
  due to
    adenovirus 480.0
    Bacterium anitratum 482.83
    Chlamydia, chlamydial 483.1
      pneumoniae 483.1
      psittaci 073.0
      specified type NEC 483.1
      trachomatis 483.1
    coccidioidomycosis 114.0
    Diplococcus (pneumoniae) 481
    Eaton's agent 483.0
    Escherichia coli (E. coli) 482.82
    Friedländer's bacillus 482.0
    fumes or vapors (chemical) (inhalation) 506.0
    fungus NEC 117.9 *[484.7]*
      coccidioidomycosis 114.0
    Hemophilus influenzae (H. influenzae) 482.2
    Herellea 482.83
    influenza 487.0
    ~~Klebsiella pneumoniae 482.0~~
    Mycoplasma (pneumoniae) 483.0
    parainfluenza virus 480.2
    pleuropneumonia-like organism (PPLO) 483.0
    Pneumococcus 481
    Pneumocystis carinii 136.3
    Proteus 482.83
    pseudomonas 482.1
    respiratory syncytial virus 480.1
    rickettsia 083.9 *[484.8]*
    specified
      bacteria NEC 482.89
      organism NEC 483.8
      virus NEC 480.8
    Staphylococcus 482.40
      aureus 482.41
      specified type NEC 482.49
    Streptococcus—*see also* Pneumonia,
        streptococcal

Pneumonia—*continued*
  pneumoniae 481
  virus (*see also* Pneumonia, viral) 480.9
  Eaton's agent 483.0
  embolic, embolism (*see also* Embolism,
    pulmonary) 415.1
  eosinophilic 518.3
  Escherichia coli (E. coli) 482.82
  Eubacterium 482.81
  fibrinous—*see* Pneumonia, lobar
  fibroid (chronic) (*see also* Fibrosis, lung) 515
  fibrous (*see also* Fibrosis, lung) 515
  Friedländer's bacillus 482.0
  Fusobacterium (nucleatum) 482.81
  gangrenous 513.0
  giant cell (*see also* Pneumonia, viral) 480.9
  gram-negative bacteria NEC 482.83
    anaerobic 482.81
  grippal 487.0
  Hemophilus influenzae (bronchial) (lobar) 482.2
  hypostatic (broncho-) (lobar) 514
  in
    actinomycosis 039.1
    anthrax 022.1 *[484.5]*
    aspergillosis 117.3 *[484.6]*
    candidiasis 112.4
    coccidioidomycosis 114.0
    cytomegalic inclusion disease 078.5 *[484.1]*
    histoplasmosis (*see also* Histoplasmosis)
      115.95
    infectious disease NEC 136.9 *[484.8]*
    measles 055.1
    mycosis, systemic NEC 117.9 *[484.7]*
    nocardiasis, nocardiosis 039.1
    ornithosis 073.0
    pneumocystosis 136.3
    psittacosis 073.0
    Q fever 083.0 *[484.8]*
    salmonellosis 003.22
    toxoplasmosis 130.4
    tularemia 021.2
    typhoid (fever) 002.0 *[484.8]*
    varicella 052.1
    whooping cough (*see also* Whooping cough)
      033.9 *[484.3]*
  infective, acquired prenatally 770.0
  influenzal (broncho) (lobar) (virus) 487.0
  inhalation (*see also* Pneumonia, aspiration)
    507.0
    fumes or vapors (chemical) 506.0
  interstitial 516.8
    with influenzal 487.0
    acute 136.3
    chronic (*see also* Fibrosis, lung) 515
    desquamative 516.8
    hypostatic 514
    lipoid 507.1
    lymphoid 516.8
    plasma cell 136.3
    pseudomonas 482.1
  intrauterine (infective) 770.0
    aspiration 770.1
  Klebsiella pneumoniae 482.0
  Legionnaires' 482.84
  lipid, lipoid (exogenous) (interstitial) 507.1
    endogenous 516.8
  lobar (diplococcal) (disseminated) (double)
    (interstitial) (pneumococcal, any type) 481
    with influenza 487.0
    bacterial 482.9
      specified type NEC 482.89

Pneumonia—*continued*
  chronic (*see also* Fibrosis, lung) 515
  Escherichia coli (E. coli) 482.82
  Friedländer's bacillus 482.0
  Hemophilus influenzae (H. influenzae) 482.2
  hypostatic 514
  influenzal 487.0
  Klebsiella 482.0
  ornithosis 073.0
  Proteus 482.83
  pseudomonas 482.1
  psittacosis 073.0
  specified organism NEC 483.8
    bacterial NEC 482.89
  staphylococcal 482.40
    aureus 482.41
    specified type NEC 482.49
  streptococcal—*see* Pneumonia, streptococcal
  viral, virus (*see also* Pneumonia, viral) 480.9
  lobular (confluent)—*see* Pneumonia, broncho-
  Löffler's 518.3
  massive—*see* Pneumonia, lobar
  meconium 770.1
  metastatic NEC 038.8 *[484.8]*
  Mycoplasma (pneumoniae) 483.0
  necrotic 513.0
  nitrogen dioxide 506.9
  orthostatic 514
  parainfluenza virus 480.2
  parenchymatous (*see also* Fibrosis, lung) 515
  passive 514
  patchy—*see* Pneumonia, broncho
  Peptococcus 482.81
  Peptostreptococcus 482.81
  plasma cell 136.3
  pleurolobar—*see* Pneumonia, lobar
  pleuropneumonia-like organism (PPLO) 483.0
  pneumococcal (broncho) (lobar) 481
  Pneumocystis (carinii) 136.3
  postinfectional NEC 136.9 *[484.8]*
  postmeasles 055.1
  postoperative 997.3
  primary atypical 486
  Proprionibacterium 482.81
  Proteus 482.83
  pseudomonas 482.1
  psittacosis 073.0
  radiation 508.0
  respiratory syncytial virus 480.1
  resulting from a procedure 997.3
  rheumatic 390 *[517.1]*
  Salmonella 003.22
  segmented, segmental—*see* Pneumonia,
    broncho-
  Serratia (marcescens) 482.83
  specified
    bacteria NEC 482.89
    organism NEC 483.8
    virus NEC 480.8
  spirochetal 104.8 *[484.8]*
  staphylococcal (broncho) (lobar) 482.40
    aureus 482.41
    specified type NEC 482.49
  static, stasis 514
  streptococcal (broncho) (lobar) NEC 482.30
    Group
      A 482.31
      B 482.32
      specified NEC 482.39
    pneumoniae 481
    specified type NEC 482.39

Pneumonia—*continued*
  Streptococcus pneumoniae 481
  traumatic (complication) (early) (secondary)
    958.8
  tuberculous (any) (*see also* Tuberculosis) 011.6
  tularemic 021.2
  TWAR agent 483.1
  varicella 052.1
  Veillonella 482.81
  viral, virus (broncho) (interstitial) (lobar) 480.9
    with influenza, flu, or grippe 487.0
    adenoviral 480.0
    parainfluenza 480.2
    respiratory syncytial 480.1
    specified type NEC 480.8
  white (congenital) 090.0
Pneumonic —*see* condition
Pneumonitis (acute) (primary) (*see also*
    Pneumonia) 486
  allergic 495.9
    specified type NEC 495.8
  aspiration 507.0
    due to fumes or gases 506.0
    newborn 770.1
    obstetric 668.0
  chemical 506.0
    due to fumes or gases 506.0
  cholesterol 516.8
  chronic (*see also* Fibrosis, lung) 515
  congenital rubella 771.0
  due to
    fumes or vapors 506.0
    inhalation
      food (regurgitated), milk, vomitus 507.0
      oils, essences 507.1
      saliva 507.0
      solids, liquids NEC 507.8
      toxoplasmosis (acquired) 130.4
        congenital (active) 771.2 *[484.8]*
  eosinophilic 518.3
  fetal aspiration 770.1
  hypersensitivity 495.9
  interstitial (chronic) (*see also* Fibrosis, lung) 515
    lymphoid 516.8
  lymphoid, interstitial 516.8
  meconium 770.1
  postanesthetic
    correct substance properly administered 507.0
    obstetric 668.0
    overdose or wrong substance given 968.4
      specified anesthetic—*see* Table of drugs
        and chemicals
  postoperative 997.3
    obstetric 668.0
  radiation 508.0
  rubella, congenital 771.0
  "ventilation" 495.7
  wood-dust 495.8
Pneumonoconiosis —*see* Pneumoconiosis
Pneumoparotid 527.8
Pneumopathy NEC 518.89
  alveolar 516.9
    specified NEC 516.8
  due to dust NEC 504
  parietoalveolar 516.9
    specified condition NEC 516.8
Pneumopericarditis (*see also* Pericarditis) 423.9
  acute 420.90

Pneumopericardium —*see also* Pericarditis
  congenital 770.2
  fetus or newborn 770.2
  traumatic (post) (*see also* Pneumothorax,
    traumatic) 860.0
    with open wound into thorax 860.1
Pneumoperitoneum 568.89
  fetus or newborn 770.2
Pneumophagia (psychogenic) 306.4
Pneumopleurisy, pneumopleuritis (*see also*
    Pneumonia) 486
Pneumopyopericardium 420.99
Pneumopyothorax (*see also* Pyopneumothorax)
    510.9
  with fistula 510.0
Pneumorrhagia 786.3
  newborn 770.3
  tuberculous (*see also* Tuberculosis, pulmonary)
    011.9
Pneumosiderosis (occupational) 503
Pneumothorax (acute) (chronic) 512.8
  congenital 770.2
  due to operative injury of chest wall or lung
    512.1
    accidental puncture or laceration 512.1
  fetus or newborn 770.2
  iatrogenic 512.1
  postoperative 512.1
  spontaneous 512.8
    fetus or newborn 770.2
    tension 512.0
  sucking 512.8
    iatrogenic 512.1
    postoperative 512.1
  tense valvular, infectional 512.0
  tension 512.0
    iatrogenic 512.1
    postoperative 512.1
    spontaneous 512.0
  traumatic 860.0
    with
      hemothorax 860.4
        with open wound into thorax 860.5
      open wound into thorax 860.1
  tuberculous (*see also* Tuberculosis) 011.7
Pocket (s)
  endocardial (*see also* Endocarditis) 424.90
  periodontal 523.8
Podagra 274.9
Podencephalus 759.89
Poikilocytosis 790.09
Poikiloderma 709.09
  Civatte's 709.09
  congenital 757.33
  vasculare atrophicans 696.2
Poikilodermatomyositis 710.3
Pointed ear 744.29
Poise imperfect 729.9
Poisoned —*see* Poisoning
Poisoning (acute)—*see also* Table of drugs and
    chemicals
  Bacillus, B.
    aertrycke (*see also* Infection, Salmonella)
      003.9
    botulinus 005.1
    cholerae (suis) (*see also* Infection,
      Salmonella) 003.9
    paratyphosus (*see also* Infection, Salmonella)
      003.9
    suipestifer (*see also* Infection, Salmonella)
      003.9

Poisoning—*continued*
  bacterial toxins NEC 005.9
  berries, noxious 988.2
  blood (general)—*see* Septicemia
  botulism 005.1
  bread, moldy, mouldy—*see* Poisoning, food
  damaged meat—*see* Poisoning, food
  death-cap (Amanita phalloides) (Amanita
    verna) 988.1
  decomposed food—*see* Poisoning, food
  diseased food—*see* Poisoning, food
  drug—*see* Table of drugs and chemicals
  epidemic, fish, meat, or other food—*see*
    Poisoning, food
  fava bean 282.2
  fish (bacterial)—*see also* Poisoning, food
    noxious 988.0
  food (acute) (bacterial) (diseased) (infected)
    NEC 005.9
    due to
      Bacillus
        aertrycke (*see also* Poisoning, food, due to
          Salmonella) 003.9
        botulinus 005.1
        cereus 005.89
        choleraesuis (*see also* Poisoning, food,
          due to Salmonella) 003.9
        paratyphosus (*see also* Poisoning, food,
          due to Salmonella) 003.9
        suipestifer (*see also* Poisoning, food, due
          to Salmonella) 003.9
      Clostridium 005.3
        botulinum 005.1
        perfringens 005.2
        welchii 005.2
      Salmonella (aertrycke) (callinarum)
        (choleraesuis) (enteritidis) (paratyphi)
        (suipestifer) 003.9
        with
          gastroenteritis 003.0
          localized infection(s) (*see also* Infection,
            Salmonella) 003.20
          septicemia 003.1
          specified manifestation NEC 003.8
      specified bacterium NEC 005.89
      Staphylococcus 005.0
      Streptococcus 005.8
      Vibrio parahaemolyticus 005.4
      Vibrio vulnificus 005.81
    noxious or naturally toxic 988.0
      berries 988.2
      fish 988.0
      mushroom 988.1
      plants NEC 988.2
  ice cream—*see* Poisoning, food
  ichthyotoxism (bacterial) 005.9
  kreotoxism, food 005.9
  malarial—*see* Malaria
  meat—*see* Poisoning, food
  mushroom (noxious) 988.1
  mussel—*see also* Poisoning, food
    noxious 988.0
  noxious foodstuffs (*see also* Poisoning, food,
    noxious) 988.9
    specified type NEC 988.8
  plants, noxious 988.2
  pork—*see also* Poisoning, food
    specified NEC 988.8
    Trichinosis 124
  ptomaine—*see* Poisoning, food
  putrefaction, food—*see* Poisoning, food

Poisoning—*continued*
  radiation 508.0
  Salmonella (*see also* Infection, Salmonella)
    003.9
  sausage—*see also* Poisoning, food
    Trichinosis 124
  saxitoxin 988.0
  shellfish—*see also* Poisoning, food
    noxious 988.0
  Staphylococcus, food 005.0
  toxic, from disease NEC 799.8
  truffles—*see* Poisoning, food
  uremic—*see* Uremia
  uric acid 274.9
Poison ivy, oak, sumac or other plant
  dermatitis 692.6
Poker spine 720.0
Policeman's disease 729.2
Polioencephalitis (acute) (bulbar) (*see also*
  Poliomyelitis, bulbar) 045.0
  inferior 335.22
  influenzal 487.8
  superior hemorrhagic (acute) (Wernicke's) 265.1
  Wernicke's (superior hemorrhagic) 265.1
Polioencephalomyelitis (acute) (anterior)
  (bulbar) (*see also* Polioencephalitis) 045.0
Polioencephalopathy, superior hemorrhagic
  265.1
  with
    beriberi 265.0
    pellagra 265.2
Poliomeningoencephalitis —*see*
  Meningoencephalitis
Poliomyelitis (acute) (anterior) (epidemic) 045.9

> *Note*—*Use the following fifth-digit*
> *subclassification with category 045:*
>
> 0 *poliovirus, unspecified type*
> 1 *poliovirus, type I*
> 2 *poliovirus, type II*
> 3 *poliovirus, type III*

  with
    paralysis 045.1
      bulbar 045.0
  abortive 045.2
  ascending 045.9
    progressive 045.9
  bulbar 045.0
  cerebral 045.0
  chronic 335.21
  congenital 771.2
  contact V01.2
  deformities 138
  exposure to V01.2
  late effect 138
  nonepidemic 045.9
  nonparalytic 045.2
  old with deformity 138
  posterior, acute 053.19
  residual 138
  sequelae 138
  spinal, acute 045.9
  syphilitic (chronic) 094.89
  vaccination, prophylactic (against) V04.0
Poliosis (eyebrow) (eyelashes) 704.3
  circumscripta (congenital) 757.4
    acquired 704.3
  congenital 757.4
Pollakiuria 788.41
  psychogenic 306.53
Pollinosis 477.0

Pollitzer's disease (hidradenitis suppurativa) 705.83
Polyadenitis (*see also* Adenitis) 289.3
  malignant 020.0
Polyalgia 729.9
Polyangiitis (essential) 446.0
Polyarteritis (nodosa) (renal) 446.0
Polyarthralgia 719.49
  psychogenic 306.0
Polyarthritis, polyarthropathy NEC 716.59
  due to or associated with other specified
    conditions—*see* Arthritis, due to or
    associated with
  endemic (*see also* Disease, Kaschin-Beck) 716.0
  inflammatory 714.9
    specified type NEC 714.89
  juvenile (chronic) 714.30
    acute 714.31
  migratory—*see* Fever, rheumatic
  rheumatic 714.0
    fever (acute)—*see* Fever, rheumatic
Polycarential syndrome of infancy 260
Polychondritis (atrophic) (chronic) (relapsing)
  733.99
Polycoria 743.46
Polycystic (congenital) (disease) 759.89
  degeneration, kidney—*see* Polycystic, kidney
  kidney (congenital) 753.12
    adult type (APKD) 753.13
    autosomal dominant 753.13
    autosomal recessive 753.14
    childhood type (CPKD) 753.14
    infantile type 753.14
  liver 751.62
  lung 518.89
    congenital 748.4
  ovary, ovaries 256.4
  spleen 759.0
Polycythemia (primary) (rubra) (vera)
  (M9950/1) 238.4
  acquired 289.0
  benign 289.0
    familial 289.6
  due to
    donor twin 776.4
    fall in plasma volume 289.0
    high altitude 289.0
    maternal-fetal transfusion 776.4
    stress 289.0
  emotional 289.0
  erythropoietin 289.0
  familial (benign) 289.6
  Gaisböck's (hypertonica) 289.0
  high altitude 289.0
  hypertonica 289.0
  hypoxemic 289.0
  neonatorum 776.4
  nephrogenous 289.0
  relative 289.0
  secondary 289.0
  spurious 289.0
  stress 289.0
Polycytosis cryptogenica 289.0
Polydactylism, polydactyly 755.00
  fingers 755.01
  toes 755.02
Polydipsia 783.5
Polydystrophic oligophrenia 277.5
Polyembryoma (M9072/3)—*see* Neoplasm, by
  site, malignant
Polygalactia 676.6

Polyglandular
  deficiency 258.9
  dyscrasia 258.9
  dysfunction 258.9
  syndrome 258.8
Polyhydramnios (*see also* Hydramnios) 657
Polymastia 757.6
Polymenorrhea 626.2
Polymicrogyria 742.2
Polymyalgia 725
  arteritica 446.5
  rheumatica 725
Polymyositis (acute) (chronic) (hemorrhagic)
  710.4
  with involvement of
    lung 710.4 *[517.8]*
    skin 710.3
  ossificans (generalisata) (progressiva) 728.19
  Wagner's (dermatomyositis) 710.3
Polyneuritis, polyneuritic (*see also*
  Polyneuropathy) 356.9
  alcoholic 357.5
    with psychosis 291.1
  cranialis 352.6
  demyelinating, chronic inflammatory 357.81
  diabetic 250.6 *[357.2]*
  due to lack of vitamin NEC 269.2 *[357.4]*
  endemic 265.0 *[357.4]*
  erythredema 985.0
  febrile 357.0
  hereditary ataxic 356.3
  idiopathic, acute 357.0
  infective (acute) 357.0
  nutritional 269.9 *[357.4]*
  postinfectious 357.0
Polyneuropathy (peripheral) 356.9
  alcoholic 357.5
  amyloid 277.3 *[357.4]*
  arsenical 357.7
  critical illness 357.82
  diabetic 250.6 *[357.2]*
  due to
    antitetanus serum 357.6
    arsenic 357.7
    drug or medicinal substance 357.6
      correct substance properly administered
        357.6
      overdose or wrong substance given or taken
        977.9
      specified drug—*see* Table of drugs and
        chemicals
    lack of vitamin NEC 269.2 *[357.4]*
    lead 357.7
    organophosphate compounds 357.7
    pellagra 265.2 *[357.4]*
    porphyria 277.1 *[357.4]*
    serum 357.6
    toxic agent NEC 357.7
  hereditary 356.0
  idiopathic 356.9
    progressive 356.4
  in
    amyloidosis 277.3 *[357.4]*
    avitaminosis 269.2 *[357.4]*
      specified NEC 269.1 *[357.4]*
    beriberi 265.0 *[357.4]*
    collagen vascular disease NEC 710.9 *[357.1]*
    deficiency
      B-complex NEC 266.2 *[357.4]*
      vitamin B 266.9 *[357.4]*
      vitamin B$_6$ 266.1 *[357.4]*

Polyneuropathy—*continued*
diabetes 250.6 *[357.2]*
diphtheria (*see also* Diphtheria) 032.89
[357.4]
disseminated lupus erythematosus 710.0
[357.1]
herpes zoster 053.13
hypoglycemia 251.2 *[357.4]*
malignant neoplasm (M8000/3) NEC 199.1
[357.3]
mumps 072.72
pellagra 265.2 *[357.4]*
polyarteritis nodosa 446.0 *[357.1]*
porphyria 277.1 *[357.4]*
rheumatoid arthritis 714.0 *[357.1]*
sarcoidosis 135 *[357.4]*
uremia 585 *[357.4]*
lead 357.7
nutritional 269.9 *[357.4]*
specified NEC 269.8 *[357.4]*
postherpetic 053.13
progressive 356.4
sensory (hereditary) 356.2
Polyonychia 757.5
Polyopia 368.2
refractive 368.15
Polyorchism, polyorchidism (three testes) 752.8
Polyorrhymenitis (peritoneal) (*see also*
Polyserositis) 568.82
pericardial 423.2
Polyostotic fibrous dysplasia 756.54
Polyotia 744.1
Polyp, polypus

---

*Note—Polyps of organs or sites that do not
appear in the list below should be coded to the
residual category for diseases of the organ or
site concerned.*

---

accessory sinus 471.8
adenoid tissue 471.0
adenomatous (M8210/0)—*see also* Neoplasm,
by site, benign
adenocarcinoma in (M8210/3)—*see*
Neoplasm, by site, malignant
carcinoma in (M8210/3)—*see* Neoplasm, by
site, malignant
multiple (M8221/0)—*see* Neoplasm, by site,
benign
antrum 471.8
anus, anal (canal) (nonadenomatous) 569.0
adenomatous 211.4
Bartholin's gland 624.6
bladder (M8120/1) 236.7
broad ligament 620.8—
cervix (uteri) 622.7
adenomatous 219.0
in pregnancy or childbirth 654.6
affecting fetus or newborn 763.89
causing obstructed labor 660.2
mucous 622.7
nonneoplastic 622.7
choanal 471.0
cholesterol 575.6
clitoris 624.6
colon (M8210/0) (*see also* Polyp, adenomatous)
211.3
corpus uteri 621.0
dental 522.0
ear (middle) 385.30
endometrium 621.0
ethmoidal (sinus) 471.8

Polyp, polypus—*continued*
fallopian tube 620.8
female genital organs NEC 624.8
frontal (sinus) 471.8
gallbladder 575.6
gingiva 523.8
gum 523.8
labia 624.6
larynx (mucous) 478.4
malignant (M8000/3)—*see* Neoplasm, by site,
malignant
maxillary (sinus) 471.8
middle ear 385.30
myometrium 621.0
nares
anterior 471.9
posterior 471.0
nasal (mucous) 471.9
cavity 471.0
septum 471.9
nasopharyngeal 471.0
neoplastic (M8210/0)—*see* Neoplasm, by site,
benign
nose (mucous) 471.9
oviduct 620.8
paratubal 620.8
pharynx 478.29
congenital 750.29
placenta, placental 674.4
prostate 600.2
pudenda 624.6
pulp (dental) 522.0
rectosigmoid 211.4
rectum (nonadenomatous) 569.0
adenomatous 211.4
septum (nasal) 471.9
sinus (accessory) (ethmoidal) (frontal)
(maxillary) (sphenoidal) 471.8
sphenoidal (sinus) 471.8
stomach (M8210/0) 211.1
tube, fallopian 620.8
turbinate, mucous membrane 471.8
ureter 593.89
urethra 599.3
uterine
ligament 620.8
tube 620.8
uterus (body) (corpus) (mucous) 621.0
in pregnancy or childbirth 654.1
affecting fetus or newborn 763.89
causing obstructed labor 660.2
vagina 623.7—
vocal cord (mucous) 478.4
vulva 624.6
Polyphagia 783.6
Polypoid —*see* condition
Polyposis —*see also* Polyp
coli (adenomatous) (M8220/0) 211.3
adenocarcinoma in (M8220/3) 153.9
carcinoma in (M8220/3) 153.9
familial (M8220/0) 211.3
intestinal (adenomatous) (M8220/0) 211.3
multiple (M8221/0)—*see* Neoplasm, by site,
benign
Polyradiculitis (acute) 357.0
Polyradiculoneuropathy (acute) (segmentally
demyelinating) 357.0
Polysarcia 278.00
Polyserositis (peritoneal) 568.82
due to pericarditis 423.2
paroxysmal (familial) 277.3

Postinfluenzal syndrome 780.79
Postlaminectomy syndrome 722.80
  cervical, cervicothoracic 722.81
  kyphosis 737.12
  lumbar, lumbosacral 722.83
  thoracic, thoracolumbar 722.82
Postleukotomy syndrome 310.0
Postlobectomy syndrome 310.0
Postmastectomy lymphedema (syndrome) 457.0
Postmaturity, postmature (fetus or newborn)
  766.2
  affecting management of pregnancy
    post term pregnancy 645.1
    prolonged pregnancy 645.2
  syndrome 766.2
Postmeasles —*see also* condition
  complication 055.8
    specified NEC 055.79
Postmenopausal
  endometrium (atrophic) 627.8
    suppurative (*see also* Endometritis) 615.9
  hormone replacement therapy V07.4
  status (age related) (natural) V49.81
Postnasal drip —*see* Sinusitis
Postnatal —*see* condition
Postoperative —*see also* condition
  confusion state 293.9
  psychosis 293.9
  status NEC (*see also* Status (post)) V45.89
Postpancreatectomy hyperglycemia 251.3
Postpartum —*see also* condition
  observation
    immediately after delivery V24.0
    routine follow-up V24.2
Postperfusion syndrome NEC 999.8
  bone marrow 996.85
Postpoliomyelitic —*see* condition
Postsurgery status NEC (*see also* Status (post))
  V45.89
Post-term (pregnancy) 645.1
  infant (294 days or more gestation) 766.2
Posttraumatic —*see* condition
Posttraumatic brain syndrome, nonpsychotic
  310.2
Post-typhoid abscess 002.0
Postures, hysterical 300.11
Postvaccinal reaction or complication —*see*
  Complications, vaccination
Postvagotomy syndrome 564.2
Postvalvulotomy syndrome 429.4
Postvasectomy sperm count V25.8
Potain's disease (pulmonary edema) 514
Potain's syndrome (gastrectasis with dyspepsia)
  536.1
Pott's
  curvature (spinal) (*see also* Tuberculosis) 015.0
    [737.43]
  disease or paraplegia (*see also* Tuberculosis)
    015.0 [730.88]
  fracture (closed) 824.4
    open 824.5
  gangrene 440.24
  osteomyelitis (*see also* Tuberculosis) 015.0
    [730.88]
  spinal curvature (*see also* Tuberculosis) 015.0
    [737.43]
  tumor, puffy (*see also* Osteomyelitis) 730.2

Potter's
  asthma 502
  disease 753.0
  facies 754.0
  lung 502
  syndrome (with renal agenesis) 753.0
Pouch
  bronchus 748.3
  Douglas'—*see* condition
  esophagus, esophageal (congenital) 750.4
    acquired 530.6
  gastric 537.1
  Hartmann's (abnormal sacculation of
    gallbladder neck) 575.8
  of intestine V44.3
    attention to V55.3
  pharynx, pharyngeal (congenital) 750.27
Poulet's disease 714.2
Poultrymen's itch 133.8
Poverty V60.2
Prader-Labhart-Willi-Fanconi syndrome
  (hypogenital dystrophy with diabetic
  tendency) 759.81
Prader-Willi syndrome (hypogenital dystrophy
  with diabetic tendency) 759.81
Preachers' voice 784.49
Pre-AIDS —*see* Human immunodeficiency virus
  (disease) (illness) (infection)
Preauricular appendage 744.1
Prebetalipoproteinemia (acquired) (essential)
  (familial) (hereditary) (primary) (secondary)
  272.1
  with chylomicronemia 272.3
Precipitate labor 661.3
  affecting fetus or newborn 763.6
Preclimacteric bleeding 627.0
  menorrhagia 627.0
Precocious
  adrenarche 259.1
  menarche 259.1
  menstruation 626.8
  pubarche 259.1
  puberty NEC 259.1
  sexual development NEC 259.1
  thelarche 259.1
Precocity, sexual (constitutional) (cryptogenic)
  (female) (idiopathic) (male) NEC 259.1
  with adrenal hyperplasia 255.2
Precordial pain 786.51
  psychogenic 307.89
Predeciduous teeth 520.2
Prediabetes, prediabetic 790.2
  complicating pregnancy, childbirth, or
    puerperium 648.8
  fetus or newborn 775.8
Predislocation status of hip, at birth (*see also*
  Subluxation, congenital, hip) 754.32
Pre-eclampsia (mild) 642.4
  with pre-existing hypertension 642.7
  affecting fetus or newborn 760.0
  severe 642.5
  superimposed on pre-existing hypertensive
    disease 642.7
Preeruptive color change, teeth, tooth 520.8
Preexcitation 426.7
  atrioventricular conduction 426.7
  ventricular 426.7
Preglaucoma 365.00

Pregnancy (single) (uterine) (without sickness)
V22.2

*Note—Use the following fifth-digit
subclassification with categories 640-648,
651-676:*

0 *unspecified as to episode of care*
1 *delivered, with or without mention of
antepartum condition*
2 *delivered, with mention of postpartum
complication*
3 *antepartum condition or complication*
4 *postpartum condition or complication*

abdominal (ectopic) 633.00
  affecting fetus or newborn 761.4
  with intrauterine pregnancy 633.01
abnormal NEC 646.9
ampullar—*see* Pregnancy, tubal
broad ligament—*see* Pregnancy, cornual
cervical—*see* Pregnancy, cornual
combined (extrauterine and intrauterine)—*see*
  Pregnancy, cornual
complicated (by) 646.9
  abnormal, abnormality NEC 646.9
    cervix 654.6
    cord (umbilical) 663.9
    glucose tolerance (conditions classifiable to
      790.2) 648.8
    pelvic organs or tissues NEC 654.9
    pelvis (bony) 653.0
    perineum or vulva 654.8
    placenta, placental (vessel) 656.7
    position
      cervix 654.4
      placenta 641.1
        without hemorrhage 641.0
      uterus 654.4
    size, fetus 653.5
    uterus (congenital) 654.0
  abscess or cellulitis
    bladder 646.6
    genitourinary tract (conditions classifiable to
      590, 595, 597, 599.0, 614-616) 646.6
    kidney 646.6
    urinary tract NEC 646.6
  air embolism 673.0
  albuminuria 646.2
    with hypertension—*see* Toxemia, of
      pregnancy
  amnionitis 658.4
  amniotic fluid embolism 673.1
  anemia (conditions classifiable to 280-285)
    648.2
  atrophy, yellow (acute) (liver) (subacute)
    646.7
  bacilluria, asymptomatic 646.5
  bacteriuria, asymptomatic 646.5
  bicornis or bicornuate uterus 654.0
  bone and joint disorders (conditions
    classifiable to 720-724 or conditions
    affecting lower limbs classifiable to
    711-719, 725-738) 648.7
  breech presentation 652.2
    with successful version 652.1
  cardiovascular disease (conditions classifiable
    to 390-398, 410-429) 648.6
    congenital (conditions classifiable to
      745-747) 648.5
  cerebrovascular disorders conditions
    (classifiable to 430-434, 436-437) 674.0

Pregnancy—*continued*
  cervicitis (conditions classifiable to 616.0)
    646.6
  chloasma (gravidarum) 646.8
  cholelithiasis 646.8
  chorea (gravidarum)—*see* Eclampsia,
    pregnancy
  contraction, pelvis (general) 653.1
    inlet 653.2
    outlet 653.3
  convulsions (eclamptic) (uremic) 642.6
    with pre-existing hypertension 642.7
  current disease or condition (nonobstetric)
    abnormal glucose tolerance 648.8
    anemia 648.2
    bone and joint (lower limb) 648.7
    cardiovascular 648.6
      congenital 648.5
    cerebrovascular 674.0
    diabetic 648.0
    drug dependence 648.3
    genital organ or tract 646.6
    gonorrheal 647.1
    hypertensive 642.2
      renal 642.1
    infectious 647.9
      specified type NEC 647.8
    liver 646.7
    malarial 647.4
    nutritional deficiency 648.9
    parasitic NEC 647.8
    renal 646.2
      hypertensive 642.1
    rubella 647.5
    specified condition NEC 648.9
    syphilitic 647.0
    thyroid 648.1
    tuberculous 647.3
    urinary 646.6
    venereal 647.2
    viral NEC 647.6
  cystitis 646.6
  cystocele 654.4
  death of fetus (near term) 656.4
    early pregnancy (before 22 completed
      weeks gestation) 632
  deciduitis 646.6
  decreased fetal movements 655.7
  diabetes (mellitus) (conditions classifiable to
    250) 648.0
  disorders of liver 646.7
  displacement, uterus NEC 654.4
  disproportion—*see* Disproportion
  double uterus 654.0
  drug dependence (conditions classifiable to
    304) 648.3
  dysplasia, cervix 654.6
  early onset of delivery (spontaneous) 644.2
  eclampsia, eclamptic (coma) (convulsions)
    (delirium) (nephritis) (uremia) 642.6
    with pre-existing hypertension 642.7
  edema 646.1
    with hypertension—*see* Toxemia, of
      pregnancy
  effusion, amniotic fluid 658.1
    delayed delivery following 658.2
  embolism
    air 673.0
    amniotic fluid 673.1
    blood-clot 673.2
    cerebral 674.0

Pregnancy—*continued*
   pulmonary NEC 673.2
   pyemic 673.3
   septic 673.3
   emesis (gravidarum)—*see* Pregnancy,
      complicated, vomiting
   endometritis (conditions classifiable to
      615.0-615.9) 646.6
   decidual 646.6
   excessive weight gain NEC 646.1
   face presentation 652.4
   failure, fetal head to enter pelvic brim 652.5
   false labor (pains) 644.1
   fatigue 646.8
   fatty metamorphosis of liver 646.7
   fetal
      death (near term) 656.4
         early (before 22 completed weeks
            gestation) 632
      deformity 653.7
      distress 656.8
   fibroid (tumor) (uterus) 654.1
   footling presentation 652.8
      with successful version 652.1
   gallbladder disease 646.8
   goiter 648.1
   gonococcal infection (conditions classifiable
      to 098) 647.1
   gonorrhea (conditions classifiable to 098)
      647.1
   hemorrhage 641.9
      accidental 641.2
      before 22 completed weeks gestation NEC
         640.9
      cerebrovascular 674.0
      due to
         afibrinogenemia or other coagulation
            defect (conditions classifiable to
            286.0-286.9) 641.3
         leiomyoma, uterine 641.8
         marginal sinus (rupture) 641.2
         premature separation, placenta 641.2
         trauma 641.8
      early (before 22 completed weeks gestation)
         640.9
      threatened abortion 640.0
      unavoidable 641.1
   hepatitis (acute) (malignant) (subacute) 646.7
      viral 647.6
   herniation of uterus 654.4
   high head at term 652.5
   hydatidiform mole (delivered) (undelivered)
      630
   hydramnios 657
   hydrocephalic fetus 653.6
   hydrops amnii 657
   hydrorrhea 658.1
   hyperemesis (gravidarum)—*see* Hyperemesis,
      gravidarum
   hypertension—*see* Hypertension,
      complicating pregnancy
   hypertensive
      heart and renal disease 642.2
      heart disease 642.2
      renal disease 642.2
   hyperthyroidism 648.1
   hypothyroidism 648.1
   hysteralgia 646.8
   icterus gravis 646.7
   incarceration, uterus 654.3
   incompetent cervix (os) 654.5

Pregnancy—*continued*
   infection 647.9
      amniotic fluid 658.4
      bladder 646.6
      genital organ (conditions classifiable to
         614-616) 646.6
      kidney (conditions classifiable to
         590.0-590.9) 646.6
      urinary (tract) 646.6
         asymptomatic 646.5
   infective and parasitic diseases NEC 647.8
   inflammation
      bladder 646.6
      genital organ (conditions classifiable to
         614-616) 646.6
      urinary tract NEC 646.6
   injury 648.9
      obstetrical NEC 665.9
   insufficient weight gain 646.8
   intrauterine fetal death (near term) NEC 656.4
      early (before 22 completed weeks'
         gestation) 632
   malaria (conditions classifiable to 084) 647.4
   malformation, uterus (congenital) 654.0
   malnutrition (conditions classifiable to
      260-269) 648.9
   malposition
      fetus—*see* Pregnancy, complicated,
         malpresentation
      uterus or cervix 654.4
   malpresentation 652.9
      with successful version 652.1
      in multiple gestation 652.6
      specified type NEC 652.8
   marginal sinus hemorrhage or rupture 641.2
   maternal obesity syndrome 646.1
   menstruation 640.8
   mental disorders (conditions classifiable to
      290-303, 305-316, 317-319) 648.4
   mentum presentation 652.4
   missed
      abortion 632
      delivery (at or near term) 656.4
      labor (at or near term) 656.4
   necrosis
      genital organ or tract (conditions classifiable
         to 614-616) 646.6
      liver (conditions classifiable to 570) 646.7
      renal, cortical 646.2
   nephritis or nephrosis (conditions classifiable
      to 580-589) 646.2
      with hypertension 642.1
   nephropathy NEC 646.2
   neuritis (peripheral) 646.4
   nutritional deficiency (conditions classifiable
      to 260-269) 648.9
   oblique lie or presentation 652.3
      with successful version 652.1
   obstetrical trauma NEC 665.9
   oligohydramnios NEC 658.0
   onset of contractions before 37 weeks 644.0
   oversize fetus 653.5
   papyraceous fetus 646.0
   patent cervix 654.5
   pelvic inflammatory disease (conditions
      classifiable to 614-616) 646.6
   placenta, placental
      abnormality 656.7
      abruptio or ablatio 641.2
      detachment 641.2
      disease 656.7

Pregnancy—*continued*
  infarct 656.7
  low implantation 641.1
    without hemorrhage 641.0
  malformation 656.7
  malposition 641.1
    without hemorrhage 641.0
  marginal sinus hemorrhage 641.2
  previa 641.1
    without hemorrhage 641.0
    separation (premature) (undelivered) 641.2
  placentitis 658.4
  polyhydramnios 657
  postmaturity
    post term 645.1
    prolonged 645.2
  prediabetes 648.8
  pre-eclampsia (mild) 642.4
    severe 642.5
    superimposed on pre-existing hypertensive
      disease 642.7
  premature rupture of membranes 658.1
    with delayed delivery 658.2
  previous
    infertility V23.0
    nonobstetric condition V23.8
    poor obstetrical history V23.49
    premature delivery V23.41
    trophoblastic disease (conditions classifiable
      to 630) V23.1
  prolapse, uterus 654.4
  proteinuria (gestational) 646.2
    with hypertension—*see* Toxemia, of
      pregnancy
  pruritus (neurogenic) 646.8
  psychosis or psychoneurosis 648.4
  ptyalism 646.8
  pyelitis (conditions classifiable to
    590.0-590.9) 646.6
  renal disease or failure NEC 646.2
    with secondary hypertension 642.1
    hypertensive 642.2
  retention, retained dead ovum 631
  retroversion, uterus 654.3
  Rh immunization, incompatibility, or
    sensitization 656.1
  rubella (conditions classifiable to 056) 647.5
  rupture
    amnion (premature) 658.1
      with delayed delivery 658.2
    marginal sinus (hemorrhage) 641.2
    membranes (premature) 658.1
      with delayed delivery 658.2
    uterus (before onset of labor) 665.0
  salivation (excessive) 646.8
  salpingo-oophoritis (conditions classifiable to
    614.0-614.2) 646.6
  septicemia (conditions classifiable to
    038.0-038.9) 647.8
    postpartum 670
    puerperal 670
  spasms, uterus (abnormal) 646.8
  specified condition NEC 646.8
  spurious labor pains 644.1
  superfecundation 651.9
  superfetation 651.9
  syphilis (conditions classifiable to 090-097)
    647.0
  threatened
    abortion 640.0
    premature delivery 644.2

Pregnancy—*continued*
  premature labor 644.0
  thrombophlebitis (superficial) 671.2
    deep 671.3
  thrombosis 671.9
    venous (superficial) 671.2
    deep 671.3
  thyroid dysfunction (conditions classifiable to
    240-246) 648.1
  thyroiditis 648.1
  thyrotoxicosis 648.1
  torsion of uterus 654.4
  toxemia—*see* Toxemia, of pregnancy
  transverse lie or presentation 652.3
    with successful version 652.1
  trauma 648.9
    obstetrical 665.9
  tuberculosis (conditions classifiable to
    010-018) 647.3
  tumor
    cervix 654.6
    ovary 654.4
    pelvic organs or tissue NEC 654.4
    uterus (body) 654.1
      cervix 654.6
    vagina 654.7
    vulva 654.8
  unstable lie 652.0
  uremia—*see* Pregnancy, complicated, renal
    disease
  urethritis 646.6
  vaginitis or vulvitis (conditions classifiable to
    616.1) 646.6
  varicose
    placental vessels 656.7
    veins (legs) 671.0
      perineum 671.1
      vulva 671.1
  varicosity, labia or vulva 671.1
  venereal disease NEC (conditions classifiable
    to 099) 647.2
  viral disease NEC (conditions classifiable to
    042, 050-055, 057-079) 647.6
  vomiting (incoercible) (pernicious)
    (persistent) (uncontrollable) (vicious)
    643.9
    due to organic disease or other cause 643.8
    early—*see* Hyperemesis, gravidarum
    late (after 22 completed weeks gestation)
      643.2
  young maternal age 659.8
complications NEC 646.9
cornual 633.80
  affecting fetus or newborn 761.4
  with intrauterine pregnancy 633.81
death, maternal NEC 646.9
delivered—*see* Delivery
ectopic (ruptured) NEC 633.90
  abdominal—*see* Pregnancy, abdominal
  affecting fetus or newborn 761.4
  combined (extrauterine and intrauterine)—*see*
    Pregnancy, cornual
  ovarian—*see* Pregnancy, ovarian
  specified type NEC 633.80
    affecting fetus or newborn 761.4
    with intrauterine pregnancy 633.81
  tubal—*see* Pregnancy, tubal
  with intrauterine pregnancy 633.91
examination, pregnancy not confirmed V72.4
extrauterine—*see* Pregnancy, ectopic
fallopian—*see* Pregnancy, tubal

Pregnancy—*continued*
false 300.11
  labor (pains) 644.1
fatigue 646.8
illegitimate V61.6
incidental finding V22.2
in double uterus 654.0
interstitial—*see* Pregnancy, cornual
intraligamentous—*see* Pregnancy, cornual
intramural—*see* Pregnancy, cornual
intraperitoneal—*see* Pregnancy, abdominal
isthmian—*see* Pregnancy, tubal
management affected by
  abnormal, abnormality
    fetus (suspected) 655.9
      specified NEC 655.8
    placenta 656.7
  advanced maternal age NEC 659.6
    multigravida 659.6
    primigravida 659.5
  antibodies (maternal)
    anti-c 656.1
    anti-d 656.1
    anti-e 656.1
    blood group (ABO) 656.2
      Rh(esus) 656.1
  elderly multigravida 659.6
  elderly primigravida 659.5
  fetal (suspected)
    abnormality 655.9
      acid-base balance 656.8
      heart rate or rhythm 659.7
      specified NEC 655.8
    acidemia 656.3
    anencephaly 655.0
    bradycardia 659.7
    central nervous system malformation 655.0
    chromosomal abnormalities (conditions
        classifiable to 758.0-758.9) 655.1
    damage from
      drugs 655.5
        obstetric, anesthetic, or sedative 655.5
      environmental toxins 655.8
      intrauterine contraceptive device 655.8
      maternal
        alcohol addiction 655.4
        disease NEC 655.4
        drug use 655.5
        listeriosis 655.4
        rubella 655.3
        toxoplasmosis 655.4
        viral infection 655.3
      radiation 655.6
    death (near term) 656.4
      early (before 22 completed weeks
          gestation) 632
    distress 656.8
    excessive growth 656.6
    growth retardation 656.5
    hereditary disease 655.2
    hydrocephalus 655.0
    intrauterine death 656.4
    poor growth 656.5
    spina bifida (with myelomeningocele) 655.0
  fetal-maternal hemorrhage 656.0
  hereditary disease in family (possibly)
      affecting fetus 655.2
  incompatibility, blood groups (ABO) 656.2
    rh(esus) 656.1
  insufficient prenatal care V23.7
  intrauterine death 656.4

Pregnancy—*continued*
  isoimmunization (ABO) 656.2
    rh(esus) 656.1
  large-for-dates fetus 656.6
  light-for-dates fetus 656.5
  meconium in liquor 656.8
  mental disorder (conditions classifiable to
      290-303, 305-316, 317-319) 648.4
  multiparity (grand) 659.4
  poor obstetric history V23.49
    pre-term labor V23.41
  postmaturity
    post term 645.1
    prolonged 645.2
  post term pregnancy 645.1
  previous
    abortion V23.2
      habitual 646.3
    cesarean delivery 654.2
    difficult delivery V23.49
    forceps delivery V23.49
    habitual abortions 646.3
    hemorrhage, antepartum or postpartum
        V23.49
    hydatidiform mole V23.1
    infertility V23.0
    malignancy NEC V23.8
    nonobstetrical conditions V23.8
    premature delivery V23.41
    trophoblastic disease (conditions in 630)
        V23.1
    vesicular mole V23.1
  prolonged pregnancy 645.2
  small-for-dates fetus 656.5
  young maternal age 659.8
maternal death NEC 646.9
mesometric (mural)—*see* Pregnancy, cornual
molar 631
  hydatidiform (*see also* Hydatidiform mole)
      630
    previous, affecting management of
        pregnancy V23.1
  previous, affecting management of pregnancy
      V23.49
multiple NEC 651.9
  with fetal loss and retention of one or more
      fetus(es) 651.6
  affecting fetus or newborn 761.5
  specified type NEC 651.8
    with fetal loss and retention of one or more
        fetus(es) 651.6
mural—*see* Pregnancy, cornual
observation NEC V22.1
  first pregnancy V22.0
  high-risk V23.9
    specified problem NEC V23.8
ovarian 633.20
  affecting fetus or newborn 761.4
  with intrauterine pregnancy 633.21
postmature
  post term 645.1
  prolonged 645.2
post term 645.1
prenatal care only V22.1
  first pregnancy V22.0
  high-risk V23.9
    specified problem NEC V23.8
prolonged 645.2
quadruplet NEC 651.2
  with fetal loss and retention of one or more
      fetus(es) 651.5

Pregnancy—*continued*
  affecting fetus or newborn 761.5
  quintuplet NEC 651.8
    with fetal loss and retention of one or more
      fetus(es) 651.6
    affecting fetus or newborn 761.5
  sextuplet NEC 651.8
    with fetal loss and retention of one or more
      fetus(es) 651.6
    affecting fetus or newborn 761.5
  spurious 300.11
  superfecundation NEC 651.9
    with fetal loss and retention of one or more
      fetus(es) 651.6
  superfetation NEC 651.9
    with fetal loss and retention of one or more
      fetus(es) 651.6
  supervision (of) (for)—*see also* Pregnancy,
    management affected by
    elderly
      multigravida V23.82
      primigravida V23.81
    high-risk V23.9
      insufficient prenatal care V23.7
      specified problem NEC V23.8
    multiparity V23.3
    normal NEC V22.1
      first V22.0
    poor
      obstetric history V23.49
        pre-term labor V23.41
      reproductive history V23.5
    previous
      abortion V23.2
      hydatidiform mole V23.1
      infertility V23.0
      neonatal death V23.5
      stillbirth V23.5
      trophoblastic disease V23.1
      vesicular mole V23.1
    specified problem NEC V23.8
    young
      multigravida V23.84
      primigravida V23.83
  triplet NEC 651.1
    with fetal loss and retention of one or more
      fetus(es) 651.4
    affecting fetus or newborn 761.5
  tubal (with rupture) 633.10
    affecting fetus or newborn 761.4
    with intrauterine pregnancy 633.11
  twin NEC 651.0
    with fetal loss and retention of one or more
      fetus(es) 651.3
    affecting fetus or newborn 761.5
  unconfirmed V72.4
  undelivered (no other diagnosis) V22.2
    with false labor 644.1
    high-risk V23.9
      specified problem NEC V23.8
  unwanted NEC V61.7
Pregnant uterus —*see* condition
Preiser's disease (osteoporosis) 733.09
Prekwashiorkor 260
Preleukemia 238.7
Preluxation of hip, congenital (*see also*
  Subluxation, congenital, hip) 754.32
Premature —*see also* condition
  beats (nodal) 427.60
    atrial 427.61
    auricular 427.61

Premature—*continued*
    postoperative 997.1
    specified type NEC 427.69
    supraventricular 427.61
    ventricular 427.69
  birth NEC 765.1
  closure
    cranial suture 756.0
    fontanel 756.0
    foramen ovale 745.8
  contractions 427.60
    atrial 427.61
    auricular 427.61
    auriculoventricular 427.61
    heart (extrasystole) 427.60
    junctional 427.60
    nodal 427.60
    postoperative 997.1
    ventricular 427.69
  ejaculation 302.75
  infant NEC 765.1
    excessive 765.0
    light-for-dates—*see* Light-for-dates
  labor 644.2
    threatened 644.0
  lungs 770.4
  menopause 256.31
  puberty 259.1
  rupture of membranes or amnion 658.1
    affecting fetus or newborn 761.1
    delayed delivery following 658.2
  senility (syndrome) 259.8
  separation, placenta (partial)—*see* Placenta,
    separation
  ventricular systole 427.69
Prematurity NEC 765.1
  extreme 765.0
Premenstrual syndrome 625.4
Premenstrual tension 625.4
Premolarization, cuspids 520.2
Premyeloma 273.1
Prenatal
  care, normal pregnancy V22.1
    first V22.0
  death, cause unknown—*see* Death, fetus
  screening—*see* Antenatal, screening
Prepartum —*see* condition
Preponderance, left or right ventricular 429.3
Prepuce —*see* condition
Presbycardia 797
  hypertensive (*see also* Hypertension, heart)
    402.90
Presbycusis 388.01
Presbyesophagus 530.89
Presbyophrenia 310.1
Presbyopia 367.4
Prescription of contraceptives NEC V25.02
  diaphragm V25.02
  oral (pill) V25.01
    repeat V25.41
  repeat V25.40
    oral (pill) V25.41
Presenile —*see also* condition
  aging 259.8
  dementia (*see also* Dementia, presenile) 290.10
Presenility 259.8
Presentation, fetal
  abnormal 652.9
    with successful version 652.1
    before labor, affecting fetus or newborn 761.7
    causing obstructed labor 660.0

Presentation—*continued*

    affecting fetus or newborn, any, except
        breech 763.1

    in multiple gestation (one or more) 652.6
        specified NEC 652.8

    arm 652.7
        causing obstructed labor 660.0

    breech (buttocks) (complete) (frank) 652.2
        with successful version 652.1
            before labor, affecting fetus or newborn
                761.7
        before labor, affecting fetus or newborn 761.7

    brow 652.4
        causing obstructed labor 660.0

    buttocks 652.2

    chin 652.4

    complete 652.2

    compound 652.8

    cord 663.0

    extended head 652.4

    face 652.4
        to pubes 652.8

    footling 652.8

    frank 652.2

    hand, leg, or foot NEC 652.8

    incomplete 652.8

    mentum 652.4

    multiple gestation (one fetus or more) 652.6

    oblique 652.3
        with successful version 652.1

    shoulder 652.8
        affecting fetus or newborn 763.1

    transverse 652.3
        with successful version 652.1

    umbilical cord 663.0

    unstable 652.0

Prespondylolisthesis (congenital) (lumbosacral) 756.11

Pressure

    area, skin ulcer (*see also* Decubitus) 707.0

    atrophy, spine 733.99

    birth, fetus or newborn NEC 767.9

    brachial plexus 353.0

    brain 348.4
        injury at birth 767.0

    cerebral—*see* Pressure, brain

    chest 786.59

    cone, tentorial 348.4
        injury at birth 767.0

    funis—*see* Compression, umbilical cord

    hyposystolic (*see also* Hypotension) 458.9

    increased
        intracranial 781.99
            due to
                benign intracranial hypertension 348.2
                hydrocephalus—*see* hydrocephalus
                injury at birth 767.8
        intraocular 365.00

    lumbosacral plexus 353.1

    mediastinum 519.3

    necrosis (chronic) (skin) (*see also* Decubitus) 707.0

    nerve—*see* Compression, nerve

    paralysis (*see also* Neuropathy, entrapment) 355.9

    sore (chronic) (*see also* Decubitus) 707.0

    spinal cord 336.9

    ulcer (chronic) (*see also* Decubitus) 707.0

    umbilical cord—*see* Compression, umbilical cord

    venous, increased 459.89

Pre-syncope 780.2

Preterm infant NEC 765.1

    extreme 765.0

Priapism (penis) 607.3

Prickling sensation (*see also* Disturbance, sensation) 782.0

Prickly heat 705.1

Primary —*see* condition

Primigravida, elderly

    affecting
        fetus or newborn 763.89
        management of pregnancy, labor, and delivery
            659.5

Primipara, old

    affecting
        fetus or newborn 763.89
        management of pregnancy, labor, and delivery
            659.5

Primula dermatitis 692.6

Primus varus (bilateral) (metatarsus) 754.52

P.R.I.N.D. 436

Pringle's disease (tuberous sclerosis) 759.5

Prinzmetal's angina 413.1

Prinzmetal-Massumi syndrome (anterior chest wall) 786.52

Prizefighter ear 738.7

Problem (with) V49.9

    academic V62.3

    acculturation V62.4

    adopted child V61.29

    aged
        in-law V61.3
        parent V61.3
        person NEC V61.8

    alcoholism in family V61.41

    anger reaction (*see also* Disturbance, conduct) 312.0

    behavior, child 312.9

    behavioral V40.9
        specified NEC V40.3

    betting V69.3

    cardiorespiratory NEC V47.2

    care of sick or handicapped person in family or household V61.49

    career choice V62.2

    communication V40.1

    conscience regarding medical care V62.6

    delinquency (juvenile) 312.9

    diet, inappropriate V69.1

    digestive NEC V47.3

    ear NEC V41.3

    eating habits, inappropriate V69.1

    economic V60.2
        affecting care V60.9
            specified type NEC V60.8

    educational V62.3

    enuresis, child 307.6

    exercise, lack of V69.0

    eye NEC V41.1

    family V61.9
        specified circumstance NEC V61.8

    fear reaction, child 313.0

    feeding (elderly) (infant) 783.3
        newborn 779.3
        nonorganic 307.50

    fetal, affecting management of pregnancy 656.9
        specified type NEC 656.8

    financial V60.2

    foster child V61.29
        specified NEC V41.8

    functional V41.9
        specified type NEC V41.8

Problem—*continued*
gambling V69.3
genital NEC V47.5
head V48.9
  deficiency V48.0
  disfigurement V48.6
  mechanical V48.2
  motor V48.2
  movement of V48.2
  sensory V48.4
  specified condition NEC V48.8
hearing V41.2
high-risk sexual behavior V69.2
influencing health status NEC V49.89
internal organ NEC V47.9
  deficiency V47.0
  mechanical or motor V47.1
interpersonal NEC V62.81
jealousy, child 313.3
learning V40.0
legal V62.5
life circumstance NEC V62.89
lifestyle V69.9
  specified NEC V69.8
limb V49.9
  deficiency V49.0
  disfigurement V49.4
  mechanical V49.1
  motor V49.2
  movement, involving
    musculoskeletal system V49.1
    nervous system V49.2
  sensory V49.3
  specified condition NEC V49.5
litigation V62.5
living alone V60.3
loneliness NEC V62.89
marital V61.10
  involving
    divorce V61.0
    estrangement V61.0
    psychosexual disorder 302.9
    sexual function V41.7
mastication V41.6
medical care, within family V61.49
mental V40.9
  specified NEC V40.2
mental hygiene, adult V40.9
multiparity V61.5
nail biting, child 307.9
neck V48.9
  deficiency V48.1
  disfigurement V48.7
  mechanical V48.3
  motor V48.3
  movement V48.3
  sensory V48.5
  specified condition NEC V48.8
neurological NEC 781.99
none (feared complaint unfounded) V65.5
occupational V62.2
parent-child V61.20
partner V61.10
personal NEC V62.89
  interpersonal conflict NEC V62.81
personality (*see also* Disorder, personality)
  301.9
phase of life V62.89
placenta, affecting management of pregnancy
  656.9
  specified type NEC 656.8

Problem—*continued*
poverty V60.2
presence of sick or handicapped person in
  family or household V61.49
psychiatric 300.9
psychosocial V62.9
  specified type NEC V62.89
relational NEC V62.81
relationship, childhood 313.3
religious or spiritual belief
  other than medical care V62.89
  regarding medical care V62.6
self-damaging behavior V69.8
sexual
  behavior, high-risk V69.2
  function NEC V41.7
sibling, relational V61.8
sight V41.0
sleep disorder, child 307.40
smell V41.5
speech V40.1
spite reaction, child (*see also* Disturbance,
  conduct) 312.0
spoiled child reaction (*see also* Disturbance,
  conduct) 312.1
swallowing V41.6
tantrum, child (*see also* Disturbance, conduct)
  312.1
taste V41.5
thumb sucking, child 307.9
tic, child 307.21
trunk V48.9
  deficiency V48.1
  disfigurement V48.7
  mechanical V48.3
  motor V48.3
  movement V48.3
  sensory V48.5
  specified condition NEC V48.8
unemployment V62.0
urinary NEC V47.4
voice production V41.4
Procedure (surgical) not done NEC V64.3
because of
  contraindication V64.1
  patient's decision V64.2
    for reasons of conscience or religion V62.6
  specified reason NEC V64.3
Procidentia
anus (sphincter) 569.1
rectum (sphincter) 569.1
stomach 537.89
uteri 618.1
Proctalgia 569.42
fugax 564.6
spasmodic 564.6
  psychogenic 307.89
Proctitis 569.49
amebic 006.8
chlamydial 099.52
gonococcal 098.7
granulomatous 555.1
idiopathic 556.2
  with ulcerative sigmoiditis 556.3
tuberculous (*see also* Tuberculosis) 014.8
ulcerative (chronic) (nonspecific) 556.2
  with ulcerative sigmoiditis 556.3
Proctocele
female (without uterine prolapse) 618.0
  with uterine prolapse 618.4
    complete 618.3

Proctocele—*continued*
  incomplete 618.2
  male 569.49
Proctocolitis, idiopathic 556.2
  with ulcerative sigmoiditis 556.3
Proctoptosis 569.1
Proctosigmoiditis 569.89
  ulcerative (chronic) 556.3
Proctospasm 564.6
  psychogenic 306.4
Prodromal-AIDS —*see* Human
  immunodeficiency virus (disease) (illness)
  (infection)
Profichet's disease or syndrome 729.9
Progeria (adultorum) (syndrome) 259.8
Prognathism (mandibular) (maxillary) 524.00
Progonoma (melanotic) (M9363/0)—*see*
  Neoplasm, by site, benign
Progressive —*see* condition
Prolapse, prolapsed
  anus, anal (canal) (sphincter) 569.1
  arm or hand, complicating delivery 652.7
    causing obstructed labor 660.0
      affecting fetus or newborn 763.1
    fetus or newborn 763.1
  bladder (acquired) (mucosa) (sphincter)
    congenital (female) (male) 756.71
    female 618.0
    male 596.8
  breast implant (prosthetic) 996.54
  cecostomy 569.69
  cecum 569.89
  cervix, cervical (stump) (hypertrophied) 618.1
    anterior lip, obstructing labor 660.2
      affecting fetus or newborn 763.1
    congenital 752.49
    postpartal (old) 618.1
  ciliary body 871.1
  colon (pedunculated) 569.89
  colostomy 569.69
  conjunctiva 372.73
  cord—*see* Prolapse, umbilical cord
  disc (intervertebral)—*see* Displacement,
    intervertebral disc
  duodenum 537.89
  eye implant (orbital) 996.59
    lens (ocular) 996.53
  fallopian tube 620.4
  fetal extremity, complicating delivery 652.8
    causing obstructed labor 660.0
    fetus or newborn 763.1
  funis—*see* Prolapse, umbilical cord
  gastric (mucosa) 537.89
  genital, female 618.9
    specified NEC 618.8
  globe 360 81
  ileostomy bud 569.69
  intervertebral disc—*see* Displacement,
    intervertebral disc
  intestine (small) 569.89
  iris 364.8
    traumatic 871.1
  kidney (*see also* Disease, renal) 593.0
    congenital 753.3
  laryngeal muscles or ventricle 478.79
  leg, complicating delivery 652.8
    causing obstructed labor 660.0
    fetus or newborn 763.1
  liver 573.8
  meatus urinarius 599.5
  mitral valve 424.0

Prolapse, prolapsed—*continued*
  ocular lens implant 996.53
  organ or site, congenital NEC—*see*
    Malposition, congenital
  ovary 620.4
  pelvic (floor), female 618.8
  perineum, female 618.8
  pregnant uterus 654.4
  rectum (mucosa) (sphincter) 569.1
    due to Trichuris trichiuria 127.3
  spleen 289.59
  stomach 537.89
  umbilical cord
    affecting fetus or newborn 762.4
    complicating delivery 663.0
  ureter 593.89
    with obstruction 593.4
  ureterovesical orifice 593.89
  urethra (acquired) (infected) (mucosa) 599.5
    congenital 753.8
  uterovaginal 618.4
    complete 618.3
    incomplete 618.2
    specified NEC 618.8
  uterus (first degree) (second degree) (third
    degree) (complete) (without vaginal wall
    prolapse) 618.1
    with mention of vaginal wall prolapse—*see*
      Prolapse, uterovaginal
    congenital 752.3
    in pregnancy or childbirth 654.4
      affecting fetus or newborn 763.1
      causing obstructed labor 660.2
        affecting fetus or newborn 763.1
    postpartal (old) 618.1
  uveal 871.1
  vagina (anterior) (posterior) (vault) (wall)
    (without uterine prolapse) 618.0
    with uterine prolapse 618.4
      complete 618.3
      incomplete 618.2
    posthysterectomy 618.5
  vitreous (humor) 379.26
    traumatic 871.1
  womb—*see* Prolapse, uterus
Prolapsus, female 618.9
Proliferative —*see* condition
Prolinemia 270.8
Prolinuria 270.8
Prolonged, prolongation
  bleeding time (*see also* Defect, coagulation)
    790.92
    "idiopathic" (in von Willebrand's disease)
      286.4
  coagulation time (*see also* Defect, coagulation)
    790.92
  gestation syndrome 766.2
  labor 662.1
    affecting fetus or newborn 763.89
    first stage 662.0
    second stage 662.2
  PR interval 426.11
  pregnancy 645.2
  prothrombin time (*see also* Defect, coagulation)
    790.92
  rupture of membranes (24 hours or more prior
    to onset of labor) 658.2
  uterine contractions in labor 661.4
    affecting fetus or newborn 763.7
Prominauris 744.29

Prominence
auricle (ear) (congenital) 744.29
  acquired 380.32
ischial spine or sacral promontory
  with disproportion (fetopelvic) 653.3
    affecting fetus or newborn 763.1
    causing obstructed labor 660.1
      affecting fetus or newborn 763.1
nose (congenital) 748.1
  acquired 738.0
Pronation
ankle 736.79
foot 736.79
  congenital 755.67
Prophylactic
administration of
  antibiotics V07.39
  antitoxin, any V07.2
  antivenin V07.2
  chemotherapeutic agent NEC V07.39
    fluoride V07.31
  diphtheria antitoxin V07.2
  gamma globulin V07.2
  immune sera (gamma globulin) V07.2
  RhoGAM V07.2
  tetanus antitoxin V07.2
chemotherapy NEC V07.39
  fluoride V07.31
immunotherapy V07.2
measure V07.9
  specified type NEC V07.8
postmenopausal hormone replacement V07.4
sterilization V25.2
Proptosis (ocular) (*see also* Exophthalmos)
  376.30
thyroid 242.0
Propulsion
eyeball 360.81
Prosecution, anxiety concerning V62.5
Prostate, prostatic —*see* condition
Prostatism 600.9
Prostatitis (congestive) (suppurative) 601.9
acute 601.0
cavitary 601.8
chlamydial 099.54
chronic 601.1
diverticular 601.8
due to Trichomonas (vaginalis) 131.03
fibrous 600.9
gonococcal (acute) 098.12
  chronic or duration of 2 months or over 098.32
granulomatous 601.8
hypertrophic 600.0
specified type NEC 601.8
subacute 601.1
trichomonal 131.03
tuberculous (*see also* Tuberculosis) 016.5
  [601.4]
Prostatocystitis 601.3
Prostatorrhea 602.8
Prostatoseminovesiculitis, trichomonal 131.03
Prostration 780.79
heat 992.5
  anhydrotic 992.3
  due to
    salt (and water) depletion 992.4
    water depletion 992.3
nervous 300.5
newborn 779.89
senile 797
Protanomaly 368.51

Protanopia (anomalous trichromat) (complete)
  (incomplete) 368.51
Protein
deficiency 260
malnutrition 260
sickness (prophylactic) (therapeutic) 999.5
Proteinemia 790.99
Proteinosis
alveolar, lung or pulmonary 516.0
lipid 272.8
Proteinosis
lipoid (of Urbach) 272.8
Proteinuria (*see also* Albuminuria) 791.0
Bence-Jones NEC 791.0
gestational 646.2
  with hypertension—*see* Toxemia, of
    pregnancy
orthostatic 593.6
postural 593.6
Proteolysis, pathologic 286.6
Protocoproporphyria 277.1
Protoporphyria (erythrohepatic) (erythropoietic)
  277.1
Protrusio acetabuli 718.65
Protrusion
acetabulum (into pelvis) 718.65
device, implant, or graft—*see* Complications,
  mechanical
ear, congenital 744.29
intervertebral disc—*see* Displacement,
  intervertebral disc
nucleus pulposus—*see* Displacement,
  intervertebral disc
Proud flesh 701.5
Prune belly (syndrome) 756.71
Prurigo (ferox) (gravis) (Hebra's) (hebrae)
  (mitis) (simplex) 698.2
agria 698.3
asthma syndrome 691.8
Besnier's (atopic dermatitis) (infantile eczema)
  691.8
eczematodes allergicum 691.8
estivalis (Hutchinson's) 692.72
Hutchinson's 692.72
nodularis 698.3
psychogenic 306.3
Pruritus, pruritic 698.9
ani 698.0
  psychogenic 306.3
conditions NEC 698.9
  psychogenic 306.3
due to Onchocerca volvulus 125.3
ear 698.9
essential 698.9
genital organ(s) 698.1
  psychogenic 306.3
gravidarum 646.8
hiemalis 698.8
neurogenic (any site) 306.3
perianal 698.0
psychogenic (any site) 306.3
scrotum 698.1
  psychogenic 306.3
senile, senilis 698.8
Trichomonas 131.9
vulva, vulvae 698.1
  psychogenic 306.3
Psammocarcinoma (M8140/3)—*see* Neoplasm,
  by site, malignant
Pseudarthrosis, pseudoarthrosis (bone) 733.82
joint following fusion V45.4

Pseudoacanthosis
nigricans 701.8
Pseudoaneurysm —*see* Aneurysm
Pseudoangina (pectoris)—*see* Angina
Pseudoangioma 452
Pseudo-Argyll-Robertson pupil 379.45
Pseudoarteriosus 747.89
Pseudoarthrosis —*see* Pseudarthrosis
Pseudoataxia 799.8
Pseudobursa 727.89
Pseudocholera 025
Pseudochromidrosis 705.89
Pseudocirrhosis, liver, pericardial 423.2
Pseudocoarctation 747.21
Pseudocowpox 051.1
Pseudocoxalgia 732.1
Pseudocroup 478.75
Pseudocyesis 300.11
Pseudocyst
lung 518.89
pancreas 577.2
retina 361.19
Pseudodementia 300.16
Pseudoelephantiasis neuroarthritica 757.0
Pseudoemphysema 518.89
Pseudoencephalitis
superior (acute) hemorrhagic 265.1
Pseudoerosion cervix, congenital 752.49
Pseudoexfoliation, lens capsule 366.11
Pseudofracture (idiopathic) (multiple)
(spontaneous) (symmetrical) 268.2
Pseudoglanders 025
Pseudoglioma 360.44
Pseudogout —*see* Chondrocalcinosis
Pseudohallucination 780.1
Pseudohemianesthesia 782.0
Pseudohemophilia (Bernuth's) (hereditary) (type
B) 286.4
type A 287.8
vascular 287.8
Pseudohermaphroditism 752.7
with chromosomal anomaly—*see* Anomaly,
chromosomal
adrenal 255.2
female (without adrenocortical disorder) 752.7
with adrenocortical disorder 255.2
adrenal 255.2
male (without gonadal disorder) 752.7
with
adrenocortical disorder 255.2
cleft scrotum 752.7
feminizing testis 257.8
gonadal disorder 257.9
adrenal 255.2
Pseudohole, macula 362.54
Pseudo-Hurler's disease (mucolipidosis III)
272.7
Pseudohydrocephalus 348.2
Pseudohypertrophic muscular dystrophy
(Erb's) 359.1
Pseudohypertrophy, muscle 359.1
Pseudohypoparathyroidism 275.49
Psuedopseudohypoparathyroidism 275.49
Pseudoinfluenza 487.1
Pseudoinsomnia 307.49
Pseudoleukemia 288.8
infantile 285.8
Pseudomembranous —*see* condition
Pseudomeningocele (cerebral) (infective)
(surgical) 349.2
spinal 349.2
Pseudomenstruation 626.8

Pseudomucinous
cyst (ovary) (M8470/0) 220
peritoneum 568.89
Pseudomyeloma 273.1
Pseudomyxoma peritonei (M8480/6) 197.6
Pseudoneuritis optic (nerve) 377.24
papilla 377.24
congenital 743.57
Pseudoneuroma —*see* Injury, nerve, by site
Pseudo-obstruction
intestine 564.89
Pseudopapilledema 377.24
Pseudoparalysis
arm or leg 781.4
atonic, congenital 358.8
Pseudopelade 704.09
Pseudophakia V43.1
Pseudopolycythemia 289.0
Pseudopolyposis, colon 556.4
Pseudoporencephaly 348.0
Pseudopseudohypoparathyroidism 275.49
Pseudopsychosis 300.16
Pseudopterygium 372.52
Pseudoptosis (eyelid) 374.34
Pseudorabies 078.89
Pseudoretinitis, pigmentosa 362.65
Pseudorickets 588.0
senile (Pozzi's) 731.0
Pseudorubella 057.8
Pseudoscarlatina 057.8
Pseudosclerema 778.1
Pseudosclerosis (brain)
Jakob's 046.1
of Westphal (-Strümpell) (hepatolenticular
degeneration) 275.1
spastic 046.1
with dementia
with behavioral disturbance 046.1 *[294.11]*
without behavioral disturbance 046.1
[294.10]
Pseudoseizure 780.39
non-psychiatric 780.39
psychiatric 300.11
Pseudotabes 799.8
diabetic 250.6 *[337.1]*
Pseudotetanus (*see also* Convulsions) 780.39
Pseudotetany 781.7
hysterical 300.11
Pseudothalassemia 285.0
Pseudotrichinosis 710.3
Pseudotruncus arteriosus 747.29
Pseudotuberculosis, pasteurella (infection)
027.2
Pseudotumor
cerebri 348.2
orbit (inflammatory) 376.11
Pseudo-Turner's syndrome 759.89
Pseudoxanthoma elasticum 757.39
Psilosis (sprue) (tropical) 579.1
Monilia 112.89
nontropical 579.0
not sprue 704.00
Psittacosis 073.9
Psoitis 728.89
Psora NEC 696.1
Psoriasis 696.1
any type, except arthropathic 696.1
arthritic, arthropathic 696.0
buccal 528.6
flexural 696.1
follicularis 696.1

Psoriasis—*continued*
  guttate 696.1
  inverse 696.1
  mouth 528.6
  nummularis 696.1
  psychogenic 316 *[696.1]*
  punctata 696.1
  pustular 696.1
  rupioides 696.1
  vulgaris 696.1
Psorospermiasis 136.4
Psorospermosis 136.4
  follicularis (vegetans) 757.39
Psychalgia 307.80
Psychasthenia 300.89
  compulsive 300.3
  mixed compulsive states 300.3
  obsession 300.3
Psychiatric disorder or problem NEC 300.9
Psychogenic —*see also* condition
  factors associated with physical conditions 316
Psychoneurosis, psychoneurotic (*see also*
    Neurosis) 300.9
  anxiety (state) 300.00
  climacteric 627.2
  compensation 300.16
  compulsion 300.3
  conversion hysteria 300.11
  depersonalization 300.6
  depressive type 300.4
  dissociative hysteria 300.15
  hypochondriacal 300.7
  hysteria 300.10
    conversion type 300.11
    dissociative type 300.15
  mixed NEC 300.89
  neurasthenic 300.5
  obsessional 300.3
  obsessive-compulsive 300.3
  occupational 300.89
  personality NEC 301.89
  phobia 300.20
  senile NEC 300.89
Psychopathic —*see also* condition
  constitution, posttraumatic 310.2
    with psychosis 293.9
  personality 301.9
    amoral trends 301.7
    antisocial trends 301.7
    asocial trends 301.7
    mixed types 301.7
  state 301.9
Psychopathy, sexual (*see also* Deviation, sexual)
    302.9
Psychophysiologic, psychophysiological
  condition—*see* Reaction, psychophysiologic
Psychose passionelle 297.8
Psychosexual identity disorder 302.6
  adult-life 302.85
  childhood 302.6
Psychosis 298.9
  acute hysterical 298.1
  affecting management of pregnancy, childbirth,
    or puerperium 648.4
  affective NEC 296.90
    drug induced 292.84
    due to or associated with physical condition
      293.83

Psychosis—*continued*

> Note—Use the following fifth-digit
> subclassification with categories 296.0-296.6:
>
> 0 unspecified
> 1 mild
> 2 moderate
> 3 severe, without mention of psychotic
>   behavior
> 4 severe, specified as with psychotic behavior
> 5 in partial or unspecified remission
> 6 in full remission

  involutional 296.2
    recurrent episode 296.3
    single episode 296.2
  manic-depressive 296.80
    circular (alternating) 296.7
      currently depressed 296.5
      currently manic 296.4
    depressed type 296.2
      atypical 296.82
      recurrent episode 296.3
      single episode 296.2
    manic 296.0
      atypical 296.81
      recurrent episode 296.1
      single episode 296.0
    mixed type NEC 296.89
    specified type NEC 296.89
  senile 290.21
  specified type NEC 296.99
  alcoholic 291.9
    with
      anxiety 291.89
      delirium tremens 291.0
      delusions 291.5
      dementia 291.2
      hallucinosis 291.3
      jealousy 291.5
      mood disturbance 291.89
      paranoia 291.5
      persisting amnesia 291.1
      sexual dysfunction 291.89
      sleep disturbance 291.89
    amnestic confabulatory 291.1
    delirium tremens 291.0
    hallucinosis 291.3
    Korsakoff's, Korsakow's 291.1
    paranoid type 291.5
    pathological intoxication 291.4
    polyneuritic 291.1
    specified type NEC 291.89
  alternating (*see also* Psychosis,
      manic-depressive, circular) 296.7
  anergastic (*see also* Psychosis, organic) 294.9
  arteriosclerotic 290.40
    with
      acute confusional state 290.41
      delirium 290.41
      delusional features 290.42
      depressive features 290.43
    depressed type 290.43
    paranoid type 290.42
    simple type 290.40
    uncomplicated 290.40
  atypical 298.9
    depressive 296.82
    manic 296.81
  borderline (schizophrenia) (*see also*
      Schizophrenia) 295.5

Psychosis—*continued*
 of childhood (*see also* Psychosis, childhood)
   299.8
  prepubertal 299.8
 brief reactive 298.8
 childhood, with origin specific to 299.9

> *Note—Use the following fifth-digit*
> *subclassification with category 299:*
>
> *0 current or active state*
> *1 residual state*

 atypical 299.8
 specified type NEC 299.8
 circular (*see also* Psychosis, manic-depressive,
   circular) 296.7
 climacteric (*see also* Psychosis, involutional)
   298.8
 confusional 298.9
  acute 293.0
  reactive 298.2
  subacute 293.1
 depressive (*see also* Psychosis, affective) 296.2
  atypical 296.82
  involutional 296.2
   recurrent episode 296.3
   single episode 296.2
  psychogenic 298.0
  reactive (emotional stress) (psychological
    trauma) 298.0
  recurrent episode 296.3
   with hypomania (bipolar II) 296.89
  single episode 296.2
 disintegrative (childhood) (*see also* Psychosis,
   childhood) 299.1
 drug 292.9
  with
   affective syndrome 292.84
   amnestic syndrome 292.83
   anxiety 292.89
   delirium 292.81
    withdrawal 292.0
   delusional syndrome 292.11
   dementia 292.82
   depressive state 292.84
   hallucinosis 292.12
   mood disturbance 292.84
   organic personality syndrome NEC 292.89
   sexual dysfunction 292.89
   sleep disturbance 292.89
   withdrawal syndrome (and delirium) 292.0
  affective syndrome 292.84
  delusional state 292.11
  hallucinatory state 292.12
  hallucinosis 292.12
  paranoid state 292.11
  specified type NEC 292.89
  withdrawal syndrome (and delirium) 292.0
 due to or associated with physical condition (*see
   also* Psychosis, organic) 293.9
 epileptic NEC 294.8
 excitation (psychogenic) (reactive) 298.1
 exhaustive (*see also* Reaction, stress, acute)
   308.9
 hypomanic (*see also* Psychosis, affective) 296.0
  recurrent episode 296.1
  single episode 296.0
 hysterical 298.8
  acute 298.1
 incipient 298.8
  schizophrenic (*see also* Schizophrenia) 295.5

Psychosis—*continued*
 induced 297.3
 infantile (*see also* Psychosis, childhood) 299.0
 infective 293.9
  acute 293.0
  subacute 293.1
 in pregnancy, childbirth, or puerperium 648.4
 interactional (childhood) (*see also* Psychosis,
   childhood) 299.1
 involutional 298.8
  depressive (*see also* Psychosis, affective)
    296.2
   recurrent episode 296.3
   single episode 296.2
  melancholic 296.2
   recurrent episode 296.3
   single episode 296.2
  paranoid state 297.2
  paraphrenia 297.2
 Korsakoff's, Korakov's, Korsakow's
   (nonalcoholic) 294.0
  alcoholic 291.1
 mania (phase) (*see also* Psychosis, affective)
   296.0
  recurrent episode 296.1
  single episode 296.0
 manic (*see also* Psychosis, affective) 296.0
  atypical 296.81
  recurrent episode 296.1
  single episode 296.0
 manic-depressive 296.80
  circular 296.7
   currently
    depressed 296.5
    manic 296.4
   mixed 296.6
  depressive 296.2
   recurrent episode 296.3
    with hypomania (bipolar II) 296.89
   single episode 296.2
  hypomanic 296.0
   recurrent episode 296.1
   single episode 296.0
  manic 296.0
   atypical 296.81
   recurrent episode 296.1
   single episode 296.0
  mixed NEC 296.89
  perplexed 296.89
  stuporous 296.89
 menopausal (*see also* Psychosis, involutional)
   298.8
 mixed schizophrenic and affective (*see also*
   Schizophrenia) 295.7
 multi-infarct (cerebrovascular) (*see also*
   Psychosis, arteriosclerotic) 290.40
 organic NEC 294.9
  due to or associated with
   addiction
    alcohol (*see also* Psychosis, alcoholic)
      291.9
    drug (*see also* Psychosis, drug) 292.9
   alcohol intoxication, acute (*see also*
     Psychosis, alcoholic) 291.9
   alcoholism (*see also* Psychosis, alcoholic)
     291.9
   arteriosclerosis (cerebral) (*see also*
     Psychosis, arteriosclerotic) 290.40
   cerebrovascular disease
    acute (psychosis) 293.0

Psychosis—*continued*
    arteriosclerotic (*see also* Psychosis,
       arteriosclerotic) 290.40
    childbirth—*see* Psychosis, puerperal
    dependence
       alcohol (*see also* Psychosis, alcoholic)
        291.9
       drug 292.9
    disease
       alcoholic liver (*see also* Psychosis,
        alcoholic) 291.9
       brain
        arteriosclerotic (*see also* Psychosis,
         arteriosclerotic) 290.40
        cerebrovascular
         acute (psychosis) 293.0
         arteriosclerotic (*see also* Psychosis,
          arteriosclerotic) 290.40
        endocrine or metabolic 293.9
         acute (psychosis) 293.0
         subacute (psychosis) 293.1
        Jakob-Creutzfeldt
         with behavioral disturbance 046.1
          [294.11]
         without behavioral disturbance 046.1
          [294.10]
        liver, alcoholic (*see also* Psychosis,
         alcoholic) 291.9
    disorder
       cerebrovascular
        acute (psychosis) 293.0
       endocrine or metabolic 293.9
        acute (psychosis) 293.0
        subacute (psychosis) 293.1
       epilepsy
        with behavioral disturbance 345.9 *[294.11]*
        without behavioral disturbance 345.9
         [294.10]
        transient (acute) 293.0
       Huntington's chorea
        with behavioral disturbance 333.4 *[294.11]*
        without behavioral disturbance 333.4
         [294.10]
    infection
       brain 293.9
        acute (psychosis) 293.0
        chronic 294.8
        subacute (psychosis) 293.1
       intracranial NEC 293.9
        acute (psychosis) 293.0
        chronic 294.8
        subacute (psychosis) 293.1
    intoxication
       alcoholic (acute) (*see also* Psychosis,
        alcoholic) 291.9
       pathological 291.4
       drug (*see also* Psychosis, drug) 292.9
    ischemia
       cerebrovascular (generalized) (*see also*
        Psychosis, arteriosclerotic) 290.40
    Jakob-Creutzfeldt disease or syndrome
       with behavioral disturbance 046.1 *[294.11]*
       without behavioral disturbance 046.1
        [294.10]
    multiple sclerosis
       with behavioral disturbance 340 *[294.11]*
       without behavioral disturbance 340
        [294.10]
    physical condition NEC 293.9
       with
        delusions 293.81

Psychosis—*continued*
        hallucinations 293.82
    presenility 290.10
    puerperium—*see* Psychosis, puerperal
    sclerosis, multiple
       with behavioral disturbance 340 *[294.11]*
       without behavioral disturbance 340
        [294.10]
    senility 290.20
    status epilepticus
       with behavioral disturbance 345.3 *[294.11]*
       without behavioral disturbance 345.3
        [294.10]
    trauma
       brain (birth) (from electrical current)
        (surgical) 293.9
        acute (psychosis) 293.0
        chronic 294.8
        subacute (psychosis) 293.1
       unspecified physical condition 293.9
        with
         delusions 293.81
         hallucinations 293.82
    infective 293.9
       acute (psychosis) 293.0
       subacute 293.1
    posttraumatic 293.9
       acute 293.0
       subacute 293.1
    specified type NEC 294.8
    transient 293.9
       with
        anxiety 293.84
        delusions 293.81
        depression 293.83
        hallucinations 293.82
       depressive type 293.83
       hallucinatory type 293.82
       paranoid type 293.81
       specified type NEC 293.89
   paranoic 297.1
   paranoid (chronic) 297.9
    alcoholic 291.5
    chronic 297.1
    climacteric 297.2
    involutional 297.2
    menopausal 297.2
    protracted reactive 298.4
    psychogenic 298.4
       acute 298.3
    schizophrenic (*see also* Schizophrenia) 295.3
    senile 290.20
   paroxysmal 298.9
    senile 290.20
   polyneuritic, alcoholic 291.1
   postoperative 293.9
   postpartum—*see* Psychosis, puerperal
   prepsychotic (*see also* Schizophrenia) 295.5
   presbyophrenic (type) 290.8
   presenile (*see also* Dementia, presenile) 290.10
   prison 300.16
   psychogenic 298.8
    depressive 298.0
    paranoid 298.4
       acute 298.3
   puerperal
    specified type—*see* categories 295-298
    unspecified type 293.89
       acute 293.0
       chronic 293.89
       subacute 293.1

Psychosis—*continued*
reactive (emotional stress) (psychological
    trauma) 298.8
  brief 298.8
  confusion 298.2
  depressive 298.0
  excitation 298.1
schizo-affective (depressed) (excited) (*see also*
    Schizophrenia) 295.7
schizophrenia, schizophrenic (*see also*
    Schizophrenia) 295.9
  borderline type 295.5
    of childhood (*see also* Psychosis, childhood)
        299.8
  catatonic (excited) (withdrawn) 295.2
  childhood type (*see also* Psychosis,
      childhood) 299.9
  hebephrenic 295.1
  incipient 295.5
  latent 295.5
  paranoid 295.3
  prepsychotic 295.5
  prodromal 295.5
  pseudoneurotic 295.5
  pseudopsychopathic 295.5
  schizophreniform 295.4
  simple 295.0
schizophreniform 295.4
senile NEC 290.20
  with
    delusional features 290.20
    depressive features 290.21
  depressed type 290.21
  paranoid type 290.20
  simple deterioration 290.20
  specified type—*see* categories 295-298
shared 297.3
situational (reactive) 298.8
symbiotic (childhood) (*see also* Psychosis,
    childhood) 299.1
toxic (acute) 293.9
Psychotic (*see also* condition) 298.9
episode 298.9
  due to or associated with physical conditions
      (*see also* Psychosis, organic) 293.9
Pterygium (eye) 372.40
central 372.43
colli 744.5
double 372.44
peripheral (stationary) 372.41
  progressive 372.42
recurrent 372.45
Ptilosis 374.55
Ptomaine (poisoning) (*see also* Poisoning, food)
    005.9
Ptosis (adiposa) 374.30
breast 611.8
cecum 569.89
colon 569.89
congenital (eyelid) 743.61
  specified site NEC—*see* Anomaly, specified
      type NEC
epicanthus syndrome 270.2
eyelid 374.30
  congenital 743.61
  mechanical 374.33
  myogenic 374.32
  paralytic 374.31
gastric 537.5
intestine 569.89

Ptosis—*continued*
kidney (*see also* Disease, renal) 593.0
  congenital 753.3
liver 573.8
renal (*see also* Disease, renal) 593.0
  congenital 753.3
splanchnic 569.89
spleen 289.59
stomach 537.5
viscera 569.89
Ptyalism 527.7
hysterical 300.11
periodic 527.2
pregnancy 646.8
psychogenic 306.4
Ptyalolithiasis 527.5
Pubalgia 848.8
Pubarche, precocious 259.1
Pubertas praecox 259.1
Puberty V21.1
abnormal 259.9
bleeding 626.3
delayed 259.0
precocious (constitutional) (cryptogenic)
    (idiopathic) NEC 259.1
  due to
    adrenal
      cortical hyperfunction 255.2
      hyperplasia 255.2
    cortical hyperfunction 255.2
    ovarian hyperfunction 256.1
      estrogen 256.0
    pineal tumor 259.8
    testicular hyperfunction 257.0
premature 259.1
  due to
    adrenal cortical hyperfunction 255.2
    pineal tumor 259.8
    pituitary (anterior) hyperfunction 253.1
Puckering, macula 362.56
Pudenda, pudendum —*see* condition
Puente's disease (simple glandular cheilitis)
    528.5
Puerperal
abscess
  areola 675.1
  Bartholin's gland 646.6
  breast 675.1
  cervix (uteri) 670
  fallopian tube 670
  genital organ 670
  kidney 646.6
  mammary 675.1
  mesosalpinx 670
  nabothian 646.6
  nipple 675.0
  ovary, ovarian 670
  oviduct 670
  parametric 670
  para-uterine 670
  pelvic 670
  perimetric 670
  periuterine 670
  retro-uterine 670
  subareolar 675.1
  suprapelvic 670
  tubal (ruptured) 670
  tubo-ovarian 670
  urinary tract NEC 646.6
  uterine, uterus 670
  vagina (wall) 646.6

Puerperal—*continued*
  vaginorectal 646.6
  vulvovaginal gland 646.6
  accident 674.9
  adnexitis 670
  afibrinogenemia, or other coagulation defect
    666.3
  albuminuria (acute) (subacute) 646.2
    pre-eclamptic 642.4
  anemia (conditions classifiable to 280-285)
    648.2
  anuria 669.3
  apoplexy 674.0
  asymptomatic bacteriuria 646.5
  atrophy, breast 676.3
  blood dyscrasia 666.3
  caked breast 676.2
  cardiomyopathy 674.8
  cellulitis—*see* Puerperal, abscess
  cerebrovascular disorder (conditions classifiable
    to 430-434, 436-437) 674.0
  cervicitis (conditions classifiable to 616.0) 646.6
  coagulopathy (any) 666.3
  complications 674.9
    specified type NEC 674.8
  convulsions (eclamptic) (uremic) 642.6
    with pre-existing hypertension 642.7
  cracked nipple 676.1
  cystitis 646.6
  cystopyelitis 646.6
  deciduitis (acute) 670
  delirium NEC 293.9
  diabetes (mellitus) (conditions classifiable to
    250) 648.0
  disease 674.9
    breast NEC 676.3
    cerebrovascular (acute) 674.0
    nonobstetric NEC (*see also* Pregnancy,
      complicated, current disease or condition)
      648.9
    pelvis inflammatory 670
    renal NEC 646.2
    tubo-ovarian 670
    Valsuani's (progressive pernicious anemia)
      648.2
  disorder
    lactation 676.9
      specified type NEC 676.8
    nonobstetric NEC (*see also* Pregnancy,
      complicated, current disease or condition)
      648.9
  disruption
    cesarean wound 674.1
    episiotomy wound 674.2
    perineal laceration wound 674.2
  drug dependence (conditions classifiable to 304)
    648.3
  eclampsia 642.6
    with pre-existing hypertension 642.7
  embolism (pulmonary) 673.2
    air 673.0
    amniotic fluid 673.1
    blood-clot 673.2
    brain or cerebral 674.0
    cardiac 674.8
    fat 673.8
    intracranial sinus (venous) 671.5
    pyemic 673.3
    septic 673.3
    spinal cord 671.5

Puerperal—*continued*
  endometritis (conditions classifiable to
    615.0-615.9) 670
  endophlebitis—*see* Puerperal, phlebitis
  endotrachelitis 646.6
  engorgement, breasts 676.2
  erysipelas 670
  failure
    lactation 676.4
    renal, acute 669.3
  fever 670
    meaning pyrexia (of unknown origin) 672
    meaning sepsis 670
  fissure, nipple 676.1
  fistula
    breast 675.1
    mammary gland 675.1
    nipple 675.0
  galactophoritis 675.2
  galactorrhea 676.6
  gangrene
    gas 670
    uterus 670
  gonorrhea (conditions classifiable to 098) 647.1
  hematoma, subdural 674.0
  hematosalpinx, infectional 670
  hemiplegia, cerebral 674.0
  hemorrhage 666.1
    brain 674.0
    bulbar 674.0
    cerebellar 674.0
    cerebral 674.0
    cortical 674.0
    delayed (after 24 hours) (uterine) 666.2
    extradural 674.0
    internal capsule 674.0
    intracranial 674.0
    intrapontine 674.0
    meningeal 674.0
    pontine 674.0
    subarachnoid 674.0
    subcortical 674.0
    subdural 674.0
    uterine, delayed 666.2
    ventricular 674.0
  hemorrhoids 671.8
  hepatorenal syndrome 674.8
  hypertrophy
    breast 676.3
    mammary gland 676.3
  induration breast (fibrous) 676.3
  infarction
    lung—*see* Puerperal, embolism
    pulmonary—*see* Puerperal, embolism
  infection
    Bartholin's gland 646.6
    breast 675.2
      with nipple 675.9
        specified type NEC 675.8
    cervix 646.6
    endocervix 646.6
    fallopian tube 670
    generalized 670
    genital tract (major) 670
      minor or localized 646.6
    kidney (bacillus coli) 646.6
    mammary gland 675.2
      with nipple 675.9
        specified type NEC 675.8
    nipple 675.0
      with breast 675.9

Puerperal—*continued*
sudden death (cause unknown) 674.9
suppuration—*see* Puerperal, abscess
syphilis (conditions classifiable to 090-097)
647.0
tetanus 670
thelitis 675.0
thrombocytopenia 666.3
thrombophlebitis (superficial) 671.2
deep 671.4
pelvic 671.4
specified site NEC 671.5
thrombosis (venous)—*see* Thrombosis,
puerperal
thyroid dysfunction (conditions classifiable to
240-246) 648.1
toxemia (*see also* Toxemia, of pregnancy) 642.4
eclamptic 642.6
with pre-existing hypertension 642.7
pre-eclamptic (mild) 642.4
with
convulsions 642.6
pre-existing hypertension 642.7
severe 642.5
tuberculosis (conditions classifiable to 010-018)
647.3
uremia 669.3
vaginitis (conditions classifiable to 616.1) 646.6
varicose veins (legs) 671.0
vulva or perineum 671.1
vulvitis (conditions classifiable to 616.1) 646.6
vulvovaginitis (conditions classifiable to 616.1)
646.6
white leg 671.4
Pulled muscle —*see* Sprain, by site
Pulmolithiasis 518.89
Pulmonary —*see* condition
Pulmonitis (unknown etiology) 486
Pulpitis (acute) (anachoretic) (chronic)
(hyperplastic) (putrescent) (suppurative)
(ulcerative) 522.0
Pulpless tooth 522.9
Pulse
alternating 427.89
psychogenic 306.2
bigeminal 427.89
fast 785.0
feeble, rapid, due to shock following injury
958.4
rapid 785.0
slow 427.89
strong 785.9
trigeminal 427.89
water-hammer (*see also* Insufficiency, aortic)
424.1
weak 785.9
Pulseless disease 446.7
Pulsus
alternans or trigeminy 427.89
psychogenic 306.2
Punch drunk 310.2
Puncta lacrimalia occlusion 375.52
Punctiform hymen 752.49
Puncture (traumatic)—*see also* Wound, open, by
site
accidental, complicating surgery 998.2
bladder, nontraumatic 596.6
by
device, implant, or graft—*see* Complications,
mechanical

Puncture—*continued*
foreign body
internal organs—*see also* Injury, internal, by
site
by ingested object—*see* Foreign body
left accidentally in operation wound 998.4
instrument (any) during a procedure,
accidental 998.2
internal organs, abdomen, chest, or pelvis—*see*
Injury, internal, by site
kidney, nontraumatic 593.89
Pupil —*see* condition
Pupillary membrane 364.74
persistent 743.46
Pupillotonia 379.46
pseudotabetic 379.46
Purpura 287.2
abdominal 287.0
allergic 287.0
anaphylactoid 287.0
annularis telangiectodes 709.1
arthritic 287.0
autoerythrocyte sensitization 287.2
autoimmune 287.0
bacterial 287.0
Bateman's (senile) 287.2
capillary fragility (hereditary) (idiopathic) 287.8
cryoglobulinemic 273.2
devil's pinches 287.2
fibrinolytic (*see also* Fibrinolysis) 286.6
fulminans, fulminous 286.6
gangrenous 287.0
hemorrhagic (*see also* Purpura,
thrombocytopenic) 287.3
nodular 272.7
nonthrombocytopenic 287.0
thrombocytopenic 287.3
Henoch's (purpura nervosa) 287.0
Henoch-Schönlein (allergic) 287.0
hypergammaglobulinemic (benign primary)
(Waldenström's) 273.0
idiopathic 287.3
nonthrombocytopenic 287.0
thrombocytopenic 287.3
infectious 287.0
malignant 287.0
neonatorum 772.6
nervosa 287.0
newborn NEC 772.6
nonthrombocytopenic 287.2
hemorrhagic 287.0
idiopathic 287.0
nonthrombopenic 287.2
peliosis rheumatica 287.0
pigmentaria, progressiva 709.09
posttransfusion 287.4
primary 287.0
primitive 287.0
red cell membrane sensitivity 287.2
rheumatica 287.0
Schönlein (-Henoch) (allergic) 287.0
scorbutic 267
senile 287.2
simplex 287.2
symptomatica 287.0
telangiectasia annularis 709.1
thrombocytopenic (congenital) (essential)
(hereditary) (idiopathic) (primary) (*see also*
Thrombocytopenia) 287.3

Purpura—*continued*
  neonatal, transitory (*see also*
    Thrombocytopenia, neonatal transitory)
    776.1
  puerperal, postpartum 666.3
  thrombotic 446.6
  thrombohemolytic (*see also* Fibrinolysis) 286.6
  thrombopenic (congenital) (essential) (*see also*
    Thrombocytopenia) 287.3
  thrombotic 446.6
  thrombocytic 446.6
  thrombocytopenic 446.6
  toxic 287.0
  variolosa 050.0
  vascular 287.0
  visceral symptoms 287.0
  Werlhof's (*see also* Purpura, thrombocytopenic)
    287.3
Purpuric spots 782.7
Purulent —*see* condition
Pus
  absorption, general—*see* Septicemia
  in
    stool 792.1
    urine 791.9
  tube (rupture) (*see also* Salpingo-oophoritis)
    614.2
Pustular rash 782.1
Pustule 686.9
  malignant 022.0
  nonmalignant 686.9
Putnam's disease (subacute combined sclerosis
  with pernicious anemia) 281.0 *[336.2]*
Putnam-Dana syndrome (subacute combined
  sclerosis with pernicious anemia) 281.0
  [336.2]
Putrefaction, intestinal 569.89
Putrescent pulp (dental) 522.1
Pyarthritis —*see* Pyarthrosis
Pyarthrosis (*see also* Arthritis, pyogenic) 711.0
  tuberculous—*see* Tuberculosis, joint
Pycnoepilepsy, pycnolepsy (idiopathic) (*see also*
  Epilepsy) 345.0
Pyelectasia 593.89
Pyelectasis 593.89
Pyelitis (congenital) (uremic) 590.80
  with
    abortion—*see* Abortion, by type, with
      specified complication NEC
    contracted kidney 590.00
    ectopic pregnancy (*see also* categories
      633.0-633.9) 639.8
    molar pregnancy (*see also* categories
      630-632) 639.8
  acute 590.10
    with renal medullary necrosis 590.11
  chronic 590.00
    with
      renal medullary necrosis 590.01
  complicating pregnancy, childbirth, or
    puerperium 646.6
    affecting fetus or newborn 760.1
  cystica 590.3
  following
    abortion 639.8
    ectopic or molar pregnancy 639.8
  gonococcal 098.19
    chronic or duration of 2 months or over 098.39
  tuberculous (*see also* Tuberculosis) 016.0
    [590.81]
Pyelocaliectasis 593.89
Pyelocystitis (*see also* Pyelitis) 590.80

Pyelohydronephrosis 591
Pyelonephritis (*see also* Pyelitis) 590.80
  acute 590.10
    with renal medullary necrosis 590.11
  chronic 590.00
  syphilitic (late) 095.4
  tuberculous (*see also* Tuberculosis) 016.0
    [590.81]
Pyelonephrosis (*see also* Pyelitis) 590.80
  chronic 590.00
Pyelophlebitis 451.89
Pyelo-ureteritis cystica 590.3
Pyemia, pyemic (purulent) (*see also* Septicemia)
  038.9
  abscess—*see* Abscess
  arthritis (*see also* Arthritis, pyogenic) 711.0
  Bacillus coli 038.42
  embolism—*see* Embolism, pyemic
  fever 038.9
  infection 038.9
  joint (*see also* Arthritis, pyogenic) 711.0
  liver 572.1
  meningococcal 036.2
  newborn 771.81
  phlebitis—*see* Phlebitis
  pneumococcal 038.2
  portal 572.1
  postvaccinal 999.3
  specified organism NEC 038.8
  staphylococcal 038.10
    aureus 038.11
    specified organism NEC 038.19
  streptococcal 038.0
  tuberculous—*see* Tuberculosis, miliary
Pygopagus 759.4
Pykno-epilepsy, pyknolepsy (idiopathic) (*see*
  also Epilepsy) 345.0
Pyle (-Cohn) disease (craniometaphyseal
  dysplasia) 756.89
Pylephlebitis (suppurative) 572.1
Pylethrombophlebitis 572.1
Pylethrombosis 572.1
Pyloritis (*see also* Gastritis) 535.5
Pylorospasm (reflex) 537.81
  congenital or infantile 750.5
  neurotic 306.4
  newborn 750.5
  psychogenic 306.4
Pylorus, pyloric —*see* condition
Pyoarthrosis —*see* Pyarthrosis
Pyocele
  mastoid 383.00
  sinus (accessory) (nasal) (*see also* Sinusitis)
    473.9
  turbinate (bone) 473.9
  urethra (*see also* Urethritis) 597.0
Pyococcal dermatitis 686.00
Pyococcide, skin 686.00
Pyocolpos (*see also* Vaginitis) 616.10
Pyocyaneus dermatitis 686.09
Pyocystitis (*see also* Cystitis) 595.9
Pyoderma, pyodermia NEC 686.00
  gangrenosum 686.01
  specified type NEC 686.09
  vegetans 686.8
Pyodermatitis 686.00
  vegetans 686.8
Pyogenic —*see* condition
Pyohemia —*see* Septicemia
Pyohydronephrosis (*see also* Pyelitis) 590.80
Pyometra 615.9
Pyometritis (*see also* Endometritis) 615.9

Pyometrium (*see also* Endometritis) 615.9
Pyomyositis 728.0
  ossificans 728.19
  tropical (bungpagga) 040.81
Pyonephritis (*see also* Pyelitis) 590.80
  chronic 590.00
Pyonephrosis (congenital) (*see also* Pyelitis)
    590.80
  acute 590.10
Pyo-oophoritis (*see also* Salpingo-oophoritis)
    614.2
Pyo-ovarium (*see also* Salpingo-oophoritis)
    614.2
Pyopericarditis 420.99
Pyopericardium 420.99
Pyophlebitis —*see* Phlebitis
Pyopneumopericardium 420.99
Pyopneumothorax (infectional) 510.9
  with fistula 510.0
  subdiaphragmatic (*see also* Peritonitis) 567.2
  subphrenic (*see also* Peritonitis) 567.2
  tuberculous (*see also* Tuberculosis, pleura)
    012.0
Pyorrhea (alveolar) (alveolaris) 523.4
  degenerative 523.5
Pyosalpingitis (*see also* Salpingo-oophoritis)
    614.2
Pyosalpinx (*see also* Salpingo-oophoritis) 614.2
Pyosepticemia —*see* Septicemia
Pyosis
  Corlett's (impetigo) 684
  Manson's (pemphigus contagiosus) 684
Pyothorax 510.9
  with fistula 510.0
  tuberculous (*see also* Tuberculosis, pleura)
    012.0
Pyoureter 593.89
  tuberculous (*see also* Tuberculosis) 016.2
Pyramidopallidonigral syndrome 332.0
Pyrexia (of unknown origin) (P.U.O.) 780.6
  atmospheric 992.0
  during labor 659.2
  environmentally-induced
    newborn 778.4
  heat 992.0
  newborn, environmentally-induced 778.4
  puerperal 672
Pyroglobulinemia 273.8
Pyromania 312.33
Pyrosis 787.1
Pyrroloporphyria 277.1
Pyuria (bacterial) 791.9

Q

Q fever 083.0
with pneumonia 083.0 *[484.8]*
Quadricuspid aortic valve 746.89
Quadrilateral fever 083.0
Quadriparesis —*see* Quadriplegia
Quadriplegia 344.00
with fracture, vertebra (process)—*see* Fracture,
     vertebra, cervical, with spinal cord injury
brain (current episode) 437.8
cerebral (current episode) 437.8
C1-C4
     complete 344.01
     incomplete 344.02
C5-C7
     complete 344.03
     incomplete 344.04
congenital or infantile (cerebral) (spastic)
     (spinal) 343.2
cortical 437.8
embolic (current episode) (*see also* Embolism,
     brain) 434.1
infantile (cerebral) (spastic) (spinal) 343.2
newborn NEC 767.0
specified NEC 344.09
thrombotic (current episode) (*see also*
     Thrombosis, brain) 434.0
traumatic—*see* Injury, spinal, cervical
Quadruplet
affected by maternal complications of
     pregnancy 761.5
healthy liveborn—*see* Newborn, multiple
pregnancy (complicating delivery) NEC 651.8
with fetal loss and retention of one or more
     fetus(es) 651.5
Quarrelsomeness 301.3
Quartan
fever 084.2
malaria (fever) 084.2
Queensland fever 083.0
coastal 083.0
seven-day 100.89
Quervain's disease 727.04
thyroid (subacute granulomatous thyroiditis)
     245.1
Queyrat's erythroplasia (M8080/2)
specified site—*see* Neoplasm, skin, in situ
unspecified site 233.5
Quincke's disease or edema —*see* Edema,
     angioneurotic
Quinquaud's disease (acne decalvans) 704.09
Quinsy (gangrenous) 475
Quintan fever 083.1
Quintuplet
affected by maternal complications of
     pregnancy 761.5
healthy liveborn—*see* Newborn, multiple
pregnancy (complicating delivery) NEC 651.2
with fetal loss and retention of one or more
     fetus(es) 651.6
Quotidian
fever 084.0
malaria (fever) 084.0

R

Rabbia 071
Rabbit fever (*see also* Tularemia) 021.9
Rabies 071
contact V01.5
exposure to V01.5
inoculation V04.5
     reaction—*see* Complications, vaccination
vaccination, prophylactic (against) V04.5
Rachischisis (*see also* Spina bifida) 741.9
Rachitic —*see also* condition
deformities of spine 268.1
pelvis 268.1
     with disproportion (fetopelvic) 653.2
     affecting fetus or newborn 763.1
     causing obstructed labor 660.1
     affecting fetus or newborn 763.1
Rachitis, rachitism —*see also* Rickets
acute 268.0
fetalis 756.4
renalis 588.0
tarda 268.0
Racket nail 757.5
Radial nerve —*see* condition
Radiation effects or sickness —*see also* Effect,
     adverse, radiation
cataract 366.46
dermatitis 692.82
sunburn (*see also* Sunburn) 692.71
Radiculitis (pressure) (vertebrogenic) 729.2
accessory nerve 723.4
anterior crural 724.4
arm 723.4
brachial 723.4
cervical NEC 723.4
due to displacement of intervertebral disc—*see*
     Neuritis, due to, displacement intervertebral
     disc
leg 724.4
lumbar NEC 724.4
lumbosacral 724.4
rheumatic 729.2
syphilitic 094.89
thoracic (with visceral pain) 724.4
Radiculomyelitis 357.0
toxic, due to
     Clostridium tetani 037
     Corynebacterium diphtheriae 032.89
Radiculopathy (*see also* Radiculitis) 729.2
Radioactive substances, adverse effect —*see*
     Effect, adverse, radioactive substance
Radiodermal burns (acute) (chronic)
     (occupational)—*see* Burn, by site
Radiodermatitis 692.82
Radionecrosis —*see* Effect, adverse, radiation
Radiotherapy session V58.0
Radium, adverse effect —*see* Effect, adverse,
     radioactive substance
Raeder-Harbitz syndrome (pulseless disease)
     446.7
Rage (*see also* Disturbance, conduct) 312.0
meaning rabies 071
Rag sorters' disease 022.1
Raillietiniasis 123.8
Railroad neurosis 300.16
Railway spine 300.16
Raised —*see* Elevation
Raiva 071
Rake teeth, tooth 524.3

Rales 786.7
Ramifying renal pelvis 753.3
Ramsay Hunt syndrome (herpetic geniculate
    ganglionitis) 053.11
  meaning dyssynergia cerebellaris myoclonica
    334.2
Ranke's primary infiltration (*see also*
  Tuberculosis) 010.0
Ranula 527.6
  congenital 750.26
Rape (*see* Injury, by site)
  alleged, observation or examination V71.5
Rapid
  feeble pulse, due to shock, following injury
    958.4
  heart (beat) 785.0
    psychogenic 306.2
  respiration 786.06
    psychogenic 306.1
  second stage (delivery) 661.3
    affecting fetus or newborn 763.6
  time-zone change syndrome 307.45
Rarefaction, bone 733.99
Rash 782.1
  canker 034.1
  diaper 691.0
  drug (internal use) 693.0
    contact 692.3
  ECHO 9 virus 078.89
  enema 692.89
  food (*see also* Allergy, food) 693.1
  heat 705.1
  napkin 691.0
  nettle 708.8
  pustular 782.1
  rose 782.1
    epidemic 056.9
    of infants 057.8
  scarlet 034.1
  serum (prophylactic) (therapeutic) 999.5
  toxic 782.1
  wandering tongue 529.1
Rasmussen's aneurysm (*see also* Tuberculosis)
  011.2
Rat-bite fever 026.9
  due to Streptobacillus moniliformis 026.1
  spirochetal (morsus muris) 026.0
Rathke's pouch tumor (M9350/1) 237.0
Raymond (-Céstan) syndrome 433.8
Raynaud's
  disease or syndrome (paroxysmal digital
    cyanosis) 443.0
  gangrene (symmetric) 443.0 *[785.4]*
  phenomenon (paroxysmal digital cyanosis)
    (secondary) 443.0
RDS 769
Reaction
  acute situational maladjustment (*see also*
    Reaction, adjustment) 309.9
  adaptation (*see also* Reaction, adjustment) 309.9
  adjustment 309.9
    with
      anxious mood 309.24
        with depressed mood 309.28
      conduct disturbance 309.3
        combined with disturbance of emotions
          309.4
      depressed mood 309.0
        brief 309.0
          with anxious mood 309.28
        prolonged 309.1

Reaction—*continued*
  elective mutism 309.83
  mixed emotions and conduct 309.4
  mutism, elective 309.83
  physical symptoms 309.82
  predominant disturbance (of)
    conduct 309.3
    emotions NEC 309.29
      mixed 309.28
    mixed, emotions and conduct 309.4
    specified type NEC 309.89
    specific academic or work inhibition 309.23
    withdrawal 309.83
  depressive 309.0
    with conduct disturbance 309.4
    brief 309.0
    prolonged 309.1
    specified type NEC 309.89
  adverse food NEC 995.7
  affective (*see also* Psychosis, affective) 296.90
    specified type NEC 296.99
  aggressive 301.3
    unsocialized (*see also* Disturbance, conduct)
      312.0
  allergic (*see also* Allergy) 995.3
    drug, medicinal substance, and
      biological—*see* Allergy, drug
    food—*see* Allergy, food
    serum 999.5
  anaphylactic—*see* Shock, anaphylactic
  anesthesia—*see* Anesthesia, complication
  anger 312.0
  antisocial 301.7
  antitoxin (prophylactic) (therapeutic)—*see*
    Complications, vaccination
  anxiety 300.00
  asthenic 300.5
  compulsive 300.3
  conversion (anesthetic) (autonomic)
    (hyperkinetic) (mixed paralytic)
    (paresthetic) 300.11
  deoxyribonuclease (DNA) (DNase)
    hypersensitivity NEC 287.2
  depressive 300.4
    acute 309.0
    affective (*see also* Psychosis, affective) 296.2
      recurrent episode 296.3
      single episode 296.2
    brief 309.0
    manic (*see also* Psychosis, affective) 296.80
    neurotic 300.4
    psychoneurotic 300.4
    psychotic 298.0
  dissociative 300.15
  drug NEC (*see also* Table of drugs and
    chemicals) 995.2
    allergic—*see* Allergy, drug
    correct substance properly administered 995.2
    obstetric anesthetic or analgesic NEC 668.9
      affecting fetus or newborn 763.5
      specified drug—*see* Table of drugs and
        chemicals
    overdose or poisoning 977.9
      specified drug—*see* Table of drugs and
        chemicals
    specific to newborn 779.4
    transmitted via placenta or breast milk—*see*
      Absorption, drug, through placenta
    withdrawal NEC 292.0
      infant of dependent mother 779.5
    wrong substance given or taken in error 977.9

Reaction—*continued*
    specified drug—*see* Table of drugs and
        chemicals
  dyssocial 301.7
  erysipeloid 027.1
  fear 300.20
    child 313.0
  fluid loss, cerebrospinal 349.0
  food—*see also* Allergy, food
    adverse NEC 995.7
    anaphylactic shock—*see* Anaphylactic shock,
        due to food
  foreign
    body NEC 728.82
      in operative wound (inadvertently left) 998.4
      due to surgical material intentionally
        left—*see* Complications, due to
        (presence of) any device, implant, or
        graft classified to 996.0-996.5 NEC
    substance accidentally left during a procedure
      (chemical) (powder) (talc) 998.7
      body or object (instrument) (sponge) (swab)
        998.4
  graft-versus-host (GVH) 996.85
  grief (acute) (brief) 309.0
    prolonged 309.1
  gross stress (*see also* Reaction, stress, acute)
    308.9
  group delinquent (*see also* Disturbance,
    conduct) 312.2
  Herxheimer's 995.0
  hyperkinetic (*see also* Hyperkinesia) 314.9
  hypochondriacal 300.7
  hypoglycemic, due to insulin 251.0
    therapeutic misadventure 962.3
  hypomanic (*see also* Psychosis, affective) 296.0
    recurrent episode 296.1
    single episode 296.0
  hysterical 300.10
    conversion type 300.11
    dissociative 300.15
  id (bacterial cause) 692.89
  immaturity NEC 301.89
    aggressive 301.3
    emotional instability 301.59
  immunization—*see* Complications, vaccination
  incompatibility
    blood group (ABO) (infusion) (transfusion)
      999.6
    Rh (factor) (infusion) (transfusion) 999.7
  inflammatory—*see* Infection
  infusion—*see* Complications, infusion
  inoculation (immune serum)—*see*
    Complications, vaccination
  insulin 995.2
  involutional
    paranoid 297.2
    psychotic (*see also* Psychosis, affective,
      depressive) 296.2
  leukemoid (lymphocytic) (monocytic)
    (myelocytic) 288.8
  LSD (*see also* Abuse, drugs, nondependent)
    305.3
  lumbar puncture 349.0
  manic-depressive (*see also* Psychosis, affective)
    296.80
    depressed 296.2
      recurrent episode 296.3
      single episode 296.2
    hypomanic 296.0
  neurasthenic 300.5

Reaction—*continued*
  neurogenic (*see also* Neurosis) 300.9
  neurotic NEC 300.9
  neurotic-depressive 300.4
  nitritoid—*see* Crisis, nitritoid
  obsessive (-compulsive) 300.3
  organic 293.9
    acute 293.0
    subacute 293.1
  overanxious, child or adolescent 313.0
  paranoid (chronic) 297.9
    acute 298.3
    climacteric 297.2
    involutional 297.2
    menopausal 297.2
    senile 290.20
    simple 297.0
  passive
    aggressive 301.84
    dependency 301.6
  personality (*see also* Disorder, personality)
    301.9
  phobic 300.20
  postradiation—*see* Effect, adverse, radiation
  psychogenic NEC 300.9
  psychoneurotic (*see also* Neurosis) 300.9
    anxiety 300.00
    compulsive 300.3
    conversion 300.11
    depersonalization 300.6
    depressive 300.4
    dissociative 300.15
    hypochondriacal 300.7
    hysterical 300.10
      conversion type 300.11
      dissociative type 300.15
    neurasthenic 300.5
    obsessive 300.3
    obsessive-compulsive 300.3
    phobic 300.20
    tension state 300.9
  psychophysiologic NEC (*see also* Disorder,
    psychosomatic) 306.9
    cardiovascular 306.2
    digestive 306.4
    endocrine 306.6
    gastrointestinal 306.4
    genitourinary 306.50
    heart 306.2
    hemic 306.8
    intestinal (large) (small) 306.4
    laryngeal 306.1
    lymphatic 306.8
    musculoskeletal 306.0
    pharyngeal 306.1
    respiratory 306.1
    skin 306.3
    special sense organs 306.7
  psychosomatic (*see also* Disorder,
    psychosomatic) 306.9
  psychotic (*see also* Psychosis) 298.9
    depressive 298.0
    due to or associated with physical condition
      (*see also* Psychosis, organic) 293.9
    involutional (*see also* Psychosis, affective)
      296.2
      recurrent episode 296.3
      single episode 296.2
  pupillary (myotonic) (tonic) 379.46
  radiation—*see* Effect, adverse, radiation

Reaction—*continued*
runaway—*see also* Disturbance, conduct
  socialized 312.2
  undersocialized, unsocialized 312.1
scarlet fever toxin—*see* Complications,
  vaccination
schizophrenic (*see also* Schizophrenia) 295.9
  latent 295.5
serological for syphilis—*see* Serology for
  syphilis
serum (prophylactic) (therapeutic) 999.5
  immediate 999.4
situational (*see also* Reaction, adjustment) 309.9
  acute, to stress 308.3
  adjustment (*see also* Reaction, adjustment)
    309.9
somatization (*see also* Disorder, psychosomatic)
  306.9
spinal puncture 349.0
spite, child (*see also* Disturbance, conduct)
  312.0
stress, acute 308.9
  bone or cartilage —*see* Fracture, stress
  with predominant disturbance (of)
    consciousness 308.1
    emotions 308.0
    mixed 308.4
    psychomotor 308.2
    specified type NEC 308.3
surgical procedure—*see* Complications,
  surgical procedure
tetanus antitoxin—*see* Complications,
  vaccination
toxin-antitoxin—*see* Complications, vaccination
transfusion (blood) (bone marrow)
  (lymphocytes) (allergic)—*see*
  Complications, transfusion
tuberculin skin test, nonspecific (without active
  tuberculosis) 795.5
  positive (without active tuberculosis) 795.5
ultraviolet—*see* Effect, adverse, ultraviolet
undersocialized, unsocialized—*see also*
  Disturbance, conduct
  aggressive (type) 312.0
  unaggressive (type) 312.1
vaccination (any)—*see* Complications,
  vaccination
white graft (skin) 996.52
withdrawing, child or adolescent 313.22
x-ray—*see* Effect, adverse, x-rays
Reactive depression (*see also* Reaction,
  depressive) 300.4
neurotic 300.4
psychoneurotic 300.4
psychotic 298.0
Rebound tenderness 789.6
Recalcitrant patient V15.81
Recanalization, thrombus —*see* Thrombosis
Recession, receding
chamber angle (eye) 364.77
chin 524.06
gingival (generalized) (localized) (postinfective)
  (postoperative) 523.2
Recklinghausen's disease (M9540/1) 237.71
bones (osteitis fibrosa cystica) 252.0
Recklinghausen-Applebaum disease
  (hemochromatosis) 275.0
Reclus' disease (cystic) 610.1
Recrudescent typhus (fever) 081.1
Recruitment, auditory 388.44
Rectalgia 569.42

Rectitis 569.49
Rectocele
female (without uterine prolapse) 618.0
  with uterine prolapse 618.4
    complete 618.3
    incomplete 618.2
in pregnancy or childbirth 654.4
  causing obstructed labor 660.2
    affecting fetus or newborn 763.1
male 569.49
vagina, vaginal (outlet) 618.0
Rectosigmoiditis 569.89
ulcerative (chronic) 556.3
Rectosigmoid junction —*see* condition
Rectourethral —*see* condition
Rectovaginal —*see* condition
Rectovesical —*see* condition
Rectum, rectal —*see* condition
Recurrent —*see* condition
Red bugs 133.8
Red cedar asthma 495.8
Redness
conjunctiva 379.93
eye 379.93
nose 478.1
Reduced ventilatory or vital capacity 794.2
Reduction
function
  kidney (*see also* Disease, renal) 593.9
  liver 573.8
  ventilatory capacity 794.2
  vital capacity 794.2
Redundant, redundancy
abdomen 701.9
anus 751.5
cardia 537.89
clitoris 624.2
colon (congenital) 751.5
foreskin (congenital) 605
intestine 751.5
labia 624.3
organ or site, congenital NEC—*see* Accessory
panniculus (abdominal) 278.1
prepuce (congenital) 605
pylorus 537.89
rectum 751.5
scrotum 608.89
sigmoid 751.5
skin (of face) 701.9
  eyelids 374.30
stomach 537.89
uvula 528.9
vagina 623.8
Reduplication —*see* Duplication
Referral
adoption (agency) V68.89
nursing care V63.8
patient without examination or treatment V68.81
social services V63.8
Reflex —*see also* condition
blink, deficient 374.45
hyperactive gag 478.29
neurogenic bladder NEC 596.54
  atonic 596.54
    with cauda equina syndrome 344.61
vasoconstriction 443.9
vasovagal 780.2
Reflux
esophageal 530.81
esophagitis 530.11
gastroesophageal 530.81

Reflux—*continued*
  mitral—*see* Insufficiency, mitral
  ureteral —*see* Reflux, vesicoureteral
  vesicoureteral 593.70
    with
      reflux nephropathy 593.73
        bilateral 593.72
        unilateral 593.71
Reformed gallbladder 576.0
Reforming, artificial openings (*see also*
  Attention to, artificial, opening) V55.9
Refractive error (*see also* Error, refractive) 367.9
Refsum's disease or syndrome (heredopathia
  atactica polyneuritiformis) 356.3
Refusal of
  food 307.59
    hysterical 300.11
  treatment because of, due to
    patient's decision NEC V64.2
    reason of conscience or religion V62.6
Regaud
  tumor (M8082/3)—*see* Neoplasm,
    nasopharynx, malignant
  type carcinoma (M8082/3)—*see* Neoplasm,
    nasopharynx, malignant
Regional —*see* condition
Regulation feeding (elderly) (infant) 783.3
  newborn 779.3
Regurgitated
  food, choked on 933.1
  stomach contents, choked on 933.1
Regurgitation
  aortic (valve) (*see also* Insufficiency, aortic)
    424.1
    congenital 746.4
    syphilitic 093.22
  food—*see also* Vomiting
    with reswallowing—*see* Rumination
    newborn 779.3
  gastric contents—*see* Vomiting
  heart—*see* Endocarditis
  mitral (valve)—*see also* Insufficiency, mitral
    congenital 746.6
  myocardial—*see* Endocarditis
  pulmonary (heart) (valve) (*see also*
    Endocarditis, pulmonary) 424.3
  stomach—*see* Vomiting
  tricuspid—*see* Endocarditis, tricuspid
  valve, valvular—*see* Endocarditis
  vesicoureteral —*see* Reflux, vesicoureteral
Rehabilitation V57.9
  multiple types V57.89
  occupational V57.21
  specified type NEC V57.89
  speech V57.3
  vocational V57.22
Reichmann's disease or syndrome
  (gastrosuccorrhea) 536.8
Reifenstein's syndrome (hereditary familial
  hypogonadism, male) 257.2
Reilly's syndrome or phenomenon (*see also*
  Neuropathy, peripheral, autonomic) 337.9
Reimann's periodic disease 277.3
Reinsertion, contraceptive device V25.42
Reiter's disease, syndrome, or urethritis 099.3
  [711.1]
Rejection
  food, hysterical 300.11
  transplant 996.80
    bone marrow 996.85
    corneal 996.51

Rejection—*continued*
  organ (immune or nonimmune cause) 996.80
    bone marrow 996.85
    heart 996.83
    intestines 996.87
    kidney 996.81
    liver 996.82
    lung 996.84
    pancreas 996.86
    specified NEC 996.89
  skin 996.52
    artificial 996.55
    decellularized allodermis 996.55
Relapsing fever 087.9
  Carter's (Asiatic) 087.0
  Dutton's (West African) 087.1
  Koch's 087.9
  louse-borne (epidemic) 087.0
  Novy's (American) 087.1
  Obermeyer's (European) 087.0
  Spirillum 087.9
  tick-borne (endemic) 087.1
Relaxation
  anus (sphincter) 569.49
    due to hysteria 300.11
  arch (foot) 734
    congenital 754.61
  back ligaments 728.4
  bladder (sphincter) 596.59
  cardio-esophageal 530.89
  cervix (*see also* Incompetency, cervix) 622.5
  diaphragm 519.4
  inguinal rings—*see* Hernia, inguinal
  joint (capsule) (ligament) (paralytic) (*see also*
    Derangement, joint) 718.90
    congenital 755.8
  lumbosacral joint 724.6
  pelvic floor 618.8
  pelvis 618.8
  perineum 618.8
  posture 729.9
  rectum (sphincter) 569.49
  sacroiliac (joint) 724.6
  scrotum 608.89
  urethra (sphincter) 599.84
  uterus (outlet) 618.8
  vagina (outlet) 618.8
  vesical 596.59
Remains
  canal of Cloquet 743.51
  capsule (opaque) 743.51
Remittent fever (malarial) 084.6
Remnant
  canal of Cloquet 743.51
  capsule (opaque) 743.51
  cervix, cervical stump (acquired)
    (postoperative) 622.8
  cystic duct, postcholecystectomy 576.0
  fingernail 703.8
    congenital 757.5
  meniscus, knee 717.5
  thyroglossal duct 759.2
  tonsil 474.8
    infected 474.00
  urachus 753.7
Remote effect of cancer —*see* Condition
Removal (of)
  catheter (urinary) (indwelling) V53.6
    from artificial opening—*see* Attention to,
      artificial, opening
    non-vascular V58.82

Removal (of)—*continued*
  vascular V58.81
  cerebral ventricle (communicating) shunt
    V53.01
  device—*see also* Fitting (of)
    contraceptive V25.42
    fixation
      external V54.89
      internal V54.0
      traction V54.89
    dressing V58.3
    ileostomy V55.2
    Kirschner wire V54.89
    non-vascular catheter V58.82
    pin V54.0
    plaster cast V54.89
    plate (fracture) V54.0
    rod V54.0
    screw V54.0
    splint, external V54.89
    subdermal implantable contraceptive V25.43
    suture V58.3
    traction device, external V54.89
    vascular catheter V58.81
Ren
  arcuatus 753.3
  mobile, mobilis (*see also* Disease, renal) 593.0
    congenital 753.3
  unguliformis 753.3
Renal —*see also* condition
  glomerulohyalinosis-diabetic syndrome 250.4
    [581.81]
Rendu-Osler-Weber disease or syndrome
  (familial hemorrhagic telangiectasia) 448.0
Reninoma (M8361/1) 236.91
Rénon-Delille syndrome 253.8
Repair
  pelvic floor, previous, in pregnancy or
    childbirth 654.4
    affecting fetus or newborn 763.89
  scarred tissue V51
Replacement by artificial or mechanical device
  or prosthesis of (*see also* Fitting (of))
  artificial skin V43.83
  bladder V43.5
  blood vessel V43.4
  breast V43.82
  eye globe V43.0
  heart V43.2
    valve V43.3
  intestine V43.89
  joint V43.60
    ankle 43.66
    elbow V43.62
    finger V43.69
    hip (partial) (total) V43.64
    knee V43.65
    shoulder V43.61
    specified NEC V43.69
    wrist V43.63
  kidney V43.89
  larynx V43.81
  lens V43.1
  limb(s) V43.7
  liver V43.89
  lung V43.89
  organ NEC V43.89
  pancreas V43.89
  skin (artificial) V43.83
  tissue NEC V43.89
Reprogramming
  cardiac pacemaker V53.31

Request for expert evidence V68.2
Reserve, decreased or low
  cardiac—*see* Disease, heart
  kidney (*see also* Disease, renal) 593.9
Residual —*see also* condition
  bladder 596.8
  foreign body—*see* Retention, foreign body
  state, schizophrenic (*see also* Schizophrenia)
    295.6
  urine 788.69
Resistance, resistant (to)

---

*Note—Use the following subclassification for
categories V09.5, V09.7, V09.8, V09.9.:*

*0 without mention of resistance to multiple
    drugs*
1 with resistance to multiple drugs

V09.5 quinolones and fluoroquinolones
V09.7 antimycobacterial agents
V09.8 specified drugs NEC
V09.9 unspecified drugs

9 multiple sites

---

  drugs by microorganisms V09.90
    Amikacin V09.4
    aminoglycosides V09.4
    Amodiaquine V09.5
    Amoxicillin V09.0
    Ampicillin V09.0
    antimycobacterial agents V09.7
    Azithromycin V09.2
    Azlocillin V09.0
    Aztreonam V09.1
    B-lactam antibiotics V09.1
    Bacampicillin V09.0
    Bacitracin V09.8
    Benznidazole V09.8
    Capreomycin V09.7
    Carbenicillin V09.0
    Cefaclor V09.1
    Cefadroxil V09.1
    Cefamandole V09.1
    Cefatetan V09.1
    Cefazolin V09.1
    Cefixime V09.1
    Cefonicid V09.1
    Cefoperazone V09.1
    Ceforanide V09.1
    Cefotaxime V09.1
    Cefoxitin V09.1
    Ceftazidine V09.1
    Ceftizoxime V09.1
    Ceftriaxone V09.1
    Cefuroxime V09.1
    Cephalexin V09.1
    Cephaloglycin V09.1
    Cephaloridine V09.1
    cephalosporins V09.1
    Cephalothin V09.1
    Cephapirin V09.1
    Cephradine V09.1
    Chloramphenicol V09.8
    Chloraquine V09.5
    Chlorguanide V09.8
    Chlorproguanil V09.8
    Chlortetracycline V09.3
    Cinoxacin V09.5
    Ciprofloxacin V09.5
    Clarithromycin V09.2

Resistance, resistant (to)—*continued*
　Clindamycin V09.8
　Clioquinol V09.5
　Clofazimine V09.7
　Cloxacillin V09.0
　Cyclacillin V09.0
　Cycloserine V09.7
　Dapsone [DZ] V09.7
　Demeclocycline V09.3
　Dicloxacillin V09.0
　Doxycycline V09.3
　Enoxacin V09.5
　Erythromycin V09.2
　Ethambutol [EMB] V09.7
　Ethionamide [ETA] V09.7
　fluoroquinolones NEC V09.5
　Gentamicin V09.4
　Halofantrine V09.8
　ImipenemV09.1
　Iodoquinol V09.5
　Isoniazid [INH] V09.7
　Kanamycin V09.4
　macrolides V09.2
　Mafenide V09.6
　Mefloquine V09.8
　Melassoprol V09.8
　Methacillin V09.0
　Methacycline V09.3
　Methenamine V09.8
　Methicillin V09.0
　Metronidazole V09.8
　Mezlocillin V09.0
　Minocycline V09.3
　Nafcillin V09.0
　Nalidixic Acid V09.5
　Natamycin V09.2
　Neomycin V09.4
　Netilmicin V09.4
　Nimorazole V09.8
　Nitrofurantoin V09.8
　Nitrofurtimox V09.8
　Norfloxacin V09.5
　Nystatin V09.2
　Ofloxacin V09.5
　Oleandomycin V09.2
　Oxacillin V09.0
　Oxytetracycline V09.3
　Para-amino salicylic acid [PAS] V09.7
　Paromomycin V09.4
　Penicillin (G)(V)(VK) V09.0
　penicillins V09.0
　Pentamidine V09.8
　Piperacillin V09.0
　Primaquine V09.5
　Proguanil V09.8
　Pyrazinamide [PZA] V09.7
　Pyrimethamine/Sulfalene V09.8
　Pyrimethamine/Sulfodoxine V09.8
　Quinacrine V09.5
　Quinidine V09.8
　Quinine V09.8
　quinolones V09.5
　Rifabutin V09.7
　Rifampin [RIF] V09.7
　Rifamycin V09.7
　Rolitetracycline V09.3
　specified drugs NEC V09.8
　Spectinomycin V09.8
　Spiramycin V09.2
　Streptomycin [SM] V09.4
　Sulfacetamide V09.6

Resistance, resistant (to)—*continued*
　Sulfacytine V90.6
　Sulfadiazine V09.6
　Sulfadoxine V09.6
　Sulfamethoxazole V09.6
　Sulfapyridine V09.6
　Sulfasalizine V09.6
　Sulfasoxazole V09.6
　sulfonamides V09.6
　Sulfoxone V09.7
　Tetracycline V09.3
　tetracyclines V09.3
　Thiamphenicol V09.8
　Ticarcillin V09.0
　Tinidazole V09.8
　Tobramycin V09.4
　Triamphenicol V09.8
　Trimethoprim V09.8
　VancomycinV09.8
Resorption
　biliary 576.8
　　purulent or putrid (*see also* Cholecystitis) 576.8
　dental (roots) 521.4
　alveoli 525.8
　septic—*see* Septicemia
　teeth (external) (internal) (pathological) (roots) 521.4
Respiration
　asymmetrical 786.09
　bronchial 786.09
　Cheyne-Stokes (periodic respiration) 786.04
　decreased, due to shock following injury 958.4
　disorder of 786.00
　　psychogenic 306.1
　　specified NEC 786.09
　failure 518.81
　　acute 518.81
　　acute and chronic 518.84
　　chronic 518.83
　　newborn 770.84
　insufficiency 786.09
　　acute 518.82
　　newborn NEC 770.89
　Kussmaul (air hunger) 786.09
　painful 786.52
　periodic 786.09
　poor 786.09
　　newborn NEC 770.89
　sighing 786.7
　　psychogenic 306.1
　wheezing 786.07
Respiratory —*see also* condition
　distress 786.09
　　acute 518.82
　　fetus or newborn NEC 770.89
　syndrome (newborn) 769
　　adult (following shock, surgery, or trauma) 518.5
　　specified NEC 518.82
　failure 518.81
　　acute 518.81
　　acute and chronic 518.84
　　chronic 518.83
Respiratory syncytial virus (RSV) 079.6
　bronchiolitis 466.11
　pneumonia 480.1
Response
　photoallergic 692.72
　phototoxic 692.72

Retinitis—*continued*
focal 363.00
  in histoplasmosis 115.92
    capsulatum 115.02
    duboisii 115.12
  juxtapapillary 363.05
  macular 363.06
  paramacular 363.06
  peripheral 363.08
  posterior pole NEC 363.07
gravidarum 646.8
hemorrhagica externa 362.12
juxtapapillary (Jensen's) 363.05
luetic—*see* Retinitis, syphilitic
metastatic 363.14
pigmentosa 362.74
proliferans 362.29
proliferating 362.29
punctata albescens 362.76
renal 585 *[363.13]*
syphilitic (secondary) 091.51
  congenital 090.0 *[363.13]*
  early 091.51
  late 095.8 *[363.13]*
syphilitica, central, recurrent 095.8 *[363.13]*
tuberculous (*see also* Tuberculous) 017.3
  [363.13]
Retinoblastoma (M9510/3) 190.5
differentiated type (M9511/3) 190.5
undifferentiated type (M9512/3) 190.5
Retinochoroiditis (*see also* Chorioretinitis)
363.20
central angiospastic 362.41
disseminated 363.10
  metastatic 363.14
  neurosyphilitic 094.83
  pigment epitheliopathy 363.15
  syphilitic 094.83
due to toxoplasmosis (acquired) (focal) 130.2
focal 363.00
  in histoplasmosis 115.92
    capsulatum 115.02
    duboisii 115.12
  juxtapapillary (Jensen's) 363.05
  macular 363.06
  paramacular 363.06
  peripheral 363.08
  posterior pole NEC 363.07
juxtapapillaris 363.05
syphilitic (disseminated) 094.83
Retinopathy (background) 362.10
arteriosclerotic 440.8 *[362.13]*
atherosclerotic 440.8 *[362.13]*
central serous 362.41
circinate 362.10
Coat's 362.12
diabetic 250.5 *[362.01]*
  proliferative 250.5 *[362.02]*
exudative 362.12
hypertensive 362.11
of prematurity 362.21
pigmentary, congenital 362.74
proliferative 362.29
  diabetic 250.5 *[362.02]*
  sickle-cell 282.60 *[362.29]*
solar 363.31
Retinoschisis 361.10
bullous 361.12
congenital 743.56
flat 361.11
juvenile 362.73
Retractile testis 752.52

Retraction
cervix (*see also* Retroversion, uterus) 621.6
drum (membrane) 384.82
eyelid 374.41
finger 736.29
head 781.0
lid 374.41
lung 518.89
mediastinum 519.3
nipple 611.79
  congenital 757.6
  puerperal, postpartum 676.0
palmar fascia 728.6
pleura (*see also* Pleurisy) 511.0
ring, uterus (Bandl's) (pathological) 661.4
  affecting fetus or newborn 763.7
sternum (congenital) 756.3
  acquired 738.3
  during respiration 786.9
substernal 738.3
supraclavicular 738.8
syndrome (Duane's) 378.71
uterus (*see also* Retroversion, uterus) 621.6
valve (heart)—*see* Endocarditis
Retrobulbar —*see* condition
Retrocaval ureter 753.4
Retrocecal —*see also* condition
appendix (congenital) 751.5
Retrocession —*see* Retroversion
Retrodisplacement —*see* Retroversion
Retroflection, retroflexion —*see* Retroversion
Retrognathia, retrognathism (mandibular)
  (maxillary) 524.06
Retrograde
ejaculation 608.87
menstruation 626.8
Retroiliac ureter 753.4
Retroperineal —*see* condition
Retroperitoneal —*see* condition
Retroperitonitis (*see also* Peritonitis) 567.9
Retropharyngeal —*see* condition
Retroplacental —*see* condition
Retroposition —*see* Retroversion
Retrosternal thyroid (congenital) 759.2
Retroversion, retroverted
cervix (*see also* Retroversion, uterus) 621.6
female NEC (*see also* Retroversion, uterus)
  621.6
iris 364.70
testis (congenital) 752.51
uterus, uterine (acquired) (acute) (adherent)
  (any degree) (asymptomatic) (cervix)
  (postinfectional) (postpartal, old) 621.6
  congenital 752.3
  in pregnancy or childbirth 654.3
    affecting fetus or newborn 763.89
    causing obstructed labor 660.2
      affecting fetus or newborn 763.1
Retrusion, premaxilla (developmental) 524.04
Rett's syndrome 330.8
Reverse, reversed
peristalsis 787.4
Reye's syndrome 331.81
Reye-Sheehan syndrome (postpartum pituitary
  necrosis) 253.2
Rh (factor)
hemolytic disease 773.0
incompatibility, immunization, or sensitization
  affecting management of pregnancy 656.1
  fetus or newborn 773.0
  transfusion reaction 999.7

Rh (factor)—*continued*
  negative mother, affecting fetus or newborn
      773.0
  titer elevated 999.7
  transfusion reaction 999.7
Rhabdomyolysis (idiopathic) 728.89
Rhabdomyoma (M8900/0)—*see also* Neoplasm,
    connective tissue, benign
  adult (M8904/0)—*see* Neoplasm, connective
      tissue, benign
  fetal (M8903/0)—*see* Neoplasm, connective
      tissue, benign
  glycogenic (M8904/0)—*see* Neoplasm,
      connective tissue, benign
Rhabdomyosarcoma (M8900/3)—*see also*
    Neoplasm connective tissue, malignant
  alveolar (M8920/3)—*see* Neoplasm, connective
      tissue, malignant
  embryonal (M8910/3)—*see* Neoplasm,
      connective tissue malignant
  mixed type (M8902/3)—*see* Neoplasm,
      connective tissue, malignant
  pleomorphic (M8901/3)—*see* Neoplasm,
      connective tissue, malignant
Rhabdosarcoma (M8900/3)—*see*
    Rhabdomyosarcoma
Rhesus (factor) (Rh) incompatibility—*see* Rh,
    incompatibility
Rheumaticosis —*see* Rheumatism
Rheumatism, rheumatic (acute NEC) 729.0
  adherent pericardium 393
  arthritis
    acute or subacute—*see* Fever, rheumatic
    chronic 714.0
      spine 720.0
  articular (chronic) NEC (*see also* Arthritis)
      716.9
    acute or subacute—*see* Fever, rheumatic
  back 724.9
  blennorrhagic 098.59
  carditis—*see* Disease, heart, rheumatic
  cerebral—*see* Fever, rheumatic
  chorea (acute)—*see* Chorea, rheumatic
  chronic NEC 729.0
  coronary arteritis 391.9
    chronic 398.99
  degeneration, myocardium (*see also*
      Degeneration, myocardium, with rheumatic
      fever) 398.0
  desert 114.0
  febrile—*see* Fever, rheumatic
  fever—*see* Fever, rheumatic
  gonococcal 098.59
  gout 274.0
  heart
    disease (*see also* Disease, heart, rheumatic)
        398.90
    failure (chronic) (congestive) (inactive) 398.91
  hemopericardium—*see* Rheumatic, pericarditis
  hydropericardium—*see* Rheumatic, pericarditis
  inflammatory (acute) (chronic) (subacute)—*see*
      Fever, rheumatic
  intercostal 729.0
    meaning Tietze's disease 733.6
  joint (chronic) NEC (*see also* Arthritis) 716.9
    acute—*see* Fever, rheumatic
  mediastinopericarditis—*see* Rheumatic,
      pericarditis
  muscular 729.0

Rheumatism, rheumatic—*continued*
  myocardial degeneration (*see also*
      Degeneration, myocardium, with rheumatic
      fever) 398.0
  myocarditis (chronic) (inactive) (with chorea)
      398.0
    active or acute 391.2
      with chorea (acute) (rheumatic)
          (Sydenham's) 392.0
  myositis 729.1
  neck 724.9
  neuralgic 729.0
  neuritis (acute) (chronic) 729.2
  neuromuscular 729.0
  nodose—*see* Arthritis, nodosa
  nonarticular 729.0
  palindromic 719.30
    ankle 719.37
    elbow 719.32
    foot 719.37
    hand 719.34
    hip 719.35
    knee 719.36
    multiple sites 719.39
    pelvic region 719.35
    shoulder (region) 719.31
    specified site NEC 719.38
    wrist 719.33
  pancarditis, acute 391.8
    with chorea (acute) (rheumatic) (Sydenham's)
        392.0
    chronic or inactive 398.99
  pericarditis (active) (acute) (with effusion) (with
      pneumonia) 391.0
    with chorea (acute) (rheumatic) (Sydenham's)
        392.0
    chronic or inactive 393
  pericardium—*see* Rheumatic, pericarditis
  pleuropericarditis—*see* Rheumatic, pericarditis
  pneumonia 390 *[517.1]*
  pneumonitis 390 *[517.1]*
  pneumopericarditis—*see* Rheumatic, pericarditis
  polyarthritis
    acute or subacute—*see* Fever, rheumatic
    chronic 714.0
  polyarticular NEC (*see also* Arthritis) 716.9
  psychogenic 306.0
  radiculitis 729.2
  sciatic 724.3
  septic—*see* Fever, rheumatic
  spine 724.9
  subacute NEC 729.0
  torticollis 723.5
  tuberculous NEC (*see also* Tuberculosis) 015.9
  typhoid fever 002.0
Rheumatoid —*see also* condition
  lungs 714.81
Rhinitis (atrophic) (catarrhal) (chronic)
    (croupous) (fibrinous) (hyperplastic)
    (hypertrophic) (membranous) (purulent)
    (suppurative) (ulcerative) 472.0
  with
    hay fever (*see also* Fever, hay) 477.9
      with asthma (bronchial) 493.0
    sore throat—*see* Nasopharyngitis
  acute 460
  allergic (nonseasonal) (seasonal) (*see also*
      Fever, hay) 477.9
    due to food 477.1
    with asthma (*see also* Asthma) 493.0
  granulomatous 472.0

Rhinitis—*continued*
  infective 460
  obstructive 472.0
  pneumococcal 460
  syphilitic 095.8
    congenital 090.0
  tuberculous (*see also* Tuberculosis) 012.8
  vasomotor (*see also* Fever, hay) 477.9
Rhinoantritis (chronic) 473.0
  acute 461.0
Rhinodacryolith 375.57
Rhinolalia (aperta) (clausa) (open) 784.49
Rhinolith 478.1
  nasal sinus (*see also* Sinusitis) 473.9
Rhinomegaly 478.1
Rhinopharyngitis (acute) (subacute) (*see also*
    Nasopharyngitis) 460
  chronic 472.2
  destructive ulcerating 102.5
  mutilans 102.5
Rhinophyma 695.3
Rhinorrhea 478.1
  cerebrospinal (fluid) 349.81
  paroxysmal (*see also* Fever, hay) 477.9
  spasmodic (*see also* Fever, hay) 477.9
Rhinosalpingitis 381.50
  acute 381.51
  chronic 381.52
Rhinoscleroma 040.1
Rhinosporidiosis 117.0
Rhinovirus infection 079.3
Rhizomelique, pseudopolyarthritic 446.5
Rhoads and Bomford anemia (refractory) 284.9
Rhus
  diversiloba dermatitis 692.6
  radicans dermatitis 692.6
  toxicodendron dermatitis 692.6
  venenata dermatitis 692.6
  verniciflua dermatitis 692.6
Rhythm
  atrioventricular nodal 427.89
  disorder 427.9
    coronary sinus 427.89
    ectopic 427.89
    nodal 427.89
  escape 427.89
  heart, abnormal 427.9
    fetus or newborn—*see* Abnormal, heart rate
  idioventricular 426.89
    accelerated 427.89
  nodal 427.89
  sleep, inversion 780.55
    nonorganic origin 307.45
Rhytidosis facialis 701.8
Rib —*see also* condition
  cervical 756.2
Riboflavin deficiency 266.0
Rice bodies (*see also* Loose, body, joint) 718.1
  knee 717.6
Richter's hernia —*see* Hernia, Richter's
Ricinism 988.2
Rickets (active) (acute) (adolescent) (adult)
    (chest wall) (congenital) (current) (infantile)
    (intestinal) 268.0
  celiac 579.0
  fetal 756.4
  hemorrhagic 267
  hypophosphatemic with nephrotic-glycosuric
    dwarfism 270.0
  kidney 588.0
  late effect 268.1

Rickets—*continued*
  renal 588.0
  scurvy 267
  vitamin D-resistant 275.3
Rickettsial disease 083.9
  specified type NEC 083.8
Rickettsialpox 083.2
Rickettsiosis NEC 083.9
  specified type NEC 083.8
  tick-borne 082.9
    specified type NEC 082.8
  vesicular 083.2
Ricord's chancre 091.0
Riddoch's syndrome (visual disorientation)
    368.16
Rider's
  bone 733.99
  chancre 091.0
Ridge, alveolus —*see also* condition
  flabby 525.2
Ridged ear 744.29
Riedel's
  disease (ligneous thyroiditis) 245.3
  lobe, liver 751.69
  struma (ligneous thyroiditis) 245.3
  thyroiditis (ligneous) 245.3
Rieger's anomaly or syndrome (mesodermal
    dysgenesis, anterior ocular segment) 743.44
Riehl's melanosis 709.09
Rietti-Greppi-Micheli anemia or syndrome
    282.4
Rieux's hernia —*see* Hernia, Rieux's
Rift Valley fever 066.3
Riga's disease (cachectic aphthae) 529.0
Riga-Fede disease (cachectic aphthae) 529.0
Riggs' disease (compound periodontitis) 523.4
Right middle lobe syndrome 518.0
Rigid, rigidity —*see also* condition
  abdominal 789.4
  articular, multiple congenital 754.89
  back 724.8
  cervix uteri
    in pregnancy or childbirth 654.6
      affecting fetus or newborn 763.89
      causing obstructed labor 660.2
        affecting fetus or newborn 763.1
  hymen (acquired) (congenital) 623.3
  nuchal 781.6
  pelvic floor
    in pregnancy or childbirth 654.4
      affecting fetus or newborn 763.89
      causing obstructed labor 660.2
        affecting fetus or newborn 763.1
  perineum or vulva
    in pregnancy or childbirth 654.8
      affecting fetus or newborn 763.89
      causing obstructed labor 660.2
        affecting fetus or newborn 763.1
  spine 724.8
  vagina
    in pregnancy or childbirth 654.7
      affecting fetus or newborn 763.89
      causing obstructed labor 660.2
        affecting fetus or newborn 763.1
Rigors 780.99
Riley-Day syndrome (familial dysautonomia)
    742.8
Ring(s)
  aorta 747.21
  Bandl's, complicating delivery 661.4
    affecting fetus or newborn 763.7

Ring(s)—*continued*
contraction, complicating delivery 661.4
  affecting fetus or newborn 763.7
esophageal (congenital) 750.3
Fleischer (-Kayser) (cornea) 275.1 *[371.14]*
hymenal, tight (acquired) (congenital) 623.3
Kayser-Fleischer (cornea) 275.1 *[371.14]*
retraction, uterus, pathological 661.4
  affecting fetus or newborn 763.7
Schatzki's (esophagus) (congenital) (lower)
  750.3
  acquired 530.3
Soemmering's 366.51
trachea, abnormal 748.3
vascular (congenital) 747.21
Vossius' 921.3
  late effect 366.21
Ringed hair (congenital) 757.4
Ringing in the ear (*see also* Tinnitus) 388.30
Ringworm 110.9
beard 110.0
body 110.5
Burmese 110.9
corporeal 110.5
foot 110.4
groin 110.3
hand 110.2
honeycomb 110.0
nails 110.1
perianal (area) 110.3
scalp 110.0
specified site NEC 110.8
Tokelau 110.5
Rise, venous pressure 459.89
Risk
factor —*see* Problem
suicidal 300.9
Ritter's disease (dermatitis exfoliativa
  neonatorum) 695.81
Rivalry, sibling 313.3
Rivalta's disease (cervicofacial actinomycosis)
  039.3
River blindness 125.3 *[360.13]*
Robert's pelvis 755.69
with disproportion (fetopelvic) 653.0
  affecting fetus or newborn 763.1
  causing obstructed labor 660.1
    affecting fetus or newborn 763.1
Robin's syndrome 756.0
Robinson's (hidrotic) ectodermal dysplasia
  757.31
Robles' disease (onchocerciasis) 125.3 *[360.13]*
Rochalimea —*see* Rickettsial disease
Rocky Mountain fever (spotted) 082.0
Rodent ulcer (M8090/3)—*see also* Neoplasm,
  skin, malignant
  cornea 370.07
Roentgen ray, adverse effect —*see* Effect,
  adverse, x-ray
Roetheln 056.9
Roger's disease (congenital interventricular
  septal defect) 745.4
Rokitansky's
disease (*see also* Necrosis, liver) 570
tumor 620.2
Rokitansky-Aschoff sinuses (mucosal
  outpouching of gallbladder) (*see also* Disease,
  gallbladder) 575.8
Rokitansky-Kuster-Hauser syndrome
  (congenital absence vagina) 752.49
Rollet's chancre (syphilitic) 091.0
Rolling of head 781.0

Romano-Ward syndrome (prolonged Q-T
  interval) 794.31
Romanus lesion 720.1
Romberg's disease or syndrome 349.89
Roof, mouth —*see* condition
Rosacea 695.3
acne 695.3
keratitis 695.3 *[370.49]*
Rosary, rachitic 268.0
Rose
cold 477.0
fever 477.0
rash 782.1
  epidemic 056.9
  of infants 057.8
Rosen-Castleman-Liebow syndrome
  (pulmonary proteinosis) 516.0
Rosenbach's erysipelatoid or erysipeloid 027.1
Rosenthal's disease (factor XI deficiency) 286.2
Roseola 057.8
infantum, infantilis 057.8
Rossbach's disease (hyperchlorhydria) 536.8
psychogenic 306.4
Rössle-Urbach-Wiethe lipoproteinosis 272.8
Ross river fever 066.3
Rostan's asthma (cardiac) (*see also* Failure,
  ventricular, left) 428.1
Rot
Barcoo (*see also* Ulcer, skin) 707.9
knife-grinders' (*see also* Tuberculosis) 011.4
Rot-Bernhardt disease 355.1
Rotation
anomalous, incomplete or insufficient—*see*
  Malrotation
cecum (congenital) 751.4
colon (congenital) 751.4
manual, affecting fetus or newborn 763.89
spine, incomplete or insufficient 737.8
tooth, teeth 524.3
vertebra, incomplete or insufficient 737.8
Röteln 056.9
Roth's disease or meralgia 355.1
Roth-Bernhardt disease or syndrome 355.1
Rothmund (-Thomson) syndrome 757.33
Rotor's disease or syndrome (idiopathic
  hyperbilirubinemia) 277.4
Rotundum ulcus —*see* Ulcer, stomach
Round
back (with wedging of vertebrae) 737.10
  late effect of rickets 268.1
hole, retina 361.31
  with detachment 361.01
ulcer (stomach)—*see* Ulcer, stomach
worms (infestation) (large) NEC 127.0
Roussy-Lévy syndrome 334.3
Routine postpartum follow-up V24.2
Roy (-Jutras) syndrome (acropachyderma) 757.39
Rubella (German measles) 056.9
complicating pregnancy, childbirth, or
  puerperium 647.5
complication 056.8
  neurological 056.00
    encephalomyelitis 056.01
    specified type NEC 056.09
  specified type NEC 056.79
congenital 771.0
contact V01.4
exposure to V01.4
maternal
  with suspected fetal damage affecting
    management of pregnancy 655.3

Rubella—*continued*
　affecting fetus or newborn 760.2
　　manifest rubella in infant 771.0
　specified complications NEC 056.79
　vaccination, prophylactic (against) V04.3
Rubeola (measles) (*see also* Measles) 055.9
　complicated 055.8
　meaning rubella (*see also* Rubella) 056.9
　scarlatinosis 057.8
Rubeosis iridis 364.42
　diabetica 250.5 *[364.42]*
Rubinstein-Taybi's syndrome (brachydactylia,
　short stature and mental retardation) 759.89
Rud's syndrome (mental deficiency, epilepsy,
　and infantilism) 759.89
Rudimentary (congenital)—*see also* Agenesis
　arm 755.22
　bone 756.9
　cervix uteri 752.49
　eye (*see also* Microphthalmos) 743.10
　fallopian tube 752.19
　leg 755.32
　lobule of ear 744.21
　patella 755.64
　respiratory organs in thoracopagus 759.4
　tracheal bronchus 748.3
　uterine horn 752.3
　uterus 752.3
　　in male 752.7
　　solid or with cavity 752.3
　vagina 752.49
Ruiter-Pompen (-Wyers) syndrome
　(angiokeratoma corporis diffusum) 272.7
Ruled out condition (*see also* Observation,
　suspected) V71.9
Rumination —*see also* Vomiting
　neurotic 300.3
　obsessional 300.3
　psychogenic 307.53
Runaway reaction —*see also* Disturbance,
　conduct
　socialized 312.2
　undersocialized, unsocialized 312.1
Runeberg's disease (progressive pernicious
　anemia) 281.0
Runge's syndrome (postmaturity) 766.2
Rupia 091.3
　congenital 090.0
　tertiary 095.9
Rupture, ruptured 553.9
　abdominal viscera NEC 799.8
　　obstetrical trauma 665.5
　abscess (spontaneous)—*see* Abscess, by site
　amnion—*see* Rupture, membranes
　aneurysm—*see* Aneurysm
　anus (sphincter)—*see* Laceration, anus
　aorta, aortic 441.5
　　abdominal 441.3
　　arch 441.1
　　ascending 441.1
　　descending 441.5
　　　abdominal 441.3
　　　thoracic 441.1
　　syphilitic 093.0
　　thoracoabdominal 441.6
　　thorax, thoracic 441.1
　　transverse 441.1
　　traumatic (thoracic) 901.0
　　　abdominal 902.0
　　valve or cusp (*see also* Endocarditis, aortic)
　　　424.1

Rupture, ruptured—*continued*
　appendix (with peritonitis) 540.0
　　traumatic—*see* Injury, internal,
　　　gastrointestinal tract
　　with peritoneal abscess 540.1
　arteriovenous fistula, brain (congenital) 430
　artery 447.2
　　brain (*see also* Hemorrhage, brain) 431
　　coronary (*see also* Infarct, myocardium) 410.9
　　heart (*see also* Infarct, myocardium) 410.9
　　pulmonary 417.8
　　traumatic (complication) (*see also* Injury,
　　　blood vessel, by site) 904.9
　bile duct, except cystic (*see also* Disease,
　　biliary) 576.3
　　cystic 575.4
　　traumatic—*see* Injury, internal,
　　　intra-abdominal
　bladder (sphincter) 596.6
　　with
　　　abortion—*see* Abortion, by type, with
　　　　damage to pelvic organs
　　　ectopic pregnancy (*see also* categories
　　　　633.0-633.9) 639.2
　　　molar pregnancy (*see also* categories
　　　　630-632) 639.2
　　following
　　　abortion 639.2
　　　ectopic or molar pregnancy 639.2
　　nontraumatic 596.6
　　obstetrical trauma 665.5
　　spontaneous 596.6
　　traumatic—*see* Injury, internal, bladder
　blood vessel (*see also* Hemorrhage) 459.0
　　brain (*see also* Hemorrhage, brain) 431
　　heart (*see also* Infarct, myocardium) 410.9
　　traumatic (complication) (*see also* Injury,
　　　blood vessel, by site) 904.9
　bone—*see* Fracture, by site
　bowel 569.89
　　traumatic—*see* Injury, internal, intestine
　Bowman's membrane 371.31
　brain
　　aneurysm (congenital) (*see also* Hemorrhage,
　　　subarachnoid) 430
　　　late effect—*see* Late effect(s) (of)
　　　　cerebrovascular disease
　　　syphilitic 094.87
　　hemorrhagic (*see also* Hemorrhage, brain) 431
　　injury at birth 767.0
　　syphilitic 094.89
　capillaries 448.9
　cardiac (*see also* Infarct, myocardium) 410.9
　cartilage (articular) (current)—*see also* Sprain,
　　by site
　　knee—*see* Tear, meniscus
　　semilunar—*see* Tear, meniscus
　cecum (with peritonitis) 540.0
　　traumatic 863.89
　　　with open wound into cavity 863.99
　　with peritoneal abscess 540.1
　cerebral aneurysm (congenital) (*see also*
　　Hemorrhage, subarachnoid) 430
　　late effect—*see* Late effect(s) (of)
　　　cerebrovascular disease
　cervix (uteri)
　　with
　　　abortion—*see* Abortion, by type, with
　　　　damage to pelvic organs
　　　ectopic pregnancy (*see also* categories
　　　　633.0-633.9) 639.2

Rupture, ruptured—*continued*
   molar pregnancy (*see also* categories
      630-632) 639.2
   following
     abortion 639.2
     ectopic or molar pregnancy 639.2
     obstetrical trauma 665.3
     traumatic—*see* Injury, internal, cervix
   chordae tendineae 429.5
   choroid (direct) (indirect) (traumatic) 363.63
   circle of Willis (*see also* Hemorrhage,
     subarachnoid) 430
     late effect—*see* Late effect(s) (of)
      cerebrovascular disease
   colon 569.89
     traumatic—*see* Injury, internal, colon
   cornea (traumatic)—*see also* Rupture, eye
     due to ulcer 370.00
   coronary (artery) (thrombotic) (*see also* Infarct,
     myocardium) 410.9
   corpus luteum (infected) (ovary) 620.1
   cyst—*see* Cyst
   cystic duct (*see also* Disease, gallbladder) 575.4
   Descemet's membrane 371.33
     traumatic—*see* Rupture, eye
   diaphragm—*see also* Hernia, diaphragm
     traumatic—*see* Injury, internal, diaphragm
   diverticulum
     bladder 596.3
     intestine (large) (*see also* Diverticula) 562.10
      small 562.00
   duodenal stump 537.89
   duodenum (ulcer)—*see* Ulcer, duodenum, with
     perforation
   ear drum (*see also* Perforation, tympanum)
     384.20
     with otitis media—*see* Otitis media
     traumatic—*see* Wound, open, ear
   esophagus 530.4
     traumatic 862.22
      with open wound into cavity 862.32
      cervical region—*see* Wound, open,
       esophagus
   eye (without prolapse of intraocular tissue) 871.0
     with
      exposure of intraocular tissue 871.1
      partial loss of intraocular tissue 871.2
      prolapse of intraocular tissue 871.1
     due to burn 940.5
   fallopian tube 620.8
     due to pregnancy—*see* Pregnancy, tubal
     traumatic—*see* Injury, internal, fallopian tube
   fontanel 767.3
   free wall (ventricle) (*see also* Infarct,
     myocardium) 410.9
   gallbladder or duct (*see also* Disease,
     gallbladder) 575.4
     traumatic—*see* Injury, internal, gallbladder
   gastric (*see also* Rupture, stomach) 537.89
     vessel 459.0
   globe (eye) (traumatic)—*see* Rupture, eye
   graafian follicle (hematoma) 620.0
   heart (auricle) (ventricle) (*see also* Infarct,
     myocardium) 410.9
     infectional 422.90
     traumatic—*see* Rupture, myocardium,
      traumatic
   hymen 623.8
   internal
     organ, traumatic—*see also* Injury, internal, by
     site

Rupture, ruptured—*continued*
   heart—*see* Rupture, myocardium, traumatic
   kidney—*see* Rupture, kidney
   liver—*see* Rupture, liver
   spleen—*see* Rupture, spleen, traumatic
   semilunar cartilage—*see* Tear, meniscus
   intervertebral disc—*see* Displacement,
     intervertebral disc
     traumatic (current)—*see* Dislocation, vertebra
   intestine 569.89
     traumatic—*see* Injury, internal, intestine
   intracranial, birth injury 767.0
   iris 364.76
     traumatic—*see* Rupture, eye
   joint capsule—*see* Sprain, by site
   kidney (traumatic) 866.03
     with open wound into cavity 866.13
     due to birth injury 767.8
     nontraumatic 593.89
   lacrimal apparatus (traumatic) 870.2
   lens (traumatic) 366.20
   ligament—*see also* Sprain, by site
     with open wound—*see* Wound, open, by site
     old (*see also* Disorder, cartilage, articular)
      718.0
   liver (traumatic) 864.04
     with open wound into cavity 864.14
     due to birth injury 767.8
     nontraumatic 573.8
   lymphatic (node) (vessel) 457.8
   marginal sinus (placental) (with hemorrhage)
     641.2
     affecting fetus or newborn 762.1
   meaning hernia—*see* Hernia
   membrana tympani (*see also* Perforation,
     tympanum) 384.20
     with otitis media—*see* Otitis media
     traumatic—*see* Wound, open, ear
   membranes (spontaneous)
     artificial
      delayed delivery following 658.3
       affecting fetus or newborn 761.1
       fetus or newborn 761.1
     delayed delivery following 658.2
      affecting fetus or newborn 761.1
     premature (less than 24 hours prior to onset of
      labor) 658.1
      affecting fetus or newborn 761.1
      delayed delivery following 658.2
      affecting fetus or newborn 761.1
   meningeal artery (*see also* Hemorrhage,
     subarachnoid) 430
     late effect—*see* Late effect(s) (of)
      cerebrovascular disease
   meniscus (knee)—*see also* Tear, meniscus
     old (*see also* Derangement, meniscus) 717.5
     site other than knee—*see* Disorder,
      cartilage, articular
     site other than knee—*see* Sprain, by site
   mesentery 568.89
     traumatic—*see* Injury, internal, mesentery
   mitral—*see* Insufficiency, mitral
   muscle (traumatic) NEC—*see also* Sprain, by
     site
     with open wound—*see* Wound, open, by site
     nontraumatic 728.83
   musculotendinous cuff (nontraumatic)
     (shoulder) 840.4
   mycotic aneurysm, causing cerebral hemorrhage
     (*see also* Hemorrhage, subarachnoid) 430

Rupture, ruptured—*continued*

late effect—*see* Late effect(s) (of) cerebrovascular disease

myocardium, myocardial (*see also* Infarct, myocardium) 410.9

traumatic 861.03

with open wound into thorax 861.13

nontraumatic (meaning hernia) (*see also* Hernia, by site) 553.9

obstructed (*see also* Hernia, by site, with obstruction) 552.9

gangrenous (*see also* Hernia, by site, with gangrene) 551.9

operation wound 998.32

internal 998.31

ovary, ovarian 620.8

corpus luteum 620.1

follicle (graafian) 620.0

oviduct 620.8

due to pregnancy—*see* Pregnancy, tubal

pancreas 577.8

traumatic—*see* Injury, internal, pancreas

papillary muscle (ventricular) 429.6

pelvic

floor, complicating delivery 664.1

organ NEC—*see* Injury, pelvic, organs

penis (traumatic)—*see* Wound, open, penis

perineum 624.8

during delivery (*see also* Laceration, perineum, complicating delivery) 664.4

pharynx (nontraumatic) (spontaneous) 478.29

pregnant uterus (before onset of labor) 665.0

prostate (traumatic)—*see* Injury, internal, prostate

pulmonary

artery 417.8

valve (heart) (*see also* Endocarditis, pulmonary) 424.3

vein 417.8

vessel 417.8

pupil, sphincter 364.75

pus tube (*see also* Salpingo-oophoritis) 614.2

pyosalpinx (*see also* Salpingo-oophoritis) 614.2

rectum 569.49

traumatic—*see* Injury, internal, rectum

retina, retinal (traumatic) (without detachment) 361.30

with detachment (*see also* Detachment, retina, with retinal defect) 361.00

rotator cuff (capsule) (traumatic) 840.4

nontraumatic, complete 727.61

sclera 871.0

semilunar cartilage, knee (*see also* Tear, meniscus) 836.2

old (*see also* Derangement, meniscus) 717.5

septum (cardiac) 410.8

sigmoid 569.89

traumatic—*see* Injury, internal, colon, sigmoid

sinus of Valsalva 747.29

spinal cord—*see also* Injury, spinal, by site

due to injury at birth 767.4

fetus or newborn 767.4

syphilitic 094.89

traumatic—*see also* Injury, spinal, by site

with fracture—*see* Fracture, vertebra, by site, with spinal cord injury

spleen 289.59

congenital 767.8

due to injury at birth 767.8

malarial 084.9

nontraumatic 289.59

Rupture, ruptured—*continued*

spontaneous 289.59

traumatic 865.04

with open wound into cavity 865.14

splenic vein 459.0

stomach 537.89

due to injury at birth 767.8

traumatic—*see* Injury, internal, stomach

ulcer—*see* Ulcer, stomach, with perforation

synovium 727.50

specified site NEC 727.59

tendon (traumatic)—*see also* Sprain, by site

with open wound—*see* Wound, open, by site

Achilles 845.09

nontraumatic 727.67

ankle 845.09

nontraumatic 727.68

biceps (long bead) 840.8

nontraumatic 727.62

foot 845.10

interphalangeal (joint) 845.13

metatarsophalangeal (joint) 845.12

nontraumatic 727.68

specified site NEC 845.19

tarsometatarsal (joint) 845.11

hand 842.10

carpometacarpal (joint) 842.11

interphalangeal (joint) 842.13

metacarpophalangeal (joint) 842.12

nontraumatic 727.63

extensors 727.63

flexors 727.64

specified site NEC 842.19

nontraumatic 727.60

specified site NEC 727.69

patellar 844.8

nontraumatic 727.66

quadriceps 844.8

nontraumatic 727.65

rotator cuff (capsule) 840.4

nontraumatic, complete 727.61

wrist 842.00

carpal (joint) 842.01

nontraumatic 727.63

extensors 727.63

flexors 727.64

radiocarpal (joint) (ligament) 842.02

radioulnar (joint), distal 842.09

specified site NEC 842.09

testis (traumatic) 878.2

complicated 878.3

due to syphilis 095.8

thoracic duct 457.8

tonsil 474.8

traumatic

with open wound—*see* Wound, open, by site

aorta—*see* Rupture, aorta, traumatic

ear drum—*see* Wound, open, ear, drum

external site—*see* Wound, open, by site

eye 871.2

globe (eye)—*see* Wound, open, eyeball

internal organ (abdomen, chest, or pelvis)—*see also* Injury, internal, by site

heart—*see* Rupture, myocardium, traumatic

kidney—*see* Rupture, kidney

liver—*see* Rupture, liver

spleen—*see* Rupture, spleen, traumatic

ligament, muscle, or tendon—*see also* Sprain, by site

with open wound—*see* Wound, open, by site

meaning hernia—*see* Hernia

Rupture, ruptured—*continued*
  tricuspid (heart) (valve)—*see* Endocarditis,
     tricuspid
  tube, tubal 620.8
    abscess (*see also* Salpingo-oophoritis) 614.2
    due to pregnancy—*see* Pregnancy, tubal
  tympanum, tympanic (membrane) (*see also*
     Perforation, tympanum) 384.20
    with otitis media—*see* Otitis media
    traumatic—*see* Wound, open, ear, drum
  umbilical cord 663.8
    fetus or newborn 772.0
  ureter (traumatic) (*see also* Injury, internal,
     ureter) 867.2
    nontraumatic 593.89
  urethra 599.84
    with
      abortion—*see* Abortion, by type, with
        damage to pelvic organs
      ectopic pregnancy (*see also* categories
        633.0-633.9) 639.2
      molar pregnancy (*see also* categories
        630-632) 639.2
    following
      abortion 639.2
      ectopic or molar pregnancy 639.2
    obstetrical trauma 665.5
    traumatic—*see* Injury, internal urethra
  uterosacral ligament 620.8
  uterus (traumatic)—*see also* Injury, internal
     uterus
    affecting fetus or newborn 763.89
    during labor 665.1
    nonpuerperal, nontraumatic 621.8
    nontraumatic 621.8
    pregnant (during labor) 665.1
     before labor 665.0
  vaginal 878.6
    complicated 878.7
    complicating delivery—*see* Laceration,
     vagina, complicating delivery
  valve, valvular (heart)—*see* Endocarditis
  varicose vein—*see* Varicose, vein
  varix—*see* Varix
  vena cava 459.0
  ventricle (free wall) (left) (*see also* Infarct,
     myocardium) 410.9
  vesical (urinary) 596.6
    traumatic—*see* Injury, internal, bladder
  vessel (blood) 459.0
    pulmonary 417.8
  viscus 799.8
  vulva 878.4
    complicated 878.5
    complicating delivery 664.0
Russell's dwarf (uterine dwarfism and
  craniofacial dysostosis) 759.89
Russell's dysentery 004.8
Russell (-Silver) syndrome (congenital
  hemihypertrophy and short stature) 759.89
Russian spring-summer type encephalitis 063.0
Rust's disease (tuberculous spondylitis) 015.0
  [720.81]
Rustitskii's disease (multiple myeloma)
  (M9730/3) 203.0
Ruysch's disease (Hirschsprung's disease) 751.3
Rytand-Lipsitch syndrome (complete
  atrioventricular block) 426.0

S

Saber
  shin 090.5
  tibia 090.5
Sac, lacrimal —*see* condition
Saccharomyces infection (*see also* Candidiasis)
  112.9
Saccharopinuria 270.7
Saccular —*see* condition
Sacculation
  aorta (nonsyphilitic) (*see also* Aneurysm, aorta)
    441.9
    ruptured 441.5
    syphilitic 093.0
  bladder 596.3
  colon 569.89
  intralaryngeal (congenital) (ventricular) 748.3
  larynx (congenital) (ventricular) 748.3
  organ or site, congenital—*see* Distortion
  pregnant uterus, complicating delivery 654.4
    affecting fetus or newborn 763.1
      causing obstructed labor 660.2
        affecting fetus or newborn 763.1
  rectosigmoid 569.89
  sigmoid 569.89
  ureter 593.89
  urethra 599.2
  vesical 596.3
Sachs (-Tay) disease (amaurotic familial idiocy)
  330.1
Sacks-Libman disease 710.0 *[424.91]*
Sacralgia 724.6
Sacralization
  fifth lumbar vertebra 756.15
  incomplete (vertebra) 756.15
Sacrodynia 724.6
Sacroiliac joint —*see* condition
Sacroiliitis NEC 720.2
Sacrum —*see* condition
Saddle
  back 737.8
  embolus, aorta 444.0
  nose 738.0
    congenital 754.0
    due to syphilis 090.5
Sadism (sexual) 302.84
Saemisch's ulcer 370.04
Saenger's syndrome 379.46
Sago spleen 277.3
Sailors' skin 692.74
Saint
  Anthony's fire (*see also* Erysipelas) 035
  Guy's dance—*see* Chorea
  Louis-type encephalitis 062.3
  triad (*see also* Hernia, diaphragm) 553.3
  Vitus' dance—*see* Chorea
Salicylism
  correct substance properly administered 535.4
  overdose or wrong substance given or taken
    965.1
Salivary duct or gland —*see also* condition
  virus disease 078.5
Salivation (excessive) (*see also* Ptyalism) 527.7
Salmonella (aertrycke) (choleraesuis)
  (enteritidis) (gallinarum) (suipestifer)
  (typhimurium) (*see also* Infection,
  Salmonella) 003.9
  arthritis 003.23
  carrier (suspected) of V02.3

Salmonella—*continued*
  meningitis 003.21
  osteomyelitis 003.24
  pneumonia 003.22
  septicemia 003.1
  typhosa 002.0
    carrier (suspected) of V02.1
Salmonellosis 003.0
  with pneumonia 003.22
Salpingitis (catarrhal) (fallopian tube) (nodular)
  (pseudofollicular) (purulent) (septic) (*see also*
  Salpingo-oophoritis) 614.2
  ear 381.50
    acute 381.51
    chronic 381.52
  Eustachian (tube) 381.50
    acute 381.51
    chronic 381.52
  follicularis 614.1
  gonococcal (chronic) 098.37
    acute 098.17
  interstitial, chronic 614.1
  isthmica nodosa 614.1
  old—*see* Salpingo-oophoritis, chronic
  puerperal, postpartum, childbirth 670
  specific (chronic) 098.37
    acute 098.17
  tuberculous (acute) (chronic) (*see also*
    Tuberculosis) 016.6
  venereal (chronic) 098.37
    acute 098.17
Salpingocele 620.4
Salpingo-oophoritis (catarrhal) (purulent)
  (ruptured) (septic) (suppurative) 614.2
  acute 614.0
    with
      abortion—*see* Abortion, by type, with sepsis
      ectopic pregnancy (*see also* categories
        633.0-633.9) 639.0
      molar pregnancy (*see also* categories
        630-632) 639.0
    following
      abortion 639.0
      ectopic or molar pregnancy 639.0
    gonococcal 098.17
    puerperal, postpartum, childbirth 670
    tuberculous (*see also* Tuberculosis) 016.6
  chronic 614.1
    gonococcal 098.37
    tuberculous (*see also* Tuberculosis) 016.6
  complicating pregnancy 646.6
    affecting fetus or newborn 760.8
  gonococcal (chronic) 098.37
    acute 098.17
  old—*see* Salpingo-oophoritis, chronic
  puerperal 670
  specific—*see* Salpingo-oophoritis, gonococcal
  subacute (*see also* Salpingo-oophoritis, acute)
    614.0
  tuberculous (acute) (chronic) (*see also*
    Tuberculosis) 016.6
  venereal—*see* Salpingo-oophoritis, gonococcal
Salpingo-ovaritis (*see also* Salpingo-oophoritis)
  614.2
Salpingoperitonitis (*see also*
  Salpingo-oophoritis) 614.2

Sarcomatosis
  meningeal (M9539/3)—*see* Neoplasm,
    meninges, malignant
  specified site NEC (M8800/3)—*see* Neoplasm,
    connective tissue, malignant
  unspecified site (M8800/6) 171.9
Sarcosinemia 270.8
Sarcosporidiosis 136.5
Saturnine —*see* condition
Saturnism 984.9
  specified type of lead—*see* Table of drugs and
    chemicals
Satyriasis 302.89
Sauriasis —*see* Ichthyosis
Sauriderma 757.39
Sauriosis —*see* Ichthyosis
Savill's disease (epidemic exfoliative dermatitis)
    695.89
SBE (subacute bacterial endocarditis) 421.0
Scabies (any site) 133.0
Scabs 782.8
Scaglietti-Dagnini syndrome (acromegalic
    macrospondylitis) 253.0
Scald, scalded —*see also* Burn, by site
  skin syndrome 695.1
Scalenus anticus (anterior) syndrome 353.0
Scales 782.8
Scalp —*see* condition
Scaphocephaly 756.0
Scaphoiditis, tarsal 732.5
Scapulalgia 733.90
Scapulohumeral myopathy 359.1
Scar, scarring (*see also* Cicatrix) 709.2
  adherent 709.2
  atrophic 709.2
  cervix
    in pregnancy or childbirth 654.6
      affecting fetus or newborn 763.89
      causing obstructed labor 660.2
        affecting fetus or newborn 763.1
  cheloid 701.4
  chorioretinal 363.30
    disseminated 363.35
    macular 363.32
    peripheral 363.34
    posterior pole NEC 363.33
  choroid (*see also* Scar, chorioretinal) 363.30
  compression, pericardial 423.9
  congenital 757.39
  conjunctiva 372.64
  cornea 371.00
    xerophthalmic 264.6
  due to previous cesarean delivery, complicating
    pregnancy or childbirth 654.2
    affecting fetus or newborn 763.89
  duodenal (bulb) (cap) 537.3
  hypertrophic 701.4
  keloid 701.4
  labia 624.4
  lung (base) 518.89
  macula 363.32
    disseminated 363.35
    peripheral 363.34
  muscle 728.89
  myocardium, myocardial 412
  painful 709.2
  papillary muscle 429.81
  posterior pole NEC 363.33
    macular—*see* Scar, macula
  postnecrotic (hepatic) (liver) 571.9

Scar, scarring—*continued*
  psychic V15.49
  retina (*see also* Scar, chorioretinal) 363.30
  trachea 478.9
  uterus 621.8
    in pregnancy or childbirth NEC 654.9
      affecting fetus or newborn 763.89
      due to previous cesarean delivery 654.2
  vulva 624.4
Scarabiasis 134.1
Scarlatina 034.1
  anginosa 034.1
  maligna 034.1
  myocarditis, acute 034.1 *[422.0]*
  old (*see also* Myocarditis) 429.0
  otitis media 034.1 *[382.02]*
  ulcerosa 034.1
Scarlatinella 057.8
Scarlet fever (albuminuria) (angina)
    (convulsions) (lesions of lid) (rash) 034.1
Schamberg's disease, dermatitis, or dermatosis
    (progressive pigmentary dermatosis) 709.09
Schatzki's ring (esophagus) (lower) (congenital)
    750.3
  acquired 530.3
Schaufenster krankheit 413.9
Schaumann's
  benign lymphogranulomatosis 135
  disease (sarcoidosis) 135
  syndrome (sarcoidosis) 135
Scheie's syndrome (mucopolysaccharidosis IS)
    277.5
Schenck's disease (sporotrichosis) 117.1
Scheuermann's disease or osteochondrosis
    732.0
Scheuthauer-Marie-Sainton syndrome
    (cleidocranialis dysostosis) 755.59
Schilder (-Flatau) disease 341.1
Schilling-type monocytic leukemia (M9890/3)
    206.9
**Schimmelbusch's disease, cystic mastitis, or hy-
    perplasia** 610.1
Schirmer's syndrome (encephalocutaneous
    angiomatosis) 759.6
Schistocelia 756.79
Schistoglossia 750.13
Schistosoma infestation —*see* Infestation,
    Schistosoma
Schistosomiasis 120.9
  Asiatic 120.2
  bladder 120.0
  chestermani 120.8
  colon 120.1
  cutaneous 120.3
  due to
    S. hematobium 120.0
    S. japonicum 120.2
    S. mansoni 120.1
    S. mattheii 120.8
  eastern 120.2
  genitourinary tract 120.0
  intestinal 120.1
  lung 120.2
  Manson's (intestinal) 120.1
  Oriental 120.2
  pulmonary 120.2
  specified type NEC 120.8
  vesical 120.0
Schizencephaly 742.4
Schizo-affective psychosis (*see also*
    Schizophrenia) 295.7
Schizodontia 520.2

Schizoid personality 301.20
  introverted 301.21
  schizotypal 301.22
Schizophrenia, schizophrenic (reaction) 295.9

Note—Use the following fifth-digit
subclassification with category 295:

0 *unspecified*
1 *subchronic*
2 *chronic*
3 *subchronic with acute exacerbation*
4 *chronic with acute exacerbation*
5 *in remission*

---

  acute (attack) NEC 295.8
    episode 295.4
  atypical form 295.8
  borderline 295.5
  catalepsy 295.2
  catatonic (type) (acute) (excited) (withdrawn)
    295.2
  childhood (type) (*see also* Psychosis,
    childhood) 299.9
  chronic NEC 295.6
  coenesthesiopathic 295.8
  cyclic (type) 295.7
  disorganized (type) 295.1
  flexibilitas cerea 295.2
  hebephrenic (type) (acute) 295.1
  incipient 295.5
  latent 295.5
  paranoid (type) (acute) 295.3
  paraphrenic (acute) 295.3
  prepsychotic 295.5
  primary (acute) 295.0
  prodromal 295.5
  pseudoneurotic 295.5
  pseudopsychopathic 295.5
  reaction 295.9
  residual (state) (type) 295.6
  restzustand 295.6
  schizo-affective (type) (depressed) (excited)
    295.7
  schizophreniform type 295.4
  simple (type) (acute) 295.0
  simplex (acute) 295.0
  specified type NEC 295.8
  syndrome of childhood NEC (*see also*
    Psychosis, childhood) 299.9
  undifferentiated 295.9
    acute 295.8
    chronic 295.6
Schizothymia 301.20
  introverted 301.21
  schizotypal 301.22
Schlafkrankheit 086.5
Schlatter's tibia (osteochondrosis) 732.4
Schlatter-Osgood disease (osteochondrosis,
  tibial tubercle) 732.4
Schloffer's tumor (*see also* Peritonitis) 567.2
Schmidt's syndrome
  sphallo-pharyngo-laryngeal hemiplegia 352.6
  thyroid-adrenocortical insufficiency 258.1
  vagoaccessory 352.6
Schmincke
  carcinoma (M8082/3)—*see* Neoplasm,
    nasopharynx, malignant
  tumor (M8082/3)—*see* Neoplasm,
    nasopharynx, malignant
Schmitz (-Stutzer) dysentery 004.0

Schmorl's disease or nodes 722.30
  lumbar, lumbosacral 722.32
  specified region NEC 722.39
  thoracic, thoracolumbar 722.31
Schneider's syndrome 047.9
Schneiderian
  carcinoma (M8121/3)
    specified site—*see* Neoplasm, by site,
      malignant
    unspecified site 160.0
  papilloma (M8121/0)
    specified site—*see* Neoplasm, by site, benign
    unspecified site 212.0
Schoffer's tumor (*see also* Peritonitis) 567.2
Scholte's syndrome (malignant carcinoid) 259.2
Scholz's disease 330.0
Scholz (-Bielschowsky-Henneberg) syndrome
  330.0
Schönlein (-Henoch) disease (primary) (purpura)
  (rheumatic) 287.0
School examination V70.3
Schottmüller's disease (*see also* Fever,
  paratyphoid) 002.9
Schroeder's syndrome (endocrine-hypertensive)
  255.3
Schüller-Christian disease or syndrome
  (chronic histiocytosis X) 277.8
Schultz's disease or syndrome (agranulocytosis)
  288.0
Schultze's acroparesthesia, simple 443.89
Schwalbe-Ziehen-Oppenheimer disease 333.6
Schwannoma (M9560/0)—*see also* Neoplasm,
  connective tissue, benign
  malignant (M9560/3)—*see* Neoplasm,
    connective tissue, malignant
Schwartz (-Jampel) syndrome 756.89
Schwartz-Bartter syndrome (inappropriate
  secretion of antidiuretic hormone) 253.6
Schweninger-Buzzi disease (macular atrophy)
  701.3
Sciatic —*see* condition
Sciatica (infectional) 724.3
  due to
    displacement of intervertebral disc 722.10
    herniation, nucleus pulposus 722.10
Scimitar syndrome (anomalous venous
  drainage, right lung to inferior vena cava)
  747.49
Sclera —*see* condition
Sclerectasia 379.11
Scleredema
  adultorum 710.1
  Buschke's 710.1
  newborn 778.1
Sclerema
  adiposum (newborn) 778.1
  adultorum 710.1
  edematosum (newborn) 778.1
  neonatorum 778.1
  newborn 778.1
Scleriasis —*see* Scleroderma
Scleritis 379.00
  with corneal involvement 379.05
  anterior (annular) (localized) 379.03
  brawny 379.06
  granulomatous 379.09
  posterior 379.07
  specified NEC 379.09
  suppurative 379.09
  syphilitic 095.0
  tuberculous (nodular) (*see also* Tuberculosis)
    017.3 [379.09]

Sclerochoroiditis (*see also* Scleritis) 379.00
Scleroconjunctivitis (*see also* Scleritis) 379.00
Sclerocystic ovary (syndrome) 256.4
Sclerodactylia 701.0
Scleroderma, sclerodermia (acrosclerotic)
    (diffuse) (generalized) (progressive)
    (pulmonary) 710.1
  circumscribed 701.0
  linear 701.0
  localized (linear) 701.0
  newborn 778.1
Sclerokeratitis 379.05
  meaning sclerosing keratitis 370.54
  tuberculous (*see also* Tuberculosis) 017.3
    [379.09]
Scleroma, trachea 040.1
Scleromalacia
  multiple 731.0
  perforans 379.04
Scleromyxedema 701.8
Scleroperikeratitis 379.05
Sclerose en plaques 340
Sclerosis, sclerotic
  adrenal (gland) 255.8
  Alzheimer's 331.0
    with dementia—*see* Alzheimer's, demential
  amyotrophic (lateral) 335.20
  annularis fibrosi
    aortic 424.1
    mitral 424.0
  aorta, aortic 440.0
    valve (*see also* Endocarditis, aortic) 424.1
  artery, arterial, arteriolar, arteriovascular—*see*
    Arteriosclerosis
  ascending multiple 340
  Baló's (concentric) 341.1
  basilar—*see* Sclerosis, brain
  bone (localized) NEC 733.99
  brain (general) (lobular) 341.9
    Alzheimer's—*see* Alzheimer's dementia
    artery, arterial 437.0
    atrophic lobar 331.0
      with dementia
        with behavioral disturbance 331.0 *[294.11]*
        without behavioral disturbance 331.0
          [294.10]
    diffuse 341.1
      familial (chronic) (infantile) 330.0
      infantile (chronic) (familial) 330.0
      Pelizaeus-Merzbacher type 330.0
    disseminated 340
    hereditary 334.2
    infantile, (degenerative) (diffuse) 330.0
    insular 340
    Krabbe's 330.0
    miliary 340
    multiple 340
    Pelizaeus-Merzbacher 330.0
    progressive familial 330.0
    senile 437.0
    tuberous 759.5
  bulbar, progressive 340
  bundle of His 426.50
    left 426.3
    right 426.4
  cardiac —*see* Arteriosclerosis, coronary
  cardiorenal (*see also* Hypertension, cardiorenal)
    404.90
  cardiovascular (*see also* Disease,
    cardiovascular) 429.2

Sclerosis, sclerotic—*continued*
  renal (*see also* Hypertension, cardiorenal)
    404.90
  centrolobar, familial 330.0
  cerebellar—*see* Sclerosis, brain
  cerebral—*see* Sclerosis, brain
  cerebrospinal 340
    disseminated 340
    multiple 340
  cerebrovascular 437.0
  choroid 363.40
    diffuse 363.56
  combined (spinal cord)—*see also* Degeneration,
    combined
    multiple 340
  concentric, Baló's 341.1
  cornea 370.54
  coronary (artery) —*see* Arteriosclerosis,
    coronary
  corpus cavernosum
    female 624.8
    male 607.89
  Dewitzky's
    aortic 424.1
    mitral 424.0
  diffuse NEC 341.1
  disease, heart —*see* Arteriosclerosis, coronary
  disseminated 340
  dorsal 340
  dorsolateral (spinal cord)—*see* Degeneration,
    combined
  endometrium 621.8
  extrapyramidal 333.90
  eye, nuclear (senile) 366.16
  Friedreich's (spinal cord) 334.0
  funicular (spermatic cord) 608.89
  gastritis 535.4
  general (vascular)—*see* Arteriosclerosis
  gland (lymphatic) 457.8
  hepatic 571.9
  hereditary
    cerebellar 334.2
    spinal 334.0
  idiopathic cortical (Garré's) (*see also*
    Osteomyelitis) 730.1
  ilium, piriform 733.5
  insular 340
    pancreas 251.8
  Islands of Langerhans 251.8
  kidney—*see* Sclerosis, renal
  larynx 478.79
  lateral 335.24
    amyotrophic 335.20
    descending 335.24
    primary 335.24
    spinal 335.24
  liver 571.9
  lobar, atrophic (of brain) 331.0
    with dementia
      with behavioral disturbance 331.0 *[294.11]*
      without behavioral disturbance 331.0
        [294.10]
  lung (*see also* Fibrosis, lung) 515
  mastoid 383.1
  mitral—*see* Endocarditis, mitral
  Mönckeberg's (medial) (*see also*
    Arteriosclerosis, extremities) 440.20
  multiple (brain stem) (cerebral) (generalized)
    (spinal cord) 340
  myocardium, myocardial —*see*
    Arteriosclerosis, coronary

Sclerosis, sclerotic—*continued*
  nuclear (senile), eye 366.16
  ovary 620.8
  pancreas 577.8
  penis 607.89
  peripheral arteries NEC (*see also*
      Arteriosclerosis, extremities) 440.20
  plaques 340
  pluriglandular 258.8
  polyglandular 258.8
  posterior (spinal cord) (syphilitic) 094.0
  posterolateral (spinal cord)—*see* Degeneration,
      combined
  prepuce 607.89
  primary lateral 335.24
  progressive systemic 710.1
  pulmonary (*see also* Fibrosis, lung) 515
    artery 416.0
    valve (heart) (*see also* Endocarditis,
        pulmonary) 424.3
  renal 587
    with
      cystine storage disease 270.0
      hypertension (*see also* Hypertension,
          kidney) 403.90
      hypertensive heart disease (conditions
          classifiable to 402) (*see also*
          Hypertension, cardiorenal) 404.90
      arteriolar (hyaline) (*see also* Hypertension,
          kidney) 403.90
      hyperplastic (*see also* Hypertension, kidney)
          403.90
  retina (senile) (vascular) 362.17
  rheumatic
    aortic valve 395.9
    mitral valve 394.9
  Schilder's 341.1
  senile—*see* Arteriosclerosis
  spinal (cord) (general) (progressive)
      (transverse) 336.8
    ascending 357.0
    combined—*see also* Degeneration, combined
      multiple 340
      syphilitic 094.89
    disseminated 340
    dorsolateral—*see* Degeneration, combined
    hereditary (Friedreich's) (mixed form) 334.0
    lateral (amyotrophic) 335.24
    multiple 340
    posterior (syphilitic) 094.0
  stomach 537.89
  subendocardial, congenital 425.3
  systemic (progressive) 710.1
    with lung involvement 710.1 [517.2]
  tricuspid (heart) (valve)—*see* Endocarditis,
      tricuspid
  tuberous (brain) 759.5
  tympanic membrane (*see also*
      Tympanosclerosis) 385.00
  valve, valvular (heart)—*see* Endocarditis
  vascular—*see* Arteriosclerosis
  vein 459.89
Sclerotenonitis 379.07
Sclerotitis (*see also* Scleritis) 379.00
  syphilitic 095.0
  tuberculous (*see also* Tuberculosis) 017.3
      [379.09]
Scoliosis (acquired) (postural) 737.30
  congenital 754.2
  due to or associated with
    Charcot-Marie-Tooth disease 356.1 [737.43]

Scoliosis—*continued*
    mucopolysaccharidosis 277.5 [737.43]
    neurofibromatosis 237.71 [737.43]
    osteitis
      deformans 731.0 [737.43]
      fibrosa cystica 252.0 [737.43]
    osteoporosis (*see also* Osteoporosis) 733.00
        [737.43]
    poliomyelitis 138 [737.43]
    radiation 737.33
    tuberculosis (*see also* Tuberculosis) 015.0
        [737.43]
  idiopathic 737.30
  infantile
    progressive 737.32
    resolving 737.31
  paralytic 737.39
  rachitic 268.1
  sciatic 724.3
  specified NEC 737.39
  thoracogenic 737.34
  tuberculous (*see also* Tuberculosis) 015.0
      [737.43]
Scoliotic pelvis 738.6
  with disproportion (fetopelvic) 653.0
    affecting fetus or newborn 763.1
    causing obstructed labor 660.1
      affecting fetus or newborn 763.1
Scorbutus, scorbutic 267
  anemia 281.8
Scotoma (ring) 368.44
  arcuate 368.43
  Bjerrum 368.43
  blind spot area 368.42
  central 368.41
  centrocecal 368.41
  paracecal 368.42
  paracentral 368.41
  scintillating 368.12
  Seidel 368.43
Scratch —*see* Injury, superficial, by site
Screening (for) V82.9
  alcoholism V79.1
  anemia, deficiency NEC V78.1
    iron V78.0
  anomaly, congenital V82.89
  antenatal V28.9
    alphafetoprotein levels, raised V28.1
    based on amniocentesis V28.2
      chromosomal anomalies V28.0
      raised alphafetoprotein levels V28.1
    fetal growth retardation using ultrasonics
        V28.4
    isoimmunization V28.5
    malformations using ultrasonics V28.3
    raised alphafetoprotein levels V28.1
    specified condition NEC V28.8
    Streptococcus B V28.6
  arterial hypertension V81.1
  arthropod-borne viral disease NEC V73.5
  asymptomatic bacteriuria V81.5
  bacterial
    conjunctivitis V74.4
    disease V74.9
      specified condition NEC V74.8
  bacteriuria, asymptomatic V81.5
  blood disorder NEC V78.9
    specified type NEC V78.8
  bronchitis, chronic V81.3
  brucellosis V74.8
  cancer—*see* Screening, malignant neoplasm

Screening (for)—*continued*
  cardiovascular disease NEC V81.2
  cataract V80.2
  Chagas' disease V75.3
  chemical poisoning V82.5
  cholera V74.0
  cholesterol level V77.91
  chromosomal
    anomalies
      by amniocentesis, antenatal V28.0
      maternal postnatal V82.4
    athletes V70.3
  condition
    cardiovascular NEC V81.2
    eye NEC V80.2
    genitourinary NEC V81.6
    neurological V80.0
    respiratory NEC V81.4
    skin V82.0
    specified NEC V82.89
  congenital
    anomaly V82.89
      eye V80.2
    dislocation of hip V82.3
    eye condition or disease V80.2
  conjunctivitis, bacterial V74.4
  contamination NEC (*see also* Poisoning) V82.5
  coronary artery disease V81.0
  cystic fibrosis V77.6
  deficiency anemia NEC V78.1
    iron V78.0
  dengue fever V73.5
  depression V79.0
  developmental handicap V79.9
    in early childhood V79.3
    specified type NEC V79.8
  diabetes mellitus V77.1
  diphtheria V74.3
  disease or disorder V82.9
    bacterial V74.9
      specified NEC V74.8
    blood V78.9
      specified type NEC V78.8
    blood-forming organ V78.9
      specified type NEC V78.8
    cardiovascular NEC V81.2
      hypertensive V81.1
      ischemic V81.0
    Chagas' V75.3
    chlamydial V73.98
      specified NEC V73.88
    ear NEC V80.3
    endocrine NEC V77.99
    eye NEC V80.2
    genitourinary NEC V81.6
    heart NEC V81.2
      hypertensive V81.1
      ischemic V81.0
    immunity NEC V77.99
    infectious NEC V75.9
    lipoid NEC V77.91
    mental V79.9
      specified type NEC V79.8
    metabolic NEC V77.99
      inborn NEC V77.7
    neurological V80.0
    nutritional NEC V77.99
    rheumatic NEC V82.2
    rickettsial V75.0
    sickle-cell V78.2
      trait V78.2

Screening (for)—*continued*
    specified type NEC V82.89
    thyroid V77.0
    vascular NEC V81.2
      ischemic V81.0
    venereal V74.5
    viral V73.99
      arthropod-borne NEC V73.5
      specified type NEC V73.89
  dislocation of hip, congenital V82.3
  drugs in athletes V70.3
  emphysema (chronic) V81.3
  encephalitis, viral (mosquito or tick borne)
    V73.5
  endocrine disorder NEC V77.99
  eye disorder NEC V80.2
    congenital V80.2
  fever
    dengue V73.5
    hemorrhagic V73.5
    yellow V73.4
  filariasis V75.6
  galactosemia V77.4
  genitourinary condition NEC V81.6
  glaucoma V80.1
  gonorrhea V74.5
  gout V77.5
  Hansen's disease V74.2
  heart disease NEC V81.2
    hypertensive V81.1
    ischemic V81.0
  heavy metal poisoning V82.5
  helminthiasis, intestinal V75.7
  hematopoietic malignancy V76.89
  hemoglobinopathies NEC V78.3
  hemorrhagic fever V73.5
  Hodgkin's disease V76.89
  hormones in athletes V70.3
  hypercholesterolemia V77.91
  hyperlipidemia V77.91
  hypertension V81.1
  immunity disorder NEC V77.99
  inborn errors of metabolism NEC V77.7
  infection
    bacterial V74.9
      specified type NEC V74.8
    mycotic V75.4
    parasitic NEC V75.8
  infectious disease V75.9
    specified type NEC V75.8
  ingestion of radioactive substance V82.5
  intestinal helminthiasis V75.7
  iron deficiency anemia V78.0
  ischemic heart disease V81.0
  lead poisoning V82.5
  leishmaniasis V75.2
  leprosy V74.2
  leptospirosis V74.8
  leukemia V76.89
  lipoid disorder NEC V77.91
  lymphoma V76.89
  malaria V75.1
  malignant neoplasm (of) V76.9
    bladder V76.3
    blood V76.89
    breast V76.10
      mammogram NEC V76.12
        for high-risk patient V76.11
      specified type NEC V76.19
    cervix V76.2
    colon V76.51

Screening (for)—*continued*
  colorectal V76.51
  hematopoietic system V76.89
  intestine V76.50
    colon V76.51
    small V76.52
  lung V76.0
  lymph (glands) V76.89
  nervous system V76.81
  oral cavity V76.42
  other specified neoplasm NEC V76.89
  ovary V76.46
  prostate V76.44
  rectum V76.41
  respiratory organs V76.0
  skin V76.43
  specified sites NEC V76.49
  testis V76.45
  vagina V76.47
    following hysterectomy for malignant
      condition V67.01
  malnutrition V77.2
  mammogram NEC V76.12
    for high-risk patient V76.11
  maternal postnatal chromosomal anomalies
    V82.4
  measles V73.2
  mental
    disorder V79.9
      specified type NEC V79.8
    retardation V79.2
  metabolic errors, inborn V77.7
  metabolic disorder NEC V77.99
  mucoviscidosis V77.6
  multiphasic V82.6
  mycosis V75.4
  mycotic infection V75.4
  nephropathy V81.5
  neurological condition V80.0
  nutritional disorder V77.99
    obesity V77.8
  obesity V77.8
  osteoporosis V82.81
  parasitic infection NEC V75.8
  phenylketonuria V77.3
  plague V74.8
  poisoning
    chemical NEC V82.5
    contaminated water supply V82.5
    heavy metal V82.5
  poliomyelitis V73.0
  postnatal chromosomal anomalies, maternal
    V82.4
  prenatal—*see* Screening, antenatal
  pulmonary tuberculosis V74.1
  radiation exposure V82.5
  renal disease V81.5
  respiratory condition NEC V81.4
  rheumatic disorder NEC V82.2
  rheumatoid arthritis V82.1
  rickettsial disease V75.0
  rubella V73.3
  schistosomiasis V75.5
  senile macular lesions of eye V80.2
  sickle-cell anemia, disease, or trait V78.2
  skin condition V82.0
  sleeping sickness V75.3
  smallpox V73.1
  special V82.9
    specified condition NEC V82.89
  specified type NEC V82.89

Screening (for)— *continued*
  spirochetal disease V74.9
    specified type NEC V74.8
  stimulants in athletes V70.3
  syphilis V74.5
  tetanus V74.8
  thyroid disorder V77.0
  trachoma V73.6
  trypanosomiasis V75.3
  tuberculosis, pulmonary V74.1
  venereal disease V74.5
  viral encephalitis
    mosquito-borne V73.5
    tick-borne V73.5
  whooping cough V74.8
  worms, intestinal V75.7
  yaws V74.6
  yellow fever V73.4
Scrofula (*see also* Tuberculosis) 017.2
Scrofulide (primary) (*see also* Tuberculosis)
  017.0
Scrofuloderma, scrofulodermia (any site)
  (primary) (*see also* Tuberculosis) 017.0
Scrofulosis (universal) (*see also* Tuberculosis)
  017.2
Scrofulosis lichen (primary) (*see also*
  Tuberculosis) 017.0
Scrofulous —*see* condition
Scrotal tongue 529.5
  congenital 750.13
Scrotum —*see* condition
Scurvy (gum) (infantile) (rickets) (scorbutic) 267
Sea-blue histiocyte syndrome 272.7
Seabright-Bantam syndrome
  (pseudohypoparathyroidism) 275.49
Seasickness 994.6
Seatworm 127.4
Sebaceous
  cyst (*see also* Cyst, sebaceous) 706.2
  gland disease NEC 706.9
Sebocystomatosis 706.2
Seborrhea, seborrheic 706.3
  adiposa 706.3
  capitis 690.11
  congestiva 695.4
  corporis 706.3
  dermatitis 690.10
    infantile 690.12
  diathesis in infants 695.89
  eczema 690.18
    infantile 690.12
  keratosis 702.19
    inflamed 702.11
  nigricans 705.89
  sicca 690.18
  wart 702.19
    inflamed 702.11
Seckel's syndrome 759.89
Seclusion pupil 364.74
Seclusiveness, child 313.22
Secondary —*see also* condition
  neoplasm—*see* Neoplasm, by site, malignant,
    secondary
Secretan's disease or syndrome (posttraumatic
  edema) 782.3
Secretion
  antidiuretic hormone, inappropriate (syndrome)
    253.6
  catecholamine, by pheochromocytoma 255.6
  hormone
    antidiuretic, inappropriate (syndrome) 253.6

Secretion—*continued*
by
  carcinoid tumor 259.2
  pheochromocytoma 255.6
  ectopic NEC 259.3
urinary
  excessive 788.42
  suppression 788.5
Section
cesarean
  affecting fetus or newborn 763.4
  post mortem, affecting fetus or newborn 761.6
  previous, in pregnancy or childbirth 654.2
    affecting fetus or newborn 763.89
nerve, traumatic—*see* Injury, nerve, by site
Seeligmann's syndrome (ichthyosis congenita)
  757.1
Segmentation, incomplete (congenital)—*see
also* Fusion
bone NEC 756.9
lumbosacral (joint) 756.15
vertebra 756.15
  lumbosacral 756.15
Seizure 780.39
akinetic (idiopathic) (*see also* Epilepsy) 345.0
  psychomotor 345.4
apoplexy, apoplectic (*see also* Disease,
  cerebrovascular, acute) 436
atonic (*see also* Epilepsy) 345.0
autonomic 300.11
brain or cerebral (*see also* Disease,
  cerebrovascular, acute) 436
convulsive (*see also* Convulsions) 780.39
cortical (focal) (motor) (*see also* Epilepsy) 345.5
epilepsy, epileptic (cryptogenic) (*see also*
  Epilepsy) 345.9
epileptiform, epileptoid 780.39
focal (*see also* Epilepsy) 345.5
febrile 780.31
heart—*see* Disease, heart
hysterical 300.11
Jacksonian (focal) (*see also* Epilepsy) 345.5
  motor type 345.5
  sensory type 345.5
newborn 779.0
paralysis (*see also* Disease, cerebrovascular,
  acute) 436
recurrent 780.39
  epileptic—*see* Epilepsy
repetitive 780.39
  epileptic—*see* Epilepsy
salaam (*see also* Epilepsy) 345.6
uncinate (*see also* Epilepsy) 345.4
Self-mutilation 300.9
Semicoma 780.09
Semiconsciousness 780.09
Seminal
vesicle—*see* condition
vesiculitis (*see also* Vesiculitis) 608.0
Seminoma (M9061/3)
anaplastic type (M9062/3)
  specified site—*see* Neoplasm, by site,
    malignant
  unspecified site 186.9
specified site—*see* Neoplasm, by site, malignant
spermatocytic (M9063/3)
  specified site—*see* Neoplasm, by site,
    malignant
  unspecified site 186.9
unspecified site 186.9
Semliki Forest encephalitis 062.8

Senear-Usher disease or syndrome (pemphigus
  erythematosus) 694.4
Senecio jacobae dermatitis 692.6
Senectus 797
Senescence 797
Senile (*see also* condition) 797
cervix (atrophic) 622.8
degenerative atrophy, skin 701.3
endometrium (atrophic) 621.8
fallopian tube (atrophic) 620.3
heart (failure) 797
lung 492.8
ovary (atrophic) 620.3
syndrome 259.8
vagina, vaginitis (atrophic) 627.3
wart 702.0
Senility 797
with
  acute confusional state 290.3
  delirium 290.3
  mental changes 290.9
  psychosis NEC (*see also* Psychosis, senile)
    290.20
premature (syndrome) 259.8
Sensation
burning (*see also* Disturbance, sensation) 782.0
  tongue 529.6
choking 784.9
loss of (*see also* Disturbance, sensation) 782.0
prickling (*see also* Disturbance, sensation) 782.0
tingling (*see also* Disturbance, sensation) 782.0
Sense loss (touch) (*see also* Disturbance,
  sensation) 782.0
smell 781.1
taste 781.1
Sensibility disturbance NEC (cortical) (deep)
  (vibratory) (*see also* Disturbance, sensation)
  782.0
Sensitive dentine 521.8
Sensitiver Beziehungswahn 297.8
Sensitivity, sensitization —*see also* Allergy
autoerythrocyte 287.2
carotid sinus 337.0
child (excessive) 313.21
cold, autoimmune 283.0
methemoglobin 289.7
suxamethonium 289.8
tuberculin, without clinical or radiological
  symptoms 795.5
Sensory
extinction 781.8
neglect 781.8
Separation
acromioclavicular—*see* Dislocation, shoulder
anxiety, abnormal 309.21
apophysis, traumatic—*see* Fracture, by site
choroid 363.70
  hemorrhagic 363.72
  serous 363.71
costochondral (simple) (traumatic)—*see*
  Dislocation, costochondral
epiphysis, epiphyseal
  nontraumatic 732.9
    upper femoral 732.2
  traumatic—*see* Fracture, by site
fracture—*see* Fracture, by site
infundibulum cardiac from right ventricle by a
  partition 746.83
joint (current) (traumatic)—*see* Dislocation, by
  site

Separation—*continued*
placenta (normally implanted)—*see* Placenta, separation
pubic bone, obstetrical trauma 665.6
retina, retinal (*see also* Detachment, retina) 361.9
  layers 362.40
    sensory (*see also* Retinoschisis) 361.10
  pigment epithelium (exudative) 362.42
    hemorrhagic 362.43
sternoclavicular (traumatic)—*see* Dislocation, sternoclavicular
symphysis pubis, obstetrical trauma 665.6
tracheal ring, incomplete (congenital) 748.3
Sepsis (generalized) (*see also* Septicemia) 038.9
  with
    abortion—*see* Abortion, by type, with sepsis
    ectopic pregnancy (*see also* categories 633.0-633.9) 639.0
    molar pregnancy (*see also* categories 630-632) 639.0
  buccal 528.3
  complicating labor 659.3
  dental (pulpal origin) 522.4
  female genital organ NEC 614.9
  fetus (intrauterine) 771.81
  following
    abortion 639.0
    ectopic or molar pregnancy 639.0
    infusion, perfusion, or transfusion 999.3
  Friedländer's 038.49
  intraocular 360.00
  localized
    in operation wound 998.59
    skin (*see also* Abscess) 682.9
  malleus 024
  nadir 038.9
  newborn (umbilical) (organism unspecified) NEC 771.81
  oral 528.3
  puerperal, postpartum, childbirth (pelvic) 670
  resulting from infusion, injection, transfusion, or vaccination 999.3
  severe 995.92
  skin, localized (*see also* Abscess) 682.9
  umbilical (newborn) (organism unspecified) 771.89
  tetanus 771.3
  urinary 599.0
Septate —*see also* Septum
Septic —*see also* condition
  adenoids 474.01
    and tonsils 474.02
  arm (with lymphangitis) 682.3
  embolus—*see* Embolism
  finger (with lymphangitis) 681.00
  foot (with lymphangitis) 682.7
  gallbladder (*see also* Cholecystitis) 575.8
  hand (with lymphangitis) 682.4
  joint (*see also* Arthritis, septic) 711.0
  kidney (*see also* Infection, kidney) 590.9
  leg (with lymphangitis) 682.6
  mouth 528.3
  nail 681.9
    finger 681.02
    toe 681.11
  shock (endotoxic) 785.59
  sore (*see also* Abscess) 682.9
    throat 034.0
      milk-borne 034.0
      streptococcal 034.0

Septic—*continued*
spleen (acute) 289.59
teeth (pulpal origin) 522.4
throat 034.0
thrombus—*see* Thrombosis
toe (with lymphangitis) 681.10
tonsils 474.00
  and adenoids 474.02
umbilical cord (newborn) (organism unspecified) 771.89
uterus (*see also* Endometritis) 615.9
Septicemia, septicemic (generalized) (suppurative) 038.9
  with
    abortion—*see* Abortion, by type, with sepsis
    ectopic pregnancy (*see also* categories 633.0-633.9) 639.0
    molar pregnancy (*see also* categories 630-632) 639.0
  Aerobacter aerogenes 038.49
  anaerobic 038.3
  anthrax 022.3
  Bacillus coli 038.42
  Bacteroides 038.3
  Clostridium 038.3
  complicating labor 659.3
  cryptogenic 038.9
  enteric gram-negative bacilli 038.40
  Enterobacter aerogenes 038.49
  Erysipelothrix (insidiosa) (rhusiopathiae) 027.1
  Escherichia coli 038.42
  following
    abortion 639.0
    ectopic or molar pregnancy 639.0
    infusion, injection, transfusion, or vaccination 999.3
  Friedländer's (bacillus) 038.49
  gangrenous 038.9
  gonococcal 098.89
  gram-negative (organism) 038.40
    anaerobic 038.3
  Hemophilus influenzae 038.41
  herpes (simplex) 054.5
  herpetic 054.5
  Listeria monocytogenes 027.0
  meningeal—*see* Meningitis
  meningococcal (chronic) (fulminating) 036.2
  navel, newborn (organism unspecified) 771.89
  newborn (umbilical) (organism unspecified) 771.81
  plague 020.2
  pneumococcal 038.2
  postabortal 639.0
  postoperative 998.59
  Proteus vulgaris 038.49
  Pseudomonas (aeruginosa) 038.43
  puerperal, postpartum 670
  Salmonella (aertrycke) (callinarum) (choleraesuis) (enteritidis) (suipestifer) 003.1
  Serratia 038.44
  Shigella (*see also* Dysentery, bacillary) 004.9
  specified organism NEC 038.8
  staphylococcal 038.10
    aureus 038.11
    specified organism NEC 038.19
  streptococcal (anaerobic) 038.0
  suipestifer 003.1
  umbilicus, newborn (organism unspecified) 771.89
  viral 079.99
  Yersinia enterocolitica 038.49

Septum, septate (congenital)—*see also*
  Anomaly, specified type NEC
  anal 751.2
  aqueduct of Sylvius 742.3
    with spina bifida (*see also* Spina bifida) 741.0
  hymen 752.49
  uterus (*see also* Double, uterus) 752.2
  vagina 752.49
    in pregnancy or childbirth 654.7
      affecting fetus or newborn 763.89
      causing obstructed labor 660.2
        affecting fetus or newborn 763.1
Sequestration
  lung (congenital) (extralobar) (intralobar) 748.5
  orbit 376.10
  pulmonary artery (congenital) 747.3
Sequestrum
  bone (*see also* Osteomyelitis) 730.1
    jaw 526.4
  dental 525.8
  jaw bone 526.4
  sinus (accessory) (nasal) (*see also* Sinusitis)
    473.9
    maxillary 473.0
Sequoiosis asthma 495.8
Serology for syphilis
  doubtful
    with signs or symptoms—*see* Syphilis, by site
      and stage
    follow-up of latent syphilis—*see* Syphilis,
      latent
  false positive 795.6
  negative, with signs or symptoms—*see*
    Syphilis, by site and stage
  positive 097.1
    with signs or symptoms—*see* Syphilis, by site
      and stage
    false 795.6
    follow-up of latent syphilis—*see* Syphilis,
      latent
    only finding—*see* Syphilis, latent
  reactivated 097.1
Seroma (postoperative) (non-infected) 998.13
  infected 998.51
Seropurulent —*see* condition
Serositis, multiple 569.89
  pericardial 423.2
  peritoneal 568.82
  pleural—*see* Pleurisy
Serotonin syndrome 333.99
Serous —*see* condition
Sertoli cell
  adenoma (M8640/0)
    specified site—*see* Neoplasm, by site, benign
    unspecified site
      female 220
      male 222.0
  carcinoma (M8640/3)
    specified site—*see* Neoplasm, by site,
      malignant
    unspecified site 186.9
  syndrome (germinal aplasia) 606.0
  tumor (M8640/0)
    with lipid storage (M8641/0)
      specified site—*see* Neoplasm, by site,
        benign
      unspecified site
        female 220
        male 222.0
    specified site—*see* Neoplasm, by site, benign

Sertoli cell—*continued*
  unspecified site
    female 220
    male 222.0
Sertoli-Leydig cell tumor (M8631/0)
  specified site—*see* Neoplasm, by site, benign
  unspecified site
    female 220
    male 222.0
Serum
  allergy, allergic reaction 999.5
    shock 999.4
  arthritis 999.5 *[713.6]*
  complication or reaction NEC 999.5
  disease NEC 999.5
  hepatitis 070.3
  intoxication 999.5
  jaundice (homologous) *see* Hepatitis, viral
  neuritis 999.5
  poisoning NEC 999.5
  rash NEC 999.5
  reaction NEC 999.5
  sickness NEC 999.5
Sesamoiditis 733.99
Seven-day fever 061
  of
    Japan 100.89
    Queensland 100.89
Sever's disease or osteochondrosis (calcaneum)
  732.5
Sex chromosome mosaics 758.81
Sextuplet
  affected by maternal complications of
    pregnancy 761.5
  healthy liveborn—*see* Newborn, multiple
  pregnancy (complicating delivery) NEC 651.8
    with fetal loss and retention of one or more
      fetus(es) 651.6
Sexual
  anesthesia 302.72
  deviation (*see also* Deviation, sexual) 302.9
  disorder (*see also* Deviation, sexual) 302.9
  frigidity (female) 302.72
  function, disorder of (psychogenic) 302.70
    specified type NEC 302.79
  immaturity (female) (male) 259.0
  impotence (psychogenic) 302.72
    organic origin NEC 607.84
  precocity (constitutional) (cryptogenic) (female)
    (idiopathic) (male) NEC 259.1
    with adrenal hyperplasia 255.2
  sadism 302.84
Sexuality, pathological (*see also* Deviation,
  sexual) 302.9
Sézary's disease, reticulosis, or syndrome
  (M9701/3) 202.2
Shadow, lung 793.1
Shaken infant syndrome 995.55
Shaking
  head (tremor) 781.0
  palsy or paralysis (*see also* Parkinsonism) 332.0
Shallowness, acetabulum 736.39
Shaver's disease or syndrome (bauxite
  pneumoconiosis) 503
Shearing
  artificial skin graft 996.55
  decellularized allodermis graft 996.55
Sheath (tendon)—*see* condition
Shedding
  nail 703.8
  teeth, premature, primary (deciduous) 520.6

Sheehan's disease or syndrome (postpartum
   pituitary necrosis) 253.2
Shelf, rectal 569.49
Shell
   shock (current) (*see also* Reaction, stress, acute)
      308.9
      lasting state 300.16
   teeth 520.5
Shield kidney 753.3
Shift, mediastinal 793.2
Shifting
   pacemaker 427.89
   sleep-work schedule (affecting sleep) 307.45
Shiga's
   bacillus 004.0
   dysentery 004.0
Shigella (dysentery) (*see also* Dysentery,
      bacillary) 004.9
   carrier (suspected) of V02.3
Shigellosis (*see also* Dysentery, bacillary) 004.9
Shingles (*see also* Herpes, zoster) 053.9
   eye NEC 053.29
Shin splints 844.9
Shipyard eye or disease 077.1
Shirodkar suture, in pregnancy 654.5
Shock 785.50
   with
      abortion—*see* Abortion, by type, with shock
      ectopic pregnancy (*see also* categories
         633.0-633.9) 639.5
      molar pregnancy (*see also* categories
         630-632) 639.5
   allergic—*see* Shock, anaphylactic
   anaclitic 309.21
   anaphylactic 995.0
      chemical—*see* Table of drugs and chemicals
      correct medicinal substance properly
         administered 995.0
      drug or medicinal substance
         correct substance properly administered
            995.0
         overdose or wrong substance given or taken
            977.9
         specified drug—*see* Table of drugs and
            chemicals
      food—*see* Anaphylactic shock, due to, food
      following sting(s) 989.5
      immunization 999.4
      serum 999.4
   anaphylactoid—*see* Shock, anaphylactic
   anesthetic
      correct substance properly administered 995.4
      overdose or wrong substance given 968.4
         specified anesthetic—*see* Table of drugs
            and chemicals
   birth, fetus or newborn NEC 779.89
   cardiogenic 785.51
   chemical substance—*see* Table of drugs and
      chemicals
   circulatory 785.59
   complicating
      abortion—*see* Abortion, by type, with shock
      ectopic pregnancy (*see also* categories
         633.0-633.9) 639.5
      labor and delivery 669.1
      molar pregnancy (*see also* categories
         630-632) 639.5
   culture 309.29

Shock—*continued*
   due to
      drug 995.0
         correct substance properly administered
            995.0
         overdose or wrong substance given or taken
            977.9
         specified drug—*see* Table of drugs and
            chemicals
      food—*see* Anaphylactic shock, due to, food
   during labor and delivery 669.1
   electric 994.8
   endotoxic 785.59
      due to surgical procedure 998.0
   following
      abortion 639.5
      ectopic or molar pregnancy 639.5
      injury (immediate) (delayed) 958.4
      labor and delivery 669.1
   gram-negative 785.59
   hematogenic 785.59
   hemorrhagic
      due to
         disease 785.59
         surgery (intraoperative) (postoperative)
            998.0
         trauma 958.4
   hypovolemic NEC 785.59
      surgical 998.0
      traumatic 958.4
   insulin 251.0
      therapeutic misadventure 962.3
   kidney 584.5
      traumatic (following crushing) 958.5
   lightning 994.0
   lung 518.5
   nervous (*see also* Reaction, stress, acute) 308.9
   obstetric 669.1
      with
         abortion—*see* Abortion, by type, with shock
         ectopic pregnancy (*see also* categories
            633.0-633.9) 639.5
         molar pregnancy (*see also* categories
            630-632) 639.5
      following
         abortion 639.5
         ectopic or molar pregnancy 639.5
   paralysis, paralytic (*see also* Disease,
      cerebrovascular, acute) 436
      late effect—*see* Late effect(s) (of)
         cerebrovascular disease
   pleural (surgical) 998.0
      due to trauma 958.4
   postoperative 998.0
      with
         abortion—*see* Abortion, by type, with shock
         ectopic pregnancy (*see also* categories
            633.0-633.9) 639.5
         molar pregnancy (*see also* categories
            630-632) 639.5
      following
         abortion 639.5
         ectopic or molar pregnancy 639.5
   psychic (*see also* Reaction, stress, acute) 308.9
      past history (of) V15.49
   psychogenic (*see also* Reaction, stress, acute)
      308.9
   septic 785.59
      with
         abortion—*see* Abortion, by type, with shock

Shock—*continued*
  ectopic pregnancy (*see also* categories
      633.0-633.9) 639.5
  molar pregnancy (*see also* categories
      630-632) 639.5
  due to
      surgical procedure 998.0
      transfusion NEC 999.8
          bone marrow 996.85
  following
      abortion 639.5
      ectopic or molar pregnancy 639.5
      surgical procedure 998.0
      transfusion NEC 999.8
          bone marrow 996.85
  spinal—*see also* Injury, spinal, by site
      with spinal bone injury—*see* Fracture,
          vertebra, by site, with spinal cord injury
  surgical 998.0
  therapeutic misadventure NEC (*see also*
      Complications) 998.89
  thyroxin 962.7
  toxic 040.82
  transfusion—*see* Complications, transfusion
  traumatic (immediate) (delayed) 958.4
Shoemakers' chest 738.3
Short, shortening, shortness
  Achilles tendon (acquired) 727.81
  arm 736.89
      congenital 755.20
  back 737.9
  bowel syndrome 579.3
  breath 786.05
  common bile duct, congenital 751.69
  cord (umbilical) 663.4
      affecting fetus or newborn 762.6
  cystic duct, congenital 751.69
  esophagus (congenital) 750.4
  femur (acquired) 736.81
      congenital 755.34
  frenulum linguae 750.0
  frenum, lingual 750.0
  hamstrings 727.81
  hip (acquired) 736.39
      congenital 755.63
  leg (acquired) 736.81
      congenital 755.30
  metatarsus (congenital) 754.79
      acquired 736.79
  organ or site, congenital NEC—*see* Distortion
  palate (congenital) 750.26
  P-R interval syndrome 426.81
  radius (acquired) 736.09
      congenital 755.26
  round ligament 629.8
  sleeper 307.49
  stature, constitutional (hereditary) 783.43
  tendon 727.81
      Achilles (acquired) 727.81
          congenital 754.79
      congenital 756.89
  thigh (acquired) 736.81
      congenital 755.34
  tibialis anticus 727.81
  umbilical cord 663.4
      affecting fetus or newborn 762.6
  urethra 599.84
  uvula (congenital) 750.26
  vagina 623.8
Shortsightedness 367.1
Shoshin (acute fulminating beriberi) 265.0
Shoulder —*see* condition

Shovel-shaped incisors 520.2
Shower, thromboembolic —*see* Embolism
Shunt (status)
  aortocoronary bypass V45.81
  arterial-venous (dialysis) V45.1
  arteriovenous, pulmonary (acquired) 417.0
      congenital 747.3
      traumatic (complication) 901.40
  cerebral ventricle (communicating) in situ V45.2
  coronary artery bypass V45.81
  surgical, prosthetic, with complications—*see*
      Complications, shunt
  vascular NEC V45.89
Shutdown
  renal 586
      with
          abortion—*see* Abortion, by type, with renal
              failure
          ectopic pregnancy (*see also* categories
              633.0-633.9) 639.3
          molar pregnancy (*see also* categories
              630-632) 639.3
      complicating
          abortion 639.3
          ectopic or molar pregnancy 639.3
      following labor and delivery 669.3
Shwachman's syndrome 288.0
Shy-Drager syndrome (orthostatic hypotension
      with multisystem degeneration) 333.0
Sialadenitis (any gland) (chronic) (suppurative)
      527.2
  epidemic—*see* Mumps
Sialadenosis, periodic 527.2
Sialaporia 527.7
Sialectasia 527.8
Sialitis 527.2
Sialoadenitis (*see also* Sialadenitis) 527.2
Sialoangitis 527.2
Sialodochitis (fibrinosa) 527.2
Sialodocholithiasis 527.5
Sialolithiasis 527.5
Sialorrhea (*see also* Ptyalism) 527.7
  periodic 527.2
Sialosis 527.8
  rheumatic 710.2
Siamese twin 759.4
Sicard's syndrome 352.6
Sicca syndrome (keratoconjunctivitis) 710.2
Sick 799.9
  cilia syndrome 759.89
  or handicapped person in family V61.49
Sickle-cell
  anemia (*see also* Disease, sickle-cell) 282.60
  disease (*see also* Disease, sickle-cell) 282.60
  hemoglobin
      C disease 282.63
      D disease 282.69
      E disease 282.69
  thalassemia 282.4
  trait 282.5
Sicklemia (*see also* Disease, sickle-cell) 282.60
  trait 282.5
Sickness
  air (travel) 994.6
  airplane 994.6
  alpine 993.2
  altitude 993.2
  Andes 993.2
  aviators' 993.2
  balloon 993.2
  car 994.6

Sickness— *continued*
compressed air 993.3
decompression 993.3
green 280.9
harvest 100.89
milk 988.8
morning 643.0
motion 994.6
mountain 993.2
acute 289.0
protein (*see also* Complications, vaccination)
999.5
radiation NEC 990
roundabout (motion) 994.6
sea 994.6
serum NEC 999.5
sleeping (African) 086.5
by Trypanosoma 086.5
gambiense 086.3
rhodesiense 086.4
Gambian 086.3
late effect 139.8
Rhodesian 086.4
sweating 078.2
swing (motion) 994.6
train (railway) (travel) 994.6
travel (any vehicle) 994.6
Sick sinus syndrome 427.81
Sideropenia (*see also* Anemia, iron deficiency)
280.9
Siderosis (lung) (occupational) 503
cornea 371.15
eye (bulbi) (vitreous) 360.23
lens 360.23
Siegal-Cattan-Mamou disease (periodic) 277.3
Siemens' syndrome
ectodermal dysplasia 757.31
keratosis follicularis spinulosa (decalvans)
757.39
Sighing respiration 786.7
Sigmoid
flexure—*see* condition
kidney 753.3
Sigmoiditis —*see* Enteritis
Silfverskiöld's syndrome 756.50
Silicosis, sillicotic (complicated) (occupational)
(simple) 502
fibrosis, lung (confluent) (massive)
(occupational) 502
non-nodular 503
pulmonum 502
Silicotuberculosis (*see also* Tuberculosis) 011.4
Silo fillers' disease 506.9
Silver's syndrome (congenital hemihypertrophy
and short stature) 759.89
Silver wire arteries, retina 362.13
Silvestroni-Bianco syndrome (thalassemia
minima) 282.4
Simian crease 757.2
Simmonds' cachexia or disease (pituitary
cachexia) 253.2
Simons' disease or syndrome (progressive
lipodystrophy) 272.6
Simple, simplex —*see* condition
Sinding-Larsen disease (juvenile osteopathia
patellae) 732.4
Singapore hemorrhagic fever 065.4
Singers' node or nodule 478.5

Single
atrium 745.69
coronary artery 746.85
umbilical artery 747.5
ventricle 745.3
Singultus 786.8
epidemicus 078.89
Sinus —*see also* Fistula
abdominal 569.81
arrest 426.6
arrhythmia 427.89
bradycardia 427.89
chronic 427.81
branchial cleft (external) (internal) 744.41
coccygeal (infected) 685.1
with abscess 685.0
dental 522.7
dermal (congenital) 685.1
with abscess 685.0
draining—*see* Fistula
infected, skin NEC 686.9
marginal, ruptured or bleeding 641.2
affecting fetus or newborn 762.1
pause 426.6
pericranii 742.0
pilonidal (infected) (rectum) 685.1
with abscess 685.0
preauricular 744.46
rectovaginal 619.1
sacrococcygeal (dermoid) (infected) 685.1
with abscess 685.0
skin
infected NEC 686.9
noninfected—*see* Ulcer, skin
tachycardia 427.89
tarsi syndrome 726.79
testis 608.89
tract (postinfectional)—*see* Fistula
urachus 753.7
Sinuses, Rokitansky-Aschoff (*see also* Disease,
gallbladder) 575.8
Sinusitis (accessory) (nasal) (hyperplastic)
(nonpurulent) (purulent) (chronic) 473.9
with influenza, flu, or grippe 487.1
acute 461.9
ethmoidal 461.2
frontal 461.1
maxillary 461.0
specified type NEC 461.8
sphenoidal 461.3
allergic (*see also* Fever, hay) 477.9
antrum—*see* Sinusitis, maxillary
due to
fungus, any sinus 117.9
high altitude 993.1
ethmoidal 473.2
acute 461.2
frontal 473.1
acute 461.1
influenzal 478.1
maxillary 473.0
acute 461.0
specified site NEC 473.8
sphenoidal 473.3
acute 461.3
syphilitic, any sinus 095.8
tuberculous, any sinus (*see also* Tuberculosis)
012.8
Sinusitis-bronchiectasis-situs inversus
(syndrome) (triad) 759.3
Sipple's syndrome (medullary thyroid
carcinoma-pheochromocytoma) 193

Sirenomelia 759.89
Siriasis 992.0
Sirkari's disease 085.0
SIRS (systemic inflammatory response
  syndrome) 995.90
  due to
    infectious disease 995.91
      with organ dysfunction 995.92
    non-infectious process 995.93
      with organ dysfunction 995.94
Siti 104.0
Sitophobia 300.29
Situation, psychiatric 300.9
Situational
  disturbance (transient) (*see also* Reaction,
    adjustment) 309.9
    acute 308.3
  maladjustment, acute (*see also* Reaction,
    adjustment) 309.9
  reaction (*see also* Reaction, adjustment) 309.9
    acute 308.3
Situs inversus or transversus 759.3
  abdominalis 759.3
  thoracis 759.3
Sixth disease 057.8
Sjögren (-Gougerot) syndrome or disease
  (keratoconjunctivitis sicca) 710.2
  with lung involvement 710.2 [517.8]
Sjögren-Larsson syndrome (ichthyosis
  congenita) 757.1
Skeletal —*see* condition
Skene's gland —*see* condition
Skenitis (*see also* Urethritis) 597.89
  gonorrheal (acute) 098.0
    chronic or duration of 2 months or over 098.2
Skerljevo 104.0
Skevas-Zerfus disease 989.5
Skin —*see also* condition
  donor V59.1
  hidebound 710.9
SLAP lesion (superior glenoid labrum) 840.7
Slate-dressers' lung 502
Slate-miners' lung 502
Sleep
  disorder 780.50
    with apnea—*see* Apnea, sleep
    child 307.40
    nonorganic origin 307.40
      specified type NEC 307.49
  disturbance 780.50
    with apnea—*see* Apnea, sleep
    nonorganic origin 307.40
      specified type NEC 307.49
  drunkenness 307.47
  paroxysmal 347
  rhythm inversion 780.55
    nonorganic origin 307.45
  walking 307.46
    hysterical 300.13
Sleeping sickness 086.5
  late effect 139.8
Sleeplessness (*see also* Insomnia) 780.52
  menopausal 627.2
  nonorganic origin 307.41
Slipped, slipping
  epiphysis (postinfectional) 732.9
    traumatic (old) 732.9
      current—*see* Fracture, by site
    upper femoral (nontraumatic) 732.2
  intervertebral disc—*see* Displacement,
    intervertebral disc

Slipped, slipping—*continued*
  ligature, umbilical 772.3
  patella 717.89
  rib 733.99
  sacroiliac joint 724.6
  tendon 727.9
  ulnar nerve, nontraumatic 354.2
  vertebra NEC (*see also* Spondylolisthesis)
    756.12
Slocumb's syndrome 255.3
Sloughing (multiple) (skin) 686.9
  abscess—*see* Abscess, by site
  appendix 543.9
  bladder 596.8
  fascia 728.9
  graft—*see* Complications, graft
  phagedena (*see also* Gangrene) 785.4
  reattached extremity (*see also* Complications,
    reattached extremity) 996.90
  rectum 569.49
  scrotum 608.89
  tendon 727.9
  transplanted organ (*see also* Rejection,
    transplant, organ, by site) 996.80
  ulcer (*see also* Ulcer, skin) 707.9
Slow
  feeding newborn 779.3
  fetal, growth NEC 764.9
    affecting management of pregnancy 656.5
Slowing
  heart 427.89
  urinary stream 788.62
Sluder's neuralgia or syndrome 337.0
Slurred, slurring, speech 784.5
Small, smallness
  cardiac reserve—*see* Disease, heart
  for dates
    fetus or newborn 764.0
      with malnutrition 764.1
      affecting management of pregnancy 656.5
    infant, term 764.0
      with malnutrition 764.1
      affecting management of pregnancy 656.5
  introitus, vagina 623.3
  kidney, unknown cause 589.9
    bilateral 589.1
    unilateral 589.0
  ovary 620.8
  pelvis
    with disproportion (fetopelvic) 653.1
      affecting fetus or newborn 763.1
    causing obstructed labor 660.1
      affecting fetus or newborn 763.1
  placenta—*see* Placenta, insufficiency
  uterus 621.8
  white kidney 582.9
Small-for-dates (*see also* Light-for-dates) 764.0
  affecting management of pregnancy 656.5
Smallpox 050.9
  contact V01.3
  exposure to V01.3
  hemorrhagic (pustular) 050.0
  malignant 050.0
  modified 050.2
  vaccination
    complications—*see* Complications,
      vaccination
    prophylactic (against) V04.1
Smith's fracture (separation) (closed) 813.41
  open 813.51
Smith-Lemli-Opitz syndrome
  (cerebrohepatorenal syndrome) 759.89

Smith-Strang disease (oasthouse urine) 270.2
Smokers'
  bronchitis 491.0
  cough 491.0
  syndrome (*see also* Abuse, drugs,
    nondependent) 305.1
  throat 472.1
  tongue 528.6
Smothering spells 786.09
Snaggle teeth, tooth 524.3
Snapping
  finger 727.05
  hip 719.65
  jaw 524.69
  knee 717.9
  thumb 727.05
Sneddon-Wilkinson disease or syndrome
  (subcorneal pustular dermatosis) 694.1
Sneezing 784.9
  intractable 478.1
Sniffing
  cocaine (*see also* Dependence) 304.2
  ether (*see also* Dependence) 304.6
  glue (airplane) (*see also* Dependence) 304.6
Snoring 786.09
Snow blindness 370.24
Snuffles (nonsyphilitic) 460
  syphilitic (infant) 090.0
Social migrant V60.0
Sodoku 026.0
Soemmering's ring 366.51
Soft —*see also* condition
  enlarged prostate 600.0
  nails 703.8
Softening
  bone 268.2
  brain (necrotic) (progressive) 434.9
    arteriosclerotic 437.0
Softening—*continued*
    congenital 742.4
    embolic (*see also* Embolism, brain) 434.1
    hemorrhagic (*see also* Hemorrhage, brain) 431
    occlusive 434.9
    thrombotic (*see also* Thrombosis, brain) 434.0
  cartilage 733.92
  cerebellar—*see* Softening, brain
  cerebral—*see* Softening, brain
  cerebrospinal—*see* Softening, brain
  myocardial, heart (*see also* Degeneration,
    myocardial) 429.1
  nails 703.8
  spinal cord 336.8
  stomach 537.89
Solar fever 061
Soldier's
  heart 306.2
  patches 423.1
Solitary
  cyst
    bone 733.21
    kidney 593.2
  kidney (congenital) 753.0
  tubercle, brain (*see also* Tuberculosis, brain)
    013.2
  ulcer, bladder 596.8
Somatization reaction, somatic reaction (*see
  also* Disorder, psychosomatic) 306.9
  disorder 300.81
Somatoform disorder 300.82
  atypical 300.82
  severe 300.81
  undifferentiated 300.82

Somnambulism 307.46
  hysterical 300.13
Somnolence 780.09
  nonorganic origin 307.43
  periodic 349.89
Sonne dysentery 004.3
Soor 112.0
Sore
  Delhi 085.1
  desert (*see also* Ulcer, skin) 707.9
  eye 379.99
  Lahore 085.1
  mouth 528.9
    canker 528.2
    due to dentures 528.9
  muscle 729.1
  Naga (*see also* Ulcer, skin) 707.9
  oriental 085.1
  pressure 707.0
    with gangrene 707.0 *[785.4]*
  skin NEC 709.9
  soft 099.0
  throat 462
    with influenza, flu, or grippe 487.1
    acute 462
    chronic 472.1
    clergyman's 784.49
    coxsackie (virus) 074.0
    diphtheritic 032.0
    epidemic 034.0
    gangrenous 462
    herpetic 054.79
    influenzal 487.1
    malignant 462
    purulent 462
    putrid 462
    septic 034.0
    streptococcal (ulcerative) 034.0
    ulcerated 462
    viral NEC 462
      Coxsackie 074.0
  tropical (*see also* Ulcer, skin) 707.9
  veldt (*see also* Ulcer, skin) 707.9
Sotos' syndrome (cerebral gigantism) 253.0
Sounds
  friction, pleural 786.7
  succussion, chest 786.7
South African cardiomyopathy syndrome 425.2
South American
  blastomycosis 116.1
  trypanosomiasis—*see* Trypanosomiasis
Southeast Asian hemorrhagic fever 065.4
Spacing, teeth, abnormal 524.3
Spade-like hand (congenital) 754.89
Spading nail 703.8
  congenital 757.5
Spanemia 285.9
Spanish collar 605
Sparganosis 123.5
Spasm, spastic, spasticity (*see also* condition)
  781.0
  accommodation 367.53
  ampulla of Vater (*see also* Disease, gallbladder)
    576.8
  anus, ani (sphincter) (reflex) 564.6
    psychogenic 306.4
  artery NEC 443.9
    basilar 435.0
    carotid 435.8
    cerebral 435.9
      specified artery NEC 435.8

Spasm, spastic, spasticity—*continued*
  retinal (*see also* Occlusion, retinal, artery)
    362.30
    vertebral 435.1
    vertebrobasilar 435.3
  Bell's 351.0
  bladder (sphincter, external or internal) 596.8
  bowel 564.9
    psychogenic 306.4
  bronchus, bronchiole 519.1
  cardia 530.0
  cardiac—*see* Angina
  carpopedal (*see also* Tetany) 781.7
  cecum 564.9
    psychogenic 306.4
  cerebral (arteries) (vascular) 435.9
    specified artery NEC 435.8
  cerebrovascular 435.9
  cervix, complicating delivery 661.4
    affecting fetus or newborn 763.7
  ciliary body (of accommodation) 367.53
  colon 564.1
    psychogenic 306.4
  common duct (*see also* Disease, biliary) 576.8
  compulsive 307.22
  conjugate 378.82
  convergence 378.84
  coronary (artery)—*see* Angina
  diaphragm (reflex) 786.8
    psychogenic 306.1
  duodenum, duodenal (bulb) 564.89
  esophagus (diffuse) 530.5
    psychogenic 306.4
  facial 351.8
  fallopian tube 620.8
  gait 781.2
  gastrointestinal (tract) 536.8
    psychogenic 306.4
  glottis 478.75
    hysterical 300.11
    psychogenic 306.1
      specified as conversion reaction 300.11
    reflex through recurrent laryngeal nerve
      478.75
  habit 307.20
    chronic 307.22
    transient of childhood 307.21
  heart—*see* Angina
  hourglass—*see* Contraction, hourglass
  hysterical 300.11
  infantile (*see also* Epilepsy) 345.6
  internal oblique, eye 378.51
  intestinal 564.9
    psychogenic 306.4
  larynx, laryngeal 478.75
    hysterical 300.11
    psychogenic 306.1
      specified as conversion reaction 300.11
  levator palpebrae superioris 333.81
  lightning (*see also* Epilepsy) 345.6
  mobile 781.0
  muscle 728.85
    back 724.8
    psychogenic 306.0
  nerve, trigeminal 350.1
  nervous 306.0
  nodding 307.3
    infantile (*see also* Epilepsy) 345.6
  occupational 300.89
  oculogyric 378.87
  ophthalmic artery 362.30

Spasm, spastic, spasticity—*continued*
  orbicularis 781.0
  perineal 625.8
  peroneo-extensor (*see also* Flat, foot) 734
  pharynx (reflex) 478.29
    hysterical 300.11
    psychogenic 306.1
      specified as conversion reaction 300.11
  pregnant uterus, complicating delivery 661.4
  psychogenic 306.0
  pylorus 537.81
    adult hypertrophic 537.0
    congenital or infantile 750.5
    psychogenic 306.4
  rectum (sphincter) 564.6
    psychogenic 306.4
  retinal artery NEC (*see also* Occlusion, retina,
    artery) 362.30
  sacroiliac 724.6
  salaam (infantile) (*see also* Epilepsy) 345.6
  saltatory 781.0
  sigmoid 564.9
    psychogenic 306.4
  sphincter of Oddi (*see also* Disease,
    gallbladder) 576.5
  stomach 536.8
    neurotic 306.4
  throat 478.29
    hysterical 300.11
    psychogenic 306.1
      specified as conversion reaction 300.11
  tic 307.20
    chronic 307.22
    transient of childhood 307.21
  tongue 529.8
  torsion 333.6
  trigeminal nerve 350.1
    postherpetic 053.12
  ureter 593.89
  urethra (sphincter) 599.84
  uterus 625.8
    complicating labor 661.4
      affecting fetus or newborn 763.7
  vagina 625.1
    psychogenic 306.51
  vascular NEC 443.9
  vasomotor NEC 443.9
  vein NEC 459.89
  vesical (sphincter, external or internal) 596.8
  viscera 789.0
Spasmodic —*see* condition
Spasmophilia (*see also* Tetany) 781.7
Spasmus nutans 307.3
Spastic —*see also* Spasm
  child 343.9
Spasticity —*see also* Spasm
  cerebral, child 343.9
Speakers' throat 784.49
Specific, specified —*see* condition
Speech
  defect, disorder, disturbance, impediment NEC
    784.5
    psychogenic 307.9
  therapy V57.3
Spells 780.39
  breath-holding 786.9
Spencer's disease (epidemic vomiting) 078.82
Spens' syndrome (syncope with heart block)
  426.9
Spermatic cord —*see* condition
Spermatocele 608.1
  congenital 752.8

Spermatocystitis 608.4
Spermatocytoma (M9063/3)
  specified site—*see* Neoplasm, by site, malignant
  unspecified site 186.9
Spermatorrhea 608.89
Sperm counts
  fertility testing V26.21
  following sterilization reversal V26.22
  postvasectomy V25.8
Sphacelus (*see also* Gangrene) 785.4
Sphenoidal —*see* condition
Sphenoiditis (chronic) (*see also* Sinusitis,
  sphenoidal) 473.3
Sphenopalatine ganglion neuralgia 337.0
Sphericity, increased, lens 743.36
Spherocytosis (congenital) (familial) (hereditary)
  282.0
  hemoglobin disease 287.7
  sickle-cell (disease) 282.60
Spherophakia 743.36
Sphincter —*see* condition
Sphincteritis, sphincter of Oddi (*see also*
  Cholecystitis) 576.8
Sphingolipidosis 272.7
Sphingolipodystrophy 272.7
Sphingomyelinosis 272.7
Spicule tooth 520.2
Spider
  finger 755.59
  nevus 448.1
  vascular 448.1
Spiegler-Fendt sarcoid 686.8
Spielmeyer-Stock disease 330.1
Spielmeyer-Vogt disease 330.1
Spina bifida (aperta) 741.9

Note—Use the following fifth-digit
subclassification with category 741:

0 *unspecified region*
1 *cervical region*
2 *dorsal [thoracic] region*
3 *lumbar region*

---

  with hydrocephalus 741.0
  fetal (suspected), affecting management of
    pregnancy 655.0
  occulta 756.17
Spindle, Krukenberg's 371.13
Spine, spinal —*see* condition
Spiradenoma (eccrine) (M8403/0)—*see*
  Neoplasm, skin, benign
Spirillosis NEC (*see also* Fever, relapsing) 087.9
Spirillum minus 026.0
Spirillum obermeieri infection 087.0
Spirochetal —*see* condition
Spirochetosis 104.9
  arthritic, arthritica 104.9 *[711.8]*
  bronchopulmonary 104.8
  icterohemorrhagica 100.0
  lung 104.8
Spitting blood (*see also* Hemoptysis) 786.3
Splanchnomegaly 569.89
Splanchnoptosis 569.89
Spleen, splenic —*see also* condition
  agenesis 759.0
  flexure syndrome 569.89
  neutropenia syndrome 288.0
  sequestration syndrome 282.60
Splenectasis (*see also* Splenomegaly) 789.2

Splenitis (interstitial) (malignant) (nonspecific)
  289.59
  malarial (*see also* Malaria) 084.6
  tuberculous (*see also* Tuberculosis) 017.7
Splenocele 289.59
Splenomegalia —*see* Splenomegaly
Splenomegalic —*see* condition
Splenomegaly 789.2
  Bengal 789.2
  cirrhotic 289.51
  congenital 759.0
  congestive, chronic 289.51
  cryptogenic 789.2
  Egyptian 120.1
  Gaucher's (cerebroside lipidosis) 272.7
  idiopathic 789.2
  malarial (*see also* Malaria) 084.6
  neutropenic 288.0
  Niemann-Pick (lipid histiocytosis) 272.7
  siderotic 289.51
  syphilitic 095.8
    congenital 090.0
  tropical (Bengal) (idiopathic) 789.2
Splenopathy 289.50
Splenopneumonia —*see* Pneumonia
Splenoptosis 289.59
Splinter —*see* Injury, superficial, by site
Split, splitting
  heart sounds 427.89
  lip, congenital (*see also* Cleft, lip) 749.10
  nails 703.8
  urinary stream 788.61
Spoiled child reaction (*see also* Disturbance,
  conduct) 312.1
Spondylarthritis (*see also* Spondylosis) 721.90
Spondylarthrosis (*see also* Spondylosis) 721.90
Spondylitis 720.9
  ankylopoietica 720.0
  ankylosing (chronic) 720.0
  atrophic 720.9
    ligamentous 720.9
  chronic (traumatic) (*see also* Spondylosis)
    721.90
  deformans (chronic) (*see also* Spondylosis)
    721.90
  gonococcal 098.53
  gouty 274.0
  hypertrophic (*see also* Spondylosis) 721.90
  infectious NEC 720.9
  juvenile (adolescent) 720.0
  Kümmell's 721.7
  Marie-Strümpell (ankylosing) 720.0
  muscularis 720.9
  ossificans ligamentosa 721.6
  osteoarthritica (*see also* Spondylosis) 721.90
  posttraumatic 721.7
  proliferative 720.0
  rheumatoid 720.0
  rhizomelica 720.0
  sacroiliac NEC 720.2
  senescent (*see also* Spondylosis) 721.90
  senile (*see also* Spondylosis) 721.90
  static (*see also* Spondylosis) 721.90
  traumatic (chronic) (*see also* Spondylosis)
    721.90
  tuberculous (*see also* Tuberculosis) 015.0
    [720.81]
  typhosa 002.0 *[720.81]*
Spondyloarthrosis (*see also* Spondylosis) 721.90

Spondylolisthesis (congenital) (lumbosacral)
    756.12
  with disproportion (fetopelvic) 653.3
    affecting fetus or newborn 763.1
    causing obstructed labor 660.1
      affecting fetus or newborn 763.1
  acquired 738.4
  degenerative 738.4
  traumatic 738.4
    acute (lumbar)—*see* Fracture, vertebra, lumbar
    site other than lumbosacral—*see* Fracture,
      vertebra, by site
Spondylolysis (congenital) 756.11
  acquired 738.4
  cervical 756.19
  lumbosacral region 756.11
    with disproportion (fetopelvic) 653.3
      affecting fetus or newborn 763.1
      causing obstructed labor 660.1
        affecting fetus or newborn 763.1
Spondylopathy
  inflammatory 720.9
    specified type NEC 720.89
  traumatic 721.7
Spondylose rhizomelique 720.0
Spondylosis 721.90
  with
    disproportion 653.3
      affecting fetus or newborn 763.1
      causing obstructed labor 660.1
        affecting fetus or newborn 763.1
    myelopathy NEC 721.91
  cervical, cervicodorsal 721.0
    with myelopathy 721.1
  inflammatory 720.9
  lumbar, lumbosacral 721.3
    with myelopathy 721.42
  sacral 721.3
    with myelopathy 721.42
  thoracic 721.2
    with myelopathy 721.41
  traumatic 721.7
Sponge
  divers' disease 989.5
  inadvertently left in operation wound 998.4
  kidney (medullary) 753.17
Spongioblastoma (M9422/3)
  multiforme (M9440/3)
    specified site—*see* Neoplasm, by site,
      malignant
    unspecified site 191.9
  polare (M9423/3)
    specified site—*see* Neoplasm, by site,
      malignant
    unspecified site 191.9
  primitive polar (M9443/3)
    specified site—*see* Neoplasm, by site,
      malignant
    unspecified site 191.9
  specified site—*see* Neoplasm, by site, malignant
  unspecified site 191.9
Spongiocytoma (M9400/3)
  specified site—*see* Neoplasm, by site, malignant
  unspecified site 191.9
Spongioneuroblastoma (M9504/3)—*see*
  Neoplasm, by site, malignant
Spontaneous —*see also* condition
  fracture—*see* Fracture, pathologic
Spoon nail 703.8
  congenital 757.5
Sporadic —*see* condition

Sporotrichosis (bones) (cutaneous)
    (disseminated) (epidermal) (lymphatic)
    (lymphocutaneous) (mucous membranes)
    (pulmonary) (skeletal) (visceral) 117.1
Sporotrichum schenckii infection 117.1
Spots, spotting
  atrophic (skin) 701.3
  Bitôt's (in the young child) 264.1
  café au lait 709.09
  cayenne pepper 448.1
  cotton wool (retina) 362.83
  de Morgan's (senile angiomas) 448.1
  Fúchs' black (myopic) 360.21
  intermenstrual
    irregular 626.6
    regular 626.5
  interpalpebral 372.53
  Koplik's 055.9
  liver 709.09
  Mongolian (pigmented) 757.33
  of pregnancy 641.9
  purpuric 782.7
  ruby 448.1
Spotted fever —*see* Fever, spotted
Sprain, strain (joint) (ligament) (muscle)
    (tendon) 848.9
  abdominal wall (muscle) 848.8
  Achilles tendon 845.09
  acromioclavicular 840.0
  ankle 845.00
    and foot 845.00
  anterior longitudinal, cervical 847.0
  arm 840.9
    upper 840.9
      and shoulder 840.9
  astragalus 845.00
  atlanto-axial 847.0
  atlanto-occipital 847.0
  atlas 847.0
  axis 847.0
  back (*see also* Sprain, spine) 847.9
  breast bone 848.40
  broad ligament—*see* Injury, internal, broad
    ligament
  calcaneofibular 845.02
  carpal 842.01
  carpometacarpal 842.11
  cartilage
    costal, without mention of injury to sternum
      848.3
      involving sternum 848.42
    ear 848.8
    knee 844.9
      with current tear (*see also* Tear, meniscus)
        836.2
    semilunar (knee) 844.8
      with current tear (*see also* Tear, meniscus)
        836.2
    septal, nose 848.0
    thyroid region 848.2
    xiphoid 848.49
  cervical, cervicodorsal, cervicothoracic 847.0
  chondrocostal, without mention of injury to
    sternum 848.3
    involving sternum 848.42
  chondrosternal 848.42
  chronic (joint)—*see* Derangement, joint
  clavicle 840.9
  coccyx 847.4
  collar bone 840.9

Sprain, strain—*continued*
  ligament 846.1
    specified site NEC 846.8
  sacrospinatus 846.2
  sacrospinous 846.2
  sacrotuberous 846.3
  scaphoid bone, ankle 845.00
  scapula(r) 840.9
  semilunar cartilage (knee) 844.8
    with current tear (*see also* Tear, meniscus)
        836.2
    old 717.5
  septal cartilage (nose) 848.0
  shoulder 840.9
    and arm, upper 840.9
    blade 840.9
  specified site NEC 848.8
  spine 847.9
    cervical 847.0
    coccyx 847.4
    dorsal 847.1
    lumbar 847.2
    lumbosacral 846.0
      chronic or old 724.6
    sacral 847.3
    sacroiliac (*see also* Sprain, sacroiliac) 846.9
      chronic or old 724.6
    thoracic 847.1
  sternoclavicular 848.41
  sternum 848.40
  subglenoid (*see also* SLAP lesion) 840.8
  subscapularis 840.5
  supraspinatus 840.6
  symphysis
    jaw 848.1
      old 524.69
    mandibular 848.1
      old 524.69
    pubis 848.5
  talofibular 845.09
  tarsal 845.10
  tarsometatarsal 845.11
  temporomandibular 848.1
    old 524.69
  teres
    ligamentum femoris 843.8
    major or minor 840.8
  thigh (proximal end) 843.9
    and hip 843.9
    distal end 844.9
  thoracic (spine) 847.1
  thorax 848.8
  thumb 842.10
  thyroid cartilage or region 848.2
  tibia (proximal end) 844.9
    distal end 845.00
  tibiofibular
    distal 845.03
    superior 844.3
  toe(s) 845.10
  trachea 848.8
  trapezoid 840.8
  ulna, ulnar (proximal end) 841.9
    collateral 841.1
    distal end 842.00
  ulnohumeral 841.3
  vertebrae (*see also* Sprain, spine) 847.9
    cervical, cervicodorsal, cervicothoracic 847.0
  wrist (cuneiform) (scaphoid) (semilunar) 842.00
  xiphoid cartilage 848.49
Sprengel's deformity (congenital) 755.52
Spring fever 309.23

Sprue 579.1
  celiac 579.0
  idiopathic 579.0
  meaning thrush 112.0
  nontropical 579.0
  tropical 579.1
Spur —*see also* Exostosis
  bone 726.91
    calcaneal 726.73
  calcaneal 726.73
  iliac crest 726.5
  nose (septum) 478.1
    bone 726.91
  septal 478.1
Spuria placenta —*see* Placenta, abnormal
Spurway's syndrome (brittle bones and blue
      sclera) 756.51
Sputum, abnormal (amount) (color) (excessive)
      (odor) (purulent) 786.4
  bloody 786.3
Squamous —*see also* condition
  cell metaplasia
    bladder 596.8
    cervix—*see* condition
  epithelium in
    cervical canal (congenital) 752.49
    uterine mucosa (congenital) 752.3
  metaplasia
    bladder 596.8
    cervix—*see* condition
Squashed nose 738.0
  congenital 754.0
Squeeze, divers' 993.3
Squint (*see also* Strabismus) 378.9
  accommodative (*see also* Esotropia) 378.00
  concomitant (*see also* Heterotropia) 378.30
Stab —*see also* Wound, open, by site
  internal organs—*see* Injury, internal, by site,
      with open wound
Staggering gait 781.2
  hysterical 300.11
Staghorn calculus 592.0
Stähl's
  ear 744.29
  pigment line (cornea) 371.11
Stähli's pigment lines (cornea) 371.11
Stain
  port wine 757.32
  tooth, teeth (hard tissues) 521.7
    due to
      accretions 523.6
      deposits (betel) (black) (green) (materia
          alba) (orange) (tobacco) 523.6
      metals (copper) (silver) 521.7
      nicotine 523.6
      pulpal bleeding 521.7
      tobacco 523.6
Stammering 307.0
Standstill
  atrial 426.6
  auricular 426.6
  cardiac (*see also* Arrest, cardiac) 427.5
  sinoatrial 426.6
  sinus 426.6
  ventricular (*see also* Arrest, cardiac) 427.5
Stannosis 503
Stanton's disease (melioidosis) 025
Staphylitis (acute) (catarrhal) (chronic)
      (gangrenous) (membranous) (suppurative)
      (ulcerative) 528.3

Staphylococcemia 038.10
  aureus 038.11
  specified organism NEC 038.19
Staphylococcus, staphylococcal —*see* condition
Staphyloderma (skin) 686.00
Staphyloma 379.11
  anterior, localized 379.14
  ciliary 379.11
  cornea 371.73
  equatorial 379.13
  posterior 379.12
  posticum 379.12
  ring 379.15
  sclera NEC 379.11
Starch eating 307.52
Stargardt's disease 362.75
Starvation (inanition) (due to lack of food) 994.2
  edema 262
  voluntary NEC 307.1
Stasis
  bile (duct) (*see also* Disease, biliary) 576.8
  bronchus (*see also* Bronchitis) 490
  cardiac (*see also* Failure, heart) 428.0
  cecum 564.89
  colon 564.89
  dermatitis (*see also* Varix, with stasis
    dermatitis) 454.1
  duodenal 536.8
  eczema (*see also* Varix, with stasis dermatitis)
    454.1
  edema (*see also* Hypertension, venous) 459.30
  foot 991.4
  gastric 536.3
  ileocecal coil 564.89
  ileum 564.89
  intestinal 564.89
  jejunum 564.89
  kidney 586
  liver 571.9
    cirrhotic—*see* Cirrhosis, liver
  lymphatic 457.8
  pneumonia 514
  portal 571.9
  pulmonary 514
  rectal 564.89
  renal 586
    tubular 584.5
  stomach 536.3
  ulcer
    with varicose veins 454.0
    without varicose veins 459.81
  urine NEC (*see also* Retention, urine) 788.20
  venous 459.81
State
  affective and paranoid, mixed, organic
    psychotic 294.8
  agitated 307.9
    acute reaction to stress 308.2
  anxiety (neurotic) (*see also* Anxiety) 300.00
    specified type NEC 300.09
  apprehension (*see also* Anxiety) 300.00
    specified type NEC 300.09
  climacteric, female 627.2
    following induced menopause 627.4
  clouded
    epileptic (*see also* Epilepsy) 345.9
    paroxysmal (idiopathic) (*see also* Epilepsy)
      345.9
  compulsive (mixed) (with obsession) 300.3
  confusional 298.9

State—*continued*
  acute 293.0
    with
      arteriosclerotic dementia 290.41
      presenile brain disease 290.11
      senility 290.3
    alcoholic 291.0
    drug-induced 292.81
    epileptic 293.0
    postoperative 293.9
    reactive (emotional stress) (psychological
      trauma) 298.2
    subacute 293.1
  constitutional psychopathic 301.9
  convulsive (*see also* Convulsions) 780.39
  depressive NEC 311
    induced by drug 292.84
    neurotic 300.4
  dissociative 300.15
  hallucinatory 780.1
    induced by drug 292.12
  hyperdynamic beta-adrenergic circulatory
    429.82
  locked-in 344.81
  menopausal 627.2
    artificial 627.4
    following induced menopause 627.4
  neurotic NEC 300.9
    with depersonalization episode 300.6
  obsessional 300.3
  oneiroid (*see also* Schizophrenia) 295.4
  panic 300.01
  paranoid 297.9
    alcohol-induced 291.5
    arteriosclerotic 290.42
    climacteric 297.2
    drug-induced 292.11
    in
      presenile brain disease 290.12
      senile brain disease 290.20
    involutional 297.2
    menopausal 297.2
    senile 290.20
    simple 297.0
  postleukotomy 310.0
  pregnant (*see also* Pregnancy) V22.2
  psychogenic, twilight 298.2
  psychotic, organic (*see also* Psychosis, organic)
    294.9
    mixed paranoid and affective 294.8
    senile or presenile NEC 290.9
    transient NEC 293.9
      with
        anxiety 293.84
        delusions 293.81
        depression 293.83
        hallucinations 293.82
  residual schizophrenic (*see also* Schizophrenia)
    295.6
  tension (*see also* Anxiety) 300.9
  transient organic psychotic 293.9
    anxiety type 293.84
    depressive type 293.83
    hallucinatory type 293.83
    paranoid type 293.81
    specified type NEC 293.89
  twilight
    epileptic 293.0
    psychogenic 298.2
  vegetative (persistent) 780.03

Status (post)

absence

epileptic (*see also* Epilepsy) 345.2

of organ, acquired (postsurgical)—*see* Absence, by site, acquired

anastomosis of intestine (for bypass) V45.3

angioplasty, percutaneous transluminal coronary V45.82

anginosus 413.9

ankle prosthesis V43.66

aortocoronary bypass or shunt V45.81

arthrodesis V45.4

artificially induced condition NEC V45.89

artificial opening (of) V44.9

gastrointestinal tract NEC V44.4

specified site NEC V44.8

urinary tract NEC V44.6

vagina V44.7

aspirator V46.0

asthmaticus (*see also* Asthma) 493.9

breast implant removal V45.83

cardiac

device (in situ) V45.00

defibrillator, automatic implantable V45.02

pacemaker V45.01

fitting or adjustment V53.3

carotid sinus V45.09

fitting or adjustment V53.3

carotid sinus stimulator V45.09

cataract extraction V45.61

chemotherapy V66.2

current V58.69

colostomy V44.3

contraceptive device V45.59

intrauterine V45.51

subdermal V45.52

convulsivus idiopathicus (*see also* Epilepsy) 345.3

coronary artery bypass or shunt V45.81

cystostomy V44.50

appendico-vesicostomy V44.52

cutaneous-vesicostomy V44.51

specified type NEC V44.59

defibrillator, automatic implantable cardiac V45.02

dental crowns V45.84

dental fillings V45.84

dental restoration V45.84

dental sealant V49.82

dialysis V45.1

donor V59.9

drug therapy or regimen V67.59

high-risk medication NEC V67.51

elbow prosthesis V43.62

enterostomy V44.4

epileptic, epilepticus (absence) (grand mal) (*see also* Epilepsy) 345.3

focal motor 345.7

partial 345.7

petit mal 345.2

psychomotor 345.7

temporal lobe 345.7

eye (adnexa) surgery V45.69

filtering bleb (eye) (postglaucoma) V45.69

with rupture or complication 997.99

postcataract extraction (complication) 997.99

finger joint prosthesis V43.69

gastrostomy V44.1

grand mal 345.3

heart valve prosthesis V43.3

hip prosthesis (joint) (partial) (total) V43.64

Status (post)—*continued*

ileostomy V44.2

intestinal bypass V45.3

intrauterine contraceptive device V45.51

jejunostomy V44.4

knee joint prosthesis V43.65

lacunaris 437.8

lacunosis 437.8

low birth weight V21.30

less than 500 grams V21.31

500-999 grams V21.32

1000-1499 grams V21.33

1500-1999 grams V21.34

2000-2500 grams V21.35

lymphaticus 254.8

malignant neoplasm, ablated or excised—*see* History, malignant neoplasm

marmoratus 333.7

nephrostomy V44.6

neuropacemaker NEC V45.89

brain V45.89

carotid sinus V45.09

neurologic NEC V45.89

organ replacement

by artificial or mechanical device or prosthesis of

artery V43.4

artificial skin V43.83

bladder V43.5

blood vessel V43.4

breast V43.82

eye globe V43.0

heart V43.2

valve V43.3

intestine V43.89

joint V43.60

ankle V43.66

elbow V43.62

finger V43.69

hip (partial) (total) V43.64

knee V43.65

shoulder V43.61

specified NEC 43.69

wrist V43.63

kidney V43.89

larynx V43.81

lens V43.1

limb(s) V43.7

liver V43.89

lung V43.89

organ NEC V43.89

pancreas V43.89

skin (artificial) V43.83

tissue NEC V43.89

vein V43.4

by organ transplant (heterologous) (homologous)—*see* Status, transplant

pacemaker

brain V45.89

cardiac V45.01

carotid sinus V45.09

neurologic NEC V45.89

specified site NEC V45.89

percutaneous transluminal coronary angioplasty V45.82

petit mal 345.2

postcommotio cerebri 310.2

postmenopausal (age related) (natural) V49.81

postoperative NEC V45.89

postpartum NEC V24.2

care immediately following delivery V24.0

Status (post)—*continued*
   routine follow-up V24.2
   postsurgical NEC V45.89
   renal dialysis V45.1
   respirator V46.1
   reversed jejunal transposition (for bypass) V45.3
   shoulder prosthesis V43.61
   shunt
     aortocoronary bypass V45.81
     arteriovenous (for dialysis) V45.1
     cerebrospinal fluid V45.2
     vascular NEC V45.89
       aortocoronary (bypass) V45.81
     ventricular (communicating) (for drainage) V45.2
   sterilization
     tubal ligation V26.51
     vasectomy V26.52
   subdermal contraceptive device V45.52
   thymicolymphaticus 254.8
   thymicus 254.8
   thymolymphaticus 254.8
   tooth extraction 525.10
   tracheostomy V44.0
   transplant
     blood vessel V42.89
     bone V42.4
       marrow V42.81
     cornea V42.5
     heart V42.1
       valve V42.2
     intestine V42.84
     kidney V42.0
     liver V42.7
     lung V42.6
     organ V42.9
       specified site NEC V42.89
     pancreas V42.83
     peripheral stem cells V42.82
     skin V42.3
     stem cells, peripheral V42.82
     tissue V42.9
       specified type NEC V42.89
     vessel, blood V42.89
   tubal ligation V26.51
   ureterostomy V44.6
   urethrostomy V44.6
   vagina, artificial V44.7
   vasectomy V26.52
   vascular shunt NEC V45.89
     aortocoronary (bypass) V45.81
   ventilator V46.1
   wrist prosthesis V43.63
Stave fracture —*see* Fracture, metacarpus, metacarpal bone(s)
Steal
   subclavian artery 435.2
   vertebral artery 435.1
Stealing, solitary, child problem (*see also* Disturbance, conduct) 312.1
Steam burn —*see* Burn, by site
Steatocystoma multiplex 706.2
Steatoma (infected) 706.2
   eyelid (cystic) 374.84
     infected 373.13
Steatorrhea (chronic) 579.8
   with lacteal obstruction 579.2
   idiopathic 579.0
     adult 579.0
     infantile 579.0
   pancreatic 579.4

Steatorrhea—*continued*
   primary 579.0
   secondary 579.8
   specified cause NEC 579.8
   tropical 579.1
Steatosis 272.8
   heart (*see also* Degeneration, myocardial) 429.1
   kidney 593.89
   liver 571.8
Steele-Richardson (-Olszewski) Syndrome 333.0
Stein's syndrome (polycystic ovary) 256.4
Stein-Leventhal syndrome (polycystic ovary) 256.4
Steinbrocker's syndrome (*see also* Neuropathy, peripheral, autonomic) 337.9
Steinert's disease 359.2
Stenocardia (*see also* Angina) 413.9
Stenocephaly 756.0
Stenosis (cicatricial)—*see also* Stricture
   ampulla of Vater 576.2
     with calculus, cholelithiasis, or stones—*see* Choledocholithiasis
   anus, anal (canal) (sphincter) 569.2
     congenital 751.2
   aorta (ascending) 747.22
     arch 747.10
     arteriosclerotic 440.0
     calcified 440.0
   aortic (valve) 424.1
     with
       mitral (valve)
         insufficiency or incompetence 396.2
         stenosis or obstruction 396.0
     atypical 396.0
     congenital 746.3
     rheumatic 395.0
       with
         insufficiency, incompetency or regurgitation 395.2
         with mitral (valve) disease 396.8
        mitral (valve)
         disease (stenosis) 396.0
         insufficiency or incompetence 396.2
         stenosis or obstruction 396.0
     specified cause, except rheumatic 424.1
     syphilitic 093.22
   aqueduct of Sylvius (congenital) 742.3
     with spina bifida (*see also* Spina bifida) 741.0
     acquired 331.4
   artery NEC 447.1
     basilar—*see* Narrowing, artery, basilar
     carotid (common) (internal)—*see* Narrowing, artery, carotid
     celiac 447.4
     cerebral 437.0
       due to
         embolism (*see also* Embolism, brain) 434.1
         thrombus (*see also* Thrombosis, brain) 434.0
     precerebral—*see* Narrowing, artery, precerebral
     pulmonary (congenital) 747.3
       acquired 417.8
     renal 440.1
     vertebral—*see* Narrowing, artery, vertebral
   bile duct or biliary passage (*see also* Obstruction, biliary) 576.2
     congenital 751.61

Stenosis—*continued*
bladder neck (acquired) 596.0
  congenital 753.6
brain 348.8
bronchus 519.1
  syphilitic 095.8
cardia (stomach) 537.89
  congenital 750.7
cardiovascular (*see also* Disease,
  cardiovascular) 429.2
carotid artery—*see* Narrowing, artery, carotid
cervix, cervical (canal) 622.4
  congenital 752.49
  in pregnancy or childbirth 654.6
    affecting fetus or newborn 763.89
    causing obstructed labor 660.2
      affecting fetus or newborn 763.1
colon (*see also* Obstruction, intestine) 560.9
  congenital 751.2
colostomy 569.62
common bile duct (*see also* Obstruction, biliary)
  576.2
  congenital 751.61
coronary (artery) —*see* Arteriosclerosis,
  coronary
cystic duct (*see also* Obstruction, gallbladder)
  575.2
  congenital 751.61
due to (presence of) any device, implant, or
  graft classifiable to 996.0-996.5—*see*
  Complications, due to (presence of) any
  device, implant, or graft classified to
  996.0-996.5 NEC
duodenum 537.3
  congenital 751.1
ejaculatory duct NEC 608.89
endocervical os—*see* Stenosis, cervix
enterostomy 569.62
esophagus 530.3
  congenital 750.3
  syphilitic 095.8
    congenital 090.5
external ear canal 380.50
  secondary to
    inflammation 380.53
    surgery 380.52
    trauma 380.51
gallbladder (*see also* Obstruction, gallbladder)
  575.2
glottis 478.74
heart valve (acquired)—*see also* Endocarditis
  congenital NEC 746.89
    aortic 746.3
    mitral 746.5
    pulmonary 746.02
    tricuspid 746.1
hepatic duct (*see also* Obstruction, biliary) 576.2
hymen 623.3
hypertrophic subaortic (idiopathic) 425.1
infundibulum cardiac 746.83
intestine (*see also* Obstruction, intestine) 560.9
  congenital (small) 751.1
    large 751.2
lacrimal
  canaliculi 375.53
  duct 375.56
    congenital 743.65
  punctum 375.52
    congenital 743.65
  sac 375.54
    congenital 743.65

Stenosis—*continued*
lacrimonasal duct 375.56
  congenital 743.65
  neonatal 375.55
larynx 478.74
  congenital 748.3
  syphilitic 095.8
    congenital 090.5
mitral (valve) (chronic) (inactive) 394.0
  with
    aortic (valve)
      disease (insufficiency) 396.1
      insufficiency or incompetence 396.1
      stenosis or obstruction 396.0
    incompetency, insufficiency or regurgitation
      394.2
      with aortic valve disease 396.8
  active or acute 391.1
    with chorea (acute) (rheumatic)
      (Sydenham's) 392.0
  congenital 746.5
  specified cause, except rheumatic 424.0
  syphilitic 093.21
myocardium, myocardial (*see also*
  Degeneration, myocardial) 429.1
  hypertrophic subaortic (idiopathic) 425.1
nares (anterior) (posterior) 478.1
  congenital 748.0
nasal duct 375.56
  congenital 743.65
nasolacrimal duct 375.56
  congenital 743.65
  neonatal 375.55
organ or site, congenital NEC—*see* Atresia
papilla of Vater 576.2
  with calculus, cholelithiasis, or stones—*see*
    Choledocholithiasis
pulmonary (artery) (congenital) 747.3
  with ventricular septal defect, dextraposition
    of aorta and hypertrophy of right ventricle
    745.2
  acquired 417.8
  infundibular 746.83
  in tetralogy of Fallot 745.2
  subvalvular 746.83
  valve (*see also* Endocarditis, pulmonary) 424.3
    congenital 746.02
  vein 747.49
    acquired 417.8
  vessel NEC 417.8
pulmonic (congenital) 746.02
  infundibular 746.83
  subvalvular 746.83
pylorus (hypertrophic) 537.0
  adult 537.0
  congenital 750.5
  infantile 750.5
rectum (sphincter) (*see also* Stricture, rectum)
  569.2
renal artery 440.1
salivary duct (any) 527.8
sphincter of Oddi (*see also* Obstruction, biliary)
  576.2
spinal 724.00
  cervical 723.0
  lumbar, lumbosacral 724.02
  nerve (root) NEC 724.9
  specified region NEC 724.09
  thoracic, thoracolumbar 724.01
stomach, hourglass 537.6

Stenosis—*continued*
  subaortic 746.81
    hypertrophic (idiopathic) 425.1
  supra (valvular)-aortic 747.22
  trachea 519.1
    congenital 748.3
    syphilitic 095.8
    tuberculous (*see also* Tuberculosis) 012.8
  tracheostomy 519.02
  tricuspid (valve) (*see also* Endocarditis,
      tricuspid) 397.0
    congenital 746.1
    nonrheumatic 424.2
  tubal 628.2
  ureter (*see also* Stricture, ureter) 593.3
    congenital 753.29
  urethra (*see also* Stricture, urethra) 598.9
  vagina 623.2
    congenital 752.49
    in pregnancy or childbirth 654.7
      affecting fetus or newborn 763.89
      causing obstructed labor 660.2
        affecting fetus or newborn 763.1
  valve (cardiac) (heart) (*see also* Endocarditis)
      424.90
    congenital NEC 746.89
      aortic 746.3
      mitral 746.5
      pulmonary 746.02
      tricuspid 746.1
      urethra 753.6
  valvular (*see also* Endocarditis) 424.90
    congenital NEC 746.89
      urethra 753.6
  vascular graft or shunt 996.1
    atherosclerosis —*see* Arteriosclerosis,
      extremities
    embolism 996.74
    occlusion NEC 996.74
    thrombus 996.74
  vena cava (inferior) (superior) 459.2
    congenital 747.49
  ventricular shunt 996.2
  vulva 624.8
Stercolith (*see also* Fecalith) 560.39
  appendix 543.9
Stercoraceous, stercoral ulcer 569.82
  anus or rectum 569.41
Stereopsis, defective
  with fusion 368.33
  without fusion 368.32
Stereotypies NEC 307.3
Sterility
  female—*see* Infertility, female
  male (*see also* Infertility, male) 606.9
Sterilization, admission for V25.2
  status
    tubal ligation V26.51
    vasectomy V26.52
Sternalgia (*see also* Angina) 413.9
Sternopagus 759.4
Sternum bifidum 756.3
Sternutation 784.9
Steroid
  effects (adverse) (iatrogenic)
    cushingoid
      correct substance properly administered
        255.0
      overdose or wrong substance given or taken
        962.0

Steroid—*continued*
  diabetes
    correct substance properly administered
      251.8
    overdose or wrong substance given or taken
      962.0
  due to
    correct substance properly administered
      255.8
    overdose or wrong substance given or taken
      962.0
  fever
    correct substance properly administered
      780.6
    overdose or wrong substance given or taken
      962.0
  withdrawal
    correct substance properly administered
      255.4
    overdose or wrong substance given or taken
      962.0
  responder 365.03
Stevens-Johnson disease or syndrome
  (erythema multiforme exudativum) 695.1
Stewart-Morel syndrome (hyperostosis frontalis
  interna) 733.3
Sticker's disease (erythema infectiosum) 057.0
Sticky eye 372.03
Stieda's disease (calcification, knee joint) 726.62
Stiff
  back 724.8
  neck (*see also* Torticollis) 723.5
Stiff-man syndrome 333.91
Stiffness, joint NEC 719.50
  ankle 719.57
  back 724.8
  elbow 719.52
  finger 719.54
  hip 719.55
  knee 719.56
  multiple sites 719.59
  sacroiliac 724.6
  shoulder 719.51
  specified site NEC 719.58
  spine 724.9
  surgical fusion V45.4
  wrist 719.53
Stigmata, congenital syphilis 090.5
Still's disease or syndrome 714.30
Still-Felty syndrome (rheumatoid arthritis with
  splenomegaly and leukopenia) 714.1
Stillbirth, stillborn NEC 779.9
Stiller's disease (asthenia) 780.79
Stilling-Türk-Duane syndrome (ocular
  retraction syndrome) 378.71
Stimulation, ovary 256.1
Sting (animal) (bee) (fish) (insect) (jellyfish)
  (Portuguese man-o-war) (wasp) (venomous)
  989.5
  anaphylactic shock or reaction 989.5
  plant 692.6
Stippled epiphyses 756.59
Stitch
  abscess 998.59
  burst (in external operation wound) 998.32
    internal 998.31
  in back 724.5
Stojano's (subcostal) syndrome 098.86
Stokes' disease (exophthalmic goiter) 242.0
Stokes-Adams syndrome (syncope with heart
  block) 426.9

Stokvis' (-Talma) disease (enterogenous
   cyanosis) 289.7
Stomach —*see* condition
Stoma malfunction
  colostomy 569.62
  cystostomy 997.5
  enterostomy 569.62
  gastrostomy 536.42
  ileostomy 569.62
  nephrostomy 997.5
  tracheostomy 519.02
  ureterostomy 997.5
Stomatitis 528.0
  angular 528.5
    due to dietary or vitamin deficiency 266.0
  aphthous 528.2
  candidal 112.0
  catarrhal 528.0
  denture 528.9
  diphtheritic (membranous) 032.0
  due to
    dietary deficiency 266.0
    thrush 112.0
    vitamin deficiency 266.0
  epidemic 078.4
  epizootic 078.4
  follicular 528.0
  gangrenous 528.1
  herpetic 054.2
  herpetiformis 528.2
  malignant 528.0
  membranous acute 528.0
  monilial 112.0
  mycotic 112.0
  necrotic 528.1
    ulcerative 101
  necrotizing ulcerative 101
  parasitic 112.0
  septic 528.0
  spirochetal 101
  suppurative (acute) 528.0
  ulcerative 528.0
    necrotizing 101
  ulceromembranous 101
  vesicular 528.0
    with exanthem 074.3
  Vincent's 101
Stomatocytosis 282.8
Stomatomycosis 112.0
Stomatorrhagia 528.9
Stone(s) —*see also* Calculus
  bladder 594.1
    diverticulum 594.0
  cystine 270.0
  heart syndrome (*see also* Failure, ventricular,
    left) 428.1
  kidney 592.0
  prostate 602.0
  pulp (dental) 522.2
  renal 592.0
  salivary duct or gland (any) 527.5
  ureter 592.1
  urethra (impacted) 594.2
  urinary (duct) (impacted) (passage) 592.9
    bladder 594.1
      diverticulum 594.0
    lower tract NEC 594.9
    specified site 594.8
  xanthine 277.2
Stonecutters' lung 502
  tuberculous (*see also* Tuberculosis) 011.4

Stonemasons'
  asthma, disease, or lung 502
    tuberculous (*see also* Tuberculosis) 011.4
  phthisis (*see also* Tuberculosis) 011.4
Stoppage
  bowel (*see also* Obstruction, intestine) 560.9
  heart (*see also* Arrest, cardiac) 427.5
  intestine (*see also* Obstruction, intestine) 560.9
  urine NEC (*see also* Retention, urine) 788.20
Storm, thyroid (apathetic) (*see also*
    Thyrotoxicosis) 242.9
Strabismus (alternating) (congenital)
    (nonparalytic) 378.9
  concomitant (*see also* Heterotropia) 378.30
    convergent (*see also* Esotropia) 378.00
    divergent (*see also* Exotropia) 378.10
  convergent (*see also* Esotropia) 378.00
  divergent (*see also* Exotropia) 378.10
  due to adhesions, scars—*see* Strabismus,
    mechanical
  in neuromuscular disorder NEC 378.73
  intermittent 378.20
    vertical 378.31
  latent 378.40
    convergent (esophoria) 378.41
    divergent (exophoria) 378.42
    vertical 378.43
  mechanical 378.60
    due to
      Brown's tendon sheath syndrome 378.61
      specified musculofascial disorder NEC
        378.62
  paralytic 378.50
    third or oculomotor nerve (partial) 378.51
      total 378.52
    fourth or trochlear nerve 378.53
    sixth or abducens nerve 378.54
  specified type NEC 378.73
  vertical (hypertropia) 378.31
Strain —*see also* Sprain, by site
  eye NEC 368.13
  heart—*see* Disease, heart
  meaning gonorrhea—*see* Gonorrhea
  physical NEC V62.89
  postural 729.9
  psychological NEC V62.89
Strands
  conjunctiva 372.62
  vitreous humor 379.25
Strangulation, strangulated 994.7
  appendix 543.9
  asphyxiation or suffocation by 994.7
  bladder neck 596.0
  bowel—*see* Strangulation, intestine
  colon—*see* Strangulation, intestine
  cord (umbilical)—*see* Compression, umbilical
    cord
  due to birth injury 767.8
  food or foreign body (*see also* Asphyxia, food)
    933.1
  hemorrhoids 455.8
    external 455.5
    internal 455.2
  hernia—*see also* Hernia, by site, with
    obstruction
    gangrenous—*see* Hernia, by site, with
      gangrene
  intestine (large) (small) 560.2
    with hernia—*see also* Hernia, by site, with
      obstruction

Strangulation, strangulated—*continued*
  gangrenous—*see* Hernia, by site, with
    gangrene
  congenital (small) 751.1
    large 751.2
  mesentery 560.2
  mucus (*see also* Asphyxia, mucus) 933.1
    newborn 770.1
  omentum 560.2
  organ or site, congenital NEC—*see* Atresia
  ovary 620.8
    due to hernia 620.4
  penis 607.89
    foreign body 939.3
  rupture (*see also* Hernia, by site, with
    obstruction) 552.9
    gangrenous (*see also* Hernia, by site, with
      gangrene) 551.9
  stomach, due to hernia (*see also* Hernia, by site,
    with obstruction) 552.9
    with gangrene (*see also* Hernia, by site, with
      gangrene) 551.9
  umbilical cord—*see* Compression, umbilical
    cord
  vesicourethral orifice 596.0
Strangury 788.1
Strawberry
  gallbladder (*see also* Disease, gallbladder) 575.6
  mark 757.32
  tongue (red) (white) 529.3
Straw itch 133.8
Streak, ovarian 752.0
Strephosymbolia 315.01
  secondary to organic lesion 784.69
Streptobacillary fever 026.1
Streptobacillus moniliformis 026.1
Streptococcemia 038.0
Streptococcicosis —*see* Infection, streptococcal
Streptococcus, streptococcal —*see* condition
Streptoderma 686.00
Streptomycosis —*see* Actinomycosis
Streptothricosis —*see* Actinomycosis
Streptothrix —*see* Actinomycosis
Streptotrichosis —*see* Actinomycosis
Stress
  fracture—*see* Fracture, stress
  polycythemia 289.0
  reaction (gross) (*see also* Reaction, stress,
    acute) 308.9
Stretching, nerve —*see* Injury, nerve, by site
Striae (albicantes) (atrophicae) (cutis distensae)
  (distensae) 701.3
Striations of nails 703.8
Stricture (*see also* Stenosis) 799.8
  ampulla of Vater 576.2
    with calculus, cholelithiasis, or stones—*see*
      Choledocholithiasis
  anus (sphincter) 569.2
    congenital 751.2
    infantile 751.2
  aorta (ascending) 747.22
    arch 747.10
    arteriosclerotic 440.0
    calcified 440.0
  aortic (valve) (*see also* Stenosis, aortic) 424.1
    congenital 746.3
  aqueduct of Sylvius (congenital) 742.3
    with spina bifida (*see also* Spina bifida) 741.0
    acquired 331.4
  artery 447.1
    basilar—*see* Narrowing, artery, basilar

Stricture—*continued*
  carotid (common) (internal)—*see* Narrowing,
    artery, carotid
  celiac 447.4
  cerebral 437.0
    congenital 747.81
    due to
      embolism (*see also* Embolism, brain)
        434.1
      thrombus (*see also* Thrombosis, brain)
        434.0
  congenital (peripheral) 747.60
    cerebral 747.81
    coronary 746.85
    gastrointestinal 747.61
    lower limb 747.64
    renal 747.62
    retinal 743.58
    specified NEC 747.69
    spinal 747.82
    umbilical 747.5
    upper limb 747.63
  coronary —*see* Arteriosclerosis, coronary
    congenital 746.85
  precerebral—*see* Narrowing, artery,
    precerebral NEC
  pulmonary (congenital) 747.3
    acquired 417.8
  renal 440.1
  vertebral—*see* Narrowing, artery, vertebral
  auditory canal (congenital) (external) 744.02
    acquired (*see also* Stricture, ear canal,
      acquired) 380.50
  bile duct or passage (any) (postoperative) (*see
    also* Obstruction, biliary) 576.2
    congenital 751.61
  bladder 596.8
    congenital 753.6
    neck 596.0
      congenital 753.6
  bowel (*see also* Obstruction, intestine) 560.9
  brain 348.8
  bronchus 519.1
    syphilitic 095.8
  cardia (stomach) 537.89
    congenital 750.7
  cardiac—*see also* Disease, heart
    orifice (stomach) 537.89
  cardiovascular (*see also* Disease,
    cardiovascular) 429.2
  carotid artery—*see* Narrowing, artery, carotid
  cecum (*see also* Obstruction, intestine) 560.9
  cervix, cervical (canal) 622.4
    congenital 752.49
    in pregnancy or childbirth 654.6
      affecting fetus or newborn 763.89
      causing obstructed labor 660.2
        affecting fetus or newborn 763.1
  colon (*see also* Obstruction, intestine) 560.9
    congenital 751.2
  colostomy 569.62
  common bile duct (*see also* Obstruction, biliary)
    576.2
    congenital 751.61
  coronary (artery) —*see* Arteriosclerosis,
    coronary
    congenital 746.85
  cystic duct (*see also* Obstruction, gallbladder)
    575.2
    congenital 751.61
  cystostomy 997.5

Stricture—*continued*
  digestive organs NEC, congenital 751.8
  duodenum 537.3
    congenital 751.1
  ear canal (external) (congenital) 744.02
    acquired 380.50
      secondary to
        inflammation 380.53
        surgery 380.52
        trauma 380.51
  ejaculatory duct 608.85
  enterostomy 569.62
  esophagus (corrosive) (peptic) 530.3
    congenital 750.3
    syphilitic 095.8
      congenital 090.5
  Eustachian tube (*see also* Obstruction,
    Eustachian tube) 381.60
    congenital 744.24
  fallopian tube 628.2
    gonococcal (chronic) 098.37
      acute 098.17
    tuberculous (*see also* Tuberculosis) 016.6
  gallbladder (*see also* Obstruction, gallbladder)
    575.2
    congenital 751.69
  glottis 478.74
  heart—*see also* Disease, heart
    congenital NEC 746.89
    valve—*see also* Endocarditis
      congenital NEC 746.89
        aortic 746.3
        mitral 746.5
        pulmonary 746.02
        tricuspid 746.1
  hepatic duct (*see also* Obstruction, biliary) 576.2
  hourglass, of stomach 537.6
  hymen 623.3
  hypopharynx 478.29
  intestine (*see also* Obstruction, intestine) 560.9
    congenital (small) 751.1
      large 751.2
    ischemic 557.1
  lacrimal
    canaliculi 375.53
      congenital 743.65
    punctum 375.52
      congenital 743.65
    sac 375.54
      congenital 743.65
  lacrimonasal duct 375.56
    congenital 743.65
    neonatal 375.55
  larynx 478.79
    congenital 748.3
    syphilitic 095.8
      congenital 090.5
  lung 518.89
  meatus
    ear (congenital) 744.02
      acquired (*see also* Stricture, ear canal,
        acquired) 380.50
    osseous (congenital) (ear) 744.03
      acquired (*see also* Stricture, ear canal,
        acquired) 380.50
    urinarius (*see also* Stricture, urethra) 598.9
      congenital 753.6
  mitral (valve) (*see also* Stenosis, mitral) 394.0
    congenital 746.5
    specified cause, except rheumatic 424.0

Stricture—*continued*
  myocardium, myocardial (*see also*
    Degeneration, myocardial) 429.1
    hypertrophic subaortic (idiopathic) 425.1
  nares (anterior) (posterior) 478.1
    congenital 748.0
  nasal duct 375.56
    congenital 743.65
    neonatal 375.55
  nasolacrimal duct 375.56
    congenital 743.65
    neonatal 375.55
  nasopharynx 478.29
    syphilitic 095.8
  nephrostomy 997.5
  nose 478.1
    congenital 748.0
  nostril (anterior) (posterior) 478.1
    congenital 748.0
  organ or site, congenital NEC—*see* Atresia
  osseous meatus (congenital) (ear) 744.03
    acquired (*see also* Stricture, ear canal,
      acquired) 380.50
  os uteri (*see also* Stricture, cervix) 622.4
  oviduct—*see* Stricture, fallopian tube
  pelviureteric junction 593.3
  pharynx (dilation) 478.29
  prostate 602.8
  pulmonary, pulmonic
    artery (congenital) 747.3
      acquired 417.8
      noncongenital 417.8
    infundibulum (congenital) 746.83
    valve (*see also* Endocarditis, pulmonary) 424.3
      congenital 746.02
    vein (congenital) 747.49
      acquired 417.8
    vessel NEC 417.8
  punctum lacrimale 375.52
    congenital 743.65
  pylorus (hypertrophic) 537.0
    adult 537.0
    congenital 750.5
    infantile 750.5
  rectosigmoid 569.89
  rectum (sphincter) 569.2
    congenital 751.2
    due to
      chemical burn 947.3
      irradiation 569.2
      lymphogranuloma venereum 099.1
    gonococcal 098.7
    inflammatory 099.1
    syphilitic 095.8
    tuberculous (*see also* Tuberculosis) 014.8
  renal artery 440.1
  salivary duct or gland (any) 527.8
  sigmoid (flexure) (*see also* Obstruction,
    intestine) 560.9
  spermatic cord 608.85
  stoma (following) (of)
    colostomy 569.62
    cystostomy 997.5
    enterostomy 569.62
    gastrostomy 536.42
    ileostomy 569.62
    nephrostomy 997.5
    tracheostomy 519.02
    ureterostomy 997.5
  stomach 537.89
    congenital 750.7

Stricture—*continued*
  hourglass 537.6
  subaortic 746.81
  hypertrophic (acquired) (idiopathic) 425.1
  subglottic 478.74
  syphilitic NEC 095.8
  tendon (sheath) 727.81
  trachea 519.1
    congenital 748.3
    syphilitic 095.8
    tuberculous (*see also* Tuberculosis) 012.8
  tracheostomy 519.02
  tricuspid (valve) (*see also* Endocarditis,
      tricuspid) 397.0
    congenital 746.1
    nonrheumatic 424.2
  tunica vaginalis 608.85
  ureter (postoperative) 593.3
    congenital 753.29
    tuberculous (*see also* Tuberculosis) 016.2
  ureteropelvic junction 593.3
    congenital 753.21
  ureterovesical orifice 593.3
    congenital 753.22
  urethra (anterior) (meatal) (organic) (posterior)
      (spasmodic) 598.9
    associated with schistosomiasis (*see also*
        Schistosomiasis) 120.9 *[598.01]*
    congenital (valvular) 753.6
    due to
      infection 598.00
        syphilis 095.8 *[598.01]*
        trauma 598.1
      gonococcal 098.2 *[598.01]*
      gonorrheal 098.2 *[598.01]*
      infective 598.00
      late effect of injury 598.1
      postcatheterization 598.2
      postobstetric 598.1
      postoperative 598.2
      specified cause NEC 598.8
      syphilitic 095.8 *[598.01]*
      traumatic 598.1
      valvular, congenital 753.6
  urinary meatus (*see also* Stricture, urethra) 598.9
    congenital 753.6
  uterus, uterine 621.5
    os (external) (internal)—*see* Stricture, cervix
  vagina (outlet) 623.2
    congenital 752.49
  valve (cardiac) (heart) (*see also* Endocarditis)
      424.90
    congenital (cardiac) (heart) NEC 746.89
      aortic 746.3
      mitral 746.5
      pulmonary 746.02
      tricuspid 746.1
      urethra 753.6
    valvular (*see also* Endocarditis) 424.90
  vascular graft or shunt 996.1
    atherosclerosis —*see* Arteriosclerosis,
        extremities
    embolism 996.74
    occlusion NEC 996.74
    thrombus 996.74
  vas deferens 608.85
    congenital 752.8
  vein 459.2
  vena cava (inferior) (superior) NEC 459.2
    congenital 747.49
  ventricular shunt 996.2

Stricture—*continued*
  vesicourethral orifice 596.0
    congenital 753.6
  vulva (acquired) 624.8
Stridor 786.1
  congenital (larynx) 748.3
Stridulous —*see* condition
Strippling of nails 703.8
Stroke (*see also* Disease, cerebrovascular, acute)
    436
  apoplectic (*see also* Disease, cerebrovascular,
      acute) 436
  brain (*see also* Disease, cerebrovascular, acute)
    436
  epileptic—*see* Epilepsy
  healed or old V12.59
  heart—*see* Disease, heart
  heat 992.0
  iatrogenic 997.02
  in evolution 435.9
  late effect—*see* Late effect(s) (of)
      cerebrovascular disease
  lightning 994.0
  paralytic (*see also* Disease, cerebrovascular,
      acute) 436
  postoperative 997.02
  progressive 435.9
Stromatosis, endometrial (M8931/1) 236.0
Strong pulse 785.9
Strongyloides stercoralis infestation 127.2
Strongyloidiasis 127.2
Strongyloidosis 127.2
Strongylus (gibsoni) infestation 127.7
Strophulus (newborn) 779.89
  pruriginosus 698.2
Struck by lightning 994.0
Struma (*see also* Goiter) 240.9
  fibrosa 245.3
  Hashimoto (struma lymphomatosa) 245.2
  lymphomatosa 245.2
  nodosa (simplex) 241.9
    endemic 241.9
    multinodular 241.1
    sporadic 241.9
    toxic or with hyperthyroidism 242.3
      multinodular 242.2
      uninodular 242.1
    toxicosa 242.3
      multinodular 242.2
      uninodular 242.1
    uninodular 241.0
  ovarii (M9090/0) 220
    and carcinoid (M9091/1) 236.2
    malignant (M9090/3) 183.0
  Riedel's (ligneous thyroiditis) 245.3
  scrofulous (*see also* Tuberculosis) 017.2
  tuberculous (*see also* Tuberculosis) 017.2
    abscess 017.2
    adenitis 017.2
    lymphangitis 017.2
    ulcer 017.2
Strumipriva cachexia (*see also*
    Hypothyroidism) 244.9
Strümpell-Marie disease or spine (ankylosing
    spondylitis) 720.0
Strümpell-Westphal pseudosclerosis
    (hepatolenticular degeneration) 275.1
Stuart's disease (congenital factor X deficiency)
    (*see also* Defect, coagulation) 286.3
Stuart-Prower factor deficiency (congenital
    factor X deficiency) (*see also* Defect,
    coagulation) 286.3

Students' elbow 727.2
Stuffy nose 478.1
Stump —*see also* Amputation
　cervix, cervical (healed) 622.8
Stupor 780.09
　catatonic (*see also* Schizophrenia) 295.2
　circular (*see also* Psychosis, manic-depressive,
　　circular) 296.7
　manic 296.89
　manic-depressive (*see also* Psychosis, affective)
　　296.89
　mental (anergic) (delusional) 298.9
　psychogenic 298.8
　reaction to exceptional stress (transient) 308.2
　traumatic NEC—*see also* Injury, intracranial
　　with spinal (cord)
　　　lesion—*see* Injury, spinal, by site
　　　shock—*see* Injury, spinal, by site
Sturge (-Weber) (-Dimitri) disease or syndrome
　(encephalocutaneous angiomatosis) 759.6
Sturge-Kalischer-Weber syndrome
　(encephalocutaneous angiomatosis) 759.6
Stuttering 307.0
Sty, stye 373.11
　external 373.11
　internal 373.12
　meibomian 373.12
Subacidity, gastric 536.8
　psychogenic 306.4
Subacute —*see* condition
Subarachnoid —*see* condition
Subclavian steal syndrome 435.2
Subcortical —*see* condition
Subcostal syndrome 098.86
　nerve compression 354.8
Subcutaneous, subcuticular —*see* condition
Subdelirium 293.1
Subdural —*see* condition
Subendocardium —*see* condition
Subependymoma (M9383/1) 237.5
Suberosis 495.3
Subglossitis —*see* Glossitis
Subhemophilia 286.0
Subinvolution (uterus) 621.1
　breast (postlactational) (postpartum) 611.8
　chronic 621.1
　puerperal, postpartum 674.8
Sublingual —*see* condition
Sublinguitis 527.2
Subluxation —*see also* Dislocation, by site
　congenital NEC—*see also* Malposition,
　　congenital
　　hip (unilateral) 754.32
　　　with dislocation of other hip 754.35
　　　bilateral 754.33
　　joint
　　　lower limb 755.69
　　　shoulder 755.59
　　　upper limb 755.59
　　lower limb (joint) 755.69
　　shoulder (joint) 755.59
　　upper limb (joint) 755.59
　lens 379.32
　　anterior 379.33
　　posterior 379.34
　rotary, cervical region of spine—*see* Fracture,
　　vertebra, cervical
Submaxillary —*see* condition
Submersion (fatal) (nonfatal) 994.1
Submissiveness (undue), in child 313.0
Submucous —*see* condition

Subnormal, subnormality
　accommodation (*see also* Disorder,
　　accommodation) 367.9
　mental (*see also* Retardation, mental) 319
　　mild 317
　　moderate 318.0
　　profound 318.2
　　severe 318.1
　temperature (accidental) 991.6
　　not associated with low environmental
　　　temperature 780.99
Subphrenic —*see* condition
Subscapular nerve —*see* condition
Subseptus uterus 752.3
Subsiding appendicitis 542
Substernal thyroid (*see also* Goiter) 240.9
　congenital 759.2
Substitution disorder 300.11
Subtentorial —*see* condition
Subtertian
　fever 084.0
　malaria (fever) 084.0
Subthyroidism (acquired) (*see also*
　Hypothyroidism) 244.9
　congenital 243
Succenturiata placenta —*see* Placenta, abnormal
Succussion sounds, chest 786.7
Sucking thumb, child 307.9
Sudamen 705.1
Sudamina 705.1
Sudanese kala-azar 085.0
Sudden
　death, cause unknown (less than 24 hours) 798.1
　　during childbirth 669.9
　　infant 798.0
　　puerperal, postpartum 674.9
　hearing loss NEC 388.2
　heart failure (*see also* Failure, heart) 428.9
　infant death syndrome 798.0
Sudeck's atrophy, disease, or syndrome 733.7
SUDS (Sudden unexplained death) 798.2
Suffocation (*see also* Asphyxia) 799.0
　by
　　bed clothes 994.7
　　bunny bag 994.7
　　cave-in 994.7
　　constriction 994.7
　　drowning 994.1
　　inhalation
　　　food or foreign body (*see also* Asphyxia,
　　　　food or foreign body) 933.1
　　　oil or gasoline (*see also* Asphyxia, food or
　　　　foreign body) 933.1
　　overlying 994.7
　　plastic bag 994.7
　　pressure 994.7
　　strangulation 994.7
　during birth 768.1
　mechanical 994.7
Sugar
　blood
　　high 790.2
　　low 251.2
　in urine 791.5
Suicide, suicidal (attempted)
　by poisoning—*see* Table of drugs and chemicals
　risk 300.9
　tendencies 300.9
　trauma NEC (*see also* nature and site of injury)
　　959.9
Suipestifer infection (*see also* Infection,
　Salmonella) 003.9

Sulfatidosis 330.0
Sulfhemoglobinemia, sulphemoglobinemia
    (acquired) (congenital) 289.7
Sumatran mite fever 081.2
Summer —*see* condition
Sunburn 692.71
    dermatitis 692.71
    due to
        other ultraviolet radiation 692.82
        tanning bed 692.82
    first degree 692.71
    second degree 692.76
    third degree 692.77
Sunken
    acetabulum 718.85
    fontanels 756.0
Sunstroke 992.0
Superfecundation 651.9
    with fetal loss and retention of one or more
        fetus(es) 651.6
Superfetation 651.9
    with fetal loss and retention of one or more
        fetus(es) 651.6
Supernumerary (congenital)
    aortic cusps 746.89
    auditory ossicles 744.04
    bone 756.9
    breast 757.6
    carpal bones 755.56
    cusps, heart valve NEC 746.89
        mitral 746.5
        pulmonary 746.09
    digit(s) 755.00
        finger 755.01
        toe 755.02
    ear (lobule) 744.1
    fallopian tube 752.19
    finger 755.01
    hymen 752.49
    kidney 753.3
    lacrimal glands 743.64
    lacrimonasal duct 743.65
    lobule (ear) 744.1
    mitral cusps 746.5
    muscle 756.82
    nipples 757.6
    organ or site NEC—*see* Accessory
    ossicles, auditory 744.04
    ovary 752.0
    oviduct 752.19
    pulmonic cusps 746.09
    rib 756.3
        cervical or first 756.2
            syndrome 756.2
    roots (of teeth) 520.2
    spinal vertebra 756.19
    spleen 759.0
    tarsal bones 755.67
    teeth 520.1
        causing crowding 524.3
    testis 752.8
    thumb 755.01
    toe 755.02
    uterus 752.2
    vagina 752.49
    vertebra 756.19
Supervision (of)
    contraceptive method previously prescribed
        V25.40
        intrauterine device V25.42
        oral contraceptive (pill) V25.41

Supervision (of)—*continued*
    specified type NEC V25.49
    subdermal implantable contraceptive V25.43
dietary (for) V65.3
    allergy (food) V65.3
    colitis V65.3
    diabetes mellitus V65.3
    food allergy intolerance V65.3
    gastritis V65.3
    hypercholesterolemia V65.3
    hypoglycemia V65.3
    intolerance (food) V65.3
    obesity V65.3
    specified NEC V65.3
lactation V24.1
pregnancy—*see* Pregnancy, supervision of
Supplemental teeth 520.1
    causing crowding 524.3
Suppression
    binocular vision 368.31
    lactation 676.5
    menstruation 626.8
    ovarian secretion 256.39
    renal 586
    urinary secretion 788.5
    urine 788.5
Suppuration, suppurative —*see also* condition
    accessory sinus (chronic) (*see also* Sinusitis)
        473.9
    adrenal gland 255.8
    antrum (chronic) (*see also* Sinusitis, maxillary)
        473.0
    bladder (*see also* Cystitis) 595.89
    bowel 569.89
    brain 324.0
        late effect 326
    breast 611.0
        puerperal, postpartum 675.1
    dental periosteum 526.5
    diffuse (skin) 686.00
    ear (middle) (*see also* Otitis media) 382.4
        external (*see also* Otitis, externa) 380.10
        internal 386.33
    ethmoidal (sinus) (chronic) (*see also* Sinusitis,
        ethmoidal) 473.2
    fallopian tube (*see also* Salpingo-oophoritis)
        614.2
    frontal (sinus) (chronic) (*see also* Sinusitis,
        frontal) 473.1
    gallbladder (*see also* Cholecystitis, acute) 575.0
    gum 523.3
    hernial sac—*see* Hernia, by site
    intestine 569.89
    joint (*see also* Arthritis, suppurative) 711.0
    labyrinthine 386.33
    lung 513.0
    mammary gland 611.0
        puerperal, postpartum 675.1
    maxilla, maxillary 526.4
        sinus (chronic) (*see also* Sinusitis, maxillary)
            473.0
    muscle 728.0
    nasal sinus (chronic) (*see also* Sinusitis) 473.9
    pancreas 577.0
    parotid gland 527.2
    pelvis, pelvic
        female (*see also* Disease, pelvis,
            inflammatory) 614.4
            acute 614.3
        male (*see also* Peritonitis) 567.2
    pericranial (*see also* Osteomyelitis) 730.2

Suppuration, suppurative—*continued*
salivary duct or gland (any) 527.2
sinus (nasal) (*see also* Sinusitis) 473.9
sphenoidal (sinus) (chronic) (*see also* Sinusitis, sphenoidal) 473.3
thymus (gland) 254.1
thyroid (gland) 245.0
tonsil 474.8
uterus (*see also* Endometritis) 615.9
vagina 616.10
wound—*see also* Wound, open, by site, complicated
dislocation—*see* Dislocation, by site, compound
fracture—*see* Fracture, by site, open
scratch or other superficial injury—*see* Injury, superficial, by site
Supraglottitis 464.50
with obstruction 464.51
Suprapubic drainage 596.8
Suprarenal (gland)—*see* condition
Suprascapular nerve —*see* condition
Suprasellar —*see* condition
Supraspinatus syndrome 726.10
Surfer knots 919.8
infected 919.9
Surgery
cosmetic NEC V50.1
following healed injury or operation V51
hair transplant V50.0
elective V50.9
breast augmentation reduction V50.1
circumcision, ritual or routine (in absence of medical indication) V50.2
cosmetic NEC V50.1
ear piercing V50.3
face-lift V50.1
following healed injury or operation V51
hair transplant V50.0
not done because of
contraindication V64.1
patient's decision V64.2
specified reason NEC V64.3
plastic
breast augmentation or reduction V50.1
cosmetic V50.1
face-lift V50.1
following healed injury or operation V51
repair of scarred tissue (following healed injury or operation) V51
specified type NEC V50.8
previous, in pregnancy or childbirth
cervix 654.6
affecting fetus or newborn 763.89
causing obstructed labor 660.2
affecting fetus or newborn 763.1
pelvic soft tissues NEC 654.9
affecting fetus or newborn 763.89
causing obstructed labor 660.2
affecting fetus or newborn 763.1
perineum or vulva 654.8
uterus NEC 654.9
affecting fetus or newborn 763.89
causing obstructed labor 660.2
affecting fetus or newborn 763.1
due to previous cesarean delivery 654.2
vagina 654.7

Surgical
abortion—*see* Abortion, legal
emphysema 998.81
kidney (*see also* Pyelitis) 590.80
operation NEC 799.9
procedures, complication or misadventure—*see* Complications, surgical procedure
shock 998.0
Suspected condition, ruled out (*see also* Observation, suspected) V71.9
specified condition NEC V71.89
Suspended uterus, in pregnancy or childbirth 654.4
affecting fetus or newborn 763.89
causing obstructed labor 660.2
affecting fetus or newborn 763.1
Sutton's disease 709.09
Sutton and Gull's disease (arteriolar nephrosclerosis) (*see also* Hypertension, kidney) 403.90
Suture
burst (in external operation wound) 998.32
internal 998.31
inadvertently left in operation wound 998.4
removal V58.3
Shirodkar, in pregnancy (with or without cervical incompetence) 654.5
Swab inadvertently left in operation wound 998.4
Swallowed, swallowing
difficulty (*see also* Dysphagia) 787.2
foreign body NEC (*see also* Foreign body) 938
Swamp fever 100.89
Swan neck hand (intrinsic) 736.09
Sweat (s), sweating
disease or sickness 078.2
excessive 780.8
fetid 705.89
fever 078.2
gland disease 705.9
specified type NEC 705.89
miliary 078.2
night 780.8
Sweeley-Klionsky disease (angiokeratoma corporis diffusum) 272.7
Sweet's syndrome (acute febrile neutrophilic dermatosis) 695.89
Swelling
abdominal (not referable to specific organ) 789.3
adrenal gland, cloudy 255.8
ankle 719.07
anus 787.99
arm 729.81
breast 611.72
Calabar 125.2
cervical gland 785.6
cheek 784.2
chest 786.6
ear 388.8
epigastric 789.3
extremity (lower) (upper) 729.81
eye 379.92
female genital organ 625.8
finger 729.81
foot 729.81
glands 785.6
gum 784.2
hand 729.81
head 784.2
inflammatory—*see* Inflammation

Swelling—*continued*
  joint (*see also* Effusion, joint) 719.0
    tuberculous—*see* Tuberculosis, joint
  kidney, cloudy 593.89
  leg 729.81
  limb 729.81
  liver 573.8
  lung 786.6
  lymph nodes 785.6
  mediastinal 786.6
  mouth 784.2
  muscle (limb) 729.81
  neck 784.2
  nose or sinus 784.2
  palate 784.2
  pelvis 789.3
  penis 607.83
  perineum 625.8
  rectum 787.99
  scrotum 608.86
  skin 782.2
  splenic (*see also* Splenomegaly) 789.2
  substernal 786.6
  superficial, localized (skin) 782.2
  testicle 608.86
  throat 784.2
  toe 729.81
  tongue 784.2
  tubular (*see also* Disease, renal) 593.9
  umbilicus 789.3
  uterus 625.8
  vagina 625.8
  vulva 625.8
  wandering, due to Gnathostoma (spinigerum)
    128.1
  white—*see* Tuberculosis, arthritis
Swift's disease 985.0
Swimmers'
  ear (acute) 380.12
  itch 120.3
Swimming in the head 780.4
Swollen —*see also* Swelling
  glands 785.6
Swyer-James syndrome (unilateral hyperlucent
  lung) 492.8
Swyer's syndrome (XY pure gonadal
  dysgenesis) 752.7
Sycosis 704.8
  barbae (not parasitic) 704.8
  contagiosa 110.0
  lupoid 704.8
  mycotic 110.0
  parasitic 110.0
  vulgaris 704.8
Sydenham's chorea —*see* Chorea, Sydenham's
Sylvatic yellow fever 060.0
Sylvest's disease (epidemic pleurodynia) 074.1
Symblepharon 372.63
  congenital 743.62
Symonds' syndrome 348.2
Sympathetic —*see* condition
Sympatheticotonia (*see also* Neuropathy,
  peripheral, autonomic) 337.9
Sympathicoblastoma (M9500/3)
  specified site—*see* Neoplasm, by site, malignant
  unspecified site 194.0
Sympathicogonioma (M9500/3)—*see*
  Sympathicoblastoma
Sympathoblastoma (M9500/3)—*see*
  Sympathicoblastoma
Sympathogonioma (M9500/3)—*see*
  Sympathicoblastoma

Symphalangy (*see also* Syndactylism) 755.10
Symptoms, specified (general) NEC 780.99
  abdomen NEC 789.9
  bone NEC 733.90
  breast NEC 611.79
  cardiac NEC 785.9
  cardiovascular NEC 785.9
  chest NEC 786.9
  development NEC 783.9
  digestive system NEC 787.99
  eye NEC 379.99
  gastrointestinal tract NEC 787.99
  genital organs NEC
    female 625.9
    male 608.9
  head and neck NEC 784.9
  heart NEC 785.9
  joint NEC 719.60
    ankle 719.67
    elbow 719.62
    foot 719.67
    hand 719.64
    hip 719.65
    knee 719.66
    multiple sites 719.69
    pelvic region 719.65
    shoulder (region) 719.61
    specified site NEC 719.68
    wrist 719.63
  larynx NEC 784.9
  limbs NEC 729.89
  lymphatic system NEC 785.9
  menopausal 627.2
  metabolism NEC 783.9
  mouth NEC 528.9
  muscle NEC 728.9
  musculoskeletal NEC 781.99
    limbs NEC 729.89
  nervous system NEC 781.99
  neurotic NEC 300.9
  nutrition, metabolism, and development NEC
    783.9
  pelvis NEC 789.9
    female 625.9
  peritoneum NEC 789.9
  respiratory system NEC 786.9
  skin and integument NEC 782.9
  subcutaneous tissue NEC 782.9
  throat NEC 784.9
  tonsil NEC 784.9
  urinary system NEC 788.9
  vascular NEC 785.9
Sympus 759.89
Synarthrosis 719.80
  ankle 719.87
  elbow 719.82
  foot 719.87
  hand 719.84
  hip 719.85
  knee 719.86
  multiple sites 719.89
  pelvic region 719.85
  shoulder (region) 719.81
  specified site NEC 719.88
  wrist 719.83
Syncephalus 759.4
Synchondrosis 756.9
  abnormal (congenital) 756.9
  ischiopubic (van Neck's) 732.1
Synchysis (senile) (vitreous humor) 379.21
  scintillans 379.22

Syncope (near) (pre-) 780.2
  anginosa 413.9
  bradycardia 427.89
  cardiac 780.2
  carotid sinus 337.0
  complicating delivery 669.2
  due to lumbar puncture 349.0
  fatal 798.1
  heart 780.2
  heat 992.1
  laryngeal 786.2
  tussive 786.2
  vasoconstriction 780.2
  vasodepressor 780.2
  vasomotor 780.2
  vasovagal 780.2
Syncytial infarct —*see* Placenta, abnormal
Syndactylism, syndactyly (multiple sites) 755.10
  fingers (without fusion of bone) 755.11
    with fusion of bone 755.12
  toes (without fusion of bone) 755.13
    with fusion of bone 755.14
Syndrome —*see also* Disease
  abdominal
    acute 789.0
    migraine 346.2
    muscle deficiency 756.79
  Abercrombie's (amyloid degeneration) 277.3
  abnormal innervation 374.43
  abstinence
    alcohol 291.81
    drug 292.0
  Abt-Letterer-Siwe (acute histiocytosis X)
    (M9722/3) 202.5
  Achard-Thiers (adrenogenital) 255.2
  acid pulmonary aspiration 997.3
    obstetric (Mendelson's) 668.0
  acquired immune deficiency 042
  acquired immunodeficiency 042
  acrocephalosyndactylism 755.55
  acute abdominal 789.0
  acute chest 282.62
  acute coronary 411.1
  Adair-Dighton (brittle bones and blue sclera,
    deafness) 756.51
  Adams-Stokes (-Morgagni) (syncope with heart
    block) 426.9
  addisonian 255.4
  Adie (-Holmes) (pupil) 379.46
  adiposogenital 253.8
  adrenal
    hemorrhage 036.3
    meningococcic 036.3
  adrenocortical 255.3
  adrenogenital (acquired) (congenital) 255.2
    feminizing 255.2
    iatrogenic 760.79
    virilism (acquired) (congenital) 255.2
  affective organic NEC 293.89
    drug-induced 292.84
  afferent loop NEC 537.89
  African macroglobulinemia 273.3
  Ahumada-Del Castillo (nonpuerperal
    galactorrhea and amenorrhea) 253.1
  air blast concussion—*see* Injury, internal, by site
  Albright (-Martin) (pseudohypoparathyroidism)
    275.49
  Albright-McCune-Sternberg (osteitis fibrosa
    disseminata) 756.59
  alcohol withdrawal 291.81
  Alder's (leukocyte granulation anomaly) 288.2

Syndrome—*continued*
  Aldrich (-Wiskott) (eczema-thrombocytopenia)
    279.12
  Alibert-Bazin (mycosis, fungoides) (M9700/3)
    202.1
  Alice in Wonderland 293.89
  Allen-Masters 620.6
  Alligator baby (ichthyosis congenita) 757.1
  Alport's (hereditary hematuria-nephropathy-
    deafness) 759.89
  Alvarez (transient cerebral ischemia) 435.9
  alveolar capillary block 516.3
  Alzheimer's 331.0
    with dementia—*see* Alzheimer's, dementia
  amnestic (confabulatory) 294.0
    alcoholic 291.1
    drug-induced 292.83
    posttraumatic 294.0
  amotivational 292.89
  amyostatic 275.1
  amyotrophic lateral sclerosis 335.20
  angina (*see also* Angina) 413.9
  ankyloglossia superior 750.0
  anterior
    chest wall 786.52
    compartment (tibial) 958.8
    spinal artery 433.8
      compression 721.1
    tibial (compartment) 958.8
  antibody deficiency 279.00
    agammaglobulinemic 279.00
    congenital 279.04
    hypogammaglobulinemic 279.00
  anticardiolipin antibody 795.79
  antimongolism 758.3
  antiphospholipid antibody 795.79
  Anton (-Babinski) (hemiasomatognosia) 307.9
  anxiety (*see also* Anxiety) 300.00
    organic 293.84
  aortic
    arch 446.7
    bifurcation (occlusion) 444.0
    ring 747.21
  Apert's (acrocephalosyndactyly) 755.55
  Apert-Gallais (adrenogenital) 255.2
  aphasia-apraxia-alexia 784.69
  "approximate answers" 300.16
  arcuate ligament (-celiac axis) 447.4
  arcus aortae 446.7
  arc-welders' 370.24
  argentaffin, argintaffinoma 259.2
  Argonz-Del Castillo (nonpuerperal galactorrhea
    and amenorrhea) 253.1
  Argyll Robertson's (syphilitic) 094.89
    nonsyphilitic 379.45
  arm-shoulder (*see also* Neuropathy, peripheral,
    autonomic) 337.9
  Arnold-Chiari (*see also* Spina bifida) 741.0
    type I 348.4
    type II 741.0
    type III 742.0
    type IV 742.2
  Arrillaga-Ayerza (pulmonary artery sclerosis
    with pulmonary hypertension) 416.0
  arteriomesenteric duodenum occlusion 537.89
  arteriovenous steal 996.73
  arteritis, young female (obliterative
    brachiocephalic) 446.7
  aseptic meningitis—*see* Meningitis, aseptic
  Asherman's 621.5
  asphyctic (*see also* Anxiety) 300.00

Syndrome—*continued*
    psychotic (*see also* Psychosis, organic) 294.9
    senile (*see also* Dementia, senile) 290.0
  branchial arch 744.41
  Brandt's (acrodermatitis enteropathica) 686.8
  Brennemann's 289.2
  Briquet's 300.81
  Brissaud-Meige (infantile myxedema) 244.9
  broad ligament laceration 620.6
  Brock's (atelectasis due to enlarged lymph
    nodes) 518.0
  Brown's tendon sheath 378.61
  Brown-Séquard 344.89
  brown spot 756.59
  Brugada 746.89
  Brugsch's (acropachyderma) 757.39
  bubbly lung 770.7
  Buchem's (hyperostosis corticalis) 733.3
  Budd-Chiari (hepatic vein thrombosis) 453.0
  Büdinger-Ludloff-Läwen 717.89
  bulbar 335.22
    lateral (*see also* Disease, cerebrovascular,
     acute) 436
  Bullis fever 082.8
  bundle of Kent (anomalous atrioventricular
    excitation) 426.7
  Bürger-Grütz (essential familial hyperlipemia)
    272.3
  Burke's (pancreatic insufficiency and chronic
    neutropenia) 577.8
  Burnett's (milk-alkali) 999.9
  Burnier's (hypophyseal dwarfism) 253.3
  burning feet 266.2
  Bywaters' 958.5
  Caffey's (infantile cortical hyperostosis) 756.59
  Calvé-Legg-Perthes (osteochondrosis, femoral
    capital) 732.1
  Caplan (-Colinet) syndrome 714.81
  capsular thrombosis (*see also* Thrombosis,
    brain) 434.0
  carcinogenic thrombophlebitis 453.1
  carcinoid 259.2
  cardiac asthma (*see also* Failure, ventricular,
    left) 428.1
  cardiacos negros 416.0
  cardiopulmonary obesity 278.8
  cardiorenal (*see also* Hypertension, cardiorenal)
    404.90
  cardiorespiratory distress (idiopathic), newborn
    769
  cardiovascular renal (*see also* Hypertension,
    cardiorenal) 404.90
  cardiovasorenal 272.7
  Carini's (ichthyosis congenita) 757.1
  carotid
    artery (internal) 435.8
    body or sinus 337.0
  carpal tunnel 354.0
  Carpenter's 759.89
  Cassidy (-Scholte) (malignant carcinoid) 259.2
  cat-cry 758.3
  cauda equina 344.60
  causalgia 355.9
    lower limb 355.71
    upper limb 354.4
  cavernous sinus 437.6
  celiac 579.0
    artery compression 447.4
    axis 447.4
  cerebellomedullary malformation (*see also*
    Spina bifida) 741.0

Syndrome—*continued*
  cerebral gigantism 253.0
  cerebrohepatorenal 759.89
  cervical (root) (spine) NEC 723.8
    disc 722.71
    posterior, sympathetic 723.2
    rib 353.0
    sympathetic paralysis 337.0
    traumatic (acute) NEC 847.0
  cervicobrachial (diffuse) 723.3
  cervicocranial 723.2
  cervicodorsal outlet 353.2
  Céstan's 344.89
  Céstan (-Raymond) 433.8
  Céstan-Chenais 344.89
  chancriform 114.1
  Charcot's (intermittent claudication) 443.9
    angina cruris 443.9
    due to atherosclerosis 440.21
  Charcot-Marie-Tooth 356.1
  Charcot-Weiss-Baker 337.0
  Cheadle (-Möller) (-Barlow) (infantile scurvy)
    267
  Chédiak-Higashi (-Steinbrinck) (congenital
    gigantism of peroxidase granules) 288.2
  chest wall 786.52
  Chiari's (hepatic vein thrombosis) 453.0
  Chiari-Frommel 676.6
  chiasmatic 368.41
  Chilaiditi's (subphrenic displacement, colon)
    751.4
  chondroectodermal dysplasia 756.55
  chorea-athetosis-agitans 275.1
  Christian's (chronic histiocytosis X) 277.8
  chromosome 4 short arm deletion 758.3
  Churg-Strauss 446.4
  Clarke-Hadfield (pancreatic infantilism) 577.8
  Claude's 352.6
  Claude Bernard-Horner (*see also* Neuropathy,
    peripheral, autonomic) 337.9
  Clérambault's
    automatism 348.8
    erotomania 297.8
  Clifford's (postmaturity) 766.2
  climacteric 627.2
  Clouston's (hidrotic ectodermal dysplasia)
    757.31
  clumsiness 315.4
  Cockayne's (microencephaly and dwarfism)
    759.89
  Cockayne-Weber (epidermolysis bullosa) 757.39
  Cogan's (nonsyphilitic interstitial keratitis)
    370.52
  cold injury (newborn) 778.2
  Collet (-Sicard) 352.6
  combined immunity deficiency 279.2
  compartment(al) (anterior) (deep) (posterior)
    (tibial) 958.8
    nontraumatic 729.9
  compression 958.5
    cauda equina 344.60
     with neurogenic bladder 344.61
  concussion 310.2
  congenital
    affecting more than one system 759.7
     specified type NEC 759.89
    facial diplegia 352.6
    muscular hypertrophy-cerebral 759.89
  congestion-fibrosis (pelvic) 625.5
  conjunctivourethrosynovial 099.3
  Conn (-Louis) (primary aldosteronism) 255.1

Syndrome—*continued*
Goldberg (-Maxwell) (-Morris) (testicular feminization) 257.8
Goldenhar's (oculoauriculovertebral dysplasia) 756.0
Goldflam-Erb 358.0
Goltz-Gorlin (dermal hypoplasia) 757.39
Goodpasture's (pneumorenal) 446.21
Gopalan's (burning feet) 266.2
Gorlin-Chaudhry-Moss 759.89
Gougerot (-Houwer) -Sjögren (keratoconjunctivitis sicca) 710.2
Gougerot-Blum (pigmented purpuric lichenoid dermatitis) 709.1
Gougerot-Carteaud (confluent reticulate papillomatosis) 701.8
Gouley's (constrictive pericarditis) 423.2
Gowers' (vasovagal attack) 780.2
Gowers-Paton-Kennedy 377.04
Gradenigo's 383.02
Gray or grey (chloramphenicol) (newborn) 779.4
Greig's (hypertelorism) 756.0
Gubler-Millard 344.89
Guérin-Stern (arthrogryposis multiplex congenita) 754.89
Guillain-Barré (-Strohl) 357.0
Gunn's (jaw-winking syndrome) 742.8
Günther's (congenital erythropoietic porphyria) 277.1
gustatory sweating 350.8
H₃O 759.81
Hadfield-Clarke (pancreatic infantilism) 577.8
Haglund-Läwen-Fründ 717.89
hairless women 257.8
Hallermann-Streiff 756.0
Hallervorden-Spatz 333.0
Hamman's (spontaneous mediastinal emphysema) 518.1
Hamman-Rich (diffuse interstitial pulmonary fibrosis) 516.3
Hand-Schüller-Christian (chronic histiocytosis X) 277.8
hand-foot 282.61
Hanot-Chauffard (-Troisier) (bronze diabetes) 275.0
Harada's 363.22
Hare's (M8010/3) (carcinoma, pulmonary apex) 162.3
Harkavy's 446.0
harlequin color change 779.89
Harris' (organic hyperinsulinism) 251.1
Hart's (pellagra-cerebellar ataxia-renal aminoaciduria) 270.0
Hayem-Faber (achlorhydric anemia) 280.9
Hayem-Widal (acquired hemolytic jaundice) 283.9
Heberden's (angina pectoris) 413.9
Hedinger's (malignant carcinoid) 259.2
Hegglin's 288.2
Heller's (infantile psychosis) (*see also* Psychosis, childhood) 299.1
H.E.L.L.P. 642.5
hemolytic-uremic (adult) (child) 283.11
Hench-Rosenberg (palindromic arthritis) (*see also* Rheumatism, palindromic) 719.3
Henoch-Schönlein (allergic purpura) 287.0
hepatic flexure 569.89
hepatorenal 572.4
due to a procedure 997.4
following delivery 674.8
hepatourologic 572.4

Syndrome—*continued*
Herrick's (hemoglobin S disease) 282.61
Herter (-Gee) (nontropical sprue) 579.0
Heubner-Herter (nontropical sprue) 579.0
Heyd's (hepatorenal) 572.4
HHHO 759.81
Hilger's 337.0
Hoffa (-Kastert) (liposynovitis prepatellaris) 272.8
Hoffmann's 244.9 *[359.5]*
Hoffmann-Bouveret (paroxysmal tachycardia) 427.2
Hoffmann-Werdnig 335.0
Holländer-Simons (progressive lipodystrophy) 272.6
Holmes' (visual disorientation) 368.16
Holmes-Adie 379.46
Hoppe-Goldflam 358.0
Horner's (*see also* Neuropathy, peripheral, autonomic) 337.9
traumatic—*see* Injury, nerve, cervical sympathetic
hospital addiction 301.51
Hunt's (herpetic geniculate ganglionitis) 053.11
dyssynergia cerebellaris myoclonica 334.2
Hunter (-Hurler) (mucopolysaccharidosis II) 277.5
hunterian glossitis 529.4
Hurler (-Hunter) (mucopolysaccharidosis II) 277.5
Hutchinson's incisors or teeth 090.5
Hutchinson-Boeck (sarcoidosis) 135
Hutchinson-Gilford (progeria) 259.8
hydralazine
correct substance properly administered 695.4
overdose or wrong substance given or taken 972.6
hydraulic concussion (abdomen) (*see also* Injury, internal, abdomen) 868.00
hyperabduction 447.8
hyperactive bowel 564.9
hyperaldosteronism with hypokalemic alkalosis (Bartter's) 255.1
hypercalcemic 275.42
hypercoagulation NEC 289.8
hypereosinophilic (idiopathic) 288.3
hyperkalemic 276.7
hyperkinetic—*see also* Hyperkinesia
heart 429.82
hyperlipemia-hemolytic anemia-icterus 571.1
hypermobility 728.5
hypernatremia 276.0
hyperosmolarity 276.0
hypersomnia-bulimia 349.89
hypersplenic 289.4
hypersympathetic (*see also* Neuropathy, peripheral, autonomic) 337.9
hypertransfusion, newborn 776.4
hyperventilation, psychogenic 306.1
hyperviscosity (of serum) NEC 273.3
polycythemic 289.0
sclerothymic 282.8
hypoglycemic (familial) (neonatal) 251.2
functional 251.1
hypokalemic 276.8
hypophyseal 253.8
hypophyseothalamic 253.8
hypopituitarism 253.2
hypoplastic left heart 746.7
hypopotassemia 276.8
hyposmolality 276.1

Syndrome—*continued*
blind loop 579.2
postpartum panhypopituitary 253.2
postperfusion NEC 999.8
    bone marrow 996.85
postpericardiotomy 429.4
postphlebitic (asymptomatic) 459.10
    with
        complications NEC 459.19
        inflammation 459.12
            and ulcer 459.13
        stasis dermatitis 459.12
            with ulcer 459.13
        ulcer 459.11
            with inflammation 459.13
postpolio (myelitis) 138
postvagotomy 564.2
postvalvulotomy 429.4
postviral (asthenia) NEC 780.79
Potain's (gastrectasis with dyspepsia) 536.1
potassium intoxication 276.7
Potter's 753.0
Prader (-Labhart) -Willi (-Fanconi) 759.81
preinfarction 411.1
preleukemic 238.7
premature senility 259.8
premenstrual 625.4
premenstrual tension 625.4
pre ulcer 536.9
Prinzmetal-Massumi (anterior chest wall
    syndrome) 786.52
Profichet's 729.9
progeria 259.8
progressive pallidal degeneration 333.0
prolonged gestation 766.2
Proteus (dermal hypoplasia) 757.39
prune belly 756.71
prurigo-asthma 691.8
pseudocarpal tunnel (sublimis) 354.0
pseudohermaphroditism-virilism-hirsutism 255.2
pseudoparalytica 358.0
pseudo-Turner's 759.89
psycho-organic 293.9
    acute 293.0
    anxiety type 293.84
    depressive type 293.83
    hallucinatory type 293.82
    nonpsychotic severity 310.1
        specified focal (partial) NEC 310.8
    paranoid type 293.81
    specified type NEC 293.89
    subacute 293.1
pterygolymphangiectasia 758.6
ptosis-epicanthus 270.2
pulmonary
    arteriosclerosis 416.0
    hypoperfusion (idiopathic) 769
    renal (hemorrhagic) 446.21
pulseless 446.7
Putnam-Dana (subacute combined sclerosis
    with pernicious anemia) 281.0 *[336.2]*
pyloroduodenal 537.89
pyramidopallidonigral 332.0
pyriformis 355.0
Q-T interval prolongation 794.31
radicular NEC 729.2
    lower limbs 724.4
    upper limbs 723.4
        newborn 767.4
Raeder-Harbitz (pulseless disease) 446.7

Syndrome—*continued*
Ramsay Hunt's
    dyssynergia cerebellaris myoclonica 334.2
    herpetic geniculate ganglionitis 053.11
rapid time-zone change 307.45
Raymond (-Céstan) 433.8
Raynaud's (paroxysmal digital cyanosis) 443.0
RDS (respiratory distress syndrome, newborn)
    769
Refsum's (heredopathia atactica
    polyneuritiformis) 356.3
Reichmann's (gastrosuccorrhea) 536.8
Reifenstein's (hereditary familial
    hypogonadism, male) 257.2
Reilly's (*see also* Neuropathy, peripheral,
    autonomic) 337.9
Reiter's 099.3
renal glomerulohyalinosis-diabetic 250.4
    [581.81]
Rendu-Osler-Weber (familial hemorrhagic
    telangiectasia) 448.0
renofacial (congenital biliary fibroangiomatosis)
    753.0
Rénon-Delille 253.8
respiratory distress (idiopathic) (newborn) 769
    adult (following shock, surgery, or trauma)
        518.5
    specified NEC 518.82
restless leg 333.99
retraction (Duane's) 378.71
retroperitoneal fibrosis 593.4
Rett's 330.8
Reye's 331.81
Reye-Sheehan (postpartum pituitary necrosis)
    253.2
Riddoch's (visual disorientation) 368.16
Ridley's (*see also* Failure, ventricular, left)
    428.1
Rieger's (mesodermal dysgenesis, anterior
    ocular segment) 743.44
Rietti-Greppi-Micheli (thalassemia minor) 282.4
right ventricular obstruction—*see* Failure heart
Riley-Day (familial dysautonomia) 742.8
Robin's 756.0
Rokitansky-Kuster-Hauser (congenital absence,
    vagina) 752.49
Romano-Ward (prolonged Q-T interval) 794.31
Romberg's 349.89
Rosen-Castleman-Liebow (pulmonary
    proteinosis) 516.0
rotator cuff, shoulder 726.10
Roth's 355.1
Rothmund's (congenital poikiloderma) 757.33
Rotor's (idiopathic hyperbilirubinemia) 277.4
Roussy-Lévy 334.3
Roy (-Jutras) (acropachyderma) 757.39
rubella (congenital) 771.0
Rubinstein-Taybi's (brachydactylia, short
    stature, and mental retardation) 759.89
Rud's (mental deficiency, epilepsy, and
    infantilism) 759.89
Ruiter-Pompen (-Wyers) (angiokeratoma
    corporis diffusum) 272.7
Runge's (postmaturity) 766.2
Russell (-Silver) (congenital hemihypertrophy
    and short stature) 759.89
Rytand-Lipsitch (complete atrioventricular
    block) 426.0
sacralization-scoliosis-sciatica 756.15
sacroiliac 724.6
Saenger's 379.46

Syndrome—*continued*
salt
  depletion (*see also* Disease, renal) 593.9
    due to heat NEC 992.8
      causing heat exhaustion or prostration
      992.4
  low (*see also* Disease, renal) 593.9
salt-losing (*see also* Disease, renal) 593.9
Sanfilippo's (mucopolysaccharidosis III) 277.5
Scaglietti-Dagnini (acromegalic
  macrospondylitis) 253.0
scalded skin 695.1
scalenus anticus (anterior) 353.0
scapulocostal 354.8
scapuloperoneal 359.1
scapulovertebral 723.4
Schaumann's (sarcoidosis) 135
Scheie's (mucopolysaccharidosis IS) 277.5
Scheuthauer-Marie-Sainton (cleidocranialis
  dysostosis) 755.59
Schirmer's (encephalocutaneous angiomatosis)
  759.6
schizophrenic, of childhood NEC (*see also*
  Psychosis, childhood) 299.9
Schmidt's
  sphallo-pharyngo-laryngeal hemiplegia 352.6
  thyroid-adrenocortical insufficiency 258.1
  vagoaccessory 352.6
Schneider's 047.9
Scholte's (malignant carcinoid) 259.2
Scholz (-Bielschowsky-Henneberg) 330.0
Schroeder's (endocrine-hypertensive) 255.3
Schüller-Christian (chronic histiocytosis X)
  277.8
Schultz's (agranulocytosis) 288.0
Schwartz (-Jampel) 756.89
Schwartz-Bartter (inappropriate secretion of
  antidiuretic hormone) 253.6
Scimitar (anomalous venous drainage, right
  lung to inferior vena cave) 747.49
sclerocystic ovary 256.4
sea-blue histiocyte 272.7
Seabright-Bantam (pseudohypoparathyroidism)
  275.49
Seckel's 759.89
Secretan's (posttraumatic edema) 782.3
secretoinhibitor (keratoconjunctivitis sicca)
  710.2
Seeligmann's (ichthyosis congenita) 757.1
Senear-Usher (pemphigus erythematosus) 694.4
senilism 259.8
serotonin 333.99
serous meningitis 348.2
Sertoli cell (germinal aplasia) 606.0
sex chromosome mosaic 758.81
Sézary's (reticulosis) (M9701/3) 202.2
shaken infant 995.55
Shaver's (bauxite pneumoconiosis) 503
Sheehan's (postpartum pituitary necrosis) 253.2
shock (traumatic) 958.4
  kidney 584.5
    following crush injury 958.5
  lung 518.5
  neurogenic 308.9
  psychic 308.9
short
  bowel 579.3
  P-R interval 426.81
shoulder-arm (*see also* Neuropathy, peripheral,
  autonomic) 337.9
shoulder-girdle 723.4

Syndrome—*continued*
shoulder-hand (*see also* Neuropathy, peripheral,
  autonomic) 337.9
Shwachman's 288.0
Shy-Drager (orthostatic hypotension with
  multisystem degeneration) 333.0
Sicard's 352.6
sicca (keratoconjunctivitis) 710.2
sick
  cell 276.1
  cilia 759.89
  sinus 427.81
sideropenic 280.8
Siemens'
  ectodermal dysplasia 757.31
  keratosis follicularis spinulosa (decalvans)
    757.39
Silfverskiöld's (osteochondrodystrophy,
  extremities) 756.50
Silver's (congenital hemihypertrophy and short
  stature) 759.89
Silvestroni-Bianco (thalassemia minima) 282.4
Simons' (progressive lipodystrophy) 272.6
sinus tarsi 726.79
sinusitis-bronchiectasis-situs inversus 759.3
Sipple's (medullary thyroid
  carcinoma-pheochromocytoma) 193
Sjögren (-Gougerot) (keratoconjunctivitis sicca)
  710.2
  with lung involvement 710.2 *[517.8]*
Sjögren-Larsson (ichthyosis congenita) 757.1
Slocumb's 255.3
Sluder's 337.0
Smith-Lemli-Opitz (cerebrohepatorenal
  syndrome) 759.89
smokers' 305.1
Sneddon-Wilkinson (subcorneal pustular
  dermatosis) 694.1
Sotos' (cerebral gigantism) 253.0
South African cardiomyopathy 425.2
spasmodic
  upward movement, eyes(s) 378.82
  winking 307.20
Spens' (syncope with heart block) 426.9
spherophakia-brachymorphia 759.89
spinal cord injury—*see also* Injury, spinal, by
  site
  with fracture, vertebra—*see* Fracture,
    vertebra, by site, with spinal cord injury
  cervical—*see* Injury, spinal, cervical
  fluid malabsorption (acquired) 331.3
splenic
  agenesis 759.0
  flexure 569.89
  neutropenia 288.0
  sequestration 282.60
Spurway's (brittle bones and blue sclera) 756.51
staphylococcal scalded skin 695.1
Stein's (polycystic ovary) 256.4
Stein-Leventhal (polycystic ovary) 256.4
Steinbrocker's (*see also* Neuropathy, peripheral,
  autonomic) 337.9
Stevens-Johnson (erythema multiforme
  exudativum) 695.1
Stewart-Morel (hyperostosis frontalis interna)
  733.3
stiff-man 333.91
Still's (juvenile rheumatoid arthritis) 714.30
Still-Felty (rheumatoid arthritis with
  splenomegaly and leukopenia) 714.1

Syndrome—*continued*
Stilling-Türk-Duane (ocular retraction
   syndrome) 378.71
Stojano's (subcostal) 098.86
Stokes (-Adams) (syncope with heart block)
   426.9
Stokvis-Talma (enterogenous cyanosis) 289.7
stone heart (*see also* Failure, ventricular, left)
   428.1
straight-back 756.19
stroke (*see also* Disease, cerebrovascular, acute)
   436
   little 435.9
Sturge-Kalischer-Weber (encephalotrigeminal
   angiomatosis) 759.6
Sturge-Weber (-Dimitri) (encephalocutaneous
   angiomatosis) 759.6
subclavian-carotid obstruction (chronic) 446.7
subclavian steal 435.2
subcoracoid-pectoralis minor 447.8
subcostal 098.86
   nerve compression 354.8
subperiosteal hematoma 267
subphrenic interposition 751.4
sudden infant death (SIDS) 798.0
Sudeck's 733.7
Sudeck-Leriche 733.7
superior
   cerebellar artery (*see also* Disease,
      cerebrovascular, acute) 436
   mesenteric artery 557.1
   pulmonary sulcus (tumor) (M8010/3) 162.3
   vena cava 459.2
suprarenal cortical 255.3
supraspinatus 726.10
swallowed blood 777.3
sweat retention 705.1
Sweet's (acute febrile neutrophilic dermatosis)
   695.89
Swyer-James (unilateral hyperlucent lung) 492.8
Swyer's (XY pure gonadal dysgenesis) 752.7
Symonds' 348.2
sympathetic
   cervical paralysis 337.0
   pelvic 625.5
syndactylic oxycephaly 755.55
syphilitic-cardiovascular 093.89
systemic
   fibrosclerosing 710.8
   inflammatory response (SIRS) 995.90
      due to
         infectious process 995.91
            with organ dysfunction 995.92
         non-infectious process 995.93
            with organ dysfunction 995.94
systolic click (-murmur) 785.2
Tabagism 305.1
tachycardia-bradycardia 427.81
Takayasu (-Onishi) (pulseless disease) 446.7
Tapia's 352.6
tarsal tunnel 355.5
Taussig-Bing (transposition, aorta and
   overriding pulmonary artery) 745.11
Taybi's (otopalatodigital) 759.89
Taylor's 625.5
teething 520.7
tegmental 344.89
telangiectasis-pigmentation-cataract 757.33
temporal 383.02
   lobectomy behavior 310.0

Syndrome—*continued*
temporomandibular joint-pain-dysfunction
   [TMJ] NEC 524.60
   specified NEC 524.69
Terry's 362.21
testicular feminization 257.8
testis, nonvirilizing 257.8
tethered (spinal) cord 742.59
thalamic 348.8
Thibierge-Weissenbach (cutaneous systemic
   sclerosis) 710.1
Thiele 724.6
thoracic outlet (compression) 353.0
thoracogenous rheumatic (hypertrophic
   pulmonary osteoarthropathy) 731.2
Thorn's (*see also* Disease, renal) 593.9
Thorson-Biörck (malignant carcinoid) 259.2
thrombopenia-hemangioma 287.3
thyroid-adrenocortical insufficiency 258.1
Tietze's 733.6
time-zone (rapid) 307.45
Tobias' (carcinoma, pulmonary apex)
   (M8010/3) 162.3
toilet seat 926.0
Tolosa-Hunt 378.55
Toni-Fanconi (cystinosis) 270.0
Touraine's (hereditary osteo-onychodysplasia)
   756.89
Touraine-Solente-Golé (acropachyderma)
   757.39
toxic
   oil 710.5
   shock 040.82
transfusion
   fetal-maternal 772.0
   twin
      donor (infant) 772.0
      recipient (infant) 776.4
Treacher Collins' (incomplete mandibulofacial
   dysostosis) 756.0
trigeminal plate 259.8
triple X female 758.81
trisomy NEC 758.5
   13 or D$_1$ 758.1
   16-18 or E 758.2
   18 or E$_3$ 758.2
   20 758.5
   21 or G (mongolism) 758.0
   22 or G (mongolism) 758.0
   G 758.0
Troisier-Hanot-Chauffard (bronze diabetes)
   275.0
tropical wet feet 991.4
Trousseau's (thrombophlebitis migrans visceral
   cancer) 453.1
Türk's (ocular retraction syndrome) 378.71
Turner's 758.6
Turner-Varny 758.6
twin-to-twin transfusion 762.3
   recipient twin 776.4
Uehlinger's (acropachyderma) 757.39
Ullrich (-Bonnevie) (-Turner) 758.6
Ullrich-Feichtiger 759.89
underwater blast injury (abdominal) (*see also*
   Injury, internal, abdomen) 868.00
universal joint, cervix 620.6
Unverricht (-Lundborg) 333.2
Unverricht-Wagner (dermatomyositis) 710.3
upward gaze 378.81
Urbach-Oppenheim (necrobiosis lipoidica
   diabeticorum) 250.8 *[709.3]*

Syndrome—*continued*
Urbach-Wiethe (lipoid proteinosis) 272.8
uremia, chronic 585
urethral 597.81
urethro-oculoarticular 099.3
urethro-oculosynovial 099.3
urohepatic 572.4
uveocutaneous 364.24
uveomeningeal, uveomeningitis 363.22
vagohypoglossal 352.6
vagovagal 780.2
van Buchem's (hyperostosis corticalis) 733.3
van der Hoeve's (brittle bones and blue sclera, deafness) 756.51
van der Hoeve-Halbertsma-Waardenburg (ptosis-epicanthus) 270.2
van der Hoeve-Waardenburg-Gualdi (ptosis-epicanthus) 270.2
van Neck-Odelberg (juvenile osteochondrosis) 732.1
vanishing twin 651.33
vascular splanchnic 557.0
vasomotor 443.9
vasovagal 780.2
VATER 759.89
velo-cardio-facial 759.89
    with chromosomal deletion 758.5
vena cava (inferior) (superior) (obstruction) 459.2
Verbiest's (claudicatio intermittens spinalis) 435.1
Vernet's 352.6
vertebral
    artery 435.1
        compression 721.1
        lumbar 724.4
        steal 435.1
vertebrogenic (pain) 724.5
vertiginous NEC 386.9
video display tube 723.8
Villaret's 352.6
Vinson-Plummer (sideropenic dysphagia) 280.8
virilizing adrenocortical hyperplasia, congenital 255.2
virus, viral 079.99
visceral larval migrans 128.0
visual disorientation 368.16
vitamin B$_6$ deficiency 266.1
vitreous touch 997.99
Vogt's (corpus striatum) 333.7
Vogt-Koyanagi 364.24
Volkmann's 958.6
von Bechterew-Strümpell (ankylosing spondylitis) 720.0
von Graefe's 378.72
von Hippel-Lindau (angiomatosis retinocerebellosa) 759.6
von Schroetter's (intermittent venous claudication) 453.8
von Willebrand (-Jürgens) (angiohemophilia) 286.4
Waardenburg-Klein (ptosis epicanthus) 270.2
Wagner (-Unverricht) (dermatomyositis) 710.3
Waldenström's (macroglobulinemia) 273.3
Waldenström-Kjellberg (sideropenic dysphagia) 280.8
Wallenberg's (posterior inferior cerebellar artery) (*see also* Disease, cerebrovascular, acute) 436
Waterhouse (-Friderichsen) 036.3
water retention 276.6

Syndrome—*continued*
Weber's 344.89
Weber-Christian (nodular nonsuppurative panniculitis) 729.30
Weber-Cockayne (epidermolysis bullosa) 757.39
Weber-Dimitri (encephalocutaneous angiomatosis) 759.6
Weber-Gubler 344.89
Weber-Leyden 344.89
Weber-Osler (familial hemorrhagic telangiectasia) 448.0
Wegener's (necrotizing respiratory granulomatosis) 446.4
Weill-Marchesani (brachymorphism and ectopia lentis) 759.89
Weingarten's (tropical eosinophilia) 518.3
Weiss-Baker (carotid sinus syncope) 337.0
Weissenbach-Thibierge (cutaneous systemic sclerosis) 710.1
Werdnig-Hoffmann 335.0
Werlhof-Wichmann (*see also* Purpura, thrombocytopenic) 287.3
Wermer's (polyendocrine adenomatosis) 258.0
Werner's (progeria adultorum) 259.8
Wernicke's (nonalcoholic) (superior hemorrhagic polioencephalitis) 265.1
Wernicke-Korsakoff (nonalcoholic) 294.0
    alcoholic 291.1
Westphal-Strümpell (hepatolenticular degeneration) 275.1
wet
    brain (alcoholic) 303.9
    feet (maceration) (tropical) 991.4
    lung
        adult 518.5
        newborn 770.6
whiplash 847.0
Whipple's (intestinal lipodystrophy) 040.2
"whistling face" (craniocarpotarsal dystrophy) 759.89
Widal (-Abrami) (acquired hemolytic jaundice) 283.9
Wilkie's 557.1
Wilkinson-Sneddon (subcorneal pustular dermatosis) 694.1
Willan-Plumbe (psoriasis) 696.1
Willebrand (-Jürgens) (angiohemophilia) 286.4
Willi-Prader (hypogenital dystrophy with diabetic tendency) 759.81
Wilson's (hepatolenticular degeneration) 275.1
Wilson-Mikity 770.7
Wiskott-Aldrich (eczema-thrombocytopenia) 279.12
withdrawal
    alcohol 291.81
    drug 292.0
    infant of dependent mother 779.5
Woakes' (ethmoiditis) 471.1
Wolff-Parkinson-White (anomalous atrioventricular excitation) 426.7
Wright's (hyperabduction) 447.8
X
    cardiac 413.9
    dysmetabolic 277.7
xiphoidalgia 733.99
XO 758.6
XXX 758.81
XXXXY 758.81
XXY 758.7
yellow vernix (placental dysfunction) 762.2
Zahorsky's 074.0

Syndrome—*continued*
  Zieve's (jaundice, hyperlipemia and hemolytic
    anemia) 571.1
  Zollinger-Ellison (gastric hypersecretion with
    pancreatic islet cell tumor) 251.5
  Zuelzer-Ogden (nutritional megaloblastic
    anemia) 281.2
Synechia (iris) (pupil) 364.70
  anterior 364.72
    peripheral 364.73
  intrauterine (traumatic) 621.5
  posterior 364.71
  vulvae, congenital 752.49
Synesthesia (*see also* Disturbance, sensation)
    782.0
Synodontia 520.2
Synophthalmus 759.89
Synorchidism 752.8
Synorchism 752.8
Synostosis (congenital) 756.59
  astragaloscaphoid 755.67
  radioulnar 755.53
  talonavicular (bar) 755.67
  tarsal 755.67
Synovial —*see* condition
Synovioma (M9040/3)—*see also* Neoplasm,
    connective tissue, malignant
  benign (M9040/3)—*see* Neoplasm, connective
    tissue, benign
Synoviosarcoma (M9040/3)—*see* Neoplasm,
    connective tissue, malignant
Synovitis 727.00
  chronic crepitant, wrist 727.2
  due to crystals—*see* Arthritis, due to crystals
  gonococcal 098.51
  gouty 274.0
  syphilitic 095.7
    congenital 090.0
  traumatic, current—*see* Sprain, by site
  tuberculous—*see* Tuberculosis, synovitis
  villonodular 719.20
    ankle 719.27
    elbow 719.22
    foot 719.27
    hand 719.24
    hip 719.25
    knee 719.26
    multiple sites 719.29
    pelvic region 719.25
    shoulder (region) 719.21
    specified site NEC 719.28
    wrist 719.23
Syphilide 091.3
  congenital 090.0
  newborn 090.0
  tubercular 095.8
    congenital 090.0
Syphilis, syphilitic (acquired) 097.9
  with lung involvement 095.1
  abdomen (late) 095.2
  acoustic nerve 094.86
  adenopathy (secondary) 091.4
  adrenal (gland) 095.8
    with cortical hypofunction 095.8
  age under 2 years NEC (*see also* Syphilis,
    congenital) 090.9
    acquired 097.9
  alopecia (secondary) 091.82
  anemia 095.8
  aneurysm (artery) (ruptured) 093.89
    aorta 093.0

Syphilis, syphilitic—*continued*
  central nervous system 094.89
    congenital 090.5
  anus 095.8
    primary 091.1
    secondary 091.3
  aorta, aortic (arch) (abdominal) (insufficiency)
      (pulmonary) (regurgitation) (stenosis)
      (thoracic) 093.89
    aneurysm 093.0
  arachnoid (adhesive) 094.2
  artery 093.89
    cerebral 094.89
    spinal 094.89
  arthropathy (neurogenic) (tabetic) 094.0 *[713.5]*
  asymptomatic—*see* Syphilis, latent
  ataxia, locomotor (progressive) 094.0
  atrophoderma maculatum 091.3
  auricular fibrillation 093.89
  Bell's palsy 094.89
  bladder 095.8
  bone 095.5
    secondary 091.61
  brain 094.89
  breast 095.8
  bronchus 095.8
  bubo 091.0
  bulbar palsy 094.89
  bursa (late) 095.7
  cardiac decompensation 093.89
  cardiovascular (early) (late) (primary)
      (secondary) (tertiary) 093.9
    specified type and site NEC 093.89
  causing death under 2 years of age (*see also*
      Syphilis, congenital) 090.9
    stated to be acquired NEC 097.9
  central nervous system (any site) (early) (late)
      (latent) (primary) (recurrent) (relapse)
      (secondary) (tertiary) 094.9
    with
      ataxia 094.0
      paralysis, general 094.1
        juvenile 090.40
      paresis (general) 094.1
        juvenile 090.40
      tabes (dorsalis) 094.0
        juvenile 090.40
      taboparesis 094.1
        juvenile 090.40
    aneurysm (ruptured) 094.87
    congenital 090.40
    juvenile 090.40
    remission in (sustained) 094.9
    serology doubtful, negative, or positive 094.9
    specified nature or site NEC 094.89
    vascular 094.89
  cerebral 094.89
    meningovascular 094.2
    nerves 094.89
    sclerosis 094.89
    thrombosis 094.89
  cerebrospinal 094.89
    tabetic 094.0
  cerebrovascular 094.89
  cervix 095.8
  chancre (multiple) 091.0
    extragenital 091.2
    Rollet's 091.0
  Charcot's joint 094.0 *[713.5]*
  choked disc 094.89 *[377.00]*
  chorioretinitis 091.51

Syphilis, syphilitic—*continued*
  interstitial keratitis 090.3
  Hutchinson's teeth 090.5
  hyalitis 095.8
  inactive—*see* Syphilis, latent
  infantum NEC (*see also* Syphilis, congenital)
    090.9
  inherited—*see* Syphilis, congenital
  internal ear 095.8
  intestine (late) 095.8
  iris, iritis (secondary) 091.52
    late 095.8 *[364.11]*
  joint (late) 095.8
  keratitis (congenital) (early) (interstitial) (late)
    (parenchymatous) (punctata profunda) 090.3
  kidney 095.4
  lacrimal apparatus 095.8
  laryngeal paralysis 095.8
  larynx 095.8
  late 097.0
    cardiovascular 093.9
    central nervous system 094.9
    latent or 2 years or more after infection
      (without manifestations) 096
      negative spinal fluid test 096
      serology positive 096
    paresis 094.1
    specified site NEC 095.8
    symptomatic or with symptoms 095.9
    tabes 094.0
  latent 097.1
    central nervous system 094.9
    date of infection unspecified 097.1
    early or less than 2 years after infection 092.9
    late or 2 years or more after infection 096
    serology
      doubtful
        follow-up of latent syphilis 097.1
          central nervous system 094.9
          date of infection unspecified 097.1
          early or less than 2 years after infection
            092.9
          late or 2 years or more after infection 096
      positive, only finding 097.1
        date of infection unspecified 097.1
        early or less than 2 years after infection
          097.1
        late or 2 years or more after infection 097.1
  lens 095.8
  leukoderma 091.3
    late 095.8
  lienis 095.8
  lip 091.3
    chancre 091.2
    late 095.8
    primary 091.2
  Lissauer's paralysis 094.1
  liver 095.3
    secondary 091.62
  locomotor ataxia 094.0
  lung 095.1
  lymphadenitis (secondary) 091.4
  lymph gland (early) (secondary) 091.4
    late 095.8
  macular atrophy of skin 091.3
    striated 095.8
  maternal, affecting fetus or newborn 760.2
    manifest syphilis in newborn—*see* Syphilis,
      congenital
  mediastinum (late) 095.8

Syphilis, syphilitic—*continued*
  meninges (adhesive) (basilar) (brain) (spinal
    cord) 094.2
  meningitis 094.2
    acute 091.81
    congenital 090.42
  meningoencephalitis 094.2
  meningovascular 094.2
    congenital 090.49
  mesarteritis 093.89
    brain 094.89
    spine 094.89
  middle ear 095.8
  mitral stenosis 093.21
  monoplegia 094.89
  mouth (secondary) 091.3
    late 095.8
  mucocutaneous 091.3
    late 095.8
  mucous
    membrane 091.3
      late 095.8
    patches 091.3
      congenital 090.0
  mulberry molars 090.5
  muscle 095.6
  myocardium 093.82
  myositis 095.6
  nasal sinus 095.8
  neonatorum NEC (*see also* Syphilis, congenital)
    090.9
  nerve palsy (any cranial nerve) 094.89
  nervous system, central 094.9
  neuritis 095.8
    acoustic nerve 094.86
  neurorecidive of retina 094.83
  neuroretinitis 094.85
  newborn (*see also* Syphilis, congenital) 090.9
  nodular superficial 095.8
  nonvenereal, endemic 104.0
  nose 095.8
    saddle back deformity 090.5
    septum 095.8
      perforated 095.8
  occlusive arterial disease 093.89
  ophthalmic 095.8 *[363.13]*
  ophthalmoplegia 094.89
  optic nerve (atrophy) (neuritis) (papilla) 094.84
  orbit (late) 095.8
  orchitis 095.8
  organic 097.9
  osseous (late) 095.5
  osteochondritis (congenital) 090.0
  osteoporosis 095.5
  ovary 095.8
  oviduct 095.8
  palate 095.8
    gumma 095.8
    perforated 090.5
  pancreas (late) 095.8
  pancreatitis 095.8
  paralysis 094.89
    general 094.1
    juvenile 090.40
  paraplegia 094.89
  paresis (general) 094.1
    juvenile 090.40
  paresthesia 094.89
  Parkinson's disease or syndrome 094.82
  paroxysmal tachycardia 093.89
  pemphigus (congenital) 090.0

Syphilis, syphilitic—*continued*
penis 091.0
  chancre 091.0
  late 095.8
pericardium 093.81
perichondritis, larynx 095.8
periosteum 095.5
  congenital 090.0
  early 091.61
  secondary 091.61
peripheral nerve 095.8
petrous bone (late) 095.5
pharynx 095.8
  secondary 091.3
pituitary (gland) 095.8
placenta 095.8
pleura (late) 095.8
pneumonia, white 090.0
pontine (lesion) 094.89
portal vein 093.89
primary NEC 091.2
  anal 091.1
  and secondary (*see also* Syphilis, secondary)
    091.9
  cardiovascular 093.9
  central nervous system 094.9
  extragenital chancre NEC 091.2
  fingers 091.2
  genital 091.0
  lip 091.2
  specified site NEC 091.2
  tonsils 091.2
prostate 095.8
psychosis (intracranial gumma) 094.89
ptosis (eyelid) 094.89
pulmonary (late) 095.1
  artery 093.89
pulmonum 095.1
pyelonephritis 095.4
recently acquired, symptomatic NEC 091.89
rectum 095.8
respiratory tract 095.8
retina
  late 094.83
  neurorecidive 094.83
retrobulbar neuritis 094.85
salpingitis 095.8
sclera (late) 095.0
sclerosis
  cerebral 094.89
  coronary 093.89
  multiple 094.89
  subacute 094.89
scotoma (central) 095.8
scrotum 095.8
secondary (and primary) 091.9
  adenopathy 091.4
  anus 091.3
  bone 091.61
  cardiovascular 093.9
  central nervous system 094.9
  chorioretinitis, choroiditis 091.51
  hepatitis 091.62
  liver 091.62
  lymphadenitis 091.4
  meningitis, acute 091.81
  mouth 091.3
  mucous membranes 091.3
  periosteum 091.61
  periostitis 091.61
  pharynx 091.3

Syphilis, syphilitic—*continued*
  relapse (treated) (untreated) 091.7
  skin 091.3
  specified form NEC 091.89
  tonsil 091.3
  ulcer 091.3
  viscera 091.69
  vulva 091.3
seminal vesicle (late) 095.8
seronegative
  with signs or symptoms—*see* Syphilis, by site
    and stage
seropositive
  with signs or symptoms—*see* Syphilis, by site
    and stage
  follow-up of latent syphilis—*see* Syphilis,
    latent
  only finding—*see* Syphilis, latent
seventh nerve (paralysis) 094.89
sinus 095.8
sinusitis 095.8
skeletal system 095.5
skin (early) (secondary) (with ulceration) 091.3
  late or tertiary 095.8
small intestine 095.8
spastic spinal paralysis 094.0
spermatic cord (late) 095.8
spinal (cord) 094.89
  with
    paresis 094.1
    tabes 094.0
spleen 095.8
splenomegaly 095.8
spondylitis 095.5
staphyloma 095.8
stigmata (congenital) 090.5
stomach 095.8
synovium (late) 095.7
tabes dorsalis (early) (late) 094.0
  juvenile 090.40
tabetic type 094.0
  juvenile 090.40
taboparesis 094.1
  juvenile 090.40
tachycardia 093.89
tendon (late) 095.7
tertiary 097.0
  with symptoms 095.8
  cardiovascular 093.9
  central nervous system 094.9
  multiple NEC 095.8
  specified site NEC 095.8
testis 095.8
thorax 095.8
throat 095.8
thymus (gland) 095.8
thyroid (late) 095.8
tongue 095.8
tonsil (lingual) 095.8
  primary 091.2
  secondary 091.3
trachea 095.8
tricuspid valve 093.23
tumor, brain 094.89
tunica vaginalis (late) 095.8
ulcer (any site) (early) (secondary) 091.3
  late 095.9
  perforating 095.9
    foot 094.0
urethra (stricture) 095.8
urogenital 095.8

Syphilis, syphilitic—*continued*
  uterus 095.8
  uveal tract (secondary) 091.50
    late 095.8 *[363.13]*
  uveitis (secondary) 091.50
    late 095.8 *[363.13]*
  uvula (late) 095.8
    perforated 095.8
  vagina 091.0
    late 095.8
  valvulitis NEC 093.20
  vascular 093.89
    brain or cerebral 094.89
  vein 093.89
    cerebral 094.89
  ventriculi 095.8
  vesicae urinariae 095.8
  viscera (abdominal) 095.2
    secondary 091.69
  vitreous (hemorrhage) (opacities) 095.8
  vulva 091.0
    late 095.8
    secondary 091.3
Syphiloma 095.9
  cardiovascular system 093.9
  central nervous system 094.9
  circulatory system 093.9
  congenital 090.5
Syphilophobia 300.29
Syringadenoma (M8400/0)—*see also*
    Neoplasm, skin, benign
  papillary (M8406/0)—*see* Neoplasm, skin,
    benign
Syringobulbia 336.0
Syringocarcinoma (M8400/3)—*see* Neoplasm,
    skin, malignant
Syringocystadenoma (M8400/0)—*see also*
    Neoplasm, skin, benign
  papillary (M8406/0)—*see* Neoplasm, skin,
    benign
Syringocystoma (M8407/0)—*see* Neoplasm,
    skin, benign
Syringoma (M8407/0)—*see also* Neoplasm,
    skin, benign
  chondroid (M8940/0)—*see* Neoplasm, by site,
    benign
Syringomyelia 336.0
Syringomyelitis 323.9
  late effect—*see* category 326
Syringomyelocele (*see also* Spina bifida) 741.9
Syringopontia 336.0
System, systemic —*see also* condition
  disease, combined—*see* Degeneration,
    combined
  fibrosclerosing syndrome 710.8
  inflammatory response syndrome (SIRS) 995.90
    due to
      infectious process 995.91
        with organ dysfunction 995.92
      non-infectious process 995.93
        with organ dysfunction 995.94
  lupus erythematosus 710.0
    inhibitor 286.5

T

Tab —*see* Tag
Tabacism 989.8
Tabacosis 989.8
Tabardillo 080
 flea-borne 081.0
 louse-borne 080
Tabes, tabetic
 with
  central nervous system syphilis 094.0
  Charcot's joint 094.0 *[713.5]*
  cord bladder 094.0
  crisis, viscera (any) 094.0
  paralysis, general 094.1
  paresis (general) 094.1
  perforating ulcer 094.0
 arthropathy 094.0 *[713.5]*
 bladder 094.0
 bone 094.0
 cerebrospinal 094.0
 congenital 090.40
 conjugal 094.0
 dorsalis 094.0
  neurosyphilis 094.0
 early 094.0
 juvenile 090.40
 latent 094.0
 mesenterica (*see also* Tuberculosis) 014.8
 paralysis insane, general 094.1
 peripheral (nonsyphilitic) 799.8
 spasmodic 094.0
  not dorsal or dorsalis 343.9
 syphilis (cerebrospinal) 094.0
Taboparalysis 094.1
Taboparesis (remission) 094.1
 with
  Charcot's joint 094.1 *[713.5]*
  cord bladder 094.1
  perforating ulcer 094.1
 juvenile 090.40
Tachyalimentation 579.3
Tachyarrhythmia, tachyrhythmia —*see also*
 Tachycardia
 paroxysmal with sinus bradycardia 427.81
Tachycardia 785.0
 atrial 427.89
 auricular 427.89
 newborn 779.82
 nodal 427.89
  nonparoxysmal atrioventricular 426.89
 nonparoxysmal atrioventricular (nodal) 426.89
 paroxysmal 427.2
  with sinus bradycardia 427.81
  atrial (PAT) 427.0
   psychogenic 316 *[427.0]*
  atrioventricular (AV) 427.0
   psychogenic 316 *[427.0]*
  essential 427.2
  junctional 427.0
  nodal 427.0
  psychogenic 316 *[427.2]*
   atrial 316 *[427.0]*
   supraventricular 316 *[427.0]*
   ventricular 316 *[427.1]*
  supraventricular 427.0
   psychogenic 316 *[427.0]*
  ventricular 427.1
   psychogenic 316 *[427.1]*
 postoperative 997.1

Tachycardia—*continued*
 psychogenic 306.2
 sick sinus 427.81
 sinoauricular 427.89
 sinus 427.89
 supraventricular 427.89
 ventricular (paroxysmal) 427.1
  psychogenic 316 *[427.1]*
Tachypnea 786.06
 hysterical 300.11
 newborn (idiopathic) (transitory) 770.6
 psychogenic 306.1
 transitory, of newborn 770.6
Taenia (infection) (infestation) (*see also*
 Infestation, taenia) 123.3
 diminuta 123.6
 echinococcal infestation (*see also*
  Echinococcus) 122.9
 nana 123.6
 saginata infestation 123.2
 solium (intestinal form) 123.0
  larval form 123.1
Taeniasis (intestine) (*see also* Infestation,
 Taenia) 123.3
 saginata 123.2
 solium 123.0
Taenzer's disease 757.4
Tag (hypertrophied skin) (infected) 701.9
 adenoid 474.8
 anus 455.9
 endocardial (*see also* Endocarditis) 424.90
 hemorrhoidal 455.9
 hymen 623.8
 perineal 624.8
 preauricular 744.1
 rectum 455.9
 sentinel 455.9
 skin 701.9
  accessory 757.39
  anus 455.9
  congenital 757.39
  preauricular 744.1
  rectum 455.9
 tonsil 474.8
 urethra, urethral 599.84
 vulva 624.8
Tahyna fever 062.5
Takayasu (-Onishi) disease or syndrome
 (pulseless disease) 446.7
Talc granuloma 728.82
Talcosis 502
Talipes (congenital) 754.70
 acquired NEC 736.79
  planus 734
 asymmetric 754.79
  acquired 736.79
 calcaneovalgus 754.62
  acquired 736.76
 calcaneovarus 754.59
  acquired 736.76
 calcaneus 754.79
  acquired 736.76
 cavovarus 754.59
  acquired 736.75
 cavus 754.71
  acquired 736.73
 equinovalgus 754.69
  acquired 736.72

Tear, torn—*continued*
  medial 836.0
    anterior horn 836.0
      old 717.1
    bucket handle 836.0
      old 717.0
    old 717.3
    posterior horn 836.0
      old 717.2
  old NEC 717.5
  site other than knee—*see* Sprain, by site
  muscle—*see also* Sprain, by site
  with open wound—*see* Wound, open by site
  pelvic
    floor, complicating delivery 664.1
    organ NEC
      with
        abortion—*see* Abortion, by type, with
          damage to pelvic organs
        ectopic pregnancy (*see also* categories
          633.0-633.9) 639.2
        molar pregnancy (*see also* categories
          630-632) 639.2
      following
        abortion 639.2
        ectopic or molar pregnancy 639.2
      obstetrical trauma 665.5
  perineum—*see also* Laceration, perineum
    obstetrical trauma 665.5
  periurethral tissue
    with
      abortion—*see* Abortion, by type, with
        damage to pelvic organs
      ectopic pregnancy (*see also* categories
        633.0-633.9) 639.2
      molar pregnancy (*see also* categories
        630-632) 639.2
    following
      abortion 639.2
      ectopic or molar pregnancy 639.2
    obstetrical trauma 665.5
  rectovaginal septum—*see* Laceration,
    rectovaginal septum
  retina, retinal (recent) (with detachment) 361.00
    without detachment 361.30
    dialysis (juvenile) (with detachment) 361.04
    giant (with detachment) 361.03
    horseshoe (without detachment) 361.32
    multiple (with detachment) 361.02
      without detachment 361.33
    old
      delimited (partial) 361.06
      partial 361.06
      total or subtotal 361.07
    partial (without detachment)
      giant 361.03
      multiple defects 361.02
      old (delimited) 361.06
      single defect 361.01
    round hole (without detachment) 361.31
    single defect (with detachment) 361.01
    total or subtotal (recent) 361.05
      old 361.07
  rotator cuff (traumatic) 840.4
    current injury 840.4
    degenerative 726.10
    nontraumatic 727.61
  semilunar cartilage, knee (*see also* Tear,
    meniscus) 836.2
    old 717.5

Tear, torn—*continued*
  tendon—*see also* Sprain, by site
    with open wound—*see* Wound, open by site
  tentorial, at birth 767.0
  umbilical cord
    affecting fetus or newborn 772.0
    complicating delivery 663.8
  urethra
    with
      abortion—*see* Abortion, by type, with
        damage to pelvic organs
      ectopic pregnancy (*see also* categories
        633.0-633.9) 639.2
      molar pregnancy (*see also* categories
        630-632) 639.2
    following
      abortion 639.2
      ectopic or molar pregnancy 639.2
    obstetrical trauma 665.5
  uterus—*see* Injury, internal, uterus
  vagina—*see* Laceration, vagina
  vessel, from catheter 998.2
  vulva, complicating delivery 664.0
Tear stone 375.57
Teeth, tooth —*see also* condition
  grinding 306.8
Teething 520.7
  syndrome 520.7
Tegmental syndrome 344.89
Telangiectasia, telangiectasis (verrucous) 448.9
  ataxic (cerebellar) 334.8
  familial 448.0
  hemorrhagic, hereditary (congenital) (senile)
    448.0
  hereditary hemorrhagic 448.0
  retina 362.15
  spider 448.1
Telecanthus (congenital) 743.63
Telescoped bowel or intestine (*see also*
  Intussusception) 560.0
Teletherapy, adverse effect NEC 990
Telogen effluvium 704.02
Temperature
  body, high (of unknown origin) (*see also*
    Pyrexia) 780.6
  cold, trauma from 991.9
    newborn 778.2
    specified effect NEC 991.8
  high
    body (of unknown origin) (*see also* Pyrexia)
      780.6
    trauma from—*see* Heat
Temper tantrum (childhood) (*see also*
  Disturbance, conduct) 312.1
Temple —*see* condition
Temporal —*see also* condition
  lobe syndrome 310.0
**Temporomandibular joint-pain-dysfunction
  syndrome** 524.60
Temporosphenoidal —*see* condition
Tendency
  bleeding (*see also* Defect, coagulation) 286.9
  homosexual, ego-dystonic 302.0
  paranoid 301.0
  suicide 300.9
Tenderness
  abdominal (generalized) (localized) 789.6
    rebound 789.6
  skin 782.0

Test(s)—*continued*
　bacterial disease NEC (*see also* Screening, by
　　name of disease) V74.9
　basal metabolic rate V72.6
　blood-alcohol V70.4
　blood-drug V70.4
　　for therapeutic drug monitoring V58.83
　developmental, infant or child V20.2
　Dick V74.8
　fertility V26.21
　genetic V26.3
　hearing V72.1
　HIV V72.6
　human immunodeficiency virus V72.6
　Kveim V82.89
　laboratory V72.6
　　for medicolegal reason V70.4
　Mantoux (for tuberculosis) V74.1
　mycotic organism V75.4
　parasitic agent NEC V75.8
　paternity V70.4
　peritoneal equilibration V56.32
　pregnancy
　　positive V22.1
　　　first pregnancy V22.0
　　unconfirmed V72.4
　preoperative V72.84
　　cardiovascular V72.81
　　respiratory V72.82
　　specified NEC V72.83
　procreative management NEC V26.29
　sarcoidosis V82.89
　Schick V74.3
　Schultz-Charlton V74.8
　skin, diagnostic
　　allergy V72.7
　　bacterial agent NEC (*see also* Screening, by
　　　name of disease) V74.9
　　Dick V74.8
　　hypersensitivity V72.7
　　Kveim V82.89
　　Mantoux V74.1
　　mycotic organism V75.4
　　parasitic agent NEC V75.8
　　sarcoidosis V82.89
　　Schick V74.3
　　Schultz-Charlton V74.8
　　tuberculin V74.1
　specified type NEC V72.85
　tuberculin V74.1
　vision V72.0
　Wassermann
　　positive (*see also* Serology for syphilis,
　　　positive) 097.1
　　false 795.6
Testicle, testicular, testis —*see also* condition
　feminization (syndrome) 257.8
Tetanus, tetanic (cephalic) (convulsions) 037
　with
　　abortion—*see* Abortion, by type, with sepsis
　　ectopic pregnancy (*see also* categories
　　　633.0-633.9) 639.0
　　molar pregnancy (*see* categories 630-632)
　　　639.0
　following
　　abortion 639.0
　　ectopic or molar pregnancy 639.0
　inoculation V03.7
　　reaction (due to serum)—*see* Complications,
　　　vaccination
　neonatorum 771.3
　puerperal, postpartum, childbirth 670

Tetany, tetanic 781.7
　alkalosis 276.3
　associated with rickets 268.0
　convulsions 781.7
　　hysterical 300.11
　functional (hysterical) 300.11
　hyperkinetic 781.7
　　hysterical 300.11
　hyperpnea 786.01
　　hysterical 300.11
　　psychogenic 306.1
　hyperventilation 786.01
　　hysterical 300.11
　　psychogenic 306.1
　hypocalcemic, neonatal 775.4
　hysterical 300.11
　neonatal 775.4
　parathyroid (gland) 252.1
　parathyroprival 252.1
　postoperative 252.1
　postthyroidectomy 252.1
　pseudotetany 781.7
　　hysterical 300.11
　　psychogenic 306.1
　　specified as conversion reaction 300.11
Tetralogy of Fallot 745.2
Tetraplegia —*see* Quadriplegia
Thailand hemorrhagic fever 065.4
Thalassanemia 282.4
Thalassemia (alpha) (beta) (disease) (Hb-C)
　(Hb-D) (Hb-E) (Hb-H) (Hb-I) (Hb-S) (high
　fetal gene) (high fetal hemoglobin)
　(intermedia) (major) (minima) (minor)
　(mixed) (sickle-cell) (trait) (with other
　hemoglobinopathy) 282.4
Thalassemic variants 282.4
Thaysen-Gee disease (nontropical sprue) 579.0
Thecoma (M8600/0) 220
　malignant (M8600/3) 183.0
Thelarche, precocious 259.1
Thelitis 611.0
　puerperal, postpartum 675.0
Therapeutic —*see* condition
Therapy V57.9
　blood transfusion, without reported diagnosis
　　V58.2
　breathing V57.0
　chemotherapy V58.1
　　fluoride V07.31
　　prophylactic NEC V07.39
　dialysis (intermittent) (treatment)
　　extracorporeal V56.0
　　peritoneal V56.8
　　renal V56.0
　　specified type NEC V56.8
　exercise NEC V57.1
　　breathing V57.0
　extracorporeal dialysis (renal) V56.0
　fluoride prophylaxis V07.31
　hemodialysis V56.0
　long term oxygen therapy V46.2
　occupational V57.21
　orthoptic V57.4
　orthotic V57.81
　peritoneal dialysis V56.8
　physical NEC V57.1
　postmenopausal hormone replacement V07.4
　radiation V58.0
　speech V57.3
　vocational V57.22
Thermalgesia 782.0
Thermalgia 782.0

Thermanalgesia 782.0
Thermanesthesia 782.0
Thermic —*see* condition
Thermography (abnormal) 793.9
  breast 793.89
Thermoplegia 992.0
Thesaurismosis
  amyloid 277.3
  bilirubin 277.4
  calcium 275.40
  cystine 270.0
  glycogen (*see also* Disease, glycogen storage)
    271.0
  kerasin 272.7
  lipoid 272.7
  melanin 255.4
  phosphatide 272.7
  urate 274.9
Thiaminic deficiency 265.1
  with beriberi 265.0
Thibierge-Weissenbach syndrome (cutaneous
    systemic sclerosis) 710.1
Thickened endometrium 793.5
Thickening
  bone 733.99
    extremity 733.99
  breast 611.79
  hymen 623.3
  larynx 478.79
  nail 703.8
    congenital 757.5
  periosteal 733.99
  pleura (*see also* Pleurisy) 511.0
  skin 782.8
  subepiglottic 478.79
  tongue 529.8
  valve, heart—*see* Endocarditis
Thiele syndrome 724.6
Thigh —*see* condition
Thinning vertebra (*see also* Osteoporosis)
    733.00
Thirst, excessive 783.5
  due to deprivation of water 994.3
Thomsen's disease 359.2
Thomson's disease (congenital poikiloderma)
    757.33
Thoracic —*see also* condition
  kidney 753.3
  outlet syndrome 353.0
  stomach—*see* Hernia, diaphragm
Thoracogastroschisis (congenital) 759.89
Thoracopagus 759.4
Thoracoschisis 756.3
Thorax —*see* condition
Thorn's syndrome (*see also* Disease, renal)
    593.9
Thornwaldt's, Tornwaldt's
  bursitis (pharyngeal) 478.29
  cyst 478.26
  disease (pharyngeal bursitis) 478.29
Thorson-Biörck syndrome (malignant
    carcinoid) 259.2
Threadworm (infection) (infestation) 127.4
Threatened
  abortion or miscarriage 640.0
    with subsequent abortion (*see also* Abortion,
      spontaneous) 634.9
    affecting fetus 762.1
  labor 644.1
    affecting fetus or newborn 761.8
    premature 644.0

Threatened—*continued*
  miscarriage 640.0
    affecting fetus 762.1
  premature
    delivery 644.2
      affecting fetus or newborn 761.8
    labor 644.0
      before 22 completed weeks gestation 640.0
Three-day fever 066.0
Threshers' lung 495.0
Thrix annulata (congenital) 757.4
Throat —*see* condition
Thrombasthenia (Glanzmann's) (hemorrhagic)
    (hereditary) 287.1
Thromboangiitis 443.1
  obliterans (general) 443.1
    cerebral 437.1
    vessels
      brain 437.1
      spinal cord 437.1
Thromboarteritis —*see* Arteritis
Thromboasthenia (Glanzmann's) (hemorrhagic)
    (hereditary) 287.1
Thrombocytasthenia (Glanzmann's) 287.1
Thrombocythemia (essential) (hemorrhagic)
    (primary) (M9962/1) 238.7
  idiopathic (M9962/1) 238.7
Thrombocytopathy (dystrophic) (granulopenic)
    287.1
Thrombocytopenia, thrombocytopenic 287.5
  with giant hemangioma 287.3
  amegakaryocytic, congenital 287.3
  congenital 287.3
  cyclic 287.3
  dilutional 287.4
  due to
    drugs 287.4
    extracorporeal circulation of blood 287.4
    massive blood transfusion 287.4
    platelet alloimmunization 287.4
  essential 287.3
  hereditary 287.3
  Kasabach-Merritt 287.3
  neonatal, transitory 776.1
    due to
      exchange transfusion 776.1
      idiopathic maternal thrombocytopenia 776.1
      isoimmunization 776.1
  primary 287.3
  puerperal, postpartum 666.3
  purpura (*see also* Purpura, thrombocytopenic)
    287.3
    thrombotic 446.6
  secondary 287.4
  sex-linked 287.3
Thrombocytosis, essential 289.9
Thromboembolism —*see* Embolism
Thrombopathy (Bernard-Soulier) 287.1
  constitutional 286.4
  Willebrand-Jürgens (angiohemophilia) 286.4
Thrombopenia (*see also* Thrombocytopenia)
    287.5
Thrombophlebitis 451.9
  antecubital vein 451.82
  antepartum (superficial) 671.2
    affecting fetus or newborn 760.3
    deep 671.3
  arm 451.89
    deep 451.83
    superficial 451.82
  breast, superficial 451.89

Thrombophlebitis—*continued*
cavernous (venous) sinus—*see*
Thrombophlebitis, intracranial venous sinus
cephalic vein 451.82
cerebral (sinus) (vein) 325
late effect—*see* category 326
nonpyogenic 437.6
in pregnancy or puerperium 671.5
late effect—*see* Late effect(s) (of)
cerebrovascular disease
due to implanted device—*see* Complications,
due to (presence of) any device, implant, or
graft classified to 996.0-996.5 NEC
during or resulting from a procedure NEC 997.2
femoral 451.11
femoropopliteal 451.19
following infusion, perfusion, or transfusion
999.2
hepatic (vein) 451.89
idiopathic, recurrent 453.1
iliac vein 451.81
iliofemoral 451.11
intracranial venous sinus (any) 325
late effect—*see* category 326
nonpyogenic 437.6
in pregnancy or puerperium 671.5
late effect—*see* Late effect(s) (of)
cerebrovascular disease
jugular vein 451.89
lateral (venous) sinus—*see* Thrombophlebitis,
intracranial venous sinus
leg 451.2
deep (vessels) 451.19
femoral vein 451.11
specified vessel NEC 451.19
superficial (vessels) 451.0
femoral vein 451.11
longitudinal (venous) sinus—*see*
Thrombophlebitis, intracranial venous sinus
lower extremity 451.2
deep (vessels) 451.19
femoral vein 451.11
specified vessel NEC 451.19
superficial (vessels) 451.0
migrans, migrating 453.1
pelvic
with
abortion—*see* Abortion, by type, with sepsis
ectopic pregnancy (*see also* categories
633.0-633.9) 639.0
molar pregnancy (*see also* categories
630-632) 639.0
following
abortion 639.0
ectopic or molar pregnancy 639.0
puerperal 671.4
popliteal vein 451.19
portal (vein) 572.1
postoperative 997.2
pregnancy (superficial) 671.2
affecting fetus or newborn 760.3
deep 671.3
puerperal, postpartum, childbirth (extremities)
(superficial) 671.2
deep 671.4
pelvic 671.4
specified site NEC 671.5
radial vein 451.83
saphenous (greater) (lesser) 451.0
sinus (intracranial)—*see* Thrombophlebitis,
intracranial venous sinus

Thrombophlebitis—*continued*
specified site NEC 451.89
tibial vein 451.19
Thrombosis, thrombotic (marantic) (multiple)
(progressive) (septic) (vein) (vessel) 453.9
with childbirth or during the puerperium—*see*
Thrombosis, puerperal, postpartum
antepartum—*see* Thrombosis, pregnancy
aorta, aortic 444.1
abdominal 444.0
bifurcation 444.0
saddle 444.0
terminal 444.0
thoracic 444.1
valve—*see* Endocarditis, aortic
apoplexy (*see also* Thrombosis, brain) 434.0
late effect—*see* Late effect(s) (of)
cerebrovascular disease
appendix, septic—*see* Appendicitis, acute
arteriolar-capillary platelet, disseminated 446.6
artery, arteries (postinfectional) 444.9
auditory, internal 433.8
basilar (*see also* Occlusion, artery, basilar)
433.0
carotid (common) (internal) (*see also*
Occlusion, artery, carotid) 433.1
with other precerebral artery 433.3
cerebellar (anterior inferior) (posterior
inferior) (superior) 433.8
cerebral (*see also* Thrombosis, brain) 434.0
choroidal (anterior) 433.8
communicating posterior 433.8
coronary (*see also* Infarct, myocardium) 410.9
due to syphilis 093.89
healed or specified as old 412
without myocardial infarction 411.81
extremities 444.22
lower 444.22
upper 444.21
femoral 444.22
hepatic 444.89
hypophyseal 433.8
meningeal, anterior or posterior 433.8
mesenteric (with gangrene) 557.0
ophthalmic (*see also* Occlusion, retina) 362.30
pontine 433.8
popliteal 444.22
precerebral—*see* Occlusion, artery,
precerebral NEC
pulmonary 415.19
iatrogenic 415.11
postoperative 415.11
renal 593.81
retinal (*see also* Occlusion, retina) 362.30
specified site NEC 444.89
spinal, anterior or posterior 433.8
traumatic (complication) (early) (*see also*
Injury, blood vessel, by site) 904.9
vertebral (*see also* Occlusion, artery,
vertebral) 433.2
with other precerebral artery 433.3
atrial (endocardial) 424.90
due to syphilis 093.89
auricular (*see also* Infarct, myocardium) 410.9
axillary (vein) 453.8
basilar (artery) (*see also* Occlusion, artery,
basilar) 433.0
bland NEC 453.9
brain (artery) (stem) 434.0
due to syphilis 094.89
iatrogenic 997.02

Thrombosis, thrombotic—*continued*
  late effect—*see* Late effect(s) (of)
    cerebrovascular disease
  postoperative 997.02
  puerperal, postpartum, childbirth 674.0
  sinus (*see also* Thrombosis, intracranial
    venous sinus) 325
  capillary 448.9
    arteriolar, generalized 446.6
  cardiac (*see also* Infarct, myocardium) 410.9
    due to syphilis 093.89
    healed or specified as old 412
    valve—*see* Endocarditis
  carotid (artery) (common) (internal) (*see also*
    Occlusion, artery, carotid) 433.1
    with other precerebral artery 433.3
  cavernous sinus (venous)—*see* Thrombosis,
    intracranial venous sinus
  cerebellar artery (anterior inferior) (posterior
    inferior) (superior) 433.8
    late effect—*see* Late effect(s) (of)
      cerebrovascular disease
  cerebral (arteries) (*see also* Thrombosis, brain)
    434.0
    late effect—*see* Late effect(s) (of)
      cerebrovascular disease
  coronary (artery) (*see also* Infarct, myocardium)
    410.9
    due to syphilis 093.89
    healed or specified as old 412
    without myocardial infarction 411.81
  corpus cavernosum 607.82
  cortical (*see also* Thrombosis, brain) 434.0
  due to (presence of) any device, implant, or
    graft classifiable to 996.0-996.5—*see*
    Complications, due to (presence of) any
    device, implant, or graft classified to
    996.0-996.5 NEC
  effort 453.8
  endocardial—*see* Infarct, myocardium
  eye (*see also* Occlusion, retina) 362.30
  femoral (vein) (deep) 453.8
    with inflammation or phlebitis 451.11
    artery 444.22
  genital organ, male 608.83
  heart (chamber) (*see also* Infarct, myocardium)
    410.9
  hepatic (vein) 453.0
    artery 444.89
    infectional or septic 572.1
  iliac (vein) 453.8
    with inflammation or phlebitis 451.81
    artery (common) (external) (internal) 444.81
  inflammation, vein—*see* Thrombophlebitis
  internal carotid artery (*see also* Occlusion,
    artery, carotid) 433.1
    with other precerebral artery 433.3
  intestine (with gangrene) 557.0
  intracranial (*see also* Thrombosis, brain) 434.0
    venous sinus (any) 325
      nonpyogenic origin 437.6
      in pregnancy or puerperium 671.5
  intramural (*see also* Infarct, myocardium) 410.9
    without
      cardiac condition 429.89
      coronary artery disease 429.89
      myocardial infarction 429.89
    healed or specified as old 412
  jugular (bulb) 453.8
  kidney 593.81
    artery 593.81

Thrombosis, thrombotic—*continued*
  lateral sinus (venous)—*see* Thrombosis,
    intracranial venous sinus
  leg 453.8
    with inflammation or phlebitis—*see*
      Thrombophlebitis
    deep (vessels) 453.8
    superficial (vessels) 453.8
  liver (venous) 453.0
    artery 444.89
    infectional or septic 572.1
    portal vein 452
  longitudinal sinus (venous)—*see* Thrombosis,
    intracranial venous sinus
  lower extremity—*see* Thrombosis, leg
  lung 415.19
    iatrogenic 415.11
    postoperative 415.11
  marantic, dural sinus 437.6
  meninges (brain) (*see also* Thrombosis, brain)
    434.0
  mesenteric (artery) (with gangrene) 557.0
    vein (inferior) (superior) 557.0
  mitral—*see* Insufficiency, mitral
  mural (heart chamber) (*see also* Infarct,
    myocardium) 410.9
    without
      cardiac condition 429.89
      coronary artery disease 429.89
      myocardial infarction 429.89
    due to syphilis 093.89
    following myocardial infarction 429.79
    healed or specified as old 412
  omentum (with gangrene) 557.0
  ophthalmic (artery) (*see also* Occlusion, retina)
    362.30
  pampiniform plexus (male) 608.83
    female 620.8
  parietal (*see also* Infarct, myocardium) 410.9
  penis, penile 607.82
  peripheral arteries 444.22
    lower 444.22
    upper 444.21
  platelet 446.6
  portal 452
    due to syphilis 093.89
    infectional or septic 572.1
  precerebral artery—*see also* Occlusion, artery,
    precerebral NEC
  pregnancy 671.9
    deep (vein) 671.3
    superficial (vein) 671.2
  puerperal, postpartum, childbirth 671.9
    brain (artery) 674.0
      venous 671.5
    cardiac 674.8
    cerebral (artery) 674.0
      venous 671.5
    deep (vein) 671.4
    intracranial sinus (nonpyogenic) (venous)
      671.5
    pelvic 671.4
    pulmonary (artery) 673.2
    specified site NEC 671.5
    superficial 671.2
  pulmonary (artery) (vein) 415.19
    iatrogenic 415.11
    postoperative 415.11
  radial vein 451.83
  renal (artery) 593.81
    vein 453.3

Thrombosis, thrombotic—*continued*
  resulting from presence of shunt or other
      internal prosthetic device—*see*
      Complications, due to (presence of) any
      device, implant, or graft classified to
      996.0-996.5 NEC
  retina, retinal (artery) 362.30
      arterial branch 362.32
      central 362.31
      partial 362.33
      vein
          central 362.35
          tributary (branch) 362.36
  scrotum 608.83
  seminal vesicle 608.83
  sigmoid (venous) sinus (*see* Thrombosis,
      intracranial venous sinus) 325
  silent NEC 453.9
  sinus, intracranial (venous) (any) (*see also*
      Thrombosis, intracranial venous sinus) 325
  softening, brain (*see also* Thrombosis, brain)
      434.0
  specified site NEC 453.8
  spermatic cord 608.83
  spinal cord 336.1
      due to syphilis 094.89
      in pregnancy or puerperium 671.5
      pyogenic origin 324.1
          late effect—*see* category 326
  spleen, splenic 289.59
      artery 444.89
  testis 608.83
  traumatic (complication) (early) (*see also*
      Injury, blood vessel, by site) 904.9
  tricuspid—*see* Endocarditis, tricuspid
  tunica vaginalis 608.83
  umbilical cord (vessels) 663.6
      affecting fetus or newborn 762.6
  vas deferens 608.83
  vena cava (inferior) (superior) 453.2
Thrombus —*see* Thrombosis
Thrush 112.0
  newborn 771.7
Thumb —*see also* condition
  gamekeeper's 842.12
  sucking (child problem) 307.9
Thygeson's superficial punctate keratitis
  370.21
Thymergasia (*see also* Psychosis, affective)
  296.80
Thymitis 254.8
Thymoma (benign) (M8580/0) 212.6
  malignant (M8580/3) 164.0
Thymus, thymic (gland)—*see* condition
Thyrocele (*see also* Goiter) 240.9
Thyroglossal —*see also* condition
  cyst 759.2
  duct, persistent 759.2
Thyroid (body) (gland)—*see also* condition
  lingual 759.2
Thyroiditis 245.9
  acute (pyogenic) (suppurative) 245.0
      nonsuppurative 245.0
  autoimmune 245.2
  chronic (nonspecific) (sclerosing) 245.8
      fibrous 245.3
      lymphadenoid 245.2
      lymphocytic 245.2
      lymphoid 245.2
  complicating pregnancy, childbirth, or
      puerperium 648.1

Thyroiditis—*continued*
  de Quervain's (subacute granulomatous) 245.1
  fibrous (chronic) 245.3
  giant (cell) (follicular) 245.1
  granulomatous (de Quervain's) (subacute) 245.1
  Hashimoto's (struma lymphomatosa) 245.2
  iatrogenic 245.4
  invasive (fibrous) 245.3
  ligneous 245.3
  lymphocytic (chronic) 245.2
  lymphoid 245.2
  lymphomatous 245.2
  pseudotuberculous 245.1
  pyogenic 245.0
  radiation 245.4
  Riedel's (ligneous) 245.3
  subacute 245.1
  suppurative 245.0
  tuberculous (*see also* Tuberculosis) 017.5
  viral 245.1
  woody 245.3
Thyrolingual duct, persistent 759.2
Thyromegaly 240.9
Thyrotoxic
  crisis or storm (*see also* Thyrotoxicosis) 242.9
  heart failure (*see also* Thyrotoxicosis) 242.9
      [425.7]
Thyrotoxicosis 242.9

---

*Note—Use the following fifth-digit
subclassification with category 242:*

0   *without mention of thyrotoxic crisis or storm*
1   *with mention of thyrotoxic crisis or storm*

---

  with
      goiter (diffuse) 242.0
          adenomatous 242.3
              multinodular 242.2
              uninodular 242.1
          nodular 242.3
              multinodular 242.2
              uninodular 242.1
      infiltrative
          dermopathy 242.0
          ophthalmopathy 242.0
          thyroid acropachy 242.0
  complicating pregnancy, childbirth, or
      puerperium 648.1
  due to
      ectopic thyroid nodule 242.4
      ingestion of (excessive) thyroid material 242.8
      specified cause NEC 242.8
  factitia 242.8
  heart 242.9 *[425.7]*
  neonatal (transient) 775.3
TIA (transient ischemic attack) 435.9
  with transient neurologic deficit 435.9
  late effect—*see* Late effect(s) (of)
      cerebrovascular disease
Tibia vara 732.4
Tic 307.20
  breathing 307.20
  child problem 307.21
  compulsive 307.22
  convulsive 307.20
  degenerative (generalized) (localized) 333.3
      facial 351.8
  douloureux (*see also* Neuralgia, trigeminal)
      350.1
      atypical 350.2

Tic —*continued*
  habit 307.20
    chronic (motor or vocal) 307.22
    transient of childhood 307.21
  lid 307.20
    transient of childhood 307.21
  motor-verbal 307.23
  occupational 300.89
  orbicularis 307.20
    transient of childhood 307.21
  organic origin 333.3
  postchoreic—*see* Chorea
  psychogenic 307.20
    compulsive 307.22
  salaam 781.0
  spasm 307.20
    chronic (motor or vocal) 307.22
    transient of childhood 307.21
Tick (-borne) fever NEC 066.1
  American mountain 066.1
  Colorado 066.1
  hemorrhagic NEC 065.3
    Crimean 065.0
    Kyasanur Forest 065.2
    Omsk 065.1
  mountain 066.1
  nonexanthematous 066.1
Tick-bite fever NEC 066.1
  African 087.1
  Colorado (virus) 066.1
  Rocky Mountain 082.0
Tick paralysis 989.5
Tics and spasms, compulsive 307.22
Tietze's disease or syndrome 733.6
Tight, tightness
  anus 564.89
  chest 786.59
  fascia (lata) 728.9
  foreskin (congenital) 605
  hymen 623.3
  introitus (acquired) (congenital) 623.3
  rectal sphincter 564.89
  tendon 727.81
    Achilles (heel) 727.81
  urethral sphincter 598.9
Tilting vertebra 737.9
Timidity, child 313.21
Tinea (intersecta) (tarsi) 110.9
  amiantacea 110.0
  asbestina 110.0
  barbae 110.0
  beard 110.0
  black dot 110.0
  blanca 111.2
  capitis 110.0
  corporis 110.5
  cruris 110.3
  decalvans 704.09
  flava 111.0
  foot 110.4
  furfuracea 111.0
  imbricata (Tokelau) 110.5
  lepothrix 039.0
  manuum 110.2
  microsporic (*see also* Dermatophytosis) 110.9
  nigra 111.1
  nodosa 111.2
  pedis 110.4
  scalp 110.0
  specified site NEC 110.8
  sycosis 110.0

Tinea—*continued*
  tonsurans 110.0
  trichophytic (*see also* Dermatophytosis) 110.9
  unguium 110.1
  versicolor 111.0
Tingling sensation (*see also* Disturbance,
    sensation) 782.0
Tin-miners' lung 503
Tinnitus (aurium) 388.30
  audible 388.32
  objective 388.32
  subjective 388.31
Tipping pelvis 738.6
  with disproportion (fetopelvic) 653.0
    affecting fetus or newborn 763.1
    causing obstructed labor 660.1
      affecting fetus or newborn 763.1
Tiredness 780.79
Tissue —*see* condition
Tobacco
  abuse (affecting health) NEC (*see also* Abuse,
    drugs, nondependent) 305.1
  heart 989.8
Tobias' syndrome (carcinoma, pulmonary apex)
    (M8010/3) 162.3
Tocopherol deficiency 269.1
Todd's
  cirrhosis—*see* Cirrhosis, biliary
  paralysis (postepileptic transitory paralysis)
    344.89
Toe —*see* condition
Toilet, artificial opening (*see also* Attention to,
    artificial, opening) V55.9
Tokelau ringworm 110.5
Tollwut 071
Tolosa-Hunt syndrome 378.55
Tommaselli's disease
  correct substance properly administered 599.7
  overdose or wrong substance given or taken
    961.4
Tongue —*see also* condition
  worms 134.1
Tongue tie 750.0
Toni-Fanconi syndrome (cystinosis) 270.0
Tonic pupil 379.46
Tonsil —*see* condition
Tonsillitis (acute) (catarrhal) (croupous)
    (follicular) (gangrenous) (infective) (lacunar)
    (lingual) (malignant) (membranous)
    (phlegmonous) (pneumococcal)
    (pseudomembranous) (purulent) (septic)
    (staphylococcal) (subacute) (suppurative)
    (toxic) (ulcerative) (vesicular) (viral) 463
  with influenza, flu, or grippe 487.1
  chronic 474.00
  diphtheritic (membranous) 032.0
  hypertrophic 474.00
  influenzal 487.1
  parenchymatous 475
  streptococcal 034.0
  tuberculous (*see also* Tuberculosis) 012.8
  Vincent's 101
Tonsillopharyngitis 465.8
Tooth, teeth —*see* condition
Toothache 525.9
Topagnosis 782.0
Tophi (gouty) 274.0
  ear 274.81
  heart 274.82
  specified site NEC 274.82
Torn —*see* Tear, torn

Tornwaldt's bursitis (disease) (pharyngeal
    bursitis) 478.29
  cyst 478.26
Torpid liver 573.9
Torsion
  accessory tube 620.5
  adnexa (female) 620.5
  aorta (congenital) 747.29
    acquired 447.1
  appendix epididymis 608.2
  bile duct 576.8
    with calculus, choledocholithiasis or
      stones—*see* Choledocholithiasis
    congenital 751.69
  bowel, colon, or intestine 560.2
  cervix (*see also* Malposition, uterus) 621.6
  duodenum 537.3
  dystonia—*see* Dystonia, torsion
  epididymis 608.2
    appendix 608.2
  fallopian tube 620.5
  gallbladder (*see also* Disease, gallbladder) 575.8
    congenital 751.69
  gastric 537.89
  hydatid of Morgagni (female) 620.5
  kidney (pedicle) 593.89
  Meckel's diverticulum (congenital) 751.0
  mesentery 560.2
  omentum 560.2
  organ or site, congenital NEC—*see* Anomaly,
    specified type NEC
  ovary (pedicle) 620.5
    congenital 752.0
  oviduct 620.5
  penis 607.89
    congenital 752.69
  renal 593.89
  spasm—*see* Dystonia, torsion
  spermatic cord 608.2
  spleen 289.59
  testicle, testis 608.2
  tibia 736.89
  umbilical cord—*see* Compression, umbilical
    cord
  uterus (*see also* Malposition, uterus) 621.6
Torticollis (intermittent) (spastic) 723.5
  congenital 754.1
    sternomastoid 754.1
  due to birth injury 767.8
  hysterical 300.11
  ocular 781.93
  psychogenic 306.0
    specified as conversion reaction 300.11
  rheumatic 723.5
  rheumatoid 714.0
  spasmodic 333.83
  traumatic, current NEC 847.0
Tortuous
  artery 447.1
  fallopian tube 752.19
  organ or site, congenital NEC—*see* Distortion
  renal vessel, congenital 747.62
  retina vessel (congenital) 743.58
    acquired 362.17
  ureter 593.4
  urethra 599.84
  vein—*see* Varicose, vein
Torula, torular (infection) 117.5
  histolytica 117.5
  lung 117.5
Torulosis 117.5

Torus
  fracture
    fibula 823.41
      with tibia 823.42
    radius 813.45
    tibia 823.40
      with fibula 823.42
  mandibularis 526.81
  palatinus 526.81
Touch, vitreous 997.99
Touraine's syndrome (hereditary
  osteo-onychodysplasia) 756.89
Touraine-Solente-Golé syndrome
  (acropachyderma) 757.39
Tourette's disease (motor-verbal tic) 307.23
Tower skull 756.0
  with exophthalmos 756.0
Toxemia 799.8
  with
    abortion—*see* Abortion, by type, with toxemia
  bacterial—*see* Septicemia
  biliary (*see also* Disease, biliary) 576.8
  burn—*see* Burn, by site
  congenital NEC 779.89
  eclamptic 642.6
    with pre-existing hypertension 642.7
  erysipelatous (*see also* Erysipelas) 035
  fatigue 799.8
  fetus or newborn NEC 779.89
  food (*see also* Poisoning, food) 005.9
  gastric 537.89
  gastrointestinal 558.2
  intestinal 558.2
  kidney (*see also* Disease, renal) 593.9
  lung 518.89
  malarial NEC (*see also* Malaria) 084.6
  maternal (of pregnancy), affecting fetus or
    newborn 760.0
  myocardial—*see* Myocarditis, toxic
  of pregnancy (mild) (pre-eclamptic) 642.4
    with
      convulsions 642.6
      pre-existing hypertension 642.7
    affecting fetus or newborn 760.0
    severe 642.5
  pre-eclamptic—*see* Toxemia, of pregnancy
  puerperal, postpartum—*see* Toxemia, of
    pregnancy
  pulmonary 518.89
  renal (*see also* Disease, renal) 593.9
  septic (*see also* Septicemia) 038.9
  small intestine 558.2
  staphylococcal 038.10
    aureus 038.11
    due to food 005.0
    specified organism NEC 038.19
  stasis 799.8
  stomach 537.89
  uremic (*see also* Uremia) 586
  urinary 586
Toxemica cerebropathia psychica
  (nonalcoholic) 294.0
  alcoholic 291.1
Toxic (poisoning)—*see also* condition
  from drug or poison—*see* Table of drugs and
    chemicals
  oil syndrome 710.5
  shock syndrome 040.82
  thyroid (gland) (*see also* Thyrotoxicosis) 242.9
Toxicemia —*see* Toxemia

Transient —*see also* condition
 alteration of awareness 780.02
 blindness 368.12
 deafness (ischemic) 388.02
 global amnesia 437.7
 person (homeless) NEC V60.0
Transitional, lumbosacral joint of vertebra
  756.19
Translocation
 autosomes NEC 758.5
  13-15 758.1
  16-18 758.2
  21 or 22 758.0
  balanced in normal individual 758.4
  D₁ 758.1
  E₃ 758.2
  G 758.0
 balanced autosomal in normal individual 758.4
 chromosomes NEC 758.89
 Down's syndrome 758.0
Translucency, iris 364.53
Transmission of chemical substances through
  the placenta
 (affecting fetus or newborn) 760.70
 alcohol 760.71
 anti-infective agents 760.74
 cocaine 760.75
 "crack" 760.75
 diethylstilbestrol [DES] 760.76
 hallucinogenic agents 760.73
 medicinal agents NEC 760.79
 narcotics 760.72
 obstetric anesthetic or analgesic drug 763.5
 specified agent NEC 760.79
 suspected, affecting management of pregnancy
  655.5
Transplant(ed)
 bone V42.4
  marrow V42.81
 complication—*see also* Complications, due to
  (presence of) any device, implant, or graft
  classified to 996.0-996.5 NEC
  bone marrow 996.85
  corneal graft NEC 996.79
   infection or inflammation 996.69
   reaction 996.51
   rejection 996.51
  organ (failure) (immune or nonimmune cause)
   (infection) (rejection) 996.80
   bone marrow 996.85
   heart 996.83
   intestines 996.87
   kidney 996.81
   liver 996.82
   lung 996.84
   pancreas 996.86
   specified NEC 996.89
  skin NEC 996.79
   infection or inflammation 996.69
   rejection 996.52
    artificial 996.55
    decellularized allodermis 996.55
 cornea V42.5
 hair V50.0
 heart V42.1
  valve V42.2
 intestine V42.84
 kidney V42.0
 liver V42.7
 lung V42.6

Transplant(ed)— *continued*
 organ V42.9
  specified NEC V42.89
 pancreas V42.83
 peripheral stem cells V42.82
 skin V42.3
 stem cells, peripheral V42.82
 tissue V42.9
  specified NEC V42.89
Transplants, ovarian, endometrial 617.1
Transposed —*see* Transposition
Transposition (congenital)—*see also*
  Malposition, congenital
 abdominal viscera 759.3
 aorta (dextra) 745.11
 appendix 751.5
 arterial trunk 745.10
 colon 751.5
 great vessels (complete) 745.10
  both originating from right ventricle 745.11
  corrected 745.12
  double outlet right ventricle 745.11
  incomplete 745.11
  partial 745.11
  specified type NEC 745.19
 heart 746.87
  with complete transposition of viscera 759.3
 intestine (large) (small) 751.5
 pulmonary veins 747.49
 reversed jejunal (for bypass) (status) V45.3
 stomach 750.7
  with general transposition of viscera 759.3
 teeth, tooth 524.3
 vessels (complete) 745.10
  partial 745.11
 viscera (abdominal) (thoracic) 759.3
Trans-sexualism 302.50
 with
  asexual history 302.51
  heterosexual history 302.53
  homosexual history 302.52
Transverse —*see also* condition
 arrest (deep), in labor 660.3
  affecting fetus or newborn 763.1
 lie 652.3
  before labor, affecting fetus or newborn 761.7
  causing obstructed labor 660.0
   affecting fetus or newborn 763.1
  during labor, affecting fetus or newborn 763.1
Transvestism, transvestitism (transvestic
  fetishism) 302.3
Trapped placenta (with hemorrhage) 666.0
 without hemorrhage 667.0
Trauma, traumatism (*see also* Injury, by site)
  959.9
 birth—*see* Birth, injury NEC
 causing hemorrhage of pregnancy or delivery
  641.8
 complicating
  abortion—*see* Abortion, by type, with damage
   to pelvic organs
  ectopic pregnancy (*see also* categories
   633.0-633.9) 639.2
  molar pregnancy (*see also* categories
   630-632) 639.2
 during delivery NEC 665.9
 following
  abortion 639.2
  ectopic or molar pregnancy 639.2
 maternal, during pregnancy, affecting fetus or
  newborn 760.5

Trauma, traumatism—*continued*
 neuroma—*see* Injury, nerve, by site
 previous major, affecting management of
  pregnancy, childbirth, or puerperium V23.8
 psychic (current)—*see also* Reaction,
  adjustment
  previous (history) V15.49
 psychologic, previous (affecting health) V15.49
 transient paralysis—*see* Injury, nerve, by site
Traumatic —*see* condition
Treacher Collins' syndrome (incomplete facial
  dysostosis) 756.0
Treitz's hernia —*see* Hernia, Treitz's
Trematode infestation NEC 121.9
Trematodiasis NEC 121.9
Trembles 988.8
Trembling paralysis (*see also* Parkinsonism)
  332.0
Tremor 781.0
 essential (benign) 333.1
 familial 333.1
 flapping (liver) 572.8
 hereditary 333.1
 hysterical 300.11
 intention 333.1
 mercurial 985.0
 muscle 728.85
 Parkinson's (*see also* Parkinsonism) 332.0
 psychogenic 306.0
  specified as conversion reaction 300.11
 senilis 797
 specified type NEC 333.1
Trench
 fever 083.1
 foot 991.4
 mouth 101
 nephritis—*see* Nephritis, acute
Treponema pallidum infection (*see also*
  Syphilis) 097.9
Treponematosis 102.9
 due to
  T. pallidum—*see* Syphilis
  T. pertenue (yaws) (*see also* Yaws) 102.9
Triad
 Kartagener's 759.3
 Reiter's (complete) (incomplete) 099.3
 Saint's (*see also* Hernia, diaphragm) 553.3
Trichiasis 704.2
 cicatricial 704.2
 eyelid 374.05
  with entropion (*see also* Entropion) 374.00
Trichinella spiralis (infection) (infestation) 124
Trichinelliasis 124
Trichinellosis 124
Trichiniasis 124
Trichinosis 124
Trichobezoar 938
 intestine 936
 stomach 935.2
Trichocephaliasis 127.3
Trichocephalosis 127.3
Trichocephalus infestation 127.3
Trichoclasis 704.2
Trichoepithelioma (M8100/0)—*see also*
  Neoplasm, skin, benign
 breast 217
 genital organ NEC—*see* Neoplasm, by site,
  benign
 malignant (M8100/3)—*see* Neoplasm, skin,
  malignant
Trichofolliculoma (M8101/0)—*see* Neoplasm,
  skin, benign

Tricholemmoma (M8102/0)—*see* Neoplasm,
  skin, benign
Trichomatosis 704.2
Trichomoniasis 131.9
 bladder 131.09
 cervix 131.09
 intestinal 007.3
 prostate 131.03
 seminal vesicle 131.09
 specified site NEC 131.8
 urethra 131.02
 urogenitalis 131.00
 vagina 131.01
 vulva 131.01
 vulvovaginal 131.01
Trichomycosis 039.0
 axillaris 039.0
 nodosa 111.2
 nodularis 111.2
 rubra 039.0
Trichonocardiosis (axillaris) (palmellina) 039.0
Trichonodosis 704.2
Trichophytid, trichophyton infection (*see also*
  Dermatophytosis) 110.9
Trichophytide —*see* Dermatophytosis
Trichophytobezoar 938
 intestine 936
 stomach 935.2
Trichophytosis —*see* Dermatophytosis
Trichoptilosis 704.2
Trichorrhexis (nodosa) 704.2
Trichosporosis nodosa 111.2
Trichostasis spinulosa (congenital) 757.4
Trichostrongyliasis (small intestine) 127.6
Trichostrongylosis 127.6
Trichostrongylus (instabilis) infection 127.6
Trichotillomania 312.39
Trichromat, anomalous (congenital) 368.59
Trichromatopsia, anomalous (congenital)
  368.59
Trichuriasis 127.3
Trichuris trichiuria (any site) (infection)
  (infestation) 127.3
Tricuspid (valve)—*see* condition
Trifid —*see also* Accessory
 kidney (pelvis) 753.3
 tongue 750.13
Trigeminal neuralgia (*see also* Neuralgia,
  trigeminal) 350.1
Trigeminoencephaloangiomatosis 759.6
Trigeminy 427.89
 postoperative 997.1
Trigger finger (acquired) 727.03
 congenital 756.89
Trigonitis (bladder) (chronic)
  (pseudomembranous) 595.3
 tuberculous (*see also* Tuberculosis) 016.1
Trigonocephaly 756.0
Trihexosidosis 272.7
Trilobate placenta —*see* Placenta, abnormal
Trilocular heart 745.8
Tripartita placenta —*see* Placenta, abnormal
Triple —*see also* Accessory
 kidneys 753.3
 uteri 752.2
 X female 758.81
Triplegia 344.89
 congenital or infantile 343.8
Triplet
 affected by maternal complications of
  pregnancy 761.5

Triplet—*continued*
  healthy liveborn—*see* Newborn, multiple
    pregnancy (complicating delivery) NEC 651.1
    with fetal loss and retention of one or more
      fetus(es) 651.4
Triplex placenta —*see* Placenta, abnormal
Triplication —*see* Accessory
Trismus 781.0
  neonatorum 771.3
  newborn 771.3
Trisomy (syndrome) NEC 758.5
  13 (partial) 758.1
  16-18 758.2
  18 (partial) 758.2
  21 (partial) 758.0
  22 758.0
  autosomes NEC 758.5
  D_1 758.1
  E_3 758.2
  G (group) 758.0
  group D_1 758.1
  group E 758.2
  group G 758.0
Tritanomaly 368.53
Tritanopia 368.53
Troisier-Hanot-Chauffard syndrome (bronze
  diabetes) 275.0
Trombidiosis 133.8
Trophedema (hereditary) 757.0
  congenital 757.0
Trophoblastic disease (*see also* Hydatidiform
  mole) 630
  previous, affecting management of pregnancy
    V23.1
Tropholymphedema 757.0
Trophoneurosis NEC 356.9
  arm NEC 354.9
  disseminated 710.1
  facial 349.89
  leg NEC 355.8
  lower extremity NEC 355.8
  upper extremity NEC 354.9
Tropical —*see also* condition
  maceration feet (syndrome) 991.4
  wet foot (syndrome) 991.4
Trouble —*see also* Disease
  bowel 569.9
  heart—*see* Disease, heart
  intestine 569.9
  kidney (*see also* Disease, renal) 593.9
  nervous 799.2
  sinus (*see also* Sinusitis) 473.9
Trousseau's syndrome (thrombophlebitis
  migrans) 453.1
Truancy, childhood —*see also* Disturbance,
  conduct
  socialized 312.2
  undersocialized, unsocialized 312.1
Truncus
  arteriosus (persistent) 745.0
  common 745.0
  communis 745.0
Trunk —*see* condition
Trychophytide —*see* Dermatophytosis
Trypanosoma infestation —*see*
  Trypanosomiasis
Trypanosomiasis 086.9
  with meningoencephalitis 086.9 *[323.2]*
  African 086.5
    due to Trypanosoma 086.5
      gambiense 086.3

Trypanosomiasis—*continued*
    rhodesiense 086.4
  American 086.2
    with
      heart involvement 086.0
      other organ involvement 086.1
    without mention of organ involvement 086.2
  Brazilian—*see* Trypanosomiasis, American
  Chagas'—*see* Trypanosomiasis, American
  due to Trypanosoma
    cruzi—*see* Trypanosomiasis, American
    gambiense 086.3
    rhodesiense 086.4
  gambiensis, Gambian 086.3
  North American—*see* Trypanosomiasis,
    American
  rhodesiensis, Rhodesian 086.4
  South American—*see* Trypanosomiasis,
    American
T-shaped incisors 520.2
Tsutsugamushi fever 081.2
Tube, tubal, tubular —*see also* condition
  ligation, admission for V25.2
Tubercle —*see also* Tuberculosis
  brain, solitary 013.2
  Darwin's 744.29
  epithelioid noncaseating 135
  Ghon, primary infection 010.0
Tuberculid, tuberculide (indurating) (lichenoid)
  (miliary) (papulonecrotic) (primary) (skin)
  (subcutaneous) (*see also* Tuberculosis) 017.0
Tuberculoma —*see also* Tuberculosis
  brain (any part) 013.2
  meninges (cerebral) (spinal) 013.1
  spinal cord 013.4
Tuberculosis, tubercular, tuberculous
  (calcification) (calcified) (caseous)
  (chromogenic acid-fast bacilli) (congenital)
  (degeneration) (disease) (fibrocaseous)
  (fistula) (gangrene) (interstitial) (isolated
  circumscribed lesions) (necrosis)
  (parenchymatous) (ulcerative) 011.9

---

*Note—Use the following fifth-digit
subclassification with categories 010-018:*

0 *unspecified*
1 *bacteriological or histological examination
   not done*
2 *bacteriological or histological examination
   unknown (at present)*
3 *tubercle bacilli found (in sputum) by
   microscopy*
4 *tubercle bacilli not found (in sputum) by
   microscopy, but found by bacterial culture*
5 *tubercle bacilli not found by bacteriological
   examination, but tuberculosis confirmed
   histologically*
6 *tubercle bacilli not found by bacteriological or
   histological examination, but tuberculosis
   confirmed by other methods [inoculation of
   animals]*

*For tuberculous conditions specified as late
effects or sequelae, see category 137.*

---

  abdomen 014.8
    lymph gland 014.8
  abscess 011.9
    arm 017.9
    bone (*see also* Osteomyelitis, due to,
      tuberculosis) 015.9 *[730.8]*

Tuberculosis, tubercular, tuberculous—*cont.*
caries (*see also* Tuberculosis, bone) 015.9
  [730.8]
cartilage (*see also* Tuberculosis, bone) 015.9
  [730.8]
  intervertebral 015.0 *[730.88]*
catarrhal (*see also* Tuberculosis, pulmonary)
  011.9
cecum 014.8
cellular tissue (primary) 017.0
cellulitis (primary) 017.0
central nervous system 013.9
  specified site NEC 013.8
cerebellum (current) 013.2
cerebral (current) 013.2
  meninges 013.0
cerebrospinal 013.6
  meninges 013.0
cerebrum (current) 013.2
cervical 017.2
  gland 017.2
  lymph nodes 017.2
cervicitis (uteri) 016.7
cervix 016.7
chest (*see also* Tuberculosis, pulmonary) 011.9
childhood type or first infection 010.0
choroid 017.3 *[363.13]*
choroiditis 017.3 *[363.13]*
ciliary body 017.3 *[364.11]*
colitis 014.8
colliers' 011.4
colliquativa (primary) 017.0
colon 014.8
  ulceration 014.8
complex, primary 010.0
complicating pregnancy, childbirth, or
  puerperium 647.3
  affecting fetus or newborn 760.2
congenital 771.2
conjunctiva 017.3 *[370.31]*
connective tissue 017.9
  bone—*see* Tuberculosis, bone
contact V01.1
converter (tuberculin skin test) (without disease)
  795.5
cornea (ulcer) 017.3 *[370.31]*
Cowper's gland 016.5
coxae 015.1 *[730.85]*
coxalgia 015.1 *[730.85]*
cul-de-sac of Douglas 014.8
curvature, spine 015.0 *[737.40]*
cutis (colliquativa) (primary) 017.0
cyst, ovary 016.6
cystitis 016.1
dacryocystitis 017.3 *[375.32]*
dactylitis 015.5
diarrhea 014.8
diffuse (*see also* Tuberculosis, miliary) 018.9
  lung—*see* Tuberculosis, pulmonary
  meninges 013.0
digestive tract 014.8
disseminated (*see also* Tuberculosis, miliary)
  018.9
  meninges 013.0
duodenum 014.8
dura (mater) 013.9
  abscess 013.8
    cerebral 013.3
    spinal 013.5
dysentery 014.8
ear (inner) (middle) 017.4

Tuberculosis, tubercular, tuberculous—*cont.*
bone 015.6
  external (primary) 017.0
  skin (primary) 017.0
elbow 015.8
emphysema—*see* Tuberculosis, pulmonary
empyema 012.0
encephalitis 013.6
endarteritis 017.9
endocarditis (any valve) 017.9 *[424.91]*
endocardium (any valve) 017.9 *[424.91]*
endocrine glands NEC 017.9
endometrium 016.7
enteric, enterica 014.8
enteritis 014.8
enterocolitis 014.8
epididymis 016.4
epididymitis 016.4
epidural abscess 013.8
  brain 013.3
  spinal cord 013.5
epiglottis 012.3
episcleritis 017.3 *[379.00]*
erythema (induratum) (nodosum) (primary)
  017.1
esophagus 017.8
Eustachian tube 017.4
exposure to V01.1
exudative 012.0
  primary, progressive 010.1
eye 017.3
  glaucoma 017.3 *[365.62]*
eyelid (primary) 017.0
  lupus 017.0 *[373.4]*
fallopian tube 016.6
fascia 017.9
fauces 012.8
finger 017.9
first infection 010.0
fistula, perirectal 014.8
Florida 011.6
foot 017.9
funnel pelvis 137.3
gallbladder 017.9
galloping (*see also* Tuberculosis, pulmonary)
  011.9
ganglionic 015.9
gastritis 017.9
gastrocolic fistula 014.8
gastroenteritis 014.8
gastrointestinal tract 014.8
general, generalized 018.9
  acute 018.0
  chronic 018.8
genital organs NEC 016.9
  female 016.7
  male 016.5
genitourinary NEC 016.9
genu 015.2
glandulae suprarenalis 017.6
glandular, general 017.2
glottis 012.3
grinders' 011.4
groin 017.2
gum 017.9
hand 017.9
heart 017.9 *[425.8]*
hematogenous—*see* Tuberculosis, miliary
hemoptysis (*see also* Tuberculosis, pulmonary)
  011.9

Tuberculosis, tubercular, tuberculous—*cont.*
hemorrhage NEC (*see also* Tuberculosis,
    pulmonary) 011.9
hemothorax 012.0
hepatitis 017.9
hilar lymph nodes 012.1
    primary, progressive 010.8
hip (disease) (joint) 015.1
    bone 015.1 *[730.85]*
hydrocephalus 013.8
hydropneumothorax 012.0
hydrothorax 012.0
hypoadrenalism 017.6
hypopharynx 012.8
ileocecal (hyperplastic) 014.8
ileocolitis 014.8
ileum 014.8
iliac spine (superior) 015.0 *[730.88]*
incipient NEC (*see also* Tuberculosis,
    pulmonary) 011.9
indurativa (primary) 017.1
infantile 010.0
infection NEC 011.9
    without clinical manifestation 010.0
infraclavicular gland 017.2
inguinal gland 017.2
inguinalis 017.2
intestine (any part) 014.8
iris 017.3 *[364.11]*
iritis 017.3 *[364.11]*
ischiorectal 014.8
jaw 015.7 *[730.88]*
jejunum 014.8
joint 015.9
    hip 015.1
    knee 015.2
    specified site NEC 015.8
    vertebral 015.0 *[730.88]*
keratitis 017.3 *[370.31]*
    interstitial 017.3 *[370.59]*
keratoconjunctivitis 017.3 *[370.31]*
kidney 016.0
knee (joint) 015.2
kyphoscoliosis 015.0 *[737.43]*
kyphosis 015.0 *[737.41]*
lacrimal apparatus, gland 017.3
laryngitis 012.3
larynx 012.3
leptomeninges, leptomeningitis (cerebral)
    (spinal) 013.0
lichenoides (primary) 017.0
linguae 017.9
lip 017.9
liver 017.9
lordosis 015.0 *[737.42]*
lung—*see* Tuberculosis, pulmonary
luposa 017.0
    eyelid 017.0 *[373.4]*
lymphadenitis—*see* Tuberculosis, lymph gland
lymphangitis—*see* Tuberculosis, lymph gland
lymphatic (gland) (vessel)—*see* Tuberculosis,
    lymph gland
lymph gland or node (peripheral) 017.2
    abdomen 014.8
    bronchial 012.1
        primary, progressive 010.8
    cervical 017.2
    hilar 012.1
        primary, progressive 010.8
    intrathoracic 012.1
        primary, progressive 010.8

Tuberculosis, tubercular, tuberculous—*cont.*
mediastinal 012.1
    primary, progressive 010.8
mesenteric 014.8
peripheral 017.2
retroperitoneal 014.8
tracheobronchial 012.1
    primary, progressive 010.8
malignant NEC (*see also* Tuberculosis,
    pulmonary) 011.9
mammary gland 017.9
marasmus NEC (*see also* Tuberculosis,
    pulmonary) 011.9
mastoiditis 015.6
maternal, affecting fetus or newborn 760.2
mediastinal (lymph) gland or node 012.1
    primary, progressive 010.8
mediastinitis 012.8
    primary, progressive 010.8
mediastinopericarditis 017.9 *[420.0]*
mediastinum 012.8
    primary, progressive 010.8
medulla 013.9
    brain 013.2
    spinal cord 013.4
melanosis, Addisonian 017.6
membrane, brain 013.0
meninges (cerebral) (spinal) 013.0
meningitis (basilar) (brain) (cerebral)
    (cerebrospinal) (spinal) 013.0
meningoencephalitis 013.0
mesentery, mesenteric 014.8
    lymph gland or node 014.8
miliary (any site) 018.9
    acute 018.0
    chronic 018.8
    specified type NEC 018.8
millstone makers' 011.4
miners' 011.4
moulders' 011.4
mouth 017.9
multiple 018.9
    acute 018.0
    chronic 018.8
muscle 017.9
myelitis 013.6
myocarditis 017.9 *[422.0]*
myocardium 017.9 *[422.0]*
nasal (passage) (sinus) 012.8
nasopharynx 012.8
neck gland 017.2
nephritis 016.0 *[583.81]*
nerve 017.9
nose (septum) 012.8
ocular 017.3
old NEC 137.0
    without residuals V12.01
omentum 014.8
oophoritis (acute) (chronic) 016.6
optic 017.3 *[377.39]*
    nerve trunk 017.3 *[377.39]*
    papilla, papillae 017.3 *[377.39]*
orbit 017.3
orchitis 016.5 *[608.81]*
organ, specified NEC 017.9
orificialis (primary) 017.0
osseous (*see also* Tuberculosis, bone) 015.9
    [730.8]
osteitis (*see also* Tuberculosis, bone) 015.9
    [730.8]

Tuberculosis, tubercular, tuberculous—*cont.*
 osteomyelitis (*see also* Tuberculosis, bone)
  015.9 *[730.8]*
 otitis (media) 017.4
 ovaritis (acute) (chronic) 016.6
 ovary (acute) (chronic) 016.6
 oviducts (acute) (chronic) 016.6
 pachymeningitis 013.0
 palate (soft) 017.9
 pancreas 017.9
 papulonecrotic (primary) 017.0
 parathyroid glands 017.9
 paronychia (primary) 017.0
 parotid gland or region 017.9
 pelvic organ NEC 016.9
  female 016.7
  male 016.5
 pelvis (bony) 015.7 *[730.85]*
 penis 016.5
 peribronchitis 011.3
 pericarditis 017.9 *[420.0]*
 pericardium 017.9 *[420.0]*
 perichondritis, larynx 012.3
 perineum 017.9
 periostitis (*see also* Tuberculosis, bone) 015.9
  [730.8]
 periphlebitis 017.9
  eye vessel 017.3 *[362.18]*
  retina 017.3 *[362.18]*
 perirectal fistula 014.8
 peritoneal gland 014.8
 peritoneum 014.0
 peritonitis 014.0
 pernicious NEC (*see also* Tuberculosis,
  pulmonary) 011.9
 pharyngitis 012.8
 pharynx 012.8
 phlyctenulosis (conjunctiva) 017.3 *[370.31]*
 phthisis NEC (*see also* Tuberculosis,
  pulmonary) 011.9
 pituitary gland 017.9
 placenta 016.7
 pleura, pleural, pleurisy, pleuritis (fibrinous)
  (obliterative) (purulent) (simple plastic)
  (with effusion) 012.0
  primary, progressive 010.1
 pneumonia, pneumonic 011.6
 pneumothorax 011.7
 polyserositis 018.9
  acute 018.0
  chronic 018.8
 potters' 011.4
 prepuce 016.5
 primary 010.9
  complex 010.0
  complicated 010.8
   with pleurisy or effusion 010.1
  progressive 010.8
   with pleurisy or effusion 010.1
  skin 017.0
 proctitis 014.8
 prostate 016.5 *[601.4]*
 prostatitis 016.5 *[601.4]*
 pulmonaris (*see also* Tuberculosis, pulmonary)
  011.9
 pulmonary (artery) (incipient) (malignant)
  (multiple round foci) (pernicious)
  (reinfection stage) 011.9
  cavitated or with cavitation 011.2
  primary, progressive 010.8
  childhood type or first infection 010.0

Tuberculosis, tubercular, tuberculous—*cont.*
 chromogenic acid-fast bacilli 795.39
 fibrosis or fibrotic 011.4
 infiltrative 011.0
  primary, progressive 010.9
 nodular 011.1
 specified NEC 011.8
 sputum positive only 795.39
 status following surgical collapse of lung
  NEC 011.9
 pyelitis 016.0 *[590.81]*
 pyelonephritis 016.0 *[590.81]*
 pyemia—*see* Tuberculosis, miliary
 pyonephrosis 016.0
 pyopneumothorax 012.0
 pyothorax 012.0
 rectum (with abscess) 014.8
  fistula 014.8
 reinfection stage (*see also* Tuberculosis,
  pulmonary) 011.9
 renal 016.0
 renis 016.0
 reproductive organ 016.7
 respiratory NEC (*see also* Tuberculosis,
  pulmonary) 011.9
  specified site NEC 012.8
 retina 017.3 *[363.13]*
 retroperitoneal (lymph gland or node) 014.8
  gland 014.8
 retropharyngeal abscess 012.8
 rheumatism 015.9
 rhinitis 012.8
 sacroiliac (joint) 015.8
 sacrum 015.0 *[730.88]*
 salivary gland 017.9
 salpingitis (acute) (chronic) 016.6
 sandblasters' 011.4
 sclera 017.3 *[379.09]*
 scoliosis 015.0 *[737.43]*
 scrofulous 017.2
 scrotum 016.5
 seminal tract or vesicle 016.5 *[608.81]*
 senile NEC (*see also* Tuberculosis, pulmonary)
  011.9
 septic NEC (*see also* Tuberculosis, miliary)
  018.9
 shoulder 015.8
  blade 015.7 *[730.8]*
 sigmoid 014.8
 sinus (accessory) (nasal) 012.8
  bone 015.7 *[730.88]*
  epididymis 016.4
 skeletal NEC (*see also* Osteomyelitis, due to
  tuberculosis) 015.9 *[730.8]*
 skin (any site) (primary) 017.0
 small intestine 014.8
 soft palate 017.9
 spermatic cord 016.5
 spinal
  column 015.0 *[730.88]*
  cord 013.4
  disease 015.0 *[730.88]*
  medulla 013.4
  membrane 013.0
  meninges 013.0
 spine 015.0 *[730.88]*
 spleen 017.7
 splenitis 017.7
 spondylitis 015.0 *[720.81]*
 spontaneous pneumothorax—*see* Tuberculosis,
  pulmonary

Tuberculosis, tubercular, tuberculous—*cont.*
  sternoclavicular joint 015.8
  stomach 017.9
  stonemasons' 011.4
  struma 017.2
  subcutaneous tissue (cellular) (primary) 017.0
  subcutis (primary) 017.0
  subdeltoid bursa 017.9
  submaxillary 017.9
    region 017.9
  supraclavicular gland 017.2
  suprarenal (capsule) (gland) 017.6
  swelling, joint (*see also* Tuberculosis, joint)
    015.9
  symphysis pubis 015.7 *[730.88]*
  synovitis 015.9 *[727.01]*
    hip 015.1 *[727.01]*
    knee 015.2 *[727.01]*
    specified site NEC 015.8 *[727.01]*
    spine or vertebra 015.0 *[727.01]*
  systemic—*see* Tuberculosis, miliary
  tarsitis (eyelid) 017.0 *[373.4]*
    ankle (bone) 015.5 *[730.87]*
  tendon (sheath)—*see* Tuberculosis,
    tenosynovitis
  tenosynovitis 015.9 *[727.01]*
    hip 015.1 *[727.01]*
    knee 015.2 *[727.01]*
    specified site NEC 015.8 *[727.01]*
    spine or vertebra 015.0 *[727.01]*
  testis 016.5 *[608.81]*
  throat 012.8
  thymus gland 017.9
  thyroid gland 017.5
  toe 017.9
  tongue 017.9
  tonsil (lingual) 012.8
  tonsillitis 012.8
  trachea, tracheal 012.8
    gland 012.1
      primary, progressive 010.8
      isolated 012.2
  tracheobronchial 011.3
    glandular 012.1
      primary, progressive 010.8
      isolated 012.2
    lymph gland or node 012.1
      primary, progressive 010.8
  tubal 016.6
  tunica vaginalis 016.5
  typhlitis 014.8
  ulcer (primary) (skin) 017.0
    bowel or intestine 014.8
    specified site NEC—*see* Tuberculosis, by site
  unspecified site—*see* Tuberculosis, pulmonary
  ureter 016.2
  urethra, urethral 016.3
  urinary organ or tract 016.3
    kidney 016.0
  uterus 016.7
  uveal tract 017.3 *[363.13]*
  uvula 017.9
  vaccination, prophylactic (against) V03.2
  vagina 016.7
  vas deferens 016.5
  vein 017.9
  verruca (primary) 017.0
  verrucosa (cutis) (primary) 017.0
  vertebra (column) 015.0 *[730.88]*
  vesiculitis 016.5 *[608.81]*
  viscera NEC 014.8

Tuberculosis, tubercular, tuberculous—*cont.*
  vulva 016.7 *[616.51]*
  wrist (joint) 015.8
    bone 015.5 *[730.83]*
Tuberculum
  auriculae 744.29
  occlusal 520.2
  paramolare 520.2
Tuberous sclerosis (brain) 759.5
Tubo-ovarian —*see* condition
Tuboplasty, after previous sterilization V26.0
Tubotympanitis 381.10
Tularemia 021.9
  with
    conjunctivitis 021.3
    pneumonia 021.2
  bronchopneumonic 021.2
  conjunctivitis 021.3
  cryptogenic 021.1
  disseminated 021.8
  enteric 021.1
  generalized 021.8
  glandular 021.8
  intestinal 021.1
  oculoglandular 021.3
  ophthalmic 021.3
  pneumonia 021.2
  pulmonary 021.2
  specified NEC 021.8
  typhoidal 021.1
  ulceroglandular 021.0
  vaccination, prophylactic (against) V03.4
Tularensis conjunctivitis 021.3
Tumefaction —*see also* Swelling
  liver (*see also* Hypertrophy, liver) 789.1
Tumor (M8000/1)—*see also* Neoplasm, by site,
  unspecified nature
  Abrikossov's (M9580/0)—*see also* Neoplasm,
    connective tissue, benign
    malignant (M9580/3)—*see* Neoplasm,
      connective tissue, malignant
  acinar cell (M8550/1)—*see* Neoplasm, by site,
    uncertain behavior
  acinic cell (M8550/1)—*see* Neoplasm, by site,
    uncertain behavior
  adenomatoid (M9054/0)—*see also* Neoplasm,
    by site, benign
    odontogenic (M9300/0) 213.1
      upper jaw (bone) 213.0
  adnexal (skin) (M8390/0)—*see* Neoplasm, skin,
    benign
  adrenal
    cortical (benign) (M8370/0) 227.0
      malignant (M8370/3) 194.0
    rest (M8671/0)—*see* Neoplasm, by site,
      benign
  alpha cell (M8152/0)
    malignant (M8152/3)
      pancreas 157.4
      specified site NEC—*see* Neoplasm, by site,
        malignant
      unspecified site 157.4
    pancreas 211.7
    specified site NEC—*see* Neoplasm, by site,
      benign
    unspecified site 211.7
  aneurysmal (*see also* Aneurysm) 442.9
  aortic body (M8691/1) 237.3
    malignant (M8691/3) 194.6
  argentaffin (M8241/1)—*see* Neoplasm, by site,
    uncertain behavior

Tumor—*continued*
  basal cell (M8090/1)—*see also* Neoplasm, skin,
    uncertain behavior
  benign (M8000/0)—*see* Neoplasm, by site,
    benign
  beta cell (M8151/0)
    malignant (M8151/3)
      pancreas 157.4
      specified site—*see* Neoplasm, by site,
        malignant
      unspecified site 157.4
    pancreas 211.7
    specified site NEC—*see* Neoplasm, by site,
      benign
    unspecified site 211.7
  blood—*see* Hematoma
  brenner (M9000/0) 220
    borderline malignancy (M9000/1) 236.2
    malignant (M9000/3) 183.0
    proliferating (M9000/1) 236.2
  Brooke's (M8100/0)—*see* Neoplasm, skin,
    benign
  brown fat (M8880/0)—*see* Lipoma, by site
  Burkitt's (M9750/3) 200.2
  calcifying epithelial odontogenic (M9340/0)
    213.1
    upper jaw (bone) 213.0
  carcinoid (M8240/1)—*see* Carcinoid
  carotid body (M8692/1) 237.3
    malignant (M8692/3) 194.5
  Castleman's (mediastinal lymph node
    hyperplasia) 785.6
  cells (M8001/1)—*see also* Neoplasm, by site,
    unspecified nature
    benign (M8001/0)—*see* Neoplasm, by site,
      benign
    malignant (M8001/3)—*see* Neoplasm, by site,
      malignant
    uncertain whether benign or malignant
      (M8001/1)—*see* Neoplasm, by site,
      uncertain nature
  cervix
    in pregnancy or childbirth 654.6
      affecting fetus or newborn 763.89
      causing obstructed labor 660.2
        affecting fetus or newborn 763.1
  chondromatous giant cell (M9230/0)—*see*
    Neoplasm, bone, benign
  chromaffin (M8700/0)—*see also* Neoplasm, by
    site, benign
    malignant (M8700/3)—*see* Neoplasm, by site,
      malignant
  Cock's peculiar 706.2
  Codman's (benign chondroblastoma)
    (M9230/0)—*see* Neoplasm, bone, benign
  dentigerous, mixed (M9282/0) 213.1
    upper jaw (bone) 213.0
  dermoid (M9084/0)—*see* Neoplasm, by site,
    benign
    with malignant transformation (M9084/3)
      183.0
  desmoid (extra-abdominal) (M8821/1)—*see
    also* Neoplasm, connective tissue, uncertain
    behavior
    abdominal (M8822/1)—*see* Neoplasm,
      connective tissue, uncertain behavior
  embryonal (mixed) (M9080/1)—*see also*
    Neoplasm, by site, uncertain behavior
    liver (M9080/3) 155.0
  endodermal sinus (M9071/3)

Tumor—*continued*
    specified site—*see* Neoplasm, by site,
      malignant
    unspecified site
      female 183.0
      male 186.9
  epithelial
    benign (M8010/0)—*see* Neoplasm, by site,
      benign
    malignant (M8010/3)—*see* Neoplasm, by site,
      malignant
  Ewing's (M9260/3)—*see* Neoplasm, bone,
    malignant
  fatty—*see* Lipoma
  fetal, causing disproportion 653.7
    causing obstructed labor 660.1
  fibroid (M8890/0)—*see* Leiomyoma
  G cell (M8153/1)
    malignant (M8153/3)
      pancreas 157.4
      specified site NEC—*see* Neoplasm, by site,
        malignant
      unspecified site 157.4
    specified site—*see* Neoplasm, by site,
      uncertain behavior
    unspecified site 235.5
  giant cell (type) (M8003/1)—*see also*
    Neoplasm, by site, unspecified nature
    bone (M9250/1) 238.0
      malignant (M9250/3)—*see* Neoplasm, bone,
        malignant
    chondromatous (M9230/0)—*see* Neoplasm,
      bone, benign
    malignant (M8003/3)—*see* Neoplasm, by site,
      malignant
    peripheral (gingiva) 523.8
    soft parts (M9251/1)—*see also* Neoplasm,
      connective tissue, uncertain behavior
      malignant (M9251/3)—*see* Neoplasm,
        connective tissue, malignant
    tendon sheath 727.02
  glomus (M8711/0)—*see also* Hemangioma, by
    site
    jugulare (M8690/1) 237.3
      malignant (M8690/3) 194.6
  gonadal stromal (M8590/1)—*see* Neoplasm, by
    site, uncertain behavior
  granular cell (M9580/0)—*see also* Neoplasm,
    connective tissue, benign
    malignant (M9580/3)—*see* Neoplasm,
      connective tissue, malignant
  granulosa cell (M8620/1) 236.2
    malignant (M8620/3) 183.0
  granulosa cell-theca cell (M8621/1) 236.2
    malignant (M8621/3) 183.0
  Grawitz's (hypernephroma) (M8312/3) 189.0
  hazard-crile (M8350/3) 193
  hemorrhoidal—*see* Hemorrhoids
  hilar cell (M8660/0) 220
  hurthle cell (benign) (M8290/0) 226
    malignant (M8290/3) 193
  hydatid (*see also* Echinococcus) 122.9
  hypernephroid (M8311/1)—*see also* Neoplasm,
    by site, uncertain behavior
  interstitial cell (M8650/1)—*see also* Neoplasm,
    by site, uncertain behavior
    benign (M8650/0)—*see* Neoplasm, by site,
      benign
    malignant (M8650/3)—*see* Neoplasm, by site,
      malignant
  islet cell (M8150/0)

Tumor—*continued*
  malignant (M8150/3)
    pancreas 157.4
    specified site—*see* Neoplasm, by site,
      malignant
    unspecified site 157.4
    pancreas 211.7
    specified site NEC—*see* Neoplasm, by site,
      benign
    unspecified site 211.7
  juxtaglomerular (M8361/1) 236.91
  Krukenberg's (M8490/6) 198.6
  Leydig cell (M8650/1)
    benign (M8650/0)
      specified site—*see* Neoplasm, by site,
        benign
      unspecified site
        female 220
        male 220.0
    malignant (M8650/3)
      specified site—*see* Neoplasm, by site,
        malignant
      unspecified site
        female 183.0
        male 186.9
    specified site—*see* Neoplasm, by site,
      uncertain behavior
    unspecified site
      female 236.2
      male 236.4
  lipid cell, ovary (M8670/0) 220
  lipoid cell, ovary (M8670/0) 220
  lymphomatous, benign (M9590/0)—*see also*
    Neoplasm, by site, benign
  Malherbe's (M8110/0)—*see* Neoplasm, skin,
    benign
  malignant (M8000/3)—*see also* Neoplasm, by
    site, malignant
    fusiform cell (type) (M8004/3)—*see*
      Neoplasm, by site, malignant
    giant cell (type) (M8003/3)—*see* Neoplasm,
      by site, malignant
    mixed NEC (M8940/3)—*see* Neoplasm, by
      site, malignant
    small cell (type) (M8002/3)—*see* Neoplasm,
      by site, malignant
    spindle cell (type) (M8004/3)—*see* Neoplasm,
      by site, malignant
  mast cell (M8740/1) 238.5
    malignant (M9740/3) 202.6
  melanotic, neuroectodermal (M9363/0)—*see*
    Neoplasm, by site, benign
  Merkel cell—*see* Neoplasm, by site, malignant
  mesenchymal
    malignant (M8800/3)—*see* Neoplasm,
      connective tissue, malignant
    mixed (M8990/1)—*see* Neoplasm, connective
      tissue, uncertain behavior
  mesodermal, mixed (M8951/3)—*see also*
    Neoplasm, by site, malignant
    liver 155.0
  mesonephric (M9110/1)—*see also* Neoplasm,
    by site, uncertain behavior
    malignant (M9110/3)—*see* Neoplasm, by site,
      malignant
  metastatic
    from specified site (M8000/3)—*see*
      Neoplasm, by site, malignant
    to specified site (M8000/6)—*see* Neoplasm,
      by site, malignant, secondary

Tumor—*continued*
  mixed NEC (M8940/0)—*see also* Neoplasm, by
    site, benign
    malignant (M8940/3)—*see* Neoplasm, by site,
      malignant
  mucocarcinoid, malignant (M8243/3)—*see*
    Neoplasm, by site, malignant
  mucoepidermoid (M8430/1)—*see* Neoplasm,
    by site, uncertain behavior
  Mullerian, mixed (M8950/3)—*see* Neoplasm,
    by site, malignant
  myoepithelial (M8982/0)—*see* Neoplasm, by
    site, benign
  neurogenic olfactory (M9520/3) 160.0
  nonencapsulated sclerosing (M8350/3) 193
  odontogenic (M9270/1) 238.0
    adenomatoid (M9300/0) 213.1
      upper jaw (bone) 213.0
    benign (M9270/0) 213.1
      upper jaw (bone) 213.0
    calcifying epithelial (M9340/0) 213.1
      upper jaw (bone) 213.0
    malignant (M9270/3) 170.1
      upper jaw (bone) 170.0
    squamous (M9312/0) 213.1
      upper jaw (bone) 213.0
  ovarian stromal (M8590/1) 236.2
  ovary
    in pregnancy or childbirth 654.4
      affecting fetus or newborn 763.89
      causing obstructed labor 660.2
        affecting fetus or newborn 763.1
  pacinian (M9507/0)—*see* Neoplasm, skin,
    benign
  Pancoast's (M8010/3) 162.3
  papillary—*see* Papilloma
  pelvic, in pregnancy or childbirth 654.9
    affecting fetus or newborn 763.89
    causing obstructed labor 660.2
      affecting fetus or newborn 763.1
  phantom 300.11
  plasma cell (M9731/1) 238.6
    benign (M9731/0)—*see* Neoplasm, by site,
      benign
    malignant (M9731/3) 203.8
  polyvesicular vitelline (M9071/3)
    specified site—*see* Neoplasm, by site,
      malignant
    unspecified site
      female 183.0
      male 186.9
  Pott's puffy (*see also* Osteomyelitis) 730.2
  Rathke's pouch (M9350/1) 237.0
  regaud's (M8082/3)—*see* Neoplasm,
    nasopharynx, malignant
  rete cell (M8140/0) 222.0
  retinal anlage (M9363/0)—*see* Neoplasm, by
    site, benign
  Rokitansky's 620.2
  salivary gland type, mixed (M8940/0)—*see also*
    Neoplasm, by site, benign
    malignant (M8940/3)—*see* Neoplasm, by site,
      malignant
  Sampson's 617.1
  Schloffer's (*see also* Peritonitis) 567.2
  Schmincke (M8082/3)—*see* Neoplasm,
    nasopharynx, malignant
  sebaceous (*see also* Cyst, sebaceous) 706.2
  secondary (M8000/6)—*see* Neoplasm, by site,
    secondary
  Sertoli cell (M8640/0)

Tumor—*continued*
  with lipid storage (M8641/0)
    specified site—*see* Neoplasm, by site,
      benign
    unspecified site
      female 220
      male 222.0
    specified site—*see* Neoplasm, by site, benign
    unspecified site
      female 220
      male 222.0
  Sertoli-Leydig cell (M8631/0)
    specified site—*see* Neoplasm, by site, benign
    unspecified site
      female 220
      male 222.0
  sex cord (-stromal) (M8590/1)—*see* Neoplasm,
    by site, uncertain behavior
  skin appendage (M8390/0)—*see* Neoplasm,
    skin, benign
  soft tissue
    benign (M8800/0)—*see* Neoplasm,
      connective tissue, benign
    malignant (M8800/3)—*see* Neoplasm,
      connective tissue, malignant
  sternomastoid 754.1
  superior sulcus (lung) (pulmonary) (syndrome)
    (M8010/3) 162.3
  suprasulcus (M8010/3) 162.3
  sweat gland (M8400/1)—*see also* Neoplasm,
    skin, uncertain behavior
    benign (M8400/0)—*see* Neoplasm, skin,
      benign
    malignant (M8400/3)—*see* Neoplasm, skin,
      malignant
  syphilitic brain 094.89
    congenital 090.49
  testicular stromal (M8590/1) 236.4
  theca cell (M8600/0) 220
  theca cell-granulosa cell (M8621/1) 236.2
  theca-lutein (M8610/0) 220
  turban (M8200/0) 216.4
  uterus
    in pregnancy or childbirth 654.1
      affecting fetus or newborn 763.89
      causing obstructed labor 660.2
        affecting fetus or newborn 763.1
  vagina
    in pregnancy or childbirth 654.7
      affecting fetus or newborn 763.89
      causing obstructed labor 660.2
        affecting fetus or newborn 763.1
  varicose (*see also* Varicose, vein) 454.9
  von Recklinghausen's (M9540/1) 237.71
  vulva
    in pregnancy or childbirth 654.8
      affecting fetus or newborn 763.89
      causing obstructed labor 660.2
        affecting fetus or newborn 763.1
  Warthin's (salivary gland) (M8561/0) 210.2
  white—*see also* Tuberculosis, arthritis
  White-Darier 757.39
  Wilms' (nephroblastoma) (M8960/3) 189.0
  yolk sac (M9071/3)
    specified site—*see* Neoplasm, by site,
      malignant
    unspecified site
      female 183.0
      male 186.9
Tumorlet (M8040/1)—*see* Neoplasm, by site,
  uncertain behavior
Tungiasis 134.1

Tunica vasculosa lentis 743.39
Tunnel vision 368.45
Turban tumor (M8200/0) 216.4
Türck's trachoma (chronic catarrhal laryngitis)
  476.0
Türk's syndrome (ocular retraction syndrome)
  378.71
Turner's
  hypoplasia (tooth) 520.4
  syndrome 758.6
  tooth 520.4
Turner-Kieser syndrome (hereditary
  osteo-onychodysplasia) 756.89
Turner-Varny syndrome 758.6
Turricephaly 756.0
Tussis convulsiva (*see also* Whooping cough)
  033.9
Twin
  affected by maternal complications of
    pregnancy 761.5
  conjoined 759.4
  healthy liveborn—*see* Newborn, twin
  pregnancy (complicating delivery) NEC 651.0
    with fetal loss and retention of one fetus 651.3
Twinning, teeth 520.2
Twist, twisted
  bowel, colon, or intestine 560.2
  hair (congenital) 757.4
  mesentery 560.2
  omentum 560.2
  organ or site, congenital NEC—*see* Anomaly,
    specified type NEC
  ovarian pedicle 620.5
    congenital 752.0
  umbilical cord—*see* Compression, umbilical
    cord
Twitch 781.0
Tylosis 700
  buccalis 528.6
  gingiva 523.8
  linguae 528.6
  palmaris et plantaris 757.39
Tympanism 787.3
Tympanites (abdominal) (intestine) 787.3
Tympanitis —*see* Myringitis
Tympanosclerosis 385.00
  involving
    combined sites NEC 385.09
      with tympanic membrane 385.03
    tympanic membrane 385.01
      with ossicles 385.02
        and middle ear 385.03
Tympanum —*see* condition
Tympany
  abdomen 787.3
  chest 786.7
Typhlitis (*see also* Appendicitis) 541
Typhoenteritis 002.0
Typhogastric fever 002.0
Typhoid (abortive) (ambulant) (any site) (fever)
  (hemorrhagic) (infection) (intermittent)
  (malignant) (rheumatic) 002.0
  with pneumonia 002.0 *[484.8]*
  abdominal 002.0
  carrier (suspected) of V02.1
  cholecystitis (current) 002.0
  clinical (Widal and blood test negative) 002.0
  endocarditis 002.0 *[421.1]*
  inoculation reaction—*see* Complications,
    vaccination
  meningitis 002.0 *[320.7]*

Typhoid—*continued*
  mesenteric lymph nodes 002.0
  myocarditis 002.0 *[422.0]*
  osteomyelitis (*see also* Osteomyelitis, due to,
    typhoid) 002.0 *[730.8]*
  perichondritis, larynx 002.0 *[478.71]*
  pneumonia 002.0 *[484.8]*
  spine 002.0 *[720.81]*
  ulcer (perforating) 002.0
  vaccination, prophylactic (against) V03.1
  Widal negative 002.0
Typhomalaria (fever) (*see also* Malaria) 084.6
Typhomania 002.0
Typhoperitonitis 002.0
Typhus (fever) 081.9
  abdominal, abdominalis 002.0
  African tick 082.1
  amarillic (*see also* Fever, Yellow) 060.9
  brain 081.9
  cerebral 081.9
  classical 080
  endemic (flea-borne) 081.0
  epidemic (louse-borne) 080
  exanthematic NEC 080
  exanthematicus SAI 080
    brillii SAI 081.1
    Mexicanus SAI 081.0
    pediculo vestimenti causa 080
    typhus murinus 081.0
  flea-borne 081.0
  Indian tick 082.1
  Kenya tick 082.1
  louse-borne 080
  Mexican 081.0
    flea-borne 081.0
    louse-borne 080
    tabardillo 080
  mite-borne 081.2
  murine 081.0
  North Asian tick-borne 082.2
  petechial 081.9
  Queensland tick 082.3
  rat 081.0
  recrudescent 081.1
  recurrent (*see also* Fever, relapsing) 087.9
  São Paulo 082.0
  scrub (China) (India) (Malaya) (New Guinea)
    081.2
  shop (of Malaya) 081.0
  Siberian tick 082.2
  tick-borne NEC 082.9
  tropical 081.2
  vaccination, prophylactic (against) V05.8
Tyrosinemia 270.2
  neonatal 775.8
Tyrosinosis (Medes) (Sakai) 270.2
Tyrosinuria 270.2
Tyrosyluria 270.2

U

Uehlinger's syndrome (acropachyderma) 757.39
Uhl's anomaly or disease (hypoplasia of
  myocardium, right ventricle) 746.84
**Ulcer, ulcerated, ulcerating, ulceration, ulcera-
  tive** 707.9
  with gangrene 707.9 *[785.4]*
  abdomen (wall) (*see also* Ulcer, skin) 707.8
  ala, nose 478.1
  alveolar process 526.5
  amebic (intestine) 006.9
    skin 006.6
  anastomotic—*see* Ulcer, gastrojejunal
  anorectal 569.41
  antral—*see* Ulcer, stomach
  anus (sphincter) (solitary) 569.41
    varicose—*see* Varicose, ulcer, anus
  aphthous (oral) (recurrent) 528.2
    genital organ(s)
      female 616.8
      male 608.89
    mouth 528.2
  arm (*see also* Ulcer, skin) 707.8
  arteriosclerotic plaque—*see* Arteriosclerosis, by
    site
  artery NEC 447.2
    without rupture 447.8
  atrophic NEC—*see* Ulcer, skin
  Barrett's (chronic peptic ulcer of esophagus)
    530.2
  bile duct 576.8
  bladder (solitary) (sphincter) 596.8
    bilharzial (*see also* Schistosomiasis) 120.9
      · *[595.4]*
    submucosal (*see also* Cystitis) 595.1
    tuberculous (*see also* Tuberculosis) 016.1
  bleeding NEC—*see* Ulcer, peptic, with
    hemorrhage
  bone 730.9
  bowel (*see also* Ulcer, intestine) 569.82
  breast 611.0
  bronchitis 491.8
  bronchus 519.1
  buccal (cavity) (traumatic) 528.9
  burn (acute)—*see* Ulcer, duodenum
  Buruli 031.1
  buttock (*see also* Ulcer, skin) 707.8
    decubitus (*see also* Ulcer, decubitus) 707.0
  cancerous (M8000/3)—*see* Neoplasm, by site,
    malignant
  cardia—*see* Ulcer, stomach
  cardio-esophageal (peptic) 530.2
  cecum (*see also* Ulcer, intestine) 569.82
  cervix (uteri) (trophic) 622.0
    with mention of cervicitis 616.0
  chancroidal 099.0
  chest (wall) (*see also* Ulcer, skin) 707.8
  Chiclero 085.4
  chin (pyogenic) (*see also* Ulcer, skin) 707.8
  chronic (cause unknown)—*see also* Ulcer, skin
    penis 607.89
  Cochin-China 085.1
  colitis —*see* Colitis, ulcerative
  colon (*see also* Ulcer, intestine) 569.82
  conjunctiva (acute) (postinfectional) 372.00

Ulcer, ulcerated, ulcerating—*continued*
  cornea (infectional) 370.00
    with perforation 370.06
    annular 370.02
    catarrhal 370.01
    central 370.03
    dendritic 054.42
    marginal 370.01
    mycotic 370.05
    phlyctenular, tuberculous (*see also*
      Tuberculosis) 017.3 *[370.31]*
    ring 370.02
    rodent 370.07
    serpent, serpiginous 370.04
    superficial marginal 370.01
    tuberculous (*see also* Tuberculosis) 017.3
      [370.31]
  corpus cavernosum (chronic) 607.89
  crural—*see* Ulcer, lower extremity
  Curling's—*see* Ulcer, duodenum
  Cushing's—*see* Ulcer, peptic
  cystitis (interstitial) 595.1
  decubitus (any site) 707.0
    with gangrene 707.0 *[785.4]*
  dendritic 054.42
  diabetes, diabetic (mellitus) 250.8 *[707.9]*
    lower limb 250.8 *[707.10]*
      ankle 250.8 *[707.13]*
      calf 250.8 *[707.12]*
      foot 250.8 *[707.15]*
      heel 250.8 *[707.14]*
      knee 250.8 *[707.19]*
      specified site NEC 250.8 *[707.19]*
      thigh 250.8 *[707.11]*
      toes 250.8 *[707.15]*
    specified site NEC 250.8 *[707.8]*
  Dieulafoy's—*see* Lesion, Dieulafoy
  due to
    infection NEC—*see* Ulcer, skin
    radiation, radium—*see* Ulcer, by site
    trophic disturbance (any region)—*see* Ulcer,
      skin
    x-ray—*see* Ulcer, by site
  duodenum, duodenal (eroded) (peptic) 532.9

> *Note—Use the following fifth-digit
> subclassification with categories 531-534:*
>
> 0 *without mention of obstruction*
> 1 *with obstruction*

    with
      hemorrhage (chronic) 532.4
        and perforation 532.6
      perforation (chronic) 532.5
        and hemorrhage 532.6
    acute 532.3
      with
        hemorrhage 532.0
          and perforation 532.2
        perforation 532.1
          and hemorrhage 532.2
    bleeding (recurrent)—*see* Ulcer, duodenum,
      with hemorrhage
    chronic 532.7
      with
        hemorrhage 532.4
          and perforation 532.6

Ulcer, ulcerated, ulcerating—*continued*
    perforation 532.5
      and hemorrhage 532.6
    penetrating—*see* Ulcer, duodenum, with
      perforation
    perforating—*see* Ulcer, duodenum, with
      perforation
  dysenteric NEC 009.0
  elusive 595.1
  endocarditis (any valve) (acute) (chronic)
    (subacute) 421.0
  enteritis —*see* Colitis, ulcerative
  enterocolitis 556.0
  epiglottis 478.79
  esophagus (peptic) 530.2
    due to ingestion
      aspirin 530.2
      chemicals 530.2
      medicinal agents 530.2
    fungal 530.2
    infectional 530.2
    varicose (*see also* Varix, esophagus) 456.1
      bleeding (*see also* Varix, esophagus,
        bleeding) 456.0
  eye NEC 360.00
    dendritic 054.42
  eyelid (region) 373.01
  face (*see also* Ulcer, skin) 707.8
  fauces 478.29
  Fenwick (-Hunner) (solitary) (*see also* Cystitis)
    595.1
  fistulous NEC—*see* Ulcer, skin
  foot (indolent) (*see also* Ulcer, lower extremity)
    707.15
    perforating 707.15
      leprous 030.1
      syphilitic 094.0
    trophic 707.15
    varicose 454.0
      inflamed or infected 454.2
  frambesial, initial or primary 102.0
  gallbladder or duct 575.8
  gall duct 576.8
  gangrenous (*see also* Gangrene) 785.4
  gastric—*see* Ulcer, stomach
  gastrocolic—*see* Ulcer, gastrojejunal
  gastroduodenal—*see* Ulcer, peptic
  gastroesophageal—*see* Ulcer, stomach
  gastrohepatic—*see* Ulcer, stomach
  gastrointestinal—*see* Ulcer, gastrojejunal
  gastrojejunal (eroded) (peptic) 534.9

Note—Use the following fifth-digit
subclassification with categories 531-534:

0 without mention of obstruction
1 with obstruction

---

    with
      hemorrhage (chronic) 534.4
        and perforation 534.6
      perforation 534.5
        and hemorrhage 534.6
    acute 534.3
      with
        hemorrhage 534.0
          and perforation 534.2
        perforation 534.1
          and hemorrhage 534.2
    bleeding (recurrent)—*see* Ulcer, gastrojejunal,
      with hemorrhage
    chronic 534.7

Ulcer, ulcerated, ulcerating—*continued*
    with
      hemorrhage 534.4
        and perforation 534.6
      perforation 534.5
        and hemorrhage 534.6
    penetrating—*see* Ulcer, gastrojejunal, with
      perforation
    perforating—*see* Ulcer, gastrojejunal, with
      perforation
  gastrojejunocolic—*see* Ulcer, gastrojejunal
  genital organ
    female 629.8
    male 608.89
  gingiva 523.8
  gingivitis 523.1
  glottis 478.79
  granuloma of pudenda 099.2
  groin (*see also* Ulcer, skin) 707.8
  gum 523.8
  gumma, due to yaws 102.4
  hand (*see also* Ulcer, skin) 707.8
  hard palate 528.9
  heel (*see also* Ulcer, lower extremity) 707.14
    decubitus (*see also* Ulcer, decubitus) 707.0
  hemorrhoids 455.8
    external 455.5
    internal 455.2
  hip (*see also* Ulcer, skin) 707.8
    decubitus (*see also* Ulcer, decubitus) 707.0
  Hunner's 595.1
  hypopharynx 478.29
  hypopyon (chronic) (subacute) 370.04
  hypostaticum—*see* Ulcer, varicose
  ileocolitis 556.1
  ileum (*see also* Ulcer, intestine) 569.82
  intestine, intestinal 569.82
    with perforation 569.83
    amebic 006.9
    duodenal—*see* Ulcer, duodenum
    granulocytopenic (with hemorrhage) 288.0
    marginal 569.82
    perforating 569.83
    small, primary 569.82
    stercoraceous 569.82
    stercoral 569.82
    tuberculous (*see also* Tuberculosis) 014.8
    typhoid (fever) 002.0
    varicose 456.8
  ischemic 707.9
    lower extremity (*see also* Ulcer, lower
      extremity) 707.10
      ankle 707.13
      calf 707.12
      foot 707.15
      heel 707.14
      knee 707.19
      specified site NEC 707.19
      thigh 707.11
      toes 707.15
  jejunum, jejunal—*see* Ulcer, gastrojejunal
  keratitis (*see also* Ulcer, cornea) 370.00
  knee—*see* Ulcer, lower extremity
  labium (majus) (minus) 616.50
  laryngitis (*see also* Laryngitis) 464.00
    with obstruction 464.01
  larynx (aphthous) (contact) 478.79
    diphtheritic 032.3
  leg—*see* Ulcer, lower extremity
  lip 528.5
  Lipschütz's 616.50

Ulcer, ulcerated, ulcerating—*continued*
  lower extremity (atrophic) (chronic)
    (neurogenic) (perforating) (pyogenic)
    (trophic) (tropical) 707.10
    with gangrene (*see also* Ulcer, lower
      extremity) 707.10 *[785.4]*
      arteriosclerotic 440.24
    ankle 707.13
    arteriosclerotic 440.23
      with gangrene 440.24
    calf 707.12
    decubitus 707.0
      with gangrene 707.0 *[785.4]*
    foot 707.15
    heel 707.14
    knee 707.19
    specified site NEC 707.19
    thigh 707.11
    toes 707.15
    varicose 454.0
      inflamed or infected 454.2
  luetic—*see* Ulcer, syphilitic
  lung 518.89
    tuberculous (*see also* Tuberculosis) 011.2
  malignant (M8000/3)—*see* Neoplasm, by site,
    malignant
  marginal NEC—*see* Ulcer, gastrojejunal
  meatus (urinarius) 597.89
  Meckel's diverticulum 751.0
  Meleney's (chronic undermining) 686.09
  Mooren's (cornea) 370.07
  mouth (traumatic) 528.9
  mycobacterial (skin) 031.1
  nasopharynx 478.29
  navel cord (newborn) 771.4
  neck (*see also* Ulcer, skin) 707.8
    uterus 622.0
  neurogenic NEC—*see* Ulcer, skin
  nose, nasal (infectional) (passage) 478.1
    septum 478.1
      varicose 456.8
    skin—*see* Ulcer, skin
    spirochetal NEC 104.8
  oral mucosa (traumatic) 528.9
  palate (soft) 528.9
  penetrating NEC—*see* Ulcer, peptic, with
    perforation
  penis (chronic) 607.89
  peptic (site unspecified) 533.9

Note—Use the following fifth-digit
subclassification with categories 531-534:

0 without mention of obstruction
1 with obstruction

---

    with
      hemorrhage 533.4
        and perforation 533.6
      perforation (chronic) 533.5
        and hemorrhage 533.6
    acute 533.3
      with
        hemorrhage 533.0
          and perforation 533.2
        perforation 533.1
          and hemorrhage 533.2
    bleeding (recurrent)—*see* Ulcer, peptic, with
      hemorrhage

Ulcer, ulcerated, ulcerating—*continued*
  chronic 533.7
    with
      hemorrhage 533.4
        and perforation 533.6
      perforation 533.5
        and hemorrhage 533.6
  penetrating—*see* Ulcer, peptic, with
    perforation
  perforating NEC (*see also* Ulcer, peptic, with
    perforation) 533.5
  skin 707.9
  perineum (*see also* Ulcer, skin) 707.8
  peritonsillar 474.8
  phagedenic (tropical) NEC—*see* Ulcer, skin
  pharynx 478.29
  phlebitis—*see* Phlebitis
  plaster (*see also* Ulcer, decubitus) 707.0
  popliteal space—*see* Ulcer, lower extremity
  postpyloric—*see* Ulcer, duodenum
  prepuce 607.89
  prepyloric—*see* Ulcer, stomach
  pressure (*see also* Ulcer, decubitus) 707.0
  primary of intestine 569.82
    with perforation 569.83
  proctitis 556.2
    with ulcerative sigmoiditis 556.3
  prostate 601.8
  pseudopeptic—*see* Ulcer, peptic
  pyloric—*see* Ulcer, stomach
  rectosigmoid 569.82
    with perforation 569.83
  rectum (sphincter) (solitary) 569.41
    stercoraceous, stercoral 569.41
    varicose—*see* Varicose, ulcer, anus
  retina (*see also* Chorioretinitis) 363.20
  rodent (M8090/3)—*see also* Neoplasm, skin,
    malignant
    cornea 370.07
  round—*see* Ulcer, stomach
  sacrum (region) (*see also* Ulcer, skin) 707.8
  Saemisch's 370.04
  scalp (*see also* Ulcer, skin) 707.8
  sclera 379.09
  scrofulous (*see also* Tuberculosis) 017.2
  scrotum 608.89
    tuberculous (*see also* Tuberculosis) 016.5
    varicose 456.4
  seminal vesicle 608.89
  sigmoid 569.82
    with perforation 569.83
  skin (atrophic) (chronic) (neurogenic)
    (non-healing) (perforating) (pyogenic)
    (trophic) 707.9
    with gangrene 707.9 *[785.4]*
    amebic 006.6
    decubitus 707.0
      with gangrene 707.0 *[785.4]*
    in granulocytopenia 288.0
    lower extremity (*see also* Ulcer, lower
      extremity) 707.10
      with gangrene 707.10 *[785.4]*
        arteriosclerotic 440.24
      ankle 707.13
      arteriosclerotic 440.23
        with gangrene 440.24
      calf 707.12
      foot 707.15
      heel 707.14
      knee 707.19
      specified site NEC 707.19

Ulcer, ulcerated, ulcerating—*continued*
    thigh 707.11
    toes 707.15
    mycobacterial 031.1
    syphilitic (early) (secondary) 091.3
    tuberculous (primary) (*see also* Tuberculosis)
        017.0
    varicose—*see* Ulcer, varicose
    sloughing NEC—*see* Ulcer, skin
    soft palate 528.9
    solitary, anus or rectum (sphincter) 569.41
    sore throat 462
      streptococcal 034.0
    spermatic cord 608.89
    spine (tuberculous) 015.0 *[730.88]*
    stasis (leg) (venous) 454.0
      inflamed or infected 454.2
      without varicose veins 459.81
    stercoral, stercoraceous 569.82
      with perforation 569.83
      anus or rectum 569.41
    stoma, stomal—*see* Ulcer, gastrojejunal
    stomach (eroded) (peptic) (round) 531.9

> *Note—Use the following fifth-digit*
> *subclassification with categories 531-534:*
>
> 0 *without mention of obstruction*
> 1 *with obstruction*

    with
      hemorrhage 531.4
        and perforation 531.6
      perforation (chronic) 531.5
        and hemorrhage 531.6
    acute 531.3
      with
        hemorrhage 531.0
          and perforation 531.2
        perforation 531.1
          and hemorrhage 531.2
    bleeding (recurrent)—*see* Ulcer, stomach,
      with hemorrhage
    chronic 531.7
      with
        hemorrhage 531.4
          and perforation 531.6
        perforation 531.5
          and hemorrhage 531.6
    penetrating—*see* Ulcer, stomach, with
      perforation
    perforating—*see* Ulcer, stomach, with
      perforation
    stomatitis 528.0
    stress—*see* Ulcer, peptic
    strumous (tuberculous) (*see also* Tuberculosis)
      017.2
    submental (*see also* Ulcer, skin) 707.8
    submucosal, bladder 595.1
    syphilitic (any site) (early) (secondary) 091.3
      late 095.9
      perforating 095.9
        foot 094.0
    testis 608.89
    thigh—*see* Ulcer, lower extremity
    throat 478.29
      diphtheritic 032.0
    toe—*see* Ulcer, lower extremity
    tongue (traumatic) 529.0
    tonsil 474.8
      diphtheritic 032.0
    trachea 519.1

Ulcer, ulcerated, ulcerating—*continued*
    trophic—*see* Ulcer, skin
    tropical NEC (*see also* Ulcer, skin) 707.9
    tuberculous—*see* Tuberculosis, ulcer
    tunica vaginalis 608.89
    turbinate 730.9
    typhoid (fever) 002.0
      perforating 002.0
    umbilicus (newborn) 771.4
    unspecified site NEC—*see* Ulcer, skin
    urethra (meatus) (*see also* Urethritis) 597.89
    uterus 621.8
      cervix 622.0
        with mention of cervicitis 616.0
      neck 622.0
        with mention of cervicitis 616.0
    vagina 616.8
    valve, heart 421.0
    varicose (lower extremity, any part) 454.0
      anus—*see* Varicose, ulcer, anus
      broad ligament 456.5
      esophagus (*see also* Varix, esophagus) 456.1
      bleeding (*see also* Varix, esophagus,
          bleeding) 456.0
      inflamed or infected 454.2
      nasal septum 456.8
      perineum 456.6
      rectum—*see* Varicose, ulcer, anus
      scrotum 456.4
      specified site NEC 456.8
      sublingual 456.3
      vulva 456.6
    vas deferens 608.89
    vesical (*see also* Ulcer, bladder) 596.8
    vulva (acute) (infectional) 616.50
      Behçet's syndrome 136.1 *[616.51]*
      herpetic 054.12
      tuberculous 016.7 *[616.51]*
    vulvobuccal, recurring 616.50
    x-ray—*see* Ulcer, by site
    yaws 102.4
Ulcerosa scarlatina 034.1
Ulcus —*see also* Ulcer
    cutis tuberculosum (*see also* Tuberculosis) 017.0
    duodeni—*see* Ulcer, duodenum
    durum 091.0
      extragenital 091.2
    gastrojejunale—*see* Ulcer, gastrojejunal
    hypostaticum—*see* Ulcer, varicose
    molle (cutis) (skin) 099.0
    serpens cornea (pneumococcal) 370.04
    ventriculi—*see* Ulcer, stomach
Ulegyria 742.4
Ulerythema
    acneiforma 701.8
    centrifugum 695.4
    ophryogenes 757.4
Ullrich (-Bonnevie) (-Turner) syndrome 758.6
Ullrich-Feichtiger syndrome 759.89
Ulnar —*see* condition
Ulorrhagia 523.8
Ulorrhea 523.8
Umbilicus, umbilical —*see also* condition
    cord necrosis, affecting fetus or newborn 762.6
Unavailability of medical facilities (at) V63.9
    due to
      investigation by social service agency V63.8
      lack of services at home V63.1
      remoteness from facility V63.0
      waiting list V63.2
    home V63.1

Unavailability of medical facilities—*continued*
outpatient clinic V63.0
specified reason NEC V63.8
Uncinaria americana infestation 126.1
Uncinariasis (*see also* Ancylostomiasis) 126.9
Unconscious, unconsciousness 780.09
Underdevelopment —*see also* Undeveloped
sexual 259.0
Undernourishment 269.9
Undernutrition 269.9
Under observation —*see* Observation
Underweight 783.22
for gestational age—*see* Light-for-dates
Underwood's disease (sclerema neonatorum)
778.1
Undescended —*see also* Malposition, congenital
cecum 751.4
colon 751.4
testis 752.51
Undetermined diagnosis or cause 799.9
Undeveloped, undevelopment —*see also*
Hypoplasia
brain (congenital) 742.1
cerebral (congenital) 742.1
fetus or newborn 764.9
heart 746.89
lung 748.5
testis 257.2
uterus 259.0
Undiagnosed (disease) 799.9
Undulant fever (*see also* Brucellosis) 023.9
Unemployment, anxiety concerning V62.0
Unequal leg (acquired) (length) 736.81
congenital 755.30
Unerupted teeth, tooth 520.6
Unextracted dental root 525.3
Unguis incarnatus 703.0
Unicornis uterus 752.3
Unicorporeus uterus 752.3
Uniformis uterus 752.3
Unilateral —*see also* condition
development, breast 611.8
organ or site, congenital NEC—*see* Agenesis
vagina 752.49
Unilateralis uterus 752.3
Unilocular heart 745.8
Uninhibited (neurogenic) bladder 596.54
with cauda equina syndrome 344.61
neurogenic—*see* Neurogenic, bladder 596.54
Union, abnormal —*see also* Fusion
divided tendon 727.89
larynx and trachea 748.3
Universal
joint, cervix 620.6
mesentery 751.4
Unknown
cause of death 799.9
diagnosis 799.9
Unna's disease (seborrheic dermatitis) 690.10
Unresponsiveness, adrenocorticotropin
(ACTH) 255.4
Unsoundness of mind (*see also* Psychosis) 298.9
Unspecified cause of death 799.9
Unstable
back NEC 724.9
colon 569.89
joint—*see* Instability, joint
lie 652.0
affecting fetus or newborn (before labor) 761.7
causing obstructed labor 660.0
affecting fetus or newborn 763.1

Unstable—*continued*
lumbosacral joint (congenital) 756.19
acquired 724.6
sacroiliac 724.6
spine NEC 724.9
Untruthfulness, child problem (*see also*
Disturbance, conduct) 312.0
Unverricht (-Lundborg) disease, syndrome, or
epilepsy 333.2
Unverricht-Wagner syndrome
(dermatomyositis) 710.3
Upper respiratory —*see* condition
Upset
gastric 536.8
psychogenic 306.4
gastrointestinal 536.8
psychogenic 306.4
virus (*see also* Enteritis, viral) 008.8
intestinal (large) (small) 564.9
psychogenic 306.4
menstruation 626.9
mental 300.9
stomach 536.8
psychogenic 306.4
Urachus —*see also* condition
patent 753.7
persistent 753.7
Uratic arthritis 274.0
Urbach's lipoid proteinosis 272.8
Urbach-Oppenheim disease or syndrome
(necrobiosis lipoidica diabeticorum) 250.8
[709.3]
Urbach-Wiethe disease or syndrome (lipoid
proteinosis) 272.8
Urban yellow fever 060.1
Urea, blood, high —*see* Uremia
Uremia, uremic (absorption) (amaurosis)
(amblyopia) (aphasia) (apoplexy) (coma)
(delirium) (dementia) (dropsy) (dyspnea)
(fever) (intoxication) (mania) (paralysis)
(poisoning) (toxemia) (vomiting) 586
with
abortion—*see* Abortion, by type, with renal
failure
ectopic pregnancy (*see also* categories
633.0-633.9) 639.3
hypertension (*see also* Hypertension, kidney)
403.91
molar pregnancy (*see also* categories
630-632) 639.3
chronic 585
complicating
abortion 639.3
ectopic or molar pregnancy 639.3
hypertension (*see also* Hypertension, kidney)
403.91
labor and delivery 669.3
congenital 779.89
extrarenal 788.9
hypertensive (chronic) (*see also* Hypertension,
kidney) 403.91
maternal NEC, affecting fetus or newborn 760.1
neuropathy 585 *[357.4]*
pericarditis 585 *[420.0]*
prerenal 788.9
pyelitic (*see also* Pyelitis) 590.80
Ureter, ureteral —*see* condition
Ureteralgia 788.0
Ureterectasis 593.89

Ureteritis 593.89
  cystica 590.3
  due to calculus 592.1
  gonococcal (acute) 098.19
    chronic or duration of 2 months or over 098.39
  nonspecific 593.89
Ureterocele (acquired) 593.89
  congenital 753.23
Ureterolith 592.1
Ureterolithiasis 592.1
Ureterostomy status V44.6
  with complication 997.5
Urethra, urethral —*see* condition
Urethralgia 788.9
Urethritis (abacterial) (acute) (allergic) (anterior)
  (chronic) (nonvenereal) (posterior) (recurrent)
  (simple) (subacute) (ulcerative)
  (undifferentiated) 597.80
  diplococcal (acute) 098.0
    chronic or duration of 2 months or over 098.2
  due to Trichomonas (vaginalis) 131.02
  gonococcal (acute) 098.0
    chronic or duration of 2 months or over 098.2
  nongonococcal (sexually transmitted) 099.40
    Chlamydia trachomatis 099.41
    Reiter's 099.3
    specified organism NEC 099.49
  nonspecific (sexually transmitted) (*see also*
    Urethritis, nongonococcal) 099.40
  not sexually transmitted 597.80
  Reiter's 099.3
  trichomonal or due to Trichomonas (vaginalis)
    131.02
  tuberculous (*see also* Tuberculosis) 016.3
  venereal NEC (*see also* Urethritis,
    nongonococcal) 099.40
Urethrocele
  female 618.0
    with uterine prolapse 618.4
      complete 618.3
      incomplete 618.2
  male 599.5
Urethrolithiasis 594.2
Urethro-oculoarticular syndrome 099.3
Urethro-oculosynovial syndrome 099.3
Urethrorectal —*see* condition
Urethrorrhagia 599.84
Urethrorrhea 788.7
Urethrostomy status V44.6
  with complication 997.5
Urethrotrigonitis 595.3
Urethrovaginal —*see* condition
Urhidrosis, uridrosis 705.89
Uric acid
  diathesis 274.9
  in blood 790.6
Uricacidemia 790.6
Uricemia 790.6
Uricosuria 791.9
Urination
  frequent 788.41
  painful 788.1
Urine, urinary —*see also* condition
  abnormality NEC 788.69
  blood in (*see also* Hematuria) 599.7
  discharge, excessive 788.42
  enuresis 788.30
    nonorganic origin 307.6
  extravasation 788.8
  frequency 788.41

Urine, urinary—*continued*
  incontinence 788.30
    active 788.30
    female 788.30
      stress 625.6
      and urge 788.33
    male 788.30
      stress 788.32
      and urge 788.33
    mixed (stress and urge) 788.33
    neurogenic 788.39
    nonorganic origin 307.6
    stress (female) 625.6
      male NEC 788.32
  intermittent stream 788.61
  pus in 791.9
  retention or stasis NEC 788.20
    bladder, incomplete emptying 788.21
    psychogenic 306.53
    specified NEC 788.29
  secretion
    deficient 788.5
    excessive 788.42
    frequency 788.41
  stream
    intermittent 788.61
    slowing 788.62
    splitting 788.61
    weak 788.62
Urinemia —*see* Uremia
Urinoma NEC 599.9
  bladder 596.8
  kidney 593.89
  renal 593.89
  ureter 593.89
  urethra 599.84
Uroarthritis, infectious 099.3
Urodialysis 788.5
Urolithiasis 592.9
Uronephrosis 593.89
Uropathy 599.9
  obstructive 599.6
Urosepsis 599.0
  meaning sepsis 038.9
  meaning urinary tract infection 599.0
Urticaria 708.9
  with angioneurotic edema 995.1
    hereditary 277.6
  allergic 708.0
  cholinergic 708.5
  chronic 708.8
  cold, familial 708.2
  dermatographic 708.3
  due to
    cold or heat 708.2
    drugs 708.0
    food 708.0
    inhalants 708.0
    plants 708.8
    serum 999.5
  factitial 708.3
  giant 995.1
    hereditary 277.6
  gigantea 995.1
    hereditary 277.6
  idiopathic 708.1
  larynx 995.1
    hereditary 277.6
  neonatorum 778.8
  nonallergic 708.1
  papulosa (Hebra) 698.2

Urticaria—*continued*
  perstans hemorrhagica 757.39
  pigmentosa 757.33
  recurrent periodic 708.8
  serum 999.5
  solare 692.72
  specified type NEC 708.8
  thermal (cold) (heat) 708.2
  vibratory 708.4
Urticarioides acarodermatitis 133.9
Use of
  nonprescribed drugs (*see also* Abuse, drugs,
    nondependent) 305.9
  patent medicines (*see also* Abuse, drugs,
    nondependent) 305.9
Usher-Senear disease (pemphigus
  erythematosus) 694.4
Uta 085.5
Uterine size-date discrepancy 646.8
Uteromegaly 621.2
Uterovaginal —*see* condition
Uterovesical —*see* condition
Uterus —*see* condition
Utriculitis (utriculus prostaticus) 597.89
Uveal —*see* condition
Uveitis (anterior) (*see also* Iridocyclitis) 364.3
  acute or subacute 364.00
    due to or associated with
      gonococcal infection 098.41
      herpes (simplex) 054.44
        zoster 053.22
      primary 364.01
      recurrent 364.02
      secondary (noninfectious) 364.04
        infectious 364.03
  allergic 360.11
  chronic 364.10
    due to or associated with
      sarcoidosis 135 *[364.11]*
      tuberculosis (*see also* Tuberculosis) 017.3
        [364.11]
Uveitis—*continued*
  due to
    operation 360.11
    toxoplasmosis (acquired) 130.2
      congenital (active) 771.2
  granulomatous 364.10
  heterochromic 364.21
  lens-induced 364.23
  nongranulomatous 364.00
  posterior 363.20
    disseminated—*see* Chorioretinitis,
      disseminated
    focal—*see* Chorioretinitis, focal
  recurrent 364.02
  sympathetic 360.11
  syphilitic (secondary) 091.50
    congenital 090.0 *[363.13]*
    late 095.8 *[363.13]*
  tuberculous (*see also* Tuberculosis) 017.3
    [364.11]
Uveoencephalitis 363.22
Uveokeratitis (*see also* Iridocyclitis) 364.3
Uveoparotid fever 135
Uveoparotitis 135
Uvula —*see* condition
Uvulitis (acute) (catarrhal) (chronic)
  (gangrenous) (membranous) (suppurative)
  (ulcerative) 528.3

V

Vaccination
complication or reaction—*see* Complications, vaccination
not done (contraindicated) V64.0
 because of patient's decision V64.2
prophylactic (against) V05.9
 arthropod-borne viral
  disease NEC V05.1
  encephalitis V05.0
 chickenpox V05.4
 cholera (alone) V03.0
  with typhoid-paratyphoid (cholera + TAB) V06.0
 common cold V04.7
 diphtheria (alone) V03.5
  with
   poliomyelitis (DTP + polio) V06.3
   tetanus V06.5
    -pertussis combined [DTP] V06.1
   typhoid-paratyphoid (DTP + TAB) V06.2
 disease (single) NEC V05.9
  bacterial NEC V03.9
   specified type NEC V03.89
  combinations NEC V06.9
   specified type NEC V06.8
  specified type NEC V05.8
 encephalitis, viral, arthropod-borne V05.0
 Hemophilus influenzae, type B [Hib] V03.81
 hepatitis, viral V05.3
 influenza V04.8
  with
   Streptococcus pneumoniae [pneumococcus] V06.6
 lileishmaniasis V05.2
 measles (alone) V04.2
  with mumps-rubella (MMR) V06.4
 mumps (alone) V04.6
  with measles and rubella (MMR) V06.4
 pertussis alone V03.6
 plague V03.3
 poliomyelitis V04.0
  with diphtheria-tetanus-pertussis (DTP + polio) V06.3
 rabies V04.5
 rubella (alone) V04.3
  with measles and mumps (MMR) V06.4
 smallpox V04.1
 Streptococcus pneumoniae [pneumococcus] V03.82
  with
   influenza V06.6
 tetanus toxoid (alone) V03.7
  with diphtheria [Td] V06.5
   with
    pertussis (DTP) V06.1
     with poliomyelitis (DTP + polio) V06.3
 tuberculosis (BCG) V03.2
 tularemia V03.4
 typhoid-paratyphoid (TAB) (alone) V03.1
  with diphtheria-tetanus-pertussis (TAB + DTP) V06.2
 varicella V05.4
 viral
  encephalitis, arthropod-borne V05.0
  hepatitis V05.3
 yellow fever V04.4

Vaccinia (generalized) 999.0
 congenital 771.2
 conjunctiva 999.3
 eyelids 999.0 *[373.5]*
 localized 999.3
 nose 999.3
 not from vaccination 051.0
  eyelid 051.0 *[373.5]*
 sine vaccinatione 051.0
 without vaccination 051.0
Vacuum
 extraction of fetus or newborn 763.3
 in sinus (accessory) (nasal) (*see also* Sinusitis) 473.9
Vagabond V60.0
Vagabondage V60.0
Vagabonds' disease 132.1
Vagina, vaginal —*see* condition
Vaginalitis (tunica) 608.4
Vaginismus (reflex) 625.1
 functional 306.51
 hysterical 300.11
 psychogenic 306.51
Vaginitis (acute) (chronic) (circumscribed) (diffuse) (emphysematous) (Hemophilus vaginalis) (nonspecific) (nonvenereal) (ulcerative) 616.10
 with
  abortion—*see* Abortion, by type, with sepsis
  ectopic pregnancy (*see also* categories 633.0-633.9) 639.0
  molar pregnancy (*see also* categories 630-632) 639.0
 adhesive, congenital 752.49
 atrophic, postmenopausal 627.3
 bacterial 616.10
 blennorrhagic (acute) 098.0
  chronic or duration of 2 months or over 098.2
 candidal 112.1
 chlamydial 099.53
 complicating pregnancy or puerperium 646.6
  affecting fetus or newborn 760.8
 congenital (adhesive) 752.49
 due to
  C. albicans 112.1
  Trichomonas (vaginalis) 131.01
 following
  abortion 639.0
  ectopic or molar pregnancy 639.0
 gonococcal (acute) 098.0
  chronic or duration of 2 months or over 098.2
 granuloma 099.2
 Monilia 112.1
 mycotic 112.1
 pinworm 127.4 *[616.11]*
 postirradiation 616.10
 postmenopausal atrophic 627.3
 senile (atrophic) 627.3
 syphilitic (early) 091.0
  late 095.8
 trichomonal 131.01
 tuberculous (*see also* Tuberculosis) 016.7
 venereal NEC 099.8
Vaginosis —*see* Vaginitis
Vagotonia 352.3
Vagrancy V60.0
Vallecula —*see* condition
Valley fever 114.0

Valsuani's disease (progressive pernicious
    anemia, puerperal) 648.2
Valve, valvular (formation)—*see also* condition
    cerebral ventricle (communicating) in situ V45.2
    cervix, internal os 752.49
    colon 751.5
    congenital NEC—*see* Atresia
    formation, congenital NEC—*see* Atresia
    heart defect—*see* Anomaly, heart, valve
    ureter 753.29
        pelvic junction 753.21
        vesical orifice 753.22
    urethra 753.6
Valvulitis (chronic) (*see also* Endocarditis)
    424.90
    rheumatic (chronic) (inactive) (with chorea)
        397.9
    active or acute (aortic) (mitral) (pulmonary)
        (tricuspid) 391.1
    syphilitic NEC 093.20
        aortic 093.22
        mitral 093.21
        pulmonary 093.24
        tricuspid 093.23
Valvulopathy —*see* Endocarditis
van Bogaert's leukoencephalitis (sclerosing)
    (subacute) 046.2
van Bogaert-Nijssen (-Peiffer) disease 330.0
van Buchem's syndrome (hyperostosis
    corticalis) 733.3
van Creveld-von Gierke disease (glycogenosis
    I) 271.0
van den Bergh's disease (enterogenous
    cyanosis) 289.7
van der Hoeve's syndrome (brittle bones and
    blue sclera, deafness) 756.51
**van der Hoeve-Halbertsma-Waardenburg
    syndrome** (ptosis-epicanthus) 270.2
van der Hoeve-Waardenburg-Gualdi syndrome
    (ptosis epicanthus) 270.2
Vanillism 692.89
Vanishing lung 492.0
Vanishing twin 651.33
van Neck (-Odelberg) disease or syndrome
    (juvenile osteochondrosis) 732.1
Vapor asphyxia or suffocation NEC 987.9
    specified agent—*see* Table of drugs and
        chemicals
Vaquez's disease (M9950/1) 238.4
Vaquez-Osler disease (polycythemia vera)
    (M9950/1) 238.4
Variance, lethal ball, prosthetic heart valve
    996.02
Variants, thalassemic 282.4
Variations in hair color 704.3
Varicella 052.9
    with
        complication 052.8
            specified NEC 052.7
        pneumonia 052.1
    vaccination and inoculation (prophylactic) V05.4
Varices —*see* Varix
Varicocele (scrotum) (thrombosed) 456.4
    ovary 456.5
    perineum 456.6
    spermatic cord (ulcerated) 456.4

Varicose
    aneurysm (ruptured) (*see also* Aneurysm) 442.9
    dermatitis (lower extremity)—*see* Varicose,
        vein, inflamed or infected
    eczema—*see* Varicose, vein
    phlebitis—*see* Varicose, vein, inflamed or
        infected
    placental vessel—*see* Placenta, abnormal
    tumor—*see* Varicose, vein
    ulcer (lower extremity, any part) 454.0
        anus 455.8
            external 455.5
            internal 455.2
        esophagus (*see also* Varix, esophagus) 456.1
            bleeding (*see also* Varix, esophagus,
                bleeding) 456.0
        inflamed or infected 454.2
        nasal septum 456.8
        perineum 456.6
        rectum—*see* Varicose, ulcer, anus
        scrotum 456.4
        specified site NEC 456.8
    vein (lower extremity) (ruptured) (*see also*
        Varix) 454.9
        with
            complications NEC 454.8
            edema 454.8
            inflammation or infection 454.1
                ulcerated 454.2
            pain 454.8
            stasis dermatitis 454.1
                with ulcer 454.2
            swelling 454.8
            ulcer 454.0
                inflamed or infected 454.2
        anus—*see* Hemorrhoids
        broad ligament 456.5
        congenital (peripheral) NEC 747.60
            gastrointestinal 747.61
            lower limb 747.64
            renal 747.62
            specified NEC 747.69
            upper limb 747.63
        esophagus (ulcerated) (*see also* Varix,
            esophagus) 456.1
            bleeding (*see also* Varix, esophagus,
                bleeding) 456.0
        inflamed or infected 454.1
            with ulcer 454.2
        in pregnancy or puerperium 671.0
            vulva or perineum 671.1
        nasal septum (with ulcer) 456.8
        pelvis 456.5
        perineum 456.6
            in pregnancy, childbirth, or puerperium
                671.1
        rectum—*see* Hemorrhoids
        scrotum (ulcerated) 456.4
        specified site NEC 456.8
        sublingual 456.3
        ulcerated 454.0
            inflamed or infected 454.2
        umbilical cord, affecting fetus or newborn
            762.6
        urethra 456.8
        vulva 456.6
            in pregnancy, childbirth, or puerperium
                671.1
    vessel—*see also* Varix
        placenta—*see* Placenta, abnormal

Varicosis, varicosities, varicosity (*see also* Varix) 454.9
Variola 050.9
  hemorrhagic (pustular) 050.0
  major 050.0
  minor 050.1
  modified 050.2
Varioloid 050.2
Variolosa, purpura 050.0
Varix (lower extremity) (ruptured) 454.9
  with
    complications NEC 454.8
    edema 454.8
    inflammation or infection 454.1
      with ulcer 454.2
    pain 454.8
    stasis dermatitis 454.1
      with ulcer 454.2
    swelling 454.8
    ulcer 454.0
      with inflammation or infection 454.2
  aneurysmal (*see also* Aneurysm) 442.9
  anus—*see* Hemorrhoids
  arteriovenous (congenital) (peripheral) NEC
    747.60
    gastrointestinal 747.61
    lower limb 747.64
    renal 747.62
    specified NEC 747.69
    spinal 747.82
    upper limb 747.63
  bladder 456.5
  broad ligament 456.5
  congenital (peripheral) NEC 747.60
  esophagus (ulcerated) 456.1
    bleeding 456.0
      in
        cirrhosis of liver 571.5 [456.20]
        portal hypertension 572.3 [456.20]
    congenital 747.69
      in
        cirrhosis of liver 571.5 [456.21]
          with bleeding 571.5 [456.20]
        portal hypertension 572.3 [456.21]
          with bleeding 572.3 [456.20]
  gastric 456.8
  inflamed or infected 454.1
    ulcerated 454.2
  in pregnancy or puerperium 671.0
    perineum 671.1
    vulva 671.1
  labia (majora) 456.6
  orbit 456.8
    congenital 747.69
  ovary 456.5
  papillary 448.1
  pelvis 456.5
  perineum 456.6
    in pregnancy or puerperium 671.1
  pharynx 456.8
  placenta—*see* Placenta, abnormal
  prostate 456.8
  rectum—*see* Hemorrhoids
  renal papilla 456.8
  retina 362.17
  scrotum (ulcerated) 456.4
  sigmoid colon 456.8
  specified site NEC 456.8
  spinal (cord) (vessels) 456.8
  spleen, splenic (vein) (with phlebolith) 456.8
  sublingual 456.3

Varix—*continued*
  ulcerated 454.0
    inflamed or infected 454.2
  umbilical cord, affecting fetus or newborn 762.6
  uterine ligament 456.5
  vocal cord 456.8
  vulva 456.6
    in pregnancy, childbirth, or puerperium 671.1
Vasa previa 663.5
  affecting fetus or newborn 762.6
  hemorrhage from, affecting fetus or newborn
    772.0
Vascular —*see also* condition
  loop on papilla (optic) 743.57
  sheathing, retina 362.13
  spasm 443.9
  spider 448.1
Vascularity, pulmonary, congenital 747.3
Vascularization
  choroid 362.16
  cornea 370.60
    deep 370.63
    localized 370.61
  retina 362.16
  subretinal 362.16
Vasculitis 447.6
  allergic 287.0
  cryoglobulinemic 273.2
  disseminated 447.6
  kidney 447.8
  leukocytoclastic 446.29
  nodular 695.2
  retinal 362.18
  rheumatic—*see* Fever, rheumatic
Vas deferens —*see* condition
Vas deferentitis 608.4
Vasectomy, admission for V25.2
Vasitis 608.4
  nodosa 608.4
  scrotum 608.4
  spermatic cord 608.4
  testis 608.4
  tuberculous (*see also* Tuberculosis) 016.5
  tunica vaginalis 608.4
  vas deferens 608.4
Vasodilation 443.9
Vasomotor —*see* condition
Vasoplasty, after previous sterilization V26.0
Vasoplegia, splanchnic (*see also* Neuropathy,
  peripheral, autonomic) 337.9
Vasospasm 443.9
  cerebral (artery) 435.9
    with transient neurologic deficit 435.9
  nerve
    arm NEC 354.9
    autonomic 337.9
    brachial plexus 353.0
    cervical plexus 353.2
    leg NEC 355.8
    lower extremity NEC 355.8
    peripheral NEC 355.9
    spinal NEC 355.9
    sympathetic 337.9
    upper extremity NEC 354.9
  peripheral NEC 443.9
  retina (artery) (*see also* Occlusion, retinal,
    artery) 362.30
Vasospastic —*see* condition
Vasovagal attack (paroxysmal) 780.2
  psychogenic 306.2
Vater's ampulla —*see* condition
VATER syndrome 759.89

Vegetation, vegetative
adenoid (nasal fossa) 474.2
consciousness (persistent) 780.03
endocarditis (acute) (any valve) (chronic)
(subacute) 421.0
heart (mycotic) (valve) 421.0
state (persistent) 780.03
Veil
Jackson's 751.4
over face (causing asphyxia) 768.9
Vein, venous —*see* condition
Veldt sore (*see also* Ulcer, skin) 707.9
Velpeau's hernia —*see* Hernia, femoral
Venereal
balanitis NEC 099.8
bubo 099.1
disease 099.9
specified nature or type NEC 099.8
granuloma inguinale 099.2
lymphogranuloma (Durand-Nicolas-Favre), any
site 099.1
salpingitis 098.37
urethritis (*see also* Urethritis, nongonococcal)
099.40
vaginitis NEC 099.8
warts 078.19
Vengefulness, in child (*see also* Disturbance,
conduct) 312.0
Venofibrosis 459.89
Venom, venomous
bite or sting (animal or insect) 989.5
poisoning 989.5
Venous —*see* condition
Ventouse delivery NEC 669.5
affecting fetus or newborn 763.3
Ventral —*see* condition
Ventricle, ventricular —*see also* condition
escape 427.69
standstill (*see also* Arrest, cardiac) 427.5
Ventriculitis, cerebral (*see also* Meningitis)
322.9
Ventriculostomy status V45.2
Verbiest's syndrome (claudicatio intermittens
spinalis) 435.1
Vernet's syndrome 352.6
Verneuil's disease (syphilitic bursitis) 095.7
Verruca (filiformis) 078.10
acuminata (any site) 078.11
necrogenica (primary) (*see also* Tuberculosis)
017.0
peruana 088.0
peruviana 088.0
plana (juvenilis) 078.19
plantaris 078.19
seborrheica 702.19
inflamed 702.11
senilis 702.0
tuberculosa (primary) (*see also* Tuberculosis)
017.0
venereal 078.19
viral NEC 078.10
Verrucosities (*see also* Verruca) 078.10
Verrucous endocarditis (acute) (any valve)
(chronic) (subacute) 710.0 *[424.91]*
nonbacterial 710.0 *[424.91]*
Verruga
peruana 088.0
peruviana 088.0
Verse's disease (calcinosis intervertebralis)
275.49 *[722.90]*

Version
before labor, affecting fetus or newborn 761.7
cephalic (correcting previous malposition) 652.1
affecting fetus or newborn 763.1
cervix (*see also* Malposition, uterus) 621.6
uterus (postinfectional) (postpartal, old) (*see
also* Malposition, uterus) 621.6
forward—*see* Anteversion, uterus
lateral—*see* Lateroversion, uterus
Vertebra, vertebral —*see* condition
Vertigo 780.4
auditory 386.19
aural 386.19
benign paroxysmal positional 386.11
central origin 386.2
cerebral 386.2
Dix and Hallpike (epidemic) 386.12
endemic paralytic 078.81
epidemic 078.81
Dix and Hallpike 386.12
Gerlier's 078.81
Pedersen's 386.12
vestibular neuronitis 386.12
epileptic—*see* Epilepsy
Gerlier's (epidemic) 078.81
hysterical 300.11
labyrinthine 386.10
laryngeal 786.2
malignant positional 386.2
Ménière's (*see also* Disease, Ménière's) 386.00
menopausal 627.2
otogenic 386.19
paralytic 078.81
paroxysmal positional, benign 386.11
Pedersen's (epidemic) 386.12
peripheral 386.10
specified type NEC 386.19
positional
benign paroxysmal 386.11
malignant 386.2
Verumontanitis (chronic) (*see also* Urethritis)
597.89
Vesania (*see also* Psychosis) 298.9
Vesical —*see* condition
Vesicle
cutaneous 709.8
seminal—*see* condition
skin 709.8
Vesicocolic —*see* condition
Vesicoperineal —*see* condition
Vesicorectal —*see* condition
Vesicourethrorectal —*see* condition
Vesicovaginal —*see* condition
Vesicular —*see* condition
Vesiculitis (seminal) 608.0
amebic 006.8
gonorrheal (acute) 098.14
chronic or duration of 2 months or over 098.34
trichomonal 131.09
tuberculous (*see also* Tuberculosis) 016.5
[608.81]
Vestibulitis (ear) (*see also* Labyrinthitis) 386.30
nose (external) 478.1
vulvar 616.10
Vestibulopathy, acute peripheral (recurrent)
386.12
Vestige, vestigial —*see also* Persistence
branchial 744.41
structures in vitreous 743.51
Vibriosis NEC 027.9
Vidal's disease (lichen simplex chronicus) 698.3
Video display tube syndrome 723.8

Vienna type encephalitis 049.8
Villaret's syndrome 352.6
Villous —*see* condition
VIN I (vulvar intraepithelial neoplasia I) 624.8
VIN II (vulvar intraepithelial neoplasia II) 624.8
VIN III (vulvar intraepithelial neoplasia III) 233.3
Vincent's
 angina 101
 bronchitis 101
 disease 101
 gingivitis 101
 infection (any site) 101
 laryngitis 101
 stomatitis 101
 tonsillitis 101
Vinson-Plummer syndrome (sideropenic
   dysphagia) 280.8
Viosterol deficiency (*see also* Deficiency,
   calciferol) 268.9
Virchow's disease 733.99
Viremia 790.8
Virilism (adrenal) (female) NEC 255.2
 with
   3-beta-hydroxysteroid dehydrogenase defect
     255.2
   11-hydroxylase defect 255.2
   21-hydroxylase defect 255.2
   adrenal
     hyperplasia 255.2
     insufficiency (congenital) 255.2
     cortical hyperfunction 255.2
Virilization (female) (suprarenal) (*see also*
   Virilism) 255.2
 isosexual 256.4
Virulent bubo 099.0
Virus, viral —*see also* condition
 infection NEC (*see also* Infection, viral) 079.99
 septicemia 079.99
Viscera, visceral —*see* condition
Visceroptosis 569.89
Visible peristalsis 787.4
Vision, visual
 binocular, suppression 368.31
 blurred, blurring 368.8
   hysterical 300.11
 defect, defective (*see also* Impaired, vision)
   369.9
 disorientation (syndrome) 368.16
 disturbance NEC (*see also* Disturbance, vision)
   368.9
   hysterical 300.11
 examination V72.0
 field, limitation 368.40
 fusion, with defective steropsis 368.33
 hallucinations 368.16
 halos 368.16
 loss 369.9
   both eyes (*see also* Blindness, both eyes) 369.3
   complete (*see also* Blindness, both eyes)
     369.00
   one eye 369.8
   sudden 368.16
 low (both eyes) 369.20
   one eye (other eye normal) (*see also* Impaired,
     vision) 369.70
   blindness, other eye 369.10
 perception, simultaneous without fusion 368.32
 tunnel 368.45
Vitality, lack or want of 780.79
 newborn 779.89
Vitamin deficiency NEC (*see also* Deficiency,
   vitamin) 269.2

Vitelline duct, persistent 751.0
Vitiligo 709.01
 due to pinta (carate) 103.2
 eyelid 374.53
 vulva 624.8
Vitium cordis —*see* Disease, heart
Vitreous —*see also* condition
 touch syndrome 997.99
Vocal cord —*see* condition
Vocational rehabilitation V57.22
Vogt's (Cecile) disease or syndrome 333.7
Vogt-Koyanagi syndrome 364.24
Vogt-Spielmeyer disease (amaurotic familial
   idiocy) 330.1
Voice
 change (*see also* Dysphonia) 784.49
 loss (*see also* Aphonia) 784.41
Volhard-Fahr disease (malignant
   nephrosclerosis) 403.00
Volhynian fever 083.1
Volkmann's ischemic contracture or paralysis
   (complicating trauma) 958.6
Voluntary starvation 307.1
Volvulus (bowel) (colon) (intestine) 560.2
 with
   hernia—*see also* Hernia, by site, with
     obstruction
   gangrenous—*see* Hernia, by site, with
     gangrene
   perforation 560.2
 congenital 751.5
 duodenum 537.3
 fallopian tube 620.5
 oviduct 620.5
 stomach (due to absence of gastrocolic
   ligament) 537.89
Vomiting 787.03
 with nausea 787.01
 allergic 535.4
 asphyxia 933.1
 bilious (cause unknown) 787.0
   following gastrointestinal surgery 564.3
 blood (*see also* Hematemesis) 578.0
 causing asphyxia, choking, or suffocation (*see
   also* Asphyxia, food) 933.1
 cyclical 536.2
   psychogenic 306.4
 epidemic 078.82
 fecal matter 569.89
 following gastrointestinal surgery 564.3
 functional 536.8
   psychogenic 306.4
 habit 536.2
 hysterical 300.11
 nervous 306.4
 neurotic 306.4
 newborn 779.3
 of or complicating pregnancy 643.9
   due to
     organic disease 643.8
     specific cause NEC 643.8
   early—*see* Hyperemesis, gravidarum
   late (after 22 completed weeks of gestation)
     643.2
 pernicious or persistent 536.2
   complicating pregnancy—*see* Hyperemesis,
     gravidarum
   psychogenic 306.4
 physiological 787.0
 psychic 306.4
 psychogenic 307.54

Vomiting—*continued*
  stercoral 569.89
  uncontrollable 536.2
    psychogenic 306.4
  uremic—*see* Uremia
  winter 078.82
von Bechterew (-Strumpell) disease or syndrome
    (ankylosing spondylitis) 720.0
von Bezold's abscess 383.01
von Economo's disease (encephalitis lethargica)
    049.8
von Eulenburg's disease (congenital
    paramyotonia) 359.2
von Gierke's disease (glycogenosis I) 271.0
von Gies' joint 095.8
von Graefe's disease or syndrome 378.72
von Hippel (-Lindau) disease or syndrome
    (retinocerebral angiomatosis) 759.6
von Jaksch's anemia or disease
    (pseudoleukemia infantum) 285.8
von Recklinghausen's
  disease or syndrome (nerves) (skin) (M9540/1)
    237.71
  bones (osteitis fibrosa cystica) 252.0
  tumor (M9540/1) 237.71
von Recklinghausen-Applebaum disease
    (hemochromatosis) 275.0
von Schroetter's syndrome (intermittent venous
    claudication) 453.8
von Willebrand (-Jürgens) (-Minot) disease or
    syndrome (angiohemophilia) 286.4
von Zambusch's disease (lichen sclerosus et
    atrophicus) 701.0
Voorhoeve's disease or dyschondroplasia 756.4
Vossius' ring 921.3
  late effect 366.21
Voyeurism 302.82
Vrolik's disease (osteogenesis imperfecta) 756.51
Vulva —*see* condition
Vulvismus 625.1
Vulvitis (acute) (allergic) (aphthous) (chronic)
    (gangrenous) (hypertrophic) (intertriginous)
    616.10
  with
    abortion—*see* Abortion, by type, with sepsis
    ectopic pregnancy (*see also* categories
      633.0-633.9) 639.0
    molar pregnancy (*see also* categories
      630-632) 639.0
  adhesive, congenital 752.49
  blennorrhagic (acute) 098.0
    chronic or duration of 2 months or over 098.2
  chlamydial 099.53
  complicating pregnancy or puerperium 646.6
  due to Ducrey's bacillus 099.0
  following
    abortion 639.0
    ectopic or molar pregnancy 639.0
  gonococcal (acute) 098.0
    chronic or duration of 2 months or over 098.2
  herpetic 054.11
  leukoplakic 624.0
  monilial 112.1
  puerperal, postpartum, childbirth 646.6
  syphilitic (early) 091.0
    late 095.8
  trichomonal 131.01
Vulvodynia 625.9
Vulvorectal —*see* condition

Vulvovaginitis (*see also* Vulvitis) 616.10
  amebic 006.8
  chlamydial 099.53
  gonococcal (acute) 098.0
    chronic or duration of 2 months or over 098.2
  herpetic 054.11
  monilial 112.1
  trichomonal (Trichomonas vaginalis) 131.01

Waardenburg's syndrome 756.89
meaning ptosis-epicanthus 270.2
Waardenburg-Klein syndrome
(ptosis-epicanthus) 270.2
Wagner's disease (colloid milium) 709.3
Wagner (-Unverricht) syndrome
(dermatomyositis) 710.3
Waiting list, person on V63.2
undergoing social agency investigation V63.8
Wakefulness disorder (*see also* Hypersomnia)
780.54
nonorganic origin 307.43
Waldenström's
disease (osteochondrosis, capital femoral) 732.1
hepatitis (lupoid hepatitis) 571.49
hypergammaglobulinemia 273.0
macroglobulinemia 273.3
purpura, hypergammaglobulinemic 273.0
syndrome (macroglobulinemia) 273.3
Waldenström-Kjellberg syndrome (sideropenic
dysphagia) 280.8
Walking
difficulty 719.7
psychogenic 307.9
sleep 307.46
hysterical 300.13
Wall, abdominal —*see* condition
Wallenberg's syndrome (posterior inferior
cerebellar artery) (*see also* Disease,
cerebrovascular, acute) 436
Wallgren's
disease (obstruction of splenic vein with
collateral circulation) 459.89
meningitis (*see also* Meningitis, aseptic) 047.9
Wandering
acetabulum 736.39
gallbladder 751.69
kidney, congenital 753.3
organ or site, congenital NEC—*see*
Malposition, congenital
pacemaker (atrial) (heart) 427.89
spleen 289.59
Wardrop's disease (with lymphangitis) 681.9
finger 681.02
toe 681.11
War neurosis 300.16
Wart (common) (digitate) (filiform) (infectious)
(juvenile) (plantar) (viral) 078.10
external genital organs (venereal) 078.19
fig 078.19
Hassall-Henle's (of cornea) 371.41
Henle's (of cornea) 371.41
juvenile 078.19
moist 078.10
Peruvian 088.0
plantar 078.19
prosector (*see also* Tuberculosis) 017.0
seborrheic 702.19
inflamed 702.11
senile 702.0
specified NEC 078.19
syphilitic 091.3
tuberculous (*see also* Tuberculosis) 017.0
venereal (female) (male) 078.19
Warthin's tumor (salivary gland) (M8561/0)
210.2
Washerwoman's itch 692.4

Wassilieff's disease (leptospiral jaundice) 100.0
Wasting
disease 799.4
due to malnutrition 261
extreme (due to malnutrition) 261
muscular NEC 728.2
palsy, paralysis 335.21
Water
clefts 366.12
deprivation of 994.3
in joint (*see also* Effusion, joint) 719.0
intoxication 276.6
itch 120.3
lack of 994.3
loading 276.6
on
brain—*see* Hydrocephalus
chest 511.8
poisoning 276.6
Waterbrash 787.1
Water-hammer pulse (*see also* Insufficiency,
aortic) 424.1
Waterhouse (-Friderichsen) disease or syndrome
036.3
Water-losing nephritis 588.8
Wax in ear 380.4
Waxy
degeneration, any site 277.3
disease 277.3
kidney 277.3 *[583.81]*
liver (large) 277.3
spleen 277.3
Weak, weakness (generalized) 780.79
arches (acquired) 734
congenital 754.61
bladder sphincter 596.59
congenital 779.89
eye muscle—*see* Strabismus
foot (double)—*see* Weak, arches
heart, cardiac (*see also* Failure, heart) 428.9
congenital 746.9
mind 317
muscle 728.9
myocardium (*see also* Failure, heart) 428.9
newborn 779.89
pelvic fundus 618.8
pulse 785.9
senile 797
valvular—*see* Endocarditis
Wear, worn, tooth, teeth (approximal) (hard
tissues) (interproximal) (occlusal) 521.1
Weather, weathered
effects of
cold NEC 991.9
specified effect NEC 991.8
hot (*see also* Heat) 992.9
skin 692.74
Web, webbed (congenital)—*see also* Anomaly,
specified type NEC
canthus 743.63
digits (*see also* Syndactylism) 755.10
esophagus 750.3
fingers (*see also* Syndactylism, fingers) 755.11
larynx (glottic) (subglottic) 748.2
neck (pterygium colli) 744.5
Paterson-Kelly (sideropenic dysphagia) 280.8
popliteal syndrome 756.89
toes (*see also* Syndactylism, toes) 755.13

Weber's paralysis or syndrome 344.89
Weber-Christian disease or syndrome (nodular nonsuppurative panniculitis) 729.30
Weber-Cockayne syndrome (epidermolysis bullosa) 757.39
Weber-Dimitri syndrome 759.6
Weber-Gubler syndrome 344.89
Weber-Leyden syndrome 344.89
Weber-Osler syndrome (familial hemorrhagic telangiectasia) 448.0
Wedge-shaped or wedging vertebra (*see also* Osteoporosis) 733.00
Wegener's granulomatosis or syndrome 446.4
Wegner's disease (syphilitic osteochondritis) 090.0
Weight
  gain (abnormal) (excessive) 783.1
    during pregnancy 646.1
      insufficient 646.8
  less than 1000 grams at birth 765.0
  loss (cause unknown) 783.21
Weightlessness 994.9
Weil's disease (leptospiral jaundice) 100.00
Weill-Marchesani syndrome (brachymorphism and ectopia lentis) 759.89
Weingarten's syndrome (tropical eosinophilia) 518.3
Weir Mitchell's disease (erythromelalgia) 443.89
Weiss-Baker syndrome (carotid sinus syncope) 337.0
Weissenbach-Thibierge syndrome (cutaneous systemic sclerosis) 710.1
Wen (*see also* Cyst, sebaceous) 706.2
Wenckebach's phenomenon, heart block (second degree) 426.13
Werdnig-Hoffmann syndrome (muscular atrophy) 335.0
Werlhof's disease (*see also* Purpura, thrombocytopenic) 287.3
Werlhof-Wichmann syndrome (*see also* Purpura, thrombocytopenic) 287.3
Wermer's syndrome or disease (polyendocrine adenomatosis) 258.0
Werner's disease or syndrome (progeria adultorum) 259.8
Werner-His disease (trench fever) 083.1
Werner-Schultz disease (agranulocytosis) 288.0
Wernicke's encephalopathy, disease or syndrome (superior hemorrhagic polioencephalitis) 265.1
Wernicke-Korsakoff syndrome or psychosis (nonalcoholic) 294.0
  alcoholic 291.1
Wernicke-Posadas disease (*see also* Coccidioidomycosis) 114.9
Wesselsbron fever 066.3
West African fever 084.8
West Nile fever 066.4
West Nile virus 066.4
Westphal-Strümpell syndrome (hepatolenticular degeneration) 275.1
Wet
  brain (alcoholic) (*see also* Alcoholism) 303.9
  feet, tropical (syndrome) (maceration) 991.4
  lung (syndrome)
    adult 518.5
    newborn 770.6
Wharton's duct —*see* condition
Wheal 709.8
Wheezing 786.07
Whiplash injury or syndrome 847.0

Whipple's disease or syndrome (intestinal lipodystrophy) 040.2
Whipworm 127.3
"Whistling face" syndrome (craniocarpotarsal dystrophy) 759.89
White —*see also* condition
  kidney
    large—*see* Nephrosis
    small 582.9
  leg, puerperal, postpartum, childbirth 671.4
    nonpuerperal 451.19
  mouth 112.0
  patches of mouth 528.6
  sponge nevus of oral mucosa 750.26
  spot lesions, teeth 521.01
White's disease (congenital) (keratosis follicularis) 757.39
Whitehead 706.2
Whitlow (with lymphangitis) 681.01
  herpetic 054.6
Whitmore's disease or fever (melioidosis) 025
Whooping cough 033.9
  with pneumonia 033.9 *[484.3]*
  due to
    Bordetella
      bronchoseptica 033.8
        with pneumonia 033.8 *[484.3]*
      parapertussis 033.1
        with pneumonia 033.1 *[484.3]*
      pertussis 033.0
        with pneumonia 033.0 *[484.3]*
    specified organism NEC 033.8
      with pneumonia 033.8 *[484.3]*
  vaccination, prophylactic (against) V03.6
Wichmann's asthma (laryngismus stridulus) 478.75
Widal (-Abrami) syndrome (acquired hemolytic jaundice) 283.9
Widening aorta (*see also* Aneurysm, aorta) 441.9
  ruptured 441.5
Wilkie's disease or syndrome 557.1
Wilkinson-Sneddon disease or syndrome (subcorneal pustular dermatosis) 694.1
Willan's lepra 696.1
Willan-Plumbe syndrome (psoriasis) 696.1
Willebrand (-Jürgens) syndrome or thrombopathy (angiohemophilia) 286.4
Willi-Prader syndrome (hypogenital dystrophy with diabetic tendency) 759.81
Willis' disease (diabetes mellitus) (*see also* Diabetes) 250.0
Wilms' tumor or neoplasm (nephroblastoma) (M8960/3) 189.0
Wilson's
  disease or syndrome (hepatolenticular degeneration) 275.1
  hepatolenticular degeneration 275.1
  lichen ruber 697.0
Wilson-Brocq disease (dermatitis exfoliativa) 695.89
Wilson-Mikity syndrome 770.7
Window —*see also* Imperfect, closure
  aorticopulmonary 745.0
Winged scapula 736.89
Winter —*see also* condition
  vomiting disease 078.82
Wise's disease 696.2
Wiskott-Aldrich syndrome (eczema-thrombocytopenia) 279.12

Withdrawal symptoms, syndrome
  alcohol 291.81
    delirium (acute) 291.0
      chronic 291.1
      newborn 760.71
  drug or narcotic 292.0
  newborn, infant of dependent mother 779.5
  steroid NEC
    correct substance properly administered 255.4
    overdose or wrong substance given or taken
      962.0
Withdrawing reaction, child or adolescent
    313.22
Witts' anemia (achlorhydric anemia) 280.9
Witzelsucht 301.9
Woakes' syndrome (ethmoiditis) 471.1
Wohlfart-Kugelberg-Welander disease 335.11
Woillez's disease (acute idiopathic pulmonary
    congestion) 518.5
Wolff-Parkinson-White syndrome (anomalous
    atrioventricular excitation) 426.7
Wolhynian fever 083.1
Wolman's disease (primary familial
    xanthomatosis) 272.7
Wood asthma 495.8
Woolly, wooly hair (congenital) (nevus) 757.4
Wool-sorters' disease 022.1
Word
  blindness (congenital) (developmental) 315.01
    secondary to organic lesion 784.61
  deafness (secondary to organic lesion) 784.69
    developmental 315.31
Worm (s) (colic) (fever) (infection) (infestation)
    (*see also* Infestation) 128.9
  guinea 125.7
  in intestine NEC 127.9
Worm-eaten soles 102.3
Worn out (*see also* Exhaustion) 780.79
"Worried well" V65.5
Wound, open (by cutting or piercing instrument)
    (by firearms) (cut) (dissection) (incised)
    (laceration) (penetration) (perforating)
    (puncture) (with initial hemorrhage, not
    internal) 879.8

*Note—For fracture with open wound, see
Fracture. For laceration, traumatic rupture,
tear or penetrating wound of internal organs,
such as heart, lung, liver, kidney, pelvic organs,
etc., whether or not accompanied by open
wound or fracture in the same region, see
Injury, internal. For contused wound, see
Contusion. For crush injury, see Crush. For
abrasion, insect bite (nonvenomous), blister, or
scratch, see Injury, superficial.*

*Complicated includes wounds with:
  delayed healing
  delayed treatment
  foreign body
  primary infection*

*For late effect of open wound, see Late, effect,
wound, open, by site.*

  abdomen, abdominal (external) (muscle) 879.2
    complicated 879.3
    wall (anterior) 879.2
      complicated 879.3
      lateral 879.4
        complicated 879.5

Wound, open—*continued*
  alveolar (process) 873.62
    complicated 873.72
  ankle 891.0
    with tendon involvement 891.2
    complicated 891.1
  anterior chamber, eye (*see also* Wound, open,
    intraocular) 871.9
  anus 879.6
    complicated 879.7
  arm 884.0
    with tendon involvement 884.2
    complicated 884.1
    forearm 881.00
      with tendon involvement 881.20
      complicated 881.10
    multiple sites—*see* Wound, open, multiple,
      upper limb
    upper 880.03
      with tendon involvement 880.23
      complicated 880.13
      multiple sites (with axillary or shoulder
        regions) 880.09
        with tendon involvement 880.29
        complicated 880.19
  artery—*see* Injury, blood vessel, by site
  auditory
    canal (external) (meatus) 872.02
      complicated 872.12
    ossicles (incus) (malleus) (stapes) 872.62
      complicated 872.72
  auricle, ear 872.01
    complicated 872.11
  axilla 880.02
    with tendon involvement 880.22
    complicated 880.12
      with tendon involvement 880.29
    involving other sites of upper arm 880.09
      complicated 880.19
  back 876.0
    complicated 876.1
  bladder—*see* Injury, internal, bladder
  blood vessel—*see* Injury, blood vessel, by site
  brain—*see* Injury, intracranial, with open
    intracranial wound
  breast 879.0
    complicated 879.1
  brow 873.42
    complicated 873.52
  buccal mucosa 873.61
    complicated 873.71
  buttock 877.0
    complicated 877.1
  calf 891.0
    with tendon involvement 891.2
    complicated 891.1
  canaliculus lacrimalis 870.8
    with laceration of eyelid 870.2
  canthus, eye 870.8
    laceration—*see* Laceration, eyelid
  cavernous sinus—*see* Injury, intracranial
  cerebellum—*see* Injury, intracranial
  cervical esophagus 874.4
    complicated 874.5
  cervix—*see* Injury, internal, cervix
  cheek(s) (external) 873.41
    complicated 873.51
    internal 873.61
      complicated 873.71
  chest (wall) (external) 875.0
    complicated 875.1

Wound, open—*continued*
  chin 873.44
    complicated 873.54
  choroid 363.63
  ciliary body (eye) (*see also* Wound, open,
    intraocular) 871.9
  clitoris 878.8
    complicated 878.9
  cochlea 872.64
    complicated 872.74
  complicated 879.9
  conjunctiva—*see* Wound, open, intraocular
  cornea (nonpenetrating) (*see also* Wound, open,
    intraocular) 871.9
  costal region 875.0
    complicated 875.1
  Descemet's membrane (*see also* Wound, open,
    intraocular) 871.9
  digit(s)
    foot 893.0
      with tendon involvement 893.2
      complicated 893.1
    hand 883.0
      with tendon involvement 883.2
      complicated 883.1
  drumhead, ear 872.61
    complicated 872.71
  ear 872.8
    canal 872.02
      complicated 872.12
    complicated 872.9
    drum 872.61
      complicated 872.71
    external 872.00
      complicated 872.10
    multiple sites 872.69
      complicated 872.79
    ossicles (incus) (malleus) (stapes) 872.62
      complicated 872.72
    specified part NEC 872.69
      complicated 872.79
  elbow 881.01
    with tendon involvement 881.21
    complicated 881.11
  epididymis 878.2
    complicated 878.3
  epigastric region 879.2
    complicated 879.3
  epiglottis 874.01
    complicated 874.11
  esophagus (cervical) 874.4
    complicated 874.5
    thoracic—*see* Injury, internal, esophagus
  Eustachian tube 872.63
    complicated 872.73
  extremity
    lower (multiple) NEC 894.0
      with tendon involvement 894.2
      complicated 894.1
    upper (multiple) NEC 884.0
      with tendon involvement 884.2
      complicated 884.1
  eye(s) (globe)—*see* Wound, open, intraocular
  eyeball NEC 871.9
    laceration (*see also* Laceration, eyeball) 871.4
    penetrating (*see also* Penetrating wound,
      eyeball) 871.7
  eyebrow 873.42
    complicated 873.52
  eyelid NEC 870.8
    laceration—*see* Laceration, eyelid

Wound, open—*continued*
  face 873.40
    complicated 873.50
    multiple sites 873.49
      complicated 873.59
    specified part NEC 873.49
      complicated 873.59
  fallopian tube—*see* Injury, internal, fallopian
    tube
  finger(s) (nail) (subungual) 883.0
    with tendon involvement 883.2
    complicated 883.1
  flank 879.4
    complicated 879.5
  foot (any part except toe(s) alone) 892.0
    with tendon involvement 892.2
    complicated 892.1
  forearm 881.00
    with tendon involvement 881.20
    complicated 881.10
  forehead 873.42
    complicated 873.52
  genital organs (external) NEC 878.8
    complicated 878.9
    internal—*see* Injury, internal, by site
  globe (eye) (*see also* Wound, open, eyeball)
    871.9
  groin 879.4
    complicated 879.5
  gum(s) 873.62
    complicated 873.72
  hand (except finger(s) alone) 882.0
    with tendon involvement 882.2
    complicated 882.1
  head NEC 873.8
    with intracranial injury—*see* Injury,
      intracranial
      due to or associated with skull fracture—*see*
        Fracture, skull
    complicated 873.9
    scalp—*see* Wound, open, scalp
  heel 892.0
    with tendon involvement 892.2
    complicated 892.1
  high-velocity (grease gun)—*see* Wound, open,
    complicated, by site
  hip 890.0
    with tendon involvement 890.2
    complicated 890.1
  hymen 878.6
    complicated 878.7
  hypochondrium 879.4
    complicated 879.5
  hypogastric region 879.2
    complicated 879.3
  iliac (region) 879.4
    complicated 879.5
  incidental to
    dislocation—*see* Dislocation, open, by site
    fracture—*see* Fracture, open, by site
    intracranial injury—*see* Injury, intracranial,
      with open intracranial wound
    nerve injury—*see* Injury, nerve, by site
  inguinal region 879.4
    complicated 879.5
  instep 892.0
    with tendon involvement 892.2
    complicated 892.1
  interscapular region 876.0
    complicated 876.1

Wound, open—*continued*
  intracranial—*see* Injury, intracranial, with open
      intracranial wound
  intraocular 871.9
    with
        partial loss (of intraocular tissue) 871.2
        prolapse or exposure (of intraocular tissue)
            871.1
    laceration (*see also* Laceration, eyeball) 871.4
    penetrating 871.7
        with foreign body (nonmagnetic) 871.6
            magnetic 871.5
    without prolapse (of intraocular tissue) 871.0
  iris (*see also* Wound, open, eyeball) 871.9
  jaw (fracture not involved) 873.44
    with fracture—*see* Fracture, jaw
    complicated 873.54
  knee 891.0
    with tendon involvement 891.2
    complicated 891.1
  labium (majus) (minus) 878.4
    complicated 878.5
  lacrimal apparatus, gland, or sac 870.8
    with laceration of eyelid 870.2
  larynx 874.01
    with trachea 874.00
        complicated 874.10
    complicated 874.11
  leg (multiple) 891.0
    with tendon involvement 891.2
    complicated 891.1
    lower 891.0
        with tendon involvement 891.2
        complicated 891.1
    thigh 890.0
        with tendon involvement 890.2
        complicated 890.1
    upper 890.0
        with tendon involvement 890.2
        complicated 890.1
  lens (eye) (alone) (*see also* Cataract, traumatic)
      366.20
    with involvement of other eye structures—*see*
        Wound, open, eyeball
  limb
    lower (multiple) NEC 894.0
        with tendon involvement 894.2
        complicated 894.1
    upper (multiple) NEC 884.0
        with tendon involvement 884.2
        complicated 884.1
  lip 873.43
    complicated 873.53
  loin 876.0
    complicated 876.1
  lumbar region 876.0
    complicated 876.1
  malar region 873.41
    complicated 873.51
  mastoid region 873.49
    complicated 873.59
  mediastinum—*see* Injury, internal, mediastinum
  midthoracic region 875.0
    complicated 875.1
  mouth 873.60
    complicated 873.70
    floor 873.64
        complicated 873.74
    multiple sites 873.69
        complicated 873.79

Wound, open—*continued*
  specified site NEC 873.69
    complicated 873.79
  multiple, unspecified site(s) 879.8

> *Note*—*Multiple open wounds of sites*
> *classifiable to the same four-digit category*
> *should be classified to that category unless they*
> *are in different limbs.*
>
> *Multiple open wounds of sites classifiable to*
> *different four-digit categories, or to different*
> *limbs, should be coded separately.*

    complicated 879.9
    lower limb(s) (one or both) (sites classifiable
        to more than one three-digit category in
        890 to 893) 894.0
        with tendon involvement 894.2
        complicated 894.1
    upper limb(s) (one or both) (sites classifiable
        to more than one three-digit category in
        880 to 883) 884.0
        with tendon involvement 884.2
        complicated 884.1
  muscle—*see* Sprain, by site
  nail
    finger(s) 883.0
        complicated 883.1
    thumb 883.0
        complicated 883.1
    toe(s) 893.0
        complicated 893.1
  nape (neck) 874.8
    complicated 874.9
    specified part NEC 874.8
        complicated 874.9
  nasal—*see also* Wound, open, nose
    cavity 873.22
        complicated 873.32
    septum 873.21
        complicated 873.31
    sinuses 873.23
        complicated 873.33
  nasopharynx 873.22
    complicated 873.32
  neck 874.8
    complicated 874.9
    nape 874.8
        complicated 874.9
    specified part NEC 874.8
        complicated 874.9
  nerve—*see* Injury, nerve, by site
  non-healing surgical 998.83
  nose 873.20
    complicated 873.30
    multiple sites 873.29
        complicated 873.39
    septum 873.21
        complicated 873.31
    sinuses 873.23
        complicated 873.33
  occipital region—*see* Wound, open, scalp
  ocular NEC 871.9
    adnexa 870.9
        specified region NEC 870.8
    laceration (*see also* Laceration, ocular) 871.4
    muscle (extraocular) 870.3
        with foreign body 870.4
        eyelid 870.1
        intraocular—*see* Wound, open, eyeball

Wound, open—*continued*
 uvula 873.69
  complicated 873.79
 vagina 878.6
  complicated 878.7
 vas deferens—*see* Injury, internal, vas deferens
 vitreous (humor) 871.2
 vulva 878.4
  complicated 878.5
 wrist 881.02
  with tendon involvement 881.22
  complicated 881.12
Wright's syndrome (hyperabduction) 447.8
 pneumonia 390 *[517.1]*
Wringer injury —*see* Crush injury, by site
Wrinkling of skin 701.8
Wrist —*see also* condition
 drop (acquired) 736.05
Wrong drug (given in error) NEC 977.9
 specified drug or substance—*see* Table of drugs
   and chemicals
Wry neck —*see also* Torticollis
 congenital 754.1
Wuchereria infestation 125.0
 bancrofti 125.0
 Brugia malayi 125.1
 malayi 125.1
Wuchereriasis 125.0
Wuchereriosis 125.0
Wuchernde struma langhans (M8332/3) 193

X

Xanthelasma 272.2
  eyelid 272.2 *[374.51]*
  palpebrarum 272.2 *[374.51]*
Xanthelasmatosis (essential) 272.2
Xanthelasmoidea 757.33
Xanthine stones 277.2
Xanthinuria 277.2
Xanthofibroma (M8831/0)—*see* Neoplasm,
  connective tissue, benign
Xanthoma (s), xanthomatosis 272.2
  with
    hyperlipoproteinemia
      type I 272.3
      type III 272.2
      type IV 272.1
      type V 272.3
  bone 272.7
  craniohypophyseal 277.8
  cutaneotendinous 272.7
  diabeticorum 250.8 *[272.2]*
  disseminatum 272.7
  eruptive 272.2
  eyelid 272.2 *[374.51]*
  familial 272.7
  hereditary 272.7
  hypercholesterinemic 272.0
  hypercholesterolemic 272.0
  hyperlipemic 272.4
  hyperlipidemic 272.4
  infantile 272.7
  joint 272.7
  juvenile 272.7
  multiple 272.7
  multiplex 272.7
  primary familial 272.7
  tendon (sheath) 272.7
  tuberosum 272.2
  tuberous 272.2
  tubo-eruptive 272.2
Xanthosis 709.09
  surgical 998.81
Xenophobia 300.29
Xeroderma (congenital) 757.39
  acquired 701.1
    eyelid 373.33
  eyelid 373.33
  pigmentosum 757.33
  vitamin A deficiency 264.8
Xerophthalmia 372.53
  vitamin A deficiency 264.7
Xerosis
  conjunctiva 372.53
    with Bitôt's spot 372.53
      vitamin A deficiency 264.1
    vitamin A deficiency 264.0
  cornea 371.40
    with corneal ulceration 370.00
      vitamin A deficiency 264.3
    vitamin A deficiency 264.2
  cutis 706.8
  skin 706.8
Xerostomia 527.7
Xiphodynia 733.90
Xiphoidalgia 733.90
Xiphoiditis 733.99
Xiphopagus 759.4
XO syndrome 758.6

X-ray
  effects, adverse, NEC 990
  of chest
    for suspected tuberculosis V71.2
    routine V72.5
XXX syndrome 758.81
XXXXY syndrome 758.81
XXY syndrome 758.7
Xyloketosuria 271.8
Xylosuria 271.8
Xylulosuria 271.8
XYY syndrome 758.81

Y

Yawning 786.09
  psychogenic 306.1
Yaws 102.9
  bone or joint lesions 102.6
  butter 102.1
  chancre 102.0
  cutaneous, less than five years after infection
    102.2
  early (cutaneous) (macular) (maculopapular)
    (micropapular) (papular) 102.2
    frambeside 102.2
    skin lesions NEC 102.2
  eyelid 102.9 *[373.4]*
  ganglion 102.6
  gangosis, gangosa 102.5
  gumma, gummata 102.4
    bone 102.6
  gummatous
    frambeside 102.4
    osteitis 102.6
    periostitis 102.6
  hydrarthrosis 102.6
  hyperkeratosis (early) (late) (palmar) (plantar)
    102.3
  initial lesions 102.0
  joint lesions 102.6
  juxta-articular nodules 102.7
  late nodular (ulcerated) 102.4
  latent (without clinical manifestations) (with
    positive serology) 102.8
  mother 102.0
  mucosal 102.7
  multiple papillomata 102.1
  nodular, late (ulcerated) 102.4
  osteitis 102.6
  papilloma, papillomata (palmar) (plantar) 102.1
  periostitis (hypertrophic) 102.6
  ulcers 102.4
  wet crab 102.1
Yeast infection (*see also* Candidiasis) 112.9
Yellow
  atrophy (liver) 570
    chronic 571.8
    resulting from administration of blood,
      plasma, serum, or other biological
      substance (within 8 months of
      administration)—*see* Hepatitis, viral
  fever—*see* Fever, yellow
  jack (*see also* Fever, yellow) 060.9
  jaundice (*see also* Jaundice) 782.4
Yersinia septica 027.8

Z

Zagari's disease (xerostomia) 527.7
Zahorsky's disease (exanthema subitum) 057.8
  syndrome (herpangina) 074.0
Zenker's diverticulum (esophagus) 530.6
Ziehen-Oppenheim disease 333.6
Zieve's syndrome (jaundice, hyperlipemia, and
  hemolytic anemia) 571.1
Zika fever 066.3
Zollinger-Ellison syndrome (gastric
  hypersecretion with pancreatic islet cell
  tumor) 251.5
Zona (*see also* Herpes, zoster) 053.9
Zoophilia (erotica) 302.1
Zoophobia 300.29
Zoster (herpes) (*see also* Herpes, zoster) 053.9
Zuelzer (-Ogden) anemia or syndrome
  (nutritional megaloblastic anemia) 281.2
Zygodactyly (*see also* Syndactylism) 755.10
Zygomycosis 117.7
Zymotic —*see* condition

SECTION 2

ALPHABETIC INDEX TO POISONING AND EXTERNAL CAUSES OF ADVERSE EFFECTS OF DRUGS AND OTHER CHEMICAL SUBSTANCES

TABLE OF DRUGS AND CHEMICALS

This table contains a classification of drugs and other chemical substances to identify poisoning states and external causes of adverse effects.

Each of the listed substances in the table is assigned a code according to the poisoning classification (960–989). These codes are used when there is a statement of poisoning, overdose, wrong substance given or taken, or intoxication.

The table also contains a listing of external causes of adverse effects. An adverse effect is a pathologic manifestation due to ingestion or exposure to drugs or other chemical substances (e.g., dermatitis, hypersensitivity reaction, aspirin gastritis). The adverse effect is to be identified by the appropriate code found in Section 1, Index to Diseases and Injuries. An external cause code can then be used to identify the circumstances involved. The table headings pertaining to external causes are defined below:

Accidental poisoning (E850–E869)—accidental overdose of drug, wrong substance given or taken, drug taken inadvertently, accidents in the usage of drugs and biologicals in medical and surgical procedures, and to show external causes of poisonings classifiable to 980–989.

Therapeutic use (E930–E949)—a correct substance properly administered in therapeutic or prophylactic dosage as the external cause of adverse effects.

Suicide attempt (E950–E952)—instances in which self–inflicted injuries or poisonings are involved.

Assault (E961–E962)—injury or poisoning inflicted by another person with the intent to injure or kill.

Undetermined (E980–E982)—to be used when the intent of the poisoning or injury cannot be determined whether it was intentional or accidental.

The American Hospital Formulary Service list numbers are included in the table to help classify new drugs not identified in the table by name. The AHFS list numbers are keyed to the continually revised American Hospital Formulary Service (AHFS).* These listings are found in the table under the main term **Drug**.

Excluded from the table are radium and other radioactive substances. The classification of adverse effects and complications pertaining to these substances will be found in Section 1, Index to Diseases and Injuries, and Section 3, Index to External Causes of Injuries.

Although certain substances are indexed with one or more subentries, the majority are listed according to one use or state. It is recognized that many substances may be used in various ways, in medicine and in industry, and may cause adverse effects whatever the state of the agent (solid, liquid, or fumes arising from a liquid). In cases in which the reported data indicates a use or state not in the table, or which is clearly different from the one listed, an attempt should be made to classify the substance in the form which most nearly expresses the reported facts.

---

*American Hospital Formulary Service, 2 vol. (Washington, DC: American Society of Hospital Pharmacists, 1959-)

Substance	Poisoning	External Cause (E-Code)				
		Accident	Therapeutic Use	Suicide Attempt	Assault	Undetermined
1–propanol	980.3	E860.4	—	E950.9	E962.1	E980.9
2–propanol	980.2	E860.3	—	E950.9	E962.1	E980.9
2, 4–D (dichlorophenoxyacetic acid)	989.4	E863.5	—	E950.6	E962.1	E980.7
2, 4–toluene diisocyanate	983.0	E864.0	—	E950.7	E962.1	E980.6
2, 4, 5–T (trichlorophenoxyacetic acid)	989.2	E863.5	—	E950.6	E962.1	E980.7
14–hydroxydihydromorphinone	965.09	E850.2	E935.2	E950.0	E962.0	E980.0
ABOB	961.7	E857	E931.7	E950.4	E962.0	E980.4
Abrus (seed)	988.2	E865.3	—	E950.9	E962.1	E980.9
Absinthe	980.0	E860.1	—	E950.9	E962.1	E980.9
beverage	980.0	E860.0	—	E950.9	E962.1	E980.9
Acenocoumarin, acenocoumarol	964.2	E858.2	E934.2	E950.4	E962.0	E980.4
Acepromazine	969.1	E853.0	E939.1	E950.3	E962.0	E980.3
Acetal	982.8	E862.4	—	E950.9	E962.1	E980.9
Acetaldehyde (vapor)	987.8	E869.8	—	E952.8	E962.2	E982.8
liquid	989.89	E866.8	—	E950.9	E962.1	E980.9
Acetaminophen	965.4	E850.4	E935.4	E950.0	E962.0	E980.0
Acetaminosalol	965.1	E850.3	E935.3	E950.0	E962.0	E980.0
Acetanilid(e)	965.4	E850.4	E935.4	E950.0	E962.0	E980.0
Acetarsol, acetarsone	961.1	E857	E931.1	E950.4	E962.0	E980.4
Acetazolamide	974.2	E858.5	E944.2	E950.4	E962.0	E980.4
Acetic						
acid	983.1	E864.1	—	E950.7	E962.1	E980.6
with sodium acetate (ointment)	976.3	E858.7	E946.3	E950.4	E962.0	E980.4
irrigating solution	974.5	E858.5	E944.5	E950.4	E962.0	E980.4
lotion	976.2	E858.7	E946.2	E950.4	E962.0	E980.4
anhydride	983.1	E864.1	—	E950.7	E962.1	E980.6
ether (vapor)	982.8	E862.4	—	E950.9	E962.1	E980.9
Acetohexamide	962.3	E858.0	E932.3	E950.4	E962.0	E980.4
Acetomenaphthone	964.3	E858.2	E934.3	E950.4	E962.0	E980.4
Acetomorphine	965.01	E850.0	E935.0	E950.0	E962.0	E980.0
Acetone (oils) (vapor)	982.8	E862.4	—	E950.9	E962.1	E980.9
Acetophenazine (maleate)	969.1	E853.0	E939.1	E950.3	E962.0	E980.3
Acetophenetidin	965.4	E850.4	E935.4	E950.0	E962.0	E980.0
Acetophenone	982.0	E862.4	—	E950.9	E962.1	E980.9
Acetorphine	965.09	E850.2	E935.2	E950.0	E962.0	E980.0
Acetosulfone (sodium)	961.8	E857	E931.8	E950.4	E962.0	E980.4
Acetrizoate (sodium)	977.8	E858.8	E947.8	E950.4	E962.0	E980.4
Acetylcarbromal	967.3	E852.2	E937.3	E950.2	E962.0	E980.2
Acetylcholine (chloride)	971.0	E855.3	E941.0	E950.4	E962.0	E980.4
Acetylcysteine	975.5	E858.6	E945.5	E950.4	E962.0	E980.4
Acetyldigitoxin	972.1	E858.3	E942.1	E950.4	E962.0	E980.4
Acetyldihydrocodeine	965.09	E850.2	E935.2	E950.0	E962.0	E980.0
Acetyldihydrocodeinone	965.09	E850.2	E935.2	E950.0	E962.0	E980.0
Acetylene (gas) (industrial)	987.1	E868.1	—	E951.8	E962.2	E981.8
incomplete combustion of — *see* Carbon monoxide, fuel, utility						
tetrachloride (vapor)	982.3	E862.4	—	E950.9	E962.1	E980.9
Acetyliodosalicylic acid	965.1	E850.3	E935.3	E950.0	E962.0	E980.0
Acetylphenylhydrazine	965.8	E850.8	E935.8	E950.0	E962.0	E980.0
Acetylsalicylic acid	965.1	E850.3	E935.3	E950.0	E962.0	E980.0
Achromycin	960.4	E856	E930.4	E950.4	E962.0	E980.4
ophthalmic preparation	976.5	E858.7	E946.5	E950.4	E962.0	E980.4
topical NEC	976.0	E858.7	E946.0	E950.4	E962.0	E980.4
Acidifying agents	963.2	E858.1	E933.2	E950.4	E962.0	E980.4
Acids (corrosive) NEC	983.1	E864.1	—	E950.7	E962.1	E980.6
Aconite (wild)	988.2	E865.4	—	E950.9	E962.1	E980.9
Aconitine (liniment)	976.8	E858.7	E946.8	E950.4	E962.0	E980.4

Substance	Poisoning	External Cause (E-Code)				
		Accident	Therapeutic Use	Suicide Attempt	Assault	Undetermined
Aconitum ferox	988.2	E865.4	—	E950.9	E962.1	E980.9
Acridine	983.0	E864.0	—	E950.7	E962.1	E980.6
vapor	987.8	E869.8	—	E952.8	E962.2	E982.8
Acriflavine	961.9	E857	E931.9	E950.4	E962.0	E980.4
Acrisorcin	976.0	E858.7	E946.0	E950.4	E962.0	E980.4
Acrolein (gas)	987.8	E869.8	—	E952.8	E962.2	E982.8
liquid	989.89	E866.8	—	E950.9	E962.1	E980.9
Actaea spicata	988.2	E865.4	—	E950.9	E962.1	E980.9
Acterol	961.5	E857	E931.5	E950.4	E962.0	E980.4
ACTH	962.4	E858.0	E932.4	E950.4	E962.0	E980.4
Acthar	962.4	E858.0	E932.4	E950.4	E962.0	E980.4
Actinomycin (C) (D)	960.7	E856	E930.7	E950.4	E962.0	E980.4
Adalin (acetyl)	967.3	E852.2	E937.3	E950.2	E962.0	E980.2
Adenosine (phosphate)	977.8	E858.8	E947.8	E950.4	E962.0	E980.4
Adhesives	989.89	E866.6	—	E950.9	E962.1	E980.9
ADH	962.5	E858.0	E932.5	E950.4	E962.0	E980.4
Adicillin	960.0	E856	E930.0	E950.4	E962.0	E980.4
Adiphenine	975.1	E855.6	E945.1	E950.4	E962.0	E980.4
Adjunct, pharmaceutical	977.4	E858.8	E947.4	E950.4	E962.0	E980.4
Adrenal (extract, cortex or medulla) (glucocorticoids) (hormones) (mineralocorticoids)	962.0	E858.0	E932.0	E950.4	E962.0	E980.4
ENT agent	976.6	E858.7	E946.6	E950.4	E962.0	E980.4
ophthalmic preparation	976.5	E858.7	E946.5	E950.4	E962.0	E980.4
topical NEC	976.0	E858.7	E946.0	E950.4	E962.0	E980.4
Adrenalin	971.2	E855.5	E941.2	E950.4	E962.0	E980.4
Adrenergic blocking agents	971.3	E855.6	E941.3	E950.4	E962.0	E980.4
Adrenergics	971.2	E855.5	E941.2	E950.4	E962.0	E980.4
Adrenochrome (derivatives)	972.8	E858.3	E942.8	E950.4	E962.0	E980.4
Adrenocorticotropic hormone	962.4	E858.0	E932.4	E950.4	E962.0	E980.4
Adrenocorticotropin	962.4	E858.0	E932.4	E950.4	E962.0	E980.4
Adriamycin	960.7	E856	E930.7	E950.4	E962.0	E980.4
Aerosol spray — see Sprays						
Aerosporin	960.8	E856	E930.8	E950.4	E962.0	E980.4
ENT agent	976.6	E858.7	E946.6	E950.4	E962.0	E980.4
ophthalmic preparation	976.5	E858.7	E946.5	E950.4	E962.0	E980.4
topical NEC	976.0	E858.7	E946.0	E950.4	E962.0	E980.4
Aethusa cynapium	988.2	E865.4	—	E950.9	E962.1	E980.9
Afghanistan black	969.6	E854.1	E939.6	E950.3	E962.0	E980.3
Aflatoxin	989.7	E865.9	—	E950.9	E962.1	E980.9
African boxwood	988.2	E865.4	—	E950.9	E962.1	E980.9
Agar (-agar)	973.3	E858.4	E943.3	E950.4	E962.0	E980.4
Agricultural agent NEC	989.89	E863.9	—	E950.6	E962.1	E980.7
Agrypnal	967.0	E851	E937.0	E950.1	E962.0	E980.1
Air contaminant(s), source or type not specified	987.9	E869.9	—	E952.9	E962.2	E982.9
specified type — see specific substance						
Akee	988.2	E865.4	—	E950.9	E962.1	E980.9
Akrinol	976.0	E858.7	E946.0	E950.4	E962.0	E980.4
Alantolactone	961.6	E857	E931.6	E950.4	E962.0	E980.4
Albamycin	960.8	E856	E930.8	E950.4	E962.0	E980.4
Albumin (normal human serum)	964.7	E858.2	E934.7	E950.4	E962.0	E980.4
Albuterol	975.7	E858.6	E945.7	E950.4	E962.0	E980.4
Alcohol	980.9	E860.9	—	E950.9	E962.1	E980.9
absolute	980.0	E860.1	—	E950.9	E962.1	E980.9
beverage	980.0	E860.0	E947.8	E950.9	E962.1	E980.9
amyl	980.3	E860.4	—	E950.9	E962.1	E980.9

Substance	Poisoning	Accident	Therapeutic Use	Suicide Attempt	Assault	Undetermined
antifreeze	980.1	E860.2	—	E950.9	E962.1	E980.9
butyl	980.3	E860.4	—	E950.9	E962.1	E980.9
dehydrated	980.0	E860.1	—	E950.9	E862.1	E980.9
beverage	980.0	E860.0	E947.8	E950.9	E962.1	E980.9
denatured	980.0	E860.1	—	E950.9	E962.1	E980.9
deterrents	977.3	E858.8	E947.3	E950.4	E962.0	E980.4
diagnostic (gastric function)	977.8	E858.8	E947.8	E950.4	E962.0	E980.4
ethyl	980.0	E860.1	—	E950.9	E962.1	E980.9
beverage	980.0	E860.0	E947.8	E950.9	E962.1	E980.9
grain	980.0	E860.1	—	E950.9	E962.1	E980.9
beverage	980.0	E860.0	E947.8	E950.9	E962.1	E980.9
industrial	980.9	E860.9	—	E950.9	E962.1	E980.9
isopropyl	980.2	E860.3	—	E950.9	E962.1	E980.9
methyl	980.1	E860.2	—	E950.9	E962.1	E980.9
preparation for consumption	980.0	E860.0	E947.8	E950.9	E962.1	E980.9
propyl	980.3	E860.4	—	E950.9	E962.1	E980.9
secondary	980.2	E860.3	—	E950.9	E962.1	E980.9
radiator	980.1	E860.2	—	E950.9	E962.1	E980.9
rubbing	980.2	E860.3	—	E950.9	E962.1	E980.9
specified type NEC	980.8	E860.8	—	E950.9	E962.1	E980.9
surgical	980.9	E860.9	—	E950.9	E962.1	E980.9
vapor (from any type of alcohol)	987.8	E869.8	—	E952.8	E962.2	E982.8
wood	980.1	E860.2	—	E950.9	E962.1	E980.9
Alcuronium chloride	975.2	E858.6	E945.2	E950.4	E962.0	E980.4
Aldactone	974.4	E858.5	E944.4	E950.4	E962.0	E980.4
Aldicarb	989.3	E863.2	—	E950.6	E962.1	E980.7
Aldomet	972.6	E858.3	E942.6	E950.4	E962.0	E980.4
Aldosterone	962.0	E858.0	E932.0	E950.4	E962.0	E980.4
Aldrin (dust)	989.2	E863.0	—	E950.6	E962.1	E980.7
Algeldrate	973.0	E858.4	E943.0	E950.4	E962.0	E980.4
Alidase	963.4	E858.1	E933.4	E950.4	E962.0	E980.4
Aliphatic thiocyanates	989.0	E866.8	—	E950.9	E962.1	E980.9
Alkaline antiseptic solution (aromatic)	976.6	E858.7	E946.6	E950.4	E962.0	E980.4
Alkalinizing agents (medicinal)	963.3	E858.1	E933.3	E950.4	E962.0	E980.4
Alkalis, caustic	983.2	E864.2	—	E950.7	E962.1	E980.6
Alkalizing agents (medicinal)	963.3	E858.1	E933.3	E950.4	E962.0	E980.4
Alka–seltzer	965.1	E850.3	E935.3	E950.0	E962.0	E980.0
Alkavervir	972.6	E858.3	E942.6	E950.4	E962.0	E980.4
Allegron	969.0	E854.0	E939.0	E950.3	E962.0	E980.3
Alleve see Naproxen						
Allobarbital, allobarbitone	967.0	E851	E937.0	E950.1	E962.0	E980.1
Allopurinol	974.7	E858.5	E944.7	E950.4	E962.0	E980.4
Allylestrenol	962.2	E858.0	E932.2	E950.4	E962.0	E980.4
Allylisopropylacetylurea	967.8	E852.8	E937.8	E950.2	E962.0	E980.2
Allylisopropylmalonylurea	967.0	E851	E937.0	E950.1	E962.0	E980.1
Allyltribromide	967.3	E852.2	E937.3	E950.2	E962.0	E980.2
Aloe, aloes, aloin	973.1	E858.4	E943.1	E950.4	E962.0	E980.4
Alosetron	973.8	E858.4	E943.8	E950.4	E962.0	E980.4
Aloxidone	966.0	E855.0	E936.0	E950.4	E962.0	E980.4
Aloxiprin	965.1	E850.3	E935.3	E950.0	E962.0	E980.0
Alpha amylase	963.4	E858.1	E933.4	E950.4	E962.0	E980.4
Alphaprodine (hydrochloride)	965.09	E850.2	E935.2	E950.0	E962.0	E980.0
Alpha tocopherol	963.5	E858.1	E933.5	E950.4	E962.0	E980.4
Alseroxylon	972.6	E858.3	E942.6	E950.4	E962.0	E980.4
Alum (ammonium) (potassium)	983.2	E864.2	—	E950.7	E962.1	E980.6
medicinal (astringent) NEC	976.2	E858.7	E946.2	E950.4	E962.0	E980.4
Aluminium, aluminum (gel) (hydroxide)	973.0	E858.4	E943.0	E950.4	E962.0	E980.4

Substance	Poisoning	Accident	Therapeutic Use	Suicide Attempt	Assault	Undetermined
acetate solution	976.2	E858.7	E946.2	E950.4	E962.0	E980.4
aspirin	965.1	E850.3	E935.3	E950.0	E962.0	E980.0
carbonate	973.0	E858.4	E943.0	E950.4	E962.0	E980.4
glycinate	973.0	E858.4	E943.0	E950.4	E962.0	E980.4
nicotinate	972.2	E858.3	E942.2	E950.4	E962.0	E980.4
ointment (surgical) (topical)	976.3	E858.7	E946.3	E950.4	E962.0	E980.4
phosphate	973.0	E858.4	E943.0	E950.4	E962.0	E980.4
subacetate	976.2	E858.7	E946.2	E950.4	E962.0	E980.4
topical NEC	976.3	E858.7	E946.3	E950.4	E962.0	E980.4
Alurate	967.0	E851	E937.0	E950.1	E962.0	E980.1
Alverine (citrate)	975.1	E858.6	E945.1	E950.4	E962.0	E980.4
Alvodine	965.09	E850.2	E935.2	E950.0	E962.0	E980.0
Amanita phalloides	988.1	E865.5	—	E950.9	E962.1	E980.9
Amantadine (hydrochloride)	966.4	E855.0	E936.4	E950.4	E962.0	E980.4
Ambazone	961.9	E857	E931.9	E950.4	E962.0	E980.4
Ambenonium	971.0	E855.3	E941.0	E950.4	E962.0	E980.4
Ambutonium bromide	971.1	E855.4	E941.1	E950.4	E962.0	E980.4
Ametazole	977.8	E858.8	E947.8	E950.4	E962.0	E980.4
Amethocaine (infiltration) (topical)	968.5	E855.2	E938.5	E950.4	E962.0	E980.4
nerve block (peripheral) (plexus)	968.6	E855.2	E938.6	E950.4	E962.0	E980.4
spinal	968.7	E855.2	E938.7	E950.4	E962.0	E980.4
Amethopterin	963.1	E858.1	E933.1	E950.4	E962.0	E980.4
Amfepramone	977.0	E858.8	E947.0	E950.4	E962.0	E980.4
Amidon	965.02	E850.1	E935.1	E950.0	E962.0	E980.0
Amidopyrine	965.5	E850.5	E935.5	E950.0	E962.0	E980.0
Aminacrine	976.0	E858.7	E946.0	E950.4	E962.0	E980.4
Aminitrozole	961.5	E857	E931.5	E950.4	E962.0	E980.4
Aminoacetic acid	974.5	E858.5	E944.5	E950.4	E962.0	E980.4
Amino acids	974.5	E858.5	E944.5	E950.4	E962.0	E980.4
Aminocaproic acid	964.4	E858.2	E934.4	E950.4	E962.0	E980.4
Aminoethylisothiourium	963.8	E858.1	E933.8	E950.4	E962.0	E980.4
Aminoglutethimide	966.3	E855.0	E936.3	E950.4	E962.0	E980.4
Aminometradine	974.3	E858.5	E944.3	E950.4	E962.0	E980.4
Aminopentamide	971.1	E855.4	E941.1	E950.4	E962.0	E980.4
Aminophenazone	965.5	E850.5	E935.5	E950.0	E962.0	E980.0
Aminophenol	983.0	E864.0	—	E950.7	E962.1	E980.6
Aminophenylpyridone	969.5	E853.8	E939.5	E950.3	E962.0	E980.3
Aminophyllin	975.7	E858.6	E945.7	E950.4	E962.0	E980.4
Aminopterin	963.1	E858.1	E933.1	E950.4	E962.0	E980.4
Aminopyrine	965.5	E850.5	E935.5	E950.0	E962.0	E980.0
Aminosalicylic acid	961.8	E857	E931.8	E950.4	E962.0	E980.4
Amiphenazole	970.1	E854.3	E940.1	E950.4	E962.0	E980.4
Amiquinsin	972.6	E858.3	E942.6	E950.4	E962.0	E980.4
Amisometradine	974.3	E858.5	E944.3	E950.4	E962.0	E980.4
Amitriptyline	969.0	E854.0	E939.0	E950.3	E962.0	E980.3
Ammonia (fumes) (gas) (vapor)	987.8	E869.8	—	E952.8	E962.2	E982.8
liquid (household) NEC	983.2	E861.4	—	E950.7	E962.1	E980.6
spirit, aromatic	970.8	E854.3	E940.8	E950.4	E962.0	E980.4
Ammoniated mercury	976.0	E858.7	E946.0	E950.4	E962.0	E980.4
Ammonium						
carbonate	983.2	E864.2	—	E950.7	E962.1	E980.6
chloride (acidifying agent)	963.2	E858.1	E933.2	E950.4	E962.0	E980.4
expectorant	975.5	E858.6	E945.5	E950.4	E962.0	E980.4
compounds (household) NEC	983.2	E861.4	—	E950.7	E962.1	E980.6
fumes (any usage)	987.8	E869.8	—	E952.8	E962.2	E982.8
industrial	983.2	E864.2	—	E950.7	E962.1	E980.6
ichthyosulfonate	976.4	E858.7	E946.4	E950.4	E962.0	E980.4

Substance	Poisoning	External Cause (E-Code) Accident Therapeutic Use	Suicide Attempt	Assault	Undetermined

Substance		Poisoning	Accident	Therapeutic Use	Suicide Attempt	Assault	Undetermined
mandelate	961.9	E857	E931.9	E950.4	E962.0	E980.4
Amobarbital	967.0	E851	E937.0	E950.1	E962.0	E980.1
Amodiaquin(e)	961.4	E857	E931.4	E950.4	E962.0	E980.4
Amopyroquin(e)	961.4	E857	E931.4	E950.4	E962.0	E980.4
Amphenidone	969.5	E853.8	E939.5	E950.3	E962.0	E980.3
Amphetamine	969.7	E854.2	E939.7	E950.3	E962.0	E980.3
Amphomycin	960.8	E856	E930.8	E950.4	E962.0	E980.4
Amphotericin B	960.1	E856	E930.1	E950.4	E962.0	E980.4
topical	976.0	E858.7	E946.0	E950.4	E962.0	E980.4
Ampicillin	960.0	E856	E930.0	E950.4	E962.0	E980.4
Amprotropine	971.1	E855.4	E941.1	E950.4	E962.0	E980.4
Amygdalin	977.8	E858.8	E947.8	E950.4	E962.0	E980.4
Amyl						
acetate (vapor)	982.8	E862.4	—	E950.9	E962.1	E980.9
alcohol	980.3	E860.4	—	E950.9	E962.1	E980.9
nitrite (medicinal)	972.4	E858.3	E942.4	E950.4	E962.0	E980.4
Amylase (alpha)	963.4	E858.1	E933.4	E950.4	E962.0	E980.4
Amylene hydrate	980.8	E860.8	—	E950.9	E962.1	E980.9
Amylobarbitone	967.0	E851	E937.0	E950.1	E962.0	E980.1
Amylocaine	968.9	E855.2	E938.9	E950.4	E962.0	E980.4
infiltration (subcutaneous)	968.5	E855.2	E938.5	E950.4	E962.0	E980.4
nerve block (peripheral) (plexus)	968.6	E855.2	E938.6	E950.4	E962.0	E980.4
spinal	968.7	E855.2	E938.7	E950.4	E962.0	E980.4
topical (surface)	968.5	E855.2	E938.5	E950.4	E962.0	E980.4
Amytal (sodium)	967.0	E851	E937.0	E950.1	E962.0	E980.1
Analeptics	970.0	E854.3	E940.0	E950.4	E962.0	E980.4
Analgesics	965.9	E850.9	E935.9	E950.0	E962.0	E980.0
aromatic NEC	965.4	E850.4	E935.4	E950.0	E962.0	E980.0
non–narcotic NEC	965.7	E850.7	E935.7	E950.0	E962.0	E980.0
specified NEC	965.8	E850.8	E935.8	E950.0	E962.0	E980.0
Anamirta cocculus	988.2	E865.3	—	E950.9	E962.1	E980.9
Ancillin	960.0	E856	E930.0	E950.4	E962.0	E980.4
Androgens (anabolic congeners)	962.1	E858.0	E932.1	E950.4	E962.0	E980.4
Androstalone	962.1	E858.0	E932.1	E950.4	E962.0	E980.4
Androsterone	962.1	E858.0	E932.1	E950.4	E962.0	E980.4
Anemone pulsatilla	988.2	E865.4	—	E950.9	E962.1	E980.9
Anesthesia, anesthetic (general) NEC	968.4	E855.1	E938.4	E950.4	E962.0	E980.4
block (nerve) (plexus)	968.6	E855.2	E938.6	E950.4	E962.0	E980.4
gaseous NEC	968.2	E855.1	E938.2	E950.4	E962.0	E980.4
halogenated hydrocarbon derivatives NEC	968.2	E855.1	E938.2	E950.4	E962.0	E980.4
infiltration (intradermal) (subcutaneous) (submucosal)	968.5	E855.2	E938.5	E950.4	E962.0	E980.4
intravenous	968.3	E855.1	E938.3	E950.4	E962.0	E980.4
local NEC	968.9	E855.2	E938.9	E950.4	E962.0	E980.4
nerve blocking (peripheral) (plexus)	968.6	E855.2	E938.6	E950.4	E962.0	E980.4
rectal NEC	968.3	E855.1	E938.3	E950.4	E962.0	E980.4
spinal	968.7	E855.2	E938.7	E950.4	E962.0	E980.4
surface	968.5	E855.2	E938.5	E950.4	E962.0	E980.4
topical	968.5	E855.2	E938.5	E950.4	E962.0	E980.4
Aneurine	963.5	E858.1	E933.5	E950.4	E962.0	E980.4
Angio–Conray	977.8	E858.8	E947.8	E950.4	E962.0	E980.4
Angininesee Glyceryl trinitrate						
Angiotensin	971.2	E855.5	E941.2	E950.4	E962.0	E980.4
Anhydrohydroxyprogesterone	962.2	E858.0	E932.2	E950.4	E962.0	E980.4
Anhydron	974.3	E858.5	E944.3	E950.4	E962.0	E980.4
Anileridine	965.09	E850.2	E935.2	E950.0	E962.0	E980.0

Substance	Poisoning	External Cause (E-Code)				
		Accident	Therapeutic Use	Suicide Attempt	Assault	Undetermined
Aniline (dye) (liquid)	983.0	E864.0	—	E950.7	E962.1	E980.6
analgesic	965.4	E850.4	E935.4	E950.0	E962.0	E980.0
derivatives, therapeutic NEC	965.4	E850.4	E935.4	E950.0	E962.0	E980.0
vapor	987.8	E869.8	—	E952.8	E962.2	E982.8
Anisindione	964.2	E858.2	E934.2	E950.4	E962.0	E980.4
Anisotropine	971.1	E855.4	E941.1	E950.4	E962.0	E980.4
Anorexic agents	977.0	E858.8	E947.0	E950.4	E962.0	E980.4
Ant (bite) (sting)	989.5	E905.5	—	E950.9	E962.1	E980.9
Antabuse	977.3	E858.8	E947.3	E950.4	E962.0	E980.4
Antacids	973.0	E858.4	E943.0	E950.4	E962.0	E980.4
Antazoline	963.0	E858.1	E933.0	E950.4	E962.0	E980.4
Anthelmintics	961.6	E857	E931.6	E950.4	E962.0	E980.4
Anthralin	976.4	E858.7	E946.4	E950.4	E962.0	E980.4
Anthramycin	960.7	E856	E930.7	E950.4	E962.0	E980.4
Antiadrenergics	971.3	E855.6	E941.3	E950.4	E962.0	E980.4
Antiallergic agents	963.0	E858.1	E933.0	E950.4	E962.0	E980.4
Antianemic agents NEC	964.1	E858.2	E934.1	E950.4	E962.0	E980.4
Antiaris toxicaria	988.2	E865.4	—	E950.9	E962.1	E980.9
Antiarteriosclerotic agents	972.2	E858.3	E942.2	E950.4	E962.0	E980.4
Antiasthmatics	975.7	E858.6	E945.7	E950.4	E962.0	E980.4
Antibiotics	960.9	E856	E930.9	E950.4	E962.0	E980.4
antifungal	960.1	E856	E930.1	E950.4	E962.0	E980.4
antimycobacterial	960.6	E856	E930.6	E950.4	E962.0	E980.4
antineoplastic	960.7	E856	E930.7	E950.4	E962.0	E980.4
cephalosporin (group)	960.5	E856	E930.5	E950.4	E962.0	E980.4
chloramphenicol (group)	960.2	E856	E930.2	E950.4	E962.0	E980.4
macrolides	960.3	E856	E930.3	E950.4	E962.0	E980.4
specified NEC	960.8	E856	E930.8	E950.4	E962.0	E980.4
tetracycline (group)	960.4	E856	E930.4	E950.4	E962.0	E980.4
Anticancer agents NEC	963.1	E858.1	E933.1	E950.4	E962.0	E980.4
antibiotics	960.7	E856	E930.7	E950.4	E962.0	E980.4
Anticholinergics	971.1	E855.4	E941.1	E950.4	E962.0	E980.4
Anticholinesterase (organophosphorus) (reversible)	971.0	E855.3	E941.0	E950.4	E962.0	E980.4
Anticoagulants	964.2	E858.2	E934.2	E950.4	E962.0	E980.4
antagonists	964.5	E858.2	E934.5	E950.4	E962.0	E980.4
Anti–common cold agents NEC	975.6	E858.6	E945.6	E950.4	E962.0	E980.4
Anticonvulsants NEC	966.3	E855.0	E936.3	E950.4	E962.0	E980.4
Antidepressants	969.0	E854.0	E939.0	E950.3	E962.0	E980.3
Antidiabetic agents	962.3	E858.0	E932.3	E950.4	E962.0	E980.4
Antidiarrheal agents	973.5	E858.4	E943.5	E950.4	E962.0	E980.4
Antidiuretic hormone	962.5	E858.0	E932.5	E950.4	E962.0	E980.4
Antidotes NEC	977.2	E858.8	E947.2	E950.4	E962.0	E980.4
Antiemetic agents	963.0	E858.1	E933.0	E950.4	E962.0	E980.4
Antiepilepsy agent NEC	966.3	E855.0	E936.3	E950.4	E962.0	E980.4
Antifertility pills	962.2	E858.0	E932.2	E950.4	E962.0	E980.4
Antiflatulents	973.8	E858.4	E943.8	E950.4	E962.0	E980.4
Antifreeze	989.89	E866.8	—	E950.9	E962.1	E980.9
alcohol	980.1	E860.2	—	E950.9	E962.1	E980.9
ethylene glycol	982.8	E862.4	—	E950.9	E962.1	E980.9
Antifungals (nonmedicinal) (sprays)	989.4	E863.6	—	E950.6	E962.1	E980.7
medicinal NEC	961.9	E857	E931.9	E950.4	E962.0	E980.4
antibiotic	960.1	E856	E930.1	E950.4	E962.0	E980.4
topical	976.0	E858.7	E946.0	E950.4	E962.0	E980.4
Antigastric secretion agents	973.0	E858.4	E943.0	E950.4	E962.0	E980.4
Antihelmintics	961.6	E857	E931.6	E950.4	E962.0	E980.4
Antihemophilic factor (human)	964.7	E858.2	E934.7	E950.4	E962.0	E980.4

Substance	Poisoning	External Cause (E-Code)				
		Accident	Therapeutic Use	Suicide Attempt	Assault	Undetermined
Antihistamine	963.0	E858.1	E933.0	E950.4	E962.0	E980.4
Antihypertensive agents NEC	972.6	E858.3	E942.6	E950.4	E962.0	E980.4
Anti–infectives NEC	961.9	E857	E931.9	E950.4	E962.0	E980.4
antibiotics	960.9	E856	E930.9	E950.4	E962.0	E980.4
specified NEC	960.8	E856	E930.8	E950.4	E962.0	E980.4
antihelmintic	961.6	E857	E931.6	E950.4	E962.0	E980.4
antimalarial	961.4	E857	E931.4	E950.4	E962.0	E980.4
antimycobacterial NEC	961.8	E857	E931.8	E950.4	E962.0	E980.4
antibiotics	960.6	E856	E930.6	E950.4	E962.0	E980.4
antiprotozoal NEC	961.5	E857	E931.5	E950.4	E962.0	E980.4
blood	961.4	E857	E931.4	E950.4	E962.0	E980.4
antiviral	961.7	E857	E931.7	E950.4	E962.0	E980.4
arsenical	961.1	E857	E931.1	E950.4	E962.0	E980.4
ENT agents	976.6	E858.7	E946.6	E950.4	E962.0	E980.4
heavy metals NEC	961.2	E857	E931.2	E950.4	E962.0	E980.4
local	976.0	E858.7	E946.0	E950.4	E962.0	E980.4
ophthalmic preparation	976.5	E858.7	E946.5	E950.4	E962.0	E980.4
topical NEC	976.0	E858.7	E946.0	E950.4	E962.0	E980.4
Anti–inflammatory agents (topical)	976.0	E858.7	E946.0	E950.4	E962.0	E980.4
Antiknock (tetraethyl lead)	984.1	E862.1	—	E950.9	E962.1	E980.9
Antilipemics	972.2	E858.3	E942.2	E950.4	E962.0	E980.4
Antimalarials	961.4	E857	E931.4	E950.4	E962.0	E980.4
Antimony (compounds) (vapor) NEC	985.4	E866.2	—	E950.9	E962.1	E980.9
anti–infectives	961.2	E857	E931.2	E950.4	E962.0	E980.4
pesticides (vapor)	985.4	E863.4	—	E950.6	E962.2	E980.7
potassium tartrate	961.2	E857	E931.2	E950.4	E962.0	E980.4
tartrated	961.2	E857	E931.2	E950.4	E962.0	E980.4
Antimuscarinic agents	971.1	E855.4	E941.1	E950.4	E962.0	E980.4
Antimycobacterials NEC	961.8	E857	E931.8	E950.4	E962.0	E980.4
antibiotics	960.6	E856	E930.6	E950.4	E962.0	E980.4
Antineoplastic agents	963.1	E858.1	E933.1	E950.4	E962.0	E980.4
antibiotics	960.7	E856	E930.7	E950.4	E962.0	E980.4
Anti–Parkinsonism agents	966.4	E855.0	E936.4	E950.4	E962.0	E980.4
Antiphlogistics	965.69	E850.6	E935.6	E950.0	E962.0	E980.0
Antiprotozoals NEC	961.5	E857	E931.5	E950.4	E962.0	E980.4
blood	961.4	E857	E931.4	E950.4	E962.0	E980.4
Antipruritics (local)	976.1	E858.7	E946.1	E950.4	E962.0	E980.4
Antipsychotic agents NEC	969.3	E853.8	E939.3	E950.3	E962.0	E980.3
Antipyretics	965.9	E850.9	E935.9	E950.0	E962.0	E980.0
specified NEC	965.8	E850.8	E935.8	E950.0	E962.0	E980.0
Antipyrine	965.5	E850.5	E935.5	E950.0	E962.0	E980.0
Antirabies serum (equine)	979.9	E858.8	E949.9	E950.4	E962.0	E980.4
Antirheumatics	965.69	E850.6	E935.6	E950.0	E962.0	E980.0
Antiseborrheics	976.4	E858.7	E946.4	E950.4	E962.0	E980.4
Antiseptics (external) (medicinal)	976.0	E858.7	E946.0	E950.4	E962.0	E980.4
Antistine	963.0	E858.1	E933.0	E950.4	E962.0	E980.4
Antithyroid agents	962.8	E858.0	E932.8	E950.4	E962.0	E980.4
Antitoxin, any	979.9	E858.8	E949.9	E950.4	E962.0	E980.4
Antituberculars	961.8	E857	E931.8	E950.4	E962.0	E980.4
antibiotics	960.6	E856	E930.6	E950.4	E962.0	E980.4
Antitussives	975.4	E858.6	E945.5	E950.4	E962.0	E980.4
Antivaricose agents (sclerosing)	972.7	E858.3	E942.7	E950.4	E962.0	E980.4
Antivenin (crotaline) (spider–bite)	979.9	E858.8	E949.9	E950.4	E962.0	E980.4
Antivert	963.0	E858.1	E933.0	E950.4	E962.0	E980.4
Antivirals NEC	961.7	E857	E931.7	E950.4	E962.0	E980.4
Ant poisons — see Pesticides						
Antrol	989.4	E863.4	—	E950.6	E962.1	E980.7

Substance	Poisoning	External Cause (E-Code)				
		Accident	Therapeutic Use	Suicide Attempt	Assault	Undetermined
fungicide	989.4	E863.6	—	E950.6	E962.1	E980.7
Apomorphine hydrochloride (emetic)	973.6	E858.4	E943.6	E950.4	E962.0	E980.4
Appetite depressants, central	977.0	E858.8	E947.0	E950.4	E962.0	E980.4
Apresoline	972.6	E858.3	E942.6	E950.4	E962.0	E980.4
Aprobarbital, aprobarbitone	967.0	E851	E937.0	E950.1	E962.0	E980.1
Apronalide	967.8	E852.8	E937.8	E950.2	E962.0	E980.2
Aqua fortis	983.1	E864.1	—	E950.7	E962.1	E980.6
Arachis oil (topical)	976.3	E858.7	E946.3	E950.4	E962.0	E980.4
cathartic	973.2	E858.4	E943.2	E950.4	E962.0	E980.4
Aralen	961.4	E857	E931.4	E950.4	E962.0	E980.4
Arginine salts	974.5	E858.5	E944.5	E950.4	E962.0	E980.4
Argyrol	976.0	E858.7	E946.0	E950.4	E962.0	E980.4
ENT agent	976.6	E858.7	E946.6	E950.4	E962.0	E980.4
ophthalmic preparation	976.5	E858.7	E946.5	E950.4	E962.0	E980.4
Aristocort	962.0	E858.0	E932.0	E950.4	E962.0	E980.4
ENT agent	976.6	E858.7	E946.6	E950.4	E962.0	E980.4
ophthalmic preparation	976.5	E858.7	E946.5	E950.4	E962.0	E980.4
topical NEC	976.0	E858.7	E946.0	E950.4	E962.0	E980.4
Aromatics, corrosive	983.0	E864.0	—	E950.7	E962.1	E980.6
disinfectants	983.0	E861.4	—	E950.7	E962.1	E980.6
Arsenate of lead (insecticide)	985.1	E863.4	—	E950.8	E962.1	E980.8
herbicide	985.1	E863.5	—	E950.8	E962.1	E980.8
Arsenic, arsenicals (compounds) (dust) (fumes) (vapor) NEC	985.1	E866.3	—	E950.8	E962.1	E980.8
anti–infectives	961.1	E857	E931.1	E950.4	E962.0	E980.4
pesticide (dust) (fumes)	985.1	E863.4	—	E950.8	E962.1	E980.8
Arsine (gas)	985.1	E866.3	—	E950.8	E962.1	E980.8
Arsphenamine (silver)	961.1	E857	E931.1	E950.4	E962.0	E980.4
Arsthinol	961.1	E857	E931.1	E950.4	E962.0	E980.4
Artane	971.1	E855.4	E941.1	E950.4	E962.0	E980.4
Arthropod (venomous) NEC	989.5	E905.5	—	E950.9	E962.1	E980.9
Asbestos	989.81	E866.8	—	E950.9	E962.1	E980.9
Ascaridole	961.6	E857	E931.6	E950.4	E962.0	E980.4
Ascorbic acid	963.5	E858.1	E933.5	E950.4	E962.0	E980.4
Asiaticoside	976.0	E858.7	E946.0	E950.4	E962.0	E980.4
Aspidium (oleoresin)	961.6	E857	E931.6	E950.4	E962.0	E980.4
Aspirin	965.1	E850.3	E935.3	E950.0	E962.0	E980.0
Astringents (local)	976.2	E858.7	E946.2	E950.4	E962.0	E980.4
Atabrine	961.3	E857	E931.3	E950.4	E962.0	E980.4
Ataractics	969.5	E853.8	E939.5	E950.3	E962.0	E980.3
Atonia drug, intestinal	973.3	E858.4	E943.3	E950.4	E962.0	E980.4
Atophan	974.7	E858.5	E944.7	E950.4	E962.0	E980.4
Atropine	971.1	E855.4	E941.1	E950.4	E962.0	E980.4
Attapulgite	973.5	E858.4	E943.5	E950.4	E962.0	E980.4
Attenuvax	979.4	E858.8	E949.4	E950.4	E962.0	E980.4
Aureomycin	960.4	E856	E930.4	E950.4	E962.0	E980.4
ophthalmic preparation	976.5	E858.7	E946.5	E950.4	E962.0	E980.4
topical NEC	976.0	E858.7	E946.0	E950.4	E962.0	E980.4
Aurothioglucose	965.69	E850.6	E935.6	E950.0	E962.0	E980.0
Aurothioglycanide	965.69	E850.6	E935.6	E950.0	E962.0	E980.0
Aurothiomalate	965.69	E850.6	E935.6	E950.0	E962.0	E980.0
Automobile fuel	981	E862.1	—	E950.9	E962.1	E980.9
Autonomic nervous system agents NEC	971.9	E855.9	E941.9	E950.4	E962.0	E980.4
Avlosulfon	961.8	E857	E931.8	E950.4	E962.0	E980.4
Avomine	967.8	E852.8	E937.8	E950.2	E962.0	E980.2
Azacyclonol	969.5	E853.8	E939.5	E950.3	E962.0	E980.3
Azapetine	971.3	E855.6	E941.3	E950.4	E962.0	E980.4

Substance		Poisoning	External Cause (E-Code)				
			Accident	Therapeutic Use	Suicide Attempt	Assault	Undetermined
Azaribine	963.1	E858.1	E933.1	E950.4	E962.0	E980.4
Azaserine	960.7	E856	E930.7	E950.4	E962.0	E980.4
Azathioprine	963.1	E858.1	E933.1	E950.4	E962.0	E980.4
Azosulfamide	961.0	E857	E931.0	E950.4	E962.0	E980.4
Azulfidine	961.0	E857	E931.0	E950.4	E962.0	E980.4
Azuresin	977.8	E858.8	E947.8	E950.4	E962.0	E980.4
Bacimycin	976.0	E858.7	E946.0	E950.4	E962.0	E980.4
ophthalmic preparation	976.5	E858.7	E946.5	E950.4	E962.0	E980.4
Bacitracin	960.8	E856	E930.8	E950.4	E962.0	E980.4
ENT agent	976.6	E858.7	E946.6	E950.4	E962.0	E980.4
ophthalmic preparation	976.5	E858.7	E946.5	E950.4	E962.0	E980.4
topical NEC	976.0	E858.7	E946.0	E950.4	E962.0	E980.4
Baking soda	963.3	E858.1	E933.3	E950.4	E962.0	E980.4
BAL	963.8	E858.1	E933.8	E950.4	E962.0	E980.4
Bamethan (sulfate)	972.5	E858.3	E942.5	E950.4	E962.0	E980.4
Bamipine	963.0	E858.1	E933.0	E950.4	E962.0	E980.4
Baneberry	988.2	E865.4	—	E950.9	E962.1	E980.9
Banewort	988.2	E865.4	—	E950.9	E962.1	E980.9
Barbenyl	967.0	E851	E937.0	E950.1	E962.0	E980.1
Barbital, barbitone	967.0	E851	E937.0	E950.1	E962.0	E980.1
Barbiturates, barbituric acid	967.0	E851	E937.0	E950.1	E962.0	E980.1
anesthetic (intravenous)	968.3	E855.1	E938.3	E950.4	E962.0	E980.4
Barium (carbonate) (chloride) (sulfate)	985.8	E866.4	—	E950.9	E962.1	E980.9
diagnostic agent	977.8	E858.8	E947.8	E950.4	E962.0	E980.4
pesticide	985.8	E863.4	—	E950.6	E962.1	E980.7
rodenticide	985.8	E863.7	—	E950.6	E962.1	E980.7
Barrier cream	976.3	E858.7	E946.3	E950.4	E962.0	E980.4
Battery acid or fluid	983.1	E864.1	—	E950.7	E962.1	E980.6
Bay rum	980.8	E860.8	—	E950.9	E962.1	E980.9
BCG vaccine	978.0	E858.8	E948.0	E950.4	E962.0	E980.4
Bearsfoot	988.2	E865.4	—	E950.9	E962.1	E980.9
Beclamide	966.3	E855.0	E936.3	E950.4	E962.0	E980.4
Bee (sting) (venom)	989.5	E905.3	—	E950.9	E962.1	E980.9
Belladonna (alkaloids)	971.1	E855.4	E941.1	E950.4	E962.0	E980.4
Bemegride	970.0	E854.3	E940.0	E950.4	E962.0	E980.4
Benactyzine	969.8	E855.8	E939.8	E950.3	E962.0	E980.3
Benadryl	963.0	E858.1	E933.0	E950.4	E962.0	E980.4
Bendrofluazide	974.3	E858.5	E944.3	E950.4	E962.0	E980.4
Bendroflumethiazide	974.3	E858.5	E944.3	E950.4	E962.0	E980.4
Benemid	974.7	E858.5	E944.7	E950.4	E962.0	E980.4
Benethamine penicillin G	960.0	E856	E930.0	E950.4	E962.0	E980.4
Benisone	976.0	E858.7	E946.0	E950.4	E962.0	E980.4
Benoquin	976.8	E858.7	E946.8	E950.4	E962.0	E980.4
Benoxinate	968.5	E855.2	E938.5	E950.4	E962.0	E980.4
Bentonite	976.3	E858.7	E946.3	E950.4	E962.0	E980.4
Benzalkonium (chloride)	976.0	E858.7	E946.0	E950.4	E962.0	E980.4
ophthalmic preparation	976.5	E858.7	E946.5	E950.4	E962.0	E980.4
Benzamidosalicylate (calcium)	961.8	E857	E931.8	E950.4	E962.0	E980.4
Benzathine penicillin	960.0	E856	E930.0	E950.4	E962.0	E980.4
Benzcarbimine	963.1	E858.1	E933.1	E950.4	E962.0	E980.4
Benzedrex	971.2	E855.5	E941.2	E950.4	E962.0	E980.4
Benzedrine (amphetamine)	969.7	E854.2	E939.7	E950.3	E962.0	E980.3
Benzene (acetyl) (dimethyl) (methyl) (solvent) (vapor)	982.0	E862.4	—	E950.9	E962.1	E980.9
hexachloride (gamma) (insecticide) (vapor)	989.2	E863.0	—	E950.6	E962.1	E980.7
Benzethonium	976.0	E858.7	E946.0	E950.4	E962.0	E980.4

Substance	Poisoning	External Cause (E-Code)				
		Accident	Therapeutic Use	Suicide Attempt	Assault	Undetermined
Benzhexol (chloride)	966.4	E855.0	E936.4	E950.4	E962.0	E980.4
Benzilonium	971.1	E855.4	E941.1	E950.4	E962.0	E980.4
Benzin(e) — see Ligroin						
Benziodarone	972.4	E858.3	E942.4	E950.4	E962.0	E980.4
Benzocaine	968.5	E855.2	E938.5	E950.4	E962.0	E980.4
Benzodiapin	969.4	E853.2	E939.4	E950.3	E962.0	E980.3
Benzodiazepines (tranquilizers) NEC	969.4	E853.2	E939.4	E950.3	E962.0	E980.3
Benzoic acid (with salicylic acid) (anti–infective)	976.0	E858.7	E946.0	E950.4	E962.0	E980.4
Benzoin	976.3	E858.7	E946.3	E950.4	E962.0	E980.4
Benzol (vapor)	982.0	E862.4	—	E950.9	E962.1	E980.9
Benzomorphan	965.09	E850.2	E935.2	E950.0	E962.0	E980.0
Benzonatate	975.4	E858.6	E945.4	E950.4	E962.0	E980.4
Benzothiadiazides	974.3	E858.5	E944.3	E950.4	E962.0	E980.4
Benzoylpas	961.8	E857	E931.8	E950.4	E962.0	E980.4
Benzperidol	969.5	E853.8	E939.5	E950.3	E962.0	E980.3
Benzphetamine	977.0	E858.8	E947.0	E950.4	E962.0	E980.4
Benzpyrinium	971.0	E855.3	E941.0	E950.4	E962.0	E980.4
Benzquinamide	963.0	E858.1	E933.0	E950.4	E962.0	E980.4
Benzthiazide	974.3	E858.5	E944.3	E950.4	E962.0	E980.4
Benztropine	971.1	E855.4	E941.1	E950.4	E962.0	E980.4
Benzyl						
acetate	982.8	E862.4	—	E950.9	E962.1	E980.9
benzoate (anti–infective)	976.0	E858.7	E946.0	E950.4	E962.0	E980.4
morphine	965.09	E850.2	E935.2	E950.0	E962.0	E980.0
penicillin	960.0	E856	E930.0	E950.4	E962.0	E980.4
Bephenium hydroxynapthoate	961.6	E857	E931.6	E950.4	E962.0	E980.4
Bergamot oil	989.89	E866.8	—	E950.9	E962.1	E980.9
Berries, poisonous	988.2	E865.3	—	E950.9	E962.1	E980.9
Beryllium (compounds) (fumes)	985.3	E866.4	—	E950.9	E962.1	E980.9
Beta–carotene	976.3	E858.7	E946.3	E950.4	E962.0	E980.4
Beta–Chlor	967.1	E852.0	E937.1	E950.2	E962.0	E980.2
Betamethasone	962.0	E858.0	E932.0	E950.4	E962.0	E980.4
topical	976.0	E858.7	E946.0	E950.4	E962.0	E980.4
Betazole	977.8	E858.8	E947.8	E950.4	E962.0	E980.4
Bethanechol	971.0	E855.3	E941.0	E950.4	E962.0	E980.4
Bethanidine	972.6	E858.3	E942.6	E950.4	E962.0	E980.4
Betula oil	976.3	E858.7	E946.3	E950.4	E962.0	E980.4
Bhang	969.6	E854.1	E939.6	E950.3	E962.0	E980.3
Bialamicol	961.5	E857	E931.5	E950.4	E962.0	E980.4
Bichloride of mercury — see Mercury, chloride						
Bichromates (calcium) (crystals) (potassium) (sodium)	983.9	E864.3	—	E950.7	E962.1	E980.6
fumes	987.8	E869.8	—	E952.8	E962.2	E982.8
Biguanide derivatives, oral	962.3	E858.0	E932.3	E950.4	E962.0	E980.4
Biligrafin	977.8	E858.8	E947.8	E950.4	E962.0	E980.4
Bilopaque	977.8	E858.8	E947.8	E950.4	E962.0	E980.4
Bioflavonoids	972.8	E858.3	E942.8	E950.4	E962.0	E980.4
Biological substance NEC	979.9	E858.8	E949.9	E950.4	E962.0	E980.4
Biperiden	966.4	E855.0	E936.4	E950.4	E962.0	E980.4
Bisacodyl	973.1	E858.4	E943.1	E950.4	E962.0	E980.4
Bishydroxycoumarin	964.2	E858.2	E934.2	E950.4	E962.0	E980.4
Bismarsen	961.1	E857	E931.1	E950.4	E962.0	E980.4
Bismuth (compounds) NEC	985.8	E866.4	—	E950.9	E962.1	E980.9
anti–infectives	961.2	E857	E931.2	E950.4	E962.0	E980.4
subcarbonate	973.5	E858.4	E943.5	E950.4	E962.0	E980.4

Substance	Poisoning	External Cause (E-Code)				
		Accident	Therapeutic Use	Suicide Attempt	Assault	Undetermined
sulfarsphenamine	961.1	E857	E931.1	E950.4	E962.0	E980.4
Bithionol	961.6	E857	E931.6	E950.4	E962.0	E980.4
Bitter almond oil	989.0	E866.8	—	E950.9	E962.1	E980.9
Bittersweet	988.2	E865.4	—	E950.9	E962.1	E980.9
Black						
flag	989.4	E863.4	—	E950.6	E962.1	E980.7
henbane	988.2	E865.4	—	E950.9	E962.1	E980.9
leaf (40)	989.4	E863.4	—	E950.6	E962.1	E980.7
widow spider (bite)	989.5	E905.1	—	E950.9	E962.1	E980.9
antivenin	979.9	E858.8	E949.9	E950.4	E962.0	E980.4
Blast furnace gas (carbon monoxide from)	986	E868.8	—	E952.1	E962.2	E982.1
Bleach NEC	983.9	E864.3	—	E950.7	E962.1	E980.6
Bleaching solutions	983.9	E864.3	—	E950.7	E962.1	E980.6
Bleomycin (sulfate)	960.7	E856	E930.7	E950.4	E962.0	E980.4
Blockain	968.9	E855.2	E938.9	E950.4	E962.0	E980.4
infiltration (subcutaneous)	968.5	E855.2	E938.5	E950.4	E962.0	E980.4
nerve block (peripheral) (plexus)	968.6	E855.2	E938.6	E950.4	E962.0	E980.4
topical (surface)	968.5	E855.2	E938.5	E950.4	E962.0	E980.4
Blood (derivatives) (natural) (plasma)						
(whole)	964.7	E858.2	E934.7	E950.4	E962.0	E980.4
affecting agent	964.9	E858.2	E934.9	E950.4	E962.0	E980.4
specified NEC	964.8	E858.2	E934.8	E950.4	E962.0	E980.4
substitute (macromolecular)	964.8	E858.2	E934.8	E950.4	E962.0	E980.4
Blue velvet	965.09	E850.2	E935.2	E950.0	E962.0	E980.0
Bone meal	989.89	E866.5	—	E950.9	E962.1	E980.9
Bonine	963.0	E858.1	E933.0	E950.4	E962.0	E980.4
Boracic acid	976.0	E858.7	E946.0	E950.4	E962.0	E980.4
ENT agent	976.6	E858.7	E946.6	E950.4	E962.0	E980.4
ophthalmic preparation	976.5	E858.7	E946.5	E950.4	E962.0	E980.4
Borate (cleanser) (sodium)	989.6	E861.3	—	E950.9	E962.1	E980.9
Borax (cleanser)	989.6	E861.3	—	E950.9	E962.1	E980.9
Boric acid	976.0	E858.7	E946.0	E950.4	E962.0	E980.4
ENT agent	976.6	E858.7	E946.6	E950.4	E962.0	E980.4
ophthalmic preparation	976.5	E858.7	E946.5	E950.4	E962.0	E980.4
Boron hydride NEC	989.89	E866.8	—	E950.9	E962.1	E980.9
fumes or gas	987.8	E869.8	—	E952.8	E962.2	E982.8
Brake fluid vapor	987.8	E869.8	—	E952.8	E962.2	E982.8
Brass (compounds) (fumes)	985.8	E866.4	—	E950.9	E962.1	E980.9
Brasso	981	E861.3	—	E950.9	E962.1	E980.9
Bretylium (tosylate)	972.6	E858.3	E942.6	E950.4	E962.0	E980.4
Brevital (sodium)	968.3	E855.1	E938.3	E950.4	E962.0	E980.4
British antilewisite	963.8	E858.1	E933.8	E950.4	E962.0	E980.4
Bromal (hydrate)	967.3	E852.2	E937.3	E950.2	E962.0	E980.2
Bromelains	963.4	E858.1	E933.4	E950.4	E962.0	E980.4
Bromides NEC	967.3	E852.2	E937.3	E950.2	E962.0	E980.2
Bromine (vapor)	987.8	E869.8	—	E952.8	E962.2	E982.8
compounds (medicinal)	967.3	E852.2	E937.3	E950.2	E962.0	E980.2
Bromisovalum	967.3	E852.2	E937.3	E950.2	E962.0	E980.2
Bromobenzyl cyanide	987.5	E869.3	—	E952.8	E962.2	E982.8
Bromodiphenhydramine	963.0	E858.1	E933.0	E950.4	E962.0	E980.4
Bromoform	967.3	E852.2	E937.3	E950.2	E962.0	E980.2
Bromophenol blue reagent	977.8	E858.8	E947.8	E950.4	E962.0	E980.4
Bromosalicylhydroxamic acid	961.8	E857	E931.8	E950.4	E962.0	E980.4
Bromo–seltzer	965.4	E850.4	E935.4	E950.0	E962.0	E980.0
Brompheniramine	963.0	E858.1	E933.0	E950.4	E962.0	E980.4
Bromural	967.3	E852.2	E937.3	E950.2	E962.0	E980.2
Brown spider (bite) (venom)	989.5	E905.1	—	E950.9	E962.1	E980.9

Substance	Poisoning	External Cause (E-Code)				
		Accident	Therapeutic Use	Suicide Attempt	Assault	Undetermined
Brucia	988.2	E865.3	—	E950.9	E962.1	E980.9
Brucine	989.1	E863.7	—	E950.6	E962.1	E980.7
Brunswick green — see Copper						
Bruten — see Ibuperofen						
Bryonia (alba) (dioica)	988.2	E865.4	—	E950.9	E962.1	E980.9
Buclizine	969.5	E853.8	E939.5	E950.3	E962.0	E980.3
Bufferin	965.1	E850.3	E935.3	E950.0	E962.0	E980.0
Bufotenine	969.6	E854.1	E939.6	E950.3	E962.0	E980.3
Buphenine	971.2	E855.5	E941.2	E950.4	E962.0	E980.4
Bupivacaine	968.9	E855.2	E938.9	E950.4	E962.0	E980.4
infiltration (subcutaneous)	968.5	E855.2	E938.5	E950.4	E962.0	E980.4
nerve block (peripheral) (plexus)	968.6	E855.2	E938.6	E950.4	E962.0	E980.4
Busulfan	963.1	E858.1	E933.1	E950.4	E962.0	E980.4
Butabarbital (sodium)	967.0	E851	E937.0	E950.1	E962.0	E980.1
Butabarbitone	967.0	E851	E937.0	E950.1	E962.0	E980.1
Butabarpal	967.0	E851	E937.0	E950.1	E962.0	E980.1
Butacaine	968.5	E855.2	E938.5	E950.4	E962.0	E980.4
Butallylonal	967.0	E851	E937.0	E950.1	E962.0	E980.1
Butane (distributed in mobile container)	987.0	E868.0	—	E951.1	E962.2	E981.1
distributed through pipes	987.0	E867	—	E951.0	E962.2	E981.0
incomplete combustion of — see Carbon monoxide, butane						
Butanol	980.3	E860.4	—	E950.9	E962.1	E980.9
Butanone	982.8	E862.4	—	E950.9	E962.1	E980.9
Butaperazine	969.1	E853.0	E939.1	E950.3	E962.0	E980.3
Butazolidin	965.5	E850.5	E935.5	E950.0	E962.0	E980.0
Butethal	967.0	E851	E937.0	E950.1	E962.0	E980.1
Butethamate	971.1	E855.4	E941.1	E950.4	E962.0	E980.4
Buthalitone (sodium)	968.3	E855.1	E938.3	E950.4	E962.0	E980.4
Butisol (sodium)	967.0	E851	E937.0	E950.1	E962.0	E980.1
Butobarbital, butobarbitone	967.0	E851	E937.0	E950.1	E962.0	E980.1
Butriptyline	969.0	E854.0	E939.0	E950.3	E962.0	E980.3
Buttercups	988.2	E865.4	—	E950.9	E962.1	E980.9
Butter of antimony — see Antimony						
Butyl						
acetate (secondary)	982.8	E862.4	—	E950.9	E962.1	E980.9
alcohol	980.3	E860.4	—	E950.9	E962.1	E980.9
carbinol	980.8	E860.8	—	E950.9	E962.1	E980.9
carbitol	982.8	E862.4	—	E950.9	E962.1	E980.9
cellosolve	982.8	E862.4	—	E950.9	E962.1	E980.9
chloral (hydrate)	967.1	E852.0	E937.1	E950.2	E962.0	E980.2
formate	982.8	E862.4	—	E950.9	E962.1	E980.9
scopolammonium bromide	971.1	E855.4	E941.1	E950.4	E962.0	E980.4
Butyn	968.5	E855.2	E938.5	E950.4	E962.0	E980.4
Butyrophenone (–based tranquilizers)	969.2	E853.1	E939.2	E950.3	E962.0	E980.3
Cacodyl, cacodylic acid — see Arsenic						
Cactinomycin	960.7	E856	E930.7	E950.4	E962.0	E980.4
Cade oil	976.4	E858.7	E946.4	E950.4	E962.0	E980.4
Cadmium (chloride) (compounds) (dust) (fumes) (oxide)	985.5	E866.4	—	E950.9	E962.1	E980.9
sulfide (medicinal) NEC	976.4	E858.7	E946.4	E950.4	E962.0	E980.4
Caffeine	969.7	E854.2	E939.7	E950.3	E962.0	E980.3
Calabar bean	988.2	E865.4	—	E950.9	E962.1	E980.9
Caladium seguinium	988.2	E865.4	—	E950.9	E962.1	E980.9
Calamine (liniment) (lotion)	976.3	E858.7	E946.3	E950.4	E962.0	E980.4
Calciferol	963.5	E858.1	E933.5	E950.4	E962.0	E980.4
Calcium (salts) NEC	974.5	E858.5	E944.5	E950.4	E962.0	E980.4

Substance	Poisoning	External Cause (E-Code)				
		Accident	Therapeutic Use	Suicide Attempt	Assault	Undetermined
acetylsalicylate	965.1	E850.3	E935.3	E950.0	E962.0	E980.0
benzamidosalicylate	961.8	E857	E931.8	E950.4	E962.0	E980.4
carbaspirin	965.1	E850.3	E935.3	E950.0	E962.0	E980.0
carbamide (citrated)	977.3	E858.8	E947.3	E950.4	E962.0	E980.4
carbonate (antacid)	973.0	E858.4	E943.0	E950.4	E962.0	E980.4
cyanide (citrated)	977.3	E858.8	E947.3	E950.4	E962.0	E980.4
dioctyl sulfosuccinate	973.2	E858.4	E943.2	E950.4	E962.0	E980.4
disodium edathamil	963.8	E858.1	E933.8	E950.4	E962.0	E980.4
disodium edetate	963.8	E858.1	E933.8	E950.4	E962.0	E980.4
EDTA	963.8	E858.1	E933.8	E950.4	E962.0	E980.4
hydrate, hydroxide	983.2	E864.2	—	E950.7	E962.1	E980.6
mandelate	961.9	E857	E931.9	E950.4	E962.0	E980.4
oxide	983.2	E864.2	—	E950.7	E962.1	E980.6
Calomel — *see* Mercury, chloride						
Caloric agents NEC	974.5	E858.5	E944.5	E950.4	E962.0	E980.4
Calusterone	963.1	E858.1	E933.1	E950.4	E962.0	E980.4
Camoquin	961.4	E857	E931.4	E950.4	E962.0	E980.4
Camphor (oil)	976.1	E858.7	E946.1	E950.4	E962.0	E980.4
Candeptin	976.0	E858.7	E946.0	E950.4	E962.0	E980.4
Candicidin	976.0	E858.7	E946.0	E950.4	E962.0	E980.4
Cannabinols	969.6	E854.1	E939.6	E950.3	E962.0	E980.3
Cannabis (derivatives) (indica) (sativa)	969.6	E854.1	E939.6	E950.3	E962.0	E980.3
Canned heat	980.1	E860.2	—	E950.9	E962.1	E980.9
Cantharides, cantharidin, cantharis	976.8	E858.7	E946.8	E950.4	E962.0	E980.4
Capillary agents	972.8	E858.3	E942.8	E950.4	E962.0	E980.4
Capreomycin	960.6	E856	E930.6	E950.4	E962.0	E980.4
Captodiame, captodiamine	969.5	E853.8	E939.5	E950.3	E962.0	E980.3
Caramiphen (hydrochloride)	971.1	E855.4	E941.1	E950.4	E962.0	E980.4
Carbachol	971.0	E855.3	E941.0	E950.4	E962.0	E980.4
Carbacrylamine resins	974.5	E858.5	E944.5	E950.4	E962.0	E980.4
Carbamate (sedative)	967.8	E852.8	E937.8	E950.2	E962.0	E980.2
herbicide	989.3	E863.5	—	E950.6	E962.1	E980.7
insecticide	989.3	E863.2	—	E950.6	E962.1	E980.7
Carbamazepine	966.3	E855.0	E936.3	E950.4	E962.0	E980.4
Carbamic esters	967.8	E852.8	E937.8	E950.2	E962.0	E980.2
Carbamide	974.4	E858.5	E944.4	E950.4	E962.0	E980.4
topical	976.8	E858.7	E946.8	E950.4	E962.0	E980.4
Carbamylcholine chloride	971.0	E855.3	E941.0	E950.4	E962.0	E980.4
Carbarsone	961.1	E857	E931.1	E950.4	E962.0	E980.4
Carbaryl	989.3	E863.2	—	E950.6	E962.1	E980.7
Carbaspirin	965.1	E850.3	E935.3	E950.0	E962.0	E980.0
Carbazochrome	972.8	E858.3	E942.8	E950.4	E962.0	E980.4
Carbenicillin	960.0	E856	E930.0	E950.4	E962.0	E980.4
Carbenoxolone	973.8	E858.4	E943.8	E950.4	E962.0	E980.4
Carbetapentane	975.4	E858.6	E945.4	E950.4	E962.0	E980.4
Carbimazole	962.8	E858.0	E932.8	E950.4	E962.0	E980.4
Carbinol	980.1	E860.2	—	E950.9	E962.1	E980.9
Carbinoxamine	963.0	E858.1	E933.0	E950.4	E962.0	E980.4
Carbitol	982.8	E862.4	—	E950.9	E962.1	E980.9
Carbocaine	968.9	E855.2	E938.9	E950.4	E962.0	E980.4
infiltration (subcutaneous)	968.5	E855.2	E938.5	E950.4	E962.0	E980.4
nerve block (peripheral) (plexus)	968.6	E855.2	E938.6	E950.4	E962.0	E980.4
topical (surface)	968.5	E855.2	E938.5	E950.4	E962.0	E980.4
Carbol–fuchsin solution	976.0	E858.7	E946.0	E950.4	E962.0	E980.4
Carbolic acid (*see also* Phenol)	983.0	E864.0	—	E950.7	E962.1	E980.6
Carbomycin	960.8	E856	E930.8	E950.4	E962.0	E980.4
Carbon						

Substance	Poisoning	Accident	Therapeutic Use	Suicide Attempt	Assault	Undetermined
			External Cause (E-Code)			
bisulfide (liquid) (vapor)	982.2	E862.4	—	E950.9	E962.1	E980.9
dioxide (gas)	987.8	E869.8	—	E952.8	E962.2	E982.8
disulfide (liquid) (vapor)	982.2	E862.4	—	E950.9	E962.1	E980.9
monoxide (from incomplete combustion of) (in) NEC	986	E868.9	—	E952.1	E962.2	E982.1
blast furnace gas	986	E868.8	—	E952.1	E962.2	E982.1
butane (distributed in mobile container)	986	E868.0	—	E951.1	E962.2	E981.1
distributed through pipes	986	E867	—	E951.0	E962.2	E981.0
charcoal fumes	986	E868.3	—	E952.1	E962.2	E982.1
coal						
gas (piped)	986	E867	—	E951.0	E962.2	E981.0
solid (in domestic stoves, fireplaces)	986	E868.3	—	E952.1	E962.2	E982.1
coke (in domestic stoves, fireplaces)	986	E868.3	—	E952.1	E962.2	E982.1
exhaust gas (motor) not in transit	986	E868.2	—	E952.0	E962.2	E982.0
combustion engine, any not in watercraft	986	E868.2	—	E952.0	E962.2	E982.0
farm tractor, not in transit	986	E868.2	—	E952.0	E962.2	E982.0
gas engine	986	E868.2	—	E952.0	E962.2	E982.0
motor pump	986	E868.2	—	E952.0	E962.2	E982.0
motor vehicle, not in transit	986	E868.2	—	E952.0	E962.2	E982.0
fuel (in domestic use)	986	E868.3	—	E952.1	E962.2	E982.1
gas (piped)	986	E867	—	E951.0	E962.2	E981.0
in mobile container	986	E868.0	—	E951.1	E962.2	E981.1
utility	986	E868.1	—	E951.8	E962.2	E981.1
in mobile container	986	E868.0	—	E951.1	E962.2	E981.1
piped (natural)	986	E867	—	E951.0	E962.2	E981.0
illuminating gas	986	E868.1	—	E951.8	E962.2	E981.8
industrial fuels or gases, any	986	E868.8	—	E952.1	E962.2	E982.1
kerosene (in domestic stoves, fireplaces)	986	E868.3	—	E952.1	E962.2	E982.1
kiln gas or vapor	986	E868.8	—	E952.1	E962.2	E982.1
motor exhaust gas, not in transit	986	E868.2	—	E952.0	E962.2	E982.0
piped gas (manufactured) (natural)	986	E867	—	E951.0	E962.2	E981.0
producer gas	986	E868.8	—	E952.1	E962.2	E982.1
propane (distributed in mobile container)	986	E868.0	—	E951.1	E962.2	E981.1
distributed through pipes	986	E867	—	E951.0	E962.2	E981.0
specified source NEC	986	E868.8	—	E952.1	E962.2	E982.1
stove gas	986	E868.1	—	E951.8	E962.2	E981.8
piped	986	E867	—	E951.0	E962.2	E981.0
utility gas	986	E868.1	—	E951.8	E962.2	E981.8
piped	986	E867	—	E951.0	E962.2	E981.0
water gas	986	E868.1	—	E951.8	E962.2	E981.8
wood (in domestic stoves, fireplaces)	986	E868.3	—	E952.1	E962.2	E982.1
tetrachloride (vapor) NEC	987.8	E869.8	—	E952.8	E962.2	E982.8
liquid (cleansing agent) NEC	982.1	E861.3	—	E950.9	E962.1	E980.9
solvent	982.1	E862.4	—	E950.9	E962.1	E980.9
Carbonic acid (gas)	987.8	E869.8	—	E952.8	E962.2	E982.8
anhydrase inhibitors	974.2	E858.5	E944.2	E950.4	E962.0	E980.4
Carbowax	976.3	E858.7	E946.3	E950.4	E962.0	E980.4
Carbrital	967.0	E851	E937.0	E950.1	E962.0	E980.1
Carbromal (derivatives)	967.3	E852.2	E937.3	E950.2	E962.0	E980.2
Cardiac						
depressants	972.0	E858.3	E942.0	E950.4	E962.0	E980.4
rhythm regulators	972.0	E858.3	E942.0	E950.4	E962.0	E980.4

Substance	Poisoning	External Cause (E-Code)				
		Accident	Therapeutic Use	Suicide Attempt	Assault	Undetermined
Cardiografin	977.8	E858.8	E947.8	E950.4	E962.0	E980.4
Cardio–green	977.8	E858.8	E947.8	E950.4	E962.0	E980.4
Cardiotonic glycosides	972.1	E858.3	E942.1	E950.4	E962.0	E980.4
Cardiovascular agents NEC	972.9	E858.3	E942.9	E950.4	E962.0	E980.4
Cardrase	974.2	E858.5	E944.2	E950.4	E962.0	E980.4
Carfusin	976.0	E858.7	E946.0	E950.4	E962.0	E980.4
Carisoprodol	968.0	E855.1	E938.0	E950.4	E962.0	E980.4
Carmustine	963.1	E858.1	E933.1	E950.4	E962.0	E980.4
Carotene	963.5	E858.1	E933.5	E950.4	E962.0	E980.4
Carphenazine (maleate)	969.1	E853.0	E939.1	E950.3	E962.0	E980.3
Carter's Little Pills	973.1	E858.4	E943.1	E950.4	E962.0	E980.4
Cascara (sagrada)	973.1	E858.4	E943.1	E950.4	E962.0	E980.4
Cassava	988.2	E865.4	—	E950.9	E962.1	E980.9
Castellani's paint	976.0	E858.7	E946.0	E950.4	E962.0	E980.4
Castor						
bean	988.2	E865.3	—	E950.9	E962.1	E980.9
oil	973.1	E858.4	E943.1	E950.4	E962.0	E980.4
Caterpillar (sting)	989.5	E905.5	—	E950.9	E962.1	E980.9
Catha (edulis)	970.8	E854.3	E940.8	E950.4	E962.0	E980.4
Cathartics NEC	973.3	E858.4	E943.3	E950.4	E962.0	E980.4
contact	973.1	E858.4	E943.1	E950.4	E962.0	E980.4
emollient	973.2	E858.4	E943.2	E950.4	E962.0	E980.4
intestinal irritants	973.1	E858.4	E943.1	E950.4	E962.0	E980.4
saline	973.3	E858.4	E943.3	E950.4	E962.0	E980.4
Cathomycin	960.8	E856	E930.8	E950.4	E962.0	E980.4
Caustic(s)	983.9	E864.4	—	E950.7	E962.1	E980.6
alkali	983.2	E864.2	—	E950.7	E962.1	E980.6
hydroxide	983.2	E864.2	—	E950.7	E962.1	E980.6
potash	983.2	E864.2	—	E950.7	E962.1	E980.6
soda	983.2	E864.2	—	E950.7	E962.1	E980.6
specified NEC	983.9	E864.3	—	E950.7	E962.1	E980.6
Ceepryn	976.0	E858.7	E946.0	E950.4	E962.0	E980.4
ENT agent	976.6	E858.7	E946.6	E950.4	E962.0	E980.4
lozenges	976.6	E858.7	E946.6	E950.4	E962.0	E980.4
Celestone	962.0	E858.0	E932.0	E950.4	E962.0	E980.4
topical	976.0	E858.7	E946.0	E950.4	E962.0	E980.4
Cellosolve	982.8	E862.4	—	E950.9	E962.1	E980.9
Cell stimulants and proliferants	976.8	E858.7	E946.8	E950.4	E962.0	E980.4
Cellulose derivatives, cathartic	973.3	E858.4	E943.3	E950.4	E962.0	E980.4
nitrates (topical)	976.3	E858.7	E946.3	E950.4	E962.0	E980.4
Centipede (bite)	989.5	E905.4	—	E950.9	E962.1	E980.9
Central nervous system						
depressants	968.4	E855.1	E938.4	E950.4	E962.0	E980.4
anesthetic (general) NEC	968.4	E855.1	E938.4	E950.4	E962.0	E980.4
gases NEC	968.2	E855.1	E938.2	E950.4	E962.0	E980.4
intravenous	968.3	E855.1	E938.3	E950.4	E962.0	E980.4
barbiturates	967.0	E851	E937.0	E950.1	E962.0	E980.1
bromides	967.3	E852.2	E937.3	E950.2	E962.0	E980.2
cannabis sativa	969.6	E854.1	E939.6	E950.3	E962.0	E980.3
chloral hydrate	967.1	E852.0	E937.1	E950.2	E962.0	E980.2
hallucinogenics	969.6	E854.1	E939.6	E950.3	E962.0	E980.3
hypnotics	967.9	E852.9	E937.9	E950.2	E962.0	E980.2
specified NEC	967.8	E852.8	E937.8	E950.2	E962.0	E980.2
muscle relaxants	968.0	E855.1	E938.0	E950.4	E962.0	E980.4
paraldehyde	967.2	E852.1	E937.2	E950.2	E962.0	E980.2
sedatives	967.9	E852.9	E937.9	E950.2	E962.0	E980.2
mixed NEC	967.6	E852.5	E937.6	E950.2	E962.0	E980.2

Substance	External Cause (E-Code)					
	Poisoning	Accident	Therapeutic Use	Suicide Attempt	Assault	Undetermined
specified NEC 967.8	E852.8	E937.8	E950.2	E962.0	E980.2
muscle–tone depressants 968.0	E855.1	E938.0	E950.4	E962.0	E980.4
stimulants 970.9	E854.3	E940.9	E950.4	E962.0	E980.4
amphetamines 969.7	E854.2	E939.7	E950.3	E962.0	E980.3
analeptics 970.0	E854.3	E940.0	E950.4	E962.0	E980.4
antidepressants 969.0	E854.0	E939.0	E950.3	E962.0	E980.3
opiate antagonists 970.1	E854.3	E940.0	E950.4	E962.0	E980.4
specified NEC 970.8	E854.3	E940.8	E950.4	E962.0	E980.4
Cephalexin 960.5	E856	E930.5	E950.4	E962.0	E980.4
Cephaloglycin 960.5	E856	E930.5	E950.4	E962.0	E980.4
Cephaloridine 960.5	E856	E930.5	E950.4	E962.0	E980.4
Cephalosporins NEC 960.5	E856	E930.5	E950.4	E962.0	E980.4
N (adicillin) 960.0	E856	E930.0	E950.4	E962.0	E980.4
Cephalothin (sodium) 960.5	E856	E930.5	E950.4	E962.0	E980.4
Cerbera (odallam) 988.2	E865.4	—	E950.9	E962.1	E980.9
Cerberin 972.1	E858.3	E942.1	E950.4	E962.0	E980.4
Cerebral stimulants 970.9	E854.3	E940.9	E950.4	E962.0	E980.4
psychotherapeutic 969.7	E854.2	E939.7	E950.3	E962.0	E980.3
specified NEC 970.8	E854.3	E940.8	E950.4	E962.0	E980.4
Cetalkonium (chloride) 976.0	E858.7	E946.0	E950.4	E962.0	E980.4
Cetoxime 963.0	E858.1	E933.0	E950.4	E962.0	E980.4
Cetrimide 976.2	E858.7	E946.2	E950.4	E962.0	E980.4
Cetylpyridinium 976.0	E858.7	E946.0	E950.4	E962.0	E980.4
ENT agent 976.6	E858.7	E946.6	E950.4	E962.0	E980.4
lozenges 976.6	E858.7	E946.6	E950.4	E962.0	E980.4
Cevadilla — see Sabadilla					
Cevitamic acid 963.5	E858.1	E933.5	E950.4	E962.0	E980.4
Chalk, precipitated 973.0	E858.4	E943.0	E950.4	E962.0	E980.4
Charcoal					
fumes (carbon monoxide) 986	E868.3	—	E952.1	E962.2	E982.1
industrial 986	E868.8	—	E952.1	E962.2	E982.1
medicinal (activated) 973.0	E858.4	E943.0	E950.4	E962.0	E980.4
Chelating agents NEC 977.2	E858.8	E947.2	E950.4	E962.0	E980.4
Chelidonium majus 988.2	E865.4	—	E950.9	E962.1	E980.9
Chemical substance 989.9	E866.9	—	E950.9	E962.1	E980.9
specified NEC 989.89	E866.8	—	E950.9	E962.1	E980.9
Chemotherapy, antineoplastic 963.1	E858.1	E933.1	E950.4	E962.0	E980.4
Chenopodium (oil) 961.6	E857	E931.6	E950.4	E962.0	E980.4
Cherry laurel 988.2	E865.4	—	E950.9	E962.1	E980.9
Chiniofon 961.3	E857	E931.3	E950.4	E962.0	E980.4
Chlophedianol 975.4	E858.6	E945.4	E950.4	E962.0	E980.4
Chloral (betaine) (formamide) (hydrate) ... 967.1	E852.0	E937.1	E950.2	E962.0	E980.2
Chloralamide 967.1	E852.0	E937.1	E950.2	E962.0	E980.2
Chlorambucil 963.1	E858.1	E933.1	E950.4	E962.0	E980.4
Chloramphenicol 960.2	E856	E930.2	E950.4	E962.0	E980.4
ENT agent 976.6	E858.7	E946.6	E950.4	E962.0	E980.4
ophthalmic preparation 976.5	E858.7	E946.5	E950.4	E962.0	E980.4
topical NEC 976.0	E858.7	E946.0	E950.4	E962.0	E980.4
Chlorate(s) (potassium) (sodium) NEC 983.9	E864.3	—	E950.7	E962.1	E980.6
herbicides 989.4	E863.5	—	E950.6	E962.1	E980.7
Chlorcyclizine 963.0	E858.1	E933.0	E950.4	E962.0	E980.4
Chlordan(e) (dust) 989.2	E863.0	—	E950.6	E962.1	E980.7
Chlordantoin 976.0	E858.7	E946.0	E950.4	E962.0	E980.4
Chlordiazepoxide 969.4	E853.2	E939.4	E950.3	E962.0	E980.3
Chloresium 976.8	E858.7	E946.8	E950.4	E962.0	E980.4
Chlorethiazol 967.1	E852.0	E937.1	E950.2	E962.0	E980.2
Chlorethyl — see Ethyl, chloride					

Substance	Poisoning	External Cause (E-Code)				
		Accident	Therapeutic Use	Suicide Attempt	Assault	Undetermined
Chloretone 967.1	967.1	E852.0	E937.1	E950.2	E962.0	E980.2
Chlorex 982.3	982.3	E862.4	—	E950.9	E962.1	E980.9
Chlorhexadol 967.1	967.1	E852.0	E937.1	E950.2	E962.0	E980.2
Chlorhexidine (hydrochloride) 976.0	976.0	E858.7	E946.0	E950.4	E962.0	E980.4
Chlorhydroxyquinolin 976.0	976.0	E858.7	E946.0	E950.4	E962.0	E980.4
Chloride of lime (bleach) 983.9	983.9	E864.3	—	E950.7	E962.1	E980.6
Chlorinated						
camphene 989.2	989.2	E863.0	—	E950.6	E962.1	E980.7
diphenyl 989.89	989.89	E866.8	—	E950.9	E962.1	E980.9
hydrocarbons NEC 989.2	989.2	E863.0	—	E950.6	E962.1	E980.7
solvent 982.3	982.3	E862.4	—	E950.9	E962.1	E980.9
lime (bleach) 983.9	983.9	E864.3	—	E950.7	E962.1	E980.6
naphthalene — see Naphthalene						
pesticides NEC 989.2	989.2	E863.0	—	E950.6	E962.1	E980.7
soda — see Sodium, hypochlorite						
Chlorine (fumes) (gas) 987.6	987.6	E869.8	—	E952.8	E962.2	E982.8
bleach 983.9	983.9	E864.3	—	E950.7	E962.1	E980.6
compounds NEC 983.9	983.9	E864.3	—	E950.7	E962.1	E980.6
disinfectant 983.9	983.9	E861.4	—	E950.7	E962.1	E980.6
releasing agents NEC 983.9	983.9	E864.3	—	E950.7	E962.1	E980.6
Chlorisondamine 972.3	972.3	E858.3	E942.3	E950.4	E962.0	E980.4
Chlormadinone 962.2	962.2	E858.0	E932.2	E950.4	E962.0	E980.4
Chlormerodrin 974.0	974.0	E858.5	E944.0	E950.4	E962.0	E980.4
Chlormethiazole 967.1	967.1	E852.0	E937.1	E950.2	E962.0	E980.2
Chlormethylenecycline 960.4	960.4	E856	E930.4	E950.4	E962.0	E980.4
Chlormezanone 969.5	969.5	E853.8	E939.5	E950.3	E962.0	E980.3
Chloroacetophenone 987.5	987.5	E869.3	—	E952.8	E962.2	E982.8
Chloroaniline 983.0	983.0	E864.0	—	E950.7	E962.1	E980.6
Chlorobenzene, chlorobenzol 982.0	982.0	E862.4	—	E950.9	E962.1	E980.9
Chlorobutanol 967.1	967.1	E852.0	E937.1	E950.2	E962.0	E980.2
Chlorodinitrobenzene 983.0	983.0	E864.0	—	E950.7	E962.1	E980.6
dust or vapor 987.8	987.8	E869.8	—	E952.8	E962.2	E982.8
Chloroethane — see Ethyl, chloride						
Chloroform (fumes) (vapor) 987.8	987.8	E869.8	—	E952.8	E962.2	E982.8
anesthetic (gas) 968.2	968.2	E855.1	E938.2	E950.4	E962.0	E980.4
liquid NEC 968.4	968.4	E855.1	E938.4	E950.4	E962.0	E980.4
solvent 982.3	982.3	E862.4	—	E950.9	E962.1	E980.9
Chloroguanide 961.4	961.4	E857	E931.4	E950.4	E962.0	E980.4
Chloromycetin 960.2	960.2	E856	E930.2	E950.4	E962.0	E980.4
ENT agent 976.6	976.6	E858.7	E946.6	E950.4	E962.0	E980.4
ophthalmic preparation 976.5	976.5	E858.7	E946.5	E950.4	E962.0	E980.4
otic solution 976.6	976.6	E858.7	E946.6	E950.4	E962.0	E980.4
topical NEC 976.0	976.0	E858.7	E946.0	E950.4	E962.0	E980.4
Chloronitrobenzene 983.0	983.0	E864.0	—	E950.7	E962.1	E980.6
dust or vapor 987.8	987.8	E869.8	—	E952.8	E962.2	E982.8
Chlorophenol 983.0	983.0	E864.0	—	E950.7	E962.1	E980.6
Chlorophenothane 989.2	989.2	E863.0	—	E950.6	E962.1	E980.7
Chlorophyll (derivatives) 976.8	976.8	E858.7	E946.8	E950.4	E962.0	E980.4
Chloropicrin (fumes) 987.8	987.8	E869.8	—	E952.8	E962.2	E982.8
fumigant 989.4	989.4	E863.8	—	E950.6	E962.1	E980.7
fungicide 989.4	989.4	E863.6	—	E950.6	E962.1	E980.7
pesticide (fumes) 989.4	989.4	E863.4	—	E950.6	E962.1	E980.7
Chloroprocaine 968.9	968.9	E855.2	E938.9	E950.4	E962.0	E980.4
infiltration (subcutaneous) 968.5	968.5	E855.2	E938.5	E950.4	E962.0	E980.4
nerve block (peripheral) (plexus) 968.6	968.6	E855.2	E938.6	E950.4	E962.0	E980.4
Chloroptic 976.5	976.5	E858.7	E946.5	E950.4	E962.0	E980.4
Chloropurine 963.1	963.1	E858.1	E933.1	E950.4	E962.0	E980.4

Substance	External Cause (E-Code)					
	Poisoning	Accident	Therapeutic Use	Suicide Attempt	Assault	Undetermined
Chloroquine (hydrochloride) (phosphate) . . .	961.4	E857	E931.4	E950.4	E962.0	E980.4
Chlorothen	963.0	E858.1	E933.0	E950.4	E962.0	E980.4
Chlorothiazide	974.3	E858.5	E944.3	E950.4	E962.0	E980.4
Chlorotrianisene	962.2	E858.0	E932.2	E950.4	E962.0	E980.4
Chlorovinyldichloroarsine	985.1	E866.3	—	E950.8	E962.1	E980.8
Chloroxylenol	976.0	E858.7	E946.0	E950.4	E962.0	E980.4
Chlorphenesin (carbamate)	968.0	E855.1	E938.0	E950.4	E962.0	E980.4
topical (antifungal)	976.0	E858.7	E946.0	E950.4	E962.0	E980.4
Chlorpheniramine	963.0	E858.1	E933.0	E950.4	E962.0	E980.4
Chlorophenoxamine	966.4	E855.0	E936.4	E950.4	E962.0	E980.4
Chlorophentermine	977.0	E858.8	E947.0	E950.4	E962.0	E980.4
Chlorproguanil	961.4	E857	E931.4	E950.4	E962.0	E980.4
Chlorpromazine	969.1	E853.0	E939.1	E950.3	E962.0	E980.3
Chlorpropamide	962.3	E858.0	E932.3	E950.4	E962.0	E980.4
Chlorprothixene	969.3	E853.8	E939.3	E950.3	E962.0	E980.3
Chlorquinaldol	976.0	E858.7	E946.0	E950.4	E962.0	E980.4
Chlortetracycline	960.4	E856	E930.4	E950.4	E962.0	E980.4
Chlorthalidone	974.4	E858.5	E944.4	E950.4	E962.0	E980.4
Chlortrianisene	962.2	E858.0	E932.2	E950.4	E962.0	E980.4
Chlor–Trimeton	963.0	E858.1	E933.0	E950.4	E962.0	E980.4
Chlorzoxazone	968.0	E855.1	E938.0	E950.4	E962.0	E980.4
Choke damp	987.8	E869.8	—	E952.8	E962.2	E982.8
Cholebrine	977.8	E858.8	E947.8	E950.4	E962.0	E980.4
Cholera vaccine	978.2	E858.8	E948.2	E950.4	E962.0	E980.4
Cholesterol–lowering agents	972.2	E858.3	E942.2	E950.4	E962.0	E980.4
Cholestyramine (resin)	972.2	E858.3	E942.2	E950.4	E962.0	E980.4
Cholic acid	973.4	E858.4	E943.4	E950.4	E962.0	E980.4
Choline						
dihydrogen citrate	977.1	E858.8	E947.1	E950.4	E962.0	E980.4
salicylate	965.1	E850.3	E935.3	E950.0	E962.0	E980.0
theophyllinate	974.1	E858.5	E944.1	E950.4	E962.0	E980.4
Cholinergics	971.0	E855.3	E941.0	E950.4	E962.0	E980.4
Cholografin	977.8	E858.8	E947.8	E950.4	E962.0	E980.4
Chorionic gonadotropin	962.4	E858.0	E932.4	E950.4	E962.0	E980.4
Chromates	983.9	E864.3	—	E950.7	E962.1	E980.6
dust or mist	987.8	E869.8	—	E952.8	E962.2	E982.8
lead	984.0	E866.0	—	E950.9	E962.1	E980.9
paint	984.0	E861.5	—	E950.9	E962.1	E980.9
Chromic acid	983.9	E864.3	—	E950.7	E962.1	E980.6
dust or mist	987.8	E869.8	—	E952.8	E962.2	E982.8
Chromium	985.6	E866.4	—	E950.9	E962.1	E980.9
compounds — *see* Chromates						
Chromonar	972.4	E858.3	E942.4	E950.4	E962.0	E980.4
Chromyl chloride	983.9	E864.3	—	E950.7	E962.1	E980.6
Chrysarobin (ointment)	976.4	E858.7	E946.4	E950.4	E962.0	E980.4
Chrysazin	973.1	E858.4	E943.1	E950.4	E962.0	E980.4
Chymar	963.4	E858.1	E933.4	E950.4	E962.0	E980.4
ophthalmic preparation	976.5	E858.7	E946.5	E950.4	E962.0	E980.4
Chymotrypsin	963.4	E858.1	E933.4	E950.4	E962.0	E980.4
ophthalmic preparation	976.5	E858.7	E946.5	E950.4	E962.0	E980.4
Cicuta maculata or virosa	988.2	E865.4	—	E950.9	E962.1	E980.9
Cigarette lighter fluid	981	E862.1	—	E950.9	E962.1	E980.9
Cinchocaine (spinal)	968.7	E855.2	E938.7	E950.4	E962.0	E980.4
topical (surface)	968.5	E855.2	E938.5	E950.4	E962.0	E980.4
Cinchona	961.4	E857	E931.4	E950.4	E962.0	E980.4
Cinchonine alkaloids	961.4	E857	E931.4	E950.4	E962.0	E980.4
Cinchophen	974.7	E858.5	E944.7	E950.4	E962.0	E980.4

Substance	Poisoning	External Cause (E-Code)				
		Accident	Therapeutic Use	Suicide Attempt	Assault	Undetermined
Cinnarizine	963.0	E858.1	E933.0	E950.4	E962.0	E980.4
Citanest	968.9	E855.2	E938.9	E950.4	E962.0	E980.4
infiltration (subcutaneous)	968.5	E855.2	E938.5	E950.4	E962.0	E980.4
nerve block (peripheral) (plexus)	968.6	E855.2	E938.6	E950.4	E962.0	E980.4
Citric acid	989.89	E866.8	—	E950.9	E962.1	E980.9
Citrovorum factor	964.1	E858.2	E934.1	E950.4	E962.0	E980.4
Claviceps purpurea	988.2	E865.4	—	E950.9	E962.1	E980.9
Cleaner, cleansing agent NEC	989.89	E861.3	—	E950.9	E962.1	E980.9
of paint or varnish	982.8	E862.9	—	E950.9	E962.1	E980.9
Clematis vitalba	988.2	E865.4	—	E950.9	E962.1	E980.9
Clemizole	963.0	E858.1	E933.0	E950.4	E962.0	E980.4
penicillin	960.0	E856	E930.0	E950.4	E962.0	E980.4
Clidinium	971.1	E855.4	E941.1	E950.4	E962.0	E980.4
Clindamycin	960.8	E856	E930.8	E950.4	E962.0	E980.4
Cliradon	965.09	E850.2	E935.2	E950.0	E962.0	E980.0
Clocortolone	962.0	E858.0	E932.0	E950.4	E962.0	E980.4
Clofedanol	975.4	E858.6	E945.4	E950.4	E962.0	E980.4
Clofibrate	972.2	E858.3	E942.2	E950.4	E962.0	E980.4
Clomethiazole	967.1	E852.0	E937.1	E950.2	E962.0	E980.2
Clomiphene	977.8	E858.8	E947.8	E950.4	E962.0	E980.4
Clonazepam	969.4	E853.2	E939.4	E950.3	E962.0	E980.3
Clonidine	972.6	E858.3	E942.6	E950.4	E962.0	E980.4
Clopamide	974.3	E858.5	E944.3	E950.4	E962.0	E980.4
Clorazepate	969.4	E853.2	E939.4	E950.3	E962.0	E980.3
Clorexolone	974.4	E858.5	E944.4	E950.4	E962.0	E980.4
Clorox (bleach)	983.9	E864.3	—	E950.7	E962.1	E980.6
Clortermine	977.0	E858.8	E947.0	E950.4	E962.0	E980.4
Clotrimazole	976.0	E858.7	E946.0	E950.4	E962.0	E980.4
Cloxacillin	960.0	E856	E930.0	E950.4	E962.0	E980.4
Coagulants NEC	964.5	E858.2	E934.5	E950.4	E962.0	E980.4
Coal (carbon monoxide from) — see also Carbon, monoxide, coal						
oil — see Kerosene						
tar NEC	983.0	E864.0	—	E950.7	E962.1	E980.6
fumes	987.8	E869.8	—	E952.8	E962.2	E982.8
medicinal (ointment)	976.4	E858.7	E946.4	E950.4	E962.0	E980.4
analgesics NEC	965.5	E850.5	E935.5	E950.0	E962.0	E980.0
naphtha (solvent)	981	E862.0	—	E950.9	E962.1	E980.9
Cobalt (fumes) (industrial)	985.8	E866.4	—	E950.9	E962.1	E980.9
Cobra (venom)	989.5	E905.0	—	E950.9	E962.1	E980.9
Coca (leaf)	970.8	E854.3	E940.8	E950.4	E962.0	E980.4
Cocaine (hydrochloride) (salt)	970.8	E854.3	E940.8	E950.4	E962.0	E980.4
topical anesthetic	968.5	E855.2	E938.5	E950.4	E962.0	E980.4
Coccidioidin	977.8	E858.8	E947.8	E950.4	E962.0	E980.4
Cocculus indicus	988.2	E865.3	—	E950.9	E962.1	E980.9
Cochineal	989.89	E866.8	—	E950.9	E962.1	E980.9
medicinal products	977.4	E858.8	E947.4	E950.4	E962.0	E980.4
Codeine	965.09	E850.2	E935.2	E950.0	E962.0	E980.0
Coffee	989.89	E866.8	—	E950.9	E962.1	E980.9
Cogentin	971.1	E855.4	E941.1	E950.4	E962.0	E980.4
Coke fumes or gas (carbon monoxide)	986	E868.3	—	E952.1	E962.2	E982.1
industrial use	986	E868.8	—	E952.1	E962.2	E982.1
Colace	973.2	E858.4	E943.2	E950.4	E962.0	E980.4
Colchicine	974.7	E858.5	E944.7	E950.4	E962.0	E980.4
Colchicum	988.2	E865.3	—	E950.9	E962.1	E980.9
Cold cream	976.3	E858.7	E946.3	E950.4	E962.0	E980.4
Colestipol	972.2	E858.3	E942.2	E950.4	E962.0	E980.4

Substance	Poisoning	External Cause (E-Code)				
		Accident	Therapeutic Use	Suicide Attempt	Assault	Undetermined
Colistimethate	960.8	E856	E930.8	E950.4	E962.0	E980.4
Colistin	960.8	E856	E930.8	E950.4	E962.0	E980.4
Collagen	977.8	E866.8	E947.8	E950.9	E962.1	E980.9
Collagenase	976.8	E858.7	E946.8	E950.4	E962.0	E980.4
Collodion (flexible)	976.3	E858.7	E946.3	E950.4	E962.0	E980.4
Colocynth	973.1	E858.4	E943.1	E950.4	E962.0	E980.4
Coloring matter — *see* Dye(s)						
Combustion gas — *see* Carbon, monoxide						
Compazine	969.1	E853.0	E939.1	E950.3	E962.0	E980.3
Compound						
42 (warfarin)	989.4	E863.7	—	E950.6	E962.1	E980.7
269 (endrin)	989.2	E863.0	—	E950.6	E962.1	E980.7
497 (dieldrin)	989.2	E863.0	—	E950.6	E962.1	E980.7
1080 (sodium fluoroacetate)	989.4	E863.7	—	E950.6	E962.1	E980.7
3422 (parathion)	989.3	E863.1	—	E950.6	E962.1	E980.7
3911 (phorate)	989.3	E863.1	—	E950.6	E962.1	E980.7
3956 (toxaphene)	989.2	E863.0	—	E950.6	E962.1	E980.7
4049 (malathion)	989.3	E863.1	—	E950.6	E962.1	E980.7
4124 (dicapthon)	989.4	E863.4	—	E950.6	E962.1	E980.7
E (cortisone)	962.0	E858.0	E932.0	E950.4	E962.0	E980.4
F (hydrocortisone)	962.0	E858.0	E932.0	E950.4	E962.0	E980.4
Congo red	977.8	E858.8	E947.8	E950.4	E962.0	E980.4
Coniine, conine	965.7	E850.7	E935.7	E950.0	E962.0	E980.0
Conium (maculatum)	988.2	E865.4	—	E950.9	E962.1	E980.9
Conjugated estrogens (equine)	962.2	E858.0	E932.2	E950.4	E962.0	E980.4
Contac	975.6	E858.6	E945.6	E950.4	E962.0	E980.4
Contact lens solution	976.5	E858.7	E946.5	E950.4	E962.0	E980.4
Contraceptives (oral)	962.2	E858.0	E932.2	E950.4	E962.0	E980.4
vaginal	976.8	E858.7	E946.8	E950.4	E962.0	E980.4
Contrast media (roentgenographic)	977.8	E858.8	E947.8	E950.4	E962.0	E980.4
Convallaria majalis	988.2	E865.4	—	E950.9	E962.1	E980.9
Copper (dust) (fumes) (salts) NEC	985.8	E866.4	—	E950.9	E962.1	E980.9
arsenate, arsenite	985.1	E866.3	—	E950.8	E962.1	E980.8
insecticide	985.1	E863.4	—	E950.8	E962.1	E980.8
emetic	973.6	E858.4	E943.6	E950.4	E962.0	E980.4
fungicide	985.8	E863.6	—	E950.6	E962.1	E980.7
insecticide	985.8	E863.4	—	E950.6	E962.1	E980.7
oleate	976.0	E858.7	E946.0	E950.4	E962.0	E980.4
sulfate	983.9	E864.3	—	E950.7	E962.1	E980.6
fungicide	983.9	E863.6	—	E950.7	E962.1	E980.6
cupric	973.6	E858.4	E943.6	E950.4	E962.0	E980.4
cuprous	983.9	E864.3	—	E950.7	E962.1	E980.6
Copperhead snake (bite) (venom)	989.5	E905.0	—	E950.9	E962.1	E980.9
Coral (sting)	989.5	E905.6	—	E950.9	E962.1	E980.9
snake (bite) (venom)	989.5	E905.0	—	E950.9	E962.1	E980.9
Cordran	976.0	E858.7	E946.0	E950.4	E962.0	E980.4
Corn cures	976.4	E858.7	E946.4	E950.4	E962.0	E980.4
Cornhusker's lotion	976.3	E858.7	E946.3	E950.4	E962.0	E980.4
Corn starch	976.3	E858.7	E946.3	E950.4	E962.0	E980.4
Corrosive	983.9	E864.4	—	E950.7	E962.1	E980.6
acids NEC	983.1	E864.1	—	E950.7	E962.1	E980.6
aromatics	983.0	E864.0	—	E950.7	E962.1	E980.6
disinfectant	983.0	E861.4	—	E950.7	E962.1	E980.6
fumes NEC	987.9	E869.9	—	E952.9	E962.2	E982.9
specified NEC	983.9	E864.3	—	E950.7	E962.1	E980.6
sublimate — *see* Mercury, chloride						
Cortate	962.0	E858.0	E932.0	E950.4	E962.0	E980.4

Substance	Poisoning	Accident	External Cause (E-Code) Therapeutic Use	Suicide Attempt	Assault	Undetermined
Cort–Dome	962.0	E858.0	E932.0	E950.4	E962.0	E980.4
ENT agent	976.6	E858.7	E946.6	E950.4	E962.0	E980.4
ophthalmic preparation	976.5	E858.7	E946.5	E950.4	E962.0	E980.4
topical NEC	976.0	E858.7	E946.0	E950.4	E962.0	E980.4
Cortef	962.0	E858.0	E932.0	E950.4	E962.0	E980.4
ENT agent	976.6	E858.7	E946.6	E950.4	E962.0	E980.4
ophthalmic preparation	976.5	E858.7	E946.5	E950.4	E962.0	E980.4
topical NEC	976.0	E858.7	E946.0	E950.4	E962.0	E980.4
Corticosteroids (fluorinated)	962.0	E858.0	E932.0	E950.4	E962.0	E980.4
ENT agent	976.6	E858.7	E946.6	E950.4	E962.0	E980.4
ophthalmic preparation	976.5	E858.7	E946.5	E950.4	E962.0	E980.4
topical NEC	976.0	E858.7	E946.0	E950.4	E962.0	E980.4
Corticotropin	962.4	E858.0	E932.4	E950.4	E962.0	E980.4
Cortisol	962.0	E858.0	E932.0	E950.4	E962.0	E980.4
ENT agent	976.6	E858.7	E946.6	E950.4	E962.0	E980.4
ophthalmic preparation	976.5	E858.7	E946.5	E950.4	E962.0	E980.4
topical NEC	976.0	E858.7	E946.0	E950.4	E962.0	E980.4
Cortisone derivatives (acetate)	962.0	E858.0	E932.0	E950.4	E962.0	E980.4
ENT agent	976.6	E858.7	E946.6	E950.4	E962.0	E980.4
ophthalmic preparation	976.5	E858.7	E946.5	E950.4	E962.0	E980.4
topical NEC	976.0	E858.7	E946.0	E950.4	E962.0	E980.4
Cortogen	962.0	E858.0	E932.0	E950.4	E962.0	E980.4
ENT agent	976.6	E858.7	E946.6	E950.4	E962.0	E980.4
ophthalmic preparation	976.5	E858.7	E946.5	E950.4	E962.0	E980.4
Cortone	962.0	E858.0	E932.0	E950.4	E962.0	E980.4
ENT agent	976.6	E858.7	E946.6	E950.4	E962.0	E980.4
ophthalmic preparation	976.5	E858.7	E946.5	E950.4	E962.0	E980.4
Cortril	962.0	E858.0	E932.0	E950.4	E962.0	E980.4
ENT agent	976.6	E858.7	E946.6	E950.4	E962.0	E980.4
ophthalmic preparation	976.5	E858.7	E946.5	E950.4	E962.0	E980.4
topical NEC	976.0	E858.7	E946.0	E950.4	E962.0	E980.4
Cosmetics	989.89	E866.7	—	E950.9	E962.1	E980.9
Cosyntropin	977.8	E858.8	E947.8	E950.4	E962.0	E980.4
Cotarnine	964.5	E858.2	E934.5	E950.4	E962.0	E980.4
Cottonseed oil	976.3	E858.7	E946.3	E950.4	E962.0	E980.4
Cough mixtures (antitussives)	975.4	E858.6	E945.4	E950.4	E962.0	E980.4
containing opiates	965.09	E850.2	E935.2	E950.0	E962.0	E980.0
expectorants	975.5	E858.6	E945.5	E950.4	E962.0	E980.4
Coumadin	964.2	E858.2	E934.2	E950.4	E962.0	E980.4
rodenticide	989.4	E863.7	—	E950.6	E962.1	E980.7
Coumarin	964.2	E858.2	E934.2	E950.4	E962.0	E980.4
Coumetarol	964.2	E858.2	E934.2	E950.4	E962.0	E980.4
Cowbane	988.2	E865.4	—	E950.9	E962.1	E980.9
Cozyme	963.5	E858.1	E933.5	E950.4	E962.0	E980.4
Crack	970.8	E854.3	E940.8	E950.4	E962.0	E980.4
Creolin	983.0	E864.0	—	E950.7	E962.1	E980.6
disinfectant	983.0	E861.4	—	E950.7	E962.1	E980.6
Creosol (compound)	983.0	E864.0	—	E950.7	E962.1	E980.6
Creosote (beechwood) (coal tar)	983.0	E864.0	—	E950.7	E962.1	E980.6
medicinal (expectorant)	975.5	E858.6	E945.5	E950.4	E962.0	E980.4
syrup	975.5	E858.6	E945.5	E950.4	E962.0	E980.4
Cresol	983.0	E864.0	—	E950.7	E962.1	E980.6
disinfectant	983.0	E861.4	—	E950.7	E962.1	E980.6
Cresylic acid	983.0	E864.0	—	E950.7	E962.1	E980.6
Cropropamide	965.7	E850.7	E935.7	E950.0	E962.0	E980.0
with crotethamide	970.0	E854.3	E940.0	E950.4	E962.0	E980.4
Crotamiton	976.0	E858.7	E946.0	E950.4	E962.0	E980.4

Substance	Poisoning	External Cause (E-Code)				
		Accident	Therapeutic Use	Suicide Attempt	Assault	Undetermined
Crotethamide	965.7	E850.7	E935.7	E950.0	E962.0	E980.0
with cropropamide	970.0	E854.3	E940.0	E950.4	E962.0	E980.4
Croton (oil)	973.1	E858.4	E943.1	E950.4	E962.0	E980.4
chloral	967.1	E852.0	E937.1	E950.2	E962.0	E980.2
Crude oil	981	E862.1	—	E950.9	E962.1	E980.9
Cryogenine	965.8	E850.8	E935.8	E950.0	E962.0	E980.0
Cryolite (pesticide)	989.4	E863.4	—	E950.6	E962.1	E980.7
Cryptenamine	972.6	E858.3	E942.6	E950.4	E962.0	E980.4
Crystal violet	976.0	E858.7	E946.0	E950.4	E962.0	E980.4
Cuckoopint	988.2	E865.4	—	E950.9	E962.1	E980.9
Cumetharol	964.2	E858.2	E934.2	E950.4	E962.0	E980.4
Cupric sulfate	973.6	E858.4	E943.6	E950.4	E962.0	E980.4
Cuprous sulfate	983.9	E864.3	—	E950.7	E962.1	E980.6
Curare, curarine	975.2	E858.6	E945.2	E950.4	E962.0	E980.4
Cyanic acid — see Cyanide(s)						
Cyanide(s) (compounds) (hydrogen)						
(potassium) (sodium) NEC	989.0	E866.8	—	E950.9	E962.1	E980.9
dust or gas (inhalation) NEC	987.7	E869.8	—	E952.8	E962.2	E982.8
fumigant	989.0	E863.8	—	E950.6	E962.1	E980.7
mercuric — see Mercury						
pesticide (dust) (fumes)	989.0	E863.4	—	E950.6	E962.1	E980.7
Cyanocobalamin	964.1	E858.2	E934.1	E950.4	E962.0	E980.4
Cyanogen (chloride) (gas) NEC	987.8	E869.8	—	E952.8	E962.2	E982.8
Cyclaine	968.5	E855.2	E938.5	E950.4	E962.0	E980.4
Cyclamen europaeum	988.2	E865.4	—	E950.9	E962.1	E980.9
Cyclandelate	972.5	E858.3	E942.5	E950.4	E962.0	E980.4
Cyclazocine	965.09	E850.2	E935.2	E950.0	E962.0	E980.0
Cyclizine	963.0	E858.1	E933.0	E950.4	E962.0	E980.4
Cyclobarbital, cyclobarbitone	967.0	E851	E937.0	E950.1	E962.0	E980.1
Cycloguanil	961.4	E857	E931.4	E950.4	E962.0	E980.4
Cyclohexane	982.0	E862.4	—	E950.9	E962.1	E980.9
Cyclohexanol	980.8	E860.8	—	E950.9	E962.1	E980.9
Cyclohexanone	982.8	E862.4	—	E950.9	E962.1	E980.9
Cyclomethycaine	968.5	E855.2	E938.5	E950.4	E962.0	E980.4
Cyclopentamine	971.2	E855.5	E941.2	E950.4	E962.0	E980.4
Cyclopenthiazide	974.3	E858.5	E944.3	E950.4	E962.0	E980.4
Cyclopentolate	971.1	E855.4	E941.1	E950.4	E962.0	E980.4
Cyclophosphamide	963.1	E858.1	E933.1	E950.4	E962.0	E980.4
Cyclopropane	968.2	E855.1	E938.2	E950.4	E962.0	E980.4
Cycloserine	960.6	E856	E930.6	E950.4	E962.0	E980.4
Cyclothiazide	974.3	E858.5	E944.3	E950.4	E962.0	E980.4
Cycrimine	966.4	E855.0	E936.4	E950.4	E962.0	E980.4
Cymarin	972.1	E858.3	E942.1	E950.4	E962.0	E980.4
Cyproheptadine	963.0	E858.1	E933.0	E950.4	E962.0	E980.4
Cyprolidol	969.0	E854.0	E939.0	E950.3	E962.0	E980.3
Cytarabine	963.1	E858.1	E933.1	E950.4	E962.0	E980.4
Cytisus						
laburnum	988.2	E865.4	—	E950.9	E962.1	E980.9
scoparius	988.2	E865.4	—	E950.9	E962.1	E980.9
Cytomel	962.7	E858.0	E932.7	E950.4	E962.0	E980.4
Cytosine (antineoplastic)	963.1	E858.1	E933.1	E950.4	E962.0	E980.4
Cytoxan	963.1	E858.1	E933.1	E950.4	E962.0	E980.4
Dacarbazine	963.1	E858.1	E933.1	E950.4	E962.0	E980.4
Dactinomycin	960.7	E856	E930.7	E950.4	E962.0	E980.4
DADPS	961.8	E857	E931.8	E950.4	E962.0	E980.4
Dakin's solution (external)	976.0	E858.7	E946.0	E950.4	E962.0	E980.4
Dalmane	969.4	E853.2	E939.4	E950.3	E962.0	E980.3

Substance	Poisoning	Accident	External Cause (E-Code) Therapeutic Use	Suicide Attempt	Assault	Undetermined
DAM	977.2	E858.8	E947.2	E950.4	E962.0	E980.4
Danilone	964.2	E858.2	E934.2	E950.4	E962.0	E980.4
Danthron	973.1	E858.4	E943.1	E950.4	E962.0	E980.4
Dantrolene	975.2	E858.6	E945.2	E950.4	E962.0	E980.4
Daphne (gnidium) (mezereum)	988.2	E865.4	—	E950.9	E962.1	E980.9
berry	988.2	E865.3	—	E950.9	E962.1	E980.9
Dapsone	961.8	E857	E931.8	E950.4	E962.0	E980.4
Daraprim	961.4	E857	E931.4	E950.4	E962.0	E980.4
Darnel	988.2	E865.3	—	E950.9	E962.1	E980.9
Darvon	965.8	E850.8	E935.8	E950.0	E962.0	E980.0
Daunorubicin	960.7	E856	E930.7	E950.4	E962.0	E980.4
DBI	962.3	E858.0	E932.3	E950.4	E962.0	E980.4
D–Con (rodenticide)	989.4	E863.7	—	E950.6	E962.1	E980.7
DDS	961.8	E857	E931.8	E950.4	E962.0	E980.4
DDT	989.2	E863.0	—	E950.6	E962.1	E980.7
Deadly nightshade	988.2	E865.4	—	E950.9	E962.1	E980.9
berry	988.2	E865.3	—	E950.9	E962.1	E980.9
Deanol	969.7	E854.2	E939.7	E950.3	E962.0	E980.3
Debrisoquine	972.6	E858.3	E942.6	E950.4	E962.0	E980.4
Decaborane	989.89	E866.8	—	E950.9	E962.1	E980.9
fumes	987.8	E869.8	—	E952.8	E962.2	E982.8
Decadron	962.0	E858.0	E932.0	E950.4	E962.0	E980.4
ENT agent	976.6	E858.7	E946.6	E950.4	E962.0	E980.4
ophthalmic preparation	976.5	E858.7	E946.5	E950.4	E962.0	E980.4
topical NEC	976.0	E858.7	E946.0	E950.4	E962.0	E980.4
Decahydronaphthalene	982.0	E862.4	—	E950.9	E962.1	E980.9
Decalin	982.0	E862.4	—	E950.9	E962.1	E980.9
Decamethonium	975.2	E858.6	E945.2	E950.4	E962.0	E980.4
Decholin	973.4	E858.4	E943.4	E950.4	E962.0	E980.4
sodium (diagnostic)	977.8	E858.8	E947.8	E950.4	E962.0	E980.4
Declomycin	960.4	E856	E930.4	E950.4	E962.0	E980.4
Deferoxamine	963.8	E858.1	E933.8	E950.4	E962.0	E980.4
Dehydrocholic acid	973.4	E858.4	E943.4	E950.4	E962.0	E980.4
DeKalin	982.0	E862.4	—	E950.9	E962.1	E980.9
Delalutin	962.2	E858.0	E932.2	E950.4	E962.0	E980.4
Delphinium	988.2	E865.3	—	E950.9	E962.1	E980.9
Deltasone	962.0	E858.0	E932.0	E950.4	E962.0	E980.4
Deltra	962.0	E858.0	E932.0	E950.4	E962.0	E980.4
Delvinal	967.0	E851	E937.0	E950.1	E962.0	E980.1
Demecarium (bromide)	971.0	E855.3	E941.0	E950.4	E962.0	E980.4
Demeclocycline	960.4	E856	E930.4	E950.4	E962.0	E980.4
Demecolcine	963.1	E858.1	E933.1	E950.4	E962.0	E980.4
Demelanizing agents	976.8	E858.7	E946.8	E950.4	E962.0	E980.4
Demerol	965.09	E850.2	E935.2	E950.0	E962.0	E980.0
Demethylchlortetracycline	960.4	E856	E930.4	E950.4	E962.0	E980.4
Demethyltetracycline	960.4	E856	E930.4	E950.4	E962.0	E980.4
Demeton	989.3	E863.1	—	E950.6	E962.1	E980.7
Demulcents	976.3	E858.7	E946.3	E950.4	E962.0	E980.4
Demulen	962.2	E858.0	E932.2	E950.4	E962.0	E980.4
Denatured alcohol	980.0	E860.1	—	E950.9	E962.1	E980.9
Dendrid	976.5	E858.7	E946.5	E950.4	E962.0	E980.4
Dental agents, topical	976.7	E858.7	E946.7	E950.4	E962.0	E980.4
Deodorant spray (feminine hygiene)	976.8	E858.7	E946.8	E950.4	E962.0	E980.4
Deoxyribonuclease	963.4	E858.1	E933.4	E950.4	E962.0	E980.4
Depressants						
appetite, central	977.0	E858.8	E947.0	E950.4	E962.0	E980.4
cardiac	972.0	E858.3	E942.0	E950.4	E962.0	E980.4

Substance	Poisoning	External Cause (E-Code)				
		Accident	Therapeutic Use	Suicide Attempt	Assault	Undetermined
central nervous system (anesthetic)	968.4	E855.1	E938.4	E950.4	E962.0	E980.4
psychotherapeutic	969.5	E853.9	E939.5	E950.3	E962.0	E980.3
Dequalinium	976.0	E858.7	E946.0	E950.4	E962.0	E980.4
Dermolate	976.2	E858.7	E946.2	E950.4	E962.0	E980.4
DES	962.2	E858.0	E932.2	E950.4	E962.0	E980.4
Desenex	976.0	E858.7	E946.0	E950.4	E962.0	E980.4
Deserpidine	972.6	E858.3	E942.6	E950.4	E962.0	E980.4
Desipramine	969.0	E854.0	E939.0	E950.3	E962.0	E980.3
Deslanoside	972.1	E858.3	E942.1	E950.4	E962.0	E980.4
Desocodeine	965.09	E850.2	E935.2	E950.0	E962.0	E980.0
Desomorphine	965.09	E850.2	E935.2	E950.0	E962.0	E980.0
Desonide	976.0	E858.7	E946.0	E950.4	E962.0	E980.4
Desoxycorticosterone derivatives	962.0	E858.0	E932.0	E950.4	E962.0	E980.4
Desoxyephedrine	969.7	E854.2	E939.7	E950.3	E962.0	E980.3
DET	969.6	E854.1	E939.6	E950.3	E962.0	E980.3
Detergents (ingested) (synthetic)	989.6	E861.0	—	E950.9	E962.1	E980.9
external medication	976.2	E858.7	E946.2	E950.4	E962.0	E980.4
Deterrent, alcohol	977.3	E858.8	E947.3	E950.4	E962.0	E980.4
Detrothyronine	962.7	E858.0	E932.7	E950.4	E962.0	E980.4
Dettol (external medication)	976.0	E858.7	E946.0	E950.4	E962.0	E980.4
Dexamethasone	962.0	E858.0	E932.0	E950.4	E962.0	E980.4
ENT agent	976.6	E858.7	E946.6	E950.4	E962.0	E980.4
ophthalmic preparation	976.5	E858.7	E946.5	E950.4	E962.0	E980.4
topical NEC	976.0	E858.7	E946.0	E950.4	E962.0	E980.4
Dexamphetamine	969.7	E854.2	E939.7	E950.3	E962.0	E980.3
Dexedrine	969.7	E854.2	E939.7	E950.3	E962.0	E980.3
Dexpanthenol	963.5	E858.1	E933.5	E950.4	E962.0	E980.4
Dextran	964.8	E858.2	E934.8	E950.4	E962.0	E980.4
Dextriferron	964.0	E858.2	E934.0	E950.4	E962.0	E980.4
Dextroamphetamine	969.7	E854.2	E939.7	E950.3	E962.0	E980.3
Dextro calcium pantothenate	963.5	E858.1	E933.5	E950.4	E962.0	E980.4
Dextromethorphan	975.4	E858.6	E945.4	E950.4	E962.0	E980.4
Dextromoramide	965.09	E850.2	E935.2	E950.0	E962.0	E980.0
Dextro pantothenyl alcohol	963.5	E858.1	E933.5	E950.4	E962.0	E980.4
topical	976.8	E858.7	E946.8	E950.4	E962.0	E980.4
Dextropropoxyphene (hydrochloride)	965.8	E850.8	E935.8	E950.0	E962.0	E980.0
Dextrorphan	965.09	E850.2	E935.2	E950.0	E962.0	E980.0
Dextrose NEC	974.5	E858.5	E944.5	E950.4	E962.0	E980.4
Dextrothyroxin	962.7	E858.0	E932.7	E950.4	E962.0	E980.4
DFP	971.0	E855.3	E941.0	E950.4	E962.0	E980.4
DHE–45	972.9	E858.3	E942.9	E950.4	E962.0	E980.4
Diabinese	962.3	E858.0	E932.3	E950.4	E962.0	E980.4
Diacetyl monoxime	977.2	E858.8	E947.2	E950.4	E962.0	E980.4
Diacetylmorphine	965.01	E850.0	E935.0	E950.0	E962.0	E980.0
Diagnostic agents	977.8	E858.8	E947.8	E950.4	E962.0	E980.4
Dial (soap)	976.2	E858.7	E946.2	E950.4	E962.0	E980.4
sedative	967.0	E851	E937.0	E950.1	E962.0	E980.1
Diallylbarbituric acid	967.0	E851	E937.0	E950.1	E962.0	E980.1
Diaminodiphenylsulfone	961.8	E857	E931.8	E950.4	E962.0	E980.4
Diamorphine	965.01	E850.0	E935.0	E950.0	E962.0	E980.0
Diamox	974.2	E858.5	E944.2	E950.4	E962.0	E980.4
Diamthazole	976.0	E858.7	E946.0	E950.4	E962.0	E980.4
Diaphenylsulfone	961.8	E857	E931.8	E950.4	E962.0	E980.4
Diasone (sodium)	961.8	E857	E931.8	E950.4	E962.0	E980.4
Diazepam	969.4	E853.2	E939.4	E950.3	E962.0	E980.3
Diazinon	989.3	E863.1	—	E950.6	E962.1	E980.7
Diazomethane (gas)	987.8	E869.8	—	E952.8	E962.2	E982.8

Substance	Poisoning	Accident	External Cause (E-Code) Therapeutic Use	Suicide Attempt	Assault	Undetermined
Diazoxide 972.5	E858.3	E942.5	E950.4	E962.0	E980.4
Dibenamine 971.3	E855.6	E941.3	E950.4	E962.0	E980.4
Dibenzheptropine 963.0	E858.1	E933.0	E950.4	E962.0	E980.4
Dibenzyline 971.3	E855.6	E941.3	E950.4	E962.0	E980.4
Diborane (gas) 987.8	E869.8	—	E952.8	E962.2	E982.8
Dibromomannitol 963.1	E858.1	E933.1	E950.4	E962.0	E980.4
Dibucaine (spinal) 968.7	E855.2	E938.7	E950.4	E962.0	E980.4
topical (surface) 968.5	E855.2	E938.5	E950.4	E962.0	E980.4
Dibunate sodium 975.4	E858.6	E945.4	E950.4	E962.0	E980.4
Dibutoline 971.1	E855.4	E941.1	E950.4	E962.0	E980.4
Dicapthon 989.4	E863.4	—	E950.6	E962.1	E980.7
Dichloralphenazone 967.1	E852.0	E937.1	E950.2	E962.0	E980.2
Dichlorodifluoromethane 987.4	E869.2	—	E952.8	E962.2	E982.8
Dichloroethane 982.3	E862.4	—	E950.9	E962.1	E980.9
Dichloroethylene 982.3	E862.4	—	E950.9	E962.1	E980.9
Dichloroethyl sulfide 987.8	E869.8	—	E952.8	E962.2	E982.8
Dichlorohydrin 982.3	E862.4	—	E950.9	E962.1	E980.9
Dichloromethane (solvent) (vapor) 982.3	E862.4	—	E950.9	E962.1	E980.9
Dichlorophen(e) 961.6	E857	E931.6	E950.4	E962.0	E980.4
Dichlorphenamide 974.2	E858.5	E944.2	E950.4	E962.0	E980.4
Dichlorvos 989.3	E863.1	—	E950.6	E962.1	E980.7
Diclofenac sodium 965.69	E850.6	E935.6	E950.0	E962.0	E980.0
Dicoumarin, dicumarol 964.2	E858.2	E934.2	E950.4	E962.0	E980.4
Dicyanogen (gas) 987.8	E869.8	—	E952.8	E962.2	E982.8
Dicyclomine 971.1	E855.4	E941.1	E950.4	E962.0	E980.4
Dieldrin (vapor) 989.2	E863.0	—	E950.6	E962.1	E980.7
Dienestrol 962.2	E858.0	E932.2	E950.4	E962.0	E980.4
Dietetics 977.0	E858.8	E947.0	E950.4	E962.0	E980.4
Diethazine 966.4	E855.0	E936.4	E950.4	E962.0	E980.4
Diethyl					
barbituric acid 967.0	E851	E937.0	E950.1	E962.0	E980.1
carbamazine 961.6	E857	E931.6	E950.4	E962.0	E980.4
carbinol 980.8	E860.8	—	E950.9	E962.1	E980.9
carbonate 982.8	E862.4	—	E950.9	E962.1	E980.9
ether (vapor) — see Ether(s)					
propion 977.0	E858.8	E947.0	E950.4	E962.0	E980.4
stilbestrol 962.2	E858.0	E932.2	E950.4	E962.0	E980.4
Diethylene					
dioxide 982.8	E862.4	—	E950.9	E962.1	E980.9
glycol (monoacetate) (monoethyl ether) . . 982.8	E862.4	—	E950.9	E962.1	E980.9
Diethylsulfone–diethylmethane 967.8	E852.8	E937.8	E950.2	E962.0	E980.2
Difencloxazine 965.09	E850.2	E935.2	E950.0	E962.0	E980.0
Diffusin 963.4	E858.1	E933.4	E950.4	E962.0	E980.4
Diflos 971.0	E855.3	E941.0	E950.4	E962.0	E980.4
Digestants 973.4	E858.4	E943.4	E950.4	E962.0	E980.4
Digitalin(e) 972.1	E858.3	E942.1	E950.4	E962.0	E980.4
Digitalis glycosides 972.1	E858.3	E942.1	E950.4	E962.0	E980.4
Digitoxin 972.1	E858.3	E942.1	E950.4	E962.0	E980.4
Digoxin 972.1	E858.3	E942.1	E950.4	E962.0	E980.4
Dihydrocodeine 965.09	E850.2	E935.2	E950.0	E962.0	E980.0
Dihydrocodeinone 965.09	E850.2	E935.2	E950.0	E962.0	E980.0
Dihydroergocristine 972.9	E858.3	E942.9	E950.4	E962.0	E980.4
Dihydroergotamine 972.9	E858.3	E942.9	E950.4	E962.0	E980.4
Dihydroergotoxine 972.9	E858.3	E942.9	E950.4	E962.0	E980.4
Dihydrohydroxycodeinone 965.09	E850.2	E935.2	E950.0	E962.0	E980.0
Dihydrohydroxymorphinone 965.09	E850.2	E935.2	E950.0	E962.0	E980.0
Dihydroisocodeine 965.09	E850.2	E935.2	E950.0	E962.0	E980.0

Substance	Poisoning	External Cause (E-Code)				
		Accident	Therapeutic Use	Suicide Attempt	Assault	Undetermined
Dihydromorphine	965.09	E850.2	E935.2	E950.0	E962.0	E980.0
Dihydromorphinone	965.09	E850.2	E935.2	E950.0	E962.0	E980.0
Dihydrostreptomycin	960.6	E856	E930.6	E950.4	E962.0	E980.4
Dihydrotachysterol	962.6	E858.0	E932.6	E950.4	E962.0	E980.4
Dihydroxyanthraquinone	973.1	E858.4	E943.1	E950.4	E962.0	E980.4
Dihydroxycodeinone	965.09	E850.2	E935.2	E950.0	E962.0	E980.0
Diiodohydroxyquin	961.3	E857	E931.3	E950.4	E962.0	E980.4
topical	976.0	E858.7	E946.0	E950.4	E962.0	E980.4
Diiodohydroxyquinoline	961.3	E857	E931.3	E950.4	E962.0	E980.4
Dilantin	966.1	E855.0	E936.1	E950.4	E962.0	E980.4
Dilaudid	965.09	E850.2	E935.2	E950.0	E962.0	E980.0
Diloxanide	961.5	E857	E931.5	E950.4	E962.0	E980.4
Dimefline	970.0	E854.3	E940.0	E950.4	E962.0	E980.4
Dimenhydrinate	963.0	E858.1	E933.0	E950.4	E962.0	E980.4
Dimercaprol	963.8	E858.1	E933.8	E950.4	E962.0	E980.4
Dimercaptopropanol	963.8	E858.1	E933.8	E950.4	E962.0	E980.4
Dimetane	963.0	E858.1	E933.0	E950.4	E962.0	E980.4
Dimethicone	976.3	E858.7	E946.3	E950.4	E962.0	E980.4
Dimethindene	963.0	E858.1	E933.0	E950.4	E962.0	E980.4
Dimethisoquin	968.5	E855.2	E938.5	E950.4	E962.0	E980.4
Dimethisterone	962.2	E858.0	E932.2	E950.4	E962.0	E980.4
Dimethoxanate	975.4	E858.6	E945.4	E950.4	E962.0	E980.4
Dimethyl						
arsine, arsinic acid — see Arsenic						
carbinol	980.2	E860.3	—	E950.9	E962.1	E980.9
diguanide	962.3	E858.0	E932.3	E950.4	E962.0	E980.4
ketone	982.8	E862.4	—	E950.9	E962.1	E980.9
vapor	987.8	E869.8	—	E952.8	E962.2	E982.8
meperidine	965.09	E850.2	E935.2	E950.0	E962.0	E980.0
parathion	989.3	E863.1	—	E950.6	E962.1	E980.7
polysiloxane	973.8	E858.4	E943.8	E950.4	E962.0	E980.4
sulfate (fumes)	987.8	E869.8	—	E952.8	E962.2	E982.8
liquid	983.9	E864.3	—	E950.7	E962.1	E980.6
sulfoxide NEC	982.8	E862.4	—	E950.9	E962.1	E980.9
medicinal	976.4	E858.7	E946.4	E950.4	E962.0	E980.4
triptamine	969.6	E854.1	E939.6	E950.3	E962.0	E980.3
tubocurarine	975.2	E858.6	E945.2	E950.4	E962.0	E980.4
Dindevan	964.2	E858.2	E934.2	E950.4	E962.0	E980.4
Dinitro (–ortho–) cresol (herbicide) (spray)	989.4	E863.5	—	E950.6	E962.1	E980.7
insecticide	989.4	E863.4	—	E950.6	E962.1	E980.7
Dinitrobenzene	983.0	E864.0	—	E950.7	E962.1	E980.6
vapor	987.8	E869.8	—	E952.8	E962.2	E982.8
Dinitro–orthocresol (herbicide)	989.4	E863.5	—	E950.6	E962.1	E980.7
insecticide	989.4	E863.4	—	E950.6	E962.1	E980.7
Dinitrophenol (herbicide) (spray)	989.4	E863.5	—	E950.6	E962.1	E980.7
insecticide	989.4	E863.4	—	E950.6	E962.1	E980.7
Dinoprost	975.0	E858.6	E945.0	E950.4	E962.0	E980.4
Dioctyl sulfosuccinate (calcium) (sodium)	973.2	E858.4	E943.2	E950.4	E962.0	E980.4
Diodoquin	961.3	E857	E931.3	E950.4	E962.0	E980.4
Dione derivatives NEC	966.3	E855.0	E936.3	E950.4	E962.0	E980.4
Dionin	965.09	E850.2	E935.2	E950.0	E962.0	E980.0
Dioxane	982.8	E862.4	—	E950.9	E962.1	E980.9
Dioxin — see herbicide						
Dioxyline	972.5	E858.3	E942.5	E950.4	E962.0	E980.4
Dipentene	982.8	E862.4	—	E950.9	E962.1	E980.9
Diphemanil	971.1	E855.4	E941.1	E950.4	E962.0	E980.4
Diphenadione	964.2	E858.2	E934.2	E950.4	E962.0	E980.4

Substance	Poisoning	External Cause (E-Code)				
		Accident	Therapeutic Use	Suicide Attempt	Assault	Undetermined
Diphenhydramine	963.0	E858.1	E933.0	E950.4	E962.0	E980.4
Diphenidol	963.0	E858.1	E933.0	E950.4	E962.0	E980.4
Diphenoxylate	973.5	E858.4	E943.5	E950.4	E962.0	E980.4
Diphenylchloroarsine	985.1	E866.3	—	E950.8	E962.1	E980.8
Diphenylhydantoin (sodium)	966.1	E855.0	E936.1	E950.4	E962.0	E980.4
Diphenylpyraline	963.0	E858.1	E933.0	E950.4	E962.0	E980.4
Diphtheria						
antitoxin	979.9	E858.8	E949.9	E950.4	E962.0	E980.4
toxoid	978.5	E858.8	E948.5	E950.4	E962.0	E980.4
with tetanus toxoid	978.9	E858.8	E948.9	E950.4	E962.0	E980.4
with pertussis component	978.6	E858.8	E948.6	E950.4	E962.0	E980.4
vaccine	978.5	E858.8	E948.5	E950.4	E962.0	E980.4
Dipipanone	965.09	E850.2	E935.2	E950.0	E962.0	E980.0
Diplovax	979.5	E858.8	E949.5	E950.4	E962.0	E980.4
Diprophylline	975.1	E858.6	E945.1	E950.4	E962.0	E980.4
Dipyridamole	972.4	E858.3	E942.4	E950.4	E962.0	E980.4
Dipyrone	965.5	E850.5	E935.5	E950.0	E962.0	E980.0
Diquat	989.4	E863.5	—	E950.6	E962.1	E980.7
Disinfectant NEC	983.9	E861.4	—	E950.7	E962.1	E980.6
alkaline	983.2	E861.4	—	E950.7	E962.1	E980.6
aromatic	983.0	E861.4	—	E950.7	E962.1	E980.6
Disipal	966.4	E855.0	E936.4	E950.4	E962.0	E980.4
Disodium edetate	963.8	E858.1	E933.8	E950.4	E962.0	E980.4
Disulfamide	974.4	E858.5	E944.4	E950.4	E962.0	E980.4
Disulfanilamide	961.0	E857	E931.0	E950.4	E962.0	E980.4
Disulfiram	977.3	E858.8	E947.3	E950.4	E962.0	E980.4
Dithiazanine	961.6	E857	E931.6	E950.4	E962.0	E980.4
Dithioglycerol	963.8	E858.1	E933.8	E950.4	E962.0	E980.4
Dithranol	976.4	E858.7	E946.4	E950.4	E962.0	E980.4
Diucardin	974.3	E858.5	E944.3	E950.4	E962.0	E980.4
Diupres	974.3	E858.5	E944.3	E950.4	E962.0	E980.4
Diuretics NEC	974.4	E858.5	E944.4	E950.4	E962.0	E980.4
carbonic acid anhydrase inhibitors	974.2	E858.5	E944.2	E950.4	E962.0	E980.4
mercurial	974.0	E858.5	E944.0	E950.4	E962.0	E980.4
osmotic	974.4	E858.5	E944.4	E950.4	E962.0	E980.4
purine derivatives	974.1	E858.5	E944.1	E950.4	E962.0	E980.4
saluretic	974.3	E858.5	E944.3	E950.4	E962.0	E980.4
Diuril	974.3	E858.5	E944.3	E950.4	E962.0	E980.4
Divinyl ether	968.2	E855.1	E938.2	E950.4	E962.0	E980.4
D–lysergic acid diethylamide	969.6	E854.1	E939.6	E950.3	E962.0	E980.3
DMCT	960.4	E856	E930.4	E950.4	E962.0	E980.4
DMSO	982.8	E862.4	—	E950.9	E962.1	E980.9
DMT	969.6	E854.1	E939.6	E950.3	E962.0	E980.3
DNOC	989.4	E863.5	—	E950.6	E962.1	E980.7
DOCA	962.0	E858.0	E932.0	E950.4	E962.0	E980.4
Dolophine	965.02	E850.1	E935.1	E950.0	E962.0	E980.0
Doloxene	965.8	E850.8	E935.8	E950.0	E962.0	E980.0
DOM	969.6	E854.1	E939.6	E950.3	E962.0	E980.3
Domestic gas — see Gas, utility						
Domiphen (bromide) (lozenges)	976.6	E858.7	E946.6	E950.4	E962.0	E980.4
Dopa (levo)	966.4	E855.0	E936.4	E950.4	E962.0	E980.4
Dopamine	971.2	E855.5	E941.2	E950.4	E962.0	E980.4
Doriden	967.5	E852.4	E937.5	E950.2	E962.0	E980.2
Dormiral	967.0	E851	E937.0	E950.1	E962.0	E980.1
Dormison	967.8	E852.8	E937.8	E950.2	E962.0	E980.2
Dornase	963.4	E858.1	E933.4	E950.4	E962.0	E980.4
Dorsacaine	968.5	E855.2	E938.5	E950.4	E962.0	E980.4

Substance		External Cause (E-Code)				
	Poisoning	Accident	Therapeutic Use	Suicide Attempt	Assault	Undetermined
Dothiepin hydrochloride 969.0		E854.0	E939.0	E950.3	E962.0	E980.3
Doxapram 970.0		E854.3	E940.0	E950.4	E962.0	E980.4
Doxepin 969.0		E854.0	E939.0	E950.3	E962.0	E980.3
Doxorubicin 960.7		E856	E930.7	E950.4	E962.0	E980.4
Doxycycline 960.4		E856	E930.4	E950.4	E962.0	E980.4
Doxylamine 963.0		E858.1	E933.0	E950.4	E962.0	E980.4
Dramamine 963.0		E858.1	E933.0	E950.4	E962.0	E980.4
Drano (drain cleaner) 983.2		E864.2	—	E950.7	E962.1	E980.6
Dromoran 965.09		E850.2	E935.2	E950.0	E962.0	E980.0
Dromostanolone 962.1		E858.0	E932.1	E950.4	E962.0	E980.4
Droperidol 969.2		E853.1	E939.2	E950.3	E962.0	E980.3
Drug 977.9		E858.9	E947.9	E950.5	E962.0	E980.5
specified NEC 977.8		E858.8	E947.8	E950.4	E962.0	E980.4
AHFS List						
4:00 antihistamine drugs 963.0		E858.1	E933.0	E950.4	E962.0	E980.4
8:04 amebacides 961.5		E857	E931.5	E950.4	E962.0	E980.4
arsenical anti–infectives 961.1		E857	E931.1	E950.4	E962.0	E980.4
quinoline derivatives 961.3		E857	E931.3	E950.4	E962.0	E980.4
8:08 anthelmintics 961.6		E857	E931.6	E950.4	E962.0	E980.4
quinoline derivatives 961.3		E857	E931.3	E950.4	E962.0	E980.4
8:12.04 antifungal antibiotics 960.1		E856	E930.1	E950.4	E962.0	E980.4
8:12.06 cephalosporins 960.5		E856	E930.5	E950.4	E962.0	E980.4
8:12.08 chloramphenicol 960.2		E856	E930.2	E950.4	E962.0	E980.4
8:12.12 erythromycins 960.3		E856	E930.3	E950.4	E962.0	E980.4
8:12.16 penicillins 960.0		E856	E930.0	E950.4	E962.0	E980.4
8:12.20 streptomycins 960.6		E856	E930.6	E950.4	E962.0	E980.4
8:12.24 tetracyclines 960.4		E856	E930.4	E950.4	E962.0	E980.4
8:12.28 other antibiotics 960.8		E856	E930.8	E950.4	E962.0	E980.4
antimycobacterial 960.6		E856	E930.6	E950.4	E962.0	E980.4
macrolides 960.3		E856	E930.3	E950.4	E962.0	E980.4
8:16 antituberculars 961.8		E857	E931.8	E950.4	E962.0	E980.4
antibiotics 960.6		E856	E930.6	E950.4	E962.0	E980.4
8:18 antivirals 961.7		E857	E931.7	E950.4	E962.0	E980.4
8:20 plasmodicides (antimalarials) 961.4		E857	E931.4	E950.4	E962.0	E980.4
8:24 sulfonamides 961.0		E857	E931.0	E950.4	E962.0	E980.4
8:26 sulfones 961.8		E857	E931.8	E950.4	E962.0	E980.4
8:28 treponemicides 961.2		E857	E931.2	E950.4	E962.0	E980.4
8:32 trichomonacides 961.5		E857	E931.5	E950.4	E962.0	E980.4
quinoline derivatives 961.3		E857	E931.3	E950.4	E962.0	E980.4
nitrofuran derivatives 961.9		E857	E931.9	E950.4	E962.0	E980.4
8:36 urinary germicides 961.9		E857	E931.9	E950.4	E962.0	E980.4
quinoline derivatives 961.3		E857	E931.3	E950.4	E962.0	E980.4
8:40 other anti–infectives 961.9		E857	E931.9	E950.4	E962.0	E980.4
10:00 antineoplastic agents 963.1		E858.1	E933.1	E950.4	E962.0	E980.4
antibiotics 960.7		E856	E930.7	E950.4	E962.0	E980.4
progestogens 962.2		E858.0	E932.2	E950.4	E962.0	E980.4
12:04 parasympathomimetic (cholinergic)						
agents 971.0		E855.3	E941.0	E950.4	E962.0	E980.4
12:08 parasympatholytic (cholinergic						
–blocking) agents 971.1		E855.4	E941.1	E950.4	E962.0	E980.4
12:12 Sympathomimetic (adrenergic)						
agents 971.2		E855.5	E941.2	E950.4	E962.0	E980.4
12:16 sympatholytic (adrenergic–						
blocking) agents 971.3		E855.6	E941.3	E950.4	E962.0	E980.4
12:20 skeletal muscle relaxants						
central nervous system muscle-tone						
depressants 968.0		E855.1	E938.0	E950.4	E962.0	E980.4

		External Cause (E-Code)				
Substance	Poisoning	Accident	Therapeutic Use	Suicide Attempt	Assault	Undetermined
myoneural blocking agents	975.2	E858.6	E945.2	E950.4	E962.0	E980.4
16:00 blood derivatives	964.7	E858.2	E934.7	E950.4	E962.0	E980.4
20:04 antianemia drugs	964.1	E858.2	E934.1	E950.4	E962.0	E980.4
20:04.04 iron preparations	964.0	E858.2	E934.0	E950.4	E962.0	E980.4
20:04.08 liver and stomach preparations	964.1	E858.2	E934.1	E950.4	E962.0	E980.4
20:12.04 anticoagulants	964.2	E858.2	E934.2	E950.4	E962.0	E980.4
20:12.08 antiheparin agents	964.5	E858.2	E934.5	E950.4	E962.0	E980.4
20:12.12 coagulants	964.5	E858.2	E934.5	E950.4	E962.0	E980.4
20:12.16 hemostatics NEC	964.5	E858.2	E934.5	E950.4	E962.0	E980.4
capillary active drugs	972.8	E858.3	E942.8	E950.4	E962.0	E980.4
24:04 cardiac drugs	972.9	E858.3	E942.9	E950.4	E962.0	E980.4
cardiotonic agents	972.1	E858.3	E942.1	E950.4	E962.0	E980.4
rhythm regulators	972.0	E858.3	E942.0	E950.4	E962.0	E980.4
24:06 antilipemic agents	972.2	E858.3	E942.2	E950.4	E962.0	E980.4
thyroid derivatives	962.7	E858.0	E932.7	E950.4	E962.0	E980.4
24:08 hypotensive agents	972.6	E858.3	E942.6	E950.4	E962.0	E980.4
adrenergic blocking agents	971.3	E855.6	E941.3	E950.4	E962.0	E980.4
ganglion blocking agents	972.3	E858.3	E942.3	E950.4	E962.0	E980.4
vasodilators	972.5	E858.3	E942.5	E950.4	E962.0	E980.4
24:12 vasodilating agents NEC	972.5	E858.3	E942.5	E950.4	E962.0	E980.4
coronary	972.4	E858.3	E942.4	E950.4	E962.0	E980.4
nicotinic acid derivatives	972.2	E858.3	E942.2	E950.4	E962.0	E980.4
24:16 sclerosing agents	972.7	E858.3	E942.7	E950.4	E962.0	E980.4
28:04 general anesthetics	968.4	E855.1	E938.4	E950.4	E962.0	E980.4
gaseous anesthetics	968.2	E855.1	E938.2	E950.4	E962.0	E980.4
halothane	968.1	E855.1	E938.1	E950.4	E962.0	E980.4
intravenous anesthetics	968.3	E855.1	E938.3	E950.4	E962.0	E980.4
28:08 analgesics and antipyretics	965.9	E850.9	E935.9	E950.0	E962.0	E980.0
antirheumatics	965.69	E850.6	E935.6	E950.0	E962.0	E980.0
aromatic analgesics	965.4	E850.4	E935.4	E950.0	E962.0	E980.0
non–narcotic NEC	965.7	E850.7	E935.7	E950.0	E962.0	E980.0
opium alkaloids	965.00	E850.2	E935.2	E950.0	E962.0	E980.0
heroin	965.01	E850.0	E935.0	E950.0	E962.0	E980.0
methadone	965.02	E850.1	E935.1	E950.0	E962.0	E980.0
specified type NEC	965.09	E850.2	E935.2	E950.0	E962.0	E980.0
pyrazole derivatives	965.5	E850.5	E935.5	E950.0	E962.0	E980.0
salicylates	965.1	E850.3	E935.3	E950.0	E962.0	E980.0
specified NEC	965.8	E850.8	E935.8	E950.0	E962.0	E980.0
28:10 narcotic antagonists	970.1	E854.3	E940.1	E950.4	E962.0	E980.4
28:12 anticonvulsants	966.3	E855.0	E936.3	E950.4	E962.0	E980.4
barbiturates	967.0	E851	E937.0	E950.1	E962.0	E980.1
benzodiazepine–based tranquilizers	969.4	E853.2	E939.4	E950.3	E962.0	E980.3
bromides	967.3	E852.2	E937.3	E950.2	E962.0	E980.2
hydantoin derivatives	966.1	E855.0	E936.1	E950.4	E962.0	E980.4
oxazolidine (derivatives)	966.0	E855.0	E936.0	E950.4	E962.0	E980.4
succinimides	966.2	E855.0	E936.2	E950.4	E962.0	E980.4
28:16.04 antidepressants	969.0	E854.0	E939.0	E950.3	E962.0	E980.3
28:16.08 tranquilizers	969.5	E853.9	E939.5	E950.3	E962.0	E980.3
benzodiazepine–based	969.4	E853.2	E939.4	E950.3	E962.0	E980.3
butyrophenone–based	969.2	E853.1	E939.2	E950.3	E962.0	E980.3
major NEC	969.3	E853.8	E939.3	E950.3	E962.0	E980.3
phenothiazine–based	969.1	E853.0	E939.1	E950.3	E962.0	E980.3
28:16.12 other psychotherapeutic agents	969.8	E855.8	E939.8	E950.3	E962.0	E980.3
28:20 respiratory and cerebral stimulants	970.9	E854.3	E940.9	E950.4	E962.0	E980.4
analeptics	970.0	E854.3	E940.0	E950.4	E962.0	E980.4
anorexigenic agents	977.0	E858.8	E947.0	E950.4	E962.0	E980.4

Substance	Poisoning	Accident	Therapeutic Use	Suicide Attempt	Assault	Undetermined
psychostimulants	969.7	E854.2	E939.7	E950.3	E962.0	E980.3
specified NEC	970.8	E854.3	E940.8	E950.4	E962.0	E980.4
28:24 sedatives and hypnotics	967.9	E852.9	E937.9	E950.2	E962.0	E980.2
barbiturates	967.0	E851	E937.0	E950.1	E962.0	E980.1
benzodiazepine–based tranquilizers	969.4	E853.2	E939.4	E950.3	E962.0	E980.3
chloral hydrate (group)	967.1	E852.0	E937.1	E950.2	E962.0	E980.2
glutethamide group	967.5	E852.4	E937.5	E950.2	E962.0	E980.2
intravenous anesthetics	968.3	E855.1	E938.3	E950.4	E962.0	E980.4
methaqualone (compounds)	967.4	E852.3	E937.4	E950.2	E962.0	E980.2
paraldehyde	967.2	E852.1	E937.2	E950.2	E962.0	E980.2
phenothiazine–based tranquilizers	969.1	E853.0	E939.1	E950.3	E962.0	E980.3
specified NEC	967.8	E852.8	E937.8	E950.2	E962.0	E980.2
thiobarbiturates	968.3	E855.1	E938.3	E950.4	E962.0	E980.4
tranquilizer NEC	969.5	E853.9	E939.5	E950.3	E962.0	E980.3
36:04 to 36:88 diagnostic agents	977.8	E858.8	E947.8	E950.4	E962.0	E980.4
40:00 electrolyte, caloric, and water balance agents NEC	974.5	E858.5	E944.5	E950.4	E962.0	E980.4
40:04 acidifying agents	963.2	E858.1	E933.2	E950.4	E962.0	E980.4
40:08 alkalinizing agents	963.3	E858.1	E933.3	E950.4	E962.0	E980.4
40:10 ammonia detoxicants	974.5	E858.5	E944.5	E950.4	E962.0	E980.4
40:12 replacement solutions	974.5	E858.5	E944.5	E950.4	E962.0	E980.4
plasma expanders	964.8	E858.2	E934.8	E950.4	E962.0	E980.4
40:16 sodium–removing resins	974.5	E858.5	E944.5	E950.4	E962.0	E980.4
40:18 potassium–removing resins	974.5	E858.5	E944.5	E950.4	E962.0	E980.4
40:20 caloric agents	974.5	E858.5	E944.5	E950.4	E962.0	E980.4
40:24 salt and sugar substitutes	974.5	E858.5	E944.5	E950.4	E962.0	E980.4
40:28 diuretics NEC	974.4	E858.5	E944.4	E950.4	E962.0	E980.4
carbonic acid anhydrase inhibitors	974.2	E858.5	E944.2	E950.4	E962.0	E980.4
mercurials	974.0	E858.5	E944.0	E950.4	E962.0	E980.4
purine derivatives	974.1	E858.5	E944.1	E950.4	E962.0	E980.4
saluretics	974.3	E858.5	E944.3	E950.4	E962.0	E980.4
thiazides	974.3	E858.5	E944.3	E950.4	E962.1	E980.4
40:36 irrigating solutions	974.5	E858.5	E944.5	E950.4	E962.0	E980.4
40:40 uricosuric agents	974.7	E858.5	E944.7	E950.4	E962.0	E980.4
44:00 enzymes	963.4	E858.1	E933.4	E950.4	E962.0	E980.4
fibrinolysis–affecting agents	964.4	E858.2	E934.4	E950.4	E962.0	E980.4
gastric agents	973.4	E858.4	E943.4	E950.4	E962.0	E980.4
48:00 expectorants and cough preparations						
antihistamine agents	963.0	E858.1	E933.0	E950.4	E962.0	E980.4
antitussives	975.4	E858.6	E945.4	E950.4	E962.0	E980.4
codeine derivatives	965.09	E850.2	E935.2	E950.0	E962.0	E980.0
expectorants	975.5	E858.6	E945.5	E950.4	E962.0	E980.4
narcotic agents NEC	965.09	E850.2	E935.2	E950.0	E962.0	E980.0
52:04 anti–infectives (EENT)						
ENT agent	976.6	E858.7	E946.6	E950.4	E962.0	E980.4
ophthalmic preparation	976.5	E858.7	E946.5	E950.4	E962.0	E980.4
52:04.04 antibiotics (EENT)						
ENT agent	976.6	E858.7	E946.6	E950.4	E962.0	E980.4
ophthalmic preparation	976.5	E858.7	E946.5	E950.4	E962.0	E980.4
52:04.06 antivirals (EENT)						
ENT agent	976.6	E858.7	E946.6	E950.4	E962.0	E980.4
ophthalmic preparation	976.5	E858.7	E946.5	E950.4	E962.0	E980.4
52:04.08 sulfonamides (EENT)						
ENT agent	976.6	E858.7	E946.6	E950.4	E962.0	E980.4
ophthalmic preparation	976.5	E858.7	E946.5	E950.4	E962.0	E980.4
52:04.12 miscellaneous anti–infectives (EENT)						
ENT agent	976.6	E858.7	E946.6	E950.4	E962.0	E980.4

Substance	Poisoning	Accident	Therapeutic Use	Suicide Attempt	Assault	Undetermined
			External Cause (E-Code)			
ophthalmic preparation 976.5	E858.7	E946.5	E950.4	E962.0	E980.4
52:08 anti–inflammatory agents (EENT)					
ENT agent 976.6	E858.7	E946.6	E950.4	E962.0	E980.4
ophthalmic preparation 976.5	E858.7	E946.5	E950.4	E962.0	E980.4
52:10 carbonic anhydrase inhibitors 974.2	E858.5	E944.2	E950.4	E962.0	E980.4
52:12 contact lens solutions 976.5	E858.7	E946.5	E950.4	E962.0	E980.4
52:16 local anesthetics (EENT) 968.5	E855.2	E938.5	E950.4	E962.0	E980.4
52:20 miotics 971.0	E855.3	E941.0	E950.4	E962.0	E980.4
52:24 mydriatics					
adrenergics 971.2	E855.5	E941.2	E950.4	E962.0	E980.4
anticholinergics 971.1	E855.4	E941.1	E950.4	E962.0	E980.4
antimuscarinics 971.1	E855.4	E941.1	E950.4	E962.0	E980.4
parasympatholytics 971.1	E855.4	E941.1	E950.4	E962.0	E980.4
spasmolytics 971.1	E855.4	E941.1	E950.4	E962.0	E980.4
sympathomimetics 971.2	E855.5	E941.2	E950.4	E962.0	E980.4
52:28 mouth washes and gargles 976.6	E858.7	E946.6	E950.4	E962.0	E980.4
52:32 vasoconstrictors (EENT) 971.2	E855.5	E941.2	E950.4	E962.0	E980.4
52:36 unclassified agents (EENT)					
ENT agent 976.6	E858.7	E946.6	E950.4	E962.0	E980.4
ophthalmic preparation 976.5	E858.7	E946.5	E950.4	E962.0	E980.4
56:04 antacids and adsorbents 973.0	E858.4	E943.0	E950.4	E962.0	E980.4
56:08 Antidiarrhea agents 973.5	E858.4	E943.5	E950.4	E962.0	E980.4
56:10 antiflatulents 973.8	E858.4	E943.8	E950.4	E962.0	E980.4
56:12 cathartics NEC 973.3	E858.4	E943.3	E950.4	E962.0	E980.4
emollients 973.2	E858.4	E943.2	E950.4	E962.0	E980.4
irritants 973.1	E858.4	E943.1	E950.4	E962.0	E980.4
56:16 digestants 973.4	E858.4	E943.4	E950.4	E962.0	E980.4
56:20 emetics and antiemetics					
antiemetics 963.0	E858.1	E933.0	E950.4	E962.0	E980.4
emetics 973.6	E858.4	E943.6	E950.4	E962.0	E980.4
56:24 lipotropic agents 977.1	E858.8	E947.1	E950.4	E962.0	E980.4
56:40 miscellaneous G.I. drugs 973.8	E858.4	E943.8	E950.4	E962.0	E980.4
60:00 gold compounds 965.69	E850.6	E935.6	E950.0	E962.0	E980.0
64:00 heavy metal antagonists 963.8	E858.1	E933.8	E950.4	E962.0	E980.4
68:04 adrenals 962.0	E858.0	E932.0	E950.4	E962.0	E980.4
68:08 androgens 962.1	E858.0	E932.1	E950.4	E962.0	E980.4
68:12 contraceptives, oral 962.2	E858.0	E932.2	E950.4	E962.0	E980.4
68:16 estrogens 962.2	E858.0	E932.2	E950.4	E962.0	E980.4
68:18 gonadotropins 962.4	E858.0	E932.4	E950.4	E962.0	E980.4
68:20 insulins and antidiabetic agents . . . 962.3	E858.0	E932.3	E950.4	E962.0	E980.4
68:20.08 insulins 962.3	E858.0	E932.3	E950.4	E962.0	E980.4
68:24 parathyroid 962.6	E858.0	E932.6	E950.4	E962.0	E980.4
68:28 pituitary (posterior) 962.5	E858.0	E932.5	E950.4	E962.0	E980.4
anterior 962.4	E858.0	E932.4	E950.4	E962.0	E980.4
68:32 progestogens 962.2	E858.0	E932.2	E950.4	E962.0	E980.4
68:34 other corpus luteum hormones					
NEC 962.2	E858.0	E932.2	E950.4	E962.0	E980.4
68:36 thyroid and antithyroid					
antithyroid 962.8	E858.0	E932.8	E950.4	E962.0	E980.4
thyroid (derivatives) 962.7	E858.0	E932.7	E950.4	E962.0	E980.4
72:00 local anesthetics NEC 968.9	E855.2	E938.9	E950.4	E962.0	E980.4
topical (surface) 968.5	E855.2	E938.5	E950.4	E962.0	E980.4
infiltration (intradermal)					
(subcutaneous) (submucosal) . . . 968.5	E855.2	E938.5	E950.4	E962.0	E980.4
nerve blocking (peripheral) (plexus)					
(regional) 968.6	E855.2	E938.6	E950.4	E962.0	E980.4
spinal 968.7	E855.2	E938.7	E950.4	E962.0	E980.4

Substance	Poisoning	External Cause (E-Code)				
		Accident	Therapeutic Use	Suicide Attempt	Assault	Undetermined
76:00 oxytocics	975.0	E858.6	E945.0	E950.4	E962.0	E980.4
78:00 radioactive agents	990	—	—	—	—	—
80:04 serums NEC	979.9	E858.8	E949.9	E950.4	E962.0	E980.4
immune gamma globulin (human)	964.6	E858.2	E934.6	E950.4	E962.0	E980.4
80:08 toxoids NEC	978.8	E858.8	E948.8	E950.4	E962.0	E980.4
diphtheria	978.5	E858.8	E948.5	E950.4	E962.0	E980.4
and tetanus	978.9	E858.8	E948.9	E950.4	E962.0	E980.4
with pertussis component	978.6	E858.8	E948.6	E950.4	E962.0	E980.4
tetanus	978.4	E858.8	E948.4	E950.4	E962.0	E980.4
and diphtheria	978.9	E858.8	E948.9	E950.4	E962.0	E980.4
with pertussis component	978.6	E858.8	E948.6	E950.4	E962.0	E980.4
80:12 vaccines	979.9	E858.8	E949.9	E950.4	E962.0	E980.4
bacterial NEC	978.8	E858.8	E948.8	E950.4	E962.0	E980.4
with						
other bacterial components	978.9	E858.8	E948.9	E950.4	E962.0	E980.4
pertussis component	978.6	E858.8	E948.6	E950.4	E962.0	E980.4
viral and rickettsial						
components	979.7	E858.8	E949.7	E950.4	E962.0	E980.4
rickettsial NEC	979.6	E858.8	E949.6	E950.4	E962.0	E980.4
with						
bacterial component	979.7	E858.8	E949.7	E950.4	E962.0	E980.4
pertussis component	978.6	E858.8	E948.6	E950.4	E962.0	E980.4
viral component	979.7	E858.8	E949.7	E950.4	E962.0	E980.4
viral NEC	979.6	E858.8	E949.6	E950.4	E962.0	E980.4
with						
bacterial component	979.7	E858.8	E949.7	E950.4	E962.0	E980.4
pertussis component	978.6	E858.8	E948.6	E950.4	E962.0	E980.4
rickettsial component	979.7	E858.8	E949.7	E950.4	E962.0	E980.4
84:04.04 antibiotics (skin and mucous membrane)	976.0	E858.7	E946.0	E950.4	E962.0	E980.4
84:04.08 fungicides (skin and mucous membrane)	976.0	E858.7	E946.0	E950.4	E962.0	E980.4
84:04.12 scabicides and pediculicides (skin and mucous membrane)	976.0	E858.7	E946.0	E950.4	E962.0	E980.4
84:04.16 miscellaneous local anti–infectives (skin and mucous membrane)	976.0	E858.7	E946.0	E950.4	E962.0	E980.4
84:06 anti–inflammatory agents (skin and mucous membrane)	976.0	E858.7	E946.0	E950.4	E962.0	E980.4
84:08 antipruritics and local anesthetics						
antipruritics	976.1	E858.7	E946.1	E950.4	E962.0	E980.4
local anesthetics	968.5	E855.2	E938.5	E950.4	E962.0	E980.4
84:12 astringents	976.2	E858.7	E946.2	E950.4	E962.0	E980.4
84:16 cell stimulants and proliferants	976.8	E858.7	E946.8	E950.4	E962.0	E980.4
84:20 detergents	976.2	E858.7	E946.2	E950.4	E962.0	E980.4
84:24 emollients, demulcents, and protectants	976.3	E858.7	E946.3	E950.4	E962.0	E980.4
84:28 keratolytic agents	976.4	E858.7	E946.4	E950.4	E962.0	E980.4
84:32 keratoplastic agents	976.4	E858.7	E946.4	E950.4	E962.0	E980.4
84:36 miscellaneous agents (skin and mucous membrane)	976.8	E858.7	E946.8	E950.4	E962.0	E980.4
86:00 spasmolytic agents	975.1	E858.6	E945.1	E950.4	E962.0	E980.4
antiasthmatics	975.7	E858.6	E945.7	E950.4	E962.0	E980.4
papaverine	972.5	E858.3	E942.5	E950.4	E962.0	E980.4
theophylline	974.1	E858.5	E944.1	E950.4	E962.0	E980.4
88:04 vitamin A	963.5	E858.1	E933.5	E950.4	E962.0	E980.4
88:08 vitamin B complex	963.5	E858.1	E933.5	E950.4	E962.0	E980.4

Substance	Poisoning	External Cause (E-Code)				
		Accident	Therapeutic Use	Suicide Attempt	Assault	Undetermined
hematopoietic vitamin	964.1	E858.2	E934.1	E950.4	E962.0	E980.4
nicotinic acid derivatives	972.2	E858.3	E942.2	E950.4	E962.0	E980.4
88:12 vitamin C	963.5	E858.1	E933.5	E950.4	E962.0	E980.4
88:16 vitamin D	963.5	E858.1	E933.5	E950.4	E962.0	E980.4
88:20 vitamin E	963.5	E858.1	E933.5	E950.4	E962.0	E980.4
88:24 vitamin K activity	964.3	E858.2	E934.3	E950.4	E962.0	E980.4
88:28 multivitamin preparations	963.5	E858.1	E933.5	E950.4	E962.0	E980.4
92:00 unclassified therapeutic agents	977.8	E858.8	E947.8	E950.4	E962.0	E980.4
Duboisine	971.1	E855.4	E941.1	E950.4	E962.0	E980.4
Dulcolax	973.1	E858.4	E943.1	E950.4	E962.0	E980.4
Duponol (C) (EP)	976.2	E858.7	E946.2	E950.4	E962.0	E980.4
Durabolin	962.1	E858.0	E932.1	E950.4	E962.0	E980.4
Dyclone	968.5	E855.2	E938.5	E950.4	E962.0	E980.4
Dyclonine	968.5	E855.2	E938.5	E950.4	E962.0	E980.4
Dydrogesterone	962.2	E858.0	E932.2	E950.4	E962.0	E980.4
Dyes NEC	989.89	E866.8	—	E950.9	E962.1	E980.9
diagnostic agents	977.8	E858.8	E947.8	E950.4	E962.0	E980.4
pharmaceutical NEC	977.4	E858.8	E947.4	E950.4	E962.0	E980.4
Dyfols	971.0	E855.3	E941.0	E950.4	E962.0	E980.4
Dymelor	962.3	E858.0	E932.3	E950.4	E962.0	E980.4
Dynamite	989.89	E866.8	—	E950.9	E962.1	E980.9
fumes	987.8	E869.8	—	E952.8	E962.2	E982.8
Dyphylline	975.1	E858.6	E945.1	E950.4	E962.0	E980.4
Ear preparations	976.6	E858.7	E946.6	E950.4	E962.0	E980.4
Echothiophate, ecothiopate	971.0	E855.3	E941.0	E950.4	E962.0	E980.4
Ectylurea	967.8	E852.8	E937.8	E950.2	E962.0	E980.2
Edathamil disodium	963.8	E858.1	E933.8	E950.4	E962.0	E980.4
Edecrin	974.4	E858.5	E944.4	E950.4	E962.0	E980.4
Edetate, disodium (calcium)	963.8	E858.1	E933.8	E950.4	E962.0	E980.4
Edrophonium	971.0	E855.3	E941.0	E950.4	E962.0	E980.4
Elase	976.8	E858.7	E946.8	E950.4	E962.0	E980.4
Elaterium	973.1	E858.4	E943.1	E950.4	E962.0	E980.4
Elder	988.2	E865.4	—	E950.9	E962.1	E980.9
berry (unripe)	988.2	E865.3	—	E950.9	E962.1	E980.9
Electrolytes NEC	974.5	E858.5	E944.5	E950.4	E962.0	E980.4
Electrolytic agent NEC	974.5	E858.5	E944.5	E950.4	E962.0	E980.4
Embramine	963.0	E858.1	E933.0	E950.4	E962.0	E980.4
Emetics	973.6	E858.4	E943.6	E950.4	E962.0	E980.4
Emetine (hydrochloride)	961.5	E857	E931.5	E950.4	E962.0	E980.4
Emollients	976.3	E858.7	E946.3	E950.4	E962.0	E980.4
Emylcamate	969.5	E853.8	E939.5	E950.3	E962.0	E980.3
Encyprate	969.0	E854.0	E939.0	E950.3	E962.0	E980.3
Endocaine	968.5	E855.2	E938.5	E950.4	E962.0	E980.4
Endrin	989.2	E863.0	—	E950.6	E962.1	E980.7
Enflurane	968.2	E855.1	E938.2	E950.4	E962.0	E980.4
Enovid	962.2	E858.0	E932.2	E950.4	E962.0	E980.4
ENT preparations (anti–infectives)	976.6	E858.7	E946.6	E950.4	E962.0	E980.4
Enzodase	963.4	E858.1	E933.4	E950.4	E962.0	E980.4
Enzymes NEC	963.4	E858.1	E933.4	E950.4	E962.0	E980.4
Epanutin	966.1	E855.0	E936.1	E950.4	E962.0	E980.4
Ephedra (tincture)	971.2	E855.5	E941.2	E950.4	E962.0	E980.4
Ephedrine	971.2	E855.5	E941.2	E950.4	E962.0	E980.4
Epiestriol	962.2	E858.0	E932.2	E950.4	E962.0	E980.4
Epilim — see Sodium valproate						
Epinephrine	971.2	E855.5	E941.2	E950.4	E962.0	E980.4
Epsom salt	973.3	E858.4	E943.3	E950.4	E962.0	E980.4
Equanil	969.5	E853.8	E939.5	E950.3	E962.0	E980.3

Substance	Poisoning	External Cause (E-Code)				
		Accident	Therapeutic Use	Suicide Attempt	Assault	Undetermined
Equisetum (diuretic)	974.4	E858.5	E944.4	E950.4	E962.0	E980.4
Ergometrine	975.0	E858.6	E945.0	E950.4	E962.0	E980.4
Ergonovine	975.0	E858.6	E945.0	E950.4	E962.0	E980.4
Ergot NEC	988.2	E865.4	—	E950.9	E962.1	E980.9
medicinal (alkaloids)	975.0	E858.6	E945.0	E950.4	E962.0	E980.4
Ergotamine (tartrate) (for migraine) NEC	972.9	E858.3	E942.9	E950.4	E962.0	E980.4
Ergotrate	975.0	E858.6	E945.0	E950.4	E962.0	E980.4
Erythrityl tetranitrate	972.4	E858.3	E942.4	E950.4	E962.0	E980.4
Erythrol tetranitrate	972.4	E858.3	E942.4	E950.4	E962.0	E980.4
Erythromycin	960.3	E856	E930.3	E950.4	E962.0	E980.4
ophthalmic preparation	976.5	E858.7	E946.5	E950.4	E962.0	E980.4
topical NEC	976.0	E858.7	E946.0	E950.4	E962.0	E980.4
Eserine	971.0	E855.3	E941.0	E950.4	E962.0	E980.4
Eskabarb	967.0	E851	E937.0	E950.1	E962.0	E980.1
Eskalith	969.8	E855.8	E939.8	E950.3	E962.0	E980.3
Estradiol (cypionate) (dipropionate) (valerate)	962.2	E858.0	E932.2	E950.4	E962.0	E980.4
Estriol	962.2	E858.0	E932.2	E950.4	E962.0	E980.4
Estrogens (with progestogens)	962.2	E858.0	E932.2	E950.4	E962.0	E980.4
Estrone	962.2	E858.0	E932.2	E950.4	E962.0	E980.4
Etafedrine	971.2	E855.5	E941.2	E950.4	E962.0	E980.4
Ethacrynate sodium	974.4	E858.5	E944.4	E950.4	E962.0	E980.4
Ethacrynic acid	974.4	E858.5	E944.4	E950.4	E962.0	E980.4
Ethambutol	961.8	E857	E931.8	E950.4	E962.0	E980.4
Ethamide	974.2	E858.5	E944.2	E950.4	E962.0	E980.4
Ethamivan	970.0	E854.3	E940.0	E950.4	E962.0	E980.4
Ethamsylate	964.5	E858.2	E934.5	E950.4	E962.0	E980.4
Ethanol	980.0	E860.1	—	E950.9	E962.1	E980.9
beverage	980.0	E860.0	—	E950.9	E962.1	E980.9
Ethchlorvynol	967.8	E852.8	E937.8	E950.2	E962.0	E980.2
Ethebenecid	974.7	E858.5	E944.7	E950.4	E962.0	E980.4
Ether(s) (diethyl) (ethyl) (vapor)	987.8	E869.8	—	E952.8	E962.2	E982.8
anesthetic	968.2	E855.1	E938.2	E950.4	E962.0	E980.4
petroleum — see Ligroin						
solvent	982.8	E862.4	—	E950.9	E962.1	E980.9
Ethidine chloride (vapor)	987.8	E869.8	—	E952.8	E962.2	E982.8
liquid (solvent)	982.3	E862.4	—	E950.9	E962.1	E980.9
Ethinamate	967.8	E852.8	E937.8	E950.2	E962.0	E980.2
Ethinylestradiol	962.2	E858.0	E932.2	E950.4	E962.0	E980.4
Ethionamide	961.8	E857	E931.8	E950.4	E962.0	E980.4
Ethisterone	962.2	E858.0	E932.2	E950.4	E962.0	E980.4
Ethobral	967.0	E851	E937.0	E950.1	E962.0	E980.1
Ethocaine (infiltration) (topical)	968.5	E855.2	E938.5	E950.4	E962.0	E980.4
nerve block (peripheral) (plexus)	968.6	E855.2	E938.6	E950.4	E962.0	E980.4
spinal	968.7	E855.2	E938.7	E950.4	E962.0	E980.4
Ethoheptazine (citrate)	965.7	E850.7	E935.7	E950.0	E962.0	E980.0
Ethopropazine	966.4	E855.0	E936.4	E950.4	E962.0	E980.4
Ethosuximide	966.2	E855.0	E936.2	E950.4	E962.0	E980.4
Ethotoin	966.1	E855.0	E936.1	E950.4	E962.0	E980.4
Ethoxazene	961.9	E857	E931.9	E950.4	E962.0	E980.4
Ethoxzolamide	974.2	E858.5	E944.2	E950.4	E962.0	E980.4
Ethyl						
acetate (vapor)	982.8	E862.4	—	E950.9	E962.1	E980.9
alcohol	980.0	E860.1	—	E950.9	E962.1	E980.9
beverage	980.0	E860.0	—	E950.9	E962.1	E980.9
aldehyde (vapor)	987.8	E869.8	—	E952.8	E962.2	E982.8
liquid	989.89	E866.8	—	E950.9	E962.1	E980.9

Substance	Poisoning	Accident	Therapeutic Use	Suicide Attempt	Assault	Undetermined
			External Cause (E-Code)			
aminobenzoate	968.5	E855.2	E938.5	E950.4	E962.0	E980.4
biscoumacetate	964.2	E858.2	E934.2	E950.4	E962.0	E980.4
bromide (anesthetic)	968.2	E855.1	E938.2	E950.4	E962.0	E980.4
carbamate (antineoplastic)	963.1	E858.1	E933.1	E950.4	E962.0	E980.4
carbinol	980.3	E860.4	—	E950.9	E962.1	E980.9
chaulmoograte	961.8	E857	E931.8	E950.4	E962.0	E980.4
chloride (vapor)	987.8	E869.8	—	E952.8	E962.2	E982.8
anesthetic (local)	968.5	E855.2	E938.5	E950.4	E962.0	E980.4
inhaled	968.2	E855.1	E938.2	E950.4	E962.0	E980.4
solvent	982.3	E862.4	—	E950.9	E962.1	E980.9
estranol	962.1	E858.0	E932.1	E950.4	E962.0	E980.4
ether — *see* Ether(s)						
formate (solvent) NEC	982.8	E862.4	—	E950.9	E962.1	E980.9
iodoacetate	987.5	E869.3	—	E952.8	E962.2	E982.8
lactate (solvent) NEC	982.8	E862.4	—	E950.9	E962.1	E980.9
methylcarbinol	980.8	E860.8	—	E950.9	E962.1	E980.9
morphine	965.09	E850.2	E935.2	E950.0	E962.0	E980.0
Ethylene (gas)	987.1	E869.8	—	E952.8	E962.2	E982.8
anesthetic (general)	968.2	E855.1	E938.2	E950.4	E962.0	E980.4
chlorohydrin (vapor)	982.3	E862.4	—	E950.9	E962.1	E980.9
dichloride (vapor)	982.3	E862.4	—	E950.9	E962.1	E980.9
glycol(s) (any) (vapor)	982.8	E862.4	—	E950.9	E962.1	E980.9
Ethylidene						
chloride NEC	982.3	E862.4	—	E950.9	E962.1	E980.9
diethyl ether	982.8	E862.4	—	E950.9	E962.1	E980.9
Ethynodiol	962.2	E858.0	E932.2	E950.4	E962.0	E980.4
Etidocaine	968.9	E855.2	E938.9	E950.4	E962.0	E980.4
infiltration (subcutaneous)	968.5	E855.2	E938.5	E950.4	E962.0	E980.4
nerve (peripheral) (plexus)	968.6	E855.2	E938.6	E950.4	E962.0	E980.4
Etilfen	967.0	E851	E937.0	E950.1	E962.0	E980.1
Etomide	965.7	E850.7	E935.7	E950.0	E962.0	E980.0
Etorphine	965.09	E850.2	E935.2	E950.0	E962.0	E980.0
Etoval	967.0	E851	E937.0	E950.1	E962.0	E980.1
Etryptamine	969.0	E854.0	E939.0	E950.3	E962.0	E980.3
Eucaine	968.5	E855.2	E938.5	E950.4	E962.0	E980.4
Eucalyptus (oil) NEC	975.5	E858.6	E945.5	E950.4	E962.0	E980.4
Eucatropine	971.1	E855.4	E941.1	E950.4	E962.0	E980.4
Eucodal	965.09	E850.2	E935.2	E950.0	E962.0	E980.0
Euneryl	967.0	E851	E937.0	E950.1	E962.0	E980.1
Euphthalmine	971.1	E855.4	E941.1	E950.4	E962.0	E980.4
Eurax	976.0	E858.7	E946.0	E950.4	E962.0	E980.4
Euresol	976.4	E858.7	E946.4	E950.4	E962.0	E980.4
Euthroid	962.7	E858.0	E932.7	E950.4	E962.0	E980.4
Evans blue	977.8	E858.8	E947.8	E950.4	E962.0	E980.4
Evipal	967.0	E851	E937.0	E950.1	E962.0	E980.1
sodium	968.3	E855.1	E938.3	E950.4	E962.0	E980.4
Evipan	967.0	E851	E937.0	E950.1	E962.0	E980.1
sodium	968.3	E855.1	E938.3	E950.4	E962.0	E980.4
Exalgin	965.4	E850.4	E935.4	E950.0	E962.0	E980.0
Excipients, pharmaceutical	977.4	E858.8	E947.4	E950.4	E962.0	E980.4
Exhaust gas — *see* Carbon, monoxide						
Ex–Lax (phenolphthalein)	973.1	E858.4	E943.1	E950.4	E962.0	E980.4
Expectorants	975.5	E858.6	E945.5	E950.4	E962.0	E980.4
External medications (skin) (mucous						
membrane)	976.9	E858.7	E946.9	E950.4	E962.0	E980.4
dental agent	976.7	E858.7	E946.7	E950.4	E962.0	E980.4
ENT agent	976.6	E858.7	E946.6	E950.4	E962.0	E980.4

Substance	Poisoning	External Cause (E-Code)				
		Accident	Therapeutic Use	Suicide Attempt	Assault	Undetermined
ophthalmic preparation	976.5	E858.7	E946.5	E950.4	E962.0	E980.4
specified NEC	976.8	E858.7	E946.8	E950.4	E962.0	E980.4
Eye agents (anti–infective)	976.5	E858.7	E946.5	E950.4	E962.0	E980.4
Factor IX complex (human)	964.5	E858.2	E934.5	E950.4	E962.0	E980.4
Fecal softeners	973.2	E858.4	E943.2	E950.4	E962.0	E980.4
Fenbutrazate	977.0	E858.8	E947.0	E950.4	E962.0	E980.4
Fencamfamin	970.8	E854.3	E940.8	E950.4	E962.0	E980.4
Fenfluramine	977.0	E858.8	E947.0	E950.4	E962.0	E980.4
Fenoprofen	965.61	E850.6	E935.6	E950.0	E962.0	E980.0
Fentanyl	965.09	E850.2	E935.2	E950.0	E962.0	E980.0
Fentazin	969.1	E853.0	E939.1	E950.3	E962.0	E980.3
Fenticlor, fentichlor	976.0	E858.7	E946.0	E950.4	E962.0	E980.4
Fer de lance (bite) (venom)	989.5	E905.0	—	E950.9	E962.1	E980.9
Ferric — *see* Iron						
Ferrocholinate	964.0	E858.2	E934.0	E950.4	E962.0	E980.4
Ferrous fumarate, gluconate, lactate, salt						
NEC, sulfate (medicinal)	964.0	E858.2	E934.0	E950.4	E962.0	E980.4
Ferrum — *see* Iron						
Fertilizers NEC	989.89	E866.5	—	E950.9	E962.1	E980.4
with herbicide mixture	989.4	E863.5	—	E950.6	E962.1	E980.7
Fibrinogen (human)	964.7	E858.2	E934.7	E950.4	E962.0	E980.4
Fibrinolysin	964.4	E858.2	E934.4	E950.4	E962.0	E980.4
Fibrinolysis–affecting agents	964.4	E858.2	E934.4	E950.4	E962.0	E980.4
Filix mas	961.6	E857	E931.6	E950.4	E962.0	E980.4
Fiorinal	965.1	E850.3	E935.3	E950.0	E962.0	E980.0
Fire damp	987.1	E869.8	—	E952.8	E962.2	E982.8
Fish, nonbacterial or noxious	988.0	E865.2	—	E950.9	E962.1	E980.9
shell	988.0	E865.1	—	E950.9	E962.1	E980.9
Flagyl	961.5	E857	E931.5	E950.4	E962.0	E980.4
Flavoxate	975.1	E858.6	E945.1	E950.4	E962.0	E980.4
Flaxedil	975.2	E858.6	E945.2	E950.4	E962.0	E980.4
Flaxseed (medicinal)	976.3	E858.7	E946.3	E950.4	E962.0	E980.4
Florantyrone	973.4	E858.4	E943.4	E950.4	E962.0	E980.4
Floraquin	961.3	E857	E931.3	E950.4	E962.0	E980.4
Florinef	962.0	E858.0	E932.0	E950.4	E962.0	E980.4
ENT agent	976.6	E858.7	E946.6	E950.4	E962.0	E980.4
ophthalmic preparation	976.5	E858.7	E946.5	E950.4	E962.0	E980.4
topical NEC	976.0	E858.7	E946.0	E950.4	E962.0	E980.4
Flowers of sulfur	976.4	E858.7	E946.4	E950.4	E962.0	E980.4
Floxuridine	963.1	E858.1	E933.1	E950.4	E962.0	E980.4
Flucytosine	961.9	E857	E931.9	E950.4	E962.0	E980.4
Fludrocortisone	962.0	E858.0	E932.0	E950.4	E962.0	E980.4
ENT agent	976.6	E858.7	E946.6	E950.4	E962.0	E980.4
ophthalmic preparation	976.5	E858.7	E946.5	E950.4	E962.0	E980.4
topical NEC	976.0	E858.7	E946.0	E950.4	E962.0	E980.4
Flumethasone	976.0	E858.7	E946.0	E950.4	E962.0	E980.4
Flumethiazide	974.3	E858.5	E944.3	E950.4	E962.0	E980.4
Flumidin	961.7	E857	E931.7	E950.4	E962.0	E980.4
Flunitrazepam	969.4	E853.2	E939.4	E950.3	E962.0	E980.3
Fluocinolone	976.0	E858.7	E946.0	E950.4	E962.0	E980.4
Fluocortolone	962.0	E858.0	E932.0	E950.4	E962.0	E980.4
Fluohydrocortisone	962.0	E858.0	E932.0	E950.4	E962.0	E980.4
ENT agent	976.6	E858.7	E946.6	E950.4	E962.0	E980.4
ophthalmic preparation	976.5	E858.7	E946.5	E950.4	E962.0	E980.4
topical NEC	976.0	E858.7	E946.0	E950.4	E962.0	E980.4
Fluonid	976.0	E858.7	E946.0	E950.4	E962.0	E980.4
Fluopromazine	969.1	E853.0	E939.1	E950.3	E962.0	E980.3

Substance	Poisoning	External Cause (E-Code)				
		Accident	Therapeutic Use	Suicide Attempt	Assault	Undetermined
Fluoracetate	989.4	E863.7	—	E950.6	E962.1	E980.7
Fluorescein (sodium)	977.8	E858.8	E947.8	E950.4	E962.0	E980.4
Fluoride(s) (pesticides) (sodium) NEC	989.4	E863.4	—	E950.6	E962.1	E980.7
hydrogen — *see* Hydrofluoric acid						
medicinal	976.7	E858.7	E946.7	E950.4	E962.0	E980.4
not pesticide NEC	983.9	E864.4	—	E950.7	E962.1	E980.6
stannous	976.7	E858.7	E946.7	E950.4	E962.0	E980.4
Fluorinated corticosteroids	962.0	E858.0	E932.0	E950.4	E962.0	E980.4
Fluorine (compounds) (gas)	987.8	E869.8	—	E952.8	E962.2	E982.8
salt — *see* Fluoride(s)						
Fluoristan	976.7	E858.7	E946.7	E950.4	E962.0	E980.4
Fluoroacetate	989.4	E863.7	—	E950.6	E962.1	E980.7
Fluorodeoxyuridine	963.1	E858.1	E933.1	E950.4	E962.0	E980.4
Fluorometholone (topical) NEC	976.0	E858.7	E946.0	E950.4	E962.0	E980.4
ophthalmic preparation	976.5	E858.7	E946.5	E950.4	E962.0	E980.4
Fluorouracil	963.1	E858.1	E933.1	E950.4	E962.0	E980.4
Fluothane	968.1	E855.1	E938.1	E950.4	E962.0	E980.4
Fluoxetine hydrochloride	969.0	E854.0	E939.0	E950.3	E962.0	E980.3
Fluoxymesterone	962.1	E858.0	E932.1	E950.4	E962.0	E980.4
Fluphenazine	969.1	E853.0	E939.1	E950.3	E962.0	E980.3
Fluprednisolone	962.0	E858.0	E932.0	E950.4	E962.0	E980.4
Flurandrenolide	976.0	E858.7	E946.0	E950.4	E962.0	E980.4
Flurazepam (hydrochloride)	969.4	E853.2	E939.4	E950.3	E962.0	E980.3
Flurbiprofen	965.61	E850.6	E935.6	E950.0	E962.0	E980.0
Flurobate	976.0	E858.7	E946.0	E950.4	E962.0	E980.4
Flurothyl	969.8	E855.8	E939.8	E950.3	E962.0	E980.3
Fluroxene	968.2	E855.1	E938.2	E950.4	E962.0	E980.4
Folacin	964.1	E858.2	E934.1	E950.4	E962.0	E980.4
Folic acid	964.1	E858.2	E934.1	E950.4	E962.0	E980.4
Follicle stimulating hormone	962.4	E858.0	E932.4	E950.4	E962.0	E980.4
Food, foodstuffs, nonbacterial or noxious	988.9	E865.9	—	E950.9	E962.1	E980.9
berries, seeds	988.2	E865.3	—	E950.9	E962.1	E980.9
fish	988.0	E865.2	—	E950.9	E962.1	E980.9
mushrooms	988.1	E865.5	—	E950.9	E962.1	E980.9
plants	988.2	E865.9	—	E950.9	E962.1	E980.9
specified type NEC	988.2	E865.4	—	E950.9	E962.1	E980.9
shellfish	988.0	E865.1	—	E950.9	E962.1	E980.9
specified NEC	988.8	E865.8	—	E950.9	E962.1	E980.9
Fool's parsley	988.2	E865.4	—	E950.9	E962.1	E980.9
Formaldehyde (solution)	989.89	E861.4	—	E950.9	E962.1	E980.9
fungicide	989.4	E863.6	—	E950.6	E962.1	E980.7
gas or vapor	987.8	E869.8	—	E952.8	E962.2	E982.8
Formalin	989.89	E861.4	—	E950.9	E962.1	E980.9
fungicide	989.4	E863.6	—	E950.6	E962.1	E980.7
vapor	987.8	E869.8	—	E952.8	E962.2	E982.8
Formic acid	983.1	E864.1	—	E950.7	E962.1	E980.6
vapor	987.8	E869.8	—	E952.8	E962.2	E982.8
Fowler's solution	985.1	E866.3	—	E950.8	E962.1	E980.8
Foxglove	988.2	E865.4	—	E950.9	E962.1	E980.9
Fox green	977.8	E858.8	E947.8	E950.4	E962.0	E980.4
Framycetin	960.8	E856	E930.8	E950.4	E962.0	E980.4
Frangula (extract)	973.1	E858.4	E943.1	E950.4	E962.0	E980.4
Frei antigen	977.8	E858.8	E947.8	E950.4	E962.0	E980.4
Freons	987.4	E869.2	—	E952.8	E962.2	E982.8
Fructose	974.5	E858.5	E944.5	E950.4	E962.0	E980.4
Frusemide	974.4	E858.5	E944.4	E950.4	E962.0	E980.4
FSH	962.4	E858.0	E932.4	E950.4	E962.0	E980.4

Substance	Poisoning	Accident	Therapeutic Use	Suicide Attempt	Assault	Undetermined
Fuel						
automobile	981	E862.1	—	E950.9	E962.1	E980.9
exhaust gas, not in transit	986	E868.2	—	E952.0	E962.2	E982.0
vapor NEC	987.1	E869.8	—	E952.8	E962.2	E982.8
gas (domestic use) — *see also* Carbon, monoxide, fuel						
utility	987.1	E868.1	—	E951.8	E962.2	E981.8
incomplete combustion of — *see* Carbon, monoxide, fuel, utility						
in mobile container	987.0	E868.0	—	E951.1	E962.2	E981.1
piped (natural)	987.1	E867	—	E951.0	E962.2	E981.0
industrial, incomplete combustion	986	E868.3	—	E952.1	E962.2	E982.1
Fugillin	960.8	E856	E930.8	E950.4	E962.0	E980.4
Fulminate of mercury	985.0	E866.1	—	E950.9	E962.1	E980.9
Fulvicin	960.1	E856	E930.1	E950.4	E962.0	E980.4
Fumadil	960.8	E856	E930.8	E950.4	E962.0	E980.4
Fumagillin	960.8	E856	E930.8	E950.4	E962.0	E980.4
Fumes (from)	987.9	E869.9	—	E952.9	E962.2	E982.9
carbon monoxide — *see* Carbon, monoxide						
charcoal (domestic use)	986	E868.3	—	E952.1	E962.2	E982.1
chloroform — *see* Chloroform						
coke (in domestic stoves, fireplaces)	986	E868.3	—	E952.1	E962.2	E982.1
corrosive NEC	987.8	E869.8	—	E952.8	E962.2	E982.8
ether — *see* Ether(s)						
freons	987.4	E869.2	—	E952.8	E962.2	E982.8
hydrocarbons	987.1	E869.8	—	E952.8	E962.2	E982.8
petroleum (liquefied)	987.0	E868.0	—	E951.1	E962.2	E981.1
distributed through pipes (pure or mixed with air)	987.0	E867	—	E951.0	E962.2	E981.0
lead — *see* Lead						
metals — *see* specified metal						
nitrogen dioxide	987.2	E869.0	—	E952.8	E962.2	E982.8
pesticides — *see* Pesticides						
petroleum (liquefied)	987.0	E868.0	—	E951.1	E962.2	E981.1
distributed through pipes (pure or mixed with air)	987.0	E867	—	E951.0	E962.2	E981.0
polyester	987.8	E869.8	—	E952.8	E962.2	E982.8
specified source, other (see also substance specified)	987.8	E869.8	—	E952.8	E962.2	E982.8
sulfur dioxide	987.3	E869.1	—	E952.8	E962.2	E982.8
Fumigants	989.4	E863.8	—	E950.6	E962.1	E980.7
Fungi, noxious, used as food	988.1	E865.5	—	E950.9	E962.1	E980.9
Fungicides (*see also* Antifungals)	989.4	E863.6	—	E950.6	E962.1	E980.7
Fungizone	960.1	E856	E930.1	E950.4	E962.0	E980.4
topical	976.0	E858.7	E946.0	E950.4	E962.0	E980.4
Furacin	976.0	E858.7	E946.0	E950.4	E962.0	E980.4
Furadantin	961.9	E857	E931.9	E950.4	E962.0	E980.4
Furazolidone	961.9	E857	E931.9	E950.4	E962.0	E980.4
Furnace (coal burning) (domestic), gas from	986	E868.3	—	E952.1	E962.2	E982.1
industrial	986	E868.8	—	E952.1	E962.2	E982.1
Furniture polish	989.89	E861.2	—	E950.9	E962.1	E980.9
Furosemide	974.4	E858.5	E944.4	E950.4	E962.0	E980.4
Furoxone	961.9	E857	E931.9	E950.4	E962.0	E980.4
Fusel oil (amyl) (butyl) (propyl)	980.3	E860.4	—	E950.9	E962.1	E980.9
Fusidic acid	960.8	E856	E930.8	E950.4	E962.0	E980.4
Gallamine	975.2	E858.6	E945.2	E950.4	E962.0	E980.4

Substance	Poisoning	Accident	External Cause (E-Code)			
			Therapeutic Use	Suicide Attempt	Assault	Undetermined
Gallotannic acid	976.2	E858.7	E946.2	E950.4	E962.0	E980.4
Gamboge	973.1	E858.4	E943.1	E950.4	E962.0	E980.4
Gamimune	964.6	E858.2	E934.6	E950.4	E962.0	E980.4
Gamma–benzene hexachloride (vapor)	989.2	E863.0	—	E950.6	E962.1	E980.7
Gamma globulin	964.6	E858.2	E934.6	E950.4	E962.0	E980.4
Gamma Hydroxy Butyrate (GHB)	968.4	E855.1	E938.4	E950.4	E962.0	E980.4
Gamulin	964.6	E858.2	E934.6	E950.4	E962.0	E980.4
Ganglionic blocking agents	972.3	E858.3	E942.3	E950.4	E962.0	E980.4
Ganja	969.6	E854.1	E939.6	E950.3	E962.0	E980.3
Garamycin	960.8	E856	E930.8	E950.4	E962.0	E980.4
ophthalmic preparation	976.5	E858.7	E946.5	E950.4	E962.0	E980.4
topical NEC	976.0	E858.7	E946.0	E950.4	E962.0	E980.4
Gardenal	967.0	E851	E937.0	E950.1	E962.0	E980.1
Gardepanyl	967.0	E851	E937.0	E950.1	E962.0	E980.1
Gas	987.9	E869.9	—	E952.9	E962.2	E982.9
acetylene	987.1	E868.1	—	E951.8	E962.2	E981.8
incomplete combustion of — see Carbon, monoxide, fuel, utility						
air contaminants, source or type not specified	987.9	E869.9	—	E952.9	E962.2	E982.9
anesthetic (general) NEC	968.2	E855.1	E938.2	E950.4	E962.0	E980.4
blast furnace	986	E868.8	—	E952.1	E962.2	E982.1
butane — see Butane						
carbon monoxide — see Carbon, monoxide						
chlorine	987.6	E869.8	—	E952.8	E962.2	E982.8
coal — see Carbon, monoxide, coal						
cyanide	987.7	E869.8	—	E952.8	E962.2	E982.8
dicyanogen	987.8	E869.8	—	E952.8	E962.2	E982.8
domestic — see Gas, utility						
exhaust — see Carbon, monoxide, exhaust gas						
from wood– or coal–burning stove or fireplace	986	E868.3	—	E952.1	E962.2	E982.1
fuel (domestic use) — see also Carbon, monoxide, fuel						
industrial use	986	E868.8	—	E952.1	E962.2	E982.1
utility	987.1	E868.1	—	E951.8	E962.2	E981.8
incomplete combustion of — see Carbon, monoxide, fuel, utility						
in mobile container	987.0	E868.0	—	E951.1	E962.2	E981.1
piped (natural)	987.1	E867	—	E951.0	E962.2	E981.0
garage	986	E868.2	—	E952.0	E962.2	E982.0
hydrocarbon NEC	987.1	E869.8	—	E952.8	E962.2	E982.8
incomplete combustion of — see Carbon, monoxide, fuel, utility						
liquefied (mobile container)	987.0	E868.0	—	E951.1	E962.2	E981.1
piped	987.0	E867	—	E951.0	E962.2	E981.0
hydrocyanic acid	987.7	E869.8	—	E952.8	E962.2	E982.8
illuminating — see Gas, utility						
incomplete combustion, any — see Carbon, monoxide						
kiln	986	E868.8	—	E952.1	E962.2	E982.1
lacrimogenic	987.5	E869.3	—	E952.8	E962.2	E982.8
marsh	987.1	E869.8	—	E952.8	E962.2	E982.8
motor exhaust, not in transit	986	E868.8	—	E952.1	E962.2	E982.1
mustard — see Mustard, gas						
natural	987.1	E867	—	E951.0	E962.2	E981.0
nerve (war)	987.9	E869.9	—	E952.9	E962.2	E982.9

Substance	Poisoning	Accident	Therapeutic Use	Suicide Attempt	Assault	Undetermined
					External Cause (E-Code)	
oils 981	E862.1	—		E950.9	E962.1	E980.9
petroleum (liquefied) (distributed in						
mobile containers) 987.0	E868.0	—		E951.1	E962.2	E981.1
piped (pure or mixed with air) 987.0	E867	—		E951.1	E962.2	E981.1
piped (manufactured) (natural) NEC . . . 987.1	E867	—		E951.0	E962.2	E981.0
producer 986	E868.8	—		E952.1	E962.2	E982.1
propane — see Propane						
refrigerant (freon) 987.4	E869.2	—		E952.8	E962.2	E982.8
not freon 987.9	E869.9	—		E952.9	E962.2	E982.9
sewer 987.8	E869.8	—		E952.8	E962.2	E982.8
specified source NEC (see also substance						
specified) 987.8	E869.8	—		E952.8	E962.2	E982.8
stove — see Gas, utility						
tear 987.5	E869.3	—		E952.8	E962.2	E982.8
utility (for cooking, heating, or lighting)						
(piped) NEC 987.1	E868.1	—		E951.8	E962.2	E981.8
incomplete combustion of — see Carbon,						
monoxide, fuel, utility						
in mobile container 987.0	E868.0	—		E951.1	E962.2	E981.1
piped (natural) 987.1	E867	—		E951.0	E962.2	E981.0
water 987.1	E868.1	—		E951.8	E962.2	E981.8
incomplete combustion of — see Carbon,						
monoxide, fuel, utility						
Gaseous substance — see Gas						
Gasoline, gasolene 981	E862.1	—		E950.9	E962.1	E980.9
vapor 987.1	E869.8	—		E952.8	E962.2	E982.8
Gastric enzymes 973.4	E858.4	E943.4		E950.4	E962.0	E980.4
Gastrografin 977.8	E858.8	E947.8		E950.4	E962.0	E980.4
Gastrointestinal agents 973.9	E858.4	E943.9		E950.4	E962.0	E980.4
specified NEC 973.8	E858.4	E943.8		E950.4	E962.0	E980.4
Gaultheria procumbens 988.2	E865.4	—		E950.9	E962.1	E980.9
Gelatin (intravenous) 964.8	E858.2	E934.8		E950.4	E962.0	E980.4
absorbable (sponge) 964.5	E858.2	E934.5		E950.4	E962.0	E980.4
Gelfilm 976.8	E858.7	E946.8		E950.4	E962.0	E980.4
Gelfoam 964.5	E858.2	E934.5		E950.4	E962.0	E980.4
Gelsemine 970.8	E854.3	E940.8		E950.4	E962.0	E980.4
Gelsemium (sempervirens) 988.2	E865.4	—		E950.9	E962.1	E980.9
Gemonil 967.0	E851	E937.0		E950.1	E962.0	E980.1
Gentamicin 960.8	E856	E930.8		E950.4	E962.0	E980.4
ophthalmic preparation 976.5	E858.7	E946.5		E950.4	E962.0	E980.4
topical NEC 976.0	E858.7	E946.0		E950.4	E962.0	E980.4
Gentian violet 976.0	E858.7	E946.0		E950.4	E962.0	E980.4
Gexane 976.0	E858.7	E946.0		E950.4	E962.0	E980.4
Gila monster (venom) 989.5	E905.0	—		E950.9	E962.1	E980.9
Ginger, Jamaica 989.89	E866.8	—		E950.9	E962.1	E980.9
Gitalin 972.1	E858.3	E942.1		E950.4	E962.0	E980.4
Gitoxin 972.1	E858.3	E942.1		E950.4	E962.0	E980.4
Glandular extract (medicinal) NEC 977.9	E858.9	E947.9		E950.5	E962.0	E980.5
Glaucarubin 961.5	E857	E931.5		E950.4	E962.0	E980.4
Globin zinc insulin 962.3	E858.0	E932.3		E950.4	E962.0	E980.4
Glucagon 962.3	E858.0	E932.3		E950.4	E962.0	E980.4
Glucochloral 967.1	E852.0	E937.1		E950.2	E962.0	E980.2
Glucocorticoids 962.0	E858.0	E932.0		E950.4	E962.0	E980.4
Glucose 974.5	E858.5	E944.5		E950.4	E962.0	E980.4
oxidase reagent 977.8	E858.8	E947.8		E950.4	E962.0	E980.4
Glucosulfone sodium 961.8	E857	E931.8		E950.4	E962.0	E980.4
Glue(s) 989.89	E866.6	—		E950.9	E962.1	E980.9

Substance	Poisoning	External Cause (E-Code)				
		Accident	Therapeutic Use	Suicide Attempt	Assault	Undetermined
Glutamic acid (hydrochloride)	973.4	E858.4	E943.4	E950.4	E962.0	E980.4
Glutathione	963.8	E858.1	E933.8	E950.4	E962.0	E980.4
Glutethimide (group)	967.5	E852.4	E937.5	E950.2	E962.0	E980.2
Glycerin (lotion)	976.3	E858.7	E946.3	E950.4	E962.0	E980.4
Glycerol (topical)	976.3	E858.7	E946.3	E950.4	E962.0	E980.4
Glyceryl						
guaiacolate	975.5	E858.6	E945.5	E950.4	E962.0	E980.4
triacetate (topical)	976.0	E858.7	E946.0	E950.4	E962.0	E980.4
trinitrate	972.4	E858.3	E942.4	E950.4	E962.0	E980.4
Glycine	974.5	E858.5	E944.5	E950.4	E962.0	E980.4
Glycobiarsol	961.1	E857	E931.1	E950.4	E962.0	E980.4
Glycols (ether)	982.8	E862.4	—	E950.9	E962.1	E980.9
Glycopyrrolate	971.1	E855.4	E941.1	E950.4	E962.0	E980.4
Glymidine	962.3	E858.0	E932.3	E950.4	E962.0	E980.4
Gold (compounds) (salts)	965.69	E850.6	E935.6	E950.0	E962.0	E980.0
Golden sulfide of antimony	985.4	E866.2	—	E950.9	E962.1	E980.9
Goldylocks	988.2	E865.4	—	E950.9	E962.1	E980.9
Gonadal tissue extract	962.9	E858.0	E932.9	E950.4	E962.0	E980.4
female	962.2	E858.0	E932.2	E950.4	E962.0	E980.4
male	962.1	E858.0	E932.1	E950.4	E962.0	E980.4
Gonadotropin	962.4	E858.0	E932.4	E950.4	E962.0	E980.4
Grain alcohol	980.0	E860.1	—	E950.9	E962.1	E980.9
beverage	980.0	E860.0	—	E950.9	E962.1	E980.9
Gramicidin	960.8	E856	E930.8	E950.4	E962.0	E980.4
Gratiola officinalis	988.2	E865.4	—	E950.9	E962.1	E980.9
Grease	989.89	E866.8	—	E950.9	E962.1	E980.9
Green hellebore	988.2	E865.4	—	E950.9	E962.1	E980.9
Green soap	976.2	E858.7	E946.2	E950.4	E962.0	E980.4
Grifulvin	960.1	E856	E930.1	E950.4	E962.0	E980.4
Griseofulvin	960.1	E856	E930.1	E950.4	E962.0	E980.4
Growth hormone	962.4	E858.0	E932.4	E950.4	E962.0	E980.4
Guaiacol	975.5	E858.6	E945.5	E950.4	E962.0	E980.4
Guaiac reagent	977.8	E858.8	E947.8	E950.4	E962.0	E980.4
Guaifenesin	975.5	E858.6	E945.5	E950.4	E962.0	E980.4
Guaiphenesin	975.5	E858.6	E945.5	E950.4	E962.0	E980.4
Guanatol	961.4	E857	E931.4	E950.4	E962.0	E980.4
Guanethidine	972.6	E858.3	E942.6	E950.4	E962.0	E980.4
Guano	989.89	E866.5	—	E950.9	E962.1	E980.9
Guanochlor	972.6	E858.3	E942.6	E950.4	E962.0	E980.4
Guanoctine	972.6	E858.3	E942.6	E950.4	E962.0	E980.4
Guanoxan	972.6	E858.3	E942.6	E950.4	E962.0	E980.4
Hair treatment agent NEC	976.4	E858.7	E946.4	E950.4	E962.0	E980.4
Halcinonide	976.0	E858.7	E946.0	E950.4	E962.0	E980.4
Halethazole	976.0	E858.7	E946.0	E950.4	E962.0	E980.4
Hallucinogens	969.6	E854.1	E939.6	E950.3	E962.0	E980.3
Haloperidol	969.2	E853.1	E939.2	E950.3	E962.0	E980.3
Haloprogin	976.0	E858.7	E946.0	E950.4	E962.0	E980.4
Halotex	976.0	E858.7	E946.0	E950.4	E962.0	E980.4
Halothane	968.1	E855.1	E938.1	E950.4	E962.0	E980.4
Halquinols	976.0	E858.7	E946.0	E950.4	E962.0	E980.4
Harmonyl	972.6	E858.3	E942.6	E950.4	E962.0	E980.4
Hartmann's solution	974.5	E858.5	E944.5	E950.4	E962.0	E980.4
Hashish	969.6	E854.1	E939.6	E950.3	E962.0	E980.3
Hawaiian wood rose seeds	969.6	E854.1	E939.6	E950.3	E962.0	E980.3
Headache cures, drugs, powders NEC	977.9	E858.9	E947.9	E950.5	E962.0	E980.9
Heavenly Blue (morning glory)	969.6	E854.1	E939.6	E950.3	E962.0	E980.3
Heavy metal						

Substance	Poisoning	External Cause (E-Code)				
		Accident	Therapeutic Use	Suicide Attempt	Assault	Undetermined
antagonists	963.8	E858.1	E933.8	E950.4	E962.0	E980.4
anti–infectives	961.2	E857	E931.2	E950.4	E962.0	E980.4
Hedaquinium	976.0	E858.7	E946.0	E950.4	E962.0	E980.4
Hedge hyssop.	988.2	E865.4	—	E950.9	E962.1	E980.9
Heet	976.8	E858.7	E946.8	E950.4	E962.1	E980.4
Helenin	961.6	E857	E931.6	E950.4	E962.0	E980.4
Hellebore (black) (green) (white)	988.2	E865.4	—	E950.9	E962.1	E980.9
Hemlock	988.2	E865.4	—	E950.9	E962.1	E980.9
Hemostatics	964.5	E858.2	E934.5	E950.4	E962.0	E980.4
capillary active drugs	972.8	E858.3	E942.8	E950.4	E962.0	E980.4
Henbane	988.2	E865.4	—	E950.9	E962.1	E980.9
Heparin (sodium)	964.2	E858.2	E934.2	E950.4	E962.0	E980.4
Heptabarbital, heptabarbitone	967.0	E851	E937.0	E950.1	E962.0	E980.1
Heptachlor	989.2	E863.0	—	E950.6	E962.1	E980.7
Heptalgin	965.09	E850.2	E935.2	E950.0	E962.0	E980.0
Herbicides	989.4	E863.5	—	E950.6	E962.1	E980.7
Heroin	965.01	E850.0	E935.0	E950.0	E962.0	E980.0
Herplex	976.5	E858.7	E946.5	E950.4	E962.0	E980.4
HES	964.8	E858.2	E934.8	E950.4	E962.0	E980.4
Hetastarch	964.8	E858.2	E934.8	E950.4	E962.0	E980.4
Hexachlorocyclohexane	989.2	E863.0	—	E950.6	E962.1	E980.7
Hexachlorophene	976.2	E858.7	E946.2	E950.4	E962.0	E980.4
Hexadimethrine (bromide)	964.5	E858.2	E934.5	E950.4	E962.0	E980.4
Hexafluorenium	975.2	E858.6	E945.2	E950.4	E962.0	E980.4
Hexa–germ	976.2	E858.7	E946.2	E950.4	E962.0	E980.4
Hexahydrophenol	980.8	E860.8	—	E950.9	E962.1	E980.9
Hexalin	980.8	E860.8	—	E950.9	E962.1	E980.9
Hexamethonium	972.3	E858.3	E942.3	E950.4	E962.0	E980.4
Hexamethyleneamine	961.9	E857	E931.9	E950.4	E962.0	E980.4
Hexamine	961.9	E857	E931.9	E950.4	E962.0	E980.4
Hexanone	982.8	E862.4	—	E950.9	E962.1	E980.9
Hexapropymate	967.8	E852.8	E937.8	E950.2	E962.0	E980.2
Hexestrol	962.2	E858.0	E932.2	E950.4	E962.0	E980.4
Hexethal (sodium)	967.0	E851	E937.0	E950.1	E962.0	E980.1
Hexetidine	976.0	E858.7	E946.0	E950.4	E962.0	E980.4
Hexobarbital, hexobarbitone	967.0	E851	E937.0	E950.1	E962.0	E980.1
sodium (anesthetic)	968.3	E855.1	E938.3	E950.4	E962.0	E980.4
soluble	968.3	E855.1	E938.3	E950.4	E962.0	E980.4
Hexocyclium	971.1	E855.4	E941.1	E950.4	E962.0	E980.4
Hexoestrol	962.2	E858.0	E932.2	E950.4	E962.0	E980.4
Hexone	982.8	E862.4	—	E950.9	E962.1	E980.9
Hexylcaine	968.5	E855.2	E938.5	E950.4	E962.0	E980.4
Hexylresorcinol	961.6	E857	E931.6	E950.4	E962.0	E980.4
Hinkle's pills	973.1	E858.4	E943.1	E950.4	E962.0	E980.4
Histalog	977.8	E858.8	E947.8	E950.4	E962.0	E980.4
Histamine (phosphate)	972.5	E858.3	E942.5	E950.4	E962.0	E980.4
Histoplasmin	977.8	E858.8	E947.8	E950.4	E962.0	E980.4
Holly berries	988.2	E865.3	—	E950.9	E962.1	E980.9
Homatropine	971.1	E855.4	E941.1	E950.4	E962.0	E980.4
Homo–tet	964.6	E858.2	E934.6	E950.4	E962.0	E980.4
Hormones (synthetic substitute) NEC	962.9	E858.0	E932.9	E950.4	E962.0	E980.4
adrenal cortical steroids	962.0	E858.0	E932.0	E950.4	E962.0	E980.4
antidiabetic agents	962.3	E858.0	E932.3	E950.4	E962.0	E980.4
follicle stimulating	962.4	E858.0	E932.4	E950.4	E962.0	E980.4
gonadotropic	962.4	E858.0	E932.4	E950.4	E962.0	E980.4
growth	962.4	E858.0	E932.4	E950.4	E962.0	E980.4
ovarian (substitutes)	962.2	E858.0	E932.2	E950.4	E962.0	E980.4

Substance	Poisoning	External Cause (E-Code)				
		Accident	Therapeutic Use	Suicide Attempt	Assault	Undetermined
parathyroid (derivatives)	962.6	E858.0	E932.6	E950.4	E962.0	E980.4
pituitary (posterior)	962.5	E858.0	E932.5	E950.4	E962.0	E980.4
anterior	962.4	E858.0	E932.4	E950.4	E962.0	E980.4
thyroid (derivative)	962.7	E858.0	E932.7	E950.4	E962.0	E980.4
Hornet (sting)	989.5	E905.3	—	E950.9	E962.1	E980.9
Horticulture agent NEC	989.4	E863.9	—	E950.6	E962.1	E980.7
Hyaluronidase	963.4	E858.1	E933.4	E950.4	E962.0	E980.4
Hyazyme	963.4	E858.1	E933.4	E950.4	E962.0	E980.4
Hycodan	965.09	E850.2	E935.2	E950.0	E962.0	E980.0
Hydantoin derivatives	966.1	E855.0	E936.1	E950.4	E962.0	E980.4
Hydeltra	962.0	E858.0	E932.0	E950.4	E962.0	E980.4
Hydergine	971.3	E855.6	E941.3	E950.4	E962.0	E980.4
Hydrabamine penicillin	960.0	E856	E930.0	E950.4	E962.0	E980.4
Hydralazine, hydrallazine	972.6	E858.3	E942.6	E950.4	E962.0	E980.4
Hydrargaphen	976.0	E858.7	E946.0	E950.4	E962.0	E980.4
Hydrazine	983.9	E864.3	—	E950.7	E962.1	E980.6
Hydriodic acid	975.5	E858.6	E945.5	E950.4	E962.0	E980.4
Hydrocarbon gas	987.1	E869.8	—	E952.8	E962.2	E982.8
incomplete combustion of — *see* Carbon, monoxide, fuel, utility						
liquefied (mobile container)	987.0	E868.0	—	E951.1	E962.2	E981.1
piped (natural)	987.0	E867	—	E951.0	E962.2	E981.0
Hydrochloric acid (liquid)	983.1	E864.1	—	E950.7	E962.1	E980.6
medicinal	973.4	E858.4	E943.4	E950.4	E962.0	E980.4
vapor	987.8	E869.8	—	E952.8	E962.2	E982.8
Hydrochlorothiazide	974.3	E858.5	E944.3	E950.4	E962.0	E980.4
Hydrocodone	965.09	E850.2	E935.2	E950.0	E962.0	E980.0
Hydrocortisone	962.0	E858.0	E932.0	E950.4	E962.0	E980.4
ENT agent	976.6	E858.7	E946.6	E950.4	E962.0	E980.4
ophthalmic preparation	976.5	E858.7	E946.5	E950.4	E962.0	E980.4
topical NEC	976.0	E858.7	E946.0	E950.4	E962.0	E980.4
Hydrocortone	962.0	E858.0	E932.0	E950.4	E962.0	E980.4
ENT agent	976.6	E858.7	E946.6	E950.4	E962.0	E980.4
ophthalmic preparation	976.5	E858.7	E946.5	E950.4	E962.0	E980.4
topical NEC	976.0	E858.7	E946.0	E950.4	E962.0	E980.4
Hydrocyanic acid — *see* Cyanide(s)						
Hydroflumethiazide	974.3	E858.5	E944.3	E950.4	E962.0	E980.4
Hydrofluoric acid (liquid)	983.1	E864.1	—	E950.7	E962.1	E980.6
vapor	987.8	E869.8	—	E952.8	E962.2	E982.8
Hydrogen	987.8	E869.8	—	E952.8	E962.2	E982.8
arsenide	985.1	E866.3	—	E950.8	E962.1	E980.8
arseniureted	985.1	E866.3	—	E950.8	E962.1	E980.8
cyanide (salts)	989.0	E866.8	—	E950.9	E962.1	E980.9
gas	987.7	E869.8	—	E952.8	E962.2	E982.8
fluoride (liquid)	983.1	E864.1	—	E950.7	E962.1	E980.6
vapor	987.8	E869.8	—	E952.8	E962.2	E982.8
peroxide (solution)	976.6	E858.7	E946.6	E950.4	E962.0	E980.4
phosphureted	987.8	E869.8	—	E952.8	E962.2	E982.8
sulfide (gas)	987.8	E869.8	—	E952.8	E962.2	E982.8
arseniureted	985.1	E866.3	—	E950.8	E962.1	E980.8
sulfureted	987.8	E869.8	—	E952.8	E962.2	E982.8
Hydromorphinol	965.09	E850.2	E935.2	E950.0	E962.0	E980.0
Hydromorphinone	965.09	E850.2	E935.2	E950.0	E962.0	E980.0
Hydromorphone	965.09	E850.2	E935.2	E950.0	E962.0	E980.0
Hydromox	974.3	E858.5	E944.3	E950.4	E962.0	E980.4
Hydrophilic lotion	976.3	E858.7	E946.3	E950.4	E962.0	E980.4
Hydroquinone	983.0	E864.0	—	E950.7	E962.1	E980.6

Substance	Poisoning	External Cause (E-Code)				
		Accident	Therapeutic Use	Suicide Attempt	Assault	Undetermined
vapor	987.8	E869.8	—	E952.8	E962.2	E982.8
Hydrosulfuric acid (gas)	987.8	E869.8	—	E952.8	E962.2	E982.8
Hydrous wool fat (lotion)	976.3	E858.7	E946.3	E950.4	E962.0	E980.4
Hydroxide, caustic	983.2	E864.2	—	E950.7	E962.1	E980.6
Hydroxocobalamin	964.1	E858.2	E934.1	E950.4	E962.0	E980.4
Hydroxyamphetamine	971.2	E855.5	E941.2	E950.4	E962.0	E980.4
Hydroxychloroquine	961.4	E857	E931.4	E950.4	E962.0	E980.4
Hydroxydihydrocodeinone	965.09	E850.2	E935.2	E950.0	E962.0	E980.0
Hydroxyethyl starch	964.8	E858.2	E934.8	E950.4	E962.0	E980.4
Hydroxyphenamate	969.5	E853.8	E939.5	E950.3	E962.0	E980.3
Hydroxyphenylbutazone	965.5	E850.5	E935.5	E950.0	E962.0	E980.0
Hydroxyprogesterone	962.2	E858.0	E932.2	E950.4	E962.0	E980.4
Hydroxyquinoline derivatives	961.3	E857	E931.3	E950.4	E962.0	E980.4
Hydroxystilbamidine	961.5	E857	E931.5	E950.4	E962.0	E980.4
Hydroxyurea	963.1	E858.1	E933.1	E950.4	E962.0	E980.4
Hydroxyzine	969.5	E853.8	E939.5	E950.3	E962.0	E980.3
Hyoscine (hydrobromide)	971.1	E855.4	E941.1	E950.4	E962.0	E980.4
Hyoscyamine	971.1	E855.4	E941.1	E950.4	E962.0	E980.4
Hyoscyamus (albus) (niger)	988.2	E865.4	—	E950.9	E962.1	E980.9
Hypaque	977.8	E858.8	E947.8	E950.4	E962.0	E980.4
Hypertussis	964.6	E858.2	E934.6	E950.4	E962.0	E980.4
Hypnotics NEC	967.9	E852.9	E937.9	E950.2	E962.0	E980.2
Hypochlorites — *see* Sodium, hypochlorite						
Hypotensive agents NEC	972.6	E858.3	E942.6	E950.4	E962.0	E980.4
Ibufenac	965.69	E850.6	E935.6	E950.0	E962.0	E980.0
Ibuprofen	965.61	E850.6	E935.6	E950.0	E962.0	E980.0
ICG	977.8	E858.8	E947.8	E950.4	E962.0	E980.4
Ichthammol	976.4	E858.7	E946.4	E950.4	E962.0	E980.4
Ichthyol	976.4	E858.7	E946.4	E950.4	E962.0	E980.4
Idoxuridine	976.5	E858.7	E946.5	E950.4	E962.0	E980.4
IDU	976.5	E858.7	E946.5	E950.4	E962.0	E980.4
Iletin	962.3	E858.0	E932.3	E950.4	E962.0	E980.4
Ilex	988.2	E865.4	—	E950.9	E962.1	E980.9
Illuminating gas — *see* Gas, utility						
Ilopan	963.5	E858.1	E933.5	E950.4	E962.0	E980.4
Ilotycin	960.3	E856	E930.3	E950.4	E962.0	E980.4
ophthalmic preparation	976.5	E858.7	E946.5	E950.4	E962.0	E980.4
topical NEC	976.0	E858.7	E946.0	E950.4	E962.0	E980.4
Imipramine	969.0	E854.0	E939.0	E950.3	E962.0	E980.3
Immu–G	964.6	E858.2	E934.6	E950.4	E962.0	E980.4
Immuglobin	964.6	E858.2	E934.6	E950.4	E962.0	E980.4
Immune serum globulin	964.6	E858.2	E934.6	E950.4	E962.0	E980.4
Immunosuppressive agents	963.1	E858.1	E933.1	E950.4	E962.0	E980.4
Immu–tetanus	964.6	E858.2	E934.6	E950.4	E962.0	E980.4
Indandione (derivatives)	964.2	E858.2	E934.2	E950.4	E962.0	E980.4
Inderal	972.0	E858.3	E942.0	E950.4	E962.0	E980.4
Indian						
hemp	969.6	E854.1	E939.6	E950.3	E962.0	E980.3
tobacco	988.2	E865.4	—	E950.9	E962.1	E980.9
Indigo carmine	977.8	E858.8	E947.8	E950.4	E962.0	E980.4
Indocin	965.69	E850.6	E935.6	E950.0	E962.0	E980.0
Indocyanine green	977.8	E858.8	E947.8	E950.4	E962.0	E980.4
Indomethacin	965.69	E850.6	E935.6	E950.0	E962.0	E980.0
Industrial						
alcohol	980.9	E860.9	—	E950.9	E962.1	E980.9
fumes	987.8	E869.8	—	E952.8	E962.2	E982.8
solvents (fumes) (vapors)	982.8	E862.9	—	E950.9	E962.1	E980.9

Substance	Poisoning	External Cause (E-Code)				
		Accident	Therapeutic Use	Suicide Attempt	Assault	Undetermined
Influenza vaccine	979.6	E858.8	E949.6	E950.4	E962.0	E982.8
Ingested substances NEC	989.9	E866.9	—	E950.9	E962.1	E980.9
INH (isoniazid)	961.8	E857	E931.8	E950.4	E962.0	E980.4
Inhalation, gas (noxious) — *see* Gas						
Ink	989.89	E866.8	—	E950.9	E962.1	E980.9
Innovar	967.6	E852.5	E937.6	E950.2	E962.0	E980.2
Inositol niacinate	972.2	E858.3	E942.2	E950.4	E962.0	E980.4
Inproquone	963.1	E858.1	E933.1	E950.4	E962.0	E980.4
Insect (sting), venomous	989.5	E905.5	—	E950.9	E962.1	E980.9
Insecticides (*see also* Pesticides)	989.4	E863.4	—	E950.6	E962.1	E980.7
chlorinated	989.2	E863.0	—	E950.6	E962.1	E980.7
mixtures	989.4	E863.3	—	E950.6	E962.1	E980.7
organochlorine (compounds)	989.2	E863.0	—	E950.6	E962.1	E980.7
organophosphorus (compounds)	989.3	E863.1	—	E950.6	E962.1	E980.7
Insular tissue extract	962.3	E858.0	E932.3	E950.4	E962.0	E980.4
Insulin (amorphous) (globin) (isophane) (Lente) (NPH) (protamine) (Semilente) (Ultralente) (zinc)	962.3	E858.0	E932.3	E950.4	E962.0	E980.4
Intranarcon	968.3	E855.1	E938.3	E950.4	E962.0	E980.4
Inulin	977.8	E858.8	E947.8	E950.4	E962.0	E980.4
Invert sugar	974.5	E858.5	E944.5	E950.4	E962.0	E980.4
Inza—*see* Naproxen						
Iodide NEC (*see also* Iodine)	976.0	E858.7	E946.0	E950.4	E962.0	E980.4
mercury (ointment)	976.0	E858.7	E946.0	E950.4	E962.0	E980.4
methylate	976.0	E858.7	E946.0	E950.4	E962.0	E980.4
potassium (expectorant) NEC	975.5	E858.6	E945.5	E950.4	E962.0	E980.4
Iodinated glycerol	975.5	E858.6	E945.5	E950.4	E962.0	E980.4
Iodine (antiseptic, external) (tincture)						
NEC	976.0	E858.7	E946.0	E950.4	E962.0	E980.4
diagnostic	977.8	E858.8	E947.8	E950.4	E962.0	E980.4
for thyroid conditions (antithyroid)	962.8	E858.0	E932.8	E950.4	E962.0	E980.4
vapor	987.8	E869.8	—	E952.8	E962.2	E982.8
Iodized oil	977.8	E858.8	E947.8	E950.4	E962.0	E980.4
Iodobismitol	961.2	E857	E931.2	E950.4	E962.0	E980.4
Iodochlorhydroxyquin	961.3	E857	E931.3	E950.4	E962.0	E980.4
topical	976.0	E858.7	E946.0	E950.4	E962.0	E980.4
Iodoform	976.0	E858.7	E946.0	E950.4	E962.0	E980.4
Iodopanoic acid	977.8	E858.8	E947.8	E950.4	E962.0	E980.4
Iodophthalein	977.8	E858.8	E947.8	E950.4	E962.0	E980.4
Ion exchange resins	974.5	E858.5	E944.5	E950.4	E962.0	E980.4
Iopanoic acid	977.8	E858.8	E947.8	E950.4	E962.0	E980.4
Iophendylate	977.8	E858.8	E947.8	E950.4	E962.0	E980.4
Iothiouracil	962.8	E858.0	E932.8	E950.4	E962.0	E980.4
Ipecac	973.6	E858.4	E943.6	E950.4	E962.0	E980.4
Ipecacuanha	973.6	E858.4	E943.6	E950.4	E962.0	E980.4
Ipodate	977.8	E858.8	E947.8	E950.4	E962.0	E980.4
Ipral	967.0	E851	E937.0	E950.1	E962.0	E980.1
Ipratropium	975.1	E858.6	E945.1	E950.4	E962.0	E980.4
Iproniazid	969.0	E854.0	E939.0	E950.3	E962.0	E980.3
Iron (compounds) (medicinal) (preparations)	964.0	E858.2	E934.0	E950.4	E962.0	E980.4
dextran	964.0	E858.2	E934.0	E950.4	E962.0	E980.4
nonmedicinal (dust) (fumes) NEC	985.8	E866.4	—	E950.9	E962.1	E980.9
Irritant drug	977.9	E858.9	E947.9	E950.5	E962.0	E980.5
Ismelin	972.6	E858.3	E942.6	E950.4	E962.0	E980.4
Isoamyl nitrite	972.4	E858.3	E942.4	E950.4	E962.0	E980.4
Isobutyl acetate	982.8	E862.4	—	E950.9	E962.1	E980.9

Substance	External Cause (E-Code)					
	Poisoning	Accident	Therapeutic Use	Suicide Attempt	Assault	Undetermined
Isocarboxazid	969.0	E854.0	E939.0	E950.3	E962.0	E980.3
Isoephedrine	971.2	E855.5	E941.2	E950.4	E962.0	E980.4
Isoetharine	971.2	E855.5	E941.2	E950.4	E962.0	E980.4
Isofluorophate	971.0	E855.3	E941.0	E950.4	E962.0	E980.4
Isoniazid (INH)	961.8	E857	E931.8	E950.4	E962.0	E980.4
Isopentaquine	961.4	E857	E931.4	E950.4	E962.0	E980.4
Isophane insulin	962.3	E858.0	E932.3	E950.4	E962.0	E980.4
Isopregnenone	962.2	E858.0	E932.2	E950.4	E962.0	E980.4
Isoprenaline	971.2	E855.5	E941.2	E950.4	E962.0	E980.4
Isopropamide	971.1	E855.4	E941.1	E950.4	E962.0	E980.4
Isopropanol	980.2	E860.3	—	E950.9	E962.1	E980.9
topical (germicide)	976.0	E858.7	E946.0	E950.4	E962.0	E980.4
Isopropyl						
acetate	982.8	E862.4	—	E950.9	E962.1	E980.9
alcohol	980.2	E860.3	—	E950.9	E962.1	E980.9
topical (germicide)	976.0	E858.7	E946.0	E950.4	E962.0	E980.4
ether	982.8	E862.4	—	E950.9	E962.1	E980.9
Isoproterenol	971.2	E855.5	E941.2	E950.4	E962.0	E980.4
Isosorbide dinitrate	972.4	E858.3	E942.4	E950.4	E962.0	E980.4
Isothipendyl	963.0	E858.1	E933.0	E950.4	E962.0	E980.4
Isoxazolyl penicillin	960.0	E856	E930.0	E950.4	E962.0	E980.4
Isoxsuprine hydrochloride	972.5	E858.3	E942.5	E950.4	E962.0	E980.4
I–thyroxine sodium	962.7	E858.0	E932.7	E950.4	E962.0	E980.4
Jaborandi (pilocarpus) (extract)	971.0	E855.3	E941.0	E950.4	E962.0	E980.4
Jalap	973.1	E858.4	E943.1	E950.4	E962.0	E980.4
Jamaica						
dogwood (bark)	965.7	E850.7	E935.7	E950.0	E962.0	E980.0
ginger	989.89	E866.8	—	E950.9	E962.1	E980.9
Jatropha	988.2	E865.4	—	E950.9	E962.1	E980.9
curcas	988.2	E865.3	—	E950.9	E962.1	E980.9
Jectofer	964.0	E858.2	E934.0	E950.4	E962.0	E980.4
Jellyfish (sting)	989.5	E905.6	—	E950.9	E962.1	E980.9
Jequirity (bean)	988.2	E865.3	—	E950.9	E962.1	E980.9
Jimson weed	988.2	E865.4	—	E950.9	E962.1	E980.9
seeds	988.2	E865.3	—	E950.9	E962.1	E980.9
Juniper tar (oil) (ointment)	976.4	E858.7	E946.4	E950.4	E962.0	E980.4
Kallikrein	972.5	E858.3	E942.5	E950.4	E962.0	E980.4
Kanamycin	960.6	E856	E930.6	E950.4	E962.0	E980.4
Kantrex	960.6	E856	E930.6	E950.4	E962.0	E980.4
Kaolin	973.5	E858.4	E943.5	E950.4	E962.0	E980.4
Karaya (gum)	973.3	E858.4	E943.3	E950.4	E962.0	E980.4
Kemithal	968.3	E855.1	E938.3	E950.4	E962.0	E980.4
Kenacort	962.0	E858.0	E932.0	E950.4	E962.0	E980.4
Keratolytics	976.4	E858.7	E946.4	E950.4	E962.0	E980.4
Keratoplastics	976.4	E858.7	E946.4	E950.4	E962.0	E980.4
Kerosene, kerosine (fuel) (solvent) NEC	981	E862.1	—	E950.9	E962.1	E980.9
insecticide	981	E863.4	—	E950.6	E962.1	E980.7
vapor	987.1	E869.8	—	E952.8	E962.2	E982.8
Ketamine	968.3	E855.1	E938.3	E950.4	E962.0	E980.4
Ketobemidone	965.09	E850.2	E935.2	E950.0	E962.0	E980.0
Ketols	982.8	E862.4	—	E950.9	E962.1	E980.9
Ketone oils	982.8	E862.4	—	E950.9	E962.1	E980.9
Ketoprofen	965.61	E850.6	E935.6	E950.0	E962.0	E980.0
Kiln gas or vapor (carbon monoxide)	986	E868.8	—	E952.1	E962.2	E982.1
Konsyl	973.3	E858.4	E943.3	E950.4	E962.0	E980.4
Kosam seed	988.2	E865.3	—	E950.9	E962.1	E980.9
Krait (venom)	989.5	E905.0	—	E950.9	E962.1	E980.9

Substance	Poisoning	Accident	Therapeutic Use	Suicide Attempt	Assault	Undetermined
			External Cause (E-Code)			

Substance	Poisoning	Accident	Therapeutic Use	Suicide Attempt	Assault	Undetermined
Kwell (insecticide)	989.2	E863.0	—	E950.6	E962.1	E980.7
anti–infective (topical)	976.0	E858.7	E946.0	E950.4	E962.0	E980.4
Laburnum (flowers) (seeds)	988.2	E865.3	—	E950.9	E962.1	E980.9
leaves	988.2	E865.4	—	E950.9	E962.1	E980.9
Lacquers	989.89	E861.6	—	E950.9	E962.1	E980.9
Lacrimogenic gas	987.5	E869.3	—	E952.8	E962.2	E982.8
Lactic acid	983.1	E864.1	—	E950.7	E962.1	E980.6
Lactobacillus acidophilus	973.5	E858.4	E943.5	E950.4	E962.0	E980.4
Lactoflavin	963.5	E858.1	E933.5	E950.4	E962.0	E980.4
Lactuca (virosa) (extract)	967.8	E852.8	E937.8	E950.2	E962.0	E980.2
Lactucarium	967.8	E852.8	E937.8	E950.2	E962.0	E980.2
Laevulose	974.5	E858.5	E944.5	E950.4	E962.0	E980.4
Lanatoside(C)	972.1	E858.3	E942.1	E950.4	E962.0	E980.4
Lanolin (lotion)	976.3	E858.7	E946.3	E950.4	E962.0	E980.4
Largactil	969.1	E853.0	E939.1	E950.3	E962.0	E980.3
Larkspur	988.2	E865.3	—	E950.9	E962.1	E980.9
Laroxyl	969.0	E854.0	E939.0	E950.3	E962.0	E980.3
Lasix	974.4	E858.5	E944.4	E950.4	E962.0	E980.4
Latex	989.82	E866.8	—	E950.9	E962.1	E980.9
Lathyrus (seed)	988.2	E865.3	—	E950.9	E962.1	E980.9
Laudanum	965.09	E850.2	E935.2	E950.0	E962.0	E980.0
Laudexium	975.2	E858.6	E945.2	E950.4	E962.0	E980.4
Laurel, black or cherry	988.2	E865.4	—	E950.9	E962.1	E980.9
Laurolinium	976.0	E858.7	E946.0	E950.4	E962.0	E980.4
Lauryl sulfoacetate	976.2	E858.7	E946.2	E950.4	E962.0	E980.4
Laxatives NEC	973.3	E858.4	E943.3	E950.4	E962.0	E980.4
emollient	973.2	E858.4	E943.2	E950.4	E962.0	E980.4
L–dopa	966.4	E855.0	E936.4	E950.4	E962.0	E980.4
L Tryptophan—*see* amino acid						
Lead (dust) (fumes) (vapor) NEC	984.9	E866.0	—	E950.9	E962.1	E980.9
acetate (dust)	984.1	E866.0	—	E950.9	E962.1	E980.9
anti–infectives	961.2	E857	E931.2	E950.4	E962.0	E980.4
antiknock compound (tetraethyl)	984.1	E862.1	—	E950.9	E962.1	E980.9
arsenate, arsenite (dust) (insecticide) (vapor)	985.1	E863.4	—	E950.8	E962.1	E980.8
herbicide	985.1	E863.5	—	E950.8	E962.1	E980.8
carbonate	984.0	E866.0	—	E950.9	E962.1	E980.9
paint	984.0	E861.5	—	E950.9	E962.1	E980.9
chromate	984.0	E866.0	—	E950.9	E962.1	E980.9
paint	984.0	E861.5	—	E950.9	E962.1	E980.9
dioxide	984.0	E866.0	—	E950.9	E962.1	E980.9
inorganic (compound)	984.0	E866.0	—	E950.9	E962.1	E980.9
paint	984.0	E861.5	—	E950.9	E962.1	E980.9
iodine	984.0	E866.0	—	E950.9	E962.1	E980.9
pigment (paint)	984.0	E861.5	—	E950.9	E962.1	E980.9
monoxide (dust)	984.0	E866.0	—	E950.9	E962.1	E980.9
paint	984.0	E861.5	—	E950.9	E962.1	E980.9
organic	984.1	E866.0	—	E950.9	E962.1	E980.9
oxide	984.0	E866.0	—	E950.9	E962.1	E980.9
paint	984.0	E861.5	—	E950.9	E962.1	E980.9
paint	984.0	E861.5	—	E950.9	E962.1	E980.9
salts	984.0	E866.0	—	E950.9	E962.1	E980.9
specified compound NEC	984.8	E866.0	—	E950.9	E962.1	E980.9
tetra–ethyl	984.1	E862.1	—	E950.9	E962.1	E980.9
Lebanese red	969.6	E854.1	E939.6	E950.3	E962.0	E980.3
Lente Iletin (insulin)	962.3	E858.0	E932.3	E950.4	E962.0	E980.4
Leptazol	970.0	E854.3	E940.0	E950.4	E962.0	E980.4

Substance	External Cause (E-Code)				
	Poisoning	Accident	Therapeutic Use	Suicide Attempt	Assault	Undetermined

Substance	Poisoning	Accident	Therapeutic Use	Suicide Attempt	Assault	Undetermined
Leritine	965.09	E850.2	E935.2	E950.0	E962.0	E980.0
Letter	962.7	E858.0	E932.7	E950.4	E962.0	E980.4
Lettuce opium	967.8	E852.8	E937.8	E950.2	E962.0	E980.2
Leucovorin (factor)	964.1	E858.2	E934.1	E950.4	E962.0	E980.4
Leukeran	963.1	E858.1	E933.1	E950.4	E962.0	E980.4
Levalbuterol	975.7	E858.6	E945.7	E950.4	E962.0	E980.4
Levallorphan	970.1	E854.3	E940.1	E950.4	E962.0	E980.4
Levanil	967.8	E852.8	E937.8	E950.2	E962.0	E980.2
Levarterenol	971.2	E855.5	E941.2	E950.4	E962.0	E980.4
Levodopa	966.4	E855.0	E936.4	E950.4	E962.0	E980.4
Levo–dromoran	965.09	E850.2	E935.2	E950.0	E962.0	E980.0
Levoid	962.7	E858.0	E932.7	E950.4	E962.0	E980.4
Levo–iso–methadone	965.02	E850.1	E935.1	E950.0	E962.0	E980.0
Levomepromazine	967.8	E852.8	E937.8	E950.2	E962.0	E980.2
Levoprome	967.8	E852.8	E937.8	E950.2	E962.0	E980.2
Levopropoxyphene	975.4	E858.6	E945.4	E950.4	E962.0	E980.4
Levorphan, levophanol	965.09	E850.2	E935.2	E950.0	E962.0	E980.0
Levothyroxine (sodium)	962.7	E858.0	E932.7	E950.4	E962.0	E980.4
Levsin	971.1	E855.4	E941.1	E950.4	E962.0	E980.4
Levulose	974.5	E858.5	E944.5	E950.4	E962.0	E980.4
Lewisite (gas)	985.1	E866.3	—	E950.8	E962.1	E980.8
Librium	969.4	E853.2	E939.4	E950.3	E962.0	E980.3
Lidex	976.0	E858.7	E946.0	E950.4	E962.0	E980.4
Lidocaine (infiltration) (topical)	968.5	E855.2	E938.5	E950.4	E962.0	E980.4
nerve block (peripheral) (plexus)	968.6	E855.2	E938.6	E950.4	E962.0	E980.4
spinal	968.7	E855.2	E938.7	E950.4	E962.0	E980.4
Lighter fluid	981	E862.1	—	E950.9	E962.1	E980.9
Lignocaine (infiltration) (topical)	968.5	E855.2	E938.5	E950.4	E962.0	E980.4
nerve block (peripheral) (plexus)	968.6	E855.2	E938.6	E950.4	E962.0	E980.4
spinal	968.7	E855.2	E938.7	E950.4	E962.0	E980.4
Ligroin(e) (solvent)	981	E862.0	—	E950.9	E962.1	E980.9
vapor	987.1	E869.8	—	E952.8	E962.2	E982.8
Ligustrum vulgare	988.2	E865.3	—	E950.9	E962.1	E980.9
Lily of the valley	988.2	E865.4	—	E950.9	E962.1	E980.9
Lime (chloride)	983.2	E864.2	—	E950.7	E962.1	E980.6
solution, sulferated	976.4	E858.7	E946.4	E950.4	E962.0	E980.4
Limonene	982.8	E862.4	—	E950.9	E962.1	E980.9
Lincomycin	960.8	E856	E930.8	E950.4	E962.0	E980.4
Lindane (insecticide) (vapor)	989.2	E863.0	—	E950.6	E962.1	E980.7
anti–infective (topical)	976.0	E858.7	E946.0	E950.4	E962.0	E980.4
Liniments NEC	976.9	E858.7	E946.9	E950.4	E962.0	E980.4
Linoleic acid	972.2	E858.3	E942.2	E950.4	E962.0	E980.4
Liothyronine	962.7	E858.0	E932.7	E950.4	E962.0	E980.4
Liotrix	962.7	E858.0	E932.7	E950.4	E962.0	E980.4
Lipancreatin	973.4	E858.4	E943.4	E950.4	E962.0	E980.4
Lipo–Lutin	962.2	E858.0	E932.2	E950.4	E962.0	E980.4
Lipotropic agents	977.1	E858.8	E947.1	E950.4	E962.0	E980.4
Liquefied petroleum gases	987.0	E868.0	—	E951.1	E962.2	E981.1
piped (pure or mixed with air)	987.0	E867	—	E951.0	E962.2	E981.0
Liquid petrolatum	973.2	E858.4	E943.2	E950.4	E962.0	E980.4
substance	989.9	E866.9	—	E950.9	E962.1	E980.9
specified NEC	989.89	E866.8	—	E950.9	E962.1	E980.9
Lirugen	979.4	E858.8	E949.4	E950.4	E962.0	E980.4
Lithane	969.8	E855.8	E939.8	E950.3	E962.0	E980.3
Lithium	985.8	E866.4	—	E950.9	E962.1	E980.9
carbonate	969.8	E855.8	E939.8	E950.3	E962.0	E980.3
Lithonate	969.8	E855.8	E939.8	E950.3	E962.0	E980.3

Substance	Poisoning	External Cause (E-Code)				
		Accident	Therapeutic Use	Suicide Attempt	Assault	Undetermined
Liver (extract) (injection) (preparations) . . .	964.1	E858.2	E934.1	E950.4	E962.0	E980.4
Lizard (bite) (venom)	989.5	E905.0	—	E950.9	E962.1	E980.9
LMD	964.8	E858.2	E934.8	E950.4	E962.0	E980.4
Lobelia	988.2	E865.4	—	E950.9	E962.1	E980.9
Lobeline	970.0	E854.3	E940.0	E950.4	E962.0	E980.4
Locorten	976.0	E858.7	E946.0	E950.4	E962.0	E980.4
Lolium temulentum	988.2	E865.3	—	E950.9	E962.1	E980.9
Lomotil	973.5	E858.4	E943.5	E950.4	E962.0	E980.4
Lomustine	963.1	E858.1	E933.1	E950.4	E962.0	E980.4
Lophophora williamsii	969.6	E854.1	E939.6	E950.3	E962.0	E980.3
Lorazepam	969.4	E853.2	E939.4	E950.3	E962.0	E980.3
Lotions NEC	976.9	E858.7	E946.9	E950.4	E962.0	E980.4
Lotronex	973.8	E858.4	E943.8	E950.4	E962.0	E980.4
Lotusate	967.0	E851	E937.0	E950.1	E962.0	E980.1
Lowila	976.2	E858.7	E946.2	E950.4	E962.0	E980.4
Loxapine	969.3	E853.8	E939.3	E950.3	E962.0	E980.3
Lozenges (throat)	976.6	E858.7	E946.6	E950.4	E962.0	E980.4
LSD (25)	969.6	E854.1	E939.6	E950.3	E962.0	E980.3
Lubricating oil NEC	981	E862.2	—	E950.9	E962.1	E980.9
Lucanthone	961.6	E857	E931.6	E950.4	E962.0	E980.4
Luminal	967.0	E851	E937.0	E950.1	E962.0	E980.1
Lung irritant (gas) NEC	987.9	E869.9	—	E952.9	E962.2	E982.9
Lutocylol	962.2	E858.0	E932.2	E950.4	E962.0	E980.4
Lutromone	962.2	E858.0	E932.2	E950.4	E962.0	E980.4
Lututrin	975.0	E858.6	E945.0	E950.4	E962.0	E980.4
Lye (concentrated)	983.2	E864.2	—	E950.7	E962.1	E980.6
Lygranum (skin test)	977.8	E858.8	E947.8	E950.4	E962.0	E980.4
Lymecycline	960.4	E856	E930.4	E950.4	E962.0	E980.4
Lymphogranuloma venereum antigen	977.8	E858.8	E947.8	E950.4	E962.0	E980.4
Lynestrenol	962.2	E858.0	E932.2	E950.4	E962.0	E980.4
Lyovac Sodium Edecrin	974.4	E858.5	E944.4	E950.4	E962.0	E980.4
Lypressin	962.5	E858.0	E932.5	E950.4	E962.0	E980.4
Lysergic acid (amide) (diethylamide) . . .	969.6	E854.1	E939.6	E950.3	E962.0	E980.3
Lysergide	969.6	E854.1	E939.6	E950.3	E962.0	E980.3
Lysine vasopressin	962.5	E858.0	E932.5	E950.4	E962.0	E980.4
Lysol	983.0	E864.0	—	E950.7	E962.1	E980.6
Lytta (vitatta)	976.8	E858.7	E946.8	E950.4	E962.0	E980.4
Mace	987.5	E869.3	—	E952.8	E962.2	E982.8
Macrolides (antibiotics)	960.3	E856	E930.3	E950.4	E962.0	E980.4
Mafenide	976.0	E858.7	E946.0	E950.4	E962.0	E980.4
Magaldrate	973.0	E858.4	E943.0	E950.4	E962.0	E980.4
Magic mushroom	969.6	E854.1	E939.6	E950.3	E962.0	E980.3
Magnamycin	960.8	E856	E930.8	E950.4	E962.0	E980.4
Magnesia magma	973.0	E858.4	E943.0	E950.4	E962.0	E980.4
Magnesium (compounds) (fumes) NEC	985.8	E866.4	—	E950.9	E962.1	E980.9
antacid	973.0	E858.4	E943.0	E950.4	E962.0	E980.4
carbonate	973.0	E858.4	E943.0	E950.4	E962.0	E980.4
cathartic	973.3	E858.4	E943.3	E950.4	E962.0	E980.4
citrate	973.3	E858.4	E943.3	E950.4	E962.0	E980.4
hydroxide	973.0	E858.4	E943.0	E950.4	E962.0	E980.4
oxide	973.0	E858.4	E943.0	E950.4	E962.0	E980.4
sulfate (oral)	973.3	E858.4	E943.3	E950.4	E962.0	E980.4
intravenous	966.3	E855.0	E936.3	E950.4	E962.0	E980.4
trisilicate	973.0	E858.4	E943.0	E950.4	E962.0	E980.4
Malathion (insecticide)	989.3	E863.1	—	E950.6	E962.1	E980.7
Male fern (oleoresin)	961.6	E857	E931.6	E950.4	E962.0	E980.4
Mandelic acid	961.9	E857	E931.9	E950.4	E962.0	E980.4

Substance	Poisoning	External Cause (E-Code)				
		Accident	Therapeutic Use	Suicide Attempt	Assault	Undetermined
Manganese compounds (fumes) NEC	985.2	E866.4	—	E950.9	E962.1	E980.9
Mannitol (diuretic) (medicinal) NEC	974.4	E858.5	E944.4	E950.4	E962.0	E980.4
hexanitrate	972.4	E858.3	E942.4	E950.4	E962.0	E980.4
mustard	963.1	E858.1	E933.1	E950.4	E962.0	E980.4
Mannomustine	963.1	E858.1	E933.1	E950.4	E962.0	E980.4
MAO inhibitors	969.0	E854.0	E939.0	E950.3	E962.0	E980.3
Mapharsen	961.1	E857	E931.1	E950.4	E962.0	E980.4
Marcaine	968.9	E855.2	E938.9	E950.4	E962.0	E980.4
infiltration (subcutaneous)	968.5	E855.2	E938.5	E950.4	E962.0	E980.4
nerve block (peripheral) (plexus)	968.6	E855.2	E938.6	E950.4	E962.0	E980.4
Marezine	963.0	E858.1	E933.0	E950.4	E962.0	E980.4
Marihuana, marijuana (derivatives)	969.6	E854.1	E939.6	E950.3	E962.0	E980.3
Marine animals or plants (sting)	989.5	E905.6	—	E950.9	E962.1	E980.9
Marplan	969.0	E854.0	E939.0	E950.3	E962.0	E980.3
Marsh gas	987.1	E869.8	—	E952.8	E962.2	E982.8
Marsilid	969.0	E854.0	E939.0	E950.3	E962.0	E980.3
Matulane	963.1	E858.1	E933.1	E950.4	E962.0	E980.4
Mazindol	977.0	E858.8	E947.0	E950.4	E962.0	E980.4
Meadow saffron	988.2	E865.3	—	E950.9	E962.1	E980.9
Measles vaccine	979.4	E858.8	E949.4	E950.4	E962.0	E980.4
Meat, noxious or nonbacterial	988.8	E865.0	—	E950.9	E962.1	E980.9
Mebanazine	969.0	E854.0	E939.0	E950.3	E962.0	E980.3
Mebaral	967.0	E851	E937.0	E950.1	E962.0	E980.1
Mebendazole	961.6	E857	E931.6	E950.4	E962.0	E980.4
Mebeverine	975.1	E858.6	E945.1	E950.4	E962.0	E980.4
Mebhydroline	963.0	E858.1	E933.0	E950.4	E962.0	E980.4
Mebrophenhydramine	963.0	E858.1	E933.0	E950.4	E962.0	E980.4
Mebutamate	969.5	E853.8	E939.5	E950.3	E962.0	E980.3
Mecamylamine (chloride)	972.3	E858.3	E942.3	E950.4	E962.0	E980.4
Mechlorethamine hydrochloride	963.1	E858.1	E933.1	E950.4	E962.0	E980.4
Meclizene (hydrochloride)	963.0	E858.1	E933.0	E950.4	E962.0	E980.4
Meclofenoxate	970.0	E854.3	E940.0	E950.4	E962.0	E980.4
Meclozine (hydrochloride)	963.0	E858.1	E933.0	E950.4	E962.0	E980.4
Medazepam	969.4	E853.2	E939.4	E950.3	E962.0	E980.3
Medicine, medicinal substance	977.9	E858.9	E947.9	E950.5	E962.0	E980.5
specified NEC	977.8	E858.8	E947.8	E950.4	E962.0	E980.4
Medinal	967.0	E851	E937.0	E950.1	E962.0	E980.1
Medomin	967.0	E851	E937.0	E950.1	E962.0	E980.1
Medroxyprogesterone	962.2	E858.0	E932.2	E950.4	E962.0	E980.4
Medrysone	976.5	E858.7	E946.5	E950.4	E962.0	E980.4
Mefenamic acid	965.7	E850.7	E935.7	E950.0	E962.0	E980.0
Megahallucinogen	969.6	E854.1	E939.6	E950.3	E962.0	E980.3
Megestrol	962.2	E858.0	E932.2	E950.4	E962.0	E980.4
Meglumine	977.8	E858.8	E947.8	E950.4	E962.0	E980.4
Meladinin	976.3	E858.7	E946.3	E950.4	E962.0	E980.4
Melanizing agents	976.3	E858.7	E946.3	E950.4	E962.0	E980.4
Melarsoprol	961.1	E857	E931.1	E950.4	E962.0	E980.4
Melia azedarach	988.2	E865.3	—	E950.9	E962.1	E980.9
Mellaril	969.1	E853.0	E939.1	E950.3	E962.0	E980.3
Meloxine	976.3	E858.7	E946.3	E950.4	E962.0	E980.4
Melphalan	963.1	E858.1	E933.1	E950.4	E962.0	E980.4
Menadiol sodium diphosphate	964.3	E858.2	E934.3	E950.4	E962.0	E980.4
Menadione (sodium bisulfate)	964.3	E858.2	E934.3	E950.4	E962.0	E980.4
Menaphthone	964.3	E858.2	E934.3	E950.4	E962.0	E980.4
Meningococcal vaccine	978.8	E858.8	E948.8	E950.4	E962.0	E980.4
Menningovax–C	978.8	E858.8	E948.8	E950.4	E962.0	E980.4
Menotropins	962.4	E858.0	E932.4	E950.4	E962.0	E980.4

| Substance | External Cause (E-Code) | | | | | |
	Poisoning	Accident	Therapeutic Use	Suicide Attempt	Assault	Undetermined
Menthol NEC 976.1		E858.7	E946.1	E950.4	E962.0	E980.4
Mepacrine 961.3		E857	E931.3	E950.4	E962.0	E980.4
Meparfynol 967.8		E852.8	E937.8	E950.2	E962.0	E980.2
Mepazine 969.1		E853.0	E939.1	E950.3	E962.0	E980.3
Mepenzolate 971.1		E855.4	E941.1	E950.4	E962.0	E980.4
Meperidine 965.09		E850.2	E935.2	E950.0	E962.0	E980.0
Mephenamin(e) 966.4		E855.0	E936.4	E950.4	E962.0	E980.4
Mephenesin (carbamate) 968.0		E855.1	E938.0	E950.4	E962.0	E980.4
Mephenoxalone 969.5		E853.8	E939.5	E950.3	E962.0	E980.3
Mephentermine 971.2		E855.5	E941.2	E950.4	E962.0	E980.4
Mephenytoin 966.1		E855.0	E936.1	E950.4	E962.0	E980.4
Mephobarbital 967.0		E851	E937.0	E950.1	E962.0	E980.1
Mepiperphenidol 971.1		E855.4	E941.1	E950.4	E962.0	E980.4
Mepivacaine 968.9		E855.2	E938.9	E950.4	E962.0	E980.4
infiltration (subcutaneous) 968.5		E855.2	E938.5	E950.4	E962.0	E980.4
nerve block (peripheral) (plexus) 968.6		E855.2	E938.6	E950.4	E962.0	E980.4
topical (surface) 968.5		E855.2	E938.5	E950.4	E962.0	E980.4
Meprednisone 962.0		E858.0	E932.0	E950.4	E962.0	E980.4
Meprobam 969.5		E853.8	E939.5	E950.3	E962.0	E980.3
Meprobamate 969.5		E853.8	E939.5	E950.3	E962.0	E980.3
Mepyramine (maleate) 963.0		E858.1	E933.0	E950.4	E962.0	E980.4
Meralluride 974.0		E858.5	E944.0	E950.4	E962.0	E980.4
Merbaphen 974.0		E858.5	E944.0	E950.4	E962.0	E980.4
Merbromin 976.0		E858.7	E946.0	E950.4	E962.0	E980.4
Mercaptomerin 974.0		E858.5	E944.0	E950.4	E962.0	E980.4
Mercaptopurine 963.1		E858.1	E933.1	E950.4	E962.0	E980.4
Mercumatilin 974.0		E858.5	E944.0	E950.4	E962.0	E980.4
Mercuramide 974.0		E858.5	E944.0	E950.4	E962.0	E980.4
Mercuranin 976.0		E858.7	E946.0	E950.4	E962.0	E980.4
Mercurochrome 976.0		E858.7	E946.0	E950.4	E962.0	E980.4
Mercury, mercuric, mercurous (compounds) (cyanide) (fumes) (nonmedicinal)						
(vapor) NEC 985.0		E866.1	—	E950.9	E962.1	E980.9
ammoniated 976.0		E858.7	E946.0	E950.4	E962.0	E980.4
anti–infective 961.2		E857	E931.2	E950.4	E962.0	E980.4
topical 976.0		E858.7	E946.0	E950.4	E962.0	E980.4
chloride (antiseptic) NEC 976.0		E858.7	E946.0	E950.4	E962.0	E980.4
fungicide 985.0		E863.6	—	E950.6	E962.1	E980.7
diuretic compounds 974.0		E858.5	E944.0	E950.4	E962.0	E980.4
fungicide 985.0		E863.6	—	E950.6	E962.1	E980.7
organic (fungicide) 985.0		E863.6	—	E950.6	E962.1	E980.7
Merethoxylline 974.0		E858.5	E944.0	E950.4	E962.0	E980.4
Mersalyl 974.0		E858.5	E944.0	E950.4	E962.0	E980.4
Merthiolate (topical) 976.0		E858.7	E946.0	E950.4	E962.0	E980.4
ophthalmic preparation 976.5		E858.7	E946.5	E950.4	E962.0	E980.4
Meruvax 979.4		E858.8	E949.4	E950.4	E962.0	E980.4
Mescal buttons 969.6		E854.1	E939.6	E950.3	E962.0	E980.3
Mescaline (salts) 969.6		E854.1	E939.6	E950.3	E962.0	E980.3
Mesoridazine besylate 969.1		E853.0	E939.1	E950.3	E962.0	E980.3
Mestanolone 962.1		E858.0	E932.1	E950.4	E962.0	E980.4
Mestranol 962.2		E858.0	E932.2	E950.4	E962.0	E980.4
Metacresylacetate 976.0		E858.7	E946.0	E950.4	E962.0	E980.4
Metaldehyde (snail killer) NEC 989.4		E863.4	—	E950.6	E962.1	E980.7
Metals (heavy) (nonmedicinal) NEC 985.9		E866.4	—	E950.9	E962.1	E980.9
dust, fumes, or vapor NEC 985.9		E866.4	—	E950.9	E962.1	E980.9
light NEC 985.9		E866.4	—	E950.9	E962.1	E980.9
dust, fumes, or vapor NEC 985.9		E866.4	—	E950.9	E962.1	E980.9

Substance	Poisoning	External Cause (E-Code)				
		Accident	Therapeutic Use	Suicide Attempt	Assault	Undetermined
pesticides (dust) (vapor) 985.9	E863.4	—	E950.6	E962.1	E980.7
Metamucil 973.3	E858.4	E943.3	E950.4	E962.0	E980.4
Metaphen 976.0	E858.7	E946.0	E950.4	E962.0	E980.4
Metaproterenol 975.1	E858.6	E945.1	E950.4	E962.0	E980.4
Metaraminol 972.8	E858.3	E942.8	E950.4	E962.0	E980.4
Metaxalone 968.0	E855.1	E938.0	E950.4	E962.0	E980.4
Metformin 962.3	E858.0	E932.3	E950.4	E962.0	E980.4
Methacycline 960.4	E856	E930.4	E950.4	E962.0	E980.4
Methadone 965.02	E850.1	E935.1	E950.0	E962.0	E980.0
Methallenestril 962.2	E858.0	E932.2	E950.4	E962.0	E980.4
Methamphetamine 969.7	E854.2	E939.7	E950.3	E962.0	E980.3
Methandienone 962.1	E858.0	E932.1	E950.4	E962.0	E980.4
Methandriol 962.1	E858.0	E932.1	E950.4	E962.0	E980.4
Methandrostenolone 962.1	E858.0	E932.1	E950.4	E962.0	E980.4
Methane gas 987.1	E869.8	—	E952.8	E962.2	E982.8
Methanol 980.1	E860.2	—	E950.9	E962.1	E980.9
vapor 987.8	E869.8	—	E952.8	E962.2	E982.8
Methantheline 971.1	E855.4	E941.1	E950.4	E962.0	E980.4
Methaphenilene 963.0	E858.1	E933.0	E950.4	E962.0	E980.4
Methapyrilene 963.0	E858.1	E933.0	E950.4	E962.0	E980.4
Methaqualone (compounds) 967.4	E852.3	E937.4	E950.2	E962.0	E980.2
Metharbital, metharbitone 967.0	E851	E937.0	E950.1	E962.0	E980.1
Methazolamide 974.2	E858.5	E944.2	E950.4	E962.0	E980.4
Methdilazine 963.0	E858.1	E933.0	E950.4	E962.0	E980.4
Methedrine 969.7	E854.2	E939.7	E950.3	E962.0	E980.3
Methenamine (mandelate) 961.9	E857	E931.9	E950.4	E962.0	E980.4
Methenolone 962.1	E858.0	E932.1	E950.4	E962.0	E980.4
Methergine 975.0	E858.6	E945.0	E950.4	E962.0	E980.4
Methiacil 962.8	E858.0	E932.8	E950.4	E962.0	E980.4
Methicillin (sodium) 960.0	E856	E930.0	E950.4	E962.0	E980.4
Methimazole 962.8	E858.0	E932.8	E950.4	E962.0	E980.4
Methionine 977.1	E858.8	E947.1	E950.4	E962.0	E980.4
Methisazone 961.7	E857	E931.7	E950.4	E962.0	E980.4
Methitural 967.0	E851	E937.0	E950.1	E962.0	E980.1
Methixene 971.1	E855.4	E941.1	E950.4	E962.0	E980.4
Methobarbital, methobarbitone 967.0	E851	E937.0	E950.1	E962.0	E980.1
Methocarbamol 968.0	E855.1	E938.0	E950.4	E962.0	E980.4
Methohexital, methohexitone (sodium) 968.3	E855.1	E938.3	E950.4	E962.0	E980.4
Methoin 966.1	E855.0	E936.1	E950.4	E962.0	E980.4
Methopholine 965.7	E850.7	E935.7	E950.0	E962.0	E980.0
Methorate 975.4	E858.6	E945.4	E950.4	E962.0	E980.4
Methoserpidine 972.6	E858.3	E942.6	E950.4	E962.0	E980.4
Methotrexate 963.1	E858.1	E933.1	E950.4	E962.0	E980.4
Methotrimeprazine 967.8	E852.8	E937.8	E950.2	E962.0	E980.2
Methoxa–Dome 976.3	E858.7	E946.3	E950.4	E962.0	E980.4
Methoxamine 971.2	E855.5	E941.2	E950.4	E962.0	E980.4
Methoxsalen 976.3	E858.7	E946.3	E950.4	E962.0	E980.4
Methoxybenzyl penicillin 960.0	E856	E930.0	E950.4	E962.0	E980.4
Methoxychlor 989.2	E863.0	—	E950.6	E962.1	E980.7
Methoxyflurane 968.2	E855.1	E938.2	E950.4	E962.0	E980.4
Methoxyphenamine 971.2	E855.5	E941.2	E950.4	E962.0	E980.4
Methoxypromazine 969.1	E853.0	E939.1	E950.3	E962.0	E980.3
Methoxypsoralen 976.3	E858.7	E946.3	E950.4	E962.0	E980.4
Methscopolamine (bromide) 971.1	E855.4	E941.1	E950.4	E962.0	E980.4
Methsuximide 966.2	E855.0	E936.2	E950.4	E962.0	E980.4
Methyclothiazide 974.3	E858.5	E944.3	E950.4	E962.0	E980.4
Methyl					

Substance	Poisoning	External Cause (E-Code)				
		Accident	Therapeutic Use	Suicide Attempt	Assault	Undetermined
acetate	982.8	E862.4	—	E950.9	E962.1	E980.9
acetone	982.8	E862.4	—	E950.9	E962.1	E980.9
alcohol	980.1	E860.2	—	E950.9	E962.1	E980.9
amphetamine	969.7	E854.2	E939.7	E950.3	E962.0	E980.3
androstanolone	962.1	E858.0	E932.1	E950.4	E962.0	E980.4
atropine	971.1	E855.4	E941.1	E950.4	E962.0	E980.4
benzene	982.0	E862.4	—	E950.9	E962.1	E980.9
bromide (gas)	987.8	E869.8	—	E952.8	E962.2	E982.8
fumigant	987.8	E863.8	—	E950.6	E962.2	E980.7
butanol	980.8	E860.8	—	E950.9	E962.1	E980.9
carbinol	980.1	E860.2	—	E950.9	E962.1	E980.9
cellosolve	982.8	E862.4	—	E950.9	E962.1	E980.9
cellulose	973.3	E858.4	E943.3	E950.4	E962.0	E980.4
chloride (gas)	987.8	E869.8	—	E952.8	E962.2	E982.8
cyclohexane	982.8	E862.4	—	E950.9	E962.1	E980.9
cyclohexanone	982.8	E862.4	—	E950.9	E962.1	E980.9
dihydromorphinone	965.09	E850.2	E935.2	E950.0	E962.0	E980.0
ergometrine	975.0	E858.6	E945.0	E950.4	E962.0	E980.4
ergonovine	975.0	E858.6	E945.0	E950.4	E962.0	E980.4
ethyl ketone	982.8	E862.4	—	E950.9	E962.1	E980.9
hydrazine	983.9	E864.3	—	E950.7	E962.1	E980.6
isobutyl ketone	982.8	E862.4	—	E950.9	E962.1	E980.9
morphine NEC	965.09	E850.2	E935.2	E950.0	E962.0	E980.0
parafynol	967.8	E852.8	E937.8	E950.2	E962.0	E980.2
parathion	989.3	E863.1	—	E950.6	E962.1	E980.7
pentynol NEC	967.8	E852.8	E937.8	E950.2	E962.0	E980.2
peridol	969.2	E853.1	E939.2	E950.3	E962.0	E980.3
phenidate	969.7	E854.2	E939.7	E950.3	E962.0	E980.3
prednisolone	962.0	E858.0	E932.0	E950.4	E962.0	E980.4
ENT agent	976.6	E858.7	E946.6	E950.4	E962.0	E980.4
ophthalmic preparation	976.5	E858.7	E946.5	E950.4	E962.0	E980.4
topical NEC	976.0	E858.7	E946.0	E950.4	E962.0	E980.4
propylcarbinol	980.8	E860.8	—	E950.9	E962.1	E980.9
rosaniline NEC	976.0	E858.7	E946.0	E950.4	E962.0	E980.4
salicylate NEC	976.3	E858.7	E946.3	E950.4	E962.0	E980.4
sulfate (fumes)	987.8	E869.8	—	E952.8	E962.2	E982.8
liquid	983.9	E864.3	—	E950.7	E962.1	E980.6
sulfonal	967.8	E852.8	E937.8	E950.2	E962.0	E980.2
testosterone	962.1	E858.0	E932.1	E950.4	E962.0	E980.4
thiouracil	962.8	E858.0	E932.8	E950.4	E962.0	E980.4
Methylated spirit	980.0	E860.1	—	E950.9	E962.1	E980.9
Methyldopa	972.6	E858.3	E942.6	E950.4	E962.0	E980.4
Methylene						
blue	961.9	E857	E931.9	E950.4	E962.0	E980.4
chloride or dichloride (solvent) NEC	982.3	E862.4	—	E950.9	E962.1	E980.9
Methylhexabital	967.0	E851	E937.0	E950.1	E962.0	E980.1
Methylparaben (ophthalmic)	976.5	E858.7	E946.5	E950.4	E962.0	E980.4
Methyprylon	967.5	E852.4	E937.5	E950.2	E962.0	E980.2
Methysergide	971.3	E855.6	E941.3	E950.4	E962.0	E980.4
Metoclopramide	963.0	E858.1	E933.0	E950.4	E962.0	E980.4
Metofoline	965.7	E850.7	E935.7	E950.0	E962.0	E980.0
Metopon	965.09	E850.2	E935.2	E950.0	E962.0	E980.0
Metronidazole	961.5	E857	E931.5	E950.4	E962.0	E980.4
Metycaine	968.9	E855.2	E938.9	E950.4	E962.0	E980.4
infiltration (subcutaneous)	968.5	E855.2	E938.5	E950.4	E962.0	E980.4
nerve block (peripheral) (plexus)	968.6	E855.2	E938.6	E950.4	E962.0	E980.4
topical (surface)	968.5	E855.2	E938.5	E950.4	E962.0	E980.4

Substance	Poisoning		External Cause (E-Code)			
		Accident	Therapeutic Use	Suicide Attempt	Assault	Undetermined
Metyrapone	977.8	E858.8	E947.8	E950.4	E962.0	E980.4
Mevinphos	989.3	E863.1	—	E950.6	E962.1	E980.7
Mezereon (berries)	988.2	E865.3	—	E950.9	E962.1	E980.9
Micatin	976.0	E858.7	E946.0	E950.4	E962.0	E980.4
Miconazole	976.0	E858.7	E946.0	E950.4	E962.0	E980.4
Midol	965.1	E850.3	E935.3	E950.0	E962.0	E980.0
Mifepristone	962.9	E858.0	E932.9	E950.4	E962.0	E980.4
Milk of magnesia	973.0	E858.4	E943.0	E950.4	E962.0	E980.4
Millipede (tropical) (venomous)	989.5	E905.4	—	E950.9	E962.1	E980.9
Miltown	969.5	E853.8	E939.5	E950.3	E962.0	E980.3
Mineral						
oil (medicinal)	973.2	E858.4	E943.2	E950.4	E962.0	E980.4
nonmedicinal	981	E862.1	—	E950.9	E962.1	E980.9
topical	976.3	E858.7	E946.3	E950.4	E962.0	E980.4
salts NEC	974.6	E858.5	E944.6	E950.4	E962.0	E980.4
spirits	981	E862.0	—	E950.9	E962.1	E980.9
Minocycline	960.4	E856	E930.4	E950.4	E962.0	E980.4
Mithramycin (antineoplastic)	960.7	E856	E930.7	E950.4	E962.0	E980.4
Mitobronitol	963.1	E858.1	E933.1	E950.4	E962.0	E980.4
Mitomycin (antineoplastic)	960.7	E856	E930.7	E950.4	E962.0	E980.4
Mitotane	963.1	E858.1	E933.1	E950.4	E962.0	E980.4
Moderil	972.6	E858.3	E942.6	E950.4	E962.0	E980.4
Mogadon—*see* Nitrazepam						
Molindone	969.3	E853.8	E939.3	E950.3	E962.0	E980.3
Monistat	976.0	E858.7	E946.0	E950.4	E962.0	E980.4
Monkshood	988.2	E865.4	—	E950.9	E962.1	E980.9
Monoamine oxidase inhibitors	969.0	E854.0	E939.0	E950.3	E962.0	E980.3
Monochlorobenzene	982.0	E862.4	—	E950.9	E962.1	E980.9
Monosodium glutamate	989.89	E866.8	—	E950.9	E962.1	E980.9
Monoxide, carbon — *see* Carbon, monoxide						
Moperone	969.2	E853.1	E939.2	E950.3	E962.0	E980.3
Morning glory seeds	969.6	E854.1	E939.6	E950.3	E962.0	E980.3
Moroxydine (hydrochloride)	961.7	E857	E931.7	E950.4	E962.0	E980.4
Morphazinamide	961.8	E857	E931.8	E950.4	E962.0	E980.4
Morphinans	965.09	E850.2	E935.2	E950.0	E962.0	E980.0
Morphine NEC	965.09	E850.2	E935.2	E950.0	E962.0	E980.0
antagonists	970.1	E854.3	E940.1	E950.4	E962.0	E980.4
Morpholinylethylmorphine	965.09	E850.2	E935.2	E950.0	E962.0	E980.0
Morrhuate sodium	972.7	E858.3	E942.7	E950.4	E962.0	E980.4
Moth balls *(see also* Pesticides)	989.4	E863.4	—	E950.6	E962.1	E980.7
naphthalene	983.0	E863.4	—	E950.7	E962.1	E980.6
Motor exhaust gas — *see* Carbon, monoxide, exhaust gas						
Mouth wash	976.6	E858.7	E946.6	E950.4	E962.0	E980.4
Mucolytic agent	975.5	E858.6	E945.5	E950.4	E962.0	E980.4
Mucomyst	975.5	E858.6	E945.5	E950.4	E962.0	E980.4
Mucous membrane agents (external)	976.9	E858.7	E946.9	E950.4	E962.0	E980.4
specified NEC	976.8	E858.7	E946.8	E950.4	E962.0	E980.4
Mumps						
immune globulin (human)	964.6	E858.2	E934.6	E950.4	E962.0	E980.4
skin test antigen	977.8	E858.8	E947.8	E950.4	E962.0	E980.4
vaccine	979.6	E858.8	E949.6	E950.4	E962.0	E980.4
Mumpsvax	979.6	E858.8	E949.6	E950.4	E962.0	E980.4
Muriatic acid — *see* Hydrochloric acid						
Muscarine	971.0	E855.3	E941.0	E950.4	E962.0	E980.4
Muscle affecting agents NEC	975.3	E858.6	E945.3	E950.4	E962.0	E980.4
oxytocic	975.0	E858.6	E945.0	E950.4	E962.0	E980.4

Substance		Poisoning	Accident	Therapeutic Use	Suicide Attempt	Assault	Undetermined
				External Cause (E-Code)			
relaxants	975.3	E858.6	E945.3	E950.4	E962.0	E980.4
central nervous system	968.0	E855.1	E938.0	E950.4	E962.0	E980.4
skeletal	975.2	E858.6	E945.2	E950.4	E962.0	E980.4
smooth	975.1	E858.6	E945.1	E950.4	E962.0	E980.4
Mushrooms, noxious	988.1	E865.5	—	E950.9	E962.1	E980.9
Mussel, noxious	988.0	E865.1	—	E950.9	E962.1	E980.9
Mustard (emetic)	973.6	E858.4	E943.6	E950.4	E962.0	E980.4
gas	987.8	E869.8	—	E952.8	E962.2	E982.8
nitrogen	963.1	E858.1	E933.1	E950.4	E962.0	E980.4
Mustine	963.1	E858.1	E933.1	E950.4	E962.0	E980.4
M–vac	979.4	E858.8	E949.4	E950.4	E962.0	E980.4
Mycifradin	960.8	E856	E930.8	E950.4	E962.0	E980.4
topical	976.0	E858.7	E946.0	E950.4	E962.0	E980.4
Mycitracin	960.8	E856	E930.8	E950.4	E962.0	E980.4
ophthalmic preparation	976.5	E858.7	E946.5	E950.4	E962.0	E980.4
Mycostatin	960.1	E856	E930.1	E950.4	E962.0	E980.4
topical	976.0	E858.7	E946.0	E950.4	E962.0	E980.4
Mydriacyl	971.1	E855.4	E941.1	E950.4	E962.0	E980.4
Myelobromal	963.1	E858.1	E933.1	E950.4	E962.0	E980.4
Myleran	963.1	E858.1	E933.1	E950.4	E962.0	E980.4
Myochrysin(e)	965.69	E850.6	E935.6	E950.0	E962.0	E980.0
Myoneural blocking agents	975.2	E858.6	E945.2	E950.4	E962.0	E980.4
Myristica fragrans	988.2	E865.3	—	E950.9	E962.1	E980.9
Myristicin	988.2	E865.3	—	E950.9	E962.1	E980.9
Mysoline	966.3	E855.0	E936.3	E950.4	E962.0	E980.4
Nafcillin (sodium)	960.0	E856	E930.0	E950.4	E962.0	E980.4
Nail polish remover	982.8	E862.4	—	E950.9	E962.1	E980.9
Nalidixic acid	961.9	E857	E931.9	E950.4	E962.0	E980.4
Nalorphine	970.1	E854.3	E940.1	E950.4	E962.0	E980.4
Naloxone	970.1	E854.3	E940.1	E950.4	E962.0	E980.4
Nandrolone (decanoate) (phenproprioate)	962.1	E858.0	E932.1	E950.4	E962.0	E980.4
Naphazoline	971.2	E855.5	E941.2	E950.4	E962.0	E980.4
Naphtha (painter's) (petroleum)	981	E862.0	—	E950.9	E962.1	E980.9
solvent	981	E862.0	—	E950.9	E962.1	E980.9
vapor	987.1	E869.8	—	E952.8	E962.2	E982.8
Naphthalene (chlorinated)	983.0	E864.0	—	E950.7	E962.1	E980.6
insecticide or moth repellent	983.0	E863.4	—	E950.7	E962.1	E980.6
vapor	987.8	E869.8	—	E952.8	E962.2	E982.8
Naphthol	983.0	E864.0	—	E950.7	E962.1	E980.6
Naphthylamine	983.0	E864.0	—	E950.7	E962.1	E980.6
Naprosyn—see Naproxen						
Naproxen	965.61	E850.6	E935.6	E950.0	E962.0	E980.0
Narcotic (drug)	967.9	E852.9	E937.9	E950.2	E962.0	E980.2
analgesic NEC	965.8	E850.8	E935.8	E950.0	E962.0	E980.0
antagonist	970.1	E854.3	E940.1	E950.4	E962.0	E980.4
specified NEC	967.8	E852.8	E937.8	E950.2	E962.0	E980.2
Narcotine	975.4	E858.6	E945.4	E950.4	E962.0	E980.4
Nardil	969.0	E854.0	E939.0	E950.3	E962.0	E980.3
Natrium cyanide — see Cyanide(s)						
Natural						
blood (product)	964.7	E858.2	E934.7	E950.4	E962.0	E980.4
gas (piped)	987.1	E867	—	E951.0	E962.2	E981.0
incomplete combustion	986	E867	—	E951.0	E962.2	E981.0
Nealbarbital, nealbarbitone	967.0	E851	E937.0	E950.1	E962.0	E980.1
Nectadon	975.4	E858.6	E945.4	E950.4	E962.0	E980.4
Nematocyst (sting)	989.5	E905.6	—	E950.9	E962.1	E980.9
Nembutal	967.0	E851	E937.0	E950.1	E962.0	E980.1

Substance	Poisoning	External Cause (E-Code)				
		Accident	Therapeutic Use	Suicide Attempt	Assault	Undetermined
Neoarsphenamine	961.1	E857	E931.1	E950.4	E962.0	E980.4
Neocinchophen	974.7	E858.5	E944.7	E950.4	E962.0	E980.4
Neomycin	960.8	E856	E930.8	E950.4	E962.0	E980.4
ENT agent	976.6	E858.7	E946.6	E950.4	E962.0	E980.4
ophthalmic preparation	976.5	E858.7	E946.5	E950.4	E962.0	E980.4
topical NEC	976.0	E858.7	E946.0	E950.4	E962.0	E980.4
Neonal	967.0	E851	E937.0	E950.1	E962.0	E980.1
Neoprontosil	961.0	E857	E931.0	E950.4	E962.0	E980.4
Neosalvarsan	961.1	E857	E931.1	E950.4	E962.0	E980.4
Neosilversalvarsan	961.1	E857	E931.1	E950.4	E962.0	E980.4
Neosporin	960.8	E856	E930.8	E950.4	E962.0	E980.4
ENT agent	976.6	E858.7	E946.6	E950.4	E962.0	E980.4
ophthalmic preparation	976.5	E858.7	E946.5	E950.4	E962.0	E980.4
topical NEC	976.0	E858.7	E946.0	E950.4	E962.0	E980.4
Neostigmine	971.0	E855.3	E941.0	E950.4	E962.0	E980.4
Neraval	967.0	E851	E937.0	E950.1	E962.0	E980.1
Neravan	967.0	E851	E937.0	E950.1	E962.0	E980.1
Nerium oleander	988.2	E865.4	—	E950.9	E962.1	E980.9
Nerve gases (war)	987.9	E869.9	—	E952.9	E962.2	E982.9
Nesacaine	968.9	E855.2	E938.9	E950.4	E962.0	E980.4
infiltration (subcutaneous)	968.5	E855.2	E938.5	E950.4	E962.0	E980.4
nerve block (peripheral) (plexus)	968.6	E855.2	E938.6	E950.4	E962.0	E980.4
Neurobarb	967.0	E851	E937.0	E950.1	E962.0	E980.1
Neuroleptics NEC	969.3	E853.8	E939.3	E950.3	E962.0	E980.3
Neuroprotective agent	977.8	E858.8	E947.8	E950.4	E962.0	E980.4
Neutral spirits	980.0	E860.1	—	E950.9	E962.1	E980.9
beverage	980.0	E860.0	—	E950.9	E962.1	E980.9
Niacin, niacinamide	972.2	E858.3	E942.2	E950.4	E962.0	E980.4
Nialamide	969.0	E854.0	E939.0	E950.3	E962.0	E980.3
Nickle (carbonyl) (compounds) (fumes) (tetracarbonyl) (vapor)	985.8	E866.4	—	E950.9	E962.1	E980.9
Niclosamide	961.6	E857	E931.6	E950.4	E962.0	E980.4
Nicomorphine	965.09	E850.2	E935.2	E950.0	E962.0	E980.0
Nicotinamide	972.2	E858.3	E942.2	E950.4	E962.0	E980.4
Nicotine (insecticide) (spray) (sulfate) NEC	989.4	E863.4	—	E950.6	E962.1	E980.7
not insecticide	989.89	E866.8	—	E950.9	E962.1	E980.9
Nicotinic acid (derivatives)	972.2	E858.3	E942.2	E950.4	E962.0	E980.4
Nicotinyl alcohol	972.2	E858.3	E942.2	E950.4	E962.0	E980.4
Nicoumalone	964.2	E858.2	E934.2	E950.4	E962.0	E980.4
Nifenazone	965.5	E850.5	E935.5	E950.0	E962.0	E980.0
Nifuraldezone	961.9	E857	E931.9	E950.4	E962.0	E980.4
Nightshade (deadly)	988.2	E865.4	—	E950.9	E962.1	E980.9
Nikethamide	970.0	E854.3	E940.0	E950.4	E962.0	E980.4
Nilstat	960.1	E856	E930.1	E950.4	E962.0	E980.4
topical	976.0	E858.7	E946.0	E950.4	E962.0	E980.4
Nimodipine	977.8	E858.8	E947.8	E950.4	E962.0	E980.4
Niridazole	961.6	E857	E931.6	E950.4	E962.0	E980.4
Nisentil	965.09	E850.2	E935.2	E950.0	E962.0	E980.0
Nitrates	972.4	E858.3	E942.4	E950.4	E962.0	E980.4
Nitrazepam	969.4	E853.2	E939.4	E950.3	E962.0	E980.3
Nitric						
acid (liquid)	983.1	E864.1	—	E950.7	E962.1	E980.6
vapor	987.8	E869.8	—	E952.8	E962.2	E982.8
oxide (gas)	987.2	E869.0	—	E952.8	E962.2	E982.8
Nitrite, amyl (medicinal) (vapor)	972.4	E858.3	E942.4	E950.4	E962.0	E980.4
Nitroaniline	983.0	E864.0	—	E950.7	E962.1	E980.6
vapor	987.8	E869.8	—	E952.8	E962.2	E982.8

Substance	Poisoning	External Cause (E-Code)				
		Accident	Therapeutic Use	Suicide Attempt	Assault	Undetermined
Nitrobenzene, nitrobenzol	983.0	E864.0	—	E950.7	E962.1	E980.6
vapor	987.8	E869.8	—	E952.8	E962.2	E982.8
Nitrocellulose	976.3	E858.7	E946.3	E950.4	E962.0	E980.4
Nitrofuran derivatives	961.9	E857	E931.9	E950.4	E962.0	E980.4
Nitrofurantoin	961.9	E857	E931.9	E950.4	E962.0	E980.4
Nitrofurazone	976.0	E858.7	E946.0	E950.4	E962.0	E980.4
Nitrogen (dioxide) (gas) (oxide)	987.2	E869.0	—	E952.8	E962.2	E982.8
mustard (antineoplastic)	963.1	E858.1	E933.1	E950.4	E962.0	E980.4
Nitroglycerin, nitroglycerol (medicinal)	972.4	E858.3	E942.4	E950.4	E962.0	E980.4
nonmedicinal	989.89	E866.8	—	E950.9	E962.1	E980.9
fumes	987.8	E869.8	—	E952.8	E962.2	E982.8
Nitrohydrochloric acid	983.1	E864.1	—	E950.7	E962.1	E980.6
Nitromersol	976.0	E858.7	E946.0	E950.4	E962.0	E980.4
Nitronaphthalene	983.0	E864.0	—	E950.7	E962.2	E980.6
Nitrophenol	983.0	E864.0	—	E950.7	E962.2	E980.6
Nitrothiazol	961.6	E857	E931.6	E950.4	E962.0	E980.4
Nitrotoluene, nitrotoluol	983.0	E864.0	—	E950.7	E962.1	E980.6
vapor	987.8	E869.8	—	E952.8	E962.2	E982.8
Nitrous	968.2	E855.1	E938.2	E950.4	E962.0	E980.4
acid (liquid)	983.1	E864.1	—	E950.7	E962.1	E980.6
fumes	987.2	E869.0	—	E952.8	E962.2	E982.8
oxide (anesthetic) NEC	968.2	E855.1	E938.2	E950.4	E962.0	E980.4
Nitrozone	976.0	E858.7	E946.0	E950.4	E962.0	E980.4
Noctec	967.1	E852.0	E937.1	E950.2	E962.0	E980.2
Noludar	967.5	E852.4	E937.5	E950.2	E962.0	E980.2
Noptil	967.0	E851	E937.0	E950.1	E962.0	E980.1
Noradrenalin	971.2	E855.5	E941.2	E950.4	E962.0	E980.4
Noramidopyrine	965.5	E850.5	E935.5	E950.0	E962.0	E980.0
Norepinephrine	971.2	E855.5	E941.2	E950.4	E962.0	E980.4
Norethandrolone	962.1	E858.0	E932.1	E950.4	E962.0	E980.4
Norethindrone	962.2	E858.0	E932.2	E950.4	E962.0	E980.4
Norethisterone	962.2	E858.0	E932.2	E950.4	E962.0	E980.4
Norethynodrel	962.2	E858.0	E932.2	E950.4	E962.0	E980.4
Norlestrin	962.2	E858.0	E932.2	E950.4	E962.0	E980.4
Norlutin	962.2	E858.0	E932.2	E950.4	E962.0	E980.4
Normison—see Benzodiazepines						
Normorphine	965.09	E850.2	E935.2	E950.0	E962.0	E980.0
Nortriptyline	969.0	E854.0	E939.0	E950.3	E962.0	E980.3
Noscapine	975.4	E858.6	E945.4	E950.4	E962.0	E980.4
Nose preparations	976.6	E858.7	E946.6	E950.4	E962.0	E980.4
Novobiocin	960.8	E856	E930.8	E950.4	E962.0	E980.4
Novocain (infiltration) (topical)	968.5	E855.2	E938.5	E950.4	E962.0	E980.4
nerve block (peripheral) (plexus)	968.6	E855.2	E938.6	E950.4	E962.0	E980.4
spinal	968.7	E855.2	E938.7	E950.4	E962.0	E980.4
Noxythiolin	961.9	E857	E931.9	E950.4	E962.0	E980.4
NPH Iletin (insulin)	962.3	E858.0	E932.3	E950.4	E962.0	E980.4
Numorphan	965.09	E850.2	E935.2	E950.0	E962.0	E980.0
Nunol	967.0	E851	E937.0	E950.1	E962.0	E980.1
Nupercaine (spinal anesthetic)	968.7	E855.2	E938.7	E950.4	E962.0	E980.4
topical (surface)	968.5	E855.2	E938.5	E950.4	E962.0	E980.4
Nutmeg oil (liniment)	976.3	E858.7	E946.3	E950.4	E962.0	E980.4
Nux vomica	989.1	E863.7	—	E950.6	E962.1	E980.7
Nydrazid	961.8	E857	E931.8	E950.4	E962.0	E980.4
Nylidrin	971.2	E855.5	E941.2	E950.4	E962.0	E980.4
Nystatin	960.1	E856	E930.1	E950.4	E962.0	E980.4
topical	976.0	E858.7	E946.0	E950.4	E962.0	E980.4
Nytol	963.0	E858.1	E933.0	E950.4	E962.0	E980.4

Substance	Poisoning	External Cause (E-Code)				
		Accident	Therapeutic Use	Suicide Attempt	Assault	Undetermined
Oblivion	967.8	E852.8	E937.8	E950.2	E962.0	E980.2
Octyl nitrite	972.4	E858.3	E942.4	E950.4	E962.0	E980.4
Oestradiol (cypionate) (dipropionate) (valerate)	962.2	E858.0	E932.2	E950.4	E962.0	E980.4
Oestriol	962.2	E858.0	E932.2	E950.4	E962.0	E980.4
Oestrone	962.2	E858.0	E932.2	E950.4	E962.0	E980.4
Oil (of) NEC	989.89	E866.8	—	E950.9	E962.1	E980.9
bitter almond	989.0	E866.8	—	E950.9	E962.1	E980.9
camphor	976.1	E858.7	E946.1	E950.4	E962.0	E980.4
colors	989.89	E861.6	—	E950.9	E962.1	E980.9
fumes	987.8	E869.8	—	E952.8	E962.2	E982.8
lubricating	981	E862.2	—	E950.9	E962.1	E980.9
specified source, other — *see* substance specified						
vitriol (liquid)	983.1	E864.1	—	E950.7	E962.1	E980.6
fumes	987.8	E869.8	—	E952.8	E962.2	E982.8
wintergreen (bitter) NEC	976.3	E858.7	E946.3	E950.4	E962.0	E980.4
Ointments NEC	976.9	E858.7	E946.9	E950.4	E962.0	E980.4
Oleander	988.2	E865.4	—	E950.9	E962.1	E980.9
Oleandomycin	960.3	E856	E930.3	E950.4	E962.0	E980.4
Oleovitamin A	963.5	E858.1	E933.5	E950.4	E962.0	E980.4
Oleum ricini	973.1	E858.4	E943.1	E950.4	E962.0	E980.4
Olive oil (medicinal) NEC	973.2	E858.4	E943.2	E950.4	E962.0	E980.4
OMPA	989.3	E863.1	—	E950.6	E962.1	E980.7
Oncovin	963.1	E858.1	E933.1	E950.4	E962.0	E980.4
Ophthaine	968.5	E855.2	E938.5	E950.4	E962.0	E980.4
Ophthetic	968.5	E855.2	E938.5	E950.4	E962.0	E980.4
Opiates, opioids, opium NEC	965.00	E850.2	E935.2	E950.0	E962.0	E980.0
antagonists	970.1	E854.3	E940.1	E950.4	E962.0	E980.4
Oracon	962.2	E858.0	E932.2	E950.4	E962.0	E980.4
Oragrafin	977.8	E858.8	E947.8	E950.4	E962.0	E980.4
Oral contraceptives	962.2	E858.0	E932.2	E950.4	E962.0	E980.4
Orciprenaline	975.1	E858.6	E945.1	E950.4	E962.0	E980.4
Organidin	975.5	E858.6	E945.5	E950.4	E962.0	E980.4
Organophosphates	989.3	E863.1	—	E950.6	E962.1	E980.7
Orimune	979.5	E858.8	E949.5	E950.4	E962.0	E980.4
Orinase	962.3	E858.0	E932.3	E950.4	E962.0	E980.4
Orphenadrine	966.4	E855.0	E936.4	E950.4	E962.0	E980.4
Ortal (sodium)	967.0	E851	E937.0	E950.1	E962.0	E980.1
Orthoboric acid	976.0	E858.7	E946.0	E950.4	E962.0	E980.4
ENT agent	976.6	E858.7	E946.6	E950.4	E962.0	E980.4
ophthalmic preparation	976.5	E858.7	E946.5	E950.4	E962.0	E980.4
Orthocaine	968.5	E855.2	E938.5	E950.4	E962.0	E980.4
Ortho–Novum	962.2	E858.0	E932.2	E950.4	E962.0	E980.4
Orthotolidine (reagent)	977.8	E858.8	E947.8	E950.4	E962.0	E980.4
Osmic acid (liquid)	983.1	E864.1	—	E950.7	E962.1	E980.6
fumes	987.8	E869.8	—	E952.8	E962.2	E982.8
Osmotic diuretics	974.4	E858.5	E944.4	E950.4	E962.0	E980.4
Ouabain	972.1	E858.3	E942.1	E950.4	E962.0	E980.4
Ovarian hormones (synthetic substitutes)	962.2	E858.0	E932.2	E950.4	E962.0	E980.4
Ovral	962.2	E858.0	E932.2	E950.4	E962.0	E980.4
Ovulation suppressants	962.2	E858.0	E932.2	E950.4	E962.0	E980.4
Ovulen	962.2	E858.0	E932.2	E950.4	E962.0	E980.4
Oxacillin (sodium)	960.0	E856	E930.0	E950.4	E962.0	E980.4
Oxalic acid	983.1	E864.1	—	E950.7	E962.1	E980.6
Oxanamide	969.5	E853.8	E939.5	E950.3	E962.0	E980.3
Oxandrolone	962.1	E858.0	E932.1	E950.4	E962.0	E980.4

Substance	External Cause (E-Code)					
	Poisoning	Accident	Therapeutic Use	Suicide Attempt	Assault	Undetermined
Oxaprozin	965.61	E850.6	E935.6	E950.0	E962.0	E980.0
Oxazepam	969.4	E853.2	E939.4	E950.3	E962.0	E980.3
Oxazolidine derivatives	966.0	E855.0	E936.0	E950.4	E962.0	E980.4
Ox bile extract	973.4	E858.4	E943.4	E950.4	E962.0	E980.4
Oxedrine	971.2	E855.5	E941.2	E950.4	E962.0	E980.4
Oxeladin	975.4	E858.6	E945.4	E950.4	E962.0	E980.4
Oxethazaine NEC	968.5	E855.2	E938.5	E950.4	E962.0	E980.4
Oxidizing agents NEC	983.9	E864.3	—	E950.7	E962.1	E980.6
Oxolinic acid	961.3	E857	E931.3	E950.4	E962.0	E980.4
Oxophenarsine	961.1	E857	E931.1	E950.4	E962.0	E980.4
Oxsoralen	976.3	E858.7	E946.3	E950.4	E962.0	E980.4
Oxtriphylline	975.7	E858.6	E945.7	E950.4	E962.0	E980.4
Oxybuprocaine	968.5	E855.2	E938.5	E950.4	E962.0	E980.4
Oxybutynin	975.1	E858.6	E945.1	E950.4	E962.0	E980.4
Oxycodone	965.09	E850.2	E935.2	E950.0	E962.0	E980.0
Oxygen	987.8	E869.8	—	E952.8	E962.2	E982.8
Oxylone	976.0	E858.7	E946.0	E950.4	E962.0	E980.4
ophthalmic preparation	976.5	E858.7	E946.5	E950.4	E962.0	E980.4
Oxymesterone	962.1	E858.0	E932.1	E950.4	E962.0	E980.4
Oxymetazoline	971.2	E855.5	E941.2	E950.4	E962.0	E980.4
Oxymetholone	962.1	E858.0	E932.1	E950.4	E962.0	E980.4
Oxymorphone	965.09	E850.2	E935.2	E950.0	E962.0	E980.0
Oxypertine	969.0	E854.0	E939.0	E950.3	E962.0	E980.3
Oxyphenbutazone	965.5	E850.5	E935.5	E950.0	E962.0	E980.0
Oxyphencyclimine	971.1	E855.4	E941.1	E950.4	E962.0	E980.4
Oxyphenisatin	973.1	E858.4	E943.1	E950.4	E962.0	E980.4
Oxyphenonium	971.1	E855.4	E941.1	E950.4	E962.0	E980.4
Oxyquinoline	961.3	E857	E931.3	E950.4	E962.0	E980.4
Oxytetracycline	960.4	E856	E930.4	E950.4	E962.0	E980.4
Oxytocics	975.0	E858.6	E945.0	E950.4	E962.0	E980.4
Oxytocin	975.0	E858.6	E945.0	E950.4	E962.0	E980.4
Ozone	987.8	E869.8	—	E952.8	E962.2	E982.8
PABA	976.3	E858.7	E946.3	E950.4	E962.0	E980.4
Packed red cells	964.7	E858.2	E934.7	E950.4	E962.0	E980.4
Paint NEC	989.89	E861.6	—	E950.9	E962.1	E980.9
cleaner	982.8	E862.9	—	E950.9	E962.1	E980.9
fumes NEC	987.8	E869.8	—	E952.8	E962.1	E982.8
lead (fumes)	984.0	E861.5	—	E950.9	E962.1	E980.9
solvent NEC	982.8	E862.9	—	E950.9	E962.1	E980.9
stripper	982.8	E862.9	—	E950.9	E962.1	E980.9
Palfium	965.09	E850.2	E935.2	E950.0	E962.0	E980.0
Palivizumab	979.9	E858.8	E949.6	E950.4	E962.0	E980.4
Paludrine	961.4	E857	E931.4	E950.4	E962.0	E980.4
PAM	977.2	E855.8	E947.2	E950.4	E962.0	E980.4
Pamaquine (naphthoate)	961.4	E857	E931.4	E950.4	E962.0	E980.4
Pamprin	965.1	E850.3	E935.3	E950.0	E962.0	E980.0
Panadol	965.4	E850.4	E935.4	E950.0	E962.0	E980.0
Pancreatic dornase (mucolytic)	963.4	E858.1	E933.4	E950.4	E962.0	E980.4
Pancreatin	973.4	E858.4	E943.4	E950.4	E962.0	E980.4
Pancrelipase	973.4	E858.4	E943.4	E950.4	E962.0	E980.4
Pangamic acid	963.5	E858.1	E933.5	E950.4	E962.0	E980.4
Panthenol	963.5	E858.1	E933.5	E950.4	E962.0	E980.4
topical	976.8	E858.7	E946.8	E950.4	E962.0	E980.4
Pantopaque	977.8	E858.8	E947.8	E950.4	E962.0	E980.4
Pantopon	965.00	E850.2	E935.2	E950.0	E962.0	E980.0
Pantothenic acid	963.5	E858.1	E933.5	E950.4	E962.0	E980.4
Panwarfin	964.2	E858.2	E934.2	E950.4	E962.0	E980.4

Substance	Poisoning	External Cause (E-Code)				
		Accident	Therapeutic Use	Suicide Attempt	Assault	Undetermined
Papain	973.4	E858.4	E943.4	E950.4	E962.0	E980.4
Papaverine	972.5	E858.3	E942.5	E950.4	E962.0	E980.4
Para–aminobenzoic acid	976.3	E858.7	E946.3	E950.4	E962.0	E980.4
Para–aminophenol derivatives	965.4	E850.4	E935.4	E950.0	E962.0	E980.0
Para–aminosalicylic acid (derivatives)	961.8	E857	E931.8	E950.4	E962.0	E980.4
Paracetaldehyde (medicinal)	967.2	E852.1	E937.2	E950.2	E962.0	E980.2
Paracetamol	965.4	E850.4	E935.4	E950.0	E962.0	E980.0
Paracodin	965.09	E850.2	E935.2	E950.0	E962.0	E980.0
Paradione	966.0	E855.0	E936.0	E950.4	E962.0	E980.4
Paraffin(s) (wax)	981	E862.3	—	E950.9	E962.1	E980.9
liquid (medicinal)	973.2	E858.4	E943.2	E950.4	E962.0	E980.4
nonmedicinal (oil)	981	E962.1	—	E950.9	E962.1	E980.9
Paraldehyde (medicinal)	967.2	E852.1	E937.2	E950.2	E962.0	E980.2
Paramethadione	966.0	E855.0	E936.0	E950.4	E962.0	E980.4
Paramethasone	962.0	E858.0	E932.0	E950.4	E962.0	E980.4
Paraquat	989.4	E863.5	—	E950.6	E962.1	E980.7
Parasympatholytics	971.1	E855.4	E941.1	E950.4	E962.0	E980.4
Parasympathomimetics	971.0	E855.3	E941.0	E950.4	E962.0	E980.4
Parathion	989.3	E863.1	—	E950.6	E962.1	E980.7
Parathormone	962.6	E858.0	E932.6	E950.4	E962.0	E980.4
Parathyroid (derivatives)	962.6	E858.0	E932.6	E950.4	E962.0	E980.4
Paratyphoid vaccine	978.1	E858.8	E948.1	E950.4	E962.0	E980.4
Paredrine	971.2	E855.5	E941.2	E950.4	E962.0	E980.4
Paregoric	965.00	E850.2	E935.2	E950.0	E962.0	E980.0
Pargyline	972.3	E858.3	E942.3	E950.4	E962.0	E980.4
Paris green	985.1	E866.3	—	E950.8	E962.1	E980.8
insecticide	985.1	E863.4	—	E950.8	E962.1	E980.8
Parnate	969.0	E854.0	E939.0	E950.3	E962.0	E980.3
Paromomycin	960.8	E856	E930.8	E950.4	E962.0	E980.4
Paroxypropione	963.1	E858.1	E933.1	E950.4	E962.0	E980.4
Parzone	965.09	E850.2	E935.2	E950.0	E962.0	E980.0
PAS	961.8	E857	E931.8	E950.4	E962.0	E980.4
PCBs	981	E862.3	—	E950.9	E962.1	E980.9
PCP (pentachlorophenol)	989.4	E863.6	—	E950.6	E962.1	E980.7
herbicide	989.4	E863.5	—	E950.6	E962.1	E980.7
insecticide	989.4	E863.4	—	E950.6	E962.1	E980.7
phencyclidine	968.3	E855.1	E938.3	E950.4	E962.0	E980.4
Peach kernel oil (emulsion)	973.2	E858.4	E943.2	E950.4	E962.0	E980.4
Peanut oil (emulsion) NEC	973.2	E858.4	E943.2	E950.4	E962.0	E980.4
topical	976.3	E858.7	E946.3	E950.4	E962.0	E980.4
Pearly Gates (morning glory seeds)	969.6	E854.1	E939.6	E950.3	E962.0	E980.3
Pecazine	969.1	E853.0	E939.1	E950.3	E962.0	E980.3
Pecilocin	960.1	E856	E930.1	E950.4	E962.0	E980.4
Pectin (with kaolin) NEC	973.5	E858.4	E943.5	E950.4	E962.0	E980.4
Pelletierine tannate	961.6	E857	E931.6	E950.4	E962.0	E980.4
Pemoline	969.7	E854.2	E939.7	E950.3	E962.0	E980.3
Pempidine	972.3	E858.3	E942.3	E950.4	E962.0	E980.4
Penamecillin	960.0	E856	E930.0	E950.4	E962.0	E980.4
Penethamate hydriodide	960.0	E856	E930.0	E950.4	E962.0	E980.4
Penicillamine	963.8	E858.1	E933.8	E950.4	E962.0	E980.4
Penicillin (any type)	960.0	E856	E930.0	E950.4	E962.0	E980.4
Penicillinase	963.4	E858.1	E933.4	E950.4	E962.0	E980.4
Pentachlorophenol (fungicide)	989.4	E863.6	—	E950.6	E962.1	E980.7
herbicide	989.4	E863.5	—	E950.6	E962.1	E980.7
insecticide	989.4	E863.4	—	E950.6	E962.1	E980.7
Pentaerythritol	972.4	E858.3	E942.4	E950.4	E962.0	E980.4
chloral	967.1	E852.0	E937.1	E950.2	E962.0	E980.2

Substance	Poisoning	External Cause (E-Code)				
		Accident	Therapeutic Use	Suicide Attempt	Assault	Undetermined
tetranitrate NEC	972.4	E858.3	E942.4	E950.4	E962.0	E980.4
Pentagastrin	977.8	E858.8	E947.8	E950.4	E962.0	E980.4
Pentalin	982.3	E862.4	—	E950.9	E962.1	E980.9
Pentamethonium (bromide)	972.3	E858.3	E942.3	E950.4	E962.0	E980.4
Pentamidine	961.5	E857	E931.5	E950.4	E962.0	E980.4
Pentanol	980.8	E860.8	—	E950.9	E962.1	E980.9
Pentaquine	961.4	E857	E931.4	E950.4	E962.0	E980.4
Pentazocine	965.8	E850.8	E935.8	E950.0	E962.0	E980.0
Penthienate	971.1	E855.4	E941.1	E950.4	E962.0	E980.4
Pentobarbital, pentobarbitone (sodium)	967.0	E851	E937.0	E950.1	E962.0	E980.1
Pentolinium (tartrate)	972.3	E858.3	E942.3	E950.4	E962.0	E980.4
Pentothal	968.3	E855.1	E938.3	E950.4	E962.0	E980.4
Pentylenetetrazol	970.0	E854.3	E940.0	E950.4	E962.0	E980.4
Pentylsalicylamide	961.8	E857	E931.8	E950.4	E962.0	E980.4
Pepsin	973.4	E858.4	E943.4	E950.4	E962.0	E980.4
Peptavlon	977.8	E858.8	E947.8	E950.4	E962.0	E980.4
Percaine (spinal)	968.7	E855.2	E938.7	E950.4	E962.0	E980.4
topical (surface)	968.5	E855.2	E938.5	E950.4	E962.0	E980.4
Perchloroethylene (vapor)	982.3	E862.4	—	E950.9	E962.1	E980.9
medicinal	961.6	E857	E931.6	E950.4	E962.0	E980.4
Percodan	965.09	E850.2	E935.2	E950.0	E962.0	E980.0
Percogesic	965.09	E850.2	E935.2	E950.0	E962.0	E980.0
Percorten	962.0	E858.0	E932.0	E950.4	E962.0	E980.4
Pergonal	962.4	E858.0	E932.4	E950.4	E962.0	E980.4
Perhexiline	972.4	E858.3	E942.4	E950.4	E962.0	E980.4
Periactin	963.0	E858.1	E933.0	E950.4	E962.0	E980.4
Periclor	967.1	E852.0	E937.1	E950.2	E962.0	E980.2
Pericyazine	969.1	E853.0	E939.1	E950.3	E962.0	E980.3
Peritrate	972.4	E858.3	E942.4	E950.4	E962.0	E980.4
Permanganates NEC	983.9	E864.3	—	E950.7	E962.1	E980.6
potassium (topical)	976.0	E858.7	E946.0	E950.4	E962.0	E980.4
Pernocton	967.0	E851	E937.0	E950.1	E962.0	E980.1
Pernoston	967.0	E851	E937.0	E950.1	E962.0	E980.1
Peronin(e)	965.09	E850.2	E935.2	E950.0	E962.0	E980.0
Perphenazine	969.1	E853.0	E939.1	E950.3	E962.0	E980.3
Pertofrane	969.0	E854	E939.0	E950.3	E962.0	E980.3
Pertussis						
immune serum (human)	964.6	E858.2	E934.6	E950.4	E962.0	E980.4
vaccine (with diphtheria toxoid) (with tetanus toxoid)	978.6	E858.8	E948.6	E950.4	E962.0	E980.4
Peruvian balsam	976.8	E858.7	E946.8	E950.4	E962.0	E980.4
Pesticides (dust) (fumes) (vapor)	989.4	E863.4	—	E950.6	E962.1	E980.7
arsenic	985.1	E863.4	—	E950.8	E962.1	E980.8
chlorinated	989.2	E863.0	—	E950.6	E962.1	E980.7
cyanide	989.0	E863.4	—	E950.6	E962.1	E980.7
kerosene	981	E863.4	—	E950.6	E962.1	E980.7
mixture (of compounds)	989.4	E863.3	—	E950.6	E962.1	E980.7
naphthalene	983.0	E863.4	—	E950.7	E962.1	E980.6
organochlorine (compounds)	989.2	E863.0	—	E950.6	E962.1	E980.7
petroleum (distillate) (products) NEC	981	E863.4	—	E950.6	E962.1	E980.7
specified ingredient NEC	989.4	E863.4	—	E950.6	E962.1	E980.7
strychnine	989.1	E863.4	—	E950.6	E962.1	E980.7
thallium	985.8	E863.7	—	E950.6	E962.1	E980.7
Pethidine (hydrochloride)	965.09	E850.2	E935.2	E950.0	E962.0	E980.0
Petrichloral	967.1	E852.0	E937.1	E950.2	E962.0	E980.2
Petrol	981	E862.1	—	E950.9	E962.1	E980.9

Substance	External Cause (E-Code)					
	Poisoning	Accident	Therapeutic Use	Suicide Attempt	Assault	Undetermined
vapor 987.1	E869.8	—	E952.8	E962.2	E982.8
Petrolatum (jelly) (ointment) 976.3	E858.7	E946.3	E950.4	E962.0	E980.4
hydrophilic 976.3	E858.7	E946.3	E950.4	E962.0	E980.4
liquid 973.2	E858.4	E943.2	E950.4	E962.0	E980.4
topical 976.3	E858.7	E946.3	E950.4	E962.0	E980.4
nonmedicinal 981	E862.1	—	E950.9	E962.1	E980.9
Petroleum (cleaners) (fuels) (products)						
NEC 981	E862.1	—	E950.9	E962.1	E980.9
benzin(e) — *see* Ligroin						
ether — *see* Ligroin						
jelly — *see* Petrolatum						
naphtha — *see* Ligroin						
pesticide 981	E863.4	—	E950.6	E962.1	E980.7
solids 981	E862.3	—	E950.9	E962.1	E980.9
solvents 981	E862.0	—	E950.9	E962.1	E980.9
vapor 987.1	E869.8	—	E952.8	E962.2	E982.8
Peyote 969.6	E854.1	E939.6	E950.3	E962.0	E980.3
Phanodorm, phanodorn 967.0	E851	E937.0	E950.1	E962.0	E980.1
Phanquinone, phanquone 961.5	E857	E931.5	E950.4	E962.0	E980.4
Pharmaceutical excipient or adjunct 977.4	E858.8	E947.4	E950.4	E962.0	E980.4
Phenacemide 966.3	E855.0	E936.3	E950.4	E962.0	E980.4
Phenacetin 965.4	E850.4	E935.4	E950.0	E962.0	E980.0
Phenadoxone 965.09	E850.2	E935.2	E950.0	E962.0	E980.0
Phenaglycodol 969.5	E853.8	E939.5	E950.3	E962.0	E980.3
Phenantoin 966.1	E855.0	E936.1	E950.4	E962.0	E980.4
Phenaphthazine reagent 977.8	E858.8	E947.8	E950.4	E962.0	E980.4
Phenazocine 965.09	E850.2	E935.2	E950.0	E962.0	E980.0
Phenazone 965.5	E850.5	E935.5	E950.0	E962.0	E980.0
Phenazopyridine 976.1	E858.7	E946.1	E950.4	E962.0	E980.4
Phenbenicillin 960.0	E856	E930.0	E950.4	E962.0	E980.4
Phenbutrazate 977.0	E858.8	E947.0	E950.4	E962.0	E980.4
Phencyclidine 968.3	E855.1	E938.3	E950.4	E962.0	E980.4
Phendimetrazine 977.0	E858.8	E947.0	E950.4	E962.0	E980.4
Phenelzine 969.0	E854.0	E939.0	E950.3	E962.0	E980.3
Phenergan 967.8	E852.8	E937.8	E950.2	E962.0	E980.2
Phenethicillin (potassium) 960.0	E856	E930.0	E950.4	E962.0	E980.4
Phenetsal 965.1	E850.3	E935.3	E950.0	E962.0	E980.0
Pheneturide 966.3	E855.0	E936.3	E950.4	E962.0	E980.4
Phenformin 962.3	E858.0	E932.3	E950.4	E962.0	E980.4
Phenglutarimide 971.1	E855.4	E941.1	E950.4	E962.0	E980.4
Phenicarbazide 965.8	E850.8	E935.8	E950.0	E962.0	E980.0
Phenindamine (tartrate) 963.0	E858.1	E933.0	E950.4	E962.0	E980.4
Phenindione 964.2	E858.2	E934.2	E950.4	E962.0	E980.4
Pheniprazine 969.0	E854.0	E939.0	E950.3	E962.0	E980.3
Pheniramine (maleate) 963.0	E858.1	E933.0	E950.4	E962.0	E980.4
Phenmetrazine 977.0	E858.8	E947.0	E950.4	E962.0	E980.4
Phenobal 967.0	E851	E937.0	E950.1	E962.0	E980.1
Phenobarbital 967.0	E851	E937.0	E950.1	E962.0	E980.1
Phenobarbitone 967.0	E851	E937.0	E950.1	E962.0	E980.1
Phenoctide 976.0	E858.7	E946.0	E950.4	E962.0	E980.4
Phenol (derivatives) NEC 983.0	E864.0	—	E950.7	E962.1	E980.6
disinfectant 983.0	E864.0	—	E950.7	E962.1	E980.6
pesticide 989.4	E863.4	—	E950.6	E962.1	E980.7
red 977.8	E858.8	E947.8	E950.4	E962.0	E980.4
Phenolphthalein 973.1	E858.4	E943.1	E950.4	E962.0	E980.4
Phenolsulfonphthalein 977.8	E858.8	E947.8	E950.4	E962.0	E980.4
Phenomorphan 965.09	E850.2	E935.2	E950.0	E962.0	E980.0

Substance	Poisoning	External Cause (E-Code)				
		Accident	Therapeutic Use	Suicide Attempt	Assault	Undetermined
Phenonyl	967.0	E851	E937.0	E950.1	E962.0	E980.1
Phenoperidine	965.09	E850.2	E935.2	E950.0	E962.0	E980.0
Phenoquin	974.7	E858.5	E944.7	E950.4	E962.0	E980.4
Phenothiazines (tranquilizers) NEC	969.1	E853.0	E939.1	E950.3	E962.0	E980.3
insecticide	989.3	E863.4	—	E950.6	E962.1	E980.7
Phenoxybenzamine	971.3	E855.6	E941.3	E950.4	E962.0	E980.4
Phenoxymethyl penicillin	960.0	E856	E930.0	E950.4	E962.0	E980.4
Phenprocoumon	964.2	E858.2	E934.2	E950.4	E962.0	E980.4
Phensuximide	966.2	E855.0	E936.2	E950.4	E962.0	E980.4
Phentermine	977.0	E858.8	E947.0	E950.4	E962.0	E980.4
Phentolamine	971.3	E855.6	E941.3	E950.4	E962.0	E980.4
Phenyl						
butazone	965.5	E850.5	E935.5	E950.0	E962.0	E980.0
enediamine	983.0	E864.0	—	E950.7	E962.1	E980.6
hydrazine	983.0	E864.0	—	E950.7	E962.1	E980.6
antineoplastic	963.1	E858.1	E933.1	E950.4	E962.0	E980.4
mercuric compounds — see Mercury						
salicylate	976.3	E858.7	E946.3	E950.4	E962.0	E980.4
Phenylephrin	971.2	E855.5	E941.2	E950.4	E962.0	E980.4
Phenylethybiguanide	962.3	E858.0	E932.3	E950.4	E962.0	E980.4
Phenylpropanolamine	971.2	E855.5	E941.2	E950.4	E962.0	E980.4
Phenylsulfthion	989.3	E863.1	—	E950.6	E962.1	E980.7
Phenyramidol, phenyramidon	965.7	E850.7	E935.7	E950.0	E962.0	E980.0
Phenytoin	966.1	E855.0	E936.1	E950.4	E962.0	E980.4
pHisoHex	976.2	E858.7	E946.2	E950.4	E962.0	E980.4
Pholcodine	965.09	E850.2	E935.2	E950.0	E962.0	E980.0
Phorate	989.3	E863.1	—	E950.6	E962.1	E980.7
Phosdrin	989.3	E863.1	—	E950.6	E962.1	E980.7
Phosgene (gas)	987.8	E869.8	—	E952.8	E962.2	E982.8
Phosphate (tricresyl)	989.89	E866.8	—	E950.9	E962.1	E980.9
organic	989.3	E863.1	—	E950.6	E962.1	E980.7
solvent	982.8	E862.4	—	E950.9	E926.1	E980.9
Phosphine	987.8	E869.8	—	E952.8	E962.2	E982.8
fumigant	987.8	E863.8	—	E950.6	E962.2	E980.7
Phospholine	971.0	E855.3	E941.0	E950.4	E962.0	E980.4
Phosphoric acid	983.1	E864.1	—	E950.7	E962.1	E980.6
Phosphorus (compounds) NEC	983.9	E864.3	—	E950.7	E962.1	E980.6
rodenticide	983.9	E863.7	—	E950.7	E962.1	E980.6
Phthalimidogluarimide	967.8	E852.8	E937.8	E950.2	E962.0	E980.2
Phthalylsulfathiazole	961.0	E857	E931.0	E950.4	E962.0	E980.4
Phylloquinone	964.3	E858.2	E934.3	E950.4	E962.0	E980.4
Physeptone	965.02	E850.1	E935.1	E950.0	E962.0	E980.0
Physostigma venenosum	988.2	E865.4	—	E950.9	E962.1	E980.9
Physostigmine	971.0	E855.3	E941.0	E950.4	E962.0	E980.4
Phytolacca decandra	988.2	E865.4	—	E950.9	E962.1	E980.9
Phytomenadione	964.3	E858.2	E934.3	E950.4	E962.0	E980.4
Phytonadione	964.3	E858.2	E934.3	E950.4	E962.0	E980.4
Picric (acid)	983.0	E864.0	—	E950.7	E962.1	E980.6
Picrotoxin	970.0	E854.3	E940.0	E950.4	E962.0	E980.4
Pilocarpine	971.0	E855.3	E941.0	E950.4	E962.0	E980.4
Pilocarpus (jaborandi) extract	971.0	E855.3	E941.0	E950.4	E962.0	E980.4
Pimaricin	960.1	E856	E930.1	E950.4	E962.0	E980.4
Piminodine	965.09	E850.2	E935.2	E950.0	E962.0	E980.0
Pine oil, pinesol (disinfectant)	983.9	E861.4	—	E950.7	E962.1	E980.6
Pinkroot	961.6	E857	E931.6	E950.4	E962.0	E980.4
Pipadone	965.09	E850.2	E935.2	E950.0	E962.0	E980.0
Pipamazine	963.0	E858.1	E933.0	E950.4	E962.0	E980.4

Substance	External Cause (E-Code)					
	Poisoning	Accident	Therapeutic Use	Suicide Attempt	Assault	Undetermined
Pipazethate	975.4	E858.6	E945.4	E950.4	E962.0	E980.4
Pipenzolate	971.1	E855.4	E941.1	E950.4	E962.0	E980.4
Piperacetazine	969.1	E853.0	E939.1	E950.3	E962.0	E980.3
Piperazine NEC	961.6	E857	E931.6	E950.4	E962.0	E980.4
estrone sulfate	962.2	E858.0	E932.2	E950.4	E962.0	E980.4
Piper cubeba	988.2	E865.4	—	E950.9	E962.1	E980.9
Piperidione	975.4	E858.6	E945.4	E950.4	E962.0	E980.4
Piperidolate	971.1	E855.4	E941.1	E950.4	E962.0	E980.4
Piperocaine	968.9	E855.2	E938.9	E950.4	E962.0	E980.4
infiltration (subcutaneous)	968.5	E855.2	E938.5	E950.4	E962.0	E980.4
nerve block (peripheral) (plexus)	968.6	E855.2	E938.6	E950.4	E962.0	E980.4
topical (surface)	968.5	E855.2	E938.5	E950.4	E962.0	E980.4
Pipobroman	963.1	E858.1	E933.1	E950.4	E962.0	E980.4
Pipradrol	970.8	E854.3	E940.8	E950.4	E962.0	E980.4
Piscidia (bark) (erythrina)	965.7	E850.7	E935.7	E950.0	E962.0	E980.0
Pitch	983.0	E864.0	—	E950.7	E962.1	E980.6
Pitkin's solution	968.7	E855.2	E938.7	E950.4	E962.0	E980.4
Pitocin	975.0	E858.6	E945.0	E950.4	E962.0	E980.4
Pitressin (tannate)	962.5	E858.0	E932.5	E950.4	E962.0	E980.4
Pituitary extracts (posterior)	962.5	E858.0	E932.5	E950.4	E962.0	E980.4
anterior	962.4	E858.0	E932.4	E950.4	E962.0	E980.4
Pituitrin	962.5	E858.0	E932.5	E950.4	E962.0	E980.4
Placental extract	962.9	E858.0	E932.9	E950.4	E962.0	E980.4
Placidyl	967.8	E852.8	E937.8	E950.2	E962.0	E980.2
Plague vaccine	978.3	E858.8	E948.3	E950.4	E962.0	E980.4
Plant foods or fertilizers NEC	989.89	E866.5	—	E950.9	E962.1	E980.9
mixed with herbicides	989.4	E863.5	—	E950.6	E962.1	E980.7
Plants, noxious, used as food	988.2	E865.9	—	E950.9	E962.1	E980.9
berries and seeds	988.2	E865.3	—	E950.9	E962.1	E980.9
specified type NEC	988.2	E865.4	—	E950.9	E962.1	E980.9
Plasma (blood)	964.7	E858.2	E934.7	E950.4	E962.0	E980.4
expanders	964.8	E858.2	E934.8	E950.4	E962.0	E980.4
Plasmanate	964.7	E858.2	E934.7	E950.4	E962.0	E980.4
Plegicil	969.1	E853.0	E939.1	E950.3	E962.0	E980.3
Podophyllin	976.4	E858.7	E946.4	E950.4	E962.0	E980.4
Podophyllum resin	976.4	E858.7	E946.4	E950.4	E962.0	E980.4
Poison NEC	989.9	E866.9	—	E950.9	E962.1	E980.9
Poisonous berries	988.2	E865.3	—	E950.9	E962.1	E980.9
Pokeweed (any part)	988.2	E865.4	—	E950.9	E962.1	E980.9
Poldine	971.1	E855.4	E941.1	E950.4	E962.0	E980.4
Poliomyelitis vaccine	979.5	E858.8	E949.5	E950.4	E962.0	E980.4
Poliovirus vaccine	979.5	E858.8	E949.5	E950.4	E962.0	E980.4
Polish (car) (floor) (furniture) (metal) (silver)	989.89	E861.2	—	E950.9	E962.1	E980.9
abrasive	989.89	E861.3	—	E950.9	E962.1	E980.9
porcelain	989.89	E861.3	—	E950.9	E962.1	E980.9
Poloxalkol	973.2	E858.4	E943.2	E950.4	E962.0	E980.4
Polyaminostyrene resins	974.5	E858.5	E944.5	E950.4	E962.0	E980.4
Polychlorinated biphenyl—see PCBs						
Polycycline	960.4	E856	E930.4	E950.4	E962.0	E980.4
Polyester resin hardener	982.8	E862.4	—	E950.9	E962.1	E980.9
fumes	987.8	E869.8	—	E952.8	E962.2	E982.8
Polyestradiol (phosphate)	962.2	E858.0	E932.2	E950.4	E962.0	E980.4
Polyethanolamine alkyl sulfate	976.2	E858.7	E946.2	E950.4	E962.0	E980.4
Polyethylene glycol	976.3	E858.7	E946.3	E950.4	E962.0	E980.4
Polyferose	964.0	E858.2	E934.0	E950.4	E962.0	E980.4
Polymyxin B	960.8	E856	E930.8	E950.4	E962.0	E980.4

Substance	Poisoning	External Cause (E-Code)				
		Accident	Therapeutic Use	Suicide Attempt	Assault	Undetermined
ENT agent	976.6	E858.7	E946.6	E950.4	E962.0	E980.4
ophthalmic preparation	976.5	E858.7	E946.5	E950.4	E962.0	E980.4
topical NEC	976.0	E858.7	E946.0	E950.4	E962.0	E980.4
Polynoxylin(e)	976.0	E858.7	E946.0	E950.4	E962.0	E980.4
Polyoxymethyleneurea	976.0	E858.7	E946.0	E950.4	E962.0	E980.4
Polytetrafluoroethylene (inhaled)	987.8	E869.8	—	E952.8	E962.2	E982.8
Polythiazide	974.3	E858.5	E944.3	E950.4	E962.0	E980.4
Polyvinylpyrrolidone	964.8	E858.2	E934.8	E950.4	E962.0	E980.4
Pontocaine (hydrochloride) (infiltration) (topical)	968.5	E855.2	E938.5	E950.4	E962.0	E980.4
nerve block (peripheral) (plexus)	968.6	E855.2	E938.6	E950.4	E962.0	E980.4
spinal	968.7	E855.2	E938.7	E950.4	E962.0	E980.4
Pot	969.6	E854.1	E939.6	E950.3	E962.0	E980.3
Potash (caustic)	983.2	E864.2	—	E950.7	E962.1	E980.6
Potassic saline injection (lactated)	974.5	E858.5	E944.5	E950.4	E962.0	E980.4
Potassium (salts) NEC	974.5	E858.5	E944.5	E950.4	E962.0	E980.4
aminosalicylate	961.8	E857	E931.8	E950.4	E962.0	E980.4
arsenite (solution)	985.1	E866.3	—	E950.8	E962.1	E980.8
bichromate	983.9	E864.3	—	E950.7	E962.1	E980.6
bisulfate	983.9	E864.3	—	E950.7	E962.1	E980.6
bromide (medicinal) NEC	967.3	E852.2	E937.3	E950.2	E962.0	E980.2
carbonate	983.2	E864.2	—	E950.7	E962.1	E980.6
chlorate NEC	983.9	E864.3	—	E950.7	E962.1	E980.6
cyanide — see Cyanide						
hydroxide	983.2	E864.2	—	E950.7	E962.1	E980.6
iodide (expectorant) NEC	975.5	E858.6	E945.5	E950.4	E962.0	E980.4
nitrate	989.89	E866.8	—	E950.9	E962.1	E980.9
oxalate	983.9	E864.3	—	E950.7	E962.1	E980.6
perchlorate NEC	977.8	E858.8	E947.8	E950.4	E962.0	E980.4
antithyroid	962.8	E858.0	E932.8	E950.4	E962.0	E980.4
permanganate	976.0	E858.7	E946.0	E950.4	E962.0	E980.4
nonmedicinal	983.9	E864.3	—	E950.7	E962.1	E980.6
Povidone–iodine (anti–infective) NEC	976.0	E858.7	E946.0	E950.4	E962.0	E980.4
Practolol	972.0	E858.3	E942.0	E950.4	E962.0	E980.4
Pralidoxime (chloride)	977.2	E858.8	E947.2	E950.4	E962.0	E980.4
Pramoxine	968.5	E855.2	E938.5	E950.4	E962.0	E980.4
Prazosin	972.6	E858.3	E942.6	E950.4	E962.0	E980.4
Prednisolone	962.0	E858.0	E932.0	E950.4	E962.0	E980.4
ENT agent	976.6	E858.7	E946.6	E950.4	E962.0	E980.4
ophthalmic preparation	976.5	E858.7	E946.5	E950.4	E962.0	E980.4
topical NEC	976.0	E858.7	E946.0	E950.4	E962.0	E980.4
Prednisone	962.0	E858.0	E932.0	E950.4	E962.0	E980.4
Pregnanediol	962.2	E858.0	E932.2	E950.4	E962.0	E980.4
Pregneninolone	962.2	E858.0	E932.2	E950.4	E962.0	E980.4
Preludin	977.0	E858.8	E947.0	E950.4	E962.0	E980.4
Premarin	962.2	E858.0	E932.2	E950.4	E962.0	E980.4
Prenylamine	972.4	E858.3	E942.4	E950.4	E962.0	E980.4
Preparation H	976.8	E858.7	E946.8	E950.4	E962.0	E980.4
Preservatives	989.89	E866.8	—	E950.9	E962.1	E980.9
Pride of China	988.2	E865.3	—	E950.9	E962.1	E980.9
Prilocaine	968.9	E855.2	E938.9	E950.4	E962.0	E980.4
infiltration (subcutaneous)	968.5	E855.2	E938.5	E950.4	E962.0	E980.4
nerve block (peripheral) (plexus)	968.6	E855.2	E938.6	E950.4	E962.0	E980.4
Primaquine	961.4	E857	E931.4	E950.4	E962.0	E980.4
Primidone	966.3	E855.0	E936.3	E950.4	E962.0	E980.4
Primula (veris)	988.2	E865.4	—	E950.9	E962.1	E980.9
Prinadol	965.09	E850.2	E935.2	E950.0	E962.0	E980.0

Substance	Poisoning	External Cause (E-Code)				
		Accident	Therapeutic Use	Suicide Attempt	Assault	Undetermined
Priscol, Priscoline	971.3	E855.6	E941.3	E950.4	E962.0	E980.4
Privet	988.2	E865.4	—	E950.9	E962.1	E980.9
Privine	971.2	E855.5	E941.2	E950.4	E962.0	E980.4
Pro–Banthine	971.1	E855.4	E941.1	E950.4	E962.0	E980.4
Probarbital	967.0	E851	E937.0	E950.1	E962.0	E980.1
Probenecid	974.7	E858.5	E944.7	E950.4	E962.0	E980.4
Procainamide (hydrochloride)	972.0	E858.3	E942.0	E950.4	E962.0	E980.4
Procaine (hydrochloride) (infiltration)						
(topical)	968.5	E855.2	E938.5	E950.4	E962.0	E980.4
nerve block (peripheral) (plexus)	968.6	E855.2	E938.6	E950.4	E962.0	E980.4
penicillin G	960.0	E856	E930.0	E950.4	E962.0	E980.4
spinal	968.7	E855.2	E938.7	E950.4	E962.0	E980.4
Procalmidol	969.5	E853.8	E939.5	E950.3	E962.0	E980.3
Procarbazine	963.1	E858.1	E933.1	E950.4	E962.0	E980.4
Prochlorperazine	969.1	E853.0	E939.1	E950.3	E962.0	E980.3
Procyclidine	966.4	E855.0	E936.4	E950.4	E962.0	E980.4
Producer gas	986	E868.8	—	E952.1	E962.2	E982.1
Profenamine	966.4	E855.0	E936.4	E950.4	E962.0	E980.4
Profenil	975.1	E858.6	E945.1	E950.4	E962.0	E980.4
Progesterones	962.2	E858.0	E932.2	E950.4	E962.0	E980.4
Progestin	962.2	E858.0	E932.2	E950.4	E962.0	E980.4
Progestogens (with estrogens)	962.2	E858.0	E932.2	E950.4	E962.0	E980.4
Progestone	962.2	E858.0	E932.2	E950.4	E962.0	E980.4
Proguanil	961.4	E857	E931.4	E950.4	E962.0	E980.4
Prolactin	962.4	E858.0	E932.4	E950.4	E962.0	E980.4
Proloid	962.7	E858.0	E932.7	E950.4	E962.0	E980.4
Proluton	962.2	E858.0	E932.2	E950.4	E962.0	E980.4
Promacetin	961.8	E857	E931.8	E950.4	E962.0	E980.4
Promazine	969.1	E853.0	E939.1	E950.3	E962.0	E980.3
Promedol	965.09	E850.2	E935.2	E950.0	E962.0	E980.0
Promethazine	967.8	E852.8	E937.8	E950.2	E962.0	E980.2
Promin	961.8	E857	E931.8	E950.4	E962.0	E980.4
Pronestyl (hydrochloride)	972.0	E858.3	E942.0	E950.4	E962.0	E980.4
Pronetalol, pronethalol	972.0	E858.3	E942.0	E950.4	E962.0	E980.4
Prontosil	961.0	E857	E931.0	E950.4	E962.0	E980.4
Propamidine isethionate	961.5	E857	E931.5	E950.4	E962.0	E980.4
Propanal (medicinal)	967.8	E852.8	E937.8	E950.2	E962.0	E980.2
Propane (gas) (distributed in mobile						
container)	987.0	E868.0	—	E951.1	E962.2	E981.1
distributed through pipes	987.0	E867	—	E951.0	E962.2	E981.0
incomplete combustion of – *see* Carbon						
monoxide, Propane						
Propanidid	968.3	E855.1	E938.3	E950.4	E962.0	E980.4
Propanol	980.3	E860.4	—	E950.9	E962.1	E980.9
Propantheline	971.1	E855.4	E941.1	E950.4	E962.0	E980.4
Proparacaine	968.5	E855.2	E938.5	E950.4	E962.0	E980.4
Propatyl nitrate	972.4	E858.3	E942.4	E950.4	E962.0	E980.4
Propicillin	960.0	E856	E930.0	E950.4	E962.0	E980.4
Propiolactone (vapor)	987.8	E869.8	—	E952.8	E962.2	E982.8
Propiomazine	967.8	E852.8	E937.8	E950.2	E962.0	E980.2
Propionaldehyde (medicinal)	967.8	E852.8	E937.8	E950.2	E962.0	E980.2
Propionate compound	976.0	E858.7	E946.0	E950.4	E962.0	E980.4
Propion gel	976.0	E858.7	E946.0	E950.4	E962.0	E980.4
Propitocaine	968.9	E855.2	E938.9	E950.4	E962.0	E980.4
infiltration (subcutaneous)	968.5	E855.2	E938.5	E950.4	E962.0	E980.4
nerve block (peripheral) (plexus)	968.6	E855.2	E938.6	E950.4	E962.0	E980.4
Propoxur	989.3	E863.2	—	E950.6	E962.1	E980.7

Substance	Poisoning	Accident	Therapeutic Use	Suicide Attempt	Assault	Undetermined
			External Cause (E-Code)			
Propoxycaine 968.9	E855.2	E938.9	E950.4	E962.0	E980.4
infiltration (subcutaneous) 968.5	E855.2	E938.5	E950.4	E962.0	E980.4
nerve block (peripheral) (plexus) 968.6	E855.2	E938.6	E950.4	E962.0	E980.4
topical (surface) 968.5	E855.2	E938.5	E950.4	E962.0	E980.4
Propoxyphene (hydrochloride) 965.8	E850.8	E935.8	E950.0	E962.0	E980.0
Propranolol 972.0	E858.3	E942.0	E950.4	E962.0	E980.4
Propyl					
alcohol 980.3	E860.4	—	E950.9	E962.1	E980.9
carbinol 980.3	E860.4	—	E950.9	E962.1	E980.9
hexadrine 971.2	E855.5	E941.2	E950.4	E962.0	E980.4
iodone 977.8	E858.8	E947.8	E950.4	E962.0	E980.4
thiouracil 962.8	E858.0	E932.8	E950.4	E962.0	E980.4
Propylene 987.1	E869.8	—	E952.8	E962.2	E982.8
Propylparaben (ophthalmic) 976.5	E858.7	E946.5	E950.4	E962.0	E980.4
Proscillaridin 972.1	E858.3	E942.1	E950.4	E962.0	E980.4
Prostaglandins 975.0	E858.6	E945.0	E950.4	E962.0	E980.4
Prostigmin 971.0	E855.3	E941.0	E950.4	E962.0	E980.4
Protamine (sulfate) 964.5	E858.2	E934.5	E950.4	E962.0	E980.4
zinc insulin 962.3	E858.0	E932.3	E950.4	E962.0	E980.4
Protectants (topical) 976.3	E858.7	E946.3	E950.4	E962.0	E980.4
Protein hydrolysate 974.5	E858.5	E944.5	E950.4	E962.0	E980.4
Prothiaden—see Dothiepin hydrochloride					
Prothionamide 961.8	E857	E931.8	E950.4	E962.0	E980.4
Prothipendyl 969.5	E853.8	E939.5	E950.3	E962.0	E980.3
Protokylol 971.2	E855.5	E941.2	E950.4	E962.0	E980.4
Protopam 977.2	E858.8	E947.2	E950.4	E962.0	E980.4
Protoveratrine(s) (A) (B) 972.6	E858.3	E942.6	E950.4	E962.0	E980.4
Protriptyline 969.0	E854.0	E939.0	E950.3	E962.0	E980.3
Provera 962.2	E858.0	E932.2	E950.4	E962.0	E980.4
Provitamin A 963.5	E858.1	E933.5	E950.4	E962.0	E980.4
Proxymetacaine 968.5	E855.2	E938.5	E950.4	E962.0	E980.4
Proxyphylline 975.1	E858.6	E945.1	E950.4	E962.0	E980.4
Prozac—see Fluoxetine hydrochloride					
Prunus					
laurocerasus 988.2	E865.4	—	E950.9	E962.1	E980.9
virginiana 988.2	E865.4	—	E950.9	E962.1	E980.9
Prussic acid 989.0	E866.8	—	E950.9	E962.1	E980.9
vapor 987.7	E869.8	—	E952.8	E962.2	E982.8
Pseudoephedrine 971.2	E855.5	E941.2	E950.4	E962.0	E980.4
Psilocin 969.6	E854.1	E939.6	E950.3	E962.0	E980.3
Psilocybin 969.6	E854.1	E939.6	E950.3	E962.0	E980.3
PSP 977.8	E858.8	E947.8	E950.4	E962.0	E980.4
Psychedelic agents 969.6	E854.1	E939.6	E950.3	E962.0	E980.3
Psychodysleptics 969.6	E854.1	E939.6	E950.3	E962.0	E980.3
Psychostimulants 969.7	E854.2	E939.7	E950.3	E962.0	E980.3
Psychotherapeutic agents 969.9	E855.9	E939.9	E950.3	E962.0	E980.3
antidepressants 969.0	E854.0	E939.0	E950.3	E962.0	E980.3
specified NEC 969.8	E855.8	E939.8	E950.3	E962.0	E980.3
tranquilizers NEC 969.5	E853.9	E939.5	E950.3	E962.0	E980.3
Psychotomimetic agents 969.6	E854.1	E939.6	E950.3	E962.0	E980.3
Psychotropic agents 969.9	E854.8	E939.9	E950.3	E962.0	E980.3
specified NEC 969.8	E854.8	E939.8	E950.3	E962.0	E980.3
Psyllium 973.3	E858.4	E943.3	E950.4	E962.0	E980.4
Pteroylglutamic acid 964.1	E858.2	E934.1	E950.4	E962.0	E980.4
Pteroyltriglutamate 963.1	E858.1	E933.1	E950.4	E962.0	E980.4
PTFE 987.8	E869.8	—	E952.8	E962.2	E982.8
Pulsatilla 988.2	E865.4	—	E950.9	E962.1	E980.9

Substance	Poisoning	External Cause (E-Code)				
		Accident	Therapeutic Use	Suicide Attempt	Assault	Undetermined
Purex (bleach)	983.9	E864.3	—	E950.7	E962.1	E980.6
Purine diuretics	974.1	E858.5	E944.1	E950.4	E962.0	E980.4
Purinethol	963.1	E858.1	E933.1	E950.4	E962.0	E980.4
PVP	964.8	E858.2	E934.8	E950.4	E962.0	E980.4
Pyrabital	965.7	E850.7	E935.7	E950.0	E962.0	E980.0
Pyramidon	965.5	E850.5	E935.5	E950.0	E962.0	E980.0
Pyrantel (pamoate)	961.6	E857	E931.6	E950.4	E962.0	E980.4
Pyrathiazine	963.0	E858.1	E933.0	E950.4	E962.0	E980.4
Pyrazinamide	961.8	E857	E931.8	E950.4	E962.0	E980.4
Pyrazinoic acid (amide)	961.8	E857	E931.8	E950.4	E962.0	E980.4
Pyrazole (derivatives)	965.5	E850.5	E935.5	E950.0	E962.0	E980.0
Pyrazolone (analgesics)	965.5	E850.5	E935.5	E950.0	E962.0	E980.0
Pyrethrins, pyrethrum	989.4	E863.4	—	E950.6	E962.1	E980.7
Pyribenzamine	963.0	E858.1	E933.0	E950.4	E962.0	E980.4
Pyridine (liquid) (vapor)	982.0	E862.4	—	E950.9	E962.1	E980.9
aldoxime chloride	977.2	E858.8	E947.2	E950.4	E962.0	E980.4
Pyridium	976.1	E858.7	E946.1	E950.4	E962.0	E980.4
Pyridostigmine	971.0	E855.3	E941.0	E950.4	E962.0	E980.4
Pyridoxine	963.5	E858.1	E933.5	E950.4	E962.0	E980.4
Pyrilamine	963.0	E858.1	E933.0	E950.4	E962.0	E980.4
Pyrimethamine	961.4	E857	E931.4	E950.4	E962.0	E980.4
Pyrogallic acid	983.0	E864.0	—	E950.7	E962.1	E980.6
Pyroxylin	976.3	E858.7	E946.3	E950.4	E962.0	E980.4
Pyrrobutamine	963.0	E858.1	E933.0	E950.4	E962.0	E980.4
Pyrrocaine	968.5	E855.2	E938.5	E950.4	E962.0	E980.4
Pyrvinium (pamoate)	961.6	E857	E931.6	E950.4	E962.0	E980.4
PZI	962.3	E858.0	E932.3	E950.4	E962.0	E980.4
Quaalude	967.4	E852.3	E937.4	E950.2	E962.0	E980.2
Quaternary ammonium derivatives	971.1	E855.4	E941.1	E950.4	E962.0	E980.4
Quicklime	983.2	E864.2	—	E950.7	E962.1	E980.6
Quinacrine	961.3	E857	E931.3	E950.4	E962.0	E980.4
Quinaglute	972.0	E858.3	E942.0	E950.4	E962.0	E980.4
Quinalbarbitone	967.0	E851	E937.0	E950.1	E962.0	E980.1
Quinestradiol	962.2	E858.0	E932.2	E950.4	E962.0	E980.4
Quinethazone	974.3	E858.5	E944.3	E950.4	E962.0	E980.4
Quinidine (gluconate) (polygalacturonate) (salts) (sulfate)	972.0	E858.3	E942.0	E950.4	E962.0	E980.4
Quinine	961.4	E857	E931.4	E950.4	E962.0	E980.4
Quiniobine	961.3	E857	E931.3	E950.4	E962.0	E980.4
Quinolines	961.3	E857	E931.3	E950.4	E962.0	E980.4
Quotane	968.5	E855.2	E938.5	E950.4	E962.0	E980.4
Rabies						
immune globulin (human)	964.6	E858.2	E934.6	E950.4	E962.0	E980.4
vaccine	979.1	E858.8	E949.1	E950.4	E962.0	E980.4
Racemoramide	965.09	E850.2	E935.2	E950.0	E962.0	E980.0
Racemorphan	965.09	E850.2	E935.2	E950.0	E962.0	E980.0
Radiator alcohol	980.1	E860.2	—	E950.9	E962.1	E980.9
Radio–opaque (drugs) (materials)	977.8	E858.8	E947.8	E950.4	E962.0	E980.4
Ranunculus	988.2	E865.4	—	E950.9	E962.1	E980.9
Rat poison	989.4	E863.7	—	E950.6	E962.1	E980.7
Rattlesnake (venom)	989.5	E905.0	—	E950.9	E962.1	E980.9
Raudixin	972.6	E858.3	E942.6	E950.4	E962.0	E980.4
Rautensin	972.6	E858.3	E942.6	E950.4	E962.0	E980.4
Rautina	972.6	E858.3	E942.6	E950.4	E962.0	E980.4
Rautotal	972.6	E858.3	E942.6	E950.4	E962.0	E980.4
Rauwiloid	972.6	E858.3	E942.6	E950.4	E962.0	E980.4
Rauwoldin	972.6	E858.3	E942.6	E950.4	E962.0	E980.4

Substance	External Cause (E-Code)					
	Poisoning	Accident	Therapeutic Use	Suicide Attempt	Assault	Undetermined
Rauwolfia (alkaloids)	972.6	E858.3	E942.6	E950.4	E962.0	E980.4
Realgar	985.1	E866.3	—	E950.8	E962.1	E980.8
Red cells, packed	964.7	E858.2	E934.7	E950.4	E962.0	E980.4
Reducing agents, industrial NEC	983.9	E864.3	—	E950.7	E962.1	E980.6
Refrigerant gas (freon)	987.4	E869.2	—	E952.8	E962.2	E982.8
not freon	987.9	E869.9	—	E952.9	E962.2	E982.9
Regroton	974.4	E858.5	E944.4	E950.4	E962.0	E980.4
Rela	968.0	E855.1	E938.0	E950.4	E962.0	E980.4
Relaxants, skeletal muscle (autonomic)	975.2	E858.6	E945.2	E950.4	E962.0	E980.4
central nervous system	968.0	E855.1	E938.0	E950.4	E962.0	E980.4
Renese	974.3	E858.5	E944.3	E950.4	E962.0	E980.4
Renografin	977.8	E858.8	E947.8	E950.4	E962.0	E980.4
Replacement solutions	974.5	E858.5	E944.5	E950.4	E962.0	E980.4
Rescinnamine	972.6	E858.3	E942.6	E950.4	E962.0	E980.4
Reserpine	972.6	E858.3	E942.6	E950.4	E962.0	E980.4
Resorcin, resorcinol	976.4	E858.7	E946.4	E950.4	E962.0	E980.4
Respaire	975.5	E858.6	E945.5	E950.4	E962.0	E980.4
Respiratory agents NEC	975.8	E858.6	E945.8	E950.4	E962.0	E980.4
Retinoic acid	976.8	E858.7	E946.8	E950.4	E962.0	E980.4
Retinol	963.5	E858.1	E933.5	E950.4	E962.0	E980.4
Rho (D) immune globulin (human)	964.6	E858.2	E934.6	E950.4	E962.0	E980.4
Rhodine	965.1	E850.3	E935.3	E950.0	E962.0	E980.0
RhoGAM	964.6	E858.2	E934.6	E950.4	E962.0	E980.4
Riboflavin	963.5	E858.1	E933.5	E950.4	E962.0	E980.4
Ricin	989.89	E866.8	—	E950.9	E962.1	E980.9
Ricinus communis	988.2	E865.3	—	E950.9	E962.1	E980.9
Rickettsial vaccine NEC	979.6	E858.8	E949.6	E950.4	E962.0	E980.4
with viral and bacterial vaccine	979.7	E858.8	E949.7	E950.4	E962.0	E980.4
Rifampin	960.6	E856	E930.6	E950.4	E962.0	E980.4
Rimifon	961.8	E857	E931.8	E950.4	E962.0	E980.4
Ringer's injection (lactated)	974.5	E858.5	E944.5	E950.4	E962.0	E980.4
Ristocetin	960.8	E856	E930.8	E950.4	E962.0	E980.4
Ritalin	969.7	E854.2	E939.7	E950.3	E962.0	E980.3
Roach killers — see Pesticides						
Rocky Mountain spotted fever vaccine	979.6	E858.8	E949.6	E950.4	E962.0	E980.4
Rodenticides	989.4	E863.7	—	E950.6	E962.1	E980.7
Rohypnol	969.4	E853.2	E939.4	E950.3	E962.0	E980.3
Rolaids	973.0	E858.4	E943.0	E950.4	E962.0	E980.4
Rolitetracycline	960.4	E856	E930.4	E950.4	E962.0	E980.4
Romilar	975.4	E858.6	E945.4	E950.4	E962.0	E980.4
Rose water ointment	976.3	E858.7	E946.3	E950.4	E962.0	E980.4
Rotenone	989.4	E863.7	—	E950.6	E962.1	E980.7
Rotoxamine	963.0	E858.1	E933.0	E950.4	E962.0	E980.4
Rough–on–rats	989.4	E863.7	—	E950.6	E962.1	E980.7
Rubbing alcohol	980.2	E860.3	—	E950.9	E962.1	E980.9
Rubella virus vaccine	979.4	E858.8	E949.4	E950.4	E962.0	E980.4
Rubelogen	979.4	E858.8	E949.4	E950.4	E962.0	E980.4
Rubeovax	979.4	E858.8	E949.4	E950.4	E962.0	E980.4
Rubidomycin	960.7	E856	E930.7	E950.4	E962.0	E980.4
Rue	988.2	E965.4	—	E950.9	E962.1	E980.9
RU486	962.9	E858.0	E932.9	E950.4	E962.0	E980.4
Ruta	988.2	E865.4	—	E950.9	E962.1	E980.9
Sabadilla (medicinal)	976.0	E858.7	E946.0	E950.4	E962.0	E980.4
pesticide	989.4	E863.4	—	E950.6	E962.1	E980.7
Sabin oral vaccine	979.5	E858.8	E949.5	E950.4	E962.0	E980.4
Saccharated iron oxide	964.0	E858.2	E934.0	E950.4	E962.0	E980.4
Saccharin	974.5	E858.5	E944.5	E950.4	E962.0	E980.4

Substance	Poisoning	Accident	Therapeutic Use	Suicide Attempt	Assault	Undetermined
			External Cause (E-Code)			
Safflower oil	972.2	E858.3	E942.2	E950.4	E962.0	E980.4
Salbutamol sulfate	975.7	E858.6	E945.7	E950.4	E962.0	E980.4
Salicylamide	965.1	E850.3	E935.3	E950.0	E962.0	E980.0
Salicylate(s)	965.1	E850.3	E935.3	E950.0	E962.0	E980.0
methyl	976.3	E858.7	E946.3	E950.4	E962.0	E980.4
theobromine calcium	974.1	E858.5	E944.1	E950.4	E962.0	E980.4
Salicylazosulfapyridine	961.0	E857	E931.0	E950.4	E962.0	E980.4
Salicylhydroxamic acid	976.0	E858.7	E946.0	E950.4	E962.0	E980.4
Salicylic acid (keratolytic) NEC	976.4	E858.7	E946.4	E950.4	E962.0	E980.4
congeners	965.1	E850.3	E935.3	E950.0	E962.0	E980.0
salts	965.1	E850.3	E935.3	E950.0	E962.0	E980.0
Saliniazid	961.8	E857	E931.8	E950.4	E962.0	E980.4
Salol	976.3	E858.7	E946.3	E950.4	E962.0	E980.4
Salt (substitute) NEC	974.5	E858.5	E944.5	E950.4	E962.0	E980.4
Saluretics	974.3	E858.5	E944.3	E950.4	E962.0	E980.4
Saluron	974.3	E858.5	E944.3	E950.4	E962.0	E980.4
Salvarsan 606 (neosilver) (silver)	961.1	E857	E931.1	E950.4	E962.0	E980.4
Sambucus canadensis	988.2	E865.4	—	E950.9	E962.1	E980.9
berry	988.2	E865.3	—	E950.9	E962.1	E980.9
Sandril	972.6	E858.3	E942.6	E950.4	E962.0	E980.4
Sanguinaria canadensis	988.2	E865.4	—	E950.9	E962.1	E980.9
Saniflush (cleaner)	983.9	E861.3	—	E950.7	E962.1	E980.6
Santonin	961.6	E857	E931.6	E950.4	E962.0	E980.4
Santyl	976.8	E858.7	E946.8	E950.4	E962.0	E980.4
Sarkomycin	960.7	E856	E930.7	E950.4	E962.0	E980.4
Saroten	969.0	E854.0	E939.0	E950.3	E962.0	E980.3
Saturnine – see Lead						
Savin (oil)	976.4	E858.7	E946.4	E950.4	E962.0	E980.4
Scammony	973.1	E858.4	E943.1	E950.4	E962.0	E980.4
Scarlet red	976.8	E858.7	E946.8	E950.4	E962.0	E980.4
Scheele's green	985.1	E866.3	—	E950.8	E962.1	E980.8
insecticide	985.1	E863.4	—	E950.8	E962.1	E980.8
Schradan	989.3	E863.1	—	E950.6	E962.1	E980.7
Schweinfurt (h) green	985.1	E866.3	—	E950.8	E962.1	E980.8
insecticide	985.1	E863.4	—	E950.8	E962.1	E980.8
Scilla — see Squill						
Sclerosing agents	972.7	E858.3	E942.7	E950.4	E962.0	E980.4
Scopolamine	971.1	E855.4	E941.1	E950.4	E962.0	E980.4
Scouring powder	989.89	E861.3	—	E950.9	E962.1	E980.9
Sea						
anemone (sting)	989.5	E905.6	—	E950.9	E962.1	E980.9
cucumber (sting)	989.5	E905.6	—	E950.9	E962.1	E980.9
snake (bite) (venom)	989.5	E905.0	—	E950.9	E962.1	E980.9
urchin spine (puncture)	989.5	E905.6	—	E950.9	E962.1	E980.9
Secbutabarbital	967.0	E851	E937.0	E950.1	E962.0	E980.1
Secbutabaritone	967.0	E851	E937.0	E950.1	E962.0	E980.1
Secobarbital	967.0	E851	E937.0	E950.1	E962.0	E980.1
Seconal	967.0	E851	E937.0	E950.1	E962.0	E980.1
Secretin	977.8	E858.8	E947.8	E950.4	E962.0	E980.4
Sedatives, nonbarbiturate	967.9	E852.9	E937.9	E950.2	E962.0	E980.2
specified NEC	967.8	E852.8	E937.8	E950.2	E962.0	E980.2
Sedormid	967.8	E852.8	E937.8	E950.2	E962.0	E980.2
Seed (plant)	988.2	E865.3	—	E950.9	E962.1	E980.9
disinfectant or dressing	989.89	E866.5	—	E950.9	E962.1	E980.9
Selenium (fumes) NEC	985.8	E866.4	—	E950.9	E962.1	E980.9
disulfide or sulfide	976.4	E858.7	E946.4	E950.4	E962.0	E980.4
Selsun	976.4	E858.7	E946.4	E950.4	E962.0	E980.4

Substance	Poisoning	Accident	Therapeutic Use	Suicide Attempt	Assault	Undetermined
			External Cause (E-Code)			

Substance	Poisoning	Accident	Therapeutic Use	Suicide Attempt	Assault	Undetermined
Senna	973.1	E858.4	E943.1	E950.4	E962.0	E980.4
Septisol	976.2	E858.7	E946.2	E950.4	E962.0	E980.4
Serax	969.4	E853.2	E939.4	E950.3	E962.0	E980.3
Serenesil	967.8	E852.8	E937.8	E950.2	E962.0	E980.2
Serenium (hydrochloride)	961.9	E857	E931.9	E950.4	E962.0	E980.4
Serepax—see Oxazepam						
Sernyl	968.3	E855.1	E938.3	E950.4	E962.0	E980.4
Serotonin	977.8	E858.8	E947.8	E950.4	E962.0	E980.4
Serpasil	972.6	E858.3	E942.6	E950.4	E962.0	E980.4
Sewer gas	987.8	E869.8	—	E952.8	E962.2	E982.8
Shampoo	989.6	E861.0	—	E950.9	E962.1	E980.9
Shellfish, nonbacterial or noxious	988.0	E865.1	—	E950.9	E962.1	E980.9
Silicones NEC	989.83	E866.8	E947.8	E950.9	E962.1	E980.9
Silvadene	976.0	E858.7	E946.0	E950.4	E962.0	E980.4
Silver (compound) (medicinal) NEC	976.0	E858.7	E946.0	E950.4	E962.0	E980.4
anti–infectives	976.0	E858.7	E946.0	E950.4	E962.0	E980.4
arsphenamine	961.1	E857	E931.1	E950.4	E962.0	E980.4
nitrate	976.0	E858.7	E946.0	E950.4	E962.0	E980.4
ophthalmic preparation	976.5	E858.7	E946.5	E950.4	E962.0	E980.4
toughened (keratolytic)	976.4	E858.7	E946.4	E950.4	E962.0	E980.4
nonmedicinal (dust)	985.8	E866.4	—	E950.9	E962.1	E980.9
protein (mild) (strong)	976.0	E858.7	E946.0	E950.4	E962.0	E980.4
salvarsan	961.1	E857	E931.1	E950.4	E962.0	E980.4
Simethicone	973.8	E858.4	E943.8	E950.4	E962.0	E980.4
Sinequan	969.0	E854.0	E939.0	E950.3	E962.0	E980.3
Singoserp	972.6	E858.3	E942.6	E950.4	E962.0	E980.4
Sintrom	964.2	E858.2	E934.2	E950.4	E962.0	E980.4
Sitosterols	972.2	E858.3	E942.2	E950.4	E962.0	E980.4
Skeletal muscle relaxants	975.2	E858.6	E945.2	E950.4	E962.0	E980.4
Skin						
agents (external)	976.9	E858.7	E946.9	E950.4	E962.0	E980.4
specified NEC	976.8	E858.7	E946.8	E950.4	E962.0	E980.4
test antigen	977.8	E858.8	E947.8	E950.4	E962.0	E980.4
Sleep–eze	963.0	E858.1	E933.0	E950.4	E962.0	E980.4
Sleeping draught (drug) (pill) (tablet)	967.9	E852.9	E937.9	E950.2	E962.0	E980.2
Smallpox vaccine	979.0	E858.8	E949.0	E950.4	E962.0	E980.4
Smelter fumes NEC	985.9	E866.4	—	E950.9	E962.1	E980.9
Smog	987.3	E869.1	—	E952.8	E962.2	E982.8
Smoke NEC	987.9	E869.9	—	E952.9	E962.2	E982.9
Smooth muscle relaxant	975.1	E858.6	E945.1	E950.4	E962.0	E980.4
Snail killer	989.4	E863.4	—	E950.6	E962.1	E980.7
Snake (bite) (venom)	989.5	E905.0	—	E950.9	E962.1	E980.9
Snuff	989.89	E866.8	—	E950.9	E962.1	E980.9
Soap (powder) (product)	989.6	E861.1	—	E950.9	E962.1	E980.9
medicinal, soft	976.2	E858.7	E946.2	E950.4	E962.0	E980.4
Soda (caustic)	983.2	E864.2	—	E950.7	E962.1	E980.6
bicarb	963.3	E858.1	E933.3	E950.4	E962.0	E980.4
chlorinated — see Sodium, hypochlorite						
Sodium						
acetosulfone	961.8	E857	E931.8	E950.4	E962.0	E980.4
acetrizoate	977.8	E858.8	E947.8	E950.4	E962.0	E980.4
amytal	967.0	E851	E937.0	E950.1	E962.0	E980.1
arsenate — see Arsenic						
bicarbonate	963.3	E858.1	E933.3	E950.4	E962.0	E980.4
bichromate	983.9	E864.3	—	E950.7	E962.1	E980.6
biphosphate	963.2	E858.1	E933.2	E950.4	E962.0	E980.4
bisulfate	983.9	E864.3	—	E950.7	E962.1	E980.6

Substance	Poisoning	External Cause (E-Code)				
		Accident	Therapeutic Use	Suicide Attempt	Assault	Undetermined
borate (cleanser)	989.6	E861.3	—	E950.9	E962.1	E980.9
bromide NEC	967.3	E852.2	E937.3	E950.2	E962.0	E980.2
cacodylate (nonmedicinal) NEC	978.8	E858.8	E948.8	E950.4	E962.0	E980.4
anti–infective	961.1	E857	E931.1	E950.4	E962.0	E980.4
herbicide	989.4	E863.5	—	E950.6	E962.1	E980.7
calcium edetate	963.8	E858.1	E933.8	E950.4	E962.0	E980.4
carbonate NEC	983.2	E864.2	—	E950.7	E962.1	E980.6
chlorate NEC	983.9	E864.3	—	E950.7	E962.1	E980.6
herbicide	983.9	E863.5	—	E950.7	E962.1	E980.6
chloride NEC	974.5	E858.5	E944.5	E950.4	E962.0	E980.4
chromate	983.9	E864.3	—	E950.7	E962.1	E980.6
citrate	963.3	E858.1	E933.3	E950.4	E962.0	E980.4
cyanide — see Cyanide(s)						
cyclamate	974.5	E858.5	E944.5	E950.4	E962.0	E980.4
diatrizoate	977.8	E858.8	E947.8	E950.4	E962.0	E980.4
dibunate	975.4	E858.6	E945.4	E950.4	E962.0	E980.4
dioctyl sulfosuccinate	973.2	E858.4	E943.2	E950.4	E962.0	E980.4
edetate	963.8	E858.1	E933.8	E950.4	E962.0	E980.4
ethacrynate	974.4	E858.5	E944.4	E950.4	E962.0	E980.4
fluoroacetate (dust) (rodenticide)	989.4	E863.7	—	E950.6	E962.1	E980.7
fluoride — see Fluoride(s)						
free salt	974.5	E858.5	E944.5	E950.4	E962.0	E980.4
glucosulfone	961.8	E857	E931.8	E950.4	E962.0	E980.4
hydroxide	983.2	E864.2	—	E950.7	E962.1	E980.6
hypochlorite (bleach) NEC	983.9	E864.3	—	E950.7	E962.1	E980.6
disinfectant	983.9	E861.4	—	E950.7	E962.1	E980.6
medicinal (anti–infective) (external)	976.0	E858.7	E946.0	E950.4	E962.0	E980.4
vapor	987.8	E869.8	—	E952.8	E962.2	E982.8
hyposulfite	976.0	E858.7	E946.0	E950.4	E962.0	E980.4
indigotindisulfonate	977.8	E858.8	E947.8	E950.4	E962.0	E980.4
iodide	977.8	E858.8	E947.8	E950.4	E962.0	E980.4
iothalamate	977.8	E858.8	E947.8	E950.4	E962.0	E980.4
iron edetate	964.0	E858.2	E934.0	E950.4	E962.0	E980.4
lactate	963.3	E858.1	E933.3	E950.4	E962.0	E980.4
lauryl sulfate	976.2	E858.7	E946.2	E950.4	E962.0	E980.4
L–triiodothyronine	962.7	E858.0	E932.7	E950.4	E962.0	E980.4
metrizoate	977.8	E858.8	E947.8	E950.4	E962.0	E980.4
monofluoroacetate (dust) (rodenticide)	989.4	E863.7	—	E950.6	E962.1	E980.7
morrhuate	972.7	E858.3	E942.7	E950.4	E962.0	E980.4
nafcillin	960.0	E856	E930.0	E950.4	E962.0	E980.4
nitrate (oxidizing agent)	983.9	E864.3	—	E950.7	E962.1	E980.6
nitrite (medicinal)	972.4	E858.3	E942.4	E950.4	E962.0	E980.4
nitroferricyanide	972.6	E858.3	E942.6	E950.4	E962.0	E980.4
nitroprusside	972.6	E858.3	E942.6	E950.4	E962.0	E980.4
para–aminohippurate	977.8	E858.8	E947.8	E950.4	E962.0	E980.4
perborate (non-medicinal) NEC	989.89	E866.8	—	E950.9	E962.1	E980.9
medicinal	976.6	E858.7	E946.6	E950.4	E962.0	E980.4
soap	989.6	E861.1	—	E950.9	E962.1	E980.9
percarbonate — see Sodium, perborate						
phosphate	973.3	E858.4	E943.3	E950.4	E962.0	E980.4
polystyrene sulfonate	974.5	E858.5	E944.5	E950.4	E962.0	E980.4
propionate	976.0	E858.7	E946.0	E950.4	E962.0	E980.4
psylliate	972.7	E858.3	E942.7	E950.4	E962.0	E980.4
removing resins	974.5	E858.5	E944.5	E950.4	E962.0	E980.4
salicylate	965.1	E850.3	E935.3	E950.0	E962.0	E980.0
sulfate	973.3	E858.4	E943.3	E950.4	E962.0	E980.4
sulfoxone	961.8	E857	E931.8	E950.4	E962.0	E980.4

Substance	Poisoning	External Cause (E-Code)				
		Accident	Therapeutic Use	Suicide Attempt	Assault	Undetermined
tetradecyl sulfate	972.7	E858.3	E942.7	E950.4	E962.0	E980.4
thiopental	968.3	E855.1	E938.3	E950.4	E962.0	E980.4
thiosalicylate	965.1	E850.3	E935.3	E950.0	E962.0	E980.0
thiosulfate	976.0	E858.7	E946.0	E950.4	E962.0	E980.4
tolbutamide	977.8	E858.8	E947.8	E950.4	E962.0	E980.4
tyropanoate	977.8	E858.8	E947.8	E950.4	E962.0	E980.4
valproate	966.3	E855.0	E936.3	E950.4	E962.0	E980.4
Solanine	977.8	E858.8	E947.8	E950.4	E962.0	E980.4
Solanum dulcamara	988.2	E865.4	—	E950.9	E962.1	E980.9
Solapsone	961.8	E857	E931.8	E950.4	E962.0	E980.4
Solasulfone	961.8	E857	E931.8	E950.4	E962.0	E980.4
Soldering fluid	983.1	E864.1	—	E950.7	E962.1	E980.6
Solid substance	989.9	E866.9	—	E950.9	E962.1	E980.9
specified NEC	989.9	E866.8	—	E950.9	E962.1	E980.9
Solvents, industrial	982.8	E862.9	—	E950.9	E962.1	E980.9
naphtha	981	E862.0	—	E950.9	E962.1	E980.9
petroleum	981	E862.0	—	E950.9	E962.1	E980.9
specified NEC	982.8	E862.4	—	E950.9	E962.1	E980.9
Soma	968.0	E855.1	E938.0	E950.4	E962.0	E980.4
Somatotropin	962.4	E858.0	E932.4	E950.4	E962.0	E980.4
Sominex	963.0	E858.1	E933.0	E950.4	E962.0	E980.4
Somnos	967.1	E852.0	E937.1	E950.2	E962.0	E980.2
Somonal	967.0	E851	E937.0	E950.1	E962.0	E980.1
Soneryl	967.0	E851	E937.0	E950.1	E962.0	E980.1
Soothing syrup	977.9	E858.9	E947.9	E950.5	E962.0	E980.5
Sopor	967.4	E852.3	E937.4	E950.2	E962.0	E980.2
Soporific drug	967.9	E852.9	E937.9	E950.2	E962.0	E980.2
specified type NEC	967.8	E852.8	E937.8	E950.2	E962.0	E980.2
Sorbitol NEC	977.4	E858.8	E947.4	E950.4	E962.0	E980.4
Sotradecol	972.7	E858.3	E942.7	E950.4	E962.0	E980.4
Spacoline	975.1	E858.6	E945.1	E950.4	E962.0	E980.4
Spanish fly	976.8	E858.7	E946.8	E950.4	E962.0	E980.4
Sparine	969.1	E853.0	E939.1	E950.3	E962.0	E980.3
Sparteine	975.0	E858.6	E945.0	E950.4	E962.0	E980.4
Spasmolytics	975.1	E858.6	E945.1	E950.4	E962.0	E980.4
anticholinergics	971.1	E855.4	E941.1	E950.4	E962.0	E980.4
Spectinomycin	960.8	E856	E930.8	E950.4	E962.0	E980.4
Speed	969.7	E854.2	E939.7	E950.3	E962.0	E980.3
Spermicides	976.8	E858.7	E946.8	E950.4	E962.0	E980.4
Spider (bite) (venom)	989.5	E905.1	—	E950.9	E962.1	E980.9
antivenin	979.9	E858.8	E949.9	E950.4	E962.0	E980.4
Spigelia (root)	961.6	E857	E931.6	E950.4	E962.0	E980.4
Spiperone	969.2	E853.1	E939.2	E950.3	E962.0	E980.3
Spiramycin	960.3	E856	E930.3	E950.4	E962.0	E980.4
Spirilene	969.5	E853.8	E939.5	E950.3	E962.0	E980.3
Spirit(s) (neutral) NEC	980.0	E860.1	—	E950.9	E962.1	E980.9
beverage	980.0	E860.0	—	E950.9	E962.1	E980.9
industrial	980.9	E860.9	—	E950.9	E962.1	E980.9
mineral	981	E862.0	—	E950.9	E962.1	E980.9
of salt — *see* Hydrochloric acid						
surgical	980.9	E860.9	—	E950.9	E962.1	E980.9
Spironolactone	974.4	E858.5	E944.4	E950.4	E962.0	E980.4
Sponge, absorbable (gelatin)	964.5	E858.2	E934.5	E950.4	E962.0	E980.4
Sporostacin	976.0	E858.7	E946.0	E950.4	E962.0	E980.4
Sprays (aerosol)	989.89	E866.8	—	E950.9	E962.1	E980.9
cosmetic	989.89	E866.7	—	E950.9	E962.1	E980.9
medicinal NEC	977.9	E858.9	E947.9	E950.5	E962.0	E980.5

Substance	Poisoning	Accident	Therapeutic Use	Suicide Attempt	Assault	Undetermined
pesticides — *see* Pesticides						
specified content — *see* substance						
specified						
Spurge flax	988.2	E865.4	—	E950.9	E962.1	E980.9
Spurges	988.2	E865.4	—	E950.9	E962.1	E980.9
Squill (expectorant) NEC	975.5	E858.6	E945.5	E950.4	E962.0	E980.4
rat poison	989.4	E863.7	—	E950.6	E962.1	E980.7
Squirting cucumber (cathartic)	973.1	E858.4	E943.1	E950.4	E962.0	E980.4
Stains	989.89	E866.8	—	E950.9	E962.1	E980.9
Stannous — *see also* Tin						
fluoride	976.7	E858.7	E946.7	E950.4	E962.0	E980.4
Stanolone	962.1	E858.0	E932.1	E950.4	E962.0	E980.4
Stanozolol	962.1	E853.0	E932.1	E950.4	E962.0	E980.4
Staphisagria or stavesacre (pediculicide)	976.0	E858.7	E946.0	E950.4	E962.0	E980.4
Stelazine	969.1	E853.0	E939.1	E950.3	E962.0	E980.3
Stemetil	969.1	E853.0	E939.1	E950.3	E962.0	E980.3
Sterculia (cathartic) (gum)	973.3	E858.4	E943.3	E950.4	E962.0	E980.4
Sternutator gas	987.8	E869.8	—	E952.8	E962.2	E982.8
Steroids NEC	962.0	E858.0	E932.0	E950.4	E962.0	E980.4
ENT agent	976.6	E858.7	E946.6	E950.4	E962.0	E980.4
ophthalmic preparation	976.5	E858.7	E946.5	E950.4	E962.0	E980.4
topical NEC	976.0	E858.7	E946.0	E950.4	E962.0	E980.4
Stibine	985.8	E866.4	—	E950.9	E962.1	E980.9
Stibophen	961.2	E857	E931.2	E950.4	E962.0	E980.4
Stilbamide, stilbamidine	961.5	E857	E931.5	E950.4	E962.0	E980.4
Stilbestrol	962.2	E858.0	E932.2	E950.4	E962.0	E980.4
Stimulants (central nervous system)	970.9	E854.3	E940.9	E950.4	E962.0	E980.4
analeptics	970.0	E854.3	E940.0	E950.4	E962.0	E980.4
opiate antagonist	970.1	E854.3	E940.1	E950.4	E962.0	E980.4
psychotherapeutic NEC	969.0	E854.0	E939.0	E950.3	E962.0	E980.3
specified NEC	970.8	E854.3	E940.8	E950.4	E962.0	E980.4
Storage batteries (acid) (cells)	983.1	E864.1	—	E950.7	E962.1	E980.6
Stovaine	968.9	E855.2	E938.9	E950.4	E962.0	E980.4
infiltration (subcutaneous)	968.5	E855.2	E938.5	E950.4	E962.0	E980.4
nerve block (peripheral) (plexus)	968.6	E855.2	E938.6	E950.5	E962.0	E980.4
spinal	968.7	E855.2	E938.7	E950.4	E962.0	E980.4
topical (surface)	968.5	E855.2	E938.5	E950.4	E962.0	E980.4
Stovarsal	961.1	E857	E931.1	E950.4	E962.0	E980.4
Stove gas — *see* Gas, utility						
Stoxil	976.5	E858.7	E946.5	E950.4	E962.0	E980.4
STP	969.6	E854.1	E939.6	E950.3	E962.0	E980.3
Stramonium (medicinal) NEC	971.1	E855.4	E941.1	E950.4	E962.0	E980.4
natural state	988.2	E865.4	—	E950.9	E962.1	E980.9
Streptodornase	964.4	E858.2	E934.4	E950.4	E962.0	E980.4
Streptoduocin	960.6	E856	E930.6	E950.4	E962.0	E980.4
Streptokinase	964.4	E858.2	E934.4	E950.4	E962.0	E980.4
Streptomycin	960.6	E856	E930.6	E950.4	E962.0	E980.4
Streptozocin	960.7	E856	E930.7	E950.4	E962.0	E980.4
Stripper (paint) (solvent)	982.8	E862.9	—	E950.9	E962.1	E980.9
Strobane	989.2	E863.0	—	E950.6	E962.1	E980.7
Strophanthin	972.1	E858.3	E942.1	E950.4	E962.0	E980.4
Strophanthus hispidus or kombe	988.2	E865.4	—	E950.9	E962.1	E980.9
Strychnine (rodenticide) (salts)	989.1	E863.7	—	E950.6	E962.1	E980.7
medicinal NEC	970.8	E854.3	E940.8	E950.4	E962.0	E980.4
Strychnos (ignatii) — *see* Strychnine						
Styramate	968.0	E855.1	E938.0	E950.4	E962.0	E980.4
Styrene	983.0	E864.0	—	E950.7	E962.1	E980.6

Substance	Poisoning	External Cause (E-Code)				
		Accident	Therapeutic Use	Suicide Attempt	Assault	Undetermined
Succinimide (anticonvulsant)	966.2	E855.0	E936.2	E950.4	E962.0	E980.4
mercuric — see Mercury						
Succinylcholine	975.2	E858.6	E945.2	E950.4	E962.0	E980.4
Succinylsulfathiazole	961.0	E857	E931.0	E950.4	E962.0	E980.4
Sucrose	974.5	E858.5	E944.5	E950.4	E962.0	E980.4
Sulfacetamide	961.0	E857	E931.0	E950.4	E962.0	E980.4
ophthalmic preparation	976.5	E858.7	E946.5	E950.4	E962.0	E980.4
Sulfachlorpyridazine	961.0	E857	E931.0	E950.4	E962.0	E980.4
Sulfacytine	961.0	E857	E931.0	E950.4	E962.0	E980.4
Sulfadiazine	961.0	E857	E931.0	E950.4	E962.0	E980.4
silver (topical)	976.0	E858.7	E946.0	E950.4	E962.0	E980.4
Sulfadimethoxine	961.0	E857	E931.0	E950.4	E962.0	E980.4
Sulfadimidine	961.0	E857	E931.0	E950.4	E962.0	E980.4
Sulfaethidole	961.0	E857	E931.0	E950.4	E962.0	E980.4
Sulfafurazole	961.0	E857	E931.0	E950.4	E962.0	E980.4
Sulfaguanidine	961.0	E857	E931.0	E950.4	E962.0	E980.4
Sulfamerazine	961.0	E857	E931.0	E950.4	E962.0	E980.4
Sulfameter	961.0	E857	E931.0	E950.4	E962.0	E980.4
Sulfamethizole	961.0	E857	E931.0	E950.4	E962.0	E980.4
Sulfamethoxazole	961.0	E857	E931.0	E950.4	E962.0	E980.4
Sulfamethoxydiazine	961.0	E857	E931.0	E950.4	E962.0	E980.4
Sulfamethoxypyridazine	961.0	E857	E931.0	E950.4	E962.0	E980.4
Sulfamethylthiazole	961.0	E857	E931.0	E950.4	E962.0	E980.4
Sulfamylon	976.0	E858.7	E946.0	E950.4	E962.0	E980.4
Sulfan blue (diagnostic dye)	977.8	E858.8	E947.8	E950.4	E962.0	E980.4
Sulfanilamide	961.0	E857	E931.0	E950.4	E962.0	E980.4
Sulfanilylguanidine	961.0	E857	E931.0	E950.4	E962.0	E980.4
Sulfaphenazole	961.0	E857	E931.0	E950.4	E962.0	E980.4
Sulfaphenylthiazole	961.0	E857	E931.0	E950.4	E962.0	E980.4
Sulfaproxyline	961.0	E857	E931.0	E950.4	E962.0	E980.4
Sulfapyridine	961.0	E857	E931.0	E950.4	E962.0	E980.4
Sulfapyrimidine	961.0	E857	E931.0	E950.4	E962.0	E980.4
Sulfarsphenamine	961.1	E857	E931.1	E950.4	E962.0	E980.4
Sulfasalazine	961.0	E857	E931.0	E950.4	E962.0	E980.4
Sulfasomizole	961.0	E857	E931.0	E950.4	E962.0	E980.4
Sulfasuxidine	961.0	E857	E931.0	E950.4	E962.0	E980.4
Sulfinpyrazone	974.7	E858.5	E944.7	E950.4	E962.0	E980.4
Sulfisoxazole	961.0	E857	E931.0	E950.4	E962.0	E980.4
ophthalmic preparation	976.5	E858.7	E946.5	E950.4	E962.0	E980.4
Sulfomyxin	960.8	E856	E930.8	E950.4	E962.0	E980.4
Sulfonal	967.8	E852.8	E937.8	E950.2	E962.0	E980.2
Sulfonamides (mixtures)	961.0	E857	E931.0	E950.4	E962.0	E980.4
Sulfones	961.8	E857	E931.8	E950.4	E962.0	E980.4
Sulfonethylmethane	967.8	E852.8	E937.8	E950.2	E962.0	E980.2
Sulfonmethane	967.8	E852.8	E937.8	E950.2	E962.0	E980.2
Sulfonphthal, sulfonphthol	977.8	E858.8	E947.8	E950.4	E962.0	E980.4
Sulfonylurea derivatives, oral	962.3	E858.0	E932.3	E950.4	E962.0	E980.4
Sulfoxone	961.8	E857	E931.8	E950.4	E962.0	E980.4
Sulfur, sulfureted, sulfuric, sulfurous,						
sulfuryl (compounds) NEC	989.89	E866.8	—	E950.9	E962.1	E980.9
acid	983.1	E864.1	—	E950.7	E962.1	E980.6
dioxide	987.3	E869.1	—	E952.8	E962.2	E982.8
ether — see Ether(s)						
hydrogen	987.8	E869.8	—	E952.8	E962.2	E982.8
medicinal (keratolytic) (ointment) NEC	976.4	E858.7	E946.4	E950.4	E962.0	E980.4
pesticide (vapor)	989.4	E863.4	—	E950.6	E962.1	E980.7
vapor NEC	987.8	E869.8	—	E952.8	E962.2	E982.8

Substance	External Cause (E-Code)					
	Poisoning	Accident	Therapeutic Use	Suicide Attempt	Assault	Undetermined
Sulkowitch's reagent	977.8	E858.8	E947.8	E950.4	E962.0	E980.4
Sulph — *see also* Sulf–						
Sulphadione	961.8	E857	E931.8	E950.4	E962.0	E980.4
Sulthiame, sultiame	966.3	E855.0	E936.3	E950.4	E962.0	E980.4
Superinone	975.5	E858.6	E945.5	E950.4	E962.0	E980.4
Suramin	961.5	E857	E931.5	E950.4	E962.0	E980.4
Surfacaine	968.5	E855.2	E938.5	E950.4	E962.0	E980.4
Surital	968.3	E855.1	E938.3	E950.4	E962.0	E980.4
Sutilains	976.8	E858.7	E946.8	E950.4	E962.0	E980.4
Suxamethoniam (bromide) (chloride)						
(iodide)	975.2	E858.6	E945.2	E950.4	E962.0	E980.4
Suxethonium (bromide)	975.2	E858.6	E945.2	E950.4	E962.0	E980.4
Sweet oil (birch)	976.3	E858.7	E946.3	E950.4	E962.0	E980.4
Sym–dichloroethyl ether	982.3	E862.4	—	E950.9	E962.1	E980.9
Sympatholytics	971.3	E855.6	E941.3	E950.4	E962.0	E980.4
Sympathomimetics	971.2	E855.5	E941.2	E950.4	E962.0	E980.4
Synagis	979.6	E858.8	E949.6	E950.4	E962.0	E980.4
Synalar	976.0	E858.7	E946.0	E950.4	E962.0	E980.4
Synthroid	962.7	E858.0	E932.7	E950.4	E962.0	E980.4
Syntocinon	975.0	E858.6	E945.0	E950.4	E962.0	E950.4
Syrosingopine	972.6	E858.3	E942.6	E950.4	E962.0	E980.4
Systemic agents (primarily)	963.9	E858.1	E933.9	E950.4	E962.0	E980.4
specified NEC	963.8	E858.1	E933.8	E950.4	E962.0	E980.4
Tablets (see also specified substance)	977.9	E858.9	E947.9	E950.5	E962.0	E980.5
Tace	962.2	E858.0	E932.2	E950.4	E962.0	E980.4
Tacrine	971.0	E855.3	E941.0	E950.4	E962.0	E980.4
Talbutal	967.0	E851	E937.0	E950.1	E962.0	E980.1
Talc	976.3	E858.7	E946.3	E950.4	E962.0	E980.4
Talcum	976.3	E858.7	E946.3	E950.4	E962.0	E980.4
Tandearil, tanderil	965.5	E850.5	E935.5	E950.0	E962.0	E980.0
Tannic acid	983.1	E864.1	—	E950.7	E962.1	E980.6
medicinal (astringent)	976.2	E858.7	E946.2	E950.4	E962.0	E980.4
Tannin — *see* Tannic acid						
Tansy	988.2	E865.4	—	E950.9	E962.1	E980.9
TAO	960.3	E856	E930.3	E950.4	E962.0	E980.4
Tapazole	962.8	E858.0	E932.8	E950.4	E962.0	E980.4
Tar NEC	983.0	E864.0	—	E950.7	E962.1	E980.6
camphor — *see* Naphthalene						
fumes	987.8	E869.8	—	E952.8	E962.2	E982.8
Taractan	969.3	E853.8	E939.3	E950.3	E962.0	E980.3
Tarantula (venomous)	989.5	E905.1	—	E950.9	E962.1	E980.9
Tartar emetic (anti–infective)	961.2	E857	E931.2	E950.4	E962.0	E980.4
Tartaric acid	983.1	E864.1	—	E950.7	E962.1	E980.6
Tartrated antimony (anti–infective)	961.2	E857	E931.2	E950.4	E962.0	E980.4
TCA — *see* Trichloroacetic acid						
TDI	983.0	E864.0	—	E950.7	E962.1	E980.6
vapor	987.8	E869.8	—	E952.8	E962.2	E982.8
Tear gas	987.5	E869.3	—	E952.8	E962.2	E982.8
Teclothiazide	974.3	E858.5	E944.3	E950.4	E962.0	E980.4
Tegretol	966.3	E855.0	E936.3	E950.4	E962.0	E980.4
Telepaque	977.8	E858.8	E947.8	E950.4	E962.0	E980.4
Tellurium	985.8	E866.4	—	E950.9	E962.1	E980.9
fumes	985.8	E866.4	—	E950.9	E962.1	E980.9
TEM	963.1	E858.1	E933.1	E950.4	E962.0	E980.4
Temazepan—*see* Benzodiazepines						
TEPA	963.1	E858.1	E933.1	E950.4	E962.0	E980.4
TEPP	989.3	E863.1	—	E950.6	E962.1	E980.7

Substance	Poisoning	Accident	External Cause (E-Code) Therapeutic Use	Suicide Attempt	Assault	Undetermined
Terbutaline	971.2	E855.5	E941.2	E950.4	E962.0	E980.4
Teroxalene	961.6	E857	E931.6	E950.4	E962.0	E980.4
Terpin hydrate	975.5	E858.6	E945.5	E950.4	E962.0	E980.4
Terramycin	960.4	E856	E930.4	E950.4	E962.0	E980.4
Tessalon	975.4	E858.6	E945.4	E950.4	E962.0	E980.4
Testosterone	962.1	E858.0	E932.1	E950.4	E962.0	E980.4
Tetanus (vaccine)	978.4	E858.8	E948.4	E950.4	E962.0	E980.4
antitoxin	979.9	E858.8	E949.9	E950.4	E962.0	E980.4
immune globulin (human)	964.6	E858.2	E934.6	E950.4	E962.0	E980.4
toxoid	978.4	E858.8	E948.4	E950.4	E962.0	E980.4
with diphtheria toxoid	978.9	E858.8	E948.9	E950.4	E962.0	E980.4
with pertussis	978.6	E858.8	E948.6	E950.4	E962.0	E980.4
Tetrabenazine	969.5	E853.8	E939.5	E950.3	E962.0	E980.3
Tetracaine (infiltration) (topical)	968.5	E855.2	E938.5	E950.4	E962.0	E980.4
nerve block (peripheral) (plexus)	968.6	E855.2	E938.6	E950.4	E962.0	E980.4
spinal	968.7	E855.2	E938.7	E950.4	E962.0	E980.4
Tetrachlorethylene—see Tetrachloroethylene						
Tetrachlormethiazide	974.3	E858.5	E944.3	E950.4	E962.0	E980.4
Tetrachloroethane (liquid) (vapor)	982.3	E862.4	—	E950.9	E962.1	E980.9
paint or varnish	982.3	E861.6	—	E950.9	E962.1	E980.9
Tetrachloroethylene (liquid) (vapor)	982.3	E862.4	—	E950.9	E962.1	E980.9
medicinal	961.6	E857	E931.6	E950.4	E962.0	E980.4
Tetrachloromethane — see Carbon, tetrachloride						
Tetracycline	960.4	E856	E930.4	E950.4	E962.0	E980.4
ophthalmic preparation	976.5	E858.7	E946.5	E950.4	E962.0	E980.4
topical NEC	976.0	E858.7	E946.0	E950.4	E962.0	E980.4
Tetraethylammonium chloride	972.3	E858.3	E942.3	E950.4	E962.0	E980.4
Tetraethyl lead (antiknock compound)	984.1	E862.1	—	E950.9	E962.1	E980.9
Tetraethyl pyrophosphate	989.3	E863.1	—	E950.6	E962.1	E980.7
Tetraethylthiuram disulfide	977.3	E858.8	E947.3	E950.4	E962.0	E980.4
Tetrahydroaminoacridine	971.0	E855.3	E941.0	E950.4	E962.0	E980.4
Tetrahydrocannabinol	969.6	E854.1	E939.6	E950.3	E962.0	E980.3
Tetrahydronaphthalene	982.0	E862.4	—	E950.9	E962.1	E980.9
Tetrahydrozoline	971.2	E855.5	E941.2	E950.4	E962.0	E980.4
Tetralin	982.0	E862.4	—	E950.9	E962.1	E980.9
Tetramethylthiuram (disulfide) NEC	989.4	E863.6	—	E950.6	E962.1	E980.7
medicinal	976.2	E858.7	E946.2	E950.4	E962.0	E980.4
Tetronal	967.8	E852.8	E937.8	E950.2	E962.0	E980.2
Tetryl	983.0	E864.0	—	E950.7	E962.1	E980.6
Thalidomide	967.8	E852.8	E937.8	E950.2	E962.0	E980.2
Thallium (compounds) (dust) NEC	985.8	E866.4	—	E950.9	E962.1	E980.9
pesticide (rodenticide)	985.8	E863.7	—	E950.6	E962.1	E980.7
THC	969.6	E854.1	E939.6	E950.3	E962.0	E980.3
Thebacon	965.09	E850.2	E935.2	E950.0	E962.0	E980.0
Thebaine	965.09	E850.2	E935.2	E950.0	E962.0	E980.0
Theobromine (calcium salicylate)	974.1	E858.5	E944.1	E950.4	E962.0	E980.4
Theophylline (diuretic)	974.1	E858.5	E944.1	E950.4	E962.0	E980.4
ethylenediamine	975.7	E858.6	E945.7	E950.4	E962.0	E980.4
Thiabendazole	961.6	E857	E931.6	E950.4	E962.0	E980.4
Thialbarbital, thialbarbitone	968.3	E855.1	E938.3	E950.4	E962.0	E980.4
Thiamine	963.5	E858.1	E933.5	E950.4	E962.0	E980.4
Thiamylal (sodium)	968.3	E855.1	E938.3	E950.4	E962.0	E980.4
Thiazesim	969.0	E854.0	E939.0	E950.3	E962.0	E980.3
Thiazides (diuretics)	974.3	E858.5	E944.3	E950.4	E962.0	E980.4
Thiethylperazine	963.0	E858.1	E933.0	E950.4	E962.0	E980.4
Thimerosal (topical)	976.0	E858.7	E946.0	E950.4	E962.0	E980.4

Substance	Poisoning	External Cause (E-Code)				
		Accident	Therapeutic Use	Suicide Attempt	Assault	Undetermined
ophthalmic preparation 976.5	E858.7	E946.5	E950.4	E962.0	E980.4	
Thioacetazone 961.8	E857	E931.8	E950.4	E962.0	E980.4	
Thiobarbiturates 968.3	E855.1	E938.3	E950.4	E962.0	E980.4	
Thiobismol 961.2	E857	E931.2	E950.4	E962.0	E980.4	
Thiocarbamide 962.8	E858.0	E932.8	E950.4	E962.0	E980.4	
Thiocarbarsone 961.1	E857	E931.1	E950.4	E962.0	E980.4	
Thiocarlide 961.8	E857	E931.8	E950.4	E962.0	E980.4	
Thioguanine 963.1	E858.1	E933.1	E950.4	E962.0	E980.4	
Thiomercaptomerin 974.0	E858.5	E944.0	E950.4	E962.0	E980.4	
Thiomerin 974.0	E858.5	E944.0	E950.4	E962.0	E980.4	
Thiopental, thiopentone (sodium) 968.3	E855.1	E938.3	E950.4	E962.0	E980.4	
Thiopropazate 969.1	E853.0	E939.1	E950.3	E962.0	E980.3	
Thioproperazine 969.1	E853.0	E939.1	E950.3	E962.0	E980.3	
Thioridazine 969.1	E853.0	E939.1	E950.3	E962.0	E980.3	
Thio–TEPA, thiotepa 963.1	E858.1	E933.1	E950.4	E962.0	E980.4	
Thiothixene 969.3	E853.8	E939.3	E950.3	E962.0	E980.3	
Thiouracil 962.8	E858.0	E932.8	E950.4	E962.0	E980.4	
Thiourea 962.8	E858.0	E932.8	E950.4	E962.0	E980.4	
Thiphenamil 971.1	E855.4	E941.1	E950.4	E962.0	E980.4	
Thiram NEC 989.4	E863.6	—	E950.6	E962.1	E980.7	
medicinal 976.2	E858.7	E946.2	E950.4	E962.0	E980.4	
Thonzylamine 963.0	E858.1	E933.0	E950.4	E962.0	E980.4	
Thorazine 969.1	E853.0	E939.1	E950.3	E962.0	E980.3	
Thornapple 988.2	E865.4	—	E950.9	E962.1	E980.9	
Throat preparation (lozenges) NEC 976.6	E858.7	E946.6	E950.4	E962.0	E980.4	
Thrombin 964.5	E858.2	E934.5	E950.4	E962.0	E980.4	
Thrombolysin 964.4	E858.2	E934.4	E950.4	E962.0	E980.4	
Thymol 983.0	E864.0	—	E950.7	E962.1	E980.6	
Thymus extract 962.9	E858.0	E932.9	E950.4	E962.0	E980.4	
Thyroglobulin 962.7	E858.0	E932.7	E950.4	E962.0	E980.4	
Thyroid (derivatives) (extract) 962.7	E858.0	E932.7	E950.4	E962.0	E980.4	
Thyrolar 962.7	E858.0	E932.7	E950.4	E962.0	E980.4	
Thyrothrophin, thyrotropin 977.8	E858.8	E947.8	E950.4	E962.0	E980.4	
Thyroxin(e) 962.7	E858.0	E932.7	E950.4	E962.0	E980.4	
Tigan 963.0	E858.1	E933.0	E950.4	E962.0	E980.4	
Tigloidine 968.0	E855.1	E938.0	E950.4	E962.0	E980.4	
Tin (chloride) (dust) (oxide) NEC 985.8	E866.4	—	E950.9	E962.1	E980.9	
anti–infectives 961.2	E857	E931.2	E950.4	E962.0	E980.4	
Tinactin 976.0	E858.7	E946.0	E950.4	E962.0	E980.4	
Tincture, iodine — see Iodine						
Tindal 969.1	E853.0	E939.1	E950.3	E962.0	E980.3	
Titanium (compounds) (vapor) 985.8	E866.4	—	E950.9	E962.1	E980.9	
ointment 976.3	E858.7	E946.3	E950.4	E962.0	E980.4	
Titroid 962.7	E858.0	E932.7	E950.4	E962.0	E980.4	
TMTD — see Tetramethylthiuram disulfide						
TNT 989.89	E866.8	—	E950.9	E962.1	E980.9	
fumes 987.8	E869.8	—	E952.8	E962.2	E982.8	
Toadstool 988.1	E865.5	—	E950.9	E962.1	E980.9	
Tobacco NEC 989.84	E866.8	—	E950.9	E962.1	E980.9	
Indian 988.2	E865.4	—	E950.9	E962.1	E980.9	
smoke, second-hand 987.8	E869.4	—	—	—	—	
Tocopherol 963.5	E858.1	E933.5	E950.4	E962.0	E980.4	
Tocosamine 975.0	E858.6	E945.0	E950.4	E962.0	E980.4	
Tofranil 969.0	E854.0	E939.0	E950.3	E962.0	E980.3	
Toilet deodorizer 989.8	E866.8	—	E950.9	E962.1	E980.9	
Tolazamide 962.3	E858.0	E932.3	E950.4	E962.0	E980.4	
Tolazoline 971.3	E855.6	E941.3	E950.4	E962.0	E980.4	

Substance	Poisoning	Accident	Therapeutic Use	Suicide Attempt	Assault	Undetermined
Tolbutamide	962.3	E858.0	E932.3	E950.4	E962.0	E980.4
sodium	977.8	E858.8	E947.8	E950.4	E962.0	E980.4
Tolmetin	965.69	E850.6	E935.6	E950.0	E962.0	E980.0
Tolnaftate	976.0	E858.7	E946.0	E950.4	E962.0	E980.4
Tolpropamine	976.1	E858.7	E946.1	E950.4	E962.0	E980.4
Tolserol	968.0	E855.1	E938.0	E950.4	E962.0	E980.4
Toluene (liquid) (vapor)	982.0	E862.4	—	E950.9	E962.1	E980.9
diisocyanate	983.0	E864.0	—	E950.7	E962.1	E980.6
Toluidine	983.0	E864.0	—	E950.7	E962.1	E980.6
vapor	987.8	E869.8	—	E952.8	E962.2	E982.8
Toluol (liquid) (vapor)	982.0	E862.4	—	E950.9	E962.1	E980.9
Tolylene–2,4–diisocyanate	983.0	E864.0	—	E950.7	E962.1	E980.6
Tonics, cardiac	972.1	E858.3	E942.1	E950.4	E962.0	E980.4
Toxaphene (dust) (spray)	989.2	E863.0	—	E950.6	E962.1	E980.7
Toxoids NEC	978.8	E858.8	E948.8	E950.4	E962.0	E980.4
Tractor fuel NEC	981	E862.1	—	E950.9	E962.1	E980.9
Tragacanth	973.3	E858.4	E943.3	E950.4	E962.0	E980.4
Tramazoline	971.2	E855.5	E941.2	E950.4	E962.0	E980.4
Tranquilizers	969.5	E853.9	E939.5	E950.3	E962.0	E980.3
benzodiazepine–based	969.4	E853.2	E939.4	E950.3	E962.0	E980.3
butyrophenone–based	969.2	E853.1	E939.2	E950.3	E962.0	E980.3
major NEC	969.3	E853.8	E939.3	E950.3	E962.0	E980.3
phenothiazine–based	969.1	E853.0	E939.1	E950.3	E962.0	E980.3
specified NEC	969.5	E853.8	E939.5	E950.3	E962.0	E980.3
Trantoin	961.9	E857	E931.9	E950.4	E962.0	E980.4
Tranxene	969.4	E853.2	E939.4	E950.3	E962.0	E980.3
Tranylcypromine (sulfate)	969.0	E854.0	E939.0	E950.3	E962.0	E980.3
Trasentine	975.1	E858.6	E945.1	E950.4	E962.0	E980.4
Travert	974.5	E858.5	E944.5	E950.4	E962.0	E980.4
Trecator	961.8	E857	E931.8	E950.4	E962.0	E980.4
Tretinoin	976.8	E858.7	E946.8	E950.4	E962.0	E980.4
Triacetin	976.0	E858.7	E946.0	E950.4	E962.0	E980.4
Triacetyloleandomycin	960.3	E856	E930.3	E950.4	E962.0	E980.4
Triamcinolone	962.0	E858.0	E932.0	E950.4	E962.0	E980.4
ENT agent	976.6	E858.7	E946.6	E950.4	E962.0	E980.4
ophthalmic preparation	976.5	E858.7	E946.5	E950.4	E962.0	E980.4
topical NEC	976.0	E858.7	E946.0	E950.4	E962.0	E980.4
Triamterene	974.4	E858.5	E944.4	E950.4	E962.0	E980.4
Triaziquone	963.1	E858.1	E933.1	E950.4	E962.0	E980.4
Tribromacetaldehyde	967.3	E852.2	E937.3	E950.2	E962.0	E980.2
Tribromoethanol	968.2	E855.1	E938.2	E950.4	E962.0	E980.4
Tribromomethane	967.3	E852.2	E937.3	E950.2	E962.0	E980.2
Trichlorethane	982.3	E862.4	—	E950.9	E962.1	E980.9
Trichlormethiazide	974.3	E858.5	E944.3	E950.4	E962.0	E980.4
Trichloroacetic acid	983.1	E864.1	—	E950.7	E962.1	E980.6
medicinal (keratolytic)	976.4	E858.7	E946.4	E950.4	E962.0	E980.4
Trichloroethanol	967.1	E852.0	E937.1	E950.2	E962.0	E980.2
Trichloroethylene (liquid) (vapor)	982.3	E862.4	—	E950.9	E962.1	E980.9
anesthetic (gas)	968.2	E855.1	E938.2	E950.4	E962.0	E980.4
Trichloroethyl phosphate	967.1	E852.0	E937.1	E950.2	E962.0	E980.2
Trichlorofluoromethane NEC	987.4	E869.2	—	E952.8	E962.2	E982.8
Trichlorotriethylamine	963.1	E858.1	E933.1	E950.4	E962.0	E980.4
Trichomonacides NEC	961.5	E857	E931.5	E950.4	E962.0	E980.4
Trichomycin	960.1	E856	E930.1	E950.4	E962.0	E980.4
Triclofos	967.1	E852.0	E937.1	E950.2	E962.0	E980.2
Tricresyl phosphate	989.89	E866.8	—	E950.9	E962.1	E980.9
solvent	982.8	E862.4	—	E950.9	E962.1	E980.9

Substance	Poisoning	External Cause (E-Code)				
		Accident	Therapeutic Use	Suicide Attempt	Assault	Undetermined
Tricyclamol	966.4	E855.0	E936.4	E950.4	E962.0	E980.4
Tridesilon	976.0	E858.7	E946.0	E950.4	E962.0	E980.4
Tridihexethyl	971.1	E855.4	E941.1	E950.4	E962.0	E980.4
Tridione	966.0	E855.0	E936.0	E950.4	E962.0	E980.4
Triethanolamine NEC	983.2	E864.2	—	E950.7	E962.1	E980.6
detergent	983.2	E861.0	—	E950.7	E962.1	E980.6
trinitrate	972.4	E858.3	E942.4	E950.4	E962.0	E980.4
Triethanomelamine	963.1	E858.1	E933.1	E950.4	E962.0	E980.4
Triethylene melamine	963.1	E858.1	E933.1	E950.4	E962.0	E980.4
Triethylenephosphoramide	963.1	E858.1	E933.1	E950.4	E962.0	E980.4
Triethylenethiophosphoramide	963.1	E858.1	E933.1	E950.4	E962.0	E980.4
Trifluoperazine	969.1	E853.0	E939.1	E950.3	E962.0	E980.3
Trifluperidol	969.2	E853.1	E939.2	E950.3	E962.0	E980.3
Triflupromazine	969.1	E853.0	E939.1	E950.3	E962.0	E980.3
Trihexyphenidyl	971.1	E855.4	E941.1	E950.4	E962.0	E980.4
Triiodothyronine	962.7	E858.0	E932.7	E950.4	E962.0	E980.4
Trilene	968.2	E855.1	E938.2	E950.4	E962.0	E980.4
Trimeprazine	963.0	E858.1	E933.0	E950.4	E962.0	E980.4
Trimetazidine	972.4	E858.3	E942.4	E950.4	E962.0	E980.4
Trimethadione	966.0	E855.0	E936.0	E950.4	E962.0	E980.4
Trimethaphan	972.3	E858.3	E942.3	E950.4	E962.0	E980.4
Trimethidinium	972.3	E858.3	E942.3	E950.4	E962.0	E980.4
Trimethobenzamide	963.0	E858.1	E933.0	E950.4	E962.0	E980.4
Trimethylcarbinol	980.8	E860.8	—	E950.9	E962.1	E980.9
Trimethylpsoralen	976.3	E858.7	E946.3	E950.4	E962.0	E980.4
Trimeton	963.0	E858.1	E933.0	E950.4	E962.0	E980.4
Trimipramine	969.0	E854.0	E939.0	E950.3	E962.0	E980.3
Trimustine	963.1	E858.1	E933.1	E950.4	E962.0	E980.4
Trinitrin	972.4	E858.3	E942.4	E950.4	E962.0	E980.4
Trinitrophenol	983.0	E864.0	—	E950.7	E962.1	E980.6
Trinitrotoluene	989.89	E866.8	—	E950.9	E962.1	E980.9
fumes	987.8	E869.8	—	E952.8	E962.2	E982.8
Trional	967.8	E852.8	E937.8	E950.2	E962.0	E980.2
Trioxide of arsenic — *see* Arsenic						
Trioxsalen	976.3	E858.7	E946.3	E950.4	E962.0	E980.4
Tripelennamine	963.0	E858.1	E933.0	E950.4	E962.0	E980.4
Triperidol	969.2	E853.1	E939.2	E950.3	E962.0	E980.3
Triprolidine	963.0	E858.1	E933.0	E950.4	E962.0	E980.4
Trisoralen	976.3	E858.7	E946.3	E950.4	E962.0	E980.4
Troleandomycin	960.3	E856	E930.3	E950.4	E962.0	E980.4
Trolnitrate (phosphate)	972.4	E858.3	E942.4	E950.4	E962.0	E980.4
Trometamol	963.3	E858.1	E933.3	E950.4	E962.0	E980.4
Tromethamine	963.3	E858.1	E933.3	E950.4	E962.0	E980.4
Tronothane	968.5	E855.2	E938.5	E950.4	E962.0	E980.4
Tropicamide	971.1	E855.4	E941.1	E950.4	E962.0	E980.4
Troxidone	966.0	E855.0	E936.0	E950.4	E962.0	E980.4
Tryparsamide	961.1	E857	E931.1	E950.4	E962.0	E980.4
Trypsin	963.4	E858.1	E933.4	E950.4	E962.0	E980.4
Tryptizol	969.0	E854.0	E939.0	E950.3	E962.0	E980.3
Tuaminoheptane	971.2	E855.5	E941.2	E950.4	E962.0	E980.4
Tuberculin (old)	977.8	E858.8	E947.8	E950.4	E962.0	E980.4
Tubocurare	975.2	E858.6	E945.2	E950.4	E962.0	E980.4
Tubocurarine	975.2	E858.6	E945.2	E950.4	E962.0	E980.4
Turkish green	969.6	E854.1	E939.6	E950.3	E962.0	E980.3
Turpentine (spirits of) (liquid) (vapor)	982.8	E862.4	—	E950.9	E962.1	E980.9
Tybamate	969.5	E853.8	E939.5	E950.3	E962.0	E980.3
Tyloxapol	975.5	E858.6	E945.5	E950.4	E962.0	E980.4

Substance	External Cause (E-Code)					
	Poisoning	Accident	Therapeutic Use	Suicide Attempt	Assault	Undetermined
Tymazoline	971.2	E855.5	E941.2	E950.4	E962.0	E980.4
Typhoid vaccine	978.1	E858.8	E948.1	E950.4	E962.0	E980.4
Typhus vaccine	979.2	E858.8	E949.2	E950.4	E962.0	E980.4
Tyrothricin	976.0	E858.7	E946.0	E950.4	E962.0	E980.4
ENT agent	976.6	E858.7	E946.6	E950.4	E962.0	E980.4
ophthalmic preparation	976.5	E858.7	E946.5	E950.4	E962.0	E980.4
Undecenoic acid	976.0	E858.7	E946.0	E950.4	E962.0	E980.4
Undecylenic acid	976.0	E858.7	E946.0	E950.4	E962.0	E980.4
Unna's boot	976.3	E858.7	E946.3	E950.4	E962.0	E980.4
Uracil mustard	963.1	E858.1	E933.1	E950.4	E962.0	E980.4
Uramustine	963.1	E858.1	E933.1	E950.4	E962.0	E980.4
Urari	975.2	E858.6	E945.2	E950.4	E962.0	E980.4
Urea	974.4	E858.5	E944.4	E950.4	E962.0	E980.4
topical	976.8	E858.7	E946.8	E950.4	E962.0	E980.4
Urethan(e) (antineoplastic)	963.1	E858.1	E933.1	E950.4	E962.0	E980.4
Urginea (maritima) (scilla) — see Squill						
Uric acid metabolism agents NEC	974.7	E858.5	E944.7	E950.4	E962.0	E980.4
Urokinase	964.4	E858.2	E934.4	E950.4	E962.0	E980.4
Urokon	977.8	E858.8	E947.8	E950.4	E962.0	E980.4
Urotropin	961.9	E857	E931.9	E950.4	E962.0	E980.4
Urtica	988.2	E865.4	—	E950.9	E962.1	E980.9
Utility gas — see Gas, utility						
Vaccine NEC	979.9	E858.8	E949.9	E950.4	E962.0	E980.4
bacterial NEC	978.8	E858.8	E948.8	E950.4	E962.0	E980.4
with						
other bacterial component	978.9	E858.8	E948.9	E950.4	E962.0	E980.4
pertussis component	978.6	E858.8	E948.6	E950.4	E962.0	E980.4
viral–rickettsial component	979.7	E858.8	E949.7	E950.4	E962.0	E980.4
mixed NEC	978.9	E858.8	E948.9	E950.4	E962.0	E980.4
BCG	978.0	E858.8	E948.0	E950.4	E962.0	E980.4
cholera	978.2	E858.8	E948.2	E950.4	E962.0	E980.4
diphtheria	978.5	E858.8	E948.5	E950.4	E962.0	E980.4
influenza	979.6	E858.8	E949.6	E950.4	E962.0	E980.4
measles	979.4	E858.8	E949.4	E950.4	E962.0	E980.4
meningococcal	978.8	E858.8	E948.8	E950.4	E962.0	E980.4
mumps	979.6	E858.8	E949.6	E950.4	E962.0	E980.4
paratyphoid	978.1	E858.8	E948.1	E950.4	E962.0	E980.4
pertussis (with diphtheria toxoid) (with tetanus toxoid)	978.6	E858.8	E948.6	E950.4	E962.0	E980.4
plague	978.3	E858.8	E948.3	E950.4	E962.0	E980.4
poliomyelitis	979.5	E858.8	E949.5	E950.4	E962.0	E980.4
poliovirus	979.5	E858.8	E949.5	E950.4	E962.0	E980.4
rabies	979.1	E858.8	E949.1	E950.4	E962.0	E980.4
respiratory syncytial virus	979.6	E858.8	E949.6	E950.4	E962.0	E980.4
rickettsial NEC	979.6	E858.8	E949.6	E950.4	E962.0	E980.4
with						
bacterial component	979.7	E858.8	E949.7	E950.4	E962.0	E980.4
pertussis component	978.6	E858.8	E948.6	E950.4	E962.0	E980.4
viral component	979.7	E858.8	E949.7	E950.4	E962.0	E980.4
Rocky mountain spotted fever	979.6	E858.8	E949.6	E950.4	E962.0	E980.4
rotavirus	979.6	E858.8	E949.6	E950.4	E962.0	E980.4
rubella virus	979.4	E858.8	E949.4	E950.4	E962.0	E980.4
sabin oral	979.5	E858.8	E949.5	E950.4	E962.0	E980.4
smallpox	979.0	E858.8	E949.0	E950.4	E962.0	E980.4
tetanus	978.4	E858.8	E948.4	E950.4	E962.0	E980.4
typhoid	978.1	E858.8	E948.1	E950.4	E962.0	E980.4
typhus	979.2	E858.8	E949.2	E950.4	E962.0	E980.4

Substance	Poisoning	External Cause (E-Code)				
		Accident	Therapeutic Use	Suicide Attempt	Assault	Undetermined
viral NEC	979.6	E858.8	E949.6	E950.4	E962.0	E980.4
with						
bacterial component	979.7	E858.8	E949.7	E950.4	E962.0	E980.4
pertussis component	978.6	E858.8	E948.6	E950.4	E962.0	E980.4
rickettsial component	979.7	E858.8	E949.7	E950.4	E962.0	E980.4
yellow fever	979.3	E858.8	E949.3	E950.4	E962.0	E980.4
Vaccinia immune globulin (human)	964.6	E858.2	E934.6	E950.4	E962.0	E980.4
Vaginal contraceptives	976.8	E858.7	E946.8	E950.4	E962.0	E980.4
Valethamate	971.1	E855.4	E941.1	E950.4	E962.0	E980.4
Valisone	976.0	E858.7	E946.0	E950.4	E962.0	E980.4
Valium	969.4	E853.2	E939.4	E950.3	E962.0	E980.3
Valmid	967.8	E852.8	E937.8	E950.2	E962.0	E980.2
Vanadium	985.8	E866.4	—	E950.9	E962.1	E980.9
Vancomycin	960.8	E856	E930.8	E950.4	E962.0	E980.4
Vapor (see also Gas)	987.9	E869.9	—	E952.9	E962.2	E982.9
kiln (carbon monoxide)	986	E868.8	—	E952.1	E962.2	E982.1
lead — see Lead						
specified source NEC (see also						
specific substance)	987.8	E869.8	—	E952.8	E962.2	E982.8
Varidase	964.4	E858.2	E934.4	E950.4	E962.0	E980.4
Varnish	989.89	E861.6	—	E950.9	E962.1	E980.9
cleaner	982.8	E862.9	—	E950.9	E962.1	E980.9
Vaseline	976.3	E858.7	E946.3	E950.4	E962.0	E980.4
Vasodilan	972.5	E858.3	E942.5	E950.4	E962.0	E980.4
Vasodilators NEC	972.5	E858.3	E942.5	E950.4	E962.0	E980.0
coronary	972.4	E858.3	E942.4	E950.4	E962.0	E980.4
Vasopressin	962.5	E858.0	E932.5	E950.4	E962.0	E980.4
Vasopressor drugs	962.5	E858.0	E932.5	E950.4	E962.0	E980.4
Venom, venomous (bite) (sting)	989.5	E905.9	—	E950.9	E962.1	E980.9
arthropod NEC	989.5	E905.5	—	E950.9	E962.1	E980.9
bee	989.5	E905.3	—	E950.9	E962.1	E980.9
centipede	989.5	E905.4	—	E950.9	E962.1	E980.9
hornet	989.5	E905.3	—	E950.9	E962.1	E980.9
lizard	989.5	E905.0	—	E950.9	E962.1	E980.9
marine animals or plants	989.5	E905.6	—	E950.9	E962.1	E980.9
millipede (topical)	989.5	E905.4	—	E950.9	E962.1	E980.9
plant NEC	989.5	E905.7	—	E950.9	E962.1	E980.9
marine	989.5	E905.6	—	E950.9	E962.1	E980.9
scorpion	989.5	E905.2	—	E950.9	E962.1	E980.9
snake	989.5	E905.0	—	E950.9	E962.1	E980.9
specified NEC	989.5	E905.8	—	E950.9	E962.1	E980.9
spider	989.5	E905.1	—	E950.9	E962.1	E980.9
wasp	989.5	E905.3	—	E950.9	E962.1	E980.9
Ventolin—see Salbutamol sulfate						
Veramon	967.0	E851	E937.0	E950.1	E962.0	E980.1
Veratrum						
album	988.2	E865.4	—	E950.9	E962.1	E980.9
alkaloids	972.6	E858.3	E942.6	E950.4	E962.0	E980.4
viride	988.2	E865.4	—	E950.9	E962.1	E980.9
Verdigris (see also Copper)	985.8	E866.4	—	E950.9	E962.1	E980.9
Veronal	967.0	E851	E937.0	E950.1	E962.0	E980.1
Veroxil	961.6	E857	E931.6	E950.4	E962.0	E980.4
Versidyne	965.7	E850.7	E935.7	E950.0	E962.0	E980.0
Viagra	972.5	E858.3	E942.5	E950.4	E962.0	E980.4
Vienna						
green	985.1	E866.3	—	E950.8	E962.1	E980.8
insecticide	985.1	E863.4	—	E950.6	E962.1	E980.7

Substance	External Cause (E-Code)					
	Poisoning	Accident	Therapeutic Use	Suicide Attempt	Assault	Undetermined
red 989.89	E866.8	—		E950.9	E962.1	E980.9
pharmaceutical dye 977.4	E858.8	E947.4		E950.4	E962.0	E980.4
Vinbarbital, vinbarbitone 967.0	E851	E937.0		E950.1	E962.0	E980.1
Vinblastine 963.1	E858.1	E933.1		E950.4	E962.0	E980.4
Vincristine 963.1	E858.1	E933.1		E950.4	E962.0	E980.4
Vinesthene, vinethene 968.2	E855.1	E938.2		E950.4	E962.0	E980.4
Vinyl						
bital 967.0	E851	E937.0		E950.1	E962.0	E980.1
ether 968.2	E855.1	E938.2		E950.4	E962.0	E980.4
Vioform 961.3	E857	E931.3		E950.4	E962.0	E980.4
topical 976.0	E858.7	E946.0		E950.4	E962.0	E980.4
Viomycin 960.6	E856	E930.6		E950.4	E962.0	E980.4
Viosterol 963.5	E858.1	E933.5		E950.4	E962.0	E980.4
Viper (venom) 989.5	E905.0	—		E950.9	E962.1	E980.9
Viprynium (embonate) 961.6	E857	E931.6		E950.4	E962.0	E980.4
Virugon 961.7	E857	E931.7		E950.4	E962.0	E980.4
Visine 976.5	E858.7	E946.5		E950.4	E962.0	E980.4
Vitamins NEC 963.5	E858.1	E933.5		E950.4	E962.0	E980.4
B$_{12}$ 964.1	E858.2	E934.1		E950.4	E962.0	E980.4
hematopoietic 964.1	E858.2	E934.1		E950.4	E962.0	E980.4
K 964.3	E858.2	E934.3		E950.4	E962.0	E980.4
Vleminckx's solution 976.4	E858.7	E946.4		E950.4	E962.0	E980.4
Voltaren—*see* Diclofenac sodium						
Warfarin (potassium) (sodium) 964.2	E858.2	E934.2		E950.4	E962.0	E980.4
rodenticide 989.4	E863.7	—		E950.6	E962.1	E980.7
Wasp (sting) 989.5	E905.3	—		E950.9	E962.1	E980.9
Water						
balance agents NEC 974.5	E858.5	E944.5		E950.4	E962.0	E980.4
gas 987.1	E868.1	—		E951.8	E962.2	E981.8
incomplete combustion of — *see* Carbon, monoxide, fuel, utility						
hemlock 988.2	E865.4	—		E950.9	E962.1	E980.9
moccasin (venom) 989.5	E905.0	—		E950.9	E962.1	E980.9
Wax (paraffin) (petroleum) 981	E862.3	—		E950.9	E962.1	E980.9
automobile 989.89	E861.2	—		E950.9	E962.1	E980.9
floor 981	E862.0	—		E950.9	E962.1	E980.9
Weed killers NEC 989.4	E863.5	—		E950.6	E962.1	E980.7
Welldorm 967.1	E852.0	E937.1		E950.2	E962.0	E980.2
White						
arsenic — *see* Arsenic						
hellebore 988.2	E865.4	—		E950.9	E962.1	E980.9
lotion (keratolytic) 976.4	E858.7	E946.4		E950.4	E962.0	E980.4
spirit 981	E862.0	—		E950.9	E962.1	E980.9
Whitewashes 989.89	E861.6	—		E950.9	E962.1	E980.9
Whole blood 964.7	E858.2	E934.7		E950.4	E962.0	E980.4
Wild						
black cherry 988.2	E865.4	—		E950.9	E962.1	E980.9
poisonous plants NEC 988.2	E865.4	—		E950.9	E962.1	E980.9
Window cleaning fluid 989.89	E861.3	—		E950.9	E962.1	E980.9
Wintergreen (oil) 976.3	E858.7	E946.3		E950.4	E962.0	E980.4
Witch hazel 976.2	E858.7	E946.2		E950.4	E962.0	E980.4
Wood						
alcohol 980.1	E860.2	—		E950.9	E962.1	E980.9
spirit 980.1	E860.2	—		E950.9	E962.1	E980.9
Woorali 975.2	E858.6	E945.2		E950.4	E962.0	E980.4
Wormseed, American 961.6	E857	E931.6		E950.4	E962.0	E980.4
Xanthine diuretics 974.1	E858.5	E944.1		E950.4	E962.0	E980.4

Substance	External Cause (E-Code)					
	Poisoning	Accident	Therapeutic Use	Suicide Attempt	Assault	Undetermined
Xanthocillin	960.0	E856	E930.0	E950.4	E962.0	E980.4
Xanthotoxin	976.3	E858.7	E946.3	E950.4	E962.0	E980.4
Xylene (liquid) (vapor)	982.0	E862.4	—	E950.9	E962.1	E980.9
Xylocaine (infiltration) (topical)	968.5	E855.2	E938.5	E950.4	E962.0	E980.4
nerve block (peripheral) (plexus)	968.6	E855.2	E938.6	E950.4	E962.0	E980.4
spinal	968.7	E855.2	E938.7	E950.4	E962.0	E980.4
Xylol (liquid) (vapor)	982.0	E862.4	—	E950.9	E962.1	E980.9
Xylometazoline	971.2	E855.5	E941.2	E950.4	E962.0	E980.4
Yellow						
fever vaccine	979.3	E858.8	E949.3	E950.4	E962.0	E980.4
jasmine	988.2	E865.4	—	E950.9	E962.1	E980.9
Yew	988.2	E865.4	—	E950.9	E962.1	E980.9
Zactane	965.7	E850.7	E935.7	E950.0	E962.0	E980.0
Zaroxolyn	974.3	E858.5	E944.3	E950.4	E962.0	E980.4
Zephiran (topical)	976.0	E858.7	E946.0	E950.4	E962.0	E980.4
ophthalmic preparation	976.5	E858.7	E946.5	E950.4	E962.0	E980.4
Zerone	980.1	E860.2	—	E950.9	E962.1	E980.9
Zinc (compounds) (fumes) (salts)						
(vapor) NEC	985.8	E866.4	—	E950.9	E962.1	E980.9
anti–infectives	976.0	E858.7	E946.0	E950.4	E962.0	E980.4
antivaricose	972.7	E858.3	E942.7	E950.4	E962.0	E980.4
bacitracin	976.0	E858.7	E946.0	E950.4	E962.0	E980.4
chloride	976.2	E858.7	E946.2	E950.4	E962.0	E980.4
gelatin	976.3	E858.7	E946.3	E950.4	E962.0	E980.4
oxide	976.3	E858.7	E946.3	E950.4	E962.0	E980.4
peroxide	976.0	E858.7	E946.0	E950.4	E962.0	E980.4
pesticides	985.8	E863.4	—	E950.6	E962.1	E980.7
phosphide (rodenticide)	985.8	E863.7	—	E950.6	E962.1	E980.7
stearate	976.3	E858.7	E946.3	E950.4	E962.0	E980.4
sulfate (antivaricose)	972.7	E858.3	E942.7	E950.4	E962.0	E980.4
ENT agent	976.6	E858.7	E946.6	E950.4	E962.0	E980.4
ophthalmic solution	976.5	E858.7	E946.5	E950.4	E962.0	E980.4
topical NEC	976.0	E858.7	E946.0	E950.4	E962.0	E980.4
undecylenate	976.0	E858.7	E946.0	E950.4	E962.0	E980.4
Zoxazolamine	968.0	E855.1	E938.0	E950.4	E962.0	E980.4
Zygadenus (venenosus)	988.2	E865.4	—	E950.9	E962.1	E980.9

Substance	External Cause (E-Code)					
	Poisoning	Accident	Therapeutic Use	Suicide Attempt	Assault	Undetermined

SECTION 3

ALPHABETIC INDEX TO EXTERNAL CAUSES
OF INJURY AND POISONING (E CODE)

This section contains the index to the codes which classify environmental events, circumstances, and other conditions as the cause of injury and other adverse effects. Where a code from the section Supplementary Classification of External Causes of Injury and Poisoning (E800-E998) is applicable, it is intended that the E code shall be used in addition to a code form the main body of the classification, Chapters 1-17.

The alphabetic index to the E codes is organized by main terms which describe the *accident, circumstance, event,* or specific *agent* which caused the injury or other adverse effect.

> *Note—Transport accidents (E800-E848) include accidents involving:*
> *aircraft and space craft (E840-E845)*
> *watercraft (E830-E838)*
> *motor vehicle (E810-E825)*
> *railway (E800-E807)*
> *other road vehicles (E826-E829)*

> *For definitions and examples related to transport accidents—see Volume 1, pages 571-585.*

> *The fourth-digit subdivisions for use with categories E800-E848 to identify the injured person are found on pages 1447-1451.*

> *For identifying the place in which an accident or poisoning occurred (circumstances classifiable to categories E850-E869 and E880-E928)— see the listing in this section under "Accident, occurring."*

See the Table of Drugs and Chemicals (Section 2 of this volume) for identifying the specific agent involved in drug overdose or a wrong substance given or taken in error, and for intoxication or poisoning by a drug or other chemical substance.

The specific adverse effect, reaction, or localized toxic effect to a correct drug or substance properly administered in therapeutic or prophylactic dosage should be classified according to the nature of the adverse effect (e.g.: allergy, dermatitis, tachycardia) listed in Section 1 of this volume.

A

Abandonment
causing exposure to weather conditions—*see*
  Exposure
child, with intent to injure or kill E968.4
helpless person, infant, newborn E904.0
  with intent to injure or kill E968.4
Abortion, criminal, injury to child E968.8
Abuse, (alleged) (suspected)
adult
  by
    child E967.4
    ex-partner E967.3
    ex-spouse E967.3
    father E967.0
    grandchild E967.7
    grandparent E967.6
    mother E967.2
    non-related caregiver E967.8
    other relative E967.7
    other specified person(s) E967.1
    partner E967.3
    sibling E967.5
    spouse E967.3
    stepfather E967.0
    stepmother E967.2
    unspecified person E967.9
child
  by
    boyfriend of parent or guardian E967.0
    child E967.4
    father E967.0
    female partner of parent or guardian
      E967.2
    girlfriend of parent or guardian E967.2
    grandchild E967.7
    grandparent E967.6
    male partner of parent or guardian E967.0
    mother E967.2
    non-related caregiver E967.8
    other relative E967.7
    other specified person(s) E967.1
    sibling E967.5
    stepfather E967.0
    stepmother E967.2
    unspecified person E967.9
Accident (to) E928.9
aircraft (in transit) (powered) E841
  at landing, take-off E840
  due to, caused by cataclysm—*see*
    categories E908, E909
  late effect of E929.1
  unpowered (*see also* Collision, aircraft,
    unpowered) E842
  while alighting, boarding E843
amphibious vehicle
  on
    land—*see* Accident, motor vehicle
    water—*see* Accident, watercraft
animal, ridden NEC E828
animal-drawn vehicle NEC E827
balloon (*see also* Collision, aircraft,
  unpowered) E842
caused by, due to
  abrasive wheel (metalworking) E919.3
  animal NEC E906.9
    being ridden (in sport or transport) E828
  avalanche NEC E909.2
  band saw E919.4
  bench saw E919.4

Accident—*continued*
bore, earth-drilling or mining (land)
  (seabed) E919.1
bulldozer E919.7
cataclysmic
  earth surface movement or eruption E909.9
  storm E908.9
chain
  hoist E919.2
    agricultural operations E919.0
    mining operations E919.1
  saw E920.1
circular saw E919.4
cold (excessive) (*see also* Cold, exposure
  to) E901.9
combine E919.0
conflagration—*see* Conflagration
corrosive liquid, substance NEC E924.1
cotton gin E919.8
crane E919.2
  agricultural operations E919.0
  mining operations E919.1
cutting or piercing instrument (*see also*
  Cut) E920.9
dairy equipment E919.8
derrick E919.2
  agricultural operations E919.0
  mining operations E919.1
drill E920.1
  earth (land) (seabed) E919.1
  hand (powered) E920.1
    not powered E920.4
  metalworking E919.3
  woodworking E919.4
earth(-)
  drilling machine E919.1
  moving machine E919.7
  scraping machine E919.7
electric
  current (*see also* Electric shock) E925.9
  motor—*see also* Accident, machine, by
    type of machine
    current (of)—*see* Electric shock
elevator (building) (grain) E919.2
  agricultural operations E919.0
  mining operations E919.1
environmental factors NEC E928.9
excavating machine E919.7
explosive material (*see also* Explosion)
  E923.9
farm machine E919.0
fire, flames—*see also* Fire
  conflagration—*see* Conflagration
firearm missile—*see* Shooting
forging (metalworking) machine E919.3
forklift (truck) E919.2
  agricultural operations E919.0
  mining operations E919.1
gas turbine E919.5
harvester E919.0
hay derrick, mower, or rake E919.0
heat (excessive) (*see also* Heat) E900.9
hoist (*see also* Accident, caused by, due
  to, lift) E919.2
  chain—*see* Accident, caused by, due to,
    chain
  shaft E919.1

Accident—*continued*
  hot
    liquid E924.0
      caustic or corrosive E924.1
      object (not producing fire or flames)
        E924.8
    substance E924.9
      caustic or corrosive E924.1
      liquid (metal) NEC E924.0
      specified type NEC E924.8
  human bite E928.3
  ignition—*see* Ignition
  internal combustion engine E919.5
  landslide NEC E909.2
  lathe (metalworking) E919.3
    turnings E920.8
    woodworking E919.4
  lift, lifting (appliances) E919.2
    agricultural operations E919.0
    mining operations E919.1
    shaft E919.1
  lightning NEC E907
  machine, machinery—*see also* Accident,
    machine
    drilling, metal E919.3
    manufacturing, for manufacture of
      beverages E919.8
      clothing E919.8
      foodstuffs E919.8
      paper E919.8
      textiles E919.8
    milling, metal E919.3
    moulding E919.4
    power press, metal E919.3
    printing E919.8
    rolling mill, metal E919.3
    sawing, metal E919.3
    specified type NEC E919.8
    spinning E919.8
    weaving E919.8
  natural factor NEC E928.9
  overhead plane E919.4
  plane E920.4
    overhead E919.4
  powered
    hand tool NEC E920.1
    saw E919.4
      hand E920.1
  printing machine E919.8
  pulley (block) E919.2
    agricultural operations E919.0
    mining operations E919.1
    transmission E919.6
  radial saw E919.4
  radiation—*see* Radiation
  reaper E919.0
  road scraper E919.7
    when in transport under its own
      power—*see* categories E810—E825
  roller coaster E919.8
  sander E919.4
  saw E920.4
    band E919.4
    bench E919.4
    chain E920.1
    circular E919.4
    hand E920.4
      powered E920.1
    powered, except hand E919.4
    radial E919.4
  sawing machine, metal E919.3

Accident—*continued*
  shaft
    hoist E919.1
    lift E919.1
    transmission E919.6
  shears E920.4
    hand E920.4
      powered E920.1
    mechanical E919.3
  shovel E920.4
    steam E919.7
  spinning machine E919.8
  steam—*see also* Burning, steam
    engine E919.5
    shovel E919.7
  thresher E919.0
  thunderbolt NEC E907
  tractor E919.0
    when in transport under its own
      power—*see* categories E810-E825
  transmission belt, cable, chain, gear,
    pinion, pulley, shaft E919.6
  turbine (gas) (water driven) E919.5
  under-cutter E919.1
  weaving machine E919.8
  winch E919.2
    agricultural operations E919.0
    mining operations E919.1
  diving E883.0
    with insufficient air supply E913.2
  glider (hang) (*see also* Collision, aircraft,
    unpowered) E842
  hovercraft
    on
      land—*see* Accident, motor vehicle
      water—*see* Accident, watercraft
  ice yacht (*see also* Accident, vehicle NEC)
    E848
  in
    medical, surgical procedure
      as, or due to misadventure—*see*
        Misadventure
      causing an abnormal reaction or later
        complication without mention of
        misadventure—*see* Reaction, abnormal
  kite carrying a person (*see also* Collision,
    aircraft, unpowered) E842
  land yacht (*see also* Accident, vehicle NEC)
    E848
  late effect of—*see* Late effect
  launching pad E845
  machine, machinery (*see also* Accident,
    caused by, due to, by specific type of
    machine) E919.9
    agricultural including animal-powered
      E919.0
    earth-drilling E919.1
    earth moving or scraping E919.7
    excavating E919.7
    involving transport under own power on
      highway or transport vehicle—*see*
      categories E810-E825, E840-E845
    lifting (appliances) E919.2
    metalworking E919.3
    mining E919.1
    prime movers, except electric motors
      E919.5
      electric motors—*see* Accident, machine,
        by specific type of machine
    recreational E919.8
    specified type NEC E919.8

Accident—*continued*
  transmission E919.6
  watercraft (deck) (engine room) (galley)
      (laundry) (loading) E836
  woodworking or forming E919.4
  motor vehicle (on public highway) (traffic)
      E819
    due to cataclysm—*see* categories E908,
        E909
    involving
      collision (*see also* Collision, motor
          vehicle) E812
      nontraffic, not on public highway—*see*
          categories E820-E825
      not involving collision—*see* categories
          E816-E819
  nonmotor vehicle NEC E829
  nonroad—*see* Accident, vehicle NEC
  road, except pedal cycle, animal-drawn
      vehicle, or animal being ridden E829
  nonroad vehicle NEC—*see* Accident, vehicle
      NEC
  not elsewhere classifiable involving
    cable car (not on rails) E847
      on rails E829
    coal car in mine E846
    hand truck—*see* Accident, vehicle NEC
    logging car E846
    sled(ge), meaning snow or ice vehicle
        E848
    tram, mine or quarry E846
    truck
      mine or quarry E846
      self-propelled, industrial E846
      station baggage E846
    tub, mine or quarry E846
    vehicle NEC E848
      snow and ice E848
      used only on industrial premises E846
    wheelbarrow E848
  occurring (at) (in)
    apartment E849.0
    baseball field, diamond E849.4
    construction site, any E849.3
    dock E849.8
      yard E849.3
    dormitory E849.7
    factory (building) (premises) E849.3
    farm E849.1
      buildings E849.1
      house E849.0
    football field E849.4
    forest E849.8
    garage (place of work) E849.3
      private (home) E849.0
    gravel pit E849.2
    gymnasium E849.4
    highway E849.5
    home (private) (residential) E849.0
      institutional E849.7
    hospital E849.7
    hotel E849.6
    house (private) (residential) E849.0
      movie E849.6
      public E849.6
    institution, residential E849.7
    jail E849.7
    mine E849.2
    motel E849.6
    movie house E849.6
    office (building) E849.6

Accident—*continued*
    orphanage E849.7
    park (public) E849.4
      mobile home E849.8
      trailer E849.8
    parking lot or place E849.8
    place
      industrial NEC E849.3
      parking E849.8
      public E849.8
        specified place NEC E849.5
      recreational NEC E849.4
      sport NEC E849.4
    playground (park) (school) E849.4
    prison E849.6
    public building NEC E849.6
    quarry E849.2
    railway
      line NEC E849.8
      yard E849.3
    residence
      home (private) E849.0
    resort (beach) (lake) (mountain)
        (seashore) (vacation) E849.4
    restaurant E849.6
    sand pit E849.2
    school (building) (private) (public) (state)
        E849.6
      reform E849.7
      riding E849.4
    seashore E849.8
      resort E849.4
    shop (place of work) E849.3
      commercial E849.6
    skating rink E849.4
    sports palace E849.4
    stadium E849.4
    store E849.6
    street E849.5
    swimming pool (public) E849.4
      private home or garden E849.0
    tennis court E849.4
    theatre, theater E849.6
    trailer court E849.8
    tunnel E849.8
      under construction E849.2
    warehouse E849.3
    yard
      dock E849.3
      industrial E849.3
      private (home) E849.0
      railway E849.3
  off-road type motor vehicle (not on public
      highway) NEC E821
    on public highway—*see* categories
        E810-E819
  pedal cycle E826
  railway E807
    due to cataclysm—*see* categories E908,
        E909
    involving
      avalanche E909.2
      burning by engine, locomotive, train (*see
          also* Explosion, railway engine) E803
      collision (*see also* Collision, railway) E800
      derailment (*see also* Derailment, railway)
          E802
      explosion (*see also* Explosion, railway
          engine) E803
      fall (*see also* Fall, from, railway rolling
          stock) E804

Accident—*continued*
    fire (*see also* Explosion, railway engine)
        E803
    hitting by, being struck by
      object falling in, on, from, rolling stock,
        train, vehicle E806
      rolling stock, train, vehicle E805
    overturning, railway rolling stock, train,
      vehicle (*see also* Derailment, railway)
      E802
    running off rails, railway (*see also*
      Derailment, railway) E802
    specified circumstances NEC E806
    train or vehicle hit by
      avalanche E909
      falling object (earth, rock, tree) E806
        due to cataclysm—*see* categories
          E908, E909
      landslide E909
  roller skate E885.1
  scooter (nonmotorized) E885.0
  skateboard E885.2
  ski(ing) E885.3
   jump E884.9
   lift or tow (with chair or gondola) E847
  snowboard E885.4
  snow vehicle, motor driven (not on public
    highway) E820
   on public highway—*see* categories
    E810-E819
  spacecraft E845
  specified cause NEC E928.8
  street car E829
  traffic NEC E819
  vehicle NEC (with pedestrian) E848
   battery powered
    airport passenger vehicle E846
    truck (baggage) (mail) E846
   powered commercial or industrial (with
    other vehicle or object within
    commercial or industrial premises)
    E846
  watercraft E838
   with
    drowning or submersion resulting from
      accident other than to watercraft E832
      accident to watercraft E830
    injury, except drowning or submersion,
      resulting from
      accident other than to watercraft—*see*
        categories E833-E838
      accident to watercraft E831
   due to, caused by cataclysm—*see*
    categories E908, E909
  machinery E836
Acid throwing E961
Acosta syndrome E902.0
Aeroneurosis E902.1
Aero-otitis media —*see* Effects of, air pressure
Aerosinusitis —*see* Effects of, air pressure
After-effect, late —*see* Late effect
Air
  blast
   in
    terrorism E979.2
    war operations E993
  embolism (traumatic) NEC E928.9
   in
    infusion or transfusion E874.1
    perfusion E874.2
  sickness E903
Alpine sickness E902.0

Altitude sickness —*see* Effects of, air pressure
Anaphylactic shock, anaphylaxis (*see also*
    Table of drugs and chemicals) E947.9
  due to bite or sting (venomous)—*see* Bite,
    venomous
Andes disease E902.0
Apoplexy heat—*see* Heat
Arachnidism E905.1
Arson E968.0
Asphyxia, asphyxiation
  by
   chemical
    in
      terrorism E979.7
      war operations E997.2
   explosion—*see* Explosion
   food (bone) (regurgitated food) (seed)
    E911
   foreign object, except food E912
   fumes
    in
      terrorism E979.7
      war operations E997.2
   gas—*see also* Table of drugs and
    chemicals
    in
      terrorism E979.7
      war operations E997.2
    legal
      execution E978
      intervention (tear) E972
    tear E972
   mechanical means (*see also* Suffocation)
    E913.9
  from
   conflagration—*see* Conflagration
   fire—*see also* Fire E899
    in
      terrorism E979.3
      war operations E990.9
   ignition—*see* Ignition
Aspiration
  foreign body—*see* Foreign body, aspiration
  mucus, not of newborn (with asphyxia,
    obstruction respiratory passage,
    suffocation) E912
  phlegm (with asphyxia, obstruction respiratory
    passage, suffocation) E912
  vomitus (with asphyxia, obstruction
    respiratory passage, suffocation) (*see also*
    Foreign body, aspiration, food) E911
Assassination (attempt) (*see also* Assault)
    E968.9
Assault (homicidal) (by) (in) E968.9
  acid E961
   swallowed E962.1
  air gun E968.6
  BB gun E968.6
  bite NEC E968.8
   of human being E968.7
  bomb ((placed in) car or house) E965.8
   antipersonnel E965.5
   letter E965.7
   petrol E965.7
  brawl (hand) (fists) (foot) E960.0
  burning, burns (by fire) E968.0
   acid E961
    swallowed E962.1
   caustic, corrosive substance E961
    swallowed E962.1

Assault—*continued*
   chemical from swallowing caustic,
      corrosive substance NEC E962.1
     hot liquid E968.3
     scalding E968.3
     vitriol E961
      swallowed E962.1
   caustic, corrosive substance E961
     swallowed E962.1
   cut, any part of body E966
   dagger E966
   drowning E964
   explosive(s) E965.9
     bomb (*see also* Assault, bomb) E965.8
     dynamite E965.8
   fight (hand) (fists) (foot) E960.0
     with weapon E968.9
      blunt or thrown E968.2
      cutting or piercing E966
      firearm—*see* Shooting, homicide
   fire E968.0
   firearm(s)—*see* Shooting, homicide
   garrotting E963
   gunshot (wound)—*see* Shooting, homicide
   hanging E963
   injury NEC E968.9
   knife E966
   late effect of E969
   ligature E963
   poisoning E962.9
     drugs or medicinals E962.0
     gas(es) or vapors, except drugs and
      medicinals E962.2
     solid or liquid substances, except drugs
      and medicinals E962.1
   puncture, any part of body E966
   pushing
     before moving object, train, vehicle
      E968.5
     from high place E968.1
   rape E960.1
   scalding E968.3
   shooting—*see* Shooting, homicide
   sodomy E960.1
   stab, any part of body E966
   strangulation E963
   submersion E964
   suffocation E963
   transport vehicle E968.5
   violence NEC E968.9
   vitriol E961
     swallowed E962.1
   weapon E968.9
     blunt or thrown E968.2
     cutting or piercing E966
     firearm—*see* Shooting, homicide
   wound E968.9
     cutting E966
     gunshot—*see* Shooting, homicide
     knife E966
     piercing E966
     puncture E966
     stab E966
Attack by animal NEC E906.9
Avalanche E909.2
   falling on or hitting
     motor vehicle (in motion) (on public
      highway) E909.2
     railway train E909.2
Aviators' disease E902.1

B

Barotitis, barodontalgia, barosinusitis,
   barotrauma (otitic) (sinus)—*see* Effects of,
   air pressure
Battered
   baby or child (syndrome)—*see* Abuse, child;
     category E967
   person other than baby or child—*see* Assault
Bayonet wound (*see also* Cut, by bayonet)
   E920.3
   in
     legal intervention E974
     terrorism E979.8
     war operations E995
Bean in nose E912
Bed set on fire NEC E898.0
Beheading (by guillotine)
   homicide E966
   legal execution E978
Bending, injury in E927
Bends E902.0
Bite
   animal (nonvenomous) NEC E906.5
     venomous NEC E905.9
   arthropod (nonvenomous) NEC E906.4
     venomous—*see* Sting
   black widow spider E905.1
   cat E906.3
   centipede E905.4
   cobra E905.0
   copperhead snake E905.0
   coral snake E905.0
   dog E906.0
   fer de lance E905.0
   gila monster E905.0
   human being
     accidental E928.3
     assault E968.7
   insect (nonvenomous) E906.4
     venomous—*see* Sting
   krait E905.0
   late effect of—*see* Late effect
   lizard E906.2
     venomous E905.0
   mamba E905.0
   marine animal
     nonvenomous E906.3
      snake E906.2
     venomous E905.6
      snake E905.0
   millipede E906.4
     venomous E905.4
   moray eel E906.3
   rat E906.1
   rattlesnake E905.0
   rodent, except rat E906.3
   serpent—*see* Bite, snake
   shark E906.3
   snake (venomous) E905.0
     nonvenomous E906.2
     sea E905.0
   spider E905.1
     nonvenomous E906.4
   tarantula (venomous) E905.1
   venomous NEC E905.9
     by specific animal—*see* category E905
   viper E905.0
   water moccasin E905.0

Blast (air)
from nuclear explosion E996
in
  terrorism E979.2
    from nuclear explosion E979.5
    underwater E979.0
  war operations E993
    from nuclear explosion E996
    underwater E992
  underwater E992
Blizzard E908.3
Blow E928.9
by law-enforcing agent, police (on duty) E975
  with blunt object (baton) (nightstick)
    (stave) (truncheon) E973
Blowing up (*see also* Explosion) E923.9
Brawl (hand) (fists) (foot) E960.0
Breakage (accidental)
cable of cable car not on rails E847
ladder (causing fall) E881.0
part (any) of
  animal-drawn vehicle E827
  ladder (causing fall) E881.0
  motor vehicle
    in motion (on public highway) E818
      not on public highway E825
  nonmotor road vehicle, except
    animal-drawn vehicle or pedal cycle
    E829
  off-road type motor vehicle (not on
    public highway) NEC E821
    on public highway E818
  pedal cycle E826
  scaffolding (causing fall) E881.1
  snow vehicle, motor-driven (not on public
    highway) E820
    on public highway E818
  vehicle NEC—*see* Accident, vehicle
Broken
glass
  fall on E888.0
  injury by E920.8
power line (causing electric shock) E925.1
Bumping against, into (accidentally)
object (moving) E917.9
  caused by crowd E917.1
    with subsequent fall E917.6
  furniture E917.3
    with subsequent fall E917.7
  in
    running water E917.2
    sports E917.0
      with subsequent fall E917.5
  stationary E917.4
    with subsequent fall E917.8
person(s) E917.9
  with fall E886.9
    in sports E886.0
  as, or caused by, a crowd E917.1
    with subsequent fall E917.6
  in sports E917.0
    with fall E886.0
Burning, burns (accidental) (by) (from) (on)
E899
acid (any kind) E924.1
  swallowed—*see* Table of drugs and
    chemicals
bedclothes (*see also* Fire, specified NEC)
  E898.0
blowlamp (*see also* Fire, specified NEC)
  E898.1

Burning, burns—*continued*
blowtorch (*see also* Fire, specified NEC)
  E898.1
boat, ship, watercraft—*see* categories E830,
  E831, E837
bonfire (controlled) E897
  uncontrolled E892
candle (*see also* Fire, specified NEC) E898.1
caustic liquid, substance E924.1
  swallowed—*see* Table of drugs and
    chemicals
chemical E924.1
  from swallowing caustic, corrosive
    substance—*see* Table of drugs and
    chemicals
  in
    terrorism E979.7
    war operations E997.2
cigar(s) or cigarette(s) (*see also* Fire,
  specified NEC) E898.1
clothes, clothing, nightdress—*see* Ignition,
  clothes
  with conflagration—*see* Conflagration
conflagration—*see* Conflagration
corrosive liquid, substance E924.1
  swallowed—*see* Table of drugs and
    chemicals
electric current (*see also* Electric shock)
  E925.9
fire, flames (*see also* Fire) E899
flare, Verey pistol E922.8
heat
  from appliance (electrical) E924.8
  in local application or packing during
    medical or surgical procedure E873.5
homicide (attempt) (*see also* Assault, burning)
  E968.0
hot
  liquid E924.0
    caustic or corrosive E924.1
  object (not producing fire or flames)
    E924.8
  substance E924.9
    caustic or corrosive E924.1
    liquid (metal) NEC E924.0
    specified type NEC E924.8
  tap water E924.2
ignition—*see also* Ignition
  clothes, clothing, nightdress—*see also*
    Ignition, clothes
    with conflagration—*see* Conflagration
  highly inflammable material (benzine)
    (fat) (gasoline) (kerosine) (paraffin)
    (petrol) E894
in
  terrorism E979.3
    from nuclear explosion E979.5
    petrol bomb E979.3
  war operations (from fire-producing
    device or conventional weapon)
    E990.9
    from nuclear explosion E996
    petrol bomb E990.0
inflicted by other person
  stated as
    homicidal, intentional (*see also* Assault,
      burning) E968.0
    undetermined whether accidental or
      intentional (*see also* Burn, stated as
      undetermined whether accidental or
      intentional) E988.1

Burning, burns—*continued*
internal, from swallowed caustic, corrosive
liquid, substance—*see* Table of drugs and
chemicals
lamp (*see also* Fire, specified NEC) E898.1
late effect of NEC E929.4
lighter (cigar) (cigarette) (*see also* Fire,
specified NEC) E898.1
lightning E907
liquid (boiling) (hot) (molten) E924.0
caustic, corrosive (external) E924.1
swallowed—*see* Table of drugs and
chemicals
local application of externally applied
substance in medical or surgical care
E873.5
machinery—*see* Accident, machine
matches (*see also* Fire, specified NEC) E898.1
medicament, externally applied E873.5
metal, molten E924.0
object (hot) E924.8
producing fire or flames—*see* Fire
oven (electric) (gas) E924.8
pipe (smoking) (*see also* Fire, specified NEC)
E898.1
radiation—*see* Radiation
railway engine, locomotive, train (*see also*
Explosion, railway engine) E803
self-inflicted (unspecified whether accidental
or intentional) E988.1
caustic or corrosive substance NEC
E988.7
stated as intentional, purposeful E958.1
caustic or corrosive substance NEC E958.7
stated as undetermined whether accidental or
intentional E988.1
caustic or corrosive substance NEC
E988.7
steam E924.0
pipe E924.8
substance (hot) E924.9
boiling or molten E924.0
caustic, corrosive (external) E924.1
swallowed—*see* Table of drugs and
chemicals
suicidal (attempt) NEC E958.1
caustic substance E958.7
late effect of E959
tanning bed E926.2
therapeutic misadventure
overdose of radiation E873.2
torch, welding (*see also* Fire, specified NEC)
E898.1
trash fire (*see also* Burning, bonfire) E897
vapor E924.0
vitriol E924.1
x-rays E926.3
in medical, surgical procedure—*see*
Misadventure, failure, in dosage,
radiation
Butted by animal E906.8

C

Cachexia, lead or saturnine E866.0
from pesticide NEC (*see also* Table of drugs
and chemicals) E863.4
Caisson disease E902.2
Capital punishment (any means) E978
Car sickness E903

Casualty (not due to war) NEC E928.9
terrorism E979.8
war (*see also* War operations) E995
Cat
bite E906.3
scratch E906.8
Cataclysmic (any injury)
earth surface movement or eruption E909.9
specified type NEC E909.8
storm or flood resulting from storm E908.9
specified type NEC E909.8
Catching fire —*see* Ignition
Caught
between
objects (moving) (stationary and moving)
E918
and machinery—*see* Accident, machine
by cable car, not on rails E847
in
machinery (moving parts of)—*see*
Accident, machine
object E918
Cave-in (causing asphyxia, suffocation (by
pressure)) (*see also* Suffocation, due to,
cave-in) E913.3
with injury other than asphyxia or suffocation
E916
with asphyxia or suffocation (*see also*
Suffocation, due to, cave-in) E913.3
struck or crushed by E916
with asphyxia or suffocation (*see also*
Suffocation, due to, cave-in) E913.3
Change(s) in air pressure—*see also* Effects of,
air pressure
sudden, in aircraft (ascent) (descent) (causing
aeroneurosis or aviators' disease) E902.1
Chilblains E901.0
due to manmade conditions E901.1
Choking (on) (any object except food or
vomitus) E912
apple E911
bone E911
food, any type (regurgitated) E911
mucus or phlegm E912
seed E911
Civil insurrection —*see* War operations
Cloudburst E908.8
Cold, exposure to (accidental) (excessive)
(extreme) (place) E901.9
causing chilblains or immersion foot E901.0
due to
manmade conditions E901.1
specified cause NEC E901.8
weather (conditions) E901.0
late effect of NEC E929.5
self-inflicted (undetermined whether
accidental or intentional) E988.3
suicidal E958.3
suicide E958.3
Colic, lead, painters', or saturnine —*see*
category E866
Collapse
building E916 (movable)
burning (uncontrolled fire) E891.8
in terrorism E979.3
private E890.8
dam E909.3
due to heat—*see* Heat
machinery—*see* Accident, machine
man-made structure E909.3
postoperative NEC E878.9

Collapse—*continued*
structure, burning NEC E891.8
burning (uncontrolled fire)
in terrorism E979.3
Collision (accidental)

> *Note—In the case of collisions between different types of vehicles, persons and objects, priority in classification is in the following order:*
>
> *Aircraft*
> *Watercraft*
> *Motor vehicle*
> *Railway vehicle*
> *Pedal Cycle*
> *Animal-drawn vehicle*
> *Animal being ridden*
> *Streetcar or other nonmotor road vehicle*
> *Other vehicle*
> *Pedestrian or person using pedestrian conveyance*
> *Object (except where falling from or set in motion by vehicle etc. listed above)*
>
> *In the listing below, the combinations are listed only under the vehicle etc. having priority. For definitions, see Volume 1, page 477.*

aircraft (with object or vehicle) (fixed) (movable) (moving) E841
with
person (while landing, taking off) (without accident to aircraft) E844
powered (in transit) (with unpowered aircraft) E841
while landing, taking off E840
unpowered E842
while landing, taking off E840
animal being ridden (in sport or transport) E828
and
animal (being ridden) (herded) (unattended) E828
nonmotor road vehicle, except pedal cycle or animal-drawn vehicle E828
object (fallen) (fixed) (movable) (moving) not falling from or set in motion by vehicle of higher priority E828
pedestrian (conveyance or vehicle) E828
animal-drawn vehicle E827
and
animal (being ridden) (herded) (unattended) E827
nonmotor road vehicle, except pedal cycle E827
object (fallen) (fixed) (movable) (moving) not falling from or set in motion by vehicle of higher priority E827
pedestrian (conveyance or vehicle) E827
streetcar E827
motor vehicle (on public highway) (traffic accident) E812
after leaving, running off, public highway (without antecedent collision) (without re-entry) E816
with antecedent collision on public highway—*see* categories E810-E815
with re-entrance collision with another motor vehicle E811
and
abutment (bridge) (overpass) E815
animal (herded) (unattended) E815

Collision—*continued*
carrying person, property E813
animal-drawn vehicle E813
another motor vehicle (abandoned) (disabled) (parked) (stalled) (stopped) E812
with, involving re-entrance (on same roadway) (across median strip) E811
any object, person, or vehicle off the public highway resulting from a noncollision motor vehicle nontraffic accident E816
avalanche, fallen or not moving E815
falling E909
boundary fence E815
culvert E815
fallen
stone E815
tree E815
falling E909.2
guard post or guard rail E815
inter-highway divider E815
landslide, fallen or not moving E815
moving E909
machinery (road) E815
moving E909.2
nonmotor road vehicle NEC E813
object (any object, person, or vehicle off the public highway resulting from a noncollision motor vehicle nontraffic accident) E815
off, normally not on, public highway resulting from a noncollision motor vehicle traffic accident E816
pedal cycle E813
pedestrian (conveyance) E814
person (using pedestrian conveyance) E814
post or pole (lamp) (light) (signal) (telephone) (utility) E815
railway rolling stock, train, vehicle E810
safety island E815
street car E813
traffic signal, sign, or marker (temporary) E815
tree E815
tricycle E813
wall of cut made for road E815
due to cataclysm—*see* categories E908, E909
not on public highway, nontraffic accident E822
and
animal (carrying person, property) (herded) (unattended) E822
animal-drawn vehicle E822
another motor vehicle (moving), except off-road motor vehicle E822
stationary E823
avalanche, fallen, not moving E823
moving E909
landslide, fallen, not moving E823
moving E909
nonmotor vehicle (moving) E822
stationary E823
object (fallen) (normally) (fixed) (movable but not in motion) (stationary) E823
moving, except when falling from, set in motion by, aircraft or cataclysm E822
pedal cycle (moving) E822

Collision—*continued*

 stationary E823
 pedestrian (conveyance) E822
 person (using pedestrian conveyance)
  E822
 railway rolling stock, train, vehicle
  (moving) E822
  stationary E823
 road vehicle (any) (moving) E822
  stationary E823
 tricycle (moving) E822
  stationary E823
 moving E909.2
off-road type motor vehicle (not on public
 highway) E821
and
 animal (being ridden) (-drawn vehicle)
  E821
 another off-road motor vehicle, except
  snow vehicle E821
 other motor vehicle, not on public
  highway E821
 other object or vehicle NEC, fixed or
  movable, not set in motion by aircraft,
  motor vehicle on highway, or snow
  vehicle, motor-driven E821
 pedal cycle E821
 pedestrian (conveyance) E821
 railway train E821
on public highway—*see* Collision, motor
 vehicle
pedal cycle E826
and
 animal (carrying person, property)
  (herded) (unherded) E826
 animal-drawn vehicle E826
 another pedal cycle E826
 nonmotor road vehicle E826
 object (fallen) (fixed) (movable) (moving)
  not falling from or set in motion by
  aircraft, motor vehicle, or railway train
  NEC E826
 pedestrian (conveyance) E826
 person (using pedestrian conveyance) E826
 street car E826
pedestrian(s) (conveyance) E917.9
 with fall E886.9
  in sports E886.0
 and
  crowd, human stampede E917.1
   with subsequent fall E917.6
  furniture E917.3
   with subsequent fall E917.7
  machinery—*see* Accident, machine
  object (fallen) (moving) not falling from
   or set in motion by any vehicle
   classifiable to E800-E848, E917.9
   caused by a crowd E917.1
    with subsequent fall E917.6
   furniture E917.3
    with subsequent fall E917.7
  in
   running water E917.2
    with drowning or submersion—*see*
     Submersion
   sports E917.0
    with subsequent fall E917.5
   stationary E917.4
    with subsequent fall E917.8
  vehicle, nonmotor, nonroad E848

Collision—*continued*

in
 running water E917.2
  with drowning or submersion—*see*
   Submersion
 sports E917.0
  with fall E886.0
person(s) (using pedestrian conveyance) (*see
 also* Collision, pedestrian) E917.9
railway (rolling stock) (train) (vehicle) (with
 (subsequent) derailment, explosion, fall or
 fire) E800
 with antecedent derailment E802
 and
  animal (carrying person) (herded)
   (unattended) E801
  another railway train or vehicle E800
  buffers E801
  fallen tree on railway E801
  farm machinery, nonmotor (in transport)
   (stationary) E801
  gates E801
  nonmotor vehicle E801
  object (fallen) (fixed) (movable) (moving)
   not falling from, set in motion by,
   aircraft or motor vehicle NEC E801
  pedal cycle E801
  pedestrian (conveyance) E805
  person (using pedestrian conveyance) E805
  platform E801
  rock on railway E801
  street car E801
snow vehicle, motor-driven (not on public
 highway) E820
and
 animal (being ridden) (-drawn vehicle)
  E820
 another off-road motor vehicle E820
 other motor vehicle, not on public
  highway E820
 other object or vehicle NEC, fixed or
  movable, not set in motion by aircraft
  or motor vehicle on highway E820
 pedal cycle E820
 pedestrian (conveyance) E820
 railway train E820
on public highway—*see* Collision, motor
 vehicle
street car(s) E829
 and
  animal, herded, not being ridden,
   unattended E829
  nonmotor road vehicle NEC E829
  object (fallen) (fixed) (movable) (moving)
   not falling from or set in motion by
   aircraft, animal-drawn vehicle, animal
   being ridden, motor vehicle, pedal
   cycle, or railway train E829
  pedestrian (conveyance) E829
  person (using pedestrian conveyance) E829
vehicle
 animal-drawn—*see* Collision,
  animal-drawn vehicle
 motor—*see* Collision, motor vehicle
 nonmotor
  nonroad E848
   and
    another nonmotor, nonroad vehicle
     E848

Collision—*continued*

object (fallen) (fixed) (movable)
(moving) not falling from or set in
motion by aircraft, animal-drawn
vehicle, animal being ridden,
motor vehicle, nonmotor road
vehicle, pedal cycle, railway train,
or streetcar E848
road, except animal being ridden,
animal-drawn vehicle, or pedal cycle
E829
and
animal, herded, not being ridden,
unattended E829
another nonmotor road vehicle, except
animal being ridden, animal-drawn
vehicle, or pedal cycle E829
object (fallen) (fixed) (movable)
(moving) not falling from or set in
motion by, aircraft, animal-drawn
vehicle, animal being ridden,
motor vehicle, pedal cycle, or
railway train E829
pedestrian (conveyance) E829
person (using pedestrian conveyance)
E829
vehicle, nonmotor, nonroad E829
watercraft E838
and
person swimming or water skiing E838
causing
drowning, submersion E830
injury except drowning, submersion E831
Combustion, spontaneous —*see* Ignition
**Complication of medical or surgical
procedure or treatment**
as an abnormal reaction—*see* Reaction,
abnormal
delayed, without mention of
misadventure—*see* Reaction, abnormal
due to misadventure—*see* Misadventure
Compression
divers' squeeze E902.2
trachea by
food E911
foreign body, except food E912
Conflagration
building or structure, except private dwelling
(barn) (church) (convalescent or
residential home) (factory) (farm
outbuilding) (hospital) (hotel) (institution)
(educational) (dormitory) (residential)
(school) (shop) (store) (theatre) E891.9
with or causing (injury due to)
accident or injury NEC E891.9
specified circumstance NEC E891.8
burns, burning E891.3
carbon monoxide E891.2
fumes E891.2
polyvinylchloride (PVC) or similar
material E891.1
smoke E891.2
causing explosion E891.0
in terrorism E979.3
not in building or structure E892
private dwelling (apartment) (boarding house)
(camping place) (caravan) (farmhouse)
(home (private)) (house) (lodging house)
(private garage) (rooming house)
(tenement) E890.9

Conflagration—*continued*

with or causing (injury due to)
accident or injury NEC E890.9
specified circumstance NEC E890.8
burns, burning E890.3
carbon monoxide E890.2
fumes E890.2
polyvinylchloride (PVC) or similar
material E890.1
smoke E890.2
causing explosion E890.0
Contact with
dry ice E901.1
liquid air, hydrogen, nitrogen E901.1
Cramp(s)
Heat—*see* Heat
swimmers (*see also* category E910) E910.2
not in recreation or sport E910.3
Cranking (car) (truck) (bus) (engine), injury
by E917.9
Crash
aircraft (in transit) (powered) E841
at landing, take-off E840
in
terrorism E979.1
war operations E994
on runway NEC E840
stated as
homicidal E968.8
suicidal E958.6
undetermined whether accidental or
intentional E988.6
unpowered E842
glider E842
motor vehicle—*see also* Accident, motor
vehicle
homicidal E968.5
suicidal E958.5
undetermined whether accidental or
intentional E988.5
Crushed (accidentally) E928.9
between
boat(s), ship(s), watercraft (and dock or
pier) (without accident to watercraft)
E838
after accident to, or collision, watercraft
E831
objects (moving) (stationary and moving)
E918
by
avalanche NEC E909.2
boat, ship, watercraft after accident to,
collision, watercraft E831
cave-in E916
with asphyxiation or suffocation (*see also*
Suffocation, due to, cave-in) E913.3
crowd, human stampede E917.1
falling
aircraft (*see also* Accident, aircraft) E841
in
terrorism E979.1
war operations E994
earth, material E916
with asphyxiation or suffocation (*see
also* Suffocation, due to, cave-in)
E913.3
object E916
on ship, watercraft E838
while loading, unloading watercraft E838
landslide NEC E909.2
lifeboat after abandoning ship E831

Crushed—*continued*
    machinery—*see* Accident, machine
    railway rolling stock, train, vehicle (part
      of) E805
    street car E829
    vehicle NEC—*see* Accident, vehicle NEC
  in
    machinery—*see* Accident, machine
    object E918
    transport accident—*see* categories
      E800-E848
  late effect of NEC E929.9
Cut, cutting (any part of body) (accidental)
    E920.9
  by
    arrow E920.8
    axe E920.4
    bayonet (*see also* Bayonet wound) E920.3
    blender E920.2
    broken glass E920.8
      following fall E888.0
    can opener E920.4
      powered E920.2
    chisel E920.4
    circular saw E919.4
    cutting or piercing instrument—*see also*
      category E920
      following fall E888.0
      late effect of E929.8
    dagger E920.3
    dart E920.8
    drill—*see* Accident, caused by drill
    edge of stiff paper E920.8
    electric
      beater E920.2
      fan E920.2
      knife E920.2
      mixer E920.2
    fork E920.4
    garden fork E920.4
    hand saw or tool (not powered) E920.4
      powered E920.1
    hedge clipper E920.4
      powered E920.1
    hoe E920.4
    ice pick E920.4
    knife E920.3
      electric E920.2
    lathe turnings E920.8
    lawn mower E920.4
      powered E920.0
      riding E919.8
    machine—*see* Accident, machine
    meat
      grinder E919.8
      slicer E919.8
    nails E920.8
    needle E920.4
      hypodermic E920.5
    object, edged, pointed, sharp—*see*
      category E920
      following fall E888.0
    paper cutter E920.4
    piercing instrument—*see also* category
      E920
      late effect of E929.8
    pitchfork E920.4
    powered
      can opener E920.2
      garden cultivator E920.1
        riding E919.8

Cut, cutting—*continued*
    hand saw E920.1
    hand tool NEC E920.1
    hedge clipper E920.1
    household appliance or implement E920.2
    lawn mower (hand) E920.0
      riding E919.8
    rivet gun E920.1
    staple gun E920.1
    rake E920.4
    saw
      circular E919.4
      hand E920.4
    scissors E920.4
    screwdriver E920.4
    sewing machine (electric) (powered)
      E920.2
      not powered E920.4
    shears E920.4
    shovel E920.4
    spade E920.4
    splinters E920.8
    sword E920.3
    tin can lid E920.8
    wood slivers E920.8
  homicide (attempt) E966
  inflicted by other person
    stated as
      intentional, homicidal E966
      undetermined whether accidental or
        intentional E986
  late effect of NEC E929.8
  legal
    execution E978
    intervention E974
  self-inflicted (unspecified whether accidental
    or intentional) E986
    stated as intentional, purposeful E956
  stated as undetermined whether accidental or
    intentional E986
  suicidal (attempt) E956
  war operations E995
  terrorism E979.8
Cyclone E908.1

D

**Death due to injury occurring one year or
  more previous** —*see* Late effect
Decapitation (accidental circumstances) NEC
  E928.9
  homicidal E966
  legal execution (by guillotine) E978
Deprivation —*see also* Privation
  homicidal intent E968.4
Derailment (accidental)
  railway (rolling stock) (train) (vehicle) (with
    subsequent collision) E802
    with
      collision (antecedent) (*see also* Collision,
        railway) E800
      explosion (subsequent) (without antecedent
        collision) E802
        antecedent collision E803
      fall (without collision (antecedent)) E802
      fire (without collision (antecedent)) E802
  street car E829
Descent
  parachute (voluntary) (without accident to
    aircraft) E844

Descent—*continued*
  due to accident to aircraft—*see* categories
    E840-E842
Desertion
  child, with intent to injure or kill E968.4
  helpless person, infant, newborn E904.0
    with intent to injure or kill E968.4
Destitution —*see* Privation
Disability, late effect or sequela of injury
  —*see* Late effect
Disease
  Andes E902.0
  aviators' E902.1
  caisson E902.2
  range E902.0
Divers' disease, palsy, paralysis, squeeze
  E902.0
Dog bite E906.0
Dragged by
  cable car (not on rails) E847
    on rails E829
  motor vehicle (on highway) E814
    not on highway, nontraffic accident E825
  street car E829
Drinking poison (accidental) —*see* Table of
  drugs and chemicals
Drowning —*see* Submersion
Dust in eye E914

E

Earth falling (on) (with asphyxia or
  suffocation (by pressure)) (*see also*
  Suffocation, due to, cave-in) E913.3
  as, or due to, a cataclysm (involving any
    transport vehicle)—*see* categories E908,
    E909
  not due to cataclysmic action E913.3
    motor vehicle (in motion) (on public
      highway) E818
      not on public highway E825
    nonmotor road vehicle NEC E829
    pedal cycle E826
    railway rolling stock, train, vehicle E806
    street car E829
    struck or crushed by E916
      with asphyxiation or suffocation E913.3
      with injury other than asphyxia,
        suffocation E916
Earthquake (any injury) E909.0
Effect(s) (adverse) of
  air pressure E902.9
    at high altitude E902.9
      in aircraft E902.1
      residence or prolonged visit (causing
        conditions classifiable to E902.0)
        E902.0
    due to
      diving E902.2
      specified cause NEC E902.8
    in aircraft E902.1
  cold, excessive (exposure to) (*see also* Cold,
    exposure to) E901.9
  heat (excessive) (*see also* Heat) E900.9
  hot
    place—*see* Heat
    weather E900.0
  insulation—*see* Heat
  late—*see* Late effect of
  motion E903

Effect(s) (adverse) of—*continued*
  nuclear explosion or weapon
    in
      terrorism E979.5
      war operations (blast) (fireball) (heat)
        (radiation) (direct) (secondary) E996
  radiation—*see* Radiation
  terrorism, secondary E979.9
  travel E903
Electric shock, electrocution (accidental)
  (from exposed wire, faulty appliance, high
  voltage cable, live rail, open socket) (by)
  (in) E925.9
  appliance or wiring
    domestic E925.0
    factory E925.2
    farm (building) E925.8
      house E925.0
    home E925.0
    industrial (conductor) (control apparatus)
      (transformer) E925.2
    outdoors E925.8
    public building E925.8
    residential institution E925.8
    school E925.8
    specified place NEC E925.8
  caused by other person
    stated as
      intentional, homicidal E968.8
      undetermined whether accidental or
        intentional E988.4
  electric power generating plant, distribution
    station E925.1
  homicidal (attempt) E968.8
  legal execution E978
  lightning E907
  machinery E925.9
    domestic E925.0
    factory E925.2
    farm E925.8
    home E925.0
  misadventure in medical or surgical procedure
    in electroshock therapy E873.4
  self-inflicted (undetermined whether
    accidental or intentional) E988.4
    stated as intentional E958.4
  stated as undetermined whether accidental or
    intentional E988.4
  suicidal (attempt) E958.4
  transmission line E925.1
Electrocution —*see* Electric shock
Embolism
  air (traumatic) NEC—*see* Air, embolism
Encephalitis
  lead or saturnine E866.0
    from pesticide NEC E863.4
Entanglement
  in
    bedclothes, causing suffocation E913.0
    wheel of pedal cycle E826
Entry of foreign body, material, any —*see*
  Foreign body
Execution, legal (any method) E978
Exhaustion
  cold—*see* Cold, exposure to
  due to excessive exertion E927
  heat—*see* Heat
Explosion (accidental) (in) (of) (on) E923.9
  acetylene E923.2
  aerosol can E921.8

Exposure (weather) (conditions) (rain) (wind)
  E904.3
  with homicidal intent E968.4
  excessive E904.3
    cold (*see also* Cold, exposure to) E901.9
      self-inflicted—*see* Cold, exposure to,
        self-inflicted
    heat (*see also* Heat) E900.9
  fire—*see* Fire
  helpless person, infant, newborn due to
    abandonment or neglect E904.0
  noise E928.1
  prolonged in deep-freeze unit or refrigerator
    E901.1
  radiation—*see* Radiation
  resulting from transport accident—*see*
    categories E800-E848
  smoke from, due to
    fire —*see* Fire
  tobacco, second-hand E869.4
  vibration E928.2

F

Fall, falling (accidental) E888.9
  building E916
    burning E891.8
      private E890.8
  down
    escalator E880.0
    ladder E881.0
      in boat, ship, watercraft E833
    staircase E880.9
    stairs, steps—*see* Fall, from, stairs
  earth (with asphyxia or suffocation (by
    pressure)) (*see also* Earth, falling) E913.3
  from, off
    aircraft (at landing, take-off) (in-transit)
      (while alighting, boarding) E843
      resulting from accident to aircraft—*see*
        categories E840-E842
    animal (in sport or transport) E828
    animal-drawn vehicle E827
    balcony E882
    bed E884.4
    bicycle E826
    boat, ship, watercraft (into water) E832
      after accident to, collision, fire on E830
        and subsequently struck by (part of)
          boat E831
      and subsequently struck by (part of) boat
        E838
      burning, crushed, sinking E830
        and subsequently struck by (part of)
          boat E831
    bridge E882
    building E882
      burning (uncontrolled fire) E891.8
        in terrorism E979.3
      private E890.8
    bunk in boat, ship, watercraft E834
      due to accident to watercraft E831
    cable car (not on rails) E847
      on rails E829
    car—*see* Fall from motor vehicle
    chair E884.2
    cliff E884.1
    commode E884.6
    curb (sidewalk) E880.1
    elevation aboard ship E834

Fall, falling—*continued*
    due to accident to ship E831
    embankment E884.9
    escalator E880.0
    fire escape E882
    flagpole E882
    furniture NEC E884.5
    gangplank (into water) (*see also* Fall,
      from, boat) E832
      to deck, dock E834
    hammock on ship E834
      due to accident to watercraft E831
    haystack E884.9
    high place NEC E884.9
      stated as undetermined whether accidental
        or intentional—*see* Jumping, from,
        high place
    horse (in sport or transport) E828
    in-line skates E885.1
    ladder E881.0
      in boat, ship, watercraft E833
        due to accident to watercraft E831
    machinery—*see also* accident, machine
      not in operation E884.9
    motor vehicle (in motion) (on public
      highway) E818
      not on public highway E825
        stationary, except while alighting,
          boarding, entering, leaving E884.9
        while alighting, boarding, entering,
          leaving E824
      stationary, except while alighting,
        boarding, entering, leaving E884.9
      while alighting, boarding, entering,
        leaving, except off-road type motor
        vehicle E817
      off-road type—*see* Fall, from, off-road
        type motor vehicle
    nonmotor road vehicle (while alighting,
      boarding) NEC E829
      stationary, except while alighting,
        boarding, entering, leaving E884.9
    off road type motor vehicle (not on
      public highway) NEC E821
      on public highway E818
        while alighting, boarding, entering,
          leaving E817
    snow vehicle—*see* Fall from snow
      vehicle, motor-driven
    one
      deck to another on ship E834
        due to accident to ship E831
      level to another NEC E884.9
        boat, ship, or watercraft E834
          due to accident to watercraft E831
    pedal cycle E826
    playground equipment E884.0
    railway rolling stock, train, vehicle (while
      alighting, boarding) E804
      with
        collision (*see also* Collision, railway)
          E800
        derailment (*see also* Derailment,
          railway) E802
        explosion (*see also* Explosion, railway
          engine) E803
    rigging (aboard ship) E834
      due to accident to watercraft E831
    roller skates E885.1
    scaffolding E881.1
    scooter (nonmotorized) E885.0

Fall, falling—*continued*
   sidewalk (curb) E880.1
      moving E885.9
   skateboard E885.2
   skis E885.3
   snowboard E885.4
   snow vehicle, motor-driven (not on public
         highway) E820
      on public highway E818
         while alighting, boarding, entering,
               leaving E817
   stairs, steps E880.9
      boat, ship, watercraft E833
         due to accident to watercraft E831
      motor bus, motor vehicle—*see* Fall, from,
            motor vehicle, while alighting, boarding
      street car E829
   stationary vehicle NEC E884.9
   stepladder E881.0
   street car (while boarding, alighting) E829
      stationary, except while boarding or
            alighting E884.9
   structure NEC E882
      burning (uncontrolled fire) E891.8
         in terrorism E979.3
   table E884.9
   toilet E884.6
   tower E882
   tree E884.9
   turret E882
   vehicle NEC—*see also* Accident, vehicle
         NEC
      stationary E884.9
   viaduct E882
   wall E882
   wheelchair E884.3
   window E882
   in, on
      aircraft (at landing, take-off) (in-transit)
            E843
         resulting from accident to aircraft—*see*
               categories E840-E842
      boat, ship, watercraft E835
         due to accident to watercraft E831
         one level to another NEC E834
         on ladder, stairs E833
      cutting or piercing instrument or machine
            E888.0
      deck (of boat, ship, watercraft) E835
         due to accident to watercraft E831
      escalator E880.0
      gangplank E835
      glass, broken E888.0
      knife E888.0
      ladder E881.0
         in boat, ship, watercraft E833
            due to accident to watercraft E831
      object
         edged, pointed or sharp E888.0
         other E888.1
      pitchfork E888.0
      railway rolling stock, train, vehicle (while
            alighting, boarding) E804
         with
            collision (*see also* Collision, railway)
                  E800
            derailment (*see also* Derailment,
                  railway) E802
            explosion (*see also* Explosion, railway
                  engine) E803
      scaffolding E881.1

Fall, falling—*continued*
   scissors E888.0
   staircase, stairs, steps (*see also* Fall,
         from, stairs) E880.9
   street car E829
   water transport (*see also* Fall, in, boat)
         E835
   into
      cavity E883.9
      dock E883.9
         from boat, ship, watercraft (*see also* Fall,
               from, boat) E832
      hold (of ship) E834
         due to accident to watercraft E831
      hole E883.9
      manhole E883.2
      moving part of machinery—*see* Accident,
            machine
      opening in surface NEC E883.9
      pit E883.9
      quarry E883.9
      shaft E883.9
      storm drain E883.2
      tank E883.9
      water (with drowning or submersion)
            E910.9
      well E883.1
   late effect of NEC E929.3
   object (*see also* Hit by, object, falling) E916
   other E888.8
   over
      animal E885.9
      cliff E884.1
      embankment E884.9
      small object E885.9
   overboard (*see also* Fall, from, boat) E832
   resulting in striking against object E888.1
      sharp E888.0
   rock E916
   same level NEC E888.9
      aircraft (any kind) E843
         resulting from accident to aircraft—*see*
               categories E840-E842
      boat, ship, watercraft E835
         due to accident to, collision, watercraft
               E831
      from
         collision, pushing, shoving, by or with
               other person(s) E886.9
            as, or caused by, a crowd E917.6
            in sports E886.0
         in-line skates E885.1
         roller skates E885.1
         scooter (nonmotorized) E885.0
         skateboard E885.2
         skis E885.3
         slipping, stumbling, tripping E885.9
         snowboard E885.4
      snowslide E916
         as avalanche E909.2
      stone E916
   through
      hatch (on ship) E834
         due to accident to watercraft E831
      roof E882
      window E882
   timber E916
   while alighting from, boarding, entering,
         leaving
      aircraft (any kind) E843

Fall, falling—*continued*
  motor bus, motor vehicle—*see* Fall, from, motor vehicle, while alighting, boarding
  nonmotor road vehicle NEC E829
  railway train E804
  street car E829
Fallen on by
  animal (horse) (not being ridden) E906.8
  being ridden (in sport or transport) E828
Fell or jumped from high place, so stated
  —*see* Jumping, from, high place
Felo-de-se (*see also* Suicide) E958.9
Fever
  heat—*see* Heat
  thermic—*see* Heat
Fight (hand) (fist) (foot) (*see also* Assault, fight) E960.0
Fire (accidental) (caused by great heat from appliance (electrical), hot object or hot substance) (secondary, resulting from explosion) E899
  conflagration—*see* Conflagration
  controlled, normal (in brazier, fireplace, furnace, or stove) (charcoal) (coal) (coke) (electric) (gas) (wood)
    bonfire E897
    brazier, not in building or structure E897
    in building or structure, except private dwelling (barn) (church) (convalescent or residential home) (factory) (farm outbuilding) (hospital) (hotel) (institution (educational) (dormitory) (residential)) (private garage) (school) (shop) (store) (theatre) E896
    in private dwelling (apartment) (boarding house) (camping place) (caravan) (farmhouse) (home (private)) (house) (lodging house) (rooming house) (tenement) E895
    not in building or structure E897
    trash E897
  forest (uncontrolled) E892
  grass (uncontrolled) E892
  hay (uncontrolled) E892
  homicide (attempt) E968.0
    late effect of E969
  in, of, on, starting in E892
    aircraft (in transit) (powered) E841
      at landing, take-off E840
      stationary E892
      unpowered (balloon) (glider) E842
    balloon E842
    boat, ship, watercraft—*see* categories E830, E831, E837
    building or structure, except private dwelling (barn) (church) (convalescent or residential home) (factory) (farm outbuilding) (hospital) (hotel) (institution (educational) (dormitory) (residential)) (school) (shop) (store) (theatre) (*see also* Conflagration, building or structure, except private dwelling) E891.9
    forest (uncontrolled) E892
    glider E842
    grass (uncontrolled) E892
    hay (uncontrolled) E892
    lumber (uncontrolled) E892
    machinery—*see* Accident, machine
    mine (uncontrolled) E892

Fire —*continued*
  motor vehicle (in motion) (on public highway) E818
    not on public highway E825
    stationary E892
  prairie (uncontrolled) E892
  private dwelling (apartment) (boarding house) (camping place) (caravan) (farmhouse) (home (private)) (house) (lodging house) (private garage) (rooming house) (tenement) (*see also* Conflagration, private dwelling) E890.9
  railway rolling stock, train, vehicle (*see also* Explosion, railway engine) E803
    stationary E892
  room NEC E898.1
  street car (in motion) E829
    stationary E892
  terrorism (by fire-producing device) E979.3
    fittings or furniture (burning building) (uncontrolled fire) E979.3
    from nuclear explosion E979.5
  transport vehicle, stationary NEC E892
  tunnel (uncontrolled) E892
  war operations (by fire-producing device or conventional weapon) E990.9
    from nuclear explosion E996
    petrol bomb E990.0
  late effect of NEC E929.4
  lumber (uncontrolled) E892
  mine (uncontrolled) E892
  prairie (uncontrolled) E892
  self-inflicted (unspecified whether accidental or intentional) E988.1
    stated as intentional, purposeful E958.1
  specified NEC E898.1
  with
    conflagration—*see* Conflagration
    ignition (of)
      clothing—*see* Ignition, clothes
      highly inflammable material (benzine) (fat) (gasoline) (kerosene) (paraffin) (petrol) E894
  started by other person
    stated as
      with intent to injure or kill E968.0
      undetermined whether or not with intent to injure or kill E988.1
  suicide (attempted) E958.1
    late effect of E959
  tunnel (uncontrolled) E892
Fireball effects from nuclear explosion in
  terrorism E979.5
  war operations E996
Fireworks (explosion) E923.0
Flash burns from explosion (*see also* Explosion) E923.9
Flood (any injury) (resulting from storm) E908.2
  caused by collapse of dam or manmade structure E909.3
Forced landing (aircraft) E840
Foreign body, object or material (entrance into (accidental))
  air passage (causing injury) E915
    with asphyxia, obstruction, suffocation E912
    food or vomitus E911

Foreign body, object or material—*continued*
  nose (with asphyxia, obstruction,
    suffocation) E912
    causing injury without asphyxia,
      obstruction, suffocation E915
  alimentary canal (causing injury) (with
    obstruction) E915
    with asphyxia, obstruction respiratory
      passage, suffocation E912
      food E911
    mouth E915
      with asphyxia, obstruction, suffocation
        E912
        food E911
    pharynx E915
      with asphyxia, obstruction, suffocation
        E912
        food E911
  aspiration (with asphyxia, obstruction
    respiratory passage, suffocation) E912
    causing injury without asphyxia,
      obstruction respiratory passage,
      suffocation E915
    food (regurgitated) (vomited) E911
      causing injury without asphyxia,
        obstruction respiratory passage,
        suffocation E915
    mucus (not of newborn) E912
    phlegm E912
  bladder (causing injury or obstruction) E915
  bronchus, bronchi—*see* Foreign body, air
    passages
  conjunctival sac E914
  digestive system—*see* Foreign body,
    alimentary canal
  ear (causing injury or obstruction) E915
  esophagus (causing injury or obstruction) (*see
    also* Foreign body, alimentary canal) E915
  eye (any part) E914
  eyelid E914
  hairball (stomach) (with obstruction) E915
  ingestion—*see* Foreign body, alimentary canal
  inhalation—*see* Foreign body, aspiration
  intestine (causing injury or obstruction) E915
  iris E914
  lacrimal apparatus E914
  larynx—*see* Foreign body, air passage
  late effect of NEC E929.8
  lung—*see* Foreign body, air passage
  mouth—*see* Foreign body, alimentary canal,
    mouth
  nasal passage—*see* Foreign body, air passage,
    nose
  nose—*see* Foreign body, air passage, nose
  ocular muscle E914
  operation wound (left in)—*see* Misadventure,
    foreign object
  orbit E914
  pharynx—*see* Foreign body, alimentary canal,
    pharynx
  rectum (causing injury or obstruction) E915
  stomach (hairball) (causing injury or
    obstruction) E915
  tear ducts or glands E914
  trachea—*see* Foreign body, air passage
  urethra (causing injury or obstruction) E915
  vagina (causing injury or obstruction) E915
Found dead, injured
  from exposure (to)—*see* Exposure
  on
    public highway E819
    railway right of way E807

Fracture (circumstances unknown or
  unspecified) E887
  due to specified external means—*see* manner
    of accident
  late effect of NEC E929.3
  occurring in water transport NEC E835
Freezing —*see* Cold, exposure to
Frostbite E901.0
  due to manmade conditions E901.1
Frozen —*see* Cold, exposure to

G

Garrotting, homicidal (attempted) E963
Gored E906.8
Gunshot wound (*see also* Shooting) E922.9

H

Hailstones, injury by E904.3
Hairball (stomach) (with obstruction) E915
Hanged himself (*see also* Hanging,
  self-inflicted) E983.0
Hang gliding E842
Hanging (accidental) E913.8
  caused by other person
    in accidental circumstances E913.8
    stated as
      intentional, homicidal E963
      undetermined whether accidental or
        intentional E983.0
  homicide (attempt) E963
  in bed or cradle E913.0
  legal execution E978
  self-inflicted (unspecified whether accidental
    or intentional) E983.0
    in accidental circumstances E913.8
    stated as intentional, purposeful E953.0
  stated as undetermined whether accidental or
    intentional E983.0
  suicidal (attempt) E953.0
Heat (apoplexy) (collapse) (cramps) (effects of)
  (excessive) (exhaustion) (fever) (prostration)
  (stroke) E900.9
  due to
    manmade conditions (listed in E900.1,
      except boat, ship, watercraft) E900.1
    weather (conditions) E900.0
  from
    electric heating apparatus causing burning
      E924.8
    nuclear explosion
      in
        terrorism E979.5
        war operations E996
  generated in, boiler, engine, evaporator, fire
    room of boat, ship, watercraft E838
  inappropriate in local application or packing
    in medical or surgical procedure E873.5
  late effect of NEC E989
Hemorrhage
  delayed following medical or surgical
    treatment without mention of
    misadventure—*see* Reaction, abnormal
  during medical or surgical treatment as
    misadventure—*see* Misadventure, cut
High
  altitude, effects E902.9
  level of radioactivity, effects—*see* Radiation

High—*continued*
  pressure effects—*see also* Effects of, air
    pressure
    from rapid descent in water (causing
      caisson or divers' disease, palsy, or
      paralysis) E902.2
  temperature, effects—*see* Heat
Hit, hitting (accidental) by
  aircraft (propeller) (without accident to
    aircraft) E844
    unpowered E842
  avalanche E909.2
  being thrown against object in or part of
    motor vehicle (in motion) (on public
      highway) E818
      not on public highway E825
    nonmotor road vehicle NEC E829
    street car E829
  boat, ship, watercraft
    after fall from watercraft E838
    damaged, involved in accident E831
    while swimming, water skiing E838
  bullet (*see also* Shooting) E922.9
    from air gun E922.4
    in
      terrorism E979.4
      war operations E991.2
        rubber E991.0
  flare, Very pistol (*see also* Shooting) E922.8
  hailstones E904.3
  landslide E909.2
  law-enforcing agent (on duty) E975
    with blunt object (baton) (night stick)
      (stave) (truncheon) E973
  machine—*see* Accident, machine
  missile
    firearm (*see also* Shooting) E922.9
    in
      terrorism —*see* Terrorism, missile
      war operations—*see* War operations,
        missile
  motor vehicle (on public highway) (traffic
    accident) E814
    not on public highway, nontraffic accident
      E822
  nonmotor road vehicle NEC E829
  object
    falling E916
      from, in, on
        aircraft E844
          due to accident to aircraft—*see*
            categories E840-E842
          unpowered E842
        boat, ship, watercraft E838
          due to accident to watercraft E831
        building E916
          burning E891.8
            in terrorism E979.3
            private E890.8
        cataclysmic
          earth surface movement or eruption
            E909.9
          storm E908.9
        cave-in E916
          with asphyxiation or suffocation (*see*
            also Suffocation, due to, cave-in)
            E913.3
        earthquake E909.0
        motor vehicle (in motion) (on public
          highway) E818
          not on public highway E825

Hit, hitting—*continued*
    stationary E916
    nonmotor road vehicle NEC E829
    pedal cycle E826
    railway rolling stock, train, vehicle E806
    street car E829
    structure, burning NEC E891.8
    vehicle, stationary E916
    moving NEC—*see* Striking against, object
    projected NEC—*see* Striking against,
      object
    set in motion by
      compressed air or gas, spring, striking,
        throwing—*see* Striking against, object
      explosion—*see* Explosion
    thrown into, on, or towards
      motor vehicle (in motion) (on public
        highway) E818
        not on public highway E825
      nonmotor road vehicle NEC E829
      pedal cycle E826
      street car E829
  off-road type motor vehicle (not on public
    highway) E821
    on public highway E814
  other person(s) E917.9
    with blunt or thrown object E917.9
      in sports E917.0
        with subsequent fall E917.5
      intentionally, homicidal E968.2
    as, or caused by, a crowd E917.1
      with subsequent fall E917.6
    in sports E917.0
  pedal cycle E826
  police (on duty) E975
    with blunt object (baton) (nightstick)
      (stave) (truncheon) E973
  railway, rolling stock, train, vehicle (part of)
    E805
  shot—*see* Shooting
  snow vehicle, motor-driven (not on public
    highway) E820
    on public highway E814
  street car E829
  vehicle NEC—*see* Accident, vehicle NEC
Homicide, homicidal (attempt) (justifiable) (*see
  also* Assault) E968.9
Hot
  liquid, object, substance, accident caused
    by—*see also* Accident, caused by, hot, by
    type of substance
    late effect of E929.8
  place, effects—*see* Heat
  weather, effects E900.0
Humidity, causing problem E904.3
Hunger E904.1
  resulting from
    abandonment or neglect E904.0
    transport accident—*see* categories
      E800-E848
Hurricane (any injury) E908.0
Hypobarism, hypobaropathy —*see* Effects of,
  air pressure
Hypothermia —*see* Cold, exposure to

I

Ictus
  caloris—*see* Heat
  solaris E900.0
Ignition (accidental)
  anesthetic gas in operating theatre E923.2
  bedclothes
    with
      conflagration—*see* Conflagration
      ignition (of)
        clothing—*see* Ignition, clothes
        highly inflammable material (benzine)
          (fat) (gasoline) (kerosene) (paraffin)
          (petrol) E894
  benzine E894
  clothes, clothing (from controlled fire) (in
    building) E893.9
    with conflagration—*see* Conflagration
    from
      bonfire E893.2
      highly inflammable material E894
      sources or material as listed in E893.8
      trash fire E893.2
      uncontrolled fire—*see* Conflagration
    in
      private dwelling E893.0
      specified building or structure, except
        private dwelling E893.1
    not in building or structure E893.2
  explosive material—*see* Explosion
  fat E894
  gasoline E894
  kerosene E894
  material
    explosive—*see* Explosion
    highly inflammable E894
      with conflagration—*see* Conflagration
      with explosion E923.2
  nightdress—*see* Ignition, clothes
  paraffin E894
  petrol E894
Immersion —*see* Submersion
Implantation of quills of porcupine E906.8
Inanition (from) E904.9
  hunger—*see* Lack of, food
  resulting from homicidal intent E968.4
  thirst—*see* Lack of, water
Inattention after, at birth E904.0
  homicidal, infanticidal intent E968.4
Infanticide (*see also* Assault)
Ingestion
  foreign body (causing injury) (with
    obstruction)—*see* Foreign body,
    alimentary canal
  poisonous substance NEC—*see* Table of
    drugs and chemicals
Inhalation
  excessively cold substance, manmade E901.1
  foreign body—*see* Foreign body, aspiration
  liquid air, hydrogen, nitrogen E901.1
  mucus, not of newborn (with asphyxia,
    obstruction respiratory passage,
    suffocation) E912
  phlegm (with asphyxia, obstruction respiratory
    passage, suffocation) E912
  poisonous gas—*see* Table of drugs and
    chemicals
  smoke from, due to
    fire —*see* Fire

Inhalation—*continued*
  tobacco, second-hand E869.4
  vomitus (with asphyxia, obstruction
    respiratory passage, suffocation) E911
Injury, injured (accidental(ly)) NEC E928.9
  by, caused by, from
    air rifle (B-B gun) E922.4
    animal (not being ridden) NEC E906.9
      being ridden (in sport or transport) E828
    assault (*see also* Assault) E968.9
    avalanche E909.2
    bayonet (*see also* Bayonet wound) E920.3
    being thrown against some part of, or
      object in
      motor vehicle (in motion) (on public
        highway) E818
        not on public highway E825
      nonmotor road vehicle NEC E829
      off-road motor vehicle NEC E821
      railway train E806
      snow vehicle, motor-driven E820
      street car E829
    bending E927
    bite, human E928.3
    broken glass E920.8
    bullet—*see* Shooting
    cave-in (*see also* Suffocation, due to,
      cave-in) E913.3
      without asphyxiation or suffocation E916
    cloudburst E908.8
    cutting or piercing instrument (*see also*
      Cut) E920.9
    cyclone E908.1
    earth surface movement or eruption
      E909.9
    earthquake E909.0
    electric current (*see also* Electric shock)
      E925.9
    explosion (*see also* Explosion) E923.9
    fire—*see* Fire
    flare, Very pistol E922.8
    flood E908.2
    foreign body—*see* Foreign body
    hailstones E904.3
    hurricane E908.0
    landslide E909.2
    law-enforcing agent, police, in course of
      legal intervention—*see* Legal
      intervention
    lightning E907
    live rail or live wire—*see* Electric shock
    machinery—*see also* Accident, machine
      aircraft, without accident to aircraft E844
      boat, ship, watercraft (deck) (engine
        room) (galley) (laundry) (loading) E836
    missile
      explosive E923.8
      firearm—*see* Shooting
      in
        terrorism —*see* Terrorism, missile
        war operations—*see* War operations,
          missile
    moving part of motor vehicle (in motion)
      (on public highway) E818
      not on public highway, nontraffic accident
        E825
      while alighting, boarding, entering,
        leaving—*see* Fall, from, motor vehicle,
        while alighting, boarding
    nail E920.8

Injury, injured—*continued*
  needle (sewing) E920.4
    hypodermic E920.5
  noise E928.1
  object
    fallen on
      motor vehicle (in motion) (on public
        highway) E818
      not on public highway E825
    falling—*see* Hit by, object, falling
  paintball gun E922.5
  radiation—*see* Radiation
  railway rolling stock, train, vehicle (part
    of) E805
    door or window E806
  rotating propeller, aircraft E844
  rough landing of off-road type motor
    vehicle (after leaving ground or rough
    terrain) E821
    snow vehicle E820
  saber (*see also* Wound, saber) E920.3
  shot—*see* Shooting
  sound waves E928.1
  splinter or sliver, wood E920.8
  storm E908.9
  straining E927
  street car (door) E829
  suicide (attempt) E958.9
  sword E920.3
  terrorism —*see* Terrorism
  third rail—*see* Electric shock
  thunderbolt E907
  tidal wave E909.4
    caused by storm E908.0
  tornado E908.1
  torrential rain E908.2
  twisting E927
  vehicle NEC—*see* Accident, vehicle NEC
  vibration E928.2
  volcanic eruption E909.1
  weapon burst, in war operations E993
  weightlessness (in spacecraft, real or
    simulated) E928.0
  wood splinter or sliver E920.8
  due to
    civil insurrection—*see* War operations
      occurring after cessation of hostilities E998
    terrorism —*see* Terrorism
    war operations—*see* War operations
      occurring after cessation of hostilities
      E998
  homicidal (*see also* Assault) E968.9
  in, on
    civil insurrection—*see* War operations
    fight E960.0
    parachute descent (voluntary) (without
      accident to aircraft) E844
      with accident to aircraft—*see* categories
      E840-E842
    public highway E819
    railway right of way E807
    terrorism —*see* Terrorism
    war operations—*see* War operations
  inflicted (by)
    in course of arrest (attempted),
      suppression of disturbance,
      maintenance of order, by
      law-enforcing agents—*see* Legal
      intervention
    law-enforcing agent (on duty)—*see* Legal
      intervention

Injury, injured—*continued*
  other person
    stated as
      accidental E928.9
      homicidal, intentional—*see* Assault
      undetermined whether accidental or
        intentional—*see* Injury, stated as
        undetermined
    police (on duty)—*see* Legal intervention
  late effect of E929.9
  purposely (inflicted) by other person(s)—*see*
    Assault
  self-inflicted (unspecified whether accidental
    or intentional) E988.9
    stated as
      accidental E928.9
      intentionally, purposely E958.9
  specified cause NEC E928.8
  stated as
    undetermined whether accidentally or
      purposely inflicted (by) E988.9
    cut (any part of body) E986
    cutting or piercing instrument (classifiable
      to E920) E986
    drowning E984
    explosive(s) (missile) E985.5
    falling from high place E987.9
      manmade structure, except residential
        E987.1
      natural site E987.2
      residential premises E987.0
    hanging E983.0
    knife E986
    late effect of E989
    puncture (any part of body) E986
    shooting—*see* Shooting, stated as
      undetermined whether accidental or
      intentional
    specified means NEC E988.8
    stab (any part of body) E986
    strangulation—*see* Suffocation, stated as
      undetermined whether accidental or
      intentional
    submersion E984
    suffocation—*see* Suffocation, stated as
      undetermined whether accidental or
      intentional
  to child due to criminal abortion E968.8
Insufficient nourishment —*see also* Lack of,
  food
  homicidal intent E968.4
Insulation, effects —*see* Heat
Interruption of respiration by
  food lodged in esophagus E911
  foreign body, except food, in esophagus E912
Intervention, legal —*see* Legal intervention
Intoxication, drug or poison —*see* Table of
  drugs and chemicals
Irradiation —*see* Radiation

J

Jammed (accidentally)
  between objects (moving) (stationary and
    moving) E918
  in object E918
Jumped or fell from high place, so stated
  —*see* Jumping, from, high place, stated as
  in undetermined circumstances

Jumping

before train, vehicle or other moving object (unspecified whether accidental or intentional) E988.0

stated as

intentional, purposeful E958.0

suicidal (attempt) E958.0

from

aircraft

by parachute (voluntarily) (without accident to aircraft) E844

due to accident to aircraft—*see* categories E840-E842

boat, ship, watercraft (into water)

after accident to, fire on, watercraft E830

and subsequently struck by (part of) boat E831

burning, crushed, sinking E830

and subsequently struck by (part of) boat E831

voluntarily, without accident (to boat) with injury other than drowning or submersion E883.0

building—*see also* Jumping, from, high place

burning (uncontrolled fire) E891.8

in terrorism E979.3

private E890.8

cable car (not on rails) E847

on rails E829

high place

in accidental circumstances or in sport—*see* categories E880-E884

stated as

with intent to injure self E957.9

man-made structures NEC E957.1

natural sites E957.2

residential premises E957.0

in undetermined circumstances E987.9

man-made structures NEC E987.1

natural sites E987.2

residential premises E987.0

suicidal (attempt) E957.9

man-made structures NEC E957.1

natural sites E957.1

residential premises E957.0

motor vehicle (in motion) (on public highway)—*see* Fall, from, motor vehicle

nonmotor road vehicle NEC E829

street car E829

structure, burning NEC E891.8 —*see also* Jumping, from, high place

burning NEC (uncontrolled fire) E891.8

in terrorism E979.3

into water

with injury other than drowning or submersion E883.0

drowning or submersion—*see* Submersion

from, off, watercraft—*see* Jumping, from, boat

Justifiable homicide —*see* Assault

K

Kicked by

animal E906.8

person(s) (accidentally) E917.9

with intent to injure or kill E960.0

as, or caused by a crowd E917.1

Kicked by—*continued*

with subsequent fall E917.6

in fight E960.0

in sports E917.0

with subsequent fall E917.5

Kicking against

object (moving) E917.9

in sports E917.0

with subsequent fall E917.5

stationary E917.4

with subsequent fall E917.8

person—*see* Striking against, person

Killed, killing (accidentally) NEC (*see also* Injury) E928.9

in

action—*see* War operations

brawl, fight (hand) (fists) (foot) E960.0

by weapon—*see also* Assault

cutting, piercing E966

firearm—*see* Shooting, homicide

self

stated as

accident E928.9

suicide—*see* Suicide

unspecified whether accidental or suicidal E988.9

Knocked down (accidentally) (by) NEC E928.9

animal (not being ridden) E906.8

being ridden (in sport or transport) E828

blast from explosion (*see also* Explosion) E923.9

crowd, human stampede E917.6

late effect of—*see* Late effect

person (accidentally) E917.9

in brawl, fight E960.0

in sports E917.5

transport vehicle—*see* vehicle involved under Hit by

while boxing E917.5

L

Laceration NEC E928.9

Lack of

air (refrigerator or closed place), suffocation by E913.2

care (helpless person) (infant) (newborn) E904.0

homicidal intent E968.4

food except as result of transport accident E904.1

helpless person, infant, newborn due to abandonment or neglect E904.0

water except as result of transport accident E904.2

helpless person, infant, newborn due to abandonment or neglect E904.0

Landslide E909.2

falling on, hitting

motor vehicle (any) (in motion) (on or off public highway) E909.2

railway rolling stock, train, vehicle E909.2

Late effect of

accident NEC (accident classifiable to E928.9) E929.9

specified NEC (accident classifiable to E910-E928.8) E929.8

assault E969

fall, accidental (accident classifiable to E880-E888) E929.3

Late effect of—*continued*
fire, accident caused by (accident classifiable
to E890-E899) E929.4
homicide, attempt (any means) E969
injury
due to terrorism E999.1
undetermined whether accidentally or
purposely inflicted (injury classifiable
to E980-E988) E989
legal intervention (injury classifiable to
E970-E976) E977
medical or surgical procedure, test or therapy
as, or resulting in, or from
abnormal or delayed reaction or
complication—*see* Reaction, abnormal
misadventure—*see* Misadventure
motor vehicle accident (accident classifiable
to E810-E825) E929.0
natural or environmental factor, accident due
to (accident classifiable to E900-E909)
E929.5
poisoning, accidental (accident classifiable to
E850-E858, E860-E869) E929.2
suicide, attempt (any means) E959
transport accident NEC (accident classifiable
to E800-E807, E826-E838, E840-E848)
E929.1
war operations, injury due to (injury
classifiable to E990-E998) E999.0
Launching pad accident E845
Legal
execution, any method E978
intervention (by) (injury from) E976
baton E973
bayonet E974
blow E975
blunt object (baton) (nightstick) (stave)
(truncheon) E973
cutting or piercing instrument E974
dynamite E971
execution, any method E973
explosive(s) (shell) E971
firearms(s) E970
gas (asphyxiation) (poisoning) (tear) E972
grenade E971
late effect of E977
machine gun E970
manhandling E975
mortar bomb E971
nightstick E973
revolver E970
rifle E970
specified means NEC E975
stabbing E974
stave E973
truncheon E973
Lifting, injury in E927
Lightning (shock) (stroke) (struck by) E907
Liquid (noncorrosive) in eye E914
corrosive E924.1
Loss of control
motor vehicle (on public highway) (without
antecedent collision) E816
with
antecedent collision on public highway
—see Collision, motor vehicle
involving any object, person or vehicle
not on public highway E816
on public highway—*see* Collision, motor
vehicle

Loss of control—*continued*
not on public highway, nontraffic accident
E825
with antecedent collision—*see* Collision,
motor vehicle, not on public highway
off-road type motor vehicle (not on public
highway) E821
on public highway—*see* Loss of control,
motor vehicle
snow vehicle, motor-driven (not on public
highway) E820
on public highway—*see* Loss of control,
motor vehicle
Lost at sea E832
with accident to watercraft E830
in war operations E995
Low
pressure, effects—*see* Effects of, air pressure
temperature, effects—*see* Cold, exposure to
**Lying before train, vehicle or other moving
object** (unspecified whether accidental or
intentional) E988.0
stated as intentional, purposeful, suicidal
(attempt) E958.0
Lynching (*see also* Assault) E968.9

M

**Malfunction, atomic power plant in water
transport** E838
Mangled (accidentally) NEC E928.9
Manhandling (in brawl, fight) E960.0
legal intervention E975
Manslaughter (nonaccidental)—*see* Assault
Marble in nose E912
Mauled by animal E906.8
Medical procedure, complication of
delayed or as an abnormal reaction without
mention of misadventure—*see* Reaction,
abnormal
due to or as a result of misadventure—*see*
Misadventure
Melting of fittings and furniture in burning
in terrorism E979.3
Minamata disease E865.2
Misadventure(s) to patient(s) during surgical or
medical care E876.9
contaminated blood, fluid, drug or biological
substance (presence of agents and toxins
as listed in E875) E875.9
administered (by) NEC E875.9
infusion E875.0
injection E875.1
specified means NEC E875.2
transfusion E875.0
vaccination E875.1
cut, cutting, puncture, perforation or
hemorrhage (accidental) (inadvertent)
(inappropriate) (during) E870.9
aspiration of fluid or tissue (by puncture
or catheterization, except heart) E870.5
biopsy E870.8
needle (aspirating) E870.5
blood sampling E870.5
catheterization E870.5
heart E870.6
dialysis (kidney) E870.2
endoscopic examination E870.4
enema E870.7
infusion E870.1

Misadventures—*continued*
  injection E870.3
  lumbar puncture E870.5
  needle biopsy E870.5
  paracentesis, abdominal E870.5
  perfusion E870.2
  specified procedure NEC E870.8
  surgical operation E870.0
  thoracentesis E870.5
  transfusion E870.1
  vaccination E870.3
excessive amount of blood or other fluid
  during transfusion or infusion E873.0
failure
  in dosage E873.9
  electroshock therapy E873.4
  inappropriate temperature (too hot or too
    cold) in local application and packing
    E873.5
  infusion
    excessive amount of fluid E873.0
    incorrect dilution of fluid E873.1
  insulin-shock therapy E873.4
  nonadministration of necessary drug or
    medicinal E873.6
  overdose—*see also* Overdose
    radiation, in therapy E873.2
  radiation
    inadvertent exposure of patient
      (receiving radiation for test or
      therapy) E873.3
    not receiving radiation for test or
      therapy—*see* Radiation
    overdose E873.2
  specified procedure NEC 873.8
  transfusion
    excessive amount of blood E873.0
  mechanical, of instrument or apparatus
    (during procedure) E874.9
  aspiration of fluid or tissue (by puncture
    or catheterization, except of heart)
    E874.4
  biopsy E874.8
    needle (aspirating) E874.4
  blood sampling E874.4
  catheterization E874.4
    heart E874.5
  dialysis (kidney) E874.2
  endoscopic examination E874.3
  enema E874.8
  infusion E874.1
  injection E874.8
  lumbar puncture E874.4
  needle biopsy E874.4
  paracentesis, abdominal E874.4
  perfusion E874.2
  specified procedure NEC E874.8
  surgical operation E874.0
  thoracentesis E874.4
  transfusion E874.1
  vaccination E874.8
  sterile precautions (during procedure)
    E872.9
  aspiration of fluid or tissue (by puncture
    or catheterization, except of heart) E872.5
  biopsy E872.8
    needle (aspirating) E872.5
  blood sampling E872.5
  catheterization E872.5
    heart E872.6
  dialysis (kidney) E872.2

Misadventures—*continued*
  endoscopic examination E872.4
  enema E872.8
  infusion E872.1
  injection E872.3
  lumbar puncture E872.5
  needle biopsy E872.5
  paracentesis, abdominal E872.5
  perfusion E872.2
  removal of catheter or packing E872.8
  specified procedure NEC E872.8
  surgical operation E872.0
  thoracentesis E872.5
  transfusion E872.1
  vaccination E872.3
  suture or ligature during surgical
    procedure E876.2
  to introduce or to remove tube or
    instrument E876.4
    foreign object left in body—*see*
      Misadventure, foreign object
foreign object left in body (during procedure)
  E871.9
  aspiration of fluid or tissue (by puncture
    or catheterization, except heart) E871.5
  biopsy E871.8
    needle (aspirating) E871.5
  blood sampling E871.5
  catheterization E871.5
    heart E871.6
  dialysis (kidney) E871.2
  endoscopic examination E871.4
  enema E871.8
  infusion E871.1
  injection E871.3
  lumbar puncture E871.5
  needle biopsy E871.5
  paracentesis, abdominal E871.5
  perfusion E871.2
  removal of catheter or packing E871.7
  specified procedure NEC E871.8
  surgical operation E871.0
  thoracentesis E871.5
  transfusion E871.1
  vaccination E871.3
hemorrhage—*see* Misadventure, cut
inadvertent exposure of patient to radiation
  (being received for test or therapy) E873.3
inappropriate
  operation performed E876.5
  temperature (too hot or too cold) in local
    application or packing E873.5
infusion—*see also* Misadventure, by specific
  type, infusion
  excessive amount of fluid E873.0
  incorrect dilution of fluid E873.1
  wrong fluid E876.1
mismatched blood in transfusion E876.0
nonadministration of necessary drug or
  medicinal E873.6
overdose—*see also* Overdose
  radiation, in therapy E873.2
perforation—*see* Misadventure, cut
performance of inappropriate operation E876.5
puncture—*see* Misadventure, cut
specified type NEC E876.8
  failure
    suture or ligature during surgical operation
      E876.2
    to introduce or to remove tube or
      instrument E876.4

Misadventures—*continued*
    foreign object left in body E871.9
  infusion of wrong fluid E876.1
  performance of inappropriate operation
    E876.5
  transfusion of mismatched blood E876.0
  wrong
    fluid in infusion E876.1
    placement of endotracheal tube during
      anesthetic procedure E876.3
  transfusion—*see also* Misadventure, by
    specific type, transfusion
    excessive amount of blood E873.0
    mismatched blood E876.0
  wrong
    drug given in error—*see* Table of drugs
      and chemicals
    fluid in infusion E876.1
    placement of endotracheal tube during
      anesthetic procedure E876.3
Motion (effects) E903
  sickness E903
Mountain sickness E902.0
**Mucus aspiration or inhalation, not of
  newborn** (with asphyxia, obstruction
  respiratory passage, suffocation) E912
Mudslide of cataclysmic nature E909.2
Murder (attempt) (*see also* Assault) E968.9

N

Nail, injury by E920.8
Needlestick (sewing needle) E920.4
  hypodermic E920.5
Neglect —*see also* Privation
  criminal E968.4
  homicidal intent E968.4
Noise (causing injury) (pollution) E928.1

O

Object
  falling
    from, in, on, hitting
      aircraft E844
        due to accident to aircraft—*see*
          categories E840-E842
      machinery—*see also* Accident, machine
        not in operation E916
      motor vehicle (in motion) (on public
        highway) E818
        not on public highway E825
        stationary E916
      nonmotor road vehicle NEC E829
      pedal cycle E826
      person E916
      railway rolling stock, train, vehicle E806
      street car E829
      watercraft E838
        due to accident to watercraft E831
  set in motion by
    accidental explosion of pressure
      vessel—*see* category E921
    firearm—*see* category E922
    machine(ry)—*see* Accident, machine
    transport vehicle—*see* categories
      E800-E848
  thrown from, in, on, towards
    aircraft E844

Object—*continued*
  cable car (not on rails) E847
    on rails E829
  motor vehicle (in motion) (on public
    highway) E818
    not on public highway E825
  nonmotor road vehicle NEC E829
  pedal cycle E826
  street car E829
  vehicle NEC—*see* Accident, vehicle NEC
Obstruction
  air passages, larynx, respiratory passages
    by
      external means NEC—*see* Suffocation
      food, any type (regurgitated) (vomited)
        E911
      material or object, except food E912
      mucus E912
      phlegm E912
      vomitus E911
  digestive tract, except mouth or pharynx
    by
      food, any type E915
      foreign body (any) E915
  esophagus
    food E911
    foreign body, except food E912
    without asphyxia or obstruction of
      respiratory passage E915
  mouth or pharynx
    by
      food, any type E911
      material or object, except food E912
  respiration—*see* Obstruction, air passages
Oil in eye E914
Overdose
  anesthetic (drug)—*see* Table of drugs and
    chemicals
  drug—*see* Table of drugs and chemicals
Overexertion (lifting) (pulling) (pushing) E927
Overexposure (accidental) (to)
  cold (*see also* Cold, exposure to) E901.9
    due to manmade conditions E901.1
  heat (*see also* Heat) E900.9
  radiation—*see* Radiation
  radioactivity—*see* Radiation
  sun, except sunburn E900.0
  weather—*see* Exposure
  wind—*see* Exposure
Overheated (*see also* Heat) E900.9
Overlaid E913.0
Overturning (accidental)
  animal-drawn vehicle E827
  boat, ship, watercraft
    causing
      drowning, submersion E830
      injury except drowning, submersion E831
  machinery—*see* Accident, machine
  motor vehicle (*see also* Loss of control,
    motor vehicle) E816
    with antecedent collision on public
      highway—*see* Collision, motor vehicle
    not on public highway, nontraffic accident
      E825
      with antecedent collision—*see* Collision,
        motor vehicle, not on public highway
  nonmotor road vehicle NEC E829
  off-road type motor vehicle—*see* Loss of
    control, off-road type motor vehicle
  pedal cycle E826

Overturning—*continued*
railway rolling stock, train, vehicle (*see also*
Derailment, railway) E802
street car E829
vehicle NEC—*see* Accident, vehicle NEC

P

Palsy, divers' E902.2
Parachuting (voluntary) (without accident to
aircraft) E844
due to accident to aircraft—*see* categories
E840-E842
Paralysis
divers' E902.2
lead or saturnine E866.0
from pesticide NEC E863.4
Pecked by bird E906.8
Phlegm aspiration or inhalation (with
asphyxia, obstruction respiratory passage,
suffocation) E912
Piercing (*see also* Cut) E920.9
Pinched
between objects (moving) (stationary and
moving) E918
in object E918
Pinned under
machine(ry)—*see* Accident, machine
Place of occurrence of accident —*see*
Accident (to), occurring (at) (in)
Plumbism E866.0
from insecticide NEC E863.4
Poisoning (accidental) (by)—*see also* Table of
drugs and chemicals
carbon monoxide
generated by
aircraft in transit E844
motor vehicle
in motion (on public highway) E818
not on public highway E825
watercraft (in transit) (not in transit) E838
caused by injection of poisons or toxins into
or through skin by plant thorns, spines, or
other mechanism E905.7
marine or sea plants E905.6
fumes or smoke due to
conflagration—*see* Conflagration
explosion or fire—*see* Fire
ignition—*see* Ignition
gas
in legal intervention E972
legal execution, by E978
on watercraft E838
used as anesthetic—*see* Table of drugs
and chemicals
in
terrorism (chemical weapons) E979.7
war operations E997.2
late effect of—*see* Late effect
legal
execution E978
intervention
by gas E972
**Pressure, external, causing asphyxia,
suffocation** (*see also* Suffocation) E913.9
Privation E904.9
food (*see also* Lack of, food) E904.1
helpless person, infant, newborn due to
abandonment or neglect E904.0
late effect of NEC E929.5

Privation— *continued*
resulting from transport accident—*see*
categories E800-E848
water (*see also* Lack of, water) E904.2
**Projected objects, striking against or struck
by** —*see* Striking against, object
Prolonged stay in
high altitude (causing conditions as listed in
E902.0) E902.0
weightless environment E928.0
Prostration
heat—*see* Heat
Pulling, injury in E927
Puncture, puncturing (*see also* Cut) E920.9
by
plant thorns or spines E920.8
toxic reaction E905.7
marine or sea plants E905.6
sea-urchin spine E905.6
Pushing (injury in) (overexertion) E927
by other person(s) (accidental) E917.9
as, or caused by, a crowd, human
stampede E917.1
with subsequent fall E917.6
before moving vehicle or object
stated as
intentional, homicidal E968.5
undetermined whether accidental or
intentional E988.8
from
high place
in accidental circumstances—*see*
categories E880-E884
stated as
intentional, homicidal E968.1
undetermined whether accidental or
intentional E987.9
man-made structure, except
residential E987.1
natural site E987.2
residential E987.0
motor vehicle (*see also* Fall, from, motor
vehicle) E818
stated as
intentional, homicidal E968.5
undetermined whether accidental or
intentional E988.8
in sports E917.0
with fall E886.0
with fall E886.9
in sports E886.0

R

Radiation (exposure to) E926.9
abnormal reaction to medical test or therapy
E879.2
arc lamps E926.2
atomic power plant (malfunction) NEC E926.9
in water transport E838
electromagnetic, ionizing E926.3
gamma rays E926.3
in
terrorism (from or following nuclear
explosion) (direct) (secondary) E979.5
laser E979.8
war operations (from or following nuclear
explosion) (direct) (secondary) E996
laser(s) E997.0
water transport E838

Radiation—*continued*
  inadvertent exposure of patient (receiving test
    or therapy) E873.3
  infrared (heaters and lamps) E926.1
    excessive heat E900.1
  ionized, ionizing (particles, artificially
    accelerated) E926.8
    electromagnetic E926.3
  isotopes, radioactive—*see* Radiation,
    radioactive isotopes
  laser(s) E926.4
    in
      terrorism E979.8
      war operations E997.0
    misadventure in medical care—*see*
      Misadventure, failure, in dosage,
      radiation
  late effect of NEC E929.8
    excessive heat from—*see* Heat
  light sources (visible) (ultraviolet) E926.2
  misadventure in medical or surgical
    procedure—*see* Misadventure, failure, in
    dosage, radiation
  overdose (in medical or surgical procedure)
    E873.2
  radar E926.0
  radioactive isotopes E926.5
    atomic power plant malfunction E926.5
      in water transport E838
    misadventure in medical or surgical
      treatment—*see* Misadventure, failure,
      in dosage, radiation
  radiobiologicals—*see* Radiation, radioactive
    isotopes
  radiofrequency E926.0
  radiopharmaceuticals—*see* Radiation,
    radioactive isotopes
  radium NEC E926.9
  sun E926.2
    excessive heat from E900.0
  tanning bed E926.2
  welding arc or torch E926.2
    excessive heat from E900.1
  x-rays (hard) (soft) E926.3
    misadventure in medical or surgical
      treatment—*see* Misadventure, failure,
      in dosage, radiation
Rape E960.1
Reaction —abnormal to or following(medical
  or surgical procedure) E879.9
  amputation (of limbs) E878.5
  anastomosis (arteriovenous) (blood vessel)
    (gastrojejunal) (skin) (tendon) (natural,
    artificial material, tissue) E878.2
    external stoma, creation of E878.3
  aspiration (of fluid) E879.4
    tissue E879.8
  biopsy E879.8
  blood
    sampling E879.7
    transfusion
      procedure E879.8
  bypass—*see* Reaction, abnormal, anastomosis
  catheterization
    cardiac E879.0
    urinary E879.6
  colostomy E878.3
  cystostomy E878.3
  dialysis (kidney) E879.1
  drugs or biologicals—*see* Table of drugs and
    chemicals

Reaction—*continued*
  duodenostomy E878.3
  electroshock therapy E879.3
  formation of external stoma E878.3
  gastrostomy E878.3
  graft—*see* Reaction, abnormal, anastomosis
  hypothermia E879.8
  implant, implantation (of)
    artificial
      internal device (cardiac pacemaker)
        (electrodes in brain) (heart valve
        prosthesis) (orthopedic) E878.1
      material or tissue (for anastomosis or
        bypass) E878.2
        with creation of external stoma E878.3
    natural tissues (for anastomosis or
      bypass) E878.2
      as transplantion—*see* Reaction, abnormal,
        transplant
      with creation of external stoma E878.3
  infusion
    procedure E879.8
  injection
    procedure E879.8
  insertion of gastric or duodenal sound E879.5
  insulin-shock therapy E879.3
  lumbar puncture E879.4
  perfusion E879.1
  procedures other than surgical operation (*see
    also* Reaction, abnormal, by specific type
    of procedure) E879.9
    specified procedure NEC E879.8
  radiological procedure or therapy E879.2
  removal of organ (partial) (total) NEC E878.6
    with
      anastomosis, bypass or graft E878.2
      formation of external stoma E878.3
      implant of artificial internal device E878.1
      transplant(ation)
        partial organ E878.4
        whole organ E878.0
  sampling
    blood E879.7
    fluid NEC E879.4
    tissue E879.8
  shock therapy E879.3
  surgical operation (*see also* Reaction,
    abnormal, by specified type of operation)
    E878.9
  restorative NEC E878.4
    with
      anastomosis, bypass or graft E878.2
      formation of external stoma E878.3
      implant(ation)—*see* Reaction, abnormal,
        implant
      transplant(ation)—*see* Reaction,
        abnormal, transplant
    specified operation NEC E878.8
  thoracentesis E879.4
  transfusion
    procedure E879.8
  transplant, transplantation (heart) (kidney)
    (liver) E878.0
    partial organ E878.4
  ureterostomy E878.3
  vaccination E879.8
Reduction in
  atmospheric pressure—*see also* Effects of, air
    pressure
    while surfacing from

Reduction in—*continued*
   deep water diving causing caisson or
      divers' disease, palsy or paralysis
      E902.2
   underground E902.8
Residual (effect)—*see* Late effect
Rock falling on or hitting (accidentally)
   motor vehicle (in motion) (on public
      highway) E818
    not on public highway E825
   nonmotor road vehicle NEC E829
   pedal cycle E826
   person E916
   railway rolling stock, train, vehicle E806
Running off, away
   animal (being ridden) (in sport or transport)
      E828
    not being ridden E906.8
   animal-drawn vehicle E827
   rails, railway (*see also* Derailment) E802
   roadway
    motor vehicle (without antecedent
      collision) E816
     nontraffic accident E825
     with antecedent collision—*see* Collision,
       motor vehicle, not on public highway
    with
     antecedent collision—*see* Collision motor
      vehicle
     subsequent collision
      involving any object, person or vehicle
       not on public highway E816
      on public highway E811
    nonmotor road vehicle NEC E829
    pedal cycle E826
Run over (accidentally) (by)
   animal (not being ridden) E906.8
    being ridden (in sport or transport) E828
   animal-drawn vehicle E827
   machinery—*see* Accident, machine
   motor vehicle (on public highway)—*see* Hit
    by, motor vehicle
   nonmotor road vehicle NEC E829
   railway train E805
   street car E829
   vehicle NEC E848

S

Saturnism E866.0
   from insecticide NEC E863.4
Scald, scalding (accidental) (by) (from) (in)
   E924.0
   acid—*see* Scald, caustic
   boiling tap water E924.2
   caustic or corrosive liquid, substance E924.1
    swallowed—*see* Table of drugs and
     chemicals
   homicide (attempt)—*see* Assault, burning
   inflicted by other person
    stated as
     intentional or homicidal E968.3
     undetermined whether accidental or
      intentional E988.2
   late effect of NEC E929.8
   liquid (boiling) (hot) E924.0
   local application of externally applied
    substance in medical or surgical care
    E873.5
   molten metal E924.0

Scald, scalding—*continued*
   self-inflicted (unspecified whether accidental
    or intentional) E988.2
    stated as intentional, purposeful E958.2
   stated as undetermined whether accidental or
    intentional E988.2
   steam E924.0
   tap water (boiling) E924.2
   transport accident—*see* categories E800-E848
   vapor E924.0
Scratch, cat E906.8
Sea
   sickness E903
Self-mutilation —*see* Suicide
Sequelae (of)
   in
    terrorism E999.1
    war operations E999.0
Shock
   anaphylactic (*see also* Table of drugs and
    chemicals) E947.9
   due to
    bite (venomous)—*see* Bite, venomous NEC
    sting—*see* Sting
   electric (*see also* Electric shock) E925.9
   from electric appliance or current (*see also*
    Electric shock) E925.9
Shooting, shot (accidental(ly)) E922.9
   air gun E922.4
   BB gun E922.4
   hand gun (pistol) (revolver) E922.0
   himself (*see also* Shooting, self-inflicted)
    E985.4
    hand gun (pistol) (revolver) E985.0
    military firearm, except hand gun E985.3
     hand gun (pistol) (revolver) E985.0
    rifle (hunting) E985.2
     military E985.3
    shotgun (automatic) E985.1
    specified firearm NEC E985.4
    Verey pistol E985.4
   homicide (attempt) E965.4
    air gun E968.6
    BB gun E968.6
    hand gun (pistol) (revolver) E965.0
    military firearm, except hand gun E965.3
     hand gun (pistol) (revolver) E965.0
    paintball gun E965.4
    rifle (hunting) E965.2
     military E965.3
    shotgun (automatic) E965.1
    specified firearm NEC E965.4
    Verey pistol E965.4
   inflicted by other person
    in accidental circumstances E922.9
     hand gun (pistol) (revolver) E922.0
     military firearm, except hand gun E922.3
      hand gun (pistol) (revolver) E922.0
     rifle (hunting) E922.2
      military E922.3
     shotgun (automatic) E922.1
     specified firearm NEC E922.8
     Verey pistol E922.8
    stated as
     intentional, homicidal E965.4
      hand gun (pistol) (revolver) E965.0
      military firearm, except hand gun E965.3
       hand gun (pistol) (revolver) E965.0
      paintball gun E965.4
      rifle (hunting) E965.2
       military E965.3

shotgun (automatic) E965.1
specified firearm E965.4
Verey pistol E965.4
undetermined whether accidental or
intentional E985.4
air gun E985.6
BB gun E985.6
hand gun (pistol) (revolver) E985.0
military firearm, except hand gun E985.3
hand gun (pistol) (revolver) E985.0
paintball gun E985.7
rifle (hunting) E985.2
shotgun (automatic) E985.1
specified firearm NEC E985.4
Verey pistol E985.4
in
terrorism —see Terrorism, shooting
war operations—see War operations,
shooting
legal
execution E978
intervention E970
military firearm, except hand gun E922.3
hand gun (pistol) (revolver) E922.0
paintball gun E922.5
rifle (hunting) 922.2
military E922.3
self-inflicted (unspecified whether accidental
or intentional) E985.4
air gun E985.6
BB gun E985.6
hand gun (pistol) (revolver) E985.0
military firearm, except hand gun E985.3
hand gun (pistol) (revolver) E985.0
paintball gun E985.7
rifle (hunting) E985.2
military E985.3
shotgun (automatic) E985.1
specified firearm NEC E985.4
stated as
accidental E922.9
hand gun (pistol) (revolver) E922.0
military firearm, except hand gun E922.3
hand gun (pistol) (revolver) E922.0
paintball gun E922.5
rifle (hunting) E922.2
military E922.3
shotgun (automatic) E922.1
specified firearm NEC E922.8
Verey pistol E922.8
intentional, purposeful E955.4
hand gun (pistol) (revolver) E955.0
military firearm, except hand gun E955.3
hand gun (pistol) (revolver) E955.0
paintball gun E955.7
rifle (hunting) E955.2
military E955.3
shotgun (automatic) E955.1
specified firearm NEC E955.4
Verey pistol E955.4
shotgun (automatic) E922.1
specified firearm NEC E922.8
stated as undetermined whether accidental or
intentional E985.4
hand gun (pistol) (revolver) E985.0
military firearm, except hand gun E985.3
hand gun (pistol) (revolver) E985.0
paintball gun E985.7
rifle (hunting) E985.2
military E985.3
shotgun (automatic) E985.1

specified firearm NEC E985.4
Verey pistol E985.4
suicidal (attempt) E955.4
air gun E955.6
BB gun E955.6
hand gun (pistol) (revolver) E955.0
military firearm, except hand gun E955.3
hand gun (pistol) (revolver) E955.0
paintball gun E955.7
rifle (hunting) E955.2
military E955.3
shotgun (automatic) E955.1
specified firearm NEC E955.4
Verey pistol E955.4
Verey pistol E922.8
Shoving (accidentally) by other person (*see
also* Pushing by other person) E917.9
Sickness
air E903
alpine E902.0
car E903
motion E903
mountain E902.0
sea E903
travel E903
Sinking (accidental)
boat, ship, watercraft (causing drowning,
submersion) E830
causing injury except drowning,
submersion E831
Siriasis E900.0
Skydiving E844
Slashed wrists (*see also* Cut, self-inflicted)
E986
Slipping (accidental)
on
deck (of boat, ship, watercraft) (icy)
(oily) (wet) E835
ice E885.9
ladder of ship E833
due to accident to watercraft E831
mud E885.9
oil E885.9
snow E885.9
stairs of ship E833
due to accident to watercraft E831
surface
slippery E885.9
wet E885.9
Sliver, wood, injury by E920.8
Smothering, smothered (*see also* Suffocation)
E913.9
Smouldering building or structure in terrorism
E979.3
Sodomy (assault) E960.1
Solid substance in eye (any part) or adnexa
E914
Sound waves (causing injury) E928.1
Splinter, injury by E920.8
Stab, stabbing E966
accidental—*see* Cut
Starvation E904.1
helpless person, infant, newborn—*see* Lack of
food
homicidal intent E968.4
late effect of NEC E929.5
resulting from accident connected with
transport—*see* categories E800-E848

Submersion— *continued*
  terrorism E979.8
  war operations E995
  water transport E832
    due to accident to boat, ship, watercraft
      E830
  landslide E909.2
  overturning boat, ship, watercraft E909.2
  sinking boat, ship, watercraft E909.2
  submersion boat, ship, watercraft E909.2
  tidal wave E909.4
    caused by storm E908.0
  torrential rain E908.2
  late effect of NEC E929.8
  quenching tank E910.8
  self-inflicted (unspecified whether accidental
    or intentional) E984
    in accidental circumstances—*see* category
      E910
    stated as intentional, purposeful E954
    stated as undetermined whether accidental or
      intentional E984
  suicidal (attempted) E954
  while
    attempting rescue of another person
      E910.3
    engaged in
      marine salvage E910.3
      underwater construction or repairs E910.3
    fishing, not from boat E910.2
    hunting, not from boat E910.2
    ice skating E910.2
    pearl diving E910.3
    placing fishing nets E910.3
    playing in water E910.2
    scuba diving E910.1
      nonrecreational E910.3
    skin diving E910.1
    snorkel diving E910.2
    spear fishing underwater E910.1
    surfboarding E910.2
    swimming (swimming pool) E910.2
    wading (in water) E910.2
    water skiing E910.0
Sucked
  into
    jet (aircraft) E844
Suffocation (accidental) (by external means)
  (by pressure) (mechanical) E913.9
  caused by other person
    in accidental circumstances—*see* category
      E913
    stated as
      intentional, homicidal E963
      undetermined whether accidental or
        intentional E983.9
      by, in
        hanging E983.0
        plastic bag E983.1
        specified means NEC E983.3
  due to, by
    avalanche E909.2
    bedclothes E913.0
    bib E913.0
    blanket E913.0
    cave-in E913.3
      caused by cataclysmic earth surface
        movement or eruption E909.9
    conflagration—*see* Conflagration
    explosion—*see* Explosion
    falling earth, other substance E913.3

Suffocation—*continued*
  fire—*see* Fire
  food, any type (ingestion) (inhalation)
    (regurgitated) (vomited) E911
  foreign body, except food (ingestion)
    (inhalation) E912
  ignition—*see* Ignition
  landslide E909.2
  machine(ry)—*see* Accident, machine
  material, object except food entering by
    nose or mouth, ingested, inhaled E912
  mucus (aspiration) (inhalation), not of
    newborn E912
  phlegm (aspiration) (inhalation) E912
  pillow E913.0
  plastic bag—*see* Suffocation, in, plastic
    bag
  sheet (plastic) E913.0
  specified means NEC E913.8
  vomitus (aspiration) (inhalation) E911
  homicidal (attempt) E963
  in
    airtight enclosed place E913.2
    baby carriage E913.0
    bed E913.0
    closed place E913.2
    cot, cradle E913.0
    perambulator E913.0
    plastic bag (in accidental circumstances)
      E913.1
      homicidal, purposely inflicted by other
        person E963
      self-inflicted (unspecified whether
        accidental or intentional) E983.1
        in accidental circumstances E913.1
        intentional, suicidal E953.1
      stated as undetermined whether
        accidentally or purposely inflicted
        E983.1
      suicidal, purposely self-inflicted E953.1
    refrigerator E913.2
  self-inflicted—*see also* Suffocation, stated as
    undetermined whether accidental or
    intentional E953.9
    in accidental circumstances—*see* category
      E913
    stated as intentional, purposeful—*see*
      Suicide, suffocation
    stated as undetermined whether accidental or
      intentional E983.9
    by, in
      hanging E983.0
      plastic bag E983.1
      specified means NEC E983.8
    suicidal—*see* Suicide, suffocation
Suicide, suicidal (attempted) (by) E958.9
  burning, burns E958.1
  caustic substance E958.7
    poisoning E950.7
    swallowed E950.7
  cold, extreme E958.3
  cut (any part of body) E956
  cutting or piercing instrument (classifiable to
    E920) E956
  drowning E954
  electrocution E958.4
  explosive(s) (classifiable to E923) E955.5
  fire E958.1
  firearm (classifiable to E922)—*see* Shooting,
    suicidal
  hanging E953.0

Suicide, suicidal—*continued*
  jumping
    before moving object, train, vehicle
      E958.0
    from high place—*see* Jumping, from,
      high place, stated as, suicidal
  knife E956
  late effect of E959
  motor vehicle, crashing of E958.5
  poisoning—*see* Table of drugs and chemicals
  puncture (any part of body) E956
  scald E958.2
  shooting—*see* Shooting, suicidal
  specified means NEC E958.8
  stab (any part of body) E956
  strangulation—*see* Suicide, suffocation
  submersion E954
  suffocation E953.9
    by, in
      hanging E953.0
      plastic bag E953.1
      specified means NEC E953.8
  wound NEC E958.9
Sunburn E926.2
Sunstroke E900.0
Supersonic waves (causing injury) E928.1
Surgical procedure, complication of
  delayed or as an abnormal reaction without
    mention of misadventure—*see* Reaction,
    abnormal
  due to or as a result of misadventure—*see*
    Misadventure
Swallowed, swallowing
  foreign body—*see* Foreign body, alimentary
    canal
  poison—*see* Table of drugs and chemicals
  substance
    caustic—*see* Table of drugs and chemicals
    corrosive—*see* Table of drugs and
      chemicals
    poisonous—*see* Table of drugs and
      chemicals
Swimmers cramp (*see also* category E910)
  E910.2
  not in recreation or sport E910.3
Syndrome, battered
  baby or child—*see* Abuse, child
  wife—*see* Assault

T

Tackle in sport E886.0
Terrorism (injury) (by) (in) E979.8
  air blast E979.2
  aircraft burned, destroyed, exploded, shot
    down E979.1
    used as a weapon E979.1
  anthrax E979.6
  asphyxia from
    chemical (weapons) E979.7
    fire, conflagration (caused by
      fire-producing device) E979.3
    from nuclear explosion E979.5
    gas or fumes E979.7
  bayonet E979.8
  biological agents E979.6
  blast (air) (effects) E979.2
    from nuclear explosion E979.5
    underwater E979.0

Terrorism—*continued*
  bomb (antipersonnel) (mortar) (explosion)
    (fragments) E979.2
  bullet(s) (from carbine, machine gun, pistol,
    rifle, shotgun) E979.4
  burn from
    chemical E979.7
    fire, conflagration (caused by
      fire-producing device) E979.3
    from nuclear explosion E979.5
    gas E979.7
  burning aircraft E979.1
  chemical E979.7
  cholera E979.6
  conflagration E979.3
  crushed by falling aircraft E979.1
  depth-charge E979.0
  destruction of aircraft E979.1
  disability, as sequelae one year or more after
    injury E999.1
  drowning E979.8
  effect
    of nuclear weapon (direct) (secondary)
      E979.5
    secondary NEC E979.9
    sequelae E999.1
  explosion (artillery shell) (breech-block)
    (cannon block) E979.2
    aircraft E979.1
    bomb (antipersonnel) (mortar) E979.2
      nuclear (atom) (hydrogen) E979.5
    depth-charge E979.0
    grenade E979.2
    injury by fragments from E979.2
    land-mine E979.2
    marine weapon E979.0
    mine (land) E979.2
      at sea or in harbor E979.0
      marine E979.0
    missile (explosive) NEC E979.2
    munitions (dump) (factory) E979.2
    nuclear (weapons) E979.5
    other direct and secondary effects of
      E979.5
    sea-based artillery shell E979.0
    torpedo E979.0
  exposure to ionizing radiation from nuclear
    explosion E979.5
  falling aircraft E979.1
  fire or fire-producing device E979.3
  firearms E979.4
  fireball effects from nuclear explosion E979.5
  fragments from artillery shell, bomb NEC,
    grenade, guided missile, land-mine, rocket,
    shell, shrapnel E979.2
  gas or fumes E979.7
  grenade (explosion) (fragments) E979.2
  guided missile (explosion) (fragments) E979.2
    nuclear E979.5
  heat from nuclear explosion E979.5
  hot substance E979.3
  hydrogen cyanide E979.7
  land-mine (explosion) (fragments) E979.2
  laser(s) E979.8
  late effect of E999.1
  lewisite E979.7
  lung irritant (chemical) (fumes) (gas) E979.7
  marine mine E979.0
  mine E979.2
    at sea E979.0
    in harbor E979.0

Terrorism—*continued*
  land (explosion) (fragments) E979.2
  marine E979.0
  missile (explosion) (fragments) (guided)
      E979.2
  marine E979.0
  nuclear E979.5
  mortar bomb (explosion) (fragments) E979.2
  mustard gas E979.7
  nerve gas E979.7
  nuclear weapons E979.5
  pellets (shotgun) E979.4
  petrol bomb E979.3
  piercing object E979.8
  phosgene E979.7
  poisoning (chemical) (fumes) (gas) E979.7
  radiation, ionizing from nuclear explosion
      E979.5
  rocket (explosion) (fragments) E979.2
  saber, sabre E979.8
  sarin E979.7
  screening smoke E979.7
  sequelae effect (of) E999.1
  shell (aircraft) (artillery) (cannon)
      (land-based) (explosion) (fragments)
      E979.2
    sea-based E979.0
  shooting E979.4
    bullet(s) E979.4
    pellet(s) (rifle) (shotgun) E979.4
  shrapnel E979.2
  smallpox E979.7
  stabbing object(s)E979.8
  submersion E979.8
  torpedo E979.0
  underwater blast E979.0
  vesicant (chemical) (fumes) (gas) E979.7
  weapon burst E979.2
Thermic fever E900.9
Thermoplegia E900.9
Thirst —*see also* Lack of water
  resulting from accident connected with
      transport—*see* categories E800-E848
Thrown (accidently)
  against object in or part of vehicle
    by motion of vehicle
      aircraft E844
      boat, ship, watercraft E838
      motor vehicle (on public highway) E818
        not on public highway E825
        off-road type (not on public highway)
            E821
          on public highway E818
        snow vehicle E820
          on public highway E818
      nonmotor road vehicle NEC E829
      railway rolling stock, train, vehicle E806
      street car E829
  from
    animal (being ridden) (in sport or
        transport) E828
    high place, homicide (attempt) E968.1
    machinery—*see* Accident, machine
    vehicle NEC—*see* Accident, vehicle NEC
    off—*see* Thrown, from
    overboard (by motion of boat, ship,
        watercraft) E832
      by accident to boat, ship, watercraft E830
Thunderbolt NEC E907
Tidal wave (any injury) E909.4
  caused by storm E908.0

Took
  overdose of drug—*see* Table of drugs and
      chemicals
  poison—*see* Table of drugs and chemicals
Tornado (any injury) E908.1
Torrential rain (any injury) E908.2
Traffic accident NEC E819
Trampled by animal E906.8
  being ridden (in sport or transport) E828
Trapped (accidentally)
  between
    objects (moving) (stationary and moving)
        E918
  by
    door of
      elevator E918
      motor vehicle (on public highway) (while
          alighting, boarding)—*see* Fall, from,
          motor vehicle, while alighting
      railway train (underground) E806
      street car E829
      subway train E806
  in object E918
Travel (effects) E903
  sickness E903
Tree
  falling on or hitting E916
    motor vehicle (in motion) (on public
        highway) E818
      not on public highway E825
    nonmotor road vehicle NEC E829
    pedal cycle E826
    person E916
    railway rolling stock, train, vehicle E806
    street car E829
Trench foot E901.0
Tripping over animal, carpet, curb, rug, or
    small object (with fall) E885.9
  without fall—*see* Striking against, object
Tsunami E909.4
Twisting, injury in E927

V

Violence, nonaccidental (*see also* Assault)
    E968.9
Volcanic eruption (any injury) E909.1
Vomitus in air passages (with asphyxia,
    obstruction or suffocation) E911

W

War operations (during hostilities) (injury)
    (by) (in) E995
  after cessation of hostilities, injury due to
      E998
  air blast E993
  aircraft burned, destroyed, exploded, shot
      down E994
  asphyxia from
    chemical E997.2
    fire, conflagration (caused by
        fire-producing device or conventional
        weapon) E990.9
      from nuclear explosion E996
      petrol bomb E990.0
    fumes E997.2
    gas E997.2
  battle wound NEC E995

War operations—*continued*
 bayonet E995
 biological warfare agents E997.1
 blast (air) (effects) E993
  from nuclear explosion E996
  underwater E992
 bomb (mortar) (explosion) E993
  after cessation of hostilities E998
  fragments, injury by E991.9
   antipersonnel E991.3
 bullet(s) (from carbine, machine gun, pistol,
   rifle, shotgun) E991.2
  rubber E991.0
 burn from
  chemical E997.2
  fire, conflagration (caused by
    fire-producing device or conventional
    weapon) E990.9
   from nuclear explosion E996
   petrol bomb E990.0
  gas E997.2
 burning aircraft E994
 chemical E997.2
 chlorine E997.2
 conventional warfare, specified form NEC
   E995
 crushing by falling aircraft E994
 depth charge E992
 destruction of aircraft E994
 disability as sequela one year or more after
   injury E999.0
 drowning E995
 effect (direct) (secondary) nuclear weapon
   E996
 explosion (artillery shell) (breech block)
   (cannon shell) E993
  after cessation of hostilities of bomb,
    mine placed in war E998
  aircraft E994
  bomb (mortar) E993
   atom E996
   hydrogen E996
   injury by fragments from E991.9
    antipersonnel E991.3
   nuclear E996
  depth charge E992
  injury by fragments from E991.9
   antipersonnel E991.3
  marine weapon E992
  mine
   at sea or in harbor E992
   land E993
    injury by fragments from E991.9
   marine E992
  munitions (accidental) (being used in
    war) (dump) (factory) E993
  nuclear (weapon) E996
  own weapons (accidental) E993
   injury by fragments from E991.9
    antipersonnel E991.3
  sea-based artillery shell E992
  torpedo E992
 exposure to ionizing radiation from nuclear
   explosion E996
 falling aircraft E994
 fire or fire-producing device E990.9
  petrol bomb E990.0
 fireball effects from nuclear explosion E996
 fragments from
  antipersonnel bomb E991.3

War operations—*continued*
  artillery shell, bomb NEC, grenade,
    guided missile, land mine, rocket,
    shell, shrapnel E991.9
 fumes E997.2
 gas E997.2
 grenade (explosion) E993
  fragments, injury by E991.9
 guided missile (explosion) E993
  fragments, injury by E991.9
  nuclear E996
 heat from nuclear explosion E996
 injury due to, but occurring after cessation of
   hostilities E998
 lacrimator (gas) (chemical) E997.2
 land mine (explosion) E993
  after cessation of hostilities E998
  fragments, injury by E991.9
 laser(s) E997.0
 late effect of E999.0
 lewisite E997.2
 lung irritant (chemical) (fumes) (gas) E997.2
 marine mine E992
 mine
  after cessation of hostilities E998
  at sea E992
  in harbor E992
  land (explosion) E993
   fragments, injury by E991.9
  marine E992
 missile (guided) (explosion) E993
  fragments, injury by E991.9
  marine E992
  nuclear E996
 mortar bomb (explosion) E993
  fragments, injury by E991.9
 mustard gas E997.2
 nerve gas E997.2
 phosgene E997.2
 poisoning (chemical) (fumes) (gas) E997.2
 radiation, ionizing from nuclear explosion
   E996
 rocket (explosion) E993
  fragments, injury by E991.9
 saber, sabre E995
 screening smoke E997.8
 shell (aircraft) (artillery) (cannon) (land
   based) (explosion) E993
  fragments, injury by E991.9
  sea-based E992
 shooting E991.2
  after cessation of hostilities E998
  bullet(s) E991.2
   rubber E991.0
  pellet(s) (rifle) E991.1
 shrapnel E991.9
 submersion E995
 torpedo E992
 unconventional warfare, except by nuclear
   weapon E997.9
  biological (warfare) E997.1
  gas, fumes, chemicals E997.2
  laser(s) E997.0
  specified type NEC E997.8
 underwater blast E992
 vesicant (chemical) (fumes) (gas) E997.2
 weapon burst E993
Washed
 away by flood—*see* Flood
 away by tidal wave—*see* Tidal wave
 off road by storm (transport vehicle) E908.9
 overboard E832

Weather exposure —*see also* Exposure
cold E901.0
hot E900.0
Weightlessness (causing injury) (effects of) (in
spacecraft, real or simulated) E928.0
Wound (accidental) NEC (*see also* Injury)
E928.9
battle (*see also* War operation) E995
bayonet E920.3
in
legal intervention E974
war operations E995
gunshot—*see* Shooting
incised—*see* Cut
saber, sabre E920.3
in war operations E995

RAILWAY ACCIDENTS (E800–E807)

The following fourth–digit subdivisions are for use with categories E800–E807 to identify the injured person.

.0 Railway employee

Any person who by virtue of his employment in connection with a railway, whether by the railway company or not, is at increased risk of involvement in a railway accident, such as:

catering staff on train	postal staff on train
driver	railway fireman
guard	shunter
porter	sleeping car attendant

.1 Passenger on railway

Any authorized person traveling on a train, except a railway employee

Excludes: intending passenger waiting at station (.8)
unauthorized rider on railway vehicle (.8)

.2 Pedestrian

See definition (r), Vol. 1, page 479

.3 Pedal cyclist

See definition (p), Vol. 1, page 479

.8 Other specified person

Intending passenger waiting at station

Unauthorized rider on railway vehicle

.9 Unspecified person

MOTOR VEHICLE TRAFFIC AND NONTRAFFIC ACCIDENTS
(E810–825)

The following fourth–digit subdivisions are for use with categories E810–E819 and E820–E825 to identify the injured person:

.0 Driver of motor vehicle other than motorcycle

> See definition (l), Vol. 1, page 479

.1 Passenger in motor vehicle other than motorcycle

> See definition (l), Vol. 1, page 479

.2 Motorcyclist

> See definition (l), Vol. 1, page 479

.3 Passenger on motorcycle

> See definition (l), Vol. 1, page 479

.4 Occupant of streetcar

.5 Rider of animal; occupant of animal–drawn vehicle

.6 Pedal cyclist

> See definition (p), Vol. 1, page 479

.7 Pedestrian

> See definition (r), Vol. 1, page 479

.8 Other specified person

> Occupant of vehicle other than above
>
> Person in railway train involved in accident
>
> Unauthorized rider of motor vehicle

.9 Unspecified person

OTHER ROAD VEHICLE ACCIDENTS (E826–E829)

(animal–drawn vehicle, streetcar, pedal cycle, and other nonmotor road vehicle accidents)

The following fourth–digit subdivisions are for use with categories E826–E829 to identify the injured person:

.0 Pedestrian

> See definition (r), Vol. 1, page 479

.1 Pedal cyclist (does not apply to codes E827, E828, E829)

> See definition (p), Vol. 1, page 479

.2 Rider of animal (does not apply to code E829)

.3 Occupant of animal–drawn vehicle (does not apply to codes E828, E829)

.4 Occupant of streetcar

.8 Other specified person

.9 Unspecified person

WATER TRANSPORT ACCIDENTS (E830–E838)

The following fourth–digit subdivisions are for use with categories E830–E838 to identify the injured person:

.0 Occupant of small boat, unpowered

.1 Occupant of small boat, powered

See definition (t), Vol. 1, page 479

Excludes: water skier (.4)

.2 Occupant of other watercraft — crew

Persons:

engaged in operation of watercraft

providing passenger services [cabin attendants, ship's physician, catering personnel]

working on ship during voyage in other capacity [musician in band, operators of shops and beauty parlors]

.3 Occupant of other watercraft — other than crew

Passenger

Occupant of lifeboat, other than crew, after abandoning ship

.4 Water skier

.5 Swimmer

.6 Dockers, stevedores

Longshoreman employed on the dock in loading and unloading ships

.8 Other specified person

Immigration and custom officials on board ship

Person:

accompanying passenger or member of crew

visiting boat

Pilot (guiding ship into port)

.9 Unspecified person

AIR AND SPACE TRANSPORT ACCIDENTS (E840–E845)

The following fourth–digit subdivisions are for use with categories E840–E845 to identify the injured person:

.0 Occupant of spacecraft

.1 Occupant of military aircraft, any

Crew	in military aircraft [air force] [army]
Passenger (civilian) (military)	[national guard] [navy]
Troops	

Excludes: occupants of aircraft operated under jurisdiction of police departments (.5)
parachutist (.7).

.2 Crew of commercial aircraft (powered) in surface to surface transport

.3 Other occupant of commercial aircraft (powered) in surface to surface transport

Flight personnel:

not part of crew
on familiarization flight

Passenger on aircraft (powered) NOS

.4 Occupant of commercial aircraft (powered) in surface to air transport

Occupant [crew] [passenger] of aircraft (powered) engaged in activities, such as:

aerial spraying (crops) (fire retardants)
air drops of emergency supplies
air drops of parachutists, except from military craft
crop dusting
lowering of construction material [bridge or telephone pole]
sky writing

.5 Occupant of other powered aircraft

Occupant [crew] [passenger] of aircraft (powered) engaged in activities, such as:

aerobatic flying
aircraft racing
rescue operation
storm surveillance
traffic surveillance

Occupant of private plane NOS

.6 Occupant of unpowered aircraft, except parachutist

Occupant of aircraft classifiable to E842

.7 Parachutist (military) (other)

Person making voluntary descent

Excludes: person making descent after accident to aircraft (.1–.6)

.8 Ground crew, airline employee

Persons employed at airfields (civil) (military) or launching pads, not occupants of aircraft

.9 Other person

| 038 | **Septicemia** | 402.91 | **With heart failure** |
| | Exclusion added | | Revised code |

038 — **Septicemia**
Exclusion added

040.82 — **Toxic shock syndrome**
New code

062.8 — **Other specified mosquito-borne viral encephalitis**
Exclusion added

066.3 — **Other mosquito-borne fever**
Description revised

066.4 — **West Nile fever**
New code

256.2 — **Postablative ovarian failure**
Description added, exclusion term revised

256.3 — **Other ovarian failure**
Description revised

277.00 — **Without mention of meconium ileus**
Description added

277.02 — **With pulmonary manifestations**
New code

277.03 — **With gastrointestinal manifestations**
New code

277.09 — **With other manifestations**
New code

277.7 — **Dysmetabolic syndrom X**
Description revised

337.3 — **Autonomic dysreflexia**
Description revised

357.8 — **Other**
Description deleted

357.81 — **Chronic inflammatory demyelinating polyneuritis**
New code

357.82 — **Critical illness polyneuropathy**
New code

357.89 — **Other inflammatory and toxic neuropathy**
New code

359.81 — **Critical illness myopathy**
New code

359.89 — **Other myopathies**
New code

365.83 — **Aqueous misdirection**
New code

368.6 — **Night blindness**
Description deleted

402 — **Hypertensive heart disease**
Description added

402.00 — **Without heart failure**
Revised code

402.01 — **With heart failure**
Revised code

402.10 — **Without heart failure**
Revised code

402.11 — **With heart failure**
Revised code

402.90 — **Without heart failure**
Revised code

402.91 — **With heart failure**
Revised code

404 — **Hypertensive heart and renal disease**
Description added, revised

411.81 — **Acute coronary occlusion without myocardial infarction**
Exclusion term revised

414.06 — **Of coronary artery of transplanted heart**
New code

414.1 — **Aneurysm and dissection of heart**
Revised code

414.10 — **Aneurysm of heart (wall)**
Revised code

414.11 — **Aneurysm of coronary vessels**
Revised code

414.12 — **Dissection of coronary artery**
New code

414.19 — **Other aneurysm of heart**
Revised code

427.89 — **Other**
Exclusion added

428 — **Heart failure**
Exclusion deleted, description added

428.0 — **Congestive heart failure, unspecified**
Revised code

428.2 — **Systolic heart failure**
New subcategory

428.20 — **Unspecified**
New code

428.21 — **Acute**
New code

428.22 — **Chronic**
New code

428.23 — **Acute on chronic**
New code

428.3 — **Diastolic heart failure**
New subcategory

428.30 — **Unspecified**
New code

428.31 — **Acute**
New code

428.32 — **Chronic**
New code

428.33 — **Acute on chronic**
New code

428.4 — **Combined systolic and diastolic heart failure**
New subcategory

428.40 — **Unspecified**
New code

428.41 — **Acute**
New code

428.42 — **Chronic**
New code

428.43 — **Acute on chronic**
New code

430-438 — **CEREBROVASCULAR DISEASE**
Exclusion added

436	**Acute, but ill-defined, cerebrovascular disease** Exclusion added		459.12	**Postphlebetic syndrome with inflammation** New code
438.6	**Alterations of sensations** New code		459.13	**Postphlebetic syndrome with ulcer and inflammation** New code
438.7	**Disturbances of vision** New code		459.19	**Postphlebetic syndrome with other complication** New code
438.83	**Facial weakness** New code		459.3	**Chronic venous hypertension (idiopathic)** New subcategory
438.84	**Ataxia** New code		459.30	**Chronic venous hypertension without complications** New code
438.85	**Vertigo** New code		459.31	**Chronic venous hypertension with ulcer** New code
440	**Atherosclerosis** Exclusion added		459.32	**Chronic venous hypertension with inflammation** New code
440.8	**Of other specified arteries** Exclusion term revised		459.33	**Chronic venous hypertension with ulcer and inflammation** New code
441.0	**Dissection of aorta** Description deleted		459.39	**Chronic venous hypertension with other complication** New code
443.2	**Other arterial dissection** New subcategory		491.2	**Obstructive chronic bronchitis** Description deleted
443.21	**Dissection of carotid artery** New code		491.20	**Without mention of acute exacerbation** Description deleted
43.22	**Dissection of iliac artery** New code		491.21	**With acute exacerbation** Description deleted
443.23	**Dissection of renal artery** New code		493.2	**Chronic obstructive asthma** Description added, exclusion added
443.24	**Dissection of vertebral artery** New code		518.81	**Acute respiratory failure** Exclusion term revised
443.29	**Dissection of other artery** New code		518.82	**Other pulmonary insufficiency, not elsewhere classified** Exclusion term revised
444	**Arterial embolism and thrombosis** Exclusion added		521.0	**Dental caries** Description deleted
445	**Atheroembolism** New category		537.84	**Dieulafoy lesion (hemorrhagic) of stomach and duodenum** New code
445.0	**Of extremities** New subcategory		569.86	**Dieulafoy lesion (hemorrhagic) of intestine** New code
445.01	**Upper extremity** New code		577.8	**Other specified diseases of pancreas** Exclusion term revised
445.02	**Lower extremity** New code		590.0	**Chronic pyelonephritis** Description added, deleted
445.8	**Of other sites** New subcategory		593.7	**Vesicoureteral reflux** Description deleted
445.81	**Kidney** New code		599.0	**Urinary tract infection, site not specified** Exclusion added
445.89	**Other site** New code		602.3	**Dysplasia of prostate** Description revised, exclusion term revised
447.6	**Arteritis, unspecified** Exclusion term revised		622.1	**Dysplasia of cervix (uteri)** Description added
454.8	**With other complications** New code		627.2	**Symptomatic menopausal or female climacteric states** Revised code
454.9	**Asymptomatic varicose veins** Revised code			
459.1	**Postphlebetic syndrome** Description added, exclusion added			
459.10	**Postphlebetic syndrome without complications** New code			
459.11	**Postphlebetic syndrome with ulcer** New code			

627.4	**Symptomatic states associated with artificial menopause** Revised code		764-779	**OTHER CONDITIONS ORIGINATING IN THE PERINATAL PERIOD** Description revised
629.0	**Hematocele, female, not elsewhere classified** Exclusion term revised		765.0	**Extreme immaturity** Revised note
633.00	**Abdominal pregnancy without intrauterine pregnancy** New code		765.1	**Other preterm infants** Revised note
633.01	**Abdominal pregnancy with intrauterine pregnancy** New code		765.2	**Weeks of gestation** New subcategory
633.10	**Tubal pregnancy without intrauterine pregnancy** New code		765.20	**Unspecfied weeks of gestation** New code
633.11	**Tubal pregnancy with intrauterine pregnancy** New code		765.21	**Less than 24 completed weeks of gestation** New code
633.20	**Ovarian pregnancy without intrauterine pregnancy** New code		765.22	**24 completed weeks of gestation** New code
633.21	**Ovarian pregnancy with intrauterine pregnancy** New code		765.23	**25-26 completed weeks of gestation** New code
633.80	**Other ectopic pregnancy without intrauterine pregnancy** New code		765.24	**27-28 completed weeks of gestation** New code
633.81	**Other ectopic pregnancy with intrauterine pregnancy** New code		765.25	**29-30 completed weeks of gestation** New code
633.90	**Unspecified ectopic pregnancy without intrauterine pregnancy** New code		765.26	**31-32 completed weeks of gestation** New code
633.91	**Unspecified ectopic pregnancy with intrauterine pregnancy** New code		765.27	**33-34 completed weeks of gestation** New code
646.6	**Infections of genitourinary tract in pregnancy** Description revised		765.28	**35-36 completed weeks of gestation** New code
674.1	**Disruption of cesarean wound** Exclusion added		765.29	**37 or more completed weeks of gestation** New code
707.1	**Ulcer of lower limbs, except decubitus** Description added		770.8	**Other respiratory problems after birth** Descriptions deleted
710	**Diffuse diseases of connective tissue** Description deleted		770.81	**Primary apnea of newborn** New code
710.1	**Systemic sclerosis** Description added		770.82	**Other apnea of newborn** New code
718.7	**Developmental dislocation of joint** Exclusion terms added, deleted		770.83	**Cyanotic attacks of newborn** New code
723.5	**Torticollis, unspecified** Exclusion added		770.84	**Respiratory failure of newborn** New code
730.1	**Chronic osteomyelitis** Description deleted		770.89	**Other respiratory problems after birth** New code
733.4	**Aseptic necrosis of bone** Exclusion term deleted		771.8	**Other infections specific to the perinatal period** Descriptions deleted
747.83	**Persistent fetal circulation** New code		771.81	**Septicemia [sepsis] of newborn** New code
751.7	**Anomalies of pancreas** Exclusion term revised		771.82	**Urinary tract infection of newborn** New code
753.0	**Renal agenesis and dysgenesis** Description deleted		771.83	**Bacteremia of newborn** New code
753.15	**Renal dysplasia** Description deleted		771.89	**Other infections specific to the perinatal period** New code
			774.5	**Perinatal jaundice from other causes** Description revised
			779.81	**Neonatal bradycardia** New code
			779.82	**Neonatal tachycardia** New code

779.89	**Other specified conditions originating in the perinatal period** New code
780.9	**Other general symptoms** Descriptions deleted
780.91	**Fussy infant (baby)** New code
780.92	**Excessive crying of infant (baby)** New code
780.99	**Other general symptoms** New code
781.93	**Ocular torticollis** New code
782.5	**Cyanosis** Exclusion term revised
785.0	**Tachycardia, unspecified** Exclusion added
786.03	**Apnea** Exclusion added
786.09	**Other** Exclusion term revised
788.3	**Incontinence of urine** Description added, deleted
790.7	**Bacteremia** Exclusion added
795.0	**Nonspecific abnormal Papanicolaou smear of cervix** Exclusion added, description deleted
795.00	**Nonspecific abnormal Papanicolaou smear of cervix, unspecified** New code
795.01	**Atypical squamous cell changes of undetermined significance favor benign (ASCUS favor benign)** New code
795.02	**Atypical squamous cell changes of undetermined significance favor dysplasia (ASCUS favor dysplasia)** New code
795.09	**Other nonspecific abnormal Papanicolaou smear of cervix** New code
795.31	**Nonspecific positive findings for anthrax** New code
795.39	**Other nonspecific positive culture findings** New code
799.1	**Respiratory arrest** Exclusion term revised
800-829	**FRACTURES** Description deleted
813.45	**Torus fracture of radius** New code
823.4	**Torus fracture** New code
959.01	**Head injury, unspecified** Exclusion added
991.6	**Hypothermia** Exclusion term revised
995.0	**Other anaphylactic shock** Description deleted

995.9	**Systemic inflammatory response syndrome (SIRS)** New subcategory
995.90	**Systemic inflammatory response syndrome, unspecified SIRS NOS** New code
995.91	**Systemic inflammatory response syndrome due to infectious process without organ dysfunction** New code
995.92	**Systemic inflammatory response syndrome due to infectious process with organ dysfunction** New code
995.93	**Systemic inflammatory response syndrome due to non-infectious process without organ dysfunction** New code
995.94	**Systemic inflammatory response syndrome due to non-infectious process with organ dysfunction** New code
996.72	**Due to other cardiac device, implant, and graft** Exclusion term revised
998.31	**Disruption of internal operation wound** New code
998.32	**Disruption of external operation wound** New code
V01-V83	**SUPPLEMENTARY CLASSIFICATION OF FACTORS INFLUENCING HEALTH STATUS AND CONTACT WITH HEALTH SERVICES (V01-V83)** Heading revised
V01.81	**Anthrax** New code
V01.89	**Other communicable diseases** New code
V13.21	**Personal history of pre-term labor** New code
V13.29	**Other genital system and obstetric disorders** New code
V23.41	**Pregnancy with history of pre-term labor** New code
V23.49	**Pregnancy with other poor obstetric history** New code
V46.2	**Supplemental oxygen** New code
V49.81	**Asymptomatic postmenopausal status (age-related) (natural)** Revised code
V54.0	**Aftercare involving removal of fracture plate or other internal fixation device** Exclusion term revised
V54.1	**Aftercare for healing traumatic fracture** New subcategory
V54.10	**Aftercare for healing traumatic fracture of arm, unspecified** New code

V54.11	Aftercare for healing traumatic fracture of upper arm New code		**V58.43**	Aftercare following surgery for injury and trauma New code
V54.12	Aftercare for healing traumatic fracture of lower arm New code		**V58.7**	Aftercare following surgery to specified body systems, not elsewhere classified New subcategory
V54.13	Aftercare for healing traumatic fracture of hip New code		**V58.71**	Aftercare following surgery of the sense organs, NEC New code
V54.14	Aftercare for healing traumatic fracture of leg, unspecified New code		**V58.72**	Aftercare following surgery of the nervous system, NEC New code
V54.15	Aftercare for healing traumatic fracture of upper ieg New code		**V58.73**	Aftercare following surgery of the circulatory system, NEC New code
V54.16	Aftercare for healing traumatic fracture of lower leg New code		**V58.74**	Aftercare following surgery of the respiratory system, NEC New code
V54.17	Aftercare for healing traumatic fracture of vertebrae New code		**V58.75**	Aftercare following surgery of the teeth, oral cavity and digestive system, NEC New code
V54.19	Aftercare for healing traumatic fracture of other bone New code		**V58.76**	Aftercare following surgery of the genitourinary system, NEC New code
V54.2	Aftercare for healing pathologic fracture New subcategory		**V58.77**	Aftercare following surgery of the skin and subcutaneous tissue, NEC New code
V54.20	Aftercare for healing pathologic fracture of arm, unspecified New code		**V58.78**	Aftercare following surgery of the musculoskeletal system, NEC New code
V54.21	Aftercare for healing pathologic fracture of upper arm New code		**V58.83**	Encounter for therapeutic drug monitoring Description added
V54.22	Aftercare for healing pathologic fracture of lower arm New code		**V70**	-V83 PERSONS WITHOUT REPORTED DIAGNOSIS ENCOUNTERED DURING EXAMINATION AND INVESTIGATION OF INDIVIDUALS AND POPULATIONS (V70-V83) Heading revised
V54.23	Aftercare for healing pathologic fracture of hip New code			
V54.24	Aftercare for healing pathologic fracture of leg, unspecified New code		**V71.8**	Observation and evaluation for other specified suspected conditions Revised code
V54.25	Aftercare for healing pathologic fracture of upper leg New code		**V71.82**	Observation and evaluation for suspected exposure to anthrax New code
V54.26	Aftercare for healing pathologic fracture of lower leg New code		**V71.83**	Observation and evaluation for suspected exposure to other biological agent New code
V54.27	Aftercare for healing pathologic fracture of vertebrae New code		**V83.8**	Other genetic carrier status New subcategory
V54.29	Aftercare for healing pathologic fracture of other bone New code		**V83.81**	Cystic fibrosis gene carrier New code
V54.8	Other orthopedic aftercare Description deleted		**V83.89**	Other genetic carrier status New code
V54.81	Aftercare following joint replacement New code		**E885.0**	Fall from (nonmotorized) scooter New code
V54.89	Other orthopedic aftercare New code		**E922.5**	Paintball gun New code
V58.4	Other aftercare following surgery Description added		**E955.7**	Paintball gun New code
V58.42	Aftercare following surgery for neoplasm New code			

E960	**-E969 HOMICIDE AND INJURY PURPOSELY INFLICTED BY OTHER PERSONS**
	Exclusion term added
E979	**Terrorism**
	New category
E979.0	**Terrorism involving explosion of marine weapons**
	New code
E979.1	**Terrorism involving destruction of aircraft**
	New code
E979.2	**Terrorism involving other explosions and fragments**
	New code
E979.3	**Terrorism involving fires, conflagration and hot substances**
	New code
E979.4	**Terrorism involving firearms**
	New code
E979.5	**Terrorism involving nuclear weapons**
	New code
E979.6	**Terrorism involving biological weapons**
	New code
E979.7	**Terrorism involving chemical weapons**
	New code
E979.8	**Terrorism involving other means**
	New code
E979.9	**Terrorism, secondary effects**
	New code
E985.7	**Paintball gun**
	New code
E999	**Late effect of injury due to war operations and terrorism**
	Revised code
E999.0	**Late effect of injury due to war operations**
	New code
E999.1	**Late effect of injury due to terrorism**
	New code

PROCEDURES: TABULAR LIST
AND
ALPHABETIC INDEX
VOLUME 3

1.   **OPERATIONS ON THE NERVOUS SYSTEM (01-05)**

- **00**   **Procedures and interventions, Not Elsewhere Classified**
  - **00.0**   **Therapeutic ultrasound**
    - **00.01** **Therapeutic ultrasound of vessels of head and neck**
      Anti-restenotic ultrasound
      Intravascular non-ablative ultrasound

      > *Excludes:* *diagnostic ultrasound of:*
      >   *eye (95.13)*
      >   *head and neck (88.71)*
      > *that of inner ear (20.79)*
      > *ultrasonic:*
      >   *angioplasty of non-coronary vessel (39.50)*
      >   *embolectomy (38.01, 38.02)*
      >   *endarterectomy (38.11, 38.12)*
      >   *thrombectomy (38.01, 38.02)*

    - **00.02** **Therapeutic ultrasound of heart**
      Anti-restenotic ultrasound
      Intravascular non-ablative ultrasound

      > *Excludes:* *diagnostic ultrasound of heart (88.72)*
      > *ultrasounic ablation of heart lesion (37.34)*
      > *ultrasonic angioplasty of coronary vessels (36.01, 36.02, 36.05, 36.09)*

    - **00.03** **Therapeutic ultrasound of peripheral vascular vessels**
      Anti-restenotic ultrasound
      Intravascular non-ablative ultrasound

      > *Excludes:* *diagnostic ultrasound of peripheral vascular system (88.77)*
      > *ultrasonic angioplasty of:*
      >   *non-coronary vessel (39.50)*

    - **00.09** **Other therapeutic ultrasound**

      > *Excludes:* *ultrasonic:*
      >   *fragmentation of urinary stones (59.95)*
      >   *percutaneous nephrostomy with fragmentation (55.04)*
      >   *physical therapy (93.35)*
      >   *transurethral guided laser induced prostatectomy (TULIP) (60.21)*

  - **00.1**   **Pharmaceuticals**
    - **00.10** **Implantation of chemotherapeutic agent**
      Brain wafer chemotherapy
      Interstitial / intracavitary

      > *Excludes:* *injection or infusion of cancer chemotherapeutic substance (99.25)*

    - **00.11** **Infusion of drotrecogin alfa (activated)**
      Infusion of recombinant protein

    - **00.12** **Administration of inhaled nitric oxide**
      Nitric oxide therapy

    - **00.13** **Injection or infusion of nesiritide**
      Human B-type natriuretic peptide (hBNP)

    - **00.14** **Injection or infusion of oxazolidinone class of antibiotics**
      Linezolid injection

  - **00.5**   **Other cardiovascular procedures**
    - **00.50** **Implantation of cardiac resynchronization pacemaker without mention of defibrillation, total system [CRT-P]**
      Biventricular pacing without internal cardiac defibrillator
      Implantation of cardiac resynchronization (biventricular) pulse generator pacing device, formation of pocket, transvenous leads including placement of lead into left ventricular coronary venous system, and intraoperative procedures for evaluation of lead signals

      > *Excludes:* *implantation of cardiac resynchronization defibrillator, total system [CRT-D] (00.51)*
      > *insertion or replacement of any type pacemaker device (37.80-37.87)*
      > *replacement of cardiac resynchronization defibrillator pulse generator only [CRT-D] (00.54)*
      > *replacement of cardiac resynchronization pacemaker pulse generator only [CRT-P] (00.53)*

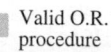 Valid O.R.
procedure

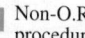 Non-O.R.
procedure

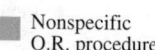 Nonspecific
O.R. procedure

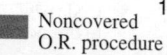 Noncovered
O.R. procedure

- **00.51 Implantation of cardiac resynchronization defibrillator, total system [CRT-D]**
  Biventricular pacing with internal cardiac defibrillator
  Implantation of a cardiac resynchronization (biventricular) pulse generator with defibrillator [AICD], formation of pocket, transvenous leads, including placement of lead into left ventricular coronary venous system, intraoperative procedures for evaluation of lead signals, and obtaining defibrillator threshold measurements

Excludes:	*implantation of cardiac resynchronization pacemaker, total system [CRT-P] (00.50)*
	implantation or replacement of automatic cardioverter/defibrillator, total system [AICD] (37.94)
	replacement of cardiac resynchronization defibrillator pulse generator only, [CRT-D] (00.54)

- **00.52 Implantation or replacement of transvenous lead [electrode] into left ventricular coronary venous system**

Excludes:	*implantation of cardiac resynchronization defibrillator, total system [CRT-D] (00.51)*
	implantation of cardiac resynchronization pacemeker, total system [CRT-P] (00.50)
	initial insertion of transvenous lead [electrode] (37.70-37.72)
	replacement of transvenous atrial and/or ventricular lead(s) [electrodes] (37.76)

- **00.53 Implantation or replacement of cardiac resynchronization pacemaker pulse generator only [CRT-P]**
  Implantation of CRT-P device with removal of any existing CRT-P or other pacemaker device

Excludes:	*implantation of cardiac resynchronization pacemaker, total system [CRT-P] (00.50)*
	implantation or replacement of cardiac resynchronization defibrillator pulse generator only [CRT-D] (00.54)
	insertion or replacement of any type pacemaker device (37.80-37.87)

- **00.54 Implantation or replacement of cardiac resynchronization defibrillator pulse generator device only [CRT-D]**
  Implantation of CRT-D device with removal of any existing CRT-D, CRT-P, pacemaker, or defibrillator device

Excludes:	*implantation of automatic cardioverter/defibrillator pulse generator only (37.96)*
	implantation of cardiac resynchronization defibrillator, total system [CRT-D] (00.51)
	implantation or replacement of cardiac resynchronization pacemaker pulse generator only [CRT-P] (00.53)

- **00.55 Insertion of drug-eluting non-coronary artery stent(s)**
  Endograft(s)
  Endovascular graft(s)
  Stent graft(s)
  Code also any non-coronary angioplasty or atherectomy (39.50)

Excludes:	*drug-coated stents, e.g., heparin coated (39.90)*
	insertion of drug-eluting coronary artery stent (36.07)
	insertion of non-drug-eluting stent(s):
	coronary artery (36.06)
	non-coronary artery (39.90)
	that for aneurysm repair (39.71-39.79)

01 Incision and excision of skull, brain, and cerebral meninges

01.0 Cranial puncture

  01.01 Cisternal puncture
  Cisternal tap

Excludes:	*pneumocisternogram (87.02)*

  01.02 Ventriculopuncture through previously implanted catheter
  Puncture of ventricular shunt tubing

● Code new to this edition   ▲ Revision of existing code   ④ ⑤ Fourth or fifth digit required

01.09 Other cranial puncture
Aspiration of
  subarachnoid space
  subdural space
Cranial aspiration NOS
Puncture of anterior fontanel
Subdural tap (through fontanel)

01.1 Diagnostic procedures on skull, brain, and cerebral meninges

01.11 Closed [percutaneous] [needle] biopsy of cerebral meninges
Burr hole approach

01.12 Open biopsy of cerebral meninges

01.13 Closed [percutaneous] [needle] biopsy of brain
Burr hole approach
Stereotactic method

01.14 Open biopsy of brain

01.15 Biopsy of skull

01.18 Other diagnostic procedures on brain and cerebral meninges

> Excludes: *cerebral:*
> *arteriography (88.41)*
> *thermography (88.81)*
> *contrast radiogram of brain (87.01-87.02)*
> *echoencephalogram (88.71)*
> *electroencephalogram (89.14)*
> *microscopic examination of specimen from nervous system and of*
> *spinal fluid (90.01-90.09)*
> *neurologic examination (89.13)*
> *phlebography of head and neck (88.61)*
> *pneumoencephalogram (87.01)*
> *radioisotope scan:*
> *cerebral (92.11)*
> *head NEC (92.12)*
> *tomography of head:*
> *C.A.T. scan (87.03)*
> *other (87.04)*

01.19 Other diagnostic procedures on skull

> Excludes: *transillumination of skull (89.16)*
> *x-ray of skull (87.17)*

01.2 Craniotomy and craniectomy

> Excludes: *decompression of skull fracture (02.02)*
> *exploration of orbit (16.01-16.09)*
> *that as operative approach—omit code*

01.21 Incision and drainage of cranial sinus

01.22 Removal of intracranial neurostimulator

> Excludes: *removal with synchronous replacement (02.93)*

01.23 Reopening of craniotomy site

01.24 Other craniotomy
Cranial:
  decompression
  exploration
  trephination
Craniotomy NOS
Craniotomy with removal of:
  epidural abscess
  extradural hematoma
  foreign body of skull

> Excludes: *removal of foreign body with incision into brain (01.39)*

01.25 Other craniectomy
Debridement of skull NOS
Sequestrectomy of skull

> Excludes: *debridement of compound fracture of skull (02.02)*
> *strip craniectomy (02.01)*

01.3 Incision of brain and cerebral meninges

01.31 Incision of cerebral meninges
Drainage of:
intracranial hygroma
subarachnoid abscess (cerebral)
subdural empyema

01.32 Lobotomy and tractotomy
Division of:
brain tissue
cerebral tracts
Percutaneous (radio frequency) cingulotomy

01.39 Other incision of brain
Amygdalohippocampotomy
Drainage of intracerebral hematoma
Incision of brain NOS

Excludes: *division of cortical adhesions (02.91)*

01.4 Operations on thalamus and globus pallidus

01.41 Operations on thalamus
Chemothalamectomy
Thalamotomy

Excludes: *that by stereotactic radiosurgery (92.30-92.39)*

01.42 Operations on globus pallidus
Pallidoansectomy
Pallidotomy

Excludes: *that by stereotactic radiosurgery (92.30-92.39)*

01.5 Other excision or destruction of brain and meninges

01.51 Excision of lesion or tissue of cerebral meninges
Decortication of (cerebral) meninges
Resection of (cerebral) meninges
Stripping of subdural membrane of (cerebral) meninges

Excludes: *biopsy of cerebral meninges (01.11-01.12)*

01.52 Hemispherectomy

01.53 Lobectomy of brain

01.59 Other excision or destruction of lesion or tissue of brain
Curettage of brain
Debridement of brain
Marsupialization of brain cyst
Transtemporal (mastoid) excision of brain tumor

Excludes: *biopsy of brain (01.13-01.14)*
that by stereotactic radiosurgery (92.30-92.39)

01.6 Excision of lesion of skull
Removal of granulation tissue of cranium

Excludes: *biopsy of skull (01.15)*
sequestrectomy (01.25)

02 Other operations on skull, brain, and cerebral meninges

02.0 Cranioplasty
Excludes: *that with synchronous repair of encephalocele (02.12)*

02.01 Opening of cranial suture
Linear craniectomy
Strip craniectomy

02.02 Elevation of skull fracture fragments
Debridement of compound fracture of skull
Decompression of skull fracture
Reduction of skull fracture

Code also any synchronous debridement of brain (01.59)

Excludes: *debridement of skull NOS (01.25)*
removal of granulation tissue of cranium (01.6)

02.03 Formation of cranial bone flap
Repair of skull with flap

● Code new
to this edition

▲ Revision of
existing code

④ ⑤ Fourth or fifth
digit required

02.04 **Bone graft to skull**
Pericranial graft (autogenous) (heterogenous)

02.05 **Insertion of skull plate**
Replacement of skull plate

02.06 **Other cranial osteoplasty**
Repair of skull NOS
Revision of bone flap of skull

02.07 **Removal of skull plate**

Excludes: removal with synchronous
replacement (02.05)

02.1 **Repair of cerebral meninges**

Excludes: marsupialization of cerebral lesion (01.59)

02.11 **Simple suture of dura mater of brain**

02.12 **Other repair of cerebral meninges**
Closure of fistula of cerebrospinal fluid
Dural graft
Repair of encephalocele including synchronous cranioplasty
Repair of meninges NOS
Subdural patch

02.13 **Ligation of meningeal vessel**
Ligation of:
longitudinal sinus
middle meningeal artery

02.14 **Choroid plexectomy**
Cauterization of choroid plexus

02.2 **Ventriculostomy**
Anastomosis of ventricle to:
cervical subarachnoid space
cisterna magna
Insertion of Holter valve
Ventriculocisternal intubation

02.3 **Extracranial ventricular shunt**
Includes: that with insertion of valve

02.31 **Ventricular shunt to structure in head and neck**
Ventricle to nasopharynx shunt
Ventriculomastoid anastomosis

02.32 **Ventricular shunt to circulatory system**
Ventriculoatrial anastomosis
Ventriculocaval shunt

02.33 **Ventricular shunt to thoracic cavity**
Ventriculopleural anastomosis

02.34 **Ventricular shunt to abdominal cavity and organs**
Ventriculocholecystostomy
Ventriculoperitoneostomy

02.35 **Ventricular shunt to urinary system**
Ventricle to ureter shunt

02.39 **Other operations to establish drainage of ventricle**
Ventricle to bone marrow shunt
Ventricular shunt to extracranial site NEC

02.4 **Revision, removal, and irrigation of ventricular shunt**

Excludes: revision of distal catheter of ventricular shunt (54.95)

▲ **02.41** **Irrigation and exploration of ventricular shunt**
Exploration of ventriculoperitoneal shunt at ventricular site

02.42 **Replacement of ventricular shunt**
Reinsertion of Holter valve
Replacement of ventricular catheter
Revision of ventriculoperitoneal shunt at ventricular site

02.43 **Removal of ventricular shunt**

	Valid O.R. procedure		Non-O.R. procedure		Nonspecific O.R. procedure		Noncovered O.R. procedure

02.9 **Other operations on skull, brain, and cerebral meninges**

> Excludes: *operations on:*
> *pineal gland (07.17, 07.51-07.59)*
> *pituitary gland [hypophysis] (07.13-07.15, 07.61-07.79)*

02.91 **Lysis of cortical adhesions**

02.92 **Repair of brain**

02.93 **Implantation of intracranial neurostimulator**
Implantation, insertion, placement, or replacement of intracranial:
brain pacemaker [neuropacemaker]
depth electrodes
electroencephalographic receiver
epidural pegs
foramen ovale electrodes
intracranial electrostimulator
subdural grids
subdural strips

02.94 **Insertion or replacement of skull tongs or halo traction device**

02.95 **Removal of skull tongs or halo traction device**

02.96 **Insertion of sphenoidal electrodes**

02.99 **Other**

> Excludes: *chemical shock therapy (94.24)*
> *electroshock therapy:*
> *subconvulsive (94.26)*
> *other (94.27)*

03 **Operations on spinal cord and spinal canal structures**
Code also any application or administration of an adhesion barrier substance (99.77)

03.0 **Exploration and decompression of spinal canal structures**

03.01 **Removal of foreign body from spinal canal**

03.02 **Reopening of laminectomy site**

03.09 **Other exploration and decompression of spinal canal**
Decompression:
laminectomy
laminotomy
Expansile laminoplasty
Exploration of spinal nerve root
Foraminotomy

> Excludes: *drainage of spinal fluid by anastomosis (03.71-03.79)*
> *laminectomy with excision of intervertebral disc (80.51)*
> *spinal tap (03.31)*
> *that as operative approach—omit code*

03.1 **Division of intraspinal nerve root**
Rhizotomy

03.2 **Chordotomy**

03.21 **Percutaneous chordotomy**
Stereotactic chordotomy

03.29 **Other chordotomy**
Chordotomy NOS
Tractotomy (one-stage) (two-stage) of spinal cord
Transection of spinal cord tracts

03.3 **Diagnostic procedures on spinal cord and spinal canal structures**

03.31 **Spinal tap**
Lumbar puncture for removal of dye

> Excludes: *lumbar puncture for injection of dye [myelogram] (87.21)*

03.32 **Biopsy of spinal cord or spinal meninges**

03.39 **Other diagnostic procedures on spinal cord and spinal canal structures**

> Excludes: *microscopic examination of specimen from nervous system or of spinal fluid (90.01-90.09)*
> *x-ray of spine (87.21-87.29)*

● Code new to this edition   ▲ Revision of existing code   ④ ⑤ Fourth or fifth digit required

03.4 **Excision or destruction of lesion of spinal cord or spinal meninges**
Curettage of spinal cord or spinal meninges
Debridement of spinal cord or spinal meninges
Marsupialization of cyst of spinal cord or spinal meninges
Resection of spinal cord or spinal meninges

Excludes: *biopsy of spinal cord or meninges (03.32)*

03.5 **Plastic operations on spinal cord structures**

03.51 **Repair of spinal meningocele**
Repair of meningocele NOS

03.52 **Repair of spinal myelomeningocele**

03.53 **Repair of vertebral fracture**
Elevation of spinal bone fragments
Reduction of fracture of vertebrae
Removal of bony spicules from spinal canal

03.59 **Other repair and plastic operations on spinal cord structures**
Repair of:
diastematomyelia
spina bifida NOS
spinal cord NOS
spinal meninges NOS
vertebral arch defect

03.6 **Lysis of adhesions of spinal cord and nerve roots**

03.7 **Shunt of spinal theca**
Includes: that with valve

03.71 **Spinal subarachnoid-peritoneal shunt**

03.72 **Spinal subarachnoid-ureteral shunt**

03.79 **Other shunt of spinal theca**
Lumbar-subarachnoid shunt NOS
Pleurothecal anastomosis
Salpingothecal anastomosis

03.8 **Injection of destructive agent into spinal canal**

03.9 **Other operations on spinal cord and spinal canal structures**

03.90 **Insertion of catheter into spinal canal for infusion of therapeutic or palliative substances**
Insertion of catheter into epidural, subarachnoid, or subdural space of spine with intermittent or continuous infusion of drug (with creation of any reservoir)
Code also any implantation of infusion pump (86.06)

03.91 **Injection of anesthetic into spinal canal for analgesia**

Excludes: *that for operative anesthesia—omit code*

03.92 **Injection of other agent into spinal canal**
Intrathecal injection of steroid
Subarachnoid perfusion of refrigerated saline

Excludes: *injection of:*
contrast material for myelogram (87.21)
destructive agent into spinal canal (03.8)

03.93 **Insertion or replacement of spinal neurostimulator**

03.94 **Removal of spinal neurostimulator**

03.95 **Spinal blood patch**

03.96 **Percutaneous denervation of facet**

03.97 **Revision of spinal thecal shunt**

03.98 **Removal of spinal thecal shunt**

03.99 **Other**

04 **Operations on cranial and peripheral nerves**

04.0 **Incision, division, and excision of cranial and peripheral nerves**

Excludes: *opticociliary neurectomy (12.79)*
sympathetic ganglionectomy (05.21-05.29)

04.01 **Excision of acoustic neuroma**
That by craniotomy

Excludes: *that by stereotactic radiosurgery (92.3)*

Valid O.R. procedure   Non-O.R. procedure   Nonspecific O.R. procedure   Noncovered O.R. procedure

04.02 Division of trigeminal nerve
Retrogasserian neurotomy

04.03 Division or crushing of other cranial and peripheral nerves

> *Excludes:* *that of:*
> *glossopharyngeal nerve (29.92)*
> *laryngeal nerve (31.91)*
> *nerves to adrenal glands (07.42)*
> *phrenic nerve for collapse of lung (33.31)*
> *vagus nerve (44.00-44.03)*

04.04 Other incision of cranial and peripheral nerves

04.05 Gasserian ganglionectomy

04.06 Other cranial or peripheral ganglionectomy

> *Excludes:* *sympathetic ganglionectomy (05.21-05.29)*

04.07 Other excision or avulsion of cranial and peripheral nerves
Curettage of peripheral nerve
Debridement of peripheral nerve
Resection of peripheral nerve
Excision of peripheral neuroma [Morton's]

> *Excludes:* *biopsy of cranial or peripheral nerve (04.11-04.12)*

04.1 Diagnostic procedures on peripheral nervous system

04.11 Closed [percutaneous] [needle] biopsy of cranial or peripheral nerve or ganglion

04.12 Open biopsy of cranial or peripheral nerve or ganglion

04.19 Other diagnostic procedures on cranial and peripheral nerves and ganglia

> *Excludes:* *microscopic examination of specimen from nervous system*
> *(90.01-90.09)*
> *neurologic examination (89.13)*

04.2 Destruction of cranial and peripheral nerves
Destruction of cranial or peripheral nerves by:
cryoanalgesia
injection of neurolytic agent
radiofrequency
Radiofrequency ablation

04.3 Suture of cranial and peripheral nerves

04.4 Lysis of adhesions and decompression of cranial and peripheral nerves

04.41 Decompression of trigeminal nerve root

04.42 Other cranial nerve decompression

04.43 Release of carpal tunnel

04.44 Release of tarsal tunnel

04.49 Other peripheral nerve or ganglion decompression or lysis of adhesions
Peripheral nerve neurolysis NOS

04.5 Cranial or peripheral nerve graft

04.6 Transposition of cranial and peripheral nerves
Nerve transplantation

04.7 Other cranial or peripheral neuroplasty

04.71 Hypoglossal-facial anastomosis

04.72 Accessory-facial anastomosis

04.73 Accessory-hypoglossal anastomosis

04.74 Other anastomosis of cranial or peripheral nerve

04.75 Revision of previous repair of cranial and peripheral nerves

04.76 Repair of old traumatic injury of cranial and peripheral nerves

04.79 Other neuroplasty

04.8 Injection into peripheral nerve

> *Excludes:* *destruction of nerve (by injection of neurolytic agent) (04.2)*

04.80 Peripheral nerve injection, not otherwise specified

● Code new
to this edition   ▲ Revision of
existing code   ④ ⑤ Fourth or fifth
digit required

04.81 Injection of anesthetic into peripheral nerve for analgesia

> Excludes: that for operative anesthesia—omit code

04.89 Injection of other agent, except neurolytic

> Excludes: injection of neurolytic agent (04.2)

04.9 Other operations on cranial and peripheral nerves

04.91 Neurectasis

04.92 Implantation or replacement of peripheral neurostimulator

04.93 Removal of peripheral neurostimulator

04.99 Other

05 Operations on sympathetic nerves or ganglia

> Excludes: paracervical uterine denervation (69.3)

05.0 Division of sympathetic nerve or ganglion

> Excludes: that of nerves to adrenal glands (07.42)

05.1 Diagnostic procedures on sympathetic nerves or ganglia

05.11 Biopsy of sympathetic nerve or ganglion

05.19 Other diagnostic procedures on sympathetic nerves or ganglia

05.2 Sympathectomy

05.21 Sphenopalatine ganglionectomy

05.22 Cervical sympathectomy

05.23 Lumber sympathectomy

05.24 Presacral sympathectomy

05.25 Periarterial sympathectomy

05.29 Other sympathectomy and ganglionectomy

Excision or avulsion of sympathetic nerve NOS
Sympathetic ganglionectomy NOS

> Excludes: biopsy of sympathetic nerve or ganglion (05.11)
> opticociliary neurectomy (12.79)
> periarterial sympathectomy (05.25)
> tympanosympathectomy (20.91)

05.3 Injection into sympathetic nerve or ganglion

> Excludes: injection of ciliary sympathetic ganglion (12.79)

05.31 Injection of anesthetic into sympathetic nerve for analgesia

05.32 Injection of neurolytic agent into sympathetic nerve

05.39 Other injection into sympathetic nerve or ganglion

05.8 Other operations on sympathetic nerves or ganglion

05.81 Repair of sympathetic nerve or ganglion

05.89 Other

05.9 Other operations on nervous system

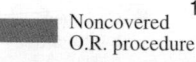

Valid O.R. procedure   Non-O.R. procedure   Nonspecific O.R. procedure   Noncovered O.R. procedure

● Code new
to this edition ▲ Revision of
existing code ④ ⑤ Fourth or fifth
digit required

2.   OPERATIONS ON THE ENDOCRINE SYSTEM (06-07)

06   Operations on thyroid and parathyroid glands
Includes: incidental resection of hyoid bone

06.0   Incision of thyroid field

> Excludes: division of isthmus (06.91)

06.01   Aspiration of thyroid field
Percutaneous or needle drainage of thyroid field

> Excludes: aspiration biopsy of thyroid (06.11)
> drainage by incision (06.09)
> postoperative aspiration of field (06.02)

06.02   Reopening of wound of thyroid field
Reopening of wound of thyroid field for:
control of (postoperative) hemorrhage
examination
exploration
removal of hematoma

06.09   Other incision of thyroid field
Drainage of hematoma by incision
Drainage of thyroglossal tract by incision
Exploration by incision:
   neck
   thyroid (field)
Removal of foreign body by incision
Thyroidotomy NOS by incision

> Excludes: postoperative exploration (06.02)
> removal of hematoma by aspiration (06.01)

06.1   Diagnostic procedures on thyroid and parathyroid glands

06.11   Closed [percutaneous] [needle] biopsy of thyroid gland
Aspiration biopsy of thyroid

06.12   Open biopsy of thyroid gland

06.13   Biopsy of parathyroid gland

06.19   Other diagnostic procedures on thyroid and parathyroid glands

> Excludes: radioisotope scan of:
> parathyroid (92.13)
> thyroid (92.01)
> soft tissue x-ray of thyroid field (87.09)

06.2   Unilateral thyroid lobectomy
Complete removal of one lobe of thyroid (with removal of isthmus or portion of other lobe)
Hemithyroidectomy

> Excludes: partial substernal thyroidectomy (06.51)

06.3   Other partial thyroidectomy

06.31   Excision of lesion of thyroid

> Excludes: biopsy of thyroid (06.11-06.12)

06.39   Other
Isthmectomy
Partial thyroidectomy NOS

> Excludes: partial substernal thyroidectomy (06.51)

06.4   Complete thyroidectomy

> Excludes: complete substernal thyroidectomy (06.52)
> that with laryngectomy (30.3-30.4)

06.5   Substernal thyroidectomy

06.50   Substernal thyroidectomy, not otherwise specified

06.51   Partial substernal thyroidectomy

06.52   Complete substernal thyroidectomy

06.6 **Excision of lingual thyroid**
Excision of thyroid by:
  submental route
  transoral route

06.7 **Excision of thyroglossal duct or tract**

06.8 **Parathyroidectomy**

  06.81 **Complete parathyroidectomy**

  06.89 **Other parathyroidectomy**
  Parathyroidectomy NOS
  Partial parathyroidectomy

  Excludes: *biopsy of parathyroid (06.13)*

06.9 **Other operations on thyroid (region) and parathyroid**

  06.91 **Division of thyroid isthmus**
  Transection of thyroid isthmus

  06.92 **Ligation of thyroid vessels**

  06.93 **Suture of thyroid gland**

  06.94 **Thyroid tissue reimplantation**
  Autotransplantation of thyroid tissue

  06.95 **Parathyroid tissue reimplantation**
  Autotransplantation of parathyroid tissue

  06.98 **Other operations on thyroid glands**

  06.99 **Other operations on parathyroid glands**

07 **Operations on other endocrine glands**
Includes: operations on:
  adrenal glands
  pineal gland
  pituitary gland
  thymus

  Excludes: *operations on:*
  aortic and carotid bodies (39.8)
  ovaries (65.0-65.99)
  pancreas (52.01-52.99)
  testes (62.0-62.99)

07.0 **Exploration of adrenal field**

  Excludes: *incision of adrenal gland (07.41)*

  07.00 **Exploration of adrenal field, not otherwise specified**

  07.01 **Unilateral exploration of adrenal field**

  07.02 **Bilateral exploration of adrenal field**

07.1 **Diagnostic procedures on adrenal glands, pituitary gland, pineal gland, and thymus**

  07.11 **Closed [percutaneous] [needle] biopsy of adrenal gland**

  07.12 **Open biopsy of adrenal gland**

  07.13 **Biopsy of pituitary gland, transfrontal approach**

  07.14 **Biopsy of pituitary gland, transsphenoidal approach**

  07.15 **Biopsy of pituitary gland, unspecified approach**

  07.16 **Biopsy of thymus**

  07.17 **Biopsy of pineal gland**

  07.19 **Other diagnostic procedures on adrenal glands, pituitary gland, pineal gland, and thymus**

  Excludes: *microscopic examination of specimen from endocrine gland (90.11-90.19)*
  radioisotope scan of pituitary gland (92.11)

07.2 **Partial adrenalectomy**

  07.21 **Excision of lesion of adrenal gland**

  Excludes: *biopsy of adrenal gland (07.11-07.12)*

  07.22 **Unilateral adrenalectomy**
  Adrenalectomy NOS

  Excludes: *excision of remaining adrenal gland (07.3)*

● Code new
to this edition
▲ Revision of
existing code
④ ⑤ Fourth or fifth
digit required

07.29 **Other partial adrenalectomy**
Partial adrenalectomy NOS

07.3 **Bilateral adrenalectomy**
Excision of remaining adrenal gland

> Excludes: bilateral partial adrenalectomy (07.29)

07.4 **Other operations on adrenal glands, nerves, and vessels**

07.41 **Incision of adrenal gland**
Adrenalotomy (with drainage)

07.42 **Division of nerves to adrenal glands**

07.43 **Ligation of adrenal vessels**

07.44 **Repair of adrenal gland**

07.45 **Reimplantation of adrenal tissue**
Autotransplantation of adrenal tissue

07.49 **Other**

07.5 **Operations on pineal gland**

07.51 **Exploration of pineal field**

> Excludes: that with incision of pineal gland (07.52)

07.52 **Incision of pineal gland**

07.53 **Partial excision of pineal gland**

> Excludes: biopsy of pineal gland (07.17)

07.54 **Total excision of pineal gland**
Pinealectomy (complete) (total)

07.59 **Other operations on pineal gland**

07.6 **Hypophysectomy**

07.61 **Partial excision of pituitary gland, transfrontal approach**
Cryohypophysectomy, partial, transfrontal approach
Division of hypophyseal stalk, transfrontal approach
Excision of lesion of pituitary [hypophysis], transfrontal approach
Hypophysectomy, subtotal, transfrontal approach
Infundibulectomy, hypophyseal, transfrontal approach

> Excludes: biopsy of pituitary gland, transfrontal approach (07.13)

07.62 **Partial excision of pituitary gland, transsphenoidal approach**

> Excludes: biopsy of pituitary gland, transsphenoidal approach (07.14)

07.63 **Partial excision of pituitary gland, unspecified approach**

> Excludes: biopsy of pituitary gland NOS (07.15)

07.64 **Total excision of pituitary gland, transfrontal approach**
Ablation of pituitary by implantation (strontium-yttrium) (Y), transfrontal approach
Cryohypophysectomy, complete, transfrontal approach

07.65 **Total excision of pituitary gland, transsphenoidal approach**

07.68 **Total excision of pituitary gland, other specified approach**

07.69 **Total excision of pituitary gland, unspecified approach**
Hypophysectomy NOS
Pituitectomy NOS

07.7 **Other operations on hypophysis**

07.71 **Exploration of pituitary fossa**

> Excludes: exploration with incision of pituitary gland (07.72)

| | Valid O.R. procedure | | Non-O.R. procedure | | Nonspecific O.R. procedure | | Noncovered O.R. procedure |

07.72 Incision of pituitary gland
Aspiration of:
craniobuccal pouch
craniopharyngioma
hypophysis
pituitary gland
Rathke's pouch

07.79 Other
Insertion of pack into sella turcica

07.8 Thymectomy

07.80 Thymectomy, not otherwise specified

07.81 Partial excision of thymus
Excludes: *biopsy of thymus (07.16)*

07.82 Total excision of thymus

07.9 Other operations on thymus

07.91 Exploration of thymus field
Excludes: *exploration with incision of thymus (07.92)*

07.92 Incision of thymus

07.93 Repair of thymus

07.94 Transplantation of thymus

07.99 Other
Thymopexy

● Code new
to this edition
▲ Revision of
existing code
④ ⑤ Fourth or fifth
digit required

3. OPERATIONS ON THE EYE (08-16)

08 Operations on eyelids
Includes: operations on the eyebrow

08.0 Incision of eyelid

    08.01 Incision of lid margin

    08.02 Severing of blepharorrhaphy

    08.09 Other incision of eyelid

08.1 Diagnostic procedures on eyelid

    08.11 Biopsy of eyelid

    08.19 Other diagnostic procedures on eyelid

08.2 Excision or destruction of lesion or tissue of eyelid
Code also any synchronous reconstruction (08.61-08.74)

    | Excludes: | *biopsy of eyelid (08.11)*

    08.20 Removal of lesion of eyelid, not otherwise specified
        Removal of meibomian gland NOS

    08.21 Excision of chalazion

    08.22 Excision of other minor lesion of eyelid
        Excision of:
            verruca
            wart

    08.23 Excision of major lesion of eyelid, partial-thickness
        Excision involving one-fourth or more of lid margin, partial-thickness

    08.24 Excision of major lesion of eyelid, full-thickness
        Excision involving one-fourth or more of lid margin, full-thickness
        Wedge resection of eyelid

    08.25 Destruction of lesion of eyelid

08.3 Repair of blepharoptosis and lid retraction

    08.31 Repair of blepharoptosis by frontalis muscle technique with suture

    08.32 Repair of blepharoptosis by frontalis muscle technique with fascial sling

    08.33 Repair of blepharoptosis by resection or advancement of levator muscle or aponeurosis

    08.34 Repair of blepharoptosis by other levator muscle techniques

    08.35 Repair of blepharoptosis by tarsal technique

    08.36 Repair of blepharoptosis by other techniques
        Correction of eyelid ptosis NOS
        Orbicularis oculi muscle sling for correction of blepharoptosis

    08.37 Reduction of overcorrection of ptosis

    08.38 Correction of lid retraction

08.4 Repair of entropion or ectropion

    08.41 Repair of entropion or ectropion by thermocauterization

    08.42 Repair of entropion or ectropion by suture technique

    08.43 Repair of entropion or ectropion with wedge resection

    08.44 Repair of entropion or ectropion with lid reconstruction

    08.49 Other repair of entropion or ectropion

08.5 Other adjustment of lid position

    08.51 Canthotomy
        Enlargement of palpebral fissure

    08.52 Blepharorrhaphy
        Canthorrhaphy
        Tarsorrhaphy

    08.59 Other
        Canthoplasty NOS
        Repair of epicanthal fold

08.6 Reconstruction of eyelid with flaps or grafts

    | Excludes: | *that associated with repair of entropion and ectropion (08.44)*

| Valid O.R. procedure | Non-O.R. procedure | Nonspecific O.R. procedure | Noncovered O.R. procedure |

08.61 **Reconstruction of eyelid with skin flap or graft**

08.62 **Reconstruction of eyelid with mucous membrane flap or graft**

08.63 **Reconstruction of eyelid with hair follicle graft**

08.64 **Reconstruction of eyelid with tarsoconjunctival flap**
Transfer of tarsoconjunctival flap from opposing lid

08.69 **Other reconstruction of eyelid with flap or graft**

08.7 **Other reconstruction of eyelid**

> Excludes: *that associated with repair of entropion and ectropion (08.44)*

08.70 **Reconstruction of eyelid, not otherwise specified**

08.71 **Reconstruction of eyelid involving lid margin, partial-thickness**

08.72 **Other reconstruction of eyelid, partial-thickness**

08.73 **Reconstruction of eyelid involving lid margin, full-thickness**

08.74 **Other reconstruction of eyelid, full-thickness**

08.8 **Other repair of eyelid**

08.81 **Linear repair of laceration of eyelid or eyebrow**

08.82 **Repair of laceration involving lid margin, partial-thickness**

08.83 **Other repair of laceration of eyelid, partial-thickness**

08.84 **Repair of laceration involving lid margin, full-thickness**

08.85 **Other repair of laceration of eyelid, full-thickness**

08.86 **Lower eyelid rhytidectomy**

08.87 **Upper eyelid rhytidectomy**

08.89 **Other eyelid repair**

08.9 **Other operations on eyelids**

08.91 **Electrosurgical epilation of eyelid**

08.92 **Cryosurgical epilation of eyelid**

08.93 **Other epilation of eyelid**

08.99 **Other**

09 **Operations on lacrimal system**

09.0 **Incision of lacrimal gland**
Incision of lacrimal cyst (with drainage)

09.1 **Diagnostic procedures on lacrimal system**

09.11 **Biopsy of lacrimal gland**

09.12 **Biopsy of lacrimal sac**

09.19 **Other diagnostic procedures on lacrimal system**

> Excludes: *contrast dacryocystogram (87.05)*
> *soft tissue x-ray of nasolacrimal duct (87.09)*

09.2 **Excision of lesion or tissue of lacrimal gland**

09.20 **Excision of lacrimal gland, not otherwise specified**

09.21 **Excision of lesion of lacrimal gland**

> Excludes: *biopsy of lacrimal gland (09.11)*

09.22 **Other partial dacryoadenectomy**

> Excludes: *biopsy of lacrimal gland (09.11)*

09.23 **Total dacryoadenectomy**

09.3 **Other operations on lacrimal gland**

09.4 **Manipulation of lacrimal passage**
Includes: removal of calculus
that with dilation

> Excludes: *contrast dacryocystogram (87.05)*

09.41 **Probing of lacrimal punctum**

09.42 **Probing of lacrimal canaliculi**

09.43 **Probing of nasolacrimal duct**

> Excludes: *that with insertion of tube or stent (09.44)*

● Code new
to this edition   ▲ Revision of
existing code   ④ ⑤ Fourth or fifth
digit required

09.44 Intubation of nasolacrimal duct
Insertion of stent into nasolacrimal duct

09.49 Other manipulation of lacrimal passage

09.5 Incision of lacrimal sac and passages

09.51 Incision of lacrimal punctum

09.52 Incision of lacrimal canaliculi

09.53 Incision of lacrimal sac

09.59 Other incision of lacrimal passages
Incision (and drainage) of nasolacrimal duct NOS

09.6 Excision of lacrimal sac and passage
Excludes: *biopsy of lacrimal sac (09.12)*

09.7 Repair of canaliculus and punctum
Excludes: *repair of eyelid (08.81-08.89)*

09.71 Correction of everted punctum

09.72 Other repair of punctum

09.73 Repair of canaliculus

09.8 Fistulization of lacrimal tract to nasal cavity

09.81 Dacryocystorhinostomy [DCR]

09.82 Conjunctivocystorhinostomy
Conjunctivodacryocystorhinostomy [CDCR]
Excludes: *that with insertion of tube or stent (09.83)*

09.83 Conjunctivorhinostomy with insertion of tube or stent

09.9 Other operations on lacrimal system

09.91 Obliteration of lacrimal punctum

09.99 Other

10 Operations on conjunctiva

10.0 Removal of embedded foreign body from conjunctiva by incision
Excludes: *removal of:*
embedded foreign body without incision (98.22)
superficial foreign body (98.21)

10.1 Other incision of conjunctiva

10.2 Diagnostic procedures on conjunctiva

10.21 Biopsy of conjunctiva

10.29 Other diagnostic procedures on conjunctiva

10.3 Excision or destruction of lesion or tissue of conjunctiva

10.31 Excision of lesion or tissue of conjunctiva
Excision of ring of conjunctiva around cornea
Excludes: *biopsy of conjunctiva (10.21)*

10.32 Destruction of lesion of conjunctiva
Excludes: *excision of lesion (10.31)*
thermocauterization for entropion (08.41)

10.33 Other destructive procedures on conjunctiva
Removal of trachoma follicles

10.4 Conjunctivoplasty

10.41 Repair of symblepharon with free graft

10.42 Reconstruction of conjunctival cul-de-sac with free graft
Excludes: *revision of enucleation socket with graft (16.63)*

10.43 Other reconstruction of conjunctival cul-de-sac
Excludes: *revision of enucleation socket (16.64)*

10.44 Other free graft to conjunctiva

10.49 Other conjunctivoplasty
Excludes: *repair of cornea with conjunctival flap (11.53)*

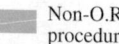 Valid O.R.
procedure   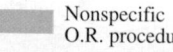 Non-O.R.
procedure   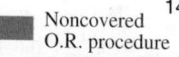 Nonspecific
O.R. procedure   Noncovered
O.R. procedure

1497

10.5 **Lysis of adhesions of conjunctiva and eyelid**
Division of symblepharon (with insertion of conformer)

10.6 **Repair of laceration of conjunctiva**
> Excludes: that with repair of sclera (12.81)

10.9 **Other operations on conjunctiva**

10.91 Subconjunctival injection

10.99 Other

11 **Operations on cornea**

11.0 **Magnetic removal of embedded foreign body from cornea**
> Excludes: that with incision (11.1)

11.1 **Incision of cornea**
Incision of cornea for removal of foreign body

11.2 **Diagnostic procedures on cornea**

11.21 Scraping of cornea for smear or culture

11.22 Biopsy of cornea

11.29 Other diagnostic procedures on cornea

11.3 **Excision of pterygium**

11.31 Transposition of pterygium

11.32 Excision of pterygium with corneal graft

11.39 Other excision of pterygium

11.4 **Excision or destruction of tissue or other lesion of cornea**

11.41 Mechanical removal of corneal epithelium
That by chemocauterization
> Excludes: that for smear or culture (11.21)

11.42 Thermocauterization of corneal lesion

11.43 Cryotherapy of corneal lesion

11.49 Other removal or destruction of corneal lesion
Excision of cornea NOS
> Excludes: biopsy of cornea (11.22)

11.5 **Repair of cornea**

11.51 Suture of corneal laceration

11.52 Repair of postoperative wound dehiscence of cornea

11.53 Repair of corneal laceration or wound with conjunctival flap

11.59 Other repair of cornea

11.6 **Corneal transplant**
> Excludes: excision of pterygium with corneal graft (11.32)

11.60 Corneal transplant, not otherwise specified
Keratoplasty NOS

11.61 Lamellar keratoplasty with autograft

11.62 Other lamellar keratoplasty

11.63 Penetrating keratoplasty with autograft
Perforating keratoplasty with autograft

11.64 Other penetrating keratoplasty
Perforating keratoplasty (with homograft)

11.69 Other corneal transplant

11.7 **Other reconstructive and refractive surgery on cornea**

~~**11.71**~~ Keratomileusis

~~**11.72**~~ Keratophakia

11.73 Keratoprosthesis

11.74 Thermokeratoplasty

~~**11.75**~~ Radial keratotomy

~~**11.76**~~ Epikeratophakia

11.79 Other

● Code new
to this edition   ▲ Revision of
existing code   ④ ⑤ Fourth or fifth
digit required

11.9 **Other operations on cornea**

    11.91 **Tattooing of cornea**

    11.92 **Removal of artificial implant from cornea**

    11.99 **Other**

12 **Operation on iris, ciliary body, sclera, and anterior chamber**

    | Excludes: | operations on cornea (11.0-11.99) |

12.0 **Removal of intraocular foreign body from anterior segment of eye**

    12.00 **Removal of intraocular foreign body from anterior segment of eye, not otherwise specified**

    12.01 **Removal of intraocular foreign body from anterior segment of eye with use of magnet**

    12.02 **Removal of intraocular foreign body from anterior segment of eye without use of magnet**

12.1 **Iridotomy and simple iridectomy**

    | Excludes: | iridectomy associated with:
        cataract extraction (13.11-13.69)
        removal of lesion (12.41-12.42)
        scleral fistulization (12.61-12.69) |

    12.11 **Iridotomy with transfixion**

    12.12 **Other iridotomy**
        Corectomy
        Discission of iris
        Iridotomy NOS

    12.13 **Excision of prolapsed iris**

    12.14 **Other iridectomy**
        Iridectomy (basal) (peripheral) (total)

12.2 **Diagnostic procedures on iris, ciliary body, sclera, and anterior chamber**

    12.21 **Diagnostic aspiration of anterior chamber of eye**

    12.22 **Biopsy of iris**

    12.29 **Other diagnostic procedures on iris, ciliary body, sclera, and anterior chamber**

12.3 **Iridoplasty and coreoplasty**

    12.31 **Lysis of goniosynechiae**
        Lysis of goniosynechiae by injection of air or liquid

    12.32 **Lysis of other anterior synechiae**
        Lysis of anterior synechiae:
          NOS
          by injection of air or liquid

    12.33 **Lysis of posterior synechiae**
        Lysis of iris adhesions NOS

    12.34 **Lysis of corneovitreal adhesions**

    12.35 **Coreoplasty**
        Needling of pupillary membrane

    12.39 **Other iridoplasty**

12.4 **Excision or destruction of lesion of iris and ciliary body**

    12.40 **Removal of lesion of anterior segment of eye, not otherwise specified**

    12.41 **Destruction of lesion of iris, nonexcisional**
        Destruction of lesion of iris by:
          cauterization
          cryotherapy
          photocoagulation

    12.42 **Excision of lesion of iris**
        | Excludes: | biopsy of iris (12.22) |

    12.43 **Destruction of lesion of ciliary body, nonexcisional**

    12.44 **Excision of lesion of ciliary body**

12.5 **Facilitation of intraocular circulation**

    12.51 **Goniopuncture without goniotomy**

    12.52 **Goniotomy without goniopuncture**

Valid O.R. procedure   Non-O.R. procedure   Nonspecific O.R. procedure   Noncovered O.R. procedure

12.53 Goniotomy with goniopuncture

12.54 Trabeculotomy ab externo

12.55 Cyclodialysis

12.59 Other facilitation of intraocular circulation

12.6 Scleral fistulization

> Excludes: exploratory sclerotomy (12.89)

12.61 Trephination of sclera with iridectomy

12.62 Thermocauterization of sclera with iridectomy

12.63 Iridencleisis and iridotasis

12.64 Trabeculectomy ab externo

12.65 Other scleral fistulization with iridectomy

12.66 Postoperative revision of scleral fistulization procedure
Revision of filtering bleb

> Excludes: repair of fistula (12.82)

12.69 Other fistulizing procedure

12.7 Other procedures for relief of elevated intraocular pressure

12.71 Cyclodiathermy

12.72 Cyclocryotherapy

12.73 Cyclophotocoagulation

12.74 Diminution of ciliary body, not otherwise specified

12.79 Other glaucoma procedures

12.8 Operations on sclera

> Excludes: those associated with:
> retinal reattachment (14.41-14.59)
> scleral fistulization (12.61-12.69)

12.81 Suture of laceration of sclera
Suture of sclera with synchronous repair of conjunctiva

12.82 Repair of scleral fistula

> Excludes: postoperative revision of scleral fistulization procedure (12.66)

12.83 Revision of operative wound of anterior segment, not elsewhere classified

> Excludes: postoperative revision of scleral fistulization procedure (12.66)

12.84 Excision or destruction of lesion of sclera

12.85 Repair of scleral staphyloma with graft

12.86 Other repair of scleral staphyloma

12.87 Scleral reinforcement with graft

12.88 Other scleral reinforcement

12.89 Other operations on sclera
Exploratory sclerotomy

12.9 Other operations on iris, ciliary body, and anterior chamber

12.91 Therapeutic evacuation of anterior chamber
Paracentesis of anterior chamber

> Excludes: diagnostic aspiration (12.21)

12.92 Injection into anterior chamber
Injection of:
air into anterior chamber
liquid into anterior chamber
medication into anterior chamber

12.93 Removal or destruction of epithelial downgrowth from anterior chamber

> Excludes: that with iridectomy (12.41-12.42)

12.97 Other operations on iris

12.98 Other operations on ciliary body

12.99 Other operations on anterior chamber

● Code new to this edition   ▲ Revision of existing code   ④ ⑤ Fourth or fifth digit required

13   Operations on lens

13.0   **Removal of foreign body from lens**

Excludes: *removal of pseudophakos (13.8)*

13.00 **Removal of foreign body from lens, not otherwise specified**

13.01 **Removal of foreign body from lens with use of magnet**

13.02 **Removal of foreign body from lens without use of magnet**

13.1   **Intracapsular extraction of lens**

Code also any synchronous insertion of pseudophakos (13.71)

13.11 **Intracapsular extraction of lens by temporal inferior route**

13.19 **Other intracapsular extraction of lens**
Cataract extraction NOS
Cryoextraction of lens
Erysiphake extraction of cataract
Extraction of lens NOS

13.2   **Extracapsular extraction of lens by linear extraction technique**

13.3   **Extracapsular extraction of lens by simple aspiration (and irrigation) technique**
Irrigation of traumatic cataract

13.4   **Extracapsular extraction of lens by fragmentation and aspiration technique**

13.41 **Phacoemulsification and aspiration of cataract**

13.42 **Mechanical phacofragmentation and aspiration of cataract by posterior route**
Code also any synchronous vitrectomy (14.74)

13.43 **Mechanical phacofragmentation and other aspiration of cataract**

13.5   **Other extracapsular extraction of lens**

Code also any synchronous insertion of pseudophakos (13.71)

13.51 **Extracapsular extraction of lens by temporal inferior route**

13.59 **Other extracapsular extraction of lens**

13.6   **Other cataract extraction**

Code also any synchronous insertion of pseudophakos (13.71)

13.64 **Discission of secondary membrane [after cataract]**

13.65 **Excision of secondary membrane [after cataract]**
Capsulectomy

13.66 **Mechanical fragmentation of secondary membrane [after cataract]**

13.69 **Other cataract extraction**

13.7   **Insertion of prosthetic lens [pseudophakos]**

13.70 **Insertion of pseudophakos, not otherwise specified**

13.71 **Insertion of intraocular lens prosthesis at time of cataract extraction, one-stage**
Code also synchronous extraction of cataract (13.11-13.69)

13.72 **Secondary insertion of intraocular lens prosthesis**

13.8   **Removal of implanted lens**
Removal of pseudophakos

13.9   **Other operations on lens**

14   Operations on retina, choroid, vitreous, and posterior chamber

14.0   **Removal of foreign body from posterior segment of eye**

Excludes: *removal of surgically implanted material (14.6)*

14.00 **Removal of foreign body from posterior segment of eye, not otherwise specified**

14.01 **Removal of foreign body from posterior segment of eye with use of magnet**

14.02 **Removal of foreign body from posterior segment of eye without use of magnet**

14.1   **Diagnostic procedures on retina, choroid, vitreous, and posterior chamber**

14.11 **Diagnostic aspiration of vitreous**

14.19 **Other diagnostic procedures on retina, choroid, vitreous, and posterior chamber**

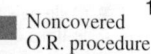

14.2 **Destruction of lesion of retina and choroid**
Includes: destruction of chorioretinopathy or isolated chorioretinal lesion

> Excludes: that for repair of retina (14.31-14.59)

    14.21 **Destruction of chorioretinal lesion by diathermy**

    14.22 **Destruction of chorioretinal lesion by cryotherapy**

    14.23 **Destruction of chorioretinal lesion by xenon arc photocoagulation**

    14.24 **Destruction of chorioretinal lesion by laser photocoagulation**

    14.25 **Destruction of chorioretinal lesion by photocoagulation of unspecified type**

    14.26 **Destruction of chorioretinal lesion by radiation therapy**

    14.27 **Destruction of chorioretinal lesion by implantation of radiation source**

    14.29 **Other destruction of chorioretinal lesion**
Destruction of lesion of retina and choroid NOS

14.3 **Repair of retinal tear**
Includes: repair of retinal defect

> Excludes: repair of retinal detachment (14.41-14.59)

    14.31 **Repair of retinal tear by diathermy**

    14.32 **Repair of retinal tear by cryotherapy**

    14.33 **Repair of retinal tear by xenon arc photocoagulation**

    14.34 **Repair of retinal tear by laser photocoagulation**

    14.35 **Repair of retinal tear by photocoagulation of unspecified type**

    14.39 **Other repair of retinal tear**

14.4 **Repair of retinal detachment with scleral buckling and implant**

    14.41 **Scleral buckling with implant**

    14.49 **Other scleral buckling**
Scleral buckling with:
    air tamponade
    resection of sclera
    vitrectomy

14.5 **Other repair of retinal detachment**
Includes: that with drainage

    14.51 **Repair of retinal detachment with diathermy**

    14.52 **Repair of retinal detachment with cryotherapy**

    14.53 **Repair of retinal detachment with xenon arc photocoagulation**

    14.54 **Repair of retinal detachment with laser photocoagulation**

    14.55 **Repair of retinal detachment with photocoagulation of unspecified type**

    14.59 **Other**

14.6 **Removal of surgically implanted material from posterior segment of eye**

14.7 **Operations on vitreous**

    14.71 **Removal of vitreous, anterior approach**
Open sky technique
Removal of vitreous, anterior approach (with replacement)

    14.72 **Other removal of vitreous**
Aspiration of vitreous by posterior sclerotomy

    14.73 **Mechanical vitrectomy by anterior approach**

    14.74 **Other mechanical vitrectomy**

    14.75 **Injection of vitreous substitute**

>   Excludes: that associated with removal (14.71-14.72)

    14.79 **Other operations on vitreous**

14.9 **Other operations on retina, choroid, and posterior chamber**

15 **Operations on extraocular muscles**

  15.0 **Diagnostic procedures on extraocular muscles or tendons**

    15.01 **Biopsy of extraocular muscle or tendon**

    15.09 **Other diagnostic procedures on extraocular muscles and tendons**

● Code new to this edition	▲ Revision of existing code	④ ⑤ Fourth or fifth digit required

15.1   **Operations on one extraocular muscle involving temporary detachment from globe**

    15.11   Recession of one extraocular muscle

    15.12   Advancement of one extraocular muscle

    15.13   Resection of one extraocular muscle

    15.19   Other operations on one extraocular muscle involving temporary detachment from globe

        | Excludes: | *transposition of muscle (15.5)* |

15.2   **Other operations on one extraocular muscle**

    15.21   Lengthening procedure on one extraocular muscle

    15.22   Shortening procedure on one extraocular muscle

    15.29   Other

15.3   **Operations on two or more extraocular muscles involving temporary detachment from globe, one or both eyes**

15.4   **Other operations on two or more extraocular muscles, one or both eyes**

15.5   **Transposition of extraocular muscles**

        | Excludes: | *that for correction of ptosis (08.31-08.36)* |

15.6   **Revision of extraocular muscle surgery**

15.7   **Repair of injury of extraocular muscle**
Freeing of entrapped extraocular muscle
Lysis of adhesions of extraocular muscle
Repair of laceration of extraocular muscle, tendon, or Tenon's capsule

15.9   **Other operations on extraocular muscles and tendon**

16   **Operations on orbit and eyeball**

    | Excludes: | *reduction of fracture of orbit (76.78-76.79)* |

16.0   **Orbitotomy**

    16.01   Orbitotomy with bone flap
        Orbitotomy with lateral approach

    16.02   Orbitotomy with insertion of orbital implant

        | Excludes: | *that with bone flap (16.01)* |

    16.09   Other orbitotomy

16.1   **Removal of penetrating foreign body from eye, not otherwise specified**

    | Excludes: | *removal of nonpenetrating foreign body (98.21)* |

16.2   **Diagnostic procedures on orbit and eyeball**

    16.21   Ophthalmoscopy

    16.22   Diagnostic aspiration of orbit

    16.23   Biopsy of eyeball and orbit

    16.29   Other diagnostic procedures on orbit and eyeball

        | Excludes: | *examination of form and structure of eye (95.11-95.16)* |
         general and subjective eye examination (95.01-95.09)
         microscopic examination of specimen from eye (90.21-90.29)
         objective functional tests of eye (95.21-95.26)
         ocular thermography (88.82)
         tonometry (89.11)
         X-ray of orbit (87.14, 87.16)

16.3   **Evisceration of eyeball**

    16.31   Removal of ocular contents with synchronous implant into scleral shell

    16.39   Other evisceration of eyeball

16.4   **Enucleation of eyeball**

    16.41   Enucleation of eyeball with synchronous implant into Tenon's capsule with attachment of muscles
        Integrated implant of eyeball

    16.42   Enucleation of eyeball with other synchronous implant

    16.49   Other enucleation of eyeball
        Removal of eyeball NOS

16.5   **Exenteration of orbital contents**

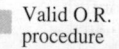 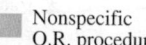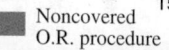

16.51 **Exenteration of orbit with removal of adjacent structures**
Radical orbitomaxillectomy

16.52 **Exenteration of orbit with therapeutic removal of orbital bone**

16.59 **Other exenteration of orbit**
Evisceration of orbit NOS
Exenteration of orbit with temporalis muscle transplant

16.6 **Secondary procedures after removal of eyeball**

> | Excludes: | *that with synchronous:*
> *enucleation of eyeball (16.41-16.42)*
> *evisceration of eyeball (16.31)*

16.61 **Secondary insertion of ocular implant**

16.62 **Revision and reinsertion of ocular implant**

16.63 **Revision of enucleation socket with graft**

16.64 **Other revision of enucleation socket**

16.65 **Secondary graft to exenteration cavity**

16.66 **Other revision of exenteration cavity**

16.69 **Other secondary procedures after removal of eyeball**

16.7 **Removal of ocular or orbital implant**

16.71 **Removal of ocular implant**

16.72 **Removal of orbital implant**

16.8 **Repair of injury of eyeball and orbit**

16.81 **Repair of wound of orbit**

> | Excludes: | *reduction of orbital fracture (76.78-76.79)*
> *repair of extraocular muscles (15.7)*

16.82 **Repair of rupture of eyeball**
Repair of multiple structures of eye

> | Excludes: | *repair of laceration of:*
> *cornea (11.51-11.59)*
> *sclera (12.81)*

16.89 **Other repair of injury of eyeball or orbit**

16.9 **Other operations on orbit and eyeball**

> | Excludes: | *irrigation of eye (96.51)*
> *prescription and fitting of low vision aids (95.31-95.33)*
> *removal of:*
> *eye prosthesis NEC (97.31)*
> *nonpenetrating foreign body from eye without incision (98.21)*

16.91 **Retrobulbar injection of therapeutic agent**

> | Excludes: | *injection of radiographic contrast material (87.14)*
> *opticociliary injection (12.79)*

16.92 **Excision of lesion of orbit**

> | Excludes: | *biopsy of orbit (16.23)*

16.93 **Excision of lesion of eye, unspecified structure**

> | Excludes: | *biopsy of eye NOS (16.23)*

16.98 **Other operations on orbit**

16.99 **Other operations on eyeball**

● Code new
to this edition   ▲ Revision of
existing code   ④ ⑤ Fourth or fifth
digit required

4.   OPERATIONS ON THE EAR (18-20)

18   Operations on external ear
Includes: operations on:
external auditory canal
skin and cartilage of:
auricle
meatus

18.0   Incision of external ear

> Excludes: removal of intraluminal foreign body (98.11)

18.01   Piercing of ear lobe
Piercing of pinna

18.02   Incision of external auditory canal

18.09   Other incision of external ear

18.1   Diagnostic procedures on external ear

18.11   Otoscopy

18.12   Biopsy of external ear

18.19   Other diagnostic procedures on external ear

> Excludes: microscopic examination of specimen from ear (90.31-90.39)

18.2   Excision or destruction of lesion of external ear

18.21   Excision of preauricular sinus
Radical excision of preauricular sinus or cyst

> Excludes: excision of preauricular remnant [appendage] (18.29)

18.29   Excision or destruction of other lesion of external ear
Cauterization of external car
Coagulation of external car
Cryosurgery of external car
Curettage of external car
Electrocoagulation of external car
Enucleation of external car
Excision of:
exostosis of external auditory canal
preauricular remnant [appendage]
Partial excision of ear

> Excludes: biopsy of external ear (18.12)
> radical excision of lesion (18.31)
> removal of cerumen (96.52)

18.3   Other excision of external ear

> Excludes: biopsy of external ear (18.12)

18.31   Radical excision of lesion of external ear

> Excludes: radical excision of preauricular sinus (18.21)

18.39   Other
Amputation of external ear

> Excludes: excision of lesion (18.21-18.29, 18.31)

18.4   Suture of laceration of external ear

18.5   Surgical correction of prominent ear
Ear:
pinning
setback

18.6   Reconstruction of external auditory canal
Canaloplasty of external auditory meatus
Construction [reconstruction] of external meatus of ear:
osseous portion
skin-lined portion (with skin graft)

18.7   Other plastic repair of external ear

18.71   Construction of auricle of ear
Prosthetic appliance for absent ear
Reconstruction:
auricle
ear

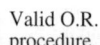 Valid O.R. procedure   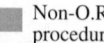 Non-O.R. procedure   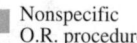 Nonspecific O.R. procedure   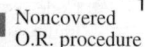 Noncovered O.R. procedure

18.72 Reattachment of amputated ear

18.79 Other plastic repair of external ear
Otoplasty NOS
Postauricular skin graft
Repair of lop ear

18.9 Other operations on external ear

> Excludes: *irrigation of ear (96.52)*
> *packing of external auditory canal (96.11)*
> *removal of:*
> *cerumen (96.52)*
> *foreign body (without incision) (98.11)*

19 Reconstructive operations on middle ear

19.0 Stapes mobilization
Division, otosclerotic: Remobilization of stapes
material   Stapediolysis
process   Transcrural stapes mobilization

> Excludes: *that with synchronous stapedectomy (19.11-19.19)*

19.1 Stapedectomy

> Excludes: *revision of previous stapedectomy (19.21-19.29)*
> *stapes mobilization only (19.0)*

19.11 Stapedectomy with incus replacement
Stapedectomy with incus:
homograft
prosthesis

19.19 Other stapedectomy

19.2 Revision of stapedectomy

19.21 Revision of stapedectomy with incus replacement

19.29 Other revision of stapedectomy

19.3 Other operations on ossicular chain
Incudectomy NOS
Ossiculectomy NOS
Reconstruction of ossicles, second stage

19.4 Myringoplasty
Epitympanic, type I
Myringoplasty by:
cauterization
graft
Tympanoplasty (type I)

19.5 Other tympanoplasty

19.52 Type II tympanoplasty
Closure of perforation with graft against incus or malleus

19.53 Type III tympanoplasty
Graft placed in contact with mobile and intact stapes

19.54 Type IV tympanoplasty
Mobile footplate left exposed with air pocket between round window and graft

19.55 Type V tympanoplasty
Fenestra in horizontal semicircular canal covered by graft

19.6 Revision of tympanoplasty

19.9 Other repair of middle ear
Closure of mastoid fistula
Mastoid myoplasty
Obliteration of tympanomastoid cavity

20 Other operations on middle and inner ear

20.0 Myringotomy

20.01 Myringotomy with insertion of tube
Myringostomy

20.09 Other myringotomy
Aspiration of middle ear NOS

20.1 Removal of tympanostomy tube

20.2 Incision of mastoid and middle ear

● Code new
to this edition   ▲ Revision of
existing code   ④ ⑤ Fourth or fifth
digit required

20.21 Incision of mastoid

20.22 Incision of petrous pyramid air cells

20.23 Incision of middle ear
Atticotomy
Division of tympanum
Lysis of adhesions of middle car

> Excludes: divisions of otosclerotic process (19.0)
> stapediolysis (19.0)
> that with stapedectomy (19.11-19.19)

20.3 Diagnostic procedures on middle and inner ear

20.31 Electrocochleography

20.32 Biopsy of middle and inner ear

20.39 Other diagnostic procedures on middle and inner ear

> Excludes: auditory and vestibular function tests (89.13, 95.41-95.49)
> microscopic examination of specimen from ear (90.31-90.39)

20.4 Mastoidectomy
Code also any:
skin graft (18.79)
tympanoplasty (19.4-19.55)

> Excludes: that with implantation of cochlear prosthetic device (20.96-20.98)

20.41 Simple mastoidectomy

20.42 Radical mastoidectomy

20.49 Other mastoidectomy
Atticoantrotomy
Mastoidectomy:
NOS
modified radical

20.5 Other excision of middle ear

> Excludes: that with synchronous mastoidectomy (20.41-20.49)

20.51 Excision of lesion of middle ear

> Excludes: biopsy of middle ear (20.32)

20.59 Other
Apicectomy of petrous pyramid
Tympanectomy

20.6 Fenestration of inner ear

20.61 Fenestration of inner ear (initial)
Fenestration of labyrinth with graft (skin) (vein)
Fenestration of semicircular canals with graft (skin) (vein)
Fenenstration of vestibule with graft (skin) (vein)

> Excludes: that with tympanoplasty type V (19.55)

20.62 Revision of fenestration of inner ear

20.7 Incision, excision, and destruction of inner ear

20.71 Endolymphatic shunt

20.72 Injection into inner ear
Destruction by injection (alcohol):
inner ear
semicircular canals
vestibule

20.79 Other incision, excision and destruction of inner ear
Decompression of labyrinth
Drainage of inner ear
Fistulization:
endolymphatic sac
labyrinth
Incision of endolymphatic sac
Labyrinthectomy (transtympanic)
Opening of bony labyrinth
Perilymphatic tap

> Excludes: biopsy of inner ear (20.32)

	Valid O.R. procedure		Non-O.R. procedure		Nonspecific O.R. procedure		Noncovered O.R. procedure

20.8 **Operations on Eustachian tube**
Catheterization of Eustachian tube
Inflation of Eustachian tube
Injection (Teflon paste) of Eustachian tube
Insufflation (boric acid-salicylic acid) of Eustachian tube
Intubation of Eustachian tube
Politzerization of Eustachian tube

20.9 **Other operations on inner and middle ear**

20.91 **Tympanosympathectomy**

20.92 **Revision of mastoidectomy**

20.93 **Repair of oval and round windows**
Closure of fistula:
oval window
perilymph
round window

20.94 **Injection of tympanum**

20.95 **Implantation of electromagnetic bearing device**
Bone conduction hearing device

> Excludes: *cochlear prosthetic device (20.96-20.98)*

20.96 **Implantation or replacement of cochlear prosthetic device, not otherwise specified**
Implantation of receiver (within skull) and insertion of electrode(s) in the cochlea
Includes: mastoidectomy

> Excludes: *electromagnetic hearing device (20.95)*

20.97 **Implantation or replacement of cochlear prosthetic device, single channel**
Implantation of receiver (within skull) and insertion of electrode in the cochlea
Includes: mastoidectomy

> Excludes: *electromagnetic hearing device (20.95)*

20.98 **Implantation or replacement of cochlear prosthetic device, multiple channel**
Implantation of receiver (within skull) and insertion of electrodes in the cochlea
Includes: mastoidectomy

> Excludes: *electromagnetic hearing device (20.95)*

20.99 **Other operations on middle and inner ear**
Repair or removal of cochlear prosthetic device (receiver) (electrode)

> Excludes: *adjustment (external components) of cochlear prosthetic device (95.49)*
> *fitting of hearing aid (95.48)*

● Code new
to this edition
▲ Revision of
existing code
④ ⑤ Fourth or fifth
digit required

5. OPERATIONS ON THE NOSE, MOUTH, AND PHARYNX (21-29)

21 Operation on nose
Includes: operations on:
bone of nose
skin of nose

21.0 Control of epistaxis

21.00 Control of epistaxis, not otherwise specified

21.01 Control of epistaxis by anterior nasal packing

21.02 Control of epistaxis by posterior (and anterior) packing

21.03 Control of epistaxis by cauterization (and packing)

21.04 Control of epistaxis by ligation of ethmoidal arteries

21.05 Control of epistaxis by (transantral) ligation of the maxillary artery

21.06 Control of epistaxis by ligation of the external carotid artery

21.07 Control of epistaxis by excision of nasal mucosa and skin grafting on septum and lateral nasal wall

21.09 Control of epistaxis by other means

21.1 Incision of nose
Chondrotomy
Incision of skin of nose
Nasal septotomy

21.2 Diagnostic procedures on nose

21.21 Rhinoscopy

21.22 Biopsy of nose

21.29 Other diagnostic procedures on nose

> Excludes: *microscopic examination of specimen from nose (90.31-90.39)*
> *nasal:*
> *function study (89.12)*
> *x-ray (87.16)*
> *rhinomanometry (89.12)*

21.3 Local excision or destruction of lesion of nose

> Excludes: *biopsy of nose (21.22)*
> *nasal fistulectomy (21.82)*

21.30 Excision or destruction of nose, not otherwise specified

21.31 Local excision or destruction of intranasal lesion
Nasal polypectomy

21.32 Local excision or destruction of other lesion of nose

21.4 Resection of nose
Amputation of nose

21.5 Submucous resection of nasal septum

21.6 Turbinectomy

21.61 Turbinectomy by diathermy or cryosurgery

21.62 Fracture of the turbinates

21.69 Other turbinectomy

> Excludes: *turbinectomy associated with sinusectomy (22.31-22.39, 22.42, 22.60-22.64)*

21.7 Reduction of nasal fracture

21.71 Closed reduction of nasal fracture

21.72 Open reduction of nasal fracture

21.8 Repair and plastic operations on the nose

21.81 Suture of laceration of nose

21.82 Closure of nasal fistula
Nasolabial fistulectomy
Nasopharyngeal fistulectomy
Oronasal fistulectomy

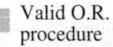 Valid O.R.
procedure

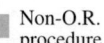 Non-O.R.
procedure

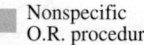 Nonspecific
O.R. procedure

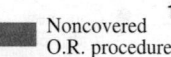 Noncovered
O.R. procedure

21.83 Total nasal reconstruction
Reconstruction of nose with:
   arm flap
   forehead flap

21.84 Revision rhinoplasty
Rhinoseptoplasty
Twisted nose rhinoplasty

21.85 Augmentation rhinoplasty
Augmentation rhinoplasty with:
   graft
   synthetic implant

21.86 Limited rhinoplasty
Plastic repair of nasolabial flaps
Tip rhinoplasty

21.87 Other rhinoplasty
Rhinoplasty NOS

21.88 Other septoplasty
Crushing of nasal septum
Repair of septal perforation
| Excludes: | *septoplasty associated with submucous resection of septum (21.5)* |

21.89 Other repair and plastic operations on nose
Reattachment of amputated nose

21.9 Other operations on nose

21.91 Lysis of adhesions of nose
Posterior nasal scrub

21.99 Other
Excludes:	*dilation of frontonasal duct (96.21)*
	irrigation of nasal passages (96.53)
	removal of:
	intraluminal foreign body without incision (98.12)
	nasal packing (97.32)
	replacement of nasal packing (97.21)

22 Operations on nasal sinuses

22.0 Aspiration and lavage of nasal sinus

22.00 Aspiration and lavage of nasal sinus, not otherwise specified

22.01 Puncture of nasal sinus for aspiration or lavage

22.02 Aspiration or lavage of nasal sinus through natural ostium

22.1 Diagnostic procedures on nasal sinus

22.11 Closed [endoscopic] [needle] biopsy of nasal sinus

22.12 Open biopsy of nasal sinus

22.19 Other diagnostic procedures on nasal sinuses
Endoscopy without biopsy
| Excludes: | *transillumination of sinus (89.35)* |
| | *x-ray of sinus (87.15-87.16)* |

22.2 Intranasal antrotomy
| Excludes: | *antrotomy with external approach (22.31-22.39)* |

22.3 External maxillary antrotomy

22.31 Radical maxillary antrotomy
Removal of lining membrane of maxillary sinus using Caldwell-Luc approach

22.39 Other external maxillary antrotomy
Exploration of maxillary antrum with Caldwell-Luc approach

22.4 Frontal sinusotomy and sinusectomy

22.41 Frontal sinusotomy

22.42 Frontal sinusectomy
Excision of lesion of frontal sinus
Obliteration of frontal sinus (with fat)
| Excludes: | *biopsy of nasal sinus (22.11-22.12)* |

22.5 Other nasal sinusotomy

● Code new
to this edition
▲ Revision of
existing code
④ ⑤ Fourth or fifth
digit required

22.50 Sinusotomy, not otherwise specified

22.51 Ethmoidotomy

22.52 Sphenoidotomy

22.53 Incision of multiple nasal sinuses

22.6 Other nasal sinusectomy
Includes: that with incidental turbinectomy

> Excludes: *biopsy of nasal sinus (22.11-22.12)*

22.60 Sinusectomy, not otherwise specified

22.61 Excision of lesion of maxillary sinus with Caldwell-Luc approach

22.62 Excision of lesion of maxillary sinus with other approach

22.63 Ethmoidectomy

22.64 Sphenoidectomy

22.7 Repair of nasal sinus

22.71 Closure of nasal sinus fist
Repair of oro-antral fistula

22.79 Other repair of nasal sinus
Reconstruction of frontonasal duct
Repair of bone of accessory sinus

22.9 Other operations on nasal sinuses
Exteriorization of maxillary sinus
Fistulization of sinus

> Excludes: *dilation of frontonasal duct (96.21)*

23 Removal and restoration of teeth

23.0 Forceps extraction of tooth

23.01 Extraction of deciduous tooth

23.09 Extraction of other tooth
Extraction of tooth NOS

23.1 Surgical removal of tooth

23.11 Removal of residual root

23.19 Other surgical extraction of tooth
Odontectomy NOS
Removal of impacted tooth
Tooth extraction with elevation of mucoperiosteal flap

23.2 Restoration of tooth by filling

23.3 Restoration of tooth by inlay

23.4 Other dental restoration

23.41 Application of crown

23.42 Insertion of fixed bridge

23.43 Insertion of removable bridge

23.49 Other

23.5 Implantation of tooth

23.6 Prosthetic dental implant
Endosseous dental implant

23.7 Apicoectomy and root canal therapy

23.70 Root canal not otherwise specified

23.71 Root canal therapy with irrigation

23.72 Root canal therapy with apicoectomy

23.73 Apicoectomy

24 Other operations on teeth, gums, and alveoli

24.0 Incision of gum or alveolar bone
Apical alveolotomy

24.1 Diagnostic procedures on teeth, gums, and alveoli

24.11 Biopsy of gum

24.12 Biopsy of alveoli

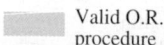 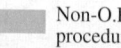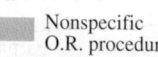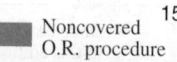

24.19 Other diagnostic procedures on teeth, gums, and alveoli

> Excludes: *dental:*
> *examination (89.31)*
> *x-ray:*
> *full-mouth (87.11)*
> *other (87.12)*
> *microscopic examination of dental specimen (90.81-90.89)*

24.2 Gingivoplasty
Gingivoplasty with bone or soft tissue graft

24.3 Other operations on gum

24.31 Excision of lesion or tissue of gum

> Excludes: *biopsy of gum (24.11)*
> *excision of odontogenic lesion (24.4)*

24.32 Suture of laceration of gum

24.39 Other

24.4 Excision of dental lesion of jaw
Excision of odontogenic lesion

24.5 Alveoloplasty
Alveolectomy (interradicular) (intraseptal) (radical) (simple) (with graft or implant)

> Excludes: *biopsy of alveolus (24.12)*
> *en bloc resection of alveolar process and palate (27.32)*

24.6 Exposure of tooth

24.7 Application of orthodontic appliance
Application, insertion, or fitting of:
arch bars
orthodontic obturator
orthodontic wiring
periodontal splint

> Excludes: *nonorthodontic dental wiring (93.55)*

24.8 Other orthodontic operation
Closure of diastema (alveolar) (dental)
Occlusal adjustment
Removal of arch bars
Repair of dental arch

> Excludes: *removal of nonorthodontic wiring (97.33)*

24.9 Other dental operations

24.91 Extension or deepening of buccolabial or lingual sulcus

24.99 Other

> Excludes: *dental:*
> *debridement (96.54)*
> *examination (89.31)*
> *prophylaxis (96.54)*
> *scaling and polishing (96.54)*
> *wiring (93.55)*
> *fitting of dental appliance [denture] (99.97)*
> *microscopic examination of dental specimen (90.81-90.89)*
> *removal of dental:*
> *packing (97.34)*
> *prosthesis (97.35)*
> *wiring (97.33)*
> *replacement of dental packing (97.22)*

25 Operations on tongue

25.0 Diagnostic procedures on tongue

25.01 Closed [needle] biopsy of tongue

25.02 Open biopsy of tongue
Wedge biopsy

25.09 Other diagnostic procedures on tongue

● Code new
to this edition   ▲ Revision of
existing code   ④ ⑤ Fourth or fifth
digit required

25.1 **Excision or destruction of lesion or tissue of tongue**

> _Excludes:_ _biopsy of tongue (25.01-25.02)_
> _frenumectomy:_
> _labial (27.41)_
> _lingual (25.92)_

25.2 **Partial glossectomy**

25.3 **Complete glossectomy**
Glossectomy NOS
Code also any neck dissection (40.40-40.42)

25.4 **Radical glossectomy**
Code also any:
neck dissection (40.40-40.42)
tracheostomy (31.1-31.29)

25.5 **Repair of tongue and glossoplasty**

25.51 **Suture of laceration of tongue**

25.59 **Other repair and plastic operations on tongue**
Fascial sling of tongue
Fusion of tongue (to lip)
Graft of mucosa or skin to tongue

> _Excludes:_ _lysis of adhesions of tongue (25.93)_

25.9 **Other operations on tongue**

25.91 **Lingual frenotomy**

> _Excludes:_ _labial frenotomy (27.91)_

25.92 **Lingual frenectomy**

> _Excludes:_ _labial frenectomy (27.41)_

25.93 **Lysis of adhesions of tongue**

25.94 **Other glossotomy**

25.99 **Other**

26 **Operations on salivary glands and ducts**
Includes: operations on:
lesser salivary gland and duct
parotid gland and duct
sublingual gland and duct
submaxillary gland and duct

Code also any neck dissection (40.40-40.42)

26.0 **Incision of salivary gland or duct**

26.1 **Diagnostic procedures on salivary glands and ducts**

26.11 **Closed [needle] biopsy of salivary gland or duct**

26.12 **Open biopsy of salivary gland or duct**

26.19 **Other diagnostic procedures on salivary glands and ducts**

> _Excludes:_ _x-ray of salivary gland (87.09)_

26.2 **Excision of lesion of salivary gland**

26.21 **Marsupialization of salivary gland cyst**

26.29 **Other excision of salivary gland lesion**

> _Excludes:_ _biopsy of salivary gland (26.11-26.12)_
> _salivary fistulectomy (26.42)_

26.3 **Sialoadenectomy**

26.30 **Sialoadenectomy, not otherwise specified**

26.31 **Partial sialoadenectomy**

26.32 **Complete sialoadenectomy**
En bloc excision of salivary gland lesion
Radical sialoadenectomy

26.4 **Repair of salivary gland or duct**

26.41 **Suture of laceration of salivary gland**

26.42 **Closure of salivary fistula**

	Valid O.R. procedure		Non-O.R. procedure		Nonspecific O.R. procedure		Noncovered O.R. procedure

26.49 Other repair and plastic operations on salivary gland or duct
Fistulization of salivary gland
Plastic repair of salivary gland or duct NOS
Transplantation of salivary duct opening

26.9 Other operations on salivary gland or duct

26.91 Probing of salivary duct

26.99 Other

27 Other operations on mouth and face
Includes: operations on:
lips
palate
soft tissue of face and mouth, except tongue and gingiva

Excludes   *operations on:*
gingiva (24.0-24.99)
tongue (25.01-25.99)

27.0 Drainage of face and floor of mouth
Drainage of:
facial region (abscess)
fascial compartment of face
Ludwig's angina

Excludes: *drainage of thyroglossal tract (06.09)*

27.1 Incision of palate

27.2 Diagnostic procedures on oral cavity

27.21 Biopsy of bony palate

27.22 Biopsy of uvula and soft palate

27.23 Biopsy of lip

27.24 Biopsy of mouth, unspecified structure

27.29 Other diagnostic procedures on oral cavity
Excludes: *soft tissue x-ray (87.09)*

27.3 Excision of lesion or tissue of bony palate

27.31 Local excision or destruction of lesion or tissue of bony palate
Local excision or destruction of palate by:
cautery
chemotherapy
cryotherapy
Excludes: *biopsy of bony palate (27.21)*

27.32 Wide excision or destruction of lesion or tissue of bony palate
En bloc resection of alveolar process and palate

27.4 Excision of other parts of mouth

27.41 Labial frenectomy
Excludes: *division of labial frenum (27.91)*

27.42 Wide excision of lesion of lip

27.43 Other excision of lesion or tissue of lip

27.49 Other excision of mouth
Excludes: *biopsy of mouth NOS (27.24)*
excision of lesion of:
palate (27.31-27.32)
tongue (25.1)
uvula (27.72)
fistulectomy of mouth (27.53)
frenectomy of:
lip (27.41)
tongue (25.92)

27.5 Plastic repair of mouth
Excludes: *palatoplasty (27.61-27.69)*

27.51 Suture of laceration of lip

27.52 Suture of laceration of other part of mouth

● Code new   ▲ Revision of   ④ ⑤ Fourth or fifth
        to this edition   existing code   digit required

27.53 **Closure of fistula of mouth**

> Excludes: fistulectomy:
>> nasolabial (21.82)
>> oro-antral (22.71)
>> oronasal (21.82)

27.54 **Repair of cleft lip**

27.55 **Full-thickness skin graft to lip and mouth**

27.56 **Other skin graft to lip and mouth**

27.57 **Attachment of pedicle or flap graft to lip and mouth**

27.59 **Other plastic repair of mouth**

27.6 **Palatoplasty**

27.61 **Suture of laceration of palate**

27.62 **Correction of cleft palate**
Correction of cleft palate by push-back operation

> Excludes: revision of cleft palate repair (27.63)

27.63 **Revision of cleft palate repair**
Secondary:
attachment of pharyngeal flap
lengthening of palate

27.69 **Other plastic repair of palate**

> Excludes: fistulectomy of mouth (27.53)

27.7 **Operations on uvula**

27.71 **Incision of uvula**

27.72 **Excision of uvula**

> Excludes: biopsy of uvula (27.22)

27.73 **Repair of uvula**

> Excludes: that with synchronous cleft palate repair (27.62)
> uranostaphylorrhaphy (27.62)

27.79 **Other operations on uvula**

27.9 **Other operations on mouth and face**

27.91 **Labial frenotomy**
Division of labial frenum

> Excludes: lingual frenotomy (25.91)

27.92 **Incision of mouth, unspecified structure**

> Excludes: incision of:
>> gum (24.0)
>> palate (27.1)
>> salivary gland or duct (26.0)
>> tongue (25.94)
>> uvula (27.71)

27.99 **Other operations on oral cavity**
Graft of buccal sulcus

> Excludes: removal of:
>> intraluminal foreign body (98.01)
>> penetrating foreign body from mouth without incision (98.22)

28 **Operations on tonsils and adenoids**

28.0 **Incision and drainage of tonsil and peritonsillar structures**
Drainage (oral) (transcervical) of:
parapharyngeal abscess
peritonsillar abscess
retropharyngeal abscess
tonsillar abscess

28.1 **Diagnostic procedures on tonsils and adenoids**

28.11 **Biopsy of tonsils and adenoids**

28.19 **Other diagnostic procedures on tonsils and adenoids**

> Excludes: soft tissue x-ray (87.09)

	Valid O.R. procedure		Non-O.R. procedure		Nonspecific O.R. procedure		Noncovered O.R. procedure

28.2	**Tonsillectomy without adenoidectomy**
28.3	**Tonsillectomy with adenoidectomy**
28.4	**Excision of tonsil tag**
28.5	**Excision of lingual tonsil**
28.6	**Adenoidectomy without tonsillectomy**

Excision of adenoid tag

28.7 **Control of hemorrhage after tonsillectomy and adenoidectomy**

28.9 **Other operations on tonsils and adenoids**

28.91 **Removal of foreign body from tonsil and adenoid by incision**

> *Excludes:* *that without incision (98.13)*

28.92 **Excision of lesion of tonsil and adenoid**

> *Excludes:* *biopsy of tonsil and adenoid (28.11)*

28.99 **Other**

29 **Operation on pharynx**

Includes: operations on:
hypopharynx
nasopharynx
oropharynx
pharyngeal pouch
pyriform sinus

29.0 **Pharyngotomy**

Drainage of pharyngeal bursa

> *Excludes:* *incision and drainage of retropharyngeal abscess (28.0)*
> *removal of foreign body (without incision) (98.13)*

29.1 **Diagnostic procedures on pharynx**

29.11 **Pharyngoscopy**

29.12 **Pharyngeal biopsy**

Biopsy of supraglottic mass

29.19 **Other diagnostic procedures on pharynx**

> *Excludes:* *x-ray of nasopharynx:*
> *contrast (87.06)*
> *other (87.09)*

29.2 **Excision of branchial cleft cyst or vestige**

> *Excludes:* *branchial cleft fistulectomy (29.52)*

29.3 **Excision or destruction of lesion or tissue of pharynx**

29.31 **Cricopharyngeal myotomy**

> *Excludes* *that with pharyngeal diverticulectomy (29.32)*

29.32 **Pharyngeal diverticulectomy**

29.33 **Pharyngectomy (partial)**

> *Excludes* *laryngopharyngectomy (30.3)*

29.39 **Other excision or destruction of lesion or tissue of pharynx**

29.4 **Plastic operation on pharynx**

Correction of nasopharyngeal atresia

> *Excludes:* *pharyngoplasty associated with cleft palate repair (27.62-27.63)*

29.5 **Other repair of pharynx**

29.51 **Suture of laceration of pharynx**

29.52 **Closure of branchial cleft fistula**

29.53 **Closure of other fistula of pharynx**

Pharyngoesophageal fistulectomy

29.54 **Lysis of pharyngeal adhesions**

29.59 **Other**

29.9 **Other operations on pharynx**

29.91 **Dilation of pharynx**

Dilation of nasopharynx

29.92 **Division of glossopharyngeal nerve**

● Code new
to this edition

▲ Revision of
existing code

④ ⑤ Fourth or fifth
digit required

29.99 **Other**

> *Excludes:* insertion of radium into pharynx and nasopharynx (92.27)
> removal of intraluminal foreign body (98.13)

	Valid O.R. procedure		Non-O.R. procedure		Nonspecific O.R. procedure		Noncovered O.R. procedure

● Code new
to this edition
▲ Revision of
existing code
④ ⑤ Fourth or fifth
digit required

6. OPERATIONS ON THE RESPIRATORY SYSTEM (30-34)

30 Excision of larynx

30.0 Excision or destruction of lesion or tissue of larynx

30.01 Marsupialization of laryngeal cyst

30.09 Other excision or destruction of lesion or tissue of larynx
Stripping of vocal cords

Excludes: *biopsy of larynx (31.43)*
laryngeal fistulectomy (31.62)
laryngotracheal fistulectomy (31.62)

30.1 Hemilaryngectomy

30.2 Other partial laryngectomy

30.21 Epiglottidectomy

30.22 Vocal cordectomy
Excision of vocal cords

30.29 Other partial laryngectomy
Excision of laryngeal cartilage

30.3 Complete laryngectomy
Block dissection of larynx (with thyroidectomy) (with synchronous tracheostomy)
Laryngopharyngectomy

Excludes: *that with radical neck dissection (30.4)*

30.4 Radical laryngectomy
Complete [total] laryngectomy with radical neck dissection (with thyroidectomy) (with synchronous tracheostomy)

31 Other operations on larynx and trachea

31.0 Injection of larynx
Injection of inert material into larynx or vocal cords

31.1 Temporary tracheostomy
Tracheotomy for assistance in breathing

31.2 Permanent tracheostomy

31.21 Mediastinal tracheostomy

31.29 Other permanent tracheostomy

Excludes: *that with laryngectomy (30.3-30.4)*

31.3 Other incision of larynx or trachea

Excludes: *that for assistance in breathing (31.1-31.29)*

31.4 Diagnostic procedures on larynx and trachea

31.41 Tracheoscopy through artificial stoma

Excludes: *that with biopsy (31.43-31.44)*

31.42 Laryngoscopy and other tracheoscopy

Excludes: *that with biopsy (31.43-31.44)*

31.43 Closed [endoscopic] biopsy of larynx

31.44 Closed [endoscopic] biopsy of trachea

31.45 Open biopsy of larynx or trachea

31.48 Other diagnostic procedures on larynx

Excludes: *contrast laryngogram (87.07)*
microscopic examination of specimen from larynx (90.31-90.39)
soft tissue x-ray of larynx NEC (87.09)

31.49 Other diagnostic procedures on trachea

Excludes: *microscopic examination of specimen from trachea (90.41-90.49)*
x-ray of trachea (87.49)

31.5 Local excision or destruction of lesion or tissue of trachea

Excludes: *biopsy of trachea (31.44-31.45)*
laryngotracheal fistulectomy (31.62)
tracheoesophageal fistulectomy (31.73)

| | Valid O.R. procedure | | Non-O.R. procedure | | Nonspecific O.R. procedure | | Noncovered O.R. procedure |

31.6 **Repair of larynx**

31.61 **Suture of laceration of larynx**

31.62 **Closure of fistula of larynx**
Laryngotracheal fistulectomy
Take-down of laryngostomy

31.63 **Revision of laryngostomy**

31.64 **Repair of laryngeal fracture**

31.69 **Other repair of larynx**
Arytenoidopexy
Graft of larynx
Transposition of vocal cords

Excludes: construction of artificial larynx (31.75)

31.7 **Repair and plastic operations on trachea**

31.71 **Suture of laceration of trachea**

31.72 **Closure of external fistula of trachea**
Closure of tracheotomy

31.73 **Closure of other fistula of trachea**
Tracheoesophageal fistulectomy

Excludes: laryngotracheal fistulectomy (31.62)

31.74 **Revision of tracheostomy**

31.75 **Reconstruction of trachea and construction of artificial larynx**
Tracheoplasty with artificial larynx

31.79 **Other repair and plastic operations on trachea**

31.9 **Other operations on larynx and trachea**

31.91 **Division of laryngeal nerve**

31.92 **Lysis of adhesions of trachea or larynx**

31.93 **Replacement of laryngeal or tracheal stent**

31.94 **Injection of locally-acting therapeutic substance into trachea**

31.95 **Tracheoesophageal fistulization**

31.98 **Other operations on larynx**
Dilation of larynx
Division of congenital web of larynx
Removal of keel or stent of larynx

Excludes: removal of intraluminal foreign body from larynx without incision
(98.14)

31.99 **Other operations on trachea**

Excludes: removal of:
intraluminal foreign body from trachea without incision (98.15)
tracheostomy tube (97.37)
replacement of tracheostomy tube (97.23)
tracheostomy toilette (96.35)

32 **Excision of lung and bronchus**
Includes: rib resection as operative approach
sternotomy as operative approach
sternum-splitting incision as operative approach
thoracotomy as operative approach
Code also any synchronous bronchoplasty (33.48)

32.0 **Local excision or destruction of lesion or tissue of bronchus**

Excludes: biopsy of bronchus (33.24-33.25)
bronchial fistulectomy (33.42)

32.01 **Endoscopic excision or destruction of lesion or tissue of bronchus**

32.09 **Other local excision or destruction of lesion or tissue of bronchus**

Excludes: that by endoscopic approach (32.01)

32.1 **Other excision of bronchus**
Resection (wide sleeve) of bronchus

Excludes: radical dissection [excision] of bronchus (32.6)

● Code new
to this edition   ▲ Revision of
existing code   ④ ⑤ Fourth or fifth
digit required

32.2   **Local excision or destruction of lesion or tissue of lung**

     32.21   **Plication of emphysematous bleb**

     32.22   **Lung volume reduction surgery**

     32.28   **Endoscopic excision or destruction of lesion or tissue of lung**

         | Excludes: | *biopsy of lung (33.26-33.27)*

     32.29   **Other local excision or destruction of lesion or tissue of lung**
         Resection of lung:
           NOS
           wedge

         | Excludes: | *biopsy of lung (33.26-33.27)*
                    that by endoscopic approach (32.28)
                    wide excision of lesion of lung (32.3)

32.3   **Segmental resection of lung**
     Partial lobectomy

32.4   **Lobectomy of lung**
     Lobectomy with segmental resection of adjacent lobes of lung

     | Excludes: | *that with radical dissection [excision] of thoracic structures (32.6)*

32.5   **Complete pneumonectomy**
     Excision of lung NOS
     Pneumonectomy (with mediastinal dissection)

32.6   **Radical dissection of thoracic structures**
     Block [en bloc] dissection of bronchus, lobe of lung, brachial plexus, intercostal structure,
     ribs (transverse process), and sympathetic nerves

32.9   **Other excision of lung**

     | Excludes: | *biopsy of lung and bronchus (33.24-33.27)*
                  pulmonary decortication (34.51)

33   **Other operations on lung and bronchus**
     Includes: rib resection as operative approach
                sternotomy as operative approach
                sternum-splitting incision as operative approach
                thoracotomy as operative approach

33.0   **Incision of bronchus**

33.1   **Incision of lung**

     | Excludes: | *puncture of lung (33.93)*

33.2   **Diagnostic procedures on lung and bronchus**

     33.21   **Bronchoscopy through artificial stoma**

         | Excludes: | *that with biopsy (33.24, 33.27)*

     33.22   **Fiber-optic bronchoscopy**

         | Excludes: | *that with biopsy (33.24. 33.27)*

     33.23   **Other bronchoscopy**

         | Excludes: | *that for:*
                   aspiration (96.05)
                   biopsy (33.24, 33.27)

     33.24   **Closed [endoscopic] biopsy of bronchus**
         Bronchoscopy (fiberoptic) (rigid) with:
           brush biopsy of "lung"
           brushing or washing for specimen collection
           excision (bite) biopsy
         Diagnostic bronchoalveolar lavage (BAL)

         | Excludes: | *closed biopsy of lung, other than brush biopsy of "lung" (33.26,*
                  33.27)
                  whole lung lavage (33.99)

     33.25   **Open biopsy of bronchus**

         | Excludes: | *open biopsy of lung (33.28)*

     33.26   **Closed [percutaneous] [needle] biopsy of lung**

         | Excludes: | *endoscopic biopsy of lung (33.27)*

33.27 Closed endoscopic biopsy of lung
Fiberoptic (flexible) bronchoscopy with fluoroscopic guidance with biopsy
Transbronchial lung biopsy

Excludes: *brush biopsy of lung (33.24)*
percutaneous biopsy of lung (33.26)

33.28 Open biopsy of lung

33.29 Other diagnostic procedures on lung and bronchus

Excludes: *contrast bronchogram:*
endotracheal (87.31)
other (87.32)
lung scan (92.15)
magnetic resonance imaging (88.92)
microscopic examination of specimen from bronchus or lung
(90.41-90.49)
routine chest x-ray (87.44)
ultrasonography of lung (88.73)
vital capacity determination (89.37)
x-ray of bronchus or lung NOS (87.49)

33.3 Surgical collapse of lung

33.31 Destruction of phrenic nerve for collapse of lung

33.32 Artificial pneumothorax for collapse of lung
Thoracotomy for collapse of lung

33.33 Pneumoperitoneum for collapse of lung

33.34 Thoracoplasty

33.39 Other surgical collapse of lung
Collapse of lung NOS

33.4 Repair and plastic operation on lung and bronchus

33.41 Suture of laceration of bronchus

33.42 Closure of bronchial fistula
Closure of bronchostomy
Fistulectomy:
bronchocutaneous
bronchoesophageal
bronchovisceral

Excludes: *closure of fistula:*
bronchomediastinal (34.73)
bronchopleural (34.73)
bronchopleuromediastinal (34.73)

33.43 Closure of laceration of lung

33.48 Other repair and plastic operation on bronchus

33.49 Other repair ad plastic operations on lung

Excludes: *closure of pleural fistula (34.73)*

33.5 Lung transplant
Code also cardiopulmonary bypass [extracorporeal circulation] [heart-lung machine]
39.61

Excludes: *Combined heart-lung transplantation (33.6)*

33.50 Lung transplantation, not otherwise specified

33.51 Unilateral lung transplantation

33.52 Bilateral lung transplantation
Double-lung transplantation
En bloc transplantation

33.6 Combined heart-lung transplantation
Code also cardiopulmonary bypass [extracorporeal circulation] [heart-lung machine]
(39.61)

33.9 Other operations on lung and bronchus

33.91 Bronchial dilation

33.92 Ligation of bronchus

33.93 Puncture of lung

Excludes: *needle biopsy (33.26)*

● Code new
to this edition
▲ Revision of
existing code
④ ⑤ Fourth or fifth
digit required

33.98 Other operations on bronchus

> Excludes: bronchial lavage (96.56)
> removal of intraluminal foreign body from bronchus without incision (98.15)

33.99 Other operations on lung
Whole lung lavage

> Excludes: other continuous mechanical ventilation (96.70-96.72)
> respiratory therapy (93.90-93.99)

34 Operations on chest wall, pleura, mediastinum, and diaphragm

> Excludes: operations on breast (85.0-85.99)

34.0 Incision of chest wall and pleura

> Excludes: that as operative approach—omit code

34.01 Incision of chest wall
Extrapleural drainage

> Excludes: incision of pleura (34.09)

34.02 Exploratory thoracotomy

34.03 Reopening of recent thoracotomy site

34.04 Insertion of intercostal catheter for drainage
Chest tube
Closed chest drainage
Revision of intercostal catheter (chest tube) (with lysis of adhesions)

34.05 Creation of pleuroperitoneal shunt

34.09 Other incision of pleura
Creation of pleural window for drainage
Intercostal stab
Open chest drainage

> Excludes: thoracoscopy (34.21)
> thoracotomy for collapse of lung (33.32)

34.1 Incision of mediastinum

> Excludes: mediastinoscopy (34.22)
> mediastinotomy associated with pneumonectomy (32.5)

34.2 Diagnostic procedures on chest wall, pleura, mediastinum, and diaphragm

34.21 Transpleural thoracoscopy

34.22 Mediastinoscopy
Code also any lymph node biopsy (40.11)

34.23 Biopsy of chest wall

34.24 Pleural biopsy

34.25 Closed [percutaneous] [needle] biopsy of mediastinum

34.26 Open biopsy of mediastinum

34.27 Biopsy of diaphragm

34.28 Other diagnostic procedures on chest wall, pleura, and diaphragm

> Excludes: angiocardiography (88.50-88.58)
> aortography (88.42)
> arteriography of:
> intrathoracic vessels NEC (88.44)
> pulmonary arteries (88.43)
> microscopic examination of specimen from chest wall. pleura, and diaphragm (90.41-90.49)
> phlebography of:
> intrathoracic vessels NEC (88.63)
> pulmonary veins (88.62)
> radiological examinations of thorax:
> C.A.T. scan (87.41)
> diaphragmatic x-ray (87.49)
> intrathoracic lymphangiogram (87.34)
> routine chest x-ray (87.44)
> sinogram of chest wall (87.38)
> soft tissue x-ray of chest wall NEC (87.39)
> tomogram of thorax NEC (87. 42)
> ultrasonography of thorax (88.73)

| | Valid O.R. procedure | | Non-O.R. procedure | | Nonspecific O.R. procedure | | Noncovered O.R. procedure |

34.29 Other diagnostic procedures on mediastinum

> | Excludes: | *mediastinal:*
> *pneumogram (87.33)*
> *x-ray NEC (87.49)*

34.3 Excision or destruction of lesion or tissue of mediastinum

> | Excludes: | *biopsy or mediastinum (34.25-34.26)*
> *mediastinal fistulectomy (34.73)*

34.4 Excision or destruction of lesion of chest wall
Excision of lesion of chest wall NOS (with excision of ribs)

> | Excludes: | *biopsy of chest wall (34.23)*
> *costectomy not incidental to thoracic procedure (77. 91)*
> *excision of lesion of:*
> *breast (85.20-85.25)*
> *cartilage (80.89)*
> *skin (86.2-86.3)*
> *fistulectomy (34. 73)*

34.5 Pleurectomy

34.51 Decortication of lung

34.59 Other excision of pleura
Excision of pleural lesion

> | Excludes: | *biopsy of pleura (34.24)*
> *pleural fistulectomy (34.73)*

34.6 Scarification of pleura
Pleurosclerosis

> | Excludes: | *injection of sclerosing agent (34.92)*

34.7 Repair of chest wall

34.71 Suture of laceration of chest wall

> | Excludes: | *suture of skin and subcutaneous tissue alone (86.59)*

34.72 Closure of thoracostomy

34.73 Closure of other fistula of thorax
Closure of:
bronchopleural fistula
bronchopleurocutaneous fistula
bronchopleuromediastinal fistula

34.74 Repair of pectus deformity
Repair of:
pectus carinatum (with implant)
pectus excavatum (with implant)

34.79 Other repair of chest wall
Repair of chest wall NOS

34.8 Operations on diaphragm

34.81 Excision of lesion or tissue of diaphragm

> | Excludes: | *biopsy of diaphragm (34.27)*

34.82 Suture of laceration of diaphragm

34.83 Closure of fistula of diaphragm
Thoracicoabdominal fistulectomy
Thoracicogastric fistulectomy
Thoracicointestinal fistulectomy

34.84 Other repair of diaphragm

> | Excludes: | *repair of diaphragmatic hernia (53.7-53.82)*

34.85 Implantation of diaphragmatic pacemaker

34.89 Other operations on diaphragm

34.9 Other operations on thorax

34.91 Thoracentesis

● Code new
to this edition   ▲ Revision of
existing code   ④ ⑤ Fourth or fifth
digit required

34.92 Injection into thoracic cavity

Chemical pleurodesis

Injection of cytotoxic agent or tetracycline

Requires additional code for any cancer chemotherapeutic substance (99.25)

Excludes: *that for collapse of lung (33.32)*

34.93 Repair of pleura

34.99 Other

Excludes: *removal of:*
mediastinal drain (97.42)
sutures (97.43)
thoracotomy tube (97.41)

Valid O.R. procedure   Non-O.R. procedure   Nonspecific O.R. procedure   Noncovered O.R. procedure

● Code new
to this edition   ▲ Revision of
existing code   ④ ⑤ Fourth or fifth
digit required

7. OPERATIONS ON THE CARDIOVASCULAR SYSTEM (35-39)

35 Operations on valves and septa of heart

Includes: sternotomy (median) (transverse) as operative approach
            thoracotomy as operative approach

Code also cardiopulmonary bypass [extracorporeal circulation] [heart-lung machine] (39.61)

35.0 Closed heart valvotomy

    | *Excludes:* | *percutaneous (balloon) valvuloplasty (35.96)*

35.00 Closed heart valvotomy, unspecified valve

35.01 Closed heart valvotomy, aortic valve

35.02 Closed heart valvotomy, mitral valve

35.03 Closed heart valvotomy, pulmonary valve

35.04 Closed heart valvotomy, tricuspid valve

35.1 Open heart valvuloplasty without replacement

Includes: open heart valvotomy

    | *Excludes:* | *that associated with repair of:*
          endocardial cushion defect (35.54, 35.63, 35.73)
          percutaneous (balloon) valvuloplasty (35.96)
          valvular defect associated with atrial and ventricular septal defects (35.54, 35.63, 35.73)

Code also cardiopulmonary bypass, if performed [extracorporeal circulation] [heart-lung machine] (39.61)

35.10 Open heart valvuloplasty without replacement, unspecified valve

35.11 Open heart valvuloplasty of aortic valve without replacement

35.12 Open heart valvuloplasty of mitral valve without replacement

35.13 Open heart valvuloplasty of pulmonary valve without replacement

35.14 Open heart valvuloplasty of tricuspid valve without replacement

35.2 Replacement of heart valve

Includes: excision of heart valve with replacement

Code also cardiopulmonary bypass [extracorporeal circulation] [heart-lung machine] (39.61)

    | *Excludes:* | *that associated with repair of:*
          endocardial cushion defect (35.54, 35.63, 35.73)
          valvular defect associated with atrial and ventricular septal defects (35.54, 35.63, 35.73)

35.20 Replacement of unspecified heart valve

Repair of unspecified heart valve with tissue graft or prosthetic implant

35.21 Replacement of aortic valve with tissue graft

Repair of aortic valve with tissue graft (autograft) (heterograft) (homograft)

35.22 Other replacement of aortic valve

Repair of aortic valve with replacement:
    NOS
    prosthetic (partial) (synthetic) (total)

35.23 Replacement of mitral valve with tissue graft

Repair of mitral valve with tissue graft (autograft) (heterograft) (homograft)

35.24 Other replacement of mitral valve

Repair of mitral valve with replacement:
    NOS
    prosthetic (partial) (synthetic) (total)

35.25 Replacement of pulmonary valve with tissue graft

Repair of pulmonary valve with tissue graft (autograft) (heterograft) (homograft)

35.26 Other replacement of pulmonary valve

Repair of pulmonary valve with replacement:
    NOS
    prosthetic (partial) (synthetic) (total)

35.27 Replacement of tricuspid valve with tissue graft

Repair of tricuspid valve with tissue graft (autograft) (heterograft) (homograft)

35.28 Other replacement of tricuspid valve
Repair of tricuspid valve with replacement:
NOS
prosthetic (partial) (synthetic) (total)

35.3 Operations on structures adjacent to heart valves
*Code also cardiopulmonary bypass [extracorporeal circulation] [heart-lung machine]
(39.61)*

35.31 Operations on papillary muscle
Division of papillary muscle
Reattachment of papillary muscle
Repair of papillary muscle

35.32 Operations on chordae tendineae
Division of chordae tendineae
Repair of chordae tendineae

35.33 Annuloplasty
Plication of annulus

35.34 Infundibulectomy
Right ventricular infundibulectomy

35.35 Operations on trabeculae carneae cordis
Division of trabeculae carneae cordis
Excision of trabeculae carneae cordis
Excision of aortic subvalvular ring

35.39 Operations on other structures adjacent to valves of heart
Repair of sinus of Valsalva (aneurysm)

35.4 Production of septal defect in heart

35.41 Enlargement of existing atrial septal defect
Rashkind procedure
Septostomy (atrial) (balloon)

35.42 Creation of septal defect in heart
Blalock-Hanlon operation

35.5 Repair of atrial and ventricular septa with prosthesis
Includes: repair of septa with synthetic implant of patch

*Code also cardiopulmonary bypass [extracorporeal circulation] [heart-lung machine]
(39.61)*

35.50 Repair of unspecified septal defect of heart with prosthesis

Excludes:	*that associated with repair of:*
	endocardial cushion defect (35.54)
	septal defect associated with valvular defect (35.54)

35.51 Repair of atrial septal defect with prosthesis, open technique
Atrioseptoplasty with prosthesis
Correction of atrial septal defect with prosthesis
Repair:
foramen ovale (patent) with prosthesis
ostium secundum defect with prosthesis

Excludes:	*that associated with repair of:*
	atrial septal defect associated with valvular and ventricular septal defects (35.54)
	endocardial cushion defect (35.54)

35.52 Repair of atrial septal defect with prosthesis, closed technique
Insertion of atrial septal umbrella [King-Mills]

35.53 Repair of ventricular septal defect with prosthesis
Correction of ventricular septal defect with prosthesis
Repair of supracristal defect with prosthesis

Excludes:	*that associated with repair of:*
	endocardial cushion defect (35.54)
	ventricular defect associated with valvular and atrial septal defects (35.54)

● Code new
to this edition   ▲ Revision of
existing code   ④ ⑤ Fourth or fifth
digit required

35.54 **Repair of endocardial cushion defect with prosthesis**
Repair:
atrioventricular canal with prosthesis (grafted to septa)
ostium primum defect with prosthesis (grafted to septa)
valvular defect associated with atrial and ventricular septal defects with prosthesis (grafted to septa)

Excludes: *repair of isolated:*
atrial septal defect (35.51-35.52)
valvular defect (35.20, 35.22, 35.24, 35.26. 35.28)
ventricular septal defect (35.53)

35.6 **Repair of atrial and ventricular septa with tissue graft**
Code also cardiopulmonary bypass [extracorporeal circulation] [heart-lung machine] (39.61)

35.60 **Repair of unspecified septal defect of heart with tissue graft**

Excludes: *that associated with repair of:*
endocardial cushion defect (35.63)
septal defect associated with valvular, defect (33.63)

35.61 **Repair of atrial septal defect with tissue graft**
Atrioseptoplasty with tissue graft
Correction of atrial septal defect with tissue graft
Repair:
foramen ovale (patent) with tissue graft
ostium secundum defect with tissue graft

Excludes: *that associated with repair of:*
atrial septal defect associated with valvular and ventricular septal defects (35.63)
endocardial cushion defect (35.63)

35.62 **Repair of ventricular septal defect with tissue graft**
Correction of ventricular septal defect with tissue graft
Repair of supracristal defect with tissue graft

Excludes: *that associated with repair of:*
endocardial cushion defect (35.63)
ventricular defect associated with valvular and atrial septal defects (35.63)

35.63 **Repair of endocardial cushion defect with tissue graft**
Repair of:
atrioventricular canal with tissue graft
ostium primum defect with tissue graft
valvular defect associated with atrial and ventricular septal defects with tissue graft

Excludes: *repair of isolated*
atrial septal defect (35.61)
valvular defect (35.20-35.21. 35.23, 35.25. 35.27)
ventricular septal defect (35.62)

35.7 **Other and unspecified repair of atrial and ventricular septa**
Code also cardiopulmonary bypass [extracorporeal circulation] [heart-lung machine] (39.61)

35.70 **Other and unspecified repair of unspecified septal defect of heart**
Repair of septal defect NOS

Excludes: *that associated with repair of:*
endocardial cushion defect (35.73)
septal defect associated with valvular defect (35.73)

	Valid O.R. procedure		Non-O.R. procedure		Nonspecific O.R. procedure		Noncovered O.R. procedure

35.71 Other and unspecified repair of atrial septal defect

Repair NOS:
  atrial septum
  foramen ovale (patent)
  ostium secundum defect

> Excludes: *that associated with repair of:*
> *atrial septal defect associated with valvular and ventricular septal*
> *defects (35.73)*
> *endocardial cushion defect (35.73)*

35.72 Other and unspecified repair of ventricular septal defect

Repair NOS:
  supracristal defect
  ventricular septum

> Excludes: *that associated with repair of:*
> *endocardial cushion defect (35.73)*
> *ventricular septal defect associated with valvular and atrial septal*
> *defects (35.73)*

35.73 Other and unspecified repair of endocardial cushion defect

Repair NOS:
  atrioventricular canal
  ostium primum defect
  valvular defect associated with atrial and ventricular septal defects

> Excludes: *repair of isolated:*
> *atrial septal defect (35.71)*
> *valvular defect (35.20, 35.22, 35.24, 35.26, 35.28)*
> *ventricular septal defect (35.72)*

35.8 Total repair of certain congenital cardiac anomalies

Note: For partial repair of defect [e.g. repair of atrial septal defect in tetralogy of Fallot]—
code to specific procedure

35.81 Total repair of tetralogy of Fallot

One-stage total correction of tetralogy of Fallot with or without:
  commissurotomy of pulmonary valve
  infundibulectomy
  outflow tract prosthesis
  patch graft of outflow tract
  prosthetic tube for pulmonary artery
  repair of ventricular septal defect (with prosthesis)
  take-down of previous systemic-pulmonary artery anastomosis

35.82 Total repair of total anomalous pulmonary venous connection

One-stage total correction of total anomalous pulmonary venous connection with or
  without:
  anastomosis between (horizontal) common pulmonary trunk and posterior wall of
    left atrium (side-to-side)
  enlargement of foramen ovale
  incision [excision] of common wall between posterior left atrium and coronary si-
    nus and roofing of resultant defect with patch graft (synthetic)
  ligation of venous connection (descending anomalous vein) (to left innominate
    vein) (to superior vena cava)
  repair of atrial septal defect (with prosthesis)

35.83 Total repair of truncus arteriosus

One-stage total correction of truncus arteriosus with or without:
  construction (with aortic homograft) (with prosthesis) of a pulmonary artery
    placed from right ventricle to arteries supplying the lung
  ligation of connections between aorta and pulmonary artery
  repair of ventricular septal defect (with prosthesis)

35.84 Total correction of transposition of great vessels, not elsewhere classified

Arterial switch operation [Jatene]
Total correction of transposition of great arteries at the arterial level by switching
  the great arteries, including the left or both coronary arteries, implanted in the
  wall of the pulmonary artery

> Excludes: *baffle operation [Mustard] [Senning] (35.91)*
> *creation of shunt between right ventricle and pulmonary artery*
> *[Rastelli] (35.92)*

● Code new
  to this edition

▲ Revision of
  existing code

④ ⑤ Fourth or fifth
  digit required

35.9 **Other operations on valves and septa of heart**

Code also cardiopulmonary bypass, if performed [extracorporeal circulation] [heart-lung machine] (39.61)

35.91 **Interatrial transposition of venous return**
Baffle:
  atrial
  interatrial
Mustard's operation
Resection of atrial septum and insertion of patch to direct systemic venous return to tricuspid valve and pulmonary venous return to mitral valve

35.92 **Creation of conduit between right ventricle and pulmonary artery**
Creation of shunt between right ventricle and (distal) pulmonary artery

  | Excludes: | *that associated with total repair of truncus arteriosus (35.83)*

35.93 **Creation of conduit between left ventricle and aorta**
Creation of apicoaortic shunt
Shunt between apex of left ventricle and aorta

35.94 **Creation of conduit between atrium and pulmonary artery**
Fontan procedure

35.95 **Revision of corrective procedure on heart**
Replacement of prosthetic heart valve poppet
Resuture or prosthesis of:
  septum
  valve

  | Excludes: | *complete revision—code to specific procedure*
    replacement of prosthesis or graft of:
      septum (35.50-35.63)
      valve (35.20-35.28)

35.96 **Percutaneous valvuloplasty**
Percutaneous balloon valvuloplasty

35.98 **Other operations on septa of heart**

35.99 **Other operations on valves of heart**

36 **Operations on vessels of heart**
Includes: sternotomy (median) (transverse) as operative approach
        thoracotomy as operative approach

Code also any injection or infusion of platelet inhibitor (99.20)

Code also cardiopulmonary bypass, if performed [extracorporeal circulation] [heart-lung machine] (39.61)

36.0 **Removal of coronary artery obstruction and insertion of stent(s)**

36.01 **Single vessel percutaneous transluminal coronary angioplasty [PTCA] or coronary atherectomy without mention of thrombolytic agent**
Code also any insertion of coronary stent(s) (36.06)
Balloon angioplasty of coronary artery
Coronary atherectomy
Percutaneous coronary angioplasty NOS
PTCA NOS

  | Excludes: | *multiple vessel percutaneous transluminal coronary angioplasty [PTCA] or coronary atherectomy performed during the same operation (36.05)*

36.02 **Single vessel percutaneous transluminal coronary angioplasty [PTCA] or coronary atherectomy with mention of thrombolytic agent**
Code also any insertion of coronary stent(s) 36.06
Balloon angioplasty of coronary artery with infusion of thrombolytic agent [streptokinase]
Coronary atherectomy

  | Excludes: | *multiple vessel percutaneous transluminal coronary angioplasty [PTCA] or coronary atherectomy performed during the same operation (36.05)*
    single vessel [PTCA] or coronary atherectomy without mention of thrombolytic agent (36.01)

Valid O.R. procedure   Non-O.R. procedure   Nonspecific O.R. procedure   Noncovered O.R. procedure

36.03 Open chest coronary artery angioplasty
Code also any insertion of coronary stent(s) 36.06
Coronary (artery):
endarterectomy (with patch graft)
thromboendarterectomy (with patch graft)
Open surgery for direct relief of coronary artery obstruction

[Excludes:] *that with coronary artery bypass graft (36.10-36.19)*

36.04 Intracoronary artery thrombolytic infusion
That by direct coronary artery injection, infusion, or catheterization
enzyme infusion
platelet inhibitor

[Excludes:] *infusion of platelet inhibitor (99.20)*
infusion of thrombolytic agent (99.10)

36.05 Multiple vessel percutaneous transluminal coronary angioplasty [PTCA] or coronary atherectomy performed during the same operation, with or without mention of thrombolytic agent
Balloon angioplasty of multiple coronary arteries
Coronary atherectomy
Code also any intracoronary artery thrombolytic infusion (36.04)
Code also any insertion of coronary artery stent(s) (36.06)

[Excludes:] *single vessel PTCA or coronary atherectomy without mention of thrombolytic agent (36.01)*
with mention of thrombolytic agent (36.02)

▲ **36.06 Insertion of non-drug-eluting coronary artery stent(s)**
Bare stent(s)
Bonded stent(s)
Drug-coated stent(s), i.e., heparin coated
Endograft(s)
Endovascular graft(s)
Stent graft(s)
Code also any open chest coronary artery angioplasty (36.03)
Code also any percutaneous transluminal coronary angioplasty [PTCA] or coronary atherectomy (36.01, 36.02, 36.05)

[Excludes:] *insertion of drug-eluting coronary artery stent(s) (36.07)*

● **36.07 Insertion of drug-eluting coronary artery stent(s)**
Endograft(s)
Endovascular graft(s)
Stent graft(s)
Code also any:
open chest coronary artery angioplasty (36.03)
percutaneous transluminal coronary angioplasty [PTCA] or coronary atherectomy (36.01, 36.02, 36.05)

[Excludes:] *drug-coated stent(s), e.g., heparin coated (36.06)*
insertion of non-drug-eluting coronary artery stent(s) (36.06)

36.09 Other removal of coronary artery obstruction
Coronary angioplasty NOS

[Excludes:] *that by open angioplasty (36.03)*
that by percutaneous transluminal coronary angioplasty [PTCA] or coronary atherectomy (36.01-36.02, 36.05)

36.1 Bypass anastomosis for heart revascularization
Code also cardiopulmonary bypass [extracorporeal circulation] [heart-lung machine] (39.61)

36.10 Aortocoronary bypass for heart revascularization, not otherwise specified
Direct revascularization with catheter stent, prosthesis, or vein graft:
cardiac
coronary
heart muscle
myocardial
Heart revascularization NOS

36.11 Aortocoronary bypass of one coronary artery

36.12 Aortocoronary bypass of two coronary arteries

36.13 Aortocoronary bypass of three coronary arteries

● Code new to this edition ▲ Revision of existing code ④ ⑤ Fourth or fifth digit required

36.14 Aortocoronary bypass of four or more coronary arteries

36.15 Single internal mammary-coronary artery bypass
Anastomosis (single):
  mammary artery to coronary artery
  thoracic artery to coronary artery

36.16 Double internal mammary-coronary artery bypass
Anastomosis (double):
  mammary artery to coronary artery
  thoracic artery to coronary artery

36.17 Abdominal-coronary artery bypass
Anastomosis:
  gastroepiploic artery to coronary artery

36.19 Other bypass anastomosis for heart revascularization

36.2 Heart revascularization by arterial implant
Implantation of:
  aortic branches [ascending aortic branches] into heart muscle
  blood vessels into myocardium
  internal mammary artery [internal thoracic artery] into:
    heart muscle
    myocardium
    ventricle
    ventricular wall
Indirect heart revascularization NOS

36.3 Other heart revascularization

36.31 Open chest transmyocardial revascularization

36.32 Other transmyocardial revascularization
Percutaneous transmyocardial revasculariztion
Thoracoscopic transmyocardial revascularization

36.39 Other heart revascularization
Abrasion of epicardium
Cardio-omentopexy
Intrapericardial poudrage
Myocardial graft:
  mediastinal fat
  omentum
  pectoral muscles

36.9 Other operations on vessels of heart

Code also cardiopulmonary bypass [extracorporeal circulation] [heart-lung machine] (39.61)

36.91 Repair of aneurysm of coronary vessel

36.99 Other operations on vessel of heart
Exploration of coronary artery
Incision of coronary artery
Ligation of coronary artery
Repair of arteriovenous fistula

37 Other operations on heart and pericardium
Code also any injection or infusion of platelet inhibitor (99.20)

37.0 Pericardiocentesis

37.1 Cardiotomy and pericardiotomy

Code also cardiopulmonary bypass [extracorporeal circulation] [heart-lung machine] (39.61)

37.10 Incision of heart, not otherwise specified
Cardiolysis NOS

37.11 Cardiotomy
Incision of:
  atrium
  endocardium
  myocardium
  ventricle

37.12 Pericardiotomy
Pericardial window operation
Pericardiolysis
Pericardiotomy

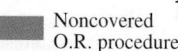

| | Valid O.R. procedure | | Non-O.R. procedure | | Nonspecific O.R. procedure | | Noncovered O.R. procedure |

37.2   Diagnostic procedures on heart and pericardium

37.21   Right heart cardiac catheterization
Cardiac catheterization NOS

Excludes: that with catheterization of left heart (37.23)

37.22   Left heart cardiac catheterization

Excludes: that with catheterization of right heart (37.23)

37.23   Combined right and left heart cardiac catheterization

37.24   Biopsy of pericardium

37.25   Biopsy of heart

37.26   Cardiac electrophysiologic stimulation and recording studies
Electrophysiologic studies (EPS)
Non-invasive programmed electrical stimulation (NIPS)
Programmed electrical stimulation

Code also any concomitant procedure

Excludes: His bundle recording (37.29)

37.27   Cardiac mapping
Code also any concomitant procedure

Excludes: electrocardiogram (89.52)
His bundle recording (37.29)

37.28   Intracardiac echocardiography [ICE]
Code also any synchronous Doppler flow mapping (88.72)

37.29   Other diagnostic procedures on heart and pericardium

Excludes: angiocardiography (88.50-88.58)
cardiac function tests (89.41-89.69)
cardiovascular radioisotopic scan and function study (92.05)
coronary arteriography (88.55-88.57)
diagnostic pericardiocentesis (37.0)
diagnostic ultrasound of heart (88.72)
x-ray of heart (87.49)

37.3   Pericardiectomy and excision of lesion of heart
Code also cardiopulmonary bypass [extracorporeal circulation] [heart-lung machine] (39.61)

37.31   Pericardiectomy
Excision of:
adhesions of pericardium
constricting scar of:
epicardium
pericardium

37.32   Excision of aneurysm of heart
Repair of aneurysm of heart

37.33   Excision or destruction of other lesion or tissue of heart

Excludes: catheter ablation of lesion or tissues of heart (37.34)

37.34   Catheter ablation of lesion or tissue of heart
Cryoablation of lesion or tissues of heart
Electrocurrent of lesion or tissues of heart
Resection of lesion or tissues of heart

37.35   Partial ventriculectomy
Ventricular reduction surgery
Ventricular remodeling

Code also any synchronous:
mitral valve repair (35.02, 35.12)
mitral valve replacement (35.23-35.24)

37.4   Repair of heart and pericardium

37.5   Heart transplantation

Excludes: combined heart-lung transplantation (33.6)

37.6   Implantation of heart assist system

37.61   Implant of pulsation balloon

● Code new
to this edition   ▲ Revision of
existing code   ④ ⑤ Fourth or fifth
digit required

37.62 Implant of other heart assist system

Insertion of:
  centrifugal pump
  heart assist system, not specified as pulsatile
  heart assist system, NOS
  heart pump

37.63 Replacement and repair of heart assist system

37.64 Removal of heart assist system

> Excludes: that with replacement of implant (37.63)
> nonoperative removal of heart assist system (97.44)

37.65 Implant of an external, pulsatile heart assist system

Note: Device not implantable (outside the body but connected to heart) with
  external circulation and pump

> Excludes: implant of pulsation balloon (37.61)

37.66 Implant of an implantable, pulsatile heart assist system

Note: Device directly connected to the heart and implanted in the upper left
  quadrant of peritoneal cavity
Transportable, implantable heart assist system

> Excludes: Implant of pulsation balloon (37.61)

37.67 Implantation of cardiomyostimulation system

Note: Two-step open procedure consisting of transfer of one end of the latissimus
  dorsi muscle; wrapping it around the heart; rib resection; implantation of
  epicardial cardiac pacing leads into the right ventricle; tunneling and pocket
  creation for the cardiomyostimulator.

**37.7 Insertion, revision, replacement, and removal of pacemaker leads; insertion of
temporary pacemaker system; or revision of pocket**

Code also any insertion and replacement of pacemaker device (37.80-37.87)

> Excludes: implantation or replacement of transvenous lead [electrode] into left ventricu-
> lar cardiac venous system (00.52)

37.70 Initial insertion of lead [electrode], not otherwise specified

> Excludes: insertion of temporary transvenous pacemaker system (37.78)
> replacement of atrial and/or ventricular lead(s) (37.76)

37.71 Initial insertion of transvenous lead [electrode] into ventricle

> Excludes: insertion of temporary transvenous pacemaker system (37.78)
> replacement of atrial and/or ventricular lead(s) (37.76)

37.72 Initial insertion of transvenous leads [electrodes] into atrium and ventricle

> Excludes: insertion of temporary transvenous pacemaker system (37.78)
> replacement of atrial and/or ventricular lead(s) (37.76)

37.73 Initial insertion of transvenous lead [electrode] into atrium

> Excludes: insertion of temporary transvenous pacemaker system (37.78)
> replacement of atrial and/or ventricular lead(s) (37.76)

37.74 Insertion or replacement of epicardial lead [electrode] into epicardium

Insertion or replacement of epicardial lead by:
  sternotomy
  thoracotomy

> Excludes: replacement of atrial and/or ventricular lead(s) (37.76)

37.75 Revision of lead [electrode]

Repair of electrode [removal with re-insertion]
Repositioning of lead [electrode]
Revision of lead NOS

> Excludes: repositioning of temporary transvenous pacemaker system—omit code

37.76 Replacement of transvenous atrial and/or ventricular lead(s) [electrode]

Removal or abandonment of existing transvenous or epicardial lead(s) with
  transvenous lead(s) replacement

> Excludes: replacement of epicardial lead [electrode] (37.74)

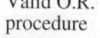 Valid O.R. procedure   Non-O.R. procedure   Nonspecific O.R. procedure   Noncovered O.R. procedure

37.77 **Removal of lead(s) [electrode] without replacement**
Removal:
epicardial lead (transthoracic approach)
transvenous lead(s)

> *Excludes:* *removal of temporary transvenous pacemaker system—omit code*
> *that with replacement of:*
> *atrial and/or ventricular lead(s) [electrode] (37.76)*
> *epicardial lead [electrode] (37.74)*

37.78 **Insertion of temporary transvenous pacemaker system**

> *Excludes:* *intraoperative cardiac pacemaker (39.64)*

37.79 **Revision or relocation of pacemaker pocket**
Debridement and reforming pocket (skin and subcutaneous tissue)
Relocation of pocket [creation of new pocket] pacemaker or CRT-P

37.8 **Insertion, replacement, removal and revision of pacemaker device**

*Code also any lead insertion, lead replacement, lead removal and/or lead revision
(37.70-37.77)*

> *Excludes:* *implantation of cardiac resynchronication pacemaker [CRT-P] (00.50)*
> *implantation or replacement of cardiac resynchronization pacemaker pulse
> generator only [CRT-P] (00.53)*

37.80 **Insertion of permanent pacemaker, initial or replacement, type of device not specified**

37.81 **Initial insertion of single-chamber device, not specified as rate responsive**

> *Excludes:* *replacement of existing pacemaker device (37.85-37.87)*

37.82 **Initial insertion of a single-chamber device, rate responsive**
Rate responsive to physiologic stimuli other than atrial rate

> *Excludes:* *replacement of existing pacemaker device (37.85-37.87)*

37.83 **Initial insertion of dual-chamber device**
Atrial ventricular sequential device

> *Excludes:* *replacement of existing pacemaker device (37.85-37.87)*

37.85 **Replacement of any type pacemaker device with single-chamber device, not specified as rate responsive**

37.86 **Replacement of any type pacemaker device with single-chamber device, rate responsive**
Rate responsive to physiologic stimuli other than atrial rate

37.87 **Replacement of any type pacemaker device with dual-chamber device**
Atrial ventricular sequential device

37.89 **Revision or removal of pacemaker device**
Removal without replacement of cardiac resynchronization pacemaker device
[CRT-P]
Repair of pacemaker device

> *Excludes:* *removal of temporary transvenous pacemaker system—omit code*
> *replacement of existing pacemaker device (37.85-37.87)*
> *replacement of existing pacemaker device with CRT-P pacemaker
> device (00.53)*

37.9 **Other operations on heart and pericardium**

37.91 **Open chest cardiac massage**

> *Excludes:* *closed chest cardiac massage (99.63)*

37.92 **Injection of therapeutic substance into heart**

37.93 **Injection of therapeutic substance into pericardium**

37.94 **Implantation or replacement of automatic cardioverter/defibrillator, total system [AICD]**
Implantation of defibrillator with leads (epicardial patches), formation of pocket
(abdominal fascia) (subcutaneous), any transvenous leads, intraoperative
procedures for evaluation of lead signals, and obtaining defibrillator thresholds
measurements
Techniques:
lateral thoracotomy
medial sternotomy
subxiphoid procedure

Code also extracorporeal circulation, if performed (39.61)

● Code new
to this edition

▲ Revision of
existing code

④ ⑤ Fourth or fifth
digit required

Code also any concomitant procedure [e.g., coronary bypass] (36.00-36.19)

| Excludes: | implantation of cardiac resynchronization defibrillator, total system [CRT-D] (00.51)

37.95 **Implantation of automatic cardioverter/defibrillator lead(s) only**

37.96 **Implantation of automatic cardioverter/defibrillator pulse generator only**

| Excludes: | *implantation or replacement of cardiac resynchronization defibrillator, pulse generator device only [CRT-D] (00.54)*

37.97 **Replacement of automatic cardioverter/defibrillator lead(s) only**

37.98 **Replacement of automatic cardioverter/defibrillator pulse generator only**

| Excludes: | *replacement of cardiac resynchronization defibrillator, pulse generator device only [CRT-D] (00.54)*

37.99 **Other**

Removal of cardioverter/defibrillator pulse generator only without replacement
Removal without replacement of cardiac resynchronization defibrillator device [CRT-D]
Repositioning of lead(s) (sensing) (pacing)[electrode]
Repositioning of pulse generator
Revision of cardioverter/defibrillator (automatic) pocket
Revision or relocation of CRT-D pocket

| Excludes: | *cardiac retraining (93.36)*
conversion of cardiac rhythm (99.60-99.69)

38 **Incision, excision, and occlusion of vessels**

Code also any application or administration of an adhesion barrier substance (99.77)
Code also cardiopulmonary bypass [extracorporeal circulation] [heart-lung machine] (39.61)

| Excludes: | *that of coronary vessels (36.01-36.99)*

The following fourth-digit subclassification is for use with appropriate categories in sections 38.0, 38.1, 38.3, 38.5, 38.6, 38.8 and 38.9, which are marked with a symbol ④ to identify the site. Valid fourth digits are in [brackets] under each code.

0 unspecified site
1 intracranial vessels
Cerebral (anterior) (middle)
Circle of Willis
Posterior communicating artery
2 other vessels of head and neck
Carotid artery (common) (external) (internal)
Jugular vein (external) (internal)
3 upper limb vessels

| Axillary | Radial |
| Brachial | Ulnar |

4 aorta
5 other thoracic vessels

| Innominate | Subclavian |
| Pulmonary (artery) (vein) | Vena cava, superior |

6 abdominal arteries

Celiac	Mesenteric
Gastric	Renal
Hepatic	Splenic
Iliac	Umbilical

| Excludes: | *abdominal aorta (4)*

7 abdominal veins

Iliac	Splenic
Portal	Vena cava(inferior)
Renal	

8 lower limb arteries
Femoral (common) (superficial)
Popliteal
Tibial
9 lower limb veins

| Femoral | Saphenous |
| Popliteal | Tibial |

| Valid O.R. procedure | Non-O.R. procedure | Nonspecific O.R. procedure | Noncovered O.R. procedure |

④ **38.0**　**Incision of vessels**
[0-9]　　Embolectomy
　　Thrombectomy

> | Excludes: | *puncture or catheterization of any:* |
> | --- | --- |
>
> 　　　　*artery (38.91, 38.98)*
> 　　　　*vein (38.92-38.95, 38.99)*

④ **38.1**　**Endarterectomy**
[0-6,8]　Endarterectomy with:
　　embolectomy
　　patch graft
　　temporary bypass during procedure
　　thrombectomy

　38.2　**Diagnostic procedures on blood vessels**

　　38.21　**Biopsy of blood vessel**

　　38.22　**Percutaneous angioscopy**

> | Excludes: | *angioscopy of eye (95.12)* |
> | --- | --- |

　　38.29　**Other diagnostic procedures on blood vessels**

> | Excludes: | *blood vessel thermography (88.86)* |
> | --- | --- |
>
> 　　　*circulatory monitoring (89.61-89.69)*
> 　　　*contrast:*
> 　　　　*angiocardiography (88.50-88.58)*
> 　　　　*arteriography (88.40-88.49)*
> 　　　　*phlebography (88.60-88.67)*
> 　　　*impedance phlebography (88.68)*
> 　　　*peripheral vascular ultrasonography (88.77)*
> 　　　*plethysmogram (89.58)*

④ **38.3**　**Resection of vessel with anastomosis**
[0-9]　　Angiectomy with anastomosis
　　Excision of:
　　aneurysm (arteriovenous) with anastomosis
　　blood vessel (lesion) with anastomosis

④ **38.4**　**Resection of vessel with replacement**
[0-9]　　Angiectomy with replacement
　　Excision of
　　aneurysm (arteriovenous) with replacement
　　blood vessel (lesion) with replacement

> | Excludes: | *endovascular repair of aneurysm (39.71-39.79)* |
> | --- | --- |

　　Requires the use of one of the following fourth-digit subclassifications to identify site:
　　0 unspecified site
　　1 intracranial vessels
　　　Cerebral (anterior) (middle)
　　　Circle of Willis
　　　Posterior communicating artery
　　2 other vessels of head and neck
　　　Carotid artery (common) (external) (internal)
　　　Jugular vein (external) (internal)
　　3 upper limb vessels
　　　Axillary　　　　Radial
　　　Brachial　　　　Ulnar
　　4 aorta, abdominal
　　　Code also any thoracic vessel involvement (thoracoabdominal procedure) (38.45)
　　5 thoracic vessel
　　　Aorta (thoracic)　　　Subclavian
　　　Innominate　　　　　Vena cava (superior)
　　　Pulmonary (artery) (vein)
　　　Code also any abdominal aorta involvement (thoracoabdominal procedure) (38.44)
　　6 abdominal arteries
　　　Celiac　　　Mesenteric
　　　Gastric　　　Renal
　　　Hepatic　　　Splenic
　　　Iliac　　　　Umbilical

> | Excludes: | *abdominal aorta (4)* |
> | --- | --- |

7 abdominal veins
Iliac
Portal
Renal
Splenic
Vena cava (inferior)

8 lower limb arteries
Femoral (common) (superficial)
Tibial

9 lower limb veins
Femoral
Popliteal
Saphenous
Tibial

④ **38.5** **Ligation and stripping of varicose veins**
[0-3,5,7,9]

> | Excludes: | ligation of varices:
> esophageal (42.91)
> gastric (44.91)

④ **38.6** **Other excision of vessels**
[0-9] Excision of blood vessel (lesion) NOS

> | Excludes: | excision of vessel for aortocoronary bypass (36.10-36.14)
> excision with:
> anastomosis (38.30-38.39)
> graft replacement (38.40-38.49)
> implant (38.40-38.49)

38.7 **Interruption of vena cava**
Insertion of implant or sieve in vena cava
Ligation of vena cava (inferior) (superior)
Plication of vena cava

④ **38.8** **Other surgical occlusion of vessels**
[0-9] Clamping of blood vessel
Division of blood vessel
Ligation of blood vessel
Occlusion of blood vessel

> | Excludes: | adrenal vessels (07.43)
> esophageal varices (42.91)
> gastric or duodenal vessel for ulcer (44.40-44.49)
> gastric varices (44.91)
> meningeal vessel (02.13)
> percutaneous transcatheter infusion embolization (99.29)
> spermatic vein for varicocele (63.1)
> surgical occlusion of vena cava (38.7)
> that for chemoembolization (99.25)
> that for control of (postoperative) hemorrhage:
> anus (49.95)
> bladder (57.93)
> following vascular procedure (39.41)
> nose (21.00-21.09)
> prostate (60.94)
> tonsil (28.7)
> thyroid vessel (06.92)

38.9 **Puncture of vessel**

> | Excludes: | that for circulatory monitoring (89.60-89.69)

38.91 **Arterial catheterization**

38.92 **Umbilical vein catheterization**

38.93 **Venous catheterization, not elsewhere classified**

> | Excludes: | that for cardiac catheterization (37.21-37.23)
> that for renal dialysis (38.95)

38.94 **Venous cutdown**

38.95 **Venous catheterization for renal dialysis**

> | Excludes: | insertion of totally implantable vascular access device [VAD] 86.07

38.98 **Other puncture of artery**

> | Excludes: | that for:
> arteriography (88.40-88.49)
> coronary arteriography (88.55-88.57)

Valid O.R.
procedure

Non-O.R.
procedure

Nonspecific
O.R. procedure

Noncovered
O.R. procedure

38.99 Other puncture of vein
Phlebotomy

Excludes: *that for:*
angiography (88.60-88.69)
extracorporeal circulation (39.61, 50.92)
injection or infusion of:
sclerosing solution (39.92)
therapeutic or prophylactic substance (99.11-99.29)
perfusion (39.96-39.97)
phlebography (88.60-88.69)
transfusion (99.01-99.09)

39 Other operations on vessels

Excludes: *those on coronary vessels (36.0-36.99)*

39.0 Systemic to pulmonary artery shunt
Descending aorta-pulmonary artery anastomosis (graft)
Left to right anastomosis (graft)
Subclavian-pulmonary anastomosis (graft)

Code also cardiopulmonary bypass [extracorporeal circulation] [heart-lung machine] (39.61)

39.1 Intra-abdominal venous shunt
Anastomosis:
mesocaval
portacaval
portal vein to inferior vena cava
splenic and renal veins
transjugular intrahepatic portosystemic shunt (TIPS)

Excludes: *peritoneovenous shunt (54.94)*

39.2 Other shunt or vascular bypass

39.21 Caval-pulmonary artery anastomosis
Code also cardiopulmonary bypass (39.61)

39.22 Aorta-subclavian-carotid bypass
Bypass (arterial):
aorta to carotid and brachial
aorta to subclavian and carotid
carotid to subclavian

39.23 Other intrathoracic vascular shunt or bypass
Intrathoracic (arterial) bypass graft NOS

Excludes: *coronary artery bypass (36.10-36.19)*

39.24 Aorta-renal bypass

39.25 Aorta-iliac-femoral bypass
Bypass:
aortofemoral
aortoiliac
aortoiliac to popliteal
aortopopliteal
iliofemoral [iliac-femoral]

39.26 Other intra-abdominal vascular shunt or bypass
Bypass:
aortoceliac
aortic-superior mesenteric
common hepatic-common iliac-renal
Intra-abdominal arterial bypass graft NOS

Excludes: *peritoneovenous shunt (54.94)*

39.27 Arteriovenostomy for renal dialysis
Anastomosis for renal dialysis
Formation of (peripheral) arteriovenous fistula for renal (kidney] dialysis
Code also any renal dialysis (39.95)

39.28 Extracranial-intracranial (EC-IC) vascular bypass

● Code new
   to this edition
▲ Revision of
   existing code
④ ⑤ Fourth or fifth
   digit required

39.29 Other (peripheral) vascular shunt or bypass

Bypass (graft):
axillary-brachial
axillary-femoral [axillofemoral] (superficial)
brachial
femoral-femoral
femoroperoneal
femoropopliteal (arteries)
femorotibial (anterior) (posterior)
popliteal
vascular NOS

> | Excludes: | peritoneovenous shunt (54.94)

39.3 Suture of vessel

Repair of laceration of blood vessel

> | Excludes: | *any other vascular puncture closure device—omit code*
> *suture of aneurysm (39.52)*
> *that for control of hemorrhage (postoperative):*
> *anus (49.95)*
> *bladder (57.93)*
> *following vascular procedure (39.41)*
> *nose (21.00-21.09)*
> *prostate (60.94)*
> *tonsil (28.7)*

39.30 Suture of unspecified blood vessel

39.31 Suture of artery

39.32 Suture of vein

39.4 Revision of vascular procedure

39.41 Control of hemorrhage following vascular surgery

> | Excludes: | *that for control of hemorrhage (postoperative):*
> *anus (49.95)*
> *bladder (57.93)*
> *nose (21.00-21.09)*
> *prostate (60.94)*
> *tonsil (28.7)*

39.42 Revision of arteriovenous shunt for renal dialysis

Conversion of renal dialysis:
end-to-end anastomosis to end-to-side
end-to-side anastomosis to end-to-end
vessel-to-vessel cannula to arteriovenous shunt
Removal of old arteriovenous shunt and creation of new shunt

> | Excludes: | *replacement of vessel-to-vessel cannula (39.94)*

39.43 Removal of arteriovenous shunt for renal dialysis

> | Excludes: | *that with replacement [revision] of shunt (39.42)*

39.49 Other revision of vascular procedure

Declotting (graft)
Revision of:
anastomosis of blood vessel
vascular procedure (previous)

39.5 Other repair of vessels

39.50 Angioplasty or atherectomy of non-coronary vessel

Percutaneous transluminal angioplasty (PTA) of non-coronary vessel:
head and neck arteries:
basilar
carotid
vertebral
lower extremity vessels
mesenteric artery
renal artery
upper extremity vessels

Code also any injection or infusion of thrombolytic agent (99.10)

Code also any insertion of non-coronary stent(s) or stent graft(s) (39.90)

39.51 Clipping of aneurysm

> Excludes: clipping of arteriovenous fistula (39.53)

39.52 Other repair of aneurysm

Repair of aneurysm by:
coagulation
electrocoagulation
filipuncture
methyl methacrylate
suture
wiring
wrapping

> Excludes: endovascular repair of aneurysm (39.71-39.79)
> re-entry operation (aorta) (39.54)
> that with:
> graft replacement (38.40-38.49)
> resection (38.30-38.49, 38.60-38.69)

39.53 Repair of arteriovenous fistula

Embolization of carotid cavernous fistula
Repair of arteriovenous fistula by:
clipping
coagulation
ligation and division

> Excludes: repair of:
> arteriovenous shunt for renal dialysis (39.42)
> head and neck vessels, endovascular approach (39.72)
> that with:
> graft replacement (38.40-38.49)
> resection (38.30-38.49, 38.60-38.69)

39.54 Re-entry operation (aorta)

Fenestration of dissecting aneurysm of thoracic aorta

Code also cardiopulmonary bypass [extracorporeal circulation] [heart-lung machine] (39.61)

39.55 Reimplantation of aberrant renal vessel

39.56 Repair of blood vessel with tissue patch graft

> Excludes: that with resection (38.40-38.49)

39.57 Repair of blood vessel with synthetic patch graft

> Excludes: that with resection (38.40-38.49)

39.58 Repair of blood vessel with unspecified type of patch graft

> Excludes: that with resection (38.40-38.49)

39.59 Other repair of vessel

Aorticopulmonary window operation
Arterioplasty NOS
Construction of venous valves (peripheral)
Plication of vein (peripheral)
Reimplantation of artery

Code also cardiopulmonary bypass [extracorporeal circulation] [heart-lung machine] (39.61)

> Excludes: interruption of the vena cava (38.7)
> reimplantation of renal artery (39.55)
> that with:
> graft (39.56-39.58)
> resection (38.30-38.49, 38.60-38.69)

39.6 Extracorporeal circulation and procedures auxiliary to heart surgery

39.61 Extracorporeal circulation auxiliary to open heart surgery

Artificial heart and lung
Cardiopulmonary bypass
Pump oxygenator

> Excludes: extracorporeal hepatic assistance (50.92)
> extracorporeal membrane oxygenation [ECMO] (39.65)
> hemodialysis (39.95)
> percutaneous cardiopulmonary bypass (39.66)

● Code new to this edition   ▲ Revision of existing code   ④ ⑤ Fourth or fifth digit required

39.62 Hypothermia (systemic) incidental to open heart surgery

39.63 Cardioplegia
Arrest:
anoxic
circulatory

39.64 Intraoperative cardiac pacemaker
Temporary pacemaker used during and immediately following cardiac surgery

39.65 Extracorporeal membrane oxygenation (ECMO)

> Excludes: *extracorporeal circulation auxiliary to open heart surgery (39.61)*
> *percutaneous cardiopulmonary bypass (39.66)*

39.66 Percutaneous cardiopulmonary bypass
Closed chest

> Excludes: *extracorporeal circulation auxiliary to open heart surgery (39.61)*
> *extracorporeal hepatic assistance (50.92)*
> *extracorporeal membrane oxygenation [ECMO] (39.65)*
> *hemodialysis (39.95)*

39.7 Endovascular repair of vessel
Endoluminal repair

> Excludes: *angioplasty or atherectomy of non-coronary vessel (39.50)*
> *insertion of non-coronary stent or stents (39.90)*
> *other repair of aneurysm (39.52)*
> *resection of abdominal aorta with replacement (38.44)*
> *resection of lower limb arteries with replacement (38.48)*
> *resection of thoracic aorta with replacement (38.45)*
> *resection of upper limb vessels with replacement (38.43)*

39.71 Endovascular implantation of graft in abdominal aorta
Endovascular repair of abdominal aortic aneurysm with graft
Stent graft(s)

● **39.72 Endovascular repair or occlusion of head and neck vessels**
Coil embolization or occlusion
Endograft(s)
Endovascular grafts(s)
Liquid tissue adhesive (glue) embolization or occlusion
Other implant or substance for repair, embolization or occlusion
That for repair of aneurysm, arteriovenous malformation [AVM] or fistula

▲ **39.79 Other endovascular repair of aneurysm of other vessels**
Coil embolization or occlusion
Endograft(s)
Endovascular graft(s)
Liquid tissue adhesive (glue) embolization or occlusion
Other implant or substance for repair, embolization or occlusion

> Excludes: *endovascular repair or occlusion of head and neck vessels (39.72)*
> *insertion of drug-eluting non-coronary artery stent(s) (00.55)*
> *insertion of non-coronary artery stent(s) (for other than aneurysm repair) (39.90)*
> *non-endovascular repair of arteriovenous fistula (39.53)*
> *other surgical occlusion of vessels—see category 38.8*
> *percutaneous transcatheter infusion (99.29)*
> *transcatheter embolization for gastric or duodenal bleeding (44.44)*

39.8 Operations on carotid body and other vascular bodies

Chemodectomy	Glomectomy, carotid
Denervation of:	Implantation into carotid body:
aortic body	electronic stimulator
carotid body	pacemaker

> Excludes: *excision of glomus jugulare (20.51)*

39.9 Other operations on vessels

▲ **39.90 Insertion of non-drug-eluting, non-coronary artery stent(s)**
Bare stent(s)
Bonded stent(s)
Drug-coated stent(s), i.e., heparin coated
Endograft(s)
Endovascular graft(s)
Endovascular recanalization techniques
Stent graft(s)

Code also any non-coronary angioplasty or atherectomy (39.50)

Valid O.R. procedure	Non-O.R. procedure	Nonspecific O.R. procedure	Noncovered O.R. procedure

| Excludes: | insertion of drug-eluting, non-coronary artery stent(s) (00.55) |
| | that for aneurysm repair (39.71-39.79) |

39.91 Freeing of vessel
Dissection and freeing of adherent tissue:
artery-vein-nerve bundle
vascular bundle

39.92 Injection of sclerosing agent into vein

Excludes:	injection:
	esophageal varices (42.33)
	hemorrhoids (49.42)

39.93 Insertion of vessel-to-vessel cannula
Formation of arteriovenous:
fistula by external cannula
shunt by external cannula
Code also any renal dialysis (39.95)

39.94 Replacement of vessel-to-vessel cannula
Revision of vessel-to-vessel cannula

39.95 Hemodialysis
Artificial kidney   Hemofiltration
Hemodiafiltration   Renal dialysis

| Excludes: | peritoneal dialysis (54.98) |

39.96 Total body perfusion
Code also substance perfused (99.21-99.29)

39.97 Other perfusion
Perfusion NOS
Perfusion, local [regional] of:
carotid artery
coronary artery
head
lower limb
neck
upper limb
Code also substance perfused (99.21-99.29)

Excludes:	perfusion of:
	kidney (55.95)
	large intestine (46.96)
	liver (50.93)
	small intestine (46.95)

39.98 Control of hemorrhage, not otherwise specified
Angiotripsy
Control of postoperative hemorrhage NOS
Venotripsy

Excludes:	control of hemorrhage (postoperative):
	anus (49.95)
	bladder (57.93)
	following vascular procedure (39.41)
	nose (21.00-21.09)
	prostate (60.94)
	tonsil (28.7)
	that by:
	ligation (38.80-38.89)
	suture (39.30-39.32)

39.99 Other operations on vessels

Excludes:	injection or infusion of therapeutic or prophylactic substance
	(99.11-99.29)
	transfusion of blood and blood components (99.01-99.09)

● Code new
to this edition   ▲ Revision of
existing code   ④ ⑤ Fourth or fifth
digit required

8.   OPERATIONS ON THE HEMIC AND LYMPHATIC SYSTEM (40-41)

40   Operations on lymphatic system

40.0   Incision of lymphatic structures

40.1   Diagnostic procedures on lymphatic structures

40.11   Biopsy of lymphatic structure

40.19   Other diagnostic procedures on lymphatic structures

> Excludes: *lymphangiogram*
> *abdominal (88.04)*
> *cervical (87.08)*
> *intrathoracic (87.34)*
> *lower limb (88.36)*
> *upper limb (88.34)*
> *microscopic examination of specimen (90.71-90.79)*
> *radioisotope scan (92.16)*
> *thermography (88.89)*

40.2   Simple excision of lymphatic structure

> Excludes: *biopsy of lymphatic structure (40.11)*

40.21   Excision of deep cervical lymph node

40.22   Excision of internal mammary lymph node

40.23   Excision of axillary lymph node

40.24   Excision of inguinal lymph mode

40.29   Simple excision of other lymphatic structure
Excision of:
cystic hygroma
lymphangioma
Simple lymphadenectomy

40.3   Regional lymph node excision
Extended regional lymph node excision
Regional lymph node excision with excision of lymphatic drainage area including skin,
subcutaneous tissue, and fat

40.4   Radical excision of cervical lymph nodes
Resection of cervical lymph nodes down to muscle and deep fascia

> Excludes: *that associated with radical laryngectomy (30.4)*

40.40   Radical neck dissection, not otherwise specified

40.41   Radical neck dissection, unilateral

40.42   Radical neck dissection, bilateral

40.5   Radical excision of other lymph nodes

> Excludes: *that associated with radical mastectomy (85.45-85.48)*

40.50   Radical excision of lymph nodes, not otherwise specified
Radical (lymph) node dissection NOS

40.51   Radical excision of axillary lymph nodes

40.52   Radical excision of periaortic lymph nodes

40.53   Radical excision of iliac lymph nodes

40.54   Radical groin dissection

40.59   Radical excision of other lymph nodes

> Excludes: *radical neck dissection (40.40-40.42)*

40.6   Operations on thoracic duct

40.61   Cannulation of thoracic duct

40.62   Fistulization of thoracic duct

40.63   Closure of fistula of thoracic duct

40.64   Ligation of thoracic duct

40.69   Other operations on thoracic duct

| Valid O.R. procedure | Non-O.R. procedure | Nonspecific O.R. procedure | Noncovered O.R. procedure |

40.9   Other operations on lymphatic structures
Anastomosis of peripheral lymphatics
Dilation of peripheral lymphatics
Ligation of peripheral lymphatics
Obliteration of peripheral lymphatics
Reconstruction of peripheral lymphatics
Repair of peripheral lymphatics
Transplantation of peripheral lymphatics
Correction of lymphedema of limb, NOS

> *Excludes:*   reduction of elephantiasis of scrotum (61.3)

41   Operations on bone marrow and spleen

41.0   Bone marrow or hematopoietic stem cell transplant

> *Excludes:*   aspiration of bone marrow from donor (41.91)

41.00   Bone marrow transplant, not otherwise specified

41.01   Autologous bone marrow transplant without purging

> *Excludes:*   that with purging (41.09)

41.02   Allogeneic bone marrow transplant with purging
Allograft of bone marrow with in vitro removal (purging) of T-cells

41.03   Allogeneic bone marrow transplant without purging
Allograft of bone marrow NOS

41.04   Autologous hematopoietic stem cell transplant without purging

> *Excludes:*   that with purging (41.07)

41.05   Allogeneic hematopoietic stem cell transplant without purging

> *Excludes:*   that with purging (41.08)

41.06   Cord blood stem cell transplant

41.07   Autologous hematopoietic stem cell transplant with purging
Cell depletion

41.08   Allogeneic hematopoietic stem cell transplant with purging
Cell depletion

41.09   Autologous bone marrow transplant with purging
With extracorporeal purging of malignant cells from marrow
Cell depletion

41.1   Puncture of spleen

> *Excludes:*   aspiration biopsy of spleen (41.32)

41.2   Splenotomy

41.3   Diagnostic procedures on bone marrow and spleen

41.31   Biopsy of bone marrow

41.32   Closed [aspiration] [percutaneous] biopsy of spleen
Needle biopsy of spleen

41.33   Open biopsy of spleen

41.38   Other diagnostic procedures on bone marrow

> *Excludes:*   microscopic examination of specimen from bone marrow
> (90.61-90.69)
> radioisotope scan (92.05)

41.39   Other diagnostic procedures on spleen

> *Excludes:*   microscopic examination of specimen from spleen (90.61-90.69)
> radioisotope scan (92.05)

41.4   Excision or destruction of lesion or tissue of spleen
Code also any application or administration of an adhesion barrier substance (99.77)

> *Excludes:*   excision of accessory spleen (41.93)

41.41   Marsupialization of splenic cyst

41.42   Excision of lesion or tissue of spleen

> *Excludes:*   biopsy of spleen (41.32-41.33)

41.43   Partial splenectomy

41.5   Total splenectomy
Splenectomy NOS
Code also any application or administration of an adhesion barrier substance (99.77)

● Code new   ▲ Revision of   ④ ⑤ Fourth or fifth
  to this edition   existing code   digit required

41.9 **Other operations on spleen and bone marrow**

Code also any application or administration of an adhesion barrier substance (99.77)

41.91 **Aspiration of bone marrow from donor for transplant**

   Excludes: *biopsy of bone marrow (41.31)*

41.92 **Injection into bone marrow**

   Excludes: *bone marrow transplant (41.00-41.03)*

41.93 **Excision of accessory spleen**

41.94 **Transplantation of spleen**

41.95 **Repair and plastic operations on spleen**

41.98 **Other operations on bone marrow**

41.99 **Other operations on spleen**

| | Valid O.R. procedure | | Non-O.R. procedure | | Nonspecific O.R. procedure | | Noncovered O.R. procedure |

● Code new
to this edition
▲ Revision of
existing code
④ ⑤ Fourth or fifth
digit required

9. OPERATIONS ON THE DIGESTIVE SYSTEM (42-54)

42 Operations on esophagus

42.0 Esophagotomy

42.01 Incision of esophageal web

42.09 Other incision of esophagus
Esophagotomy NOS

Excludes: *esophagomyotomy (42.7)*
esophagostomy (42.10-42.19)

42.1 Esophagostomy

42.10 Esophagostomy, not otherwise specified

42.11 Cervical esophagostomy

42.12 Exteriorization of esophageal pouch

42.19 Other external fistulization of esophagus
Thoracic esophagostomy
Code also any resection (42.40-42.42)

42.2 Diagnostic procedures on esophagus

42.21 Operative esophagoscopy by incision

42.22 Esophagoscopy through artificial stoma

Excludes: *that with biopsy (42.24)*

42.23 Other esophagoscopy

Excludes: *that with biopsy (42.24)*

42.24 Closed [endoscopic] biopsy of esophagus
Brushing or washing for specimen collection
Esophagoscopy with biopsy
Suction biopsy of the esophagus

Excludes: *esophagogastroduodenoscopy [EGD] with closed biopsy (45.16)*

42.25 Open biopsy of esophagus

42.29 Other diagnostic procedures on esophagus

Excludes: *barium swallow (87.61)*
esophageal manometry (89.32)
microscopic examination of specimen from esophagus (90.81-90.89)

42.3 Local excision or destruction of lesion or tissue of esophagus

42.31 Local excision of esophageal diverticulum

42.32 Local excision of other lesion or tissue of esophagus

Excludes: *biopsy of esophagus (42.24-42.25)*
esophageal fistulectomy (42.84)

42.33 Endoscopic excision or destruction of lesion or tissue of esophagus
Ablation of esophageal neoplasm by endoscopic approach
Control of esophageal bleeding by endoscopic approach
Esophageal polypectomy by endoscopic approach
Esophageal varices by endoscopic approach
Injection of esophageal varices by endoscopic approach

Excludes: *biopsy of esophagus (42.24-42.25)*
fistulectomy (42.84)
open ligation of esophageal varices (42.91)

42.39 Other destruction of lesion or tissue of esophagus

Excludes: *that by endoscopic approach (42.33)*

42.4 Excision of esophagus

Excludes: *esophagogastrectomy NOS (43.99)*

42.40 Esophagectomy, not otherwise specified

	Valid O.R. procedure		Non-O.R. procedure		Nonspecific O.R. procedure		Noncovered O.R. procedure

42.41 Partial esophagectomy

Code also any synchronous:
anastomosis other than end-to-end (42.51-42.69)
esophagostomy (42.10-42.19)
gastrostomy (43.11-43.19)

42.42 Total esophagectomy

Code also any synchronous:
gastrostomy (43.11-43.19)
interposition or anastomosis other than end-to-end (42.51-42.69)

Excludes: *esophagogastrectomy (43.99)*

42.5 Intrathoracic anastomosis of esophagus

Code also any synchronous:
esophagectomy (42.40-42.42)
gastrostomy (43.1)

42.51 Intrathoracic esophagoesophagostomy

42.52 Intrathoracic esophagogastrostomy

42.53 Intrathoracic esophageal anastomosis with interposition of small bowel

42.54 Other intrathoracic esophagoenterostomy
Anastomosis of esophagus to intestinal segment NOS

42.55 Intrathoracic esophageal anastomosis with interposition of colon

42.56 Other intrathoracic esophagocolostomy
Esophagocolostomy NOS

42.58 Intrathoracic esophageal anastomosis with other interposition
Construction of artificial esophagus
Retrosternal formation of reversed gastric tube

42.59 Other intrathoracic anastomosis of esophagus

42.6 Antesternal anastomosis of esophagus

Code also any synchronous:
esophagectomy (42.40-42.42)
gastrostomy (43.1)

42.61 Antesternal esophagoesophagostomy

42.62 Antesternal esophagogastrostomy

42.63 Antesternal esophageal anastomosis with interposition of small bowel

42.64 Other antesternal esophagoenterostomy
Antethoracic:
esophagoenterostomy
esophagoileostomy
esophagojejunostomy

42.65 Antesternal esophageal anastomosis with interposition of colon

42.66 Other antesternal esophagocolostomy
Antethoracic esophagocolostomy

42.68 Other antesternal esophageal anastomosis with interposition

42.69 Other antesternal anastomosis of esophagus

42.7 Esophagomyotomy

42.8 Other repair of esophagus

42.81 Insertion of permanent tube into esophagus

42.82 Suture of laceration of esophagus

42.83 Closure of esophagostomy

42.84 Repair of esophageal fistula, not elsewhere classified

Excludes: *repair of fistula:*
bronchoesophageal (33.42)
esophagopleurocutaneous (34.73)
pharyngoesophageal (29.53)
tracheoesophageal (31.73)

42.85 Repair of esophageal stricture

42.86 Production of subcutaneous tunnel without esophageal anastomosis

● Code new
to this edition
▲ Revision of
existing code
④ ⑤ Fourth or fifth
digit required

42.87 Other graft of esophagus

> *Excludes:* *antesternal esophageal anastomosis with interposition of:*
> *colon (42.65)*
> *small bowel (42.63)*
> *antesternal esophageal anastomosis with other interposition (42.68)*
> *intrathoracic esophageal anastomosis with interposition of:*
> *colon (42.55)*
> *small bowel (42.53)*
> *intrathoracic esophageal anastomosis with other interposition (42.58)*

42.89 Other repair of esophagus

42.9 Other operations on esophagus

42.91 Ligation of esophageal varices

> *Excludes:* *that by endoscopic approach (42.33)*

42.92 Dilation of esophagus
Dilation of cardiac sphincter

> *Excludes:* *intubation of esophagus (96.03, 96.06-96.08)*

42.99 Other

> *Excludes:* *insertion of Sengstaken tube (96.06)*
> *intubation of esophagus (96.03, 96.06-96.08)*
> *removal of intraluminal foreign body from esophagus without incision (98.02)*
> *tamponade of esophagus (96.06)*

43 Incision and excision of stomach

Code also any application or administration of an adhesion barrier substance (99.77)

43.0 Gastrotomy

> *Excludes:* *gastrostomy (43.11-43.19)*
> *that for control of hemorrhage (44.49)*

43.1 Gastrostomy

43.11 Percutaneous [endoscopic] gastrostomy [PEG]
Percutaneous transabdominal gastrostomy

43.19 Other gastrostomy

> *Excludes:* *percutaneous [endoscopic] gastrostomy [PEG] (43.11)*

43.3 Pyloromyotomy

43.4 Local excision or destruction of lesion or tissue of stomach

43.41 Endoscopic excision or destruction of lesion or tissue of stomach
Gastric polypectomy by endoscopic approach
Gastric varices by endoscopic approach

> *Excludes:* *biopsy of stomach (44.14-44.15)*
> *control of hemorrhage (44.43)*
> *open ligation of gastric varices (44.91)*

43.42 Local excision of other lesion or tissue of stomach

> *Excludes:* *biopsy of stomach (44.14-44.15)*
> *gastric fistulectomy (44.62-44.63)*
> *partial gastrectomy (43.5-43.89)*

43.49 Other destruction of lesion or tissue of stomach

> *Excludes:* *that by endoscopic approach (43.41)*

43.5 Partial gastrectomy with anastomosis to esophagus
Proximal gastrectomy

43.6 Partial gastrectomy with anastomosis to duodenum
Billroth I operation
Distal gastrectomy
Gastropylorectomy

43.7 Partial gastrectomy with anastomosis to jejunum
Billroth II operation

43.8 Other partial gastrectomy

43.81 Partial gastrectomy with jejunal transposition
Henley jejunal transposition operation

Code also any synchronous intestinal resection (45.51)

	Valid O.R. procedure		Non-O.R. procedure		Nonspecific O.R. procedure		Noncovered O.R. procedure

43.89 **Other**
Partial gastrectomy with bypass gastrogastrostomy
Sleeve resection of stomach

43.9 **Total gastrectomy**

43.91 **Total gastrectomy with intestinal interposition**

43.99 **Other total gastrectomy**
Complete gastroduodenectomy
Esophagoduodenostomy with complete gastrectomy
Esophagogastrectomy NOS
Esophagojejunostomy with complete gastrectomy
Radical gastrectomy

44 **Other operations on stomach**
Code also any application or administration of an adhesion barrier substance (99.77)

44.0 **Vagotomy**

44.00 **Vagotomy, not otherwise specified**
Division of vagus nerve NOS

44.01 **Truncal vagotomy**

44.02 **Highly selective vagotomy**
Parietal cell vagotomy
Selective proximal vagotomy

44.03 **Other selective vagotomy**

44.1 **Diagnostic procedures on stomach**

44.11 **Transabdominal gastroscopy**
Intraoperative gastroscopy

Excludes: *that with biopsy (44.14)*

44.12 **Gastroscopy through artificial stoma**

Excludes: *that with biopsy (44.14)*

44.13 **Other gastroscopy**

Excludes: *that with biopsy (44.14)*

44.14 **Closed [endoscopic] biopsy of stomach**
Brushing or washing for specimen collection

Excludes: *esophagogastroduodenoscopy [EGD] with closed biopsy (45.16)*

44.15 **Open biopsy of stomach**

44.19 **Other diagnostic procedures on stomach**

Excludes: *gastric lavage (96.33)*
microscopic examination of specimen from stomach (90.81-90.89)
upper GI series (87.62)

44.2 **Pyloroplasty**

44.21 **Dilation of pylorus by incision**

44.22 **Endoscopic dilation of pylorus**
Dilation with balloon endoscope
Endoscopic dilation of gastrojejunostomy site

44.29 **Other pyloroplasty**
Pyloroplasty NOS
Revision of pylorus

44.3 **Gastroenterostomy without gastrectomy**

44.31 **High gastric bypass**
Printen and Mason gastric bypass

44.32 **Percutaneous [endoscopic] gastrojejunostomy**
Endoscopic conversion of gastrostomy to jejunostomy

44.39 **Other gastroenterostomy**
Bypass:
gastroduodenostomy
gastroenterostomy
gastrogastrostomy
Gastrojejunostomy without gastrectomy NOS

44.4 **Control of hemorrhage and suture of ulcer of stomach or duodenum**

44.40 **Suture of peptic ulcer, not otherwise specified**

● Code new
to this edition
▲ Revision of
existing code
④ ⑤ Fourth or fifth
digit required

44.41 **Suture of gastric ulcer site**

> Excludes: ligation of gastric varices (44.91)

44.42 **Suture of duodenal ulcer site**

44.43 **Endoscopic control of gastric or duodenal bleeding**

44.44 **Transcatheter embolization for gastric or duodenal bleeding**

> Excludes: surgical occlusion of abdominal vessels (38.86-38.87)

44.49 **Other control of hemorrhage of stomach or duodenum**
That with gastrotomy

44.5 **Revision of gastric anastomosis**
Closure of:
  gastric anastomosis
  gastroduodenostomy
  gastrojejunostomy
Pantaloon operation

44.6 **Other repair of stomach**

44.61 **Suture of laceration of stomach**

> Excludes: that of ulcer site (44.41)

44.62 **Closure of gastrostomy**

44.63 **Closure of other gastric fistula**
Closure of:
  gastrocolic fistula
  gastrojejunocolic fistula

44.64 **Gastropexy**

44.65 **Esophagogastroplasty**
Belsey operation
Esophagus and stomach cardioplasty

44.66 **Other procedures for creation of esophagogastric sphincteric competence**
Fundoplication
Gastric cardioplasty
Nissen's fundoplication
Restoration of cardio-esophageal angle

44.69 **Other**
Inversion of gastric diverticulum
Repair of stomach NOS

44.9 **Other operations on stomach**

44.91 **Ligation of gastric varices**

> Excludes: that by endoscopic approach (43.41)

44.92 **Intraoperative manipulation of stomach**
Reduction of gastric volvulus

44.93 **Insertion of gastric bubble [balloon]**

44.94 **Removal of gastric bubble [balloon]**

44.99 **Other**

> Excludes: change of gastrostomy tube (97.02)
> dilation of cardiac sphincter (42.92)
> gastric:
>   cooling (96.31)
>   freezing (96.32)
>   gavage (96.35)
>   hypothermia (96.31)
>   lavage (96.33)
> insertion of nasogastric tube (96.07)
> irrigation of gastrostomy (96.36)
> irrigation of nasogastric tube (96.34)
> removal of:
>   gastrostomy tube (97.51)
>   intraluminal foreign body from stomach without incision (98.03)
> replacement of:
>   gastrostomy tube (97.02)
>   (naso-)gastric tube (97.01)

Valid O.R.
procedure

Non-O.R.
procedure

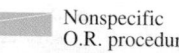
Nonspecific
O.R. procedure

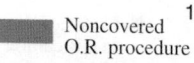
Noncovered
O.R. procedure

45 **Incision, excision, and anastomosis of intestine**

Code also any application or administration of an adhesion barrier substance (99.77)

45.0 **Enterotomy**

Excludes:	duodenocholedochotomy (51.41-51.42, 51.51)
	that for destruction of lesion (45.30-45.34)
	that of exteriorized intestine (46.14, 46.24, 46.31)

45.00 **Incision of intestine, not otherwise specified**

45.01 **Incision of duodenum**

45.02 **Other incision of small intestine**

45.03 **Incision of large intestine**

> Excludes: *proctotomy (48.0)*

45.1 **Diagnostic procedures on small intestine**

Code also any laparotomy (54.11-54.19)

45.11 **Transabdominal endoscopy of small intestine**
Intraoperative endoscopy of small intestine

> Excludes: *that with biopsy (45.14)*

45.12 **Endoscopy of small intestine through artificial stoma**

> Excludes: *that with biopsy (45.14)*

45.13 **Other endoscopy of small intestine**
Esophagogastroduodenoscopy [EGD]

> Excludes: *that with biopsy (45.14, 45.16)*

45.14 **Closed [endoscopic] biopsy of small intestine**
Brushing or washing for specimen collection

> Excludes: *esophagogastroduodenoscopy [EGD] with closed biopsy (45.16)*

45.15 **Open biopsy of small intestine**

45.16 **Esophagogastroduodenoscopy [EGD] with closed biopsy**
Biopsy of one or more sites involving esophagus, stomach, and/or duodenum

45.19 **Other diagnostic procedures on small intestine**

> Excludes: *microscopic examination of specimen from small intestine*
> *(90.91-90.99)*
> *radioisotope scan (92.04)*
> *ultrasonography (88.74)*
> *x-ray (87.61-87.69)*

45.2 **Diagnostic procedures on large intestine**

Code also any laparotomy (54.11-54.19)

45.21 **Transabdominal endoscopy of large intestine**
Intraoperative endoscopy of large intestine

> Excludes: *that with biopsy (45.25)*

45.22 **Endoscopy of large intestine through artificial stoma**

> Excludes: *that with biopsy (45.25)*

45.23 **Colonoscopy**
Flexible fiberoptic colonoscopy

> Excludes: *endoscopy of large intestine through artificial stoma (45.22)*
> *flexible sigmoidoscopy (45.24)*
> *rigid proctosigmoidoscopy (48.23)*
> *transabdominal endoscopy of large intestine (45.21)*

45.24 **Flexible sigmoidoscopy**
Endoscopy of descending colon

> Excludes: *rigid proctosigmoidoscopy (48.23)*

45.25 **Closed [endoscopic] biopsy of large intestine**
Biopsy, closed, of unspecified intestinal site
Brushing or washing for specimen collection
Colonoscopy with biopsy

> Excludes: *proctosigmoidoscopy with biopsy (48.24)*

45.26 **Open biopsy of large intestine**

45.27 **Intestinal biopsy, site unspecified**

● Code new
to this edition ▲ Revision of
existing code ④ ⑤ Fourth or fifth
digit required

45.28 Other diagnostic procedures on large intestine

45.29 Other diagnostic procedures on intestine, site unspecified

> | *Excludes:* | *microscopic examination of specimen (90.91-90.99)* |
> | --- | --- |
> | | *scan and radioisotope function study (92.04)* |
> | | *ultrasonography (88.74)* |
> | | *x-ray (87.61-87.69)* |

45.3 Local excision or destruction of lesion or tissue of small intestine

45.30 Endoscopic excision or destruction of lesion of duodenum

> | *Excludes:* | *biopsy of duodenum (45.14-45.15)* |
> | --- | --- |
> | | *control of hemorrhage (44.43)* |
> | | *fistulectomy (46.72)* |

45.31 Other local excision of lesion of duodenum

> | *Excludes:* | *biopsy of duodenum (45.14-45.15)* |
> | --- | --- |
> | | *fistulectomy (46.72)* |
> | | *multiple segmental resection (45.61)* |
> | | *that by endoscopic approach (45.30)* |

45.32 Other destruction of lesion of duodenum

> | *Excludes:* | *that by endoscopic approach (45.30)* |
> | --- | --- |

45.33 Local excision of lesion or tissue of small intestine, except duodenum
Excision of redundant mucosa of ileostomy

> | *Excludes:* | *biopsy of small intestine (45.14-45.15)* |
> | --- | --- |
> | | *fistulectomy (46.74)* |
> | | *multiple segmental resection (45.61)* |

45.34 Other destruction of lesion of small intestine, except duodenum

45.4 Local excision or destruction of lesion or tissue of large intestine

45.41 Excision of lesion or tissue of large intestine
Excision of redundant mucosa of colostomy

> | *Excludes:* | *biopsy of large intestine (45.25-45.27)* |
> | --- | --- |
> | | *endoscopic polypectomy of large intestine (45.42)* |
> | | *fistulectomy (46.76)* |
> | | *multiple segmental resection (45.71)* |
> | | *that by endoscopic approach (45.42-45.43)* |

45.42 Endoscopic polypectomy of large intestine

> | *Excludes:* | *that by open approach (45.41)* |
> | --- | --- |

45.43 Endoscopic destruction of other lesion or tissue of large intestine
Endoscopic ablation of tumor of large intestine
Endoscopic control of colonic bleeding

> | *Excludes:* | *endoscopic polypectomy of large intestine (45.42)* |
> | --- | --- |

45.49 Other destruction of lesion of large intestine

> | *Excludes:* | *that by endoscopic approach (45.43)* |
> | --- | --- |

45.5 Isolation of intestinal segment

Code also any synchronous:
anastomosis other than end-to-end (45.90-45.94)
enterostomy (46.10-46.39)

45.50 Isolation of intestinal segment not otherwise specified
Isolation of intestinal pedicle flap
Reversal of intestinal segment

45.51 Isolation of segment of small intestine
Isolation of ileal loop
Resection of small intestine for interposition

45.52 Isolation of segment of large intestine
Resection of colon for interposition

1555

	Valid O.R. procedure		Non-O.R. procedure		Nonspecific O.R. procedure		Noncovered O.R. procedure

45.6   **Other excision of small intestine**

> *Code also any synchronous:*
> anastomosis other than end-to-end (45.90-45.93, 45.95)
> colostomy (46.10-46.13)
> enterostomy (46.10-46.39)

> | Excludes: | cecectomy (45.72)
> | | enterocolectomy (45.79)
> | | gastroduodenectomy (43.6-43.99)
> | | ileocolectomy (45.73)
> | | pancreatoduodenectomy (52.51-52.7)

45.61   **Multiple segmental resection of small intestine**
Segmental resection for multiple traumatic lesions of small intestine

45.62   **Other partial resection of small intestine**
Duodenectomy   Jejunectomy
Ileectomy

> | Excludes: | duodenectomy with synchronous pancreatectomy (52.51-52.7)
> | | resection of cecum and terminal ileum (45.72)

45.63   **Total removal of small intestine**

45.7   **Partial excision of large intestine**

> *Code also any synchronous:*
> anastomosis other than end-to-end (45.92-45.94)
> enterostomy (46.10-46.39)

45.71   **Multiple segmental resection of large intestine**
Segmental resection for multiple traumatic lesions of large intestine

45.72   **Cecectomy**
Resection of cecum and terminal ileum

45.73   **Right hemicolectomy**
Ileocolectomy
Right radical colectomy

45.74   **Resection of transverse colon**

45.75   **Left hemicolectomy**

> | Excludes: | proctosigmoidectomy (48.41-48.69)
> | | second stage Mikulicz operation (46.04)

45.76   **Sigmoidectomy**

45.79   **Other partial excision of large intestine**
Enterocolectomy NEC

45.8   **Total intra-abdominal colectomy**
Excision of cecum, colon, and sigmoid

> | Excludes: | coloproctectomy (48.41-48.69)

45.9   **Intestinal anastomosis**

> *Code also any synchronous resection (45.31-45.8, 48.41-48.69)*

> | Excludes: | end-to-end anastomosis – omit code

45.90   **Intestinal anastomosis, not otherwise specified**

45.91   **Small-to-small intestinal anastomosis**

45.92   **Anastomosis of small intestine to rectal stump**
Hampton procedure

45.93   **Other small-to-large intestinal anastomosis**

45.94   **Large-to-large intestinal anastomosis**

> | Excludes: | rectorectostomy (48.74)

45.95   **Anastomosis to anus**
Formation of endorectal ileal pouch (J-pouch) (H-pouch) (S-pouch) with
anastomosis of small intestine to anus

46   **Other operations on intestine**

> *Code also any application or administration of an adhesion barrier substance (99.77)*

46.0   **Exteriorization of intestine**
Includes: loop enterostomy
multiple stage resection of intestine

46.01   **Exteriorization of small intestine**
Loop ileostomy

● Code new
to this edition   ▲ Revision of
existing code   ④ ⑤ Fourth or fifth
digit required

46.02 **Resection of exteriorized segment of small intestine**

46.03 **Exteriorization of large intestine**
Exteriorization of intestine NOS
First stage Mikulicz exteriorization of intestine
Loop colostomy

46.04 **Resection of exteriorized segment of large intestine**
Resection of exteriorized segment of intestine NOS
Second stage Mikulicz operation

46.1 **Colostomy**
Code also any synchronous resection (45.49, 45.71-45.79, 45.8)

> Excludes: *loop colostomy (46.03)*
> *that with abdominoperineal resection of rectum (48.5)*
> *that with synchronous anterior rectal resection (48.62)*

46.10 **Colostomy, not otherwise specified**

46.11 **Temporary colostomy**

46.13 **Other permanent colostomy**

46.14 **Delayed opening of colostomy**

46.2 **Ileostomy**
Code also any synchronous resection (45.34, 45.61-45.63)

> Excludes: *loop ileostomy (46.01)*

46.20 **Ileostomy, not otherwise specified**

46.21 **Temporary ileostomy**

46.22 **Continent ileostomy**

46.23 **Other permanent ileostomy**

46.24 **Delayed opening of ileostomy**

46.3 **Other enterostomy**
Code also any synchronous resection (45.61-45.8)

46.31 **Delayed opening of other enterostomy**

46.32 **Percutaneous [endoscopic] jejunostomy [PEJ]**

46.39 **Other**
Duodenostomy
Feeding enterostomy

46.4 **Revision of intestinal stoma**

46.40 **Revision of intestinal stoma, not otherwise specified**
Plastic enlargement of intestinal stoma
Reconstruction of stoma of intestine
Release of scar tissue of intestinal stoma

> Excludes: *excision of redundant mucosa (45.41)*

46.41 **Revision of stoma of small intestine**

> Excludes: *excision of redundant mucosa (45.33)*

46.42 **Repair of pericolostomy hernia**

46.43 **Other revision of stoma of large intestine**

> Excludes: *excision of redundant mucosa (45.41)*

46.5 **Closure of intestinal stoma**
Code also any synchronous resection (45.34, 45.49, 45.61-45.8)

46.50 **Closure of intestinal stoma, not otherwise specified**

46.51 **Closure of stoma of small intestine**

46.52 **Closure of stoma of large intestine**
Closure or take-down of:
cecostomy
colostomy
sigmoidostomy

46.6 **Fixation of intestine**

46.60 **Fixation of intestine, not otherwise specified**
Fixation of intestine to abdominal wall

46.61 **Fixation of small intestine to abdominal wall**
Ileopexy

	Valid O.R. procedure		Non-O.R. procedure		Nonspecific O.R. procedure		Noncovered O.R. procedure	1557

46.62 **Other fixation of small intestine**
Noble plication of small intestine
Plication of jejunum

46.63 **Fixation of large intestine to abdominal wall**
Cecocoloplicopexy
Sigmoidopexy (Moschowitz)

46.64 **Other fixation of large intestine**
Cecofixation
Colofixation

46.7 **Other repair of intestine**

> Excludes: closure of:
> ulcer of duodenum (44.42)
> vesicoenteric fistula (57.83)

46.71 **Suture of laceration of duodenum**

46.72 **Closure of fistula of duodenum**

46.73 **Suture of laceration of small intestine, except duodenum**

46.74 **Closure of fistula of small intestine, except duodenum**

> Excludes: closure of:
> artificial stoma (46.51)
> vaginal fistula (70.74)
> repair of gastrojejunocolic fistula (44.63)

46.75 **Suture of laceration of large intestine**

46.76 **Closure of fistula of large intestine**

> Excludes: closure of:
> gastrocolic fistula (44.63)
> rectal fistula (48.73)
> sigmoidovesical fistula (57.83)
> stoma (46.52)
> vaginal fistula (70.72-70.73)
> vesicocolic fistula (57.83)
> vesicosigmoidovaginal fistula (57.83)

46.79 **Other repair of intestine**
Duodenoplasty

46.8 **Dilation and manipulation of intestine**

46.80 **Intra-abdominal manipulation of intestine, not otherwise specified**
Correction of intestinal malrotation
Reduction of:
intestinal torsion
intestinal volvulus
intussusception

> Excludes: reduction of intussusception with:
> fluoroscopy (96.29)
> ionizing radiation enema (96.29)
> ultrasonography guidance (96.29)

46.81 **Intra-abdominal manipulation of small intestine**

46.82 **Intra-abdominal manipulation of large intestine**

46.85 **Dilation of intestine**
Dilation (balloon) of duodenum
Dilation (balloon) of jejunum
Endoscopic dilation (balloon) of large intestine
That through rectum or colostomy

46.9 **Other operations on intestines**

46.91 **Myotomy of sigmoid colon**

46.92 **Myotomy of other parts of colon**

46.93 **Revision of anastomosis of small intestine**

46.94 **Revision of anastomosis of large intestine**

46.95 **Local perfusion of small intestine**
Code also substance perfused (99.21-99.29)

46.96 **Local perfusion of large intestine**
Code also substance perfused (99.21-99.29)

46.97 Transplant of intestine

46.99 Other
Ileoentectropy

> | Excludes: | *diagnostic procedures on intestine (45.11-45.29)*
> | | *dilation of enterostomy stoma (96.24)*
> | | *intestinal intubation (96.08)*
> | | *removal of:*
> | | *intraluminal foreign body from intestine without incision (98.04)*
> | | *intraluminal foreign body from small intestine without incision (98.03)*
> | | *tube from large intestine (97.53)*
> | | *tube from small intestine (97.52)*
> | | *replacement of:*
> | | *large intestine tube or enterostomy device (97.04)*
> | | *small intestine tube or enterostomy device (97.03)*

47 Operations on appendix
Includes: appendiceal stump

Code also any application or administration of an adhesion barrier substance (99.77)

47.0 Appendectomy

> | Excludes: | *incidental appendectomy, so described (47.11, 47.19)*

47.01 Laparoscopic appendectomy

47.09 Other appendectomy

47.1 Incidental appendectomy

47.11 Laparoscopic incidental appendectomy

47.19 Other incidental appendectomy

47.2 Drainage of appendiceal abscess

> | Excludes: | *that with appendectomy (47.0)*

47.9 Other operations on appendix

47.91 Appendicostomy

47.92 Closure of appendiceal fistula

47.99 Other
Anastomosis of appendix

> | Excludes: | *diagnostic procedures on appendix (45.21-45.29)*

48 Operations on rectum, rectosigmoid, and perirectal tissue
Code also any application or administration of an adhesion barrier substance (99.77)

48.0 Proctotomy
Decompression of imperforate anus
Panas' operation [linear proctotomy]

> | Excludes: | *incision of perirectal tissue (48.81)*

48.1 Proctostomy

48.2 Diagnostic procedures on rectum, rectosigmoid, and perirectal tissue

48.21 Transabdominal proctosigmoidoscopy
Intraoperative proctosigmoidoscopy

> | Excludes: | *that with biopsy (48.24)*

48.22 Proctosigmoidoscopy through artificial stoma

> | Excludes: | *that with biopsy (48.24)*

48.23 Rigid proctosigmoidoscopy

> | Excludes: | *flexible sigmoidoscopy (45.24)*

48.24 Closed [endoscopic] biopsy of rectum
Brushing or washing for specimen collection
Proctosigmoidoscopy with biopsy

48.25 Open biopsy of rectum

48.26 Biopsy of perirectal tissue

48.29 Other diagnostic procedures on rectum, rectosigmoid and perirectal tissue

> | Excludes: | *digital examination of rectum (89.34)*
> | | *lower GI series (87.64)*
> | | *microscopic examination of specimen from rectum (90.91-90.99)*

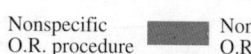

| | Valid O.R. procedure | | Non-O.R. procedure | | Nonspecific O.R. procedure | | Noncovered O.R. procedure |

48.3   Local excision or destruction of lesion or tissue of rectum

    48.31   Radical electrocoagulation of rectal lesion or tissue

    48.32   Other electrocoagulation of rectal lesion or tissue

    48.33   Destruction of rectal lesion or tissue by laser

    48.34   Destruction of rectal lesion or tissue by cryosurgery

    48.35   Local excision of rectal lesion or tissue

> | *Excludes:* | *biopsy of rectum (48.24-48.25)* |
> | --- | --- |
> | | *[endoscopic] polypectomy of rectum (48.36)* |
> | | *excision of perirectal tissue (48.82)* |
> | | *hemorrhoidectomy (49.46)* |
> | | *rectal fistulectomy (48.73)* |

    48.36   [Endoscopic] polypectomy of rectum

48.4   Pull-through resection of rectum
Code also any synchronous anastomosis other than end-to-end (45.90, 45.92-45.95)

    48.41   Soave submucosal resection of rectum
    Endorectal pull-through operation

    48.49   Other pull-through resection of rectum
    Abdominoperineal pull-through
    Altemeier operation
    Swenson proctectomy

> | *Excludes:* | *Duhamel abdominoperineal pull-through (48.65)* |
> | --- | --- |

48.5   Abdominoperineal resection of rectum
Combined abdominoendorectal resection
Complete proctectomy
Includes: with synchronous colostomy
Code also any synchronous anastomosis other than end-to-end (45.90, 45.92-45.95)

> | *Excludes:* | *Duhamel abdominoperineal pull-through (48.65)* |
> | --- | --- |
> | | *that as part of pelvic exenteration (68.8)* |

48.6   Other resection of rectum
Code also any synchronous anastomosis other than end-to-end (45.90, 45.92-45.95)

    48.61   Transsacral rectosigmoidectomy

    48.62   Anterior resection of rectum with synchronous colostomy

    48.63   Other anterior resection of rectum

> | *Excludes:* | *that with synchronous colostomy (48.62)* |
> | --- | --- |

    48.64   Posterior resection of rectum

    48.65   Duhamel resection of rectum
    Duhamel abdominoperineal pull-through

    48.69   Other
    Partial proctectomy
    Rectal resection NOS

48.7   Repair of rectum

> | *Excludes:* | *repair of:* |
> | --- | --- |
> | | *current obstetric laceration (75.62)* |
> | | *vaginal rectocele (70.50, 70.52)* |

    48.71   Suture of laceration of rectum

    48.72   Closure of proctostomy

    48.73   Closure of other rectal fistula

> | *Excludes:* | *fistulectomy:* |
> | --- | --- |
> | | *perirectal (48.93)* |
> | | *rectourethral (58.43)* |
> | | *rectovaginal (70.73)* |
> | | *rectovesical (57.83)* |
> | | *rectovesicovaginal (57.83)* |

    48.74   Rectorectostomy
    Rectal anastomosis NOS

    48.75   Abdominal proctopexy
    Frickman procedure
    Ripstein repair of rectal prolapse

  ● Code new
to this edition
  ▲ Revision of
existing code
  ④ ⑤ Fourth or fifth
digit required

48.76 **Other proctopexy**
Delorme repair of prolapsed rectum
Proctosigmoidopexy
Puborectalis sling operation

Excludes: manual reduction of rectal prolapse (96.26)

48.79 **Other repair of rectum**
Repair of old obstetric laceration of rectum

Excludes: anastomosis to:
large intestine (45.94)
small intestine (45.92-45.93)
repair of:
current obstetrical laceration (75.62)
vaginal rectocele (70.50, 70.52)

48.8 **Incision or excision of perirectal tissue or lesion**
Includes: pelvirectal tissue
rectovaginal septum

48.81 **Incision of perirectal tissue**
Incision of rectovaginal septum

48.82 **Excision of perirectal tissue**

Excludes: perirectal biopsy (48.26)
perirectofistulectomy (48.93)
rectal fistulectomy (48.73)

48.9 **Other operations on rectum and perirectal tissue**

48.91 **Incision of rectal stricture**

48.92 **Anorectal myectomy**

48.93 **Repair of perirectal fistula**

Excludes: that opening into rectum (48.73)

48.99 **Other**

Excludes: digital examination of rectum (89.34)
dilation of rectum (96.22)
insertion of rectal tube (96.09)
irrigation of rectum (96.38-96.39)
manual reduction of rectal prolapse (96.26)
proctoclysis (96.37)
rectal massage (99.93)
rectal packing (96.19)
removal of:
impacted feces (96.38)
intraluminal foreign body from rectum without incision (98.05)
rectal packing (97.59)
transanal enema (96.39)

49 **Operations on anus**
Code also any application or administration of an adhesion barrier substance (99.77)

49.0 **Incision or excision of perianal tissue**

49.01 **Incision of perianal abscess**

49.02 **Other incision of perianal tissue**
Undercutting of perianal tissue

Excludes: anal fistulotomy (49.11)

49.03 **Excision of perianal skin tags**

49.04 **Other excision of perianal tissue**

Excludes: anal fistulectomy (49.12)
biopsy of perianal tissue (49.22)

49.1 **Incision or excision of anal fistula**

Excludes: closure of anal fistula (49.73)

49.11 **Anal fistulotomy**

49.12 **Anal fistulectomy**

49.2 **Diagnostic procedures on anus and perianal tissue**

49.21 **Anoscopy**

49.22 **Biopsy of perianal tissue**

| Valid O.R. procedure | Non-O.R. procedure | Nonspecific O.R. procedure | Noncovered O.R. procedure |

49.23 Biopsy of anus

49.29 Other diagnostic procedures on anus and perianal tissue

> *Excludes:* *microscopic examination of specimen from anus (90.91-90.99)*

49.3 Local excision or destruction of other lesion or tissue of anus
Anal cryptotomy
Cauterization of lesion of anus

> *Excludes:* *biopsy of anus (49.23)*
> *control of (postoperative) hemorrhage of anus (49.95)*
> *hemorrhoidectomy (49.46)*

49.31 Endoscopic excision or destruction of lesion or tissue of anus

49.39 Other local excision or destruction of lesion or tissue of anus

> *Excludes:* *that by endoscopic approach (49.31)*

49.4 Procedures on hemorrhoids

49.41 Reduction of hemorrhoids

49.42 Injection of hemorrhoids

49.43 Cauterization of hemorrhoids
Clamp and cautery of hemorrhoids

49.44 Destruction of hemorrhoids by cryotherapy

49.45 Ligation of hemorrhoids

49.46 Excision of hemorrhoids
Hemorrhoidectomy NOS

49.47 Evacuation of thrombosed hemorrhoids

49.49 Other procedures on hemorrhoids
Lord procedure

49.5 Division of anal sphincter

49.51 Left lateral anal sphincterotomy

49.52 Posterior anal sphincterotomy

49.59 Other anal sphincterotomy
Division of sphincter NOS

49.6 Excision of anus

49.7 Repair of anus

> *Excludes:* *repair of current obstetric laceration (75.62)*

49.71 Suture of laceration of anus

49.72 Anal cerclage

49.73 Closure of anal fistula

> *Excludes:* *excision of anal fistula (49.12)*

49.74 Gracilis muscle transplant for anal incontinence

● **49.75 Implantation or revision of artificial anal sphincter**
Removal with subsequent replacement
Replacement during same or subsequent operative episode

● **49.76 Removal of artificial anal sphincter**
Explanation or removal without replacement

> *Excludes:* *revision with implantation during same operative episode (49.75)*

49.79 Other repair of anal sphincter
Repair of old obstetric laceration of anus

> *Excludes:* *anoplasty with synchronous*
> *hemorrhoidectomy (49.46)*
> *repair of current obstetric laceration (75.62)*

49.9 Other operations on anus

> *Excludes:* *dilation of anus (sphincter) (96.23)*

49.91 Incision of anal septum

49.92 Insertion of subcutaneous electrical anal stimulator

● Code new
to this edition
▲ Revision of
existing code
④ ⑤ Fourth or fifth
digit required

49.93 Other incision of anus
Removal of:
  foreign body from anus with incision
  seton from anus

| Excludes: | *anal fistulotomy (49.11)* |

removal of intraluminal foreign body without incision (98.05)

49.94 Reduction of anal prolapse

| Excludes: | *manual reduction of rectal prolapse (96.26)* |

49.95 Control of (postoperative) hemorrhage of anus

49.99 Other

50 Operations on liver
Code also any application or administration of an adhesion barrier substance (99.77)

50.0 Hepatotomy
Incision of abscess of liver
Removal of gallstones from liver
Stromeyer-Little operation

50.1 Diagnostic procedures on liver

50.11 Closed (percutaneous) [needle] biopsy of liver
Diagnostic aspiration of liver

50.12 Open biopsy of liver
Wedge biopsy

50.19 Other diagnostic procedures on liver

| Excludes: | *liver scan and radioisotope function study (92.02)* |

microscopic examination of specimen from liver (91.01-91.09)

50.2 Local excision or destruction of liver tissue or lesion

50.21 Marsupialization of lesion of liver

50.22 Partial hepatectomy
Wedge resection of liver

| Excludes: | *biopsy of liver, (50.11-50.12)* |

hepatic lobectomy (50.3)

50.29 Other destruction of lesion of liver
Cauterization of hepatic lesion
Enucleation of hepatic lesion
Evacuation of hepatic lesion

| Excludes: | *percutaneous aspiration of lesion (50.91)* |

50.3 Lobectomy of liver
Total hepatic lobectomy with partial excision of other lobe

50.4 Total hepatectomy

50.5 Liver transplant

50.51 Auxiliary liver transplant
Auxiliary hepatic transplantation leaving patient's own liver in situ

50.59 Other transplant of liver

50.6 Repair of liver

50.61 Closure of laceration of liver

50.69 Other repair of liver
Hepatopexy

50.9 Other operations on liver

| Excludes: | *lysis of adhesions (54.5)* |

50.91 Percutaneous aspiration of liver

| Excludes: | *percutaneous biopsy (50.11)* |

50.92 Extracorporeal hepatic assistance
Liver dialysis

50.93 Localized perfusion of liver

50.94 Other injection of therapeutic substance into liver

50.99 Other

| | Valid O.R. procedure | | Non-O.R. procedure | | Nonspecific O.R. procedure | | Noncovered O.R. procedure |

51   Operations on gallbladder and biliary tract

Includes: operations on:
>   ampulla of Vater
>   common bile duct
>   cystic duct
>   hepatic duct
>   intrahepatic bile duct
>   sphincter of Oddi

Code also any application or administration of an adhesion barrier substance (99.77)

51.0   Cholecystotomy and cholecystostomy

51.01   Percutaneous aspiration of gallbladder
Percutaneous cholecystotomy for drainage
That by: needle or catheter

> Excludes: *needle biopsy (51.12)*

51.02   Trocar cholecystostomy

51.03   Other cholecystostomy

51.04   Other cholecystotomy
Cholelithotomy NOS

51.1   Diagnostic procedures on biliary tract

> Excludes: *that for endoscopic procedures classifiable to 51.64, 51.84-51.88, 52.14, 52.21, 52.93-52.94, 52.97-52.98*

51.10   Endoscopic retrograde cholangiopancreatography [ERCP]

> Excludes: *endoscopic retrograde:*
> *cholangiography [ERC] (51.11)*
> *pancreatography [ERP] (52.13)*

51.11   Endoscopic retrograde cholangiography [ERC]
Laparoscopic exploration of common bile duct

> Excludes: *endoscopic retrograde:*
> *cholangiopancreatography [ERCP] (51.10)*
> *pancreatography [ERP] (52.13)*

51.12   Percutaneous biopsy of gallbladder or bile ducts
Needle biopsy of gallbladder

51.13   Open biopsy of gallbladder or bile ducts

51.14   Other closed [endoscopic] biopsy of biliary duct or sphincter of Oddi
Brushing or washing for specimen collection
Closed biopsy of biliary duct or sphincter of Oddi by procedures classifiable to 51.10-51.11, 52.13

51.15   Pressure measurement of sphincter of Oddi
Pressure measurement of sphincter by procedures classifiable to 51.10-51.11, 52.13

51.19   Other diagnostic procedures on biliary tract

> Excludes: *biliary tract x-ray (87.51-87.59)*
> *microscopic examination of specimen from biliary tract (91.01-91.09)*

51.2   Cholecystectomy

51.21   Other partial cholecystectomy
Revision of prior cholecystectomy

> Excludes: *that by laparoscope (51.24)*

51.22   Cholecystectomy

> Excludes: *laparoscopic cholecystectomy (51.23)*

51.23   Laparoscopic cholecystectomy
That by laser

51.24   Laparoscopic partial cholecystectomy

51.3   Anastomosis of gallbladder or bile duct

> Excludes: *resection with end-to-end anastomosis (51.61-51.69)*

51.31   Anastomosis of gallbladder to hepatic ducts

51.32   Anastomosis of gallbladder to intestine

51.33   Anastomosis of gallbladder to pancreas

51.34   Anastomosis of gallbladder to stomach

● Code new
to this edition   ▲ Revision of
existing code   ④ ⑤ Fourth or fifth
digit required

51.35 **Other gallbladder anastomosis**
Gallbladder anastomosis NOS

51.36 **Choledochoenterostomy**

51.37 **Anastomosis of hepatic duct to gastrointestinal tract**
Kasai portoenterostomy

51.39 **Other bile duct anastomosis**
Anastomosis of bile duct NOS
Anastomosis of unspecified bile duct to:
intestine
liver
pancreas
stomach

51.4 **Incision of bile duct for relief of obstruction**

51.41 **Common duct exploration for removal of calculus**
Excludes: *percutaneous extraction (51.96)*

51.42 **Common duct exploration for relief of other obstruction**

51.43 **Insertion of choledochohepatic tube for decompression**
Hepatocholedochostomy

51.49 **Incision of other bile ducts for relief of obstruction**

51.5 **Other incision of bile duct**
Excludes: *that for relief of obstruction (51.41-51.49)*

51.51 **Exploration of common duct**
Incision of common bile duct

51.59 **Incision of other bile duct**

51.6 **Local excision or destruction of lesion or tissue of biliary ducts and sphincter of Oddi**
Code also anastomosis other than end-to-end (51.31, 51.36-51.39)
Excludes: *biopsy of bile duct (51.12-51.13)*

51.61 **Excision of cystic duct remnant**

51.62 **Excision of ampulla of Vater (with reimplantation of common duct)**

51.63 **Other excision of common duct**
Choledochectomy
Excludes: *fistulectomy (51.72)*

51.64 **Endoscopic excision or destruction of lesion of biliary ducts or sphincter of Oddi**
Excision or destruction of lesion of biliary duct by procedures classifiable to
51.10-51.11, 52.13

51.69 **Excision of other bile duct**
Excision of lesion of bile duct NOS
Excludes: *fistulectomy (51.79)*

51.7 **Repair of bile ducts**

51.71 **Simple suture of common bile duct**

51.72 **Choledochoplasty**
Repair of fistula of common bile duct

51.79 **Repair of other bile ducts**
Closure of artificial opening of bile duct NOS
Suture of bile duct NOS
Excludes: *operative removal of prosthetic device (51.95)*

51.8 **Other operations on biliary ducts and sphincter of Oddi**

51.81 **Dilation of sphincter of Oddi**
Dilation of ampulla of Vater
Excludes: *that by endoscopic approach (51.84)*

51.82 **Pancreatic sphincterotomy**
Incision of pancreatic sphincter
Transduodenal ampullary sphincterotomy
Excludes: *that by endoscopic approach (51.85)*

51.83 **Pancreatic sphincteroplasty**

51.84 **Endoscopic dilation of ampulla and biliary duct**
Dilation of ampulla and biliary duct by procedures classifiable to 51.10-51.11, 52.13

Valid O.R.
procedure

Non-O.R.
procedure

Nonspecific
O.R. procedure

Noncovered
O.R. procedure

51.85 Endoscopic sphincterotomy and papillotomy
Sphincterotomy and papillotomy by procedures classifiable to 51.10-51.11, 52.13

51.86 Endoscopic insertion of nasobiliary drainage tube
Insertion of nasobiliary tube by procedures classifiable to 51.10-51.11, 52.13

51.87 Endoscopic insertion of stent (tube) into bile duct
Endoprosthesis of bile duct
Insertion of stent into bile duct by procedures classifiable to 51.10-51.11, 52.13

> Excludes: *nasobiliary drainage tube (51.86)*
> *replacement of stent (tube) (97.05)*

51.88 Endoscopic removal of stone(s) from biliary tract
Laparoscopic removal of stone(s) from biliary tract
Removal of biliary tract stone(s) by procedures classifiable to 51.10-51.11, 52.13

> Excludes: *percutaneous extraction of common duct stones (51.96)*

51.89 Other operations on sphincter of Oddi

51.9 Other operations on biliary tract

51.91 Repair of laceration of gallbladder

51.92 Closure of cholecystostomy

51.93 Closure of other biliary fistula
Cholecystogastroenteric fistulectomy

51.94 Revision of anastomosis of biliary tract

51.95 Removal of prosthetic device from bile duct

> Excludes: *nonoperative removal (97.55)*

51.96 Percutaneous extraction of common duct stones

51.98 Other percutaneous procedures on biliary tract
Percutaneous biliary endoscopy via existing T-tube or other tract for:
dilation of biliary duct stricture
exploration (postoperative)
removal of stone(s) except common duct stone
Percutaneous transhepatic biliary drainage

> Excludes: *percutaneous aspiration of gallbladder (51.01)*
> *percutaneous biopsy and/or collection of specimen by brushing or*
> *washing (51.12)*
> *percutaneous removal of common duct stone(s) (51.96)*

51.99 Other
Insertion or replacement of biliary tract prosthesis

> Excludes: *biopsy of gallbladder (51.12-51.13)*
> *irrigation of cholecystostomy and other biliary tube (96.41)*
> *lysis of peritoneal adhesions (54.5)*
> *nonoperative removal of:*
> *cholecystostomy tube (97.54)*
> *tube from biliary tract or liver (97.55)*

52 Operations on pancreas
Includes: operations on pancreatic duct
Code also any application or administration of an adhesion barrier substance (99.77)

52.0 Pancreatotomy

52.01 Drainage of pancreatic cyst by catheter

52.09 Other pancreatotomy
Pancreatolithotomy

> Excludes: *drainage by anastomosis (52.4, 52.96)*
> *incision of pancreatic sphincter (51.82)*
> *marsupialization of cyst (52.3)*

52.1 Diagnostic procedures on pancreas

52.11 Closed [aspiration] [needle] [percutaneous] biopsy of pancreas

52.12 Open biopsy of pancreas

● Code new
to this edition   ▲ Revision of
existing code   ④ ⑤ Fourth or fifth
digit required

52.13 **Endoscopic retrograde pancreatography [EPR]**

Excludes: *endoscopic retrograde:*
cholangiography [ERC] (51.11)
cholangiopancreatography [ERCP] (51.10)
that for procedures classifiable to 51.14-51.15, 51.64, 51.84-51.88,
52.14, 52.21, 52.92-52.94, 52.97-52.98

52.14 **Closed [endoscopic] biopsy of pancreatic duct**
Closed biopsy of pancreatic duct by procedures classifiable to 51.10-51.11, 52.13

52.19 **Other diagnostic procedure on pancreas**

Excludes: *contrast pancreatogram (87.66)*
endoscopic retrograde pancreatography [ERP] (52.13))
microscopic examination of specimen from pancreas (91.01-91.09)

52.2 **Local excision or destruction of pancreas and pancreatic duct**

Excludes: *biopsy of pancreas (52.11-52.12, 52.14)*
pancreatic fistulectomy (52.95)

52.21 **Endoscopic excision or destruction of lesion or tissue of pancreatic duct**
Excision or destruction of lesion or tissue of pancreatic duct by procedures
classifiable to 51.10-51.11, 52.13

52.22 **Other excision or destruction of lesion or tissue of pancreas or pancreatic duct**

52.3 **Marsupialization of pancreatic cyst**

Excludes: *drainage of cyst by catheter (52.01)*

52.4 **Internal drainage of pancreatic cyst**
Pancreaticocystoduodenostomy
Pancreaticocystogastrostomy
Pancreaticocystojejunostomy

52.5 **Partial pancreatectomy**

Excludes: *pancreatic fistulectomy (52.95)*

52.51 **Proximal pancreatectomy**
Excision of head of pancreas (with part of body)
Proximal pancreatectomy with synchronous duodenectomy

52.52 **Distal pancreatectomy**
Excision of tail of pancreas (with part of body)

52.53 **Radical subtotal pancreatectomy**

52.59 **Other partial pancreatectomy**

52.6 **Total pancreatectomy**
Pancreatectomy with synchronous duodenectomy

52.7 **Radical pancreaticoduodenectomy**
One-stage pancreaticoduodenal resection with choledochojejunal anastomosis,
pancreaticojejunal anastomosis, and gastrojejunostomy
Two-stage pancreaticoduodenal resection (first stage) (second stage)
Radical resection of the pancreas
Whipple procedure

Excludes: *radical subtotal pancreatectomy (52.53)*

52.8 **Transplant of pancreas**

52.80 **Pancreatic transplant, not otherwise specified**

52.81 **Reimplantation of pancreatic tissue**

52.82 **Homotransplant of pancreas**

52.83 **Heterotransplant of pancreas**

52.84 **Autotransplantation of cells of Islets of Langerhans**
Homotransplantation of islet cells of pancreas

52.85 **Allotransplantation of cells of Islets of Langerhans**
Heterotransplantation of islet cells of pancreas

52.86 **Transplantation of cells of Islets of Langerhans, not otherwise specified**

52.9 **Other operations on pancreas**

52.92 **Cannulation of pancreatic duct**

Excludes: *that by endoscopic approach (52.93)*

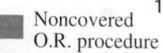

Valid O.R.
procedure

Non-O.R.
procedure

Nonspecific
O.R. procedure

Noncovered
O.R. procedure

52.93 **Endoscopic insertion of stent (tube) into pancreatic duct**
Insertion of cannula or stent into pancreatic duct by procedures classifiable to 51.10-51.11, 52.13

> Excludes: *endoscopic insertion of nasopancreatic drainage tube (52.97)*
> *replacement of stent (tube) (97.05)*

52.94 **Endoscopic removal of stone(s) from pancreatic duct**
Removal of stone(s) from pancreatic duct by procedures classifiable to 51.10-51.11, 52.13

52.95 **Other repair of pancreas**
Fistulectomy of pancreas
Simple suture of pancreas

52.96 **Anastomosis of pancreas**
Anastomosis of pancreas (duct) to:
  intestine
  jejunum
  stomach

> Excludes: *anastomosis to:*
> *bile duct (51.39)*
> *gallbladder (51.33)*

52.97 **Endoscopic insertion of nasopancreatic drainage tube**
Insertion of nasopancreatic drainage tube by procedures classifiable to 51.10-51.11, 52.13

> Excludes: *drainage of pancreatic cyst by catheter (52.01)*
> *replacement of stent (tube) (97.05)*

52.98 **Endoscopic dilation of pancreatic duct**
Dilation of Wirsung's duct by procedures classifiable to 51.10-51.11,52.13

52.99 **Other**
Dilation of pancreatic [Wirsung's] duct by open approach
Repair of pancreatic [Wirsung's] duct by open approach

> Excludes: *irrigation of pancreatic tube (96.42)*
> *removal of pancreatic tube (97.56)*

53 Repair of hernia
Includes: hernioplasty
      herniorrhaphy
      herniotomy

Code also any application or administration of an adhesion barrier substance (99.77)

> Excludes: *manual reduction of hernia (96.27)*

53.0 **Unilateral repair of inguinal hernia**

53.00 **Unilateral repair of inguinal hernia, not otherwise specified**
Inguinal herniorrhaphy NOS

53.01 **Repair of direct inguinal hernia**

53.02 **Repair of indirect inguinal hernia**

53.03 **Repair of direct inguinal hernia with graft or prosthesis**

53.04 **Repair of indirect inguinal hernia with graft or prosthesis**

53.05 **Repair of inguinal hernia with graft or prosthesis, not otherwise specified**

53.1 **Bilateral repair of inguinal hernia**

53.10 **Bilateral repair of inguinal hernia, not otherwise specified**

53.11 **Bilateral repair of direct inguinal hernia**

53.12 **Bilateral repair of indirect inguinal hernia**

53.13 **Bilateral repair of inguinal hernia, one direct and one indirect**

53.14 **Bilateral repair of direct inguinal hernia with graft or prosthesis**

53.15 **Bilateral repair of indirect inguinal hernia with graft or prosthesis**

53.16 **Bilateral repair of inguinal hernia, one direct and one indirect, with graft or prosthesis**

53.17 **Bilateral inguinal hernia repair with graft or prosthesis, not otherwise specified**

53.2 **Unilateral repair of femoral hernia**

53.21 Unilateral repair of femoral hernia with graft or prosthesis

53.29 Other unilateral femoral herniorrhaphy

53.3 Bilateral repair of femoral hernia

53.31 Bilateral repair of femoral hernia with graft or prosthesis

53.39 Other bilateral femoral herniorrhaphy

53.4 Repair of umbilical hernia

> Excludes: repair of gastroschisis (54.71)

53.41 Repair of umbilical hernia with prosthesis

53.49 Other umbilical herniorrhaphy

53.5 Repair of other hernia of anterior abdominal wall (without graft or prosthesis)

53.51 Incisional hernia repair

53.59 Repair of other hernia of anterior abdominal wall
Repair of hernia:
epigastric
hypogastric
spigelian
ventral

53.6 Repair of other hernia of anterior abdominal wall with graft or prosthesis

53.61 Incisional hernia repair with prosthesis

53.69 Repair of other hernia of anterior abdominal wall with prosthesis

53.7 Repair of diaphragmatic hernia, abdominal approach

53.8 Repair of diaphragmatic hernia, thoracic approach

53.80 Repair of diaphragmatic hernia with thoracic approach, not otherwise specified
Thoracoabdominal repair of diaphragmatic hernia

53.81 Plication of the diaphragm

53.82 Repair of parasternal hernia

53.9 Other hernia repair
Repair of hernia:
ischiatic   omental
ischiorectal   retroperitoneal
lumbar   sciatic
obturator

> Excludes: relief of strangulated hernia with exteriorization of intestine (46.01, 46.03)
> repair of pericolostomy hernia (46.42)
> repair of vaginal enterocele (70.92)

54 Other operations on abdominal region
Includes: operations on:
epigastric region   male pelvic cavity
flank   mesentery
groin region   omentum
hypochondrium   peritoneum
inguinal region   retroperitoneal tissue space
loin region

Code also any application or administration of an adhesion barrier substance (99.77)

> Excludes: female pelvic cavity (69.01- 70.92)
> hernia repair (53.00-53.9)
> obliteration of cul-de-sac (70.92)
> retroperitoneal tissue dissection (59.00-59.09)
> skin and subcutaneous tissue of abdominal wall (86.01-86.99)

54.0 Incision of abdominal wall
Drainage of:
abdominal wall
extraperitoneal abscess
retroperitoneal abscess

> Excludes: incision of peritoneum (54.95)
> laparotomy (54.11-54.19)

54.1 Laparotomy

54.11 Exploratory laparotomy

> Excludes: exploration incidental to intra-abdominal surgery—omit code

	Valid O.R. procedure		Non-O.R. procedure		Nonspecific O.R. procedure		Noncovered O.R. procedure

54.12 Reopening of recent laparotomy site
Reopening of recent laparotomy site for:
control of hemorrhage
exploration
incision of hematoma

54.19 Other laparotomy
Drainage of intraperitoneal abscess or hematoma

> Excludes: *culdocentesis (70.0)*
> *drainage of appendiceal abscess (47.2)*
> *exploration incidental to intra-abdominal surgery—omit code*
> *Ladd operation (54.95)*
> *percutaneous drainage of abdomen (54.91)*
> *removal of foreign body (54.92)*

54.2 Diagnostic procedures of abdominal region

54.21 Laparoscopy
Peritoneoscopy

> Excludes: *laparoscopic cholecystectomy (51.23)*
> *that incidental to destruction of fallopian tubes (66.21-66.29)*

54.22 Biopsy or abdominal wall or umbilicus

54.23 Biopsy of peritoneum
Biopsy of:
mesentery
omentum
peritoneal implant

> Excludes: *closed biopsy of:*
> *omentum (54.24)*
> *peritoneum (54.24)*

54.24 Closed [percutaneous] [needle] biopsy of intra-abdominal mass
Closed biopsy of:
omentum
peritoneal implant
peritoneum

> Excludes: *that of:*
> *fallopian tube (66.11)*
> *ovary (65.11)*
> *uterine ligaments (68.15)*
> *uterus (68.16)*

54.25 Peritoneal lavage
Diagnostic peritoneal lavage

> Excludes: *peritoneal dialysis (54.98)*

54.29 Other diagnostic procedures on abdominal region

> Excludes: *abdominal lymphangiogram (88.04)*
> *abdominal x-ray NEC (88.19)*
> *angiocardiography of venae cavae (88.51)*
> *C.A.T. scan of abdomen (88.01)*
> *contrast x-ray of abdominal cavity (88.11-88.15)*
> *intra-abdominal arteriography NEC (88.47)*
> *microscopic examination of peritoneal and retroperitoneal specimen*
> *(91.11-91.19)*
> *phlebography of:*
> *intra-abdominal vessels NEC (88.65)*
> *portal venous system (88.64)*
> *sinogram of abdominal wall (88.03)*
> *soft tissue x-ray of abdominal wall NEC (88.09)*
> *tomography of abdomen NEC(88.02)*
> *ultrasonography of abdomen and retroperitoneum (88.76)*

54.3 Excision or destruction of lesion or tissue of abdominal wall or umbilicus
Debridement of abdominal wall
Omphalectomy

> Excludes: *biopsy of abdominal wall or umbilicus (54.22)*
> *size reduction operation (86.83)*
> *that of skin of abdominal wall (86.22, 86.26, 86.3)*

54.4 **Excision or destruction of peritoneal tissue**
Excision of:
    appendices epiploicae
    falciform ligament
    gastrocolic ligament
    lesion of:
        mesentery
        omentum
        peritoneum
    presacral lesion NOS
    retroperitoneal lesion NOS

> Excludes: *biopsy of peritoneum (54.23)*
> *endometrectomy of cul-de-sac (70.32)*

54.5 **Lysis of peritoneal adhesions**
Freeing of adhesions of:
    biliary tract
    intestines
    liver
    pelvic peritoneum
    peritoneum
    spleen
    uterus

> Excludes: *lysis of adhesions of:*
> *bladder (59.11)*
> *fallopian tube and ovary (65.81, 65.89)*
> *kidney (59.02)*
> *ureter (59.01-59.02)*

54.51 **Laparoscopic lysis of peritoneal adhesions**

54.59 **Other lysis of peritoneal adhesions**

54.6 **Suture of abdominal wall and peritoneum**

54.61 **Reclosure of postoperative disruption of abdominal wall**

54.62 **Delayed closure of granulating abdomen wound**
Tertiary subcutaneous wound closure

54.63 **Other suture of abdominal wall**
Suture of laceration of abdominal wall

> Excludes: *closure of operative wound—omit code*

54.64 **Suture of peritoneum**
Secondary suture of peritoneum

> Excludes: *closure of operative wound—omit code*

54.7 **Other repair of abdominal wall and peritoneum**

54.71 **Repair of gastroschisis**

54.72 **Other repair of abdominal wall**

54.73 **Other repair of peritoneum**
Suture of gastrocolic ligament

54.74 **Other repair of omentum**
Epiplorrhaphy
Graft of omentum
Omentopexy
Reduction of torsion of omentum

> Excludes: *cardio-omentopexy (36.39)*

54.75 **Other repair of mesentery**
Mesenteric plication
Mesenteropexy

54.9 **Other operations of abdominal region**

> Excludes: *removal of ectopic pregnancy (69.11, 74.3)*

54.91 **Percutaneous abdominal drainage**
Paracentesis

> Excludes: *creation of cutaneoperitoneal fistula (54.93)*

54.92 **Removal of foreign body from peritoneal cavity**

54.93 **Creation of cutaneoperitoneal fistula**

| | Valid O.R. procedure | | Non-O.R. procedure | | Nonspecific O.R. procedure | | Noncovered O.R. procedure |

54.94 **Creation of peritoneovascular shunt**
Peritoneovenous shunt

54.95 **Incision of peritoneum**
Exploration of ventriculoperitoneal shunt at peritoneal site
Ladd operation
Revision of distal catheter of ventricular shunt
Revision of ventriculoperitoneal shunt at peritoneal site

Excludes: *that incidental to laparotomy (54.11-54.19)*

54.96 **Injection of air into peritoneal cavity**
Pneumoperitoneum

Excludes: *that for:*
collapse of lung (33.33)
radiography (88.12-88.13, 88.15)

54.97 **Injection of locally-acting therapeutic substance into peritoneal cavity**

Excludes: *peritoneal dialysis (54.98)*

54.98 **Peritoneal dialysis**

Excludes: *peritoneal lavage (diagnostic) (54.25)*

54.99 **Other**

Excludes: *removal of:*
abdominal wall sutures (97.83)
peritoneal drainage device (97.82)
retroperitoneal drainage device (97.81)

● Code new
to this edition
▲ Revision of
existing code
④ ⑤ Fourth or fifth
digit required

10. OPERATIONS ON THE URINARY SYSTEM (55-59)

55 Operations on kidney
Includes: operations on renal pelvis

Code also any application or administration of an adhesion barrier substance (99.77)

> Excludes: *perirenal tissue (59.00-59.09, 59.21-59.29, 59.91-59.92)*

55.0 Nephrotomy and nephrostomy

> Excludes: *drainage by:*
> *anastomosis (55.86)*
> *aspiration (55.92)*
> *incision of kidney pelvis (55.11-55.12)*

55.01 Nephrotomy
Evacuation of renal cyst
Exploration of kidney
Nephrolithotomy

55.02 Nephrostomy

55.03 Percutaneous nephrostomy without fragmentation
Nephrostolithotomy, percutaneous (nephroscopic)
Percutaneous removal of kidney stone(s) by:
basket extraction
forceps extraction (nephroscopic)
Pyelostolithotomy, percutaneous (nephroscopic)
With placement of catheter down ureter

> Excludes: *percutaneous removal by fragmentation (55.04)*
> *repeat nephroscopic removal during current episode (55.92)*

55.04 Percutaneous nephrostomy with fragmentation
Percutaneous nephrostomy with disruption of kidney stone by ultrasonic energy and
extraction (suction) through endoscope
With placement of catheter down ureter
With fluoroscopic guidance

> Excludes: *repeat fragmentation during current episode (59.95)*

55.1 Pyelotomy and pyelostomy

> Excludes: *drainage by anastomosis (55.86)*
> *percutaneous pyelostolithotomy (55.03)*
> *removal of calculus without incision (56.0)*

55.11 Pyelotomy
Exploration of renal pelvis
Pyelolithotomy

55.12 Pyelostomy
Insertion of drainage tube into renal pelvis

55.2 Diagnostic procedures on kidney

55.21 Nephroscopy

55.22 Pyeloscopy

55.23 Closed [percutaneous] [needle] biopsy of kidney
Endoscopic biopsy via existing nephrostomy, nephrotomy, pyelostomy, or
pyelotomy

55.24 Open biopsy of kidney

55.29 Other diagnostic procedures on kidney

> Excludes: *microscopic examination of specimen from kidney (91.21-91.29)*
> *pyelogram:*
> *intravenous (87.73)*
> *percutaneous (87.75)*
> *retrograde (87.74)*
> *radioisotope scan (92.03)*
> *renal arteriography (88.45)*
> *tomography:*
> *C.A.T. scan (87.71)*
> *other (87.72)*

55.3 Local excision or destruction of lesion or tissue of kidney

55.31 Marsupialization of kidney lesion

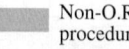 Valid O.R.
procedure

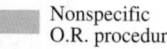 Non-O.R.
procedure

Nonspecific
O.R. procedure

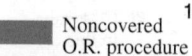 Noncovered
O.R. procedure

55.39   Other local destruction or excision of renal lesion or tissue
Obliteration of calyceal diverticulum

> *Excludes:*   *biopsy of kidney (55.23-55.24)*
> *partial nephrectomy (55.4)*
> *percutaneous aspiration of kidney (55.92)*
> *wedge resection of kidney (55.4)*

55.4   Partial nephrectomy
Calycectomy
Wedge resection of kidney
Code also any synchronous resection of ureter (56.40-56.42)

55.5   Complete nephrectomy
Code also any synchronous excision of:
bladder segment (57.6)
lymph nodes (40.3, 40.52-40.59)

55.51   Nephroureterectomy
Nephroureterectomy with bladder cuff
Total nephrectomy (unilateral)

> *Excludes:*   *removal of transplanted kidney (55.53)*

55.52   Nephrectomy of remaining kidney
Removal of solitary kidney

> *Excludes:*   *removal of transplanted kidney (55.53)*

55.53   Removal of transplanted or rejected kidney

55.54   Bilateral nephrectomy

> *Excludes:*   *complete nephrectomy NOS (55.51)*

55.6   Transplant of kidney

55.61   Renal autotransplantation

55.69   Other kidney transplantation

55.7   Nephropexy
Fixation or suspension of movable [floating] kidney

55.8   Other repair of kidney

55.81   Suture of laceration of kidney

55.82   Closure of nephrostomy and pyelostomy

55.83   Closure of other fistula of kidney

55.84   Reduction of torsion of renal pedicle

55.85   Symphysiotomy for horseshoe kidney

55.86   Anastomosis of kidney
Nephropyeloureterostomy
Pyeloureterovesical anastomosis
Ureterocalyceal anastomosis

> *Excludes:*   *nephrocystanastomosis NOS (56.73)*

55.87   Correction of ureteropelvic junction

55.89   Other

55.9   Other operations on kidney

> *Excludes:*   *lysis of perirenal adhesions (59.02)*

55.91   Decapsulation of kidney
Capsulectomy of kidney
Decortication of kidney

55.92   Percutaneous aspiration of kidney (pelvis)
Aspiration of renal cyst
Renipuncture

> *Excludes:*   *percutaneous biopsy of kidney (55.23)*

55.93   Replacement of nephrostomy tube

55.94   Replacement of pyelostomy tube

55.95   Local perfusion of kidney

55.96   Other Injection of therapeutic substance into kidney
Injection into renal cyst

● Code new
to this edition   ▲ Revision of
existing code   ④ ⑤ Fourth or fifth
digit required

55.97 Implantation or replacement of mechanical kidney

55.98 Removal of mechanical kidney

55.99 Other

> *Excludes:* *removal of pyelostomy or nephrostomy tube (97.61)*

56 Operations on ureter

Code also any application or administration of an adhesion barrier substance (99.77)

56.0 Transurethral removal of obstruction from ureter and renal pelvis
Removal of:
  blood clot from ureter or renal pelvis without incision
  calculus from ureter or renal pelvis without incision
  foreign body from ureter or renal pelvis without incision

> *Excludes:* *manipulation without removal of obstruction (59.8)*
> *that by incision (55.11, 56.2)*
> *transurethral insertion of ureteral stent for passage of calculus (59.8)*

56.1 Ureteral meatotomy

56.2 Ureterotomy
Incision of ureter for:
  drainage
  exploration
  removal of calculus

> *Excludes:* *cutting of ureterovesical orifice (56.1)*
> *removal of calculus without incision (56.0)*
> *transurethral insertion of ureteral stent for passage of calculus (59.8)*
> *urinary diversion (56.51-56.79)*

56.3 Diagnostic procedures on ureter

56.31 Ureteroscopy

56.32 Closed percutaneous biopsy of ureter

> *Excludes:* *endoscopic biopsy of ureter (56.33)*

56.33 Closed endoscopic biopsy of ureter
Cystourethroscopy with ureteral biopsy
Transurethral biopsy of ureter
Ureteral endoscopy with biopsy through ureterotomy
Ureteroscopy with biopsy

> *Excludes:* *percutaneous biopsy of ureter (56.32)*

56.34 Open biopsy of ureter

56.35 Endoscopy (cystoscopy) (looposcopy) of ileal conduit

56.39 Other diagnostic procedures on ureter

> *Excludes:* *microscopic examination of specimen from ureter (91.21-91.29)*

56.4 Ureterectomy

Code also anastomosis other than end-to-end (56.51-56.79)

> *Excludes:* *fistulectomy (56.84)*
> *nephroureterectomy (55.51-55.54)*

56.40 Ureterectomy, not otherwise specified

56.41 Partial ureterectomy
Excision of lesion of ureter
Shortening of ureter with reimplantation

> *Excludes:* *biopsy of ureter (56.32-56.34)*

56.42 Total ureterectomy

56.5 Cutaneous uretero-ileostomy

56.51 Formation of cutaneous uretero-ileostomy
Construction of ileal conduit
External ureteral ileostomy
Formation of open ileal bladder
Ileal loop operation
Ileoureterostomy (Bricker's) (ileal bladder)
Transplantation of ureter into ileum with external diversion

> *Excludes:* *closed ileal bladder (57.87)*
> *replacement of ureteral defect by ileal segment (56.89)*

| | Valid O.R. procedure | | Non-O.R. procedure | | Nonspecific O.R. procedure | | Noncovered O.R. procedure |

56.52 Revision of cutaneous uretero-ileostomy

56.6 Other external urinary diversion

56.61 Formation of other cutaneous ureterostomy
Anastomosis of ureter to skin
Ureterostomy NOS

56.62 Revision of other cutaneous ureterostomy
Revision of ureterostomy stoma

Excludes: nonoperative removal of ureterostomy tube (97.62)

56.7 Other anastomosis or bypass of ureter

Excludes: ureteropyelostomy (55.86)

56.71 Urinary diversion to intestine
Anastomosis of ureter to intestine
Internal urinary diversion NOS

Code also any synchronous colostomy (46.10-46.13)

Excludes: external ureteral ileostomy (56.51)

56.72 Revision of ureterointestinal anastomosis

Excludes: revision of external ureteral ileostomy (56.52)

56.73 Nephrocystanastomosis, not otherwise specified

56.74 Ureteroneocystostomy
Replacement of ureter with bladder flap
Ureterovesical anastomosis

56.75 Transureteroureterostomy

Excludes: ureteroureterostomy associated with partial resection (56.41)

56.79 Other

56.8 Repair of ureter

56.81 Lysis of intraluminal adhesions of ureter

Excludes: lysis of periureteral adhesions (59.01-59.02)
ureterolysis (59.01-59.02)

56.82 Suture of laceration of ureter

56.83 Closure of ureterostomy

56.84 Closure of other fistula of ureter

56.85 Ureteropexy

56.86 Removal of ligature from ureter

56.89 Other repair of ureter
Graft of ureter
Replacement of ureter with ileal segment implanted into bladder
Ureteroplication

56.9 Other operations on ureter

56.91 Dilation of ureteral meatus

56.92 Implantation of electronic ureteral stimulator

56.93 Replacement of electronic ureteral stimulator

56.94 Removal of electronic ureteral stimulator

Excludes: that with synchronous replacement (56.93)

56.95 Ligation of ureter

56.99 Other

Excludes: removal of ureterostomy tube and ureteral catheter (97.62)
ureteral catheterization (59.8)

57 Operations on urinary bladder

Code also any application or administration of an adhesion barrier substance (99.77)

Excludes: perivesical tissue (59.11-59.29, 59.91-59.92)
ureterovesical orifice (56.0-56.99)

● Code new
to this edition   ▲ Revision of
existing code   ④ ⑤ Fourth or fifth
digit required

57.0 **Transurethral clearance of bladder**
Drainage of bladder without incision
Removal of:
  blood clots from bladder without incision
  calculus from bladder without incision
  foreign body from bladder without incision

  Excludes: *that by incision (57.19)*

57.1 **Cystotomy and cystostomy**

  Excludes: *cystotomy and cystostomy as operative approach—omit code*

  57.11 **Percutaneous aspiration of bladder**

  57.12 **Lysis of intraluminal adhesion with incision into bladder**

  Excludes: *transurethral lysis of intraluminal adhesions (57.41)*

  57.17 **Percutaneous cystostomy**
  Closed cystostomy
  Percutaneous suprapubic cystostomy

  Excludes: *removal of cystostomy tube (97.63)*
  replacement of cystostomy tube (59.94)

  57.18 **Other suprapubic cystostomy**

  Excludes *percutaneous cystostomy (57.17)*
  removal of cystostomy tube (97.63)
  replacement of cystostomy tube (59.94)

  57.19 **Other cystotomy**
  Cystolithotomy

  Excludes: *percutaneous cystostomy (57.17)*
  suprapubic cystostomy (57.18)

57.2 **Vesicostomy**

  Excludes: *percutaneous cystostomy (57.17)*
  suprapubic cystostomy (57.18)

  57.21 **Vesicostomy**
  Creation of permanent opening from bladder to skin using a bladder flap

  57.22 **Revision or closure of vesicostomy**

  Excludes: *closure of cystostomy (57.82)*

57.3 **Diagnostic procedures on bladder**

  57.31 **Cystoscopy through artificial stoma**

  57.32 **Other cystoscopy**
  Transurethral cystoscopy

  Excludes: *cystourethroscopy with ureteral biopsy (56.33)*
  retrograde pyelogram (87.74)
  that for control of hemorrhage (postoperative):
    bladder (57.93)
    prostate (60.94)

  57.33 **Closed [transurethral] biopsy of bladder**

  57.34 **Open biopsy of bladder**

  57.39 **Other diagnostic procedures on bladder**

  Excludes: *cystogram NEC (87.77)*
  microscopic examination of specimen from bladder (91.31-91.39)
  retrograde cystourethrogram (87.76)
  therapeutic distention of bladder (96.25)

57.4 **Transurethral excision or destruction of bladder tissue**

  57.41 **Transurethral lysis of intraluminal adhesions**

  57.49 **Other transurethral excision or destruction of lesion or tissue of bladder**
  Endoscopic resection of bladder lesion

  Excludes: *transurethral biopsy of bladder (57.33)*
  transurethral fistulectomy (57.83-57.84)

57.5 **Other excision or destruction of bladder tissue**

  Excludes: *that with transurethral approach (57.41-57.49)*

| | Valid O.R. procedure | | Non-O.R. procedure | | Nonspecific O.R. procedure | | Noncovered O.R. procedure |

57.51 Excision of urachus
Excision of urachal sinus of bladder

> Excludes: excision of urachal cyst of abdominal wall (54.3)

57.59 Open excision or destruction of other lesion or tissue of bladder
Endometrectomy of bladder
Suprapubic excision of bladder lesion

> Excludes: biopsy of bladder (57.33-57.34)
> fistulectomy of bladder (57.83-57.84)

57.6 Partial cystectomy
Excision of bladder dome
Trigonectomy
Wedge resection of bladder

57.7 Total cystectomy
Includes: total cystectomy with urethrectomy

57.71 Radical cystectomy
Pelvic exenteration in male
Removal of bladder, prostate, seminal vesicles, and fat
Removal of bladder, urethra, and fat in a female

> Code also any:
> lymph node dissection (40.3, 40.5)
> urinary diversion (56.51-56.79)

> Excludes: that as part of pelvic exenteration in female (68.8)

57.79 Other total cystectomy

57.8 Other repair of urinary bladder

> Excludes: repair of:
> current obstetric laceration (75.61)
> cystocele (70.50-70.51)
> that for stress incontinence (59.3-59.79)

57.81 Suture of laceration of bladder

57.82 Closure of cystostomy

57.83 Repair of fistula involving bladder and intestine
Rectovesicovaginal fistulectomy
Vesicosigmoidovaginal fistulectomy

57.84 Repair of other fistula of bladder
Cervicovesical fistulectomy
Urethroperineovesical fistulectomy
Uterovesical fistulectomy
Vaginovesical fistulectomy

> Excludes: vesicoureterovaginal fistulectomy (56.84)

57.85 Cystourethroplasty and plastic repair of bladder neck
Plication of sphincter of urinary bladder
V-Y plasty of bladder neck

57.86 Repair of bladder exstrophy

57.87 Reconstruction of urinary bladder
Anastomosis of bladder with isolated segment of ileum
Augmentation of bladder
Replacement of bladder with ileum or sigmoid [closed ileal bladder]

> Code also resection of intestine (45.50-45.52)

57.88 Other anastomosis of bladder
Anastomosis of bladder to intestine NOS
Cystocolic anastomosis

> Excludes: formation of closed ileal bladder (5787)

57.89 Other repair of bladder
Bladder suspension, not elsewhere classified
Cystopexy NOS
Repair of old obstetric laceration of bladder

> Excludes: repair of current obstetric laceration (75.61)

57.9 Other operations on bladder

57.91 Sphincterotomy of bladder
Division of bladder neck

● Code new
  to this edition   ▲ Revision of
  existing code   ④ ⑤ Fourth or fifth
  digit required

57.92 Dilation of bladder neck

57.93 Control of (postoperative) hemorrhage of bladder

57.94 Insertion of indwelling urinary catheter

57.95 Replacement of indwelling urinary catheter

57.96 Implantation of electronic bladder stimulator

57.97 Replacement of electronic bladder stimulator

57.98 Removal of electronic bladder stimulator

> Excludes: *that with synchronous replacement (57.97)*

57.99 Other

> Excludes: *irrigation of:*
> *cystostomy (96.47)*
> *other indwelling urinary catheter (96.48)*
> *lysis of external adhesions (59.11)*
> *removal of:*
> *cystostomy tube (97.63)*
> *other urinary drainage device (97.64)*
> *therapeutic distention of bladder (96.25)*

58 Operations on urethra

Code also any application or administration of an adhesion barrier substance (99.77)
Includes: operations on:
bulbourethral gland [Cowper's gland]
periurethral tissue

58.0 Urethrotomy
Excision of urethral septum
Formation of urethrovaginal fistula
Perineal urethrostomy
Removal of calculus from urethra by incision

> Excludes: *drainage of bulbourethral gland or periurethral tissue (58.91)*
> *internal urethral meatotomy (58.5)*
> *removal of urethral calculus without incision (58.6)*

58.1 Urethral meatotomy

> Excludes: *internal urethral meatotomy (58.5)*

58.2 Diagnostic procedures on urethra

58.21 Perineal urethroscopy

58.22 Other urethroscopy

58.23 Biopsy of urethra

58.24 Biopsy of periurethral tissue

58.29 Other diagnostic procedures on urethra and periurethral tissue

> Excludes: *microscopic examination of specimen from urethra (91.31-91.39)*
> *retrograde cystourethrogram (87.76)*
> *urethral pressure profile (89.25)*
> *urethral sphincter electromyogram (89.23)*

58.3 Excision or destruction of lesion or tissue of urethra

> Excludes: *biopsy of urethra (58.23)*
> *excision of bulbourethral gland (58.92)*
> *fistulectomy (58.43)*
> *urethrectomy as part of:*
> *complete cystectomy (57.79)*
> *pelvic evisceration (68.8)*
> *radical cystectomy (57.71)*

58.31 Endoscopic excision or destruction of lesion or tissue of urethra
Fulguration of urethral lesion

58.39 Other local excision or destruction of lesion or tissue of urethra
Excision of:
congenital valve of urethra
lesion of urethra
stricture of urethra
Urethrectomy

> Excludes: *that by endoscopic approach (58.31)*

| | Valid O.R. procedure | | Non-O.R. procedure | | Nonspecific O.R. procedure | | Noncovered O.R. procedure |

58.4 Repair of urethra

[Excludes:] *repair of current obstetric laceration (75.61)*

58.41 Suture of laceration of urethra

58.42 Closure of urethrostomy

58.43 Closure of other fistula of urethra

[Excludes:] *repair of urethroperineovesical fistula (57.84)*

58.44 Reanastomosis of urethra
Anastomosis of urethra

58.45 Repair of hypospadias or epispadias

58.46 Other reconstruction of urethra
Urethral construction

58.47 Urethral meatoplasty

58.49 Other repair of urethra
Benenenti rotation of bulbous urethra
Repair of old obstetric laceration of urethra
Urethral plication

[Excludes:] *repair of:*
current obstetric laceration (75.61)
urethrocele (70.50-70.51)

58.5 Release of urethral stricture
Cutting of urethra] sphincter
Internal urethral meatotomy
Urethrolysis

58.6 Dilation of urethra
Dilation of urethrovesical junction
Passage of sounds through urethra
Removal of calculus from urethra without incision

[Excludes:] *urethral calibration (89.29)*

58.9 Other operations on urethra and periurethral tissue

58.91 Incision of periurethral tissue
Drainage of bulbourethral gland

58.92 Excision of periurethral tissue

[Excludes:] *biopsy of periurethral tissue (58.24)*
lysis of periurethral adhesions (59.11-59.12)

58.93 Implantation of artificial urinary sphincter [AUS]
Placement of inflatable:
bladder sphincter
urethral sphincter
Removal with replacement of sphincter device [AUS]
With pump and/or reservoir

58.99 Other
Removal of inflatable urinary sphincter without replacement
Repair of inflatable sphincter pump and/or reservoir
Surgical correction of hydraulic pressure of inflatable sphincter device

[Excludes:] *removal of:*
intraluminal foreign body from urethra without incision (98.19)
urethral stent (97.65)

59 Other operations on urinary tract
Code also any application or administration of an adhesion barrier substance (99.77)

59.0 Dissection of retroperitoneal tissue

59.00 Retroperitoneal dissection, not otherwise specified

59.02 Other lysis of perirenal or periureteral adhesions

[Excludes:] *that by laparoscope (59.03)*

59.03 Laparoscopic lysis of perirenal or periureteral adhesions

59.09 Other incision of perirenal or periureteral tissue
Exploration of perinephric area
Incision of perirenal abscess

59.1 Incision of perivesical tissue

● Code new to this edition ▲ Revision of existing code ④ ⑤ Fourth or fifth digit required

59.11 Other lysis of perivesical adhesions

59.12 Laparoscopic lysis of perivesical adhesions

59.19 Other incision of perivesical tissue
Exploration of perivesical tissue
Incision of hematoma of space of Retzius
Retropubic exploration

59.2 Diagnostic procedures on perirenal and perivesical tissue

59.21 Biopsy of perirenal or perivesical tissue

59.29 Other diagnostic procedures on perirenal tissue, perivesical tissue, and retroperitoneum

Excludes: *microscopic examination of specimen from:*
perirenal tissue (91.21-91.29)
perivesical tissue (91.31-91.39)
retroperitoneum NEC (91.11-91.19)
retroperitoneal x-ray (88.14-88.16)

59.3 Plication of urethrovesical junction
Kelly-Kennedy operation on urethra
Kelly-Stoeckel urethral plication

59.4 Suprapubic sling operation
Goebel-Frangenheim-Stoeckel urethrovesical suspension
Millin-Read urethrovesical suspension
Oxford operation for urinary incontinence
Urethrocystopexy by suprapubic suspension

59.5 Retropubic urethral suspension
Burch procedure
Marshall-Marchetti-Krantz operation
Suture of periurethral tissue to symphysis pubis
Urethral suspension NOS

59.6 Paraurethral suspension
Pereyra paraurethral suspension
Periurethral suspension

59.7 Other repair of urinary stress incontinence

59.71 Levator muscle operation for urethrovesical suspension
Cystourethropexy with levator muscle sling
Gracilis muscle transplant for urethrovesical suspension
Pubococcygeal sling

59.72 Injection of implant into urethra and/or bladder neck
Collagen implant
Endoscopic injection of implant
Fat implant
Polytef implant

59.79 Other
Anterior urethropexy
Augmentation urethroplasty
Repair of stress incontinence NOS
Tudor "rabbit ear" urethropexy

59.8 Ureteral catheterization
Drainage of kidney by catheter
Insertion of ureteral stent
Ureterovesical orifice dilation

Code also any synchronous ureterotomy (56.2)

Excludes: *that for:*
retrograde pyelogram (87.74)
transurethral removal of calculus or clot from ureter and renal pelvis (56.0)

59.9 Other operations on urinary system

Excludes: *nonoperative removal of therapeutic device (97.61-97.69)*

59.91 Excision of perirenal or perivesical tissue

Excludes: *biopsy of perirenal or perivesical tissue (59.21)*

59.92 Other operations on perirenal or perivesical tissue

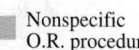 Valid O.R.
procedure

Non-O.R.
procedure

Nonspecific
O.R. procedure

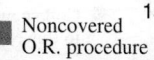 Noncovered
O.R. procedure

59.93 **Replacement of ureterostomy tube**
Change of ureterostomy tube
Reinsertion of ureterostomy tube

Excludes: *nonoperative removal of ureterostomy tube (97.62)*

59.94 **Replacement of cystostomy tube**

Excludes: *nonoperative removal of cystostomy tube (97.63)*

59.95 **Ultrasonic fragmentation of urinary stones**
Shattered urinary stones

Excludes: *percutaneous nephrostomy with fragmentation (55.04)*
shockwave disintegration (98.51)

59.99 **Other**

Excludes: *instillation of medication into urinary tract (96.49)*
irrigation of urinary tract (96.45-96.48)

● Code new
to this edition   ▲ Revision of
existing code   ④ ⑤ Fourth or fifth
digit required

11.   OPERATIONS ON THE MALE GENITAL ORGANS (60-64)

60   Operations on prostate and seminal vesicles
Includes: operations on periprostatic tissue

Code also any application or administration of an adhesion barrier substance (99.77)

Excludes: *that associated with radical cystectomy (57.71)*

60.0   Incision of prostate
Drainage of prostatic abscess
Prostatolithotomy

Excludes: *drainage of periprostatic tissue only (60.81)*

60.1   Diagnostic procedures on prostate and seminal vesicles

60.11   Closed [percutaneous] [needle] biopsy of prostate
Approach:
transrectal
transurethral
Punch biopsy

60.12   Open biopsy of prostate

60.13   Closed [percutaneous] biopsy of seminal vesicles
Needle biopsy of seminal vesicles

60.14   Open biopsy of seminal vesicles

60.15   Biopsy of periprostatic tissue

60.18   Other diagnostic procedures on prostate and periprostatic tissue

Excludes: *microscopic examination of specimen from prostate (91.31-91.39)*
x-ray of prostate (87.92)

60.19   Other diagnostic procedures on seminal vesicles

Excludes: *microscopic examination of specimen from seminal vesicles*
(91.31-91.39)
x-ray:
contrast seminal vesiculogram (87.91)
other (87.92)

60.2   Transurethral prostatectomy

Excludes: *local excision of lesion of prostate (60.61)*

60.21   Transurethral (ultrasound) guided laser induced prostatectomy (TULIP)
Ablation (contact) (noncontact) by laser

60.29   Other transurethral prostatectomy
Excision of median bar by transurethral approach
Transurethral electrovaporization of prostate (TEVAP)
Transurethral enucleative procedure
Transurethral prostatectomy NOS
Transurethral resection of prostate (TURP)

60.3   Suprapubic prostatectomy
Transvesical prostatectomy

Excludes: *local excision of lesion of prostate (60.61)*
radical prostatectomy (60.5)

60.4   Retropubic prostatectomy

Excludes: *local excision of lesion of prostate (60.61)*
radical prostatectomy (60.5)

60.5   Radical prostatectomy
Prostatovesiculectomy
Radical prostatectomy by any approach

Excludes: *cystoprostatectomy (57.71)*

60.6   Other prostatectomy

60.61   Local excision of lesion of prostate
Excision of prostatic lesion by any approach

Excludes: *biopsy of prostate (60.11-60 12)*

| | Valid O.R. procedure | | Non-O.R. procedure | | Nonspecific O.R. procedure | | Noncovered O.R. procedure |

60.62 **Perineal prostatectomy**
Cryoablation of prostate
Cryoprostatectomy
Cryosurgery of prostate
Radical cryosurgical ablation of prostate (RCSA)

> Excludes: local excision of lesion of prostate (60.61)

60.69 **Other**

60.7 **Operations on seminal vesicles**

60.71 **Percutaneous aspiration of seminal vesicle**

> Excludes: needle biopsy of seminal vesicle (60.13)

60.72 **Incision of seminal vesicle**

60.73 **Excision of seminal vesicle**
Excision of Mullerian duct cyst
Spermatocystectomy

> Excludes: biopsy of seminal vesicle (60.13-60.14)
> prostatovesiculectomy (60.5)

60.79 **Other operations on seminal vesicles**

60.8 **Incision or excision of periprostatic tissue**

60.81 **Incision of periprostatic tissue**
Drainage of periprostatic abscess

60.82 **Excision of periprostatic tissue**
Excision of lesion of periprostatic tissue

> Excludes: biopsy of periprostatic tissue (60.15)

60.9 **Other operations on prostate**

60.91 **Percutaneous aspiration of prostate**

> Excludes: needle biopsy of prostate (60.11)

60.92 **Injection into prostate**

60.93 **Repair of prostate**

60.94 **Control of (postoperative) hemorrhage of prostate**
Coagulation of prostatic bed
Cystoscopy for control of prostate hemorrhage

60.95 **Transurethral balloon dilation of the prostatic urethra**

60.96 **Transurethral destruction of prostate tissue by microwave thermotherapy**
Transurethral microwave thermotherapy (TUMT) of prostate

> Excludes: Prostatectomy:
> other (60.61-60.69)
> radical (60.5)
> retropubic (60.4)
> suprapubic (60.3)
> transurethral (60.21-60.29)

60.97 **Other transurethral destruction of prostate tissue by other thermotherapy**
Radiofrequency thermotherapy
Transurethral needle ablation (TUNA) of prostate

> Excludes: Prostatectomy:
> other (60.61-60.69)
> radical (60.5)
> retropubic (60.4)
> suprapubic (60.3)
> transurethral (60.21-60.29)

60.99 **Other**

> Excludes: prostatic massage (99.94)

61 **Operations on scrotum and tunica vaginalis**

61.0 **Incision and drainage of scrotum and tunica vaginalis**

> Excludes: percutaneous aspiration of hydrocele (61.91)

61.1 **Diagnostic procedures on scrotum and tunica vaginalis**

61.11 **Biopsy of scrotum or tunica vaginalis**

61.19 **Other diagnostic procedures on scrotum and tunica vaginalis**

● Code new
to this edition ▲ Revision of
existing code ④ ⑤ Fourth or fifth
digit required

61.2 **Excision of hydrocele (of tunica vaginalis)**
Bottle repair of hydrocele of tunica vaginalis

Excludes: percutaneous aspiration of hydrocele (61.91)

61.3 **Excision or destruction of lesion or tissue of scrotum**
Fulguration of lesion of scrotum
Reduction of elephantiasis of scrotum
Partial scrotectomy of scrotum

Excludes: biopsy of scrotum (61.11)
scrotal fistulectomy (61.42)

61.4 **Repair of scrotum and tunica vaginalis**

61.41 **Suture of laceration of scrotum and tunica vaginalis**

61.42 **Repair of scrotal fistula**

61.49 **Other repair of scrotum and tunica vaginalis**
Reconstruction with rotational or pedicle flaps

61.9 **Other operations on scrotum and tunica vaginalis**

61.91 **Percutaneous aspiration of tunics vaginalis**
Aspiration of hydrocele of tunica vaginalis

61.92 **Excision of lesion of tunica vaginalis other than hydrocele**
Excision of hematocele of tunica vaginalis

61.99 **Other**

Excludes: removal of foreign body from scrotum without incision (98.24)

62 **Operations on testes**

62.0 **Incision of testis**

62.1 **Diagnostic procedures on testes**

62.11 **Closed [percutaneous] [needle] biopsy of testis**

62.12 **Open biopsy or testis**

62.19 **Other diagnostic procedures on testes**

62.2 **Excision or destruction of testicular lesion**
Excision of appendix testis
Excision of cyst of Morgagni in the male

Excludes: biopsy of testis (62.11-62.12)

62.3 **Unilateral orchiectomy**
Orchidectomy (with epididymectomy) NOS

62.4 **Bilateral orchiectomy**
Male castration
Radical bilateral orchiectomy (with epididymectomy)
Code also any synchronous lymph node dissection (40.3, 40.5)

62.41 **Removal of both testes at same operative episode**
Bilateral orchidectomy NOS

62.42 **Removal of remaining testis**
Removal of solitary testis

62.5 **Orchiopexy**
Mobilization and replacement of testis in scrotum
Orchiopexy with detorsion of testis
Torek (-Bevan) operation (orchidopexy) (first stage) (second stage)
Transplantation to and fixation of testis in scrotum

62.6 **Repair of testes**

Excludes: reduction of torsion (63.52)

62.61 **Suture of laceration of testis**

62.69 **Other repair of testis**
Testicular graft

62.7 **Insertion of testicular prosthesis**

62.9 **Other operations on testis**

62.91 **Aspiration of testis**

Excludes: percutaneous biopsy of testis (62.11)

62.92 **Injection of therapeutic substance into testis**

62.99 **Other**

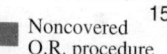

	Valid O.R. procedure		Non-O.R. procedure		Nonspecific O.R. procedure		Noncovered O.R. procedure

63   Operations on spermatic cord, epididymis, and vas deferens

63.0   Diagnostic procedures on spermatic cord, epididymis and vas deferens

63.01   Biopsy of spermatic cord, epididymis, or vas deferens

63.09   Other diagnostic procedures on spermatic cord, epididymis, and vas deferens

Excludes: *contrast epididymogram (87.93)*
contrast vasogram (87.94)
other x-ray of epididymis and vas deferens (87.95)

63.1   Excision of varicocele and hydrocele of spermatic cord
High ligation of spermatic vein
Hydrocelectomy of canal of Nuck

63.2   Excision of cyst of epididymis
Spermatocelectomy

63.3   Excision of other lesion or tissue of spermatic cord and epididymis
Excision of appendix epididymis

Excludes: *biopsy of spermatic cord or epididymis (63.01)*

63.4   Epididymectomy

Excludes: *that synchronous with orchiectomy (62.3-62.42)*

63.5   Repair of spermatic cord and epididymis

63.51   Suture of laceration of spermatic cord and epididymis

63.52   Reduction of torsion of testis or spermatic cord

Excludes: *that associated with orchiopexy (62.5)*

63.53   Transplantation of spermatic cord

63.59   Other repair of spermatic cord and epididymis

63.6   Vasotomy
Vasostomy

63.7   Vasectomy and ligation of vas deferens

63.70   Male sterilization procedure not otherwise specified

63.71   Ligation of vas deferens
Crushing of vas deferens
Division of vas deferens

63.72   Ligation of spermatic cord

63.73   Vasectomy

63.8   Repair of vas deferens and epididymis

63.81   Suture of laceration of vas deferens and epididymis

63.82   Reconstruction of surgically divided vas deferens

63.83   Epididymovasostomy

63.84   Removal of ligature from vas deferens

63.85   Removal of valve from vas deferens

63.89   Other repair of vas deferens and epididymis

63.9   Other operations on spermatic cord, epididymis and vas deferens

63.91   Aspiration of spermatocele

63.92   Epididymotomy

63.93   Incision of spermatic cord

63.94   Lysis of adhesions of spermatic cord

63.95   Insertion of valve in vas deferens

63.99   Other

64   Operations on penis
Includes: operations on:
corpora cavernosa
glans penis
prepuce

64.0   Circumcision

64.1   Diagnostic procedures on the penis

64.11   Biopsy of penis

64.19   Other diagnostic procedures on penis

● Code new
to this edition   ▲ Revision of
existing code   ④ ⑤ Fourth or fifth
digit required

64.2 **Local excision or destruction of lesion of penis**

> *Excludes:* *biopsy of penis (64.11)*

64.3 **Amputation of penis**

64.4 **Repair and plastic operation on penis**

64.41 **Suture of laceration of penis**

64.42 **Release of chordee**

64.43 **Construction of penis**

64.44 **Reconstruction of penis**

64.45 **Replantation of penis**
Reattachment of amputated penis

64.49 **Other repair of penis**

> *Excludes:* *repair of epispadias and hypospadias (58.45)*

64.5 **Operations for sex transformation, not otherwise classified.**

64.9 **Other operations on male genital organs**

64.91 **Dorsal or lateral slit of prepuce**

64.92 **Incision of penis**

64.93 **Division of penile adhesions**

64.94 **Fitting of external prosthesis of penis**
Penile prosthesis NOS

64.95 **insertion or replacement of non-inflatable penile prosthesis**
Insertion of semi-rigid rod prosthesis into shaft of penis

> *Excludes:* *external penile prosthesis (64.94)*
> *inflatable penile prosthesis (64.97)*
> *plastic repair, penis (64.43-64.49)*
> *that associated with:*
> *construction (64.43)*
> *reconstruction (64.44)*

64.96 **Removal of internal prosthesis of penis**
Removal without replacement of non-inflatable or inflatable penile prosthesis

64.97 **Insertion or replacement or inflatable penile prosthesis**
Insertion of cylinders into shaft of penis and placement of pump and reservoir

> *Excludes:* *external penile prosthesis (64.94)*
> *non-inflatable penile prosthesis (64.95)*
> *plastic repair, penis (64.43-64.49)*

64.98 **Other operations on penis**
Corpora cavernosa-corpus spongiosum shunt
Corpora-saphenous shunt
Irrigation of corpus cavernosum

> *Excludes:* *removal of foreign body:*
> *intraluminal (98.19)*
> *without incision (98.24)*
> *stretching of foreskin (99.95)*

64.99 **Other**

> *Excludes:* *collection of sperm for artificial insemination (99.96)*

	Valid O.R. procedure		Non-O.R. procedure		Nonspecific O.R. procedure		Noncovered O.R. procedure

● Code new
   to this edition

▲ Revision of
   existing code

④ ⑤ Fourth or fifth
   digit required

12. OPERATIONS ON THE FEMALE GENITAL ORGANS (65-71)

65 Operations on ovary

Code also any application or administration of an adhesion barrier substance (99.77)

65.0 Oophorotomy
Salpingo-oophorotomy

65.01 Laparoscopic oophorotomy

65.09 Other oophorotomy

65.1 Diagnostic procedures on ovaries

65.11 Aspiration biopsy of ovary

65.12 Other biopsy of ovary

65.13 Laparoscopic biopsy of ovary

65.14 Other laparoscopic diagnostic procedures on ovaries

65.19 Other diagnostic procedure on ovaries

> Excludes: *microscopic examination of specimen from ovary (91.41-91-49)*

65.2 Local excision or destruction of ovarian lesion or tissue

65.21 Marsupialization of ovarian cyst

> Excludes: *that by laparoscope (65.23)*

65.22 Wedge resection of ovary

> Excludes: *that by laparoscope (65.24)*

65.23 Laparoscopic marsupialization of ovarian cyst

65.24 Laparoscopic wedge resection of ovary

65.25 Other laparoscopic local excision or destruction of ovary

65.29 Other local excision or destruction of ovary
Bisection of ovary
Cauterization of ovary
Partial excision of ovary

> Excludes: *biopsy of ovary (65.11-65.13)*
> *that by laparoscope (65.25)*

65.3 Unilateral oophorectomy

65.31 Laparoscopic unilateral oophorectomy

65.39 Other unilateral oophorectomy

> Excludes: *that by laparoscope (65.31)*

65.4 Unilateral salpingo-oophorectomy

65.41 Laparoscopic unilateral salpingo-oophorectomy

65.49 Other unilateral salpingo-oophorectomy

65.5 Bilateral oophorectomy

65.51 Other removal of both ovaries at same operative episode
Female castration

> Excludes: *that by laparoscope (65.53)*

65.52 Other removal of remaining ovary
Removal of solitary ovary

> Excludes: *that by laparoscope (65.54)*

65.53 Laparoscopic removal of both ovaries at same operative episode

65.54 Laparoscopic removal of remaining ovary

65.6 Bilateral salpingo-oophorectomy

65.61 Other removal of both ovaries and tubes at same operative episode

> Excludes: *that by laparoscope (65.63)*

65.62 Other removal of remaining ovary and tube
Removal of solitary ovary and tube

> Excludes: *that by laparoscope (65.64)*

65.63 Laparoscopic removal of both ovaries and tubes at same operative episode

65.64 Laparoscopic removal of remaining ovary and tube

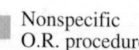

	Valid O.R. procedure		Non-O.R. procedure		Nonspecific O.R. procedure		Noncovered O.R. procedure

65.7 **Repair of ovary**

> Excludes: *salpingo-oophorostomy (66.72)*

> **65.71** **Other simple suture of ovary**
>
> > Excludes: *that by laparoscope (65.74)*

> **65.72** **Other reimplantation of ovary**
>
> > Excludes: *that by laparoscope (65.75)*

> **65.73** **Other salpingo-oophoroplasty**
>
> > Excludes: *that by laparoscope (65.76)*

> **65.74** **Laparoscopic simple suture of ovary**

> **65.75** **Laparoscopic reimplantation of ovary**

> **65.76** **Laparoscopic salpingo-oophoroplasty**

> **65.79** **Other repair of ovary**
> Oophoropexy

65.8 **Lysis of adhesions of ovary and fallopian tube**

> **65.81** **Laparoscopic lysis of adhesions of ovary and fallopian tube**

> **65.89** **Other lysis of adhesions of ovary and fallopian tube**
>
> > Excludes: *that by laparoscope (65.81)*

65.9 **Other operations on ovary**

> **65.91** **Aspiration of ovary**
>
> > Excludes: *aspiration biopsy of ovary (65.11)*

> **65.92** **Transplantation of ovary**
>
> > Excludes: *reimplantation of ovary (65.72, 65.75)*

> **65.93** **Manual rupture of ovarian cyst**

> **65.94** **Ovarian denervation**

> **65.95** **Release of torsion of ovary**

> **65.99** **Other**

66 **Operations on fallopian tubes**
 Code also any application or administration of an adhesion barrier substance (99.77)

66.0 **Salpingotomy and salpingostomy**

> **66.01** **Salpingotomy**

> **66.02** **Salpingostomy**

66.1 **Diagnostic procedures on fallopian tubes**

> **66.11** **Biopsy of fallopian tube**

> **66.19** **Other diagnostic procedures on fallopian tubes**
>
> > Excludes: *microscopic examination of specimen from fallopian tubes (91.41-91.49)*
> > *radiography of fallopian tubes (87.82-87.83, 87.85)*
> > *Rubin's test (66.8)*

66.2 **Bilateral endoscopic destruction or occlusion of fallopian tubes**
 Includes: bilateral endoscopic destruction or occlusion of fallopian tubes by:
 culdoscopy
 endoscopy
 hysteroscopy
 laparoscopy
 peritoneoscopy
 endoscopic destruction of solitary fallopian tube

> **66.21** **Bilateral endoscopic ligation and crushing of fallopian tubes**

> **66.22** **Bilateral endoscopic ligation and division of fallopian tubes**

> **66.29** **Other bilateral endoscopic destruction or occlusion of fallopian tubes**

66.3 **Other bilateral destruction or occlusion of fallopian tubes**
 Includes: destruction of solitary fallopian tube

> Excludes: *endoscopic destruction or occlusion of fallopian tubes (66.21-66.29)*

> **66.31** **Other bilateral ligation and crushing of fallopian tubes**

● Code new
 to this edition

▲ Revision of
 existing code

④ ⑤ Fourth or fifth
 digit required

66.32 Other bilateral ligation and division of fallopian tubes
Pomeroy operation

66.39 Other bilateral destruction or occlusion of fallopian tubes
Female sterilization operation NOS

66.4 Total unilateral salpingectomy

66.5 Total bilateral salpingectomy

Excludes: *bilateral partial salpingectomy for sterilization (66.39)*
that with oophorectomy (65.61-65.64)

66.51 Removal of both fallopian tubes at same operative episode

66.52 Removal of remaining fallopian tube
Removal of solitary fallopian tube

66.6 Other salpingectomy
Includes: salpingectomy by:
cauterization
coagulation
electrocoagulation
excision

Excludes: *fistulectomy (66.73)*

66.61 Excision or destruction of lesion of fallopian tube

Excludes: *biopsy of fallopian tube (66.11)*

66.62 Salpingectomy with removal of tubal pregnancy
Code also any synchronous oophorectomy (65.31, 65.39)

66.63 Bilateral partial salpingectomy, not otherwise specified

66.69 Other partial salpingectomy

66.7 Repair of fallopian tube

66.71 Simple suture of fallopian tube

66.72 Salpingo-oophorostomy

66.73 Salpingo-salpingostomy

66.74 Salpingo-uterostomy

66.79 Other repair of fallopian tube
Graft of fallopian tube
Reopening of divided fallopian tube
Salpingoplasty

66.8 Insufflation of fallopian tube
Insufflation of fallopian tube with:
air
dye
gas
saline
Rubin's test

Excludes: *insufflation of therapeutic agent (66.95)*
that for hysterosalpingography (87.82-87.83)

66.9 Other operations on fallopian tubes

66.91 Aspiration of fallopian tube

66.92 Unilateral destruction or occlusion of fallopian tube

Excludes: *that of solitary tube (66.21-66.39)*

66.93 Implantation or replacement of prosthesis of fallopian tube

66.94 Removal of prosthesis of fallopian tube

66.95 Insufflation of therapeutic agent into fallopian tubes

66.96 Dilation of fallopian tube

66.97 Burying of fimbriae in uterine wall

66.99 Other

Excludes: *lysis of adhesions of ovary and tube (65.81, 65.89)*

67 Operations on cervix
Code also any application or administration of an adhesion barrier substance (99.77)

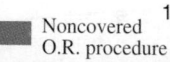

Valid O.R.
procedure

Non-O.R.
procedure

Nonspecific
O.R. procedure

Noncovered
O.R. procedure

67.0   **Dilation of cervical canal**

> *Excludes:* *dilation and curettage (69.01-69.09)*
> *that for induction of labor (73.1)*

67.1   **Diagnostic procedures on cervix**

   67.11 **Endocervical biopsy**

> *Excludes:* *conization of cervix (67.2)*

   67.12 **Other cervical biopsy**
Punch biopsy of cervix NOS

> *Excludes:* *conization of cervix (67.2)*

   67.19 **Other diagnostic procedures on cervix**

> *Excludes:* *microscopic examination of specimen from cervix (91.41-91.49)*

67.2   **Conization of cervix**

> *Excludes:* *that by:*
> *cryosurgery (67.33)*
> *electrosurgery (67.32)*

67.3   **Other excision or destruction of lesion or tissue of cervix**

   67.31 **Marsupialization of cervical cyst**

   67.32 **Destruction of lesion of cervix by cauterization**
Electroconization of cervix
LEEP (loop electrosurgical excision procedure)
LLETZ (large loop excision of the transformation zone)

   67.33 **Destruction of lesion of cervix by cryosurgery**
Cryoconization of cervix

   67.39 **Other excision or destruction of lesion or tissue of cervix**

> *Excludes:* *biopsy of cervix (67.11-67.12)*
> *cervical fistulectomy (67.62)*
> *conization of cervix (67.2)*

67.4   **Amputation of cervix**
Cervicectomy with synchronous colporrhaphy

67.5   **Repair of internal cervical os**

   67.51 **Transabdominal cerclage of cervix**

   67.59 **Other repair of internal cervical os**
Cerclage of isthmus uteri
McDonald operation
Shirodkar operation
Transvaginal cerclage

> *Excludes:* *transabdominal cerclage of cervix (67.51)*

67.6   **Other repair of cervix**

> *Excludes:* *repair of current obstetric laceration (75.51)*

   67.61 **Suture of laceration of cervix**

   67.62 **Repair of fistula of cervix**
Cervicosigmoidal fistulectomy

> *Excludes:* *fistulectomy:*
> *cervicovesical (57.84)*
> *ureterocervical (56.84)*
> *vesicocervicovaginal (57.84)*

   67.69 **Other repair of cervix**
Repair of old obstetric laceration of cervix

68 **Other incision and excision of uterus**

Code also any application or administration of an adhesion barrier substance (99.77)

68.0 **Hysterotomy**
Hysterotomy with removal of hydatidiform mole

> *Excludes:* *hysterotomy for termination of pregnancy (74.91)*

68.1   **Diagnostic procedures on uterus and supporting structures**

● Code new
  to this edition
   ▲ Revision of
    existing code
   ④ ⑤ Fourth or fifth
     digit required

68.11 Digital examination of uterus

> Excludes: *pelvic examination, so described (89.26)*
> *postpartal manual exploration of uterine cavity (75.7)*

68.12 Hysteroscopy

> Excludes: *that with biopsy (68.16)*

68.13 Open biopsy of uterus

> Excludes: *closed biopsy of uterus (68.16)*

68.14 Open biopsy of uterine ligaments

> Excludes: *closed biopsy of uterine ligaments (68.15)*

68.15 Closed biopsy of uterine ligaments
Endoscopic (laparoscopy) biopsy of uterine adnexa, except ovary and fallopian tube

68.16 Closed biopsy of uterus
Endoscopic (laparoscopy) (hysteroscopy) biopsy of uterus

> Excludes: *open biopsy of uterus (68.13)*

68.19 Other diagnostic procedures on uterus and supporting structures

> Excludes: *diagnostic:*
> *aspiration curettage (69.59)*
> *dilation and curettage (69.09)*
> *microscopic examination of specimen from uterus (91.41-91.49)*
> *pelvic examination (89.26)*
> *radioisotope scan of:*
> *placenta (92.17)*
> *uterus (92.19)*
> *ultrasonography of uterus (88.78-88.79)*
> *x-ray of uterus (87.81-87.89)*

68.2 Excision or destruction of lesion or tissue of uterus

68.21 Division of endometrial synechiae
Lysis of intraluminal uterine adhesions

68.22 Incision or excision of congenital septum of uterus

68.23 Endometrial ablation
Dilation and curettage
Hysteroscopic endometrial ablation

68.29 Other excision or destruction of lesion of uterus
Uterine myomectomy

> Excludes: *biopsy of uterus (68.13)*
> *uterine fistulectomy (69.42)*

68.3 Subtotal abdominal hysterectomy
Supracervical hysterectomy

68.4 Total abdominal hysterectomy
Hysterectomy:
extended

Code also any synchronous removal of tubes and ovaries (65.3-65.6)

68.5 Vaginal hysterectomy

Code also any synchronous:
removal of tubes and ovaries (65.31-65.64)
repair of cystocele or rectocele (70.50-70.52)
repair of pelvic floor (70.79)

68.51 Laparoscopically assisted vaginal hysterectomy (LAVH)

68.59 Other vaginal hysterectomy

> Excludes: *laparoscopically assisted vaginal hysterectomy (LAVH) (68.51)*
> *radical vaginal hysterectomy (68.7)*

68.6 Radical abdominal hysterectomy
Modified radical hysterectomy
Wertheim's operation

Code also any synchronous:
lymph gland dissection (40.3, 40.5)
removal of tubes and ovaries (65.61-65.64)

> Excludes: *pelvic evisceration (68.8)*

Valid O.R. procedure   Non-O.R. procedure   Nonspecific O.R. procedure   Noncovered O.R. procedure

68.7   **Radical vaginal hysterectomy**
Schauta operation

Code also any synchronous:
lymph gland dissection (40.3, 40.5)
removal of tubes and ovaries (65.61-65.64)

68.8   **Pelvic evisceration**
Removal of ovaries, tubes, uterus, vagina, bladder and urethra (with removal of sigmoid colon and rectum)

Code also any synchronous:
colostomy (46.12-46.13)
lymph gland dissection (40.3, 40.5)
urinary diversion (56.51-56.79)

68.9   **Other and unspecified hysterectomy**
Hysterectomy NOS

> *Excludes:*   abdominal hysterectomy, any approach (68.3, 68.4, 68.6)
> vaginal hysterectomy, any approach (68.51, 68.59, 68.7)

69   **Other operations on uterus and supporting structures**
Code also any application or administration of an adhesion barrier substance (99.77)

69.0   **Dilation and curettage of uterus**

> *Excludes:*   aspiration curettage of uterus (69.51-69.59)

   69.01   **Dilation and curettage for termination of pregnancy**

   69.02   **Dilation and curettage following delivery or abortion**

   69.09   **Other dilation and curettage**
Diagnostic D and C

69.1   **Excision or destruction of lesion or tissue of uterus and supporting structures**

   69.19   **Other excision or destruction of uterus and supporting structures**

> *Excludes:*   biopsy of uterine ligament (68.14)

69.2   **Repair of uterine supporting structures**

   69.21   **Interposition operation**
Watkins procedure

   69.22   **Other uterine suspension**
Hysteropexy
Manchester operation
Plication of uterine ligament

   69.23   **Vaginal repair of chronic inversion of uterus**

   69.29   **Other repair of uterus and supporting structures**

69.3   **Paracervical uterine denervation**

69.4   **Uterine repair**

> *Excludes:*   repair of current obstetric laceration (75.50-75.52)

   69.41   **Suture of laceration of uterus**

   69.42   **Closure of fistula of uterus**

> *Excludes:*   uterovesical fistulectomy (57.84)

   69.49   **Other repair of uterus**
Repair of old obstetric laceration of uterus

69.5   **Aspiration curettage of uterus**

> *Excludes:*   menstrual extraction (69.6)

   69.51   **Aspiration curettage of uterus for termination of pregnancy**
Therapeutic abortion NOS

   69.52   **Aspiration curettage following delivery or abortion**

   69.59   **Other aspiration curettage of uterus**

69.6   **Menstrual extraction or regulation**

69.7   **Insertion of intrauterine contraceptive device**

69.9   **Other operations on uterus, cervix, and supporting structures**

> *Excludes:*   obstetric dilation or incision of cervix (73.1, 73.93)

● Code new
to this edition   ▲ Revision of
existing code   ④ ⑤ Fourth or fifth
digit required

69.91 Insertion of therapeutic device into uterus

> *Excludes:*   insertion of:
> > *intrauterine contraceptive device (69.7)*
> > *laminaria (69.93)*
> > *obstetric insertion of bag, bougie, or pack (73.1)*

69.92 Artificial insemination

69.93 Insertion of laminaria

69.94 Manual replacement of inverted uterus

> *Excludes:*   *that in immediate postpartal period (75.94)*

69.95 Incision of cervix

> *Excludes:*   *that to assist delivery (73.93)*

69.96 Removal of cerclage material from cervix

69.97 Removal of other penetrating foreign body from cervix

> *Excludes:*   *removal of intraluminal foreign body from cervix (98.16)*

69.98 Other operations on supporting structures of uterus

> *Excludes:*   *biopsy of uterine ligament (68.14)*

69.99 Other operations on cervix and uterus

> *Excludes:*   removal of:
> > *foreign body (98.16)*
> > *intrauterine contraceptive device (97.71)*
> > *obstetric bag, bougie, or pack (97.72)*
> > *packing (97.72)*

70   Operations on vagina and cul-de-sac
Code also any application or administration of an adhesion barrier substance (99.77)

70.0 Culdocentesis

70.1 Incision of vagina and cul-de-sac

70.11 Hymenotomy

70.12 Culdotomy

70.13 Lysis of intraluminal adhesion of vagina

70.14 Other vaginotomy
Division of vaginal septum
Drainage of hematoma of vaginal cuff

70.2 Diagnostic procedures on vagina and cul-de-sac

70.21 Vaginoscopy

70.22 Culdoscopy

70.23 Biopsy of cul-de-sac

70.24 Vaginal biopsy

70.29 Other diagnostic procedures on vagina and cul-de-sac

70.3 Local excision or destruction of vagina and cul-de-sac

70.31 Hymenectomy

70.32 Excision or destruction of lesion of cul-de-sac
Endometrectomy of cul-de-sac

> *Excludes:*   *biopsy of cul-de-sac (70.23)*

70.33 Excision or destruction of lesion of vagina

> *Excludes:*   *biopsy of vagina (70.24)*
> > *vaginal fistulectomy (70.72-70.75)*

70.4 Obliteration and total excision of vagina
Vaginectomy

> *Excludes:*   *obliteration of vaginal vault (70.8)*

70.5 Repair of cystocele and rectocele

70.50 Repair of cystocele and rectocele

70.51 Repair of cystocele
Anterior colporrhaphy (with urethrocele repair)

| | Valid O.R. procedure | | Non-O.R. procedure | | Nonspecific O.R. procedure | | Noncovered O.R. procedure |

70.52 Repair of rectocele
Posterior colporrhaphy

70.6 Vaginal construction and reconstruction

70.61 Vaginal construction

70.62 Vaginal reconstruction

70.7 Other repair of vagina

> Excludes: *lysis of intraluminal adhesions (70.13)*
> *repair of current obstetric laceration (75.69)*
> *that associated with cervical amputation (67.4)*

70.71 Suture of laceration of vagina

70.72 Repair of colovaginal fistula

70.73 Repair of rectovaginal fistula

70.74 Repair of other vaginoenteric fistula

70.75 Repair of other fistula of vagina

> Excludes: *repair of fistula:*
> *rectovesicovaginal (57.83)*
> *ureterovaginal (56.84)*
> *urethrovaginal (58.43)*
> *uterovaginal (69.42)*
> *vesicocervicovaginal (57.84)*
> *vesicosigmoidovaginal (57.83)*
> *vesicoureterovaginal (56.84)*
> *vesicovaginal (57.84)*

70.76 Hymenorrhaphy

70.77 Vaginal suspension and fixation

70.79 Other repair of vagina
Colpoperineoplasty
Repair of old obstetric laceration of vagina

70.8 Obliteration of vaginal vault
LeFort operation

70.9 Other operations on vagina and cul-de-sac

70.91 Other operations on vagina

> Excludes: *insertion of:*
> *diaphragm (96.17)*
> *mold (96.15)*
> *pack (96.14)*
> *pessary (96.18)*
> *suppository (96.49)*
> *removal of:*
> *diaphragm (97.73)*
> *foreign body (98.17)*
> *pack (97.75)*
> *pessary (97.74)*
> *replacement of:*
> *diaphragm (97.24)*
> *pack (97.26)*
> *pessary (97.25)*
> *vaginal dilation (96.16)*
> *vaginal douche (96.44)*

70.92 Other operations on cul-de-sac
Obliteration of cul-de-sac
Repair of vaginal enterocele

71 Operations on vulva and perineum
Code also any application or administration of an adhesion barrier substance (99.77)

71.0 Incision of vulva and perineum

71.01 Lysis of vulvar adhesions

71.09 Other incision of vulva and perineum
Enlargement of introitus NOS

> Excludes: *removal of foreign body without incision (98.23)*

● Code new
to this edition

▲ Revision of
existing code

④ ⑤ Fourth or fifth
digit required

71.1   Diagnostic procedures on vulva

    71.11   Biopsy of vulva

    71.19   Other diagnostic procedures on vulva

71.2   Operations on Bartholin's gland

    71.21   Percutaneous aspiration of Bartholin's gland (cyst)

    71.22   Incision of Bartholin's gland (cyst)

    71.23   Marsupialization of Bartholin's gland (cyst)

    71.24   Excision or other destruction of Bartholin's gland (cyst)

    71.29   Other operations on Bartholin's gland

71.3   Other local excision or destruction of vulva and perineum
Division of Skene's gland

> Excludes: *biopsy of vulva (71.11)*
> *vulvar fistulectomy (71.72)*

71.4   Operations on clitoris
Amputation of clitoris
Clitoridotomy
Female circumcision

71.5   Radical vulvectomy
Code also any synchronous lymph gland dissection (40.3, 40.5)

71.6   Other vulvectomy

    71.61   Unilateral vulvectomy

    71.62   Bilateral vulvectomy
Vulvectomy NOS

71.7   Repair of vulva and perineum

> Excludes: *repair of current obstetric laceration (75.69)*

    71.71   Suture of laceration of vulva or perineum

    71.72   Repair of fistula of vulva or perineum

> > Excludes: *repair of fistula:*
> > *urethroperineal (58.43)*
> > *urethroperineovesical (57.84)*
> > *vaginoperineal (70.75)*

    71.79   Other repair of vulva and perineum
Repair of old obstetric laceration of vulva or perineum

71.8   Other operations on vulva

> Excludes: *removal of:*
> *foreign body without incision (98.23)*
> *packing (97.75)*
> *replacement of packing (97.26)*

71.9   Other operations on female genital organs

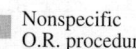
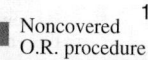

| | Valid O.R. procedure | | Non-O.R. procedure | | Nonspecific O.R. procedure | | Noncovered O.R. procedure |

● Code new
to this edition

▲ Revision of
existing code

④ ⑤ Fourth or fifth
digit required

13. OBSTETRICAL PROCEDURES (72-75)

72 Forceps, vacuum, and breech delivery

72.0 Low forceps operation
Outlet forceps operation

72.1 Low forceps operation with episiotomy
Outlet forceps operation with episiotomy

72.2 Mid forceps operation

72.21 Mid forceps operation with episiotomy

72.29 Other mid forceps operation

72.3 High forceps operation

72.31 High forceps operation with episiotomy

72.39 Other high forceps operation

72.4 Forceps rotation of fetal head
DeLee maneuver
Key-in-lock rotation
Kielland rotation
Scanzoni's maneuver
Code also any associated forceps extraction (72.0-72.39)

72.5 Breech extraction

72.51 Partial breech extraction with forceps to aftercoming head

72.52 Other partial breech extraction

72.53 Total breech extraction with forceps to aftercoming head

72.54 Other total breech extraction

72.6 Forceps application to aftercoming head
Piper forceps operation

> *Excludes:* partial breech extraction with forceps to aftercoming head (72.51)
> total breech extraction with forceps to aftercoming head (72.53)

72.7 Vacuum extraction
Includes: Malström's extraction

72.71 Vacuum extraction with episiotomy

72.79 Other vacuum extraction

72.8 Other specified instrumental delivery

72.9 Unspecified instrumental delivery

73 Other procedures inducing or assisting delivery

73.0 Artificial rupture of membranes

73.01 Induction of labor by artificial rupture of membranes
Surgical induction NOS

> *Excludes:* artificial rupture of membranes after onset of labor (73.09)

73.09 Other artificial rupture of membranes
Artificial rupture of membranes at time of delivery

73.1 Other surgical induction of labor
Induction by cervical dilation

> *Excludes:* injection for abortion (75.0)
> insertion of suppository for abortion (96.49)

73.2 Internal and combined version and extraction

73.21 Internal and combined version without extraction
Version NOS

73.22 Internal and combined version with extraction

73.3 Failed forceps
Application of forceps without delivery
Trial forceps

73.4 Medical induction of labor

> *Excludes:* medication to augment active labor—omit code

73.5 Manually assisted delivery

73.51 Manual rotation of fetal head

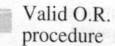 Valid O.R. procedure
 Non-O.R. procedure
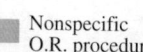 Nonspecific O.R. procedure
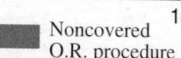 Noncovered O.R. procedure

73.59 Other manually assisted delivery
Assisted spontaneous delivery
Crede maneuver

73.6 Episiotomy
Episioproctotomy
Episiotomy with subsequent episiorrhaphy

| Excludes: | *that with:* |

high forceps (72.31)
low forceps (72.1)
mid forceps (72.21)
outlet forceps (72.1)
vacuum extraction (72.71)

73.8 Operations on fetus to facilitate delivery
Clavicotomy on fetus
Destruction of fetus
Needling of hydrocephalic head

73.9 Other operations assisting delivery

73.91 External version

73.92 Replacement of prolapsed umbilical cord

73.93 Incision of cervix to assist delivery
Dührssen's incisions

73.94 Pubiotomy to assist delivery
Obstetrical symphysiotomy

73.99 Other

| Excludes: | *dilation of cervix obstetrical, to induce labor (73.1)* |

insertion of bag or bougie to induce labor (73.1)
removal of cerclage material (69.96)

74 Cesarean section and removal of fetus
Code also any synchronous:
hysterectomy (68.3-68.4, 68.6, 68.8)
myomectomy (68.29)
sterilization (66.31-66.39, 66.63)

74.0 Classical cesarean section
Transperitoneal classical cesarean section

74.1 Low cervical cesarean section
Lower uterine segment cesarean section

74.2 Extraperitoneal cesarean section
Supravesical cesarean section

74.3 Removal of extratubal ectopic pregnancy
Removal of:
ectopic abdominal pregnancy
fetus from peritoneal or extraperitoneal cavity following uterine or tubal rupture

| Excludes: | *that by salpingostomy (66.02)* |

that by salpingotomy (66.01)
that with synchronous salpingectomy (66.62)

74.4 Cesarean section of other specified type
Peritoneal exclusion cesarean section
Transperitoneal cesarean section NOS
Vaginal cesarean section

74.9 Cesarian section of unspecified type

74.91 Hysterotomy to terminate pregnancy
Therapeutic abortion by hysterotomy

74.99 Other cesarean section of unspecified type
Cesarean section NOS
Obstetrical abdominouterotomy
Obstetrical hysterotomy

● Code new
to this edition   ▲ Revision of
existing code   ④ ⑤ Fourth or fifth
digit required

75   Other obstetric operations

75.0   Intra-amniotic injection for abortion
Injection of:
   prostaglandin for induction of abortion
   saline for induction of abortion
Termination of pregnancy by intrauterine injection

> Excludes: *insertion of prostaglandin suppository for abortion (96.49)*

75.1   Diagnostic amniocentesis

75.2   Intrauterine transfusion
Exchange transfusion in utero
Insertion of catheter into abdomen of fetus for transfusion
Code also any hysterotomy approach (68.0)

75.3   Other Intrauterine operations on fetus and amnion
Code also any hysterotomy approach (68.0)

75.31   Amnioscopy
Fetoscopy
Laparoamnioscopy

75.32   Fetal EKG (scalp)

75.33   Fetal blood sampling and biopsy

75.34   Other fetal monitoring
Fetal monitoring, not otherwise specified

> Excludes: *fetal pulse oximetry (75.38)*

75.35   Other diagnostic procedures on fetus and amnion
Intrauterine pressure determination

> Excludes: *amniocentesis (75.1)*
> *diagnostic procedures on gravid uterus and placenta (87.81, 88.46, 88.78, 92.17)*

75.36   Correction of fetal defect

75.37   Amnioinfusion
Code also injection of antibiotic (99.21)

75.38   Fetal pulse oximetry
Transcervical fetal oxygen saturation monitoring
Transcervical fetal SpO$_2$ monitoring

75.4   Manual removal of retained placenta

> Excludes: *aspiration curettage (69.52)*
> *dilation and curettage (69.02)*

75.5   Repair of current obstetric laceration of uterus

75.50   Repair of current obstetric laceration of uterus not otherwise specified

75.51   Repair of current obstetric laceration of cervix

75.52   Repair of current obstetric laceration of corpus uteri

75.6   Repair of other current obstetric laceration

75.61   Repair of current obstetric laceration of bladder and urethra

75.62   Repair of current obstetric laceration of rectum and sphincter ani

75.69   Repair of other current obstetric laceration
Episioperineorrhaphy
Repair of:
   pelvic floor
   perineum
   vagina
   vulva
Secondary repair of episiotomy

> Excludes: *repair of routine episiotomy (73.6)*

75.7   Manual exploration of uterine cavity, postpartum

75.8   Obstetric tamponade of uterus or vagina

> Excludes: *antepartum tamponade (73.1)*

75.9   Other obstetric operations

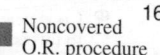

| | Valid O.R. procedure | | Non-O.R. procedure | | Nonspecific O.R. procedure | | Noncovered O.R. procedure |

75.91 Evacuation of obstetrical incision hematoma of perineum
    Evacuation of hematoma of:
      episiotomy
      perineorrhaphy

75.92 Evacuation of other hematoma of vulva or vagina

75.93 Surgical correction of inverted uterus
    Spintelli operation

> Excludes: *vaginal repair of chronic inversion of uterus (69.23)*

75.94 Manual replacement of inverted uterus

75.99 Other

  ● Code new
    to this edition
    ▲ Revision of
      existing code
    ④ ⑤ Fourth or fifth
      digit required

14. OPERATIONS ON THE MUSCULOSKELETAL SYSTEM (76-84)

76 Operations on facial bones and joints

> | Excludes: | accessory sinuses (22.00-22.9)
> nasal bones (21.00-21.99)
> skull (01.01-02.99)

76.0 Incision of facial bone without division

76.01 Sequestrectomy of facial bone
Removal of necrotic bone chip from facial bone

76.09 Other incision of facial bone
Reopening of osteotomy site of facial bone

> | Excludes: | osteotomy associated with orthognathic surgery (76.61-76.69)
> removal of internal fixation device (76.97)

76.1 Diagnostic procedures on facial bones and joints

76.11 Biopsy of facial bone

76.19 Other diagnostic procedures on facial bones and joints

> | Excludes: | contrast arthrogram of temporomandibular joint (87.13)
> other x-ray (87.11-87.12 87.14-87.16)

76.2 Local excision or destruction of lesion of facial bone

> | Excludes: | biopsy of facial bone (76.11)
> excision of odontogenic lesion (24.4)

76.3 Partial ostectomy of facial bone

76.31 Partial mandibulectomy
Hemimandibulectomy

> | Excludes: | that associated with temporomandibular arthroplasty (76.5)

76.39 Partial ostectomy of other facial bone
Hemimaxillectomy (with bone graft or prosthesis)

76.4 Excision and reconstruction of facial bones

76.41 Total mandibulectomy with synchronous reconstruction

76.42 Other total mandibulectomy

76.43 Other reconstruction of mandible

> | Excludes: | genioplasty (76.67-76.68)
> that with synchronous total mandibulectomy (76.41)

76.44 Total ostectomy of other facial bone with synchronous reconstruction

76.45 Other total ostectomy of other facial bone

76.46 Other reconstruction of other facial bone

> | Excludes: | that with synchronous total ostectomy (76.44)

76.5 Temporomandibular arthroplasty

76.6 Other facial bone repair and orthognathic surgery

Code also any synchronous:
bone graft (76.91)
synthetic implant (76.92)

> | Excludes: | reconstruction of facial bones (76.41-76.46)

76.61 Closed osteoplasty [osteotomy] of mandibular ramus
Gigli saw osteotomy

76.62 Open osteoplasty [osteotomy] of mandibular ramus

76.63 Osteoplasty [osteotomy] of body of mandible

76.64 Other orthognathic surgery on mandible
Mandibular osteoplasty NOS
Segmental or subapical osteotomy

76.65 Segmental osteoplasty [osteotomy] of maxilla
Maxillary osteoplasty NOS

76.66 Total osteoplasty [osteotomy] of maxilla

76.67 Reduction genioplasty
Reduction mentoplasty

76.68 **Augmentation genioplasty**
Mentoplasty:
NOS
with graft or implant

76.69 **Other facial bone repair**
Osteoplasty of facial bone NOS

76.7 **Reduction of facial fracture**
Includes: internal fixation

Code also any synchronous:
bone graft (76.91)
synthetic implant (76.92)

Excludes: *that of nasal bones (21.71-21.72)*

76.70 **Reduction of facial fracture, not otherwise specified**

76.71 **Closed reduction of malar and zygomatic fracture**

76.72 **Open reduction of malar and zygomatic fracture**

76.73 **Closed reduction of maxillary fracture**

76.74 **Open reduction of maxillary fracture**

76.75 **Closed reduction of mandibular fracture**

76.76 **Open reduction of mandibular fracture**

76.77 **Open reduction of alveolar fracture**
Reduction of alveolar fracture with stabilization of teeth

76.78 **Other closed reduction of facial fracture**
Closed reduction of orbital fracture

Excludes: *nasal bone (21.71)*

76.79 **Other open reduction of facial fracture**
Open reduction of orbit rim or wall

Excludes: *nasal bone (21.72)*

76.9 **Other operations on facial bones and joints**

76.91 **Bone graft to facial bone**
Autogenous graft to facial bone
Bone bank graft to facial bone
Heterogenous graft to facial bone

76.92 **Insertion of synthetic implant in facial bone**
Alloplastic implant to facial bone

76.93 **Closed reduction of temporomandibular dislocation**

76.94 **Open reduction of temporomandibular dislocation**

76.95 **Other manipulation of temporomandibular joint**

76.96 **Injection of therapeutic substance into temporomandibular joint**

76.97 **Removal of internal fixation device from facial bone**

Excludes: *removal of:*
dental wiring (97.33)
external mandibular fixation device NEC (97.36)

76.99 **Other**

77 **Incision, excision, and division of other bones**

Excludes: *laminectomy for decompression (03.09)*
operations on:
accessory sinuses (22.00-22.9)
ear ossicles (19.0-19.55)
facial bones (76.01-76.99)
joint structures (80.00-81.99)
mastoid (19.9-20.99)
nasal bones (21.00-21.99)
skull (01.01-02.99)

● Code new
to this edition
▲ Revision of
existing code
④ ⑤ Fourth or fifth
digit required

The following fourth-digit subclassification is for use with appropriate categories in section 77, marked with a symbol to identify the site. Valid fourth-digit categories are in [brackets] under each code.

0   **unspecified site**
1   **scapula, clavicle, and thorax [ribs and sternum]**
2   **humerus**
3   **radius and ulna**
4   **carpals and metacarpals**
5   **femur**
6   **patella**
7   **tibia and fibula**
8   **tarsals and metatarsals**
9   **other**
      Pelvic bones
      Phalanges (of foot) (of hand)
      Vertebrae

④ **77.0**   **Sequestrectomy**
[0-9]

④ **77.1**   **Other incision of bone without division**
[0-9]   Reopening of osteotomy site

> Excludes: *aspiration of bone marrow (41.31, 41.91)*
>   *removal of internal fixation device (78.60-78.69)*

④ **77.2**   **Wedge osteotomy**
[0-9]   > Excludes: *that for hallux valgus (77.51)*

④ **77.3**   **Other division of bone**
[0-9]   Osteoarthrotomy

> Excludes: *clavicotomy of fetus (73.8)*
>   *laminotomy or incision of vertebra (03.01-03.09)*
>   *pubiotomy to assist delivery (73.94)*
>   *sternotomy incidental to thoracic operation—omit code*

④ **77.4**   **Biopsy of bone**
[0-9]

77.5   **Excision and repair of bunion and other toe deformities**

    77.51   **Bunionectomy with soft tissue correction and osteotomy of the first metatarsal**

    77.52   **Bunionectomy with soft tissue correction and arthrodesis**

    77.53   **Other bunionectomy with soft tissue correction**

    77.54   **Excision or correction of bunionette**
        That with osteotomy

    77.56   **Repair of hammer toe**
        Fusion of hammer toe
        Phalangectomy (partial) of hammer toe
        Filleting of hammer toe

    77.57   **Repair of claw toe**
        Fusion of claw toe
        Phalangectomy (partial) of claw toe
        Capsulotomy of claw toe
        Tendon lengthening of claw toe

    77.58   **Other excision, fusion, and repair of toes**
        Cockup toe repair
        Overlapping toe repair
        That with use of prosthetic materials

    77.59   **Other bunionectomy**
        Resection of hallux valgus joint with insertion of prosthesis

④ **77.6**   **Local excision of lesion or tissue of bone**
[0-9]   > Excludes: *biopsy of bone (77.40-77.49)*
>   *debridement of compound fracture (79.60-79.69)*

④ **77.7**   **Excision of bone for graft**
[0-9]

	Valid O.R. procedure		Non-O.R. procedure		Nonspecific O.R. procedure		Noncovered O.R. procedure

④ **77.8** **Other partial ostectomy**
[0-9] Condylectomy

> Excludes: *amputation (84.00-84.19,84.91)*
> *arthrectomy (80.90-80.99)*
> *excision of bone ends associated with:*
> *arthrodesis (81.00-81.29)*
> *arthroplasty (81.51-81.59, 81.71-81.81, 81.84)*
> *excision of cartilage (80.5-80.6, 80.80-80.99)*
> *excision of head of femur with synchronous replacement (81.51-81.53)*
> *hemilaminectomy (03.01-03.09)*
> *laminectomy (03.01-03.09)*
> *ostectomy for hallux valgus (77.51-77.59)*
> *partial amputation:*
> *finger (84.01)*
> *thumb (84.02)*
> *toe (84.11)*
> *resection of ribs incidental to thoracic operation—omit code*
> *that incidental to other operation—omit code*

④ **77.9** **Total ostectomy**
[0-9]
> Excludes: *amputation of limb (84.00-84.19, 84.91)*
> *that incidental to other operation—omit code*

78 **Other operations on bones, except facial bones**

> Excludes: *operations on:*
> *accessory sinuses (22.00-22.9)*
> *facial bones (76.01-76.99)*
> *joint structures (80.00-81.99)*
> *nasal bones (21.00-21.99)*
> *skull (01.01-02.99)*

The following fourth-digit subclassification is for use with categories in section 78 to identify the site. Valid fourth-digit categories are in [brackets] under each code.

0 unspecified site
1 scapula, clavicle, and thorax (ribs and sternum)
2 humerus
3 radius and ulna
4 carpals and metacarpals
5 femur
6 patella
7 tibia and fibulas
8 tarsals and metatarsals
9 other
   Pelvic bones
   Phalanges (of foot) (of hand)
   Vertebrae

④ **78.0** **Bone graft**
[0-9] Bone:
   bank graft
   graft (autogenous) (heterogenous)
That with debridement of bone graft site (removal of sclerosed, fibrous, or necrotic bone or tissue)
Transplantation of bone
Code also any excision of bone for graft (77.70-77.79)

> Excludes: *that for bone lengthening (78.30-78.39)*

④ **78.1** **Application of external fixation device**
[0-9] Minifixator with insertion of pins/wires/screws into bone

> Excludes: *other immobilization, pressure, and attention to wound (93.51-93.59)*

④ **78.2** **Limb shortening procedures**
[0,2-5,7-9] Epiphyseal stapling
   Open epiphysiodesis
   Percutaneous epiphysiodesis
   Resection/osteotomy

④ **78.3** **Limb lengthening procedures**
[0,2-5,7-9] Bone graft with or without internal fixation devices or osteotomy
   Distraction technique with or without corticotomy/osteotomy
   Code also any application of an external fixation device (78.10-78.19)

● Code new   ▲ Revision of   ④ ⑤ Fourth or fifth
   to this edition   existing code   digit required

④ **78.4 Other repair or plastic operations on bone**
[0-9]   Other operation on bone NEC
    Repair of malunion or nonunion fracture NEC

> *Excludes:*   *application of external fixation device (78.10-78.19)*
> *limb lengthening procedures (78.30-78.39)*
> *limb shortening procedures (78.20-78.29)*
> *osteotomy (77.3)*
> *reconstruction of thumb (82.61-82.69)*
> *repair of pectus deformity (34.74)*
> *repair with bone graft (78.00-78.09)*

④ **78.5 Internal fixation of bone without fracture reduction**
[0-9]   Internal fixation of bone (prophylactic)
    Reinsertion of internal fixation device
    Revision of displaced or broken fixation device

> *Excludes:*   *arthroplasty and arthrodesis (81.00-81.85)*
> *bone graft (78.00-78.09)*
> *limb shortening procedures (78.20-78.29)*
> *that for fracture reduction (79.10-79.19, 79.30-79.59)*

④ **78.6 Removal of implanted devices from bone**
[0-9]   External fixator device (invasive)
    Internal fixation device
    Removal of bone growth stimulator (invasive)

> *Excludes:*   *removal of cast, splint, and traction device (Kirschner wire) (Steinmann pin) (97.88)*
> *removal of skull tongs or halo traction device (02.95)*

④ **78.7 Osteoclasis**
[0-9]

④ **78.8 Diagnostic procedures on bone, not elsewhere classified**
[0-9]   *Excludes:*   *biopsy of bone (77.40-77.49)*

> *magnetic resonance imaging (88.94)*
> *microscopic examination of specimen from bone (91.51-91.59)*
> *radioisotope scan (92.14)*
> *skeletal x-ray (87.21-87.29, 87.43, 88.21-88.33)*
> *thermography (88.83)*

④ **78.9 Insertion of bone growth stimulator**
(0-9)   Insertion of:
      bone stimulator (electrical) to aid bone healing
      osteogenic electrodes for bone growth stimulation
      totally implanted device (invasive)

> *Excludes:*   *non-invasive (transcutaneous) (surface) stimulator (99.86)*

79 Reduction of fracture and dislocation
    Includes: application of cast or splint
             reduction with insertion of traction device (Kirschner wire) (Steinmann pin)

Code also any application of external fixation device (78.10-78.19)

> *Excludes:*   *external fixation alone for immobilization of fracture (93.51-93.56, 93.59)*
> *internal fixation without reduction of fracture (78.50-78.59)*
> *operations on:*
>   *facial bones (76.70-76.79)*
>   *nasal bones (21.71-21.72)*
>   *orbit (76.78-76.79)*
>   *skull (02.02)*
>   *vertebrae (03.53)*
> *removal of cast or splint (97.88)*
> *replacement of cast or splint (97.11-97.14)*
> *traction alone for reduction of fracture (93.41-93.46)*

The following fourth-digit subclassification is for use with appropriate categories in section 79, marked with a symbol to identify the site. Valid fourth-digit codes are in [brackets] under each code.

    0 unspecified site
    1 humerus
    2 radius and ulna
        Arm NOS
    3 carpals and metacarpals
        Hand NOS
    4 phalanges of hand
    5 femur
    6 tibia and fibula
        Leg NOS
    7 tarsals and metatarsals
        Foot NOS
    8 phalanges of foot
    9 other specified bone

④ **79.0** **Closed reduction of fracture without internal fixation**
[0-9]   *Excludes:*   *that for separation of epiphysis (79.40-79.49)*

④ **79.1** **Closed reduction of fracture with internal fixation**
[0-9]   *Excludes:*   *that for separation of epiphysis (79.40-79.49)*

④ **79.2** **Open reduction of fracture without internal fixation**
[0-9]   *Excludes:*   *that for separation of epiphysis (79.50-79.59)*

④ **79.3** **Open reduction of fracture with internal fixation**
[0-9]   *Excludes:*   *that for separation of epiphysis (79.50-79.59)*

④ **79.4** **Closed reduction of separated epiphysis**
[0-2,5,6,9] Reduction with or without internal fixation

④ **79.5** **Open reduction of separated epiphysis**
[0-2,5,6,9] Reduction with or without internal fixation

④ **79.6** **Debridement of open fracture site**
[0-9]   Debridement of compound fracture

79.7 **Closed reduction of dislocation**
    Includes: closed reduction (with external traction device)

    Excludes: *closed reduction of dislocation of temporomandibular joint (76.93)*

    79.70 **Closed reduction of dislocation of unspecified site**
    79.71 **Closed reduction of dislocation of shoulder**
    79.72 **Closed reduction of dislocation of elbow**
    79.73 **Closed reduction of dislocation of wrist**
    79.74 **Closed reduction of dislocation of hand and finger**
    79.75 **Closed reduction of dislocation of hip**
    79.76 **Closed reduction of dislocation of knee**
    79.77 **Closed reduction of dislocation of ankle**
    79.78 **Closed reduction of dislocation of foot and toe**
    79.79 **Closed reduction of dislocation of other specified sites**

79.8 **Open reduction of dislocation**
    Includes: open reduction (with internal and external fixation devices)

    Excludes: *open reduction of dislocation of temporomandibular joint (76.94)*

    79.80 **Open reduction of dislocation of unspecified site**
    79.81 **Open reduction of dislocation of shoulder**
    79.82 **Open reduction of dislocation of elbow**
    79.83 **Open reduction of dislocation of wrist**
    79.84 **Open reduction of dislocation of hand and finger**
    79.85 **Open reduction of dislocation of hip**
    79.86 **Open reduction of dislocation of knee**
    79.87 **Open reduction of dislocation of ankle**
    79.88 **Open reduction of dislocation of foot and toe**

   ● Code new to this edition   ▲ Revision of existing code   ④ ⑤ Fourth or fifth digit required

79.89 Open reduction or dislocation of other specified sites

④ **79.9** Unspecified operation on bone injury
[0-9]

80   **Incision and excision of joint structures**
Includes: operations on:
capsule of joint
cartilage
condyle
ligament
meniscus
synovial membrane

Excludes: cartilage of:
ear (18.01-18.9)
nose (21.00-21.99)
temporomandibular joint (76.01-76.99)

The following fourth-digit subclassification is for use with appropriate categories in section 80,
that are marked with a symbol to identify the site:
0 unspecified site
1 shoulder
2 elbow
3 wrist
4 hand and finger
5 hip
6 knee
7 ankle
8 foot and toe
9 other specified sites
Spine

④ **80.0** **Arthrotomy for removal of prosthesis**
Includes: cement spacer

④ **80.1** **Other arthrotomy**
Arthrostomy

Excludes: that for:
arthrography (88.32)
arthroscopy (80.20-80.29)
injection of drug (81.92)
operative approach—omit code

④ **80.2** **Arthroscopy**

④ **80.3** **Biopsy of joint structure**
Aspiration biopsy

④ **80.4** **Division of joint capsule, ligament, or cartilage**
Goldner clubfoot release
Heyman-Herndon(-Strong) correction of metatarsus varus
Release of:
adherent or constrictive joint capsule
joint
ligament

Excludes: symphysiotomy to assist delivery (73.94)
that for:
carpal tunnel syndrome (04.43)
tarsal tunnel syndrome (04.44)

80.5 **Excision or destruction of intervertebral disc**

80.50 **Excision or destruction of intervertebral disc, unspecified**
Unspecified as to excision or destruction

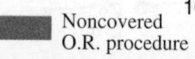

Valid O.R.
procedure

Non-O.R.
procedure

Nonspecific
O.R. procedure

Noncovered
O.R. procedure

80.51 Excision of intervertebral disc
Diskectomy
Levels:
cervical
lumbar (lumbosacral)
thoracic
Removal of herniated nucleus pulposus
That by laminotomy or hemilaminectomy
That with decompression of spinal nerve root at same level
Requires additional code for any concomitant decompression of spinal nerve root at different level from excision site

Code also any concurrent spinal fusion (81.00-81.09)

[Excludes:] *intervertebral chemonucleolysis (80.52)*
laminectomy for exploration of intraspinal canal (03.09)
laminotomy for decompression of spinal nerve root only (03.09)

80.52 Intervertebral chemonucleolysis
Injection of proteolytic enzyme into intervertebral space (chymopapain)
With aspiration of disc fragments
With diskography

[Excludes:] *injection of anesthetic substance (03.91)*
injection of other substances (03.92)

80.59 Other destruction of intervertebral disc
Destruction NEC
That by laser

80.6 Excision of semilunar cartilage of knee
Excision of meniscus of knee

④ **80.7 Synovectomy**
Complete or partial resection of synovial membrane

[Excludes:] *excision of Baker's cyst (83.39)*

④ **80.8 Other local excision or destruction of lesion of joint**

④ **80.9 Other excision of joint**

[Excludes:] *cheilectomy of joint (77.80-77.89)*
excision of bone ends (77.80-77.89)

81 Repair and plastic operations on joint structures

81.0 Spinal fusion
Includes: arthrodesis of spine with:
bone graft
internal fixation

Code also any 360 degree spinal fusion by a single incision (81.61)

Code also any insertion of interbody spinal fusion device (84.51)

Code also any insertion of recombinant bone morphogenetic protein (84.52)

[Excludes:] *correction of pseudarthrosis of spine (81.30-81.39)*
refusion of spine (81.30-81.39)

81.00 Spinal fusion, not otherwise specified

81.01 Atlas-axis spinal fusion
Craniocervical fusion by anterior transoral or posterior technique
C1-C2 fusion by anterior transoral or posterior technique
Occiput-C2 fusion by anterior transoral or posterior technique

81.02 Other cervical fusion, anterior technique
Arthrodesis of C2 level or below:
anterior (interbody) technique
anterolateral technique

81.03 Other cervical fusion, posterior technique
Arthrodesis of C2 level or below:
posterior (interbody) technique
posterolateral technique

81.04 Dorsal and dorsolumbar fusion, anterior technique
Arthrodesis of thoracic or thoracolumbar region:
anterior (interbody) technique
anterolateral technique

● Code new to this edition ▲ Revision of existing code ④ ⑤ Fourth or fifth digit required

81.05 Dorsal and dorsolumbar fusion, posterior technique
Arthrodesis of thoracic or thoracolumbar region:
posterior (interbody) technique
posterolateral technique

81.06 Lumbar and lumbosacral fusion, anterior technique
Arthrodesis of lumbar or lumbosacral region:
anterior (interbody) technique
anterolateral technique

81.07 Lumbar and lumbosacral fusion, lateral transverse process technique

81.08 Lumbar and lumbosacral fusion, posterior technique
Arthrodesis of lumbar or lumbosacral region:
posterior (interbody) technique
posterolateral technique

81.1 Arthrodesis of foot and ankle
Includes: arthrodesis of foot and ankle with:
bone graft
external fixation device

81.11 Ankle fusion
Tibiotalar fusion

81.12 Triple arthrodesis
Talus to calcaneus and calcaneus to cuboid and navicular

81.13 Subtalar fusion

81.14 Midtarsal fusion

81.15 Tarsometatarsal fusion

81.16 Metatarsophalangeal fusion

81.17 Other fusion of foot

81.2 Arthrodesis of other joint
Includes: arthrodesis with:
bone graft
external fixation device
excision of bone ends and compression

81.20 Arthrodesis of unspecified joint

81.21 Arthrodesis of hip

81.22 Arthrodesis of knee

81.23 Arthrodesis of shoulder

81.24 Arthrodesis of elbow

81.25 Carporadial fusion

81.26 Metacarpocarpal fusion

81.27 Metacarpophalangeal fusion

81.28 Interphalangeal fusion

81.29 Arthrodesis of other specified joints

81.3 Refusion of spine
Includes: arthrodesis of spine with:
bone graft
internal fixation
correction of pseudarthrosis of spine
Code also any 360 degree spinal fusion by a single incision (81.61)
Code also any insertion of interbody spinal fusion device (84.51)
Code also any insertion of recombinant bone morphogenetic protein (84.52)

81.30 Refusion of spine, not otherwise specified

81.31 Refusion of atlas-axis spine
Craniocervical fusion by anterior, transoral or posterior technique
C1-C2 fusion by anterior, transoral or posterior technique
Occiput C2 fusion by anterior, transoral or posterior technique

81.32 Refusion of other cervical spine, anterior technique
Arthrodesis of C2 level or below:
anterior (interbody) technique
anterolateral technique

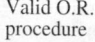 Valid O.R.
procedure

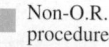 Non-O.R.
procedure

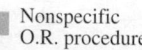 Nonspecific
O.R. procedure

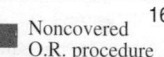 Noncovered
O.R. procedure

81.33 Refusion of other cervical spine, posterior technique
Arthrodesis of C2 level or below:
   posterior (interbody) technique
   posterolateral technique

81.34 Refusion of dorsal and dorsolumbar spine, anterior technique
Arthrodesis of thoracic or thoracolumbar region:
   anterior (interbody) technique
   anterolateral technique

81.35 Refusion of dorsal and dorsolumbar spine, posterior technique
Arthrodesis of thoracic and thoracolumbar region:
   posterior (interbody) technique
   posterolateral technique

81.36 Refusion of lumbar and lumbosacral spine, anterior technique
Arthrodesis of lumbar or lumbosacral region:
   anterior (interbody) technique
   anterolateral technique

81.37 Refusion of lumbar and lumbosacral spine, lateral transverse process technique

81.38 Refusion of lumbar and lumbosacral spine, posterior technique
Arthrodesis of lumbar or lumbosacral region:
   posterior (interbody) technique
   posterolateral technique

81.39 Refusion of spine, not elsewhere classified

81.4 Other repair of joint of lower extremity
Includes: arthroplasty of lower extremity with:
      external traction or fixation
      graft of bone chips or cartilage
      internal fixation device

81.40 Repair of hip, not elsewhere classified

81.42 Five-in-one repair of knee
Medial meniscectomy, medial collateral ligament repair, vastus medialis
   advancement, semitendinosus advancement, and pes anserinus transfer

81.43 Triad knee repair
Medial meniscectomy with repair of the anterior cruciate ligament and the medial
   collateral ligament
O'Donoghue procedure

81.44 Patellar stabilization
Roux-Goldthwait operation for recurrent dislocation of patella

81.45 Other repair of the cruciate ligaments

81.46 Other repair of the collateral ligaments

81.47 Other repair of knee

81.49 Other repair of ankle

81.5 Joint replacement of lower extremity
Includes: arthroplasty of lower extremity with:
      external traction or fixation
      graft of bone (chips) or cartilage
      internal fixation device or prosthesis
      removal of cement spacer

81.51 Total hip replacement
Replacement of both femoral head and acetabulum by prosthesis
Total reconstruction of hip

81.52 Partial hip replacement
Bipolar endoprosthesis

81.53 Revision of hip replacement
Partial
Total

81.54 Total knee replacement
Bicompartmental
Tricompartmental
Unicompartmental (hemijoint)

81.55 Revision of knee replacement
Excludes: arthrodesis of knee (81.22)

81.56 Total ankle replacement

  ● Code new
   to this edition
     ▲ Revision of
      existing code
     ④ ⑤ Fourth or fifth
       digit required

81.57 Replacement of joint of foot and toe

81.59 Revision of joint replacement of lower extremity, not elsewhere classified

● **81.6** Other procedures on spine

● **81.61** 360 degree spinal fusion, single incision approach
That by a single incision but fusing or refusing both anterior and posterior spine
Code also refusion of spine (81.30-81.39)
Code also spinal fusion (81.00-81.08)

81.7 Arthroplasty and repair of hand, fingers, and wrist
Includes: arthroplasty of hand and finger with:
external traction or fixation
graft of bone (chips) or cartilage
internal fixation device or prosthesis

| Excludes: | *operations on muscle, tendon, and fascia of hand (82.01-82.99)* |

81.71 Arthroplasty of metacarpophalangeal and interphalangeal joint with implant

81.72 Arthroplasty of metacarpophalangeal and interphalangeal joint without implant

81.73 Total wrist replacement

81.74 Arthroplasty of carpocarpal or carpometacarpal joint with implant

81.75 Arthroplasty of carpocarpal or carpometacarpal joint without implant

81.79 Other repair of hand, fingers, and wrist

81.8 Arthroplasty and repair of shoulder and elbow
Includes: arthroplasty of upper limb NEC with:
external traction or fixation
graft of bone (chips) or cartilage
internal fixation device or prosthesis

81.80 Total shoulder replacement

81.81 Partial shoulder replacement

81.82 Repair of recurrent dislocation of shoulder

81.83 Other repair of shoulder
Revision of arthroplasty of shoulder

81.84 Total elbow replacement

81.85 Other repair of elbow

81.9 Other operations on joint structures

81.91 Arthrocentesis
Joint aspiration

| Excludes: | *that for:*
arthrography (88.32)
biopsy of joint structure (80.30-80.39)
injection of drug (81.92) |

81.92 Injection of therapeutic substance into joint or ligament

81.93 Suture of capsule or ligament of upper extremity

| Excludes: | *that associated with arthroplasty (81.71-81.75, 81.80-81.81, 81.84)* |

81.94 Suture of capsule or ligament of ankle and foot

| Excludes: | *that associated with arthroplasty (81.56-81.59)* |

81.95 Suture of capsule or ligament of other lower extremity

| Excludes: | *that associated with arthroplasty (81.51-81.55, 81.59)* |

81.96 Other repair of joint

81.97 Revision of joint replacement of upper extremity
Partial
Total
Includes: removal of cement spacer

81.98 Other diagnostic procedures on joint structures

| Excludes: | *arthroscopy (80.20-80.29)*
biopsy of joint structure (80.30-80.39)
microscopic examination of specimen from joint (91.51-91.59)
thermography (88.83)
x-ray (87.21-87.29, 88.21-88.33) |

81.99 Other

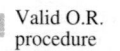 Valid O.R. procedure

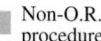 Non-O.R. procedure

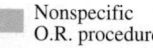 Nonspecific O.R. procedure

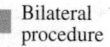 Bilateral procedure

82   Operations on muscle, tendon, and fascia of hand

Includes: operations on:
aponeurosis
synovial membrane (tendon sheath)
tendon sheath

82.0   Incision of muscle, tendon, fascia, and bursa of hand

82.01   Exploration of tendon sheath of hand
Incision of tendon sheath of hand
Removal of rice bodies in tendon sheath of hand

> *Excludes:*   *division of tendon (82.11)*

82.02   Myotomy of hand

> *Excludes:*   *myotomy for division (82.19)*

82.03   Bursotomy of hand

82.04   Incision and drainage of palmar or thenar space

82.09   Other incision of soft tissue of hand

> *Excludes:*   *incision of skin and subcutaneous tissue alone (86.01-86.09)*

82.1   Division of muscle, tendon, and fascia of hand

82.11   Tenotomy of hand
Division of tendon of hand

82.12   Fasciotomy of hand
Division of fascia of hand

82.19   Other division of soft tissue of hand
Division of muscle of hand

82.2   Excision of lesion of muscle, tendon, and fascia of hand

82.21   Excision of lesion of tendon sheath of hand
Ganglionectomy of tendon sheath (wrist)

82.22   Excision of lesion of muscle of hand

82.29   Excision of other lesion of soft tissue of hand

> *Excludes:*   *excision of lesion of skin and subcutaneous tissue (86.21-86.3)*

82.3   Other excision of soft tissue of hand
Code also any skin graft (86.61-86.62, 86.73)

> *Excludes:*   *excision of skin and subcutaneous tissue (86.21-86.3)*

82.31   Bursectomy of hand

82.32   Excision of tendon of hand for graft

82.33   Other tenonectomy of hand
Tenosynovectomy of hand

> *Excludes:*   *excision of lesion of:*
> *tendon (82.29)*
> *sheath (82.21)*

82.34   Excision of muscle or fascia of hand for graft

82.35   Other fasciectomy of hand
Release of Dupuytren's contracture

> *Excludes:*   *excision of lesion of fascia (82.29)*

82.36 Other myectomy of hand

> *Excludes:*   *excision of lesion of muscle (82.22)*

82.39 Other excision of soft tissue of hand

> *Excludes:*   *excision of skin (86.21-86.3)*
> *excision of soft tissue lesion (82.29)*

82.4   Suture of muscle, tendon, and fascia of hand

82.41   Suture of tendon sheath of hand

82.42   Delayed suture of flexor tendon of hand

82.43   Delayed suture of other tendon of hand

82.44   Other suture of flexor tendon of hand

> *Excludes:*   *delayed suture of flexor tendon of hand (82.42)*

● Code new
to this edition   ▲ Revision of
existing code   ④ ⑤ Fourth or fifth
digit required

82.45 Other suture of other tendon of hand

> Excludes: delayed suture of other tendon of hand (82.43)

82.46 Suture of muscle or fascia of hand

82.5 Transplantation of muscle and tendon of hand

82.51 Advancement of tendon of hand

82.52 Recession of tendon of hand

82.53 Reattachment of tendon of hand

82.54 Reattachment of muscle of hand

82.55 Other change in hand muscle or tendon length

82.56 Other hand tendon transfer or transplantation

> Excludes: pollicization of thumb (82.61)
> transfer of finger, except thumb (82.81)

82.57 Other hand tendon transposition

82.58 Other hand muscle transfer or transplantation

82.59 Other hand muscle transposition

82.6 Reconstruction of thumb

Includes: digital transfer to act as thumb

Code also any amputation for digital transfer (84.01, 84.11)

82.61 Pollicization operation carrying over nerves and blood supply

82.69 Other reconstruction of thumb

"Cocked-hat" procedure [skin flap and bone]
Grafts:
bone to thumb
skin (pedicle) to thumb

82.7 Plastic operation on hand with graft or implant

82.71 Tendon pulley reconstruction

Reconstruction for opponensplasty

82.72 Plastic operation on hand with graft of muscle or fascia

82.79 Plastic operation on hand with other graft or implant

Tendon graft to hand

82.8 Other plastic operations on hand

82.81 Transfer of finger, except thumb

> Excludes: pollicization of thumb (82.61)

82.82 Repair of cleft hand

82.83 Repair of macrodactyly

82.84 Repair of mallet finger

82.85 Other tenodesis of hand

Tendon fixation of hand NOS

82.86 Other tenoplasty of hand

Myotenoplasty of hand

82.89 Other plastic operations on hand

Plication of fascia
Repair of fascial hernia

> Excludes: that with graft or implant (82.71-82.79)

82.9 Other operations on muscle, tendon, and fascia of hand

> Excludes: diagnostic procedures on soft tissue of hand (83.21-83.29)

82.91 Lysis of adhesions of hand

Freeing of adhesions of fascia, muscle, and tendon of hand

> Excludes: decompression of carpal tunnel (04.43)
> that by stretching or manipulation only (93.26)

82.92 Aspiration of bursa of hand

82.93 Aspiration of other soft tissue of hand

> Excludes: skin and subcutaneous tissue (86.01)

82.94 Injection of therapeutic substance into bursa of hand

82.95 Injection of therapeutic substance into tendon of hand

Valid O.R.
procedure

Non-O.R.
procedure

Nonspecific
O.R. procedure

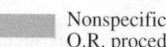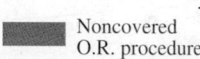

Noncovered
O.R. procedure

82.96 Other injection of locally-acting therapeutic substance into soft tissue of hand

> Excludes: *subcutaneous or intramuscular injection (99.11-99.29)*

82.99 Other operations on muscle, tendon, and fascia of hand

83 **Operations on muscle, tendon, fascia, and bursa, except hand**

Includes: operations on:
aponeurosis
synovial membrane of bursa and tendon sheaths
tendon sheaths

> Excludes: *diaphragm (34.81-34.89)*
> *hand (82.01-82.99)*
> *muscles of eye (15.01-15.9).*

83.0 Incision of muscle, tendon, fascia, and bursa

83.01 Exploration of tendon sheath
Incision of tendon sheath
Removal of rice bodies from tendon sheath

83.02 Myotomy

> Excludes: *cricopharyngeal myotomy (29.31)*

83.03 Bursotomy
Removal of calcareous deposit of bursa

> Excludes: *aspiration of bursa (percutaneous) (83.94)*

83.09 Other incision of soft tissue
Incision of fascia

> Excludes: *incision of skin and subcutaneous tissue alone (86.01-86.09)*

83.1 Division of muscle, tendon, and fascia

83.11 Achillotenotomy

83.12 Adductor tenotomy of hip

83.13 Other tenotomy
Aponeurotomy
Division of tendon
Tendon release
Tendon transection
Tenotomy for thoracic outlet decompression

83.14 Fasciotomy
Division of fascia
Division of iliotibial band
Fascia stripping
Release of Volkmann's contracture by fasciotomy

83.19 Other division of soft tissue
Division of muscle
Muscle release
Myotomy for thoracic outlet decompression
Myotomy with division
Scalenotomy
Transection of muscle

83.2 Diagnostic procedures on muscle, tendon, fascia, and bursa, including that of hand

83.21 Biopsy of soft tissue

> Excludes: *biopsy of chest wall (34.23)*
> *biopsy of skin and subcutaneous tissue (86.11)*

83.29 Other diagnostic procedures on muscle, tendon, fascia, and bursa, including that of hand

> Excludes: *microscopic examination of specimen (91.51-91.59)*
> *soft tissue x-ray (87.09, 87.38-87.39, 88.09, 88.35, 88.37)*
> *thermography of muscle (88.84)*

83.3 Excision of lesion of muscle, tendon, fascia, and bursa

> Excludes: *biopsy of soft tissue (83.21)*

83.31 Excision of lesion of tendon sheath
Excision of ganglion of tendon sheath, except of hand

● Code new
to this edition ▲ Revision of
existing code ④ ⑤ Fourth or fifth
digit required

83.32 **Excision of lesion of muscle**
Excision of:
heterotopic bone
muscle scar for release of Volkmann's contracture
myositis ossificans

83.39 **Excision of lesion of other soft tissue**
Excision of Baker's cyst

> Excludes: bursectomy (83.5)
> excision of lesion of skin and subcutaneous tissue (86.3)
> synovectomy (80.70-80.79)

83.4 **Other excision of muscle, tendon, and fascia**

83.41 **Excision of tendon for graft**

83.42 **Other tenonectomy**
Excision of:
aponeurosis
tendon sheath
Tenosynovectomy

83.43 **Excision of muscle or fascia for graft**

83.44 **Other fasciectomy**

83.45 **Other myectomy**
Debridement of muscle NOS
Scalenectomy

83.49 **Other excision of soft tissue**

83.5 **Bursectomy**

83.6 **Suture of muscle, tendon, and fascia**

83.61 **Suture of tendon sheath**

83.62 **Delayed suture of tendon**

83.63 **Rotator cuff repair**

83.64 **Other suture of tendon**
Achillorrhaphy
Aponeurorrhaphy

> Excludes: delayed suture of tendon (83.62)

83.65 **Other suture of muscle or fascia**
Repair of diastasis recti

83.7 **Reconstruction of muscle and tendon**

> Excludes: reconstruction of muscle and tendon associated with arthroplasty

83.71 **Advancement of tendon**

83.72 **Recession of tendon**

83.73 **Reattachment of tendon**

83.74 **Reattachment of muscle**

83.75 **Tendon transfer or transplantation**

83.76 **Other tendon transposition**

83.77 **Muscle transfer or transplantation**
Release of Volkmann's contracture by muscle transplantation

83.79 **Other muscle transposition**

83.8 **Other plastic operations on muscle, tendon, and fascia**

> Excludes: plastic operations on muscle, tendon, and fascia associated with arthroplasty

83.81 **Tendon graft**

83.82 **Graft of muscle or fascia**

83.83 **Tendon pulley reconstruction**

83.84 **Release of clubfoot, not elsewhere classified**
Evans operation on clubfoot

83.85 **Other change in muscle or tendon length**
Hamstring lengthening
Heel cord shortening
Plastic achillotenotomy
Tendon plication

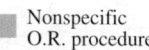 Valid O.R.
procedure

Non-O.R.
procedure

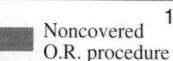 Nonspecific
O.R. procedure

Noncovered
O.R. procedure

83.86 Quadricepsplasty

83.87 **Other plastic operations on muscle**
Musculoplasty
Myoplasty

83.88 **Other plastic operations on tendon**
Myotenoplasty
Tendon fixation
Tenodesis
Tenoplasty

83.89 **Other plastic operations on fascia**
Fascia lengthening
Fascioplasty
Plication of fascia

83.9 **Other operations on muscle, tendon, fascia, and bursa**

| Excludes: | nonoperative:
manipulation (93.25-93.29)
stretching (93.27-93.29)

83.91 **Lysis of adhesions of muscle, tendon, fascia,and bursa**

| Excludes: | that for tarsal tunnel syndrome (04.44)

83.92 **Insertion or replacement of skeletal muscle stimulator**
Implantation, insertion, placement, or replacement of skeletal muscle:
electrodes
stimulator

83.93 **Removal of skeletal muscle stimulator**

83.94 **Aspiration of bursa**

83.95 **Aspiration of other soft tissue**

| Excludes: | that of skin and subcutaneous tissue (86.01)

83.96 **Injection of therapeutic substance into bursa**

83.97 **Injection of therapeutic substance into tendon**

83.98 **Injection of locally-acting therapeutic substance into other soft tissue**

| Excludes: | subcutaneous or intramuscular injection (99.11-99.29)

83.99 **Other operations on muscle, tendon, fascia and bursa**
Suture of bursa

84 **Other procedures on musculoskeletal system**

84.0 **Amputation of upper limb**

| Excludes: | revision of amputation stump (84.3)

84.00 **Upper limb amputation, not otherwise specified**
Closed flap amputation of upper limb NOS
Kineplastic amputation of upper limb NOS
Open or guillotine amputation of upper limb NOS
Revision of current traumatic amputation of upper limb NOS

84.01 **Amputation and disarticulation of finger**

| Excludes: | ligation of supernumerary finger (86.26)

84.02 **Amputation and disarticulation of thumb**

84.03 **Amputation through hand**
Amputation through carpals

84.04 **Disarticulation of wrist**

84.05 **Amputation through forearm**
Forearm amputation

84.06 **Disarticulation of elbow**

84.07 **Amputation through humerus**
Upper arm amputation

84.08 **Disarticulation of shoulder**

84.09 **Interthoracoscapular amputation**
Forequarter amputation

84.1 **Amputation of lower limb**

● Code new
  to this edition
▲ Revision of
  existing code
④ ⑤ Fourth or fifth
  digit required

> *Excludes:* revision of amputation stump (84.3)

84.10 Lower limb amputation, not otherwise specified
Closed flap amputation of lower limb NOS
Kineplastic amputation of lower limb NOS
Open or guillotine amputation of lower limb NOS
Revision of current traumatic amputation of lower limb NOS

84.11 Amputation of toe
Amputation through metatarsophalangeal joint
Disarticulation of toe
Metatarsal head amputation
Ray amputation of foot (disarticulation of the metatarsal head of the toe extending
across the forefoot just proximal to the metatarsophalangeal crease)

> *Excludes:* ligation of supernumerary toe (86.26)

84.12 Amputation through foot
Amputation of forefoot
Amputation through middle of foot
Chopart's amputation
Midtarsal amputation
Transmetatarsal amputation (amputation of the forefoot, including all the toes)

> *Excludes:* ray amputation of foot (84.11)

84.13 Disarticulation of ankle

84.14 Amputation of ankle through malleoli of tibia and fibula

84.15 Other amputation below knee
Amputation of leg through tibia and fibula NOS

84.16 Disarticulation of knee
Batch, Spitler, and McFaddin amputation
Mazet amputation
S.P. Roger's amputation

84.17 Amputation above knee
Amputation of leg through femur
Amputation of thigh
Conversion of below-knee amputation into above-knee amputation
Supracondylar above-knee amputation

84.18 Disarticulation of hip

84.19 Abdominopelvic amputation
Hemipelvectomy
Hindquarter amputation

84.2 Reattachment of extremity

84.21 Thumb reattachment

84.22 Finger reattachment

84.23 Forearm, wrist, or hand reattachment

84.24 Upper arm reattachment
Reattachment of arm NOS

84.25 Toe reattachment

84.26 Foot reattachment

84.27 Lower leg or ankle reattachment
Reattachment of leg NOS

84.28 Thigh reattachment

84.29 Other reattachment

84.3 Revision of amputation stump
Reamputation of stump
Secondary closure of stump
Trimming of stump

> *Excludes:* revision of current traumatic amputation [revision by further amputation of
> current injury] (84.00-84.19, 84.91)

84.4 Implantation or fitting of prosthetic limb device

84.40 Implantation or fitting of prosthetic limb device not otherwise specified

84.41 Fitting of prosthesis of upper arm and shoulder

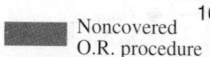

| Valid O.R. procedure | Non-O.R. procedure | Nonspecific O.R. procedure | Noncovered O.R. procedure |

84.42 **Fitting of prosthesis of lower arm and hand**

84.43 **Fitting of prosthesis of arm, not otherwise specified**

84.44 **Implantation of prosthetic device of arm**

84.45 **Fitting of prosthesis above knee**

84.46 **Fitting of prosthesis below knee**

84.47 **Fitting of prosthesis of leg, not otherwise specified**

84.48 **Implantation of prosthetic device of leg**

● 84.5 **Implantation of other musculoskeletal devices and substances**

● 84.51 **Insertion of interbody spinal fusion device**
Insertion of:
cages (carbon, ceramic, metal, plastic, or titanium)
interbody fusion cage
synthetic cages or spacers
threaded bone dowels

Code also refusion of spine (81.30-81.39)

Code also spinal fusion (81.00-81.08)

● 84.52 **Insertion of recombinant bone morphogenetic protein rhBMP**
That via collagen sponge, coral, ceramic and other carriers

Code also primary procedure performed:
fracture repair (79.00-79.99)
spinal fusion (81.00-81.08)
spinal refusion (81.30-81.39)

84.9 **Other operations on musculoskeletal system**

Excludes: *nonoperative manipulation (93.25-93.29)*

84.91 **Amputation, not otherwise specified**

84.92 **Separation of equal conjoined twins**

84.93 **Separation of unequal conjoined twins**
Separation of conjoined twins NOS

84.99 **Other**

● Code new
to this edition

▲ Revision of
existing code

④ ⑤ Fourth or fifth
digit required

15. OPERATIONS ON THE INTEGUMENTARY SYSTEM (85-86)

85 Operations on the breast

Includes: operations on the skin and subcutaneous tissue of:
> breast, female or male
> previous mastectomy site, female or male
> revision of previous mastectomy site, female or male

85.0 Mastotomy
Incision of breast (skin)
Mammotomy

> Excludes: aspiration of breast (85.91)
> removal of implant (85.94)

85.1 Diagnostic procedures on breast

85.11 Closed [percutaneous] [needle] biopsy of breast

85.12 Open biopsy of breast

85.19 Other diagnostic procedures on breast

> Excludes: mammary ductogram (87.35)
> mammography NEC (87.37)
> manual examination (89.36)
> microscopic examination of specimen (91.61-91.69)
> thermography (88.85)
> ultrasonography (88.73)
> xerography (87.36)

85.2 Excision or destruction of breast tissue

> Excludes: mastectomy (85.41-85.48)
> reduction mammoplasty (85.31-85.32)

85.20 Excision or destruction of breast tissue, not otherwise specified

85.21 Local excision of lesion of breast
Lumpectomy
Removal of area of fibrosis from breast

> Excludes: biopsy of breast (85.11-8.5.12)

85.22 Resection of quadrant of breast

85.23 Subtotal mastectomy

> Excludes: quadrant resection (85.22)

85.24 Excision of ectopic breast tissue
Excision of accessory nipple

85.25 Excision of nipple

> Excludes: excision of accessory nipple (85.24)

85.3 Reduction mammoplasty and subcutaneous mammectomy

85.31 Unilateral reduction mammoplasty
Unilateral:
> amputative mammoplasty
> size reduction mammoplasty

85.32 Bilateral reduction mammoplasty
Amputative mammoplasty
Reduction mammoplasty (for gynecomastia)

85.33 Unilateral subcutaneous mammectomy with synchronous implant

> Excludes: that without synchronous implant (85.34)

85.34 Other unilateral subcutaneous mammectomy
Removal of breast tissue with preservation of skin and nipple
Subcutaneous mammectomy NOS

85.35 Bilateral subcutaneous mammectomy with synchronous implant

> Excludes: that without synchronous implant (85.36)

85.36 Other bilateral subcutaneous mammectomy

85.4 Mastectomy

85.41 Unilateral simple mastectomy
Mastectomy:
NOS
complete

85.42 Bilateral simple mastectomy
Bilateral complete mastectomy

85.43 Unilateral extended simple mastectomy
Extended simple mastectomy NOS
Modified radical mastectomy
Simple mastectomy with excision of regional lymph nodes

85.44 Bilateral extended simple mastectomy

85.45 Unilateral radical mastectomy
Excision of breast, pectoral muscles, and regional lymph nodes [axillary, clavicular, supraclavicular]
Radical mastectomy NOS

85.46 Bilateral radical mastectomy

85.47 Unilateral extended radical mastectomy
Excision of breast, muscles, and lymph nodes [axillary, clavicular, supraclavicular, internal mammary, and mediastinal]
Extended radical mastectomy NOS

85.48 Bilateral extended radical mastectomy

85.5 Augmentation mammoplasty

Excludes: *that associated with subcutaneous mammectomy (85.33, 85.35)*

85.50 Augmentation mammoplasty, not otherwise specified

85.51 Unilateral injection into breast for augmentation

85.52 Bilateral injection into breast for augmentation
Injection into breast for augmentation NOS

85.53 Unilateral breast implant

85.54 Bilateral breast implant
Breast implant NOS

85.6 Mastopexy

85.7 Total reconstruction of breast

85.8 Other repair and plastic operations on breast

Excludes: *that for:*
augmentation (85.50-85.54)
reconstruction (85.7)
reduction (85.31-85.32)

85.81 Suture of laceration of breast

85.82 Split-thickness graft to breast

85.83 Full-thickness graft to breast

85.84 Pedicle graft to breast

85.85 Muscle flap graft to breast

85.86 Transposition of nipple

85.87 Other repair or reconstruction of nipple

85.89 Other mammoplasty

85.9 Other operations on the breast

85.91 Aspiration of breast

Excludes: *percutaneous biopsy of breast (85.11)*

85.92 Injection of therapeutic agent into breast

Excludes: *that for augmentation of breast (85.51-85.52)*

85.93 Revision of implant of breast

85.94 Removal of implant of breast

85.95 Insertion of breast tissue expander
Insertion (soft tissue) of tissue expander (one or more) under muscle or platysma to develop skin flaps for donor use

85.96 Removal of breast tissue expander(s)

● Code new to this edition   ▲ Revision of existing code   ④ ⑤ Fourth or fifth digit required

85.99 Other

86 **Operations on skin and subcutaneous tissue**
Includes: operations on:
hair follicles
male perineum
nails
sebaceous glands
subcutaneous fat pads
sudoriferous glands
superficial fossae

Excludes: *those on skin of:*
anus (49.01-49.99)
breast (mastectomy site) (85.0-85.99)
ear (18.01-18.9)
eyebrow (08.01-08.99)
eyelid (08.01-08.99)
female perineum (71.01-71.9)
lips (27.0-27.99)
nose (21.00-21.99)
penis (64.0-64.99)
scrotum (61.0-61.99)
vulva (71.01-71.9)

86.0 **Incision of skin and subcutaneous tissue**

86.01 **Aspiration of skin and subcutaneous tissue**
Aspiration of:
abscess of nail, skin, or subcutaneous tissue
hematoma of nail, skin, or subcutaneous tissue
seroma of nail, skin, or subcutaneous tissue

86.02 **Injection or tattooing of skin lesion or defect**
Injection of filling material
Insertion of filling material
Pigmenting of skin

86.03 **Incision of pilonidal sinus or cyst**
Excludes: *marsupialization (86.21)*

86.04 **Other incision with drainage of skin and subcutaneous tissue**
Excludes: *drainage of:*
fascial compartments of face and mouth (27.0)
palmar or thenar space (82.04)
pilonidal sinus or cyst (86.03)

86.05 **Incision with removal of foreign body from skin and subcutaneous tissue**
Removal of loop recorder
Removal of tissue expander(s) from skin or soft tissue other than breast tissue
Excludes: *removal of foreign body without incision (98.20-98.29)*

86.06 **Insertion of totally implantable infusion pump**
Code also any associated catheterization
Excludes: *insertion of totally implantable vascular access device (86.07)*

86.07 **Insertion of totally implantable vascular access device [VAD]**
Totally implanted port
Excludes: *insertion of totally implantable infusion pump (86.06)*

86.09 **Other incision of skin and subcutaneous tissue**
Creation of loop recorder pocket, new site and insertion/relocation of device
Creation of pocket for implantable, patient-activated cardiac event recorder and
insertion/relocation of device
Creation of thalamic stimulator pulse generator pocket, new site
Escharotomy
Exploration:
sinus tract, skin
superficial fossa
Undercutting of hair follicle
Excludes: *that of cardiac pacemaker pocket, new site (37.79)*
that of fascial compartments of face and mouth (27.0)

| | Valid O.R.
procedure | | Non-O.R.
procedure | | Nonspecific
O.R. procedure | | Noncovered
O.R. procedure |

86.1 **Diagnostic procedures on skin and subcutaneous tissue**

    86.11 **Biopsy of skin and subcutaneous tissue**

    86.19 **Other diagnostic procedures on skin and subcutaneous tissue**

        | Excludes: | *microscopic examination of specimen from skin and subcutaneous tissue (91.61-91.79)*

86.2 **Excision or destruction of lesion or tissue of skin and subcutaneous tissue**

    86.21 **Excision of pilonidal cyst or sinus**
        Marsupialization of cyst

        | Excludes: | *incision of pilonidal cyst or sinus (86.03)*

    86.22 **Excisional debridement of wound, infection, or burn**
        Removal by excision of:
          devitalized tissue
          necrosis
          slough

        | Excludes: | *debridement of:*
                abdominal all (wound) (54.3)
                bone (77.60-77.69)
                muscle (83.45) of hand (82.36)
                nail (bed) (fold) (86.27)
                nonexcisional debridement of wound, infection, or burn (86.28)
                open fracture site (79.60-79.69)
                pedicle or flap graft (86.75)

    86.23 **Removal of nail, nailbed, or nail fold**

    86.24 **Chemosurgery of skin**
        Chemical peel of skin

    86.25 **Dermabrasion**
        That with laser

        | Excludes: | *dermabrasion of wound to remove embedded debris (86.28)*

    86.26 **Ligation of dermal appendage**

        | Excludes: | *excision of preauricular appendage (18.29)*

    86.27 **Debridement of nail, nail bed, or nail fold**
        Removal of:
          necrosis
          slough

        | Excludes: | *removal of nail, nail bed, or nail fold (86.23)*

    86.28 **Nonexcisional debridement of wound, infection, or burn**
        Debridement NOS
        Maggot therapy
        Removal of devitalized tissue, necrosis, and slough by such methods as:
          brushing
          irrigation (under pressure)
          scrubbing
          washing

86.3 **Other local excision or destruction of lesion or tissue of skin and subcutaneous tissue**
    Destruction of skin by:
      cauterization
      cryosurgery
      fulguration
      laser beam
    That with Z-plasty

    | Excludes: | *adipectomy (86.83)*
           biopsy of skin (86.11)
           wide or radical excision of skin (86.4)
           Z-plasty without excision (86.84)

86.4 **Radical excision of skin lesion**
    Wide excision of skin lesion involving underlying or adjacent structure
    Code also any lymph node dissection (40.3-40.5)

86.5 **Suture or other closure of skin and subcutaneous tissue**

    86.51 **Replantation of scalp**

● Code new   ▲ Revision of   ④ ⑤ Fourth or fifth
      to this edition   existing code   digit required

86.59 Closure of skin and subcutaneous tissue of other sites
Adhesives (surgical) (tissue)
Staples
Sutures

> *Excludes:* *application of adhesive strips (butterfly)—omit code*

86.6 Free skin graft
Includes: excision of skin for autogenous graft

> *Excludes:* *construction or reconstruction of:*
> *penis (64.43-64.44)*
> *trachea (31.75)*
> *vagina (70.61-70.62)*

86.60 Free skin graft, not otherwise specified

86.61 Full-thickness skin graft to hand

> *Excludes:* *heterograft (86.65)*
> *homograft (86.66)*

86.62 Other skin graft to hand

> *Excludes:* *heterograft (86.65)*
> *homograft (86.66)*

86.63 Full-thickness skin graft to other sites

> *Excludes:* *heterograft (86.65)*
> *homograft (86.66)*

86.64 Hair transplant

> *Excludes:* *hair follicle transplant to eyebrow or eyelash (08.63)*

86.65 Heterograft to skin
Pigskin graft
Porcine graft

> *Excludes:* *application of dressing only (93.57)*

86.66 Homograft to skin
Graft to skin of:
amnionic membrane from donor
skin from donor

86.67 Dermal regenerative graft
Artificial skin, NOS
Creation of "neodermis"
Decellularized allodermis
Integumentary matrix implants
Prosthetic implant of dermal layer of skin
Regenerate dermal layer of skin

> *Excludes:* *heterograft to skin (86.65)*
> *homograft to skin (86.66)*

86.69 Other skin graft to other sites

> *Excludes:* *heterograft (86.65)*
> *homograft (86.66)*

86.7 Pedicle grafts or flaps

> *Excludes:* *construction or reconstruction of:*
> *penis (64.43-64.44)*
> *trachea (31.75)*
> *vagina (70.61-70.62)*

86.70 Pedicle or flap graft, not otherwise specified

86.71 Cutting and preparation of pedicle grafts or flaps
Elevation of pedicle from its bed
Flap design and raising
Partial cutting of pedicle or tube
Pedicle delay

> *Excludes:* *pollicization or digital transfer (82.61, 82.81)*
> *revision of pedicle (86.75)*

86.72 Advancement of pedicle graft

86.73 Attachment of pedicle or flap graft to hand

> *Excludes:* *pollicization or digital transfer (82.61, 82.81)*

| | Valid O.R. procedure | | Non-O.R. procedure | 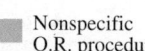 Nonspecific O.R. procedure | 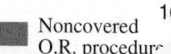 Noncovered O.R. procedure |

86.74 Attachment of pedicle or flap graft to other sites
Attachment by: Attachment by:
  advanced flap   rotating flap
  double pedicled flap   sliding flop
  pedicle graft   tube graft

86.75 Revision of pedicle or flap graft
Debridement of pedicle or flap graft
Defatting of pedicle or flap graft

86.8 Other repair and reconstruction of skin and subcutaneous tissue

86.81 Repair for facial weakness

86.82 Facial rhytidectomy
Face lift

> *Excludes:* *rhytidectomy of eyelid (08.86-08.87)*

86.83 Size reduction plastic operation
Liposuction
Reduction of adipose tissue of:
  abdominal wall (pendulous)
  arms (batwing)
  buttock
  thighs (trochanteric lipomatosis)

> *Excludes:* *breast (85.31-85.32)*

86.84 Relaxation of scar or web contracture of skin
Z-plasty of skin

> *Excludes:* *Z-plasty with excision of lesion (86.3)*

86.85 Correction of syndactyly

86.86 Onychoplasty

86.89 Other repair and reconstruction of skin and subcutaneous tissue

> *Excludes:* *mentoplasty (76.67-76.68)*

86.9 Other operations on skin and subcutaneous tissue

86.91 Excision of skin for graft
Excision of skin with closure of donor site

> *Excludes:* *that with graft at same operative episode (86.60-86.69)*

86.92 Electrolysis and other epilation of skin

> *Excludes:* *epilation of eyelid (08.91-08.93)*

86.93 Insertion of tissue expander
Insertion (subcutaneous) (soft tissue) of expander (one or more) in scalp (subgaleal
  space), face, neck, trunk except breast, and upper and lower extremities for
  development of skin flaps for donor use

> *Excludes:* *flap graft preparation (86.71)*
> *tissue expander, breast (85.95)*

86.99 Other

> *Excludes:* *removal of sutures from:*
> *abdomen (97.83)*
> *head and neck (97.38)*
> *thorax (97.43)*
> *trunk NEC (97.84)*
> *wound catheter:*
> *irrigation (96.58)*
> *replacement (97.15)*

● Code new   ▲ Revision of   ④ ⑤ Fourth or fifth
  to this edition   existing code   digit required

16. MISCELLANEOUS DIAGNOSTIC AND THERAPEUTIC PROCEDURES (87-99)

87   Diagnostic Radiology

87.0   Soft tissue x-ray of face, head, and neck

> Excludes: *angiography (88.40-88.68)*

87.01   Pneumoencephalogram

87.02   Other contrast radiogram of brain and skull
Pneumocisternogram
Pneumoventriculogram
Posterior fossa myelogram

87.03   Computerized axial tomography of bead
C.A.T. scan of head

87.04   Other tomography of bead

87.05   Contrast dacryocystogram

87.06   Contrast radiogram of nasopharynx

87.07   Contrast laryngogram

87.08   Cervical lymphangiogram

87.09   Other soft tissue x-ray of face, head, and neck
Noncontrast x-ray of:
adenoid
larynx
nasolacrimal duct
nasopharynx
salivary gland
thyroid region
uvula

> Excludes: *x-ray study of eye (95.14)*

87.1   Other x-ray of face, head, and neck

> Excludes: *angiography (88.40-88.68)*

87.11   Full-mouth x-ray of teeth

87.12   Other dental x-ray
Orthodontic cephalogram or cephalometrics
Panorex examination of mandible
Root canal x-ray

87.13   Temporomandibular contrast arthrogram

87.14   Contrast radiogram of orbit

87.15   Contrast radiogram of sinus

87.16   Other x-ray of facial bones
X-ray of:
frontal area
mandible
maxilla
nasal sinuses
nose
orbit
supraorbital area
symphysis menti
zygomaticomaxillary complex

87.17   Other x-ray of skull
Lateral projection of skull
Sagittal projection of skull
Tangential projection of skull

87.2   X-ray of spine

87.21   Contrast myelogram

87.22   Other x-ray of cervical spine

87.23   Other x-ray of thoracic spine

87.24   Other x-ray of lumbosacral spine
Sacrococcygeal x-ray

87.29   Other x-ray of spine
Spinal x-ray NOS

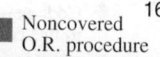

Valid O.R. procedure   Non-O.R. procedure   Nonspecific O.R. procedure   Noncovered O.R. procedure

87.3   Soft tissue x-ray of thorax

> *Excludes:*   *angiocardiography (88.50-88.58)*
> *angiography (88.40-88.68)*

87.31   Endotracheal bronchogram

87.32   Other contrast bronchogram
Transcricoid bronchogram

87.33   Mediastinal pneumogram

87.34   Intrathoracic lymphangiogram

87.35   Contrast radiogram of mammary ducts

87.36   Xerography of breast

87.37   Other mammography

87.38   Sinogram of chest wall
Fistulogram of chest wall

87.39   Other soft tissue x-ray of chest wall

87.4   Other x-ray of thorax

> *Excludes:*   *angiocardiography (88.50-88.58)*
> *angiography (88.40-88.68)*

87.41   Computerized axial tomography of thorax
C.A.T. scan of thorax
Crystal linea scan of x-ray beam of thorax
Electronic substraction of thorax
Photoelectric response of thorax
Tomography with use of computer, x-rays, and camera of thorax

87.42   Other tomography of thorax
Cardiac tomogram

87.43   X-ray of ribs, sternum, and clavicle
Examination for:
cervical rib
fracture

87.44   Routine chest x-ray, so described
X-ray of chest NOS

87.49   Other chest x-ray
X-ray of:
bronchus NOS
diaphragm NOS
heart NOS
lung NOS
mediastinum NOS
trachea NOS

87.5   Biliary tract x-ray

87.51   Percutaneous hepatic cholangiogram

87.52   Intravenous cholangiogram

87.53   Intraoperative cholangiogram

87.54   Other cholangiogram

87.59   Other biliary tract x-ray
Cholecystogram

87.6   Other x-ray of digestive system

87.61   Barium swallow

87.62   Upper GI series

87.63   Small bowel series

87.64   Lower GI series

87.65   Other x-ray of intestine

87.66   Contrast pancreatogram

87.69   Other digestive tract x-ray

87.7   X-ray of urinary system

> *Excludes:*   *angiography of renal vessels (88.45, 88.65)*

● Code new
to this edition   ▲ Revision of
existing code   ④ ⑤ Fourth or fifth
digit required

87.71 **Computerized axial tomography of kidney**
C.A.T. scan of kidney

87.72 **Other nephrotomogram**

87.73 **Intravenous pyelogram**
Diuretic infusion pyelogram

87.74 **Retrograde pyelogram**

87.75 **Percutaneous pyelogram**

87.76 **Retrograde cystourethrogram**

87.77 **Other cystogram**

87.78 **Ileal conduitogram**

87.79 **Other x-ray of the urinary system**
KUB x-ray

87.8 **X-ray of female genital organs**

87.81 **X-ray of gravid uterus**
Intrauterine cephalometry by x-ray

87.82 **Gas contrast hysterosalpingogram**

87.83 **Opaque dye contrast hysterosalpingogram**

87.84 **Percutaneous hysterogram**

87.85 **Other x-ray of fallopian tubes and uterus**

87.89 **Other x-ray of female genital organs**

87.9 **X-ray of male genital organs**

87.91 **Contrast seminal vesiculogram**

87.92 **Other x-ray of prostate and seminal vesicles**

87.93 **Contrast epididymogram**

87.94 **Contrast vasogram**

87.95 **Other x-ray of epididymis and vas deferens**

87.99 **Other x-ray of male genital organs**

88 **Other diagnostic radiology and related techniques**

88.0 **Soft tissue x-ray of abdomen**

> *Excludes:* angiography (88.40-88.68)

88.01 **Computerized axial tomography of abdomen**
C.A.T. scan of abdomen

> *Excludes:* C.A.T. scan of kidney (87.71)

88.02 **Other abdomen tomography**

> *Excludes:* nephrotomogram (87.72)

88.03 **Sinogram of abdominal wall**
Fistulogram of abdominal wall

88.04 **Abdominal lymphangiogram**

88.09 **Other soft tissue x-ray of abdominal wall**

88.1 **Other x-ray of abdomen**

88.11 **Pelvic opaque dye contrast radiography**

88.12 **Pelvic gas contrast radiography**
Pelvic pneumoperitoneum

88.13 **Other peritoneal pneumogram**

88.14 **Retroperitoneal fistulogram**

88.15 **Retroperitoneal pneumogram**

88.16 **Other retroperitoneal x-ray**

88.19 **Other x-ray of abdomen**
Flat plate of abdomen

88.2 **Skeletal x-ray of extremities and pelvis**

> *Excludes:* contrast radiogram of joint (88.32)

88.21 **Skeletal x-ray of shoulder and upper arm**

88.22 **Skeletal x-ray of elbow and forearm**

88.23 **Skeletal x-ray of wrist and hand**

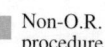 Valid O.R. procedure   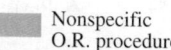 Non-O.R. procedure   Nonspecific O.R. procedure   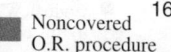 Noncovered O.R. procedure

88.24 Skeletal x-ray of upper limb, not otherwise specified

88.25 Pelvimetry

88.26 Other skeletal x-ray of pelvis and hip

88.27 Skeletal x-ray of thigh, knee, and lower leg

88.28 Skeletal x-ray of ankle and foot

88.29 Skeletal x-ray of lower limb, not otherwise specified

88.3 Other x-ray

88.31 Skeletal series
X-ray of whole skeleton

88.32 Contrast arthrogram

> Excludes: *that of temporomandibular joint (87.13)*

88.33 Other skeletal x-ray

> Excludes: *skeletal x-ray of:*
> *extremities and pelvis (88.21-88.29)*
> *face, head, and neck (87.11-87.17)*
> *spine (87.21-87.29)*
> *thorax (87.43)*

88.34 Lymphangiogram of upper limb

88.35 Other soft tissue x-ray of upper limb

88.36 Lymphangiogram of lower limb

88.37 Other soft tissue x-ray of lower limb

> Excludes: *femoral angiography (88.48, 88.66)*

88.38 Other computerized axial tomography
C.A.T. scan NOS

> Excludes: *C.A.T. scan of:*
> *abdomen (88.01)*
> *head (87.03)*
> *kidney (87.71)*
> *thorax (87.41)*

88.39 X-ray, other and unspecified

88.4 Arteriography using contrast material
Includes: angiography of arteries
arterial puncture for injection of contrast material
radiography of arteries (by fluoroscopy)
retrograde arteriography
Note: The fourth-digit subclassification identifies the site to be viewed, not the site of
injection.

> Excludes: *arteriography using:*
> *radioisotopes or radionuclides (92.01-92.19)*
> *ultrasound (88.71-88.79)*
> *fluorescein angiography of eye (95.12)*

88.40 Arteriography using contrast material, unspecified site

88.41 Arteriography of cerebral arteries
Angiography of:
basilar artery
carotid (internal)
posterior cerebral circulation
vertebral artery

88.42 Aortography
Arteriography of aorta and aortic arch

88.43 Arteriography of pulmonary arteries

88.44 Arteriography of other intrathoracic vessels

> Excludes: *angiocardiography (88.50-88.58)*
> *arteriography of coronary arteries (88.55-88.57)*

88.45 Arteriography of renal arteries

88.46 Arteriography of placenta
Placentogram using contrast material

88.47 Arteriography of other intra-abdominal arteries

88.48 Arteriography of femoral and other lower extremity arteries

● Code new
to this edition   ▲ Revision of
existing code   ④ ⑤ Fourth or fifth
digit required

88.49 Arteriography of other specified sites

88.5 Angiocardiography using contrast material

Includes: arterial puncture and insertion of arterial catheter for injection of contrast material
cineangiocardiography
selective angiocardiography

Code also synchronous cardiac catheterization (37.21-37.23)

Excludes: *angiography of pulmonary vessels (88.43, 88.62)*

88.50 Angiocardiography, not otherwise specified

88.51 Angiocardiography of venae cavae
Interior vena cavography
Phlebography of vena cava (inferior) (superior)

88.52 Angiocardiography of right heart structures
Angiocardiography of:
pulmonary valve
right atrium
right ventricle (outflow tract)

Excludes: *that combined with left heart angiocardiography (88.54)*

88.53 Angiocardiography of left heart structures
Angiocardiography of:
aortic valve
left atrium
left ventricle (outflow tract)

Excludes: *that combined with right heart angiocardiography (88.54)*

88.54 Combined right and left heart angiocardiography

88.55 Coronary arteriography using a single catheter
Coronary arteriography by Sones technique
Direct selective coronary arteriography using a single catheter

88.56 Coronary arteriography using two catheters
Coronary arteriography by:
Judkins technique
Ricketts and Abrams technique
Direct selective coronary arteriography using two catheters

88.57 Other and unspecified coronary arteriography
Coronary arteriography NOS

88.58 Negative-contrast cardiac roentgenography
Cardiac roentgenography with injection of carbon dioxide

88.6 Phlebography

Includes: angiography of veins
radiography of veins (by fluoroscopy)
retrograde phlebography
venipuncture for injection of contrast material
venography using contrast material

Note: The fourth-digit subclassification (88.60-88.67) identifies the site to be viewed, not the site of injection.

Excludes: *angiography using:*
radioisotopes or radionuclides (92.01-92.19)
ultrasound (88.71-88.79)
fluorescein angiography of eye (95.12)

88.60 Phlebography using contrast material, unspecified site

88.61 Phlebography of veins of head and neck using contrast material

88.62 Phlebography of pulmonary veins using contrast material

88.63 Phlebography of other intrathoracic veins using contrast material

88.64 Phlebography of the portal venous system using contrast material
Splenoportogram (by splenic arteriography)

88.65 Phlebography of other intra-abdominal veins using contrast material

88.66 Phlebography of femoral and other lower extremity veins using contrast material

88.67 Phlebography of other specified sites using contrast material

88.68 Impedance phlebography

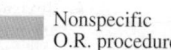 Valid O.R. procedure   Non-O.R. procedure   Nonspecific O.R. procedure   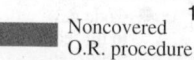 Noncovered O.R. procedure

88.7 **Diagnostic ultrasound**
Includes: echography
ultrasonic angiography
ultrasonography

> Excludes: *therapeutic ultrasound (00.01-00.09)*

88.71 **Diagnostic ultrasound of head and neck**
Determination of midline shift of brain
Echoencephalography

> Excludes: *eye (95.13)*

88.72 **Diagnostic ultrasound of heart**
Echocardiography
Intravascular ultrasound of heart

88.73 **Diagnostic ultrasound of other sites of thorax**
Aortic arch ultrasonography
Breast ultrasonography
Lung ultrasonography

88.74 **Diagnostic ultrasound of digestive system**

88.75 **Diagnostic ultrasound of urinary system**

88.76 **Diagnostic ultrasound of abdomen and retroperitoneum**

88.77 **Diagnostic ultrasound of peripheral vascular system**
Deep vein thrombosis ultrasonic scanning

88.78 **Diagnostic ultrasound of gravid uterus**
Intrauterine cephalometry:
echo
ultrasonic
Placental localization by ultrasound

88.79 **Other diagnostic ultrasound**
Ultrasonography of:
multiple sites
nongravid uterus
total body

88.8 **Thermography**

88.81 **Cerebral thermography**

88.82 **Ocular thermography**

88.83 **Bone thermography**
Osteoarticular thermography

88.84 **Muscle thermography**

88.85 **Breast thermography**

88.86 **Blood vessel thermography**
Deep vein thermography

88.89 **Thermography of other sites**
Lymph gland thermography
Thermography NOS

88.9 **Other diagnostic imaging**

88.90 **Diagnostic imaging, not elsewhere classified**

88.91 **Magnetic resonance imaging of brain and brain stem**

> Excludes: *intraoperative magnetic resonance imaging (88.96)*
> *real-time magnetic resonance imaging (88.96)*

88.92 **Magnetic resonance imaging of chest and myocardium**
For evaluation of hilar and mediastinal lymphadenopathy

88.93 **Magnetic resonance imaging of spinal canal**
Levels:
cervical
lumbar (lumbosacral)
thoracic
Spinal cord
Spine

88.94 **Magnetic resonance imaging of musculoskeletal**
Bone marrow blood supply
Extremities (upper) (lower)

88.95 **Magnetic resonance imaging of pelvis, prostate, and bladder**

● Code new ▲ Revision of ④ ⑤ Fourth or fifth
to this edition existing code digit required

- **88.96 Other intraoperative magnetic resonance imaging**
  iMRI
  Real-time magnetic resonance imaging

88.97 Magnetic resonance imaging of other and unspecified sites

abdomen	neck
face	eye orbit

88.98 Bone mineral density studies
Dual photon absorptiometry
Quantitative computed tomography (CT) studies
Radiographic densitometry
Single photon absorptiometry

89 Interview, evaluation, consultation, and examination

89.0 Diagnostic interview, consultation, and evaluation

> Excludes: psychiatric diagnostic interview (94.11-94.19)

89.01 Interview and evaluation, described as brief
Abbreviated history and evaluation

89.02 Interview and evaluation, described as limited
Interval history and evaluation

89.03 Interview and evaluation, described as comprehensive
History and evaluation of new problem

89.04 Other interview and evaluation

89.05 Diagnostic interview and evaluation, not otherwise specified

89.06 Consultation, described as limited
Consultation on a single organ system

89.07 Consultation, described as comprehensive

89.08 Other consultation

89.09 Consultation, not otherwise specified

89.1 Anatomic and physiologic measurements and manual examinations—nervous system and sense organs

> Excludes: ear examination (95.41-95.49)
> eye examination (95.01-95.26)
> the listed procedures when done as part of a general physical examination (89.7)

89.10 Intracarotid amobarbital test
Wada test

89.11 Tonometry

89.12 Nasal function study
Rhinomanometry

89.13 Neurologic examination

89.14 Electroencephalogram

> Excludes: that with polysomnogram (89.17)

89.15 Other nonoperative neurologic function tests

89.16 Transillumination of newborn skull

89.17 Polysomnogram
Sleep recording

89.18 Other sleep disorder function tests
Multiple sloop latency test [MSLT]

89.19 Video and radio-telemetered electroencephalographic monitoring
Radiographic EEG monitoring
Video EEG monitoring

89.2 Anatomic and physiologic measurements and manual examinations—genitourinary system

> Excludes: the listed procedures when done as part of a general physical examination (89.7)

89.21 Urinary manometry
Manometry through:
  indwelling urethral catheter
  nephrostomy
  pyelostomy
  ureterostomy

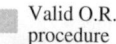 Valid O.R. procedure 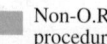 Non-O.R. procedure 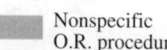 Nonspecific O.R. procedure 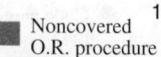 Noncovered O.R. procedure

89.22 Cystometrogram

89.23 Urethral sphincter electromyogram

89.24 Uroflowmetry [UFR]

89.25 Urethral pressure profile [UPP]

89.26 Gynecological examination
Pelvic examination

89.29 Other nonoperative genitourinary system measurements
Bioassay of urine
Renal clearance
Urine chemistry

89.3 Other anatomic and physiologic measurements and manual examinations

> Excludes: the listed procedures when done as part of a general physical examination (89.7)

89.31 Dental examination
Oral mucosal survey
Periodontal survey

89.32 Esophageal manometry

89.33 Digital examination of enterostomy stoma
Digital examination of colostomy stoma

89.34 Digital examination of rectum

89.35 Transillumination of nasal sinuses

89.36 Manual examination of breast

89.37 Vital capacity determination

89.38 Other nonoperative respiratory measurements
Plethysmography for measurement of respiratory function
Thoracic impedance plethysmography

89.39 Other nonoperative measurements and examinations
Basal metabolic rate [BMR]
14 C-Urea breath test
Gastric:
    analysis
    function NEC

> Excludes: body measurements (93.07)
> cardiac tests (89.41-89.69)
> fundus photography (95.11)
> limb length measurement (93.06)

89.4 Cardiac stress tests and pacemaker checks

89.41 Cardiovascular stress test using treadmill

89.42 Masters' two-step stress test

89.43 Cardiovascular stress test using bicycle ergometer

89.44 Other cardiovascular stress test
Thallium stress test with or without transesophageal pacing

89.45 Artificial pacemaker rate check
Artificial pacemaker function check NOS

89.46 Artificial pacemaker artifact wave form check

89.47 Artificial pacemaker electrode impedance check

89.48 Artificial pacemaker voltage or amperage threshold check

89.5 Other nonoperative cardiac and vascular diagnostic procedures

> Excludes: fetal EKG (75.32)

89.50 Ambulatory cardiac monitoring
Analog devices [Holter-type]

89.51 Rhythm electrocardiogram
Rhythm EKG (with one to three leads)

89.52 Electrocardiogram
ECG NOS
EKG (with 12 or more leads)

89.53 Vectorcardiogram (with ECG)

89.54 Electrographic monitoring
Telemetry

● Code new
to this edition   ▲ Revision of
existing code   ④ ⑤ Fourth or fifth
digit required

> *Excludes:*   *ambulatory cardiac monitoring (89.50)*
> *electrographic monitoring during surgery—omit code*

89.55 **Phonocardiogram with ECG lead**

89.56 **Carotid pulse tracing with ECG lead**

> *Excludes:*   *oculoplethysmography (89.58)*

89.57 **Apexcardiogram (with ECG lead)**

89.58 **Plethysmogram**
Penile plethysmography with nerve stimulation

> *Excludes:*   *plethysmography (for):*
>   *measurement of respiratory function (89.38)*
>   *thoracic impedance (89.38)*

89.59 **Other nonoperative cardiac and vascular measurements**

89.6   **Circulatory monitoring**

> *Excludes:*   *electrocardiographic monitoring during surgery—omit code*

● **89.60** **Continuous intra-arterial blood gas monitoring**
Insertion of blood gas monitoring system and continuous monitoring of blood gases through an intra-arterial sensor

89.61 **Systemic arterial pressure monitoring**

89.62 **Central venous pressure monitoring**

89.63 **Pulmonary artery pressure monitoring**

> *Excludes:*   *pulmonary artery wedge monitoring (89.64)*

89.64 **Pulmonary artery wedge monitoring**
Pulmonary capillary wedge [PCW] monitoring
Swan-Ganz catheterization

89.65 **Measurement of systemic arterial blood gases**

> *Excludes:*   *continuous intra-arterial blood gas monitoring (89.60)*

89.66 **Measurement of mixed venous blood gases**

89.67 **Monitoring of cardiac output by oxygen consumption technique**
Fick method

89.68 **Monitoring of cardiac output by other technique**
Cardiac output monitor by thermodilution indicator

89.69 **Monitoring of coronary blood flow**
Coronary blood flow monitoring by coincidence counting technique

89.7   **General physical examination**

89.8   **Autopsy**

90   **Microscopic examination—I**
The following fourth-digit subclassification is for use with categories in section 90 to identify type of examination:
    1 bacterial smear
    2 culture
    3 culture and sensitivity
    4 parasitology
    5 toxicology
    6 cell block and Papanicolaou smear
    9 other microscopic examination

④ **90.0**   **Microscopic examination of specimen from nervous system and of spinal fluid**

④ **90.1**   **Microscopic examination of specimen from endocrine gland, not elsewhere classified**

④ **90.2**   **Microscopic examination of specimen from eye**

④ **90.3**   **Microscopic examination of specimen from ear, nose, throat, and larynx**

④ **90.4**   **Microscopic examination of specimen from trachea, bronchus, pleura, lung, and other thoracic specimen, and of sputum**

④ **90.5**   **Microscopic examination of blood**

④ **90.6**   **Microscopic examination of specimen from spleen and of bone marrow**

④ **90.7**   **Microscopic examination of specimen from lymph node and of lymph**

④ **90.8**   **Microscopic examination of specimen from upper gastrointestinal tract and of vomitus**

④ **90.9**   **Microscopic examination of specimen from lower gastrointestinal tract and of stool**

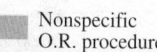

91 Microscopic examination—II

The following fourth-digit subclassification is for use with categories in section 91 to identify type of examination:

    1 bacterial smear
    2 culture
    3 culture and sensitivity
    4 parasitology
    5 toxicology
    6 cell block and Papanicolaou smear
    9 other microscopic examination

④ **91.0 Microscopic examination of specimen from liver, biliary trace and pancreas**

④ **91.1 Microscopic examination of peritoneal and retroperitoneal specimen**

④ **91.2 Microscopic examination of specimen from kidney, ureter, perirenal and periureteral tissue**

④ **91.3 Microscopic examination of specimen from bladder, urethra, prostate, seminal vesicle, perivesical tissue, and of urine and semen**

④ **91.4 Microscopic examination of specimen from female genital tract**
    Amnionic sac
    Fetus

④ **91.5 Microscopic examination of specimen from musculoskeletal system and of joint fluid**
    Microscopic examination of:
        bone   ligament
        bursa   muscle
        cartilage   synovial membrane
        fascia   tendon

④ **91.6 Microscopic examination of specimen from skin and other integument**
    Microscopic examination of:
        hair
        nails
        skin

    | Excludes: | mucous membrane—code to organ site that of operative wound (91.70-91.79)

④ **91.7 Microscopic examination of specimen from operative wound**

④ **91.8 Microscopic examination of specimen from other site**

④ **91.9 Microscopic examination of specimen from unspecified site**

92 Nuclear Medicine

   92.0 Radioisotope scan and function study

      92.01 Thyroid scan and radioisotope function studies
            Iodine-131 uptake
            Protein-bound iodine
            Radio-iodine uptake

      92.02 Liver scan and radioisotope function study

      92.03 Renal scan and radioisotope function study
            Renal clearance study

      92.04 Gastrointestinal scan and radioisotope function study
            Radio-cobalt B_{12} Schilling test
            Radio-iodinated triolein study

      92.05 Cardiovascular and hematopoietic scan and radioisotope function study
            Bone marrow scan or function study
            Cardiac output scan or function study
            Circulation time scan or function study
            Radionuclide cardiac ventriculogram scan or function study
            Spleen scan or function study

      92.09 Other radioisotope function studies

   92.1 Other radioisotope scan

      92.11 Cerebral scan
            Pituitary

      92.12 Scan of other sites of head
            | Excludes: | eye (95.16)

      92.13 Parathyroid scan

      92.14 Bone scan

      92.15 Pulmonary scan

● Code new   ▲ Revision of   ④ ⑤ Fourth or fifth
      to this edition   existing code   digit required

92.16   **Scan of lymphatic system**

92.17   **Placental scan**

92.18   **Total body scan**

92.19   **Scan of other sites**

92.2   **Therapeutic radiology and nuclear medicine**

> Excludes: that for:
>> ablation of pituitary gland (07.64-07.69)
>> destruction of chorioretinal lesion (14.26-14.27)

92.21   **Superficial radiation**
Contact radiation [up to 150 KVP]

92.22   **Orthovoltage radiation**
Deep radiation [200-300 KVP]

92.23   **Radioisotopic teleradiotherapy**
Teleradiotherapy using:
  cobalt-60
  iodine-125
  radioactive cesium

92.24   **Teleradiotherapy using photons**
Megavoltage NOS
Supervoltage NOS
Use of:
  Betatron
  linear accelerator

92.25   **Teleradiotherapy using electrons**
Beta particles

92.26   **Teleradiotherapy of other particulate radiation**
Neutrons   Protons NOS

92.27   **Implantation or insertion of radioactive elements**
Intravascular brachytherapy
Code also incision of site

92.28   **Injection or instillation of radioisotopes**
Intracavitary injection or instillation
Intravenous injection or instillation

92.29   **Other radiotherapeutic procedure**

92.3   **Stereotactic radiosurgery**

> Excludes: stereotactic biopsy

Code also stereotactic head frame application (93.59)

92.30   **Stereotactic radiosurgery, not otherwise specified**

92.31   **Single source photon radiosurgery**
High energy x-rays
Linear accelerator (LINAC)

92.32   **Multi-source photon radiosurgery**
Cobalt 60 radiation
Gamma irradiation

92.33   **Particulate radiosurgery**
Particle beam radiation (cyclotron)
Proton accelerator

92.39   **Stereotactic radiosurgery, not elsewhere classified**

93   **Physical therapy, respiratory therapy, rehabilitation, and related procedures**

93.0   **Diagnostic physical therapy**

93.01   **Functional evaluation**

93.02   **Orthotic evaluation**

93.03   **Prosthetic evaluation**

93.04   **Manual testing of muscle function**

93.05   **Range of motion testing**

93.06   **Measurement of limb length**

93.07   **Body measurement**
Girth measurement
Measurement of skull circumference

Valid O.R. procedure	Non-O.R. procedure	Nonspecific O.R. procedure	Noncovered O.R. procedure

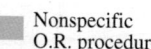
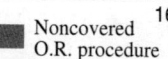

1637

93.08 Electromyography

> Excludes: *eye EMG (95.25)*
> *that with polysomnogram (89.17)*
> *urethral sphincter EMG (89.23)*

93.09 Other diagnostic physical therapy procedure

93.1 Physical therapy exercises

93.11 Assisting exercise

> Excludes: *assisted exercise in pool (93.31)*

93.12 Other active musculoskeletal exercise

93.13 Resistive exercise

93.14 Training in joint movements

93.15 Mobilization of spine

93.16 Mobilization of other joints

> Excludes: *manipulation of temporomandibular joint (76.95)*

93.17 Other passive musculoskeletal exercise

93.18 Breathing exercise

93.19 Exercise, not elsewhere classified

93.2 Other physical therapy musculoskeletal manipulation

93.21 Manual and mechanical traction

> Excludes: *skeletal traction (93.43-93.44)*
> *skin traction (93.45-93.46)*
> *spinal traction (93.41-93.42)*

93.22 Ambulation and gait training

93.23 Fitting of orthotic device

93.24 Training in use of prosthetic or orthotic device
Training in crutch walking

93.25 Forced extension of limb

93.26 Manual rupture of joint adhesions

93.27 Stretching of muscle or tendon

93.28 Stretching of fascia

93.29 Other forcible correction of deformity

93.3 Other physical therapy therapeutic procedures

93.31 Assisted exercise in pool

93.32 Whirlpool treatment

93.33 Other hydrotherapy

93.34 Diathermy

93.35 Other heat therapy
Acupuncture with smouldering moxa
Hot packs
Hyperthermia NEC
Infrared irradiation
Moxibustion
Paraffin bath

> Excludes: *hyperthermia for treatment of cancer (99.85)*

93.36 Cardiac retraining

93.37 Prenatal training
Training for natural childbirth

93.38 Combined physical therapy without mention of the components

93.39 Other physical therapy

93.4 Skeletal traction and other traction

93.41 Spinal traction using skull device
Traction using:
caliper tongs
Crutchfield tongs
halo device
Vinke tongs

● Code new
to this edition
▲ Revision of
existing code
④ ⑤ Fourth or fifth
digit required

> Excludes: insertion of tongs or halo traction device (02.94)

93.42 Other spinal traction
Cotrel's traction

> Excludes: cervical collar (93.52)

93.43 Intermittent skeletal traction

93.44 Other skeletal traction
Bryant's traction
Dunlop's traction
Lyman Smith traction
Russell's traction

93.45 Thomas' splint traction

93.46 Other skin traction of limbs
Adhesive tape traction
Boot traction
Buck's traction
Gallows traction

93.5 Other immobilization, pressure, and attention to wound

> Excludes: wound cleansing (96.58-96.59)

93.51 Application of plaster jacket

> Excludes: Minerva jacket (93.52)

93.52 Application of neck support
Application of:
cervical collar
Minerva jacket
molded neck support

93.53 Application of other cast

93.54 Application of splint
Plaster splint   Tray splint

> Excludes: periodontal splint (24.7)

93.55 Dental wiring

> Excludes: that for orthodontia (24.7)

93.56 Application of pressure dressing
Application of:
Gibney bandage
Robert Jones' bandage
Shanz dressing

93.57 Application of other wound dressing
Porcine wound dressing

93.58 Application of pressure trousers
Application of:
anti-shock trousers
MAST trousers
vasopneumatic device

93.59 Other immobilization, pressure, and attention to wound
Elastic stockings
Electronic gaiter
Intermittent pressure device
Oxygenation of wound (hyperbaric)
Stereotactic head frame application
Velpeau dressing

93.6 Osteopathic manipulative treatment

93.61 Osteopathic manipulative treatment for general mobilization
General articulatory treatment

93.62 Osteopathic manipulative treatment using high-velocity low-amplitude forces
Thrusting forces

93.63 Osteopathic manipulative treatment using low-velocity high-amplitude forces
Springing forces

93.64 Osteopathic manipulative treatment using isotonic, isometric forces

93.65 Osteopathic manipulative treatment using indirect forces

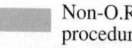 Valid O.R. procedure

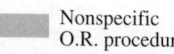 Non-O.R. procedure

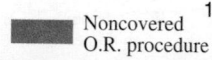 Nonspecific O.R. procedure

Noncovered O.R. procedure

93.66 **Osteopathic manipulative treatment to move tissue fluids**
Lymphatic pump

93.67 **Other specified osteopathic manipulative treatment**

93.7 **Speech and reading rehabilitation and rehabilitation of the blind**

93.71 **Dyslexia training**

93.72 **Dysphasia training**

93.73 **Esophageal speech training**

93.74 **Speech defect training**

93.75 **Other speech training and therapy**

93.76 **Training in use of lead dog for the blind**

93.77 **Training in braille or Moon**

93.78 **Other rehabilitation for the blind**

93.8 **Other rehabilitation therapy**

93.81 **Recreation therapy**
Diversional therapy
Play therapy

> Excludes: *play psychotherapy (94.36)*

93.82 **Educational therapy**
Education of bed-bound children
Special schooling for the handicapped

93.83 **Occupational therapy**
Daily living activities therapy

> Excludes: *training in activities of daily living for the blind (93.78)*

93.84 **Music therapy**

93.85 **Vocational rehabilitation**
Sheltered employment
Vocational:
assessment
retraining
training

93.89 **Rehabilitation, not elsewhere classified**

93.9 **Respiratory therapy**

> Excludes: *insertion of airway (96.01-96.05)*
> *other continuous mechanical ventilation (96.70-96.72)*

93.90 **Continuous positive airway pressure [CPAP]**

93.91 **Intermittent positive pressure breathing [IPPB]**

93.93 **Nonmechanical methods of resuscitation**
Artificial respiration
Manual resuscitation
Mouth-to-mouth resuscitation

93.94 **Respiratory medication administered by nebulizer**
Mist therapy

93.95 **Hyperbaric oxygenation**

> Excludes: *oxygenation of wound (93.59)*

93.96 **Other oxygen enrichment**
Catalytic oxygen therapy
Cytoreductive effect
Oxygenators
Oxygen therapy

> Excludes: *oxygenation of wound (93.59)*

93.97 **Decompression chamber**

93.98 **Other control of atmospheric pressure and composition**
Antigen-free air conditioning
Helium therapy

> Excludes: *inhaled nitric oxide therapy (INO) (00.12)*

93.99 **Other respiratory procedures**
Continuous negative pressure ventilation [CNP]
Postural drainage

● Code new
to this edition ▲ Revision of
existing code ④ ⑤ Fourth or fifth
digit required

94   Procedures related to the psyche

94.0   Psychologic evaluation and testing

94.01   Administration of intelligence test
Administration of:
Stanford-Binet
Wechsler Adult Intelligence Scale
Wechsler Intelligence Scale for Children

94.02   Administration of psychologic test
Administration of:
Bender Visual - Motor Gestalt Test
Benton Visual Retention Test
Minnesota Multiphasic Personality Inventory
Wechsler Memory Scale

94.03   Character analysis

94.08   Other psychologic evaluation and testing

94.09   Psychologic mental status determination, not otherwise specified

94.1   Psychiatric interviews, consultations, and evaluations

94.11   Psychiatric mental status determination
Clinical psychiatric mental status determination
Evaluation for criminal responsibility
Evaluation for testimentary capacity
Medicolegal mental status determination
Mental status determination NOS

94.12   Routine psychiatric visit, not otherwise specified

94.13   Psychiatric commitment evaluation
Pre-commitment interview

94.19   Other psychiatric interview and evaluation
Follow-up psychiatric interview NOS

94.2   Psychiatric somatotherapy

94.21   Narcoanalysis
Narcosynthesis

94.22   Lithium therapy

94.23   Neuroleptic therapy

94.24   Chemical shock therapy

94.25   Other psychiatric drug therapy

94.26   Subconvulsive electroshock therapy

94.27   Other electroshock therapy
Electroconvulsive therapy (ECT)
EST

94.29   Other psychiatric somatotherapy

94.3   Individual psychotherapy

94.31   Psychoanalysis

94.32   Hypnotherapy
Hypnodrome
Hypnosis

94.33   Behavior therapy
Aversion therapy
Behavior modification
Desensitization therapy
Extinction therapy
Relaxation training
Token economy

94.34   Individual therapy for psychosexual dysfunction
Excludes: that performed in group setting (94.41)

94.35   Crisis intervention

94.36   Play psychotherapy

94.37   Exploratory verbal psychotherapy

94.38   Supportive verbal psychotherapy

94.39   Other individual psychotherapy
Biofeedback

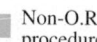 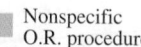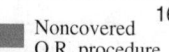

94.4   **Psychotherapy and counselling**

     94.41   **Group therapy for psychosexual dysfunction**

     94.42   **Family therapy**

     94.43   **Psychodrama**

     94.44   **Other group therapy**

     94.45   **Drug addiction counselling**

     94.46   **Alcoholism counselling**

     94.49   **Other counselling**

94.5   **Referral for psychologic rehabilitation**

     94.51   **Referral for psychotherapy**

     94.52   **Referral for psychiatric aftercare**
         That in:
           halfway house
           outpatient (clinic) facility

     94.53   **Referral for alcoholism rehabilitation**

     94.54   **Referral for drug addiction rehabilitation**

     94.55   **Referral for vocational rehabilitation**

     94.59   **Referral for other psychologic rehabilitation**

94.6   **Alcohol and drug rehabilitation and detoxification**

     94.61   **Alcohol rehabilitation**

     94.62   **Alcohol detoxification**

     94.63   **Alcohol rehabilitation and detoxification**

     94.64   **Drug rehabilitation**

     94.65   **Drug detoxification**

     94.66   **Drug rehabilitation and detoxification**

     94.67   **Combined alcohol and drug rehabilitation**

     94.68   **Combined alcohol and drug detoxification**

     94.69   **Combined alcohol and drug rehabilitation and detoxification**

95   **Ophthalmologic and otologic diagnosis and treatment**

95.0   **General and subjective eye examination**

     95.01   **Limited eye examination**
         Eye examination with prescription of spectacles

     95.02   **Comprehensive eye examination**
         Eye examination covering all aspects of the visual system

     95.03   **Extended ophthalmologic work-up**
         Examination (for):
           glaucoma
           neuro-ophthalmology
           retinal disease

     95.04   **Eye examination under anesthesia**
         Code also type of examination

     95.05   **Visual field study**

     95.06   **Color vision study**

     95.07   **Dark adaptation study**

     95.09   **Eye examination, not otherwise specified**
         Vision check NOS

95.1   **Examinations of form and structure of eye**

     95.11   **Fundus photography**

     95.12   **Fluorescein angiography or angioscopy of eye**

     95.13   **Ultrasound study of eye**

     95.14   **X-ray study of eye**

     95.15   **Ocular motility study**

     95.16   **P^{32} and other tracer studies of eye**

95.2   **Objective functional tests of eye**

     Excludes: *that with polysomnogram (89.17)*

● Code new
to this edition
     ▲ Revision of
existing code
     ④ ⑤ Fourth or fifth
digit required

95.21 **Electroretinogram [ERG]**

95.22 **Electro-oculogram [EOG]**

95.23 **Visual evoked potential [VEP]**

95.24 **Electronystagmogram [ENG]**

95.25 **Electromyogram of eye [EMG]**

95.26 **Tonography, provocative tests, and other glaucoma testing**

95.3 **Special vision services**

95.31 **Fitting and dispensing of spectacles**

95.32 **Prescription, fitting, and dispensing of contact lens**

95.33 **Dispensing of other low vision aids**

95.34 **Ocular prosthetics**

95.35 **Orthoptic training**

95.36 **Ophthalmologic counselling and instruction**
Counselling in:
adaptation to visual loss
use of low vision aids

95.4 **Nonoperative procedures related to hearing**

95.41 **Audiometry**
Békésy 5-tone audiometry
Impedance audiometry
Stapedial reflex response
Subjective audiometry
Tympanogram

95.42 **Clinical test of hearing**
Tuning fork test
Whispered speech test

95.43 **Audiological evaluation**
Audiological evaluation by:
Barany noise machine
blindfold test
delayed feedback
masking
Weber lateralization

95.44 **Clinical vestibular function tests**
Thermal test of vestibular function

95.45 **Rotation tests**
Barany chair

95.46 **Other auditory and vestibular function tests**

95.47 **Hearing examination, not otherwise specified**

95.48 **Fitting of hearing aid**
> Excludes: implantation of electromagnetic hearing device (20.95)

95.49 **Other nonoperative procedures related to hearing**
Adjustment (external components) of cochlear prosthetic device

96 **Nonoperative intubation and irrigation**

96.0 **Nonoperative intubation of gastrointestinal and respiratory tracts**

96.01 **Insertion of nasopharyngeal airway**

96.02 **Insertion of oropharyngeal airway**

96.03 **Insertion of esophageal obturator airway**

96.04 **Insertion of endotracheal tube**

96.05 **Other intubation of respiratory tract**

96.06 **Insertion of Sengstaken tube**
Esophageal tamponade

96.07 **Insertion of other (naso-)gastric tube**
Intubation for decompression
> Excludes: that for enteral infusion of nutritional substances (96.6)

96.08 **Insertion of (naso-)intestinal tube**
Miller-Abbott tube (for decompression)

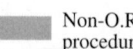 Valid O.R. procedure

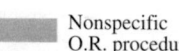 Non-O.R. procedure Nonspecific O.R. procedure

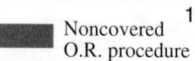 Noncovered O.R. procedure

96.09 Insertion of rectal tube
Replacement of rectal tube

96.1 Other nonoperative insertion

> Excludes: *nasolacrimal intubation (09.44)*

96.11 Packing of external auditory canal

96.14 Vaginal packing

96.15 Insertion of vaginal mold

96.16 Other vaginal dilation

96.17 Insertion of vaginal diaphragm

96.18 Insertion of other vaginal pessary

96.19 Rectal packing

96.2 Nonoperative dilation and manipulation

96.21 Dilation of frontonasal duct

96.22 Dilation of rectum

96.23 Dilation of anal sphincter

96.24 Dilation and manipulation of enterostomy stoma

96.25 Therapeutic distention of bladder
Intermittent distention of bladder

96.26 Manual reduction of rectal prolapse

96.27 Manual reduction of hernia

96.28 Manual reduction of enterostomy prolapse

96.29 Reduction with intussusception of alimentary tract
With:
Fluoroscopy
Ionizing radiation enema
Ultrasonography guidance
Hydrostatic reduction
Pneumantic reduction

> Excludes: *intra-abdominal manipulation of intestine, not otherwise specified (46.80)*

96.3 Nonoperative alimentary tract irrigation, cleaning, and local instillation

96.31 Gastric cooling
Gastric hypothermia

96.32 Gastric freezing

96.33 Gastric lavage

96.34 Other irrigation of (naso-)gastric tube

96.35 Gastric gavage

96.36 Irrigation of gastrostomy or enterostomy

96.37 Proctoclysis

96.38 Removal of impacted feces
Removal of impaction:
by flushing
manually

96.39 Other transanal enema
Rectal irrigation

> Excludes: *reduction of intussusception of alimentary tract by ionizing radiation enema (96.29)*

96.4 Nonoperative irrigation, cleaning, and local instillation of other digestive and genitourinary organs

96.41 Irrigation of cholecystostomy and other biliary tube

96.42 Irrigation of pancreatic tube

96.43 Digestive tract instillation, except gastric gavage

96.44 Vaginal douche

96.45 Irrigation of nephrostomy and pyelostomy

96.46 Irrigation of ureterostomy and ureteral catheter

96.47 Irrigation of cystostomy

96.48 Irrigation of other indwelling urinary catheter

● Code new
to this edition

▲ Revision of
existing code

④ ⑤ Fourth or fifth
digit required

96.49 Other genitourinary instillation
Insertion of prostaglandin suppository

96.5 Other nonoperative irrigation and cleaning

96.51 Irrigation of eye
Irrigation of cornea

> Excludes: *irrigation with removal of foreign body (98.21)*

96.52 Irrigation of ear
Irrigation with removal of cerumen

96.53 Irrigation of nasal passages

96.54 Dental scaling, polishing, and debridement
Dental prophylaxis
Plaque removal

96.55 Tracheostomy toilette

96.56 Other lavage of bronchus and trachea

> Excludes: *diagnostic bronchoalveolar lavage (BAL) (33.24)*
> *whole lung lavage (33.99)*

96.57 Irrigation of vascular catheter

96.58 Irrigation of wound catheter

96.59 Other irrigation of wound
Wound cleaning NOS

> Excludes: *debridement (86.22, 86.27-86.28)*

96.6 Enteral infusion of concentrated nutritional substances

96.7 Other continuous mechanical ventilation
Includes: Endotracheal respiratory assistance
Intermittent mandatory ventilation [IMV]
Positive end expiratory pressure [PEEP]
Pressure support ventilation [PSV]
That by tracheostomy
Weaning of an intubated (endotracheal tube) patient

> Excludes: *bi-level airway pressure (93.90)*
> *continuous negative pressure ventilation [CNP] (iron lung) (cuirass) (93.99)*
> *continuous positive airway pressure [CPAP] (93.90)*
> *intermittent positive pressure breathing [IPPB] (93.91)*
> *that by face mask (93.90-93.99)*
> *that by nasal cannula (93.90-93.99)*
> *that by nasal catheter (93.90-93.99)*

Code also any associated:
endotracheal tube insertion (96.04)
tracheostomy (31.1-31.29)

Note: Endotracheal Intubation
To calculate the number of hours (duration) of continuous mechanical ventilation during a hospitalization, begin the count from the start of the (endotracheal) intubation. The duration ends with (endotracheal) extubation.

If the patient is intubated prior to admission, begin counting the duration from the time of admission. If a patient is transferred (discharged) while intubated, the duration would end at the time of transfer (discharge).

For patients who begin on (endotracheal) intubation and subsequently have a tracheostomy performed for mechanical ventilation, the duration begins with the (endotracheal) intubation and ends when the mechanical ventilation is turned off (after the weaning period).

Tracheostomy
To calculate the number of hours of continuous mechanical ventilation during a hospitalization, begin counting the duration when mechanical ventilation is started. The duration ends when the mechanical ventilator is turned off (after the weaning period).

If a patient has received a tracheostomy prior to admission and is on mechanical ventilation at the time of admission, begin counting the duration from the time of admission. If a patient is transferred (discharged) while still on mechanical ventilation via tracheostomy, the duration would end at the time of the transfer (discharge).

96.70 Continuous mechanical ventilation of unspecified duration
Mechanical ventilation NOS

96.71 Continuous mechanical ventilation for less than 96 consecutive hours

	Valid O.R. procedure		Non-O.R. procedure		Nonspecific O.R. procedure		Noncovered O.R. procedure

96.72 Continuous mechanical ventilation for 96 consecutive hours or more

97 **Replacement and removal of therapeutic appliances**

97.0 Nonoperative replacement of gastrointestinal appliance

97.01 Replacement of (naso-)gastric or esophagostomy tube

97.02 Replacement of gastrostomy tube

97.03 Replacement of tube or enterostomy device of small intestine

97.04 Replacement of tube or enterostomy device of large intestine

97.05 Replacement of stent (tube) in biliary or pancreatic duct

97.1 Nonoperative replacement of musculoskeletal and integumentary system appliance

97.11 Replacement of cast on upper limb

97.12 Replacement of cast on lower limb

97.13 Replacement of other cast

97.14 Replacement of other device for musculoskeletal immobilization

97.15 Replacement of wound catheter

97.16 Replacement of wound packing or drain

> Excludes: *repacking of:*
> *dental wound (97.22)*
> *vulvar wound (97.26)*

97.2 Other nonoperative replacement

97.21 Replacement of nasal packing

97.22 Replacement of dental packing

97.23 Replacement of tracheostomy tube

97.24 Replacement and refitting of vaginal diaphragm

97.25 Replacement of other vaginal pessary

97.26 Replacement of vaginal or vulvar packing or drain

97.29 Other nonoperative replacements

97.3 Nonoperative removal of therapeutic device from head and neck

97.31 Removal of eye prosthesis

> Excludes: *removal of ocular implant (16.71)*
> *removal of orbital implant (16.72)*

97.32 Removal of nasal packing

97.33 Removal of dental wiring

97.34 Removal of dental packing

97.35 Removal of dental prosthesis

97.36 Removal of other external mandibular fixation device

97.37 Removal of tracheostomy tube

97.38 Removal of sutures from head and neck

97.39 Removal of other therapeutic device from head and neck

> Excludes: *removal of skull tongs (02.94)*

97.4 Nonoperative removal of therapeutic device from thorax

97.41 Removal of thoracotomy tube or pleural cavity drain

97.42 Removal of mediastinal drain

97.43 Removal of sutures from thorax

97.44 Nonoperative removal of heart ssist system
Intra-aortic balloon pump [IABP]

97.49 Removal of other device from thorax

97.5 Nonoperative removal of therapeutic device from digestive system

97.51 Removal of gastrostomy tube

97.52 Removal of tube from small intestine

97.53 Removal of tube from large intestine or appendix

97.54 Removal of cholecystostomy tube

97.55 Removal of T-tube, other bile duct tube, or liver tube
Removal of bile duct stent

● Code new
   to this edition
▲ Revision of
   existing code
④ ⑤ Fourth or fifth
   digit required

97.56 Removal of pancreatic tube or drain

97.59 Removal of other device from digestive system
Removal of rectal packing

97.6 Nonoperative removal of therapeutic device from urinary system

97.61 Removal of pyelostomy and nephrostomy tube

97.62 Removal of ureterostomy tube and ureteral catheter

97.63 Removal of cystostomy tube

97.64 Removal of other urinary drainage device
Removal of indwelling urinary catheter

97.65 Removal of urethral stent

97.69 Removal of other device from urinary system

97.7 Nonoperative removal of therapeutic device from genital system

97.71 Removal of intrauterine contraceptive device

97.72 Removal of intrauterine pack

97.73 Removal of vaginal diaphragm

97.74 Removal of other vaginal pessary

97.75 Removal of vaginal or vulva packing

97.79 Removal of other device from genital tract
Removal of sutures

97.8 Other nonoperative removal of therapeutic device

97.81 Removal of retroperitoneal drainage device

97.82 Removal of peritoneal drainage device

97.83 Removal of abdominal wall sutures

97.84 Removal of sutures from trunk, not elsewhere classified

97.85 Removal of packing from trunk, not elsewhere classified

97.86 Removal of other device from abdomen

97.87 Removal of other device from trunk

97.88 Removal of external immobilization device
Removal of:
brace
cast
splint

97.89 Removal of other therapeutic device

98 Nonoperative removal of foreign body or calculus

98.0 Removal of intraluminal foreign body from digestive system without incision
| Excludes: | removal of therapeutic device (97.51-97.59) |

98.01 Removal of intraluminal foreign body from mouth without incision

98.02 Removal of intraluminal foreign body from esophagus without incision

98.03 Removal of intraluminal foreign body from stomach and small intestine without incision

98.04 Removal of intraluminal foreign body from large intestine without incision

98.05 Removal of intraluminal foreign body from rectum and anus without incision

98.1 Removal of intraluminal foreign body from other sites without incision
| Excludes: | removal of therapeutic device (97.31-97.49, 97.61-97.89) |

98.11 Removal of intraluminal foreign body from ear without incision

98.12 Removal of intraluminal foreign body from nose without incision

98.13 Removal of intraluminal foreign body from pharynx without incision

98.14 Removal of intraluminal foreign body from larynx without incision

98.15 Removal of intraluminal foreign body from trachea and bronchus without incision

98.16 Removal of intraluminal foreign body from uterus without incision
| Excludes: | removal of intrauterine contraceptive device (97.71) |

98.17 Removal of intraluminal foreign body from vagina without incision

98.18 Removal of intraluminal foreign body from artificial stoma without incision

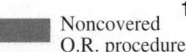

Valid O.R. procedure · Non-O.R. procedure · Nonspecific O.R. procedure · Noncovered O.R. procedure

98.19 Removal of intraluminal foreign body from urethra without incision

98.2 **Removal of other foreign body without incision**

Excludes: *removal of intraluminal foreign body (98.01-98.19)*

98.20 Removal of foreign body, not otherwise specified

98.21 Removal of superficial foreign body from eye without incision

98.22 Removal of other foreign body without incision from head and neck
Removal of embedded foreign body from eyelid or conjunctiva without incision

98.23 Removal of foreign body from vulva without incision

98.24 Removal of foreign body from scrotum or penis without incision

98.25 Removal of other foreign body without incision from trunk except scrotum, penis, or vulva

98.26 Removal of foreign body from hand without incision

98.27 Removal of foreign body without incision from upper limb, except hand

98.28 Removal of foreign body from foot without incision

98.29 Removal of foreign body without incision from lower limb, except foot

98.5 **Extracorporeal shockwave lithotripsy [ESWL]**
Lithotriptor tank procedure
Disintegration of stones by extracorporeal induced shockwaves
That with insertion of stent

98.51 **Extracorporeal shockwave lithotripsy [ESWL] of the kidney, ureter and/or bladder**

98.52 **Extracorporeal shockwave lithotripsy [ESWL] of the gallbladder and/or bile duct**

98.59 **Extracorporeal shockwave lithotripsy of other sites**

99 **Other nonoperative procedures**

99.0 **Transfusion of blood and blood components**
Use additional code for that done via catheter or cutdown (38.92-38.94)

99.00 **Perioperative autologous transfusion of whole blood or blood components**
Intraoperative blood collection
Postoperative blood collection
Salvage

99.01 **Exchange transfusion**
Transfusion:
exsanguination
replacement

99.02 **Transfusion of previously collected autologous blood**
Blood component

99.03 **Other transfusion of whole blood**
Transfusion:
NOS
blood NOS
hemodilution

99.04 **Transfusion of packed cells**

99.05 **Transfusion of platelets**
Transfusion of thrombocytes

99.06 **Transfusion of coagulation factors**
Transfusion of antihemophilic factor

99.07 **Transfusion of other serum**
Transfusion of plasma

Excludes: *injection [transfusion] of:*
antivenin (99.16)
gamma globulin (99.14)

99.08 **Transfusion of blood expander**
Transfusion of Dextran

99.09 **Transfusion of other substance**
Transfusion of:
blood surrogate
granulocytes

Excludes: *transplantation [transfusion] of bone marrow (41.0)*

● Code new
to this edition

▲ Revision of
existing code

④ ⑤ Fourth or fifth
digit required

99.1   Injection or Infusion of therapeutic or prophylactic substance
Includes: injection or infusion given:
hypodermically, acting locally or systemically
intramuscularly, acting locally or systemically
intravenously, acting locally or systemically

99.10   Injection or infusion of thromboblytic agent
Streptokinase
Tissue plasminogen activator (TPA)
Urokinase

Excludes: *aspirin—omit code*
GP IIB/IIIa platelet inhibitors (99.20)
heparin (99.19)
single vessel percutaneous transluminal coronary angioplasty [PTCA]
or coronary atherectomy with mention of thrombolytic agent
(36.02)
warfarin—omit code

99.11   Injection of Rh immune globulin
Injection of:
Anti-D (Rhesus) globulin
RhoGAM

99.12   Immunization for allergy
Desensitization

99.13   Immunization for autoimmune disease

99.14   Injection of gamma globulin
Injection of immune sera

99.15   Parenteral infusion of concentrated nutritional substances
Hyperalimentation
Peripheral parenteral nutrition [PPN]
Total parenteral nutrition [TPN]

99.16   Injection of antidote
Injection of:
antivenin
heavy metal antagonist

99.17   Injection of insulin

99.18   Injection or infusion of electrolytes

99.19   Injection of anticoagulant

Excludes: *infusion of drotrecogin alfa (activated) (00.11)*

99.2   Injection or infusion of other therapeutic or prophylactic substance
Includes: injection or infusion given:
hypodermically acting locally or systemically
intramuscularly acting locally or systemically
intravenously acting locally or systemically
Use additional code for:
injection (into):
breast (85.92)
bursa (82.94, 83.96)
intraperitoneal (cavity) (54.97)
intrathecal (03.92)
joint (76.96, 81.92)
kidney (55.96)
liver (50.94)
orbit (16.91)
other sites—see Alphabetic Index
perfusion:
NOS (39.97)
intestine (46.95, 46.96)
kidney (55.95)
liver (50.93)
total body (39.96)

99.20   Injection or infusion of platelet inhibitor
Glycoprotein IIB/IIIa inhibitor
GP IIB/IIIa inhibitor
GP IIB-IIIa inhibitor

Excludes: *infusion of heparin (99.19)*
injection or infusion of thrombolytic agent (99.10)

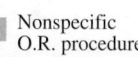 Valid O.R.
procedure   Non-O.R.
procedure   Nonspecific
O.R. procedure   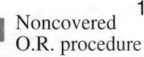 Noncovered
O.R. procedure

99.21 **Injection of antibiotic**

> | Excludes: | *injection or infusion of oxazolidinone class of antibiotics (00.14)*

99.22 **Injection of other anti-infective**

> | Excludes: | *injection or infusion of oxazolidinone class of antibiotics (00.14)*

99.23 **Injection of steroid**
Injection of cortisone
Subdermal implantation of progesterone

99.24 **Injection of other hormone**

99.25 **Injection or infusion of cancer chemotherapeutic substance**
Chemoembolization
Injection or infusion of antineoplastic agent

> | Excludes: | *immunotherapy, antineoplastic (99.28)*
> *implantation of chemotherapeutic agent (00.10)*
> *injection or infusion of biological response modifier [BRM] as an antineoplastic agent (99.28)*
> *injection of radioisotopes (92.28)*

99.26 **Injection of tranquilizer**

99.27 **Iontophoresis**

99.28 **Injection or infusion of biological response modifier [BRM] as an antineoplastic agent**
High-dose interleukin-2 (IL-2) therapy
Immunotherapy, antineoplastic
Interleukin therapy
Tumor vaccine

99.29 **Injection or infusion of other therapeutic or prophylactic substance**

> | Excludes: | *administration of neuroprotective agent (99.75)*
> *immunization (99.31-99.59)*
> *injection of sclerosing agent into:*
>   *esophageal varices (42.33)*
>   *hemorrhoids (49.42)*
>   *veins (39.92)*
> *injection or infusion of human B-type natriuretic peptide (hBNP) (00.13)*
> *injection or infusion of nesiritide (00.13)*
> *injection or infusion of platelet inhibitor (99.20)*
> *injection or infusion of thrombolytic agent (99.10)*

99.3 **Prophylactic vaccination and inoculation against certain bacterial diseases**

99.31 **Vaccination against cholera**

99.32 **Vaccination against typhoid and paratyphoid fever**
Administration of TAB vaccine

99.33 **Vaccination against tuberculosis**
Administration of BCG vaccine

99.34 **Vaccination against plague**

99.35 **Vaccination against tularemia**

99.36 **Administration of diphtheria toxoid**

> | Excludes: | *administration of:*
> *diphtheria antitoxin (99.58)*
> *diphtheria-tetanus-pertussis combined (99.39)*

99.37 **Vaccination against pertussis**

> | Excludes: | *administration of diphtheria-tetanus-pertussis, combined (99.39)*

99.38 **Administration of tetanus toxoid**

> | Excludes: | *administration of:*
> *diphtheria-tetanus-pertussis combined (99.39)*
> *tetanus antitoxin (99.56)*

99.39 **Administration of diphtheria-tetanus-pertussis, combined**

99.4 **Prophylactic vaccination and inoculation against certain viral diseases**

99.41 **Administration of poliomyelitis vaccine**

99.42 **Vaccination against smallpox**

99.43 **Vaccination against yellow fever**

● Code new
to this edition   ▲ Revision of
existing code   ④ ⑤ Fourth or fifth
digit required

99.44 Vaccination against rabies

99.45 Vaccination against measles

> | Excludes: | administration of measles-mumps-rubella vaccine (99.48)

99.46 Vaccination against mumps

> | Excludes: | administration of measles-mumps-rubella vaccine (99.48)

99.47 Vaccination against rubella

> | Excludes: | administration of measles-mumps-rubella vaccine (99.48)

99.48 Administration of measles-mumps-rubella vaccine

99.5 Other vaccination and inoculation

99.51 Prophylactic vaccination against the common cold

99.52 Prophylactic vaccination against influenza

99.53 Prophylactic vaccination against arthropod-borne viral encephalitis

99.54 Prophylactic vaccination against other arthropod-borne viral diseases

99.55 Prophylactic administration of vaccine against other disease
Vaccination against:
anthrax
brucellosis
Rocky Mountain spotted fever
Staphylococcus
Streptococcus
typhus

99.56 Administration of tetanus antitoxin

99.57 Administration of botulism antitoxin

99.58 Administration of other antitoxins
Administration of:
diphtheria antitoxin
gas gangrene antitoxin
scarlet fever antitoxin

99.59 Other vaccination and inoculation
Vaccination NOS

> | Excludes: | injection of:
>   gamma globulin (99.14)
>   Rh immune globulin (99.11)
>   immunization for:
>   allergy (99.12)
>   autoimmune disease (99.13)

99.6 Conversion of cardiac rhythm

> | Excludes: | open chest cardiac:
>   electric stimulation (37.91)
>   massage (37.91)

99.60 Cardiopulmonary resuscitation, not otherwise specified

99.61 Atrial cardioversion

99.62 Other electric countershock of heart
Cardioversion:
NOS
external
Conversion to sinus rhythm
Defibrillation
External electrode stimulation

99.63 Closed chest cardiac massage
Cardiac massage NOS
Manual external cardiac massage

99.64 Carotid sinus stimulation

99.69 Other conversion of cardiac rhythm

99.7 Therapeutic apheresis or other injection, administration, or infusion of other therapeutic or prophylactic substance

99.71 Therapeutic plasmapheresis

> | Excludes: | extracorporeal immunoadsorption [ECI] (99.76)

Valid O.R. procedure   Non-O.R. procedure   Nonspecific O.R. procedure   Noncovered O.R. procedure

99.72 Therapeutic leukopheresis
Therapeutic leukocytapheresis

99.73 Therapeutic erythrocytapheresis
Therapeutic erythropheresis

99.74 Therapeutic plateletpheresis

99.75 Administration of neuroprotective agent

● **99.76 Extracorporeal immunoadsorption**
Removal of antibodies from plasma with protein A columns

● **99.77 Application or administraion of adhesion barrier substance**

99.79 Other
Apheresis (harvest) of stem cells
Leech therapy

99.8 Miscellaneous physical procedures

99.81 Hypothermia (central) (local)

Excludes:	*gastric cooling (96.31)*
	gastric freezing (96.32)
	that incidental to open heart surgery (39.62)

99.82 Ultraviolet light therapy
Actinotherapy

99.83 Other phototherapy
Phototherapy of the newborn

Excludes:	*extracorporeal photochemotherapy (99.88)*
	photocoagulation of retinal lesion (14.23-14.25, 14.33-14.35,
	14.53-14.55)

99.84 Isolation
Isolation after contact with infectious disease
Protection of individual from his surroundings
Protection of surroundings from individual

99.85 Hyperthermia for treatment of cancer
Hyperthermia (adjunct therapy) induced by microwave, ultrasound, low energy
radiofrequency, probes (interstitial), or other means in the treatment of cancer

Code also any concurrent chemotherapy or radiation therapy

99.86 Non-invasive placement of bone growth stimulator
Transcutaneous (surface) placement of pads or patches for stimulation to aid bone
healing

Excludes:	*insertion of invasive or semi-invasive bone growth stimulators (device)*
	(percutaneous electrodes) (78.90-78.99)

99.88 Therapeutic photopheresis
Extracorporeal photochemotherapy
Extracorporeal photopheresis

Excludes:	*other phototherapy (99.83)*
	ultraviolet light therapy (99.82)

99.9 Other miscellaneous procedures

99.91 Acupuncture for anesthesia

99.92 Other acupuncture

Excludes:	*that with smouldering moxa (93.35)*

99.93 Rectal massage (for levator spasm)

99.94 Prostatic massage

99.95 Stretching of foreskin

99.96 Collection of sperm for artificial insemination

99.97 Fitting of denture

99.98 Extraction of milk from lactating breast

99.99 Other
Leech therapy

● Code new
to this edition   ▲ Revision of
existing code   ④ ⑤ Fourth or fifth
digit required

A

Amputation—*continued*
nose 21.4
penis (circle) (complete) (flap) (partial) (radical)
64.3
Pirogoff's (ankle amputation through malleoli
of tibia and fibula) 84.14
ray
finger 84.01
foot 84.11
toe (metatarsal head) 84.11
root (tooth) (apex) 23.73
with root canal therapy 23.72
shoulder (disarticulation) 84.08
Sorondo-Ferré (hindquarter) 84.19
S.P. Rogers (knee disarticulation) 84.16
supracondylar, above-knee 84.17
supramalleolar, foot 84.14
Syme's (ankle amputation through malleoli of
tibia and fibula) 84.14
thigh 84.17
thumb 84.02
toe (through metatarsophalangeal joint) 84.11
transcarpal 84.03
transmetatarsal 84.12
upper limb NEC (*see also* Amputation, arm)
84.00
wrist (disarticulation) 84.04
Amygdalohippocampotomy 01.39
Amygdalotomy 01.39
Analysis
character 94.03
gastric 89.39
psychologic 94.31
transactional
group 94.44
individual 94.39
Anastomosis
abdominal artery to coronary artery 36.17
accessory-facial nerve 04.72
accessory-hypoglossal nerve 04.73
anus (with formation of endorectal deal pouch)
45.95
aorta (descending)—pulmonary (artery) 39.0
aorta-renal artery 39.24
aorta-subclavian artery 39.22
aortoceliac 39.26
aorto(ilio)femoral 39.25
aortomesenteric 39.26
appendix 47.99
arteriovenous NEC 39.29
for renal dialysis 39.27
artery (suture of distal to proximal end) 39.31
with
bypass graft 39.29
extracranial-intracranial [EC-IC] 39.28
excision or resection of vessel—*see*
Arteriectomy, with anastomosis, by site
revision 39.49
bile ducts 51.39
bladder NEC 57.88
with
isolated segment of intestine 57.87 *[45.50]*
colon (sigmoid) 57.87 *[45.52]*
ileum 57.87 *[45.51]*
open loop of ileum 57.87 *[45.51]*
to intestine 57.88
ileum 57.87 *[45.51]*
bowel—(*see also* Anastomosis, intestine) 45.90
bronchotracheal 33.48
bronchus 33.48
carotid-subclavian artery 39.22

Anastomosis—*continued*
caval-mesenteric vein 39.1
caval-pulmonary artery 39.21
cervicoesophageal 42.59
colohypopharyngeal (intrathoracic) 42.55
antesternal or antethoracic 42.65
common bile duct 51.39
common pulmonary trunk and left atrium
(posterior wall) 35.82
cystic bile duct 51.39
cystocolic 57.88
epididymis to vas deferens 63.83
esophagocolic (intrathoracic) NEC 42.56
with interposition 42.55
antesternal or antethoracic NEC 42.66
with interposition 42.65
esophagocologastric (intrathoracic) 42.55
antesternal or antethoracic 42.65
esophagoduodenal (intrathoracic) NEC 42.54
with interposition 42.53
esophagoenteric (intrathoracic) NEC *see also*
Anastomosis, esophagus to intestinal
segment) 42.54
antesternal or antethoracic NEC (*see also*
Anastomosis, esophagus, antesternal, to
intestinal segment) 42.64
esophagoesophageal (intrathoracic) 42.51
antesternal or antethoracic 42.61
esophagogastric (intrathoracic) 42.52
antesternal or antethoracic 42.62
esophagus (intrapleural) (intrathoracic)
(retrosternal) NEC 42.59
with
gastrectomy (partial) 43.5
complete or total 43.99
interposition (of) NEC 42.58
colon 42.55
jejunum 42.53
small bowel 42.53
antesternal or antethoracic NEC 42.69
with
interposition (of) NEC 42.68
colon 42.65
jejunal loop 42.63
small bowel 42.63
rubber tube 42.68
to intestinal segment NEC 42.64
with interposition 42.68
colon NEC 42.66
with interposition 42.65
small bowel NEC 42.64
with interposition 42.63
to intestinal segment (intrathoracic) NEC
42.54
with interposition 42.58
antesternal or antethoracic NEC 42.64
with interposition 42.68
colon (intrathoracic) NEC 42.56
with interposition 42.55
antesternal or antethoracic 42.66
with interposition 42.65
small bowel NEC 42.54
with interposition 42.53
antesternal or antethoracic 42.64
with interposition 42.63
facial-accessory nerve 04.72
facial-hypoglossal nerve 04.71
fallopian tube 66.73
by reanastomosis 66.79
gallbladder 51.35
to

Anastomosis—*continued*
    hepatic ducts 51.31
    intestine 51.32
    pancreas 51.33
    stomach 51.34
  gastroepiploic artery (to)
    coronary artery 36.17
  hepatic duct 51.39
  hypoglossal-accessory nerve 04.73
  hypoglossal-facial nerve 04.71
  ileal loop to bladder 57.87 *[45.51]*
  ileoanal 45.95
  ileorectal 45.93
  inferior vena cava and portal vein 39.1
  internal mammary artery (to)
    coronary artery (single vessel) 36.15
      double vessel 36.16
    myocardium 36.2
  intestine 45.90
    large-to-anus 45.95
    large-to-large 45.94
    large-to-rectum 45.94
    large-to-small 45.93
    small-to-anus 45.95
    small-to-large 45.93
    small-to-rectal stump 45.92
    small-to-small 45.91
  intrahepatic 51.79
  intrathoracic vessel NEC 39.23
  kidney (pelvis) 55.86
  lacrimal sac to conjunctiva 09.82
  left-to-right (systemic-pulmonary artery) 39.0
  lymphatic (channel) (peripheral) 40.9
  mesenteric-caval 39.1
  mesocaval 39.1
  nasolacrimal 09.81
  nerve (cranial) (peripheral) NEC 04.74
    accessory-facial 04.72
    accessory-hypoglossal 04.73
    hypoglossal-facial 04.71
  pancreas (duct) (to) 52.96
    bile duct 51.39
    gall bladder 51.33
    intestine 52.96
    jejunum 52.96
    stomach 52.96
  pleurothecal (with valve) 03.79
  portacaval 39.1
  portal vein to inferior vena cava 39.1
  pulmonary-aortic (Pott's) 39.0
  pulmonary artery and superior vena cava 39.21
  pulmonary-innominate artery (Blalock) 39.0
  pulmonary-subclavian artery (Blalock-Taussig) 39.0
  pulmonary vein and azygos vein 39.23
  pyeloileocutaneous 56.51
  pyeloureterovesical 55.86
  radial artery 36.19
  rectum, rectal NEC 48.74
    stump to small intestine 45.92
  renal (pelvis) 55.86
    vein and splenic vein 39.1
  renoportal 39.1
  salpingothecal (with valve) 03.79
  splenic to renal veins 39.1
  splenorenal (venous) 39.1
    arterial 39.26
  subarachnoid-peritoneal (with valve) 03.71
  subarachnoid-ureteral (with valve) 03.72
  subclavian-aortic 39.22
  superior vena cava to pulmonary artery 39.21

Anastomosis—*continued*
  systemic-pulmonary artery 39.0
  thoracic artery (to)
    coronary artery (single) 36.15
      double 36.16
    myocardium 36.2
  ureter (to) NEC 56.79
    bladder 56.74
    colon 56.71
    ileal pouch (bladder) 56.51
    ileum 56.71
    intestine 56.71
    skin 56.61
  ureterocalyceal 55.86
  ureterocolic 56.71
  ureterovesical 56.74
  urethra (end-to-end) 58.44
  vas deferens 63.82
  veins (suture of proximal to distal end) (with bypass graft) 39.29
    with excision or resection of vessel—*see* Phlebectomy, with anastomosis, by site
    mesenteric to vena cava 39.1
    portal to inferior vena cava 39.1
    revision 39.49
    splenic and renal 39.1
  ventricle, ventricular (intracerebral) (with valve)
    (*see also* Shunt, ventricular) 02.2
  ventriculoatrial (with valve) 02.32
  ventriculocaval (with valve) 02.32
  ventriculomastoid (with valve) 02.31
  ventriculopleural (with valve) 02.33
  vesicle—*see* Anastomosis, bladder
Anderson operation (tibial lengthening) 78.37
Anel operation (dilation of lacrimal duct) 09.42
Anesthesia
  acupuncture for 99.91
  cryoanalgesia
  nerve (cranial) (peripheral) 04.2
  spinal —*omit code*
Aneurysmectomy 38.60
  with
    anastomosis 38.30
      abdominal
        artery 38.36
        vein 38.37
      aorta (arch) (ascending) (descending) 38.34
      head and neck NEC 38.32
      intracranial NEC 38.31
      lower limb
        artery 38.38
        vein 38.39
      thoracic NEC 38.35
      upper limb (artery) (vein) 38.33
    graft replacement (interposition) 38.40
      abdominal
        aorta 38.44
        artery 38.46
        vein 38.47
      aorta (arch) (ascending) (descending thoracic)
        abdominal 38.44
        thoracic 38.45
        thoracoabdominal 38.45 *[38.44]*
      head and neck NEC 38.42
      intracranial NEC 38.41
      lower limb
        artery 38.48
        vein 38.49
      thoracic NEC 38.45
      upper limb (artery) (vein) 38.43

Angiorrhaphy 39.30
  artery 39.31
  vein 39.32
Angioscopy, percutaneous 38.22
  eye (fluorescein) 95.12
Angiotomy 38.00
  abdominal
    artery 38.06
    vein 38.07
  aorta (arch) (ascending) (descending) 38.04
  head and neck NEC 38.02
  intracranial NEC 38.01
  lower limb
    artery 38.08
    vein 38.09
  thoracic NEC 38.05
  upper limb (artery) (vein) 38.03
Angiotripsy 39.98
Ankylosis, production of —*see* Arthrodesis
Annuloplasty (heart) (posteromedial) 35.33
Anoplasty 49.79
  with hemorrhoidectomy 49.46
Anoscopy 49.21
Antibiogram —*see* Examination, microscopic
Antiembolic filter, vena cava 38.7
Antiphobic treatment 94.39
Antrectomy
  mastoid 20.49
  maxillary 22.39
    radical 22.31
  pyloric 43.6
Antrostomy —*see* Antrotomy
Antrotomy (exploratory) (nasal sinus) 22.2
  Caldwell-Luc (maxillary sinus) 22.39
    with removal of membrane lining 22.31
  intranasal 22.2
    with external approach (Caldwell-Luc) 22.39
      radical 22.31
  maxillary (simple) 22.2
    with Caldwell-Luc approach 22.39
      with removal of membrane lining 22.31
    external (Caldwell-Luc approach) 22.39
      with removal of membrane lining 22.31
    radical (with removal of membrane lining) 22.31
Antrum window operation —*see* Antrotomy,
    maxillary
Aorticopulmonary window operation 39.59
Aortogram, aortography (abdominal)
    (retrograde) (selective) (translumbar) 88.42
Aortoplasty (aortic valve) (gusset type) 35.11
Aortotomy 38.04
Apexcardiogram (with ECG lead) 89.57
Apheresis, therapeutic —*see category* 99.7
Apicectomy
  lung 32.3
  petrous pyramid 20.59
  tooth (root) 23.73
    with root canal therapy 23.72
Apicoectomy 23.73
  with root canal therapy 23.72
Apicolysis (lung) 33.39
Apicostomy, alveolar 24.0
Aponeurectomy 83.42
  hand 82.33
Aponeurorrhaphy (*see also* Suture, tendon)
    83.64
  hand (*see also* Suture, tendon, hand) 82.45
Aponeurotomy 83.13
  hand 82.11
Appendectomy (with drainage) 47.09
  incidental 47.19

Appendectomy—*continued*
  laparoscopic 47.11
  laparoscopic 47.01
Appendicectomy (with drainage) 47.09
  incidental 47.19
  laparoscopic 47.11
  laparoscopic 47.01
Appendicocecostomy 47.91
Appendicoenterostomy 47.91
Appendicolysis 54.59
  with appendectomy 47.01, 47.09
  laparoscopic 54.51
Appendicostomy 47.91
  closure 47.92
Appendicotomy 47.2
Application
  adhesion barrier substance 99.77
  anti-shock trousers 93.58
  arch bars (orthodontic) 24.7
    for immobilization (fracture) 93.55
  barrier substance, adhesion 99.77
  Barton's tongs (skull) (with synchronous
      skeletal traction) 02.94
  bone growth stimulator (surface)
      (transcutaneous) 99.86
  bone morphogenetic protein (recombinant)
      (rhBMP) 84.52
  Bryant's traction 93.44
    with reduction of fracture or dislocation—*see*
      Reduction, fracture and Reduction,
      dislocation
  Buck's traction 93.46
  caliper tongs (skull) (with synchronous skeletal
      traction) 02.94
  cast (fiberglass) (plaster) (plastic) NEC 93.53
    with reduction of fracture or dislocation—*see*
      Reduction, fracture and Reduction,
      dislocation
    spica 93.51
  cervical collar 93.52
    with reduction of fracture or dislocation—*see*
      Reduction, fracture and Reduction,
      dislocation
  clamp, cerebral aneurysm (Crutchfield)
      (Silverstone) 39.51
  croupette, croup tent 93.94
  crown (artificial) 23.41
  Crutchfield tongs (skull) (with synchronous
      skeletal traction) 02.94
  Dunlop's traction 93.44
    with reduction of fracture or dislocation—*see*
      Reduction, fracture and Reduction,
      dislocation
  elastic stockings 93.59
  electronic gaiter 93.59
  external fixation device (bone) 78.10
    carpal, metacarpal 78.14
    clavicle 78.11
    femur 78.15
    fibula 78.17
    humerus 78.12
    patella 78.16
    pelvic 78.19
    phalanges (foot) (hand) 78.19
    radius 78.13
    scapula 78.11
    specified site NEC 78.19
    tarsal, metatarsal 78.18
    thorax (ribs) (sternum) 78.11
    tibia 78.17
    ulna 78.13

Arthrotomy 80.10
  as operative approach—*omit code*
  with
    arthrography—*see* Arthrogram
    arthroscopy—*see* Arthroscopy
    injection of drug 81.92
    removal of prosthesis (*see also* Removal,
      prosthesis, joint structures) 80.00
  ankle 80.17
  elbow 80.12
  foot and toe 80.18
  hand and finger 80.14
  hip 80.15
  knee 80.16
  shoulder 80.11
  specified site NEC 80.19
  spine 80.19
  wrist 80.13
Artificial
  insemination 69.92
  kidney 39.95
  rupture of membranes 73.09
Arytenoidectomy 30.29
Arytenoidopexy 31.69
Asai operation (larynx) 31.75
Aspiration
  abscess—*see* Aspiration, by site
  anterior chamber, eye (therapeutic) 12.91
    diagnostic 12.21
  aqueous (eye) (humor) (therapeutic) 12.91
    diagnostic 12.21
  ascites 54.91
  Bartholin's gland (cyst) (percutaneous) 71.21
  biopsy—*see* Biopsy, by site
  bladder (catheter) 57.0
    percutaneous (needle) 57.11
  bone marrow (for biopsy) 41.31
    from donor for transplant 41.91
    stem cell 99.79
  branchial cleft cyst 29.0
  breast 85.91
  bronchus 96.05
    with lavage 96.56
  bursa (percutaneous) 83.94
    hand 82.92
  calculus, bladder 57.0
  cataract 13.3
    with
      phacoemulsification 13.41
      phacofragmentation 13.43
        posterior route 13.42
  chest 34.91
  cisternal 01.01
  cranial (puncture) 01.09
  craniobuccal pouch 07.72
  craniopharyngioma 07.72
  cul-de-sac (abscess) 70.0
  curettage, uterus 69.59
    after abortion or delivery 69.52
    diagnostic 69.59
    to terminate pregnancy 69.51
  cyst—*see* Aspiration, by site
  diverticulum, pharynx 29.0
  endotracheal 96.04
    with lavage 96.56
  extradural 01.09
  eye (anterior chamber) (therapeutic) 12.91
    diagnostic 12.21
  fallopian tube 66.91
  fascia 83.95
    hand 82.93

Aspiration—*continued*
  gallbladder (percutaneous) 51.01
  hematoma—*see also* Aspiration, by site
    obstetrical 75.92
      incisional 75.91
  hydrocele, tunica vaginalis 61.91
  hygroma—*see* Aspiration, by site
  hyphema 12.91
  hypophysis 07.72
  intracranial space (epidural) (extradural)
      (subarachnoid) (subdural) (ventricular) 01.09
    through previously implanted catheter or
      reservoir (Ommaya) (Rickham) 01.02
  joint 81.91
    for arthrography—*see* Arthrogram
  kidney (cyst) (pelvis) (percutaneous)
      (therapeutic) 55.92
    diagnostic 55.23
  liver (percutaneous) 50.91
  lung (percutaneous) (puncture) (needle) (trocar)
      33.93
  middle ear 20.09
    with intubation 20.01
  muscle 83.95
    hand 82.93
  nail 86.01
  nasal sinus 22.00
    by puncture 22.01
    through natural ostium 22.02
  nasotracheal 96.04
    with lavage 96.56
  orbit, diagnostic 16.22
  ovary 65.91
  percutaneous—*see* Aspiration, by site
  pericardium (wound) 37.0
  pituitary gland 07.72
  pleural cavity 34.91
  prostate (percutaneous) 60.91
  Rathke's pouch 07.72
  seminal vesicles 60.71
  seroma—*see* Aspiration, by site
  skin 86.01
  soft tissue NEC 83.95
    hand 82.93
  spermatocele 63.91
  spinal (puncture) 03.31
  spleen (cyst) 41.1
  stem cell 99.79
  subarachnoid space (cerebral) 01.09
  subcutaneous tissue 86.01
  subdural space (cerebral) 01.09
  tendon 83.95
    hand 82.93
  testis 62.91
  thymus 07.92
  thyroid (field) (gland) 06.01
    postoperative 06.02
  trachea 96.04
    with lavage 96.56
    percutaneous 31.99
  tunica vaginalis (hydrocele) (percutaneous)
      61.91
  vitreous (and replacement) 14.72
    diagnostic 14.11
Assessment
  fitness to testify 94.11
  mental status 94.11
  nutritional status 89.39
  personality 94.03
  temperament 94.02
  vocational 93.85

Assistance
  cardiac—(*see also* Resuscitation, cardiac
      extracorporeal circulation) 39.61
  endotracheal respiratory—*see* category 96.7
  hepatic, extracorporeal 50.92
  respiratory (endotracheal) (mechanical)—*see*
      ventilation, mechanical
  respiratory (mechanical) (endotracheal) NEC
      93.92
Astragalectomy 77.98
Asymmetrogammagram —*see* Scan,
      radioisotope
Atherectomy
  coronary—*see* angioplasty
  peripheral 39.50
Atriocommissuropexy (mitral valve) 35.12
Atrioplasty NEC 37.99
  combined with repair of valvular and ventricular
      septal defects—*see* Repair, endocardial
      cushion defect
  septum (heart) NEC 35.71
Atrioseptopexy (*see also* Repair, atrial septal
      defect) 35.71
Atrioseptoplasty (*see also* Repair, atrial
      septal defect) 35.71
Atrioseptostomy (balloon) 35.41
Atriotomy 37.11
Atrioventriculostomy (cerebral-heart) 02.32
Attachment
  eye muscle
      orbicularis oculi to eyebrow 08.36
      rectus to frontalis 15.9
  pedicle (flap) graft 86.74
      hand 86.73
      lip 27.57
      mouth 27.57
  pharyngeal flap (for cleft palate repair) 27.62
      secondary or subsequent 27.63
  retina—*see* Reattachment, retina
Atticoantrostomy (ear) 20.49
Atticoantrotomy (ear) 20.49
Atticotomy (ear) 20.23
Audiometry (Békésy 5-tone) (impedance)
      (stapedial reflex response) (subjective) 95.41
Augmentation
  bladder 57.87
  breast—*see* Mammoplasty, augmentation
  buttock ("fanny-lift") 86.89
  chin 76.68
  genioplasty 76.68
  mammoplasty—*see* Mammoplasty,
      augmentation
  outflow tract (pulmonary valve) (gusset
      type) 35.26
      in total repair of tetralogy or Fallot 35.81
  vocal cord(s) 31.0
Auriculectomy 18.39
Autograft —*see* Graft
Autologous —*see* Blood, transfusion
Autopsy 89.8
Autotransfusion (whole blood)—*see* Blood,
      transfusion
Autotransplant, autotransplantation —*see also*
      Reimplantation
  adrenal tissue (heterotopic) (orthotopic) 07.45
  kidney 55.61
  lung —*see* Transplant, transplantation, lung
  ovary 65.72
      laparoscopic 65.75
  pancreatic tissue 52.81

Autotransplant(ation)— *continue*
  parathyroid tissue (heterotopic) (orthotopic)
      06.95
  thyroid tissue (heterotopic) (orthotopic) 06.94
  tooth 23.5
Avulsion, nerve (cranial) (peripheral) NEC 04.07
  acoustic 04.01
  phrenic 33.31
  sympathetic 05.29
Azygography 88.63

B

Bacterial smear —*see* Examination, microscopic
Baffes operation (interatrial transposition of venous return) 35.91
Baffle, atrial or interatrial 35.91
Balanoplasty 64.49
Baldy-Webster operation (uterine suspension) 69.22
Ballistocardiography 89.59
Balloon
  angioplasty—*see* Angioplasty, balloon
  dilation of pylorus 44.22
  pump, intra-aortic 37.61
  systostomy (atrial) 35.41
  valvuloplasty, percutaneous 35.96
Ball operation
  herniorrhaphy—*see* Repair, hernia, inguinal
  undercutting 49.02
Bandage 93.57
  elastic 93.56
Banding, pulmonary artery 38.85
Bankhart operation (capsular repair into glenoid, for shoulder dislocation) 81.82
Bardenheurer operation (ligation of innominate artery) 38.85
Barium swallow 87.61
Barkan operation (goniotomy) 12.52
  with goniopuncture 12.53
Barr operation (transfer of tibialis posterior tendon) 83.75
Barsky operation (closure of cleft hand) 82.82
Basal metabolic rate 89.39
Basiotripsy 73.8
Bassett operation (vulvectomy with inguinal lymph node dissection) 71.5 *[40.3]*
Bassini operation —*see* Repair, hernia, inguinal
Batch-Spittler-McFaddin operation (knee disarticulation) 84.16
Batista operation (partial ventriculectomy) (ventricular reduction) (ventricular remodeling) 37.35
Beck operation
  aorta-coronary sinus shunt 36.39
  epicardial poudrage 36.39
Beck-Jianu operation (permanent gastrostomy) 43.19
Behavior modification 94.33
Bell-Beuttner operation (subtotal abdominal hysterectomy) 68.3
Belsey operation (esophagogastric sphincter) 44.65
Benenenti operation (rotation of bulbous urethra) 58.49
Berke operation (levator resection of eyelid) 08.33
Bicuspidization of heart valve 35.10
  aortic 35.11
  mitral 35.12
Bicycle dynamometer 93.01
Biesenberger operation (size reduction of breast, bilateral) 85.32
  unilateral 85.31
Bifurcation, bone (*see also* Osteotomy) 77.30
Bigelow operation (litholapaxy) 57.0
Bililite therapy (ultraviolet) 99.82
Billroth I operation (partial gastrectomy with gastroduodenostomy) 43.6
Billroth II operation (partial gastrectomy with gastrojejunostomy) 43.7
Binnie operation (hepatopexy) 50.69

Biofeedback, psychotherapy 94.39
Biopsy
  abdominal wall 54.22
  adenoid 28.11
  adrenal gland NEC 07.11
    closed 07.11
    open 07.12
    percutaneous (aspiration) (needle) 07.11
  alveolus 24.12
  anus 49.23
  appendix 45.26
  artery (any site) 38.21
  aspiration—*see* Biopsy, by site
  bile ducts 51.14
    closed (endoscopic) 51.14
    open 51.13
    percutaneous (needle) 51.12
  bladder 57.33
    closed 57.33
    open 57.34
    transurethral 57.33
  blood vessel (any site) 38.21
  bone 77.40
    carpal, metacarpal 77.44
    clavicle 77.41
    facial 76.11
    femur 77.45
    fibula 77.47
    humerus 77.42
    marrow 41.31
    patella 77.46
    pelvic 77.49
    phalanges (foot) (hand) 77.49
    radius 77.43
    scapula 77.41
    specified site NEC 77.49
    tarsal, metatarsal 77.48
    thorax (ribs) (sternum) 77.41
    tibia 77.47
    ulna 77.43
    vertebrae 77.49
  bowel—*see* Biopsy, intestine
  brain NEC 01.13
    closed 01.13
    open 01.14
    percutaneous (needle) 01.13
  breast 85.11
    blind 85.11
    closed 85.11
    open 85.12
    percutaneous (needle) (Vimm-Silverman) 85.11
  bronchus NEC 33.24
    brush 33.24
    closed (endoscopic) 33.24
    washings 33.24
    open 33.25
  bursa 83.21
  cardioesophageal (junction) 44.14
    closed (endoscopic) 44.14
    open 44.15
  cecum 45.25
    brush 45.25
    closed (endoscopic) 45.25
    open 45.26
  cerebral meninges NEC 01.11
    closed 01.11
    open 01.12

Blepharoplasty (*see also* Reconstruction, eyelid) 08.70
 extensive 08.44
Blepharorrhaphy 08.52
 division or severing 08.02
Blepharotomy 08.09
Blind rehabilitation therapy NEC 93.78
Block
 caudal—*see* Injection, spinal
 celiac ganglion or plexus 05.31
 dissection
  breast
   bilateral 85.46
   unilateral 85.45
  bronchus 32.6
  larynx 30.3
  lymph nodes 40.50
  neck 40.40
  vulva 71.5
 epidural, spinal—*see* Injection, spinal
 gasserian ganglion 04.81
 intercostal nerves 04.81
 intrathecal—*see* Injection, spinal
 nerve (cranial) (peripheral) NEC 04.81
 paravertebral stellate ganglion 05.31
 peripheral nerve 04.81
 spinal nerve root (intrathecal)—*see* Injection, spinal
 stellate (ganglion) 05.31
 subarachnoid, spinal—*see* Injection, spinal
 sympathetic nerve 05.31
 trigeminal nerve 04.81
Blood
 flow study, Doppler-type (ultrasound)—*see* Ultrasonography
 patch, spine (epidural) 03.95
 transfusion
  antihemophilic factor 99.06
  autologous
   collected prior to surgery 99.02
   intraoperative 99.00
   perioperative 99.00
   postoperative 99.00
   previously collected 99.02
   salvage 99.00
  blood expander 99.08
  blood surrogate 99.09
  coagulation factors 99.06
  exchange 99.01
  granulocytes 99.09
  hemodilution 99.03
  other substance 99.09
  packed cells 99.04
  plasma 99.07
  platelets 99.05
  serum, other 99.07
  thrombocytes 99.05
Blount operation
 femoral shortening (with blade plate) 78.25
 by epiphyseal stapling 78.25
Boari operation (bladder flap) 56.74
Bobb operation (cholelithotomy) 51.04
Bone
 age studies 88.33
 mineral density study 88.98
Bonney operation (abdominal hysterectomy) 68.4
Borthen operation (iridotasis) 12.63
Boot operation
 plantar dissection 80.48
 radiocarpal fusion 81.26

Bosworth operation
 arthroplasty for acromioclavicular separation 81.83
 fusion of posterior lumbar and lumbosacral spine 81.08
  for pseudarthrosis 81.38
 resection of radial head ligaments (for tennis elbow) 80.92
 shelf procedure, hip 81.40
Bottle repair of hydrocele, tunics vaginalis 61.2
Boyd operation (hip disarticulation) 84.18
Brachytherapy intravascular 92.27
Brauer operation (cardiolysis) 37.10
Breech extraction —*see* Extraction, breech
Bricker operation (ileoureterostomy) 56.51
Brisement (force) 93.26
Bristow operation (repair of shoulder dislocation) 81.82
Brock operation (pulmonary valvotomy) 35.03
Brockman operation (soft tissue release for clubfoot) 83.84
Bronchogram, bronchography 87.32
 endotracheal 87.31
 transcricoid 87.32
Bronchoplasty 33.48
Bronchorrhaphy 33.41
Bronchoscopy NEC 33.23
 with biopsy 33.24
  lung 33.27
  brush 33.24
 fiberoptic 33.22
  with biopsy 33.24
   lung 33.27
   brush 33.24
 through tracheostomy 33.21
  with biopsy 33.24
   lung 33.27
   brush 33.24
Bronchospirometry 89.38
Bronchostomy 33.0
 closure 33.42
Bronchotomy 33.0
Browne (Denis) operation (hypospadias repair) 58.45
Brunschwig operation (temporary gastrostomy) 43.19
Buckling, scleral 14.49
 with
  air tamponade 14.49
  implant (silicone) (vitreous) 14.41
  resection of sclera 14.49
  vitrectomy 14.49
  vitreous implant (silicone) 14.41
Bunionectomy (radical) 77.59
 with
  arthrodesis 77.52
  osteotomy of first metatarsal 77.51
  resection of joint with prosthetic implant 77.59
  soft tissue correction NEC 77.53
Bunnell operation (tendon transfer) 82.56
Burch procedure (retropubic urethral suspension for urinary stress incontinence) 59.5
Burgess operation (amputation of ankle) 84.14
Burn dressing 93.57
Burr holes 01.24
Bursectomy 83.5
 hand 82.31
Bursocentesis 83.94
 hand 82.92
Bursotomy 83.03
 hand 82.03
Burying of fimbriae in uterine wall 66.97

Cesarean section—*continued*
peritoneal exclusion 74.4
specified type NEC 74.4
supravesical 74.2
transperitoneal 74.4
classical 74.0
low cervical 74.1
upper uterine segment 74.0
vaginal 74.4
Waters 74.2
Chandler operation (hip fusion) 81.21
Change —*see also* Replacement
cast NEC 97.13
lower limb 97.12
upper limb 97.11
cystostomy catheter or tube 59.94
gastrostomy tube 97.02
length
bone—*see either category* 78.2 Shortening,
bone *or category* 78.3 Lengthening, bone
muscle 83.85
hand 82.55
tendon 83.85
hand 82.55
nephrostomy catheter or tube 55.93
pyelostomy catheter or tube 55.94
tracheostomy tube 97.23
ureterostomy catheter or tube 59.93
urethra] catheter, indwelling 57.95
Character analysis, psychologic 94.03
Charles operation (correction of lymphedema)
40.9
Charnley operation (compression arthrodesis)
ankle 81.11
hip 81.21
knee 81.22
Cheatle-Henry operation —*see* Repair, hernia,
femoral
Check
pacemaker, artificial (cardiac) (function) (rate)
89.45
amperage threshold 89.48
artifact wave form 89.46
electrode impedance 89.47
voltage threshold 89.48
vision NEC 95.09
Cheiloplasty 27.59
Cheilorrhaphy 27.51
Cheilostomatoplasty 27.59
Cheilotomy 27.0
Chemical peel, skin 86.24
Chemocauterization —*see also* Destruction,
lesion, by site
corneal epithelium 11.41
palate 27.31
Chemodectomy 39.8
Chemoembolization 99.25
Chemolysis
nerve (peripheral) 04.2
spinal canal structure 03.8
Chemoneurolysis 04.2
Chemonucleolysis (nucleus pulposus) 80.52
Chemopallidectomy 01.42
Chemopeel (skin) 86.24
Chemosurgery
esophagus 42.39
endoscopic 42.33
Mohs' 86.24
skin (superficial) 86.24
stomach 43.49
endoscopic 43.41
Chemothalamectomy 01.41

Chemotherapy —*see also* Immunotherapy
Antabuse 94.25
for cancer NEC 99.25
brain wafer implantation 00.10
implantation of chemotherapeutic agent 00.10
interstitial implantation 00.10
intracavitary implantation 00.10
wafer chemotherapy 00.10
lithium 94.22
methadone 94.25
palate (bony) 27.31
Chevalier-Jackson operation (partial
laryngectomy) 30.29
Child operation (radical subtotal
pancreatectomy) 52.53
Cholangiocholangiostomy 51.39
Cholangiocholecystocholedochectomy 51.22
Cholangio-enterostomy 51.39
Cholangiogastrostomy 51.39
Cholangiogram 87.54
endoscopic retrograde (ERC) 51.11
intraoperative 87.53
intravenous 87.52
percutaneous hepatic 87.51
transhepatic 87.53
Cholangiography (*see also* Cholangiogram)
87.54
Cholangiojejunostomy (intrahepatic) 51.39
Cholangiopancreatography
endoscopic retrograde 51.10
Cholangiostomy 51.59
Cholangiotomy 51.59
Cholecystectomy (total) 51.22
laparoscopic 51.23
partial 51.21
laparoscopic 51.24
percutaneous 51.01
Cholecystenterorrhaphy 51.91
Cholecystocecostomy 51.32
Cholecystocholangiogram 87.59
Cholecystocolostomy 51.32
Cholecystoduodenostomy 51.32
Cholecystoenterostomy (Winiwater) 51.32
Cholecystogastrostomy 51.34
Cholecystogram 87.59
Cholecystoileostomy 51.32
Cholecystojejunostomy (Roux-en-Y) (with
jejunojejunostomy) 51.32
Cholecystopancreatostomy 51.33
Cholecystopexy 51.99
Cholecystorrhaphy 51.91
Cholecystostomy NEC 51.03
by trocar 51.02
Cholecystotomy 51.04
Choledochectomy 51.63
Choledochoduodenostomy 51.36
Choledochoenterostomy 51.36
Choledochojejunostomy 51.36
Choledocholithotomy 51.41
endoscopic 51.88
Choledocholithotripsy 51.41
endoscopic 51.88
Choledochopancreatostomy 51.39
Choledochoplasty 51.72
Choledochorrhaphy 51.71
Choledochoscopy 51.11
Choledochostomy 51.51
Choledochotomy 51.51
Cholelithotomy 51.04

Chondrectomy 80.90
  ankle 80.97
  elbow 80.92
  foot and toe 80.98
  hand and finger 80.94
  hip 80.95
  intervertebral cartilage *see category* 80.5
  knee (semilunar cartilage) 80.6—
  nasal (submucous) 21.5
  semilunar cartilage (knee) 80.6
  shoulder 80.91
  specified site NEC 80.99
  spine *see category* 80.5
  wrist 80.93
Chondroplasty —*see* Arthroplasty
Chondrosternoplasty (for pectus excavatum
    repair) 34.74
Chondrotomy (*see also* Division, cartilage) 80.40
  nasal 21.1
Chopart operation (midtarsal amputation) 84.12
Chordectomy, vocal 30.22
Chordotomy (spinothalmic) (anterior) (posterior)
    NEC 03.29
  percutaneous 03.21
  stereotactic 03.21
Ciliarotomy 12.55
Ciliectomy (ciliary body) 12.44
  eyelid margin 08.20
Cinch, cinching
  for scleral buckling (*see also* Buckling, scleral)
    14.49
  ocular muscle (oblique) (rectus) 15.22
    multiple (two or more muscles) 15.4
Cineangiocardiography (*see also*
    Angiocardiography) 88.50
Cineplasty, cineplastic prosthesis
  amputation—*see* Amputation
  arm 84.44
  biceps 84.44
  extremity 84.40
    lower 84.48
    upper 84.44
  leg 84.48
Cineradiography —*see* Radiography
Cingulumotomy (brain) (percutaneous radio
    frequency) 01.32
Circumcision (male) 64.0
  female 71.4
Clagett operation (closure of chest wall
    following open flap drainage) 34.72
Clamp and cautery, hemorrhoids 49.43
Clamping
  aneurysm (cerebral) 39.51
  blood vessel—*see* Ligation, blood vessel
  ventricular shunt 02.43
Clavicotomy 77.31
  fetal 73.8
Claviculectomy (partial) 77.81
  total 77.91
Clayton operation (resection of metatarsal heads
    and bases of phalanges) 77.88
Cleaning, wound 96.59
Clearance
  bladder (transurethral) 57.0
  pelvic
    female 68.8
    male 57.71
  prescalene fat pad 40.21
  renal pelvis (transurethral) 56.0
  ureter (transurethral) 56.0
Cleidotomy 77.31
  fetal 73.8

Clipping
  aneurysm (basilar) (carotid) (cerebellar)
    (cerebellopontine) (communicating artery)
    (vertebral) 39.51
  arteriovenous fistula 39.53
  frenulum, frenum
    labia (lips) 27.91
    lingual (tongue) 25.91
  tip of uvula 27.72
Clitoridectomy 71.4
Clitoridotomy 71.4
Clivogram 87.02
Closure —*see also* Repair
  abdominal wall 54.63
    delayed (granulating wound) 54.62
    secondary 54.61
    tertiary 54.62
  amputation stump, secondary 84.3
  aorticopulmonary fenestration (fistula) 39.59
  appendicostomy 47.92
  artificial opening
    bile duct 51.79
    bladder 57.82
    bronchus 33.42
    common duct 51.72
    esophagus 42.83
    gallbladder 51.92
    hepatic duct 51.79
    intestine 46.50
      large 46.52
      small 46.51
    kidney 55.82
    larynx 31.62
    rectum 48.72
    stomach 44.62
    thorax 34.72
    trachea 31.72
    ureter 56.83
    urethra 58.42
  atrial septal defect (*see also* Repair, atrial septal
      defect) 35.71
    with umbrella device (King-Mills type) 35.52
    combined with repair of valvular and
        ventricular septal defects—*see* Repair,
        endocardial cushion defect
  bronchostomy 33.42
  cecostomy 46.52
  cholecystostomy 51.92
  cleft hand 82.82
  colostomy 46.52
  cystostomy 57.82
  diastema (alveolar) (dental) 24.8
  disrupted abdominal wall (postoperative) 54.61
  duodenostomy 46.51
  encephalocele 02.12
  endocardial cushion defect (*see also* Repair,
      endocardial cushion defect) 35.73
  enterostomy 46.50
  esophagostomy 42.83
  fenestration
    aorticopulmonary 39.59
    septal, heart (*see also* Repair, heart, septum)
        35.70
  filtering bleb, corneoscleral (postglaucoma)
      12.66
  fistula
    abdominothoracic 34.83
    anorectal 48.73
    anovaginal 70.73
    antrobuccal 22.71
    anus 49.73

Closure—*continued*
  aorticopulmonary (fenestration) 39.59
  aortoduodenal 39.59
  appendix 47.92
  biliary tract 51.79—
  bladder NEC 57.84
  branchial cleft 29.52
  bronchocutaneous 33.42
  bronchoesophageal 33.42
  bronchomediastinal 34.73
  bronchopleural 34.73
  bronchopleurocutaneous 34.73
  bronchopleuromediastinal 34.73
  bronchovisceral 33.42
  bronchus 33.42
  cecosigmoidal 46.76
  cerebrospinal fluid 02.12
  cervicoaural 18.79
  cervicosigmoidal 67.62
  cervicovesical 57.84
  cervix 67.62
  cholecystocolic 51.93
  cholecystoduodenal 51.93
  cholecystoenteric 51.93
  cholecystogastric 51.93
  cholecystojejunal 51.93
  cisterna chyli 40.63
  colon 46.76
  colovaginal 70.72
  common duct 51.72
  cornea 11.49
    with lamellar graft (homograft) 11.62
      autograft 11.61
  diaphragm 34.83
  duodenum 46.72
  ear, middle 19.9
  ear drum 19.4
  enterocolic 46.74
  enterocutaneous 46.74
  enterouterine 69.42
  enterovaginal 70.74
  enterovesical 57.83
  esophagobronchial 33.42
  esophagocutaneous 42.84
  esophagopleurocutaneous 34.73
  esophagotracheal 31.73
  esophagus NEC 42.84
  fecal 46.79
  gallbladder 51.93
  gastric NEC 44.63
  gastrocolic 44.63
  gastroenterocolic 44.63
  gastroesophageal 42.84
  gastrojejunal 44.63
  gastrojejunocolic 44.63
  heart valve—*see* Repair, heart, valve
  hepatic duct 51.79
  hepatopleural 34.73
  hepatopulmonary 34.73
  ileorectal 46.74
  ileosigmoidal 46.74
  ileovesical 57.83
  ileum 46.74
  in ano 49.73
  intestine 46.79
    large 46.76
    small NEC 46.74
  intestinocolonic 46.74
  intestinoureteral 56.84
  intestinouterine 69.42
  intestinovaginal 70.74

Closure—*continued*
  intestinovesical 57.83
  jejunum 46.74
  kidney 55.83
  lacrimal 09.99
  laryngotracheal 31.62
  larynx 31.62
  lymphatic duct, left (thoracic) 40.63
  mastoid (antrum) 19.9
  mediastinobronchial 34.73
  mediastinocutaneous 34.73
  mouth (external) 27.53
  nasal 21.82
    sinus 22.71
  nasolabial 21.82
  nasopharyngeal 21.82
  oroantral 22.71
  oronasal 21.82
  oval window (ear) 20.93
  pancreaticoduodenal 52.95
  perilymph 20.93
  perineorectal 48.73
  perineosigmoidal 46.76
  perineourethroscrotal 58.43
  perineum 71.72
  perirectal 48.93
  pharyngoesophageal 29.53
  pharynx NEC 29.53
  pleura, pleural NEC 34.93
  pleurocutaneous 34.73
  pleuropericardial 37.4
  pleuroperitoneal 34.83
  pulmonoperitoneal 34.83
  rectolabial 48.73
  rectoureteral 56.84
  rectourethral 58.43
  rectovaginal 70.73
  rectovesical 57.83
  rectovesicovaginal 57.83
  rectovulvar 48.73
  rectum NEC 48.73
  renal 55.83
  reno-intestinal 55.83
  round window 20.93
  salivary (gland) (duct) 26.42
  scrotum 61.42
  sigmoidovaginal 70.74
  sigmoidovesical 57.83
  splenocolic 41.95
  stomach NEC 44.63
  thoracic duct 40.63
  thoracoabdominal 34.83
  thoracogastric 34.83
  thoracointestinal 34.83
  thorax NEC 34.71
  trachea NEC 31.73
  tracheoesophageal 31.73
  tympanic membrane (*see also*
    Tympanoplasty) 19.4
  umbilicourinary 57.51
  ureter 56.84
  ureterocervical 56.84
  ureterorectal 56.84
  ureterosigmoidal 56.84
  ureterovaginal 56.84
  ureterovesical 56.84
  urethra 58.43
  urethroperineal 58.43
  urethroperineovesical 57.84
  urethrorectal 58.43
  urethroscrotal 58.43

Control
  atmospheric pressure and composition NEC
      93.98
    antigen-free air conditioning 93.98
    decompression chamber 93.97
    mountain sanatorium 93.98
  epistaxis 21.00
    by
      cauterization (and packing) 21.03
      coagulation (with packing) 21.03
      electrocoagulation (with packing) 21.03
      excision of nasal mucosa with grafting 21.07
      ligation of artery 21.09
        ethmoidal 21.04
        external carotid 21.06
        maxillary (transantral) 21.05
      packing (nasal) (anterior) 21.01
        posterior (and anterior) 21.02
      specified means NEC 21.09
  hemorrhage 39.98
    abdominal cavity 54.19
    adenoids (postoperative) 28.7
    anus (postoperative) 49.95
    bladder (postoperative) 57.93
    chest 34.09
    colon 45.49
      endoscopic 45.43
    duodenum (ulcer) 44.49
      by
        embolization (transcatheter) 44.44
        suture (ligation) 44.42
      endoscopic 44.43
    esophagus 42.39
      endoscopic 42.33
    gastric (ulcer) 44.49
      by
        embolization (transcatheter) 44.44
        suture (ligation) 44.41
      endoscopic 44.43
    intrapleural 34.09
      postoperative (recurrent) 34.03
    laparotomy site 54.12
    nose (*see also* Control, epistaxis) 21.00
    peptic (ulcer) 44.49
      by
        embolization (transcatheter) 44.44
        suture (ligation) 44.40
      endoscopic 44.43
    pleura, pleural cavity 34.09
      postoperative (recurrent) 34.03
    postoperative NEC 39.98
    postvascular surgery 39.41
    prostate 60.94
    specified site NEC 39.98
    stomach (*see* Control, hemorrhage, gastric)
    thorax NEC 34.09
      postoperative (recurrent) 34.03
    thyroid (postoperative) 06.02
    tonsils (postoperative) 28.7
Conversion
  anastomosis—*see* Revision, anastomosis
  cardiac rhythm NEC 99.69
    to sinus rhythm 99.62
  gastrostomy to jejunostomy (endoscopic) 44.32
  obstetrical position—*see* Version
Cooling, gastric 96.31
Cordectomy, vocal 30.22
Cordopexy, vocal 31.69

Cordotomy
  spinal (bilateral) NEC 03.29
    percutaneous 03.21
  vocal 31.3
Corectomy 12.12
Corelysis 12.35
Coreoplasty 12.35
Corneoconjunctivoplasty 11.53
Correction —*see also* Repair
  atresia
    esophageal 42.85
      by magnetic forces 42.99
    external meatus (ear) 18.6
    nasopharynx, nasopharyngeal 29.4
    rectum 48.0
    tricuspid 35.94
  atrial septal defect (*see also* Repair, atrial septal
      defect) 35.71
    combined with repair of valvular and
        ventricular septal defects—*see* Repair,
        endocardial cushion defect
  blepharoptosis (*see also* Repair, blepharoptosis)
      08.36
  bunionette (with osteotomy) 77.54
  chordee 64.42
  claw toe 77.57
  cleft
    lip 27.54
    palate 27.62
  clubfoot NEC 83.84
  coarctation of aorta
    with
      anastomosis 38.34
      graft replacement 38.44
  cornea NEC 11.59
    refractive NEC 11.79
      epikeratophakia 11.76
      keratomileusis 11.71
      keratophakia 11.72
      radial keratotomy 11.75
  esophageal atresia 42.85
    by magnetic forces 42.99
  everted lacrimal punctum 09.71
  eyelid
    ptosis (*see also* Repair, blepharoptosis) 08.36
    retraction 08.38
  fetal defect 75.36
  forcible, of musculoskeletal deformity
      NEC 93.29
  hammer toe 77.56
  hydraulic pressure, open surgery (for) penile
      prosthesis, inflatable 64.99
    urinary sphincter, artificial 58.99
  intestinal malrotation 46.80
    large 46.82
    small 46.81
  inverted uterus—*see* Repair, inverted uterus
  lymphedema (of limb) 40.9
    excision with graft 40.9
    obliteration of lymphatics 40.9
    transplantation of autogenous lymphatics 40.9
  nasopharyngeal atresia 29.4
  overlapping toes 77.58
  palate (cleft) 27.62
  prognathism NEC 76.64
  prominent ear 18.5
  punctum (everted) 09.71
  spinal pseudarthrosis —*see* Refusion, spinal
  syndactyly 86.85

Correction—*continued*
  tetralogy of Fallot
    one-stage 35.81
    partial—*see specific procedure*
    total 35.81
  total anomalous pulmonary venous connection
    one-stage 35.82
    partial—*see specific procedure*
    total 35.82
  transposition, great arteries, total 35.84
  tricuspid atresia 35.94
  truncus arteriosus
    one-stage 35.83
    partial—*see specific procedure*
    total 35.83
  ureteropelvic junction 55.87
  ventricular septal defect (*see also* Repair,
      ventricular septal defect) 35.72
    combined with repair of valvular and atrial
        septal defects—*see* Repair, endocardial
        cushion defect
Costectomy 77.91
  with lung excision—*see* Excision, lung
  associated with thoracic operation—*omit code*
Costochondrectomy 77.91
  associated with thoracic operation—*omit code*
Costosternoplasty (pectus excavatum repair)
    34.74
Costotomy 77.31
Costotransversectomy 77.91
  associated with thoracic operation—*omit code*
Counseling (for) NEC 94.49
  alcoholism 94.46
  drug addiction 94.45
  employers 94.49
  family (medical) (social) 94.49
  marriage 94.49
  ophthalmologic (with instruction) 95.36
  pastoral 94.49
Countershock, cardiac NEC 99.62
Coventry Operation (tibial wedge osteotomy)
    77.27
CPAP (continuous positive airway pressure)
    93.90
Craniectomy 01.25
  linear (opening of cranial suture) 02.01
  reopening of site 01.23
  strip (opening of cranial suture) 02.01
Cranioclasis, fetal 73.8
Cranioplasty 02.06
  with synchronous repair of encephalocele 02.12
Craniotomy 01.24
  as operative approach—*omit code*
  fetal 73.8
  for decompression of fracture 02.02
  reopening of site 01.23
Craterization, bone (*see also* Excision, lesion,
    bone) 77.60
Crawford operation (tarso-frontalis sling of
    eyelid) 08.32
Creation —*see also* Formation
  cardiac pacemaker pocket
    with initial insertion of pacemaker—*omit code*
    new site (skin) (subcutaneous) 37.79
  conduit
    ileal (urinary) 56.51
    left ventricle and aorta 35.93
    right atrium and pulmonary artery 35.94
    right ventricle and pulmonary (distal) artery
        35.92

Creation—*continued*
  in repair of
    pulmonary artery atresia 35.92
    transposition of great vessels 35.92
    truncus arteriosus 35.83
  endorectal ileal pouch (J-pouch) (H-pouch)
      (S-pouch) (with anastomosis to anus) 45.95
  esophagogastric sphincteric competence NEC
      44.66
  Hartmann pouch—*see* Colectomy, by site
  interatrial fistula 35.42
  pericardial window 37.12
  pleural window, for drainage 34.09
  pocket
    cardiac pacemaker
      with initial insertion of pacemaker—*omit
          code*
      new site (skin) (subcutaneous) 37.79
    loop recorder 86.09
    thalamic stimulator pulse generator
      with initial insertion of battery package
          —omit code
      new site (skin) (subcutaneous) 86.09
  shunt—*see also* Shunt
    arteriovenous fistula, for dialysis 39.93
    left-to-right (systemic to pulmonary
        circulation) 39.0
  subcutaneous tunnel for esophageal anastomosis
      42.86
    with anastomosis—*see* Anastomosis,
        esophagus, antesternal
  syndactyly (ringer) (toe) 86.89
  thalamic stimulator pulse generator pocket
    with initial insertion of battery package—*omit
        code*
    new site (skin) (subcutaneous) 86.09
  tracheoesophageal fistula 31.95
  window
    pericardial 37.12
    pleura, for drainage 34.09
Credé maneuver 73.59
Cricoidectomy 30.29
Cricothyreotomy (for assistance in breathing)
    31.1
Cricothyroidectomy 30.29
Cricothyrostomy 31.1
Cricothyrotomy (for assistance in breathing) 31.1
Cricotomy (for assistance in breathing) 31.1
Cricotracheotomy (for assistance in breathing)
    31.1
Crisis Intervention 94.35
Croupette, croup tent 93.94
Crown, dental (ceramic) (gold) 23.41
Crushing
  bone—*see category* 78.4
  calculus
    bile (hepatic) passage 51.49
      endoscopic 51.88
    bladder (urinary) 57.0
    pancreatic duct 52.09
      endoscopic 52.94
  fallopian tube (*see also* Ligation, fallopian tube)
      66.39
  ganglion—*see* Crushing, nerve
  hemorrhoids 49.45
  nasal septum 21.88
  nerve (cranial) (peripheral) NEC 04.03
    acoustic 04.01
    auditory 04.01
    phrenic 04.03
      for collapse of lung 33.31

Crushing—*continued*
    sympathetic 05.0
    trigeminal 04.02
    vestibular 04.01
  vas deferens 63.71
Cryoablation —*see* Ablation
Cryoanalgesia
  nerve (cranial) (peripheral) 04.2
Cryoconization, cervix 67.33
Cryodestruction —*see* Destruction, lesion, by
  site
Cryoextraction, lens (*see also* Extraction,
  cataract, intracapsular) 13.19
Cryohypophysectomy (complete) (total) (*see
  also* Hypophysectomy) 07.69
Cryoleucotomy 01.32
Cryopexy, retinal —*see* Cryotherapy, retina
Cryoprostatectomy 60.62
Cryoretinopexy (for)
  reattachment 14.52
  repair of tear or defect 14.32
Cryosurgery —*see* Cryotherapy
Cryothalamectomy 01.41
Cryotherapy —*see also* Destruction, lesion, by
  site
  bladder 57.59
  brain 01.59
  cataract 13.19
  cervix 67.33
  choroid—*see* Cryotherapy, retina
  ciliary body 12.72
  corneal lesion (ulcer) 11.43
    to reshape cornea 11.79
  ear
    external 18.29
    inner 20.79
  esophagus 42.39
    endoscopic 42.33
  eyelid 08.25
  hemorrhoids 49.44
  iris 12.41
  nasal turbinates 21.61
  palate (bony) 27.31
  prostate 60.62
  retina (for)
    destruction of lesion 14.22
    reattachment 14.52
    repair of tear 14.32
  skin 86.3
  stomach 43.49
    endoscopic 43.41
  subcutaneous tissue 86.3
  turbinates (nasal) 21.61
  warts 86.3
    genital 71.3
Cryptectomy (anus) 49.39
  endoscopic 49.31
Cryptorchidectomy (unilateral) 62.3
  bilateral 62.41
Cryptotomy (anus) 49.39
  endoscopic 49.31
Cuirass 93.99
Culdocentesis 70.0
Culdoplasty 70.92
Culdoscopy (exploration) (removal of foreign
  body or lesion) 70.22
Culdotomy 70.12
Culp-Deweerd operation (spiral flap
  pyeloplasty) 55.87
Culp-Scardino operation (ureteral flap
  pyeloplasty) 55.87

Culture (and sensitivity)—*see* Examination,
  microscopic
Curettage (with packing) (with secondary
  closure)—*see also* Dilation and curettage
  adenoids 28.6
  anus 49.39
    endoscopic 49.31
  bladder 57.59
    transurethral 57.49
  bone (*see also* Excision, lesion, bone) 77.60
  brain 01.59
  bursa 83.39
    hand 82.29
  cartilage (*see also* Excision, lesion, joint) 80.80
  cerebral meninges 01.51
  chalazion 08.25
  conjunctiva (trachoma follicles) 10.33
  corneal epithelium 11.41
    for smear or culture 11.21
  ear, external 18.29
  eyelid 08.25
  joint (*see also* Excision, lesion, joint) 80.80
  meninges (cerebral) 01.51
    spinal 03.4
  muscle 83.32
    hand 82.22
  nerve (peripheral) 04.07
    sympathetic 05.29
  sclera 12.84
  skin 86.3
  spinal cord (meninges) 03.4
  subgingival 24.31
  tendon 83.39
    hand 82.29
    sheath 83.31
      hand 82.21
  uterus (with dilation) 69.09
    aspiration (diagnostic) NEC 69.59
      after abortion or delivery 69.52
      to terminate pregnancy 69.51
    following delivery or abortion 69.02
Curette evacuation, lens 13.2
Curtis operation (interphalangeal joint
  arthroplasty) 81.72
Cutaneolipectomy 86.83
Cutdown, venous 38.94
Cutting
  nerve (crania]) (peripheral) NEC 04.03
    acoustic 04.01
    auditory 04.01
    root, spinal 03.1
    sympathetic 05.0
    trigeminal 04.02
    vestibular 04.01
  pedicle (flap) graft 86.71
  pylorus (with wedge resection) 43.3
  spinal nerve root 03.1
  ureterovesical orifice 56.1
  urethral sphincter 58.5
CVP (central venous pressure monitoring) 89.62
Cyclectomy (ciliary body) 12.44
  eyelid margin 08.20
Cyclicotomy 12.55
Cycloanemization 12.74
Cyclocryotherapy 12.72
Cyclodialysis (initial) (subsequent) 12.55
Cyclodiathermy (penetrating) (surface) 12.71
Cycloelectrolysis 12.71
Cyclophotocoagulation 12.73
Cyclotomy 12.55

D

Destruction—*continued*
  excision 71.24
  incision 71.22
  marsupialization 71.23
 biliary ducts 51.69
  endoscopic 51.64
 bladder 57.59
  transurethral 57.49
 bone—*see* Excision, lesion, bone
 bowel—*see* Destruction, lesion, intestine
 brain (transtemporal approach) NEC 01.59
  by stereotactic radiosurgery 92.30
   cobalt 60 92.32
   linear accelerator (LINAC) 92.31
   multi-source 92.32
   particle beam (92.33)
   particulate (92.33)
   radiosurgery NEC (92.39)
   single source photon (92.31)
 breast NEC 85.20
 bronchus NEC 32.09
  endoscopic 32.01
 cerebral NEC 01.59
  meninges 01.51
 cervix 67.39
  by
   cauterization 67.32
   cryosurgery, cryoconization 67.33
   electroconization 67.32
 choroid 14.29
  by
   cryotherapy 14.22
   diathermy 14.21
   implantation of radiation source 14.27
   photocoagulation 14.25
    laser 14.24
    xenon arc 14.23
   radiation therapy 14.26
 ciliary body (nonexcisional) 12.43
  by excision 12.44
 conjunctiva 10.32
  by excision 10.31
 cornea NEC 11.49
  by
   cryotherapy 11.43
   electrocauterization 11.42
   thermocauterization 11.42
 cul-de-sac 70.32
 duodenum NEC 45.32
  by excision 45.31
   endoscopic 45.30
  endoscopic 45.30
 esophagus (chemosurgery) (cryosurgery)
   (electroresection) (fulguration) NEC 42.39
  by excision 42.32
   endoscopic 42.33
  endoscopic 42.33
 eye NEC 16.93
 eyebrow 08.25
 eyelid 08.25
  excisional—*see* Excision, lesion, eyelid
 heart 37.33
  by catheter ablation 37.34
 intestine (large) 45.49
  by excision 45.41
   endoscopic 45.43
    polypectomy 45.42
  endoscopic 45.43
   polypectomy 45.42
  small 45.34
   by excision 45.33

Destruction—*continued*
  intranasal 21.31
  iris (nonexcisional) NEC 12.41
   by excision 12.42
  kidney 55.39
   by marsupialization 55.31
  lacrimal sac 09.6
  larynx 30.09
  liver 50.29
  lung 32.29
   endoscopic 32.28
  meninges (cerebral) 01.51
   spinal 03.4
  nerve (peripheral) 04.07
   sympathetic 05.29
  nose 21.30
   intranasal 21.31
   specified NEC 21.32
  ovary
   by aspiration 65.91
   by excision 65.29
    laparoscopic 65.25
   cyst by rupture (manual) 65.93
  palate (bony) (local) 27.31
   wide 27.32
  pancreas 52.22
   by marsupialization 52.3
   endoscopic 52.21
  pancreatic duct 52.22
   endoscopic 52.21
  penis 64.2
  pharynx (excisional) 29.39
  pituitary gland
   by stereotactic radiosurgery 92.30
    cobalt 60 92.32
    linear accelerator (LINAC) 92.31
    multi-source 92.32
    particle beam 92.33
    particulate 92.33
    radiosurgery NEC 92.39
    single source photon 92.31
  rectum (local) 48.32
   by
    cryosurgery 48.34
    electrocoagulation 48.32
    excision 48.35
    fulguration 48.32
    laser (Argon) 48.33
    polyp 48.36
    radical 48.31
  retina 14.29
   by
    cryotherapy 14.22
    diathermy 14.21
    implantation of radiation source 14.27
    photocoagulation 14.25
     laser 14.24
     xenon arc 14.23
    radiation therapy 14.26
  salivary gland NEC 26.29
   by marsupialization 26.21
  sclera 12.84
  scrotum 61.3
  skin NEC 86.3
  sphincter of Oddi 51.69
   endoscopic 51.64
  spinal cord (meninges) 03.4
  spleen 41.42
   by marsupialization 41.41
  stomach NEC 43.49
   by excision 43.42

Destruction—*continued*
   endoscopic 43.41
   endoscopic 43.41
   subcutaneous tissue NEC 86.3
   testis 62.2
   tongue 25.1
   urethra (excisional) 58.39
     endoscopic 58.31
   uterus 68.29
   nerve (cranial) (peripheral) (by cryoanalgesia)
     (by radio frequency) 04.2
   sympathetic, by injection of neurolytic agent
     05.32
   neuroma 04.07
    acoustic
     by craniotomy 04.01
     by radiosurgery 04.07
    cranial 04.07
    Morton's 04.07
    peripheral
     Morton's 04.07
  neuroma
    acoustic 04.01
    by craniotomy 04.01
    by stereotactic radiosurgery 92.30
     cobalt 60 92.32
     linear accelerator (LINAC) 92.31
     multi-source 92.32
     particle beam 92.33
     particulate 92.33
     radiosurgery NEC 92.39
     single source photon 92.31
   prostate (prostatic tissue)
    by
     cryotherapy 60.62
     microwave 60.96
     radiofrequency 60.97
     transurethral microwave thermotherapy
      (TUMT) 60.96
     transurethral needle ablation (TUNA) 60.97
     TULIP (transurethral (ultrasound) guided
      laser induced prostatectomy) 60.21
     TUMT (transurethral microwave
      thermotherapy) 60.96
     TUNA (transurethral needle ablation) 60.97
   semicircular canals, by injection 20.72
   vestibule, by injection 20.72
Detachment, uterosacral ligaments 69.3
Determination
   mental status (clinical) (medicolegal)
    (psychiatric) NEC 94.11
   psychologic NEC 94.09
   vital capacity (pulmonary) 89.37
Detorsion
   intestine (twisted) (volvulus) 46.80
    large 46.82
     endoscopic (balloon) 46.85
    small 46.81
   kidney 55.84
   ovary 65.95
   spermatic cord 63.52
    with orchiopexy 62.5
   testis 63.52
    with orchiopexy 62.5
   volvulus 46.80
    endoscopic (balloon) 46.85
Detoxification therapy 94.25
   alcohol 94.62
    with rehabilitation 94.63
    combined alcohol and drug 94.68
     with rehabilitation 94.69

Detoxification therapy—*continued*
   drug 94.65
    with rehabilitation 94.66
    combined alcohol and drug 94.68
     with rehabilitation 94.69
Devascularization, stomach 44.99
Dewebbing
   esophagus 42.01
   syndactyly (fingers) (toes) 86.85
Dextrorotation —*see* Reduction, torsion
Dialysis
   hemodiafiltration, hemofiltration
    (extracorporeal) 39.95
   kidney (extracorporeal) 39.95
   liver 50.92
   peritoneal 54.98
   renal (extracorporeal) 39.95
Diaphanoscopy
   nasal sinuses 89.35
   skull (newborn) 89.16
Diaphysectomy —*see category* 77.8
Diathermy 93.34
   choroid—*see* Diathermy, retina
   nasal turbinates 21.61
   retina
    for
     destruction of lesion 14.21
     reattachment 14.51
     repair of tear 14.31
   surgical—*see* Destruction, lesion, by site
   turbinates (nasal) 21.61
Dickson operation (fascial transplant) 83.82
Dickson-Diveley operation (tendon transfer and
   arthrodesis to correct claw toe) 77.57
Dieffenbach operation (hip disarticulation) 84.18
Dilation
   achalasia 42.92
   ampulla of Vater 51.81
    endoscopic 51.84
   anus, anal (sphincter) 96.23
   biliary duct
    endoscopic 51.84
    pancreatic duct 52.99
     endoscopic 52.98
    percutaneous (endoscopy) 51.98
    sphincter
     of Oddi 51.81
      endoscopic 51.84
     pancreatic 51.82
      endoscopic 51.85
   bladder 96.25
    neck 57.92
   bronchus 33.91
   cervix (canal) 67.0
    obstetrical 73.1
    to assist delivery 73.1
   choanae (nasopharynx) 29.91
   colon, (endoscopic) (balloon) 46.85
   colostomy stoma 96.24
   duodenum,(endoscopic) (balloon) 46.85
   endoscopic—*see* Dilation, by site
   enterostomy stoma 96.24
   esophagus (by bougie) (by sound) 42.92
   fallopian tube 66.96
   foreskin (newborn) 99.95
   frontonasal duct 96.21
   gastrojejunostomy site, endoscopic 44.22
   heart valve—*see* Valvulotomy, heart
   ileostomy stoma 96.24
   ileum (endoscopic) (balloon) 46.85
   intestinal stoma (artificial) 96.24

Dilation—*continued*
  intestine (endoscopic) (balloon) 46.85
  jejunum (endoscopic) (balloon) 46.85
  lacrimal
    duct 09.42
    punctum 09.41
  larynx 31.98
  lymphatic structure(s) (peripheral) 40.9
  nares 21.99
  nasolacrimal duct (retrograde) 09.43
    with insertion of tube or stent 09.44
  nasopharynx 29.91
  pancreatic duct 52.99
    endoscopic 52.98
  pharynx 29.91
  prostatic urethra (transurethral) (balloon) 60.95
  punctum, lacrimal papilla 09.41
  pylorus
    by incision 44.21
    endoscopic 44.22
  rectum 96.22
  salivary duct 26.91
  sphenoid ostia 22.52
  sphincter
    anal 96.23
    cardiac 42.92
    of Oddi 51.81
      endoscopic 51.84
    pancreatic 51.82
      endoscopic 51.85
    pylorus (endoscopic) 44.22
      by incision 44.21
  Stenson's duct 26.91
  trachea 31.99
  ureter 59.8
    meatus 56.91
  ureterovesical orifice 59.8
  urethra 58.6
    prostatic (transurethral))balloon) 60.95
  urethrovesical junction 58.6
  vagina (instrumental) (manual) NEC 96.16
  vesical neck 57.92
  Wharton's duct 26.91
  Wirsung's duct 52.99
    endoscopic 52.98
Dilation and curettage, uterus (diagnostic) 69.09
  after
    abortion 69.02
    delivery 69.02
  to terminate pregnancy 69.01
Diminution, ciliary body 12.74
Disarticulation 84.91
  ankle 84.13
  elbow 84.06
  finger, except thumb 84.01
    thumb 84.02
  hip 84.18
  knee 84.16
  shoulder 84.08
  thumb 84.02
  toe 84.11
  wrist 84.04
Discission
  capsular membrane 13.64
  cataract (Wheeler knife) (Ziegler knife) 13.2
    congenital 13.69
    secondary membrane 13.64
  iris 12.12
  lens (capsule) (Wheeler knife) (Ziegler knife)
    (with capsulotomy) 13.2

Discission—*continued*
  orbitomaxillary, radical 16.51
  pupillary 13.2
  secondary membrane (after cataract) 13.64
  vitreous strands (posterior approach) 14.74
    anterior approach 14.73
Discogram, diskogram 87.21
Discolysis (by injection) 80.52
Diskectomy, intervertebral 80.51
  herniated (nucleus pulposus) 80.51
    percutaneous 80.59
Dispensing (with fitting)
  contact lens 95.32
  low vision aids NEC 95.33
  spectacles 95.31
Dissection —*see also* Excision
  aneurysm 38.60
  artery-vein-nerve bundle 39.91
  branchial cleft fistula or sinus 29.52
  bronchus 32.1
  femoral hernia 53.29
  groin, radical 40.54
  larynx block (en bloc) 30.3
  mediastinum with pneumonectomy 32.5
  neck, radical 40.40
    with laryngectomy 30.4
    bilateral 40.42
    unilateral 40.41
  orbital fibrous bands 16.92
  pterygium (with reposition) 11.31
  radical neck—*see* Dissection, neck, radical
  retroperitoneal NEC 59.00
  thoracic structures (block) (en bloc) (radical)
    (brachial plexus, bronchus, lobe of lung,
    ribs, and sympathetic nerves) 32.6
  vascular bundle 39.91
Distention, bladder (therapeutic) (intermittent)
  96.25
Diversion, urinary
  cutaneous 56.61
  ileal conduit 56.51
  internal NEC 56.71
  ureter to
    intestine 56.71
    skin 56.61
  uretero-ileostomy 56.51
Diversional therapy 93.81
Diverticulectomy
  bladder (suprapubic) 57.59
    transurethral approach 57.49
  duodenum 45.31
    endoscopic 45.30
  esophagus 42.31
    endoscopic 42.33
  esophagomyotomy 42.7
  hypopharyngeal (by cricopharyngeal myotomy)
    29.32
  intestine
    large 45.41
      endoscopic 45.43
    small 45.33
  kidney 55.39
  Meckel's 45.33
  pharyngeal (by cricopharyngeal myotomy) 29.32
  pharyngoesophageal (by cricopharyngeal
    myotomy) 29.32
  stomach 43.42
    endoscopic 43.41
  urethra 58.39
    endoscopic 58.31

Division—*continued*
  nerve root 03.1
  symblepharon (with insertion of conformer) 10.5
  synechiae
    endometrial 68.21
    iris (posterior) 12.33
      anterior 12.32
  tarsorrhaphy 08.02
  tendon 83.13
    Achilles 83.11
    adductor (hip) 83.12
    hand 82.11
  trabeculae carneae cordis (heart) 35.35
  tympanum 20.23
  uterosacral ligaments 69.3
  vaginal septum 70.14
  vas deferens 63.71
  vein (with ligation) 38.80
    abdominal 38.87
    head and neck NEC 38.82
    intracranial NEC 38.81
    lower limb 38.89
      varicose 38.59
    thoracic NEC 38.85
    upper limb 38.83
    varicose 38.50
      abdominal 38.57
      head and neck NEC 38.52
      intracranial NEC 38.51
      lower limb 38.59
      thoracic NEC 38.55
      upper limb 39.53
  vitreous, cicatricial bands (posterior approach) 14.74
    anterior approach 14.73
Doleris operation (shortening of round ligaments) 69.22
D'Ombrain operation (excision of pterygium with corneal graft) 11.32
Domestic tasks therapy 93.83
Dopplergram, Doppler flow mapping —*see also* Ultrasonography
  aortic arch 88.73
  head and neck 88.71
  heart 88.72
  thorax NEC 88.73
Dorrance operation (push-back operation for cleft palate) 27.62
Dotter operation (transluminal angioplasty) 39.59
Douche, vagina 96.44
Douglas operation (suture of tongue to lip for micrognathia) 25.59
Doyle operation (paracervical uterine denervation) 69.3
Drainage
  by
    anastomosis—*see* Anastomosis
    aspiration—*see* Aspiration
    incision—*see* Incision
  abdomen 54.19
    percutaneous 54.91
  abscess—*see also* Drainage, by site and Incision, by site
    appendix 47.2
      with appendectomy 47.09
        laparoscopic 47.01
    parapharyngeal (oral) (transcervical) 28.0
    peritonsillar (oral) (transcervical) 28.0
    retropharyngeal (oral) (transcervical) 28.0

Drainage—*continued*
  thyroid (field) (gland) 06.09
    percutaneous (needle) 06.01
    postoperative 06.02
  tonsil, tonsillar (oral) (transcervical) 28.0
  antecubital fossa 86.04
  appendix 47.91
    with appendectomy 47.09
      laparoscopic 47.01
    abscess 47.2
      with appendectomy 47.09
        laparoscopic 47.01
  axilla 86.04
  bladder (without incision) 57.0
    by indwelling catheter 57.94
      percutaneous suprapubic (closed) 57.17
      suprapubic NEC 57.18
  buccal space 27.0
  bursa 83.03
    by aspiration 83.94
      hand 82.92
    hand 82.03
      by aspiration 82.92
    radial 82.03
    ulnar 82.03
  cerebrum, cerebral (meninges) (ventricle) (incision) (trephination) 01.39
    by
      anastomosis—*see* Shunt, ventricular
      aspiration 01.09
      through previously implanted catheter 01.02
  chest (closed) 34.04
    open (by incision) 34.09
  crania] sinus (incision) (trephination) 01.21
    by aspiration 01.09
  cul-de-sac 70.12
    by aspiration 70.0
  cyst—*see also* Drainage, by site and incision, by site
    pancreas (by catheter) 52.01
      by marsupialization 52.3
      internal (anastomosis) 52.4
    pilonidal 86.03
    spleen, splenic (by marsupialization) 41.41
  duodenum (tube) 46.39
    by incision 45.01
  ear
    external 18.09
    inner 20.79
    middle (by myringotomy) 20.09
      with intubation 20.01
  epidural space, cerebral (incision) (trephination) 01.24
    by aspiration 01.09
  extradural space, cerebral (incision) (trephination) 01.24
    by aspiration 01.09
  extraperitoneal 54.0
  facial region 27.0
  fascial compartments, head and neck 27.0
  fetal hydrocephalic head (needling) (trocar) 73.8
  gallbladder 51.04
    by
      anastomosis 51.35
      aspiration 51.01
      incision 51.04
  groin region (abdominal wall) (inguinal) 54.0
    skin 86.04
    subcutaneous tissue 86.04

Drainage—*continued*
  hematoma—*see* Drainage, by site and Incision, by site
  hydrocephalic head (needling) (trocar) 73.8
  hypochondrium 54.0
    intra-abdominal 54.19
  iliac fossa 54.0
  infratemporal fossa 27.0
  intracranial space (epidural) (extradural) (incision) (trephination) 01.24
    by aspiration 01.09
    subarachnoid or subdural (incision) (trephination) 01.31
      by aspiration 01.09
  intraperitoneal 54.19
    percutaneous 54.91
  kidney (by incision) 55.01
    by
      anastomosis 55.86
      catheter 59.8
    pelvis (by incision) 55.11
  liver 50.0
    by aspiration 50.91
  Ludwig's angina 27.0
  lung (by incision) 33.1
    by punch (needle) (trocar) 33.93
  midpalmar space 82.04
  mouth floor 27.0
  mucocele, nasal sinus 22.00
    by puncture 22.01
    through natural ostium 22.02
  omentum 54.19
    percutaneous 54.91
  ovary (aspiration) 65.91
    by incision 65.09
      laparoscopic 65.01
  palmar space (middle) 82.04
  pancreas (by catheter) 52.01
    by anastomosis 52.96
  parapharyngeal 28.0
  paronychia 86.04
  parotid space 27.0
  pelvic peritoneum (female) 70.12
    male 54.19
  pericardium 37.0
  perigastric 54.19
    percutaneous 54.91
  perineum
    female 71.09
    male 86.04
  perisplenic tissue 54.19
    percutaneous 54.91
  peritoneum 54.19
    pelvic (female) 70.12
    percutaneous 54.91
  peritonsillar 28.0
  pharyngeal space, lateral 27.0
  pilonidal cyst or sinus 86.03
  pleura (closed) 34.04
    open (by incision) 34.09
  popliteal space 86.04
  postural 93.99
  postzygomatic space 27.0
  pseudocyst, pancreas 52.3
    by anastomosis 52.4
  pterygopalatine fossa 27.0
  retropharyngeal 28.0
  scrotum 61.0
  skin 86.04

Drainage—*continued*
  spinal (canal) (cord) 03.09
    by anastomosis—*see* Shunt, spinal
    diagnostic 03.31
  spleen 41.2
    cyst (by marsupialization) 41.41
  subarachnoid space, cerebral (incision) (trephination) 01.31
    by aspiration 01.09
  subcutaneous tissue 86.04
  subdiaphragmatic 54.91
    percutaneous 54.91
  subdural space, cerebral (incision) (trephination) 01.31
    by aspiration 01.09
  subhepatic space 54.19
    percutaneous 54.91
  sublingual space 27.0
  submental space 27.0
  subphrenic space 54.19
    percutaneous 54.91
  supraclavicular fossa 86.04
  temporal pouches 27.0
  tendon (sheath) 83.01
    hand 82.01
  thenar space 82.04
  thorax (closed) 34.04
    open (by incision) 34.09
  thyroglossal tract (by incision) 06.09
    by aspiration 06.01
  thyroid (field) (gland) (by incision) 06.09
    by aspiration 06.01
    postoperative 06.02
  tonsil 28.0
  tunica vaginalis 61.0
  ureter (by catheter) 59.8
    by
      anastomosis NEC (*see also* Anastomosis, ureter) 56.79
      incision 56.2
  ventricle (cerebral) (incision) NEC 02.39
    by
      anastomosis—*see* Shunt, ventricular
      aspiration 01.09
      through previously implanted catheter 01.02
  vertebral column 03.09
Drawing test 94.08
Dressing
  burn 93.57
  ulcer 93.56
  wound 93.57
Drilling, bone (*see also* Incision, bone) 77.10
Ductogram, mammary 87.35
Duhamel operation (abdominoperineal pull-through) 48.65
Dührssen's
  incisions (cervix, to assist delivery) 73.93
  operation (vaginofixation of uterus) 69.22
Dunn operation (triple arthrodesis) 81.12
Duodenectomy 45.62
  with
    gastrectomy—*see* Gastrectomy
    pancreatectomy—*see* Pancreatectomy
Duodenocholedochotomy 51.51
Duodenoduodenostomy 45.91
  proximal to distal segment 45.62
Duodenoileostomy 45.91
Duodenojejunostomy 45.91
Duodenoplasty 46.79
Duodenorrhaphy 46.71

E

Eagleton operation (extrapetrosal drainage) 20.22
ECG —*see* Electrocardiogram
Echocardiography 88.72
  intracardiac (ICE) 37.28
  transesophageal 88.72
    monitoring (Doppler) (ultrasound) 89.68
Echoencephalography 88.71
Echography —*see* Ultrasonography
Echogynography 88.79
Echoplacentogram 88.78
ECMO (extracorporeal membrane oxygenation) 39.65
Eden-Hybinette operation (glenoid bone block) 78.01
Educational therapy (bed-bound children) (handicapped) 93.82
EEG (electroencephalogram) 89.14
  monitoring (radiographic) (video) 89.19
Effler operation (heart) 36.2
Effleurage 93.39
EGD (esophagogastroduodenoscopy) 45.13
  with closed biopsy 45.16
Eggers operation
  tendon release (patellar retinacula) 83.13
  tendon transfer (biceps femoris tendon) (hamstring tendon) 83.75
EKG (*see also* Electrocardiogram) 89.52
Elastic hosiery 93.59
Electrocardiogram (with 12 or more leads) 89.52
  with vectorcardiogram 89.53
  fetal (scalp), intrauterine 75.32
  rhythm (with one to three leads) 89.51
Electrocautery —*see also* Cauterization
  cervix 67.32
  corneal lesion (ulcer) 11.42
  esophagus 42.39
    endoscopic 42.33
Electrocoagulation —*see also* Destruction, lesion, by site
  aneurysm (cerebral) (peripheral vessels) 39.52
  cervix 67.32
  cystoscopic 57.49
  ear
    external 18.29
    inner 20.79
    middle 20.51
  fallopian tube (lesion) 66.61
    for tubal ligation—*see* Ligation, fallopian tube
  gasserian ganglion 04.02
  nasal turbinates 21.61
  nose, for epistaxis (with packing) 21.03
  ovary 65.29
    laparoscopic 65.25
  prostatic bed 60.94
  rectum (polyp) 48.32
    radical 48.31
  retina (for)
    destruction of lesion 14.21
    reattachment 14.51
    repair of tear 14.31
  round ligament 69.19
  semicircular canals 20.79
  urethrovesical junction, transurethral 57.49
  uterine ligament 69.19
  uterosacral ligament 69.19
  uterus 68.29
  vagina 70.33
  vulva 71.3

Electrocochleography 20.31
Electroconization, cervix 67.32
Electroconvulsive therapy (ECT) 94.27
Electroencephalogram (EEG) 89.14
  monitoring (radiographic) (video) 89.19
Electrogastrogram 44.19
Electrokeratotomy 11.49
Electrolysis
  ciliary body 12.71
  hair follicle 86.92
  retina (for)
    destruction of lesion 14.21
    reattachment 14.51
    repair of tear 14.31
  skin 86.92
  subcutaneous tissue 86.92
Electromyogram, electromyography (EMG) muscle) 93.08
  eye 95.25
  urethral sphincter 89.23
Electronarcosis 94.29
Electronic gaiter 93.59
Electronystagmogram (ENG) 95.24
Electrooculogram (EOG) 95.22
Electroresection —*see also* Destruction, lesion, by site
  bladder neck (transurethral) 57.49
  esophagus 42.39
    endoscopic 42.33
  prostate (transurethral) 60.29
  stomach 43.49
    endoscopic 43.41
Electroretinogram (ERG) 95.21
Electroshock therapy (EST) 94.27
  subconvulsive 94.26
Elevation
  bone fragments (fractured)
    orbit 76.79
    sinus (nasal)
      frontal 22.79
      maxillary 22.79
    skull (with debridement) 02.02
    spinal 03.53
  pedicle graft 86.71
Elliot operation (scleral trephination with iridectomy) 12.61
Ellis Jones operation (repair of peroneal tendon) 83.88
Ellison operation (reinforcement of collateral ligament) 81.44
Elmslie-Cholmeley operation (tarsal wedge osteotomy) 77.28
Eloesser operation
  thoracoplasty 33.34
  thoracostomy 34.09
Elongation —*see* Lengthening
Embolectomy 38.00
  with endarterectomy—*see* Endarterectomy
  abdominal
    artery 38.06
    vein 38.07
  aorta (arch) (ascending) (descending) 38.04
  head and neck NEC 38.02
  intracranial NEC 38.01
  lower limb
    artery 38.08

Endoscopy—*continued*
 urethra 58.22
 uterus 68.12
 vagina 70.21
Enema (transanal) NEC 96.39
 for removal of impacted feces 96.38
ENG (electronystagmogram) 95.24
Enlargement
 aortic lumen, thoracic 38.14
 atrial septal defect (pre-existing) 35.41
  in repair of total anomalous pulmonary
   venous connection 35.82
 eye socket 16.64
 foramen ovale (pre-existing) 35.41
  in repair of total anomalous pulmonary
   venous connection 35.82
 intestinal stoma 46.40
  large intestine 46.43
  small intestine 46.41
 introitus 96.16
 orbit (eye) 16.64
 palpebral fissure 08.51
 punctum 09.41
 sinus tract (skin) 86.89
Enterectomy NEC 45.63
Enteroanastomosis
 large-to-large intestine 45.94
 small-to-large intestine 45.93
 small-to-small intestine 45.91
Enterocelectomy 53.9
 female 70.92
 vaginal 70.92
Enterocentesis 45.00
 duodenum 45.01
 large intestine 45.03
 small intestine NEC 45.02
Enterocholecystostomy 51.32
Enteroclysis (small bowel) 96.43
Enterocolectomy NEC 45.79
Enterocolostomy 45.93
Enteroentectropy 46.99
Enteroenterostomy 45.90
 small-to-large intestine 45.93
 small-to-small intestine 45.91
Enterogastrostomy 44.39
Enterolithotomy 45.00
Enterolysis 54.59
 laparoscopic 54.51
Enteropancreatostomy 52.96
Enterorrhaphy 46.79
 large intestine 46.75
 small intestine 46.73
Enterostomy NEC 46.39
 cecum (*see also* Colostomy) 46.10
 colon (transverse) (*see also* Colostomy) 46.10
  loop 46.03
 delayed opening 46.31
 duodenum 46.39
  loop 46.01
 feeding NEC 46.39
  percutaneous (endoscopic) 46.32
 ileum (Brooke) (Dragstedt) 46.20
  loop 46.01
 jejunum (feeding) 46.39
  loop 46.01
  percutaneous (endoscopic) 46.32
 sigmoid colon (*see also* Colostomy) 46.10
  loop 46.03
 transverse colon (*see also* Colostomy) 46.10
  loop 46.03

Enterotomy 45.00
 large intestine 45.03
 small intestine 45.02
Enucleation —*see also* Excision, lesion, by site
 cyst
  broad ligament 69.19
  dental 24.4
  liver 50.29
  ovarian 65.29
   laparoscopic 65.25
  parotid gland 26.29
  salivary gland 26.29
  skin 86.3
  subcutaneous tissue 86.3
 eyeball 16.49
  with implant (into Tenon's capsule) 16.42
   with attachment of muscles 16.41
EOG (electro-oculogram) 95.22
Epicardiectomy 36.39
Epididymectomy 63.4
 with orchidectomy (unilateral) 62.3
  bilateral 62.41
Epididymogram 87.93
Epididymoplasty 63.59
Epididymorrhaphy 63.81
Epididymotomy 63.92
Epididymovasostomy 63.83
Epiglottidectomy 30.21
Epikeratophakia 11.76
Epilation
 eyebrow (forceps) 08.93
  cryosurgical 08.92
  electrosurgical 08.91
 eyelid (forceps) NEC 08.93
  cryosurgical 08.92
  electrosurgical 08.91
 skin 86.92
Epiphysiodesis (*see also* Arrest, bone growth)-
 see category 78.2
Epiphysiolysis (*see also* Arrest, bone growth)-
 see 78.2
Epiploectomy 54.4
Epiplopexy 54.74
Epiplorrhaphy 54.74
Episioperineoplasty 71.79
Episioperineorrhaphy 71.71
 obstetrical 75.69
Episioplasty 71.79
Episioproctotomy 73.6
Episiorrhaphy 71.71
 following routine episiotomy—*see* Episiotomy
 for obstetrical laceration 75.69
Episiotomy (with subsequent episiorrhaphy) 73.6
 high forceps 72.31
 low forceps 72.1
 mid forceps 72.21
 nonobstetrical 71.09
 outlet forceps 72.1
EPS (electrophysiologic stimulation) 37.26
Eptifibatide, infusion 99.20
Equalization, leg
 lengthening—*see* category 78.3
 shortening—*see* category 78.2
Equilibration (occlusal) 24.8
Equiloudness balance 95.43
ERC (endoscopic) retrograde cholangiography
 51.11
ERCP (endoscopic retrograde
 cholangiopancreatography) 51.10
 cannulation of pancreatic duct 52.93
ERG (electroretinogram) 95.21

ERP (endoscopic retrograde pancreatography) 52.13
Eruption, tooth, surgical 24.6
Erythrocytapheresis, therapeutic 99.73
Escharectomy 86.22
Escharotomy 86.09
Esophageal voice training (postlaryngectomy) 93.73
Esophagectomy 42.40
  abdominothoracocervical (combined) (synchronous) 42.42
  partial or subtotal 42.41
  total 42.42
Esophagocologastrostomy (intrathoracic) 42.55
  antesternal or antethoracic 42.65
Esophagocolostomy (intrathoracic) NEC 42.56
  with interposition of Colon 42.55
  antesternal or antethoracic NEC 42.66
    with interposition of colon 42.65
Esophagoduodenostomy (intrathoracic) NEC 42.54
  with
    complete gastrectomy 43.99
    interposition of small bowel 42.53
Esophagoenterostomy (intrathoracic) NEC (*see also* Anastomosis, esophagus, to intestinal segment) 42.54
  antesternal or antethoracic (*see also* Anastomosis, esophagus, antesternal, to intestinal segment) 42.64
Esophagoesophagostomy (intrathoracic) 42.51
  antesternal or antethoracic 42.61
Esophagogastrectomy 43.99
Esophagogastroduodenoscopy (EGD) 45.13
  with closed biopsy 45.16
  through stoma (artificial) 45.12
  transabdominal (operative) 45.11
Esophagogastromyotomy 42.7
Esophagogastropexy 44.65
Esophagogastroplasty 44.65
Esophagogastroscopy NEC 44.13
  through stoma (artificial) 44.12
  transabdominal (operative) 44.11
Esophagogastrostomy (intrathoracic) 42.52
  with partial gastrectomy 43.5
  antesternal or antethoracic 42.62
Esophagoileostomy (intrathoracic) NEC 42.54
  with interposition of small bowel 42.53
  antesternal or antethoracic NEC 42.64
    with interposition of small bowel 42.63
Esophagojejunostomy (intrathoracic) NEC 42.54
  with
    complete gastrectomy 43.99
    interposition of small bowel 42.53
  antesternal or antethoracic NEC 42.64
    with interposition of small bowel 42.63
Esophagomyotomy 42.7
Esophagoplasty NEC 42.89
Esophagorrhaphy 42.82
Esophagoscopy NEC 42.23
  with closed biopsy 42.24
  by incision (operative) 42.21
  through stoma (artificial) 42.22
  transabdominal (operative) 42.21
Esophagostomy 42.10
  cervical 42.11
  thoracic 42.19
Esophagotomy NEC 42.09
Estes operation (ovary) 65.72
  laparoscopic 65.75
Estlander operation (thoracoplasty) 33.34

ESWL (extracorporeal shock wave lithotripsy) NEC 98.59
  bile duct 98.52
  bladder 98.51
  gallbladder 98.52
  kidney 98.51
  Kock pouch (urinary diversion) 98.51
  renal pelvis 98.51
  specified site NEC 98.59
  ureter 98.51
Ethmoidectomy 22.63
Ethmoidotomy 22.51
Evacuation
  abscess—*see* Drainage, by site
  anterior chamber (eye) (aqueous) (hyphema) 12.91
  cyst—*see also* Excision, lesion, by site
    breast 85.91
    kidney 55.01
    liver 50.29
  hematoma—*see also* Incision, hematoma
    obstetrical 75.92
      incisional 75.91
  hemorrhoids (thrombosed) 49.47
  pelvic blood clot (by incision) 54.19
    by
      culdocentesis 70.0
      culdoscopy 70.22
  retained placenta
    with curettage 69.02
    manual 75.4
  streptothrix from lacrimal duct 09.42
Evaluation (of)
  audiological 95.43
  criminal responsibility, psychiatric 94.11
  functional (physical therapy) 93.01
  hearing NEC 95.49
  orthotic (for brace fitting) 93.02
  prosthetic (for artificial limb fitting) 93.03
  psychiatric NEC 94.19
    commitment 94.13
  psychologic NEC 94.08
  testimentary capacity, psychiatric 94.11
Evans operation (release of clubfoot) 83.84
Evisceration
  eyeball 16.39
    with implant (into scleral shell) 16.31
  ocular contents 16.39
    with implant (into scleral shell) 16.31
  orbit (*see also* Exenteration, orbit) 16.59
  pelvic (anterior) (posterior) (partial) (total) (female) 68.8
    male 57.71
Evulsion
  nail (bed) (fold) 86.23
  skin 86.3
  subcutaneous tissue 86.3
Examination (for)
  breast
    manual 89.36
    radiographic NEC 87.37
    thermographic 88.85
    ultrasonic 88.73
  cervical rib (by x-ray) 87.43
  colostomy stoma (digital) 89.33
  dental (oral mucosa) (peridontal) 89.31
    radiographic NEC 87.12
  enterostomy stoma (digital) 89.33
  eye 95.09
    color vision 95.06
    comprehensive 95.02

Examination—*continued*
  dark adaptation 95.07
  limited (with prescription of spectacles) 95.01
  under anesthesia 95.04
fetus, intrauterine 75.35
general physical 89.7
glaucoma 95.03
gynecological 89.26
hearing 95.47
microscopic (specimen) (of) 91.9

Note—Use the following fourth-digit
subclassification with categories 90-91 to
identify type of examination:

1 bacterial smear
2 culture
3 culture and sensitivity
4 parasitology
5 toxicology
6 cell block and Papanicolaou smear
9 other microscopic examination

---

  adenoid 90.3
  adrenal gland 90.1
  amnion 91.4
  anus 90.9
  appendix 90.9
  bile ducts 91.0
  bladder 91.3
  blood 90.5
  bone 91.5
    marrow 90.6
  brain 90.0
  breast 91.6
  bronchus 90.4
  bursa 91.5
  cartilage 91.5
  cervix 91.4
  chest wall 90.4
  chorion 91.4
  colon 90.9
  cul-de-sac 91.1
  dental 90.8
  diaphragm 90.4
  duodenum 90.8
  ear 90.3
  endocrine gland NEC 90.1
  esophagus 90.8
  eye 90.2
  fallopian tube 91.4
  fascia 91.5
  female genital tract 91.4
  fetus 91.4
  gallbladder 91.0
  hair 91.6
  ileum 90.9
  jejunum 90.9
  joint fluid 91.5
  kidney 91.2
  large intestine 90.9
  larynx 90.3
  ligament 91.5
  liver 91.0
  lung 90.4
  lymph (node) 90.7
  meninges 90.0
  mesentery 91.1
  mouth 90.8
  muscle 91.5
  musculoskeletal system 91.5
  nails 91.6

Examination—*continued*
  nerve 90.0
  nervous system 90.0
  nose 90.3
  omentum 91.1
  operative wound 91.7
  ovary 91.4
  pancreas 91.0
  parathyroid gland 90.1
  penis 91.3
  perirenal tissue 91.2
  peritoneum (fluid) 91.1
  periureteral tissue 91.2
  perivesical (tissue) 91.3
  pharynx 90.3
  pineal gland 90.1
  pituitary gland 90.1
  placenta 91.4
  pleura (fluid) 90.4
  prostate 91.3
  rectum 90.9
  retroperitoneum 91.1
  semen 91.3
  seminal vesicle 91.3
  sigmoid 90.9
  skin 91.6
  small intestine 90.9
  specified site NEC 91.8
  spinal fluid 90.0
  spleen 90.6
  sputum 90.4
  stomach 90.8
  stool 90.9
  synovial membrane 91.5
  tendon 91.5
  thorax NEC 90.4
  throat 90.3
  thymus 90.1
  thyroid gland 90.1
  tonsil 90.3
  trachea 90.4
  ureter 91.2
  urethra 91.3
  urine 91.3
  uterus 91.4
  vagina 91.4
  vas deferens 91.3
  vomitus 90.8
  vulva 91.4
neurologic 89.13
neuro-ophthalmology 95.03
ophthalmoscopic 16.21
panorex, mandible 87.12
pelvic (manual) 89.26
  instrumental (by pelvimeter) 88.25
  pelvimetric 88.25
physical, general 89.7
postmortem 89.8
rectum (digital) 89.34
  endoscopic 48.23
    through stoma (artificial) 48.22
    transabdominal 48.21
retinal disease 95.03
specified type (manual) NEC 89.39
thyroid field, postoperative 06.02
uterus (digital) 68.11
  endoscopic 68.12
vagina 89.26
  endoscopic 70.21
visual field 95.05

Exchange transfusion 99.01
   intrauterine 75.2
Excision
   aberrant tissue—*see* Excision, lesion, by site of
      tissue origin
   abscess—*see* Excision, lesion, by site
   accessory tissue—*see also* Excision, lesion, by
      site of tissue origin
     lung 32.29
      endoscopic 32.28
     spleen 41.93
   adenoids (tag) 28.6
     with tonsillectomy 28.3
   adenoma—*see* Excision, lesion, by site
   adrenal gland (*see also* Adrenalectomy) 07.22
   ampulla of Vater (with reimplantation of
      common duct) 51.62
   anal papilla 49.39
     endoscopic 49.31
   aneurysm (arteriovenous) (*see also*
      Aneurysmectomy) 38.60
     coronary artery 36.91
     heart 37.32
     myocardium 37.32
     sinus of Valsalva 35.39
     ventricle (heart) 37.32
   anus (complete) (partial) 49.6
   aortic subvalvular ring 35.35
   apocrine gland 86.3
   aponeurosis 83.42
     hand 82.33
   appendiceal stump 47.01-47.09
   appendices epiploicae 54.4
   appendix (*see also* Appendectomy) 47.01, 47.09
     epididymis 63.3
     testis 62.2
   arcuate ligament (spine)—*omit code*
   arteriovenous fistula (*see also*
      Aneurysmectomy) 38.60
   artery (*see also* Arteriectomy) 38.60
   Baker's cyst, knee 83.39
   Bartholin's gland 71.24
   basal ganglion 01.59
   bile duct 51.69
     endoscopic 51.64
   bladder—*see also* Cystectomy
   bleb (emphysematous), lung 32.29
     endoscopic 32.28
   blood vessel (*see also* Angiectomy) 38.60
   bone (ends) (partial), except facial—*see*
      category 77.8
     facial NEC 76.39
      total 76.45
       with reconstruction 76.44
     for graft (autograft) (homograft)—*see*
      category 77.7
     fragments (chips) (*see also* Incision, bone)
      77.10
     joint (*see also* Arthrotomy) 80.10
     necrotic (*see also* Sequestrectomy, bone)
      77.00
     heterotopic, from
      muscle 83.32
       hand 82.22
      skin 86.3
      tendon 83.31
       hand 82.21
     mandible 76.31
      with arthrodesis—*see* Arthrodesis
      total 76.42
       with reconstruction 76.41

Excision—*continued*
   spur—*see* Excision, lesion, bone
   total, except facial—*see category* 77.9
     facial NEC 76.45
      with reconstruction 76.44
     mandible 76.42
   with reconstruction 76.41
   brain 01.59
     hemisphere 01.52
     lobe 01.53
   branchial cleft cyst or vestige 29.2
   breast (*see also* Mastectomy) 85.41
     aberrant tissue 85.24
     accessory 85.24
     ectopic 85.24
     nipple 85.25
      accessory 85.24
     segmental 85.23
     supernumerary 85.24
     wedge 85.21
   broad ligament 69.19
   bronchogenic cyst 32.09
     endoscopic 32.01
   bronchus (wide sleeve) NEC 32.1
   buccal mucosa 27.49
   bulbourethral gland 58.92
   bulbous tuberosities (mandible) (maxilla)
      (fibrous) (osseous) 24.31
   bunion (*see also* Bunionectomy) 77.59
   bunionette (with osteotomy) 77.54
   bursa 83.5
     hand 82.31
   canal of Nuck 69.19
   cardioma 37.33
   carotid body (lesion) (partial) (total) 39.8
   cartilage (*see also* Chondrectomy) 80.90
     intervertebral *see category* 80.5
     knee (semilunar) 80.6
     larynx 30.29
     nasal (submucous) 21.5
   caruncle, urethra 58.39
     endoscopic 58.31
   cataract (*see also* Extraction, cataract) 13.19
     secondary membrane (after cataract) 13.65
   cervical
     rib 77.91
     stump 67.4
   cervix (stump) NEC 67.4
     cold (knife) 67.2
     conization 67.2
     cryoconization 67.33
     electroconization 67.32
   chalazion (multiple) (single) 08.21
   cholesteatoma—*see* Excision, lesion, by site
   choroid plexus 02.14
   cicatrix (skin) 86.3
   cilia base 08.20
   ciliary body, prolapsed 12.98
   clavicle (head) (partial) 77.81
     total (complete) 77.91
   clitoris 71.4
   coarctation of aorta (end-to-end anastomosis)
      38.64
     with
      graft replacement (interposition)
       abdominal 38.44
       thoracic 38.45
       thoracoabdominal 38.45 *[38.44]*
   common
     duct 51.63

Excision—*continued*

    wall between posterior and coronary sinus
    (with roofing of resultant defect with patch
      graft) 35.82

  condyle—*see category* 77.8
    mandible 76.5

  conjunctival ring 10.31

  cornea 11.49
    epithelium (with chemocauterization) 11.41
      for smear or culture 11.21

  costal cartilage 80.99

  cul-de-sac (Douglas) 70.92

  cusp, heart valve 35.10
    aortic 35.11
    mitral 35.12
    tricuspid 35.14

  cyst—*see also* Excision, lesion, by site
    apical (tooth) 23.73
      with root canal therapy 23.72
    Baker's (popliteal) 83.39
    breast 85.21
    broad ligament 69.19
    bronchogenic 32.09
      endoscopic 32.01
    cervix 67.39
    dental 24.4
    dentigerous 24.4
    epididymis 63.2
    fallopian tube 66.61
    Gartner's duct 70.33
    hand 82.29
    labia 71.3
    lung 32.29
      endoscopic 32.28
    mesonephric duct 69.19
    Morgagni
      female 66.61
      male 62.2
    mullerian duct 60.73
    nasolabial 27.49
    nasopalatine 27.31
      by wide excision 27.32
    ovary 65.29
      laparoscopic 65.25
    parovarian 69.19
    pericardium 37.31
    periodontal (apical) (lateral) 24.4
    popliteal (Baker's), knee 83.39
    radicular 24.4
    spleen 41.42
    synovial (membrane) 83.39
    thyroglossal (with resection of hyoid bone)
      06.7
    urachal (bladder) 57.51
      abdominal wall 54.3
    vagina (Gartner's duct) 70.33

  cystic
    duct remnant 51.61
    hygroma 40.29

  dentinoma 24.4

  diaphragm 34.81

  disc, intervertebral NOS 80.50
    herniated (nucleus pulposus) 80.51
    other specified (diskectomy) 80.51

  diverticulum
    ampulla of Vater 51.62
    anus 49.39
      endoscopic 49.31
    bladder 57.59
      transurethral 57.49
    duodenum 45.31

Excision—*continued*

    endoscopic 45.30
    esophagus (local) 42.31
      endoscopic 42.33
    hypopharyngeal (by cricopharyngeal
      myotomy) 29.32
    intestine
      large 45.41
        endoscopic 45.43
      small NEC 45.33
    Meckel's 45.33
    pharyngeal (by cricopharyngeal myotomy)
      29.32
    pharyngoesophageal (by cricopharyngeal
      myotomy) 29.32
    stomach 43.42
      endoscopic 43.41
    urethra 58.39
      endoscopic 58.31
    ventricle, heart 37.33

  duct
    mullerian 69.19
    paramesonephric 69.19
    thyroglossal (with resection of hyoid bone)
      06.7

  ear, external (complete) NEC 18.39
    partial 18.29
    radical 18.31

  ectopic
    abdominal fetus 74.3
    tissue—*see also* Excision, lesion, by site of
      tissue origin
      bone, from muscle 83.32
      breast 85.24
      lung 32.29
        endoscopic 32.28
      spleen 41.93

  empyema pocket, lung 34.09

  epididymis 63.4

  epiglottis 30.21

  epithelial downgrowth, anterior chamber (eye)
    12.93

  epulis (gingiva) 24.31

  esophagus (*see also* Esophagectomy) 42.40

  exostosis (*see also* Excision, lesion, bone) 77.60
    auditory canal, external 18.29
    facial bone 76.2
    first metatarsal (hallux valgus repair)—*see*
      Bunionectomy

  eye 16.49
    with implant (into Tenon's capsule) 16.42
      with attachment of muscles 16.41

  eyelid 08.20
    redundant skin 08.86

  falciform ligament 54.4

  fallopian tube—*see* Salpingectomy

  fascia 83.44
    for graft 83.43
      hand 82.34
    hand 82.35
      for graft 82.34

  fat pad NEC 86.3
    knee (infrapatellar) (prepatellar) 86.3
    scalene 40.21

  fibroadenoma, breast 85.21

  fissure, anus 49.39
    endoscopic 49.31

  fistula—*see also* Fistulectomy
    anal 49.12
    arteriovenous (*see also* Aneurysmectomy)
      38.60

Excision—*continued*
  ileorectal 46.74
  lacrimal
    gland 09.21
    sac 09.6
  rectal 48.73
  vesicovaginal 57.84
  frenulum, frenum
    labial (lip) 27.41
    lingual (tongue) 25.92
  ganglion (hand) (tendon sheath) (wrist) 82.21
    gasserian 04.05
    site other than hand or nerve 83.31
    sympathetic nerve 05.29
    trigeminal nerve 04.05
  gastrocolic ligament 54.4
  gingiva 24.31
  glomus jugulare tumor 20.51
  goiter—*see* Thyroidectomy
  gum 24.31
  hamartoma, mammary 85.21
  hallux valgus—*see also* Bunionectomy with
    prosthetic implant 77.59
  hematocele, tunica vaginalis 61.92
  hematoma—*see* Drainage, by site
  hemorrhoids (external) (internal) (tag) 49.46
  heterotopic bone, from
    muscle 83.32
      hand 82.22
    skin 86.3
    tendon 83.31
      hand 82.21
  hydatid of Morgagni
    female 66.61
    male 62.2
  hydatid cyst, liver 50.29
  hydrocele
    canal of Nuck (female) 69.19
    male 63.1
    round ligament 69.19
    spermatic cord 63.1
    tunica vaginalis 61.2
  hygroma, cystic 40.29
  hymen (tag) 70.31
  hymeno-urethral fusion 70.31
  intervertebral disc--*see* Excision, disc,
    intervertebral (NOS) 80.50
  intestine (*see also* Resection, intestine) 45.8
    for interposition 45.50
      large 45.52
      small 45.51
    large (total) 45.8
      for interposition 45.52
      local 45.41
        endoscopic 45.43
      segmental 45.79
        multiple 45.71
    small (total) 45.63
      for interposition 45.51
      local 45.33
      partial 45.62
      segmental 45.62
        multiple 45.61
  intraductal papilloma 85.21
  iris prolapse 12.13
  joint (*see also* Arthrectomy) 80.90
  keloid (scar), skin 86.3
  labia—*see* Vulvectomy
  lacrimal
    gland 09.20
      partial 09.22

Excision—*continued*
    total 09.23
    passage 09.6
  sac 09.6
  lesion (local)
    abdominal wall 54.3
    accessory sinus—*see* Excision, lesion, nasal
      sinus
    adenoids 28.92
    adrenal gland(s) 07.21
    alveolus 24.4
    ampulla of Vater 51.62
    anterior chamber (eye) NEC 12.40
    anus 49.39
      endoscopic 49.31
    apocrine gland 86.3
    artery 38.60
      abdominal 38.66
      aorta (arch) (ascending) (descending
        thoracic) 38.64
        with end-to-end anastomosis 38.45
          abdominal 38.44
          thoracic 38.45
          thoracoabdominal 38.45 *[38.44]*
        with interposition graft replacement 38.45
          abdominal 38.44
          thoracic 38.45
          thoracoabdominal 38.45 *[38.44]*
      head and neck NEC 38.62
      intracranial NEC 38.61
      lower limb 38.68
      thoracic NEC 38.65
      upper limb 38.63
    atrium 37.33
    auditory canal or meatus, external 18.29
      radical 18.31
    auricle, ear 18.29
      radical 18.31
    biliary ducts 51.69
      endoscopic 51.64
    bladder (transurethral) 57.49
      open 57.59
      suprapubic 57.59
    blood vessel 38.60
      abdominal
        artery 38.66
        vein 38.67
      aorta (arch) (ascending) (descending) 38.64
      head and neck NEC 38.62
      intracranial NEC 38.61
      lower limb
        artery 38.68
        vein 38.69
      thoracic NEC 38.65
      upper limb (artery) (vein) 38.63
    bone 77.60
      carpal, metacarpal 77.64
      clavicle 77.61
      facial 76.2
      femur 77.65
      fibula 77.67
      humerus 77.62
      jaw 76.2
        dental 24.4
      patella 77.66
      pelvic 77.69
      phalanges (foot) (hand) 77.69
      radius 77.63
      scapula 77.61
      skull 01.6
      specified site NEC 77.69

Excision—*continued*

tarsal, metatarsal 77.68
thorax (ribs) (sternum) 77.61
tibia 77.67
ulna 77.63
vertebrae 77.69
brain (transtemporal approach) NEC 01.59
by stereotactic radiosurgery 92.30
cobalt 60 92.32
linear accelerator (LINAC) 92.31
multi-source 92.32
particle beam 92.33
particulate 92.33
radiosurgery NEC 92.39
single source photon 92.31
breast (segmental) (wedge) 85.21
broad ligament 69.19
bronchus NEC 32.09
endoscopic 32.01
cerebral (cortex) NEC 01.59
meninges 01.51
cervix (myoma) 67.39
chest wall 34.4
choroid plexus 02.14
ciliary body 12.44
colon 45.41
endoscopic NEC 45.43
polypectomy 45.42
conjunctive 10.31
cornea 11.49
cranium 01.6
cul-de-sac (Douglas) 70.32
dental (jaw) 24.4
diaphragm 34.81
duodenum (local) 45.31
endoscopic 45.30
ear, external 18.29
radical 18.31
endometrium 68.29
epicardium 37.31
epididymis 63.3
epiglottis 30.09
esophagus NEC 42.32
endoscopic 42.33
eye, eyeball 16.93
anterior segment NEC 12.40
eyebrow (skin) 08.20
eyelid 08.20
by
halving procedure 08.24
wedge resection 08.24
major
full-thickness 08.24
partial-thickness 08.23
minor 08.22
fallopian tube 66.61
fascia 83.39
hand 82.29
groin region (abdominal wall) (inguinal) 54.3
skin 86.3
subcutaneous tissue 86.3
gum 24.31
heart 37.33
hepatic duct 51.69
inguinal canal 54.3
intestine
large 45.41
endoscopic NEC 45.43
polypectomy 45.42
small NEC 45.33
intracranial NEC 01.59

Excision—*continued*

intranasal 21.31
intraspinal 03.4
iris 12.42
jaw 76.2
dental 24.4
joint 80.80
ankle 80.87
elbow 80.82
foot and toe 80.88
hand and finger 80.84
hip 80.85
knee 80.86
shoulder 80.81
specified site NEC 80.89
spine 80.89
wrist 80.83
kidney 55.39
with partial nephrectomy 55.4
labia 71.3
lacrimal
gland (frontal approach) 09.21
passage 09.6
sac 09.6
larynx 30.09
ligament (joint) (*see also* Excision, lesion,
joint) 80.80
broad 69.19
round 69.19
uterosacral 69.19
lip 27.43
by wide excision 27.42
liver 50.29
lung NEC 32.29
by wide excision 32.3
endoscopic 32.28
lymph structure(s) (channel) (vessel) NEC
40.29
node—*see* Excision, lymph, node
mammary duct 85.21
mastoid (bone) 20.49
mediastinum 34.3
meninges (cerebral) 01.51
spinal 03.4
mesentery 54.4
middle ear 20.51
mouth NEC 27.49
muscle 83.32
hand 82.22
ocular 15.13
myocardium 37.33
nail 86.23
nasal sinus 22.60
antrum 22.62
with Caldwell-Luc approach 22.61
specified approach NEC 22.62
ethmoid 22.63
frontal 22.42
maxillary 22.62
with Caldwell-Luc approach 22.61
specified approach NEC 22.62
sphenoid 22.64
nasopharynx 29.3
nerve (cranial) (peripheral) 04.07
sympathetic 05.29
nonodontogenic 24.31
nose 21.30
intranasal 21.31
polyp 21.31
skin 21.32
specified site NEC 21.32

Excision—*continued*
  odontogenic 24.4
  omentum 54.4
  orbit 16.92
  ovary 65.29
    by wedge resection 65.22
      laparoscopic 65.24
    that by laparoscope 65.25
  palate (bony) 27.31
    by wide excision 27.32
    soft 27.49
  pancreas (local) 52.22
    endoscopic 52.21
  parathyroid 06.89
  parotid gland or duct NEC 26.29
  pelvic wall 54.3
  pelvirectal tissue 48.82
  penis 64.2
  pericardium 37.31
  perineum (female) 71.3
    male 86.3
  periprostatic tissue 60.82
  perirectal tissue 48.82
  perirenal tissue 59.91
  peritoneum 54.4
  perivesical tissue 59.91
  pharynx 29.39
    diverticulum 29.32
  pineal gland 07.53
  pinna 18.29
    radical 18.31
  pituitary (gland) (*see also* Hypophysectomy,
    partial) 07.63
    by stereotactic radiosurgery 92.30
      cobalt 60 92.32
      linear accelerator (LINAC) 92.31
      multi-source 92.32
      particle beam 92.33
      particulate 92.33
      radiosurgery NEC 92.39
      single source photon 92.31
  pleura 34.59
  pouch of Douglas 70.32
  preauricular (ear) 18.21
  presacral 54.4
  prostate (transurethral) 60.61
  pulmonary (fibrosis) 32.29
    endoscopic 32.28
  rectovaginal septum 48.82
  rectum 48.35
    polyp (endoscopic) 48.36
  retroperitoneum 54.4
  salivary gland or duct NEC 26.29
    en bloc 26.32
  sclera 12.84
  scrotum 61.3
  sinus (nasal)—*see* Excision, lesion, nasal sinus
  Skene's gland 71.3
  skin 86.3
    breast 85.21
    nose 21.32
    radical (wide) (involving underlying or
      adjacent structure) (with flap closure)
      86.4
    scrotum 61.3
  skull 01.6
  soft tissue NEC 83.39
    hand 82.29
  spermatic cord 63.3
  sphincter of Oddi 51.62
    endoscopic 51.64

Excision—*continued*
  spinal cord (meninges) 03.4
  spleen (cyst) 41.42
  stomach NEC 43.42
    endoscopic 43.41
      polyp 43.41
    polyp (endoscopic) 43.41
  subcutaneous tissue 86.3
    breast 85.21
  subgingival 24.31
  sweat gland 86.3
  tendon 83.39
    hand 82.29
    ocular 15.13
    sheath 83.31
      hand 82.21
  testis 62.2
  thorax 34.4
  thymus 07.81
  thyroid 06.31
    substernal or transsternal route 06.51
  tongue 25.1
  tonsil 28.92
  trachea 31.5
  tunica vaginalis 61.92
  ureter 56.41
  urethra 58.39
    endoscopic 58.31
  uterine ligament 69.19
  uterosacral ligament 69.19
  uterus 68.29
  vagina 70.33
  vein 38.60
    abdominal 38.67
    head and neck NEC 38.62
    intracranial NEC 38.61
    lower limb 38.69
    thoracic NEC 38.65
    upper limb 38.63
  ventricle (heart) 37.33
  vocal cords 30.09
  vulva 71.3
  ligament (*see also* Arthrectomy) 80.90
    broad 69.19
    round 69.19
    uterine 69.19
    uterosacral 69.19
  ligamentum flavum (spine)—*omit code*
  lingual tonsil 28.5
  lip 27.43
  liver (partial) 50.22
  loose body
    bone—*see* Sequestrectomy, bone
    joint 80.10
  lung (complete) (with mediastinal dissection)
    32.5
    accessory or ectopic tissue 32.29
      endoscopic 32.28
    segmental 32.3
    specified type NEC 32.29
      endoscopic 32.28
    volume reduction surgery 32.22
    wedge 32.29
  lymph, lymphatic
    drainage area 40.29
      radical—*see* Excision, lymph, node, radical
      regional (with lymph node, skin,
        subcutaneous tissue, and fat) 40.3
    node (simple) NEC 40.29
      with

Excision—*continued*
　septum 68.22
　uvula 27.72
　vagina (total) 70.4
　varicocele, spermatic cord 63.1
　vein (*see also* Phlebectomy) 38.60
　　varicose 38.50
　　　abdominal 38.57
　　　head and neck NEC 38.52
　　　intracranial NEC 38.51
　　　lower limb 38.59
　　　ovarian 38.67
　　　thoracic NEC 38.55
　　　upper limb 38.53
　verruca—*see also* Excision, lesion, by site
　　eyelid 08.22
　vesicovaginal septum 70.33
　vitreous opacity 14.74
　　anterior approach 14.73
　vocal cord(s) (submucous) 30.22
　vulva (bilateral) (simple) (*see also* Vulvectomy)
　　71.62
　wart—*see also* Excision, lesion, by site
　　eyelid 08.22
　wolffian duct 69.19
　xanthoma (tendon sheath, hand) 82.21
　　site other than hand 83.31
Excisional biopsy —*see* Biopsy
Exclusion, pyloric 44.39
Exenteration
　ethmoid air cells 22.63
　orbit 16.59
　　with
　　　removal of adjacent structures 16.51
　　　temporalis muscle transplant 16.59
　　　therapeutic removal of bone 16.52
　　pelvic (organs) (female) 68.8
　　male 57.71
　petrous pyramid air cells 20.59
Exercise (physical therapy) NEC 93.19
　active musculoskeletal NEC 93.12
　assisting 93.11
　　in pool 93.31
　breathing 93.18
　musculoskeletal
　　active NEC 93.12
　　passive NEC 93.17
　neurologic 89.13
　passive musculoskeletal NEC 93.17
　resistive 93.13
Exfoliation, skin, by chemical 86.24
Exostectomy (*see also* Excision, lesion, bone)
　77.60
　first metatarsal (hallux valgus repair)—*see*
　　Bunionectomy
　hallux valgus repair (with wedge
　　osteotomy)—*see* Bunionectomy
Expiratory flow rate 89.38
Exploration —*see also* Incision
　abdomen 54.11
　abdominal wall 54.0
　adrenal (gland) 07.41
　　field 07.00
　　　bilateral 07.02
　　　unilateral 07.01
　artery 38.00
　　abdominal 38.06
　　aorta (arch) (ascending) (descending) 38.04
　　head and neck NEC 38.02
　　intracranial NEC 38.01
　　lower limb 38.08

Exploration—*continued*
　　thoracic NEC 38.05
　　upper limb 38.03
　auditory canal, external 18.02
　axilla 86.09
　bile duct(s) 51.59
　　common duct 51.51
　　　endoscopic 51.11
　　　for relief of obstruction 51.42
　　　　endoscopic 51.84
　　　for removal of calculus 51.41
　　　　endoscopic 51.88
　　　laparoscopic 51.11
　　for relief of obstruction 51.49
　　　endoscopic 51.84
　bladder (by incision) 57.19
　　endoscopic 57.32
　　　through stoma (artificial) 57.31
　bone (*see also* Incision, bone) 77.10
　brain (tissue) 01.39
　breast 85.0
　bronchus 33.0
　　endoscopic—*see* Bronchoscopy
　bursa 83.03
　　hand 82.03
　carotid body 39.8
　carpal tunnel 04.43
　choroid 14.9
　ciliary body 12.44
　colon 45.03
　common bile duct 51.51
　　endoscopic 51.11
　　for
　　　relief of obstruction 51.42
　　　　endoscopic 51.84
　　　removal of calculus 51.41
　　　　endoscopic 51.88
　coronary artery 36.99
　cranium 01.24
　cul-de-sac 70.12
　　endoscopic 70.22
　disc space 03.09
　duodenum 45.01
　endoscopic—*see* Endoscopy, by site
　epididymis 63.92
　esophagus (by incision) NEC 42.09
　　endoscopic—*see* Esophagoscopy
　ethmoid sinus 22.51
　eyelid 08.09
　fallopian tube 66.01
　fascia 83.09
　　hand 82.09
　flank 54.0
　fossa (superficial) NEC 86.09
　　pituitary 07.71
　frontal sinus 22.41
　frontonasal duct 96.21
　gallbladder 51.04
　groin (region) (abdominal wall) (inguinal) 54.0
　　skin and subcutaneous tissue 86.09
　heart 37.11
　hepatic duct 51.59
　hypophysis 07.72
　ileum 45.02
　inguinal canal (groin) 54.0
　intestine (by incision) NEC 45.00
　　large 45.03
　　small 45.02
　intrathoracic 34.02
　jejunum 45.02

F

Face lift 86.82
Facetectomy 77.89
Facilitation, Intraocular circulation NEC 12.59
Failed (trial) forceps 73.3
Family
  counselling (medical) (social) 94.49
  therapy 94.42
Farabeuf operation (ischiopubiotomy) 77.39
Fasanella-Servatt operation
  (blepharoptosis repair) 08.35
Fasciaplasty —*see* Fascioplasty
Fascia sling operation —*see* Operation, sling
Fasciectomy 83.44
  for graft 83.43
    hand 82.34
  hand 82.35
    for graft 82.34
  palmar (release of Dupuytren's contracture)
    82.35
Fasciodesis 83.89
  hand 82.89
Fascioplasty (*see also* Repair, fascia) 83.89
  hand (*see also* Repair, fascia, hand) 82.89
Fasciorrhaphy —*see* Suture, fascia
Fasciotomy 83.14
  Dupuytren's 82.12
    with excision 82.35
  Dwyer 83.14
  hand 82.12
  Ober-Yount 83.14
  orbital (*see also* Orbitotomy) 16.09
  palmar (release of Dupuytren's
    contracture) 82.12
    with excision 82.35
Fenestration
  aneurysm (dissecting), thoracic aorta 39.54
  aortic aneurysm 39.54
  cardiac valve 35.10
  chest wall 34.01
  ear
    inner (with graft) 20.61
      revision 20.62
    tympanic 19.55
  labyrinth (with graft) 20.61
  Lempert's (endaural) 19.9
  operation (aorta) 39.54
  oval window, ear canal 19.55
  palate 27.1
  pericardium 37.12
  semicircular canals (with graft) 20.61
  stapes foot plate (with vein graft) 19.19
    with incus replacement 19.11
  tympanic membrane 19.55
  vestibule (with graft) 20.61
Ferguson operation (hernia repair) 53.00
Fetography 87.81
Fetoscopy 75.31
Fiberoscopy —*see* Endoscopy, by site
Fibroidectomy, uterine 68.29
Fick operation (perforation of foot plate) 19.0
Filipuncture (aneurysm) (cerebral) 39.52
Filleting
  hammer toe 77.56
  pancreas 52.3
Filling, tooth (amalgam) (plastic) (silicate) 23.2
  root canal (*see also* Therapy, root canal) 23.70

Fimbriectomy (*see also* Salpingectomy, partial)
  66.69
  Uchida (with tubal ligation) 66.32
Finney operation (pyloroplasty) 44.29
Fissurectomy, anal 49.39
  endoscopic 49.31
  skin (subcutaneous tissue) 49.04
Fistulectomy —*see also* Closure, fistula, by site
  abdominothoracic 34.83
  abdominouterine 69.42
  anus 49.12
  appendix 47.92
  bile duct 51.79
  biliary tract NEC 51.79
  bladder (transurethral approach) 57.84
  bone (*see also* Excision, lesion, bone) 77.60
  branchial cleft 29.52
  bronchocutaneous 33.42
  bronchoesophageal 33.42
  bronchomediastinal 34.73
  bronchopleural 34.73
  bronchopleurocutaneous 34.73
  bronchopleuromediastinal 34.73
  bronchovisceral 33.42
  cervicosigmoidal 67.62
  cholecystogastroenteric 51.93
  cornea 11.49
  diaphragm 34.83
  enterouterine 69.42
  esophagopleurocutaneous 34.73
  esophagus NEC 42.84
  fallopian tube 66.73
  gallbladder 51.93
  gastric NEC 44.63
  hepatic duct 51.79
  hepatopleural 34.73
  hepatopulmonary 34.73
  intestine
    large 46.76
    small 46.74
  intestinouterine 69.42
  joint (*see also* Excision, lesion, joint) 80.80
  lacrimal
    gland 09.21
    sac 09.6
  laryngotracheal 31.62
  larynx 31.62
  mediastinocutaneous 34.73
  mouth NEC 27.53
  nasal 21.82
    sinus 22.71
  nasolabial 21.82
  nasopharyngeal 21.82
  oroantral 22.71
  oronasal 21.82
  pancreas 52.95
  perineorectal 71.72
  perineosigmoidal 71.72
  perirectal, not opening into rectum 48.93
  pharyngoesophageal 29.53
  pharynx NEC 29.53
  pleura 34.73
  rectolabial 71.72
  rectourethral 58.43
  rectouterine 69.42
  rectovaginal 70.73
  rectovesical 57.83
  rectovulvar 71.72

Fistulectomy—*continued*
rectum 48.73
salivary (duct) (gland) 26.42
scrotum 61.42
skin 86.3
stomach NEC 44.63
subcutaneous tissue 86.3
thoracoabdominal 34.83
thoracogastric 34.83
thoracointestinal 34.83
thorax NEC 34.73
trachea NEC 31.73
tracheoesophageal 31.73
ureter 56.84
urethra 58.43
uteroenteric 69.42
uterointestinal 69.42
uterorectal 69.42
uterovaginal 69.42
vagina 70.75
vesicosigmoidovaginal 57.83
vocal cords 31.62
vulvorectal 71.72
Fistulization
appendix 47.91
arteriovenous 39.27
cisterna chyli 40.62
endolymphatic sac (for decompression) 20.79
esophagus, external 42.10
cervical 42.11
specified technique NEC 42.19
interatrial 35.41
labyrinth (for decompression) 20.79
lacrimal sac into nasal cavity 09.81
larynx 31.29
lymphatic duct, left (thoracic) 40.62
orbit 16.09
peritoneal 54.93
salivary gland 26.49
sclera 12.69
by trephination 12.61
with iridectomy 12.65
sinus, nasal NEC 22.9
subarachnoid space 02.2
thoracic duct 40.62
trachea 31.29
tracheoesophageal 31.95
urethrovaginal 58.0
ventricle, cerebral (*see also* Shunt, ventricular)
02.2
Fistulogram
abdominal wall 88.03
chest wall 87.38
retroperitoneum 88.14
Fistulotomy, anal 49.11
Fitting
arch bars (orthodontic) 24.7
for immobilization (fracture) 93.55
artificial limb 84.40
contact lens 95.32
denture (total) 99.97
bridge (fixed) 23.42
removable 23.43
partial (fixed) 23.42
removable 23.43
hearing aid 95.48
obturator (orthodontic) 24.7
ocular prosthetics 95.34
orthodontic
appliance 24.7
obturator 24.7

Fitting—*continued*
wiring 24.7
orthotic device 93.23
periodontal splint (orthodontic) 24.7
prosthesis, prosthetic device
above knee 84.45
arm 84.43
lower (and hand) 84.42
upper (and shoulder) 84.41
below knee 84.46
hand (and lower arm) 84.42
leg 84.47
above knee 84.45
below knee 84.46
limb NEC 84.40
ocular 95.34
penis (external) 64.94
shoulder (and upper arm) 84.41
spectacles 95.31
Five-in-one repair, knee 81.42
Fixation
bone
external, without reduction 93.59
with fracture reduction—*see* Reduction,
fracture
cast immobilization NEC 93.53
splint 93.54
traction (skeletal) NEC 93.44
intermittent 93.43
internal (without fracture-reduction) 78.50
with fracture-reduction—*see* Reduction,
fracture
carpal, metacarpal 78.54
clavicle 78.51
femur 78.55
fibula 78.57
humerus 78.52
patella 78.56
pelvic 78.59
phalanges (foot) (hand) 78.59
radius 78.53
scapula 78.51
specified site NEC 78.59
tarsal, metatarsal 78.58
thorax (ribs) (sternum) 78.51
tibia 78.57
ulna 78.53
vertebrae 78.59
breast (pendulous) 85.6
cardinal ligaments 69.22
duodenum 46.62
to abdominal wall 46.61
external (without manipulation for reduction)
93.59
with fracture-reduction—*see* Reduction,
fracture
cast immobilization NEC 93.53
pressure dressing 93.56
splint 93.54
traction (skeletal) NEC 93.44
intermittent 93.43
hip 81.40
ileum 46.62
to abdominal wall 46.61
internal
with fracture-reduction—*see* Reduction,
fracture
without fracture-reduction—*see* Fixation,
bone, internal
intestine 46.60

Fixation—*continued*
  large 46.64
    to abdominal wall 46.63
  small 46.62
    to abdominal wall 46.61
    to abdominal wall 46.60
  iris (bombé) 12.11
  jejunum 46.62
    to abdominal wall 46.61
  joint—*see* Arthroplasty
  kidney 55.7
  ligament
    cardinal 69.22
    palpebrae 08.36
  omentum 54.74
  parametrial 69.22
  rectum (sling) 48.76
  spine, with fusion (*see also* Fusion, spinal) 81.00
  spleen 41.95
  tendon 83.88
    hand 82.85
  testis in scrotum 62.5
  tongue 25.59
  urethrovaginal (to Cooper's ligament) 70.77
  uterus (abdominal) (vaginal) (ventrofixation)
    69.22
  vagina 70.77
Flooding (psychologic desensitization) 94.33
Flowmetry, Doppler (ultrasonic)—*see also*
  Ultrasonography
  aortic arch 88.73
  head and neck 88.71
  heart 88.72
  thorax NEC 88.73
Fluoroscopy —*see* Radiography
Fog therapy (respiratory) 93.94
Folding, eye muscle 15.22
  multiple (two or more muscles) 15.4
Foley operation (pyeloplasty) 55.87
Fontan operation (creation of conduit between
  right atrium and pulmonary artery) 35.94
Foraminotomy 03.09
Forced extension, limb 93.25
Forceps delivery —*see* Delivery, forceps
Formation
  adhesions
    pericardium 36.39
    pleura 34.6
  anus, artificial (*see also* Colostomy) 46.13
    duodenostomy 46.39
    ileostomy (*see also* Ileostomy) 46.23
    jejunostomy 46.39
      percutaneous (endoscopic) (PEJ) 46.32
  arteriovenous fistula (for kidney dialysis)
    (peripheral) (shunt) 39.27
    external cannula 39.93
  bone flap, cranial 02.03
  cardiac pacemaker pocket
    with initial insertion of pacemaker—*omit code*
    new site (skin) (subcutaneous) 37.79
  colostomy (*see also* Colostomy) 46.13
  conduit
    ileal (urinary) 56.51
    left ventricle and aorta 35.93
    right atrium and pulmonary artery 35.94
    right ventricle and pulmonary (distal) artery
      35.92
      in repair of
        pulmonary artery atresia 35.92
        transposition of great vessels 35.92

Formation—*continued*
    truncus arteriosus 35.83
  endorectal ileal pouch (J-pouch) (H-pouch)
    (S-pouch) (with anastomosis to anus) 45.95
  fistula
    arteriovenous (for kidney dialysis) (peripheral
      shunt) 39.27
      external cannula 39.93
    bladder to skin NEC 57.18
      with bladder flap 57.21
      percutaneous 57.17
    cutaneoperitoneal 54.93
    gastric 43.19
      percutaneous (endoscopic)
        (transabdominal) 43.11
    mucous (Sec also Colostomy) 46.13
    rectovaginal 48.99
    tracheoesophageal 31.95
    tubulovalvular (Beck-Jianu) (Frank's)
      (Janeway) (Spivack's)
      (Ssabanejew-Frank) 43.19
    urethrovaginal 58.0
  ileal
    bladder
      closed 57.87 *[45.51]*
      open 56.51
    conduit 56.51
  interatrial fistula 35.42
  mucous fistula (*see also* Colostomy) 46.13
  pericardial
    baffle, interatrial 35.91
    window 37.12
  pleural window (for drainage) 34.09
  pocket
    cardiac pacemaker
      with initial insertion of pacemaker —*omit*
        code
      new site (skin) (subcutaneous) 37.79
    thalamic stimulator pulse generator
      with initial insertion of battery
        package—*omit code*
      new site (skin) (subcutaneous) 86.09
  pupil 12.39
    by iridectomy 12.14
  rectovaginal fistula 48.99
  reversed gastric tube (intrathoracic)
    (retrosternal) 42.58
    antesternal or antethoracic 42.68
  septal defect, interatrial 35.42
  shunt
    abdominovenous 54.94
    arteriovenous 39.93
    peritoneojugular 54.94
    peritoneo-vascular 54.94
    pleuroperitoneal 34.05
    transjugular intrahepatic portosystemic (TIPS)
      39.1
  subcutaneous tunnel
    esophageal 42.86
      with anastomosis—*see* Anastomosis,
        esophagus, antesternal
    pulse generator lead wire 86.99
      with initial procedure —*omit code*
    thalamic stimulator pulse generator pocket
      with insertion of battery package—*omit code*
      new site (skin) (subcutaneous) 86.09
  syndactyly (finger) (toe) 86.89
  tracheoesophageal 31.95
  tubulovalvular fistula (Beck-Jianu) (Frank's)
    (Janeway) (Spivack's) (Ssabanejew-Frank)
    43.19

G

Goebel-Frangenheim-Stoeckel operation
(urethrovesical suspension) 59.4
Goldner operation (clubfoot release) 80.48
Goldthwaite operation
ankle stabilization 81.11
patellar stabilization 81.44
tendon transfer for stabilization of patella 81.44
Gonadectomy
ovary
bilateral 65.51
laparoscopic 65.53
unilateral 65.39
laparoscopic 65.31
testis 62.3
Goniopuncture 12.51
with goniotomy 12.53
Gonioscopy 12.29
Goniopasis 12.59
Goniotomy (Barkan's) 12.52
with goniopuncture 12.53
Goodal-Power operation (vagina) 70.8
Gordon-Taylor operation (hindquarter
amputation) 84.19
GP IIB/IIIa inhibitor, infusion 99.20
Graber-Duvernay operation (drilling of
femoral head) 77.15
Graft, grafting
aneurysm 39.52
endovascular
abdominal aorta 39.71
lower extremity artery(s) 39.79
thoracic aorta 39.79
upper extremity artery(s) 39.79
artery, arterial (patch) 39.58
with
excision or resection of vessel—see
Arteriectomy, with graft replacement
synthetic patch (Dacron) (Teflon) 39.57
tissue patch (vein) (autogenous) (homograft)
39.56
blood vessel (patch) 39.58
with
excision or resection of vessel—see
Angiectomy, with graft replacement
synthetic patch (Dacron) (Teflon) 39.57
tissue patch (vein) (autogenous) (homograft)
39.56
bone (autogenous) (bone bank) (dual onlay)
(heterogenous) (inlay) (massive onlay)
(multiple) (osteoperiosteal) (peg)
(subperiosteal) (with metallic fixation) 78.00
with
arthrodesis—see Arthrodesis
arthroplasty—see Arthroplasty
gingivoplasty 24.2
lengthening—see Lengthening, bone
carpals, metacarpals 78.04
clavicle 78.01
facial NEC 76.91
with total ostectomy 76.44
femur 78.05
fibula 78.07
humerus 78.02
joint—see Arthroplasty
mandible 76.91
with total mandibulectomy 76.41
marrow—see Transplant, bone, marrow
nose—see Graft, nose
patella 78.06
pelvic 78.09
pericranial 02.04

Graft, grafting—continued
phalanges (foot) (hand) 78.09
radius 78.03
scapula 78.01
skull 02.04
specified site NEC 78.09
spine 78.09
with fusion—see Fusion, spinal
tarsal, metatarsal 78.08
thorax (ribs) (sternum) 78.01
thumb (with transfer of skin nap) 82.69
tibia 78.07
ulna 78.03
vertebrae 78.09
with fusion—see Fusion, spinal
breast (see also Mammoplasty) 85.89
buccal sulcus 27.99
cartilage (joint)—see also Arthroplasty
nose—see Graft, nose
chest wall (mesh) (silastic) 34.79
conjunctiva (free) (mucosa) 10.44
for symblepharon repair 10.41
cornea (see also Keratoplasty) 11.60
dermal-fat 86.69
dermal regenerative 86.67
dura 02.12
ear
auricle 18.79
external auditory meatus 18.6
inner 20.61
pedicle preparation 86.71
esophagus NEC 42.87
with interposition (intrathoracic) NEC 42.58
antesternal or antethoracic NEC 42.68
colon (intrathoracic) 42.55
antesternal or antethoracic 42.65
small bowel (intrathoracic) 42.53
antesternal or antethoracic 42.63
eyebrow (see also Reconstruction, eyelid, with
graft) 08.69
eyelid (see also Reconstruction, eyelid, with
graft) 08.69
free mucous membrane 08.62
eye socket (skin) (cartilage) (bone) 16.63
fallopian tube 66.79
fascia 83.82
with hernia repair—see Repair, hernia
eyelid 08.32
hand 82.72
tarsal cartilage 08.69
fat pad NEC 86.89
with skin graft—see Graft, skin, full-thickness
flap (advanced) (rotating) (sliding)—see also
Graft, skin, pedicle
tarsoconjunctival 08.64
hair-bearing skin 86.64
hand
fascia 82.72
free skin 86.62
muscle 82.72
pedicle (flap) 86.73
tendon 82.79
heart, for revascularization—see category 36.3
joint—see Arthroplasty
larynx 31.69
lip 27.56
full-thickness 27.55
lymphatic structure(s) (channel) (node) (vessel)
40.9
mediastinal fat to myocardium 36.39
meninges (cerebral) 02.12

H

Hydrotherapy 93.33
  assisted exercise in pool 93.31
  whirlpool 93.32
Hymenectomy 70.31
Hymenoplasty 70.76
Hymenorrhaphy 70.76
Hymenotomy 70.11
Hyperalimentation 99.15
Hyperbaric oxygenation 93.95
  wound 93.59
Hyperextension, joint 93.25
Hyperthermia NEC 93.35
  for cancer treatment (interstitial) (local)
      (radiofrequency) (regional) (ultrasound)
      (whole-body) 99.85
Hypnodrama, psychiatric 94.32
Hypnosis (psychotherapeutic) 94.32
  for anesthesia—*omit code*
Hypnotherapy 94.32
Hypophysectomy (complete) (total) 07.69
  partial or subtotal 07.63
    transfrontal approach 07.61
    transsphenoidal approach 07.62
  specified approach NEC 07.68
  transfrontal approach (complete) (total) 07.64
    partial 07.61
  transsphenoidal approach (complete) (total)
      07.65
    partial 07.62
Hypothermia (central) (local) 99.81
  gastric (cooling) 96.31
    freezing 96.32
  systemic (in open heart surgery) 39.62
Hypotympanotomy 20.23
Hysterectomy 68.9
  abdominal 68.4
    partial or subtotal (supracervical)
        (supravaginal) 68.3
    radical (modified) (Wertheim's) 68.6
  vaginal (complete) (partial) (subtotal) (total)
      68.59
    laparoscopically assisted (LAVH) 68.51
    radical (Schauta) 68.7
Hysterocolpectomy (radical) (vaginal) 68.7
  abdominal 68.6
Hysterogram NEC 87.85
  percutaneous 87.84
Hysterolysis 54.59
  laparoscopic 54.51
Hysteromyomectomy 68.29
Hysteropexy 69.22
Hysteroplasty 69.49
Hysterorrhaphy 69.41
Hysterosalpingography
  gas (contrast) 87.82
  opaque dye (contrast) 87.83
Hysterosalpingostomy 66.74
Hysteroscopy 68.12
  ablation
    endometrial 68.23
  with biopsy 68.16
Hysterotomy (with removal of foreign body)
      (with removal of hydatidiform mole) 68.0
  for intrauterine transfusion 75.2
  obstetrical 74.99
    for termination of pregnancy 74.91
Hysterotrachelectomy 67.4
Hysterotracheloplasty 69.49
Hysterotrachelorrhaphy 69.41
Hysterotrachelotomy 69.95

I

Implant, implantation—*continued*
    total repair of tetralogy of Fallot 35.81
    penile (non-inflatable) (internal) 64.95
      inflatable (internal) 64.97
    skin (dermal regenerative) (matrix) 86.67
    testicular (bilateral) (unilateral) 62.7
    pulsation balloon (phase-shift) 37.61
    pump, infusion 86.06
    radial artery 36.19
    radioactive isotope 92.27
    radium (radon) 92.27
    retinal attachment 14.41
      with buckling 14.41
    Rickham reservoir 02.2
    silicone
      breast (bilateral) 85.54
        unilateral 85.53
      skin (for filling of defect) 86.02
        for augmentation NEC 86.89
    stimoceiver
      brain 02.93
      intracranial 02.93
      peripheral nerve 04.92
      spine 03.93
    subdural
      grids 02.93
      strips 02.93
    Swanson prosthesis (joint) (silastic) NEC 81.96
      carpocarpal, carpometacarpal 81.74
      finger 81.71
      hand (metacarpophalangeal) (interphalangeal) 81.71
      interphalangeal 81.71
      knee (partial) (total) 81.54
        revision 81.55
      metacarpophalangeal 81.71
      toe 81.57
        for hallux valgus repair 77.59
      wrist (partial) 81.74
        total 81.73
    systemic arteries into myocardium (Vineberg type operation) 36.2
    testicular prosthesis (bilateral) (unilateral) 62.7
    tissue expander (skin) NEC 86.93
      breast 85.95
    tissue mandril (for vascular graft) 39.99
      with
        blood vessel repair 39.56
        vascular bypass or shunt—*see* Bypass, vascular
    tooth (bud) (germ) 23.5
      prosthetic 23.6
    umbrella, vena cava 38.7
    ureters into
      bladder 56.74
      intestine 56.71
        external diversion 56.51
      skin 56.61
    urethan sphincter, artificial (inflatable) 58.93
    urethra
      for repair of urinary stress incontinence
        collagen 59.72
        fat 59.72
        polytef 59.72
    urinary sphincter, artificial (inflatable) 58.93
    vascular access device 86.07
    vitreous (silicone) 14.75
      for retinal reattachment 14.41
        with buckling 14.41
    vocal cord(s) (paraglottic) 31.98
Implosion (psychologic desensitization) 94.33

Incision (and drainage)
    with
      exploration—*see* Exploration
      removal of foreign body—*see* Removal, foreign body
    abdominal wall 54.0
    as operative approach—*omit code*
    abscess—*see also* Incision, by site
      appendix 47.2
        with appendectomy 47.09
          laparoscopic 47.01
      extraperitoneal 54.0
      ischiorectal 49.01
      lip 27.0
      omental 54.19
      perianal 49.01
      perigastric 54.19
      perisplenic 54.19
      peritoneal NEC 54.19
        pelvic (female) 70.12
      retroperitoneal 54.0
      sclera 12.89
      skin 86.04
      subcutaneous tissue 86.04
      subdiaphragmatic 54.19
      subhepatic 54.19
      subphrenic 54.19
      vas deferens 63.6
    adrenal gland 07.41
    alveolus, alveolar bone 24.0
    antecubital fossa 86.09
    anus NEC 49.93
      fistula 49.11
      septum 49.91
    appendix 47.2
    artery 38.00
      abdominal 38.06
      aorta (arch) (ascending) (descending) 38.04
      head and neck NEC 38.02
      intracranial NEC 38.01
      lower limb 38.08
      thoracic NEC 38.05
      upper limb 38.03
    atrium (heart) 37.11
    auditory canal or meatus, external 18.02
    auricle 18.09
    axilla 86.09
    Bartholin's gland or cyst 71.22
    bile duct (with T or Y tube insertion) NEC 51.59
      common (exploratory) 51.51
        for
          relief of obstruction NEC 51.42
          removal of calculus 51.41
      for
        exploration 51.59
        relief of obstruction 51.49
    bladder 57.19
      neck (transurethral) 57.91
      percutaneous suprapubic (closed) 57.17
      suprapubic NEC 57.18
    blood vessel (*see also* Angiotomy) 38.00
    bone 77.10
      alveolus, alveolar 24.0
      carpals, metacarpals 77.14
      clavicle 77.11
      facial 76.09
      femur 77.15
      fibula 77.17
      humerus 77.12
      patella 77.16

Incision—*continued*
    pelvic 77.19
    phalanges (foot) (hand) 77.19
    radius 77.13
    scapula 77.11
    skull 01.24
    specified site NEC 77.19
    tarsals, metatarsals 77.18
    thorax (ribs) (sternum) 77.11
    tibia 77.17
    ulna 77.13
    vertebrae 77.19
  brain 01.39
    cortical adhesions 02.91
  breast (skin) 85.0
    with removal of tissue expander 85.96
  bronchus 33.0
  buccal space 27.0
  bulbourethral gland 58.91
  bursa 83.03
    hand 82.03
    pharynx 29.0
  carotid body 39.8
  cerebral (meninges) 01.39
    epidural or extradural space 01.24
    subarachnoid or subdural space 01.31
  cerebrum 01.39
  cervix 69.95
    to
      assist delivery 73.93
      replace inverted uterus 75.93
  chalazion 08.09
    with removal of capsule 08.21
  cheek 86.09
  chest wall (for extrapleural drainage) (for
    removal of foreign body) 34.01
    as operative approach—*omit code*
  common bile duct (for exploration) 51.51
    for
      relief of obstruction 51.42
      removal of calculus 51.41
  common wall between posterior left atrium and
    coronary sinus (with roofing of resultant
    defect with patch graft) 35.82
  conjunctiva 10.1
  cornea 11.1
    radial (refractive) 11.75
  cranial sinus 01.21
  craniobuccal pouch 07.72
  cul-de-sac 70.12
  cyst
    dentigerous 24.0
    radicular (apical) (periapical) 24.0
  Dührssen's (cervix, to assist delivery) 73.93
  duodenum 45.01
  ear
    external 18.09
    inner 20.79
    middle 20.23
  endocardium 37.11
  endolymphatic sac 20.79
  epididymis 63.92
  epidural space, cerebral 01.24
  epigastric region 54.0
    intra-abdominal 54.19
  esophagus, esophageal NEC 42.09
    web 42.01
  exploratory—*see* Exploration
  extradural space (cerebral) 01.24
  extrapleural 34.01
  eyebrow 08.09

Incision—*continued*
  eyelid 08.09
    margin (trichiasis) 08.01
  face 86.09
  fallopian tube 66.01
  fascia 83.09
    with division 83.14
      hand 82.12
    hand 82.09
      with division 82.12
  fascial compartments, head and neck 27.0
  fistula, anal 49.11
  flank 54.0
  furuncle—*see* Incision, by site
  gallbladder 51.04
  gingiva 24.0
  gluteal 86.09
  groin region (abdominal wall) (inguinal) 54.0
    skin 86.09
    subcutaneous tissue 86.09
  gum 24.0
  hair follicles 86.09
  heart 37.10
    valve—*see* Valvulotomy
  hematoma—*see also* Incision, by site
    axilla 86.04
    broad ligament 69.98
    ear 18.09
    episiotomy site 75.91
    fossa (superficial) NEC 86.04
    groin region (abdominal wall) (inguinal) 54.0
      skin 86.04
      subcutaneous tissue 86.04
    laparotomy site 54.12
    mediastinum 34.1
    perineum (female) 71.09
      male 86.04
    popliteal space 86.04
    scrotum 61.0
    skin 86.04
    space of Retzius 59.19
    subcutaneous tissue 86.04
    vagina (cuff) 70.14
      episiotomy site 75.91
      obstetrical NEC 75.92
  hepatic ducts 51.59
  hordeolum 08.09
  hygroma—*see also* Incision, by site
    cystic 40.0
  hymen 70.11
  hypochondrium 54.0
    intra-abdominal 54.19
  hypophysis 07.72
  iliac fossa 54.0
  infratemporal fossa 27.0
  ingrown nail 86.09
  intestine 45.00
    large 45.03
    small 45.02
  intracerebral 01.39
  intracranial (epidural space) (extradural space)
    01.24
    subarachnoid or subdural space 01.31
  intraperitoneal 54.19
  ischiorectal tissue 49.02
    abscess 49.01
  joint structures (*see also* Arthrotomy) 80.10
  kidney 55.01
    pelvis 55.11
  labia 71.09
  lacrimal

Incision—*continued*
  canaliculus 09.52
  gland 09.0
  passage NEC 09.59
  punctum 09.51
  sac 09.53
  larynx NEC 31.3
  ligamentum flavum (spine)—*omit code*
  liver 50.0
  lung 33.1
  lymphangioma 40.0
  lymphatic structure (channel) (node) (vessel)
    40.0
  mastoid 20.21
  mediastinum 34.1
  meibomian gland 08.09
  meninges (cerebral) 01.31
    spinal 03.09
  midpalmar space 82.04
  mouth NEC 27.92
    floor 27.0
  muscle 83.02
    with division 83.19
      hand 82.19
    hand 82.02
      with division 82.19
  myocardium 37.11
  nailbed or nailfold 86.09
  nasolacrimal duct (stricture) 09.59
  neck 86.09
  nerve (cranial) (peripheral) NEC 04.04
    root (spinal) 03.1
  nose 21.1
  omentum 54.19
  orbit (*see also* Orbitotomy) 16.09
  ovary 65.09
    laparoscopic 65.01
  palate 27.1
  palmar space (middle) 82.04
  pancreas 52.09
  pancreatic sphincter 51.82
    endoscopic 51.85
  parapharyngeal (oral) (transcervical) 28.0
  paronychia 86.09
  parotid
    gland or duct 26.0
    space 27.0
  pelvirectal tissue 48.81
  penis 64.92
  perianal (skin) (tissue) 49.02
    abscess 49.01
  perigastric 54.19
  perineum (female) 71.09
    male 86.09
  peripheral vessels
    lower limb
      artery 38.08
      vein 38.09
    upper limb (artery) (vein) 38.03
  periprostatic tissue 60.81
  perirectal tissue 48.81
  perirenal tissue 59.09
  perisplenic 54.19
  peritoneum 54.95
    by laparotomy 54.19
    pelvic (female) 70.12
      male 54.19
  periureteral tissue 59.09
  periurethral tissue 58.91
  perivesical tissue 59.19

Incision—*continued*
  petrous pyramid (air cells) (apex)
    (mastoid) 20.22
  pharynx, pharyngeal (bursa) 29.0
  space, lateral 27.0
  pilonidal sinus (cyst) 86.03
  pineal gland 07.52
  pituitary (gland) 07.72
  pleura NEC 34.09
  popliteal space 86.09
  postzygomatic space 27.0
  pouch of Douglas 70.12
  prostate (perineal approach) (transurethral
    approach) 60.0
  pterygopalatine fossa 27.0
  pulp canal (tooth) 24.0
  Rathke's pouch 07.72
  rectovaginal septum 48.81
  rectum 48.0
    stricture 48.91
  renal pelvis 55.11
  retroperitoneum 54.0
  retropharyngeal (oral) (transcervical) 28.0
  salivary gland or duct 26.0
  sclera 12.89
  scrotum 61.0
  sebaceous cyst 86.04
  seminal vesicle 60.72
  sinus—*see* Sinusotomy
  Skene's duct or gland 71.09
  skin 86.09
    with drainage 86.04
    breast 85.0
    cardiac pacemaker pocket, new site 37.79
    ear 18.09
    nose 21.1
    subcutaneous tunnel for pulse generator lead
      wire 86.99
      with initial procedure—*omit code*
    thalamic stimulator pulse generator pocket,
      new site 86.09
      with initial insertion of battery
        package—*omit code*
    tunnel, subcutaneous for pulse generator lead
      wire 86.99
      with initial procedure —*omit code*
  skull (bone) 01.24
  soft tissue NEC 83.09
    with division 83.19
      hand 82.19
    hand 82.09
      with division 82.19
  space of Retzius 59.19
  spermatic cord 63.93
  sphincter of Oddi 51.82
    endoscopic 51.85
  spinal
    cord 03.09
    nerve root 03.1
  spleen 41.2
  stomach 43.0
  stye 08.09
  subarachnoid space, cerebral 01.31
  subcutaneous tissue 86.09
    with drainage 86.04
    tunnel
      esophageal 42.86
        with anastomosis—*see* Anastomosis,
          esophagus, antesternal
      pulse generator lead wire 86.99
        with initial procedure—*omit code*

Injection—*continued*
  anterior chamber, eye (air) (liquid) (medication) 12.92
  antibiotic 99.21
    oxazolidinone class 00.14
  anticoagulant 99.19
  anti-D (Rhesus) globulin 99.11
  antidote NEC 99.16
  anti-infective NEC 99.22
  antineoplastic agent (chemotherapeutic) NEC 99.25
    biological response modifier [BRM] 99.28
    high-dose interleukin-2 99.28
  antivenin 99.16
  barrier substance, adhesion 99.77
  BCG
    for chemotherapy 99.25
    vaccine 99.33
  biological response modifier [BRM], antineoplastic agent 99.28
    high-dose interleukin-2 99.28
  bone marrow 41.92
    transplant—*see* Transplant, bone, marrow
  breast (therapeutic agent) 85.92
    inert material (silicone) (bilateral) 85.52
      unilateral 85.51
  bursa (therapeutic agent) 83.96
    hand 82.94
  cancer chemotherapeutic agent 99.25
  caudal—*see* Injection, spinal
  cortisone 99.23
  costochondral junction 81.92
  dinoprost-tromethine, intra-amniotic 75.0
  ear, with alcohol 20.72
  electrolytes 99.18
  enzymes, thrombolytic (streptokinase) (tissue plasminogen activator) (TPA) (urokinase)
    direct coronary artery 36.04
    intravenous 99.10
  epidural, spinal—*see* Injection, spinal
  esophageal varices or blood vessel (endoscopic)(sclerosing agent) 42.33
  Eustachian tube (inert material) 20.8
  eye (orbit) (retrobulbar) 16.91
    anterior chamber 12.92
    subconjunctival 10.91
  fascia 83.98
    hand 82.96
  gamma globulin 99.14
  ganglion, sympathetic 05.39
    ciliary 12.79
    paravertebral stellate 05.39
  gel, adhesion barrier—*see* Injection, adhesion barrier substance
  globulin
    anti-D (Rhesus) 99.11
    gamma 99.14
    Rh immune 99.11
  heart 37.92
  heavy metal antagonist 99.16
  hemorrhoids (sclerosing agent) 49.42
  hormone NEC 99.24
  human B-type natriuretic peptide (hBNP) 00.13
  immune sera 99.14
  inert material—*see* Implant, inert material
  inner ear, for destruction 20.72
  insulin 99.17
  intervertebral space for herniated disc 80.52
  intra-amniotic
    for induction of
      abortion 75.0

Injection—*continued*
    labor 73.1
  intrathecal—*see* Injection, spinal
  joint (therapeutic agent) 81.92
    temporomandibular 76.96
  kidney (cyst) (therapeutic substance) NEC 55.96
  larynx 31.0
  ligament (joint) (therapeutic substance) 81.92
  liver 50.94
  lung, for surgical collapse 33.32
  Methotrexate, for cancer chemotherapy 99.25
  nerve (cranial) (peripheral) 04.80
    agent NEC 04.89
      alcohol 04.2
      anesthetic for analgesia 04.81
        for operative anesthesia—*omit code*
      neurolytic 04.2
      phenol 04.2
    laryngeal (external) (recurrent) (superior) 31.91
    optic 16.91
    sympathetic 05.39
      alcohol 05.32
      anesthetic for analgesia 05.31
      neurolytic agent 05.32
      phenol 05.32
  nesiritide 00.13
  neuroprotective agent 99.75
  nimodipine 99.75
  orbit 16.91
  pericardium 37.93
  peritoneal cavity
    air 54.96
    locally-acting therapeutic substance 54.97
  platelet inhibitor
    direct coronary artery 36.04
    intravenous 99.20
  prophylactic substance NEC 99.29
  prostate 60.92
  radioisotopes (intracavitary) (intravenous) 92.28
  renal pelvis (cyst) 55.96
  retrobulbar (therapeutic substance) 16.91
    for anesthesia—*omit code*
  Rh immune globulin 99.11
  RhoGAM 99.11
  sclerosing agent NEC 99.29
    esophageal varices 42.33
    hemorrhoids 49.42
    pleura 34.92
      treatment of malignancy (cytotoxic agent) 34.92 *[99.25]*
        with tetracycline 34.92 *[99.21]*
    varicose vein 39.92
    vein NEC 39.92
  semicircular canals, for destruction 20.72
  silicone—*see* Implant, inert material
  skin (sclerosing agent) (filling material) 86.02
  soft tissue 83.98
    hand 82.96
  spinal (canal) NEC 03.92
    alcohol 03.8
    anesthetic agent for analgesia 03.91
      for operative anesthesia—*omit code*
    contrast material (for myelogram) 87.21
    destructive agent NEC 03.8
    neurolytic agent NEC 03.8
    phenol 03.8
    proteolytic enzyme (chemopapain) (chemodiactin) 80.52
    saline (hypothermic) 03.92
    steroid 03.92

Injection—*continued*

  spinal nerve root (intrathecal)—*see* Injection, spinal

  steroid NEC 99.23

  subarachnoid, spinal—*see* Injection, spinal

  subconjunctival 10.91

  tendon 83.97

    hand 82.95

  testis 62.92

  therapeutic agent NEC 99.29

  thoracic cavity 34.92

  thrombolytic agent (enzyme) (streptokinase) 99.10

    with percutaneous transluminal angioplasty

      coronary (single vessel) 36.02

        multiple vessels 36.05

      direct intracoronary artery 36.04

      non-coronary vessel(s) 39.50

      specified site NEC 39.50

  trachea 31.94

  tranquilizer 99.26

  tunica vaginalis (with aspiration) 61.91

  tympanum 20.94

  urethra (inert material)

    for repair of urinary stress incontinence

      collagen implant 59.72

      endoscopic injection of implant 59.72

      fat implant 59.72

      polytef implant 59.72

  vaccine

    tumor 99.28

  varices, esophagus (endoscopic) (sclerosing agent) 42.33

  varicose vein (sclerosing agent) 39.92

    esophagus 42.33

  vestibule, for destruction 20.72

  vitreous substitute (silicone) 14.75

    for reattachment of retina 14.59

  vocal cords 31.0

Inlay, tooth 23.3

Inoculation

  antitoxins—*see* Administration, antitoxins

  toxoids—*see* Administration, toxoids

  vaccine—*see* Administration, vaccine

Insemination, artificial 69.92

Insertion

  airway

    esophageal obturator 96.03

    nasopharynx 96.01

    oropharynx 96.02

  Allen-Brown cannula 39.93

  arch bars (orthodontic) 24.7

    for immobilization (fracture) 93.55

  atrial septal umbrella 35.52

  Austin-Moore prosthesis 81.52

  baffle, heart (atrial) (interatrial) (intra-atrial) 35.91

  bag, cervix (nonobstetrical) 67.0

    after delivery or abortion 75.8

    to assist delivery or induce labor 73.1

  Baker's (tube) (for stenting) 46.85

  balloon

    gastric 44.93

    heart (pulsation-type) (Kantrowitz) 37.61

    intestine (for decompression) (for dilation) 46.85

  Barton's tongs (skull) (with synchronous skeletal traction) 02.94

  bipolar endoprosthesis (femoral head) 81.52

  bladder sphincter, artificial (inflatable) 58.93

  Blakemore-Sengstaken tube 96.06

Insertion—*continued*

  bone growth stimulator (invasive) (percutaneous) (semi-invasive)—*see category* 78.9

  bone morphogenetic protein (recombinant) (rhBMP) 84.52

  bougie, cervix, nonobstetrical 67.0

    to assist delivery or induce labor 73.1

  breast implant (for augmentation) (bilateral) 85.54

    unilateral 85.53

  bridge (dental) (fixed) 23.42

    removable 23.43

  bubble (balloon), stomach 44.93

  caliper tongs (skull) (with synchronous skeletal traction) 02.94

  cannula

    Allen-Brown 39.93

    for extracorporeal membrane oxygenation (ECMO)—*omit code*

    nasal sinus (by puncture) 22.01

      through natural ostium 22.02

    pancreatic duct 52.92

      endoscopic 52.93

    vessel to vessel 39.93

  cardiac resynchronization device

    defibrillator (CRT-D) (total system) 00.51

      left ventricular coronary venous lead only 00.52

      pulse generator only 00.54

    pace maker (CRT-P) (total system) 00.50

      left ventricular coronary venous lead only 00.52

      pulse generator only 00.53

  catheter

    abdomen of fetus, for intrauterine transfusion 75.2

    anterior chamber (eye), for permanent drainage (glaucoma) 12.79

    artery 38.91

    bile duct(s) 51.59

      common 51.51

        endoscopic 51.87

      endoscopic 51.87

    bladder, indwelling 57.94

      suprapubic 57.18

        percutaneous (closed) 57.17

    bronchus 96.05

      with lavage 96.56

    central venous NEC 38.93

      for

        hemodialysis 38.95

        pressure monitoring 89.62

      peripherally inserted central catheter (PICC) 38.93

    chest 34.04

      revision (with lysis of adhesions) 34.04

    esophagus (nonoperative) 96.06

      permanent tube 42.81

    intercostal (with water seal), for drainage 34.04

      revision (with lysis of adhesions) 34.04

    spinal canal space (epidural) (subarachnoid) (subdural) for infusion of therapeutic or palliative substances 03.90

    Swan-Ganz (pulmonary) 89.64

    transtracheal for oxygenation 31.99

    vein NEC 38.93

      for renal dialysis 38.95

  chest tube 34.04

Insertion—*continued*

choledochohepatic tube (for decompression) 51.43
endoscopic 51.87
cochlear prosthetic device-*see* Implant, cochlea, prosthetic device
contraceptive device (intrauterine) 69.7
cordis cannula 54.98
coronary (artery)
stent(s) (stent graft) 36.06
Crosby-Cooney button 54.98
CRT-D (cardiac resynchronization defibrillator) 00.51
left ventricular coronary venous lead only 00.52
pulse generator only 00.54
CRT-P (cardiac resynchronization pacemaker) 00.50
left ventricular coronary venous lead only 00.52
pulse generator only 00.53
Crutchfield tongs (skull) (with synchronous skeletal traction) 02.94
Davidson button 54.98
denture (total) 99.97
device, vascular access 86.07
diaphragm, vagina 96.17
drainage tube
kidney 55.02
pelvis 55.12
renal pelvis 55.12
elbow prosthesis (total) 81.84
revision 81.97
electrode(s)
bone growth stimulator (invasive) (percutaneous) (semi-invasive)—*see category* 78.9
brain 02.93
depth 02.93
foramen ovale 02.93
sphenoidal 02.96
depth 02.93
foramen ovale 02.93
heart (initial) (transvenous) 37.70
atrium (initial) 37.73
replacement 37.76
atrium and ventricle (initial) 37.72
replacement 37.76
epicardium (sternotomy or thoracotomy approach) 37.74
left ventricular coronary venous system 00.52
temporary transvenous pacemaker system 37.78
during and immediately following cardiac surgery 39.64
ventricle (initial) 37.71
replacement 37.76
intracranial 02.93
osteogenic (for bone growth stimulation)—*see category* 78.9
peripheral nerve 04.92
sphenoidal 02.96
spine 03.93
electroencephalographic receiver—*see* Implant, electroencephalographic receiver, by site
electronic stimulator—*see* Implant, electronic stimulator, by site
electrostimulator—*see* Implant, electronic stimulator, by site

Insertion—*continued*

endograft(s), endovascular graft(s)
endovascular, head and neck vessels 39.72
endovascular, other vessels (for aneurysm) 39.79
endoprosthesis
bile duct 51.87
femoral head (bipolar) 81.52
pancreatic duct 52.93
epidural pegs 02.93
external fixation device (bone)—*see category* 78.1
facial bone implant (alloplastic) (synthetic) 76.92
filling material, skin (filling of defect) 86.02
filter
vena cava (inferior) (superior) (transvenous) 38.7
fixator, mini device (bone)—*see category* 78.1
frame (stereotactic)
for radiosurgery 93.59
Gardner Wells tongs (skull) (with synchronous skeletal traction) 02.94
gastric bubble (balloon) 44.93
globe, into eye socket 16.69
Greenfield filter 38.7
halo device (skull) (with synchronous skeletal traction) 02.94
Harrington rod—*see also* Fusion, spinal, by level
with dorsal, dorsolumbar fusion 81.05
Harris pin 79.15
heart
pacemaker—*see* Insertion, pacemaker, cardiac
pump (Kantrowitz) 37.62
valve—*see* Replacement, heart valve
hip prosthesis (partial) 81.52
revision 81.53
total 81.51
revision 81.53
Holter valve 02.2
Hufnagel valve—*see* Replacement, heart valve
implant—*see* Insertion, prosthesis
infusion pump 86.06
intercostal catheter (with water seal) for drainage 34.04
intra-arterial blood gas monitoring system 89.60
intrauterine
contraceptive device 69.7
radium (intracavitary) 69.91
tamponade (nonobstetric) 69.91
Kantrowitz
heart pump 37.62
pulsation balloon (phase-shift) 37.61
keratoprosthesis 11.73
King-Mills umbrella device (heart) 35.52
Kirschner wire 93.44
with reduction of fracture or dislocation—*see* Reduction, fracture *and* Reduction, dislocation
laminaria, cervix 69.93
larynx, valved tube 31.75
leads (cardiac)—*see* Insertion, electrode(s), heart
lens, prosthetic (intraocular) 13.70
with cataract extraction, one-stage 13.71
secondary (subsequent to cataract extraction) 13.72
loop recorder 86.09
metal staples into epiphyseal plate (*see also* Stapling, epiphyseal plate) 78.20
minifixator device (bone)—*see category* 78.1

Insertion—*continued*
Mobitz-Uddin umbrella, vena cava 38.7
mold, vagina 96.15
Moore (cup) 81.52
myringotomy device (button) (tube) 20.01
  with intubation 20.01
nasobiliary drainage tube (endoscopic) 51.86
nasogastric tube
  for
    decompression, intestinal 96.07
    feeding 96.6
naso-intestinal tube 96.08
nasolacrimal tube or stent 09.44
nasopancreatic drainage tube (endoscopic) 52.97
neuropacemaker—*see* Implant,
  neuropacemaker, by site
neurostimulator—*see* Implant, neurostimulator,
  by site
non-coronary vessel stent(s) (stent graft) 39.90
  with angioplasty or atherectomy 39.50
non-invasive (transcutaneous) (surface)
  stimulator 99.86
obturator (orthodontic) 24.7
ocular implant
  with synchronous
    enucleation 16.42
      with muscle attachment to implant 16.41
    evisceration 16.31
  following or secondary to
    enucleation 16.61
    evisceration 16.61
Ommaya reservoir 02.2
orbital implant (stent) (outside muscle cone)
  16.69
  with orbitotomy 16.02
orthodontic appliance (obturator) (wiring) 24.7
outflow tract prosthesis (gusset type) (heart)
  in
    pulmonary valvuloplasty 35.26
    total repair of tetralogy of Fallot 35.81
pacemaker
  brain 02.93
  cardiac (device) (initial) (permanent)
    (replacement) 37.80
      dual-chamber device (initial) 37.83
        replacement 37.87
      during and immediately following cardiac
        surgery 39.64
      resynchronization (CRT-P) (device)
        device only (initial) (replacement) 00.53
        total system 00.50
        transvenous lead into left ventricular
          coronary venous system 00.52
      single-chamber device (initial) 37.81
        rate responsive 37.82
        replacement 37.85
          rate responsive 37.86
      temporary transvenous pacemaker system
        37.78
      during and immediately following cardiac
        surgery 39.64
  carotid 39.8
  heart—*see* Insertion, pacemaker, cardiac
  intracranial 02.93
  neural
    brain 02.93
    intracranial 02.93
    peripheral nerve 04.92
    spine 03.93
  peripheral nerve 04.92
  spine 03.93

Insertion—*continued*
  pacing catheter—*see* Insertion, pacemaker,
    cardiac
  pack
    auditory canal, external 96.11
    cervix (nonobstetrical) 67.0
      after delivery or abortion 75.8
      to assist delivery or induce labor 73.1
    rectum 96.19
    sella turcica 07.79
    vagina (nonobstetrical) 96.14
      after delivery or abortion 75.8
  penis, prosthetic (non-inflatable) (internal) 64.95
    inflatable (internal) 64.97
  peridontal splint (orthodontic) 24.7
  peripheral blood vessel —*see* non-coronary
  pessary
    cervix 96.18
      to assist delivery or induce labor 73.1
    vagina 96.18
  pharyngeal valve, artificial 31.75
  port, vascular access 86.07
  prostaglandin suppository (for abortion) 96.49
  prosthesis, prosthetic device
    acetabulum (partial) 81.52
      revision 81.53
    ankle (total) 81.56
    arm (bioelectric) (cineplastic) (kineplastic)
      84.44
    biliary tract 51.99
    breast (bilateral) 85.54
      unilateral 85.53
    chin (polyethylene) (silastic) 76.68
    elbow (total) 81.84
      revision 81.97
    extremity (bioelectric) (cineplastic)
      (kineplastic) 84.40
      lower 84.48
      upper 84.44
    fallopian tube 66.93
    femoral head (Austin-Moore) (bipolar)
      (Eicher) (Thompson) 81.52
    hip (partial) 81.52
      revision 81.53
      total 81.51
        revision 81.53
    joint—*see* Arthroplasty
    knee (partial) (total) 81.54
      revision 81.55
    leg (bioelectric) (cineplastic) (kineplastic)
      84.48
    ocular (secondary) 16.61
      with orbital exenteration 16.42
    outflow tract (gusset type) (heart)
      in
        pulmonary valvuloplasty 35.26
        total repair of tetralogy of Fallot 35.81
    penile (non-inflatable) (internal) 64.95
      inflatable (internal) 64.97
      with
        construction 64.43
        reconstruction 64.44
    Rosen (for urinary incontinence) 59.79
    Shoulder
      partial 81.81
        revision 81.97
      total 81.80
    testicular (bilateral) (unilateral) 62.7
    toe 81.57
      for hallux valgus repair 77.59
  pseudophakos (*see also* Insertion, lens) 13.70

Irrigation—*continued*
  cholecystostomy 96.41
  cornea 96.51
    with removal of foreign body 98.21
  corpus cavernosum 64.98
  cystostomy 96.47
  ear (removal of cerumen) 96.52
  enterostomy 96.36
  eye 96.51
    with removal of foreign body 98.21
  gastrostomy 96.36
  lacrimal
    canaliculi 09.42
    punctum 09.41
  muscle 83.02
    hand 82.02
  nasal
    passages 96.53
    sinus 22.00
  nasolacrimal duct 09.43
    with insertion of tube or stent 09.44
  nephrostomy 96.45
  peritoneal 54.25
  pyelostomy 96.45
  rectal 96.39
  stomach 96.33
  tendon (sheath) 83.01
    hand 82.01
  trachea NEC 96.56
  traumatic cataract 13.3
  tube
    biliary NEC 96.41
    nasogastric NEC 96.34
    pancreatic 96.42
  ureterostomy 96.46
  ventricular shunt 02.41
  wound (cleaning) NEC 96.59
Irving operation (tubal ligation) 66.32
Irwin operation (*see also* Osteotomy) 77.30
Ischiectomy (partial) 77.89
  total 77.99
Ischiopubiotomy 77.39
Isolation
  after contact with infectious disease 99.84
  ileal loop 45.51
  intestinal segment or pedicle nap
    large 45.52
    small 45.51
Isthmectomy, thyroid (*see also* Thyroidectomy,
  partial) 06.39

J-K

Jaboulay operation (gastroduodenostomy) 44.39
Janeway operation (permanent gastrostomy) 43.19
Jatene operation (arterial switch) 35.84
Jejunectomy 45.62
Jejunocecostomy 45.93
Jejunocholecystostomy 51.32
Jejunocolostomy 45.93
Jejunoileostomy 45.91
Jejunojejunostomy 45.91
Jejunopexy 46.61
Jejunorrhaphy 46.73
Jejunostomy (feeding) 46.39
  delayed opening 46.31
  loop 46.01
  percutaneous (endoscopic) (PEJ) 46.32
  revision 46.41
Jejunotomy 45.02
Johanson operation (urethral reconstruction) 58.46
Jones operation
  claw toe (transfer of extensor hallucis longus tendon) 77.57
    modified (with arthrodesis) 77.57
  dacryocystorhinostomy 09.81
  hammer toe (interphalangeal fusion) 77.56
    modified (tendon transfer with arthrodesis) 77.57
  repair of peroneal tendon 83.88
Joplin operation (exostectomy with tendon transfer) 77.53

Kader operation (temporary gastrostomy) 43.19
Kasai portoenterostomy 51.37
Kaufman operation (for urinary stress incontinence) 59.79
Kazanjiian operation (buccal vestibular sulcus extension) 24.91
Kehr operation (hepatopexy) 50.69
Keller operation (bunionectomy) 77.59
Kelly (Kennedy) operation (urethrovesical plication) 59.3
Kelly-Stoeckel operation (urethrovesical plication) 59.3
Kelotomy 53.9
Keratectomy (complete) (partial) (superficial) 11.49
  for pterygium 11.39
    with corneal graft 11.32
Keratocentesis (for hyphema) 12.91
Keratomileusis 11.71
Keratophakia 11.72
Keratoplasty (tectonic) (with autograft) (with homograft) 11.60
  lamellar (nonpenetrating) (with homograft) 11.62
    with autograft 11.61
  penetrating (full-thickness) (with homograft) 11.64
    with autograft 11.63
  perforating—see Keratoplasty, penetrating
  refractive 11.71
  specified type NEC 11.69
Keratoprosthesis 11.73
Keratotomy (delimiting) (posterior) 11.1
  radial (refractive) 11.75
Kerr operation (low cervical cesarean section) 74.1
Kessler operation (arthroplasty, carpometacarpal joint) 81.74
Kidner operation (excision of accessory navicular bone) (with tendon transfer) 77.98
Killian operation (frontal sinusotomy) 22.41
Kineplasty —see Cineplasty
King-Steelquist operation (hindquarter amputation) 84.19
Kirk operation (amputation through thigh) 84.17
Kock pouch operation
  bowel anastomosis—omit code
  continent ileostomy 46.22
  cutaneous uretero-ileostomy 56.51
  ESWL (extracorporeal shockwave lithotripsy) 98.51
  removal, calculus 57.19
  revision, cutaneous uretero-ileostomy 56.52
  urinary diversion procedure 56.51
Kondoleon operation (correction of lymphedema) 40.9
Krause operation (sympathetic denervation) 05.29
Kroener operation (partial salpingectomy) 66.69
Kroenlein operation (lateral orbitotomy) 16.01
Krönig operation (low cervical cesarean section) 74.1
Krukenberg operation (reconstruction of below-elbow amputation) 82.89
Kuhnt-Szymanowski operation (ectropion repair with lid reconstruction) 08.44

L

Note:
  blunt — omit code
  digital — omit code
  manual — omit code
  mechanical — omit code
  without instrumentation — omit code

M

Myoclasis 83.99
  hand 82.99
Myomectomy (uterine) 68.29
  broad ligament 69.19
Myoplasty (*see also* Repair, muscle) 83.87
  hand (*see also* Repair, muscle, hand) 82.89
  mastoid 19.9
Myorrhaphy 83.65
  hand 82.46
Myosuture 83.65
  hand 82.46
Myotasis 93.27
Myotenontoplasty (*see also* Repair, tendon)
    83.88
  hand 82.86
Myotenoplasty (*see also* Repair, tendon) 83.88
  hand 82.86
Myotenotomy 83.13
  hand 82.11
Myotomy 83.02
  with division 83.19
    hand 82.19
  colon NEC 46.92
    sigmoid 46.91
  cricopharyngeal 29.31
    that for pharyngeal (pharyngoesophageal)
       diverticulectomy 29.32
  esophagus 42.7
  eye (oblique) (rectus) 15.21
    multiple (two or more muscles) 15.4
  hand 82.02
    with division 82.19
  levator palpebrae 08.38
  sigmoid (colon) 46.91
Myringectomy 20.59
Myringodectomy 20.59
Myringomalleolabyrinthopexy 19.52
Myringoplasty (epitympanic, type I) (by
    cauterization) (by graft) 19.4
  revision 19.6
Myringostapediopexy 19.53
Myringostomy 20.01
Myringotomy (with aspiration) (with drainage)
    20.09
  with insertion of tube or drainage device
    (button) (grommet) 20.01

N

O

Operation—*continued*
  undercutting 49.02
Bankhart (capsular repair into glenoid, for
    shoulder dislocation) 81.82
Bardenheurer (ligation of innominate artery)
    38.85
Barkan (goniotomy) 12.52
  with goniopuncture 12.53
Barr (transfer of tibialis posterior tendon) 83.75
Barsky (closure of cleft hand) 82.82
Bassett (vulvectomy with inguinal lymph node
    dissection) 71.5 *[40.3]*
Bassini (herniorrhaphy)—*see* Repair, hernia,
    inguinal
Batch-Spittler-McFaddin (knee disarticulation)
    84.16
Batista (partial ventriculectomy) (ventricular
    reduction) (ventricular remodeling) 37.35
Beck I (epicardial poudrage) 36.39
Beck II (aorta-coronary sinus shunt) 36.39
Beck-Jianu (permanent gastrostomy) 43.19
Bell-Beuttner (subtotal abdominal
    hysterectomy) 68.3
Belsey (esophagogastric sphincter) 44.65
Benenenti (rotation of bulbous urethra) 58.49
Berke (levator resection eyelid) 08.33
Biesenberger (size reduction of breast, bilateral)
    85.32
  unilateral 85.31
Bigelow (litholapaxy) 57.0
biliary (duct) (tract) NEC 51.99
Billroth I (partial gastrectomy with
    gastroduodenostomy) 43.6
Billroth II (partial gastrectomy with
    gastrojejunostomy) 43.7
Binnie (hepatopexy) 50.69
Bischoff (ureteroneocystostomy) 56.74
bisection hysterectomy 68.3
Bishoff (spinal myelotomy) 03.29
bladder NEC 57.99
  flap 56.74
Blalock (systemic-pulmonary anastomosis) 39.0
Blalock-Hanlon (creation of atrial septal defect)
    35.42
Blalock-Taussig (subclavian-pulmonary
    anastomosis) 39.0
Blascovic (resection and advancement of
    levator palpebrae superioris) 08.33
blood vessel NEC 39.99
Blount
  femoral shortening (with blade plate) 78.25
  by epiphyseal stapling 78.25
Boari (bladder flap) 56.74
Bobb (cholelithotomy) 51.04
bone NEC—*see category* 78.4
  facial 76.99
  injury NEC—*see category* 79.9
  marrow NEC 41.98
  skull NEC 02.99
Bonney (abdominal hysterectomy) 68.4
Borthen (iridotasis) 12.63
Bost
  plantar dissection 80.48
  radiocarpal fusion 81.26
Bosworth
  arthroplasty for acromioclavicular separation
    81.83
  fusion of posterior lumbar spine 81.08
    for pseudarthrosis 81.38
  resection of radial head ligaments (for tennis
    elbow) 80.92

Operation—*continued*
  shelf procedure, hip 81.40
bottle (repair of hydrocele of tunica vaginalis)
    61.2
Boyd (hip disarticulation) 84.18
brain NEC 02.99
Brauer (cardiolysis) 37.10
breast NEC 85.99
Bricker (ileoureterostomy) 56.51
Bristow (repair of shoulder dislocation) 81.82
Brock (pulmonary valvulotomy) 35.03
Brockman (soft tissue release for clubfoot) 83.84
bronchus NEC 33.98
Browne (Denis) (hypospadias repair) 58.45
Brunschwig (temporary gastrostomy) 43.19
buccal cavity NEC 27.99
Bunnell (tendon transfer) 82.56
Burch procedure (retropubic urethral suspension
    for urinary stress incontinence) 59.5
Burgess (amputation of ankle) 84.14
bursa NEC 83.99
  hand 82.99
bypass—*see* Bypass
Caldwell (sulcus extension) 24.91
Caldwell-Luc (maxillary sinusotomy) 22.39
  with removal of membrane lining 22.31
Callander (knee disarticulation) 84.16
Campbell
  bone block, ankle 81.11
  fasciotomy (iliac crest) 83.14
  reconstruction of anterior cruciate ligaments
    81.45
canthus NEC 08.99
cardiac NEC 37.99
  septum NEC 35.98
  valve NEC 35.99
carotid body or gland NEC 39.8
Carroll and Taber (arthroplasty proximal
    interphalangeal joint) 81.72
Cattell (herniorrhaphy) 53.51
cecum NEC 46.99
cerebral (meninges) NEC 02.99
cervix NEC 69.99
Chandler (hip fusion) 81.21
Charles (correction of lymphedema) 40.9
Charnley (compression arthrodesis)
  ankle 81.11
  hip 81.21
  knee 81.22
Cheatle-Henry—*see* Repair, hernia, femoral
chest cavity NEC 34.99
Chevalier-Jackson (partial laryngectomy) 30.29
Child (radical subtotal pancreatectomy) 52.53
Chopart (midtarsal amputation) 84.12
chordae tendineae NEC 35.32
choroid NEC 14.9
ciliary body NEC 12.98
cisterna chyli NEC 40.69
Clagett (closure of chest wall following open
    flap drainage) 34.72
Clayton (resection of metatarsal heads and
    bases of phalanges) 77.88
clitoris NEC 71.4
cocked hat (metacarpal lengthening and transfer
    of local flap) 82.69
Cockett (varicose vein)
  lower limb 38.59
  upper limb 38.53
Cody tack (perforation of footplate) 19.0

Operation—*continued*

Coffey (uterine suspension) (Meigs' modification) 69.22
Cole (anterior tarsal wedge osteotomy) 77.28
Collis-Nissen (hiatal hernia repair) 53.80
colon NEC 46.99
Colonna
  adductor tenotomy (first stage) 83.12
  hip arthroplasty (second stage) 81.40
  reconstruction of hip (second stage) 81.40
commando (radical glossectomy) 25.4
conjunctive NEC 10.99
  destructive NEC 10.33
cornea NEC 11.99
Coventry (tibial wedge osteotomy) 77.27
Crawford (tarso-frontalis sling of eyelid) 08.32
cul-de-sac NEC 70.92
Culp-Deweerd (spiral flap pyeloplasty) 55.87
Culp-Scardino (ureteral flap pyeloplasty) 55.87
Curtis (interphalangeal joint arthroplasty) 81.72
cystocele NEC 70.51
Dahlman (excision of esophageal diverticulum) 42.31
Dana (posterior rhizotomy) 03.1
Danforth (fetal) 73.8
Darrach (ulnar resection) 77.83
Davis (intubated ureterotomy) 56.2
de Grandmont (tarsectomy) 08.35
Delorme
  pericardiectomy 37.31
  proctopexy 48.76
  repair of prolapsed rectum 48.76
  thoracoplasty 33.34
Denker (radical maxillary antrotomy) 22.31
Dennis-Varco (herniorrhaphy)—*see* Repair, hernia, femoral
Denonvillier (limited rhinoplasty) 21.86
dental NEC 24.99
  orthodontic NEC 24.8
Derlacki (tympanoplasty) 19.4
diaphragm NEC 34.89
Dickson (fascial transplant) 83.82
Dickson-Diveley (tendon transfer and arthrodesis to correct claw toe) 77.57
Dieffenbach (hip disarticulation) 84.18
digestive tract NEC 46.99
Doleris (shortening of round ligaments) 69.22
D'Ombrain (excision of pterygium with corneal graft) 11.32
Dorrance (push-back operation for cleft palate) 27.62
Dotter (transluminal angioplasty) 39.59
Douglas (suture of tongue to lip for micrognathia) 25.59
Doyle (paracervical uterine denervation) 69.3
Duhamel (abdominoperineal pull-through) 48.65
Duhrssen (vaginofixation of uterus) 69.22
Dunn (triple arthrodesis) 81.12
duodenum NEC 46.99
Dupuytren
  fasciectomy 82.35
  fasciotomy 82.12
    with excision 82.35
  shoulder disarticulation 84.08
Durham (Caldwell) (transfer of biceps femoris tendon) 83.75
DuToit and Roux (staple capsulorrhaphy of shoulder) 81.82
DuVries (tenoplasty) 83.88
Dwyer
  fasciotomy 83.14

Operation—*continued*

soft tissue release NEC 83.84
  wedge osteotomy, calcaneus 77.28
Eagleton (extrapetrosal drainage) 20.22
ear (external) NEC 18.9
  middle or inner NEC 20.99
Eden-Hybinette (glenoid bone block) 78.01
Effler (heart) 36.2
Eggers
  tendon release (patellar retinacula) 83.13
  tendon transfer (biceps femoris tendon) (hamstring tendon) 83.75
Elliot (scleral trephination with iridectomy) 12.61
Ellis Jones (repair of peroneal tendon) 83.88
Ellison (reinforcement of collateral ligament) 81.44
Elmslie-Cholmeley (tarsal wedge osteotomy) 77.28
Eloesser
  thoracoplasty 33.34
  thoracostomy 34.09
Emmet (cervix) 67.61
endorectal pull-through 48.41
epididymis NEC 63.99
esophagus NEC 42.99
Estes (ovary) 65.72
  laparoscopic 65.75
Estlander (thoracoplasty) 33.34
Evans (release of clubfoot) 83.84
extraocular muscle NEC 15.9
  multiple (two or more muscles) 15.4
    with temporary detachment from globe 15.3
  revision 15.6
  single 15.29
    with temporary detachment from globe 15.19
eyeball NEC 16.99
eyelid(s) NEC 08.99
face NEC 27.99
facial bone or joint NEC 76.99
fallopian tube NEC 66.99
Farabeuf (ischiopubiotomy) 77.39
Fasanella-Servatt (blepharoptosis repair) 08.35
fascia NEC 83.99
  hand 82.99
female (genital organs) NEC 71.9
  hysterectomy NEC 68.9
fenestration (aorta) 39.54
Ferguson (hernia repair) 53.00
Fick (perforation of footplate) 19.0
filtering (for glaucoma) 12.79
  with iridectomy 12.65
Finney (pyloroplasty) 44.2
fistulizing, sclera NEC 12.69
Foley (pyeloplasty) 55.87
Fontan (creation of conduit between right atrium and pulmonary artery) 35.94
Fothergill (Donald) (uterine suspension) 69.22
Fowler
  arthroplasty of metacarpophalangeal joint 81.72
  release (mallet finger repair) 82.84
  tenodesis (hand) 82.85
  thoracoplasty 33.34
Fox (entropion repair with wedge resection) 08.43
Franco (suprapubic cystotomy) 57.19
Frank (permanent gastrostomy) 43.19
Frazier (Spiller) (subtemporal trigeminal rhizotomy) 04.02

Operation—*continued*

  Kessler (arthroplasty, carpometacarpal joint) 81.74

  Kidner (excision of accessory navicular bone) (with tendon transfer) 77.98

  kidney NEC 55.99

  Killian (frontal sinusotomy) 22.41

  King-Steelquist (hindquarter amputation) 84.19

  Kirk (amputation through thigh) 84.17

  Kock pouch

    bowel anastomosis —*omit code*

    continent ileostomy 46.22

    cutaneous uretero-ileostomy 56.51

    ESWL (extracorporeal shockwave lithotripsy) 98.51

    removal, calculus 57.19

    revision, cutaneous uretero-ileostomy 56.52

    urinary diversion procedure 56.51

  Kondoleon (correction of lymphedema) 40.9

  Krause (sympathetic denervation) 05.29

  Kroener (partial salpingectomy) 66.69

  Kroenlein (lateral orbitotomy) 16.01

  Kronig (low cervical cesarean section) 74.1

  Krukenberg (reconstruction of below-elbow amputation) 82.89

  Kuhnt-Szymanowski (ectropion repair with lid reconstruction) 08.44

  Labbe (gastrotomy) 43.0

  labia NEC 71.8

  lacrimal

    gland 09.3

    system NEC 09.99

  Ladd (mobilization of intestine) 54.95

  Lagrange (iridosclerectomy) 12.65

  Lambrinudi (triple arthrodesis) 81.12

  Langenbeck (cleft palate repair) 27.62

  Lapidus (bunionectomy with metatarsal osteotomy) 77.51

  Larry (shoulder disarticulation) 84.08

  larynx NEC 31.98

  Lash (internal cervical Os repair) 67.59

  Latzko

    cesarean section, extraperitoneal 74.2

    colpocleisis 70.8

  Leadbetter (urethral reconstruction) 58.46

  Leadbetter-Politano (ureteroneocystostomy) 56.74

  Le Fort (colpocleisis) 70.8

  LeMesurier (cleft lip repair) 27.54

  lens NEC 13.9

  Leriche (periarterial sympathectomy) 05.25

  levator muscle sling

    eyelid ptosis repair 08.33

    urethrovesical suspension 59.71

    urinary stress incontinence 59.71

  lid suture (blepharoptosis) 08.31

  ligament NEC 81.99

    broad NEC 69.98

    round NEC 69.98

    uterine NEC 69.98

  Lindholm (repair of ruptured tendon) 83.88

  Linton (varicose vein) 38.59

  lip NEC 27.99

  Lisfranc

    foot amputation 84.12

    shoulder disarticulation 84.08

  Littlewood (forequarter amputation) 84.09

  liver NEC 50.99

  Lloyd-Davies (abdominoperineal resection) 48.5

  Longmire (bile duct anastomosis) 51.39

Operation—*continued*

  Lord

    dilation of anal canal for hemorrhoids 49.49

    hemorrhoidectomy 49.49

    orchidopexy 62.5

  Lucas and Murray (knee arthrodesis with plate) 81.22

  lung NEC 33.99

  lung volume reduction 32.22

  lymphatic structure(s) NEC 40.9

    duct, left (thoracic) NEC 40.69

  Madlener (tubal ligation) 66.31

  Magnuson (Stack) (arthroplasty for recurrent shoulder dislocation) 81.82

  male genital organs NEC 64.99

  Manchester (Donald) (Fothergill), (uterine suspension) 69.22

  mandible NEC 76.99

    orthognathic 76.64

  Marckwald (cervical os repair) 67.59

  Marshall-Marchetti (Krantz) (retropubic urethral suspension) 59.5

  Matas (aneurysmorrhaphy) 39.52

  Mayo

    bunionectomy 77.59

    herniorrhaphy 53.49

    vaginal hysterectomy 68.59

    laparoscopically assisted (LAVH) 68.51

  Mazet (knee disarticulation) 84.16

  McBride (bunionectomy with soft tissue correction) 77.53

  McBurney—*see* Repair, hernia, inguinal

  McCall (enterocele repair) 70.92

  McCauley (release of clubfoot) 83.84

  McDonald (encirclement suture, cervix) 67.59

  McIndoe (vaginal construction) 70.61

  McKeever (fusion of first metatarsophalangeal joint for hallux valgus repair) 77.52

  McKissock (breast reduction) 85.33

  McReynolds (transposition of pterygium) 11.31

  McVay

    femoral hernia—*see* Repair, hernia, femoral

    inguinal hernia—*see* Repair, hernia, inguinal

  meninges (spinal) NEC 03.99

    cerebral NEC 02.99

  mesentery NEC 54.99

  Mikulicz (exteriorization of intestine) (first stage) 46.03

    second stage 46.04

  Miles (complete proctectomy) 48.5

  Millard (cheiloplasty) 27.54

  Miller

    midtarsal arthrodesis 81.14

    urethrovesical suspension 59.4

  Millin-Read (urethrovesical suspension) 59.4

  Mitchell (hallux valgus repair) 77.51

  Mohs (chemosurgical excision of skin) 86.24

  Moore (arthroplasty) 81.52

  Moschowitz

    enterocele repair 70.92

    herniorrhaphy—*see* Repair, hernia, femoral

    sigmoidopexy 46.63

  mouth NEC 27.99

  Muller (banding of pulmonary artery) 38.85

  Mumford (partial claviculectomy) 77.81

  muscle NEC 83.99

    extraocular—*see* Operation, extraocular

    hand NEC 82.99

    papillary heart NEC 35.31

  musculoskeletal system NEC 84.99

Operation—*continued*

Mustard (interatrial transposition of venous return) 35.91
nail (finger) (toe) NEC 86.99
nasal sinus NEC 22.9
nasopharynx NEC 29.99
nerve (cranial) (peripheral) NEC 04.99
  adrenal NEC 07.49
  sympathetic NEC 05.89
nervous system NEC 05.9
Nicola (tenodesis for recurrent dislocation of shoulder) 81.82
nipple NEC 85.99
Nissen (fundoplication of stomach) 44.66
Noble (plication of small intestine) 46.62
node (lymph) NEC 40.9
Norman Miller (vaginopexy) 70.77
Norton (extraperitoneal cesarean operation) 74.2
nose, nasal NEC 21.99
  sinus NEC 22.9
Ober (Yount) (gluteal-iliotibial fasciotomy) 83.14
obstetric NEC 75.99
ocular NEC 16.99
  muscle—*see* Operation, extraocular muscle
O'Donoghue (triad knee repair) 81.43
Olshausen (uterine suspension) 69.22
omentum NEC 54.99
ophthalmologic NEC 16.99
oral cavity NEC 27.99
orbicularis muscle sling 08.36
orbit NEC 16.98
oropharynx NEC 29.99
orthodontic NEC 24.8
orthognathic NEC 76.69
Oscar Miller (midtarsal arthrodesis) 81.14
Osmond-Clark (soft tissue release with peroneus brevis tendon transfer) 83.75
ovary NEC 65.99
Oxford (for urinary incontinence) 59.4
palate NEC 27.99
palpebral ligament sling 08.36
Panas (linear proctotomy) 48.0
Pancoast (division of trigeminal nerve at foramen ovale) 04.02
pancreas NEC 52.99
pantaloon (revision of gastric anastomosis) 44.5
papillary muscle (heart) NEC 35.31
Paquin (ureteroneocystostomy) 56.74
parathyroid gland(s) NEC 06.99
parotid gland or duct NEC 26.99
Partsch (marsupialization of dental cyst) 24.4
Pattee (auditory canal) 18.6
Peet (splanchnic resection) 05.29
Pemberton
  osteotomy of ilium 77.39
  rectum (mobilization and fixation for prolapse repair) 48.76
penis NEC 64.98
Pereyra (paraurethral suspension) 59.6
pericardium NEC 37.99
perineum (female) NEC 71.8
  male NEC 86.99
perirectal tissue NEC 48.99
perirenal tissue NEC 59.92
peritoneum NEC 54.99
periurethral tissue NEC 58.99
perivesical tissue NEC 59.92
pharyngeal flap (cleft palate repair) 27.62
  secondary or subsequent 27.63
pharynx, pharyngeal (pouch) NEC 29.99

Operation—*continued*

pineal gland NEC 07.59
Pinsker (obliteration of nasoseptal telangiectasia) 21.07
Piper (forceps) 72.6
Pirogoff (ankle amputation through malleoli of tibia and fibula) 84.14
pituitary gland NEC 07.79
plastic—*see* Repair, by site
pleural cavity NEC 34.99
Politano-Leadbetter (ureteroneocystostomy) 56.74
pollicization (with nerves and blood supply) 82.61
Polya (gastrectomy) 43.7
Pomeroy (ligation and division of fallopian tubes) 66.32
Poncet
  lengthening of Achilles tendon 83.85
  urethrostomy, perineal 58.0
Porro (cesarean section) 74.99
posterior chamber (eye) NEC 14.9
Potts-Smith (descending aorta-left pulmonary artery anastomosis) 39.0
Printen and Mason (high gastric bypass) 44.31
prostate NEC (*see also* Prostatectomy) 60.69
  specified type 60.99
pterygium 11.39
  with corneal graft 11.32
Puestow (pancreaticojejunostomy) 52.96
pull-through NEC 48.49
pulmonary NEC 33.99
push-back (cleft palate repair) 27.62
Putti-Platt (capsulorrhaphy of shoulder for recurrent dislocation) 81.82
pyloric exclusion 44.39
pyriform sinus NEC 29.99
"rabbit ear" (anterior urethropexy) (Tudor) 59.79
Ramadier (intrapetrosal drainage) 20.22
Ramstedt (pyloromyotomy) (with wedge resection) 43.3
Rankin
  exteriorization of intestine 46.03
  proctectomy (complete) 48.5
Rashkind (balloon septostomy) 35.41
Rastelli (creation of conduit between right ventricle and pulmonary artery) 35.92
  in repair of
    pulmonary artery atresia 35.92
    transposition of great vessels 35.92
    truncus arteriosus 35.83
Raz-Pereyra procedure (bladder neck suspension) 59.79
rectal NEC 48.99
rectocele NEC 70.52
re-entry (aorta) 39.54
renal NEC 55.99
respiratory (tract) NEC 33.99
retina NEC 14.9
Ripstein (repair of rectal prolapse) 48.75
Rodney Smith (radical subtotal pancreatectomy) 52.53
Roux-en-Y
  bile duct 51.36
  cholecystojejunostomy 51.32
  esophagus (intrathoracic) 42.54
  pancreaticojejunostomy 52.96
Roux-Goldthwait (repair of patellar dislocation) 81.44
Roux-Herzen-Judine (jejunal loop interposition) 42.63

Operation—*continued*

Ruiz-Mora (proximal phalangectomy for hammer toe) 77.99

Russe (bone graft of scaphoid) 78.04

Saemisch (corneal section) 11.1

salivary gland or duct NEC 26.99

Salter (innominate osteotomy) 77.39

Sauer-Bacon (abdominoperineal resection) 48.5

Schanz (femoral osteotomy) 77.35

Schauta (Amreich) (radical vaginal hysterectomy) 68.7

Schede (thoracoplasty) 33.34

Scheie

  cautery of sclera 12.62

  sclerostomy 12.62

Schlatter (total gastrectomy) 43.99

Schroeder (endocervical excision) 67.39

Schuchardt (nonobstetrical episiotomy) 71.09

Schwartze (simple mastoidectomy) 20.41

sclera NEC 12.89

Scott

  intestinal bypass for obesity 45.93

  jejunocolostomy (bypass) 45.93

scrotum NEC 61.99

Seddon-Brooks (transfer of pectoralis major tendon) 83.75

Semb (apicolysis of lung) 33.39

seminal vesicle NEC 60.79

Senning (correction of transposition of great vessels) 35.91

Sever (division of soft tissue of arm) 83.19

Sewell (heart) 36.2

sex transformation NEC 64.5

Sharrard (iliopsoas muscle transfer) 83.77

shelf (hip arthroplasty) 81.40

Shirodkar (encirclement suture, cervix) 67.59

sigmoid NEC 46.99

Silver (bunionectomy) 77.59

Sistrunk (excision of thyroglossal cyst) 06.7

Skene's gland NEC 71.8

skin NEC 86.99

skull NEC 02.99

sling

  eyelid

    fascia lata, palpebral 08.36

    frontalis fascial 08.32

    levator muscle 08.33

    orbicularis muscle 08.36

    palpebrae ligament, fascia lata 08.36

    tarsus muscle 08.35

  fascial (fascia lata)

    eye 08.32

    for facial weakness (trigeminal nerve paralysis) 86.81

    palpebral ligament 08.36

    tongue 25.59

  tongue (fascial) 25.59

  urethra (suprapubic) 59.4

    retropubic 59.5

  urethrovesical 59.5

Slocum (pes anserinus transfer) 81.47

Sluder (tonsillectomy) 28.2

Smith (open osteotomy of mandible) 76.62

Smith-Peterson (radiocarpal arthrodesis) 81.25

Smithwick (sympathectomy) 05.29

Soave (endorectal pull-through) 48.41

soft tissue NEC 83.99

  hand 82.99

Sonneberg (inferior maxillary neurectomy) 04.07

Sorondo-Ferré (hindquarter amputation) 84.19

Operation—*continued*

Soutter (iliac crest fasciotomy) 83.14

Spalding-Richardson (uterine suspension) 69.22

spermatic cord NEC 63.99

sphincter of Oddi NEC 51.89

spinal (canal) (cord) (structures) NEC 03.99

Spinelli (correction of inverted uterus) 75.93

Spivack (permanent gastrostomy) 43.19

spleen NEC 41.99

S.P. Rogers (knee disarticulation) 84.16

Ssabanejew-Frank (permanent gastrostomy) 43.19

Stacke (simple mastoidectomy) 20.41

Stallard (conjunctivocystorhinostomy) 09.82

  with insertion of tube or stent 09.83

Stamm (Kader) (temporary gastrostomy) 43.19

Steinberg 44.5

Steindler

  fascia stripping (for cavus deformity) 83.14

  flexorplasty (elbow) 83.77

  muscle transfer 83.77

sterilization NEC

  female (*see also* specific operation) 66.39

  mate (*see also* Ligation, vas deferens) 63.70

Stewart (renal plication with pyeloplasty) 55.87

stomach NEC 44.99

Stone (anoplasty) 49.79

Strassman (metroplasty) 69.49

  metroplasty (Jones modification) 69.49

  uterus 68.22

Strayer (gastrocnemius recession) 83.72

stress incontinence—*see* Repair, stress incontinence

Stromeyer-Little (hepatotomy) 50.0

Strong (unbridling of celiac artery axis) 39.91

Sturmdorf (conization of cervix) 67.2

subcutaneous tissue NEC 86.99

sublingual gland or duct NEC 26.99

submaxillary gland or duct NEC 26.99

Summerskill (dacryocystorhinostomy by intubation) 09.81

Surmay (jejunostomy) 46.39

Swenson

  bladder reconstruction 57.87

  proctectomy 48.49

Swinney (urethral reconstruction) 58.46

Syme

  ankle amputation through malleoli of tibia and fibula 84.14

  urethrotomy, external 58.0

sympathetic nerve NEC 05.89

Taarnhoj (trigeminal nerve root decompression) 04.41

Tack (sacculotomy) 20.79

Talma-Morison (omentopexy) 54.74

Tanner (devascularization of stomach) 44.99

TAPVC NEC 35.82

tarsus NEC 08.99

  muscle sling 08.35

tendon NEC 83.99

  extraocular NEC 15.9

  hand NEC 82.99

testis NEC 62.99

tetralogy of Fallot

  partial repair—*see specific procedure*

  total (one-stage) 35.81

Thal (repair of esophageal stricture) 42.85

thalamus (stereotactic) 01.41

  by stereotactic radiosurgery 92.32

    cobalt 60 92.32

    linear accelerator (LINAC) 92.31

Operation—*continued*
  capsuloplasty 81.72
  tendon transfer (biceps) 82.56
  Ziegler (iridectomy) 12.14
Operculectomy 24.6
Ophthalmectomy 16.49
  with implant (into Tenon's capsule) 16.42
  with attachment of muscles 16.41
Ophthalmoscopy 16.21
Opponensplasty (hand) 82.56
Orbitomaxillectomy, radical 16.51
Orbitotomy (anterior) (frontal) (temporofrontal)
  (transfrontal) NEC 16.09
  with
    bone flap 16.01
    insertion of implant 16.02
    Kroenlein (lateral) 16.01
    lateral 16.01
Orchidectomy (with epididymectomy)
  (unilateral) 62.3
  bilateral (radical) 62.41
  remaining or solitary testis 62.42
Orchidopexy 62.5
Orchidoplasty 62.69
Orchidorrhaphy 62.61
Orchidotomy 62.0
Orchiectomy (with epididymectomy) (unilateral)
  62.3
  bilateral (radical) 62.41
  remaining or solitary testis 62.42
Orchiopexy 62.5
Orchioplasty 62.69
Orthoroentgenography —*see* Radiography
Oscar Miller operation (midtarsal arthrodesis)
  81.14
Osmond-Clark operation (soft tissue release
  with peroneus brevis tendon transfer) 83.75
Ossiculectomy NEC 19.3
  with
    stapedectomy (*see also* Stapedectomy) 19.19
    stapes mobilization 19.0
    tympanoplasty 19.53
     revision 19.6
Ossiculotomy NEC 19.3
Ostectomy (partial), except facial—*see also*
  category 77.8
  facial NEC 76.39
    total 76.45
     with reconstruction 76.44
  first metatarsal head—*see* Bunionectomy
  for graft (autograft) (homograft)—*see also*
    category 77.7
  mandible 76.31
    total 76.42
     with reconstruction 76.41
  total, except facial—*see also category* 77.9
    facial NEC 76.45
     with reconstruction 76.44
    mandible 76.42
     with reconstruction 76.41
Osteoarthrotomy (*see also* Osteotomy) 77.30
Osteoclasis 78.70
  carpal, metacarpal 78.74
  clavicle 78.71
  ear 20.79
  femur 78.75
  fibula 78.77
  humerus 78.72
  patella 78.76
  pelvic 78.79
  phalanges (foot) (hand) 78.79

Osteoclasis—*continued*
  radius 78.73
  scapula 78.71
  specified site NEC 78.79
  tarsal, metatarsal 78.78
  thorax (ribs) (sternum) 78.71
  tibia 78.77
  ulna 78.73
  vertebrae 78.79
Osteolysis —*see category* 78.4
Osteopathic manipulation (*see also*
  Manipulation, osteopathic) 93.67
Osteoplasty NEC—*see category* 78.4
  with bone graft—*see* Graft, bone
  for
    bone lengthening—*see* Lengthening, bone
    bone shortening—*see* Shortening, bone
    repair of malunion or nonunion of
     fracture—*see* Repair, fracture, malunion
     or nonunion
  carpal, metacarpal 78.44
  clavicle 78.41
  cranium NEC 02.06
    with
     flap (bone) 02.03
     graft (bone) 02.04
  facial bone NEC 76.69
  femur 78.45
  fibula 78.47
  humerus 78.42
  mandible, mandibular NEC 76.64
    body 76.63
    ramus (open) 76.62
     closed 76.61
  maxilla (segmental) 76.65
    total 76.66
  nasal bones 21.89
  patella 78.46
  pelvic 78.49
  phalanges (foot) (hand) 78.49
  radius 78.43
  scapula 78.41
  skull NEC 02.06
    with
     flap (bone) 02.03
     graft (bone) 02.04
  specified site NEC 78.49
  tarsal, metatarsal 78.48
  thorax (ribs) (sternum) 78.41
  tibia 78.47
  ulna 78.43
  vertebrae 78.49
Osteorrhaphy (*see also* Osteoplasty) 78.40
Osteosynthesis (fracture) —*see* Reduction,
  fracture
Osteotomy (adduction) (angulation) (block)
  (derotational) (displacement) (partial)
  (rotational) 77.30
  carpals, metacarpals 77.34
    wedge 77.24
  clavicle 77.31
    wedge 77.21
  facial bone NEC 76.69
  femur 77.35
    wedge 77.25
  fibula 77.37
    wedge 77.27
  humerus 77.32
    wedge 77.22
  mandible (segmental) (subapical) 76.64
    angle (open) 76.62

P

Pacemaker
cardiac—*see also* Insertion, pacemaker, cardiac
  intraoperative (temporary) 39.64
  temporary (during and immediately following
    cardiac surgery) 39.64
Packing —*see also* Insertion, pack
auditory canal 96.11
nose, for epistaxis (anterior) 21.01
  posterior (and anterior) 21.02
rectal 96.19
sella turcica 07.79
vaginal 96.14
Palatoplasty 27.69
for cleft palate 27.62
  secondary or subsequent 27.63
Palatorrhaphy 27.61
for cleft palate 27.62
Pallidectomy 01.42
Pallidoansotomy 01.42
Pallidotomy 01.42
by stereotactic radiosurgery 92.32
  cobalt 60 92.32
  linear accelerator (LINAC) 92.31
  multi-source 92.32
  particle beam 92.33
  particulate 92.33
  radiosurgery NEC 92.39
  single source proton 92.31
Panas operation (linear proctotomy) 48.0
Pancoast operation (division of trigeminal nerve
  at foramen ovale) 04.02
Pancreatectomy (total) (with synchronous
  duodenectomy) 52.6
partial NEC 52.59
  distal (tail) (with part of body) 52.52
  proximal (head) (with part of body) (with
    synchronous duodenectomy) 52.51
  radical 52.53
    subtotal 52.53
  radical 52.7
    subtotal 52.53
Pancreaticocystoduodenostomy 52.4
Pancreaticocystoenterostomy 52.4
Pancreaticocystogastrostomy 52.4
Pancreaticocystojejunostomy 52.4
Pancreaticoduodenectomy (total) 52.6
partial NEC 52.59
  proximal 52.51
  radical subtotal 52.53
radical (one-stage) (two-stage) 52.7
  subtotal 52.53
Pancreaticoduodenostomy 52.96
Pancreaticoenterostomy 52.96
Pancreaticogastrostomy 52.96
Pancreaticoileostomy 52.96
Pancreaticojejunostomy 52.96
Pancreatoduodenectomy (total) 52.6
partial NEC 52.59
radical (one-stage) (two-stage) 52.7
  subtotal 52.53
Pancreatogram 87.66
endoscopic retrograde (ERP) 52.13
Pancreatolithotomy 52.09
endoscopic 52.94
Pancreatotomy 52.09
Pancreatolithotomy 52.09
endoscopic 52.94

Panendoscopy 57.32
specified site, other than bladder—*see*
  Endoscopy, by site
through artificial stoma 57.31
Panhysterectomy (abdominal) 68.4
vaginal 68.59
  laparoscopically assisted (LAVH) 68.51
Panniculectomy 86.83
Panniculotomy 86.83
Pantaloon operation (revision of gastric
  anastomosis) 44.5
Papillectomy, anal 49.39
endoscopic 49.31
Papillotomy (pancreas) 51.82
endoscopic 51.85
Paquin operation (ureteroneocystostomy) 56.74
Paracentesis
abdominal (percutaneous) 54.91
anterior chamber, eye 12.91
bladder 57.11
cornea 12.91
eye (anterior chamber) 12.91
thoracic, thoracis 34.91
tympanum 20.09
  with intubation 20.01
Parasitology *see* Examination, microscopic
Parathyroidectomy (partial) (subtotal) NEC
  06.89
complete 06.81
ectopic 06.89
global removal 06.81
mediastinal 06.89
total 06.81
Parenteral nutrition, total 99.15
peripheral 99.15
Parotidectomy 26.30
complete 26.32
partial 26.31
radical 26.32
Partsch operation (marsupialization of dental
  cyst) 24.4
Passage —*see* Insertion and Intubation
Passage of sounds, urethra 58.6
Patch
blood, spinal (epidural) 03.95
graft—*see* Graft
spinal, blood (epidural) 03.95
subdural, brain 02.12
Patellapexy 78.46
Patellaplasty NEC 78.46
Patellectomy 77.96
partial 77.86
Pattee operation (auditory canal) 18.6
Pectenotomy (*see also* Sphincterotomy, anal)
  49.59
Pedicle flap —*see* Graft, skin, pedicle
Peet operation (splanchnic resection) 05.29
PEG (percutaneous endoscopic gastrostomy)
  43.11
PEJ (percutaneous endoscopic jejunostomy)
  46.32
Pelvectomy, kidney (partial) 55.4
Pelvimetry 88.25
gynecological 89.26
Pelviolithotomy 55.11
Pelvioplasty, kidney 55.87
Pelviostomy 55.12
closure 55.82

Q-R

Quadrant resection of breast 85.22
Quadricepsplasty (Thompson) 83.86
Quarantine 99.84
Quenuthoracoplasty 77.31
Quotient, respiratory 89.38

Rachicentesis 03.31
Rachitomy 03.09
Radiation therapy —*see also* Therapy, radiation
   teleradiotheraphy—*see* Teleradiotherapy
Radical neck dissection —*see* Dissection, neck
Radicotomy 03.1
Radiculectomy 03.1
Radiculotomy 03.1
Radiography (diagnostic) NEC 88.39
  abdomen, abdominal (flat plate) NEC 88.19
    wall (soft tissue) NEC 88.09
  adenoid 87.09
  ankle (skeletal) 88.28
    soft tissue 88.37
  bone survey 88.31
  bronchus 87.49
  chest (routine) 87.44
    wall NEC 87.39
  clavicle 87.43
  contrast (air) (gas) (radio-opaque substance)
    NEC
    abdominal wall 88.03
    arteries (by fluoroscopy)—*see* Arteriography
    bile ducts NEC 87.54
    bladder NEC 87.77
    brain 87.02
    breast 87.35
    bronchus NEC (transcricoid) 87.32
      endotracheal 87.31
    epididymis 87.93
    esophagus 87.61
    fallopian tubes
      gas 87.82
      opaque dye 87.83
    fistula (sinus tract)—*see also* Radiography,
      contrast, by site
      abdominal wall 88.03
      chest wall 87.38
    gallbladder NEC 87.59
    intervertebral disc(s) 87.21
    joints 88.32
    larynx 87.07
    lymph—*see* Lymphangiogram
    mammary ducts 87.35
    mediastinum 87.33
    nasal sinuses 87.15
    nasolacrimal ducts 87.05
    nasopharynx 87.06
    orbit 87.14
    pancreas 87.66
    pelvis
      gas 88.12
      opaque dye 88.11
    peritoneum NEC 88.13
    retroperitoneum NEC 88.15
    seminal vesicles 87.91
    sinus tract—*see also* Radiography, contrast,
      by site
      abdominal wall 88.03
      chest wall 87.38
      nose 87.15
    skull 87.02
    spinal disc(s) 87.21
    trachea 87.32
    uterus
      gas 87.82
      opaque dye 87.83

Radiography—*continued*
  vas deferens 87.94
  veins (by fluoroscopy)—*see* Phlebography
  vena cava (inferior) (superior) 88.51
  dental NEC 87.12
  diaphragm 87.49
  digestive tract NEC 87.69
    barium swallow 87.61
    lower GI series 87.64
    small bowel series 87.63
    upper GI series 87.62
  elbow (skeletal) 88.22
    soft tissue 88.35
  epididymis NEC 87.95
  esophagus 87.69
    barium-swallow 87.61
  eye 95.14
  face, head, and neck 87.09
  facial bones 87.16
  fallopian tubes 87.85
  foot 88.28
  forearm (skeletal) 88.22
    soft tissue 88.35
  frontal area, facial 87.16
  genital organs
    female NEC 87.89
    male NEC 87.99
  hand (skeletal) 88.23
    soft tissue 88.35
  head NEC 87.09
  heart 87.49
  hip (skeletal) 88.26
    soft tissue 88.37
  intestine NEC 87.65
  kidney-ureter-bladder (KUB) 87.79
  knee (skeletal) 88.27
    soft tissue 88.37
  KUB (kidney-ureter-bladder) 87.79
  larynx 87.09
  lower leg (skeletal) 88.27
    soft tissue 88.37
  lower limb (skeletal) NEC 88.29
    soft tissue NEC 88.37
  lung 87.49
  mandible 87.16
  maxilla 87.16
  mediastinum 87.49
  nasal sinuses 87.16
  nasolacrimal duct 87.09
  nasopharynx 87.09
  neck NEC 87.09
  nose 87.16
  orbit 87.16
  pelvis (skeletal) 88.26
    pelvimetry 88.25
    soft tissue 88.19
  prostate NEC 87.92
  retroperitoneum NEC 88.16
  ribs 87.43
  root canal 87.12
  salivary gland 87.09
  seminal vesicles NEC 87.92
  shoulder (skeletal) 88.21
    soft tissue 88.35
  skeletal NEC 88.33
    series (whole or complete) 88.31
  skull (lateral, sagittal or tangential projection) NEC 87.17
  spine NEC 87.29
    cervical 87.22
    lumbosacral 87.24

Radiography—*continued*
    sacrococcygeal 87.24
    thoracic 87.23
  sternum 87.43
  supraorbital area 87.16
  symphysis menti 87.16
  teeth NEC 87.12
    full-mouth 87.11
  thigh (skeletal) 88.27
    soft tissue 88.37
  thyroid region 87.09
  tonsils and adenoids 87.09
  trachea 87.49
  ultrasonic—*see* Ultrasonography
  upper arm (skeletal) 88.21
    soft tissue 88.35
  upper limb (skeletal) NEC 88.24
    soft tissue NEC 88.35
  urinary system NEC 87.79
  uterus NEC 87.85
    gravid 87.81
  uvula 87.09
  vas deferens NEC 87.95
  wrist 88.23
  zygomaticomaxillary complex 87.16
Radioisotope
  scanning—*see* Scan, radioisotope
  therapy—*see* Therapy, radioisotope
Radiology
  diagnostic—*see* Radiography
  therapeutic—*see* Therapy, radiation
Radiosurgery, stereotactic 92.30
  cobalt 60 92.32
  linear accelerator (LINAC) 92.31
  multi-source 92.32
  particle beam 92.33
  particulate 92.33
  radiosurgry NEC 92.39
  single source photon 92.31
Raising, pedicle graft 86.71
Ramadier operation (intrapetrosal drainage) 20.22
Ramisection (sympathetic) 05.0
Ramstedt operation (pyeloromyotomy) (with wedge resection) 43.3
Range of motion testing 93.05
Rankin operation
  exteriorization of intestine 46.03
  proctectomy (complete) 48.5
Rashkind operation (balloon septostomy) 35.41
Rastelli operation (creation of conduit between right ventricle and pulmonary artery) 35.92
  in repair of
    pulmonary artery atresia 35.92
    transposition of great vessels 35.92
    truncus arteriosus 35.83
Raz-Pereyra procedure (Bladder neck suspension) 59.79
RCSA (radical cryosurgical ablation) of prostate 60.62
Readjustment —*see* Adjustment
Reamputation, stump 84.3
Reanastomosis —*see* Anastomosis
Reattachment
  amputated ear 18.72
  ankle 84.27
  arm (upper) NEC 84.24
  choroid and retina NEC 14.59
    by
      cryotherapy 14.52
      diathermy 14.51

Reduction—*continued*
  phalanges
    foot (closed) 79.08
      with internal fixation 79.18
      open 79.28
        with internal fixation 79.38
    hand (closed) 79.04
      with internal fixation 79.14
      open 79.24
        with internal fixation 79.34
    radius (closed) 79.02
      with internal fixation 79.12
      open 79.22
        with internal fixation 79.32
    skull 02.02
    specified site (closed) NEC 79.09
      with internal fixation 79.19
      open 79.29
        with internal fixation 79.39
    spine 03.53
    tarsal, metatarsal (closed) 79.07
      with internal fixation 79.17
      open 79.27
        with internal fixation 79.37
    tibia (closed) 79.06
      with internal fixation 79.16
      open 79.26
        with internal fixation 79.36
    ulna (closed) 79.02
      with internal fixation 79.12
      open 79.22
        with internal fixation 79.32
    vertebra 03.53
    zygoma, zygomatic arch (closed) 76.71
      open 76.72
  fracture-dislocation—*see* Reduction, fracture
  heart volume 37.35
  hemorrhoids (manual) 49.41
  hernia—*see also* Repair, hernia
    manual 96.27
  intussusception (open) 46.80
    with
      fluoroscopy 96.29
      ionizing radiation enema 96.29
      ultrasonography guidance 96.29
    hydrostatic 96.29
    large intestine 46.82
      endoscopic (balloon) 46.85
    pneumatic 96.29
    small intestine 46.81
  lung volume 32.22
  malrotation, intestine (manual) (surgical) 46.80
    large 46.82
      endoscopic (balloon) 46.85
    small 46.81
  mammoplasty (bilateral) 85.32
    unilateral 85.31
  prolapse
    anus (operative) 49.94
    colostomy (manual) 96.28
    enterostomy (manual) 96.28
    ileostomy (manual) 96.28
    rectum (manual) 96.26
    uterus
      by pessary 96.18
      surgical 69.22
  ptosis overcorrection 08.37
  retroversion, uterus by pessary 96.18
  separation, epiphysis (with internal fixation)
    (closed) 79.40
    femur (closed) 79.45

Reduction—*continued*
    open 79.55
    fibula (closed) 79.46
      open 79.56
    humerus (closed) 79.41
      open 79.51
    open 79.50
    specified site (closed) NEC—*see also*
      category 79.4
      open—*see category* 79.5
    tibia (closed) 79.46
      open 79.56
  size
    abdominal wall (adipose) (pendulous) 86.83
    arms (adipose) (batwing) 86.83
    breast (bilateral) 85.32
      unilateral 85.31
    buttocks (adipose) 86.83
    finger (macrodactyly repair) 82.83
    skin 86.83
    subcutaneous tissue 86.83
    thighs (adipose) 86.83
  torsion
    intestine (manual) (surgical) 46.80
      large 46.82
        endoscopic (balloon) 46.85
      small 46.81
    kidney pedicle 55.84
    omentum 54.74
    spermatic cord 63.52
      with orchiopexy 62.5
    testis 63.52
      with orchiopexy 62.5
    uterus NEC 69.98
      gravid 75.99
    ventricular 37.35
  volvulus
    intestine 46.80
      large 46.82
        endoscopic (balloon) 46.85
      small 46.81
    stomach 44.92
Reefing, joint capsule (*see also* Arthroplasty)
  81.96
Re-entry operation (aorta) 39.54
Re-establishment, continuity —*see also*
  Anastomosis
  bowel 46.50
  fallopian tube 66.79
  vas deferens 63.82
Referral (for)
  psychiatric aftercare (halfway house) (outpatient
    clinic) 94.52
  psychotherapy 94.51
  rehabilitation
    alcoholism 94.53
    drug addiction 94.54
    psychologic NEC 94.59
    vocational 94.55
Reformation
  cardiac pacemaker pocket, new site (skin)
    (subcutaneous) 37.79
  cardioverter/defibrillator (automatic) pocket,
    new site (skin) (subcutaneous) 37.99
  chamber of eye 12.99
Refracture
  bone (for faulty union) (*see also* Osteoclasis)
    78.70
  nasal bones 21.88

Removal—*continued*
    scapula 78.61
    specified site NEC 78.69
    tarsal metatarsal 78.68
    thorax (ribs) (sternum) 78.61
    tibia 78.67
    ulna 78.63
    vertebrae 78.69
  foreign body NEC (*see also* Incision, by site) 98.20
    abdominal (cavity) 54.92
      wall 54.0
    adenoid 98.13
      by incision 28.91
    alveolus, alveolar bone 98.22
      by incision 24.0
    antecubital fossa 98.27
      by incision 86.05
    anterior chamber 12.00
      by incision 12.02
        with use of magnet 12.01
    anus (intraluminal) 98.05
      by incision 49.93
    artificial stoma (intraluminal) 98.18
    auditory canal, external 18.02
    axilla 98.27
      by incision 86.05
    bladder (without incision) 57.0
      by incision 57.19
    bone, except fixation device (*see also* Incision, bone) 77.10
      alveolus, alveolar 98.22
        by incision 24.0
    brain 01.39
      without incision into brain 01.24
    breast 85.0
    bronchus (intraluminal) 98.15
      by incision 33.0
    bursa 83.03
      hand 82.03
    canthus 98.22
      by incision 08.51
    cerebral meninges 01.31
    cervix (intraluminal) NEC 98.16
      penetrating 69.97
    choroid (by incision) 14.00
      with use of magnet 14.01
      without use of magnet 14.02
    ciliary body (by incision) 12.00
      with use of magnet 12.01
      without use of magnet 12.02
    conjunctiva (by magnet) 98.22
      by incision 10.0
    cornea 98.21
      by incision 11.1
      by magnet 11.0
    duodenum 98.03
      by incision 45.01
    ear (intraluminal) 98.11
      with incision 18.09
    epididymis 63.92
    esophagus (intraluminal) 98.02
      by incision 42.09
    extrapleural (by incision) 34.01
    eye, eyeball (by magnet) 98.21
      anterior segment (by incision) 12.00
        with use of magnet 12.01
        without use of magnet 12.02
      posterior segment (by incision) 14.00
        with use of magnet 14.01
        without use of magnet 14.02

Removal—*continued*
    superficial 98.21
    eyelid 98.22
      by incision 08.09
    fallopian tube
      by salpingostomy 66.02
      by salpingotomy 66.01
    fascia 83.09
      hand 82.09
    foot 98.28
    gall bladder 51.04
    groin region (abdominal wall) (inguinal) 54.0
    gum 98.22
      by incision 24.0
    hand 98.26
    head and neck NEC 98.22
    heart 37.11
    internal fixation, device—*see* Removal, fixation device, internal
    intestine
      by incision 45.00
      large (intraluminal) 98.04
        by incision 45.03
      small (intraluminal) 98.03
        by incision 45.02
    intraocular (by incision) 12.00
      with use of magnet 12.01
      without use of magnet 12.02
    iris (by incision) 12.00
      with use of magnet 12.01
      without use of magnet 12.02
    joint structure (*see also* Arthrotomy) 80.10
    kidney (transurethral) (by endoscopy) 56.0
      by incision 55.01
      pelvis (transurethral) 56.0
        by incision 55.11
    labia 98.23
      by incision 71.09
    lacrimal
      canaliculi 09.42
        by incision 09.52
      gland 09.3
        by incision 09.0
      passage(s) 09.49
        by incision 09.59
      punctum 09.41
        by incision 09.51
      sac 09.49
        by incision 09.53
    large intestine (intraluminal) 98.04
      by incision 45.03
    larynx (intraluminal) 98.14
      by incision 31.3
    lens 13.00
      by incision 13.02
      with use of magnet 13.01
    liver 50.0
    lower limb, except foot 98.29
      foot 98.28
    lung 33.1
    mediastinum 34.1
    meninges (cerebral) 01.31
      spinal 03.01
    mouth (intraluminal) 98.01
      by incision 27.92
    muscle 83.02
      hand 82.02
    nasal sinus 22.50
      antrum 22.2
        with Caldwell-Luc approach 22.39
      ethmoid 22.51

Removal—*continued*
    frontal 22.41
    maxillary 22.2
      with Caldwell-Luc approach 22.39
    sphenoid 22.52
  nerve (cranial) (peripheral) NEC 04.04
    root 03.01
  nose (intraluminal) 98.12
    by incision 21.1
  oral cavity (intraluminal) 98.01
    by incision 27.92
  orbit (by magnet) 98.21
    by incision 16.1
  palate (penetrating) 98.22
    by incision 27.1
  pancreas 52.09
  penis 98.24
    by incision 64.92
  pericardium 37.12
  perineum (female) 98.23
    by incision 71.09
    male 98.25
      by incision 86.05
  perirenal tissue 59.09
  peritoneal cavity 54.92
  perivesical tissue 59.19
  pharynx (intraluminal) 98.13
    by pharyngotomy 29.0
  pleura (by incision) 34.09
  popliteal space 98.29
    by incision 86.05
  rectum (intraluminal) 98.05
    by incision 48.0
  renal pelvis (transurethral) 56.0
    by incision 56.1
  retina (by incision) 14.00
    with use of magnet 14.01
    without use of magnet 14.02
  retroperitoneum 54.92
  sclera (by incision) 12.00
    with use of magnet 12.01
    without use of magnet 12.02
  scrotum 98.24
    by incision 61.0
  sinus (nasal) 22.50
    antrum 22.2
      with Caldwell-Luc approach 22.39
    ethmoid 22.51
    frontal 22.41
    maxillary 22.2
      with Caldwell-Luc approach 22.39
    sphenoid 22.52
  skin NEC 98.20
    by incision 86.05
  skull 01.24
    with incision into brain 01.39
  small intestine (intraluminal) 98.03
    by incision 45.02
  soft tissue NEC 83.09
    hand 82.09
  spermatic cord 63.93
  spinal (canal) (cord) (meninges) 03.01
  stomach (intraluminal) 98.03
    bubble (balloon) 44.94
    by incision 43.0
  subconjunctival (by magnet) 98.22
    by incision 10.0
  subcutaneous tissue NEC 98.20
    by incision 86.05
  supraclavicular fossa 98.27
    by incision 86.05

Removal—*continued*
  tendon (sheath) 83.01
    hand 82.01
  testis 62.0
  thorax (by incision) 34.09
  thyroid (field) (gland) (by incision) 06.09
  tonsil 98.13
    by incision 28.91
  trachea (intraluminal) 98.15
    by incision 31.3
  trunk NEC 98.25
  tunica vaginalis 98.24
  upper limb, except hand 98.27
    hand 98.26
  ureter (transurethral) 56.0
    by incision 56.2
  urethra (intraluminal) 98.19
    by incision 58.0
  uterus (intraluminal) 98.16
  vagina (intraluminal) 98.17
    by incision 70.14
  vas deferens 63.6
  vitreous (by incision) 14.00
    with use of magnet 14.01
    without use of magnet 14.02
  vulva 98.23
    by incision 71.09
gallstones
  bile duct (by incision) NEC 51.49
    endoscopic 51.88
  common duct (by incision) 51.41
    endoscopic 51.88
    percutaneous 51.96
  duodenum 45.01
  gallbladder 51.04
    endoscopic 51.88
    laparoscopic 51.88
  hepatic ducts 51.49
    endoscopic 51.88
  intestine 45.00
    large 45.03
    small NEC 45.02
  liver 50.0
Gardner Wells tongs (skull) 02.95
  with synchronous replacement 02.94
gastric bubble (balloon) 44.94
granulation tissue—*see also* Excision, lesion, by
    site
  with repair—*see* Repair, by site
  cranial 01.6
  skull 01.6
halo traction device (skull) 02.95
  with synchronous replacement 02.94
heart assist system 37.64
  with replacement 37.63
  intra-aortic balloon pump (IABP) 97.44
  nonoperative 97.44
hematoma—*see* Drainage, by site
Hoffman minifixator device (bone)—*see*
    category 78.6
hydatidiform mole 68.0
impacted
  feces (rectum) (by flushing) (manual) 96.38
  tooth 23.19
    from nasal sinus (maxillary) 22.61
implant
  breast 85.94
  cochlear prosthetic device 20.99
  cornea 11.92
  lens (prosthetic) 13.8
  middle ear NEC 20.99

Removal—*continued*
  ocular 16.71
    posterior segment 14.6
    orbit 16.72
    retina 14.6
    tympanum 20.1
  internal fixation device—*see* Removal, fixation
    device, internal
  intra-aortic balloon pump (IABP) 97.44
  intrauterine contraceptive device (IUD) 97.71
  joint (structure) NOS 80.90
    ankle 80.97
    elbow 80.92
    foot and toe 80.98
    hand and finger 80.94
    hip 80.95
    knee 80.96
    other specified sites 80.99
    shoulder 80.91
    spine 80.99
    toe 80.98
    wrist 80.93
  Kantrowitz heart pump 37.64
    nonoperative 97.44
  keel (tantalum plate), larynx 31.98
  kidney—*see also* Nephrectomy
    mechanical 55.98
    transplanted or rejected 55.53
  laminaria (tent), uterus 97.79
  leads (cardiac)—*see* Removal, electrodes,
    cardiac pacemaker
  lesion—*see* Excision, lesion, by site
  ligamentum flavum (spine)—*omit code*
  ligature
    fallopian tube 66.79
    ureter 56.86
    vas deferens 63.84
  loop recorder 86.05
  loose body
    bone—*see* Sequestrectomy, bone
    joint 80.10
  mesh (surgical)—*see* Removal, foreign body,
    by site
  lymph node—*see* Excision, lymph, node
  minifixator device (bone)—*see category* 78.6
    external fixation device 97.88
  Mulligan hood, fallopian tube 66.94
    with synchronous replacement 66.93
  muscle stimulator (skeletal) 83.93
    with replacement 83.92
  myringotomy device or tube 20.1
  nail (bed) (fold) 86.23
    internal fixation device—*see* Removal,
      fixation device, internal
  necrosis
    skin 86.28
      excisional 86.22
  neuropacemaker
    brain 01.22
      with synchronous replacement 02.93
    intracranial 01.22
      with synchronous replacement 02.93
    peripheral nerve 04.93
      with synchronous replacement 04.92
    spinal 03.94
      with synchronous replacement 03.93
  neurostimulator
    brain 01.22
      with synchronous replacement 02.93
    intracranial 01.22
      with synchronous replacement 02.93

Removal—*continued*
  peripheral nerve 04.93
    with synchronous replacement 04.92
  spinal 03.94
    with synchronous replacement 03.93
  nonabsorbable surgical material NEC—*see*
    Removal, foreign body, by site
  odontoma (tooth) 24.4
  orbital implant 16.72
  osteocartilaginous loose body, joint structures
    (*see also* Arthrotomy) 80.10
  outer attic wall (middle ear) 20.59
  ovo-testis (unilateral) 62.3
    bilateral 62.41
  pacemaker
    brain (intracranial) 01.22
      with synchronous replacement 02.93
    cardiac (device) (initial) (permanent)
      37.89
      with replacement
        dual-chamber device 37.87
        single-chamber device 37.85
          rate responsive 37.86
      electrodes (atrial) (transvenous)
        (ventricular) 37.77
        with replacement 37.76
      epicardium (myocardium) 37.77
        with replacement (by)
          atrial and/or ventricular lead(s)
            (electrode) 37.76
          epicardial lead 37.74
      temporary transvenous pacemaker
        system—*omit code*
    intracranial 01.22
      with synchronous replacement 02.93
    neural
      brain 01.22
        with synchronous replacement 02.93
      peripheral nerve 04.93
        with synchronous replacement 4.92
      spine 03.94
        with synchronous replacement 03.93
      spinal 03.94
        with synchronous replacement 03.93
  pack, packing
    dental 97.34
    intrauterine 97.72
    nasal 97.32
    rectum 97.59
    trunk NEC 97.85
    vagina 97.75
    vulva 97.75
  pantopaque dye, spinal canal 03.31
  patella (complete) 77.96
    partial 77.86
  pectus deformity implant device 34.01
  pelvic viscera, en masse (female) 68.8
    male 57.71
  pessary, vagina NEC 97.74
  pharynx (partial) 29.33
  phlebolith—*see* Removal, embolus
  placenta (by)
    aspiration curettage 69.52
    D and C 69.02
    manual 75.4
  plaque, dental 96.54
  plate, skull 02.07
    with synchronous replacement 02.05
  polyp—*see also* Excision, lesion, by site
    esophageal 42.32
      endoscopic 42.33

Removal—*continued*
  gastric (endoscopic) 43.41
  intestine 45.41
    endoscopic 45.42
    nasal 21.31
  prosthesis
    bile duct 51.95
      nonoperative 97.55
    cochlear prosthetic device 20.99
    dental 97.35
    eye 97.31
    facial bone 76.99
    fallopian tue 66.94
      with synchronous replacement 66.93
    joint structures 80.00
      ankle 80.07
      elbow 80.02
      foot and toe 80.08
      hand and finger 80.04
      hip 80.05
      knee 80.06
      shoulder 80.01
      specified site NEC 80.09
      spine 80.09
      wrist 80.03
    lens 13.8
    penis (internal) without replacement 64.96
    Rosen (urethra) 59.99
    testicular, by incision 62.0
    urinary sphincter, artificial 58.99
      with replacement 58.93
  pseudophakos 13.8
  pterygium 11.39
    with corneal graft 11.32
  pulse generator
    cardiac pacemaker 37.86
    cardioverter/defibrillator 37.99
  pump assist device, heart 37.64
    with replacement 37.63
    nonoperative 97.44
  radioactive material—*see* Removal, foreign
      body, by site
  redundant skin, eyelid 08.86
  rejected organ
    kidney 55.53
    testis 62.42
  reservoir, ventricular (Ommaya) (Rickham)
      02.43
    with synchronous replacement 02.42
  retained placenta (by)
    aspiration curettage 69.52
    D and C 69.02
    manual 75.4
  retinal implant 14.6
  rhinolith 21.31
  rice bodies, tendon sheaths 83.01
    hand 82.01
  Roger-Anderson minifixator device (bone) *see*
      category 78.6
  root, residual (tooth) (buried) (retained) 23.11
  Rosen prosthesis (urethra) 59.99
  Scribner shunt 39.43
  scleral buckle or implant 14.6
  secondary membranous cataract (with
      iridectomy) 13.65
  secundines (by)
    aspiration curettage 69.52
    D and C 69.02
    manual 75.4
  sequestrum—*see* Sequestrectomy
  seton, anus 49.93

Removal—*continued*
  Shepard's tube (ear) 20.1
  Shirodkar suture, cervix 69.96
  shunt
    arteriovenous 39.43
      with creation of new shunt 39.42
    lumbar-subarachnoid NEC 03.98
    pleurothecal 03.98
    salpingothecal 03.98
    spinal (thecal) NEC 03.98
    subarachnoid-peritoneal 03.98
    subarachnoid-ureteral 03.98
  silastic tubes
    ear 20.1
    fallopian tubes 66.94
      with synchronous replacement 66.93
  skin
    necrosis or slough 86.28
      excisional 86.22
    superficial layer (by dermabrasion) 86.25
  skull tongs 02.95
    with synchronous replacement 02.94
  splint 97.88
  stent
    bile duct 97.55
    larynx 31.98
    ureteral 97.62
    urethral 97.65
  stimoceiver (brain) (intracranial) 01.22
    with synchronous replacement 02.93
  subdural
    grids 01.22
    strips 01.22
  supernumerary digit(s) 86.26
  suture(s) NEC 97.89
    abdominal wall 97.83
    by incision—*see* Incision, by site
    genital tract 97.79
    head and neck 97.38
    thorax 97.43
    trunk NEC 97.84
  symblepharon—*see* Repair, symblepharon
  temporary transvenous pacemaker
      system—*omit code*
  testis (unilateral) 62.3
    bilateral 62.41
    remaining or solitary 62.42
  thrombus 38.00
    with endarterectomy—*see* Endarterectomy
    abdominal
      artery 38.06
      vein 38.07
    aorta (arch) (ascending) (descending) 38.04
    arteriovenous shunt or cannula 39.49
    bovine graft 39.49
    coronary artery 36.09
    head and neck vessel NEC 38.02
    intracranial vessel NEC 38.01
    lower limb
      artery 38.08
      vein 38.09
    pulmonary (artery) (vein) 38.05
    thoracic vessel NEC 38.05
    upper limb (artery) (vein) 38.0
  tissue expander (skin) NEC 86.05
    breast 85.96
  toes, supernumerary 86.26
  tongs, skull 02.95
    with synchronous replacement 02.94
  tonsil tag 28.4
  tooth (by forceps) (multiple) (single NEC 23.09

Repair—*continued*
  cisterna chyli 40.69
  claw toe 77.57
  cleft
    hand 82.82
    laryngotracheal 31.69
    lip 27.54
    palate 27.62
      secondary or subsequent 27.63
  coarctation of aorta—*see* Excision, coarctation
    of aorta
  cochlear prosthetic device 20.99
    external components only 95.49
  cockup toe 77.58
  colostomy 46.43
  conjunctiva NEC 10.49
    with scleral repair 12.81
    laceration 10.6
      with repair of sclera 12.81
  late effect of trachoma 10.49
  cornea NEC 11.59
    with
      conjunctiva flap 11.53
      transplant—*see* Keratoplasty
    postoperative dehiscence 11.52
  coronary artery NEC 36.99
    by angioplasty—*see* Angioplasty, coronary
    by atherectomy—*see* Angioplasty, coronary
  cranium NEC 02.06
    with
      flap (bone) 02.03
      graft (bone) 02.04
  cusp, valve—*see* Repair, heart, valve
  cystocele 70.51
    and rectocele 70.50
  dental arch 24.8
  diaphragm NEC 34.84
  diastasis recti 83.65
  diastematomyelia 03.59
  ear (external) 18.79
    auditory canal or meatus 18.6
    auricle NEC 18.79
    cartilage NEC 18.79
    laceration (by suture) 18.4
    lop ear 18.79
    middle NEC 19.9
    prominent or protruding 18.5
  ectropion 08.49
    by or with
      lid reconstruction 08.44
      suture (technique) 08.42
      thermocauterization 08.41
      wedge resection 08.43
  encephalocele (cerebral) 02.12
  endocardial cushion defect 35.73
    with
      prosthesis (grafted to septa) 35.54
      tissue graft 35.63
  enterocele (female) 70.92
    male 53.9
  enterostomy 46.40
  entropion 08.49
    by or with
      lid reconstruction 08.44
      suture (technique) 08.42
      thermocauterization 08.41
      wedge resection 08.43
  epicanthus (fold) 08.59
  epididymis (and spermatic cord) NEC 63.59
    with vas deferens 63.89
  epiglottis 31.69

Repair—*continued*
  episiotomy
    routine following delivery—*see* Episiotomy
    secondary 75.69
  epispadias 58.45
  esophagus, esophageal NEC 42.89
    fistula NEC 42.84
    stricture 42.85
  exstrophy of bladder 57.86
  eye, eyeball 16.89
    multiple structures 16.82
    rupture 16.82
    socket 16.64
      with graft 16.63
  eyebrow 08.89
    linear 08.81
  eyelid 08.89
    full-thickness 08.85
      involving lid margin 08.84
    laceration 08.81
      full-thickness 08.85
      involving lid margin 08.84
      partial-thickness 08.83
      involving lid margin 08.82
    linear 08.81
    partial-thickness 08.83
      involving lid margin 08.82
    retraction 08.38
  fallopian tube (with prosthesis) 66.79
    by
      anastomosis 66.73
      reanastomosis 66.79
      reimplantation into
        ovary 66.72
        uterus 66.74
      suture 66.71
  false aneurysm—*see* Repair, aneurysm
  fascia 83.89
    by or with
      arthroplasty—*see* Arthroplasty
      graft (fascial) (muscle) 83.82
        hand 82.72
        tendon 83.81
          hand 82.79
      suture (direct) 83.65
        hand 82.46
    hand 82.89
      by
        graft NEC 82.79
          fascial 82.72
          muscle 82.72
        suture (direct) 82.46
    joint—*see* Arthroplasty
  filtering bleb (corneal) (scleral) (by excision)
    12.82
    by
      corneal graft (*see also* Keratoplasty) 11.60
      scleroplasty 12.82
      suture 11.51
    with conjunctival flap 11.53
  fistula—*see also* Closure, fistula
    anovaginal 70.73
    arteriovenous 39.53
      clipping 39.53
      coagulation 39.53
        endovascular approach 39.79
          head and neck 39.72
      division 39.53
      excision or resection—*see also*
        Aneurysmectomy, by site
        with

Repair—*continued*
    anastomosis—*see* Aneurysmectomy,
      with anastomosis, by site
    graft replacement—*see*
      Aneurysmectomy, with graft
      replacement, by site
    ligation 39.53
      coronary artery 36.99
    occlusion 39.53
      endovascular approach 39.79
      head and neck 39.72
    suture 39.53
    cervicovesical 57.84
    cervix 67.62
    choledochoduodenal 51.72
    colovaginal 70.72
    enterovaginal 70.74
    enterovesical 57.83
    esophagocutaneous 42.84
    ileovesical 57.83
    intestinovaginal 70.74
    intestinovesical 57.83
    oroantral 22.71
    perirectal 48.93
    pleuropericardial 37.4
    rectovaginal 70.73
    rectovesical 57.83
    rectovesicovaginal 57.83
    scrotum 61.42
    sigmoidovaginal 70.74
    sinus
      nasal 22.71
      of Valsalva 35.39
    splenocolic 41.95
    urethroperineovesical 57.84
    urethrovesical 57.84
    urethrovesicovaginal 57.84
    uterovesical 57.84
    vagina NEC 70.75
    vaginocutaneous 70.75
    vaginoenteric NEC 70.74
    vaginoileal 70.74
    vaginoperineal 70.75
    vaginovesical 57.84
    vesicocervicovaginal 57.84
    vesicocolic 57.83
    vesicocutaneous 57.84
    vesicoenteric 57.83
    vesicointestinal 57.83
    vesicometrorectal 57.83
    vesicoperineal 57.84
    vesicorectal 57.83
    vesicosigmoidal 57.83
    vesicosigmoidovaginal 57.83
    vesicourethral 57.84
    vesicourethrorectal 57.83
    vesicouterine 57.84
    vesicovaginal 57.84
    vulva 71.72
    vulvorectal 48.73
   foramen ovale (patent) 35.71
    with
      prosthesis (open heart technique) 35.51
        closed heart technique 35.52
      tissue graft 35.61
   fracture—*see also* Reduction, fracture
    larynx 31.64
    malunion or nonunion (delayed) NEC—*see*
      category 78.4
      with
        graft—*see* Graft, bone

Repair—*continued*
   insertion (of)
    bone growth stimulator (invasive)—*see*
      category 78.9
    internal fixation device 78.5
   manipulation for realignment—*see*
    Reduction, fracture, by site, closed
   osteotomy
    with
      correction of alignment—*see category*
      77.3
      with internal fixation device—*see*
        categories 77.3 *[78.5]*
      with intramedullary rod—*see*
        categories 77.3 *[78.5]*
   replacement arthroplasty—*see*
    Arthroplasty
   sequestrectomy—*see category* 77.0
   Sofield type procedure—*see* categories
    77.3 *[78.5]*
   synostosis technique—*see* Arthrodesis
   vertebra 03.53
  funnel chest (with implant) 34.74
  gallbladder 51.91
  gastroschisis 54.71
  great vessels NEC 39.59
   laceration (by suture) 39.30
    artery 39.31
    vein 39.32
  hallux valgus NEC 77.59
   resection of joint with prosthetic implant 77.59
  hammer toe 77.56
  hand 82.89
   with graft or implant 82.79
    fascia 82.72
    muscle 82.72
    tendon 82.79
  heart 37.4
   assist system 37.63
   septum 35.70
    with
      prosthesis 35.50
      tissue graft 35.60
    atrial 35.71
     with
      prosthesis (open heart technique) 35.51
       closed heart technique 35.52
      tissue graft 35.61
     combined with repair of valvular and
      ventricular septal defects—*see* Repair,
      endocardial cushion defect
     in total repair of
      tetralogy of Fallot 35.81
      total anomalous pulmonary venous
       connection 35.82
      truncus arteriosus 35.83
    combined with repair of valvular
      defect—*see* Repair, endocardial cushion
      defect
    ventricular 35.72
     with
      prosthesis 35.53
      tissue graft 35.62
     combined with repair of valvular and atrial
      septal defects—*see* Repair,
      endocardial cushion defect
     in total repair of
      tetralogy of Fallot 35.81
      total anomalous pulmonary venous
       connection 35.82
      truncus arteriosus 35.83

Repair—*continued*
  lacrimal system NEC 09.99
    canaliculus 09.73
    punctum 09.72
      for eversion 09.71
  laryngostomy 31.62
  laryngotracheal cleft 31.69
  larynx 31.69
    fracture 31.64
    laceration 31.61
  leads (cardiac) NEC 37.75
  ligament (*see also* Arthroplasty) 81.96
    broad 69.29
    collateral, knee NEC 81.46
    cruciate, knee NEC 81.45
    round 69.29
    uterine 69.29
  lip NEC 27.59
    cleft 27.54
    laceration (by suture) 27.51
  liver NEC 50.69
    laceration 50.61
  lop ear 18.79
  lung NEC 33.49
  lymphatic (channel) (peripheral) NEC 40.9
    duct, left (thoracic) NEC 40.69
  macrodactyly 82.83
  mallet finger 82.84
  mandibular ridge 76.64
  mastoid (antrum) (cavity) 19.9
  meninges (cerebral) NEC 02.12
    spinal NEC 03.59
      meningocele 03.51
      myelomeningocele 03.52
  meningocele (spinal) 03.51
    cranial 02.12
  mesentery 54.75
  mouth NEC 27.59
    laceration NEC 27.52
  muscle NEC 83.87
    by
      graft or implant (fascia) (muscle) 83.82
        hand 82.72
      tendon 83.81
        hand 82.79
      suture (direct) 83.65
        hand 82.46
      transfer or transplantation (muscle) 83.77
        hand 82.58
    hand 82.89
    by
      graft or implant NEC 82.79
        fascia 82.72
      suture (direct) 82.46
      transfer or transplantation (muscle) 82.58
  musculotendinous cuff, shoulder 83.63
  myelomeningocele 03.52
  nasal
    septum (perforation) NEC 21.88
    sinus NEC 22.79
    fistula 22.71
  nasolabial flaps (plastic) 21.86
  nasopharyngeal atresia 29.4
  nerve (cranial) (peripheral) NEC 04.79
    old injury 04.76
    revision 04.75
    sympathetic 05.81
  nipple NEC 85.87
  nose (external) (internal) (plastic) NEC (*see also* Rhinoplasty) 21.89
    laceration (by suture) 21.81

Repair—*continued*
  notched lip 27.59
  omentum 54.74
  omphalocele 53.49
    with prosthesis 53.41
  orbit 16.89
    wound 16.81
  ostium
    primum defect 35.73
      with prosthesis 35.54
      with tissue graft 35.63
    secundum defect 35.71
      with
        prosthesis (open heart technique) 35.51
          closed heart technique 35.52
        tissue graft 35.61
  ovary 65.79
    with tube 65.73
      laparoscopic 65.76
  overlapping toe 77.58
  pacemaker
    cardiac
      device (permanent) 37.89
      electrode(s) (lead) NEC 37.75
      pocket (skin) (subcutaneous) 37.79
  palate NEC 27.69
    cleft 27.62
      secondary or subsequent 27.63
    laceration (by suture) 27.61
  pancreas NEC 52.95
    Wirsung's duct 52.99
  papillary muscle (heart) 35.31
  patent ductus arteriosus 38.85
  pectus deformity (chest) (carinatum) (excavatum) 34.74
  pelvic floor NEC 70.79
    obstetric laceration (current) 75.69
    old 70.79
  penis NEC 64.49
    for episadias or hypospadias 58.45
    inflatable prosthesis 64.99
    laceration 64.41
  pericardium 37.4
  perineum (female) 71.79
    laceration (by suture) 71.71
      obstetric (current) 75.69
      old 71.79
    male NEC 86.89
      laceration (by suture) 86.59
  peritoneum NEC 54.73
    by suture 54.64
  pharynx NEC 29.59
    laceration (by suture) 29.51
    plastic 29.4
  pleura 34.93
  postcataract wound dehiscence 11.52
    with conjunctival flap 11.53
  pouch of Douglas 70.52
  primum ostium defect 35.73
    with
      prosthesis 35.54
      tissue graft 35.63
  prostate 60.93
  ptosis, eyelid—*see* Repair, blepharoptosis
  punctum, lacrimal NEC 09.72
    for correction of eversion 09.71
  quadriceps (mechanism) 83.86
  rectocele (posterior colporrhaphy) 70.52
    and cystocele 70.50
  rectum NEC 48.79
    laceration (by suture) 48.71

Replacement—*continued*

  left ventricular coronary venous lead only
    00.52

  pulse generator only 00.54

  CRT-P (cardiac resynchronization pacemaker)
    00.50

  left ventricular coronary venous lead only
    00.52

  pulse generator only 00.53

  Crutchfield tongs (skull) 02.94

  cystostomy tube (catheter) 59.94

  diaphragm, vagina 97.24

  drain—*see also* Replacement, tube

    vagina 97.26

    vulva 97.26

    wound, musculoskeletal or skin 97.16

  ear (prosthetic) 18.71

  elbow (joint), total 81.84

  electrode(s)—*see* Implant, electrode or lead, by
    site or name of device

  brain

    depth 02.93

    foramen ovale 02.93

    sphenoidal 02.96

  depth 02.93

  foramen ovale 02.93

  sphenoidal 02.96

  electroencephalographic receiver (brain)
    (intracranial) 02.93

  electronic

    cardioverter/defibrillator—*see* Replacement,
      cardioverter/defibrillator

    leads (electrodes) —*see* Replacement,
      pacemaker, electrodes, cardiac

    stimulator—*see also* Implant, electronic
      stimulator, by site

      bladder 57.97

      muscle (skeletal) 83.92

      ureter 56.93

  electrostimulator—*see* Implant, electronic
    stimulator, by site

  enterostomy device (tube)

    large intestine 97.04

    small intestine 97.03

  epidural pegs 02.93

  femoral head, by prosthesis 81.52

    revision 81.53

  Gardner Wells tongs (skull) 02.94

  graft—*see* Graft

  halo traction device (skull) 02.94

  Harrington rod (with refusion of spine)—*see*
    Refusion, spinal

  heart

    artificial 37.63

    valve (with prosthesis) (with tissue graft)
      35.20

      aortic (with prosthesis) 35.22

        with tissue graft 35.21

      mitral (with prosthesis) 35.24

        with tissue graft 35.23

      poppet (prosthetic) 35.95

      pulmonary (with prosthesis) 35.26

        with tissue graft 35.25

        in total repair of tetralogy of Fallot 35.81

      tricuspid (with prosthesis) 35.28

        with tissue graft 35.27

  hip (partial) (with fixation device) (with
    prosthesis) (with traction) 81.52

    acetabulum 81.52

      revision 81.53

    femoral head 81.52

Replacement—*continued*

    revision 81.53

    total 81.51

      revision 81.53

  inverted uterus—*see* Repair, inverted uterus

  iris NEC 12.39

  kidney, mechanical 55.97

  knee, (bicompartmental) (hemijoint) (partial)
    (total) (tricompartmental)
    (unicompartmental) 81.54

    revision 81.55

  laryngeal stent 31.93

  leads (electrode) (s)—*see* Replacement,
    pacemaker, electrode(s), cardiac

  mechanical kidney 55.97

  mitral valve (with prosthesis) 35.24

    with tissue graft 35.23

  Mulligan hood, fallopian tube 66.93

  muscle stimulator (skeletal) 83.92

  nephrostomy tube 55.93

  neuropacemaker—*see* Implant,
    neuropacemaker, by site

  neurostimulator—*see also* Implant,
    neurostimulator, by site

    peripheral nerve 04.92

    skeletal muscle 83.92

  pacemaker

    brain 02.93

    cardiac device (initial) (permanent)

      dual-chamber device 37.87

      single-chamber device 37.85

      rate responsive 37.86

      resynchronization—*see* Replacement,
        CRT-P

    electrode(s), cardiac (atrial) (transvenous)
      (ventricular) 37.76

      epicardium (myocardium) 37.74

      left ventricular coronary venous system
        00.52

    intracranial 02.93

    neural

      brain 02.93

      intracranial 02.93

      peripheral nerve 04.92

    spine 03.93

    spine 03.93

    temporary transvenous pacemaker system
      37.78

  pack or bag

    nose 97.21

    teeth, tooth 97.22

    vagina 97.26

    vulva 97.26

    wound 97.16

  pessary, vagina NEC 97.25

  prosthesis

    acetabulum 81.53

    arm (bioelectric) (cineplastic) (kineplastic)
      84.44

    biliary tract 51.99

    cochlear 20.96

    channel (single) 20.97

      multiple 20.98

    elbow 81.97

    extremity (bioelectric) (cineplastic)
      (kineplastic) 84.40

      lower 84.48

      upper 84.44

    fallopian tube (Mulligan hood) (stent) 66.93

    femur 81.53

    knee 81.55

Replacement—*continued*
  leg (bioelectric) (cineplastic) (kineplastic)
    84.48
  penis (non-inflatable) (internal) 64.95
    inflatable (internal) 64.97
  shoulder NEC 81.83
    partial 81.81
    total 81.80
  urinary sphincter, artificial 58.93
  pulmonary valve (with prosthesis) 35.26
    with tissue graft 35.25
    in total repair tetrology of Fallot 35.81
  pyelostomy tube 55.94
  rectal tube 96.09
  shoulder NEC 81.83
    partial 81.81
    total 81.80
  skull
    plate 02.05
    tongs 02.94
  specified appliance or device NEC 97.29
  stent
    bile duct 97.05
    fallopian tube 66.93
    larynx 31.93
    pancreatic duct 97.05
    trachea 31.93
  stimoceiver—*see* Implant, stimoceiver, by site
  subdural
    grids 02.93
    strips 02.93
  testis in scrotum 62.5
  tongs, skull 02.94
  tracheal stent 31.93
  tricuspid valve (with prosthesis) 35.28
    with tissue graft 35.27
  tube
    bile duct 97.05
    bladder 57.95
    cystostomy 59.94
    esophagostomy 97.01
    gastrostomy 97.02
    large intestine 97.04
    nasogastric 97.01
    nephrostomy 55.93
    pancreatic duct 97.05
    pyelostomy 55.94
    rectal 96.09
    small intestine 97.03
    tracheostomy 97.23
    ureterostomy 59.93
    ventricular (cerebral) 02.42
  umbilical cord, prolapsed 73.92
  ureter (with)
    bladder flap 56.74
    ileal segment implanted into bladder 56.89
      [45.51]
  ureterostomy tube 59.93
  urethral sphincter, artificial 58.93
  urinary sphincter, artificial 58.93
  valve
    heart—*see also* Replacement, heart valve
      poppet (prosthetic) 35.95
    ventricular (cerebral) 02.42
  ventricular shunt (catheter) (valve) 02.42
  Vinke tongs (skull) 02.94
  vitreous (silicone) 14.75
    for retinal reattachment 14.59

Replant, replantation —*see also* Reattachment
  extremity—*see* Reattachment, extremity
  penis 64.45
  scalp, 86.51
  tooth 23.5
Reposition
  cardiac pacemaker
    electrode(s) (atrial) (transvenous) (ventricular)
      37.75
    pocket 37.79
  cardioverter/defibrillator
    lead(s) (sensing) (pacing) (epicardial patch)
      37.99
    pocket 37.99
    pulse generator 37.99
  cilia base 08.71
  iris 12.39
  renal vessel, aberrant 39.55
  thyroid tissue 06.94
  tricuspid valve (with plication) 35.14
Resection —*see also* Excision, by site
  abdominoendorectal (combined) 48.5
  abdominoperineal (rectum) 48.5
    pull-through (Altmeier) (Swenson) NEC 48.49
      Duhamel type 48.65
  alveolar process and palate (en bloc) 27.32
  aneurysm—*see* Aneurysmectomy
  aortic valve (for subvalvular stenosis) 35.11
  artery—*see* Arteriectomy
  bile duct NEC 51.69
    common duct NEC 51.63
  bladder (partial) (segmental) (transvesical)
    (wedge) 57.6
    complete or total 57.79
    lesion NEC 57.59
      transurethral approach 57.49
    neck 57.59
      transurethral approach 57.49
  blood vessel—*see* Angiectomy
  brain 01.59
    by
      stereotactic radiosurgery 92.30
        cobalt 60 92.32
        linear accelerator (LINAC) 92.31
        multi-source 92.32
        particle beam 92.33
        particulate 92.33
        radiosurgery NEC 92.39
        single source photon 92.31
    hemisphere 01.52
    lobe 01.53
  breast—*see also* Mastectomy
    quadrant 85.22
    segmental 85.23
  broad ligament 69.19
  bronchus (sleeve) (wide sleeve) 32.1
  block (en bloc) (with radical dissection of
    brachial plexus, bronchus, lobe of lung, ribs,
    and sympathetic nerves) 32.6
  bursa 83.5
    hand 82.31
  cecum (and terminal ileum) 45.72
  cerebral meninges 01.51
  chest wall 34.4
  clavicle 77.81
  clitoris 71.4
  colon (partial) (segmental) 45.79
    ascending (cecum and terminal ileum) 45.72
    cecum (and terminal ileum) 45.72
    complete 45.8

Resection—*continued*
  descending (sigmoid) 45.76
  for interposition 45.52
  Hartmann 45.75
  hepatic flexure 45.73
  left radical (hemicolon) 45.75
  multiple segmental 45.71
  right radical (hemicolon) (ileocolectomy)
    45.73
  segmental NEC 45.79
    multiple 45.71
  sigmoid 45.76
  splenic flexure 45.75
  total 45.8
  transverse 45.74
conjunctiva, for pterygium 11.39
  corneal graft 11.32
cornual (fallopian tube) (unilateral) 66.69
  bilateral 66.63
diaphragm 34.81
endaural 20.79
endorectal (pull-through) (Soave) 48.41
  combined abdominal 48.5
esophagus (partial) (subtotal) (*see also*
    Esophagectomy) 42.41
  total 42.42
exteriorized intestine—*see* Resection, intestine,
    exteriorized
fascia 83.44
  for graft 83.43
    hand 82.34
  hand 82.35
    for graft 82.34
gallbladder (total) 51.22
gastric (partial) (sleeve) (subtotal) NEC (*see
    also* Gastrectomy) 43.89
  with anastomosis NEC 43.89
    esophagogastric 43.5
    gastroduodenal 43.6
    gastrogastric 43.89
    gastrojejunal 43.7
  complete or total NEC 43.99
    with intestinal interposition 43.91
  radical NEC 43.99
    with intestinal interposition 43.91
  wedge 43.42
  endoscopic 43.41
hallux valgus (joint)—*see also* Bunionectomy
  with prosthetic implant 77.59
hepatic
  duct 51.69
  flexure (colon) 45.73
infundibula, heart (right) 35.34
intestine (partial) NEC 45.79
  cecum (with terminal ileum) 45.72
  exteriorized (large intestine) 46.04
    small intestine 46.02
  for interposition 45.50
    large intestine 45.52
    small intestine 45.51
  hepatic flexure 45.73
  ileum 45.62
    with cecum 45.72
  large (partial) (segmental) NEC 45.79
    for interposition 45.52
    multiple segmental 45.71
    total 45.8
  left hemicolon 45.75
  multiple segmental (large intestine) 45.71
    small intestine 45.61
  right hemicolon 45.73

Resection—*continued*
  segmental (large intestine) 45.79
    multiple 45.71
    small intestine 45.62
      multiple 45.61
  sigmoid 45.76
  small (partial) (segmental) NEC 45.62
    for interposition 45.51
    multiple segmental 45.61
    total 45.63
  total
    large intestine 45.8
    small intestine 45.63
joint structure NEC (*see also* Arthrectomy)
    80.90
kidney (segmental) (wedge) 55.4
larynx—*see also* Laryngectomy
  submucous 30.29
lesion—*see* Excision, lesion, by site
levator palpebrae muscle 08.33
ligament (*see also* Arthrectomy) 80.90
  broad 69.19
  round 69.19
  uterine 69.19
lip (wedge) 27.43
liver (partial) (wedge) 50.22
  lobe (total) 50.3
  total 50.4
lung (wedge) NEC 32.29
  endoscopic 32.28
  segmental (any part) 32.3
  volume reduction 32.22
meninges (cerebral) 01.51
  spinal 03.4
mesentery 54.4
muscle 83.45
  extraocular 15.13
    with
      advancement or recession of other eye
        muscle 15.3
      suture of original insertion 15.13
    levator palpebrae 08.33
    Müller's for blepharoptosis 08.35
    orbicularis oculi 08.20
    tarsal, for blepharoptosis 08.35
  for graft 83.43
    hand 82.34
  hand 82.36
    for graft 82.34
  ocular—*see* Resection, muscle, extraocular
myocardium 37.33
nasal septum (submucous) 21.5
nerve (cranial) (peripheral) NEC 04.07
  phrenic 04.03
    for collapse of lung 33.31
  sympathetic 05.29
  vagus—*see* Vagotomy
nose (complete) (extended) (partial)
    (radical) 21.4
omentum 54.4
orbitomaxillary, radical 16.51
ovary—(*see also* Oophorectomy
  wedge 65.22
    laparoscopic 65.24
palate (bony) (local) 27.31
  by wide excision 27.32
  soft 27.49
pancreas (total) (with synchronous
    duodenectomy) 52.6
  partial NEC 52.59
    distal (tail) (with part of body) 52.52

Resuscitation—*continued*
  cardiopulmonary 99.60
  endotracheal intubation 96.04
  manual 93.93
  mouth-to-mouth 93.93
  pulmonary 93.93
Resuture
  abdominal wall 54.61
  cardiac septum prosthesis 35.95
  chest wall 34.71
  heart valve prosthesis (poppet) 35.95
  wound (skin and subcutaneous tissue) (without
    graft) NEC 86.59
Retavase, infusion 99.10
Reteplase, infusion 99.10
Retinaculotomy NEC (*see also* Division,
    ligament) 80.40
  carpal tunnel (flexor) 04.43
Retraining
  cardiac 93.36
  vocational 93.85
Retrogasserian neurotomy 04.02
Revascularization
  cardiac (heart muscle) (myocardium) (direct)
    36.10
  with
    bypass anastomosis
      abdominal artery to coronary artery 36.17
      aortocoronary (catheter stent) (homograft)
        (prosthesis) (saphenous vein graft)
        36.10
      one coronary vessel 36.11
      two coronary vessels 36.12
      three coronary vessels 36.13
      four coronary vessels 36.14
      gastroepiploic artery to coronary artery
        36.17
      internal mammary-coronary artery (single
        vessel) 36.15
        double vessel 36.16
      specified type NEC 36.19
      thoracic artery-coronary artery (single
        vessel) 36.15
        double vessel 36.16
    implantation of artery into heart (muscle)
      (myocardium) (ventricle) 36.2
  indirect 36.2
  specified type NEC 36.39
  transmyocardial
    open chest 36.31
    percutaneous 36.32
    specified type NEC 36.32
    thoracoscopic 36.32
Reversal, intestinal segment 45.50
  large 45.52
  small 45.51
Revision
  amputation stump 84.3
    current traumatic—*see* Amputation
  anastomosis
    biliary tract 51.94
    blood vessel 39.49
    gastric, gastrointestinal (with jejunal
      interposition) 44.5
    intestine (large) 46.94
      small 46.93
    pleurothecal 03.97
    pyelointestinal 56.72
    salpingothecal 03.97
    subarachnoid-peritoneal 03.97
    subarachnoid-ureteral 03.97

Revision—*continued*
    ureterointestinal 56.72
  ankle replacement (prosthesis) 81.59
  anterior segment (eye) wound (operative) NEC
    12.83
  arteriovenous shunt (cannula) (for dialysis)
    39.42
  arthroplasty—*see* Arthroplasty
  bone flap, skull 02.06
  breast implant 85.93
  bronchostomy 33.42
  bypass graft (vascular) 39.49
    abdominal-coronary artery 36.17
    aortocoronary (catheter stent) (with
      prosthesis) (with saphenous vein graft)
      (with vein graft) 36.10
    one coronary vessel 36.11
    two coronary vessels 36.12
    three coronary vessels 36.13
    four coronary vessels 36.14
    CABG—*see* Revision, aortocoronary bypass
      graft
    chest tube—*see* intercostal catheter
    coronary artery bypass graft (CABG)—*see*
      Revision, aortocoronary bypass graft,
      abdominal-coronary artery bypass, and
      internal mammary-coronary artery bypass
    intercostal catheter (with lysis of adhesions)
      34.04
    internal mammary-coronary artery (single)
      36.15
    double vessel 36.16
  cannula, vessel-to-vessel (arteriovenous) 39.94
  canthus, lateral 08.59
  cardiac pacemaker
    device (permanent) 37.89
    electrode(s) (atrial) (transvenous) (ventricular)
      37.75
    pocket 37.79
  cardioverter/defibrillator (automatic) pocket
    37.99
  cholecystostomy 51.99
  cleft palate repair 27.63
  colostomy 46.43
  conduit, urinary 56.52
  cystostomy (stoma) 57.22
  elbow replacement (prosthesis) 81.97
  enterostomy (stoma) 46.40
    large intestine 46.43
    small intestine 46.41
  enucleation socket 16.64
    with graft 16.63
  esophagostomy 42.83
  exenteration cavity 16.66
    with secondary graft 16.65
  extraocular muscle surgery 15.6
  fenestration, inner ear 20.62
  filtering bleb 12.66
  fixation device (broken) (displaced) (*see also*
    Fixation, bone, internal) 78.50
  flap or pedicle graft (skin) 86.75
  foot replacement (prosthesis) 81.59
  gastric anastomosis (with jejunal interposition)
    44.5
  gastroduodenostomy (with jejunal interposition)
    44.5
  gastrointestinal anastomosis (with jejunal
    interposition) 44.5
  gastrojejunostomy 44.5
  gastrostomy 44.69
  hand replacement (prosthesis) 81.97

Revision—*continued*
  heart procedure NEC 35.95
  hip replacement (acetabulum) (femoral head)
      (partial) (total) 81.53
  Holter (Spitz) valve 02.42
  ileal conduit 56.52
  ileostomy 46.41
  jejunoileal bypass 46.93
  jejunostomy 46.41
  joint replacement 81.59
    acetabulum 81.53
    ankle 81.59
    elbow 81.97
    femoral head 81.53
    foot 81.59
    hand 81.97
    hip (partial) (total) 81.53
    knee 81.55
    lower extremity NEC 81.59
    toe 81.59
    upper extremity 81.97
    wrist 81.97
  knee replacement (prosthesis) 81.55
  laryngostomy 31.63
  lateral canthus 08.59
  mallet finger 82.84
  mastoid antrum 19.9
  mastoidectomy 20.92
  nephrostomy 55.89
  neuroplasty 04.75
  ocular implant 16.62
  orbital implant 16.62
  pocket
    cardiac pacemaker
      with initial insertion of pacemaker—*omit
          code*
      new site (skin) (subcutaneous) 37.79
    thalamic stimulator pulse generator
      with initial insertion of battery
          package—*omit code*
      new site (skin) (subcutaneous) 86.09
  previous mastectomy site—*see categories*
      85.0-85.99
  proctostomy 48.79
  prosthesis
    acetabulum
      hip 81.53
    ankle 81.59
    breast 85.93
    elbow 81.97
    femoral head 81.53
    foot 81.59
    hand 81.97
    heart valve (poppet) 35.95
    hip (partial) (total) 81.53
    knee 81.55
    lower extremity NEC 81.59
    shoulder 81.97
    toe 81.59
    upper extremity 81.97
    wrist 81.97
  ptosis overcorrection 08.37
  pyelostomy 55.12
  pyloroplasty 44.29
  rhinoplasty 21.84
  scar
    skin 86.84
      with excision 86.3
  scleral fistulization 12.66
  shoulder replacement (prosthesis) 81.97
  shunt

Revision—*continued*
    arteriovenous (cannula) (for dialysis) 39.42
    lumbar-subarachnoid NEC 03.97
    peritoneojugular 54.99
    peritoneovascular 54.99
    pleurothecal 03.97
    salpingothecal 03.97
    spinal (thecal) NEC 03.97
    subarachnoid-peritoneal 03.97
    subarachnoid-ureteral 03.97
    ventricular (cerebral) 02.42
    ventriculoperitoneal
      at peritoneal site 54.95
      at ventricular site 02.42
  stapedectomy NEC 19.29
    with incus replacement (homograft)
        (prosthesis) 19.21
  stoma
    bile duct 51.79
    bladder (vesicostomy) 57.22
    bronchus 33.42
    common duct 51.72
    esophagus 42.89
    gallbladder 51.99
    hepatic duct 51.79
    intestine 46.40
      large 46.43
      small 46.41
    kidney 55.89
    larynx 31.63
    rectum 48.79
    stomach 44.69
    thorax 34.79
    trachea 31.74
    ureter 56.62
    urethra 58.4
  tack operation 20.79
  toe replacement (prosthesis) 81.59
  tracheostomy 31.74
  tunnel
    pulse generator lead wire 86.99
      with initial procedure—*omit code*
  tympanoplasty 19.6
  uretero-ileostomy, cutaneous 56.52
  ureterostomy (cutaneous) (stoma) NEC 56.62
    ileal 56.52
  urethrostomy 58.49
  urinary conduit 56.52
  vascular procedure (previous) NEC 39.49
  ventricular shunt (cerebral) 02.42
  vesicostomy stoma 57.22
  wrist replacement (prosthesis) 81.97
Rhinectomy 21.4
Rhinocheiloplasty 27.59
  cleft lip 27.54
Rhinomanometry 89.12
Rhinoplasty (external) (internal) NEC 21.87
  augmentation (with graft) (with synthetic
      implant) 21.85
  limited 21.86
  revision 21.84
  tip 21.86
  twisted nose 21.84
Rhinorrhaphy (external) (internal) 21.81
  for epistaxis 21.09
Rhinoscopy 21.21
Rhinoseptoplasty 21.84
Rhinotomy 21.1
Rhizotomy (radio frequency) (spinal) 03.1
  acoustic 04.01
  trigeminal 04.02

Rhytidectomy (facial) 86.82
  eyelid
    lower 08.86
    upper 08.87
Rhytidoplasty (facial) 86.82
Ripstein operation (repair of prolapsed rectum)
  48.75
Rodney Smith operation (radical subtotal
  pancreatectomy) 52.53
Roentgenography —*see also* Radiography
  cardiac, negative contrast 88.58
Rolling of conjunctiva 10.33
Root
  canal (tooth) (therapy) 23.70
    with
      apicoectomy 23.72
      irrigation 23.71
  resection (tooth) (apex) 23.73
    with root canal therapy 23.72
    residual or retained 23.11
Rotation of fetal head
  forceps (instrumental) (Kielland) (Scanzoni)
    (key-in-lock) 72.4
  manual 73.51
Routine
  chest x-ray 87.44
  psychiatric visit 94.12
Roux-en-Y operation
  bile duct 51.36
  cholecystojejunostomy 51.32
  esophagus (intrathoracic) 42.54
  pancreaticojejunostomy 52.96
Roux-Goldthwait operation (repair of recurrent
  patellar dislocation) 81.44
Roux-Herzen-Judine operation (jejunal loop
  interposition) 42.63
Rubin test (insufflation of fallopian tube) 66.8
Ruiz-Mora operation (proximal phalangectomy
  for hammer toe) 77.99
Rupture
  esophageal web 42.01
  joint adhesions, manual 93.26
  membranes, artificial 73.09
    for surgical induction of labor 73.01
  ovarian cyst, manual 65.93
Russe operation (bone graft of scaphoid) 78.04

S

Scintiphotography —*see* Scan, radioisotope
Scintiscan —*see* Scan, radioisotope
Sclerectomy (punch) (scissors) 12.65
for retinal reattachment 14.49
Holth's 12.65
trephine 12.61
with implant 14.41
Scleroplasty 12.89
Sclerostomy (Scheie's) 12.62
Sclerotherapy
esophageal varices (endoscopic) 42.33
hemorrhoids 49.42
pleura 34.92
treatment of malignancy (cytotoxic agent) 34.92 [99.25]
with tetracycline 34.92 [99.21]
varicose vein 39.92
vein NEC 39.92
Sclerotomy (exploratory) 12.89
anterior 12.89
with
iridectomy 12.65
removal of vitreous 14.71
posterior 12.89
with
iridectomy 12.65
removal of vitreous 14.72
Scott operation
intestinal bypass for obesity 45.93
jejunocolostomy (bypass) 45.93
Scraping
corneal epithelium 11.41
for smear or culture 11.21
trachoma follicles 10.33
Scrotectomy (partial) 61.3
Scrotoplasty 61.49
Scrotorrhaphy 61.41
Scrototomy 61.0
Scrub, posterior nasal (adhesions) 21.91
Sculpturing, heart valve —*see* Valvuloplasty, heart
Section —*see also* Division *and* Incision
cesarean—*see* Cesarean section
ganglion, sympathetic 05.0
hypophyseal stalk (*see also* Hypophysectomy, partial) 07.63
ligamentum flavum (spine)—*omit code*
nerve (cranial) (peripheral) NEC 04.03
acoustic 04.01
spinal root (posterior) 03.1
sympathetic 05.0
trigeminal tract 04.02
Saemisch (corneal) 11.1
spinal ligament 80.49
arcuate—*omit code*
flavum—*omit code*
tooth (impacted) 23.19
Seddon-Brooks operation (transfer of pectoralis major tendon) 83.75
Semb operation (apicolysis of lung) 33.39
Senning operation (correction of transposition of great vessels) 35.91
Separation
twins (attached) (conjoined) (Siamese) 84.93
asymmetrical (unequal) 84.93
symmetrical (equal) 84.92
Septectomy
atrial (closed) 35.41
open 35.42
transvenous method (balloon) 35.41
submucous (nasal) 21.5

Septoplasty NEC 21.88
with submucous resection of septum 21.5
Septorhinoplasty 21.84
Septostomy (atrial) (balloon) 35.41
Septotomy, nasal 21.1
Sequestrectomy
bone 77.00
carpals, metacarpals 77.04
clavicle 77.01
facial 76.01
femur 77.05
fibula 77.07
humerus 77.02
nose 21.32
patella 77.06
pelvic 77.09
phalanges (foot) (hand) 77.09
radius 77.03
scapula 77.01
skull 01.25
specified site NEC 77.09
tarsals, metatarsals 77.08
thorax (ribs) (sternum) 77.01
tibia 77.07
ulna 77.03
vertebrae 77.09
nose 21.32
skull 01.25
Sesamoidectomy 77.98
Setback, ear 18.5
Sever operation (division of soft tissue of arm) 83.19
Severing of blepharorrhaphy 08.02
Sewell operation (heart) 36.2
Sharrard operation (iliopsoas muscle transfer) 83.77
Shaving
bone (*see also* Excision, lesion, bone) 77.60
cornea (epithelium) 11.41
for smear or culture 11.21
patella 77.66
Shelf operation (hip arthroplasty) 81.40
Shirodkar operation (encirclement suture, cervix) 67.59
Shock therapy
chemical 94.24
electroconvulsive 94.27
electrotonic 94.27
insulin 94.24
subconvulsive 94.26
Shortening
bone (fusion) 78.20
femur 78.25
specified site NEC (*see category* 78.2)
tibia 78.27
ulna 78.23
endopelvic fascia 69.22
extraocular muscle NEC 15.22
multiple (two or more muscles) 15.4
eyelid margin 08.71
eye muscle NEC 15.22
multiple (two or more muscles) (with lengthening) 15.4
finger (macrodactyly repair) 82.83
heel cord 83.85
levator palpebrae muscle 08.33
ligament—*see also* Arthroplasty
round 69.22
uterosacral 69.22

Shortening—*continued*
  muscle 83.85
    extraocular 15.22
      multiple (two or more muscles) 15.4
    hand 82.55
  sclera (for repair of retinal detachment) 14.59
    by scleral buckling (*see also* Buckling,
      scleral) 14.49
  tendon 83.85
    hand 82.55
  ureter (with reimplantation) 56.41
Shunt —*see also* Anastomosis *and* Bypass,
  vascular
  abdominovenous 54.94
  aorta-coronary sinus 36.39
  aorta (descending) pulmonary (artery) 39.0
  aortocarotid 39.22
  aortoceliac 39.26
  aortofemoral 39.25
  aortoiliac 39.25
  aortoiliofemoral 39.25
  aortomesenteric 39.26
  aorto-myocardial (graft) 36.2
  aortorenal 39.24
  aortosubclavian 39.22
  apicoaortic 35.93
  arteriovenous NEC 39.29
    for renal dialysis (by)
      anastomosis 39.27
      external cannula 39.93
  ascending aorta to pulmonary artery
    (Waterston) 39.0
  axillary-femoral 39.29
  carotid-carotid 39.22
  carotid-subclavian 39.22
  caval-mesenteric 39.1
  corpora cavernosa-corpus spongiosum 64.98
  corpora-saphenous 64.98
  descending aorta to pulmonary artery
    (Potts-Smith) 39.0
  endolymphatic (subarachnoid) 20.71
  endolymph-perilymph 20.71
  extracranial-intracranial (EC-IC) 39.28
  femoroperoneal 39.29
  femoropopliteal 39.29
  iliofemoral 39.25
  ilioiliac 39.25
  intestinal
    large-to-large 45.94
    small-to-large 45.93
    small-to-small 45.91
  left subclavian to descending aorta
    (Blalock-Park) 39.0
  left-to-right (systemic-pulmonary artery) 39.0
  left ventricle (heart) (apex) and aorta 35.93
  lienorenal 39.1
  lumbar-subarachnoid (with valve) NEC 03.79
  mesocaval 39.1
  peritoneal-jugular 54.94
  peritoneo-vascular 54.94
  peritoneovenous 54.94
  pleuroperitoneal 34.05
  pleurothecal (with valve) 03.79
  portacaval (double) 39.1
  portal-systemic 39.1
  portal vein to vena cava 39.1
  pulmonary-innominate 39.0
  pulmonary vein to atrium 35.82
  renoportal 39.1
  right atrium and pulmonary artery 35.94

Shunt—*continued*
  right ventricle and pulmonary artery (distal)
    35.92
  in repair of
    pulmonary artery atresia 35.92
    transposition of great vessels 35.92
    truncus arteriosus 35.83
  salpingothecal (with valve) 03.79
  semicircular-subarachnoid 20.71
  spinal (thecal) (with valve) NEC 03.79
  subarachnoid-peritoneal 03.71
  subarachnoid-ureteral 03.72
  splenorenal (venous) 39.1
    arterial 39.26
  subarachnoid-peritoneal (with valve) 03.71
  subarachnoid-ureteral (with valve) 03.72
  subclavian-pulmonary 39.0
  subdural-peritoneal (with valve) 02.34
  superior mesenteric-caval 39.1
  systemic-pulmonary artery 39.0
  transjugular intrahepatic portosystemic (TIPS)
    39.1
  vena cava to pulmonary artery (Green) 39.21
  ventricular (cerebral) (with valve) 02.2
    to
      abdominal cavity or organ 02.34
      bone marrow 02.39
      cervical subarachnoid space 02.2
      circulatory system 02.32
      cisterna magna 02.2
      extracranial site NEC 02.39
      gallbladder 02.34
      head or neck structure 02.31
      intracerebral site NEC 02.2
      lumbar site 02.39
      mastoid 02.31
      nasopharynx 02.31
      thoracic cavity 02.33
      ureter 02.35
      urinary system 02.35
      venous system 02.32
  ventriculoatrial (with valve) 02.32
  ventriculocaval (with valve) 02.32
  ventriculocisternal (with valve) 02.2
  ventriculolumbar (with valve) 02.39
  ventriculomastoid (with valve) 02.31
  ventriculonasopharyngeal 02.31
  ventriculopleural (with valve) 02.33
Sialoadenectomy (parotid) (sublingual)
  (submaxillary) 26.30
  complete 26.32
  partial 26.31
  radical 26.32
Sialoadenolithotomy 26.0
Sialoadenotomy 26.0
Sialodochoplasty NEC 26.49
Sialogram 87.09
Sialolithotomy 26.0
Sieve, vena cava 38.7
Sigmoid bladder 57.87 *[45.52]*
Sigmoidectomy 45.76
Sigmoidomyotomy 46.91
Sigmoidopexy (Moschowitz) 46.63
Sigmoidoproctectomy (*see also* Resection,
  rectum) 48.69
Sigmoidoproctostomy 45.94
Sigmoidorectostomy 45.94
Sigmoidorrhaphy 46.75

Suture—*continued*
  nose (external) (internal) 21.81
    for epistaxis 21.09
  obstetric laceration NEC 75.69
    bladder 75.61
    cervix 75.51
    corpus uteri 75.52
    pelvic floor 75.69
    perineum 75.69
    rectum 75.62
    sphincter ani 75.62
    urethra 75.61
    uterus 75.50
    vagina 75.69
    vulva 75.69
  omentum 54.64
  ovary 65.71
    laparoscopic 65.74
  palate 27.61
    cleft 27.62
  palpebral fissure 08.59
  pancreas 52.95
  pelvic floor 71.71
    obstetric laceration (current) 75.69
  penis 64.41
  peptic ulcer (bleeding) (perforated) 44.40
  pericardium 37.4
  perineum (female) 71.71
    after delivery 75.69
      episiotomy repair—*see* Episiotomy
    male 86.59
  periosteum 78.20
    carpal, metacarpal 78.24
    femur 78.25
    fibula 78.27
    humerus 78.22
    pelvic 78.29
    phalanxes (foot) (hand) 78.29
    radius 78.23
    specified site NEC 78.29
    tarsal metatarsal 78.28
    tibia 78.27
    ulna 78.23
    vertebrae 78.29
  peritoneum 54.64
  periurethral tissue to symphysis pubis 59.5
  pharynx 29.51
  pleura 34.93
  rectum 48.71
    obstetric laceration (current) 75.62
  retina (for reattachment) 14.59
  sacrouterine ligament 69.29
  salivary gland 26.41
  scalp 86.59
    replantation 86.51
  sclera (with repair of conjunctive) 12.81
  scrotum (skin) 61.41
  secondary
    abdominal wall 54.61
    episiotomy 75.69
    peritoneum 54.64
  sigmoid 46.75
  skin (mucous membrane) (without graft) 86.59
    with graft—*see* Graft, skin
    breast 85.81
    ear 18.4
    eyebrow 08.81
    eyelid 08.81
    nose 21.81
    penis 64.41
    scalp 86.59

Suture—*continued*
    replantation 86.51
   scrotum 61.41
   vulva 71.71
  specified site NEC—*see* Repair, by site
  spermatic cord 63.51
  sphincter ani 49.71
    obstetric laceration (current) 75.62
    old 49.79
  spinal meninges 03.59
  spleen 41.95
  stomach 44.61
    ulcer (bleeding) (perforated) 44.41
      endoscopic 44.43
  subcutaneous tissue (without skin graft) 86.59
    with graft—*see* Graft, skin
  tendon (direct) (immediate) (primary) 83.64
    delayed (secondary) 83.62
      hand NEC 82.43
      flexors 82.42
    hand NEC 82.45
      delayed (secondary) 82.43
      flexors 82.44
      delayed (secondary) 82.42
    ocular 15.7
    rotator cuff 83.63
    sheath 83.61
      hand 82.41
    supraspinatus (rotator cuff repair) 83.63
    to skeletal attachment 83.88
      hand 82.85
  Tenon's capsule 15.7
  testis 62.61
  thymus 07.93
  thyroid gland 06.93
  tongue 25.51
  tonsillar fossa 28.7
  trachea 31.71
  tunics vaginalis 61.41
  ulcer (bleeding) (perforated) (peptic) 44.40
    duodenum 44.42
      endoscopic 44.43
    gastric 44.41
      endoscopic 44.43
    intestine 46.79
    skin 86.59
    stomach 44.41
      endoscopic 44.43
  ureter 56.82
  urethra 58.41
    obstetric laceration (current) 75.61
  uterosacral ligament 69.29
  uterus 69.41
    obstetric laceration (current) 75.50
    old 69.49
  uvula 27.73
  vagina 70.71
    obstetric laceration (current) 75.69
    old 70.79
  vas deferens 63.81
  vein 39.32
  vulva 71.71
    obstetric laceration (current) 75.69
    old 71.79
Suture-ligation —*see also* Ligation
  blood vessel—*see* Ligation, blood vessel
Sweep, anterior iris 12.97
Swenson operation
  bladder reconstruction 57.87
  proctectomy 48.49
Swinney operation (urethral reconstruction) 58.46

T

Tenoplasty (*see also* Repair, tendon) 83.88
  hand (*see also* Repair, tendon, hand) 82.86
Tenorrhaphy (*see also* Suture, tendon) 83.64
  hand (*see also* Suture, tendon, hand) 82.45
  to skeletal attachment 83.88
    hand 82.85
Tenosuspension 83.88
  hand 82.86
Tenosuture (*see also* Suture, tendon) 83.64
  hand (*see also* Suture, tendon, hand) 82.45
  to skeletal attachment 83.88
    hand 82.85
Tenosynovectomy 83.42
  hand 82.33
Tenotomy 83.13
  Achilles tendon 83.11
  adductor (hip) (subcutaneous) 83.12
  eye 15.12
    levator palpebrae 08.38
    multiple (two or more tendons) 15.4
  hand 82.11
  levator palpebrae 08.38
  pectoralis minor tendon (decompression
    thoracic outlet) 83.13
  stapedius 19.0
  tensor tympani 19.0
Tenovaginotomy —*see* Tenotomy
Tensing, orbicularis oculi 08.59
Termination of pregnancy
  by
    aspiration curettage 69.51
    dilation and curettage 69.01
    hysterectomy—*see* Hysterectomy
    hysterotomy 74.91
    intra-amniotic injection (saline) 75.0
Test, testing (for)
  auditory function NEC 95.46
  Bender Visual-Motor Gestalt 94.02
  Benton Visual Retention 94.02
  14 C-Urea breath 89.39
  cardiac (vascular)
    function NEC 89.59
    stress 89.44
      bicycle ergometer 89.43
      Masters' two-step 89.42
      treadmill 89.41
  Denver developmental (screening) 94.02
  fetus, fetal
    nonstress (fetal activity acceleration
      determinations) 75.35
    oxytocin challenge (contraction stress) 75.35
    sensitivity (to oxytocin)—*omit code*
  function
    cardiac NEC 89.59
    hearing NEC 95.46
    muscle (by)
      electromyography 93.08
      manual 93.04
    neurologic NEC 89.15
    vestibular 95.46
      clinical 95.44
  glaucoma NEC 95.26
  hearing 95.47
    clinical NEC 95.42
  intelligence 94.01
  internal jugular-subclavian venous reflux 89.62
  intracarotid amobarbital (Wada) 89.10
  Masters' two-step stress (cardiac) 89.42
  muscle function (by)
    electromyography 93.08
    manual 93.04

Test, testing—*continued*
  neurologic function NEC 89.15
  nocturnal penile tumescence 89.29
  provocative, for glaucoma 95.26
  psychologic NEC 94.08
  psychometric 94.01
  radio-cobalt B$_{12}$ Schilling 92.04
  range of motion 93.05
  rotation (Barany chair) (hearing) 95.45
  sleep disorder function—*see categories*
    89.17-89.18
  Stanford-Binet 94.01
  Thallium stress (transesophageal pacing) 89.44
  tuning fork (hearing) 95.42
  Urea breath, (14 C) 89.39
  vestibular function NEC 95.46
    thermal 95.44
  Wada (hemispheric function) 89.10
  whispered speech (hearing) 95.42
TEVAP (transurethral electrovaporization of
  prostate) 60.29
Thalamectomy 01.41
Thalamotomy 01.41
  by stereotactic radiosurgery 92.32
    cobalt 60 92.32
    linear accelerator (LINAC) 92.31
    multi-source 92.32
    particle beam 92.33
    particulate 92.33
    radiosurgery NEC 92.39
    single source proton 92.31
Thai operation (repair of esophageal stricture)
  42.85
Theleplasty 85.87
Therapy
  Antabuse 94.25
  art 93.89
  aversion 94.33
  behavior 94.33
  Bennett respirator—*see category* 96.7
  blind rehabilitation NEC 93.78
  Byrd respirator—*see category* 96.7
  carbon dioxide 94.25
  cobalt-60 92.23
  conditioning, psychiatric 94.33
  continuous positive airway pressure (CPAP)
    93.90
  croupette, croup tent 93.94
  daily living activities 93.83
    for the blind 93.78
  dance 93.89
  desensitization 94.33
  detoxification 94.25
  diversional 93.81
  domestic tasks 93.83
    for the blind 93.78
  educational (bed-bound children) (handicapped)
    93.82
  electroconvulsive (ECT) 94.27
  electroshock (EST) 94.27
    subconvulsive 94.26
  electrotonic (ETT) 94.27
  encounter group 94.44
  extinction 94.33
  family 94.42
  fog (inhalation) 93.94
  gamma ray 92.23
  group NEC 94.44
    for psychosexual dysfunction 94.41
  hearing NEC 95.49

Therapy—*continued*
heat NEC 93.35
  for cancer treatment 99.85
helium 93.98
hot pack(s) 93.35
hyperbaric oxygen 93.95
  wound 93.59
hyperthermia NEC 93.35
  for cancer treatment 99.85
individual, psychiatric NEC 94.39
  for psychosexual dysfunction 94.34
industrial 93.89
infrared irradiation 93.35
inhalation NEC 93.96
  nitric oxide 00.12
insulin shock 94.24
intermittent positive pressure breathing (IPPB)
  93.91
IPPB (intermittent positive pressure breathing)
  93.91
leech 99.99
lithium 94.22
maggot 86.28
manipulative, osteopathic (*see also*
  Manipulation, osteopathic) 93.67
manual arts 93.81
methadone 94.25
mist (inhalation) 93.94
music 93.84
nebulizer 93.94
neuroleptic 94.23
nitric oxide 00.12
occupational 93.83
oxygen 93.96
  catalytic 93.96
  hyperbaric 93.95
    wound 93.59
  wound (hyperbaric) 93.59
paraffin bath 93.35
physical NEC 93.39
  combined (without mention of components)
    93.38
  diagnostic NEC 93.09
play 93.81
  psychotherapeutic 94.36
positive and expiratory pressure—*see* category
  96.7
psychiatric NEC 94.39
  drug NEC 94.25
    lithium 94.22
radiation 92.29
  contact (150 KVP or less) 92.21
  deep (200-300 KVP) 92.22
  high voltage (200-300 KVP) 92.22
  low voltage (150 KVP or less) 92.21
  megavoltage 92.24
  orthovoltage 92.22
  particle source NEC 92.26
  photon 92.24
  radioisotope (teleradiotherapy) 92.23
  retinal lesion 14.26
  superficial (150 KVP or less) 92.21
  supervoltage 92.24
radioisotope, radioisotopic NEC 92.29
  implantation or insertion 92.27
  injection or instillation 92.28
  teleradiotherapy 92.23
radium (radon) 92.23
recreational 93.81
rehabilitation NEC 93.89
respiratory NEC 93.99

Therapy—*continued*
bi-level airway pressure 93.90
continuous positive airway pressure [CPAP]
  93.90
endotracheal respiratory assistance—*see*
  category 96.7
intermittent mandatory ventilation
  [IMV]—*see* category 96.7
intermittent positive pressure breathing
  [IPPB] 93.91
negative pressure (continuous) [CNP] 93.99
nitric oxide 00.12
other continuous (unspecified duration) 96.70
  for less than 96 consecutive hours 96.71
  for 96 consecutive hours or more 96.72
positive and expiratory pressure [PEEP]—*see*
  category 96.7
pressure support ventilation [PSV]—*see*
  category 96.7
root canal 23.70
  with
    apicoectomy 23.72
    irrigation 23.71
shock
  chemical 94.24
  electric 94.27
    subconvulsive 94.26
  insulin 94.24
speech 93.75
  for correction of defect 93.74
ultrasound
  heat therapy 93.35
  hyperthermia for cancer treatment 99.85
  physical therapy 93.35
  therapeutic—*see* Ultrasound
ultraviolet light 99.82
Thermocautery —*see* Cauterization
Thermography 88.89
blood vessel 88.86
bone 88.83
breast 88.85
cerebral 88.81
eye 88.82
lymph gland 88.89
muscle 88.84
ocular 88.82
osteoarticular 88.83
specified site NEC 88.89
vein, deep 88.86
Thermokeratoplasty 11.74
Thermosclerectomy 12.62
Thermotherapy (hot packs) (paraffin bath) NEC
  93.35
prostate
  by
    microwave 60.96
    radiofrequency 60.97
  transurethral microwave thermotherapy
    (TUMT) 60.96
  transurethral needle ablation (TUNA) 60.97
  TUMT (transurethral microwave
    thermotherapy) 60.96
  TUNA (transurethral needle ablation) 60.97
Thiersch operation
anus 49.79
skin graft 86.69
  hand 86.62
Thompson operation
cleft lip repair 27.54
correction of lymphedema 40.9
quadricepsplasty 83.86
thumb apposition with bone graft 82.69

Thoracectomy 34.09
  for lung collapse 33.34
Thoracentesis 34.91
Thoracocentesis 34.91
Thoracolysis (for collapse of lung) 33.39
Thoracoplasty (anterior) (extrapleural)
  (paravertebral) (posterolateral) (complete)
  (partial) 33.34
Thoracoscopy, transpleural (for exploration)
  34.21
Thoracostomy 34.09
  for lung collapse 33.32
Thoracotomy (with drainage) 34.09
  exploratory 34.02
Three-snip operation, punctum 09.51
Thrombectomy 38.00
  with endarterectomy—*see*
    Endarterectomy
  abdominal
    artery 38.06
    vein 38.07
  aorta (arch) (ascending) (descending) 38.04
  bovine graft 39.49
  coronary artery 36.09
  head and neck vessel NEC 38.02
  intracranial vessel NEC 38.01
  lower limb
    artery 38.08
    vein 38.09
  pulmonary vessel 38.05
  thoracic vessel NEC 38.05
  upper limb (artery) (vein) 38.03
Thromboendarterectomy 38.10
  abdominal 38.16
  aorta (arch) (ascending) (descending) 38.14
  coronary artery 36.09
    open chest approach 36.03
  head and neck NEC 38.12
  intracranial NEC 38.11
  lower limb 38.18
  thoracic NEC 38.15
  upper limb 38.13
Thymectomy 07.80
  partial 07.81
  total 07.82
Thymopexy 07.99
Thyrochondrotomy 31.3
Thyrocricoidectomy 30.29
Thyrocricotomy (for assistance in breathing)
  31.1
Thyroidectomy NEC 06.39
  by mediastinotomy (*see also* Thyroidectomy,
    substernal) 06.50
  with laryngectomy—*see* Laryngectomy
  complete or total 06.4
    substernal (by mediastinotomy) (transsternal
      route) 06.52
    transoral route (lingual) 06.6
  lingual (complete) (partial) (subtotal) (total) 06.6
  partial or subtotal NEC 06.39
    with complete removal of remaining lobe 06.2
    submental route (lingual) 06.6
    substernal (by mediastinotomy) (transsternal
      route) 06.51
  remaining tissue 06.4
  submental route (lingual) 06.6
  substernal (by mediastinotomy)
    (transsternal route) 06.50
    complete or total 06.52
    partial or subtotal 06.51
  transoral route (lingual) 06.6

Thyroidectomy—*continued*
  transsternal route (*see also* Thyroidectomy,
    substernal) 06.50
  unilateral (with removal of isthmus) (with
    removal of portion of other lobe) 06.2
Thyroidorrhaphy 06.93
Thyroidotomy (field) (gland) NEC 06.09
  postoperative 06.02
Thyrotomy 31.3
  with tantalum plate 31.69
Tirofiban (HCl), infusion 99.20
Toilette
  skin—*see* Debridement, skin or subcutaneous
    tissue
  tracheostomy 96.55
Token economy (behavior therapy) 94.33
Tomkins operation (metroplasty) 69.49
Tomography —*see also* Radiography
  abdomen NEC 88.02
  cardiac 87.42
  computerized axial NEC 88.38
    abdomen 88.01
    bone 88.38
      quantitative 88.98
    brain 87.03
    head 87.03
    kidney 87.71
    skeletal 88.38
      quantitative 88.98
    thorax 87.41
  head NEC 87.04
  kidney NEC 87.72
  lung 87.42
  thorax NEC 87.42
Tongue tie operation 25.91
Tonography 95.26
Tonometry 89.11
Tonsillectomy 28.2
  with adenoidectomy 28.3
Tonsillotomy 28.0
Topectomy 01.32
Torek (Bevan) operation (orchidopexy) (first
  stage) (second stage) 62.5
Torkildsen operation (ventriculocisternal shunt)
  02.2
Torpin operation (cul-de-sac resection) 70.92
Toti operation (dacryocystorhinostomy) 09.81
Touchas operation 86.83
Touroff operation (ligation of subclavian artery)
  38.85
Toxicology —*see* Examination, microscopic
TPN (total parenteral nutrition) 99.15
Trabeculectomy ab externo 12.64
Trabeculodialysis 12.59
Trabeculotomy ab externo 12.54
Trachelectomy 67.4
Trachelopexy 69.22
Tracheloplasty 67.69
Trachelorrhaphy (Emmet) (suture) 67.61
  obstetrical 75.51
Trachelotomy 69.95
  obstetrical 73.93
Tracheocricotomy (for assistance breathing) 31.1
Tracheofissure 31.1
Tracheography 87.32
Trachelaryngotomy (emergency) 31.1
  permanent opening 31.29
Tracheoplasty 31.79
  with artificial larynx 31.75
Tracheorrhaphy 31.71
Tracheoscopy NEC 31.42
  through tracheotomy (stoma) 31.41

Tracheostomy (emergency) (temporary) (for
assistance in breathing) 31.1
  mediastinal 31.21
  permanent NEC 31.29
  revision 31.74
Tracheotomy (emergency) (temporary) (for
assistance in breathing) 31.1
  permanent 31.29
Tracing, carotid pulse with ECG lead 89.56
Traction
  with reduction of fracture or dislocation—*see*
      Reduction, fracture *and* Reduction,
      dislocation
  adhesive tape (skin) 93.46
  boot 93.46
  Bryant's (skeletal) 93.44
  Buck's 93.46
  caliper tongs 93.41
    with synchronous insertion of device 02.94
  Cortel's (spinal) 93.42
  Crutchfield tongs 93.41
    with synchronous insertion of device 02.94
  Dunlop's (skeletal) 93.44
  gallows 93.46
  Gardner Wells 93.41
    with synchronous insertion of device 02.94
  halo device, skull 93.41
    with synchronous insertion of device 02.94
  Lyman Smith (skeletal) 93.44
  manual, intermittent 93.21
  mechanical, intermittent 93.21
  Russell's (skeletal) 93.44
  skeletal NEC 93.44
    intermittent 93.43
  skin, limbs NEC 93.46
  spinal NEC 93.42
    with skull device (halo) (caliper) (Crutchfield)
        (Gardner Wells) (Vinke) (tongs) 93.41
      with synchronous insertion of device 02.94
  Thomas' splint 93.45
  Vinke tongs 93.41
    with synchronous insertion of device 02.94
Tractotomy
  brain 01.32
  medulla oblongata 01.32
  mesencephalon 01.32
  percutaneous 03.21
  spinal cord (one-stage) (two-stage) 03.29
  trigeminal (percutaneous) (radio frequency)
      04.02
Training (for) (in)
  ADL (activities of daily living) 93.83
    for the blind 93.78
  ambulation 93.22
  braille 93.77
  crutch walking 93.24
  dyslexia 93.71
  dysphasia 93.72
  esophageal speech (postlaryngectomy) 93.73
  gait 93.22
  joint movements 93.14
  lip reading 93.75
  Moon (blind reading) 93.77
  orthoptic 95.35
  prenatal (natural childbirth) 93.37
  prosthetic or orthotic device usage 93.24
  relaxation 94.33
  speech NEC 93.75
    esophageal 93.73
    for correction of defect 93.74
  use of lead dog for the blind 93.76
  vocational 93.85

TRAM (transverse rectus abdominis
musculocutaneous) flap of breast 85.7
Transactional analysis
  group 94.44
  individual 94.39
Transection —*see also* Division
  artery (with ligation) (*see also* Division, artery)
      38.80
    renal, aberrant (with reimplantation) 39.55
  bone (*see also* Osteotomy) 77.30
  fallopian tube (bilateral) (remaining)
      (solitary) 66.39
    by endoscopy 66.22
    unilateral 66.92
  isthmus, thyroid 06.91
  muscle 83.19
    eye 15.13
      multiple (two or more muscles) 15.3
    hand 82.19
  nerve (cranial) (peripheral) NEC 04.03
    acoustic 04.01
    root (spinal) 03.1
    sympathetic 05.0
    tracts in spinal cord 03.29
    trigeminal 04.02
    vagus (transabdominal) (*see also* Vagotomy)
        44.00
  pylorus (with wedge resection) 43.3
  renal vessel, aberrant (with reimplantation)
      39.55
  spinal
    cord tracts 03.29
    nerve root 03.1
  tendon 83.13
    hand 82.11
  uvula 27.71
  vas deferens 63.71
  vein (with ligation) (*see also* Division, vein)
      38.80
    renal, aberrant (with reimplantation) 39.55
    varicose (lower limb) 38.59
Transfer, transference
  bone shaft, fibula into tibia 78.47
  digital (to replace absent thumb) 82.69
    finger (to thumb) (same hand) 82.61
      to
        finger, except thumb 82.81
        opposite hand (with amputation) 82.69
            [84.01]
    toe (to thumb) (with amputation) 82.69 *[84.11]*
      to finger, except thumb 82.81 *[84.11]*
  fat pad NEC 86.89
    with skin graft—*see* Graft, skin, full-thickness
  finger (to replace absent thumb) (same hand)
      82.61
    to
      finger, except thumb 82.81
      opposite hand (with amputation) 82.69
          [84.01]
  muscle origin 83.77
    hand 82.58
  nerve (cranial) (peripheral) (radial anterior)
      (ulnar) 04.6
  pedicle graft 86.74
  pes anserinus (tendon) (repair of knee) 81.47
  tarsoconjunctival flap, from opposing lid 08.64
  tendon 83.75
    hand 82.56
    pes anserinus (repair of knee) 81.47
  toe-to-thumb (free) (pedicle) (with amputation)
      82.69 *[84.11]*

Transfixion —*see also* Fixation
  iris (bombe) 12.11
Transfusion (of) 99.03
  antihemophilic factor 99.06
  antivenin 99.16
  autologous blood
    collected prior to surgery 99.02
    intraoperative 99.00
    perioperative 99.00
    postoperative 99.00
    previously collected 99.02
    salvage 99.00
  blood (whole) NOS 99.03
    expander 99.08
    surrogate 99.09
  bone marrow 41.00
    allogeneic 41.03
      with purging 41.02
    allograft 41.03
      with purging 41.02
    autograft 41.01
      with purging 41.09
    autologous 41.01
      with purging 41.09
  coagulation factors 99.06
  Dextran 99.08
  exchange 99.01
    intraperitoneal 75.2
    in utero (with hysterotomy) 75.2
  exsanguination 99.01
  gamma globulin 99.14
  granulocytes 99.09
  hemodilution 99.03
  intrauterine 75.2
  packed cells 99.04
  plasma 99.07
  platelets 99.05
  replacement, total 99.01
  serum NEC 99.07
  substitution 99.01
  thrombocytes 99.05
Transillumination
  nasal sinuses 89.35
  skull (newborn) 89.16
Translumbar aortogram 88.42
Transplant, transplantation
  artery 39.59
    renal, aberrant 39.55
  autotransplant—*see* Reimplantation
  blood vessel 39.59
    renal, aberrant 39.55
  bone (*see also* Graft, bone) 78.00
    marrow 41.00
      allogeneic 41.03
        with purging 41.02
      allograft 41.03
        with purging 41.02
      autograft 41.01
        with purging 41.09
      autologous 41.01
        with purging 41.09
    stem cell
      allogeneic (hematopoietic) 41.05
        with purging 41.08
      autologous (hematopoietic) 41.04
        with purging 41.07
      cord blood 41.06
    stem cell
      allogeneic (hematopoietic) 41.05
        with purging 41.08
      autologous (hematopoietic) 41.04

Transplant, transplantation—*continued*
      with purging 41.07
    cord blood 41.06
  combined heart-lung 33.6
  conjunctiva, for pterygium 11.39
  corneal (*see also* Keratoplasty) 11.60
  dura 02.12
  fascia 83.82
    hand 82.72
  finger (replacing absent thumb) (same hand)
    82.61
    to
      finger, except thumb 82.81
      opposite hand (with amputation) 82.69
        [84.01]
  gracilis muscle (for) 83.77
    anal incontinence 49.74
    urethrovesical suspension 59.71
  hair follicles
    eyebrow 08.63
    eyelid 08.63
    scalp 86.64
  heart (orthotopic) 37.5
    combined with lung 33.6
  ileal stoma to new site 46.23
  intestine 46.97
  Islets of Langerhans (cells) 52.86
    allotransplantation of cells 52.85
    autotransplantation of cells 52.84
    heterotransplantation 52.85
    homotransplantation 52.84
  kidney NEC 55.69
  liver 50.59
    auxiliary (permanent) (temporary) (recipient's
      liver in situ) 50.51
    cells into spleen via percutaneous
      catheterization 38.91
  lung 33.50
    bilateral 33.52
    combined with heart 33.6
    double 33.52
    single 33.51
    unilateral 33.51
  lymphatic structure(s) (peripheral) 40.9
  mammary artery to myocardium or ventricular
    wall 36.2
  muscle 83.77
    gracilis (for) 83.77
      anal incontinence 49.74
      urethrovesical suspension 59.71
    hand 82.58
    temporalis 83.77
      with orbital exenteration 16.59
  nerve (cranial) (peripheral) 04.6
  ovary 65.92
  pancreas 52.80
    heterotransplant 52.83
    homotransplant 52.82
    Islets of Langerhans (cells) 52.86
      allotransplantation of cells 52.85
      autotransplantation of cells 52.84
      heterotransplantation of cells 52.85
      homotransplantation of cells 52.84
    reimplantation 52.81
  pes anserinus (tendon) (repair of knee) 81.47
  renal NEC 55.69
    vessel, aberrant 39.55
  salivary duct opening 26.49
  skin—*see* Graft, skin
  spermatic cord 63.53
  spleen 41.94

Transplant, transplantation—*continued*
  stem cell
    allogeneic (hematopoietic) 41.05
      with purging 41.08
      autologous (hematopoietic) 41.04
      with purging 41.07
    cord blood 41.06
  tendon 83.75
    hand 82.56
    pes anserinus (repair of knee) 81.47
    superior rectus (blepharoptosis) 08.36
  testis to scrotum 62.5
  thymus 07.94
  thyroid tissue 06.94
  toe (replacing absent thumb) (with amputation)
    82.69 *[84.11]*
    to finger, except thumb 82.81 *[84.11]*
  tooth 23.5
  ureter to
    bladder 56.74
    ileum (external diversion) 56.51
      internal diversion only 56.71
    intestine 56.71
    skin 56.61
  vein (peripheral) 39.59
    renal, aberrant 39.55
  vitreous 14.72
    anterior approach 14.71
Transposition
  extraocular muscles 15.5
  eyelash naps 08.63
  eye muscle (oblique) (rectus) 15.5
  finger (replacing absent thumb) (same hand)
    82.61
    to
      finger, except thumb 82.81
      opposite hand (with amputation) 82.69
        [84.01]
  interatrial venous return 35.91
  jejunal (Henley) 43.81
  joint capsule (*see also* Arthroplasty) 81.96
  muscle NEC 83.79
    extraocular 15.5
    hand 82.59
  nerve (cranial) (peripheral) (radial anterior)
    (ulnar) 04.6
  nipple 85.86
  pterygium 11.31
  tendon NEC 83.76
    hand 82.57
  vocal cords 31.69
Transureteroureterostomy 56.75
Transversostomy (*see also* Colostomy) 46.10
Trapping, aneurysm (cerebral) 39.52
Trauner operation (lingual sulcus extension)
  24.91
Trephination, trephining
  accessory sinus—*see* Sinusotomy
  corneoscleral 12.89
  cranium 01.24
  nasal sinus—*see* Sinusotomy
  sclera (with iridectomy) 12.61
Trial (failed) forceps 73.3
Trigonectomy 57.6
Trimming, amputation stump 84.3
Triple arthrodesis 81.12
Trochanterplasty 81.40
Tsuge operation (macrodactyly repair) 82.83
Tuck, tucking —*see also* Plication
  eye muscle 15.22
    multiple (two or more muscles) 15.4
  levator palpebrae, for blepharoptosis 08.34

Tudor "rabbit ear" operation (anterior
  urethropexy) 59.79
Tuffier operation
  apicolysis of lung 33.39
  vaginal hysterectomy 68.59
    laparoscopically assisted (LAVH) 68.51
TULIP (transurethral ultrasound guided laser
  induced prostatectomy) 60.21
TUMT (transurethral microwave thermotherapy)
  of prostate 60.96
TUNA (transurethral needle ablation) of prostate
  60.97
TURP (transurethral resection of prostate) 60.29
Tunnel, subcutaneous (antethoracic) 42.86
  esophageal 42.86
    with anastomosis—*see* Anastomosis,
      esophagus, antesternal
  pulse generator lead wire 86.99
    with initial procedure—*omit code*
Turbinectomy (complete) (partial) NEC 21.69
  by
    cryosurgery 21.61
    diathermy 21.61
  with sinusectomy—*see* Sinusectomy
Turco operation (release of joint capsules in
  clubfoot) 80.48
Tylectomy (breast) (partial) 85.21
Tympanectomy 20.59
  with tympanoplasty—*see* Tympanoplasty
Tympanogram 95.41
Tympanomastoidectomy 20.42
Tympanoplasty (type I) (with graft) 19.4
  with
    air pocket over round window 19.54
    fenestra in semicircular canal 19.55
    graft against
      incus or malleus 19.52
      mobile and intact stapes 19.53
    incudostapediopexy 19.52
  epitympanic, type I 19.4
  revision 19.6
  type
    II (graft against incus or malleus) 19.52
    III (graft against mobile and intact stapes)
      19.53
    IV (air pocket over round window) 19.54
    V (fenestra in semicircular canal) 19.55
Tympanosympathectomy 20.91
Tympanotomy 20.09
  with intubation 20.01

U

Uchida operation (tubal ligation with or without fimbriectomy) 66.32
UFR (uroflowmetry) 89.24
Ultrasonography
abdomen 88.76
aortic arch 88.73
biliary tract 88.74
breast 88.73
deep vein thrombosis 88.77
digestive system 88.74
eye 95.13
head and neck 88.71
heart (intravascular) 88.72
intestine 88.74
lung 88.73
midline shift, brain 88.71
multiple sites 88.79
peripheral vascular system 88.77
retroperitoneum 88.76
therapeutic—*see* Ultrasound
thorax NEC 88.73
total body 88.79
urinary system 88.75
uterus 88.79
gravid 88.78
Ultrasound
diagnostic—*see* Ultrasonography
fragmentation (of)
cataract (with aspiration) 13.41
urinary calculus, stones (Kock pouch) 59.95
heart (intravascular) 88.72
inner ear 20.79
therapeutic
head 00.01
heart 00.02
neck 00.01
other therapeutic ultrasound 00.09
peripheral vascular vessels 00.03
vessels of head and neck 00.01
therapy 93.35
Umbilectomy 54.3
Unbridling
blood vessel, peripheral 39.91
celiac artery axis 39.91
Uncovering —*see* Incision, by site
Undercutting
hair follicle 86.09
perianal tissue 49.02
Unroofing —*see also* Incision, by site
external
auditory canal 18.02
ear NEC 18.09
kidney cyst 55.39
UPP (urethral pressure profile) 89.25
UPPP (uvulopalatopharyngoplasty) 27.69 *[29.4]*
Upper GI series (x-ray) 87.62
Uranoplasty (for cleft palate repair) 27.62
Uranorrhaphy (for cleft palate repair) 27.62
Uranostaphylorrhaphy 27.62
Urban operation (mastectomy) (unilateral) 85.47
bilateral 85.48
Ureterectomy 56.40
with nephrectomy 55.51
partial 56.41
total 56.42
Ureterocecostomy 56.71
Ureterocelectomy 56.41
Ureterocolostomy 56.71
Ureterocystostomy 56.74

Ureteroenterostomy 56.71
Ureteroileostomy (internal diversion) 56.71
external diversion 56.51
Ureterolithotomy 56.2
Ureterolysis 59.02
with freeing or repositioning of ureter 59.02
laparoscopic 59.03
Ureteroneocystostomy 56.74
Ureteropexy 56.85
Ureteroplasty 56.89
Ureteroplication 56.89
Ureteroproctostomy 56.71
Ureteropyelography (intravenous) (diuretic infusion) 87.73
percutaneous 87.75
retrograde 87.74
Ureteropyeloplasty 55.87
Ureteropyelostomy 55.86
Ureterorrhaphy 56.82
Ureteroscopy 56.31
with biopsy 56.33
Ureterosigmoidostomy 56.71
Ureterostomy (cutaneous) (external) (tube) 56.61
closure 56.83
ileal 56.51
Ureterotomy 56.2
Ureteroureterostomy (crossed) 56.75
lumbar 56.41
resection with end-to-end anastomosis 56.41
spatulated 56.41
Urethral catheterization, indwelling 57.94
Urethral pressure profile (UPP) 89.25
Urethrectomy (complete) (partial) (radical) 58.39
with
complete cystectomy 57.79
pelvic exenteration 68.8
radical cystectomy 57.71
Urethrocystography (retrograde) (voiding) 87.76
Urethrocystopexy (by) 59.79
levator muscle sling 59.71
retropubic suspension 59.5
suprapubic suspension 59.4
Urethrolithotomy 58.0
Urethrolysis 58.5
Urethropexy 58.49
anterior 59.79
Urethroplasty 58.49
augmentation 59.79
collagen implant 59.72
fat implant 59.72
injection (endoscopic) of implant into urethra 59.72
polytef implant 59.72
Urethrorrhaphy 58.41
Urethroscopy 58.22
for control of hemorrhage of prostate 60.94
perineal 58.21
Urethrostomy (perineal) 58.0
Urethrotomy (external) 58.0
internal (endoscopic) 58.5
Uroflowmetry (UFR) 89.24
Urography (antegrade) (excretory) (intravenous) 87.73
retrograde 87.74
Uteropexy (abdominal approach) (vaginal approach) 69.22
UVP (uvulopalatopharyngoplasty) 27.69 *[29.4]*
Uvulectomy 27.72

V

Ventriculectomy, heart partial 37.35
Ventriculocholecystostomy 02.34
Ventriculocisternostomy 02.2
Ventriculocordectomy 30.29
Ventriculogram, Ventriculography (cerebral)
87.02
  cardiac
    left ventricle (outflow tract) 88.53
      combined with right heart 88.54
    right ventricle (outflow tract) 88.52
      combined with left heart 88.54
  radionuclide cardiac 92.05
Ventriculomyocardiotomy 37.11
Ventriculoperitoneostomy 02.34
Ventriculopuncture 01.09
  through previously implanted catheter or
    reservoir (Ommaya) (Rickham) 01.02
Ventriculoseptopexy (*see also* Repair,
  ventricular septal defect) 35.72
Ventriculoseptoplasty (*see also* Repair,
  ventricular septal defect) 35.72
Ventriculostomy 02.2
Ventriculotomy
  cerebral 02.2
  heart 37.11
Ventriculoureterostomy 02.35
Ventriculovenostomy 02.32
Ventrofixation, uterus 69.22
Ventrohysteropexy 69.22
Ventrosuspension, uterus 69.22
VEP (visual evoked potential) 95.23
Version, obstetrical (bimanual) (cephalic)
  (combined) (internal) (podalic) 73.21
  with extraction 73.22
  Braxton Hicks 73.21
    with extraction 73.22
  external (bipolar) 73.91
  Potter's (podalic) 73.21
    with extraction 73.22
  Wigand's (external) 73.91
  Wright's (cephalic) 73.21
    with extraction 73.22
Vesicolithotomy (suprapubic) 57.19
Vesicostomy 57.21
Vesicourethroplasty 57.85
Vesiculectomy 60.73
  with radical prostatectomy 60.5
Vesiculogram, seminal 87.92
  contrast 87.91
Vesiculotomy 60.72
Vestibuloplasty (buccolabial) (lingual) 24.91
Vestibulotomy 20.79
Vicq D'azyr operation (larynx) 31.1
Vidal operation (varicocele ligation) 63.1
Vidianectomy 05.21
Villusectomy (*see also* Synovectomy) 80.70
Vision check 95.09
Visual evoked potential (VEP) 95.23
Vitrectomy (mechanical) (posterior approach)
14.74
  with scleral buckling 14.49
  anterior approach 14.73
Vocational
  assessment 93.85
  retraining 93.85
  schooling 93.82
Voice training (postlaryngectomy) 93.73
von Kraske operation (proctectomy) 48.64
Voss operation (hanging hip operation) 83.19
Vulpius (-Compere) operation (lengthening of
  gastrocnemius muscle) 83.85

Vulvectomy (bilateral) (simple) 71.62
  partial (unilateral) 71.61
  radical (complete) 71.5
  unilateral 71.61
V-Y operation (repair)
  bladder 57.89
    neck 57.85
  ectropion 08.44
  lip 27.59
  skin (without graft) 86.89
  subcutaneous tissue (without skin graft) 86.89
  tongue 25.59

W

X

Y

Z

SUMMARY OF ADDITIONS, DELETIONS AND REVISIONS
TO VOLUME 3 IN 2003

00   Procedures and interventions, not elsewhere classified
New category

00.0   Therapeutic ultrasound
New subcategory

00.01   Therapeutic ultrasound of vessels of head and neck
New code

00.02   Therapeutic ultrasound of heart
New code

00.03   Therapeutic ultrasound of peripheral vascular vessels
New code

00.09   Other therapeutic ultrasound
New code

00.1   Pharmaceuticals
New subcategory

00.10   Implantation of chemotherapeutic agent
New code

00.11   Infusion of drotrecogin alfa (activated)
New code

00.12   Administration of inhaled nitric oxide
New code

00.13   Injection or infusion of nesiritide
New code

00.14   Injection or infusion of oxazolidinone class of antibiotics
New code

00.5   Other cardiovascular procedures
New subcategory

00.50   Implantation of cardiac resynchronization pacemaker without mention of defibrillation, total system [CRT-P]
New code

00.51   Implantation of cardiac resynchronization defibrillator, total system [CRT-D]
New code

00.52   Implantation or replacement of transvenous lead [electrode] into left ventricular coronary venous system
New code

00.53   Implantation or replacement of cardiac resynchronization pacemaker pulse generator only [CRT-P]
New code

00.54   Implantation or replacement of cardiac resynchronization defibrillator pulse generator device only [CRT-D]
New code

00.55   Insertion of drug-eluting non-coronary artery stent(s)
New code

02.41   Irrigation and exploration of ventricular shunt
Revised code

03   Operations on spinal cord and spinal canal structures
Add "Code also" instructions

03.09   Other exploration and decompression of spinal canal
Inclusion term added

04.2   Destruction of cranial and peripheral nerves
Inclusion terms added

33.24   Closed [endoscopic] biopsy of bronchus
Inclusion, exclusion terms added

33.99   Other operations on lung
Inclusion term added

36.06   Insertion of non-drug-eluting coronary artery stent(s)
Revised code and inclusion terms added

36.07   Insertion of drug-eluting coronary artery stent(s)
New code

37.26   Cardiac electrophysiologic stimulation and recording studies
Inclusion term added

37.7   Insertion, revision, replacement, and removal of pacemaker leads; insertion of temporary pacemaker system; or revision of pocket
Exclusion term added

37.79   Revision or relocation of pacemaker pocket
Inclusion term revised

37.8   Insertion, replacement, removal, and revision of pacemaker device
Exclusion term added

37.89   Revision or removal of pacemaker device
Inclusion term added

37.94   Implantation or replacement of automatic cardioverter/defibrillator, total system [AICD]
Exclusion term added

37.96   Implantation of automatic cardioverter/defibrillator pulse generator only
Exclusion term added

37.98   Replacement of automatic cardioverter/defibrillator pulse generator only
Exclusion term added

37.99   Other
Inclusion terms added

38   Incision, excision, and occlusion of vessels
Add "Code also" instructions

38.9   Puncture of vessel
Exclusion term revised

39.53   Repair of arteriovenous fistula
Exclusion term revised

39.72 **Endovascular repair or occlusion of head and neck vessels**
New code

39.79 **Other endovascular repair of aneurysm of other vessels**
Revised code

39.90 **Insertion of non-drug-eluting, non-coronary artery stent(s)**
Revised code

41.4 **Excision or destruction of lesion or tissue of spleen**
Add "Code also" instructions

41.5 **Total splenectomy**
Add "Code also" instructions

41.9 **Other operations on spleen and bone marrow**
Add "Code also" instructions

43 **Incision and excision of stomach**
Add "Code also" instructions

44 **Other operations on stomach**
Add "Code also" instructions

44.32 **Percutaneous [endoscopic] gastrojejunostomy**
Inclusion term(s) added

45 **Incision, excision, and anastomosis of intestine**
Add "Code also" instructions

46 **Other operations on intestine**
Add "Code also" instructions

46.32 **Percutaneous [endoscopic] jejunostomy**
Inclusion term deleted

46.79 **Other repair of intestine**
Inclusion term(s) added

47 **Operations on appendix**
Add "Code also" instructions

48 **Operations on rectum, rectosigmoid, and perirectal tissue**
Add "Code also" instructions

49 **Operations on anus**
Add "Code also" instructions

49.75 **Implantation or revision of artificial anal sphincter**
New code

49.76 **Removal of artificial anal sphincter**
New code

50 **Operations on liver**
Add "Code also" instructions

51 **Operations on gallbladder and biliary tract**
Add "Code also" instructions

51.01 **Percutaneous aspiration of gallbladder**
Inclusion term(s) added

51.37 **Anastomosis of hepatic duct to gastrointestinal tract**
Inclusion term(s) added

52 **Operations on pancreas**
Add "Code also" instructions

53 **Repair of hernia**
Add "Code also" instructions

54 **Other operations on abdominal region**
Add "Code also" instructions

54.95 **Incision of peritoneum**
Inclusion term(s) added

55 **Operations on kidney**
Add "Code also" instructions

56 **Operations on ureter**
Add "Code also" instructions

57 **Operations on urinary bladder**
Add "Code also" instructions

58 **Operations on urethra**
Add "Code also" instructions

59 **Other operations on urinary tract**
Add "Code also" instructions

60 **Operations on prostate and seminal vesicles**
Add "Code also" instructions

65 **Operations on ovary**
Add "Code also" instructions

66 **Operations on fallopian tubes**
Add "Code also" instructions

67 **Operations on cervix**
Add "Code also" instructions

68 **Other incision and excision of uterus**
Add "Code also" instructions

69 **Other operations on uterus and supporting structures**
Add "Code also" instructions

70 **Operations on vagina and cul-de-sac**
Add "Code also" instructions

71 **Operations on vulva an perineum**
Add "Code also" instructions

81.0 **Spinal fusion**
Add "Code also" instructions

81.3 **Refusion of spine**
Inclusion term(s) added

81.6 **Other procedures on spine**
New subcategory

81.61 **360 degree spinal fusion, single incision approach**
New code

84.5 **Implantation of other musculoskeletal devices and substances**
New subcategory

84.51 **Insertion of interbody spinal fusion device**
New code

84.52 **Insertion of recombinant bone morphogenetic protein**
New code

86.28 **Nonexcisional debridement of wound, infection, or burn**
Inclusion term(s) added

86.65 **Heterograft to skin**
Exclusion term(s) added

88.7 **Diagnostic ultrasound**
Exclusion term(s) added

88.91 **Magnetic resonance imaging of brain and brain stem**
Exclusion term(s) added

88.96 **Other intraoperative magnetic resonance imaging**
New code

89.60 **Continuous intra-arterial blood gas monitoring**
New code

89.65 **Measurement of systemic arterial blood gases**
Exclusion term(s) added

93.57 **Application of other wound dressing**
Inclusion term(s) added

93.98 **Other control of atmospheric pressure and composition**
Inclusion term(s) added, deleted

96.56 **Other lavage of bronchus and trachea**
Exclusion term(s) added

99.19 **Injection of anticoagulant**
Exclusion term(s) added

99.21 **Injection of antibiotic**
Exclusion term(s) added

99.22 **Injection of other anti-infective**
Exclusion term(s) added

99.25 **Injection or infusion of cancer chemotherapeutic substance**
Exclusion term(s) added

99.28 **Injection or infusion of biological response modifier [BRM] as an antineoplastic agent**
Inclusion term(s) added

99.29 **Injection or infusion of other therapeutic or prophylactic substance**
Exclusion term added

99.71 **Therapeutic plasmapheresis**
Exclusion term(s) added

99.76 **Extracorporeal immunoadsorption**
New code

99.77 **Application or administration of adhesion barrier substance**
New code

99.99 **Other**
Inclusion term(s) added

1815

1817